D1126989

Comprehensive Vascular and Endovascular Surgery

Comprehensive Vascular and Endovascular Surgery

Second Edition

John W. Hallett Jr, MD, FACS
Medical Director and Vascular Surgeon
Clinical Professor of Surgery
Medical University of South Carolina
Roper St Francis Heart and Vascular Center
Charleston, South Carolina, USA

Joseph L. Mills Sr, MD, FACS
Professor of Surgery
Chief, Division of Vascular and Endovascular Surgery
University of Arizona Health Sciences Center
Tucson, Arizona, USA

Jonothan J. Earnshaw, DM, FRCS
Consultant Surgeon
Department of Vascular Surgery
Gloucestershire Royal Hospital
Gloucestershire, United Kingdom

Jim A. Reekers, MD, PhD
Professor of Interventional Radiology
Department of Radiology
Academic Medical Center
University of Amsterdam
Amsterdam, The Netherlands

Thom W. Rooke, MD
Krehbiel Professor of Vascular Medicine
Department of Cardiovascular Diseases
Gonda Vascular Center
Mayo Clinic
Rochester, Minnesota, USA

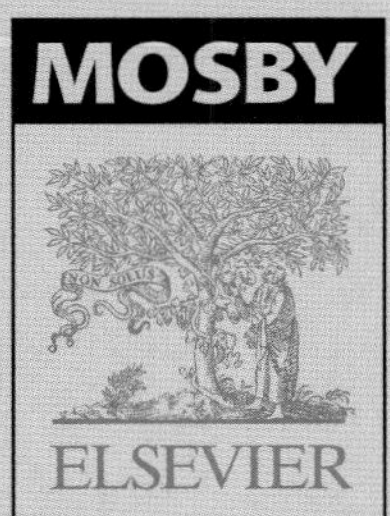

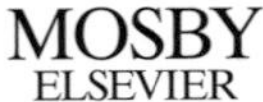

1600 John F. Kennedy Blvd.
Ste 1800
Philadelphia, PA 19103-2899

COMPREHENSIVE VASCULAR AND ENDOVASCULAR
SURGERY, SECOND EDITION
ISBN: 978-0-323-05726-4

Notice

Knowledge and best practice in this field are constantly changing. As new research and experience broaden our knowledge, changes in practice, treatment, and drug therapy may become necessary or appropriate. Readers are advised to check the most current information provided (i) on procedures featured or (ii) by the manufacturer of each product to be administered, to verify the recommended dose or formula, the method and duration of administration, and contraindications. It is the responsibility of the practitioner, relying on their own experience and knowledge of the patient, to make diagnoses, to determine dosages and the best treatment for each individual patient, and to take all appropriate safety precautions. To the fullest extent of the law, neither the Publisher nor the Editors assume any liability for any injury and/or damage to persons or property arising out of or related to any use of the material contained in this book.

The Publisher

Library of Congress Cataloging-in-Publication Data

Comprehensive vascular and endovascular surgery/[edited by] John W. Hallett … [et al.]. -- 2nd ed.
p. ; cm.
Includes bibliographical references and index.
ISBN 978-0-323-05726-4
1. Blood-vessels--Surgery. 2. Blood-vessels--Endoscopic surgery. I. Hallett, John W.
[DNLM: 1. Vascular Surgical Procedures. 2. Endoscopy--methods. 3. Vascular Diseases--surgery. WG 170 C7377 2009]

RD598.5.C644 2009
617.4'130597--dc22
2009008603

Acquisitions Editor: Judith Fletcher
Developmental Editor: Lisa Barnes
Project Manager: Mary Stermel
Marketing Manager: Radha Mawrie

Printed in China

Last digit is the print number: 9 8 7 6 5 4 3 2 1

Contributors

DONALD T. BARIL, MD
Fellow, Vascular and Endovascular Surgery
Division of Vascular Surgery
Department of Surgery
University of Pittsburgh Medical Center
Pittsburgh, Pennsylvania, USA

GINGER BARTHEL, RN, MA, FACHE
Vice President, Clinical Operations
Advocate Lutheran General Hospital
Park Ridge, Illinois, USA

B. TIMOTHY BAXTER, MD
Professor
Department of Surgery
University of Nebraska
Omaha, Nebraska, USA

JONATHAN D. BEARD, FRCS, ChM, Med
Professor of Surgical Education
University of Sheffield
Consultant Vascular Surgeon
Sheffield Vascular Institute
Northern General Hospital
Sheffield, United Kingdom

JEAN-PIERRE BECQUEMIN, MD, FRCS
Professor of Vascular Surgery
University of Paris XII
Head of the "Pole"
Cardiac Vascular and Thoracic
Henri Mondor Hospital
Creteil, France

MICHAEL BELKIN, MD
Associate Professor of Surgery
Harvard Medical School
Chief, Division of Vascular and Endovascular Surgery
Brigham and Women's Hospital
Boston, Massachusetts, USA

THOMAS C. BOWER, MD
Professor of Surgery
Mayo Clinic College of Medicine
Consultant
Division of Vascular and Endovascular Surgery
Mayo Clinic
Rochester, Minnesota, USA

KEVIN G. BURNAND, MBBS, MS, FRCS
Professor, Academic Surgery
King's College London
Professor, Academic Surgery
St. Thomas Hospital
London, United Kingdom

JAAP BUTH, MD, PhD
Consultant Vascular Surgeon
Department of Vascular Surgery
Catharina Hospital
Eind Hovem, The Netherlands

JOHN BYRNE, MCh FRCSI (GEN)
Assistant Professor of Surgery
Division of Vascular Surgery
Albany Medical Center
Albany, New York, USA

RICHARD P. CAMBRIA, MD, FACS
Professor of Surgery
Harvard Medical School
Chief, Division of Vascular and Endovascular Surgery
Massachusetts General Hospital
Boston, Massachusetts, USA

CHRISTOPHER G. CARSTEN, MD
Assistant Program Director
Academic Department of Surgery
Greenville Hospital System University Medical Center
Greenville, South Carolina, USA

KENNETH J. CHERRY Jr, MD
Head, Division of Vascular Surgery
Department of Surgery
Professor of Surgery
Chair, Vascular Surgery
University of Virginia Hospital
Charlottesville, Virginia, USA

W. DARRIN CLOUSE, MD, FACS
Associate Professor of Surgery
The Uniformed Services University of the Health Sciences
Bethesda, Maryland, USA
Chief, Division of Vascular and Endovascular Surgery
San Antonio Military Medical Center
San Antonio, Texas, USA

MARC COGGIA, MD
Professor of Vascular Surgery
Versailles Saint-Quentin-en-Yvelines University
Versailles, France
Vascular Surgeon
Department of Vascular Surgery
Ambroise Pare University Hospital
Boulogne-Billancourt, France

MATTHEW A. CORRIERE, MD
Fellow
Section on Vascular and Endovascular Surgery
Wake Forest University School of Medicine
Winston-Salem, North Carolina, USA

DAVID L. CULL, MD
Vice Chairman, Surgical Research
Academic Department of Surgery
Greenville Hospital System University Medical Center
Greenville, South Carolina, USA

PHILIPPE CUYPERS, MD, PhD
Consultant Vascular Surgeon
Department of Vascular Surgery
Catharina Hospital
Eindhovem, The Netherlands

MICHAEL D. DAKE, MD
Chairman
Department of Radiology
University of Virginia Health System
Charlottesville, Virginia, USA

ALUN H. DAVIES, MA, DM, FRCS, ILTM
Imperial College
Imperial Vascular Unit
Charing Cross Hospital
London, United Kingdom

MAGRUDER C. DONALDSON, MD
Associate Professor of Surgery
Harvard Medical School
Boston, Massachusetts, USA
Chairman
Adjunct Staff
Department of Surgery
Metro West Medical Center
Framingham, Massachusetts, USA
Department of Surgery
Brigham and Women's Hospital
Boston, Massachusetts, USA

JOSÉE DUBOIS, MD
Professor
Department of Radiology, Radio-Oncology, and Nuclear Medicine
University of Montreal
Chair
Department of Medical Imaging
CHU Sainte-Justine
Montreal, Quebec, Canada

WALTER N DURÁN, PhD
Professor of Physiology and Surgery
Director, Program in Vascular Biology
Department of Pharmacology and Physiology
New Jersey Medical School
University of Medicine and Dentistry of New Jersey Medical School
Newark, New Jersey, USA

JONOTHAN J. EARNSHAW, DM, FRCS
Consultant Surgeon
Department of Vascular Surgery
Gloucestershire Royal Hospital
Gloucestershire, United Kingdom

JAMES M. EDWARDS, MD
Professor of Surgery
Portland Veterans Affairs Medical Center
Oregon Health and Science University
Department of Surgery
Division of Vascular Surgery
Portland, Oregon, USA

MATTHEW S. EDWARDS, MD
Associate Professor of Surgery
Department of Vascular and Endovascular Surgery
Wake Forest University Health Sciences
Assistant Professor of Surgery
Department of Vascular and Endovascular Surgery
Wake Forest University Baptist Medical Center
Winston-Salem, North Carolina, USA

JULIE FREISCHLAG, MD
Chair
Department of Surgery
Surgeon-in-Chief
Johns Hopkins Medical Institution
Baltimore, Maryland, USA

MARY E. GISWOLD, MD
Staff Surgeon
Kaiser Permanente
Sunnybrook Medical Office
Clackamas, Oregon, USA

PETER GLOVICZKI, MD, FACS
Professor of Surgery
Mayo Clinic College of Medicine
Chair
Division of Vascular and Endovascular Surgery
Director
Gonda Vascular Center
Mayo Clinic
Rochester, Minnesota, USA

OLIVIER GOËAU-BRISSONNIÈRE, MD, PhD
Professor of Vascular Surgery
Versailles Saint-Quentin-en–Yvelines University
Versailles, France
Head
Department of Vascular Surgery
Ambroise Pare University Hospital
Boulogne-Billancourt, France

MANJ S. GOHEL, MD, MRCS
Honorary Research Fellow
Faculty of Medicine
Imperial College London
Specialist Registrar
Department of Vascular Surgery
Charing Cross Hospital
London, United Kingdom

BRUCE H. GRAY, DO
GHS Clinical Professor of Surgery
Department of Surgery
Medical University of South Carolina
Director of Endovascular Services
Department of Vascular Surgery
Greenville, South Carolina, USA

MARCELO GUIMARAES, MD
Assistant Professor
Department of Radiology—Heart and Vascular Center
Medical University of South Carolina
Charleston, South Carolina, USA

MAHER HAMISH, MD, FRCS
Senior Clinical Fellow
Imperial Vascular Unit
Charing Cross Hospital
London, United Kingdom

KIMBERLEY J. HANSEN, MD
Professor of Surgery and Section Head
Section of Vascular and Endovascular Surgery
Division of Surgical Sciences
Wake Forest University School of Medicine
Winston-Salem, North Carolina, USA

PAUL N. HARDEN, MB, ChB, FRCP
Consultant Nephrologist
Oxford Kidney Unit
The Churchill Hospital
Oxford, United Kingdom

JOHANNA M. HENDRIKS, MD, PhD
Consultant
Department of Vascular Surgery
Erasmus University
Rotterdam, The Netherlands

NORMAN R. HERTZER, MD, FACS
Emeritus Chairman
Department of Vascular Surgery
The Cleveland Clinic
Cleveland, Ohio, USA

WALTER HUDA, PhD
Professor
Department of Radiology
Medical University of South Carolina
Charleston, South Carolina, USA

GLENN C. HUNTER, MD
Staff Surgeon
Department of Surgery
Tucson Medical Center
Tucson, Arizona, USA

DANIEL M. IHNAT, MD, FACS
Assistant Professor of Clinical Surgery
Department of Surgery
University of Arizona
Tucson, Arizona, USA

JEFFREY A. KALISH, MD
Clinical Fellow in Vascular and Endovascular Surgery
Beth Israel Deaconess Medical Center
Boston, Massachusetts, USA

MANJU KALRA, MBBS
Associate Professor of Surgery
Mayo Clinic College of Medicine
Mayo Clinic
Consultant
Division of Vascular and Endovascular Surgery
Rochester, Minnesota, USA

EDOUARD KIEFFER, MD
Professor of Vascular Surgery and Chief
Department of Vascular Surgery
Pitie-Salpetriere University Hospital
Paris, France

CONSTANTINOS KYRIAKIDES, MD, FRCS
Consultant Vascular Surgeon
Department of Surgery
Barts and the London NHS Trust
The Royal London Hospital
Whitechapel, London, United Kingdom

FRANK A. LEDERLE, MD
Professor of Medicine
Veteran Affairs Medical Center
Minneapolis, Minnesota, USA

LUIS R. LEON Jr, MD, RVT, FACS
Chief of Vascular Surgery
Department of Vascular and Endovascular Surgery
Southern Arizona Veterans Affairs Health Care System
Associate Professor of Surgery
Department of Vascular and Endovascular Surgery
University of Arizona Medical Center
Tucson, Arizona, USA

BENJAMIN LINDSEY, MB BS, FRCSE
Department of Vascular Surgery
Royal Cornwall Hospital
Cornwall, United Kingdom

NICK J.M. LONDON, MD, FRCS, FRCP
Professor of Surgery
Vascular Surgery Group
University of Leicester
Hon. Consultant Vascular/Endocrine Surgeon
Vascular Surgery
UHoL, Leicester Royal Infirmary
Leicester, United Kingdom

WILLIAM C. MACKEY, MD, FACS
Andrews Professor and Chairman
Department of Surgery
Tufts University School of Medicine
Surgeon-in-Chief
Tufts New England Medical Center
Boston, Massachusetts, USA

JASON MacTAGGART, MD
Fellow in Vascular Surgery
University of California, San Francisco
San Francisco, California, USA

JOVAN N. MARKOVIC, MD
Postdoctorate
Department of Surgery
Duke University Medical Center
Durham, North Carolina, USA

CATHARINE L. McGUINNESS, MS, FRCS
Consultant Vascular Surgeon
Royal Surrey County Hospital
Guildford, Surrey, United Kingdom

MARK H. MEISSNER, MD
Professor
Department of Surgery
University of Washington School of Medicine
Seattle, Washington, USA

MATTHEW T. MENARD, MD
Instructor in Surgery
Harvard Medical School
Co-Director, Endovascular Surgery
Division of Vascular and Endovascular Surgery
Brigham and Women's Hospital
Boston, Massachusetts, USA

VIRGINIA M. MILLER, PhD
Professor
Departments of Surgery and Physiology and Biomedical Engineering
Mayo Clinic College of Medicine
Rochester, Minnesota, USA

JOSEPH L. MILLS Sr, MD, FACS
Professor of Surgery
Department of Surgery
University of Arizona Health Sciences Center
Chief of Vascular and Endovascular Surgery
Division of Vascular Surgery
University Medical Center
Tucson, Arizona, USA

GREGORY L. MONETA, MD
Professor of Surgery
Department of Surgery
Oregon Health and Science University
Chief of Vascular Surgery
Oregon Health and Science University Hospital
Portland Department of Veterans Affairs Hospital
Portland, Oregon, USA

JONATHAN G. MOSS, MBChB, FRCS, FRCR
Professor of Interventional Radiology
University of Glasgow
North Glasgow University Hospitals
Glasgow Scotland, United Kingdom

JOSEPH J. NAOUM, MD
Division of Vascular Surgery
The Methodist Hospital
Cardiovascular Surgery Associates
Houston, Texas, USA

A. ROSS NAYLOR, MBChB, MD, FRCS
Professor of Vascular Surgery
Department of Vascular Surgery
Leicester Royal Infirmary
Leicester, United Kingdom

GUSTAVO S. ODERICH, MD
Assistant Professor of Surgery
Mayo Clinic College of Medicine
Consultant
Division of Vascular and Endovascular Surgery
Mayo Clinic
Rochester, Minnesota, USA

PATRICK J. O'HARA, MD, FACS
Professor of Surgery
Cleveland Clinic Lerner College of Medicine
Staff Vascular Surgeon
Department of Vascular Surgery
The Cleveland Clinic Foundation
Cleveland, Ohio, USA

VINCENT L. OLIVA, MD
Professor of Radiology
Department of Radiology
University of Montreal
Assistant Chief
Department of Radiology
Centre Hospitalier de l'Université de Montreal
Chief of Vascular and Interventional Radiology Division
Department of Radiology
Centre Hospitalier de l'Université de Montreal
Montreal, Quebec, Canada

FRANK PADBERG Jr, MD
Professor of Surgery
Division of Vascular Surgery
Department of Surgery
New Jersey Medical School
University of Medicine and Dentistry of New Jersey
Attending Vascular Surgeon
Department of Vascular Surgery
University Hospital
Newark, New Jersey, USA
Chief, Section of Vascular Surgery
Department of Surgery
Veterans Affairs, New Jersey Health Care System
East Orange, New Jersey, USA

LUIGI PASCARELLA, MD
Resident
Department of Surgery
Duke University Medical Center
Durham, North Carolina, USA

FRANK B. POMPOSELLI Jr, MD
Associate Professor of Surgery
Harvard Medical School
Chief of Vascular and Endovascular Surgery
Beth Israel Deaconess Medical Center
Boston, Massachusetts, USA

BRENDON QUINN, MD
Vascular Fellow
Academic Department of Surgery
Division of Vascular Surgery
Greenville Hospital System University Medical Center
Greenville, South Carolina, USA

TODD E. RASMUSSEN, MD
Associate Professor of Surgery
Norman M. Rich Department of Surgery
The Uniformed Services University of the Health Sciences
Bethesda, Maryland, USA
Chief, San Antonio Military Vascular Surgery
Wilford Hall United States Air Force Medical Center
Lackland Air Force Base, Texas, USA
Chief, San Antonio Military Vascular Surgery
Brooke Army Medical Center
Fort Sam Houston, Texas, USA

JOHN E. RECTENWALD, MD
Assistant Professor of Surgery
Department of Surgery
University of Michigan
Ann Arbor, Michigan, USA

AMY B. REED, MD
Director, Vascular Surgery Fellowship
Division of Vascular Surgery
Department of Surgery
Staff Vascular Surgeon
University Hospital
Department of Surgery
Cincinnati, Ohio, USA

LINDA M. REILLY, MD
Professor of Surgery
Department of Surgery—Vascular Division
University of California, San Francisco
Professor of Surgery
Department of Surgery
University of California, San Francisco Medical Center
Professor of Surgery
Department of Surgery
San Francisco VA Medical Center
San Francisco, California, USA

ROBERT Y. RHEE, MD
Clinical Director
Division of Vascular Surgery
Department of Surgery
University of Pittsburgh Medical Center
Pittsburgh, Pennsylvania, USA

JEFFREY M. RHODES, MD
Attending Physician
Department of Vascular Surgery
Rochester General Hospital
Rochester, New York, USA

JOSEPH J. RICOTTA II, MD
Assistant Professor of Surgery
Mayo Clinic College of Medicine
Consultant
Division of Vascular and Endovascular Surgery
Mayo Clinic
Rochester, Minnesota, USA

DAVID RIGBERG, MD
Assistant Professor of Surgery
Division of Vascular Surgery
University of California, Los Angeles
Los Angeles, California, USA

CLAUDIO SCHÖNHOLZ, MD
Professor of Radiology
Radiology Heart and Vascular Center
Medical University of South Carolina
Charleston, South Carolina, USA

PARITOSH SHARMA, MRCS
Vascular Research Fellow
Department of Surgery
Barts and the London NHS Trust
The Royal London Hospital
Whitechapel, London, United Kingdom

AMANDA SHEPHERD, MRCS
Doctor
Imperial Vascular Unit
Imperial College
London, United Kingdom

CYNTHIA SHORTELL, MD, FACS
Professor of Surgery
Chief of Vascular Surgery
Program Director, Vascular Residency
Division of Surgery
Duke University Medical Center
Durham, North Carolina, USA

FRANK C.T. SMITH, BSc, MD, FRCS
Reader and Consultant Vascular Surgeon
University of Bristol
Bristol Royal Infirmary
Bristol, United Kingdom

GILLES SOULEZ, MD, MSc
Professor
Department of Radiology
University de Montreal
Interventional Radiologist, Director of Research
Department of Radiology
Centre Hospitalier de l'Universite de Montreal
Montreal, Quebec, Canada

JAMES C. STANLEY, MD
Professor of Surgery
Department of Surgery
University of Michigan Medical School
Director
Cardiovascular Center
University of Michigan
Ann Arbor, Michigan, USA

KONG TENG TAN, MD
Assistant Professor of Radiology
Interventional Radiology
University of Toronto
Toronto, Ontario, Canada

DESAROM TESO, MD
Fellow in Vascular Surgery
Section of Vascular Surgery
Tufts Medical Center
Boston, Massachusetts, USA

STEPHEN C. TEXTOR, MD
Professor of Medicine
Departments of Nephrology and Hypertension
Mayo Clinic College of Medicine
Consultant
Departments of Nephrology and Hypertension
Rochester Methodist Hospital
Consultant
Saint Mary's Hospital
Rochester, Minnesota, USA

BRAD H. THOMPSON, MD
Associate Professor of Radiology
Department of Radiology
Roy J. and Lucille A. Carver College of Medicine
Department of Radiology
University of Iowa Hospitals and Clinics
Iowa City, Iowa, USA

RENAN UFLACKER, MD
Professor of Radiology
Department of Radiology—Heart and Vascular Center
Medical University of South Carolina
Charleston, South Carolina, USA

GILBERT R. UPCHURCH Jr, MD
Professor of Surgery
Section of Vascular Surgery
Department of Surgery
University of Michigan
Ann Arbor, Michigan, USA

EDWIN J.R. VAN BEEK, MD, PhD
Professor of Radiology, Medicine, and Biomedical Engineering
Department of Radiology
Carver College of Medicine
Iowa City, Iowa, USA

MARC R.H.M. VAN SAMBEEK, MD, PhD
Associate Professor
Department of Anesthesiology
Erasmus University
Rotterdam, The Netherlands
Consultant Vascular Surgeon
Department of Vascular Surgery
Catharina Hospital
Eindhovem, The Netherlands

FRANK C. VANDY, MD
Resident
Department of Vascular Surgery
University of Michigan Medical Center
Ann Arbor, Michigan, USA

DIERK VORWERK, MD
Professor
Department of Radiology
University of Technology
Chairman
Department of Diagnostic and Interventional Radiology
Klinikum Ingolstadt
Ingolstadt, Germany

THOMAS W. WAKEFIELD, MD
S. Martin Lindeanuer Professor of Vascular Surgery
Section Head
Department of Vascular Surgery
University of Michigan Medical Center
Ann Arbor, Michigan, USA

NICOLE WHEELER, MD
Vascular Surgery Bidwell Fellow
Oregon Health and Science University
Portland, Oregon, USA

JOHN V. WHITE, MD
Clinical Professor
Department of Surgery
University of Illinois
Chicago, Illinois, USA
Chairman
Department of Surgery
Advocate Lutheran General Hospital
Park Ridge, Illinois, USA

CHRISTOPHER L. WIXON, MD, FACS
Assistant Professor of Surgery and Radiology
Mercer University School of Medicine
Director and Chairman
Department of Cardiovascular Medicine and Surgery
Memorial Health University Medical Center
Savannah, Georgia, USA

KENNETH R. WOODBURN, MB ChB, MD FRCSG (GEN)
Honorary University Fellow
Peninsula College of Medicine and Dentistry
University of Plymouth
Plymouth, United Kingdom
Consultant Vascular and Endovascular Surgeon
Vascular Unit
Royal Cornwall Hospitals Trust
Truro, Cornwall, United Kingdom

KENNETH J. WOODSIDE, MD
Clinical Lecturer in Surgery
Division of Transplantation
Department of Surgery
University of Michigan Health System
Ann Arbor, Michigan, USA

Preface

Something happens with the first edition of a textbook that leads to a second edition. Something must have succeeded. Someone has to understand the success to ensure that the next edition meets the expectations of the readers. As we planned this new edition of *Comprehensive Vascular and Endovascular Surgery*, the original four editors and our editorial staff discussed that "something" in great detail.

What have we heard about the first edition that sets this textbook apart from others? First, we chose a comprehensive but concise approach to cover all the main topics in vascular disease. Detailed discussions of rare topics were left to other, more encyclopedic, books. In other words, our readers commented that they could read this textbook cover-to-cover in a reasonable period of time. Second, we chose authors who are clinical experts in both open surgical and endovascular techniques. Consequently, the first edition revealed a balance in open and endovascular options for every clinical problem.

Some other features of the first textbook appealed to our readers, too. The consistency in simply designed anatomical drawings and reproductions of vascular imaging was considered a strength. Next, and perhaps as important, the CD-ROM collection of all illustrations and tables helped our readers to quickly assemble PowerPoint presentations for teaching. This innovation with the book may have done more to advance vascular disease education than any other feature of the first edition.

This newest edition of *Comprehensive Vascular and Endovascular Surgery* sustains the features that our readers acknowledged so graciously with the first textbook. With this edition, all of the text, illustrations, and study questions will be available on a special website. In other words, you will have the textbook at your fingertips on the Internet at any location where you may need to refresh your knowledge or prepare a PowerPoint presentation. In addition, we have advanced this new edition with several new features. First, Dr Thom Rooke, an internationally recognized cardiovascular medicine specialist at the Mayo Clinic, joins our editorial team. We recognize that cardiologists and vascular internists are venturing more into medical and interventional management of peripheral vascular disease. Dr Rooke's input represents their interests. Second, we have updated every chapter and added several new erudite discussions of other topics, such as vascular imaging and radiation safety, vascular infections, and aortic dissections. Finally, we have added a bank of study questions to assist with review and preparation for board examinations.

We hope that this second edition of *Comprehensive Vascular and Endovascular Surgery* provides a practical and user-friendly reference for the care of your patients. Again, we welcome your feedback to improve future editions. Stay in touch. Share your experience and knowledge with us and with your colleagues who are dedicated to vascular care.

John (Jeb) Hallett

Joseph Mills

Jonathan Earnshaw

Jim Reekers

Thom Rooke

Contents

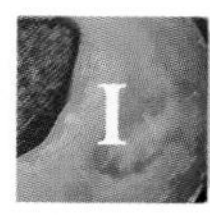

Background

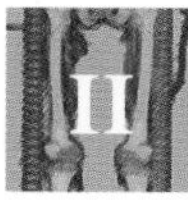

Chronic Lower Extremity Ischemia

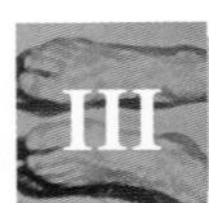

III Acute Limb Ischemia

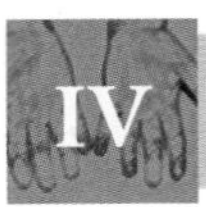

IV Upper Extremity Problems

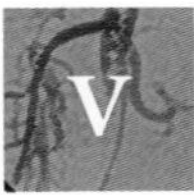

V Mesenteric Vascular Disease

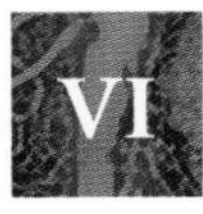

VI Renovascular Disease

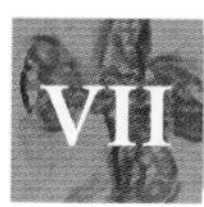

VII Aneurysmal Disease

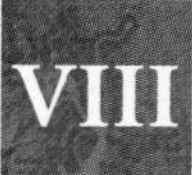

VIII Cerebrovascular Disease

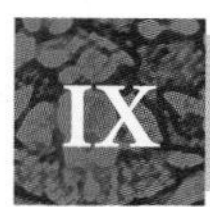

IX Vascular Complications

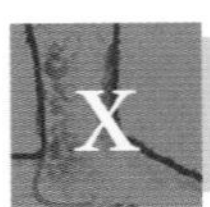

X Venous Disease and Lymphedema

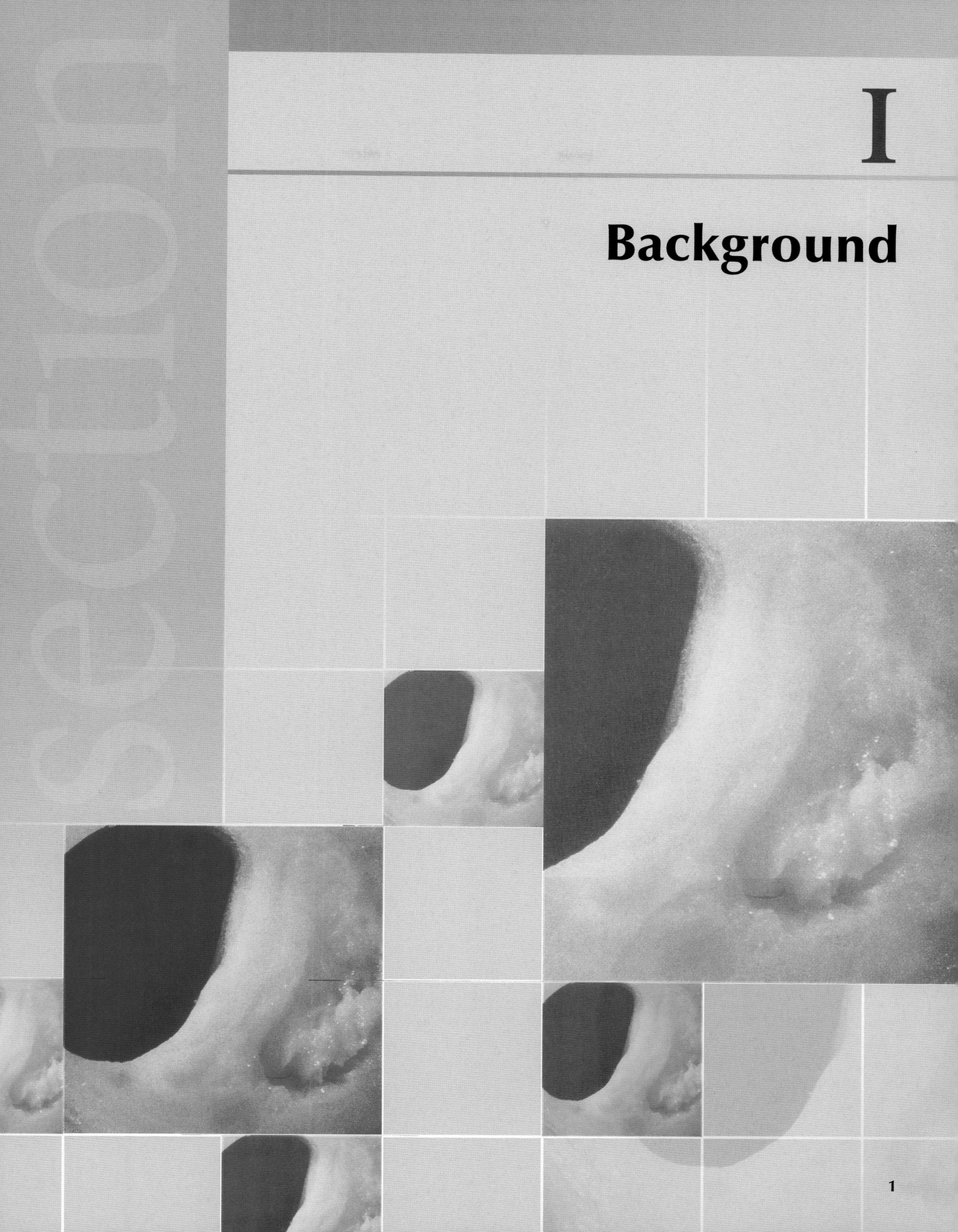

Section I

Background

chapter

1

Historical Perspectives in Vascular Surgery: The Evolution of Modern Trends

Todd E. Rasmussen, MD • Kenneth J. Cherry Jr, MD

Key Points

- Military vascular surgery
- The beginnings of aortic surgery
- Peripheral arterial reconstruction
- Aortic thromboendarterectomy
- Development of aortic prostheses
- Thoracoabdominal aortic aneurysms and aortic dissections
- Mesenteric occlusive disease
- Carotid arterial reconstruction
- Evolution of endovascular procedures
- Conclusion

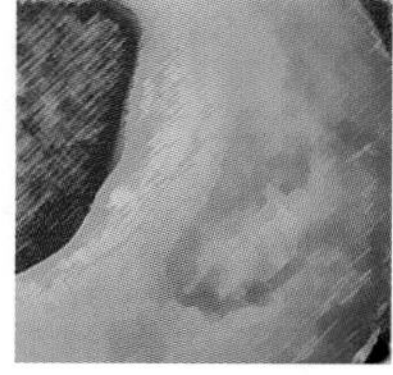

This chapter focuses on the evolution of interesting and important trends in the history of vascular surgery and endovascular therapy. We emphasize that a comprehensive history of vascular surgery is beyond the scope of this chapter for several reasons. Foremost, attempts to account for all of the contributions of Antyllus, Paré, Lambert, Eck, Murphy, the Hunters, Cooper, Mott, Matas, Halstead, Carrel, Exner, Goyanes, and other pioneers of surgery and medicine would fail to do them justice. Furthermore, a comprehensive and modern historical account would incorporate the contributions of transplant and cardiovascular surgery, venous surgery, vascular medicine and pharmacology, diagnostic and therapeutic radiology, and noninvasive vascular testing. Such breadth would surely require more text than the editors are willing to spare.

Consequently, this chapter represents not a complete history of vascular surgery but rather a selective perspective—a perspective of those people and advances of the modern era that have sparked or perpetuated an evolution of vascular care. The omission of certain surgeons and reports may dismay some readers, and the inclusion of others will undoubtedly cause similar discord. Other interpretations and appraisals of our history are as valid as this one; therefore, this effort can be seen as a starting point for collegial discussion.

MILITARY VASCULAR SURGERY

Hippocrates is credited with the phrase "He who wishes to be a surgeon should go to war." Consequently, no history of vascular surgery would be complete without examination of the contributions made by military surgeons. This notion is especially relevant today with the global war on terror in Afghanistan and Iraq. These conflicts have provided the environment in which advances in vascular and endovascular surgery are being made under the most challenging conditions and with the most devastating injuries seen since the Vietnam War. Claudius Galen, one of the greatest surgeons of antiquity, was known for his treatment of traumatic wounds.[1] As a surgeon to the gladiators of the second century, he cared for orthopedic, abdominal, and vascular injuries using sutures, dressings, and splints. The use of heat or cautery was paramount in the treatment of bleeding at the time and was often achieved using boiling oil.[2] In the sixteenth century, the French physician Ambrose Paré advocated a method other than cautery to control hemorrhage. Specifically, Paré introduced the ligature for control of bleeding in a battle in which he had exhausted the supply

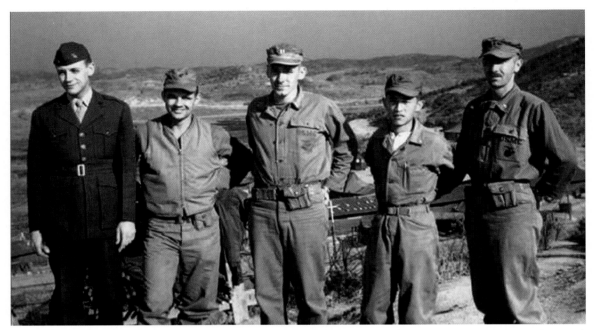

Figure 1-1. Members of Easy Medical Company, a U.S. Marine Corps unit in the First Marine Division in Korea in 1952. Frank Spencer is standing second from the left. (From Spencer FC. *J Trauma* 2006;60:906-909.)

of boiling oil.[2] Ligation of vascular injuries as documented by Paré would remain the treatment of choice until 1952.

Another French surgeon, Dominique Jean Larrey, was the surgeon-in-chief of the Napoleonic armies (1797 to 1815) and is widely regarded as the first modern military surgeon. Larrey's greatest contribution was the "flying ambulance," which was a horse-drawn vehicle designed to transport wounded soldiers from the battlefield to hospitals in the rear for surgical care. Larrey's legacy of rapid casualty movement was fully realized nearly 150 years later when use of helicopters was implemented during the Korean War.

World War I

During World War I, George Makins, the British surgeon general, reported great experience with the treatment of vascular injuries in his paper "On Gunshot Injuries of the Blood Vessels."[3] In this report, Makins reviewed more than 1000 vascular injuries and described the preferred treatment as *ligation.* In contrast, the German surgeon Jaeger began attempts to repair, instead of ligate, arterial injuries in an effort to avoid amputation.[1,4] The German literature reported successful vascular repairs during World War I. Unfortunately, these successes were largely ignored, and enthusiasm for arterial repair waned.

World War II

Despite improvements in mobile surgical units, antibiotics, and whole blood transfusions, World War II did little to advance the treatment of battlefield vascular injuries beyond the principle of ligation. In their classic review of nearly 2500 cases of arterial wounds treated in World War II, Michael DeBakey and Fiorindo Simeone found only 81 instances of suture repair.[5] The amputation rate in this "highly selective group" of patients with "minimal wounds" was 36%, as compared with an amputation rate of 49% following ligation. The poor results of vascular repair led the authors to acknowledge that ligation of vascular injury during wartime was "one of necessity," although repair would be ideal. The major obstacle to vascular repair was prolonged evacuation time, which averaged more than 10 hours, practically precluding successful arterial repair and limb salvage.[4,5] Although the concept of bringing the surgeon close to the battlefield was explored, it was considered unworkable to provide definitive operative care of vascular injuries at forward echelons.

Korean War

Following World War II, military doctrine prohibited attempts at vascular repair in the battlefield, although a program to explore this possibility was initiated at Walter Reed Army Hospital in 1949. At the onset of the Korean War, a U.S. Navy surgeon, Frank C. Spencer, was deployed with "Easy Medical Company," a unit of the First Marine Division (Figure 1-1).[6] In 1952, Spencer challenged warfare doctrine mandating ligation and repaired an arterial injury with a cadaveric femoral artery (i.e., arterial homograft). The Pentagon sent Army surgeons to verify Spencer's achievements, which were eventually reported in 1955. Col. Carl Hughes visited Spencer in Korea and not only verified his clinical experience but also aided in the delivery of badly needed surgical tools to accomplish vascular reconstruction.

Soon a new policy of vascular reconstruction to restore or maintain perfusion to injured extremities was begun under the guidance of Hughes, Edward Janke, and S.F. Seeley.[1,4] This program and the clinical successes of Easy Medical Company represented the first deviation from the practice of ligation started by Paré more than a century earlier. By using the techniques of direct anastomosis, lateral repair, and interposition graft placement, the initial limb salvage rates were encouraging.[7,8]

Subsequently, a contingent of Army surgeons returned to Korea armed with additional surgical techniques at the same time that the medical evacuation helicopter was being fully implemented. The combination of these events provided the momentum for vascular repair to begin in earnest in the mobile Army surgical hospitals (MASHs). Amputation rates associated with extremity vascular injury declined dramatically. In his landmark review of more than 300 major arterial repairs performed during the Korean War, Hughes reported a 13% amputation rate.[4,9,10]

Vietnam War

The experience of DeBakey during World War II and the achievements of Hughes and others in Korea were advanced in the Vietnam War. Foremost, the importance of rapid transport of the wounded soldier to surgical care was realized. In one report, 95% of wounded patients reached surgical attention by helicopter within 2 hours of injury.[11] Recognizing the opportunity, Norman Rich and Hughes initiated the Vietnam Vascular Registry in 1966 to document and analyze vascular injuries.[12] In a review of more than 1000 arterial injuries treated during the Vietnam War, Rich and Hughes reported a limb salvage rate of 87%.[13] The Vietnam Vascular Registry also provided vital information related to venous injuries, missile emboli, concomitant bony and vascular injuries, type of bypass material (prosthetic versus autogenous), and utility of continuous wave Doppler to assess perfusion of the injured extremity.[14-16]

Global War on Terror (2001 to Present)

Contemporary experience with wartime vascular injury has confirmed and extended past military contributions. Modern successes are based on the premise established by Larrey 200 years ago of rapid transport of the injured to surgical expertise. Operations in Iraq and Afghanistan represent the first in which defined forward surgical capability has been used for a prolonged period during different phases of warfare. Deployment of level 2 surgical teams (general and orthopedic surgeons with anesthesia and corpsman support) near the site of injury, in combination with rapid casualty evacuation, means that most wartime injuries are now treated within 1 hour of wounding.[17]

The broad use of commercially engineered tourniquets and body armor has prevented immediate death in many injured soldiers.[17] But, the result has been a three- to fivefold increase in the rate of vascular injury seen on the modern battlefield. Contemporary success with vascular injury management is also based on the near-exclusive use of autologous vein for conduit, as well as an aggressive approach to repair of extremity venous injuries. Interestingly, the importance of the continuous wave Doppler first advocated by Lavenson, Rich, and Strandness to assess perfusion of injured extremities in wartime has been further validated in current military endeavors.[18]

Novel or groundbreaking perspectives have also stemmed from current wartime experience.[19,20] These innovations include the effectiveness of temporary vascular shunts to restore or maintain perfusion until vascular reconstruction can occur. While this technique was first described in the 1950s during the French-Algerian War and again by the Israelis in the early 1970s, the use of temporary vascular shunts in Iraq has been more extensive.[4,21] Current observations have allowed clinical study and discernment of vascular injury patterns most amenable to this damage control adjunct versus those best treated with the time-honored technique of ligation.[19]

Another first in warfare management of vascular injuries has been endovascular capabilities introduced to diagnose and treat select injury patterns.[22] While catheter-based procedures are not common in wartime, this capability has been shown to extend the diagnostic and therapeutic armamentarium of the surgeon during wartime. In some cases, endovascular therapy has provided the preferred or standard therapy (e.g., coil embolization of pelvic fracture or solid organ injury and placement of covered stents).

Another major advance has been negative pressure wound therapy, or VAC (KCI, San Antonio, Texas), which has revolutionized the management of complex soft-tissue wounds associated with vascular injury.[23,24] This closed wound management strategy was not available during previous military conflicts, and its rapid acceptance and common use has made it a standard now used in some phase of nearly all battle-related soft-tissue wounds.

Finally, contemporary wartime experience has prompted a historic reevaluation of the resuscitation strategy applied to the most severely injured. Damage control resuscitation is based on the use of blood products with a high ratio of fresh frozen plasma to packed red blood cells, minimal crystalloid, and selective use of recombinant factor VII.[25] This relatively new strategy has increased survival in injured patients who arrive with markers of severe physiological compromise (e.g., hypotension, hypothermia, anemia, acidosis, or coagulopathy).

BEGINNINGS OF AORTIC SURGERY

The first operations on the aorta took place in the early 1800s and were for aneurysmal disease, invariably due to syphilis, in young to middle-aged men. In 1817, Sir Astley Cooper, a student of John Hunter, ligated the aortic bifurcation in a 38-year-old man who had suffered a ruptured iliac artery aneurysm.[26] The patient died soon after the operation. Keen, Tillaux, Morris, and Halstead reported similar attempts to ligate aortic and iliac artery aneurysms without patient survival in the 100 years following Cooper's initial report.[1]

In 1888, during the era of arterial ligation for aneurysmal disease, Rudolph Matas revived the dormant but centuries-old concept of endoaneurysmorrhaphy. Nearly 16 centuries earlier, Antyllus had introduced the concept of opening and evacuating the contents of the arterial aneurysm sac. Matas successfully performed the technique on a brachial artery aneurysm, after an initial attempt at proximal ligation had failed, in a patient named Manuel Harris, who had a traumatic aneurysm following a shotgun injury to his arm.[27] Although in this instance the technique was successful, Matas was reluctant to apply this method broadly during the era when aneurysm ligation was the prevailing dogma. The technique of open endoaneurysmorrhaphy was not used for more than a decade following Matas's original description.

In 1923, while professor of surgery and the chief of the Department of Surgery at Tulane University, Matas was the first to ligate successfully the abdominal aorta for aneurysmal disease with survival of his patient.[28] He reported this technique again in 1940.[29] Matas eventually improved and refined the technique of open endoaneurysmorrhaphy, described in three forms: obliterative, restorative, and reconstructive. The reconstructive form allowed for maintenance of arterial

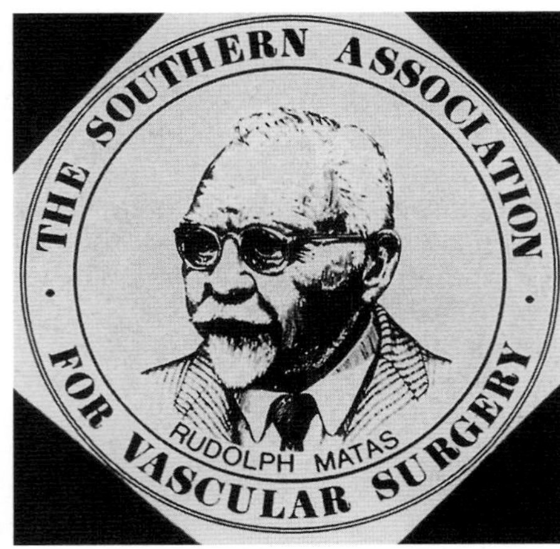

Figure 1-2. Official seal of the Southern Association for Vascular Surgery. (From Ochsner J. *J Vasc Surg* 2001;34:387-392.)

patency. In all, Matas operated on more than 600 abdominal aortic aneurysms, with remarkably low morbidity and mortality rates. In 1940, at the age of 80 years, he presented his experience with the operative treatment of abdominal aortic aneurysms to the American Surgical Association.[30] Through his success and pioneering techniques, Matas demonstrated the efficacy of a direct operative approach to the aorta and began the era of aortic reconstruction.

Matas is widely held as the father of American vascular surgery. In 1977, during the organization of the Southern Association for Vascular Surgery, a likeness of Matas was chosen as the new society's logo (Figure 1-2).[31] In one of his most significant addresses, "The Soul of the Surgeon," he established and emphasized the qualities of a surgeon to which we all should aspire.[32]

PERIPHERAL ARTERIAL RECONSTRUCTION

During this same era, vascular reconstruction of the peripheral arteries was developing rapidly. The first attempts to place venous autografts into the peripheral circulation were described by Alfred Exner in Austria and Alexis Carrel in France at the beginning of the twentieth century.[1] Separately, these two individuals pioneered the vascular anastomosis. Exner used techniques with Erwin Payr's magnesium tubes, while Carrel used segments of vein. Carrel and Charles Guthrie developed the model of the arterial anastomosis in dogs at the Hull Physiological Laboratory in Chicago.[33] In 1912, Carrel was awarded the Nobel Prize in Physiology and Medicine in "recognition of his work on vascular suture and the transplantation of blood vessels and organs."

Guthrie, who was born in Missouri, returned to Washington University in St. Louis as professor. He eventually joined the faculty at the University of Pittsburgh as the chairman of physiology and pharmacology. A likeness of Guthrie was designated as the logo for the Midwestern Vascular Surgical Society during its first annual meeting at the Drake Hotel in Chicago in 1977 (Figure 1-3).[34]

The first use of a venous autograft in the human arterial circulation was performed by the Spanish surgeon José Goyanes in 1906, following resection of a syphilitic popliteal aneurysm.

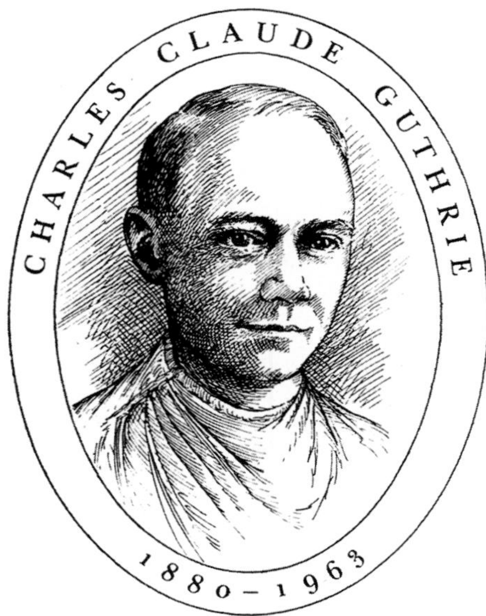

Figure 1-3. Charles Guthrie, as illustrated in the official logo of the Midwestern Vascular Surgical Society. (From Pfeifer JR, et al.[34])

One year later, a German surgeon, Erich Lexer, used a reversed greater saphenous vein as an interposition graft in the axillary position of the arm.[1]

The modern technique of venous grafting fell out of favor following these initial reports until revived by Jean Kunlin with dramatic success in 1948 in Paris. One of Kunlin's first patients was initially under the care of his close associate René Leriche. The patient had persistent ischemic gangrene following sympathectomy and femoral arteriectomy. Kunlin performed a greater saphenous vein bypass from the femoral to the popliteal artery in his patient, employing end-to-side anastomotic techniques at the proximal and distal aspects of the bypass. The concept of end-to-side anastomosis was important as it allowed for preservation of side branches. In 1951, Kunlin reported his results of 17 such bypass operations.[35] In 1955, Robert Linton, from Massachusetts General Hospital, popularized use of the reversed greater saphenous as a bypass conduit in the leg, when he reported his experience.[36]

Heparin was first discovered in 1916 by Jay Maclean and reported in 1918.[37] However, heparin remained too toxic for clinical use until Best and Scott reported the purification of heparin in 1933.[38] Four years later, in 1937, Murray demonstrated that heparin could prevent thrombosis in venous bypass grafts.[39] Murray and Best noted that the use of this novel anticoagulant was important not only during repair of blood vessels but also in treatment of venous thrombosis.[39,40] The availability of heparin emboldened surgeons to attempt vascular reconstructions that had been complicated previously by high rates of thrombosis.

AORTIC THROMBOENDARTERECTOMY

In the early 1900s, Severeanu, Jianu, and Delbet first described thromboendarterectomy. These attempts were before the discovery of heparin and generally resulted in failure due to early thrombosis.[1] Subsequently, the technique was abandoned until the mid-1940s, when John Cid Dos Santos performed the first successful thromboendarterectomy of the aortoiliac

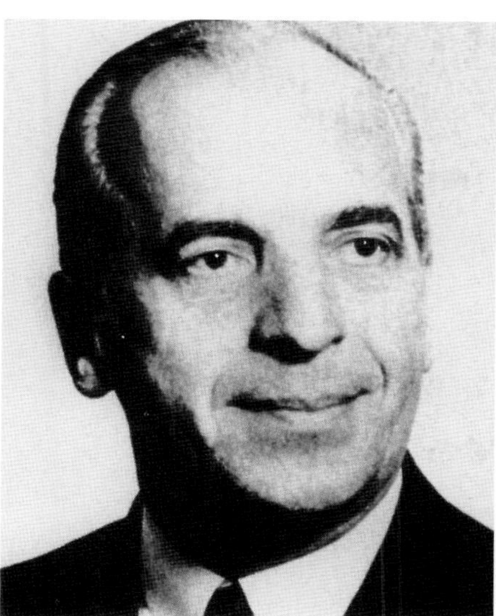

Figure 1-4. Charles Dubost. (From Friedman SG. *J Vasc Surg* 2001;33:895-898.)

segment using an ophthalmic spatula and a gallstone scoop.[8] Edwin Wylie in San Francisco and others soon took up and perfected the technique of aortic thromboendarterectomy in the United States.[41,42] Wylie and colleagues developed and extended endarterectomy techniques to the great vessels, aorta, mesenteric arteries, and renal arteries. The technique of thromboendarterectomy was also used briefly for the management of some abdominal aortic aneurysms, as described by Wylie, who reported the use of fascia lata to wrap an aneurysmal aorta following thromboendarterectomy and tailoring of the vessel.[43]

DEVELOPMENT OF AORTIC PROSTHESES

Successful operations for aortic coarctation in the 1940s by Clarence Crafoord in Sweden and Robert Gross in the United States stimulated interest in arterial homografts that might be used when primary aortic repair could not be accomplished.[44,45] In 1948, Gross and colleagues reported the use of preserved arterial grafts in humans with cyanotic heart disease and aortic coarctation.[46]

Initial successes with arterial homografts in pediatric and cardiac surgery led to their use in the operative treatment of aortoiliac occlusive disease and aortic aneurysms. In 1950, Jacques Oudot replaced a thrombosed aortic bifurcation with an arterial homograft. One year later, another French vascular surgeon, Charles Dubost (Figure 1-4), did the same following resection of an abdominal aortic aneurysm.[47,48]

Arterial homografts seemed initially to be an effective substitute for the thoracic and abdominal aorta. At first, fresh grafts were used; then, Tyrode solution, a preservative, was used to preserve grafts for short periods. Development of the techniques of freezing and lyophilization allowed for the establishment of artery banks.[49,50] Despite early successes, arterial homografts did not provide a durable bypass conduit for the aorta due to aneurysmal degeneration or fibrotic occlusions. A satisfactory aortic substitute was still lacking.

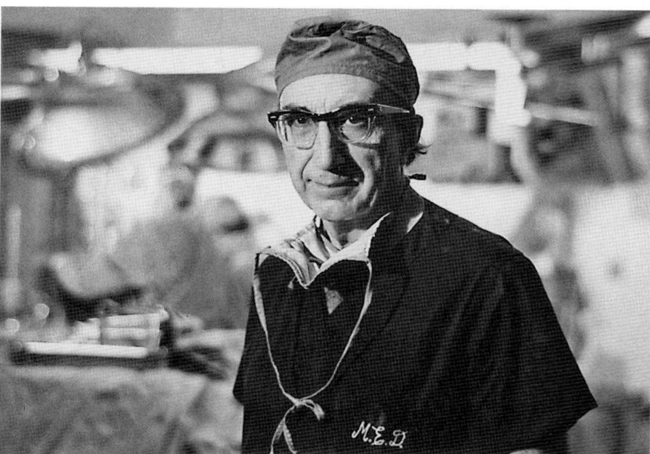

Figure 1-5. Michael DeBakey, MD. (From McCollum CH. *J Vasc Surg* 2000;31:406-409.)

The eventual development of synthetic grafts propelled aortic surgery to its current maturity. As a surgical research fellow at Columbia University under the mentorship of Arthur Blakemore, Arthur Voorhees made a fortuitous observation in 1947. Voorhees recognized that a silk suture inadvertently placed in the ventricle of the dog became "coated in endocardium" after a period in vivo. His observation caused him to speculate that a "cloth tube acting as a lattice work of threads might indeed serve as an arterial prosthesis."[1]

In 1948, during an assignment to Brooke Army Medical Center in San Antonio, Texas, Voorhees fashioned synthetic grafts from parachute material and placed them in the aortic position of the dog. Although few of the initial prostheses lasted for more than a week, Voorhees remained optimistic and returned to Columbia in 1950 to resume his surgical residency. Alfred Jaretzki joined Voorhees and Blakemore in 1951, and their collaboration resulted in a report in 1952 of cloth prostheses in the animal aortic position.[1,51] Having established the efficacy of such in the animal model, the group reported the use of vinyon-N cloth tubes used to replace the abdominal aorta in 17 patients with abdominal aortic aneurysms in 1954.[1,52] Unfortunately, the early synthetic fabrics available were subject to degenerative problems, as well as failure to be incorporated.

DeBakey's (Figure 1-5) introduction of knitted Dacron in 1957 allowed widespread application of the prosthetic graft replacement technique for large- and medium-sized arteries, and modern conventional aortic surgery began in earnest.[53] Modifications of the knitted Dacron graft were provided initially by Cooley and Sauvage and later by others; these modifications improved the original knitted Dacron that DeBakey provided.[54]

THORACOABDOMINAL AORTIC ANEURYSMS AND AORTIC DISSECTIONS

Samuel Etheredge performed the first successful repair of a thoracoabdominal aortic aneurysm in 1954.[55] Etheredge used a plastic tube or shunt, first proposed by Schaffer in 1951, to maintain distal aortic perfusion as he moved the clamp down the graft after each successive visceral anastomosis had been completed. DeBakey and colleagues used modifications of Etheredge's technique and extended the use of graft replacement and bypass to visceral arteries in patients with thoracoabdominal aortic aneurysms. In 1956, DeBakey, Creech, and Morris reported a series of complicated thoracoabdominal aneurysm repairs involving the renal and mesenteric arteries.[56]

In the late 1960s and early 1970s, Wylie and Ronald Stoney in San Francisco popularized the long, spiral thoracoabdominal incision for the approach of thoracoabdominal aortic aneurysms.[33] In his discussion of Wylie and Stoney's paper, Etheredge made reference to the polyethylene bypass tube that he had used as a shunt during his original aneurysm resection. Etheredge noted that he had "fashioned the tube over his gas kitchen stove with a spoon for shaping." Also during the discussion, Etheredge showed pictures of the original thoracoabdominal aortic aneurysm repair, including a picture of the patient 18 years after operation.[57]

Extending the work of Matas and Carrel, DeBakey's younger partner, E. Stanley Crawford, provided the greatest advancement in the operative management of thoracoabdominal aortic aneurysms. Crawford introduced a direct approach to the aneurysm, where the aorta was clamped above and below the aneurysm and then opened longitudinally throughout the aneurysm's length.[58,59] A fabric graft was then sewn into the lumen of the proximal and distal aorta into nonaneurysmal artery. Inclusion of major groups of intercostal or visceral vessels were then sewn into the wall of the fabric graft using modifications of Carrel's patch method of anastomosis, sometimes referred to as a "Crawford window."[58,59]

The ability to handle aortic dissections operatively was first reported by DeBakey with primary resection, as well as fenestration. DeBakey himself underwent operation for aortic dissection in his 90s; he died several years later at the age of 99 (2008). In recent years, aortic stent grafts have become important in managing both thoracic aortic dissections (type B) and descending and some arch aneurysms.

MESENTERIC OCCLUSIVE DISEASE

In 1936, Dunphy first recognized the clinical and anatomical entity known now as chronic mesenteric ischemia. He reviewed autopsy results of patients dying of gut infarction from mesenteric artery occlusions and documented that most patients had the prodrome of abdominal pain and weight loss associated with this syndrome.[60] Robert Shaw and E.P. Maynard III, from Massachusetts General Hospital, first reported thromboendarterectomy of the paravisceral aorta and superior mesenteric artery for treatment of chronic intestinal ischemia in 1958.[61] Following this report, Morris et al. described the use of a retrograde aortomesenteric bypass using knitted Dacron in the treatment of chronic mesenteric ischemia.[62] Although this technique avoided exposure of the midaorta, it was associated with tortuosity and kinking of the retrograde grafts.

The early experience with retrograde grafts and the problem with tortuosity led Wylie and Stoney to develop other techniques to establish visceral flow.[57,63] Wylie's technique evolved from experience doing renal endarterectomy and was facilitated by the thoracoretroperitoneal approach that he had championed for the exposure of thoracoabdominal aortic aneurysms.[57,63] Transaortic endarterectomy was accomplished through a trapdoor aortotomy and eversion endarterectomy of the mesenteric vessels. This technique is now applied transabdominally after medial visceral rotation to avoid the morbidity of the thoracoabdominal incision.

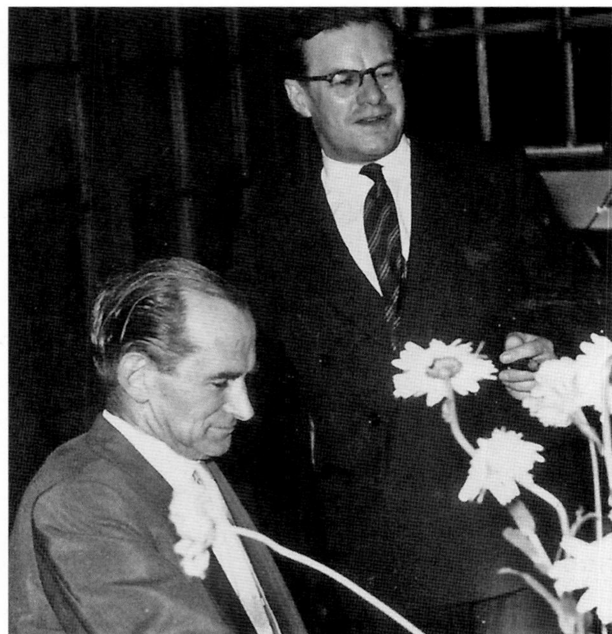

Figure 1-6. Charles Rob and Felix Eastcott, 1960. (From Rosenthal D. *J Vasc Surg* 2002;36:430-436.)

CAROTID ARTERIAL RECONSTRUCTION

The prevailing thought at the turn of the twentieth century was that the major cause of stroke was intracranial vascular disease. A neurologist, Ramsay Hunt, was one of the first to assert that the extracranial carotid circulation was a potential source of cerebral infarcts. In an address to the American Neurological Association in 1913, he recommended the routine examination of the carotid arteries in patients with cerebral symptoms.[64]

Egas Moniz described the first cerebral arteriography in 1927, originally as a technique to diagnose cerebral tumors.[1] In 1950, a neurologist from Massachusetts General Hospital, Miller Fisher reported the results of postmortem examinations of the brains of patients who had died from cerebral vascular occlusive disease. In his observations, Fisher found that a minority of strokes were caused by primary hemorrhagic disease, and he concluded that the majority of strokes were caused by embolic disease.[65,66]

Three years after Fisher proclaimed that "it is conceivable that some day vascular surgery will find a way to bypass the occluded portion of the artery,"[1] DeBakey performed the first carotid endarterectomy in the United States. He performed a thromboendarterectomy on the patient, a 53-year-old man with a symptomatic carotid stenosis; closed the artery primarily; and confirmed patency with an intraoperative arteriogram.[67] Nine months later, Felix Eastcott, George Pickering, and Charles Rob (Figure 1-6) successfully treated a patient with a symptomatic carotid stenosis by means of a carotid bulb resection and primary end-to-end anastomosis of the internal and common carotid arteries.[68]

Figure 1-7. Thomas Fogarty. (Courtesy Thomas Fogarty.)

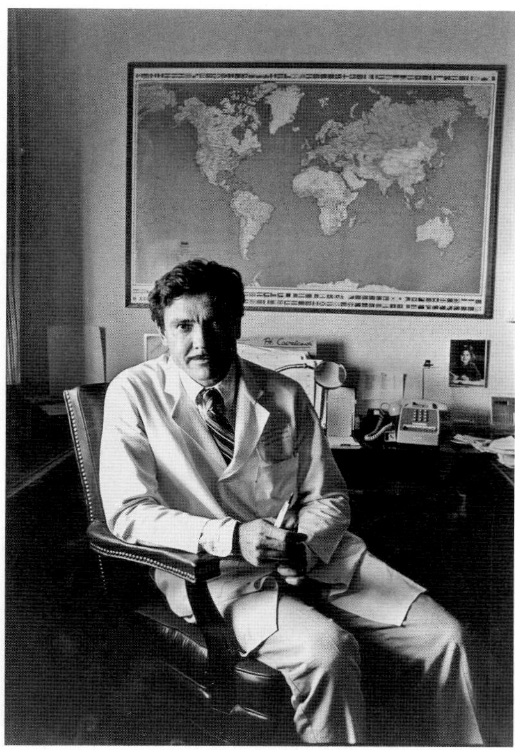

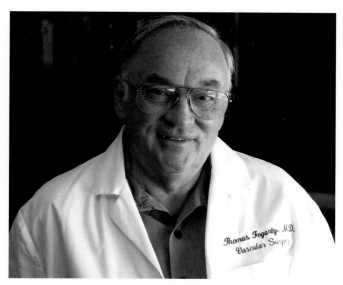

Figure 1-9. Andreas Gruntzig. (Courtesy Emory University School of Medicine, Atlanta.)

In 1961, Yates and Hutchinson further emphasized the importance of extracranial carotid occlusive disease as a cause of stroke.[69] Jack Whisnant, from the Mayo Clinic, identified the risk of stroke in the presence of transient ischemic attacks and provided additional basis for operation on symptomatic disease of the carotid arteries and great vessels, which was becoming widely accepted.[70] Endarterectomy or "disobliteration" of not only symptomatic carotid lesions but also lesions of the subclavian and innominate arteries was advanced by investigators such as Jesse Thompson in Dallas, Wylie in San Francisco, and Inahara in Portland, Oregon. These investigators, as well as others, refined techniques, determined the range of uses, and clarified indications and contraindications. The origins of prophylactic carotid endarterectomy for asymptomatic disease, a topic of debate today, can be traced to Jesse Thompson and colleagues in Dallas in the mid-1970s.[71]

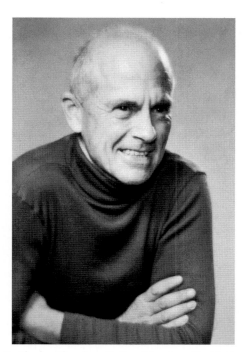

Figure 1-8. Charles Theodore Dotter. (Courtesy The Dotter Interventional Institute, Portland, Ore.)

EVOLUTION OF ENDOVASCULAR PROCEDURES

A Swedish radiologist, Sven-Ivar Seldinger (1921 to 1998), described a minimally invasive access technique to the artery in 1953.[72] Seldinger's technique used a catheter passed over a wire that in turn was introduced through the primary arterial puncture site. The wire was advanced to the desired site, and then the appropriate catheter was advanced over the wire. Previous to Seldinger's technique, arteriography was limited and performed using a single needle at the puncture site in the artery for the injection of contrast material.

One decade after Seldinger's technique had been described, Thomas Fogarty (Figure 1-7) and colleagues reported the use of the thromboembolectomy catheter. That report in 1963, while Fogarty was a surgical resident, detailed the use of a balloon-tipped catheter to extract thrombus, embolus, or both from a vessel lumen without having to open the vessel.[73] A year later, Charles Theodore Dotter (Figure 1-8) reported the use of a rigid Teflon dilator passed through a large radiopaque catheter sheath to perform the first transluminal treatment of diseased arteries.[74]

Five years after his original report, Dotter elaborated on a technique for percutaneous transluminal placement of tubes

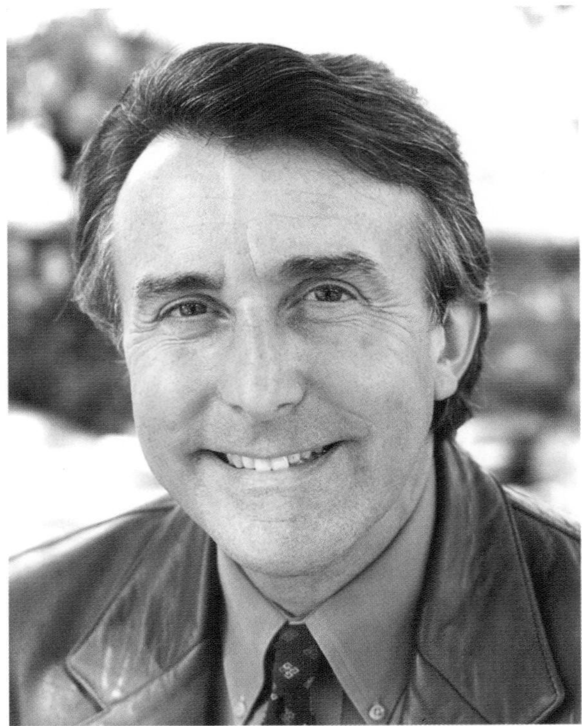

Figure 1-10. Julio Palmaz. (Courtesy Julio Palmaz.)

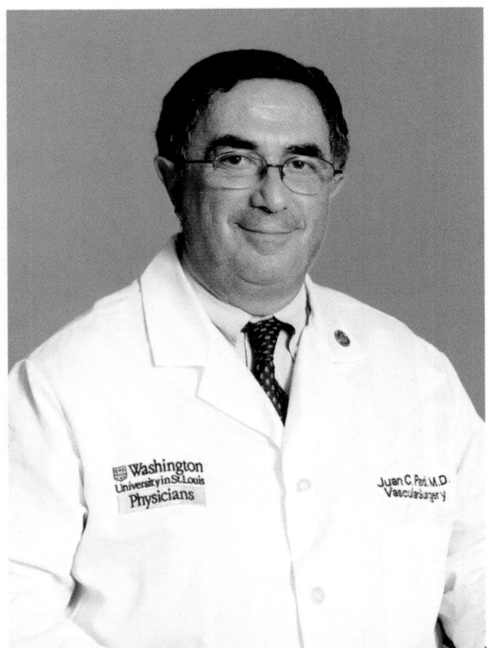

Figure 1-11. Juan Parodi. (Courtesy Washington University, St. Louis.)

within arteries to relieve obstructed arteries and restore blood flow.[75] Together, the work of Fogarty and Dotter in the early to mid-1960s heralded an evolution from diagnostic to diagnostic and therapeutic endovascular procedures.

Silastic balloons were later introduced by a Swiss radiologist, Andreas Gruntzig (Figure 1-9), who extended the work of Fogarty and Dotter and in 1974 reported that percutaneous transluminal angioplasty with a silastic balloon could be performed in different vascular beds, including coronary, renal, iliac, and femoral.[76] Metallic stents in various designs followed percutaneous balloon angioplasty, beginning with the stent developed by Julio Palmaz (Figure 1-10) in 1985.[77] Arguably the greatest advance in transluminal endovascular interventions came when Juan Parodi (Figure 1-11) performed the first endovascular abdominal aortic aneurysm repair.[78] His repair merged the old and the new by attaching a woven Dacron graft to a Palmaz stent and delivering it through a large-bore sheath placed via surgical exposure of the femoral artery.

CONCLUSION

The management of patients with peripheral vascular disease has evolved such that effective treatments often can be performed not only with minimal morbidity but also with short—and, in many cases, no—hospital stay. We have evolved such that the effectiveness of a procedure or treatment is critically assessed in clinical research studies in thousands of patients and measured by single-digit percentages. The pathophysiology and genetic basis of vascular disease are now understood so well in some cases that disease processes are managed effectively with nonoperative means. The rapidity with which the treatment of peripheral vascular disease has evolved over the past century is remarkable. We can only imagine how the practice of vascular surgery will look during the next 50 years if such great progress continues.

References

1. Friedman SG. *A history of vascular surgery*. New York: Futura; 1989.
2. Wangensteen WO, Wangensteen SD, Klinger CF. Wound management of Ambrose Paré and Dominique Larrey, great French military surgeons of the 16th and 19th centuries. *Bull Hist Med* 1972;46:207.
3. Makins GH. *On gunshot injuries to the blood vessels*. Bristol, UK: John Wright & Sons; 1919.
4. Rich NM, Rhee P. An historical tour of vascular injury management: from its inception to the new millennium. *Surg Clin North Am* 2001;81: 1199-1215.
5. DeBakey ME, Simeone FA. Battle injuries of arteries in World War II: an analysis of 2471 cases. *Ann Surg* 1946;123:534-579.
6. Spencer FC. Historical vignette: the introduction of arterial repair into the US Marine Corps, US Naval Hospital, in July-August 1952. *J Trauma* 2006;60:906-909.
7. Jahnke EJ, Seeley SF. Acute vascular injuries in the Korean War: an analysis of 77 consecutive cases. *Ann Surg* 1953;138:158.
8. Hughes CW. The primary repair of wounds of major arteries. *Ann Surg* 1955;141:297.
9. Hughes CW. Arterial repair during the Korean War. *Ann Surg* 1958;147:155.
10. Jahnke EJ. Late structural and functional results of arterial injuries primarily repaired. *Surgery* 1958;43:175.
11. Rich NM. Vietnam missile wound evacuation in 750 patients. *Mil Med* 1968;133:9.
12. Rich NM, Hughes CW. Vietnam vascular registry: a preliminary report. *Surgery* 1969;65:218.
13. Rich NM, Baugh JH, Hughes CW. Acute arterial injuries in Vietnam: 1000 cases. *J Trauma* 1970;10:359-369.
14. Rich NM, Hughes CW, Baugh JH. Management of venous injuries. *Ann Surg* 1970;171:724-730.
15. Rich NM. Vascular trauma. *Surg Clin North Am* 1973;53:1367-1392.
16. Rich NM, Collins Jr GJ, Anderson CA, et al. Missile emboli. *J Trauma* 1978;18:236-239.

17. Rasmussen TE, Clouse WD, Jenkins DH, et al. Echelons of care and the management of wartime vascular injury: a report from the 332nd EMDG/Air Force Theater Hospital Balad Air Base Iraq. *Persp Vasc Surg Endovasc Ther* 2006;10:1-9.
18. Lavenson Jr GS, Rich NM, Strandness Jr DE. Ultrasonic flow detector value in combat vascular injuries. *Arch Surg* 1971;103:644-647.
19. Rasmussen TE, Clouse WD, Jenkins DH, et al. The use of temporary vascular shunts as a damage control adjunct in the management of wartime vascular injury. *J Trauma* 2006;61(1):8-12.
20. Chambers LW, Rhee P, Baker BC, et al. Initial experience of US Marine Corps forward resuscitative surgical system during Operation Iraqi Freedom. *Arch Surg* 2005;140:26-32.
21. Eger M, Golcman L, Goldstein A, et al. The use of a temporary shunt in the management of arterial vascular injuries. *Surg Gyn Obst* 1971;32: 67-70.
22. Rasmussen TE, Clouse WD, Peck MA, et al. Development and implementation of endovascular capabilities in wartime. *J Trauma* 2008;64:1169-1176.
23. Leininger BE, Rasmussen TE, Smith DL, et al. Experience with wound VAC and delayed primary closure of contaminated soft tissue injuries in Iraq. *J Trauma* 2006;61:1207-1211.
24. Peck MA, Clouse WD, Cox MW, et al. The complete management of extremity vascular injury in a local population: a wartime report from the 332nd Expeditionary Medical Group/Air Force Theater Hospital, Balad Air Base, Iraq. *J Vasc Surg* 2007;45:1197-1204.
25. Fox CJ, Gillespie DL, Cox ED, et al. The effectiveness of a damage control resuscitation strategy for vascular injury in a combat support hospital: results of a case control study. *J Trauma* 2008;64(Suppl 2):S99-S106.
26. Brock RC. The life and work of Sir Astley Cooper. *Ann R Coll Surg Engl* 1969;44:1-2.
27. Matas R. Traumatic aneurism of the left brachial artery. *Med News* 1888;53:462.
28. Matas R. Ligation of the abdominal aorta: report of the ultimate result, one year, five months and nine days after ligation of the abdominal aorta for aneurysm of the bifurcation. *Ann Surg* 1925;81:457.
29. Matas R. Aneurysm of the abdominal aorta at its bifurcation into the common iliac arteries. *Ann Surg* 1940;112:909.
30. Matas R. Personal experiences in vascular surgery: a statistical synopsis. *Ann Surg* 1940;112:802.
31. Ernst CB. The Southern Association for Vascular Surgery: the beginning. *J Vasc Surg* 2001;34:381-383.
32. Matas R. The soul of the surgeon. *Tr Miss M Assoc* 1915;48:149.
33. Carrel A, Guthrie CC. Results of biterminal transplantation of veins. *Am J Med Sci* 1906;132:415.
34. Pfeifer JR, Stanley JC. The Midwestern Vascular Surgical Society: the formative years, 1976 to 1981. *J Vasc Surg* 2002;35:837-840.
35. Kunlin J. Le traitement de l'ischemie arteritique par la greffe veineuse longeu. *Rev Chir* 1951;70:206.
36. Linton RR. Some practical considerations in surgery of blood vessels. *Surgery* 1955;38:817.
37. Howell WH. Two new factors in blood coagulation: heparin and proantithrombin. *Am J Physiol* 1918;47:328-341.
38. Best CH, Scott C. The purification of heparin. *J Biol Chem* 1933;102:425.
39. Murray DWG, Best CH. The use of heparin in thrombosis. *Ann Surg* 1938;108:163.
40. Murray DWG. Heparin in surgical treatment of blood vessels. *Arch Surg* 1940;40:307.
41. Wylie EJ. Thromboendarterectomy for atherosclerotic thrombosis of major arteries. *Surgery* 1952;32:275.
42. Freeman NE, Gilfillan RS. Regional heparinization after thromboendarterectomy in the treatment of obliterative arterial disease: preliminary report based on 12 cases. *Surgery* 1952;31:115.
43. Wylie Jr EJ, Kerr E, Davies O. Experimental and clinical experience with the use of fascia lata applied as a graft about major arteries after thromboendarterectomy and aneurysmorrhaphy. *Surg Gynecol Obstet* 1951;93:257.
44. Crafoord C, Nylin G. Congenital coarctation of the aorta and its surgical treatment. *J Thorac Surg* 1945;14:347-361.
45. Gross RE. Treatment of certain aortic coarctations by homologous grafts: a report of nineteen cases. *Ann Surg* 1951;134:753.
46. Gross RE, Hurwitt ES, Bill Jr AH, et al. Preliminary observations on the use of human arterial grafts in the treatment of certain cardiovascular defects. *N Engl J Med* 1948;239:578-579.
47. Oudot J, Beaconsfield P. Thrombosis of the aortic bifurcation treated by resection and homograft replacement: report of five cases. *Arch Surg* 1953;66:365-370.
48. Dubost C, Allary M, Oeconomos N. Resection of an aneurysm of the abdominal aorta: re-establishment of the continuity by a preserved human arterial graft, with results after five months. *Arch Surg* 1952;64:405-408.
49. Deterling Jr RA, Coleman CC, Parshley MS. Experimental studies on the frozen homologous aortic graft. *Surgery* 1951;29:419.
50. Marangoni AG, Cecchini LP. Homotransplantation of arterial segments by the freeze-drying method. *Ann Surg* 1951;134:977.
51. Voorhees Jr AB, Jaretzki A III, Blakemore AH. Use of tubes constructed from vinyon-N cloth bridging arterial defects. *Ann Surg* 1952;135:332.
52. Blakemore A, Voorhees Jr AB. The use of tubes constructed from vinyon-N cloth in bridging arterial defects: experimental and clinical. *Ann Surg* 1954;140:324-334.
53. DeBakey ME, Cooley DA, Crawford ES, et al. Clinical application of a new flexible knitted Dacron arterial substitute. *Arch Surg* 1958;77:713.
54. Sauvage G, Berger KE, Wood SJ, et al. An external velour surface for porous arterial prosthesis. *Surgery* 1971;70:940-953.
55. Etheredge SN, Yee JY, Smith JV, et al. Successful resection of a large aneurysm of the upper abdominal aorta and replacement with homograft. *Surgery* 1955;38:1071.
56. DeBakey ME, Creech O, Morris GC. Aneurysm of the thoracoabdominal aorta involving the celiac, mesenteric and renal arteries: report of four cases treated by resection and homograft replacement. *Ann Surg* 1956;144:549-573.
57. Stoney RJ, Wylie EJ. Surgical management of arterial lesions of the thoracoabdominal aorta. *Am J Surg* 1973;126:157-164.
58. DeBakey ME, Crawford ES, Garrett HE, et al. Surgical considerations in the treatment of aneurysms of the thoracoabdominal aorta. *Ann Surg* 1965;162:350-362.
59. Crawford ES. Thoraco-abdominal aortic aneurysms involving renal, superior mesenteric and celiac arteries. *Ann Surg* 1974;179:763-772.
60. Dunphy JE. Abdominal pains of vascular origins. *Am J Med Sci* 1936;192:109.
61. Shaw RS, Maynard EP. Acute and chronic thrombosis of the mesenteric arteries associated with malabsorption. *N Engl J Med* 1958;258:874.
62. Morris GC, Crawford ES, Cooley DA, et al. Revascularization of the celiac and superior mesenteric arteries. *Arch Surg* 1962;84:95-107.
63. Stoney RJ, Ehrenfeld WK, Wylie EJ. Revascularization methods in chronic visceral ischemia. *Ann Surg* 1977;186:468-476.
64. Hunt JR. The role of the carotid arteries in the causation of vascular lesions of the brain with remarks on certain special features of the symptomatology. *Am J Med Sci* 1914;147:704-713.
65. Fisher M. Occlusion of the internal carotid artery. *Arch Neurol Psychiat* 1951;65:346-377.
66. Fisher M, Adams RD. Observation on brain embolism with special reference to the mechanism of hemorrhagic infarction. *J Neuropath Exp Neurol* 1951;10:92.
67. DeBakey ME. Successful carotid endarterectomy for cerebral vascular insufficiency: nineteen year follow up. *JAMA* 1975;233:1083-1085.
68. Eastcott HHG, Pickering GW, Rob C. Reconstruction of internal carotid artery in a patient with intermittent attacks of hemiplegia. *Lancet* 1954; 2:994-996.
69. Yates PO, Hutchinson EC. Cerebral infarction: the role of stenosis of the extracranial arteries. *Med Res Council Spec Report (London)* 1961;300:1.
70. Whisnant JP, Matsumoto N, Elveback LR. Transient cerebral ischemic attacks in a community: Rochester, Minnesota, 1955 through 1969. *Mayo Clin Proc* 1973;48:194-198.
71. Thompson JE, Patman RD, Talkington CM. Asymptomatic carotid bruit. *Ann Surg* 1978;188:308-316.
72. Seldinger S. Catheter placement of the needle in percutaneous arteriography: a new technique. *Acta Radiol* 1953;39:368.
73. Fogarty T, Cranley J, Krause R, et al. A method for extraction of arterial emboli and thrombi. *Surg Gynecol Obstet* 1963;116:241.
74. Dotter CT, Judkins MP. Transluminal treatment of arteriosclerotic obstruction. *Circulation* 1964;30:654-670.
75. Dotter CT. Transluminally placed coilspring endarterial tube grafts: long-term patency in canine popliteal artery. *Invest Radiol* 1969;4:329-332.
76. Gruntzig A, Hopff H. Perkutane rekanalisation chronischer arterieller verschlusse mit einem neuen dilatationskatheter: modifikation der dotter-technik. *Dtsch Med Wochenschr* 1974;99:2502-2510.
77. Palmaz J, Sibbitt R, Reuter S, et al. Expandable intraluminal graft: a preliminary study. *Radiology* 1985;156:72-77.
78. Parodi JC, Palmaz JC, Barone HD. Transfemoral intraluminal graft implantation for abdominal aortic aneurysms. *Ann Vasc Surg* 1991;5: 491-499.

chapter

2

Vascular Biology

Virginia M. Miller, PhD

Key Points

- Endovascular and vascular surgeons are largely concerned with correction of degenerative vascular disease, explained by the abnormal biology (or pathology) of blood vessels.
- Biological responses of blood vessels to vascular and endovascular procedures limit the long-term success of mechanical intervention.
- Understanding vascular biology may lead to the development of new medical and interventional techniques.
- The balance in production and release of endothelium-derived relaxing and contracting factors affects how injured and grafted blood vessels heal.
- Production and release of endothelium-derived factors are influenced by hemodynamic changes, sex steroid hormones, infection, and aging.
- Growth factors and enzymes released from blood elements interacting with the blood vessel wall promote development of intimal hyperplasia.
- Monogenic vascular disorders are uncommon, but they provide valuable insight into mechanisms of vascular disease.
- Growth factors, together with extracellular matrix cues, regulate the growth of new blood vessels. Growth factors can be used as adjuncts for revascularization and recovery of tissue loss.
- Sex, hormonal status, and immunological competence are confounding factors that modulate vascular healing.

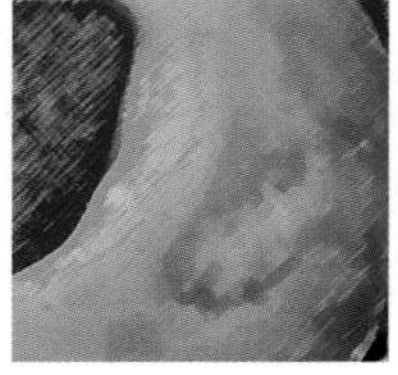

Many contemporary challenges faced by vascular and endovascular surgeons have their basis in vascular pathology, or abnormal vascular biology. The success of endovascular aneurysm repair depends partly on the absence of endoleak through lumbar and other vessels and arresting the process of aortic dilatation at the aneurysm neck. The success of peripheral bypass surgery depends on the limitation of anastomotic hyperplasia and controlling the progression of atherosclerosis in inflow and outflow vessels. Intimal hyperplasia with recurrent stenosis is a common consequence of femoral angioplasty. In other cases, tissue loss and absence of vessels for reconstruction make amputation the logical treatment choice. Advances in vascular biology can be harnessed by vascular and endovascular specialists to improve the results of their intervention.

BASIC ANATOMY

The blood vessel wall consists of a single layer of endothelial cells that provides an interface between the blood and the smooth muscle forming the medial layer. The adventia contains undifferentiated dendritic cells, connective tissue (through which course the autonomic innervation to the vascular wall), and the vasa vasorum. The thickness of the medial layer and the density of innervation differ among blood vessels in various anatomical locations within the body (e.g., arteries have thicker media compared to veins and arterioles and cutaneous veins are more highly innervated than conduit arteries and capacitance veins). In terms of physiological control, vascular smooth muscle is layered between two regulatory systems. The first of these regulators is the *endothelium,* which influences the tone and growth of the underlying smooth muscle through inhibitory and stimulatory factors released in response to blood flow, oxygen tension, hormones, and cytokines and chemokines in the blood. The second regulator, *autonomic innervation,* responds to activation of peripheral baroreceptors, chemoreceptors, and temperature receptors; this causes higher brain centers to trigger neurotransmitter release, causing contraction of medial smooth muscle cells. In the periphery, the primary innervation is sympathetic adrenergic neurotransmission (Figure 2-1). Although endothelium-dependent relaxation was first described in response to acetylcholine, no evidence exists that muscarinic neurons innervate peripheral arteries or veins such as the

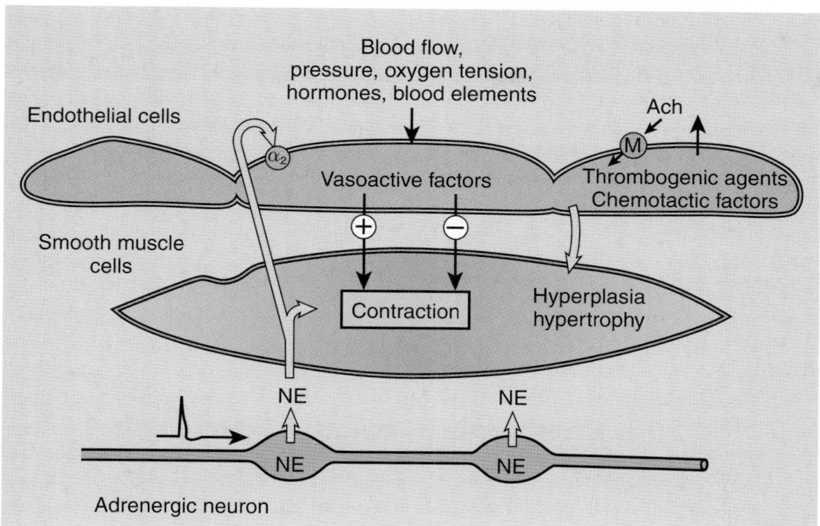

Figure 2-1. Basic components of the vascular wall. Endothelial cells act as sensors of the local environment, releasing vasoactive and mitogenic factors in response to changes in blood flow, pressure, oxygen tension, circulating cytokines, and hormones and in response to physical attachment of blood elements to their surface or to cytokines that they might release. Endothelium-derived factors released toward the underlying vascular smooth muscle regulate contraction, proliferation, and migration; those released into the blood affect adhesion and activation of circulating blood elements. The endothelial cells contain receptors for various agonists, including neurotransmitters of the sympathetic (α_2-adrenergic) and parasympathetic (muscarinic receptor) nervous system: norepinephrine and acetylcholine, respectively. The major innervation to peripheral arteries is from the sympathetic nervous system. Therefore, the vascular smooth muscle is layered between two regulators: the autonomic nervous system that signals from peripheral receptors and brain and the endothelium that signals from the local environment.

saphenous vein. However, receptors for adrenergic (α_2) and muscarinic neurotransmitters are located on the endothelium of peripheral arteries and the saphenous vein. Stimulation of these receptors normally leads to the release of endothelium-derived relaxing factors, which would functionally antagonize the contraction initiated by both types of receptors on the medial smooth muscle of these blood vessels.

These two regulatory systems enable vascular tone to be modulated in response to "central command" and to be individualized at each vascular bed in response to local changes in the immediate environment. However, manipulation of the blood vessels, such as dissection and transplantation, disrupts innervation and shifts the balance of control of vascular tone and remodeling to the endothelium.

VASCULAR RESPONSE TO INJURY

Endothelial Dysfunction

In health, the endothelium provides an antithrombotic surface for blood flow by releasing endothelium-derived factors. The primary factor is nitric oxide, which inhibits adhesion and coagulation of blood elements on the endothelial surface and inhibits contraction of the underlying smooth muscle. In addition to nitric oxide, cyclooxygenase products of arachidonic acid—prostacyclin and thromboxane—affect the adherent surface and smooth muscle tone. Prostacyclin inhibits platelet adhesion and aggregation, proliferation and migration of vascular smooth muscle and dendrite cells, and promotes vasodilatation, and thromboxane has the opposite effect (Figure 2-2). A potent vasoconstrictor, endothelin-1, is also produced in endothelial cells and acts to antagonize actions of nitric oxide. These factors are released in response to stimuli such as shear stress of the blood flowing over the surface of the cells, hormones, cytokines, and changes in oxygen tension. Furthermore, the relative proportion of endothelium-derived relaxing compared to contracting factors differs among vascular beds. In general, endothelium-derived relaxing factors predominate in arteries while contracting factors dominate in veins. The endothelium can be damaged by mechanical (physical) forces; by biochemical factors, such as overproduction of oxygen-derived free radicals by abnormal lipid metabolism, tobacco smoke-associated particulate matter and carbon monoxide, infection-associated lipopolysaccharide and cytokines (including those associated with transplant rejection); or by a combination of physical and biochemical exposure as occurs during cardiopulmonary bypass.[1,2] Dysfunction of the endothelium is considered an initiating step in development of atherosclerosis as the balance of endothelium-derived factors is shifted from one that inhibits contraction and proliferation of migratory cells to one that promotes these actions.[3]

The endothelium is fragile: even the most careful dissection of any blood vessel causes some damage to the endothelium. Physical or chemical injury to the endothelium facilitates the adhesion of platelets, leukocytes, and monocytes to the vessel wall. Stimuli facilitating chemical injury to the endothelium include lipids, oxidized lipids, cytokines released from damaged organs, and infection. Increased generation of oxygen-derived free radicals can inactivate nitric oxide, thus reducing its bioavailability.[4] Furthermore, the resulting compound, peroxynitrite, initiates an inflammatory phenotype and triggers apoptosis in endothelial cells. Various populations of lipoproteins (i.e., low-density versus high-density lipoproteins) stimulate expression of adhesion molecules on endothelial cells. Chronic infection may produce and exacerbate other types of endothelial injury.[5,6] (For example, the vascular effects of periodontal disease may be different in an otherwise healthy person from in a smoker with elevated low-density lipoproteins.) These chronic inflammatory conditions affect vascular healing in response to endovascular procedures or grafting. Activated endothelial cells allow adherence of leukocytes, which secrete enzymes and growth factors that facilitate their migration into the vessel wall and in doing so damage the subendothelium. Once resident in the endothelium, these cells (macrophages) alter their phenotype, a process accelerated by oxidant stress. The expression of specific cell surface receptors permits the uptake of oxidized lipids and cholesterol, particularly oxidized low-density lipoproteins. The altered pattern of gene expression of growth factors, chemoattractants, and proteases causes the proliferation and migration of underlying smooth muscle cells into the intima. The stage is set for the development of intimal pathology: atherosclerosis and intimal hyperplasia (Figure 2-3).

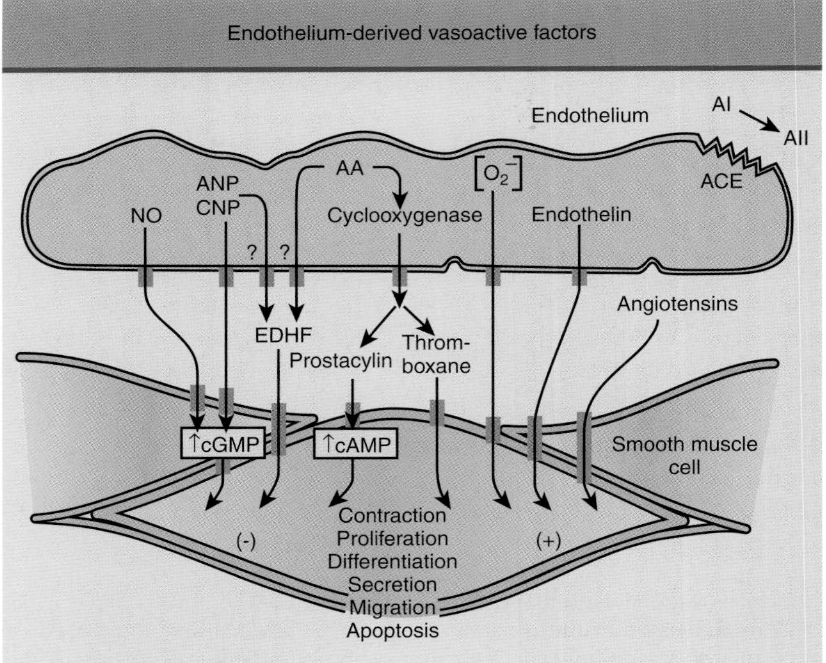

Figure 2-2. Vasoactive factors are produced by the endothelium. AA, arachidonic acid; ACE, angiotensin converting enzyme; A1 and AII, angiotension I and II; ANP, atrial natriuretic peptide; cAMP, cyclic adenosine monophosphate; cGMP, cyclic guanosine monophosphate; CNP, c-type natriuretic peptide; EDHF, endothelium-derived hyperpolarizing factors, which include CNP and various other metabolites of arachidonic acid by lipoxygenase; O_2^-, oxygen-derived free radicals.

Even when the endothelium is relatively undisturbed, dissection of the adventia can interrupt the innervation[7-10] and vasa vasorum, resulting in migration of cells into the intima and a hyperplastic response.[11-14] This situation occurs with transplanted organs and blood vessels removed for grafting.

Endothelium as Mechanosensors

The hemodynamic forces affecting endothelial cells can be divided into two principal forces: shear stress and pressure. Shear stress is the frictional force acting at the interface between the circulating blood and the endothelial surface. Pressure, which acts perpendicular to the vessel wall, imposes circumferential deformation on blood vessels. Therefore, it becomes convenient to address the vascular biology of hemodynamic forces in two parts: the effect of shear stress, where the endothelial monolayer transduces mechanical signals into biological responses, and circumferential stretch and deformation, which impose different, usually pathological, biological responses. Endothelial cells orient in parallel with the direction of laminar flow. Disruption of laminar flow as occurs at bifurcations, at branches, in regions of arterial narrowing, in areas of extreme curvature (as at the carotid bulb), and at valves results in turbulent flow patterns, reversal of flow, and areas of flow stagnation. In these regions, endothelial cells appear as flattened cobblestones. Abnormal hemodynamic stresses also occur during angioplasty, in the fashioning of vein grafts, and with other endovascular and vascular interventions.

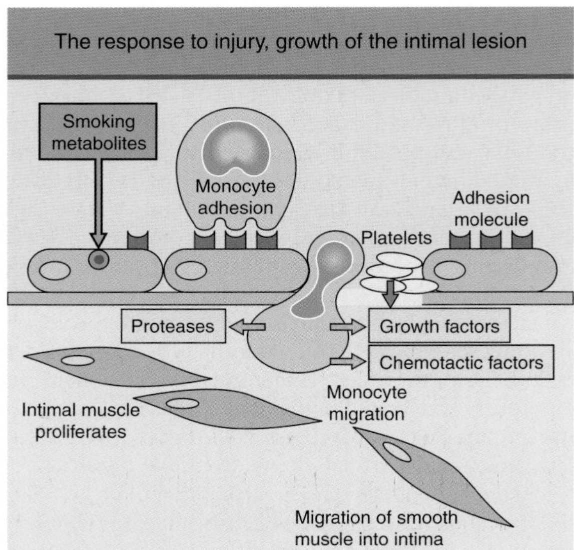

Figure 2-3. The response to injury and development of intimal hyperplasia.

Steady laminar blood flow maintains release of nitric oxide and other antithrombotic, antiadhesive, and growth-inhibitory endothelium-derived factors. In contrast, abnormal flow promotes thrombosis, along with the recruitment and adhesion of monocytes that in turn create foci for development of intimal hyperplasia and conditions focal atherosclerosis.[15] The mechanosensors on the endothelium that sense changes in blood flow and shear stress are poorly defined at the molecular level, but at the cellular level a time-scale of cell-signaling pathways has been carefully described. One of the important molecules involved in the regulation of blood vessels in response to altered flow is nitric oxide, and reactive hyperemia on release of a tourniquet provides an elegant physiological example of this phenomenon. After release of a limb tourniquet, blood flow suddenly increases. This response, called *reactive hyperemia,* can be monitored by changes in brachial artery diameter using ultrasound or by changes in arterial tonometry and blood flow in the finger.[16-18]

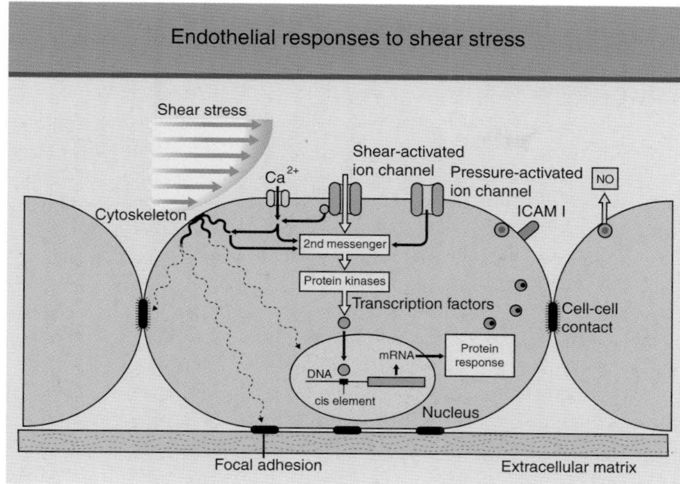

Figure 2-4. How shear stress activates intracellular signaling in endothelial cells.

Rapid increases in blood flow over the endothelial surface stimulates both the synthesis and the release of nitric oxide and causes the dilatation of numerous blood vessels, resulting in hyperemia of the limb. The endothelium responds to sudden increases in shear stress within milliseconds, with changes in membrane potential and an increase in intracellular calcium concentration, probably achieved through calcium influx. These changes in intracellular calcium concentration drive changes in potassium channel activation, generation of inositol triphosphate and diacylglycerol, and changes in G protein activation to inform the cell-signaling cascades within the endothelial cells. These signaling cascades within the endothelial cell are activated over a period of several minutes to 1 hour and include activation of the mitogen-activated protein kinase–signaling cascade and the translocation of the transcription factor NFκB from the cytosol into the nucleus (Figure 2-4).[19] In addition, changes occur within the cytoskeleton of the cell and the cell membrane, both of which are likely to facilitate the release of nitric oxide and other vasodilators, including prostacyclin. These immediate changes in response to dramatic changes in shear stress are followed within a few hours by changes in the regulation of a subset of genes comprising up to 3% of the repertoire of expressed genes within the endothelium.[20] Specific examples include increased synthesis of nitric oxide synthase, tissue plasminogen activator, intercellular adhesion molecule-1, monocyte chemoattractant protein-1, and platelet-derived growth factor–B. Some of these genes have a particular consensus of nucleotides in the 5′ (promoter) region of the gene, which is known to be a shear stress responsive element. Mutation of this limited cassette of bases can result in the loss of sensitivity of gene expression in response to shear stress. Genes may be downregulated, as well as upregulated. The genes that are downregulated in response to increased shear stress include thrombomodulin and the vasoconstrictor endothelin-1. Later, within several hours, further changes to the cytoskeleton and focal adhesion sites allow the cells to become more aligned with blood flow.

The totality of these changes affects the anticoagulant and antiadhesive nature of the endothelial cell surface. While these changes may explain much of the pathology observed by the vascular surgeon, these same responses of the endothelium to shear stress partly control the adaptation of a vein graft to arterial flow. The range of blood flow within the graft influences (by way of the endothelium) the rate of development and magnitude of intimal hyperplasia.[21] However, for the vein graft, the clinician has to consider not only the primary hemodynamic force of shear stress but also the circumferential deformation.[22] Some changes observed in vein grafts or dialysis fistulae, particularly some proadhesive changes, might occur more rapidly in response to changes in pressure and circumferential deformation than to changes in shear stress. These changes in pressure or circumferential deformation also control the cytoskeletal biology of the underlying smooth muscle cell. Permeability changes resulting from pressure are thought to increase exposure to oxygen radicals such as superoxide. The oxidation of lipids results in changes of smooth muscle cell gene expression, with increased secretion of the growth factors and proteases that predispose to intimal hyperplasia (the migration of proliferative smooth muscle cells into the intima).

These changes are likely to be influenced by early changes in cellular calcium concentration and activity of cation channels in the cell membrane. The earliest responses that have been observed include increases in the C-fos gene, increase of apoptotic markers, and changes in the expression of genes associated with the reorganization of actin filaments. These changes have been more difficult to elucidate experimentally than the changes in the endothelium; cultured endothelial cells retain a phenotype similar to that of the native endothelium, while cultured smooth muscle cells rapidly lose the contractile phenotype they have in the arterial wall and acquire the synthetic phenotype of the smooth muscle cells observed in intimal lesions.

Because much of the pathology of vein grafts has been associated with abnormal smooth muscle cell proliferation and elaboration of a dense extracellular matrix, there has been considerable focus on how pressure or circumferential deformation alters the replicative activity of the smooth muscle cell. Most of this work has explored how the high intraluminal pressures associated with angioplasty alter the replicative activity of smooth muscle cells and, in doing so, provides a rationale for the development of drug-eluting stents.[23,24]

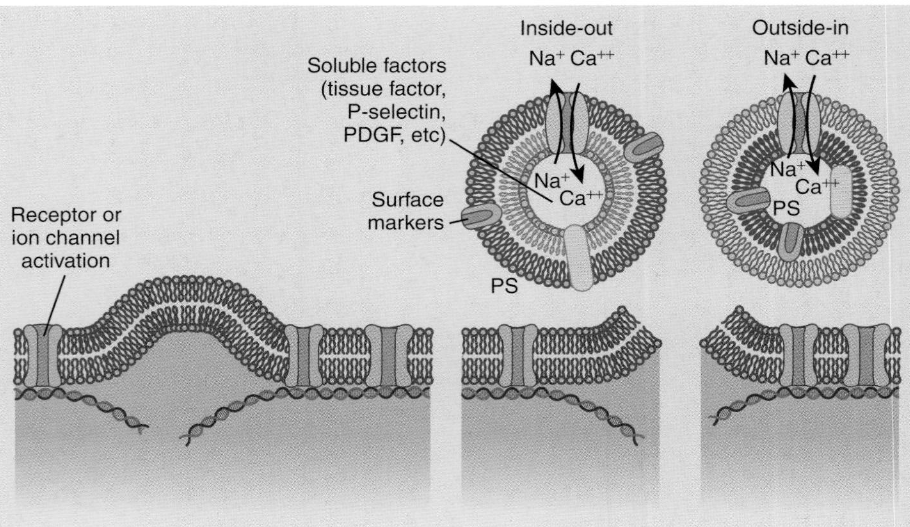

Figure 2-5. Formation of microparticles or vesicles from activated cells. In response to a specific stimulus, a growth factor, enzymatic digestion may occur, which disrupts the integrity of the cell wall and releases blebs of membrane. These blebs may have a configuration in which cell-specific proteins are expressed on their surface. Once in the circulation, these microvesicles can activate their cell of origin or other cells; they can also transfer soluble material such as tissue factor or growth factors such as platelet-derived growth factors to other cells.

Cell-Derived Microvesicles or Microparticles

Following activation or during apoptosis, a series of calcium-dependent enzymatic pathways is activated. These pathways disrupt the outer membrane of endothelial (and other cells), resulting in the release of membrane fragments that form vesicles varying in size from 100 to 1000 nm (Figure 2-5).[25] The orientation of some of these released vesicles is such that they bear on their surface phosphatidylserine and other protein markers of their cell of origin. The content of these vesicles can vary, but most contain soluble factors such as tissue factor, P-selectin, and platelet-derived growth factor, which are subsequently released or transferred to other cells such as platelets or leukocytes. Elevated numbers of circulating microvesicles are associated with end-stage renal disease, atherosclerosis, atrial fibrillation, gestational hypertension, and clotting disorders.[26-30] Because microvesicles promote endothelial dysfunction[31] and thrombin generation,[31] they have the potential to affect vascular healing in response to grafting and endovascular procedures. However, how these microvesicles relate to specific vascular surgical outcomes has not been explored.

Reendothelialization

Endothelium can repopulate segments of blood vessels that have undergone mechanical endothelial denudation. This process was usually considered as proceeding from in-growth of dividing cells around the perimeter of the damage, such as at a site of vascular anastamoses. However, evidence suggests that the bone marrow–derived endothelial progenitor cells also circulate in the blood and adhere to damaged surfaces. The number of these progenitor cells varies, but in general increased healing is associated with increased numbers of these cells.[32-37] Hormonal status modulates the number of these circulating cells such that an estrogen replete condition is associated with increased number and survival of these cells, this accounting perhaps partly for the decreased incident of cardiovascular disease in premenopausal women compared to age-matched men.[38-40]

In spite of the ability of the endothelium to repopulate an area of injury, experimental evidence suggested that the regenerated endothelium may not have functional recovery,[41-44] thus affecting long-term remodeling and patency of stented arteries, vascular grafts, and arteries in transplanted organs.[1]

Revascularization

New blood vessels can develop by (1) sprouting of existing vessels in response to growth factor stimuli, (2) maturation of bone marrow–derived endothelial cell progenitors (angioblasts), or (3) growth of arteries from arterioles. These three forms of vessel growth are known as angiogenesis, vasculogenesis, and arteriogenesis.[45] Various growth factors (and cytokines) coordinate the reprogramming of endothelial cells, mesenchymal cells, and monocytes associated with new vessel formation; these include vascular endothelial growth factor, basic fibroblast growth factor, platelet-derived growth factor, granulocyte–monocyte colony-stimulating factor, transforming growth factor-β, and monocyte chemoattractant protein-1. Growth factors interact with specific cell surface receptors.

Binding of the growth factor to the receptor results in changes in the shape and/or phosphorylation of the receptor tail on the inside of the cell. This in turn leads to the recruitment of various adaptor proteins or a sequence of enzyme phosphorylations. Both processes eventually lead to the altered transcription of the cellular genes, permitting the cell to migrate, proliferate, or change its phenotype. These processes involve platelets, endothelium-derived progenitor cells, and dendritic cells resident in the vascular wall.[46-49]

These cell systems are being explored as "cell based" therapies to improve circulation to ischemic areas.[50-56] However, much remains to be explored regarding the utility of these therapies in large artery and reconstructive disease.

GENETIC CONSIDERATIONS FOR VASCULAR DISEASE AND HEALING

Sex-Based Medicine

In the era of personalized medicine, the most fundamental genetic difference among individuals is the presence of an XX or XY chromosome that defines biological sex. In 2001,

Table 2-1
Genetic Variation in Vascular Mechanisms and Disease*

	Pathophysiological Implications
Receptors	
α-Adrenergic	
α_{1a}-Adrenergic	Increased risk for coronary events
α_{2b}-Adrenergic	Ethnic differences in the development of hypertension: risk of heart failure
α_{2c}-Adrenergic	Increased risk for pregnancy-induced hypertension
Angiotensin II type I	Idiopathic dilated cardiomyopathy
β_1-Adrenergic	Synergistic interaction with α1c-adrenergic receptor to increase risk of heart failure in blacks
β_2-Adrenergic	Family history of hypertension: risk of obesity
B_2-Bradykinin	Increased risk for hypertension in some ethnic populations
Enzymes	
Angiotensin-converting enzyme (ACE)	Increased risk for atherosclerotic disease, heart failure, and response to ACE inhibitors
CYP3A4	ACE inhibitors (losartan): calcium channel blockers (amlodipine, diltiazem, felodipine, lercanidipine, nicardipine, nifedipine, nimodipine, nisoldipine, nitrendipine, verapamil) and HMG-CoA inhibitors or statins (atorvastatin, lovastatin, pravastatin, simvastatin, fluvastatin)
CYP2D6	Beta blockers (propranolol, S-metoprolol)
CYP2C9	ACE inhibitors (losartan): HMG-CoA inhibitor (fluvastatin)
Endothelial nitric oxide synthase	Increased risk for cardiovascular events, including myocardial infarction, thrombosis, and hypertension

From Schaefer BM, Caracciolo V, Frishman WH, et al. *Heart Dis* 2003;5:129.
*CYP, cytochrome P450; HMG-CoA, 3-hydroxy-3-methylglutaryl-coenzyme A.

the Institute of Medicine released the report "Exploring the Biological Contributions to Human Health: Does Sex Matter?"[57] The major conclusion of this report is that sex matters in ways that have previously been unrecognized and unexplored related to etiology, diagnosis, and treatment of disease. In terms of vascular biology, the best illustration of how sex matters is that the incidence of cardiovascular disease in men exceeds that of age-matched women until the age of menopause in women, when the incidence in women increases exponentially and eventually exceeds that of men.[58] This observation forms the basis for investigations into the actions of sex steroid hormones on the vascular wall. Indeed, sex steroid hormones influence all components and functions of the vascular wall, including endothelium, smooth muscle, release and uptake of transmitter from neuronal varicosities, cells in the adventitia, and cellular elements in the blood. In general, the female sex hormone 17β-estradiol promotes functions that maintain vasodilatation, including increases in release of nitric oxide from endothelial cells, increases in endothelial cell proliferation, and inhibition of smooth muscle cell proliferation.[59-61] For these reasons, estrogen treatments given close to the time of ovariectomy or menopause slow progression of cardiovascular disease.[62,63] Endogenous estrogen also seems to contribute to cardiovascular health in men, as a man deficient in one of two estrogen receptors (estrogen receptor-α) had accelerated atherosclerosis.[64,65] Additional genetic studies suggest that polymorphisms in estrogen receptor-α are associated with increased cardiovascular disease in men.[66-68]

Vascular effects of testosterone have not been studied as extensively as those of estrogen.[69,70] The direct effects on the vascular wall are confounded partly because of the endogenous conversion of testosterone to 17β-estradiol; polymorphisms in the enzymes mediating this conversion are just beginning to be explored.[70-75]

Genetic Implications of Drug Metabolism

Differences in response to pharmacological agents are documented among men and women and among people of different ethnicities.[76-79] In terms of vascular physiology, in addition to the variation mentioned earlier regarding steroid hormone metabolism, genetic variations affect responsiveness to adrenergic neurotransmitters, endothelium-derived factors, enzymes involved in the synthesis of endogenous vasoactive substances, and enzymes that metabolize pharmacological agents used to treat various cardiovascular diseases (Table 2-1). As the science of pharmacogenomics advances and testing for genetic polymorphisms becomes more affordable, it will be possible to tailor pharmacological interventions for the individual to provide maximal benefit with minimal harm.

Genetic Components of Aneurysmal Disease

At least two rare monogenic disorders are associated with the development of aortic and/or arterial aneurysms before the onset of "middle age." In both Marfan syndrome and Ehlers-Danlos syndrome type IV, deletions, mutations, or both occur in genes encoding the extracellular matrix proteins essential for coordinating cellular metabolism and directly contributing to the mechanical and elastic properties of arteries. The Marfan gene is for fibrillin, a key component of microfibrils forming the elastic scaffold, while the Ehlers-Danlos type IV gene is for type III collagen. Mutations in these genes are not associated with the common form of "atherosclerotic" abdominal aortic aneurysm (AAA), which has a prevalence of about 5% in men older than 60 years. However, many AAAs are found in familial clusters, and 20% to 30% of the brothers of patients with AAA also develop an AAA. This observation has directed attention at the genes of other major extracellular

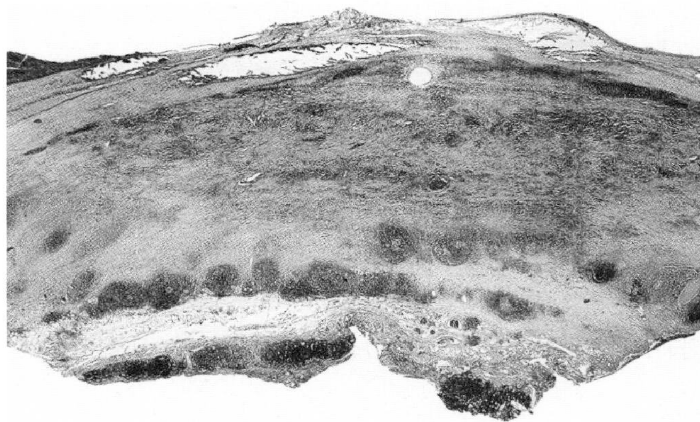

Figure 2-6. Section through an inflammatory abdominal aortic aneurysm stained with hematoxylin and eosinophil (×1; lumen at the top of the slide). There is dense lymphocytic infiltrates within the densely fibrotic adventitia and periadventitial tissues. The media is thin, whereas the intima is thickened with areas of calcification.

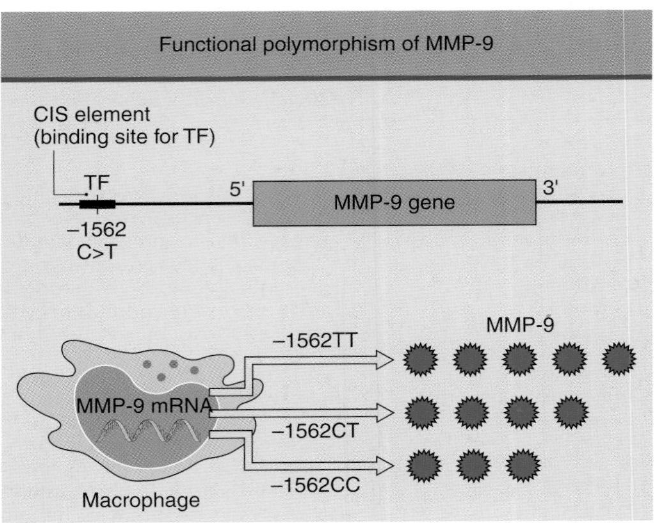

Figure 2-7. Functional polymorphism of matrix metalloproteinase-9 (MMP-9). The −1562T allele is associated with increased MMP-9 production. TF, transcription factor.

matrix components in aorta, including elastin and type I collagen. Interestingly, elastin gene mutations give rise to a rare form of stenosing arterial disease, supravalvular aortic stenosis, rather than to aneurysms. No evidence links mutations in the type I collagen gene to AAA. Nevertheless, aneurysmal disease is characterized by thinning of the extracellular matrix in the aortic media with elastin destruction, loss of smooth muscle cells, and transmural ingress of inflammatory cells (Figure 2-6). This has focused attention on a family of enzymes, the matrix metalloproteinases (MMPs), which have the ability to break down the extracellular matrix of the arterial wall.[80]

MMPs are a family of structurally related, zinc-containing enzymes that have their activity regulated at several levels, including transcription (how much messenger RNA is produced), activation (proteolytic processing of the inactive form or zymogen produced in cells), and inhibition (principally by tissue inhibitors of MMPs). Regulation of both of these families of enzymes provides a regulatory or balancing mechanism to prevent excessive degradation of extracellular matrix. One of the members of this MMP family, MMP-9, has the ability to degrade elastin, denatured collagen, type IV collagen, fibronectin, and other matrix components; this activity has been specifically linked with AAA disease. MMP-9 is an enzyme produced by macrophages and other cells in the aneurysm wall. The amount of MMP-9 that is synthesized by a cell depends on the binding of regulatory transcription factors to the 5′-noncoding sequence (promoter) of the gene. A single nucleotide polymorphism 1562 bases from the start of the MMP-9 gene (−1562 C > T) influences the rate of MMP-9 messenger RNA transcription.[81] This type of single nucleotide polymorphism is known as a functional polymorphism and can be used to gain insight into mechanisms of disease. Functions of promoter polymorphisms usually are investigated in cultured cells. For example, in one region of the gene, the −1562T allele supports binding of a transcription factor, allows the gene to be transcribed (Figure 2-7). Patients with the −1562T allele appear to be more likely to have severe coronary artery atherosclerosis, whereas another region of the MMP-9 gene affecting transcription is linked to intracranial aneurysms.[81,82] The investigation of functional polymorphisms is likely to be one of the most useful approaches to complex genetic traits such as AAA. Furthermore, inhibitors of the MMPs are being tested as therapeutic approaches to limit aneurysm expansion, reduce development of intimal hyperplasia, and improve patency in vein grafts.[80]

Varicose Disease

In addition to their contribution to formation of aneurysms, an imbalance in MMPs, particularly MMP-2, MMP-9, and MMP-13, and tissue inhibitors of MMPs is implicated in development of varicose veins.[80] However, factors contributing to their dysregulation are not known. Although pregnancy is known to upregulate expression of MMPs, the specific mechanism by which hormones (i.e., estrogen, progesterone, or other pregnancy-associated hormones) provide the primary stimulus for venous remodeling is unclear. In addition to hormones, changes in production of growth factors such as transforming growth factor-β1, nitric oxide, matrix Gla protein, and dysregulation of the cell cycle (resulting in inhibition of apoptosis) have been implicated in development of varicose veins.[83-86] While physical factors such as gravitational hydrostatic force and hydrodynamic muscle contractile forces are also implicated in development of varicose veins,[87] no consistent relationship between development of varicose veins and any particular lifestyle factors has been identified.[88] Chronic venous insufficiency and varicosities seem to have an inheritable component, but the exact gene or genes contributing to the disorder remain to be defined.[89,90] One potential genetic contributor is related to forkhead transcription factor FOXC2, which has also been implicated in embryonic vascular development, including lymphangiogenesis.[91-93] In the future, improved understanding of the factors regulating development of venous remodeling may lead to new therapies to prevent or limit their development in susceptible individuals. Furthermore, insight may be gained into factors contributing to hyperplastic occlusive diseases related to other vascular reconstruction.

References

1. Perrault LP, Carrier M. The central role of the endothelium in graft coronary vasculopathy and heart transplantation. *Can J Cardiol* 2005;21:1077.
2. Stevens LM, Fortier S, Aubin MC, et al. Effect of tetrahydrobiopterin on selective endothelial dysfunction of epicardial porcine coronary arteries induced by cardiopulmonary bypass. *Eur J Cardiothorac Surg* 2006;30:464.
3. Splawinska B, Furmaga W, Kuzniar J, et al. Formation of prostacyclin-sensitive platelet aggregates in human whole blood in vitro. II. The occurrence of the phenomenon in males suffering from acute myocardial infarction. *Scand J Clin Lab Invest* 1987;47:125.
4. Wolin MS. Interactions of oxidants with vascular signaling systems. *Arterioscler Thromb Vasc Biol* 2000;20:1430.
5. Muhlestein JB. Bacterial infections and atherosclerosis. *J Investig Med* 1998;46:396.
6. Ford PJ, Yamazaki K, Seymour GJ. Cardiovascular and oral disease interactions: what is the evidence? *Prim Dent Care* 2007;14:59.
7. Abel TJ, Richards AM, Nakamura M, et al. Endothelin-induced changes in intracellular calcium concentration in rat vascular smooth muscle cells: effects of extracellular calcium and atrial natriuretic factor. *Heart Vessels* 1992;7:31.
8. Branco D, Teixeira AA, Azevedo I, et al. Structural and functional alterations caused at the extraneuronal level by sympathetic denervation of blood vessels. *Naunyn Schmiedebergs Arch Pharmacol* 1984;326:302.
9. Mangiarua EI, Bevan RD. Altered endothelium-mediated relaxation after denervation of growing rabbit ear artery. *Eur J Pharmacol* 1986;122:149.
10. Miller MD, Scott TM. The effect of perivascular denervation on endothelium-dependent relaxation to acetylcholine. *Artery* 1990;17:233.
11. Barker SGE, Talbert A, Cottam S, et al. Arterial intimal hyperplasia after occlusion of the adventitial vasa vasorum in the pig. *Arterioscler Thromb* 1993;13:70.
12. Crotty TP. The roles of turbulence and vasa vasorum in the aetiology of varicose veins. *Med Hypotheses* 1991;34:41.
13. McGeachie JK, Meagher S, Prendergast FJ. Vein-to-artery grafts: the long-term development of neo-intimal hyperplasia and its relationship to vasa vasorum and sympathetic innervation. *Aust NZ J Surg* 1989;59:59.
14. Stefanadis C, Vlachopoulos C, Karayannacos P, et al. Effect of vasa vasorum flow on structure and function of the aorta in experimental animals. *Circulation* 1995;91:2669.
15. Miller VM, Aarhus LL, Vanhoutte PM. Modulation of endothelium-dependent responses by chronic alterations of blood flow. *Am J Physiol* 1986;251. H520.
16. Engelke KA, Dietz NM, Proctor DN, et al. Contribution of endothelial vasodilating factors to reactive hyperemia in the human forearm. *J Appl Physiol* 1996;81:1807.
17. Gerhard-Herman M, Hurley S, Mitra D, et al. Assessment of endothelial function (nitric oxide) at the tip of a finger. *Circulation* 2002;106:170.
18. Bonetti PO, Pumper GM, Higano ST, et al. Noninvasive identification of patients with early coronary atherosclerosis by assessment of digital reactive hyperemia. *J Am Coll Cardiol* 2004;44:2137.
19. Traub O, Berk BC. Laminar shear stress: mechanisms by which endothelial cells transduce an atheroprotective force. *Arterioscler Thromb Vasc Biol* 1998;18:677.
20. Garcia-Cardena G, Comander J, Anderson KR, et al. Biomechanical activation of vascular endothelium as a determinant of its functional phenotype. *Proc Natl Acad Sci USA* 2001;98:4478.
21. Cambria RA, Lowell RC, Gloviczki P, et al. Chronic changes in blood flow alter endothelium-dependent responses in autogenous vein grafts in dogs. *J Vasc Surg* 1994;20:765.
22. Seiler C, Pohl T, Wustmann K, et al. Promotion of collateral growth by granulocyte–macrophage colony-stimulating factor in patients with coronary artery disease: a randomized, double-blind, placebo-controlled study. *Circulation* 2001;104:2012.
23. Kumbhani DJ, Bavry AA, Kamdar AR, et al. The effect of drug-eluting stents on intermediate angiographic and clinical outcomes in diabetic patients: insights from randomized clinical trials. *Am Heart J* 2008;155:640.
24. Nakazawa G, Finn AV, John MC, et al. The significance of preclinical evaluation of sirolimus-, paclitaxel-, and zotarolimus-eluting stents. *Am J Cardiol* 2007;100:36M.
25. Piccin A, Murphy WG, Smith OP. Circulating microparticles: pathophysiology and clinical implications. *Blood Rev* 2007;21:157-171.
26. Hugel B, Socie G, Vu T, et al. Elevated levels of circulating procoagulant microparticles in patients with paroxysmal nocturnal hemoglobinuria and aplastic anemia. *Blood* 1999;93:3451-3456.
27. Seelig MS. Interrelationship of magnesium and estrogen in cardiovascular and bone disorders, eclampsia, migraine and premenstrual syndrome. *J Am Coll Nutr* 1993;12:442.
28. Tan KT, Tayebjee MH, Lim HS, et al. Clinically apparent atherosclerotic disease in diabetes is associated with an increase in platelet microparticle levels. *Diabet Med* 2005;22:1657.
29. Amabile N, Guerin AP, Leroyer A, et al. Circulating endothelial microparticles are associated with vascular dysfunction in patients with end-stage renal failure. *J Am Soc Nephrol* 2005;16:3381.
30. Wang JM, Huang YJ, Wang Y, et al. Increased circulating $CD31^+/CD42^-$ microparticles are associated with impaired systemic artery elasticity in healthy subjects. *Am J Hypertens* 2007;20:957.
31. Berckmans RJ, Neiuwland R, Boing AN, et al. Cell-derived microparticles circulate in healthy humans and support low grade thrombin generation. *Thromb Haemost* 2001;85:639.
32. Vasa M, Fichtlscherer S, Alexandra A, et al. Number and migratory activity of circulating endothelial progenitor cells inversely correlate with risk factors for coronary artery disease. *Circ Res* 2001;89. e1.
33. Goldschmidt-Clermont PJ. Loss of bone marrow–derived vascular progenitor cells leads to inflammation and atherosclerosis. *Am Heart J* 2003;146. S5.
34. Ballard VL, Edelberg JM. Stem cells and the regeneration of the aging cardiovascular system. *Circ Res* 2007;100:1116.
35. Hoenig MR, Campbell GR, Campbell JH. Vascular grafts and the endothelium. *Endothelium* 2006;13:385.
36. Schmidt-Lucke C, Rossig L, Fichtlscherer S, et al. Reduced number of circulating endothelial progenitor cells predicts future cardiovascular events: proof of concept for the clinical importance of endogenous vascular repair. *Circulation* 2005;111:2981.
37. Dome B, Dobos J, Tovari J, et al. Circulating bone marrow–derived endothelial progenitor cells: characterization, mobilization, and therapeutic considerations in malignant disease. *Cytometry A* 2008;73:186.
38. Strehlow K, Werner N, Berweiler J, et al. Estrogen increases bone marrow–derived endothelial progenitor cell production and diminishes neointima formation. *Circulation* 2003;107:3059.
39. Dalal S, Zhukovsky DS. Pathophysiology and management of hot flashes. *J Support Oncol* 2006;4:315.
40. Imanishi T, Hano T, Nishio I. Estrogen reduces endothelial progenitor cell senescence through augmentation of telomerase activity. *J Hypertens* 2005;23:1699.
41. Shimokawa H, Aarhus LL, Vanhoutte PM. Porcine coronary arteries with regenerated endothelium have a reduced endothelium-dependent responsiveness to aggregating platelets and serotonin. *Circ Res* 1987;61:256.
42. Shimokawa H, Vanhoutte PM. Angiographic demonstration of hyperconstriction induced by serotonin and aggregating platelets in porcine coronary arteries with regenerated endothelium. *J Am Coll Cardiol* 1991; 17:1197.
43. Perrault LP, Bidouard JP, Janiak P, et al. Impairment of G protein–mediated signal transduction in the porcine coronary endothelium during rejection after heart transplantation. *Cardiovasc Res* 1999;43:457.
44. Fournet-Bourguignon M-P, Castedo-Delrieu M, Bidouard J-P, et al. Phenotypic and functional changes in regenerated porcine coronary endothelial cells: increased uptake of modified LDL and reduced production of NO. *Circ Res* 2000;86:854.
45. Semenza GL. Vasculogenesis, angiogenesis, and arteriogenesis: mechanisms of blood vessel formation and remodeling. *J Cell Biochem* 2007;102:840.
46. Velazquez OC. Angiogenesis and vasculogenesis: inducing the growth of new blood vessels and wound healing by stimulation of bone marrow–derived progenitor cell mobilization and homing. *J Vasc Surg* 2007;45(Suppl A): A39.
47. Sozzani S, Rusnati M, Riboldi E, et al. Dendritic cell–endothelial cell cross-talk in angiogenesis. *Trends Immunol* 2007;28:385.
48. Czirok A, Zamir EA, Szabo A, et al. Multicellular sprouting during vasculogenesis. *Curr Top Dev Biol* 2008;81:269.
49. Rafii DC, Psaila B, Butler J, et al. Regulation of vasculogenesis by platelet-mediated recruitment of bone marrow–derived cells. *Arterioscler Thromb Vasc Biol* 2008;28:217.
50. Boodhwani M, Sodha NR, Sellke FW. Biologically based myocardial regeneration: is there a role for the surgeon? *Curr Opin Cardiol* 2006;21:589.
51. Nikol S. Therapeutic angiogenesis for peripheral artery disease: gene therapy. *Vasa* 2007;36:165.
52. Zhou B, Poon MC, Pu WT, et al. Therapeutic neovascularization for peripheral arterial diseases: advances and perspectives. *Histol Histopathol* 2007;22:677.

53. Napoli C, Maione C, Schiano C, et al. Bone marrow cell–mediated cardiovascular repair: potential of combined therapies. *Trends Mol Med* 2007;13:278.
54. Koshikawa M, Shimodaira S, Yoshioka T, et al. Therapeutic angiogenesis by bone marrow implantation for critical hand ischemia in patients with peripheral arterial disease: a pilot study. *Curr Med Res Opin* 2006;22:793.
55. Shaffer RG, Greene S, Arshi A, et al. Flow cytometric measurement of circulating endothelial cells: the effect of age and peripheral arterial disease on baseline levels of mature and progenitor populations. *Cytometry B Clin Cytom* 2006;70:56.
56. Szmitko PE, Fedak PW, Weisel RD, et al. Endothelial progenitor cells: new hope for a broken heart. *Circulation* 2003;107:3093.
57. Wizemann TM, Pardue M-L. *Exploring the biological contributions to human health: does sex matter?* Washington, DC: Institute of Medicine; 2001. Board on Health Sciences Policy.
58. Thom T, Haase N, Rosamond WD, et al. Heart disease and stroke statistics, 2006 update: a report from the American Heart Association Statistics Committee and Stroke Statistics Subcommittee. *Circulation* 2006;113:85.
59. O'Rourke S, Vanhoutte PM, Miller VM. Vascular pharmacology. In: Creager MA, Dzau VJ, Loscalzo J, eds. Vascular medicine: a companion to Braunwald's Heart Disease. Philadelphia: Elsevier; 2006:71.
60. Miller VM, Mulvagh SL. Sex steroids and endothelial function: translating basic science to clinical practice. *Trends Pharmacol Sci* 2007;28: 263.
61. Miller VM, Duckles SP. Vascular actions of estrogens: functional implications. *Pharmacol Rev* 2008;60:210-248.
62. Harman SM, Brinton EA, Cedars M, et al. KEEPS: the Kronos Early Estrogen Prevention Study. *Climacteric* 2005;8:3.
63. Clarkson TB. Estrogen effects on arteries vary with stage of reproductive life and extent of subclinical atherosclerosis progression. *Menopause* 2007;14:373.
64. Sudhir K, Chou TM, Messina LM, et al. Endothelial dysfunction in a man with disruptive mutation in oestrogen-receptor gene. *Lancet* 1997;349:1146.
65. Sudhir K, Chou TM, Chatterjee K, et al. Premature coronary artery disease associated with a disruptive mutation in the estrogen receptor gene in a man. *Circulation* 1997;96:3774.
66. Shearman AM, Cupples LA, Demissie S, et al. Association between estrogen receptor a gene variation and cardiovascular disease. *JAMA* 2003;290:2263.
67. Peter ISA, Zucker DR, Schmid CH, et al. Variation in estrogen-related genes and cross-sectional and longitudinal blood pressure in the Framingham Heart Study. *J Hypertens* 2005;23:2193.
68. Shearman AM, Cooper JA, Kotwinski PJ, et al. Estrogen receptor-α gene variation and the risk of stroke. *Stroke* 2005;36:2281.
69. Weidemann W, Hanke H. Cardiovascular effects of androgens. *Cardiovasc Drug Rev* 2002;20:175.
70. Liu PY, Death AK, Handelsman DJ. Androgens and cardiovascular disease. *Endocr Rev* 2003;24:313.
71. Catelli MG, Ramachandran C, Gauthier Y, et al. Development regulation of murine mammary-gland 90 kDa heat-shock proteins. *Biochem J* 1989;258:895.
72. Ling S, Dai A, Williams MRI, et al. Testosterone (T) enhances apoptosis-related damage in human vascular endothelial cells. *Endocrinology* 2002;143:1119.
73. Dunajska K, Milewicz A, Szymczak J, et al. Evaluation of sex hormone levels and some metabolic factors in men with coronary atherosclerosis. *Aging Male* 2004;7:197.
74. Muller M, van den Beld AW, Bots ML, et al. Endogenous sex hormones and progression of carotid atherosclerosis in elderly men. *Circulation* 2004;109:2074.
75. Bunck MC, Toorians AW, Lips P, et al. The effects of the aromatase inhibitor anastrozole on bone metabolism and cardiovascular risk indices in ovariectomized, androgen-treated female-to-male transsexuals. *Eur J Endocrinol* 2006;154:569.
76. Schaefer BM, Caracciolo V, Frishman WH, et al. Gender, ethnicity and genetics in cardiovascular disease. I. Basic principles. *Heart Dis* 2003;5:129.
77. Sowers MR, Wilson AL, Karvonen-Gutierrez CA, et al. Sex steroid hormone pathway genes and health-related measures in women of 4 races/ethnicities: the Study of Women's Health across the Nation (SWAN). *Am J Med* 2006;119:S103.
78. Sowers MR, Wilson AL, Kardia SR, et al. CYP1A1 and CYP1B1 polymorphisms and their association with estradiol and estrogen metabolites in women who are premenopausal and perimenopausal. *Am J Med* 2006;119:S44.
79. Sowers MR, Jannausch ML, McConnell DS, et al. Endogenous estradiol and its association with estrogen receptor gene polymorphisms. *Am J Med* 2006;119:S16.
80. Raffetto JD, Khalil RA. Matrix metalloproteinases and their inhibitors in vascular remodeling and vascular disease. *Biochem Pharmacol* 2008;75:346.
81. Zhang B, Ye S, Herrmann SM, et al. Functional polymorphism in the regulatory region of gelatinase B gene in relation to severity of coronary atherosclerosis. *Circulation* 1999;99:1788.
82. Peters DG, Kassam A, St Jean PL, et al. Functional polymorphism in the matrix metalloproteinase-9 promoter as a potential risk factor for intracranial aneurysm. *Stroke* 1999;30:2612.
83. Ascher E, Jacob T, Hingorani A, et al. Programmed cell death (apoptosis) and its role in the pathogenesis of lower extremity varicose veins. *Ann Vasc Surg* 2000;14:24.
84. Cario-Toumaniantz C, Boularan C, Schurgers LJ, et al. Identification of differentially expressed genes in human varicose veins: involvement of matrix Gla protein in extracellular matrix remodeling. *J Vasc Res* 2007;44:444.
85. Jacob T, Hingorani A, Ascher E. Overexpression of transforming growth factor-β1 correlates with increased synthesis of nitric oxide synthase in varicose veins. *J Vasc Surg* 2005;41:523.
86. Pascual G, Mendieta C, Garcia-Honduvilla N, et al. TGF-β1 upregulation in the aging varicose vein. *J Vasc Res* 2007;44:192.
87. Gloviczki P. Handbook of venous disorders: guidelines of the American Venous Forum. London: Hodder Arnold, 2009.
88. Lee AJ, Evans CJ, Allan PL, et al. Lifestyle factors and the risk of varicose veins: Edinburgh Vein Study. *J Clin Epidemiol* 2003;56:171.
89. Guo Q, Guo C. Genetic analysis of varicose vein of lower extremities. *Zhonghua Yi Xue Yi Chuan Xue Za Zhi* 1998;15:221.
90. Pistorius MA. Chronic venous insufficiency: the genetic influence. *Angiology* 2003;54(Suppl 1):S5.
91. Ji RC. Lymphatic endothelial cells, lymphangiogenesis, and extracellular matrix. *Lymphat Res Biol* 2006;4:83.
92. Matousek V, Prerovsky I. A contribution to the problem of the inheritance of primary varicose veins. *Hum Hered* 1974;24:225.
93. Seo S, Fujita H, Nakano A, et al. The forkhead transcription factors, Foxc1 and Foxc2, are required for arterial specification and lymphatic sprouting during vascular development. *Dev Biol* 2006;294:458.

chapter 3

Thrombosis and Hemostasis

Frank C. Vandy, MD • Thomas W. Wakefield, MD

Key Points

- Hemostasis requires the interaction of platelets, coagulation and fibrinolytic factors, endothelium, proinflammatory and anti-inflammatory mediators, and leukocytes.
- Clot formation is typically initiated by vascular injury in which a platelet plug forms and is reinforced with fibrin produced via the extrinsic pathway.
- Physiological anticoagulants such as antithrombin III and activated protein C oppose thrombosis, serving to localize it to sites of vascular injury.
- Under normal conditions, clot formation is balanced by plasmin-mediated fibrinolysis, resulting in the formation of D-dimers and other fibrin degradation products.
- Endothelium normally sustains an antithrombotic environment, but during states of injury or dysfunction it produces various prothrombotic and proinflammatory agents that augment clot formation.
- Thrombosis and inflammation are interrelated processes; during thrombosis, leukocytes, as well as platelets and endothelial cells, are activated and subsequently release tissue factor–rich procoagulant microparticles, further augmenting thrombosis.
- Arterial thrombosis may be the result of plaque rupture and release of thrombogenic material into the bloodstream, as well as platelet accumulation along points of high shear forces at stenoses.
- Hypercoagulability, stasis, and endothelial injury contribute to venous thrombosis with augmentation by inflammation.
- Factor V Leiden, elevated levels of factor VIII, prothrombin 20210A, and hyperhomocysteinemia are the most common causes of primary venous thrombosis.
- Von Willebrand disease is the most common inherited bleeding disorder. Congenital hemophilias, platelet defects, and disorders of fibrinolysis are less common.
- Anticoagulation for the treatment and prevention of venous thromboembolism currently uses not only heparin and warfarin but also direct thrombin and Xa inhibitors.

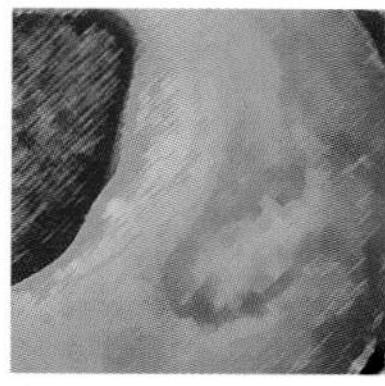

Normal hemostasis relies on the balanced interaction of multiple components of blood. These include the coagulation factors critical to the production of cross-linked fibrin as an end product of the clotting cascade, as well as the physiological anticoagulant and fibrinolytic mechanisms necessary to keep the thrombotic process localized to the area of injury. Also central to normal thrombosis are platelets, which not only are necessary for the formation of the initial hemostatic "plug" through aggregation at sites of vessel wall injury but also provide a phospholipid surface for enzymatic reactions of the coagulation cascade.

Other factors are important in hemostasis. Depending on their state of activation, endothelial cells have been shown to express procoagulant and anticoagulant activity, platelet proaggregation factors, vasoconstrictor and vasodilatory substances, as well as adhesion molecules important for trafficking leukocytes and facilitating the inflammatory response. Through these mechanisms and others, thrombosis and inflammation are closely linked, especially in the venous circulation. Thrombosis is known to directly elicit an inflammatory response.

However, only recently have the molecular and cellular events occurring at the thrombus–vessel wall interface been elucidated. A host of cytokines, including tumor necrosis factor (TNF) and the interleukins IL-6, IL-8, and IL-10, have been identified not only as amplifiers of inflammation but also as promoters of thrombosis.

COAGULATION MECHANISMS

Hemostasis is typically initiated by damage to the vessel wall and disruption of the endothelium, although it may originate in the absence of vessel wall damage. This injury results in the exposure of subendothelial collagen to circulating platelets. Ultimately, platelets bind to these exposed sites and become activated. Vessel wall damage simultaneously results in release of tissue factor (TF), a cell membrane protein, from injured cells and the activation of the extrinsic pathway of the coagulation cascade. These two events are critical to the activation and acceleration of thrombosis.

The role of TF extends beyond the initiation of the extrinsic pathway. TF has been shown to contribute to thrombus propagation, migration and proliferation of vascular smooth muscle cells, development of embryonic blood vessels, tumor neovascularization, and proinflammatory response.[1] TF is expressed constitutively by subendothelial cells such as vascular smooth muscle cells, pericytes, and adventitial fibroblasts.[1-3] Under normal physiological conditions, cells that express TF are not in contact with blood. However, vascular wall injury not only exposes underlying TF but also causes upregulation and expression.[2-3] TF binds with factor VII, forming an activated factor VII complex (TF-VIIa). This complex heralds the initiation of the extrinsic pathway. The presence of TF in other cells types, such as platelets, monocytes, and endothelial cells, is of undetermined significance. TF expression in the aforementioned cell types may be related to a proinflammatory response rather than to hemostasis and thrombosis. TF antigen and procoagulant activity also exist independently in cell-free plasma as microparticles. These microparticles are small membrane fragments shed from leukocytes, endothelial cells, vascular smooth muscle cells, platelets, and atherosclerotic plaques.[1-3] TF-positive microparticles are elevated in disease states such as cardiovascular disease, diabetes, cancer, and endotoxemia and may be a marker of procoagulant activity.[3-4]

The adhesion of platelets to exposed collagen is the first step in the formation of an effective hemostatic "platelet plug," resulting in platelet activation. This interaction is mediated by von Willebrand factor (VWF), whose platelet receptor is glycoprotein (Gp) Ib.[5] Similarly, fibrinogen forms bridges between platelets by binding to the GpIIb/IIIa receptor on adjacent platelets, resulting in platelet aggregation.[6,7] Activation of platelets leads to the "release reaction" in which the prothrombotic contents of platelet granules (dense bodies and α-granules) are secreted in response to transmembrane signals and a subsequent influx of calcium.[8] These granules are rich in receptors for coagulation factors Va and VIIIa,[9,10] as well as fibrinogen, VWF, and adenosine diphosphate, a potent activator of other platelets. Platelet activation also leads to the elaboration of arachidonic acid metabolites such as thromboxane A2, a powerful initiator of platelet aggregation.[8] Simultaneous contraction of platelets during activation results in a dramatic shape change from one that is initially discoid to that of a "spiny" sphere with long pseudopodia.[8] This shape change leads to the externalization of negatively charged procoagulant phospholipids (phosphatidylserine and phosphatidylinositol), normally located within the inner leaflet of the platelet membrane.[11] This special surface facilitates the assembly of the coagulation factors, accelerating their reactions.[12]

Fibrin is critical in stabilizing the initial platelet plug. The formation of fibrin involves several enzymatic steps leading to the formation of thrombin, which converts fibrinogen to fibrin (Figure 3-1).[13] Following the binding of TF with factor VII, the TF-VIIa complex then activates factors IX and X to IXa and Xa in the presence of calcium (Ca^{2+}).[14] Feedback amplification is achieved because factors VIIa, IXa, and Xa are all capable of activating factor VII to VIIa, especially when bound to TF.[15] Factor Xa is also capable of activating factor V to Va (on the platelet phospholipid surface).[15] Factors Xa, Va, and II (prothrombin) form on the platelet phospholipid surface in the presence of Ca^{2+} to initiate the prothrombinase complex, which catalyzes the formation of thrombin from prothrombin.[12] Thrombin feedback amplifies the system by activating not only factor V to Va but also factor VIII (normally circulating bound to VWF) to VIIIa and factor XI to XIa. After activation, factor VIIIa dissociates from VWF and assembles with factors IXa and X on the platelet surface in the presence of Ca^{2+} to form a complex called the Xase complex, which catalyzes the activation of factor X to Xa.[12] This further facilitates thrombin production through amplified activity of the prothrombinase complex.

Thrombin is central to all coagulation. Its action occurs through the cleavage and release of fibrinopeptide A from the α-chain of fibrinogen and fibrinopeptide B from the β-chain of fibrinogen.[16] This leaves newly formed fibrin monomers, which then covalently cross-link, leading to fibrin polymerization. This cross-linking strengthens and stabilizes the clot. Thrombin also activates factor XIII to XIIIa, which catalyzes this cross-linking of fibrin, as well as that of other plasma proteins such as fibronectin and α2-antitrypsin, resulting in their incorporation into the clot and the formation of a "stronger" clot less likely to undergo thrombolysis.[17] In addition, factor XIIIa activates platelets, as well as factors V and VIII, further amplifying thrombin production.[12]

The extrinsic pathway, via TF exposure, is the main mechanism by which coagulation is initiated in vivo in response to trauma or tissue damage. Alternatively, coagulation can be activated through the intrinsic pathway, whose true physiological role remains to be clarified. This route requires activation of factor XI to XIa, which subsequently converts factor IX to IXa,[18] promoting formation of the Xase complex and ultimately thrombin (Figure 3-1). One mechanism by which this occurs in vitro is through the contact activation system, in which factor XII (Hageman factor) is activated to XIIa when complexed to prekallikrein and high-molecular-weight kininogen on a negatively charged surface; factor XIIa then activates factor XI to XIa. Both thrombin and factor XIa (in an autocatalytic manner) are also capable of activating factor XI.[19] The physiological importance of the intrinsic pathway is not completely clear, as patients deficient in factor XII, prekallikrein, or high-molecular-weight kininogen usually have no difficulties with bleeding, whereas deficiency of factor XI leads to a moderately severe bleeding disorder.[17] The contact activation system is most important in extracorporeal bypass

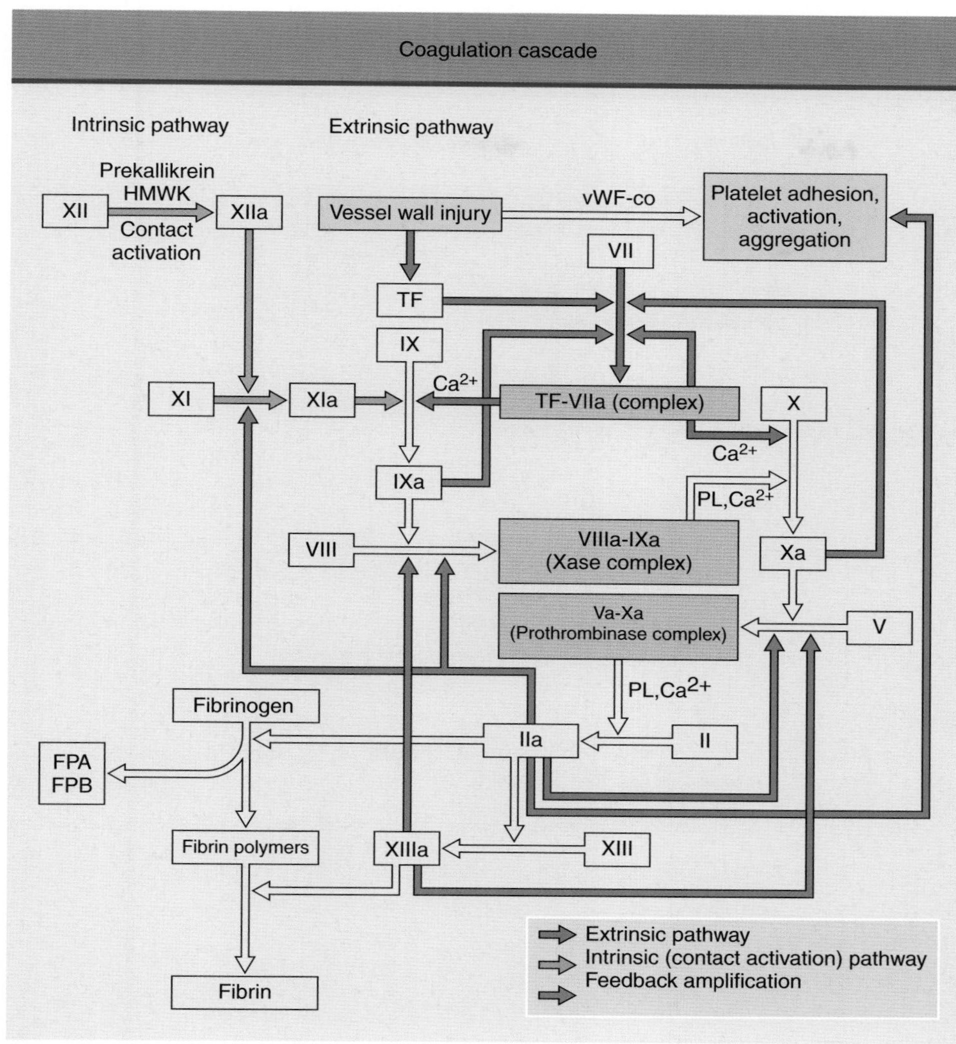

Figure 3-1. Coagulation cascade. Coagulation is initiated by formation of a platelet plug and release of tissue factor (TF) from injured cells, resulting in fibrin production through the extrinsic pathway. Alternatively, activation of factor XII on negatively charged surfaces leads to clot production via the intrinsic pathway. Thrombin (IIa) and other activated factors (VIIa, IXa, Xa, and XIIIa) are capable of amplifying coagulation through multiple positive feedback pathways. co, collagen; FPA, fibrinopeptide A; FPB, fibrinopeptide B; HMWK, high-molecular-weight kininogen; PL, phospholipid; VWF, von Willebrand factor.

circuits, such as cardiopulmonary bypass and extracorporeal membrane oxygenation.

PHYSIOLOGICAL ANTICOAGULANT MECHANISMS

Physiological anticoagulants oppose further thrombin formation and localize thrombotic activity to sites of vascular injury, therefore maintaining hemostatic balance. Just as thrombin is essential to normal coagulation, antithrombin III (ATIII) is the central anticoagulant protein. ATIII acts by binding to and "trapping" thrombin. This interferes with coagulation by three major mechanisms (Figure 3-2). First, inhibition of thrombin prevents the removal of fibrinopeptide A and fibrinopeptide B from fibrinogen, a thrombin substrate, thus limiting fibrin formation.[20] Second, thrombin becomes unavailable for factor V and VIII activation, slowing the coagulation cascade. Third, thrombin-mediated platelet activation and aggregation are inhibited. In the presence of heparin, this inhibition of thrombin by ATIII is markedly accelerated, resulting in systemic anticoagulation. ATIII also has been shown to directly inhibit factors VIIa, IXa, Xa, XIa, and XIIa.[13,21,22]

A second natural anticoagulant is activated protein C (APC). It is produced on the surface of intact endothelium when thrombin binds to its receptor, thrombomodulin (Figure 3-3). This thrombin–thrombomodulin complex not only inhibits the actions of thrombin but also activates protein C to APC.[23-25] APC, in the presence of its cofactor, protein S, inactivates factors Va and VIIIa, therefore reducing Xase and prothrombinase activity.[26-28] APC also increases fibrinolysis by inactivation of an inhibitor of tissue plasminogen activator (tPA).[29]

Another innate anticoagulant is tissue factor pathway inhibitor. As it is mostly bound to low-density lipoproteins in plasma, it has also been termed lipoprotein-associated coagulation inhibitor. This protein binds the TF-VIIa complex, thus inhibiting the activation of factor X to Xa and formation of the prothrombinase complex.[17] Interestingly, factor IX activation is not inhibited. Finally, heparin cofactor II is another inhibitor of thrombin,[30] whose action appears to be focused in the extravascular compartment. The activity of heparin cofactor II is augmented by both heparin (in a manner analogous to ATIII) and dermatan sulfate.[31] Its role in physiological hemostasis is not yet fully understood.

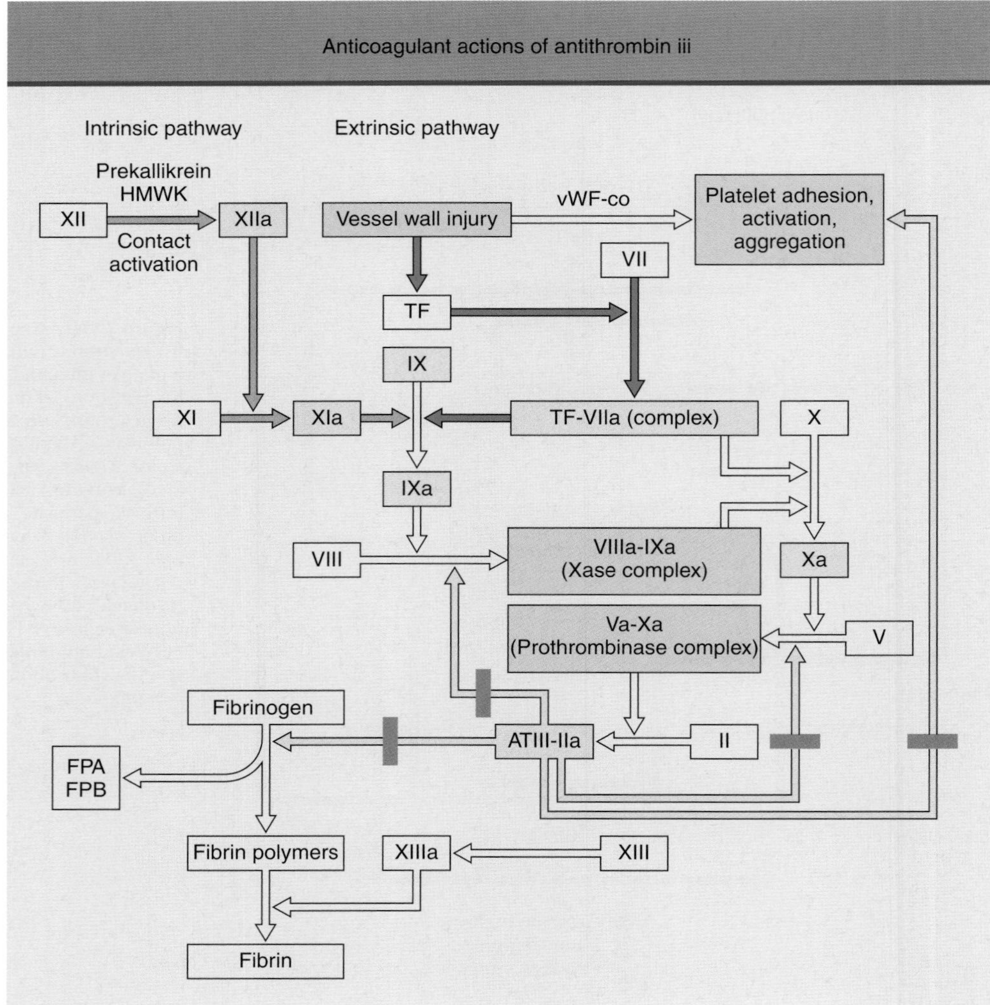

Figure 3-2. Anticoagulant actions of antithrombin III (ATIII). ATIII acts by binding to and "trapping" thrombin. This not only prevents the formation of fibrin from fibrinogen but also inhibits multiple positive feedback pathways that normally amplify coagulation, including platelet aggregation. ATIII also directly inhibits factors VIIa, IXa, Xa, XIa, and XIIa. The actions of ATIII are accelerated by heparin. FPA, fibrinopeptide A; FPB, fibrinopeptide B, TF, tissue factor.

FIBRINOLYTIC MECHANISMS

In addition to these natural anticoagulants, physiological clot formation is balanced by a constant process of thrombolysis that prevents pathological intravascular thrombosis. The central fibrinolytic enzyme is plasmin, a serine protease generated by the proteolytic cleavage of the proenzyme plasminogen. Its main substrates include fibrin, fibrinogen, and other coagulation factors. Plasmin also interferes with VWF-mediated platelet adhesion by proteolysis of GpIb.[32]

Activation of plasminogen occurs through four major mechanisms. In the presence of thrombin, vascular endothelial cells produce and release tPA, as well as α2-antiplasmin, a natural inhibitor of excess fibrin-bound plasmin. As a clot is formed, plasminogen, tPA, and α2-antiplasmin become incorporated into the fibrin clot.[12] In contrast to free-circulating tPA, fibrin-bound tPA is an efficient activator of plasminogen. A second endogenous pathway leading to the activation of plasminogen involves the urokinase-type plasminogen activator (uPA), also produced by endothelial cells but with less affinity for fibrin.[33] The activation of uPA in vivo is not completely understood. It is hypothesized that plasmin, in small amounts (produced through tPA), activates uPA, leading to further plasminogen activation and amplification of fibrinolysis.[34] The third mechanism for plasminogen activation involves factors of the contact activation system; activated forms of factor XII, kallikrein, and factor XI can each independently convert plasminogen to plasmin.[35] These activated factors may also catalyze the release of bradykinin from high-molecular-weight kininogen, which further augments tPA secretion. Finally, APC has been found to proteolytically inactivate plasminogen activator inhibitor type-1 (PAI-1), an inhibitor of tPA released by endothelial cells in the presence of thrombin, thus promoting tPA activity and fibrinolysis.[36]

The degradation of fibrin polymers by plasmin ultimately results in the creation of fragment E and two molecules of fragment D, which, during physiological thrombolysis, are released as a covalently linked dimer (D-dimer).[12] Clinically, detection of D-dimer in the circulation is a marker for ongoing clot formation and fibrinolysis. In contrast, during

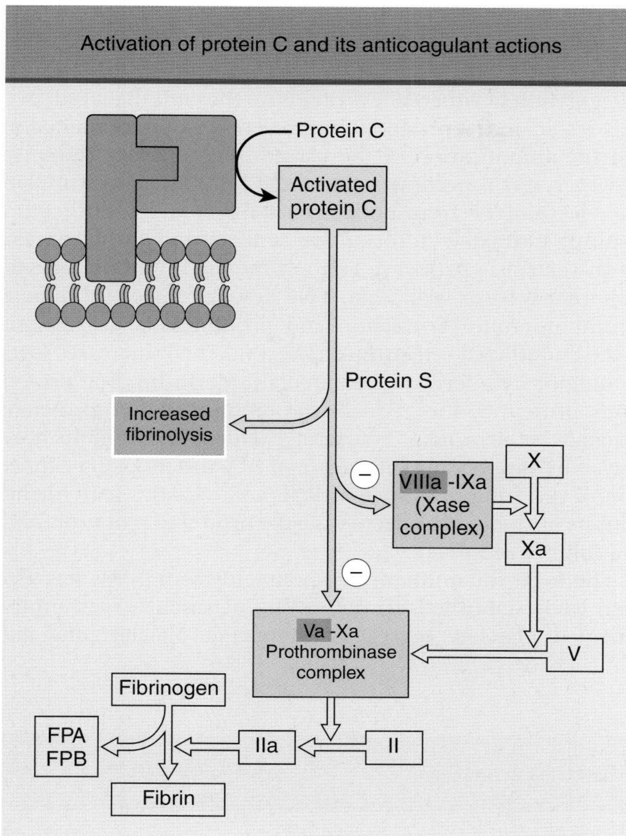

Figure 3-3. Activation of protein C and its anticoagulant actions. Protein C is activated by the thrombin–thrombomodulin complex on the surface of endothelium. In the presence of protein S, activated protein C inactivates factors Va and VIIIa. It also inhibits plasminogen activator inhibitor-1 (PAI-1), therefore increasing fibrinolysis. FPA, fibrinopeptide A; FPB, fibrinopeptide B.

therapeutic administration of thrombolytics and other systemic fibrinolytic states, circulating fibrinogen becomes a second target for plasmin in addition to clot-associated fibrin (Figure 3-4). This circulating plasmin is not inhibited by α2-antiplasmin. Furthermore, in fibrinogenolysis, circulating fibrinogen is degraded by plasmin through the removal of fibrinopeptide B, as well as the carboxy-terminal portion of its α-chain, producing fragment X.[37] Fragment X is then further broken down to one molecule of fragment D and one molecule of fragment Y. Finally, fragment Y is degraded to one molecule of fragment E and two molecules of fragment D, as monomers[12]; no D-dimer is formed. Fragments Y and D are potent inhibitors of fibrin formation.

ENDOTHELIUM AND HEMOSTASIS

Through its ability to express procoagulants and anticoagulants, vasoconstrictors and vasodilators, and key cell adhesion molecules and cytokines, the endothelial cell has emerged as one of the pivotal regulators of hemostasis. Under normal conditions, vascular endothelium sustains a vasodilatory and local fibrinolytic state in which coagulation, platelet adhesion, and activation, as well as inflammation and leukocyte activation, are suppressed (Figure 3-5). Vasodilatory endothelial products include adenosine, nitric oxide, and prostacyclin.[38] A nonthrombogenic endothelial surface is maintained through four main mechanisms: (1) endothelial production of thrombomodulin and subsequent activation of protein C; (2) endothelial expression of surface heparin sulfate and dermatan sulfate, with acceleration of ATIII and heparin cofactor II activity; (3) constitutive expression of tissue factor pathway inhibitor by endothelium (which is markedly accelerated in response to heparin); and (4) local production of tPA and uPA. Finally, the elaboration of nitric oxide and IL-10 by endothelium inhibits the adhesion and activation of leukocytes.[38]

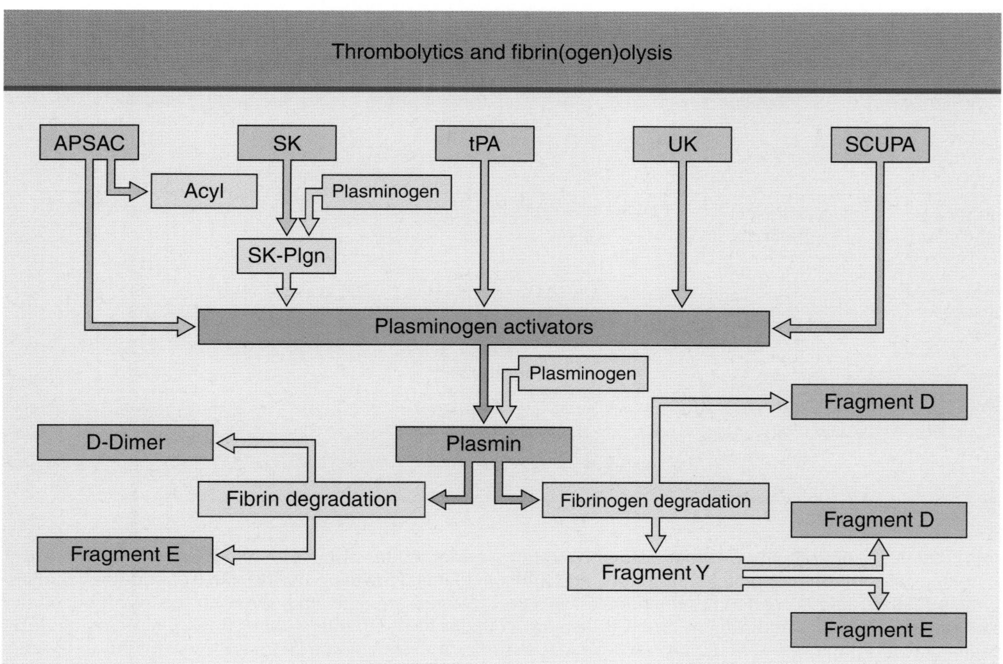

Figure 3-4. Thrombolytics and fibrin(ogen)olysis. Thrombolytics are activators of plasminogen. The three main agents are streptokinase (SK), tissue plasminogen activator (tPA), and urokinase (UK). SK must complex with plasminogen before activating other plasminogen molecules, while the other agents act directly. Single-chain urokinase-type plasminogen activator (SCUPA) and anisoylated plasminogen–streptokinase activator complex (APSAC) are fibrin-selective forms of UK and SK, respectively. APSAC requires in vivo deacylation before acquiring activity. As opposed to fibrinogenolysis, fibrinolysis results in the production of D-dimers.

During states of endothelial disturbances, whether physical (e.g., vascular trauma) or functional (e.g., sepsis), a prothrombotic and proinflammatory state of vasoconstriction is supported by the endothelial surface (Figure 3-5).[38] Endothelial release of platelet-activating factor and endothelin-1 promotes vasoconstriction.[39] Furthermore, during prothrombotic conditions endothelial cells increase production of VWF, TF, and PAI-1, as well as factor V, to augment thrombosis.[38] Lastly, in response to endothelial injury, endothelial cells are "activated," resulting in increased surface expression of certain cell adhesion molecules (such as P-selectin or E-selectin) and promoting the adhesion and activation of leukocytes. This initiates and amplifies inflammation and thrombosis.

THROMBOSIS AND INFLAMMATION

Growing evidence shows that thrombosis and inflammation are interrelated. This relationship now appears to be bidirectional. States of systemic inflammation, such as sepsis, result in the elaboration of cytokines that also activate coagulation. More recently, however, the inflammatory response has been shown to play a major role in the amplification of thrombosis. In response to a toxic stimulus, such as endotoxin in the case of sepsis, stimulated macrophages release both TNF and IL-1. These cytokines are well known for their ability to stimulate leukocyte–endothelial adhesion and activation through the upregulation of adherence proteins on the endothelial surface. This results in the production of several secondary mediators and the amplification of the classic inflammatory response. However, it is now known that these cytokines also stimulate the release of TF from both macrophages and endothelium, resulting ultimately in formation of thrombin and fibrin clot via the extrinsic pathway. TNF promotes thrombosis in several other ways as well. First, TNF downregulates endothelial thrombomodulin expression and promotes its degradation at the endothelial cell surface.[40] Second, TNF increases C4b-binding protein levels; since circulating C4b-binding protein binds protein S, this reduces the amount of free protein S available as the protein C cofactor.[41] Third, TNF inhibits fibrinolysis by suppressing the release of tPA and inducing expression of tPA inhibitors such as PAI-1.[42-47] Lastly, TNF further inhibits fibrinolysis by decreasing the production of protein C, an inhibitor of PAI-1.

The local inflammatory response to thrombosis has also been well established. In the setting of vascular wall injury, activated platelets aggregate to form a platelet plug and

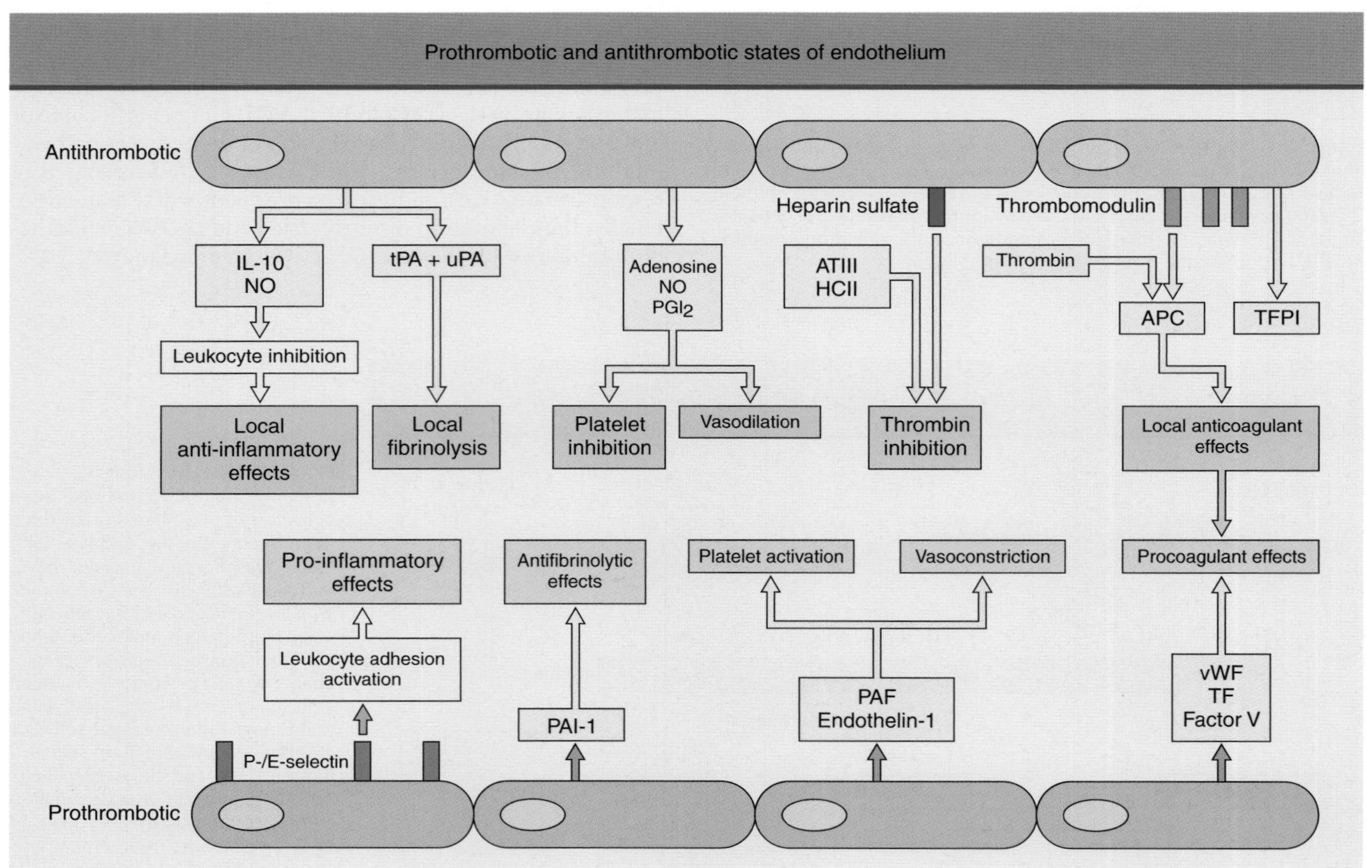

Figure 3-5. Prothrombotic and antithrombotic states of endothelium. Under normal conditions, endothelium sustains an antithrombotic environment through the local production of certain cytokines, thrombolytics, platelet inhibitors, and anticoagulants. However, during states of endothelial injury or dysfunction, a prothrombotic and proinflammatory state is created in which leukocytes and platelets are activated, thrombolysis is inhibited, and procoagulants are released. APC, activated protein C; ATIII, antithrombin III; HCII, heparin cofactor II; IL-10, interleukin-10; NO, nitric oxide; PAF, platelet-activating factor; PAI-1, plasminogen activator inhibitor-1; PGI2, prostacyclin; TF, tissue factor; TFPI, tissue factor pathway inhibitor; tPA, tissue plasminogen activator; uPA, urokinase-type plasminogen activator; VWF, von Willebrand factor.

fibrin clot formation occurs in response to the release of TF. Circulating neutrophils and monocytes then interact with these platelets through P-selectin and with the endothelium through P-selectin and E-selectin, together with other cell adhesion molecules, becoming well incorporated into the clot at the thrombus–vessel wall interface (Figure 3-6). This not only generates a local inflammatory response but also amplifies thrombosis through further monocyte TF expression and induction of endothelial TF expression. Activated platelets release certain chemoattractants, such as platelet factor IV and neutrophil-activating peptide-2, that increase leukocyte recruitment.[38,41]

ARTERIAL VERSUS VENOUS THROMBOSIS

Classically, the elements required for the initiation of thrombosis were described by Rudolf Virchow more than a century ago as the triad of stasis, endothelial injury, and hypercoagulability of the blood. In the arterial circulation, endothelial injury (whether acute or chronic) is central to thrombosis. This is most clearly demonstrated by the typical atherosclerotic plaque, often the result of long-term intimal injury. In advanced lesions, the lipid core of the plaque is rich in inflammatory cells (often apoptotic), cholesterol crystals, and TF (generated by activated macrophages within the plaque). Ulceration or fissuring of the plaque, as in acute coronary syndromes, results in exposure of the highly thrombogenic lipid core to the bloodstream, with activation of the coagulation cascade, platelet aggregation and activation, and deposition of clot (Figure 3-7).[48] Contributing to this is the increased platelet deposition that occurs at the apex of stenoses, the points of maximal shear forces. Thrombosis in the venous circulation differs significantly. Although direct endothelial injury, blood stasis, and changes in its composition leading to hypercoagulable states are known risk factors in venous thrombosis, the inciting event involves the formation of thrombus from local procoagulant events, such as small endothelial disruptions

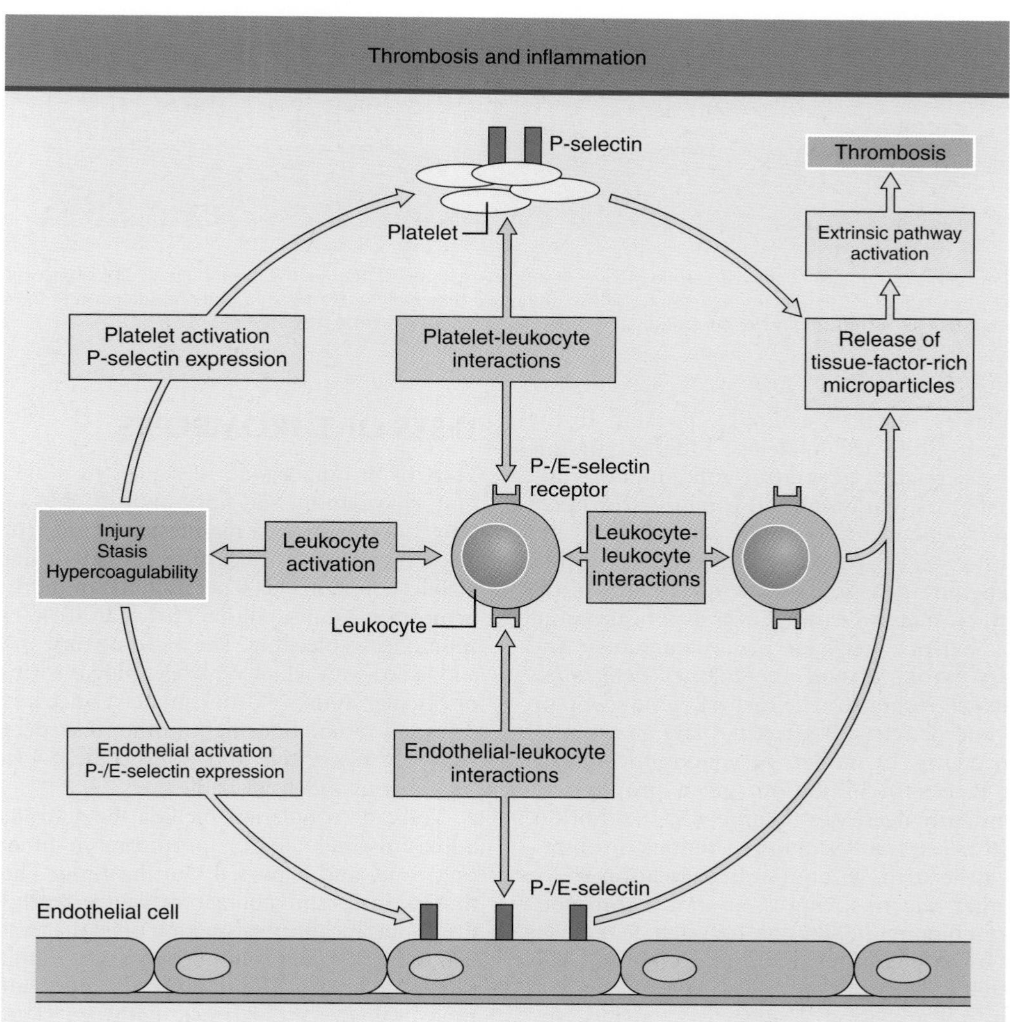

Figure 3-6. Thrombosis and inflammation. In response to vascular injury, stasis, or hypercoagulability, leukocytes, platelets, and endothelial cells are activated. This results in expression of surface P-selectin and E-selectin on platelets and endothelium, which not only increases local inflammation but also leads to the release of tissue factor–rich procoagulant microparticles, thus augmenting thrombosis.

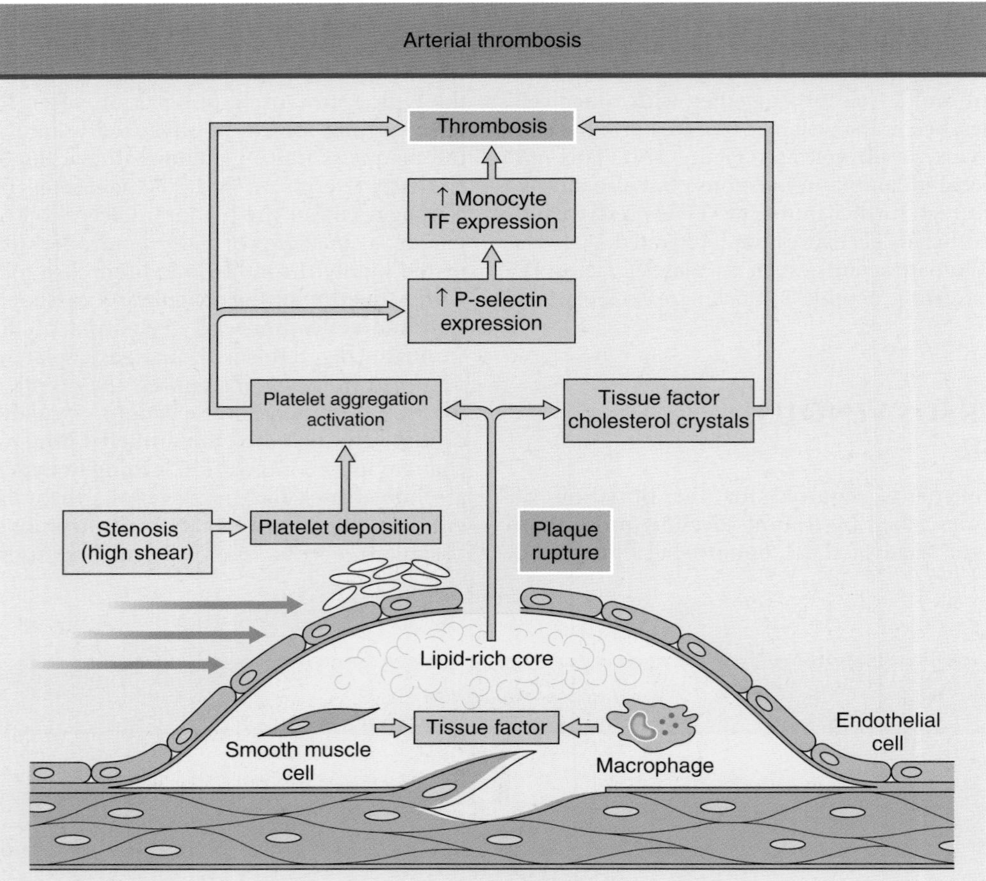

Figure 3-7. Arterial thrombosis. Rupture of atherosclerotic plaques results in exposure of their highly thrombogenic lipid contents to the bloodstream. This leads to platelet aggregation and P-selectin expression, further monocyte tissue–factor expression, and amplification of thrombosis. In addition, arterial flow across the stenosis results in platelet deposition at its apex, the point of maximal shear force.

at venous confluences, saccules, and valve pockets. In the second stage, neutrophils and platelets adherent to this thrombus become activated, generating inflammatory and procoagulant mediators that amplify thrombosis further.[49] With progression, leukocytes (initially neutrophils and subsequently monocytes) extravasate into the vein wall in response to the chemokine gradient generated by the initial thrombotic event, ultimately resulting in transmural venous inflammation. A balance between proinflammatory and anti-inflammatory cytokines and chemokines determines the ultimate vein wall response. The earliest elevated Gp on endothelial cells and platelets, P-selectin, plays an essential role in thrombogenesis. In models of venous thrombosis in the primate, P-selectin inhibition, given prophylactically, dose-dependently decreases thrombosis. In addition, P-selectin inhibitors can treat established venous thrombosis as effectively as heparin, without anticoagulation.[50,51] It is hypothesized that selectins, expressed after a thrombogenic stimulus, facilitate interactions between leukocytes and endothelial cells, leukocytes and leukocytes, and leukocytes and platelets (Figure 3-6). TF-rich procoagulant microparticles are released from leukocytes, platelets, and endothelium, further amplifying coagulation. In addition, TF released from the vein wall contributes to thrombosis when direct vein wall injury occurs.[52]

TESTS OF THROMBOSIS

Tests of thrombosis are designed to evaluate platelet function, coagulation, and fibrinolysis (Table 3-1). Platelet function abnormalities are manifested by mucocutaneous bleeding or excessive hemorrhage after surgery or trauma.[13] Usually, a platelet count of 50,000 per milliliter or more ensures adequate hemostasis, while a count of less than 10,000 per milliliter risks spontaneous bleeding. The bleeding time measures the ability and speed with which a platelet plug is formed in vivo at sites of vascular injury.[53] Unfortunately, since it is operator dependent and often abnormal in other disorders, it is considered relatively insensitive and nonspecific.[54] Platelet aggregation tests are not widely available.

Tests of coagulation include the activated partial thromboplastin time (aPTT), prothrombin time, thrombin clotting time, and activated clotting time. The aPTT evaluates the intrinsic and contact activation pathways of coagulation—specifically, the function of all the factors except factors VII and XIII—and is important in the monitoring of heparin therapy. The prothrombin time or international normalized ratio evaluates the extrinsic pathway: factors VII, X, V, II, and fibrinogen. This test remains the most common mode of monitoring patients on the oral anticoagulant warfarin. The activated clotting time measures the ability of the whole blood

Table 3-1
Laboratory Tests of Thrombosis*

Test	Description	Normal Values†
Platelet Function		
Platelet count	Is increased in some myeloproliferative disorders; is decreased in autoimmune disorders, in response to drugs, and during extracorporeal circulation	150,000-450,000 per milliliter
Peripheral smear	Assesses platelet and blood cell morphology; requires interpretation	
Bleeding time	Measures the ability and speed of platelet-plug formation in vivo at sites of vascular injury	2.5-9.5 minutes
Aggregation	Measures response to agonists that cause aggregation; requires interpretation	
Coagulation		
aPTT	Evaluates the intrinsic coagulation system; is used to monitor heparin	21-34 seconds
PT	Evaluates the extrinsic coagulation system; is used to monitor warfarin	9-11 seconds
INR	Standardizes PT values among laboratories	1.0
TCT	Gives the time necessary for conversion of fibrinogen to fibrin by exogenous thrombin; is specific for fibrinogen deficiencies and monitoring heparin	7.7-9.3 seconds
ACT	Tests whole blood clotting following activation of the contact pathway	70-120 seconds
Fibrinolysis		
Fibrin(ogen) degradation products	Identifies conditions of fibrinolysis and fibrinogenolysis	>8 mg/dl
D-dimer	Detects circulating cross-linked fibrin fragments; is a marker for clot production and lysis and for DIC	<0.20 mg/ml
Plasminogen activity	Measures plasma plasminogen function; plasminogen antigen levels may also be measured	81-151%

*ACT, activated clotting time; aPTT, activated partial thromboplastin time; DIC, disseminated intravascular coagulation; INR, international normalized ratio; PT, prothrombin time; TCT, thrombin clotting time.
†Normal values are based on University of Michigan Laboratory reference ranges.

to clot and therefore is an indicator of platelet function and the coagulation cascade together. It is often used to monitor heparin-based anticoagulation intraoperatively during peripheral vascular procedures and while on cardiopulmonary bypass. In terms of fibrinolysis, fibrin and fibrinogen degradation products result from the proteolytic effects of plasmin. During states of fibrinolysis, the D-dimer fragment is formed and serves as a marker for ongoing clot formation and plasmin-mediated breakdown. During fibrinogenolysis, no D-dimer is formed; rather, fragment E and two fragment D monomers are formed. Other tests of fibrinolysis are less well characterized. Plasminogen, plasminogen activator, and antiplasmin levels can be measured and are often useful in evaluating patients with recurrent thrombosis and suspected fibrinolytic abnormalities.

HYPERCOAGULABLE STATES

Several conditions can result in a hypercoagulable state and subsequent vascular thrombosis. Our understanding of these conditions has recently expanded, with the three most common causes for thrombosis being recognized within the past few years. These disorders can be classified according to their severity (Table 3-2). Components of the appropriate hypercoagulable screen are listed in Table 3-3. Not every patient with a thrombotic event should be screened, but patients with strong family histories, young patients with arterial and venous thrombosis of unclear cause, and patients with multiple episodes of thrombosis should undergo such screening. Although anticoagulation with heparin and warfarin is used most often as treatment for these conditions, novel antithrombotic agents that target specific points in the coagulation cascade, platelets, and the inflammatory component of thrombosis are in development (Table 3-4 and Figures 3-8 and 3-9).

Defects with High Risk for Thrombosis

ATIII deficiency exists on both a congenital basis and an acquired basis and accounts for 1% to 2% of venous thromboses.[55] Produced in the liver, ATIII inhibits thrombin plus factors VIIa, IXa, Xa, XIa, and XIIa. The congenital syndrome usually occurs by age 50. The diagnosis should be suspected

Table 3-2
Hypercoagulable Disorders*

Severity	Frequency (%)	Sites of Thrombosis
High Risk for Thrombosis		
Antithrombin III deficiency	1-2	Venous > arterial
Protein C deficiency	3-5	Venous > arterial
Protein S deficiency	2-3	Venous > arterial
Lower Risk for Thrombosis		
Factor V Leiden	20-60	Venous > arterial
Hyperhomocysteinemia	10	Venous and arterial
Prothrombin 20210A	4-5	Venous
Dysplasminogenemia	<1	Venous and arterial
Dysfibrinogenemia	1-3	Venous and arterial
Variable Risk for Thrombosis		
Elevated factor VIII level	20	Venous
HIT or HITTS	1-30†	Venous and arterial
Lupus anticoagulant	8-12	Venous and arterial
Abnormal platelet aggregation	Not known	Arterial > venous

*HIT, heparin-induced thrombocytopenia; HITTS, heparin-induced thrombocytopenia and thrombosis syndrome.
†Frequency of patients who develop HIT or HITTS among patients in whom heparin is administered.

Table 3-3
Components of the Hypercoagulable Screen*

Standard coagulation tests (i.e., aPTT, TCT, ACT)
Mixing studies (if aPTT elevated)
Antithrombin III antigen level and activity assay
Protein C antigen level and activity assay
Protein S antigen level
APC resistance assay and factor V Leiden genetic analysis
Prothrombin 20210A gene analysis
Homocysteine level
Factor VIII level
Antiphospholipid and anticardiolipin antibody screen
Platelet count, platelet aggregation tests (if available)
Functional plasminogen assay (or some test of fibrinolysis)

*ACT, activated clotting time; APC, activated protein C; aPTT, activated partial thromboplastin time; TCT, thrombin clotting time.

Table 3-4
Future Antithrombotic Agents*

Drug	Mechanism of Action
Oral Heparins	
SNAC–UFH SNAD–LMWH	Heparin is bound noncovalently to carrier proteins, enabling passage through GI mucosa.
Direct Thrombin Inhibitors	
Recombinant hirudin and analogues Desirudin Lepirudin Bivalirudin Argatroban Dabigatran	Hirudin and analogues bind to thrombin and inhibit its activity directly without need for cofactors (e.g., ATIII). Dabigatran is administered orally, while other agents are given intravenously.
Ancrod (defibrination agent)	This serine protease that cleaves fibrinopeptide A from fibrinogen, resulting in less stable fibrin clot more easily degraded by plasmin.
P-selectin inhibitors (rPSGL-1)	These inhibitors decrease amplification of thrombosis by reducing inflammatory response.
Factor VIIa inhibitors	Inhibitors compete with factor VIIa for TF binding.
Tissue factor pathway inhibitor	This inhibits the factor VIIa–TF complex.
Activated protein C	This inactivates factors Va and VIIIa, as well as inhibitors of tPA.
Fondaparinux (synthetic pentasaccharide)	Fondaparinux augments ATIII inhibition of factor Xa without inhibiting thrombin (synthetic pentasaccharide).
Idraparinux	Idraparinux is a factor Xa inhibitor with a 130-hour half-life.
Rivaroxaban	Rivaroxaban is an oral factor Xa inhibitor.

*ATIII, antithrombin III; GI, gastrointestinal; rPSGL-1, recombinant P-selectin glycoprotein ligand-1; SNAC–UFH, N-(8-[2-hydroxybenzoyl]amino)caprylate unfractionated heparin; SNAD–LMWH, sodium N-(10-[2-hydroxybenzoyl]amino)decanoate low-molecular-weight heparin; TF, tissue factor; tPA, tissue plasminogen activator.

in a patient who cannot be adequately anticoagulated with heparin or who develops a thrombosis while on heparin. Episodes of native arterial and arterial graft thrombosis have also been described with this deficiency.[56] The diagnosis is made by measuring ATIII antigen and activity levels while off

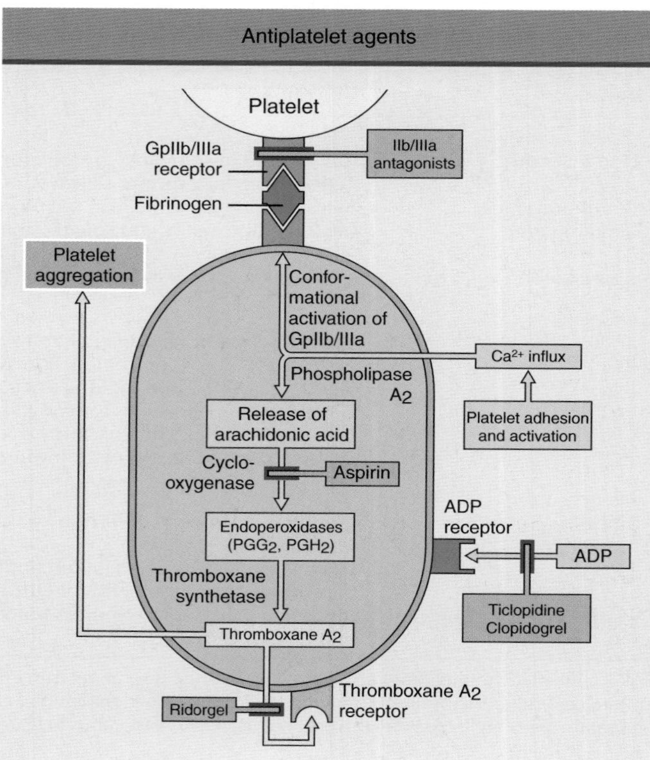

Figure 3-8. Antiplatelet agents. Antiplatelet agents include inhibitors of cyclooxygenase (e.g., aspirin), which inhibit the production of thromboxane A2, a potent platelet activator and vasoconstrictor. Adenosine diphosphate, thromboxane A2, and glycoprotein (Gp) IIb/IIIa receptor antagonists have also been developed. PGG2, prostaglandin G2; PGH2, prostaglandin H2.

anticoagulation, as heparin may decrease levels by 30% for up to 10 days following its cessation and warfarin increases ATIII levels. Homozygote individuals usually die in utero, while heterozygotes usually have ATIII levels of less than 70%. Treatment requires administration of fresh frozen plasma (containing ATIII) with heparin, followed by oral anticoagulation. ATIII concentrates are also available.[57] Additional acquired causes of ATIII deficiency (as a result of protein loss, consumption, or decreased production) include liver disease, disseminated intravascular coagulation, malnutrition, and nephrotic syndrome.

Protein C deficiency accounts for 3% to 5% of venous thromboses.[55] Protein C with its cofactor protein S inactivates factors Va and VIIIa and promotes fibrinolysis. Both protein C and protein S are made in the liver. Although venous thrombosis is most common in protein C deficiency, arterial thrombosis has also been described, especially in patients 50 years or younger.[58] Thrombosis usually occurs between 15 and 30 years of age. When homozygous, patients usually die in infancy from a disseminated intravascular coagulation–like state termed *purpura fulminans.* The diagnosis is made by measuring protein C antigen and activity levels. Heterozygotes usually have antigenic levels less than 60%.[12] Acquired deficiency may also result from liver disease, disseminated intravascular coagulation, and nephrotic syndrome. Protein S deficiency accounts for 2% to 3% of venous thromboses and clinically presents and behaves like protein C deficiency. However, in addition to the already-mentioned acquired causes,

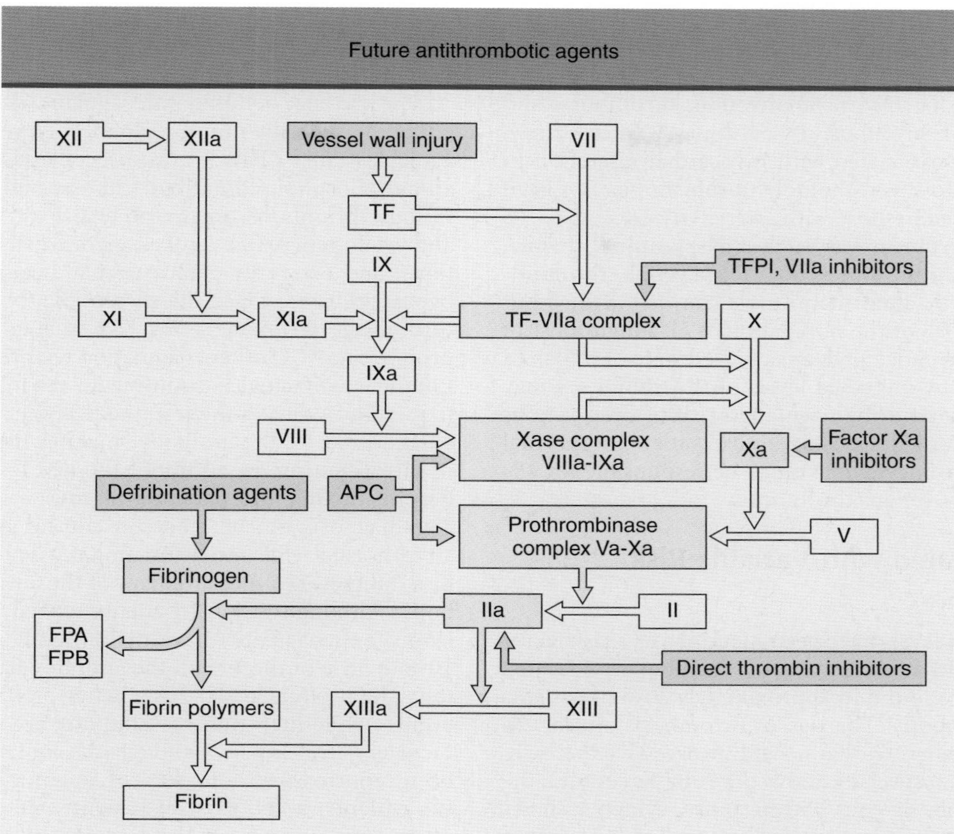

Figure 3-9. Future antithrombotic agents. Agents that target various points in the coagulation cascade are in development. Indications for their use include intolerance to conventional anticoagulants (e.g., in heparin-induced thrombocytopenia) and, in certain settings, need for prophylaxis and treatment of venous thromboembolic disease. APC, activated protein C; FPA, fibrinopeptide A; FPB, fibrinopeptide B; TF, tissue factor; TFPI, tissue factor pathway inhibitor.

inflammatory diseases such as systemic lupus erythematosus that result in elevated levels of C4b-binding protein can lead to a relative protein S deficiency by depleting the free protein S supply. Protein S deficiency can be diagnosed by measuring free protein S antigen levels. Treatment of both protein S and protein C deficiency is heparin followed by lifelong oral anticoagulation. However, in both deficiencies, treatment should be instituted only after the first episode of thrombosis, as many heterozygotes remain asymptomatic.[55] Since protein C and protein S are vitamin K–dependent factors with short half-lives relative to other liver-produced factors (II, IX, X), initiation of warfarin before complete anticoagulation with heparin may result in an initial hypercoagulable state, microcirculatory thrombosis, and the syndrome of warfarin-induced skin necrosis in patients diagnosed with venous thromboembolism.[59]

Defects with Lower Risk for Thrombosis

Resistance to APC (factor V Leiden) has been reported in 20% to 60% of all cases of venous thrombosis.[60] The defect is due to resistance to inactivation of factor Va by APC, most commonly secondary to a mutation resulting in a Glu/Arg amino acid substitution at position 506 of the factor V gene.[61] Thrombotic manifestations have been found in both the arterial and the venous circulation, although the latter predominate. Both homozygous and heterozygous forms exist. Although the homozygous form is not lethal in infancy, the relative risk for thrombosis is increased eightyfold.[62] In the heterozygous form, the relative risk is increased only sevenfold, but in the setting of other risk factors, such as oral contraceptive use or the presence of other hypercoagulable defects (such as protein C or protein S deficiency), this risk increases markedly. The diagnosis of factor V Leiden is made by genetic analysis, as well as by a functional assay in which exogenous APC is added to the plasma; if the aPTT is not prolonged, factor V may be abnormal, suggesting the Leiden mutation.[55] However, the genetic analysis is critical to differentiate homozygous from heterozygous forms. Although treatment for this disorder involves heparin and warfarin anticoagulation, the relatively low risk for recurrent thrombosis in heterozygotes suggests that not all patients require long-term anticoagulation after the first episode.

Hyperhomocysteinemia, a known risk factor for atherosclerosis, has also been found to be a risk factor for venous thrombosis, accounting for 10% of venous thromboses overall.[55] As with other hypercoagulable states, the combination of hyperhomocysteinemia with other disorders such as factor V Leiden increases the risk of thrombosis further. The mechanism of thrombosis may relate to decreased availability or production of nitric oxide (hindering vasodilation), a direct toxic effect on vascular endothelium, as well as reduced protein C and plasminogen activation.[63-68] Treatment is directed to reducing homocysteine levels using folic acid, vitamin B_6, and vitamin B_{12}.

The recently identified prothrombin 20210A polymorphism, in which the prothrombin gene is altered at position 20210 by a Glu/Arg substitution, results in a hypercoagulable state that accounts for 4% to 5% of venous thromboses and increases the risk of thrombosis by 5.4 times.[69] Interestingly, this abnormality is associated with myocardial infarction in younger women. However, the polymorphism has not been found to be increased in those with arterial disease.

Known defects in fibrinolysis, such as dysplasminogenemia, are quite rare, accounting for less than 1% of venous thromboses. Other fibrinolytic abnormalities are less well defined but may affect up to 10% of the population.[70] Although most of these conditions are congenital, an acquired state of impaired fibrinolysis caused by increased levels of tPA inhibitors may account for the temporarily heightened risk of deep venous thrombosis (DVT) in the postoperative patient. Abnormal fibrinogens (dysfibrinogenemias) may be responsible for 1% to 3% of episodes of venous thrombosis.

Defects Associated with Variable Risk for Thrombosis

Elevated factor VIII levels have been identified as a risk factor for both primary and recurrent venous thrombosis.[71] Elevated factor VIII levels are found in approximately 20% of patients with venous thrombosis. The risk of thrombosis appears to increase dose dependently; that is, with progressive increases in factor VIII levels (especially above the 90th percentile), the incidence of thrombosis rises. Furthermore, evidence shows that this abnormality may be genetically inherited.[72] The exact mechanism by which high factor VIII levels result in thrombosis is still not clear. Treatment includes oral anticoagulation following the first episode of thrombosis. The optimal duration of anticoagulation remains to be determined, although the high risk of recurrence (37% at 2 years) argues for extended prophylaxis with warfarin.[71]

Heparin-induced thrombocytopenia (HIT) occurs in 1% to 30% of patients on heparin.[55] A more severe form of HIT associated with thrombosis—heparin-induced thrombocytopenia and thrombosis syndrome—is much less common. This syndrome is caused by a heparin-dependent immunoglobulin G antibody that results in platelet aggregation during heparin administration. This antibody binds to the heparin–platelet factor IV complex. It then binds by its Fc portion to a platelet Fc receptor. This results in platelet activation, aggregation, and release of cytokines, catecholamines, and microparticles. This also leads to the deposition of complement and immunoglobulins on the endothelial surface, stimulating the release of TF and resulting in arterial or venous thrombosis.[73] The syndrome should be suspected in patients who develop thrombosis while on heparin, especially when there is a fall in the platelet count to less than 100,000 per milliliter, or by 50% from its baseline preheparin level. It usually begins 3 to 14 days after heparin exposure. The illness may vary from isolated thrombocytopenia to thrombosis, embolic episodes, and death. Both standard unfractionated heparin and low-molecular-weight heparin (LMWH) may cause HIT. The diagnosis can be made by the serotonin release assay, a platelet aggregation assay, a fluorescence-activated cell sorter analysis for platelet microparticles, and, more recently, an enzyme-linked immunosorbent assay (ELISA) to detect the antibody.[74-76] Treatment involves stopping heparin, initiating an alternative anticoagulant (such as hirudin or argatroban), and under its protection, initiating warfarin.

The presence of lupus anticoagulant with antiphospholipid antibodies, usually immunoglobulin G, results in a hypercoagulable state.[77] This syndrome consists of the presence of an antiphospholipid antibody in association with arterial or venous thrombosis, recurrent fetal loss, thrombocytopenia, and livedo reticularis. Strokes, myocardial and visceral infarctions, and extremity gangrene may occur. Arterial vascular bypass grafts are especially susceptible to failure, with a 50% thrombosis rate in one series.[78] The diagnosis is suggested by a prolonged aPTT; other coagulation tests remain normal. This finding is artifactual, accounting for the misleading syndrome name, since, during the test, the necessary phospholipids are antagonized by the antibody, making them unavailable for in vitro clotting. In addition, the aPTT remains prolonged despite mixing the patient's plasma with normal plasma. The diagnosis can be made on clinical grounds with either an abnormal clot-based functional assay off anticoagulants or a direct ELISA measurement of the antiphospholipid antibody. Although 80% of patients with a positive aPTT test (lupus anticoagulant) have the antibody by an ELISA, only 10% to 50% of those with the antibody have a positive aPTT test. The prolonged aPTT is a better predictor of thrombotic events, while high titers of antibody are more predictive of recurrent fetal loss.[79] Although the lupus anticoagulant has been reported in 5% to 40% of systemic lupus erythematosus patients, it can exist in patients without systemic lupus erythematosus and can also be induced in patients by infection, drugs, and cancer. Possible mechanisms responsible for the thrombotic effects of this syndrome include inhibition of endothelial prostacyclin production, inhibition of protein C activation, increased PAI-1 levels, direct platelet activation, direct endothelial activation by antiphospholipid antibodies, increased monocyte TF expression, and decreased free protein S levels.[80-85] No one dominant mechanism has emerged, suggesting a multifactorial cause of thrombosis. Treatment consists of long-term anticoagulation. As the aPTT is artifactually prolonged, heparin therapy should be monitored with the thrombin clotting time or antifactor Xa level.

Abnormal platelet aggregation has been associated with thrombosis in the setting of advanced malignancy of the lung and uterus and after carotid endarterectomy. "Hyperactive" platelets have also been seen in the setting of graft thrombosis following peripheral vascular reconstructions. Diabetes mellitus, known to be associated with hyperactive platelets, may contribute to these conditions. Sophisticated tests of platelet function, and specifically aggregation, are not uniformly available. Thus, relatively little is known about the influence of platelet aggregation on hypercoagulable states.

BLEEDING DISORDERS

Coagulation Factor Deficiency

Von Willebrand disease (VWD), a deficiency of VWF, is the most common inherited coagulation disorder affecting an estimated 1% of the population.[86] The role of VWF in primary hemostasis is multifaceted. It serves as an adhesive protein binding platelets to platelets, as well as platelets to the vascular subendothelium.[87-88] In addition, VWF is a carrier protein for factor VIII. In the absence of VWF, factor VIII has been shown to exist at an abnormally low concentration with a shortened half-life.[89] VWF-bound factor VIII increases the half-life of factor VIII from about 2 hours to 20 to 40 hours.[90] This complex is protective against the proteolytic degradation of activated factor VIII by activated protein C in the presence of protein S. Normally, VWF is produced by endothelial cells and megakaryocytes with posttranslational modification into dimers and multimers occurring in the endoplasmic reticulum and Golgi complex.[91-93] VWF is stored in both endothelial cells and platelets as Weibel-Palade bodies and α-granules, respectively.[94,95] These secretory granules can be stimulated to release their contents upon their interaction with prothrombotic agents such as thrombin and fibrin.[96] VWF also exists in the plasma at varying concentrations dependent on blood type.[97] In its extracellular form, VWF must be activated, presumably by high shear stress, such that binding sites for the platelet GpIb receptor are exposed.[98] It is during this period of activation through conformational change that large multimers of VWF are cleaved by the metalloproteinase ADAMTS13 to smaller forms. This proteolysis prevents the formation of large platelet aggregates and thrombosis of the microcirculation.[99]

Symptoms of VWD vary, respective of subtypes, from minor postoperative bleeding to severe spontaneous hemorrhage into the soft tissues and joints.[100] Type 1 VWD, the most common subtype, is an autosomal dominant disease in which there is a quantitative deficiency of VWF. Symptoms may include easy bruising, epistaxis, menorrhagia in females, and prolonged bleeding following surgery. However, in those who do not undergo surgery, the course may be asymptomatic.[101] Type 3 VWD, an autosomal recessive disorder, carries an incidence of 1 in 1 million and is the most severe form of VWD.[102] It is characterized by an absence of detectable VWF. The lack of VWF gives symptoms of severe bleeding of the mucous membranes and skin not unlike type 1 VWD but also resembles hemophilia A (as explained later) secondary to decreased factor VIII. Type 2 VWD is further subdivided into four classifications: types 2A, 2B, 2M, and 2N. In all subtypes, the defect in VWF is qualitative rather than quantitative. Of special note, in type 2N VWD, the only autosomal recessive type 2 subtype, a defect in the binding site for factor VIII causes a presentation consistent with hemophilia A, as VWF is otherwise normal.[103]

The diagnosis of VWD can often be suggested from a clinical and family history of prolonged or increased episodes of bleeding. Suspicion of VWD can be confirmed with simple laboratory tests evaluating aPTT, VWF levels, VWF activity, and factor VIII activity. Classic bleeding time has fallen out of favor, as the results can be inconsistent secondary to operator variability.[104] Factor VIII activity is decreased in VWD due to its shortened half-life and indirectly prolongs aPTT. VWF levels are evaluated using plasma VWF antigen and an ELISA. VWF activity is evaluated by testing the ability of VWF to cause platelet aggregation in the presence of ristocetin. Both activity and levels are decreased in VWD.[105] More recently, a platelet function analyzer assay has been used to screen for VWD with mixed results.[106]

The current therapeutic approach to the patient with VWD emphasizes desmopressin acetate (DDAVP) and VWF–factor VIII plasma-derived concentrates.[107] Cryoprecipitate is rarely used as it presents the potential risk of viral transmission associated with transfusion. DDAVP is the treatment of choice for mild bleeding in the quantitative deficient type 1 VWD as it causes a release of VWF from the cellular compartments. DDAVP is also effective in types 2A and 2B VWD. However, in types 2M, 2N, and 3 VWD, as well as individuals unresponsive to DDAVP, substitutive therapy with VWF–factor VIII concentrates is necessary. Unlike cryoprecipitate, VWF–factor VIII does not carry the infectious risks of transfusion. In the rare patient with type 3 VWD who develops antibodies to VWF concentrate and is in need of emergent surgery, recombinant factor VIII has been used.[108] However, in the absence of VWF, the short half-life of factor VIII is limited and often a continuous infusion is needed. Recombinant activated factor VII has also been used. However, it and recombinant factor VIII have been associated with an increased risk of thrombosis.[109]

Although classic VWD is genetic in etiology, acquired VWD is associated with various disease states and pharmacological agents. Most commonly, acquired VWD is found in systemic lupus erythematous as an autoimmune process.[110] However, VWD has also been reported in multiple myeloma, both myeloproliferative and lymphoproliferative disorders, hypothyroidism, cirrhosis, and pancreatitis.[111] In addition, valproic acid and dextrans have been shown to be associated with acquired VWD.[112,113]

Hemophilia A is a sex-linked recessive deficiency of factor VIII, occurring in 1 in 10,000 births.[41] Epistaxis and hematuria are common. Findings in severe forms include joint, intramuscular, and retroperitoneal bleeding. The aPTT is prolonged, and factor VIII levels are decreased. The minimum level required for hemostasis is 30%, and spontaneous bleeding is uncommon with levels greater than 5% to 10%.[114] Treatment originally consisted of factor VIII concentrates and cryoprecipitate, but this resulted in widespread transmission of human immunodeficiency virus in the 1980s. Introduction of recombinant factor VIII has eliminated this risk. However, development of neutralizing anti-factor-VIII antibodies, occurring in 10% to 15% of patients, remains a problem. To combat this, new forms of factor VIII are being investigated.

Hemophilia B is a similar sex-linked recessive deficiency of factor IX. Clinically indistinguishable from hemophilia A, it also presents with a prolonged aPTT. Treatment consists of factor IX concentrates and vitamin K.[113]

Other factor deficiencies are much rarer. Most are autosomal recessive and may be treated with fresh frozen plasma, specific factor concentrates, or vitamin K when appropriate. Fibrinolytic abnormalities leading to bleeding include α2-antiplasmin deficiency, as well as PAI-1 deficiency. Patients may present with bleeding after trauma or surgery, which may not present until 24 to 36 hours later.

Platelet Disorders

Inherited and acquired platelet disorders are less common but still important causes of bleeding. Normal platelet function is mediated through the binding interactions of platelet Gp receptors (GpIa/IIa, GpIIb/IIIa, etc.) with the components of the subendothelium (VWF, collagen, fibrinogen, etc.).[115] This interaction leads to platelet activation, which is characterized by a conformational change in platelet shape and the release of platelet granules, furthering the development of a platelet aggregate. In Glanzmann thrombasthenia, an autosomal recessive disorder, a loss of the GpIIb/IIIa receptor occurs on the platelet membrane. This receptor binds fibrinogen, which contains two GpIIb/IIIa binding sites, and allows for platelet linkage and aggregation. Clinically, patients with Glanzmann thrombasthenia have persistent mucocutaneous bleeding in spite of a normal platelet count.[116] GpIIb/IIIa inhibitors abciximab and eptifibatide create a clinical picture of acquired Glanzmann thrombasthenia. Platelet transfusion is the cornerstone of treatment; however, recombinant factor VII may be lifesaving in those refractory to platelet transfusions.[117]

Bernard-Soulier syndrome, an autosomal recessive disease occurring in 1 in 1 million births, is caused by a defect in the platelet receptor for VWF.[118] The clinical presentation of Bernard-Soulier syndrome is similar to that of VWD. However, this syndrome is also associated with thrombocytopenia and giant platelets.[119] Also like VWD, Bernard-Soulier syndrome platelets do not aggregate in response to ristocetin. Again, platelet transfusion is the treatment of choice, but a trial of DDVAP for mild bleeds and recombinant factor VII for emergent bleeding should be considered.[118]

Dysfunction of platelet granules represents an exceedingly rare and often difficult to diagnose condition.[118,120] Deficiency of the α-granules or dense granules is referred to as a storage pool disorder; these include the gray platelet syndrome, Wiskott-Aldrich syndrome, and Chediak-Higashi syndrome. Malfunctions of platelet storage granule release in the face of an appropriate amount of both α-granules and dense granules are referred to as platelet release disorders. Other congenital platelet disorders include collagen receptor deficiency and the hereditary macrothrombocytopenias.[120,121] Traditional platelet aggregation studies can often distinguish among the platelet functional disorders.

Acquired platelet disorders may be seen in liver disease and cardiopulmonary bypass, independent of the thrombocytopenia that both conditions are known to cause. Platelet dysfunction has also been shown in multiple myeloma and Waldenström macroglobulinemia. In addition, the use of aspirin, abciximab, eptifibatide, clopidogrel, or dipyridamole causes platelet dysfunction.[122]

ANTICOAGULATION

The incidence of venous thromboembolism (VTE, which includes DVT and pulmonary embolism) is approximately 900,000 events per year in the United States.[123] Of this number, approximately one third are fatal.[124,125] Most of these events have been either treated or prevented with the traditional anticoagulants unfractionated heparin (UFH) and warfarin. UFH, given subcutaneously or intravenously, binds to ATIII and accelerates its inhibitory action on thrombin (IIa), the final enzyme in the clotting pathway, as well as factors Xa, IXa, XIa, and XII. While this reaction occurs physiologically in the absence of heparin, the presence of heparin may increase the speed of this reaction by 4000-fold.[126] The effects of heparin may be reversed with protamine. The oral drug warfarin mediates its anticoagulation effects by inhibiting the vitamin K–dependent γ-carboxylation of coagulation factors II, VII, IX, and X, rendering these factors biologically inactive. The effects of warfarin may be reversed with vitamin K and, when necessary, fresh frozen plasma. Although both warfarin and UFH have been effective in treating and preventing VTE, their use is not without limitations.[127,128] The use of either UFH or warfarin carries the burden of a narrow therapeutic window, a variable dose response among individuals, the need for constant laboratory monitoring, and a significant bleeding risk. Heparin, which must be given intravenously, has been associated with HIT, as well as heparin-induced osteoporosis and alopecia. In addition, warfarin can induce a transient hypercoagulable state following initiation of therapy.[128] These negative aspects have prompted the development of new anticoagulants.

The development of the LMWHs in the early 1980s provided an advantage over UFH in that they had a higher bioavailability, a longer half-life, and a more predictable dose response, which allowed for subcutaneous dosing one to two times a day with a response equivalent to intravenous UFH.[129,130] In addition, LMWH has been shown to be superior to UFH in the recurrence of VTE and in decreasing major hemorrhage and mortality in certain patient groups totally.[131] However, unlike UFH, the effects of LMWH cannot be reversed with the use of protamine. In addition, LMWH shares cross-reactivity with HIT antibodies and must be used with caution in renal failure as it is totally excreted by the kidneys.[129,130] LMWH acts more selectively on the clotting cascade by primarily inhibiting factor Xa and to a lesser extent inhibiting factors IIa, IXa, and XIa. The effect of LMWH can be monitored by checking antifactor Xa levels.[128-130] Factor Xa, the start of the common coagulation pathway, has been an attractive target for anticoagulation; it has been hypothesized that selective inhibition of Xa may allow small amounts of thrombin to remain active and thus lead to a more favorable safety profile with respect to bleeding.[129]

Selective Xa inhibitors have been developed for either oral or subcutaneous use.[132,133] The inhibition of Xa may be direct, or it may be mediated indirectly through a selective Xa binding site on antithrombin.[134] Fondaparinux, the first subcutaneous selective Xa inhibitor approved by the U.S. Food and Drug Administration for prevention and treatment of VTE works through an indirect mechanism. Fondaparinux shows no cross-reactivity with HIT antibodies, has a half-life of 17 hours, and can be given once a day.[128] The efficacy of fondaparinux in prevention of VTE has been studied extensively in the orthopedic literature, specifically those undergoing knee or hip replacement. A meta-analysis of 7344 patients undergoing major orthopedic surgery of the lower extremities demonstrated that fondaparinux significantly decreased the incidence of VTE by day 11 as compared to enoxaparin.[135] Although the incidence of clinically relevant bleeding was similar in both groups, the incidence of major bleeding was significantly higher in those receiving fondaparinux. However, in those undergoing major abdominal surgery, fondaparinux was at least as effective as dalteparin in prevention of VTE.[133] Fondaparinux performed equally as well as UFH and enoxaparin for the initial treatment of pulmonary embolism and DVT, respectively.[136,137] The anticoagulant effects of fondaparinux can be partially reversed with recombinant factor VII.[138]

Idraparinux, an indirect selective Xa inhibitor with a half-life of 130 hours, has been evaluated for once-weekly subcutaneous dosing for the prevention of VTE.[139,140] A comparison between once-weekly idraparinux and standard therapy of heparin followed by warfarin revealed no significant difference in the recurrence of DVT at 3 and 6 months.[139] However, despite its effectiveness in DVT prevention, the use of idraparinux in the treatment and prevention of recurrent pulmonary embolism was found to be inferior to heparin followed by warfarin. Clinically relevant bleeding was significantly less in the idraparinux group at 3 months and equal in both groups at 6 months. Long-term use of idraparinux has been shown to be associated with increased risk of clinically relevant bleeding.[140] Thus, disadvantages of this agent are its bleeding potential and the nonexistence of a reversal agent. The use of a new biotinylated idraparinux, which can be reversed by avidin, is currently undergoing trials.

Oral Xa inhibitors that mediate their effects by direct inhibition of factor Xa are being developed. Rivaroxaban (BAY 59-7939), one such inhibitor, has shown promising results in phase II trials when compared to enoxaparin for the prevention of VTE in those undergoing major orthopedic surgery.[132] Phase III trials are under way.

Acting one step farther down the coagulation pathway than Xa inhibitors, direct thrombin inhibitors have been developed for both oral and parental use. Unlike heparin, the direct thrombin inhibitors have the ability to inactivate fibrin-bound thrombin.[127] Direct thrombin inhibitors such as argatroban and lepirudin have also been shown to be effective anticoagulants in patients with HIT.[129,141,142] Argatroban has a relatively short half-life, is dosed using the aPTT, and is cleared by the liver. Severe hepatic dysfunction is a relative contraindication for the use of argatroban; however, it is the preferred anticoagulant in HIT patients with renal insufficiency.[143] Lepirudin is cleared renally, has a slightly longer half-life, and is also dosed with the aPTT.[144] Severe renal insufficiency is a relative contraindication for the use of lepirudin, and it is the preferred anticoagulant in patients with hepatic insufficiency. Both argatroban and lepirudin were as effective as historical controls in the prevention and treatment of VTE in HIT-positive patients.[145,146] A third parental thrombin inhibitor, bivalirudin, is used in patients with unstable angina who are undergoing percutaneous cardiac intervention.

Ximelagatran, a renally cleared anticoagulant with a half-life of 5 hours, was the first oral thrombin inhibitor developed. This drug is given twice daily, and unlike warfarin, there is no need for coagulation monitoring. Early trials performed in those undergoing total knee replacements demonstrated superior efficacy over warfarin at preventing VTE.[147,148] The rate of bleeding was similar in both groups. In a comparison of ximelagatran and enoxaparin followed by warfarin for the initial treatment of acute VTE, no difference was seen in recurrent DVT.[149] Bleeding and mortality rates were similar within both groups. Successful results were also demonstrated in a comparison of ximlagatran and warfarin for the prevention of stroke in patients with atrial fibrillation.[150] Despite promising results and the approval of ximelagatran in Europe, it was not approved for use by the U.S. Food and Drug Administration because of concerns of hepatotoxicity.[151] Subsequently, its European approval was withdrawn and the manufacturer withdrew ximelagatran from the market.

More recently, an oral thrombin inhibitor in the same family, dabigatran, has been studied in individuals undergoing major orthopedic surgery for the prevention and treatment of VTE and in those with atrial fibrillation for the prevention of stroke, as well as for treatment and secondary prevention in those with acute VTE.[129] Results of a large phase II trial comparing dabigatran to enoxaparin for VTE prevention in those undergoing hip replacement demonstrated noniferiority to enoxaparin.[152] Ongoing trials are also comparing dabigatran to warfarin.[153] Thus far, there have been no increased bleeding rates, nor have there been any potentially dangerous side effects discovered, including hepatotoxicity.

SUMMARY

Normal hemostasis requires the interaction of platelets, coagulation and fibrinolysis factors, endothelium, proinflammatory and anti-inflammatory mediators, and leukocytes. Clot formation is typically initiated by vascular injury, in which a platelet plug forms and is reinforced with fibrin. Clot formation is balanced by plasmin-mediated fibrinolysis and the action of physiological anticoagulants. Endothelium is capable of sustaining either a prothrombotic or an antithrombotic environment in response to various local factors. Arterial thrombosis may be the result of plaque rupture and release of thrombogenic material into the bloodstream, as well as platelet accumulation along points of high shear forces at stenoses. Hypercoagulability, stasis, and endothelial injury, along with local and systemic inflammatory mediators, contribute to venous thrombosis. Factor V Leiden, elevated levels of factor VIII, prothrombin 20210A, and hyperhomocysteinemia are the most common causes of primary venous thrombosis. Von Willebrand disease is the most common inherited bleeding disorder. Congenital hemophilias, platelet defects, and disorders of fibrinolysis are less common. Anticoagulation has traditionally been accomplished with the heparins and warfarin. More recently, direct thrombin and Xa inhibitors are being used.

The authors wish to acknowledge Tamer N. Boules, MD, who was a co-author of Chapter 3 in the first edition of *Comprehensive Vascular and Endovascular Surgery.*

References

1. Monroe DM, Key NS. The tissue factor–factor VIIa complex: procoagulant activity, regulation, and multitasking. *J Thromb Haemost* 2007;5:1097-1105.
2. Wiiger MT, Prydz H. The changing faces of tissue factor biology: a personal tribute to the understanding of the "extrinsic coagulation activation." *Thromb Haemost* 2007;98:38-42.
3. Mackman N, Tilley RE, Key NS. Role of the extrinsic pathway of blood coagulation in hemostasis and thrombosis. *Arterioscler Thromb Vasc Biol* 2007;27:1687-1693.
4. Hron G, Kollars M, Weber H, et al. Tissue factor–positive microparticles: cellular origin and association with coagulation activation in patients with colorectal cancer. *Thromb Haemost* 2007;97:119-123.
5. Hickey MJ, Williams SA, Roth GJ. Human platelet glycoprotein IX: an adhesive prototype of leucine rich glycoproteins with flank–center–flank structures. *Proc Natl Acad Sci USA* 1989;86:6773-6777.
6. Bennett JS, Vilaire G, Cines DB. Identification of the fibrinogen receptor on human platelets by photoaffinity labeling. *J Biol Chem* 1982;257:8049-8054.
7. Savage B, Ruggeri ZM. Selective recognition of adhesive sites in surface-bound fibrinogen by glycoprotein IIb/IIIa on nonactivated platelets. *J Biol Chem* 1991;266:11227-11233.
8. Shapiro AD. Platelet function disorders. *Haemophilia* 2000;6(Suppl 1):120-127.
9. Sims PJ, Faioni EM, Wiedmer T, et al. Complement proteins C5b-9 cause release of membrane vesicles from the platelet surface that are enriched in the membrane receptor for coagulation factor Va and express prothrombinase activity. *J Biol Chem* 1988;263:18205-18212.
10. Gilbert GE, Sims PJ, Wiedmer T, et al. Platelet-derived microparticles express high affinity receptors for factor VIII. *J Biol Chem* 1991;266:17261-17268.
11. Ferguson JJ, Waly HM, Wilson JM. Fundamentals of coagulation and glycoprotein IIb/IIIa receptor inhibition. *Eur Heart J* 1998;19(Suppl D):D3-D9.
12. Hassouna HI. Laboratory evaluation of hemostatic disorders. *Hematol Oncol Clin North Am* 1993;7:1161-1249.

13. Triplett DA. Coagulation and bleeding disorders: review and update. *Clin Chem* 2000;46:1260-1269.
14. Zur M, Radcliffe RD, Oberdick J, et al. The dual role of factor VII in blood coagulation: initiation and inhibition of a proteolytic system by a zymogen. *J Biol Chem* 1982;257:5623-5631.
15. Dahlbäck B. Blood coagulation. *Lancet* 2000;355:1627-1632.
16. Blomback B, Blomback M. The molecular structure of fibrinogen. *Ann NY Acad Sci* 1972;202:77-97.
17. Davie EW, Fujikawa K, Kisiel W. The coagulation cascade: initiation, maintenance, and regulation. *Biochemistry* 1991;30:10363-10370.
18. DiScipio RG, Kurachi K, Davie EW. Activation of human factor IX (Christmas factor). *J Clin Invest* 1978;61:1528-1538.
19. Naito K, Fujikawa K. Activation of human blood coagulation factor XI independent of factor XII: factor XI is activated by thrombin and factor XIa in the presence of negatively charged surfaces. *J Biol Chem* 1991;266:7353-7358.
20. Rosenberg RD, Damus PS. The purification and mechanism of action of human antithrombin–heparin cofactor. *J Biol Chem* 1973;248: 6490-6505.
21. Kurachi K, Fujikawa K, Schmer G, et al. Inhibition of bovine factor IXa and factor Xab by antithrombin III. *Biochemistry* 1976;15:373-377.
22. Kurachi K, Davie EW. Activation of factor XI (plasma thromboplastin antecedent) by factor XIIa (activated Hageman factor). *Biochemistry* 1977;16:5831-5839.
23. Esmon CT, Owen WG. Identification of an endothelial cell cofactor for thrombin-catalyzed activation of protein C. *Proc Natl Acad Sci USA* 1981;78:2249-2252.
24. Owen WG, Esmon CT. Functional properties of an endothelial cell cofactor for thrombin-catalyzed activation of protein C. *J Biol Chem* 1981;256:5532-5535.
25. Esmon NL, Owen WG, Esmon CT. Isolation of a membrane-bound cofactor for thrombin-catalyzed activation of protein C. *J Biol Chem* 1982;257:859-864.
26. Kisiel W, Canfield WM, Ericsson LH, et al. Anticoagulant properties of bovine plasma protein C following activation by thrombin. *Biochemistry* 1977;16:5824-5831.
27. Marlar RA, Kleiss AJ, Griffin JH. Mechanism of action of human activated protein C, a thrombin dependent anticoagulant enzyme. *Blood* 1982;59:1067-1072.
28. Vehar GA, Davie EW. Preparation and properties of bovine factor VIII (antihemophilic factor). *Biochemistry* 1980;19:401-410.
29. Greenfield LJ, Proctor MC, Wakefield TW. Coagulation cascade and thrombosis. In: Ernst CB, Stanley JC, eds. *Current therapy in vascular surgery*. 4th ed. St. Louis: Mosby; 2001:813-817.
30. Tollefsen DM, Majerus PW, Blank MK. Heparin cofactor II: purification and properties of a heparin-dependent inhibitor of thrombin in human plasma. *J Biol Chem* 1982;257:2162-2169.
31. Geiger M, Krebs M, Jerabek I, et al. Protein C inhibitor (PCI) and heparin cofactor II (HCII): possible alternative roles of these heparin-binding serpins outside the hemostatic system. *Immunopharmacology* 1997;36:279-284.
32. Adelman B, Michelson AD, Loscalzo J, et al. Plasmin effect on platelet glycoprotein Ib–von Willebrand factor interactions. *Blood* 1985;65:32-40.
33. Gurewich V, Pannell R. Fibrin binding and zymogenic properties of single-chain urokinase (pro-urokinase). *Semin Thromb Hemost* 1987;13:146-151.
34. Sidelmann JJ, Gram J, Jesperson J, et al. Fibrin clot formation and lysis: basic mechanisms. *Semin Thromb Hemost* 2000;26:605-618.
35. Hajjar KA, Nachman RL. Endothelial cell–mediated conversion of Glu-plasminogen to Lys-plasminogen: further evidence for assembly of the fibrinolytic system on the endothelial cell surface. *J Clin Invest* 1988;82:1769-1778.
36. Esmon CT. The regulation of natural anticoagulant pathways. *Science* 1987;235:1348-1352.
37. Schmaier AH. Disseminated intravascular coagulation: pathogenesis and management. *J Intensive Care Med* 1991;6:209-228.
38. Becker BF, Heindl B, Kupatt C, et al. Endothelial function and hemostasis. *Z Kardiol* 2000;89:160-167.
39. Gross PL, Aird WC. The endothelium and thrombosis. *Semin Thromb Hemost* 2000;26:463-478.
40. Esmon NL, Esmon CT. Protein C and the endothelium. *Semin Thromb Hemost* 1988;14:210-215.
41. Wakefield TW. Hemostasis. In: Greenfield LJ, Mulholland MW, Oldham KT, eds. *Surgery: scientific principles and practice.* 3rd ed. Philadelphia: Lippincott Williams & Wilkins; 2001:88-111.
42. Nawroth PP, Stern DM. Modulation of endothelial cell hemostatic properties by tumor necrosis factor. *J Exp Med* 1986;163:740-745.
43. Bevilacqua MP, Pober JS, Majeau GR, et al. Recombinant tumor necrosis factor induces procoagulant activity in cultured human vascular endothelium: characterization and comparison with the actions of interleukin-1. *Proc Natl Acad Sci USA* 1986;83:4533-4537.
44. Conway EM, Bach R, Rosenberg RD, et al. Tumor necrosis factor enhances expression of tissue factor mRNA in endothelial cells. *Thromb Res* 1989;53:231-241.
45. Schleef RR, Bevilacqua MP, Sawdey M, et al. Cytokine activation of vascular endothelium: effects on tissue-type plasminogen activator and type I plasminogen inhibitor. *J Biol Chem* 1988;263:5797-5803.
46. Van Hinsbergh VW, Kooistra T, van den Berg EA, et al. Tumor necrosis factor increases production of plasminogen activator inhibitor in human endothelial cells in vitro and rats in vivo. *Blood* 1988;72: 1467-1473.
47. Medina R, Schocher SH, Han JH. Interleukin-1, endotoxin, or tumor necrosis factor/cachectin enhance the level of plasminogen activator messenger RNA in bovine aortic endothelial cells. *Thromb Res* 1989;54:41-52.
48. Rauch U, Osende JI, Fuster V, et al. Thrombus formation on atherosclerotic plaques: pathogenesis and clinical consequences. *Ann Intern Med* 2001;134:224-238.
49. Stewart GJ. Neutrophils and deep venous thrombosis. *Haemostasis* 1993;23:127-140.
50. Myers Jr DD, Schaub R, Wrobleski SK, et al. P-Selectin antagonism causes dose-dependent venous thrombosis inhibition. *Thromb Haemost* 2001;85:423-429.
51. Myers D, Wrobleski S, Londy F, et al. New and effective treatment of experimentally induced venous thrombosis with anti-inflammatory rPSGL-Ig. *Thromb Haemost* 2002;87:374-382.
52. Day SM, Reeve JL, Pedersen B, et al. Macrovascular thrombosis is driven by tissue factor derived primarily from the blood vessel wall. *Blood* 2005;105:192-198.
53. Mielke CH. Measurement of the bleeding time. *Thromb Haemost* 1984;52:210-211.
54. Rodgers RP, Levin J. A critical reappraisal of the bleeding time. *Semin Thromb Haemost* 1990;16:1-20.
55. Henke PK, Schmaier A, Wakefield TW. Vascular thrombosis due to hypercoagulable states. In: Rutherford RB, ed. *Vascular surgery.* 6th ed. Philadelphia: Elsevier; 2005:560-578.
56. Towne JB, Bandyk DF, Hussey CV, et al. Antithrombin deficiency: a cause of unexplained thrombosis in vascular surgery. *Surgery* 1981;89:735-742.
57. Menache D. Antithrombin III concentrates. *Hematol Oncol Clin North Am* 1992;6:1115-1120.
58. Eldrup-Jorgensen J, Flanigan DP, Brace L, et al. Hypercoagulable states and lower limb ischemia in young adults. *J Vasc Surg* 1989;9:334-341.
59. Cole MS, Minifee PK, Wolma FJ. Coumadin necrosis: a review of the literature. *Surgery* 1988;103:271-277.
60. Svensson PJ, Dahlbäck B. Resistance to activated protein C as a basis for venous thrombosis. *N Engl J Med* 1994;330:517-522.
61. Kalafatis M, Mann KG. Factor V Leiden and thrombophilia. *Arterioscler Thromb Vasc Biol* 1997;17:620-627.
62. Rosendaal FR, Koster T, Vandenbroucke JP, et al. High risk of thrombosis in patients homozygous for factor V Leiden (activated protein C resistance). *Blood* 1995;85:1504-1508.
63. Loscalzo J. The oxidant stress of hyperhomocyst(e)inemia. *J Clin Invest* 1996;98:5-7.
64. Tawakol A, Omland T, Gerhard M, et al. Hyperhomocyst(e)inemia is associated with impaired endothelium-dependent vasodilation in humans. *Circulation* 1997;95:1119-1121.
65. Upchurch GR, Welch GN, Randev N, et al. The effect of homocysteine on endothelial nitric oxide production (abstract). *FASEB J* 1995;9 A876.
66. Starkebaum G, Harlan JM. Endothelial cell injury due to copper-catalyzed hydrogen peroxide generation from homocysteine. *J Clin Invest* 1986;77:1370-1376.
67. Graeber JE, Slott JH, Ulane RE, et al. Effect of homocysteine and homocystine on platelet and vascular arachidonic acid metabolism. *Pediatr Res* 1982;16:490-493.
68. Nehler MR, Taylor Jr LM, Porter JM. Homocysteinemia as a risk factor for atherosclerosis: a review. *Cardiovasc Surg* 1997;5:559-567.
69. Cumming AM, Keeney S, Salden A, et al. The prothrombin gene G20210A variant: prevalence in a UK anticoagulant clinic population. *Br J Haematol* 1997;98:353-355.

70. Towne JB, Bandyk DF, Hussey CV, et al. Abnormal plasminogen: a genetically determined cause of hypercoagulability. *J Vasc Surg* 1984;1:896-902.
71. Kyrle PA, Minar E, Hirschl M, et al. High plasma levels of factor VIII and the risk of recurrent venous thromboembolism. *N Engl J Med* 2000;343:457-462.
72. Kraaijenhagen RA, in't Anker PS, Koopman MMW, et al. High plasma concentration of factor VIIIc is a major risk factor for venous thromboembolism. *Thromb Haemost* 2000;83:5-9.
73. Cancio LC, Cohen DJ. Heparin-induced thrombocytopenia and thrombosis. *J Am Coll Surg* 1998;186:76-91.
74. Sheridan D, Carter C, Kelton JG. A diagnostic test for heparin-induced thrombocytopenia. *Blood* 1986;67:27-30.
75. Jackson MR, Krishnamurti C, Aylesworth CA, et al. Diagnosis of heparin-induced thrombocytopenia in the vascular surgery patient. *Surgery* 1997;121:419-424.
76. Lee DH, Warkentin TE, Hayward CP, et al. The development and evaluation of a novel test for heparin induced thrombocytopenia (abstract). *Blood* 1994;84:188a.
77. Greenfield LJ. Lupus-like anticoagulants and thrombosis. *J Vasc Surg* 1988;7:818-819.
78. Ahn SS, Kalunian K, Rosove M, et al. Postoperative thrombotic complications in patients with the lupus anticoagulant: increased risk after vascular procedures. *J Vasc Surg* 1988;7:749-756.
79. Lynch A, Marlar R, Murphy J, et al. Antiphospholipid antibodies in predicting adverse pregnancy outcome: a prospective study. *Ann Intern Med* 1994;120:470-475.
80. Carreras LO, Defreyn G, Machin SJ, et al. Arterial thrombosis, intrauterine death, and "lupus" anticoagulant: detection of immunoglobulin interfering with prostacyclin formation. *Lancet* 1981;1:244-246.
81. Comp PC, DeBault LE, Esmon NL, et al. Human thrombomodulin is inhibited by IgG from two patients with non-specific anticoagulants (abstract). *Blood* 1983;62;(Suppl 1):299a.
82. Violi F, Ferro D, Valesini G, et al. Tissue plasminogen activator inhibitor in patients with systemic lupus erythematosus and thrombosis. *BMJ* 1990;300:1099-1102.
83. Vermylen J, Blockmans D, Spitz B, et al. Thrombosis and immune disorders. *Clin Haematol* 1986;15:393-412.
84. Ferro D, Pittoni V, Quintarelli C, et al. Coexistence of antiphospholipid antibodies and endothelial perturbation in systemic lupus erythematosus patients with ongoing prothrombotic state. *Circulation* 1997;95: 1425-1432.
85. Reverter JC, Tassies D, Font J, et al. Hypercoagulable state in patients with antiphospholipid syndrome is related to high induced tissue factor expression on monocytes and to low free protein S. *Arterioscler Thromb Vasc Biol* 1996;16:1319-1326.
86. Murray EW, Lillicrap D. Von Willebrand disease: pathogenesis, classification, and management. *Transfus Med Rev* 1996;10:93-110.
87. Ruggeri ZM, Ware J. Von Willebrand factor. *FASEB J* 1993;7:308-316.
88. Ruggeri ZM. The role of von Willebrand factor in thrombus formation. *Thromb Res* 2007;120(Suppl 1):S5-S9.
89. Brinkhous KM, Sandberg H, Garris JB, et al. Purified human factor VIII procoagulant protein: comparative hemostatic response after infusion into hemophilic and von Willebrand disease dogs. *Proc Natl Acad Sci USA* 1985;82:8752-8756.
90. Fay PJ, Coumans JV, Walker FJ. Von Willebrand factor mediates protection of factor VIII from activated protein C–catalyzed inactivation. *J Biol Chem* 1991;266:2172-2177.
91. Hollestelle MJ, Thinnes T, Crain K, et al. Tissue distribution of factor VIII gene expression in vivo: a closer look. *Thromb Haemost* 2001;86:855-861.
92. Wagner DD. Cell biology of von Willebrand factor. *Annu Rev Cell Biol* 1990;6:217-246.
93. Carew JA, Browning PJ, Lynch DC. Sulfation of von Willebrand factor. *Blood* 1990;76:2530-2539.
94. Wagner DD, Olmstead JB, Marder VJ. Immunolocalization of von Willebrand protein in Weibel-Palade bodies of human endothelial cells. *J Cell Biol* 1982;95:355-360.
95. Cramer EM, Meyer D, le Menn R, Breton-Gorius J. Eccentric localization of von Willebrand factor in an internal structure of platelet α-granule resembling that of Weibel-Palade bodies. *Blood* 1985;66:710-713.
96. Wagner DD, Bonfanti R. Von Willebrand factor and the endothelium. *Mayo Clin Proc* 1991;66:621-627.
97. Gill JC, Endres-Brooks J, Bauer PJ, et al. The effect of ABO blood group on the diagnosis of von Willebrand disease. *Blood* 1987; 69:1691-1695.
98. Siedlecki CA, Lestini BJ, Kottke-Marchant KK, et al. Shear dependent changes in the three-dimensional structure of human von Willebrand factor. *Blood* 1996;88:2939-2950.
99. Tsai H. Thrombotic thrombocytopenic purpura: a thrombotic disorder caused by ADAMTS13 deficiency. *Hematol Oncol North Am* 2007;21:609-632.
100. Sadler JE. A revised classification of von Willebrand disease: for the Subcommittee on von Willebrand Factor of the Scientific and Standardization Committee of the International Society on Thrombosis and Haemostasis. *Thromb Haemost* 1994;71:520-525.
101. Werner EJ. Von Willebrand disease in children and adolescents. *Pediatr Clin North Am* 1996;43:683-707.
102. Mannucci PM, Bloom AL, Larrieu MJ, et al. Atherosclerosis and von Willebrand factor: prevalence of severe von Willebrand's disease in western Europe and Israel. *Br J Haematol* 1984;57:163-169.
103. Nishino M, Girma JP, Rothschild C, et al. New variant of von Willebrand disease with defective binding to factor VIII. *Blood* 1989;74: 1591-1599.
104. Peterson P, Hayes TE, Arkin CF, et al. The preoperative bleeding time test lacks clinical benefit: College of American Pathologists' and American Society of Clinical Pathologists' position article. *Arch Surg* 1998;133:134-139.
105. Favaloro EJ, Smith J, Petinos P, et al. Laboratory testing for von Willebrand's disease: an assessment of current diagnostic practice and efficacy by means of a multi-laboratory survey. RCPA Quality Assurance Program (QAP) in Haematology Haemostasis Scientific Advisory Panel. *Thromb Haemost* 1999;82:1276-1282.
106. Posan E, McBane RD, Grill DE, et al. Comparison of PFA-100 testing and bleeding time for detecting platelet hypofunction and von Willebrand disease in clinical practice. *Thromb Haemost* 2003;90:483-490.
107. Michiels JJ, van Vliet H, Berneman Z, et al. Intravenous DDAVP and factor VIII–von Willebrand factor concentrate for the treatment and prophylaxis of bleedings in patients with von Willebrand disease type 1,2 and 3. *Clin Applied Thromb Hemost* 2007;13:14-34.
108. Ciavarella N, Schiavoni M, Valenzano E, et al. Use of recombinant factor VIIa (Novoseven) in the treatment of two patient with type III von Willebrand disease and an inhibitor against von Willebrand factor. *Haemostasis* 1996;26:150-154.
109. Federici AB. Management of inherited von Willebrand disease in 2006. *Semin Thromb Hemost* 2006;32:616-620.
110. Simone JV, Cornet JA, Abildgaard CF. Acquired von Willebrand's syndrome and thrombopathy in systemic lupus erythematosus. *Blood* 1968;31:806-812.
111. Franchini M, Lippi G. Acquired von Willebrand's syndrome: an update. *Am J Hematol* 2007;82:368-375.
112. Kreuz W, Linde R, Funk M, et al. Valproate therapy induces von Willebrand disease type I. *Epilepsia* 1992;33:178-184.
113. Jonville-Bera AP, Autret-Leca E, Gruel Y. Acquired type I von Willebrand's disease associated with highly substituted hydroxyethyl starch. *N Engl J Med* 2001;345:622-623.
114. Collins JA. Blood transfusion and disorders of surgical bleeding. In: Sabiston DC, ed. Textbook of surgery. 14th ed. Philadelphia: WB Saunders; 1991:85-102.
115. Ruggeri ZM, Mendolicchio GL. Adhesion mechanisms in platelet function. *Circ Res* 2007;100:1673-1685.
116. Bellucci S, Caen J. Molecular basis of Glanzmann's thrombasthenia and current strategies in treatment. *Blood Rev* 2002;16:193-202.
117. Poon MC, D'Oiron R, Von Depka M, et al. Prophylactic and therapeutic recombinant factor VIIa administration to patients with Glanzmann's thrombasthenia: results of an international survey. *J Thromb Haemost* 2004;2:1096-1103.
118. Handin RI. Inherited platelet disorders. *Hematology Am Soc Hematol Educ Program* 2005:396-402.
119. Lopez JA, Andrews RK. Bernard-Soulier syndrome. *Blood* 1998;91: 4397-4418.
120. Bolton Maggs PH, Chalmers EA, Collins PW, et al. A review of inherited platelet disorders with guidelines for their management on behalf of the UKHCDO. *Br J Haematol* 2006;135:603-633.
121. Rodriguez V, Nichols WL, Charlesworth JE, et al. Sebastian platelet syndrome: hereditary macrothrombocytopenia. *Mayo Clin Proc* 2003;78:1416-1421.
122. Shen YM, Frenkel EP. Acquired platelet dysfunction. *Hematol Oncol Clin North Am* 2007;21:647-661.
123. Wakefield TW, Myers DD, Henke PK. Mechanisms of venous thrombosis and resolution. *Arterioscler Thromb Vasc Biol* 2008;28:387-391.

124. White RH. The epidemiology of venous thromboembolism. *Circulation* 2003;107:I4-I8.
125. Heit JA, Silverstein MD, Mohr DN, et al. Predictors of survival after deep vein thrombosis and pulmonary embolism: a population-based, cohort study. *Arch Intern Med* 1999;159:445-453.
126. Perry DJ. Antithrombin and its inherited deficiencies. *Blood Rev* 1994;8:37-55.
127. Ansell J, Hirsh J, Poller L, et al. The pharmacology and management of the vitamin K antagonist: the seventh ACCP conference on antithrombotic and thrombolytic therapy. *Chest* 2004;126:204S-233S.
128. Hirsh J, O'Donnell M, Eikelboom JW. Beyond unfractionated heparin and warfarin: current and future advances. *Circulation* 2007;116: 552-560.
129. Bauer KA. New anticoagulants. *Hematology Am Soc Hematol Educ Program* 2006:450-456.
130. Hirsh J, Ranschke R. Heparin and low-molecular weight heparin: the seventh ACCP conference on antithrombotic and thrombolytic therapy. *Chest* 2004;126:188S-203S.
131. Mismetti P, LaPorte S, Darmon JY, et al. Meta-analysis of low molecular weight heparin in the prevention of venous thromboembolism in general surgery. *Br J Surg* 2001;88:913-930.
132. Laux V, Perzborn E, Kubitza D, et al. Preclinical and clinical characteristics of rivaroxaban: a novel oral direct factor Xa inhibitor. *Semin Thromb Hemost* 2007;33:515-523.
133. Agnelli G, Bergqvist A, Cohen AT, et al. Randomized clinical trial of postoperative fondaparinux versus perioperative dalteparin for prevention of venous thromboembolism in high-risk abdominal surgery. *Br J Surg* 2005;92:1212-1220.
134. Hirsh J, O'Donnel M, Weitz JI. New anticoagulants. *Blood* 2005;105: 453-463.
135. Turpie AGG, Bauer KA, Eriksson BI, et al. Fondaparinux vs enoxaparin for the prevention of venous thromboembolism in major orthopedic surgery: a meta-analysis of 4 randomized major double blind studies. *Arch Intern Med* 2002;163:1833-1840.
136. Buller HR, Davidson BL, Decousus H, et al. Fondaparinux or enoxaparin for the initial treatment of symptomatic deep venous thrombosis: a randomized trial. *Ann Intern Med* 2004;140:867-873.
137. Buller HR, Davidson BL, Decousus H, et al. Subcutaneous fondaparinux versus intravenous unfractionated heparin in the initial treatment of pulmonary embolism. *N Engl J Med* 2003;349:1695-1702.
138. Bijsterveld NR, Moons AH, Boekholdt SM, et al. Ability of recombinant factor VIIa to reverse the anticoagulant effect of the pentasacchardie fondaparinux in healthy volunteers. *Circulation* 2002;106:2550-2554.
139. van Gogh Investigators Buller HR, Cohen AT, et al. Extended prophylaxis of venous thromboembolism with idraparinux. *N Engl J Med* 2007;357:1105-1112.
140. van Gogh Investigators Buller HR, Cohen AT, et al. Idraparinux versus standard therapy for venous thromboembolism disease. *N Engl J Med* 2007;357:1094-1104.
141. Jang IK, Brown DF, Giugliano RP, et al. and MINT Investigators. A multicenter, randomized study of argatroban versus heparin as adjunct to tissue plasminogen activator (tPA) in acute myocardial infarction: myocardial infarction with Novastan and tPA (MINT) study. *J Am Coll Cardiol* 1999;33:1879-1885.
142. Greinacher A, Volpel H, Janssens V, et al. Recombinant hirudin (lepirudin) provides safe and effective anticoagulation in patients with heparin-induced thrombocytopenia: a prospective study. *Circulation* 1999;99:73-80.
143. Swan SK, Hurstings MJ. The pharmacokinetics and pharmacodynamics of argatroban: effects of age, gender, and hepatic or renal dysfunction. *Pharmacotherapy* 2000;20:318-329.
144. Schiele F, Vuillemenot A, Kramarz P, et al. Use of recombinant hirudin as antithrombotic treatment in patients with heparin- induced thrombocytopenia. *Am J Hematol* 1995;50:20-25.
145. Begelman SM, Hursting MJ, Aghababian RV, et al. Heparin-induced thrombocytopenia from venous thromboembolism treatment. *J Intern Med* 2005;258:563-572.
146. Hassan Y, Awaisu A, Aziz NA, et al. Heparin-induced thrombocytopenia and recent advances in its therapy. *J Clin Pharm Ther* 2007;32: 535-544.
147. Francis CW, Berkowitz SD, Comp PC, et al. Comparison of ximelagatran with warfarin for the prevention of venous thromboembolism after total knee replacement. *N Engl J Med* 2003;349:1703-1712.
148. Colwell Jr CW, Berkowitz SD, Lieberman JR, et al. Oral direct thrombin inhibitor ximelagatran compared with warfarin for the prevention of venous thromboembolism after total knee arthroplasty. *J Bone Joint Surg Am* 2005;87:2169-2177.
149. Feissinger JN, Huisman MV, Davidson BL, et al. Ximelagatran vs low-molecular weight heparin and warfarin for the treatment of deep vein thrombosis: a randomized trial. *JAMA* 2005;293:681-689.
150. Olsson SB. Stroke prevention with the oral direct thrombin inhibitor ximelagatran compared with warfarin in patients with non-valvular atrial fibrillation (SPORTIF III): randomized controlled trial. *Lancet* 2003;362:1691-1698.
151. Gurewich. V. Ximelagatran: promises and concerns. *JAMA* 2005;293: 736-739.
152. Eriksson BI, Dahl OE, Rosencher N, et al. and RE-NOVATE Study Group. Dabigatran etexilate versus enoxaparin for prevention of venous thromboembolism after total hip replacement: a randomized, double-blind, non-inferiority trial. *Lancet* 2007;370:949-956.
153. Turpie AG. New oral anticoagulation in atrial fibrillation. *Eur Heart J* 2008;29:155-165.

chapter

4

Vascular Hemodynamics

Christopher L. Wixon, MD, FACS

Key Points

- Basic concepts of vascular surgery pertain to the fields of vessel wall mechanics and vascular hemodynamics.
- Physical properties govern physiological and pathophysiological conditions, interventions, and technologies.

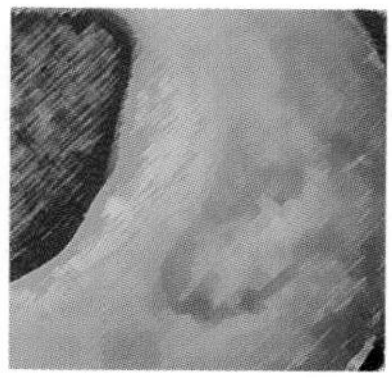

Although a patient may possess a constellation of vascular lesions unique to the individual, each lesion must obey the principles of physics and fluid dynamics. As such, an individual's response to a change in hemodynamic pattern should be orderly and predictable.

The field of hemodynamics represents a series of mathematical formulas that describe the interaction between blood and the vessels through which it travels. Such models may be created for nearly all physiological and pathophysiological observations within the vascular system. The importance of a clear understanding of vascular physics and hemodynamics cannot be overestimated as these rules dictate the manner in which a diverse patient population responds to an intervention (Table 4-1).

The field of vascular physics can be broken into two generalized areas: vessel wall mechanics and vascular hemodynamics. The area of vessel wall mechanics is based upon classical Newtonian concepts and describes the physical properties and interactions of the elements that compose the blood vessel wall and their responses when exposed to an external force. Vascular hemodynamics describes the properties of blood in motion and characterizes energy gradients that exist within the vascular system in the form of pressure, thermal, potential, or kinetic energy.

The purpose of this chapter is to review vessel wall and fluid mechanics from a conceptual basis as they pertain to the daily clinical work of a practicing physician. These considerations are helpful in the understanding normal physiology of the arterial system and the expected consequences of circulatory perturbations. Substantial effort was made to present concepts in the most fundamental manner with the hope that such a broad approach provides stimulus for deeper insights. Quantitative formulation is beyond the scope of the current discussion, and I defer to more comprehensive texts for further consideration.[1-4]

HISTORICAL PERSPECTIVE

If I have seen further, it is by standing on the shoulders of giants.

Although often attributed to Sir Isaac Newton, this quote was probably first recorded by Bernard of Chartres in the twelfth century as a reference to the emerging Enlightenment. Newton popularized the phrase in a written response to Robert Hooke, who had publicly criticized Newton's ideas regarding optics. It is said that Newton was so offended by Hooke's criticism that he withdrew from public debate and the two remained enemies until Hooke's death. Newton's choice to use the phrase is of particular interest when taken in the context that Hooke was a slight man who suffered from a combination of severe scoliosis and Pott's disease, making Hooke a hunchback. The field of vascular physics is founded upon Newton's concepts of mass, acceleration, and viscosity, presented in his opus magnus, *Philosophiae Naturalis Principia Mathematica* (1687).[5] The elegance and simplicity of Newton's laws of motion are worth reproducing as they continue to form the basis for classical mechanics (Table 4-2).

Newton's laws of motion described the acceleration of massive particles and provided a quantitative explanation for a range of physical phenomena within a worldview that philosophized "instantaneous action at a distance" between material particles. He was prepared for criticism, and it was in this context that he appended the second edition of *The Principia* (1713), in which he stated the famous phrase "hypotheses non fingo" (I feign no hypotheses).[1] It was his answer to those who had publicly challenged him to give an explanation for the *causes* of gravity rather than simply imparting the

1. "I have not as yet been able to discover the reason for these properties of gravity from phenomena, and I do not feign hypotheses. For whatever is not deduced from the phenomena must be called a hypothesis; and hypotheses, whether metaphysical or physical, or based on occult qualities, or mechanical, have no place in experimental philosophy. In this philosophy, particular propositions are inferred from the phenomena, and afterwards rendered general by induction." Newton I. *Philosophiae naturalis principia mathematica: general scholium.* 2nd ed. Cambridge University Press; 1713.

Table 4-1
Governing Principles of Vascular Physics That Allow the Physician to Optimize Care

Early recognition of physiological and pathophysiological conditions
Critical evaluation and application of new technologies
Sound treatment decisions
Foundation upon which future innovations may be based

mathematical principles of kinetics. The phrase represents a departure from the Aristotelian hypothetic-deductive method of natural philosophy.

Having defined the relationship of force, mass, and velocity, it became possible to understand simple interactions of objects when external forces were applied upon these objects. While the discipline of geometry had been well established, broader application required Pierre-Simon de Laplace's translation of classical mechanics to one based upon calculus in his five-volume work *Exposition du Système du Monde* and the *Mécanique Céleste (Celestial Mechanics)*.[6] The next major development in the scientific community was an understanding of the concept of conservation of energy as described by Daniel Bernoulli in *Hydrodynamique (Hydrodynamica)*, in 1738.[7] These principles provide the basis for the field of fluid dynamics and patterns associated with the motion of blood from an area of high energy to one of low energy.

BASIC CONCEPTS

Mechanics is the field of physics dealing with the basic physical units. The basic units are those of mass, length, and time. All mechanical quantities can be expressed in terms of these three quantities:

Length ÷ Time = Velocity (m/sec)

↓

Velocity ÷ Time = Acceleration (m/sec^2)

↓

Acceleration Mass = Force ([kg m]/sec^2, newtons, N)

↓

Force Length = Work (N × m, joules, J)

↓

Work ÷ Time = Power (J/sec, watts)

↓

Force ÷ Area = Pressure (N/m^2, pascal), or $\frac{kg}{m \cdot s^2}$

Table 4-2
Newton's Laws of Motion

First Law
A physical body will remain at rest, or continue to move at a constant velocity, unless an outside net force acts upon it. If no net force acts on a particle, then it is possible to select a set of reference frames, observed from which the particle moves without any change in velocity.

Second Law
Rate of change of momentum is proportional to the resultant force producing it and takes place in the direction of that force. The net force on a particle is proportional to the time rate of change of its linear momentum: $F = d(mv)/dt$. Momentum, mv, is the product of mass and velocity. When the mass is constant, this law is often stated as $F = ma$.

Third Law
To every action there is an equal and opposite reaction. Whenever a particle, *A*, exerts a force on another particle, *B*, *B* simultaneously exerts a force on *A* with the same magnitude in the opposite direction.

From Newton I. *The principia.* Cohen IB, Whitman A, trans. Berkeley: University of California Press; 1999.

CONCEPTS OF PRESSURE

When a fluid contains energy, it is able to exert a force upon another object and, therefore, perform work. In vascular physiology, it is most convenient to consider the *concentration of energy* contained within the fluid in terms of pressure, rather than in terms of quantity of energy. Pressure in a fluid can be considered a measure of energy per unit volume by means of the definition of work (*work* = $F \times d$, *volume* = *area* $\times d$). For a force exerted on a fluid, this can be seen from the definition of pressure:

$$\text{Pressure} = \frac{\text{Force}}{\text{Unit Area}} = \frac{F}{A} = \frac{F \times d}{A \times d} = \frac{\text{Energy}}{\text{Volume}}$$

Alternatively, pressure is defined as force per unit area. In other words, when a similar force is applied to devices of different cross-sectional areas, the energy per unit area (pressure) is substantially greater in the device of smaller cross-sectional area (Figure 4-1). The standard unit for pressure is the pascal, which is a newton per square meter ($kg/m \cdot s^2$).

Although the mercury containing sphygmomanometer has largely been replaced by digital instruments, in clinical practice we continue to express pressure in units of millimeters of mercury, which is defined as the hydrostatic pressure for a column of fluid:

$$\text{Pressure} = \rho g h$$

where:
ρ = Density of the fluid
g = Gravitational force
h = Height of the fluid column

These units may be converted to standard units of pressure that may be more familiar in the setting of bioengineering (Table 4-3).

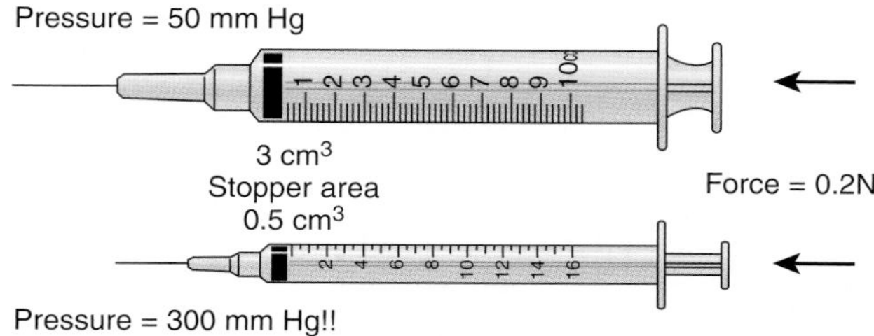

Figure 4-1. For two syringes in which equal force is applied, the force per unit area developed in the syringe of smaller diameter achieves a significantly higher pressure. Given similar forces, the ratio of the cross-sectional area is inversely proportional to the ratio of the pressure generated by each syringe.

While the concept of generating pressure within a fluid through the application of an external force is rather straightforward, the idea that a pressurized fluid contains a discrete and quantifiable energy is less intuitive. On the molecular level, the hydrostatic pressure energy contained in a fluid represents the sum total of particle interaction energies that exist when compressed beyond their resting state.

The concept of pressure is best illustrated by the relationship between pressure and volume, which is exhibited by an ideal gas as defined by Boyle's law:

$$P_iV_i = P_fV_f$$

In this model, when an ideal gas is pressurized, the density increases by overcoming the particle-to-particle repelling forces. The sum total of microscopic energies created from the particle-to-particle repelling forces divided by the total volume of the compressed gas is equivalent to the pressure of the gas.

The change in density associated with pressurization of a liquid is poorly understood (Figure 4-2). Although water is usually considered a poorly compressible liquid, small changes in density may occur, creating strain in the hydrogen bonds that bind the molecules together. For most liquids, the change in density of a liquid and can be expressed by the following equation:

$$\rho 1 = \rho 0\ [1 - (P_1 - P_0)/E]$$

where:
E = Bulk modulus fluid elasticity (N/m^2)
P_1 = Final pressure (N/m^2)
P_0 = Initial pressure (N/m^2)

Due to the rigid elastic modulus (more on this subject later) of a water molecule ($E = 2.15 \times 10^9$ N/m^2), only small changes in volume or density occur within the physiological range of pressures.[2] Nonetheless, as these small changes in density occur, the increased particle–particle interaction can be thought to store energy that may later be released much in the way a coiled spring is able to release its energy upon another object.

Although most energy within the vascular system exists in the form of pressure, other forms of energy likewise exist: kinetic energy, thermal energy, and potential energy. We recognize these other forms of energy density in the forms of velocity and temperature and in less recognizable forms such as the elongation of an elastin fiber beyond its resting length. Although energy is constantly transferred from one form to another, the sum total energy (kinetic, potential, pressure, thermal) must remain constant (Figure 4-3). Accordingly, in the absence of any external source (or loss) of energy, as blood traverses the vascular system, losses observed in one form of energy must be accompanied by a gain in a different form of energy.

2. The percent volume change of water during the physiological pressure range of 0-150 mm Hg is approximately 0.001%.

Table 4-3
Conversion of Standard Units of Pressure

1 Pa	=	1 N/m^2	=	10 dynes/cm^2
1 cm H_2O	=	980 dynes/cm^2		
1 mm Hg	=	1333 dynes/cm^2		
1 atmosphere	=	760 mm Hg	=	1033 cm H_2O

VESSEL WALL MECHANICS

The density of energy contained within the blood is well recognized to the practicing physician as pressure, and the energy contained therein has the ability to do work. The heart imparts discrete quanta of energy to the vascular system through rhythmic contraction and relaxation, thereby creating regional pressure gradients. The vascular system comprises a complex network of vessels with unique properties that allow the vessel to insulate, conduct, resist, and store energy as it traverses the vascular system.

Blood vessels function as viscoelastic tubes and respond to a transmural pressure gradient as a function of the composition of the blood vessel wall. As the vessel wall is subjected to a transmural pressure gradient, a portion of the intraluminal energy is used to stretch the fibers within the wall, thereby converting pressure energy to that of stored energy in a manner similar to the work performed when exerting a force upon a spring. The energy stored within the blood vessel fibers is later released back into the system upon closure of the aortic valve. As intraluminal pressure oscillates, the constant loading and unloading

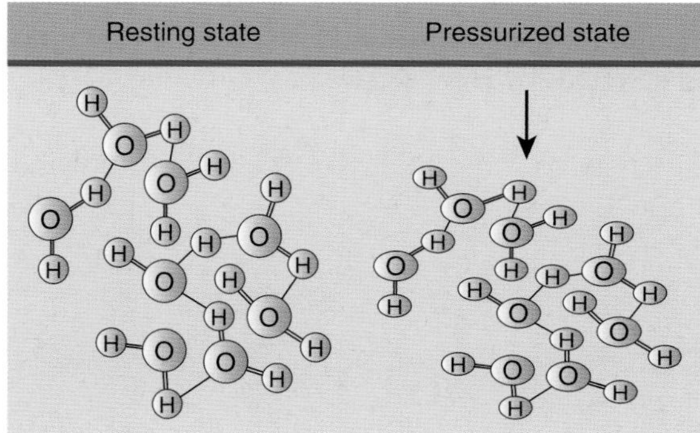

Figure 4-2. A liquid can be thought to be a network of molecules arranged in a three-dimensional lattice that, when placed under an external pressure, stores energy through strain of molecular bonds comprising the lattice. Water is a poorly compressible fluid in that only small changes in volume occur when exposed to an external pressure. Nonetheless, the strain created between the hydrogen bonds stores large amounts of energy, much like a stiff spring is able to store significant amounts of energy with little displacement. The stored energy may be released when no longer confined, much like a spring is able to release its energy upon an external object. The sum total energy created from the strain on the individual molecules divided by the volume is equivalent to the energy density or pressure in the sac.

Figure 4-3. Energy is introduced into the arterial system via the left ventricular stroke volume. After its introduction, energy may be converted from one form to another. In general, when energy is converted to thermal energy through frictional interactions, it is not recoverable; the system gradually loses energy as heat dissipates.

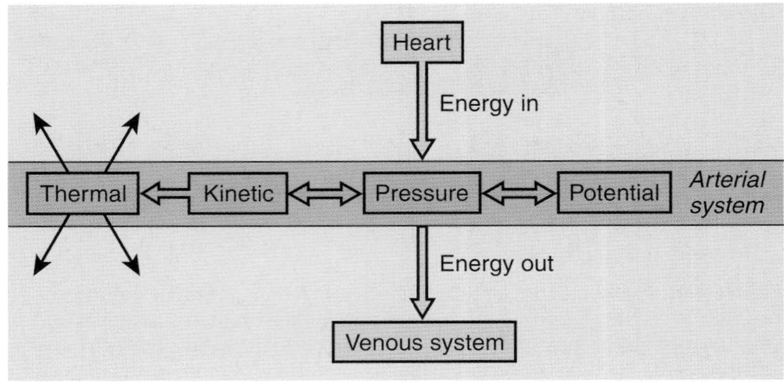

of the fibers in the vessel wall result in a change in diameter of the blood vessel, which is noted clinically as a palpable pulse.

The resultant change in blood vessel diameter is a function of the blood vessel elastic modulus and is determined by the relative quantities of collagen and elastin within the vascular wall. Over the range of physiological pressures, individual elastin fibers may be stretched by 50% to 70% of their resting length, while collagen fibers stretch only by 2% to 4% of their resting length. When the transmural pressures are sufficiently low (less than 25 mm Hg), the vessel remains passively collapsed and distensible. At intermediate transmural pressures, the elastic lamellae of the media begin to straighten and confer their individual elastic modulus to the vessel wall. At pressures greater than 100 mm Hg, the arteries become increasingly stiff as the elastic lamellae approach their fully distended state and recruitment of the relatively nondistensible collagen fibers occurs.

Both elastin and collagen fibers demonstrate the property of elasticity—that is, fibers stretch under an external stress and return to their original shape when the stress is removed. A spring is an example of an elastic object—when the spring is stretched, it exerts a restoring force that tends to bring it back to its original length. This restoring force is generally proportional to the amount of stretch. The relationship between applied force and change in fiber length is a function of the physical property of the material. In mechanics, this relationship is described by Hooke's law:

$$F_{\text{spring}} = (-k)x$$

where:
F_{spring} = Force applied to the spring
x = Distance that the spring moves
k = Coefficient defined by the "stiffness" of the spring

In the simplest terms, the relationship between applied force and distance is linear. That is, if a spring requires a force to move a particular distance, then the application of two times the force would be expected to move the spring two times the distance (Figure 4-4).

The amount of deformation is the strain (Δ diameter/diameter), and elastic modulus is the mathematical description of the tendency to be deformed elastically (i.e., nonpermanently) when a force is applied to it. The elastic modulus of an object is defined as the slope of its stress–strain curve in the elastic deformation region (Figure 4-5). Both collagen and elastin demonstrate linear stress–strain relationships; however, the amalgam of collagen and elastin contained in the blood vessel wall produces a nonlinear elastic modulus. The slope of the stress–strain curve therefore changes with the transmural pressure gradient.

When the architecture of the blood vessel is evaluated with regard to anatomical location, a relative change in the number of elastic lamellae and collagen fibers is noted. These structural changes confer a unique elastic modulus based upon the relative concentrations of elastin and collagen. The relatively high concentration of elastin within central vessels (like the thoracic and abdominal aorta) confers considerable distensibility at low transmural pressure gradients. Conversely, more peripheral arteries containing proportionally less elastin (relative

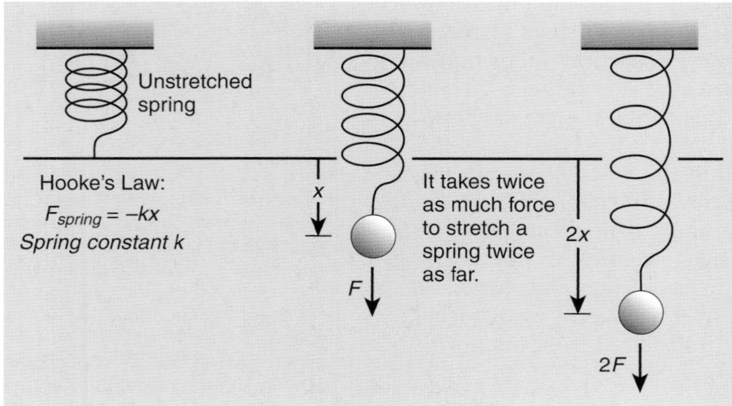

Figure 4-4. The linear dependence of displacement upon stretching force is called Hooke's law.

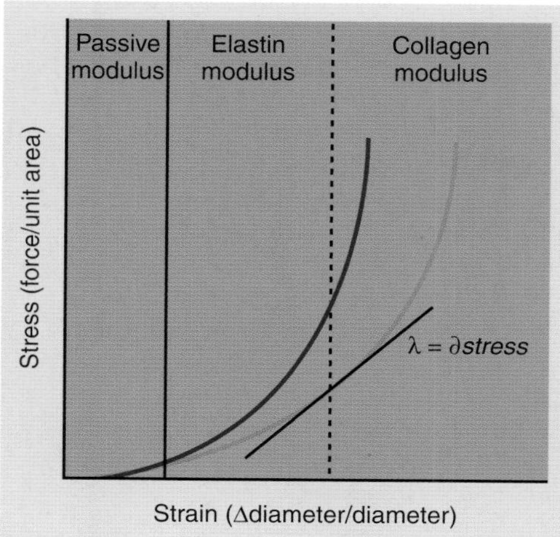

Figure 4-5. The relationship between stress and strain for a blood vessel is nonlinear, as the bimodal composition of the blood vessel (elastin and collagen) displays a unique modulus at different transmural pressures. The resultant elastic modulus for a blood vessel wall is therefore nonlinear.

to collagen) become increasingly stiff at similar transmural gradients (Figure 4-6).

The elastic modulus of the more central vessels provides the unique ability to store energy during the systolic phase of the cardiac cycle as the elastic fibers are "loaded." This energy may later be released to the vascular system during the diastolic phase when the aortic valve closes and no further energy is being supplied to the vascular system. In contrast, peripheral vessels contain little elastin and therefore store little energy. As such, most energy supplied to the peripheral arteries is expressed as pure pressure energy; this energy increases the amplitude of the systolic waveform as it proceeds peripherally—a phenomenon known as systolic amplification (Figure 4-7A). This observation provides the rationale for the resting ankle–brachial index to be greater than 1.0 in normal individuals.

The transiently higher pressure in the more peripheral arteries is responsible for the reversal of blood flow (in a more central direction) during early diastole. Retrograde flow quickly yields to antegrade flow as the stored energy in the more central blood vessels is released back to the system. Thus, the mechanical properties of the blood vessels help explain the triphasic waveform observed on Doppler evaluation (Figure 4-7B).

As a patient ages, vessels become more rigid due to progressive loss in elastin and gradual dilation, which causes the collagen fibers to become load bearing at progressively smaller pressures. Hence, a significant tendency exists for people to gravitate toward hypertension as they age. Conversely, given the relatively rich concentration of elastin in the blood vessels of children, the presence of hypertension at a young age should prompt further investigation.

Tensile strength of a material is the maximum amount of stress that the material can be subjected to before failure (Figure 4-8). *Yield strength* represents the stress at which material strain changes from elastic deformation to plastic

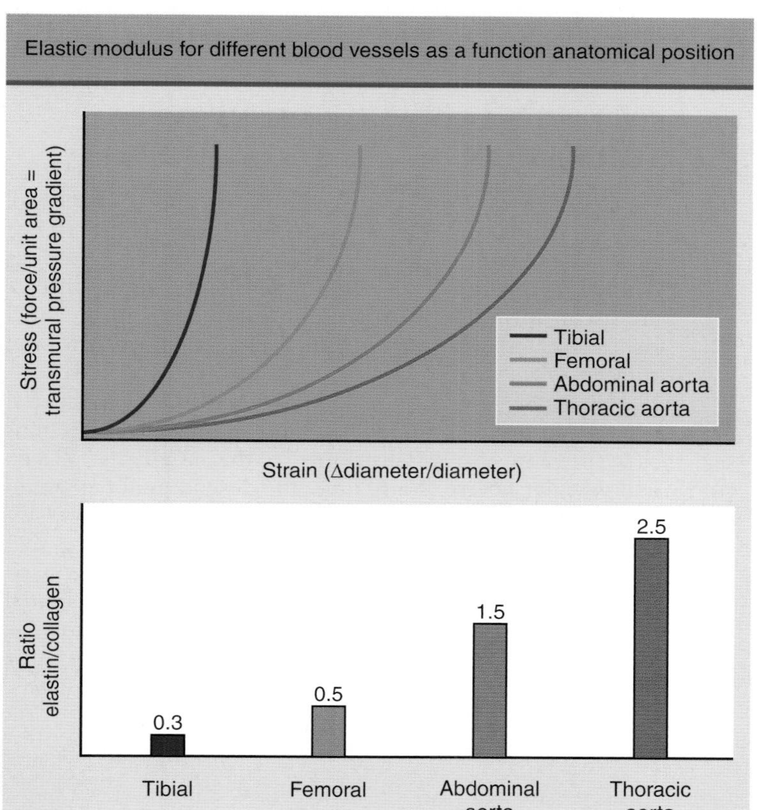

Figure 4-6. Elastic modulus for different blood vessels as a function anatomical position.

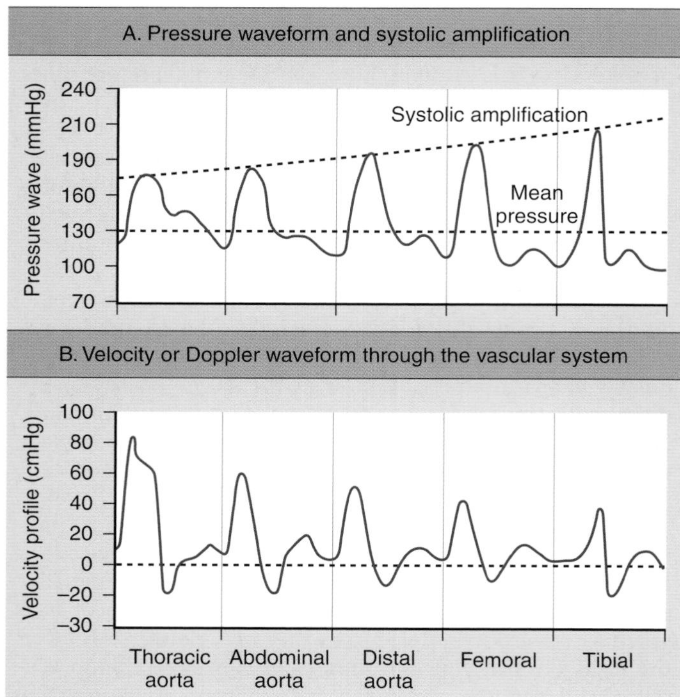

Figure 4-7. **A,** Pressure waveform and systolic amplification. **B,** Velocity or Doppler waveform through the vascular system.

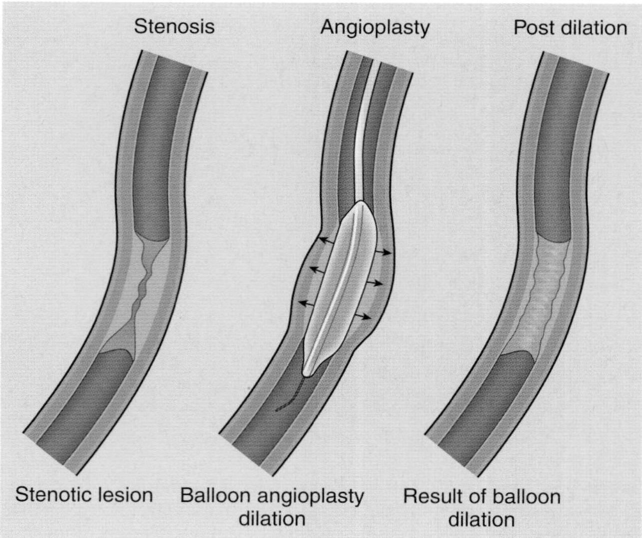

Figure 4-9. The property of blood vessel plasticity is observed during balloon angioplasty. Below a certain stress known as the elastic limit, or the yield strength, the blood vessel demonstrates elastic recoil. As transmural pressure exceeds the elastic limit, the vessel demonstrates irreversible deformation. Elastic limit is a function of the lesion. Typically calcified lesions have low elastic limits as the brittle calcifications yield to moderate angioplasty pressures. Collagen-rich areas of myointimal hyperplasia have high elastic limits and require large transmural pressures to overcome the elastic limit.

deformation, causing it to deform permanently. *Breaking strength* is the stress coordinate on the stress–strain curve at the point of rupture.

In contrast to elasticity, plasticity occurs when stress exceeds the object's elastic limit, resulting in irreversible deformation of the object. Although blood vessels do not exhibit plasticity at physiological transmural pressure gradients, the application of high intramural pressure during a percutaneous balloon angioplasty procedure is one physiological example of plasticity (Figure 4-9). If intraluminal pressure remains below the yield strength of the vessel, elastic recoil of the lesion is observed. As pressure exceeds yield strength, permanent changes in the blood vessel are observed. If pressure exceeds tensile strength for the material, rupture occurs.

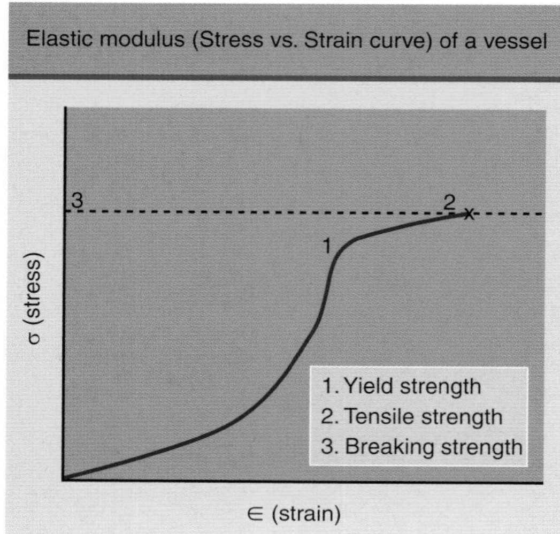

Figure 4-8. Elastic modulus (stress versus strain curve) of a vessel: 1. yield strength; 2. tensile strength; 3. breaking strength.

LAPLACE'S LAW AND ANEURYSM FORMATION

Laplace's law describes the changes in the blood vessel wall tension, radius, and thickness associated with the transfer of intramural energy to that stored in the blood vessel wall as defined by the blood vessel elastic modulus. These concepts are useful in understanding the development and potential risk associated with aneurysmal deformation, growth, and rupture.

When a blood vessel is exposed to a transmural gradient, it distends in both circumferential and longitudinal directions as the pressure energy is distributed to the underlying collagen and vascular fibers. At any time, the distending force within a blood vessel is at equilibrium with the retractile forces of the vessel wall. Physiologically, the longitudinal changes that occur in native cylindrical vessels are negligible in comparison to change in the radial direction. The circumferential distending force within the tube is simply the product of the transmural pressure gradient and the area over which the force is exerted:

$$F_{\text{distending}} = \text{Pt} \times A$$

or

$$F_{\text{distending}} = \text{P}_{\text{t}} \times (\text{D}_{\text{i}} \times L)$$

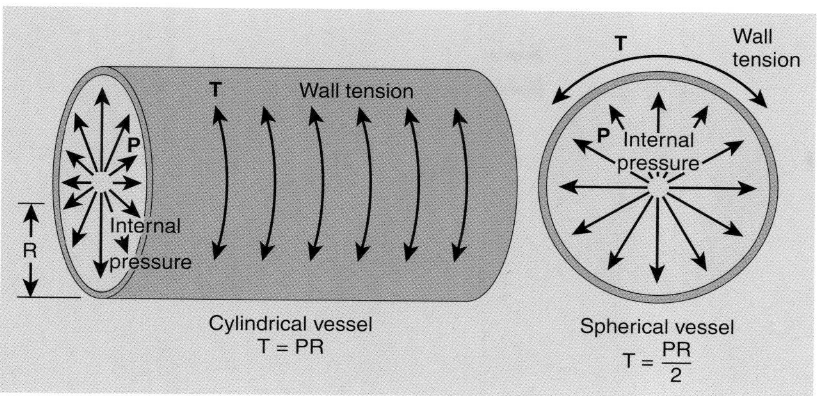

Figure 4-10. For a given vessel radius and internal pressure, a spherical vessel has half the wall tension of a cylindrical vessel.

where:
$F_{\text{distending}}$ = Distending force
P_t = Transmural pressure gradient
A = Area
D_i = Internal diameter
L = Length of the tube

Given the cylindrical morphology of a blood vessel, the two walls exert an opposing retractile force in the circumferential direction:

$$F_{\text{retractile}} = \partial \times 2 \times (h \times L)$$

where:
$F_{\text{retractile}}$ = Opposing retractile force
∂= Circumferential wall stress
h = Thickness of the vessel
L = Length of the vessel

In the steady state, the distending force and the retractile forces are equal and you can set the two equations equal and solve for wall stress:

$$\partial = (P_t \times D_i)/2h$$

or

$$\partial = (P_t \times r_i)/h$$

where r_i is the internal radius.

This calculation yields the force per unit area for the vessel wall at rest. For a vessel of infinitely thinness, the equation becomes the familiar Laplace's law:

$$T = P_t \times r$$

where T is the wall tension and r is the radius.

Wall tension is the driving force behind conformational changes in aneurysm morphology. When wall tension exceeds blood vessel tensile strength, rupture occurs. These factors directly affect the behavior of aneurysms, as degradation of collagen and elastin fibers leads to gradual dilation. The change in geometrical configuration associated with aneurysm formation (in which a cylindrical vessel becomes spherical) distributes wall tension in a longitudinal direction, as well as a radial direction, and reduces the risk of rupture (Figure 4-10).

More sophisticated measures of wall tension can be performed by considering the geometry of an aneurysm sac, as significant differences in effective radius generate differences in wall tension for different parts of the aneurysm. The variation is described by Laplace's law: the larger the radius, the larger the wall tension required to withstand a given internal fluid pressure (Figure 4-11). The inflection point represents the area of infinite radius and is the area most prone to mechanical failure. Sophisticated modeling of specific aneurysm geometry using finite element analysis can help predict risk of rupture.

Concepts of Endotension

The advent of endovascular aneurysm repair has heightened interest in the interaction between endotension and the aneurysm sac. This interaction is described by Pascal's principle, which states that a change in the pressure of an enclosed incompressible fluid is conveyed undiminished to every part of the fluid and to the surfaces of its container. In this manner, a small source of energy (pressure) generates systemic pressure in a larger space, assuming the enclosed space is of

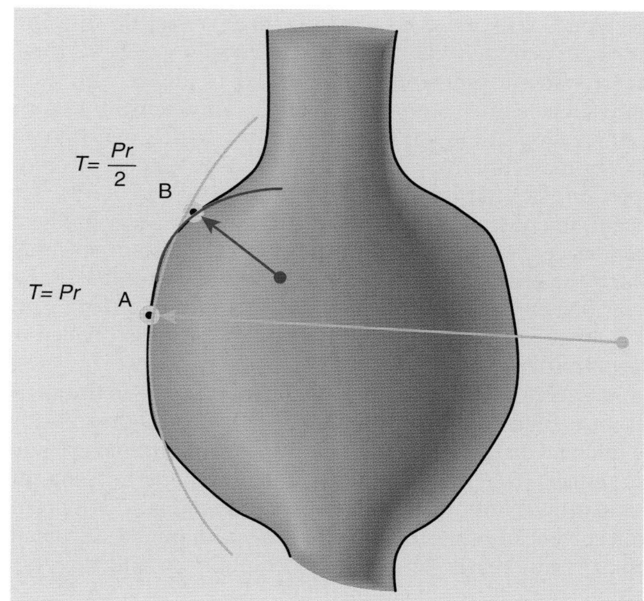

Figure 4-11. Laplace's law states that the larger the vessel radius, the larger the wall tension required to withstand a given internal fluid pressure. As such, the wall tension is a function of the effective radius. The area where the effective radius is large *(point A)* experiences maximum wall tension, while the area of effective radius that is much smaller *(point B)* experiences smaller wall tension. In addition, the spherical shape of the aneurysm at point B allows the wall tension to be distributed in both longitudinal and radial directions.

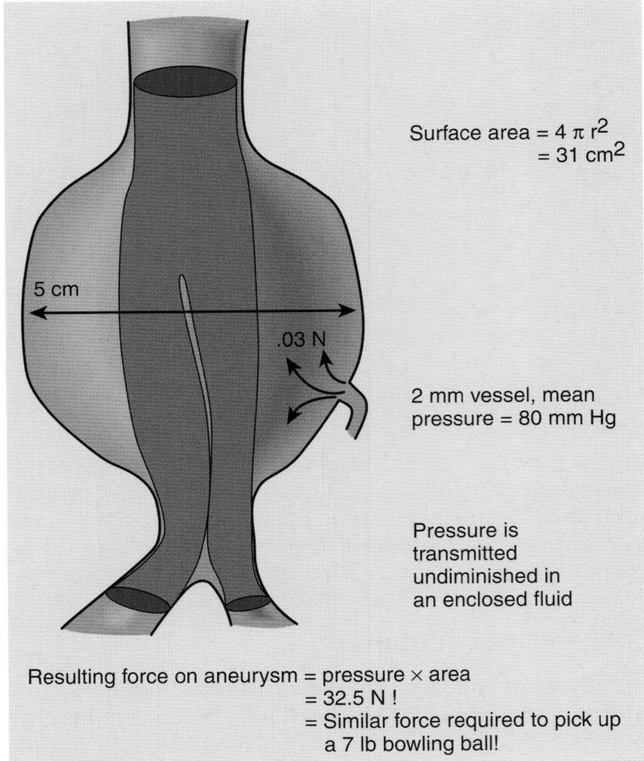

Figure 4-12. According to Pascal's principle, an isolated Type 2 endoleak can exert significant forces on the aneurysm sac.

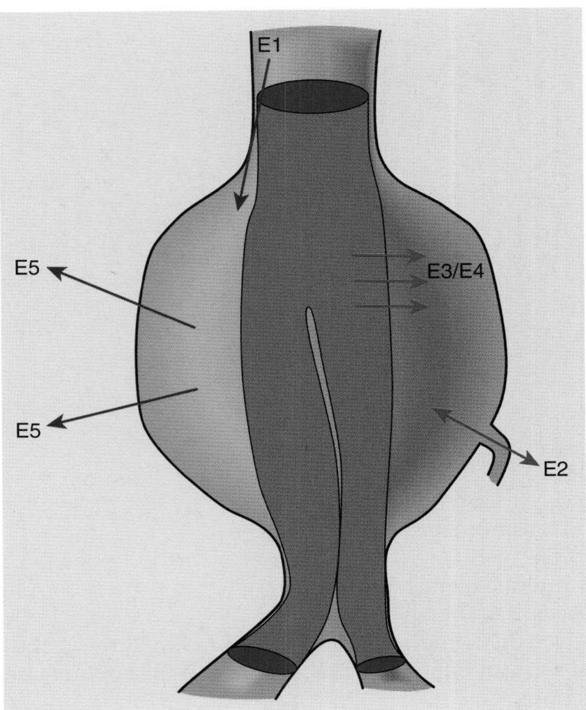

Figure 4-13. Endotension and energy flux into and out of an excluded aneurysm sac. Energy fluxes across a membrane according to the energy gradient that exists across the membrane, the surface area of the membrane, and the permittivity of the membrane. E1, E3, and E4 are energy offered by a type I, type III, and type IV endoleak, respectively; E2 is energy offered by (or removed from) a type II endoleak; and E5 is the pressure that dissipates across the aortic wall. At equilibrium, the sum total of energy in the aneurysm sac divided by the volume is equal to the energy density, which is equivalent to the pressure or endotension.

static volume. Pascal's principle makes it possible for a large multiplication of force (as occurs with a hydraulic press) and explains why even a type II endoleak can be problematic. If the type II leak exists as a small, single vessel flowing into the aneurysm sac (with no associated outflow vessel), it may confer systemic pressure, undiminished, to the sac with resultant wall tension of a nontreated aneurysm (Figure 4-12).

In reality, an aneurysm sac is not a static environment. Energy may flux into, or out of, the aneurysm sac by multiple sources after endoluminal exclusion (Figure 4-13). The magnitude of energy flux is a function of the energy gradient, the surface area, and the permittivity of the substance through which the energy must pass. The condition is similar to that described by Gauss's law, which states that the electric flux out of a closed surface is equal to the charge enclosed divided by the permittivity.

As energies reach equilibrium, the total energy in the aneurysm sac divided by the volume of the sac could theoretically be calculated and used to determine the intraluminal pressure of the sac. Given the dynamics of the system, performing this calculation is not practical. However, it remains an important concept because it explains why all endoluminal aneurysm repairs must reach some state of equilibrium and therefore exhibit some degree of endotension.

Occasionally, a patient's aneurysm sac increases in size without a demonstrable endoleak. Permeability of graft material—even if microscopic—has been implicated. Because the endograft is deployed in a blood-filled sac, tissue ingrowth has little opportunity to occur. As such, endovascular grafts have a tendency to permit the transmission of serum and energy through micropores that exist in the membrane. According to Pascal's principle, when this condition exists in *the absence* of an associated type II leak, the conditions of a static environment are satisfied and the dangerous scenario of systemic pressure may arise—so-called endotension. I have observed seroma formation within the aneurysm sac that displayed systemic pressure waveforms (Figure 4-14). While these cases have typically been treated by relining the older graft material with a new device (resolving the permeability issue), I have treated one individual by percutaneously accessing and rupturing the sac with a 4-mm angioplasty balloon—a so-called sac fenestration procedure—to allow the energy to dissipate into the retroperitoneal space rather than allow it to accumulate in the sac, where it may act upon the aneurysm wall. Subsequent computed tomography imaging has demonstrated aneurysm sac shrinkage at 6 and 12 months. In this manner, the presence of a type II leak may actually be beneficial if it functions to disperse the accumulation of energy in the aneurysm sac. Likewise, aneurysm sacs that have ruptured and required treatment in the emergent setting may demonstrate increased rates of sac shrinkage after successful endoluminal exclusion.

It has been suggested that an aneurysm sac may contain regional pressure gradients. In a static environment, Pascal's principle would imply this not to be the case. However, given the dynamics of the vascular system, significant energy gradients may exist within the sac. Consider the regional energy released across a type III endoleak (graft defect): as

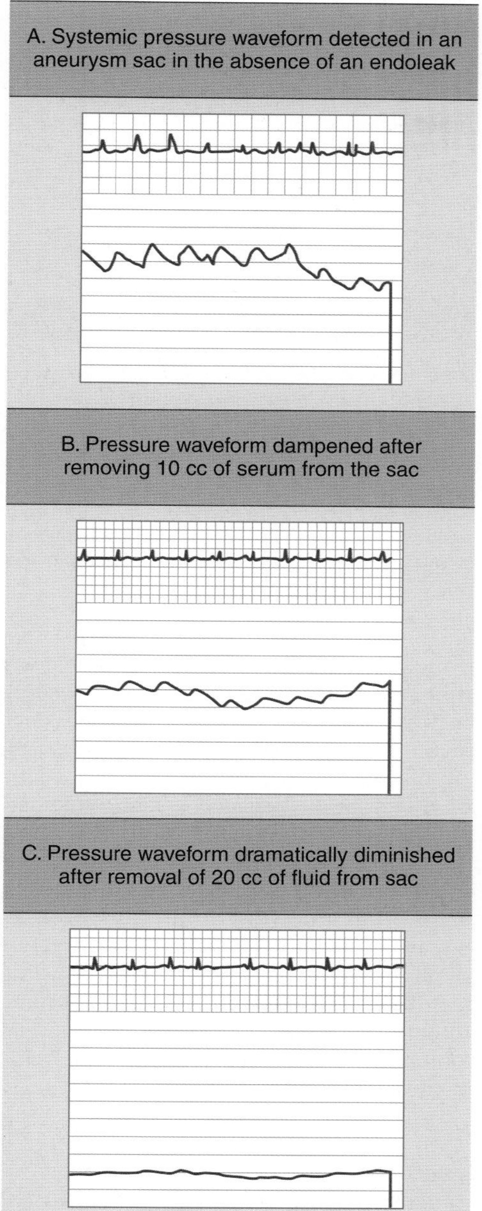

Figure 4-14. A, Systemic pressure waveform detected in an aneurysm sac in the absence of an endoleak. **B,** Pressure waveform dampened after removing 10 cc of serum from the sac. **C,** Pressure waveform dramatically diminished after removal of 20 cc of fluid from sac.

energy dissipates from areas of high energy density to areas of lower energy, significant energy density gradients are likely. In the dynamics of a changing aneurysm sac, wherein multiple sources of energy flux occur both into and out of the aneurysm sac, significant energy density and pressure gradients may permit regional areas of high pressure to develop within the aneurysm sac.

The potential impact of laminated thrombus within an aneurysm sac has long been a controversial subject. From a physical viewpoint, thrombus offers little protective effect; it functions as a poorly organized semisolid that offers negligible tensile strength to oppose the intramural pressure and readily permits undiminished pressure to be exerted upon the aneurysm wall. However, in a nonstatic environment, intramural thrombus may indeed affect the manner in which the energy is transferred within the aneurysm sac and may influence regional energy density gradients.

Finally, although it has been suggested that aneurysm sac growth may be *independent* of intraluminal pressure, I am not inclined to agree. Barring any change in the composition and mechanical properties of the aneurysm sac, a well-defined stress–strain curve exists for the blood vessel. Failure to acknowledge the fundamental relationship between intramural pressure and aneurysm sac diameter is a rejection of the basic relationship of pressure and radius as established by Laplace.

Role of Peripheral Vascular Resistance

Collectively, the arterioles provide most peripheral vascular resistance. In the absence of significant atherosclerotic disease, little energy is lost to friction. Energy dissipates as the arterioles permit it to escape into the large venous reservoir; therefore, the large capacitance of the venous system is where most energy is lost.

In the venous system, blood is no longer confined to its smaller (arterial) volume. The strained molecules return to their resting state and expand back to their resting volume and density. In the process, the blood accelerates and gains kinetic energy. Because velocity is created without vector, turbulence occurs as the heterogeneous velocities are channeled into a single outflow vein. In the process, pressure energy is converted to kinetic energy, which is eventually converted to thermal energy through frictional losses.

Recalling the concept of pressure as a form of energy density, the arterioles regulate the amount of energy that dissipates into the large capacitance venous system, much like a faucet. Assuming no significant change in effective volume within the arterial system, blood pressure increases when energy is introduced at a rate that exceeds dissipation to venous system. Small vessels can constrict flow to one part of the body while enhancing the flow to another to meet changing demands for oxygen and nutrients. Small changes in arteriole diameter can create large changes in volume flow rate. Maintenance of proper blood pressure and perfusion patterns within the systemic circulation is tightly regulated by multiple feedback mechanisms.

Failure of peripheral vascular resistance occurs during sepsis when loss of arteriolar tone permits large amounts of energy to dissipate into the venous system. In this condition, the heart attempts to maintain energy density balance by increasing cardiac output through both increased force of contraction and increased rate of contraction.

Likewise, the creation of an arteriovenous fistula creates similar perturbations within the vascular system. In general, blood flow through a fistula remains a function of the diameter of the inflow artery, rather than a function of the diameter of the outflow vein (Figure 4-15). Placing the large capacitance of the venous system in juxtaposition to the artery often exceeds the capacity of the inflow artery to provide sufficient energy to satisfy both the fistula and the peripheral vascular beds. The ischemic steal syndrome occurs when peripheral perfusion is insufficient to satisfy the metabolic requirements of the distal extremity.

Were it not for the concomitant development of a robust collateral network, the ischemic steal syndrome would occur more often. Failure to generate sufficient collateral circulation

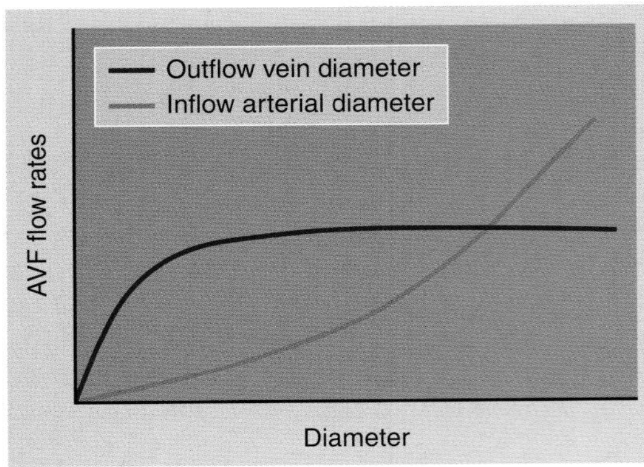

Figure 4-15. Plot with fistula flow and diameter of inflow artery and outflow vein. For high flow arteriovenous fistula in the absence of venous obstruction, flow remains a function of arterial diameter.

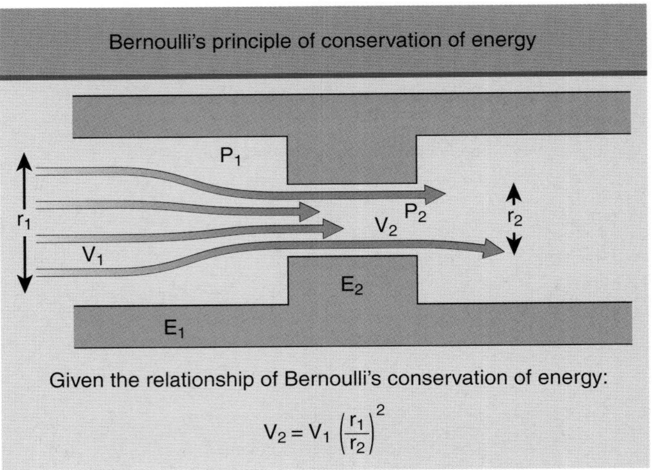

Figure 4-16. Bernoulli's principle of conservation of energy. Due to the increased velocity and increase in kinetic energy within an area of stenosis, Bernoulli's law dictates that the pressure within the area of stenosis must decrease relative to that in the area of larger diameter.

leads to distal limb ischemia as the fistula continues to mature. The concept of pressure as a form of energy density is fundamental to understanding the mechanisms by which the ischemic steal syndrome occurs.

The presence of a pressure sink at the level of the arteriovenous anastomosis remains poorly understood. In the simplest terms, the loss of pressure energy at the level of an arteriovenous anastomosis is similar to that which occurs in a hydroelectric plant. As water is dammed, it accumulates significant hydrostatic energy *(ρgh)* that may be released in the form of kinetic energy, which is used to turn a turbine and generate electrical energy.

Similarly, as pressure energy leaks from the arterial system into the high-capacity venous system, pressure energy is converted to kinetic energy. The blood accelerates randomly, and large amounts of the kinetic energy succumb to frictional losses. As velocity increases, the conditions satisfy the Reynolds criteria and kinetic energy continues to be lost to friction.

The ischemic steal syndrome occurs when the fistula permits energy to dissipate into the venous system such that inadequate energy is available to sustain positive blood flow to the more distal vascular beds of the extremity.

During reconstructive distal revascularization, interval ligation, and proximalization operations, the high-capacitance venous system is separated from the arterial circulation by an intervening segment that offers both low resistance and low capacity.[8] This segment separates the location of the pressure sink from the arterial system, thereby improving the perfusion pressure available to serve the distal vascular beds of the extremity. Therefore, patients who undergo placement of an arteriovenous graft develop the ischemic steal syndrome less often.

FLUID DYNAMICS

Hemodynamics defines blood in motion. In the most basic terms, blood flow between two points in the vascular system occurs as a result of an energy gradient between the two points. With each contraction, the heart serves as the source of energy, delivering a sinusoidal pattern of energy from the left ventricle to the peripheral vascular system. The energy delivered to the vascular system may exist in multiple forms, including pressure, thermal, kinetic, and potential energy. In different portions of the vascular system, energy forms may be transformed from one to another. The only energy that is "lost" within the vascular system is frictional energy. Due to the efficiency of the vascular system, little of this energy is lost as flow remains laminar under most physiological conditions.

The law of conservation of energy states that the total amount of energy in any isolated system remains constant, although it may change forms (e.g., friction turns kinetic energy into thermal energy). Bernoulli's principle states that, for an inviscid flow, an increase in the speed of the fluid occurs simultaneously with a decrease in pressure or a decrease in the fluid's gravitational potential energy (Figure 4-16). Thus, the sum of all forms of mechanical energy in a fluid along a streamline is the same at all points on that streamline.

According to Bernoulli's principle of conservation of energy, as blood enters the area of stenosis the velocity must increase by the square of the radius:

$$\Delta v = (1/\Delta r)^2$$

where v is the velocity and r is the radius.

In this manner, even small changes in radius generate significant changes in velocity. Assuming no frictional losses, Bernoulli's law implies that the hydrostatic pressure in the region of the stenosis must be smaller than the pressure in the more proximal portion of the vessel. Bernoulli's principle provides the explanation for the measure of negative pressure within the anastomosis of an arteriovenous fistula.

Bernoulli's principle is most relevant to vascular physiology as it relates to the progression of aortic dissection. When a discrete entry point generates a false passage within the media of the blood vessel wall, a blind cul-de-sac develops. When this fails to enter the true lumen, a pressure gradient is created that causes the false lumen to increase in size while compromising the true lumen (Figure 4-17).

Energy Losses Due to Friction

As blood traverses the vascular system, frictional energy losses convert small portions of the total energy into heat. Therefore, as blood travels along the circulatory pathway, the sum

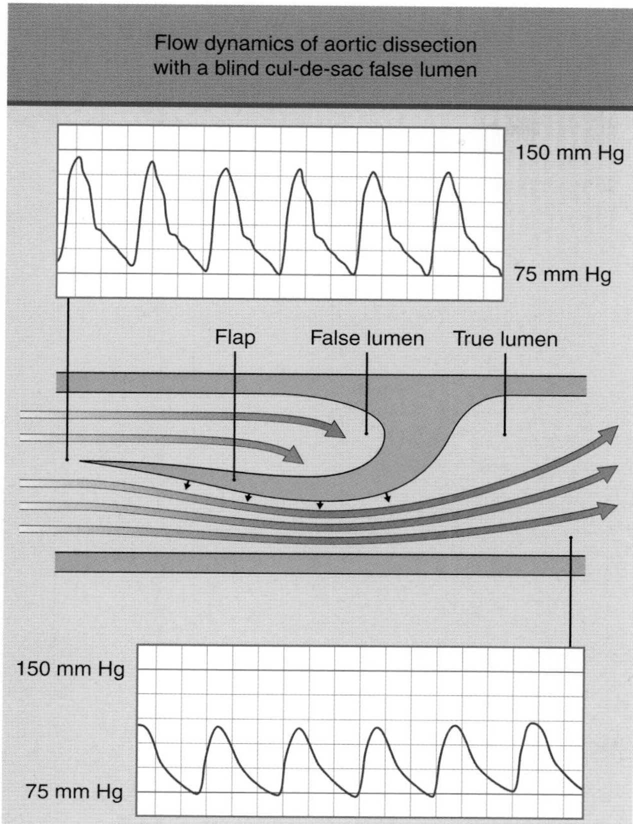

Figure 4-17. Flow dynamics of an aortic dissection with a blind cul-de-sac false lumen. The increased flow velocity through the true lumen generates significant kinetic energy that does not exist within the false lumen. Bernoulli's law dictates that the loss of kinetic energy in the false lumen must create a higher pressure to preserve total energy. The resultant pressure gradient that develops between the true lumen and the false lumen further "draws" the dissection flap into the true lumen, thereby reducing the distal perfusion. From a physiological standpoint, the true lumen is generally the smaller of the two lumens and possesses a lower pressure.

total of energy continuously diminishes. One aspect of frictional energy losses occurs due to interaction of moving particles along the stationary vessel wall secondary to attraction of adhesion molecules expressed on the endothelial surface. The particles that are immediately adjacent to the vessel wall experience the greatest degree of attraction and travel at infinitely low velocities.

Frictional energy also occurs due to particle–particle interactions. Under normal blood flow conditions, blood flows so that concentric laminae of blood move with a particular velocity profile (Figure 4-18).The more central laminae are furthest from the covalent interactions with the blood vessel wall and therefore have the weakest attraction and travel with the highest velocity.

A gradient of velocity occurs as liquid moves away from the vessel wall, and the liquid tends to move in layers with successively higher speed. This is called laminar flow. A liquid's resistance to flow can be characterized in terms of the viscosity. Viscous resistance to flow can be modeled for laminar flow, but if the laminae break up into turbulence, it is difficult to characterize the fluid flow. A common example of laminar flow is the smooth flow of a viscous liquid through a tube. The velocity of flow varies from zero at the wall to a maximum along the centerline of the vessel. The profile of laminar flow through a tube can be calculated by dividing the flow into thin cylindrical elements to create a parabolic velocity profile.

Poiseuille's Law

In large vessels frictional energy losses are negligible, but in smaller vessels energy losses are large. Additional factors such as length of the tube, viscosity of the blood (largely a function of the hemoglobin concentration), or velocity of the blood (as in the case of an arteriovenous fistula) must be considered.

While frictional energy losses within large blood vessels are negligible, the smaller-diameter blood vessels in the microcirculation create frictional energy losses that are important; most intraluminal energy (pressure) is dissipated at the level of the arteriole. Jean Léonard Marie Poiseuille first noted this phenomenon in the late 1840s. From his observations, he correctly predicted that the pressure gradient occurring across a vessel varies directly with the flow of blood, the viscosity of the blood, and the length of the tube and varies inversely with the radius of the vessel. He also noted that the relationship with the radius was nonlinear.

Mathematically, this was not solved until 1860, when Eduard Haganbach correctly expressed the relationship of a pressure gradient to blood flow, fluid viscosity, length of the conduit, and radius of the conduit:

$$\Delta P = 8\, QL\mu / \pi r^4$$

where:
ΔP = Pressure gradient
Q = Flow
L = Length
μ = Viscosity
r = Radius
Stated otherwise:

$$\Delta P = QR$$

where R is the resistance equal to $8\, L\mu/\pi r^4$.

It should be noted that the Poiseuille-Haganbach equation holds true for an ideal fluid traveling at constant laminar flow in a rigid tube of uniform bore. While blood does indeed function as an ideal fluid in vessels of diameter greater than 100 μm, predicting energy losses during conditions of dynamic flow and within vessels of changing diameter and direction requires the application of differential equations and computational analysis.

From a clinical standpoint, the importance of defining a critical stenosis—that is, a lesion that produces a reduction of perfusion pressure beyond the stenosis—is evident. A lesion of the abdominal aorta does not become hemodynamically significant until 90% cross-sectional luminal narrowing exists. For smaller arteries, such as the iliac, renal, or carotid, hemodynamic changes occur at smaller cross-sectional luminal narrowing (70% to 90%). Of particular importance is differentiation between cross-sectional luminal narrowing and percent diameter narrowing. In general, a 50% reduction in diameter narrowing produces a 75% cross-sectional narrowing and a 66% diameter reduction produces a 90%

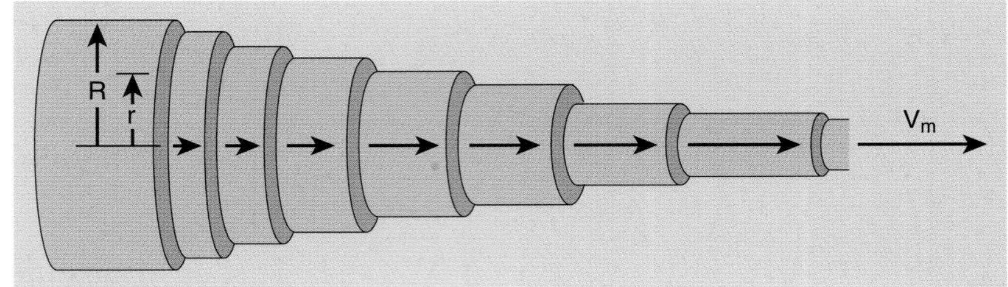

Figure 4-18. Underconditions of laminar flow in a viscous fluid, the velocity increases toward the center of a tube.

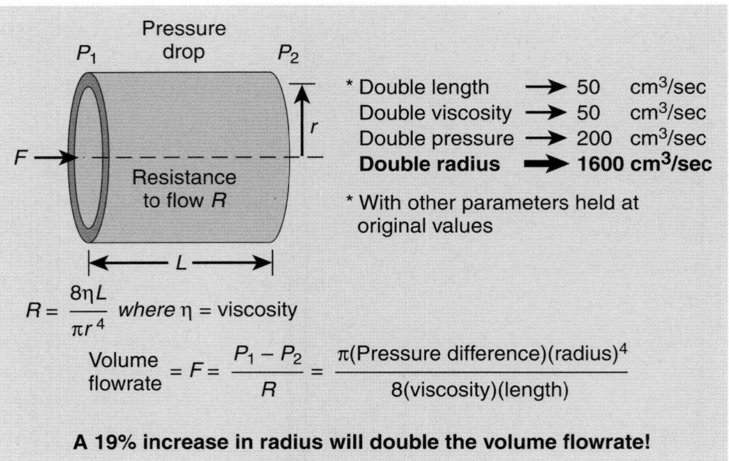

Figure 4-19. Parameters that affect flow.

cross-sectional luminal narrowing. Traditional parameters of hemodynamic significance have generally been set at a diameter reduction greater than 60%.

While traditional standards that use the percentage of diameter narrowing are sufficient in most circumstances, several conditions exist for which traditional parameters of hemodynamic significance do not apply (Figure 4-19). These include conditions in which velocity profiles in the locations of the stenosis are elevated, such as iliac artery stenosis proximal to a fem–fem bypass or subclavian artery stenosis proximal to a patent arteriovenous fistula (Figure 4-20). In these situations, traditional parameters of hemodynamic significance may not be applicable to lesions of less than 50% diameter reduction and actual measurements of the pressure gradient across the lesion should be considered. In contrast, the individual with vasculogenic claudication who demonstrates normal ankle–brachial index pressures at rest offers an example of failure to identify hemodynamic lesions in low-flow situations. The principle serves as a basis for the correct interpretation of postexercise ankle–brachial index testing and for intravascular pressure monitoring after hyperemic challenge.

Shear stress (ω) is a product of velocity and velocity gradient (Figure 4-21) and is defined as the cumulative tangential drag generated upon the blood vessel wall as blood flows over the endothelial surface. It may be calculated by the Poiseuille equation:

$$\omega = 4\eta Q / \pi r^3$$

where:
ω = Sheer stress
η = Blood viscosity
Q = Blood flow
r = Radius of the blood vessel

Thus, for a given rate of blood flow, shear stress changes with the diameter of the blood vessel. The effect of shear forces on the blood vessel wall was noted by Donald Fry, who demonstrated an increased permeability within endothelial cells that are subjected to varying shear stresses.[9] When pulsatile flow in an arterial segment is smooth and undisturbed, the development of myointimal hyperplasia and atherosclerosis is rare. However, varying blood vessel diameter, blood vessel tortuosity, and points of bifurcation produces changes in mural blood flow velocity that generate shear stress values, triggering

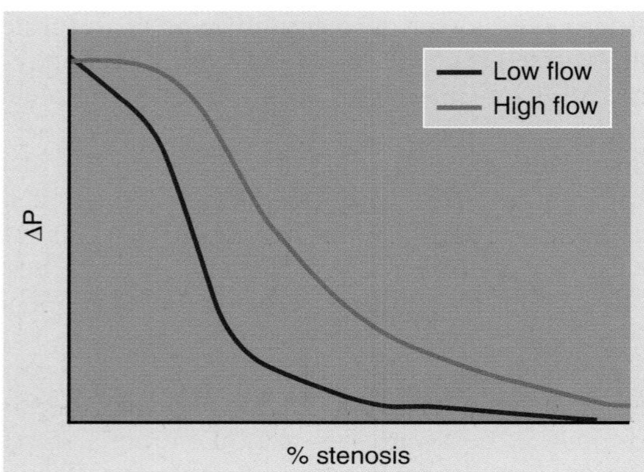

Figure 4-20. Hemodynamic significance of a stenosis depends on flow velocity of blood across the stenosis.

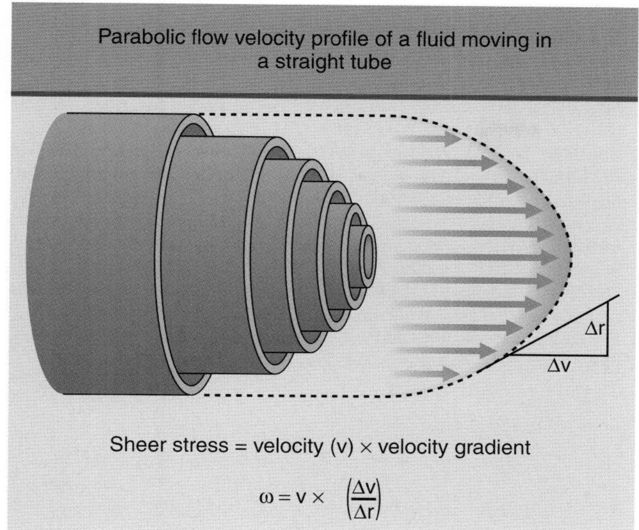

Figure 4-21. Parabolic velocity profile and shear stress.

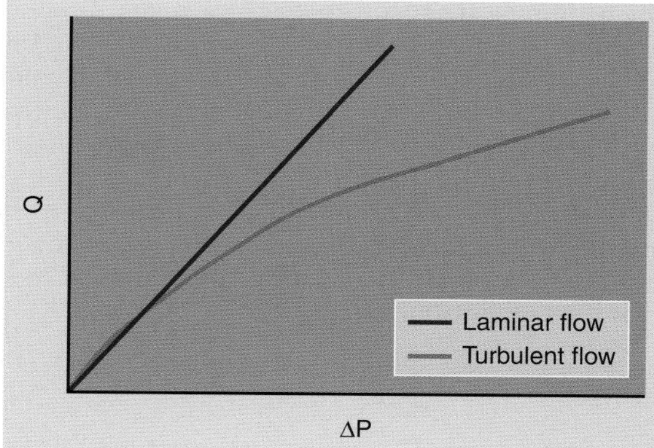

Figure 4-22. Turbulent flow generates more significant energy losses and, therefore, greater pressure gradients than would have been predicted by the Poiseuille equation.

the endothelial cell to release prostaglandins and stimulate the underlying smooth muscle cell.

While it was initially proposed that areas of high shear stress were injurious to the endothelium, it is now recognized that areas of low shear stress or areas of high shear stress predispose a patient to myointimal hyperplasia and atherosclerosis. These locations, which often exist in regions of flow separation, cause downstream vortex formation. This predisposes to a patient prolonged particle residence times, which exposes the luminal surface to circulating atherogenic agents for prolonged intervals.

This mechanism may predispose the infrarenal aorta to the development of atherosclerosis. Because a high percentage of blood delivered to the abdominal aorta is diverted to the visceral and renal circulations, blood flow through the infrarenal aorta is relatively low. When coupled with the anatomical bifurcation, this location is favored for the deposition of atherosclerotic particles. Another factor that may exacerbate this condition is sedentary lifestyle, because blood flow through the infrarenal segment largely depends on the muscular activity of the lower extremities. Finally, the slow degenerative process of loss of collagen and elastin fibers with aging causes the infrarenal segment to dilate, reducing velocity and increasing particle resonance time.

The development of an abdominal aortic aneurysm dramatically predisposes a patient to atherosclerosis, as the large-caliber aneurysm causes mural blood flow to slow considerably. Thus, although the etiology of aneurysm formation is often described as atherosclerotic, it is more plausible that the atherosclerosis develops as a secondary consequence of increased diameter and lower shear stress. Finally, shear stress appears to be an important factor in the maintenance of blood vessel luminal diameter. Endothelial cells remain sensitive to such changes and cause the blood vessel to either dilate or contract in an attempt to normalize shear stress. Accordingly, the artery proximal to a patent arteriovenous fistula dilates, while the artery proximal to an amputated or atrophic limb is significantly smaller in caliber when compared to the corresponding blood vessel of the contralateral limb. This also explains the development of a rich collateral network in response to an exercise program in the individual with lower extremity claudication.

Turbulent Blood Flow

The Reynolds number is an experimental number used in fluid flow to predict the critical flow velocity at which turbulence occurs. It is defined by the following relationship:

$$V_{\text{critical}} = R\eta / 2\rho r$$

where:

V_{critical} = Critical flow velocity
R = Critical Reynolds number at which turbulence occurs (≈2000)
η = Viscosity of the fluid
ρ = Density of the fluid
r = Radius of the vessel

Another approach is to define a variable Reynolds number in terms of the maximum velocity for laminar flow in a tube:

$$R = 2v\rho r / \eta$$

When the Reynolds number exceeds 2000, blood flow is said to be turbulent and the physical sign of a bruit or thrillt may be present. In general, the viscosity of blood is approximately 3.5 times that of water and the density of blood is similar to water—both of which remain constant. As such, the diameter of the blood vessel and the velocity with which the blood travels are the primary determinants of turbulence. From the standpoint of energy consumption, turbulent flow is important because the loss of energy occurring between two points exceeds that predicted by the Poiseuille equation (Figure 4-22).

Within the complexities of the circulatory system, additional factors predispose a patient to turbulent flow, and turbulent flow likely occurs at lower Reynolds number values. These factors include pulsatile flow, changes in vessel diameter, and directional changes in flow. Clinical conditions associated with turbulence include the aortic root after periods of exercise, the carotid bifurcation, and arteriovenous fistula anastomoses. In addition, blood flow may demonstrate turbulence during the systolic phase in which blood is accelerating.

The area distal to a stenosis is another location that is predisposed to turbulent flow. As blood traverses the stenosis, the velocity within the stenosis increases by a factor of the square of the change in radius. Beyond the stenosis, the velocity jet enters a blood vessel of normal diameter. The combination of increased velocity and large vessel diameter provides conditions that satisfy the Reynolds criteria and result in turbulence in the area beyond the stenosis. This is manifest clinically as a bruit or thrill. The vibrations and energy released from the enhanced particle–particle interaction increases the shear stress in the adjacent artery and stimulates the vessel to dilate in the process of poststenotic dilation.

References

1. Strandness DE, Sumner DS. *Hemodynamics for surgeons.* New York: Grune & Stratton; 1975.
2. McDonald DA. *Blood flow in arteries.* 2nd ed. Baltimore: Williams & Wilkins; 1974.
3. Nichols WW, O'Rourke MF. *McDonald's blood flow in arteries.* Philadelphia: Lua & Febiger; 1990.
4. Lee BY, Trainor FS. *Peripheral vascular surgery: hemodynamics of arterial pulsatile flow.* New York: Meredith; 1973.
5. Newton I. *The principia.* In: Cohen IB, Whitman A, eds. trans. Berkeley: University of California Press; 1999.
6. Bowditch, N, trans. *Mécanique céleste.* 4 vols. Boston: Little and Wilkins; 1829-1839. *Celestial mechanics.* 5 vols, including the original French. Boston: Reprint Services; 1966-1969.
7. Bernoulli D. *Hydrodynamica, sive de viribus et motibus fluidorum commentarii (Hydrodynamics, or commentaries on forces and motions of fluids).* Strasbourg: J.R. Dulsecker; 1738.
8. Wixon CL, Hughes JD, Mills JL. Understanding strategies for the treatment of vascular steal syndrome. *J Am Coll Surg* 2000;191(3):301-310.
9. Fry DL. Acute vascular endothelial changes associated with the increased blood velocity gradients. *Circ Res* 1967;22:165-197.

chapter

5

Evidence-Based Medicine: Basic Concepts, Population Dynamics, and Outcomes Analysis

John V. White, MD • Ginger Barthel, RN, MA, FACHE

Key Points

- Despite the use of rigorous methodologies, the value of trials may be limited if results are applied inappropriately.
- The case report, as a method for communicating outcomes, has limitations due to the lack of an established research protocol and the high likelihood of investigator bias.
- Case-control studies provide well-defined inclusion and exclusion criteria, as well as consecutive patients with matched criteria, yielding information that can be applied to the community.
- Randomized, prospective, blinded clinical trials provide the strongest link between cause and effect and to the presence or absence of differences produced by a treatment modality.
- Meta-analysis uses data from carefully selected, published studies to produce a rigorous, systematic, and quantitative review of available information.
- Markov analysis is a computer-based analytical tool used to determine whether one event in a sequence of events is related to another, such as treatment to outcome.
- Monte Carlo simulation is a computer tool that attempts to use probabilities for the occurrence of events to predict outcomes.
- Validated, generic quality-of-life survey instruments have value in assessing overall health status.
- Disease-specific questionnaires focus on a patient's underlying disease, its impact on general health, and the benefit and adverse effects of the treatment.
- Not all published data are equivalent, and it is essential for the surgeon to recognize the strength of the evidence presented in a report before incorporating that diagnostic or therapeutic modality in the realm of patient care.

match are based on the control variables of the disease. The match should use patient characteristics or descriptors that need to be controlled but are not the subject of the study.[10] Age, gender, ethnic background, and race are often used as matching criteria. For example, to study the impact of diabetes on lower extremity arterial occlusive disease in men, a group of age-matched men might be used as the control group. The target group and the controls may be selected from a hospital

spective study, many well-recognized limitations exist. The inclusion of only specialized sites of treatment may yield clear results on efficacy but not on effectiveness. Efficacy is defined as the performance of a diagnostic or therapeutic endeavor under carefully controlled conditions, such as U.S. Food and Drug Administration trials; effectiveness is the performance of that test or intervention when broadly applied to the community (generalizability).[16] Kempczinski and colleagues

"Every hospital should follow every patient it treats long enough to determine whether the treatment has been successful, and then to inquire 'if not why not' with a view to preventing similar failures in the future."

Ernest Codman, MD, 1914

Surgery is a specialty of inherent com-

data regarding diagnosis and treatment are gathered and evaluated critically. Conclusions about the best approach to patient care are developed and applied; the process is one of continuous learning and quality improvement. To incorporate evidence-based practice into patient care, surgeons must be familiar not only with current data but also with its strength and the manner in which it can be applied.

demonstrated the differences in these two concepts (although they did so through a retrospective, large database study, not a randomized, prospective trial). Evaluating carotid endarterectomy done in the community, they found that the combined morbidity and mortality of this procedure was significantly different in community hospitals (effectiveness) compared with university centers (efficacy).[17]

Large, randomized, experimental studies are quite time consuming and costly. The development of a detailed protocol for the conduct of the study and the collection of data may require years. During this time, improved diagnostic and therapeutic regimens may be developed that render the impact of the study limited. This was true, for example, with the Asymptomatic Carotid Atherosclerosis Study.[18,19] The study randomized patients with a 50% or greater stenosis of the carotid artery to surgery or medical therapy. No stratification by degree of stenosis was made. After the onset of data collection in this randomized study, methods for the improved noninvasive detection and quantification of carotid artery stenoses were developed and subsets of patients with differing degrees of stenosis could more easily be identified. Since the methodology of the study was set and could not be changed, the study was conducted with less than ideal diagnostic criteria, limiting its value. Although the surgical group demonstrated a reduction in ipsilateral neurological events, no reduction occurred in the combined endpoint of stroke and death.

Inclusion and exclusion criteria for patient enrollment in a randomized study can also be controversial.[20] Broad inclusion criteria permit the rapid enrollment of numerous patients who may be dissimilar, whereas definitive exclusion criteria may slow enrollment but can enhance the comparability of the patients. In addition, patient cooperation may decrease over time. Many patients prefer the option to choose their own form of treatment even if the scientific basis for that treatment may not be established.

SECONDARY STUDY DESIGN

Meta-analysis is an analytical tool that permits the evaluation of a diagnostic or therapeutic modality through the appropriate use of previously published smaller studies.[21] Meta-analysis is not the simple pooling of data reported in numerous small studies, a notion that has often caused investigational errors. The simple pooling of data from multiple small studies often compounds biases and may further reduce the ability to detect important differences among study groups.[22] A meta-analysis of available data is a rigorous, systematic, and quantitative review. To undertake a meta-analysis to address a research question or hypothesis, the investigator must first define the appropriate study population and methodology. The literature is then reviewed exhaustively for the identification of all relevant studies that meet the established criteria. These studies are then evaluated critically to determine and correct for possible bias in data collection. Reports in which data collection did not adhere to the established meta-analysis criteria, or in which an unquantified bias was introduced, are not included. The raw data from the selected studies are then combined and analyzed. This methodology permits the detection of statistically significant differences among study groups that may not have been possible in individual reports due to their small size.

COMPUTER ANALYSIS AND SIMULATION

A Markov analysis is a computer-based analysis designed to determine whether one event is related to another in a sequence of events. It can analyze the likelihood of future changes in health states of a person or population.[23] A state transition diagram is created that lists all possible health state transitions (outcomes) after an event.[24] The probability of each health state transition is entered into the computer. Although it would be possible to calculate the health state transitions after a single event by hand, calculations become more complex with each change in health state. The Markov analysis can identify the likelihood of future changes in health states. For example, the possible health states after lower extremity bypass include an improvement in health, a worsening of health, or death. It may be possible to predict the likelihood of outcomes after a bypass through manual calculation. Adding another event, such as angioplasty after failure of a bypass, adds another series of outcomes and probabilities. The incremental complexities are handled easily through Markov analysis. A well-performed analysis provides excellent insight into outcomes and is a valuable tool for extending the impact of available data. For example, Michaels and Galland used Markov analysis to determine the best approach for treatment of patients with a popliteal aneurysm.[25] The study concluded that the best treatment is elective surgery, which produces better results 1 to 2 years after presentation than does conservative management. The authors emphasized that the values used for the rate of development of symptoms, limb loss, and mortality in the analysis were crucial in determining its outcome.

A Monte Carlo simulation is a computer tool that attempts to simulate possible real-life outcomes by randomly selecting from a range of acceptable values for several variables and predicting final outcomes.[26] The simulation calculates numerous outcome scenarios, rather than just one, and the probabilities of obtaining that outcome. The use of multiple probabilities makes simple hand calculations impossible. Because this computer analytical tool and Markov analysis use probabilities obtained from acceptable studies reported in the literature, they provide excellent methods for evaluating treatments and technologies.

POPULATION DYNAMICS

Population Subgroups

Few populations are uniform, and disease processes do not manifest uniformly in all populations. Population dynamics can significantly affect the outcomes of studies. Therefore, even a prospective, randomized, controlled trial can produce results that are not broadly applicable in all patients if recruitment does not reflect the prevalence of the disease process and responses to treatment in the general population. Race, genetics, or subtle unmeasured differences in study subjects, such as place of birth and dietary influences, may cause variations in the manifestation of a disease or the response to treatment and may alter the results of a clinical trial. White and colleagues examined the age-adjusted incidence of first ischemic stroke among whites, Hispanics, and blacks in Manhattan.[27] They noted an incidence of 88 per 100,000 in whites, 149 per 100,000 in Hispanics, and 191 per 100,000 in blacks, confirming that cerebrovascular disease does not equally affect all subgroups within a population. Incidence and prevalence studies would clearly have skewed results if a given subgroup were excluded or excessively recruited. Elkins and Johnston developed a model to predict ischemic stroke deaths in the United States until 2032.[28] The death rate of blacks from ischemic stroke was 61.7 per 100,000 person-years in 2002. This was significantly higher than the overall rate from ischemic stroke of 47.6 per 100,000 person-years, or the rate among whites of 45.9 per 100,000 person-years. The investigators calculated that by 2032 there will be a decrease in ischemic stroke-related deaths but that rates among blacks will remain significantly higher than those for the overall population.[28] Therefore, population dynamics could lead to an overestimation or underestimation of mortality related to ischemic stroke in a study, depending on the subgroups recruited.

The results of studies reporting the response to treatment may also be influenced by population subgroups. Dardik and colleagues examined the impact of race on the outcome of carotid endarterectomy performed in nonfederal acute care hospitals in Maryland from 1990 to 1995.[29] They noted that, while the in-hospital stroke rate among white patients of 1.6% was consistent with other studies reported in the literature, the rate among blacks was 3.1%. Clearly, the in-hospital stroke risk of a carotid endarterectomy trial would be skewed by the percentage of blacks included in the trial. These findings were confirmed by Kennedy and associates, who examined the impact of race on the outcome of carotid endarterectomy in a population study of patients treated in California. Nonwhites had a statistically significantly greater risk of postoperative stroke than whites.[30]

Such population variations are not limited to the United States. Sundquist and Li examined the relationship between country of birth and death from coronary artery disease.[31] They noted that coronary artery disease and death from ischemic cardiac disease were more prevalent in first- and second-generation immigrants to Sweden compared to native Swedes. Similar findings were reported by Wild and colleagues, who analyzed the presence of cardiac and peripheral vascular disease in citizens of England and Wales, stratified by country of birth.[32] Using census and mortality data for 2001 to 2003, these investigators found that death rates from myocardial infarction or stroke were significantly higher among those born in Ireland, Scotland, and Africa compared to those born in England and Wales. In light of the innate heterogeneity of nearly all major populations worldwide, subsets may influence even large clinical trials. Although randomized and prospective, a trial from a single institution may have findings that are skewed by population dynamics. Large clinical trials that involve multiple centers in diverse geographical areas of the country or world are less likely to be influenced by population dynamics, since the composition of both the study group and the control group should be similarly affected.

Gender

Gender differences can also affect the conclusions of many studies. Failure to include both men and women in clinical trials in proportion to the incidence of the disease in each gender may lead to incorrect conclusions and the application of unsubstantiated treatments. This is nowhere more evident than in the treatment with aspirin. One of the first compelling studies to endorse the recommendation of aspirin to reduce the risk of myocardial infarction was the Physicians' Health Study.[33] Released in 1988, this prospective analysis of risk reduction in 22,071 male physicians noted a 44% reduction in first myocardial infarction. Subsequently, support grew for aspirin use for the prevention of myocardial infarction in both men and women. In a meta-analysis published in 2003, Eidelman and associates examined data from five major, prospective, randomized clinical trials that included 11,466 women and 44,114 men greater than 40 years of age.[34] Of the five trials, however, women were recruited into only two. The investigators noted a statistically significant 32% reduction in first myocardial infarction but no significant impact on stroke for both men and women. Their conclusions supported the American Heart Association recommendations that aspirin be considered for myocardial infarction risk reduction in both men and women at moderate cardiovascular risk.[35]

Although unintentional, the lack of uniform recruitment of women in three of the five major trials resulted in methodological bias and incorrect conclusions. This error was subsequently demonstrated in another large trial recruiting only women. In 1992, the Women's Health Study began to enroll volunteers into a randomized, prospective, double-blind, placebo-controlled trial of aspirin for the prevention of myocardial infarction and stroke.[36] The study followed 39,876 women for a mean of 10 years. Overall, a statistically significant 24% reduction in ischemic stroke was documented, but no significant reduction in nonfatal or fatal myocardial infarction was found. Including this large study into a meta-analysis with the previously mentioned five major trials, Berger and colleagues noted a statistically significant advantage for aspirin in women to reduce the risk of ischemic stroke and in men to reduce the risk of myocardial infarction.[37] The differing conclusions of these two major meta-analyses confirmed the potential impact of gender bias. As with other forms of population dynamics, recruitment into trials should reflect the incidence of the disease process in each gender.

Levels of Evidence and Data Analysis

To ensure that patient care decisions are based on the strongest available evidence, physicians must be able to identify the best studies. This is perhaps the greatest challenge of evidence-based medicine. The escalating volume of literature has made the acquisition of information more difficult. Important and vital advances in patient care can become buried in mounds of literature that are of limited value. This has led to a significant effort to evaluate scientific publications on the strength of their hypothesis, methodology, data analysis, and conclusions.[38] Although there remains controversy about the optimal methods for establishing the strength of data contained in a publication, most have adopted some variation of the levels of evidence set forth by the Canadian Task Force on Periodic Health Examination (Table 5-2).[39]

It is accepted that the randomized, controlled trial is the best method for identifying the presence or absence of differences among treatment effects with least investigator bias.

Table 5-2
Levels of Evidence

Level	Type of Evidence
I	Evidence obtained from at least one properly randomized controlled trial
II-1	Evidence obtained from well-designed controlled trials without randomization
II-2	Evidence obtained from well-designed cohort or case-control analytical studies, preferably from more than one center or research group
II-3	Evidence obtained from comparisons among times or places with or without the intervention; dramatic results in uncontrolled experiments could also be included in this category
III	Opinions of respected authorities, based on clinical experience, descriptive studies, or reports of expert committees

From Canadian Task Force on Periodic Health Examination. The periodic health examination. *Can Med Assoc J* 1979;121:1193-1254.

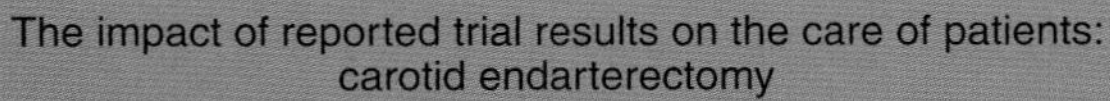

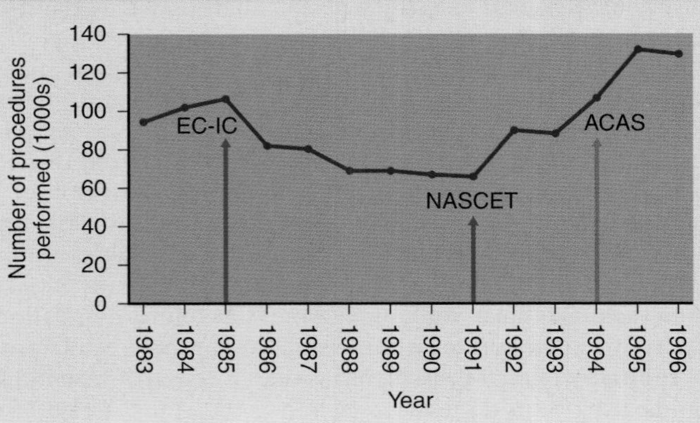

Figure 5-1. The impact of reported trial results on the care of patients: carotid endarterectomy. ACAS, Asymptomatic Carotid Atherosclerosis Study; EC–IC, Extracranial–Intracranial Bypass Study; NASCET, North American Symptomatic Carotid Endarterectomy Trial.

This concept stems from a landmark publication by Sacks and colleagues, which reported that observational studies were far less likely to identify the new or target treatment to be effective than were randomized, controlled studies.[13] More recent evidence, however, indicates this may not always be true. Comparisons between the findings of observational (case-control and cohort) and randomized trials evaluating the type of anesthesia used for carotid endarterectomy, for example, have demonstrated that observational studies do not overestimate the treatment effect.[40]

Many surgical techniques cannot be tested appropriately in randomized clinical trials.[8] Observational studies may be more suitable for emergency treatments or comparing disparate therapies, such as aortic stent-grafting versus open aneurysm repair. Therefore, the evaluation of a diagnostic test or the indications for treatment may best be tested in large, randomized, prospective studies, but surgical technology and techniques may sometimes be better assessed through large observational studies.

Vascular surgeons must be aware of the available evidence, its strength, and the appropriate application of the evidence if they are to care for the individual patient. Even with the use of rigorous methodologies, the value of trials may be limited if physicians apply the results inappropriately.

Carotid endarterectomy has been one of the most rigorously evaluated vascular surgical interventions. As the technique of endarterectomy became standardized and results improved, the procedure was performed with increasing frequency. Nevertheless, after results of the randomized, prospective trial on extracranial–intracranial bypass failed to demonstrate benefit to that procedure, physicians referred fewer patients for extracranial carotid endarterectomy.[41,42] This represents the inappropriate extrapolation of the results of the study. Subsequently, vascular surgeons and neurologists organized the North American Symptomatic Carotid Endarterectomy Trial.[43] This well-designed trial clearly demonstrated the benefit of the surgical procedure in a subset of patients. The result was an increase in referrals for carotid endarterectomy, with procedures increasing 3.4% per month for the first 6 months after the release of the data (Figure 5-1).[44] Similarly, after publication of the Asymptomatic Carotid Atherosclerosis Study data, the carotid endarterectomy rate increased 7.3% over the first 7 months.

Despite the completion of more than seven major trials, the indications for carotid endarterectomy remain somewhat controversial (Table 5-3).[45] This may be because no trial is flawless and no data analysis and interpretation are beyond question. The application of evidence is rarely uniform among all practitioners. This may be the result of regional differences in patient populations, the availability of services or specialists.[46] Finally, the results of the major trials indicate that validity of the data depends on the achievement of a low morbidity and mortality rate. This suggests that each surgeon must assess his or her own skills when applying information to specific patients.

Outcomes Assessment

Even large clinical trials or epidemiological studies with significant levels of evidence do not always provide an accurate assessment of appropriate patient care. Perhaps as important

Table 5-3
Indications for Carotid Endarterectomy

Best Indications
- Stenosis ≥70%
- Overall good general health
- Hemispherical transient ischemic attacks
- Tandem extracranial and intracranial occlusive lesions
- Evidence for lack of collateral vessels

Acceptable Indications but with Higher Risk
- Widespread leukoaraiosis*
- Contralateral internal carotid artery occlusion
- Intraluminal thrombus

Acceptable Indications but with Lesser Benefit
- Lacunar stroke
- Nearly occluded internal carotid artery

From Inzitari D. Leukoaraiosis: an independent risk factor for stroke? *Stroke* 2003;34:2067-2071.

*Bilateral patchy or diffuse areas of low attenuation on computed tomography or hyperintense T_2 magnetic resonance areas.

as the type of clinical trial is the recording of meaningful outcomes. The adequacy of patient treatment is not described only in terms of graft patency, morbidity, and mortality. The ultimate value of a therapeutic intervention is its ability to improve a patient's quality of life (QOL) and personal productivity. Although it is generally presumed that complete cure of the disease accomplishes this, few vascular procedures directly affect the underlying arterial occlusive or aneurysmal process.

Endarterectomy, reconstruction, and revascularization procedures do little to affect the progress of the underlying atherosclerotic occlusive disease. Both recurrent and progressive distal atherosclerosis can reduce the hemodynamic benefit of vascular intervention.[47-49] Life expectancy of patients with lower extremity ischemia remains severely reduced despite successful revascularization.[50,51] Similarly, aneurysm repair does not alter the metabolic pathways that weaken the aortic wall. Continued growth of the aneurysm neck after aortic stent grafting and recurrent aneurysm formation above the graft after open surgery occur occasionally.[52,53]

Vascular procedures are designed to reduce the complications of arterial and venous disease and to improve a patient's QOL, rather than directly affect the disease process. Appropriate assessment of vascular interventions and proof of their benefit therefore requires evaluation of not only the technical outcomes, but also the impact on QOL. This perspective was stressed by the U.S. Congress when it created the Agency for Health Care Policy and Research, now known as the Agency for Healthcare Research and Quality, in 1989.[54] Since that time, significant effort has been devoted to developing methods to assess the outcomes of diagnostic and therapeutic interventions. The Agency for Healthcare Research and Quality emphasizes that treatments should be evaluated on the basis of outcomes that directly affect the patient, such as physical functioning, pain, and psychological well-being, rather than on the basis of intermediate parameters, such as laboratory tests.[55]

The need for more complete outcomes assessment is clear. Mounting evidence shows that vascular laboratory values do not accurately describe the impact of the disease on the patient. Feinglass and associates assessed the ankle–brachial index (ABI) and patient-reported limitations in 555 patients with lower limb ischemia.[56] They noted only a modest correlation between these two sets of data. Many patients with significant reductions in ABI to the range of 0.4 to 0.6 experienced minimal limitations on their daily activities, whereas some patients with ABI values in the range of 0.8 to 0.9 felt they were limited. Similar findings were reported by Chetter and colleagues, who evaluated 235 patients with lower limb ischemia by means of ABI measurement, treadmill walking distance, and a survey on QOL.[57] They found that increasing ischemia was associated with worsening QOL but that the correlation of laboratory values and QOL scores was tenuous. Barletta and associates evaluated 251 claudicants and 89 age-matched controls with treadmill walking distance and QOL as reported on a general health survey.[58] They noted a reduction in physical, emotional, and social functioning in claudicants compared with the controls, but the level of reduction of these QOL parameters did not correlate with walking distance. Thus, while the vascular laboratory can provide the physician with a quantitative assessment of blood flow, it does not indicate the degree of impairment experienced by the patient.

Anatomical and vascular laboratory studies also fail to assess the complete impact of vascular intervention on the patient. This has been demonstrated by numerous investigators. Currie and colleagues noted significant improvements in physical function and pain assessed by a general health survey in 34 patients undergoing surgery and 74 patients undergoing angioplasty for claudication.[59] The improvements reported by the patients, however, did not correlate with increases in ABI. In another study, 150 consecutive patients with limb-threatening ischemia who underwent vascular intervention were evaluated pre- and postoperatively with regard to surgical outcome and QOL by Johnson and associates.[60] There were six treatment subgroups: angioplasty, thrombolysis or thrombectomy, bypass, primary amputation, amputation after failed revascularization, and primary bilateral amputation. These investigators found that reconstructive surgery significantly improved mobility, pain, anxiety, depression, lifestyle, and self-care ability. The benefits of angioplasty were similar, but this treatment modality did not reduce anxiety or depression. The other interventions demonstrated even less positive impact on the patient's general health.

Several investigators have noted a discrepancy between an excellent clinical outcome and a patient-reported improvement. Gibbons and colleagues evaluated activities of daily living, mental well-being, and symptoms of vascular disease in 156 patients with limb-threatening ischemia.[61] Although limb salvage was 97% at 6 months, only 45% of patients reported feeling "back to normal." Nicoloff and colleagues evaluated the functional status in 112 patients who had undergone infrainguinal bypass 5 to 7 years previously.[62] These investigators found that 30% of patients who were ambulatory preoperatively were not walking at the time of evaluation. Only 14.3% experienced an "ideal" surgical result of an uncomplicated operation with long-term symptom relief, maintenance of functional, status and no repeat operations.

Even an aggressive policy of graft surveillance to maintain graft patency may have a variable impact on the patient. Ronayne documented greater anxieties and less satisfaction among patients requiring repeat vascular surgical interventions compared to those undergoing their first procedure.[63] Seabrook and colleagues reported a persistently decreased ability to perform activities of daily living, such as distance walking, performing household chores, bathing, and participating in social activities, in patients who had undergone successful revascularization.[64] Despite this, patients with a patent graft did experience an improvement in their sense of well-being. The benefits and adverse effects of vascular surgical interventions should also be defined by their impact on the patient's QOL and quantity of life, not simply by clinical parameters. To accomplish this, both generic and disease-specific QOL evaluations should be undertaken.

The Transatlantic Intersociety Consensus group, comprising representatives from the major vascular societies of North America and Europe, attempted to embrace this concept and address the need for more complete assessment of vascular therapy for arterial occlusive disease.[65] The group recommended that the outcome of vascular treatment of the lower extremity be based on a combination of hemodynamic, anatomical, and patient-reported assessment of symptomatic improvement and QOL. The multiple components provide a complete evaluation of not only the underlying disease process but also the impact of the disease on the patient, potential

Table 5-4
Recommended Outcome Measures in Peripheral Arterial Disease

- Objective or hemodynamic assessment of the limb
- Patency of the treated segment
- Symptomatic status of the limb
- General quality of life of the patient
- Value assessment of quality of life of the patient

From Dormandy JA, Rutherford RB. Management of peripheral arterial disease (pad): transatlantic intersociety consensus. *J Vasc Surg* 2000;31(Pt 2):S1-S288.

benefits, and adverse effects (Table 5-4). For assessment of improvements in QOL, the use of both generic health and disease-specific patient survey tools is recommended.

Generic Quality-of-Life Survey Instruments

Several generic health surveys that assess overall health status have been developed and standardized in large populations of patients (Table 5-5).[66-70] These instruments obtain important data directly from patients in four major categories:

- Functional status
- Perceived health
- Psychological well-being
- Role function

Functional status provides insight into how well patients perform basic physical tasks important in the activities of daily living. Perceived health indicates how healthy or ill patients believe they are. Psychological well-being reveals the degree to which patients are distressed, anxious, or depressed about the illness. Role function demonstrates the extent to which the disease affects a patient's ability to work and to care for family or resources.

Each of the listed instruments has proven reliability and validity.[71] Reliability indicates that each person with the same overall health condition will interpret and answer the questions in the survey in the same way. Validity indicates that each question actually measures what is intended and that the answers given by a patient to similar questions are consistent within a survey and over time, if there has been no change in general health status. These demonstrated characteristics of a survey tool are crucial. Therefore, questionnaires that have not been subjected to rigorous reliability and validity testing should not be used, and their results in publications should be taken with a strong measure of skepticism.

In the United States, efforts to describe a patient's health status and the outcomes of that patient's interaction with the health-care system began to coalesce in the 1980s with the Medical Outcomes Study.[69] The study undertook the development of a patient assessment tool that could determine the following:

- How patients with the same health problem fare over time despite different treatments
- How the lives of patients with different health problems were affected by those conditions
- How the benefits on the patients' lives of treatments compared across conditions

The result of the study was the development of a general health outcomes assessment tool: the short form–36 (SF-36). This survey tool, which is completed by the patient, obtains information about eight areas of the patient's life (Table 5-6). An overall general health score can be calculated, and each of the domains can be scored individually and tracked.

Table 5-5
Generic Quality-of-Life Survey Instruments

- Nottingham Health Profile[66]
- EuroQol[67]
- Sickness Impact Profile[68]
- Medical Outcomes Study (short form–36)[69]
- Quality of Well-Being Scale[70]

Table 5-6
Domains of the Short Form–36 Survey

- Perception of health
- Psychological well-being
- Role limitations due to physical health problems
- Role limitations due to mental health problems
- Physical function
- Social relations
- Pain
- Fatigue

The value of survey tools such as the SF-36 lies in their standardization in large populations of patients over time in a manner similar to laboratory studies. They are capable of demonstrating the impact of any disease that may extend far beyond physiological parameters, especially for chronic illnesses such as diabetes, hypertension, and angina. This is certainly true of claudication as assessed by the SF-36 (Figure 5-2).[72] Generic QOL instruments may also guide the establishment of appropriate treatment goals. Johnson and colleagues studied QOL in patients who had either revascularization or amputation for limb-threatening ischemia.[73] They noted that successful revascularization resulted in better mobility, self-care, and lifestyle than amputation. However, a subset of patients undergoing amputation (22%) had scores equivalent to those who had a bypass. Treatment goals, therefore, may have been different for these individuals.

Because generic QOL instruments are not disease specific, they reflect only changes in the overall health status of the patient. Perception of health may not be altered significantly by the treatment of only one of several comorbid conditions, as noted by Duggan and colleagues. They studied 17 patients with patent lower extremity bypasses and found continued decline in perceived health over an 18-month interval.[74] Cook and Galland identified a reduction in perceived health in 24 claudicants despite an improvement in walking distance maintained for 1 year after angioplasty.[75] This reduction was due to the development or worsening of comorbid conditions. Similar data have been demonstrated in patients undergoing carotid endarterectomy for symptomatic disease. Dardik and colleagues noted an improvement in overall general health scores 3 months after a successful surgery but not when complications occurred.[76] When used with objective and hemodynamic assessments, the generic health surveys provide the vascular specialist with invaluable insight into the specific

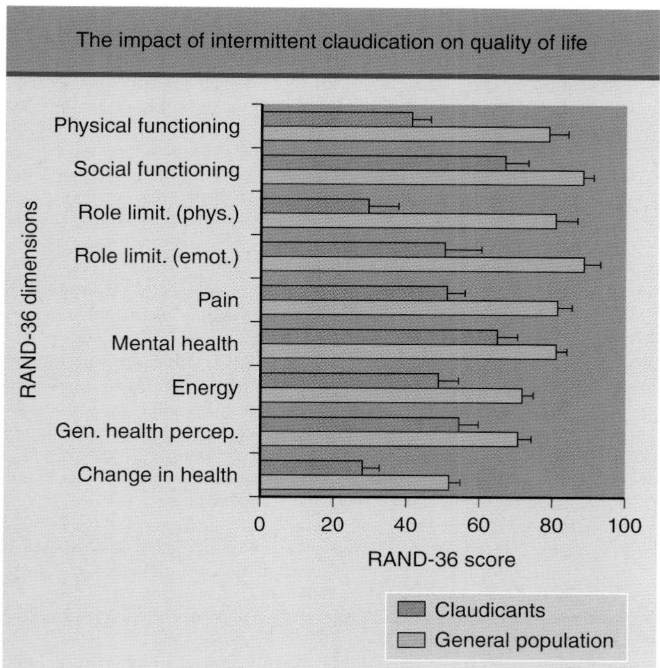

Figure 5-2. The impact of intermittent claudication on quality of life as indicated by the short form–36 survey. Note the differences in domain scores and overall change in health of patients with intermittent claudication compared with the general population.

effects of the vascular disease and comorbid conditions on a patient's life and the impact of therapy on the level of functioning. They do not, however, provide information on the impact of a specific disease on QOL; for this, a disease-specific survey instrument must be used.

Disease-Specific Quality-of-Life Survey Instruments

The quest for disease-specific instruments has focused on symptomatic arterial occlusive disease of the lower extremity. Ideally, such a tool would permit documentation of the presence of peripheral arterial disease, its impact on a patient's general health, and the response to treatment. The tool should be able to detect improvement or deterioration in health caused by the disease and its treatment, independent from that caused by comorbid conditions. Rose developed one of the first questionnaires to identify patients with claudication.[77] Although used widely, this questionnaire lacked sensitivity. Subsequently, Regensteiner and colleagues developed the Walking Impairment Questionnaire (WIQ) to define more clearly the presence and impact of claudication on the patient.[78] It attempts to assess the reason for difficulty in walking, the degree of pain, the walking distance and speed, and stair-climbing ability. It also is useful for the documentation of the benefits of treatment. Unlike the tenuous relationship between patient-reported improvement and ABI, the WIQ scores do improve with increased walking distance. This was demonstrated by Regensteiner and colleagues, who noted that after a 24-week supervised exercise therapy program, claudicants had WIQ score improvement that paralleled the increase in treadmill walking distance.[78]

Several other disease-specific questionnaires have been developed for the assessment of patients with lower extremity arterial occlusive disease (Table 5-7).[79-81] Significant progress is being made toward evaluating these instruments in large populations in the setting of various comorbid conditions. Continued evaluation of these tools is essential for improved assessments of the benefits and adverse effects of treatment for arterial occlusive disease of the leg.

Table 5-7
Disease-Specific Survey Instruments for Leg Ischemia

- Rose questionnaire[77]
- Walking Impairment Questionnaire[78]
- King's College Hospital Vascular Quality of Life Questionnaire[79]
- Intermittent Claudication Questionnaire[80]
- Claudication Scale (CLAU-S) Quality-of-Life Questionnaire[81]

CHALLENGES FOR THE FUTURE

QOL and disease-specific instruments that clearly identify a patient's underlying disease, the impact on their general health, and the outcomes of treatment have demonstrated their value. The SF-36 has established the adverse effects of various symptomatic disorders on a patient's general health. Disease-specific instruments such as the WIQ are valuable for the assessment of the impact of symptomatic arterial occlusive disease and its treatment, independent of comorbid conditions. However, several vascular disorders are life-threatening but lack significant symptoms. These include asymptomatic aortic aneurysms and asymptomatic carotid artery stenoses. Appropriate tools are needed to better describe vascular disease and its treatment in asymptomatic patients.

Current instruments such as the SF-36 have been used to assess small groups of patients with asymptomatic infrarenal aortic aneurysms. Perkins and colleagues used the SF-36 to study changes in QOL in 59 consecutive patients undergoing elective aneurysm repair.[82] They noted improvement in QOL scores between 6 weeks and 3 months postoperatively. Using the SF-36, Lloyd and associates evaluated the QOL in 82 patients 6 months after undergoing elective aneurysm repair by either open or endovascular methods.[83] They noted that physical function and vitality scores were still lower than preoperative levels. In similar studies, patients have been noted to have overall scores return to baseline levels by 8 weeks or to exceed baseline levels by 3 months.[84,85] The discrepancy in the results of these studies most likely occurs because the SF-36 does not discriminate between the impact of the target disease and that of comorbid conditions. Therefore, more disease-specific instruments, especially those with sensitivity to asymptomatic conditions, must be developed.

As the economic burden of health-care continues to escalate, greater effort must be made to identify those diagnostic and therapeutic modalities that are of greatest benefit in improving QOL and productivity. For vascular surgery, this will require both generic and disease-specific survey tools that demonstrate clearly the impact of vascular disease on the patient and document the benefits of therapy.

References

1. Blakemore AH, Voorhees Jr AB. Use of tubes constructed from vinyon "N" cloth in bridging arterial defects: experimental and clinical results. *Ann Surg* 1954;140:324-334.
2. Baker JD. The vascular laboratory. In: Rutherford RB, ed. *Vascular surgery.* 5th ed. Philadelphia: WB Saunders; 2000:127-139.
3. Evidence-Based Medicine Working Group. Evidence-based medicine. *JAMA* 1992;268:2420-2425.
4. Passaro Jr E, Organ Jr CH, Codman EA. The improper Bostonian. *Bull Am Coll Surg* 1999;84:16-22.
5. US Congress. Office of Technology Assessment. The development of clinical practice guidelines. In: *Identifying health technologies that work: searching for evidence.* Washington, DC: U.S. Government Printing Office; 1994:145-171.
6. US Congress. Office of Technology Assessment. The impact of clinical guidelines on practice. In: Identifying health technologies that work: searching for evidence. Washington, DC: U.S. Government Printing Office; 1994:173-198.
7. Fung EK, Lore Jr JM. Randomized controlled trials for evaluating surgical questions. *Arch Otolaryngol Head Neck Surg* 2002;128:631-634.
8. Solomon MJ, McLeod RS. Should we be performing more randomized controlled trials evaluating surgical operations? *Surgery* 1995;118:459-467.
9. US Congress. Office of Technology Assessment. *Identifying health technologies that work: searching for evidence.* Washington, DC: U.S. Government Printing Office; 1994:601.
10. Wacholder S, Silverman DT, McLaughlin JK, Mandel JS. Selection of controls in case-control studies. *Am J Epidemiol* 1992;135:1042-1050.
11. White E, Hunt JR, Casso D. Exposure measurement in cohort studies: the challenges of prospective data collection. *Epidemiol Rev* 1998;20:43-56.
12. Kannel WB. The Framingham study: historical insight on the impact of cardiovascular risk factors in men versus women. *J Gend Specif Med* 2002;5:27-37.
13. Sacks H, Chalmers TC, Smith Jr H. Randomized versus historical controls for clinical trials. *Am J Med* 1982;72:233-240.
14. Chalmers TC, Smith Jr H, Blackburn B, et al: A method for assessing the quality of a randomized control trial. *Control Clin Trials* 1981;2:31-49.
15. Buring JE, Jonas MA, Hennekens CH. Large and simple randomized trials. In: *Tools for evaluating health technologies.* Washington, DC: U.S. Government Printing Office; 1995:83-87.
16. US Congress. Office of Technology Assessment. *Identifying health technologies that work: searching for evidence.* Washington, DC: U.S. Government Printing Office; 1994:4.
17. Kempczinski RF, Brott TG, Labutta RJ. The influence of surgical specialty and caseload on the results of carotid endarterectomy. *J Vasc Surg* 1986;3:911-916.
18. Asymptomatic Carotid Atherosclerosis Study Group. Study design for randomized prospective trial of carotid endarterectomy for asymptomatic atherosclerosis. *Stroke* 1989;20:844-849.
19. Hobson II RW, Weiss DG, Fields WS, et al. Efficacy of carotid endarterectomy for asymptomatic carotid stenosis: the veterans affairs cooperative study group. *N Engl J Med* 1993;328:221-227.
20. Buring JE, Jonas MA, Hennekens CH. Large and simple randomized trials. In: *Tools for evaluating health technologies.* Washington, DC: U.S. Government Printing Office; 1995:72-73.
21. L'Abbe KA, Detsky AS, O'Rourke K. Meta-analysis in clinical research. *Ann Intern Med* 1987;107:224-233.
22. Jones DR. Meta-analysis: weighing the evidence. *Stat Med* 1995;14:137-149.
23. Sonnenberg FA, Beck JR. Markov models in medical decision making: a practical guide. *Med Decis Making* 1993;13:322-338.
24. Detsky AS, Naglie G, Krahn MD, et al. Primer on medical decision analysis. II. Building a tree. *Med Decis Making* 1998;17:126-135.
25. Michaels JA, Galland RB. Management of asymptomatic popliteal aneurysms: the use of a Markov decision tree to determine the criteria for a conservative approach. *Eur J Vasc Surg* 1993;7:136-143.
26. Concato J, Feinstein AR. Monte Carlo methods in clinical research: applications in multivariable analysis. *J Investig Med* 1997;45:394-400.
27. White H, Boden-Albala B, Wang C, et al. Ischemic stroke subtype incidence among whites, blacks, and Hispanics: the northern Manhattan study. *Circulation* 2005;111:1327-1331.
28. Elkins JS, Johnston SC. Thirty-year projections for deaths from ischemic stroke in the United States. *Stroke* 2003;34:2109-2113.
29. Dardik A, Bowman HM, Gordon TA, Hsieh G, Perler BA. Impact of race on outcome of carotid endarterectomy. *Ann Surg* 2000;232:704-709.
30. Kennedy B, Fortmann SP, Stafford RS. Elective and isolated carotid endarterectomy: health disparities in utilization and outcomes but not readmission. *J Natl Med Assoc* 2007;99:480-488.
31. Sundquist K, Li X. Coronary heart disease risks in first- and second-generation immigrants in Sweden: a follow-up study. *J Intern Med* 2006;259:418-427.
32. Wild SH, Fischbacher C, Brock A, Griffiths C, Bhopal R. Mortality from all causes and circulatory disease by country of birth in England and Wales, 2001-2003. *J Public Health (Oxf)* 2007;29:191-198.
33. The Steering Committee of the Physicians' Health Study Research Group. Findings from the aspirin component of the ongoing Physicians' Health Study. *N Engl J Med* 1988;318:262-264.
34. Eidelman RS, Hebert PR, Weisman SM, Hennekens CH. An update on aspirin in the primary prevention of cardiovascular disease. *Arch Intern Med* 2003;163:2006-2010.
35. Pearson TA, Blair SN, Daniels SR, et al. AHA guidelines for primary prevention of cardiovascular disease and stroke: 2002 update—consensus panel guide to comprehensive risk reduction for adult patients without coronary or other atherosclerotic vascular disease. *Circulation* 2002;106:388-391.
36. Ridker PM, Cook NR, Lee IM, et al. A randomized trial of low-dose aspirin in the primary prevention of cardiovascular disease in women. *N Engl J Med* 2005;352:1293-1304.
37. Berger JS, Roncaglione MC, Avanzini F, Pangrazzi I, Tognoni G, Brown DL. Aspirin for the primary prevention of cardiovascular events in women and men. *JAMA* 2006;295:306-313.
38. Meakins JL. Innovations in surgery: the rules of evidence. *Am J Surg* 2002;183:399-405.
39. Canadian Task Force on Periodic Health Examination. The periodic health examination. *Can Med Assoc J* 1979;121:1193-1254.
40. Benson K, Hartz AJ. A comparison of observational studies and randomized, controlled trials. *N Engl J Med* 2000;342:1878-1886.
41. The EC–IC Bypass Study Group. Failure of extracranial–intracranial arterial bypass to reduce the risk of ischemic stroke: results of an international randomized trial. *N Engl J Med* 1985;313:1191-2000.
42. Cronenwett JL, Birkmeyer JD, eds. *The Dartmouth atlas of vascular health care.* Chicago: AHA Press; 2000:42-43.
43. Executive Committee for the Asymptomatic Carotid Atherosclerosis Study. Endarterectomy for asymptomatic carotid artery stenosis. *JAMA* 1995;273:1421-1428.
44. Gross CP, Steiner CA, Bass EB, Powe NR. Relation between prepublication release of clinical trial results and the practice of carotid endarterectomy. *JAMA* 2000;284:2886-2893.
45. Barnett HJ, Meldrum HE, Eliasziw M, et al. The appropriate use of carotid endarterectomy. *CMAJ* 2002;166:1169-1179.
46. Glasziou PP, Irwig LM. An evidence based approach to individualizing treatment. *BMJ* 1995;311:1356-1359.
47. Robb JV, Wylie EJ. Factors contributing to recurrent lower limb ischemia following bypass surgery for aortoiliac occlusive disease, and their management. *Ann Surg* 1981;193:346-352.
48. Valentine RJ, Myers SI, Hagino RT, Clagett GP. Late outcome of patients with premature carotid atherosclerosis after carotid endarterectomy. *Stroke* 1996;27:1502-1506.
49. Dawson I, van Bockel JH. Reintervention and mortality after infrainguinal reconstructive surgery for leg ischaemia. *Br J Surg* 1999;86:38-44.
50. Dawson I, Keller BP, Brand R, et al. Late outcomes of limb loss after failed infrainguinal bypass. *J Vasc Surg* 1995;21:613-622.
51. Abou-Zamzam AM, Lee RW, Moneta GL, et al. Functional outcome after infrainguinal bypass for limb salvage. *J Vasc Surg* 1997;25:287-295.
52. Plate G, Hollier LA, O'Brien P, et al. Recurrent aneurysms and late vascular complications following repair of abdominal aortic aneurysms. *Arch Surg* 1985;120:590-594.
53. Matsumura JS, Pearce WH, Cabellon A, et al. Reoperative aortic surgery. *Cardiovasc Surg* 1999;7:614-621.
54. US Congress. Office of Technology Assessment. *Identifying health technologies that work: searching for evidence.* Washington, DC: U.S. Government Printing Office; 1994:33.
55. US Congress. Office of Technology Assessment. *Identifying health technologies that work: searching for evidence.* Washington, DC: U.S. Government Printing Office; 1994:34.
56. Feinglass J, McCarthy WJ, Slavensky R, et al. Effect of lower extremity blood pressure on physical functioning in patients who have intermittent claudication. *J Vasc Surg* 1996;24:503-512.
57. Chetter IC, Dolan P, Spark JI, et al. Correlating clinical indicators of lower-limb ischaemia with quality of life. *Cardiovasc Surg* 1997;5:361-366.

58. Barletta G, Brevetti G, O'Boyle C, et al. Quality of life in patients with intermittent claudication: relationship with laboratory exercise performance. *Vasc Med* 1996;1:1-3.
59. Currie IC, Lamont PM, Baird RN, Wilson YG. Treatment of intermittent claudication: the impact on quality of life. *Eur J Vasc Endovasc Surg* 1995;10:356-361.
60. Johnson BF, Singh S, Evans L, et al. A prospective study of the effect of limb-threatening ischaemia and its surgical treatment on the quality of life. *Eur J Vasc Endovasc Surg* 1997;13:306-314.
61. Gibbons GW, Burgess AM, Guadagnoli E, et al. Return to well-being and function after infrainguinal revascularization. *J Vasc Surg* 1995;21:35-44.
62. Nicoloff AD, Taylor LM, McLafferty RB, et al. Patient recovery after infrainguinal bypass grafting for limb salvage. *J Vasc Surg* 1998;27:256-263.
63. Ronayne R. Feelings and attitudes during early convalescence following vascular surgery. *J Adv Nurs* 1985;10:435-441.
64. Seabrook GR, Cambria RA, Freischlag JA, Towne JB. Health-related quality of life and functional outcome following arterial reconstruction for limb salvage. *Cardiovasc Surg* 1999;7:279-286.
65. Dormandy JA, Rutherford RB. Management of peripheral arterial disease (PAD): Transatlantic Intersociety Consensus. *J Vasc Surg* 2000;31 (Pt 2):S1-S288.
66. Hunt SM, Mcewen J, McKenna SP, eds. *Measuring health status.* Dover, NH: Croom Helm; 1986.
67. EuroQol Group. EuroQol: a new facility for the measurement of health-related quality of life. *Health Policy* 1990;16:199-208.
68. Bergner M, Bobbitt RA, Carter WB, et al. The Sickness Impact Profile: development and final revision of a health status measure. *Med Care* 1981;19:787-805.
69. Ware JE, Sherbourne CD. The MOS 36-item short-form health survey (SF-36). I. Conceptual framework and item selection. *Med Care* 1992;30:473-483.
70. Kaplan RM, Bush JW. Health-related quality of life measurement for evaluation and research and policy analysis. *Health Psychol* 1982;1:61-71.
71. Fowler FJ. Using patients' reports to evaluate medical outcomes. In: *Tools for evaluating health technologies.* Washington, DC: U.S. Government Printing Office; 1995:14-16.
72. Bosch JL, Hunink MGM. The relationship between descriptive and valuational quality-of-life measures in patients with intermittent claudication. *Med Decis Making* 1996;16:217-225.
73. Johnson BF, Evans L, Drury R, et al. Surgery for limb-threatening ischaemia: a reappraisal of the costs and benefits. *Eur J Vasc Endovasc Surg* 1995;9:181-188.
74. Duggan MM, Woodson J, Scott TE, et al. Functional outcomes in limb salvage vascular surgery. *Am J Surg* 1994;168:188-191.
75. Cook TA, Galland RB. Quality of life changes after angioplasty for claudication: medium-term results affected by comorbid conditions. *Cardiovasc Surg* 1997;5:424-426.
76. Dardik A, Minor J, Watson C, Hands LJ. Improved quality of life among patients with symptomatic carotid artery disease undergoing carotid endarterectomy. *J Vasc Surg* 2001;33:329-333.
77. Rose GA. The diagnosis of ischemic heart pain and intermittent claudication in field surveys. *Bull World Health Organ* 1962;27:645-658.
78. Regensteiner JG, Steiner JF, Panzer RJ, Hiatt WR. Evaluation of walking impairment by questionnaire in patients with peripheral arterial disease. *J Vasc Med Biol* 1990;2:142-156.
79. Morgan MB, Crayford T, Murrin B, Fraser SC. Developing the Vascular Quality Of Life Questionnaire: a new disease-specific quality of life measure for use in lower limb ischemia. *J Vasc Surg* 2001;33:679-687.
80. Chong PF, Garratt AM, Golledge J, et al. The Intermittent Claudication Questionnaire: a patient-assessed condition-specific health outcome measure. *J Vasc Surg* 2002;36:764-771.
81. Marquis P, Comte S, Lehert P. International validation of the CLAU-S Quality-of-Life Questionnaire for use in patients with intermittent claudication. *Pharmacoeconomics* 2001;19:667-677.
82. Perkins JM, Magee TR, Hands LJ, et al. Prospective evaluation of quality of life after conventional abdominal aortic aneurysm repair. *Eur J Vasc Surg* 1998;16:203-207.
83. Lloyd AJ, Boyle J, Bell PR, Thompson MM. Comparison of cognitive function and quality of life after endovascular or conventional aortic aneurysm repair. *Br J Surg* 2000;87:443-447.
84. Aquino RV, Jones MA, Zullo TG, et al. Quality of life assessment in patients undergoing endovascular or conventional AAA repair. *J Endovasc Ther* 2001;8:521-528.
85. Malina M, Nilsson M, Brunkwall J, et al. Quality of life before and after endovascular and open repair of asymptomatic AAAs: a prospective study. *J Endovasc Ther* 2000;7:372-379.

chapter 6

Vascular Laboratory Evaluation of Lower Extremity Arterial Occlusive Disease

Gregory L. Moneta, MD • Nicole Wheeler, MD • Mary E. Giswold, MD

Key Points

- The noninvasive vascular laboratory is useful to confirm the presence and quantify the hemodynamic significance of lower extremity peripheral arterial disease (PAD).
- Plethysmography and applications of Doppler ultrasound are the two most commonly used techniques to evaluate PAD.
- Plethysmography is primarily used to evaluate digital arterial waveforms and pressures; these measurements are especially applicable to diabetic patients with medial calcinosis and suprasystolic ankle pressures.
- The ankle–brachial index is simple, is reproducible, and allows categorization of PAD into severity subgroups that are of prognostic and clinical importance.
- Exercise testing is useful to quantify the hemodynamics of patients with intermittent claudication caused by PAD but is especially useful in differentiating vasculogenic from neurogenic claudication.
- Arterial duplex scanning allows the physician to localize the anatomical site of a stenosis and quantify its hemodynamic significance based on systolic velocity ratios. It also can differentiate stenosis from occlusion and can be used to plan potential intervention (angioplasty or surgical reconstruction).
- Noninvasive testing provides essential, quantitative, objective physiological data that are the scientific basis for modern therapeutic approaches to PAD patients.

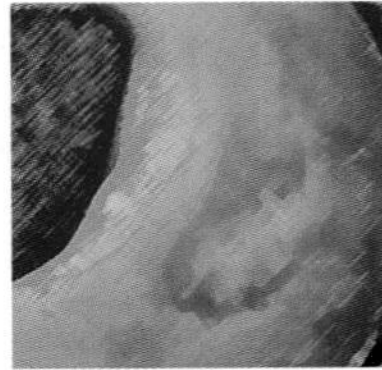

Because the differential diagnosis of chronic leg pain is quite broad, the ability to confirm the presence of arterial obstruction and quantify the hemodynamic and physiological significance of detected lesions is of paramount importance. The noninvasive vascular laboratory has a critical role as an adjunct to the history and physical examination in providing an objective, quantitative diagnosis of lower extremity arterial occlusive disease and the functional abnormalities resulting from a decrease in limb blood flow.

HISTORY AND PHYSICAL EXAMINATION

The clinical history provides valuable information regarding the evaluation of patients with chronic lower-extremity pain. In many patients, the clinical history, including questioning for coexistent atherosclerotic risk factors, coupled with the physical examination, is all that is necessary to firmly establish the diagnosis of exercise-induced muscular ischemia, intermittent claudication, or ischemic extremity pain at rest. It must be remembered that palpation of pulses is quite subjective and poorly reproducible. Whenever possible, the pulse examination in a patient suspected of having arterial disease should be confirmed with objective testing in the noninvasive vascular laboratory. It has also recently been recognized that many patients with peripheral arterial disease (PAD) have atypical leg symptoms or are asymptomatic. Such patients appear to have the same adverse natural history with regard to an increased risk of cardiovascular death as patients with typical symptoms of intermittent claudication, and they experience levels of functional decline over time similar to those experienced by patients with more classic symptoms of intermittent claudication. Recognition of this group of patients has led to an increased emphasis on vascular laboratory or office screening for the presence of PAD in patients with atypical leg symptoms of uncertain etiology and in patients with atherosclerotic risk factors.

Patients with exercise-induced leg or buttock pain should be specifically asked the location of the pain, its relationship to walking, the duration and severity of the symptoms, and the symptomatic progression over time. Only exercise-induced muscular pain of the calf, thigh, or buttock, relieved within a few minutes of rest and reliably reproduced by further walking, can confidently be improved by lower extremity revascularization. No data exist on the response of atypical leg symptoms to revasculazation in patients with evidence of PAD and less than typical signs and symptoms of intermittent claudication or critical limb ischemia. Almost all patients with intermittent claudication have diminished or absent lower-extremity pulses. Occasionally, however, a patient may give a classic history of intermittent claudication yet have palpable pedal pulses at rest. Under these circumstances, exercise testing with postexercise Doppler-measured ankle–brachial systolic blood pressure ratios is crucial to confirm the diagnosis of intermittent claudication secondary to an arterial disease (discussed later).

Ischemic rest pain should be suspected when a patient complains of pain, numbness, or both in the forefoot, toes, or instep. Ischemic rest pain is typically aggravated by elevating the leg and improved by placing the leg in a dependent position. It usually is worsened by exercise. Nocturnal leg cramps, which are often associated with lower extremity arterial occlusive disease, are themselves not manifestations of ischemic rest pain. However, true ischemic rest pain is often worse at night. Afflicted patients often describe the need to sleep in a chair to keep the involved foot dependent; a position that provides some relief from ischemic pain because of the gravitational-induced increase in arterial blood flow. Because of the need to maintain the foot in a dependent position, many patients with chronic ischemic pain develop significant edema of the symptomatic extremity. It is important to note that edema is not a classic feature of arterial insufficiency but rather reflects prolonged dependency of the ischemic extremity rather than ischemia itself.

In addition to an absence of pedal pulses, patients with rest pain often have thin, atrophic skin of the foot and lower leg, often with dependent rubor and pallor in elevation, and ultimately areas of cutaneous gangrene and ulceration. If the findings on physical examination are not consistent with ischemic pain, the physician should carefully inquire about a history of diabetes, thyroid disorders, vitamin deficiencies, or alcoholism, all of which can produce neuropathy with nocturnal foot dysesthetic discomfort similar to ischemic rest pain.

While the history and physical examination are clearly important in establishing the diagnosis of lower extremity arterial occlusive disease, the information obtained is by nature subjective and depends on the skill of the observer. The location and hemodynamic significance of various atherosclerotic lesions can only be grossly approximated by history and physical examination alone. This is clearly inadequate for monitoring individual lesions and for predicting the magnitude and complexity of any revascularization procedure. For these reasons, together with an increasing appreciation of the importance of arterial hemodynamics in determining and following the outcome of reconstructive procedures, the noninvasive vascular laboratory has assumed a pivotal role in the modern practice of peripheral arterial surgery.

PERIPHERAL VASCULAR LABORATORY

The objectives of modern noninvasive testing of patients with known or suspected lower-extremity PAD are to confirm the presence of arterial ischemia, to provide quantitative and reproducible physiological data concerning its severity, and to document the location and hemodynamic significance of individual arterial lesions. Two broad categories of noninvasive techniques are used to evaluate lower extremity arterial occlusive disease: plethysmography and various applications of Doppler ultrasound. Each technique has advantages and disadvantages. Understanding what the tests can and cannot do is required for the optimal and cost-effective use of the vascular laboratory.

PLETHYSMOGRAPHY

Plethysmography preceded ultrasound in the evaluation of lower extremity ischemia. Plethysmography is based on the detection of volume changes in the limb in response to arterial inflow. In addition to volume flow, the basic technology can be modified to produce pulse waveforms and determine digital pressures. Mercury strain gauge plethysmography, air plethysmography (pulse volume recordings), and photoplethysmography all have been used clinically.

Volume Flow

Calf or foot blood flow can be conveniently recorded with a mercury-in-silastic strain gauge. Measurements are based on detection of minute changes in the electrical resistance of the mercury column, which depend on its length. Unfortunately, neither calf nor foot blood flow at rest differ between normal subjects and patients with even rather severe degrees of arterial insufficiency.[1] Hyperemic flow may be decreased in patients with arterial ischemia when compared with normal subjects, but these changes in volume flow are not routinely used to quantify precise differences in severity of arterial occlusive lesions.[2] Therefore, measurements of volume flow have not proven useful in the evaluation of chronic lower-extremity ischemia.

Pulse Volume Recordings

Air plethysmography can be used clinically to demonstrate pulse volume waveforms.[3] These pulse volume recordings are obtained with partially inflated segmental blood pressure cuffs

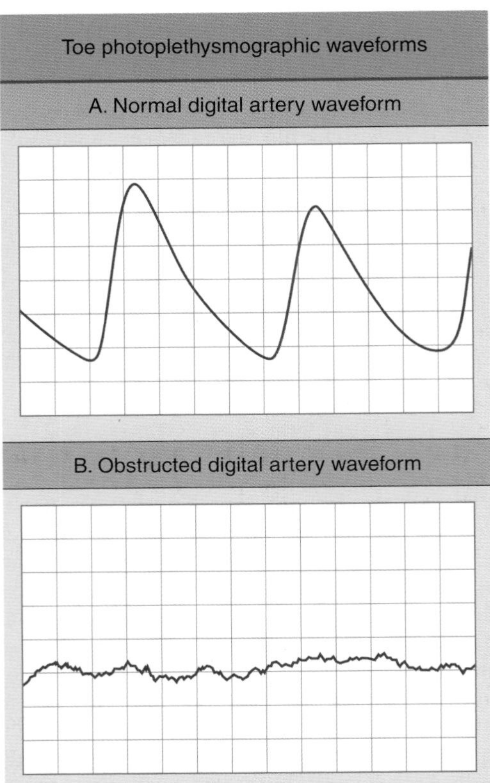

Figure 6-1. Toe photoplethysmographic waveforms. **A,** Normal digital artery waveform. **B,** Obstructed digital artery waveform.

that detect volume changes sequentially down a limb. Volume changes beneath the cuffs resulting from systole and diastole cause small pressure changes within the cuffs, which, with the use of appropriate transducers, can be displayed as arterial waveforms. A normal pulse volume waveform is characterized by a sharp systolic upstroke and peak and a prominent dicrotic notch on the downward portion of the curve. Such a waveform reflects normal arterial inflow to the portion of the extremity under the cuff. With increasing proximal arterial occlusion, the dicrotic notch is lost and the pulse peak wave becomes rounded, with loss of amplitude, and upstroke and downstroke times are nearly equal. With severe proximal occlusive disease, the pulse wave may be absent.[4] Pulse volume waveforms are generally evaluated qualitatively based on the shape of the curve, with flat, dampened curves considered severely abnormal. Although quantitative interpretive criteria have been proposed, these criteria, which are based on amplitude and contour changes of the pulse volume curves, are not in widespread clinical use.[5] The lack of reliable, reproducible, quantitative data in pulse volume recordings limits the utility of air plethysmography in the modern practice of vascular surgery.

Digital Measurements

Perhaps the greatest current role for plethysmography is in the evaluation of digital pressures and waveforms. Air plethysmography, strain gauge plethysmography, and photoplethysmography can all be adapted for this purpose. Strictly speaking, photoplethysmography is not a method to record volume change; rather, a photoelectrode is used to detect changes in cutaneous blood flow. This allows the technique to be readily used, in combination with pneumatic cuffs, to detect digital systolic pressures. These techniques are particularly useful in patients with pedal artery occlusive disease or highly calcified vessels, in whom Doppler-derived ankle blood pressures may not accurately reflect true intraluminal arterial pressure because of the relative incompressibility of the arterial walls. The presence of normal digital waveforms in patients with calcified proximal vessels indicates minimal restriction to blood flow despite the calcific arterial disease. Conversely, an obstructive digital waveform in the presence of normal ankle pulses often indicates pedal artery occlusive disease, a situation often encountered in patients with diabetes or with distal atheroembolism (Figure 6-1).

DOPPLER ULTRASOUND TECHNIQUES

Ultrasound has proved to be the most important modality in the noninvasive evaluation of lower extremity ischemia. Ultrasound techniques are based on the principle that sound waves emitted from a transducer are reflected at the interface of two surfaces with different acoustic properties. By coupling the transducer with a receiver, and by knowing the transmitting frequency and the acoustical characteristics of the transmitting medium, the reflected ultrasound waves can be analyzed for energy loss and frequency shift by the receiver. With appropriate technology, these reflected waves can then be processed to produce a picture (B-mode image) or a velocity waveform. The generation of velocity waveforms is based on the observation that an ultrasound wave undergoes a frequency shift proportional to the velocity of any moving object (e.g., red blood cells) encountered, the Doppler principle. The reflected waves can be processed into audible signals (continuous-wave Doppler) or displayed as an analog waveform similar to the plethysmographically derived waveforms. If the angle between the transmitting ultrasound beam and the flowing blood is known, quantitative measurements of systolic and diastolic blood flow velocities can be derived from the analog waveforms by using the Doppler equation.

Ankle–Brachial Index

The ankle-to-brachial systolic pressure ratio is the simplest application of Doppler ultrasound to the noninvasive vascular laboratory and is perhaps also the most useful. It compares systolic blood pressures determined at the ankle with brachial artery systolic pressures. With a patient supine and resting, a pneumatic pressure cuff placed just above the ankle is inflated to suprasystolic levels. As the cuff is deflated, a handheld continuous-wave Doppler probe positioned over the posterior tibial or dorsalis pedis artery distal to the cuff is used to determine the systolic pressure—the cuff pressure at which distal blood flow, using the Doppler probe, is first heard as the cuff is deflated. These values are then compared with the highest brachial artery systolic pressure, also obtained with the Doppler device. Some controversy exists as to the best method to calculate an ankle–brachial index (ABI). However, for clinical purposes, the higher ipsilateral dorsal pedal or posterior tibial pressure is divided by the higher Doppler-determined brachial artery systolic pressure, yielding an ABI for that lower extremity. Changes in systolic pressure are used because

Table 6-1
Correlation between Ankle–Brachial Index (ABI) and Severity of Arterial Ischemia

ABI	Clinical Status
>1.4	Abnormal, significant arterial wall calcification
1.1 ± 0.1	Normal
0.6 ± 0.2	Intermittent claudication
0.3 ± 0.1	Ischemic rest pain
0.1 ± 0.1	Impending tissue necrosis

they are more sensitive to the presence of arterial occlusive disease than are changes in diastolic or mean pressure and because only systolic pressure can be accurately determined with the handheld Doppler probe. By comparing ankle systolic pressure with brachial artery systolic pressure, the test is relatively independent of day-to-day variations in arterial blood pressure, permitting quantitative comparison by serial examinations.

The ABI serves as an excellent indicator of the overall arterial supply of each lower extremity. A normal ABI is 1.0 to 1.2, with progressively lower values corresponding to worsening arterial disease (Table 6-1). This test, however, has several distinct limitations. Significant bilateral subclavian or axillary artery occlusive disease may result in a falsely elevated ABI. In addition, patients with longstanding renal failure or diabetes may have medial calcinosis of the popliteal and tibial arteries. Such calcific arteries may be inadequately compressed by the ankle pressure cuff, resulting in a falsely elevated (suprasystolic) ankle pressure or ABI. Indeed, an ABI greater than 1.4 should also be considered abnormal in that it indicates significant arterial disease and such patients have an increased risk of cardiovascular death. Under such circumstances, qualitative analysis of Doppler-derived analog or plethysmographic waveforms or measurement of digital systolic pressures is more appropriate. In the presence of severe arterial occlusive disease, no arterial Doppler signal may be audible at the ankle. Under such circumstances, venous signals may be confused with arterial signals. ABI is also relatively insensitive to certain patterns of progression of arterial disease. For example, a patient may occlude a tibial artery without a change in ABI if the remaining tibial vessels remain patent. Also, a more proximal high-grade stenosis may progress to occlusion without a change in ABI.

Segmental Limb Pressures

Multiple pneumatic cuffs may be used on the leg to determine the arterial blood pressure in different segments of the limb. These segmental leg pressures are compared with one another and with the higher brachial artery systolic pressure. Most laboratories prefer a four-cuff technique. Cuffs are placed (1) as far proximal on the thigh as possible, (2) immediately above the knee, (3) just below the knee, and (4) just proximal to the malleolus. Theoretically, each cuff width should be 20% greater than the diameter of the limb at the point of application.[6] This would in most cases necessitate a single, wide, thigh cuff. Use of two cuffs above the knee, however, may permit a determination of iliac artery inflow, as well as superficial femoral artery disease. Narrower cuffs may be associated with the measurement of artifactually high pressures. It is important to recognize that when four cuffs are used the most proximal

Abnormal segmental limb pressures

	RIGHT		LEFT	
	Pressure	Leg/arm ratio	Pressure	Leg/arm ratio
Arm	152		150	
Upper thigh	156	1.02	122	0.80
Above knee	144	0.94	120	0.79
Below knee	124	0.81	90	0.59
Ankle D.P.	136	0.89	96	0.63
P.T.	144	0.94	96	0.63
Toe	88	0.57	66	0.43

Figure 6-2. Abnormal segmental limb pressures. The left limb has an iliac or common femoral artery lesion, as well as a popliteal lesion. The right limb has a popliteal lesion.

thigh cuff is often theoretically too narrow and an artificially elevated pressure in the proximal thigh is expected. Normally, therefore, the high thigh index, comparing the proximal thigh pressure to the brachial pressure, is about 1.4 with the four-cuff technique and 1.0 to 1.1 with the three-cuff technique. An awareness of this problem helps avoid confusion in the interpretation of segmental limb pressures.

The examination is performed by using the handheld Doppler probe to detect the most prominent Doppler signal at the ankle. First, the high-thigh cuff is inflated until the Doppler signal at the ankle is no longer audible. The cuff is then deflated, and the cuff pressure at which return of the Doppler signal at the ankle occurs is the high-thigh pressure. The above-knee, below-knee, and ankle pressures are similarly determined. If no Doppler signal is audible at the ankle, the popliteal artery is examined with the Doppler probe. Under such circumstances, only high-thigh and above-knee pressures can be determined. By comparing the pressures at various levels in the leg, the physician can predict with reasonable accuracy the location of the arterial occlusive lesions (Figure 6-2 and Table 6-2).

Several potential problems and significant limitations arise in the interpretation of segmental limb pressures. In addition to cuff-induced artifacts, the high-thigh pressure is subject to

Table 6-2
Gradient Location and Corresponding Anatomical Location

Gradient Location	Corresponding Anatomical Location	Normal Vertical Gradient
Brachial–high thigh	Aorta, iliac artery, common femoral and superficial femoral arteries	+35-46 mm Hg
High thigh–above knee	Superficial femoral artery	−5-13 mm Hg
Above knee–high calf	Distal superficial femoral artery, popliteal artery	−12 mm Hg
High calf–ankle	Trifurcation vessels	−10-11 mm Hg
Ankle–toes	Pedal or digital arteries	−10 mm Hg

particular difficulties in interpretation. Ideally, the high-thigh pressure should reflect iliac artery inflow to the groin. A diminished high-thigh pressure should indicate a pressure-reducing stenosis in the ipsilateral common or external iliac artery. A diminished high-thigh pressure, however, may also reflect a significant common femoral stenosis or tandem pressure-reducing lesions in both the profunda femoris and the proximal superficial femoral artery. As noted, calcified arteries may also result in artificially elevated pressures. In patients with multilevel disease, diminished proximal pressures may mask gradients that exist farther down the leg. Finally, segmental pressure gradients give no information as to the nature of the pressure-reducing lesion. No differentiation is possible between short- and long-segment occlusions or between occluded versus patent but highly stenotic arteries.

Exercise Testing

Measurement of Doppler-determined pressures can be combined with treadmill exercise testing, assuming the patient does not have a significant medical contraindication to exercise. After determination of supine resting ankle pressures and the ABI, the patient is asked to walk continuously on a treadmill with a 10% incline at a predetermined rate, usually 1.5 miles per hour. The test lasts for 5 minutes or until the patient is forced to stop because of claudication symptoms. The time to onset of symptoms, as well as the location of the symptoms, is recorded. At completion of the test, the patient is immediately placed supine and the ABIs are determined. If the ABI has dropped from the resting measurement, ABIs are determined every 30 seconds until they return to normal. The greater the drop in the ABI with exercise, and the longer the time required to return to baseline, the more severe the patient's arterial occlusive disease (Figure 6-3).

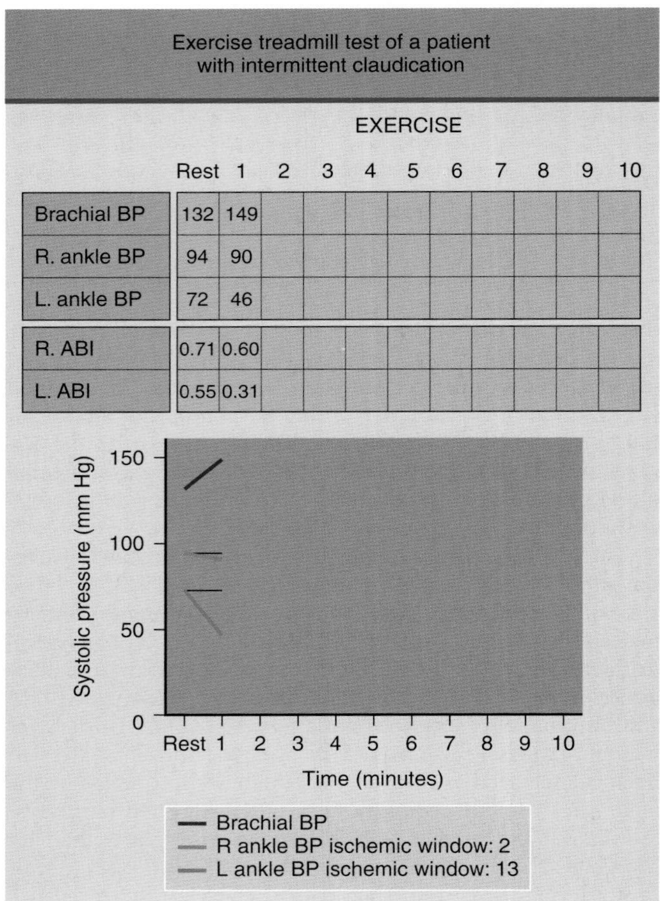

Figure 6-3. Exercise treadmill test of a patient with intermittent claudication. The ankle–brachial index drops significantly after 1 minute of exercise.

Whereas many laboratories perform exercise testing in all patients with suspected lower limb arterial insufficiency, the examination in most patients only confirms the diagnosis suspected by history and physical examination. A patient with classic symptoms of claudication and absent peripheral pulses, combined with a diminished ABI at rest in the appropriate lower extremity, does not require routine exercise testing for the determination of ABI decrease and recovery. Exercise testing may be helpful in following postoperative patients and documenting a physiological response to revascularization. The postexercise recovery of ankle pressure can provide an objective assessment of the potential postoperative physiological benefit.

Exercise testing is particularly useful in the occasional patient with symptoms of claudication who has palpable pedal pulses at rest and a normal or near-normal ABI. Patients with claudication secondary to arterial insufficiency show a significant decrease in the postexercise ABI. The exact endpoints and techniques of exercise testing are controversial. Some laboratories exercise patients at low speeds with no inclination of the treadmill, while others use various inclines and graded increases in treadmill velocity. Both initial and absolute claudication distances can be determined. The initial claudication distance is the point at which the patient first experiences claudication type pain. The absolute claudication distance is that point at which the patient can no longer continue the examination. In our clinical vascular laboratory, patients are exercised with zero incline of the treadmill at 1.5 mph and absolute claudication distance is the endpoint.

The criteria for a positive exercise treadmill test include a decrease in the absolute ankle pressure of 20 mm Hg, or 20%, or a decrease in the ABI of 0.2 in the symptomatic extremity after exercise testing. With the exception of the rare patient with buttock claudication secondary to isolated internal iliac disease, failure of the ABI to decrease 20% with exercise, in association with a normal resting ABI, substantially rules out arterial insufficiency as the cause of the patient's exercise-induced leg pain. The oft-encountered condition of spinal stenosis and neurogenic claudication may be confused with arterial ischemia. These patients also typically present with symptoms of exercise-induced leg or calf pain, but careful questioning reveals atypical characteristics, including occurrence of the pain with standing, occasional pain relief by leaning forward, worsening with coughing, and prolonged time requirement for pain abatement after exercise. In these patients, exercise testing reveals normal ankle pressures that do not decrease with exercise despite the onset of symptoms. Failure of the ankle pressures to decrease with exercise may also be a clue to the presence of other uncommon conditions, such as venous claudication and chronic exercise-induced compartment syndromes. Another, more common indication for exercise testing is to try and document an arterial ischemic response to exercise in patients with PAD and multiple other common conditions that may limit their ability to walk. Patients with chronic obstructive pulmonary disease, arthritis, venous disease, and PAD are often more limited in their walking ability by these coexisting conditions than by their PAD. If the patients cannot complete a treadmill examination but no ischemic pressure response to exercise occurs, it is highly unlikely their walking ability would be improved by a revascularization procedure.

Doppler Analog Waveform Analysis

Doppler analog waveforms may be obtained using a continuous-wave Doppler probe and may be analyzed qualitatively analogous to plethysmographic waveforms. Normal lower-extremity Doppler waveforms are triphasic, with a reverse flow component in early diastole and low end-diastolic forward flow. The reverse flow component and low overall diastolic velocities reflect a relatively high end-organ resistance to blood flow in the resting extremity. With increasing proximal stenosis, the shape of the waveform changes. Initially, the reverse flow component is lost. With more severe degrees of stenosis, the rate of rise of the systolic upstroke is decreased, the amplitude of the waveform is diminished, and diastolic flow increases relative to systolic flow.

The primary clinical application of qualitative Doppler waveform analysis has been in assessing the adequacy of iliac artery inflow to the common femoral artery. An attenuated waveform recorded from the common femoral artery indicates proximal disease. Unfortunately, the technique cannot quantify stenosis or distinguish between iliac stenosis and occlusion. In addition, attenuated waveforms may be caused by superficial femoral artery disease or a combination of superficial femoral and aortoiliac disease.

Peripheral Arterial Duplex Scanning

Arterial duplex scanning provides detailed anatomical and hemodynamic information that cannot be determined by the indirect noninvasive tests (pulse volume recording, segmental pressures, ABI). Duplex scanning uses both B-mode ultrasound and pulsed Doppler ultrasound. The combination of color Doppler and B-mode ultrasound allows assessment of anatomical and hemodynamic abnormalities from the infrarenal aorta to the distal tibial vessels. B-mode imaging alone cannot reliably distinguish hemodynamically significant soft plaque and thrombus from blood. However, Doppler ultrasound is able to detect the flow disturbances created by these lesions. B-mode ultrasound visualizes calcified plaque and localizes the artery of interest. This permits the precise placement of the Doppler sample volume at a known angle to the artery being examined. Knowledge of the angle of insonation allows quantitative determination of frequency shifts. Blood flow velocities can be calculated from the frequency shift to determine the degree of stenosis of an arterial lesion. Arterial duplex scanning has been prospectively compared with angiography to establish standard criteria for normal and diseased arteries.[7] In this study, the sensitivity of the duplex examination for detecting the presence of a hemodynamically significant lesion (>50%) ranged from 89% at the iliac artery to 68% at the popliteal artery. Overall sensitivities for predicting interruption of patency were 90% for the anterior tibial, 90% for the posterior tibial, and 82% for the peroneal artery. The sensitivity of arterial duplex mapping is not heavily influenced by the severity of atherosclerotic disease (Figure 6-4).

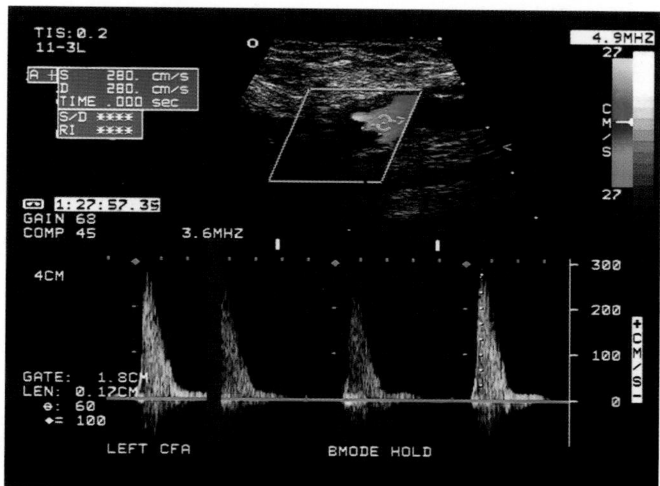

Figure 6-4. Arterial duplex of a left common femoral artery stenosis. The velocity is elevated, and there is loss of the triphasic waveform.

Examination, Equipment, and Personnel

Color-flow imaging facilitates the duplex examination by aiding in rapid identification of the arteries, thereby decreasing the overall time for the examination. Color flow is particularly useful for evaluating the iliac arteries, the popliteal trifurcation, and the tibial vessels. Also, color flow can identify the presence and length of an arterial occlusion, as well as the distal site of reconstitution. Color-flow changes are not used to determine specific percent degrees of stenosis other than occlusion. The degree of stenosis of a subocclusive lesion is determined with velocity waveform analysis.

Lower extremity arterial duplex examination requires various transducers. A 2-MHz or 3-MHz transducer is required for evaluating the iliac vessels. Infrainguinal vessels can be examined with a 5-MHz transducer. Examining the superficial femoral artery in patients with large legs occasionally requires a lower-frequency transducer. Conversely, the tibial vessels are best examined with a higher-frequency transducer.

Using angle-corrected velocity recordings is of practical necessity when examining peripheral arteries. Varying body habitus and depth of vessels makes it impossible to insonate all portions of the peripheral arteries using a constant angle with the currently available technology. Although 60 degrees is considered the ideal angle of insonation, angles between 30 and 70 degrees are sufficiently accurate for the peripheral arterial examination.[8]

The complete lower-extremity arterial duplex examination includes evaluation of the infrarenal aorta; the common and external iliac arteries; the profunda origin; the proximal, middle, and distal superficial femoral arteries; the popliteal artery; and the tibial vessels. The tibial arteries should be evaluated from the popliteal trifurcation to the level of the ankle. Examining patients after a fast of 8 to

Table 6-3
Duplex Ultrasound Blood Flow Velocities (Mean ± Standard Deviation) of Normal Lower Extremity Arterial Segments

Artery	Peak Systolic Velocity (cm/sec)
External iliac	119 ± 21
Common femoral	114 ± 25
Superficial femoral	91 ± 14
Popliteal	69 ± 14

12 hours reduces abdominal gas and facilitates examination of the intra-abdominal vessels. The entire examination is performed with the patient in the supine position, except for the popliteal artery, which is best examined in the prone or lateral position.

Velocities should be routinely recorded from several sites along a vessel and from any site where a flow disturbance is identified. Areas both of high velocity, suggestive of a hemodynamically significant stenosis, and of low velocity, indicating a more proximal stenosis or occlusion, should be noted. Table 6-3 demonstrates the expected duplex ultrasound velocities of normal arterial segments.

The lower extremity arterial duplex study is most efficient when it follows a physical examination, determination of segmental pressures, and exercise testing. If these tests are normal, arterial duplex is generally not indicated. Abnormalities in the physical examination, the segmental pressures, or both can guide the technologist to examine certain areas with more detail. A complete arterial duplex study in a patient with complicated arterial anatomy may require 1 to 1.5 hours (Figure 6-5).

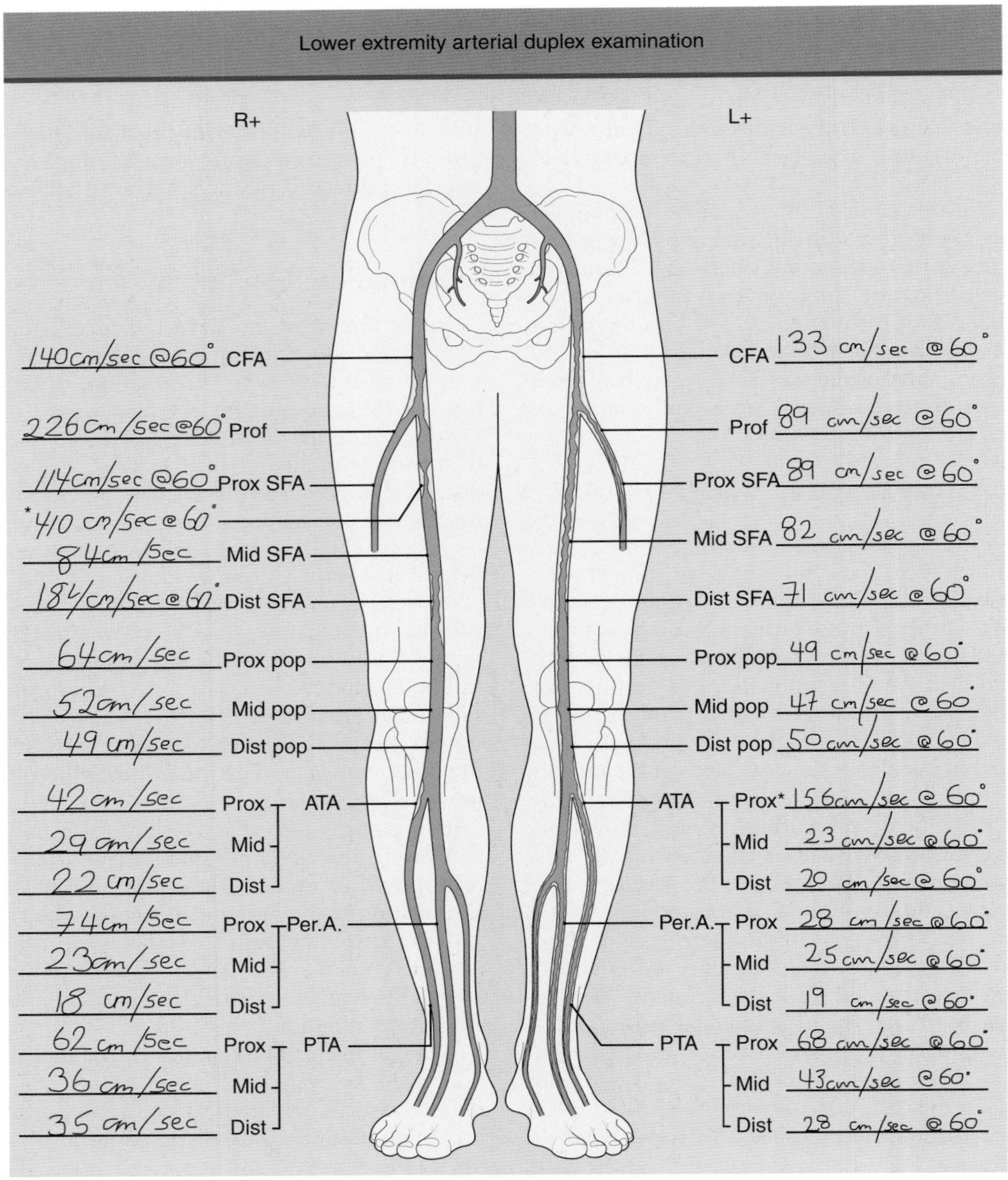

Figure 6-5. Lower extremity arterial duplex examination. This patient has diffuse arteriosclerosis of the left lower extremity and a right superficial femoral artery stenosis.

Velocity Patterns and Classifications of Stenosis

Duplex-derived velocity waveforms of normal resting peripheral arteries are triphasic with a short reverse flow component at the end of systole. End-diastolic flow is near zero because of the high end-organ resistance associated with the peripheral circulation. The triphasic waveform is maintained throughout the leg, but the peak systolic velocities (PSVs) decrease steadily from the iliac to the tibial vessels.

The hemodynamic significance of a given lesion is determined by analysis of duplex velocity waveforms. Important features that signify disease include the absence of the reverse flow component and an elevated PSV. Traditionally, a 50% reduction in arterial diameter (equivalent to a cross-sectional surface area reduction of 75%) is considered to be associated with a significant drop in blood pressure across the lesion.

The original classification criteria derived for the noninvasive quantification of peripheral arterial stenosis were developed at the University of Washington (Table 6-4). This classification system uses spectral broadening to discriminate between lesions of 1% to 19% stenosis and those of 20% to 49% stenosis.[9] The assessment of spectral broadening, however, requires a constant Doppler angle, which is often not possible in peripheral duplex scanning. Therefore, analysis of varying degrees of spectral broadening has practical limitations in the evaluation of PAD.

The PSV ratio is also a widely accepted tool for grading the degree of stenosis. This ratio is based on the principle that the total flow at a lesion must be the same as the immediate pre- and poststenotic area; therefore, a change in velocity is directly proportional to a change in cross-sectional area. The main advantage of the PSV ratio is that it is independent of changes in blood pressure, cardiac output, and vascular compliance. Typically, the velocity within a stenosis is compared with the velocity just proximal to the stenosis. Grading of stenoses using the PSV ratio has been found to be highly reproducible.[10,11] A 50% stenosis in the lower extremity has been considered by different investigators to correlate with a PSV ratio from 1.4 to 3.0,[7,12-15] although a velocity ratio of 2.0 is used by most vascular laboratories as indicative of a 50% lesion.

Table 6-4
University of Washington Duplex Criteria for Determination of Peripheral Arterial Stenosis

Degree of Stenosis (%)	Criteria
0	Normal waveform velocities
1-19	Normal waveform velocities with spectral broadening
20-49	Marked spectral broadening, 30% increase in peak systolic velocity
50-99	Marked spectral broadening, 100% increase in peak systolic velocity, loss of reverse diastolic flow component of waveform
Occluded	No detectable flow signal in well-visualized artery

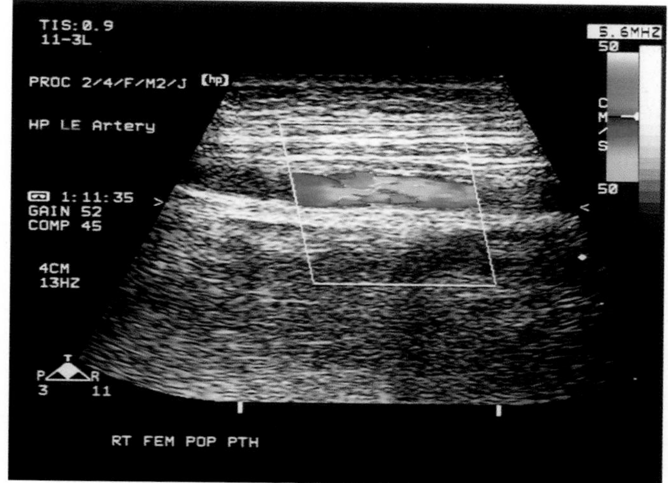

Figure 6-6. Arterial duplex of a right femoral popliteal reverse vein graft.

Clinical Applications

For the past decade, research efforts have focused on the ability of lower extremity duplex to replace contrast arteriography in the preoperative assessment of candidates for arterial intervention. Arterial duplex is clearly less invasive, less expensive, and safer than arteriography; however, this technology is highly operator dependent. Also, the technical success rate of imaging the infrapopliteal arteries is reported to be 82% to 90%.[7] Nevertheless, in selected centers, successful lower-extremity revascularization either by open arterial bypass grafting or with catheter-based techniques can be completed using only arterial duplex in a high percentage of cases.[16-18] Overall, the limiting factor with preoperative arterial duplex is the ability to accurately identify the best site for the distal anastomosis of a bypass graft, especially when the distal anastomotic site is below the knee.[19]

The role of duplex ultrasound scanning in the surveillance of lower extremity vein grafts has been well documented (Figures 6-6 and 6-7). Detection and repair of graft-threatening

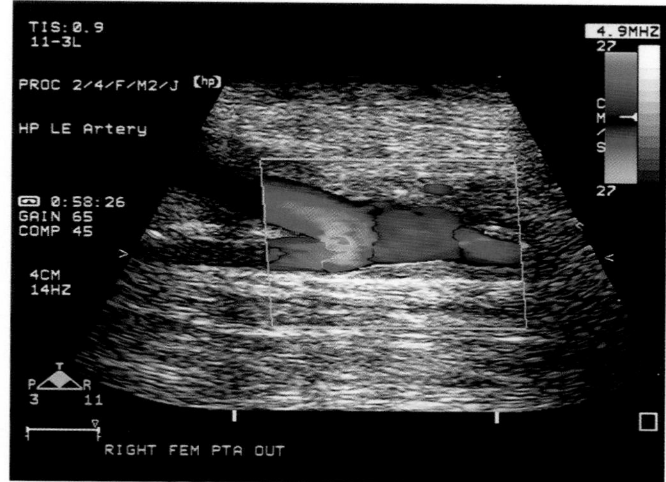

Figure 6-7. Arterial duplex of the distal anastomosis of a right femoral posterior tibial vein graft.

stenoses improve graft patency.[20-23] Of vein grafts, 20% to 30% develop a stenosis, which requires revision.[24] These lesions are readily identified and monitored for progression by duplex ultrasound. The recommended regimen for vein graft duplex surveillance is every 3 months for the first year and every 6 months thereafter. Approximately 80% of vein graft stenoses develop in the first postoperative year, but because lesions can develop at any time, surveillance is generally recommended for the life of the graft. The examination involves insonation of the proximal inflow artery, proximal anastomosis, midgraft, distal anastomosis, and distal outflow artery. A PSV ratio of 4, or a PSV above 300 cm/sec, indicates a critical graft stenosis, and repair of the lesion by open or catheter-based techniques should be considered.[25] If the PSV ratio is between 2 and 4, the patient should be reevaluated in 3 months with a duplex examination.

SUMMARY

The noninvasive vascular laboratory provides critically important, objective information to supplement a careful history and physical examination in the evaluation of patients with chronic lower-extremity ischemia. Optimal utilization of vascular testing will always depend on a sophisticated knowledge of vascular disease and detailed knowledge of the individual patient. A keen awareness of the limitations of each form of testing and potential sources of error is mandatory. Noninvasive vascular testing allows quantitative, physiological assessment of lower extremity ischemia and provides the scientific basis for modern therapeutic approaches to the care of patients with arterial occlusive disease. Clearly, the vascular laboratory provides the objective diagnostic foundation on which the modern practice of vascular surgery is built.

References

1. Yao JST, Nedham TN, Gourmos C. A comparative study of strain gauge plethysmography and Doppler ultrasound in the assessment of occlusive arterial disease of the lower extremities. *Surgery* 1972;71:4-9.
2. Yao JST, Flinn WR. Plethysmography. In: Kempczinski RF, Yao JST, eds. *Practical noninvasive vascular diagnosis.* Chicago: Yearbook Medical Publishers; 1987:80-94.
3. Darling RC, Raines JK, Brener BF. Quantitative segmental pulse volume recorder: a clinical tool. *Surgery* 1972;72:873-887.
4. Strandness DE. *Peripheral arterial disease: a physiologic approach.* Boston: Little, Brown; 1969:112-130.
5. Kempczinski RF. Segmental volume plethysmography: the pulse volume recorder. In: Kempczinski RF, Yao JST, eds. *Practical noninvasive vascular diagnosis.* Chicago: Yearbook Medical Publishers; 1987: 140-153.
6. Krikendall WM, Burton AC, Epstein FH, et al. Recommendations for human blood pressure determination by sphygmomanometers: report of a subcommittee of the postgraduate education committee, American Heart Association. *Circulation* 1967;36:980-988.
7. Moneta GL, Yeager RA, Antonovic R, et al. Accuracy of lower extremity arterial duplex mapping. *J Vasc Surg* 1992;15:275-284.
8. Rizzo RJ, Sandager G, Astleford P, et al. Mesenteric flow velocity variations as a function of angle of insonation. *J Vasc Surg* 1990;11:688-694.
9. Jager KA, Ricketts HJ, Strandness DE. Duplex scanning for evaluation of lower limb arterial disease. In: Bernstein EF, ed. *Noninvasive diagnostic techniques in vascular disease.* St Louis: Mosby; 1985:619-631.
10. Whyman MR, Hoskins PR, Leng GC, et al. Accuracy and reproducibility of duplex ultrasound imaging in a phantom model of femoral artery stenosis. *J Vasc Surg* 1993;17:524-530.
11. Leng GC, Whyman MR, Donnan PT, et al. Accuracy and reproducibility of duplex ultrasonography in grading femoropopliteal stenoses. *J Vasc Surg* 1993;17:510-517.
12. Sacks D, Robinson ML, Marinelli DL, Perlmutter GS. Peripheral arterial Doppler ultrasonography: diagnostic criteria. *J Ultrasound Med* 1992;11:95-103.
13. Jager KA, Phillips DJ, Martin RL, et al. Noninvasive mapping of lower limb arterial lesions. *Ultrasound Med Biol* 1985;11:515-521.
14. Sensier Y, Hartshorne T, Thrush A, Nydahl S, Bolia A, London NJ. A prospective comparison of lower limb colour-coded duplex scanning with arteriography. *Eur J Vasc Endovasc Surg* 1996;11:170-175.
15. de Smet AA, Ermers EJ, Kitslaar PJ. Duplex velocity characteristics of aortoiliac stenoses. *J Vasc Surg* 1996;23:628-636.
16. Elsman BH, Legemate DA, van der Heijden FH, de Vos HJ, Mali WP, Eikelboom BC. Impact of ultrasonographic duplex scanning on therapeutic decision making in lower-limb arterial disease. *Br J Surg* 1995;82: 630-633.
17. Ascher E, Mazzariol F, Hingorani A, Salles-Cunha S, Gade P. The use of duplex ultrasound arterial mapping as an alternative to conventional arteriography for primary and secondary infrapopliteal bypasses. *Am J Surg* 1999;178:162-165.
18. Mazzariol F, Ascher E, Salles-Cunha SX, Gade P, Hingorani A. Values and limitations of duplex ultrasonography as the sole imaging method of preoperative evaluation for popliteal and infrapopliteal bypasses. *Ann Vasc Surg* 1999;13:1-10.
19. Larch E, Minar E, Ahmadi R, et al. Value of color duplex sonography for evaluation of tibioperoneal arteries in patients with femoropopliteal obstruction: a prospective comparison with anterograde intra-arterial digital subtraction angiography. *J Vasc Surg* 1997;25:629-636.
20. Landry GJ, Moneta GL, Taylor Jr LM, Edwards JM, Yeager RA, Porter JM. Patency and characteristics of lower extremity vein grafts requiring multiple revisions. *J Vasc Surg* 2000;32:23-31.
21. Johnson BL, Bandyk DF, Back MR, Avino AJ, Roth SM. Intraoperative duplex monitoring of infrainguinal vein bypass procedures. *J Vasc Surg* 2000;31:678-690.
22. Idu MM, Blankenstein JD, de Gier P, Truyen E, Buth J. Impact of a color-flow duplex surveillance program on infrainguinal vein graft patency: a five-year experience. *J Vasc Surg* 1993;17:42-52. discussion, 52-53.
23. Lundell A, Lindblad B, Bergqvist D, Hansen F. Femoropopliteal-crural graft patency is improved by an intensive surveillance program: a prospective randomized study. *J Vasc Surg* 1995;21:26-33. discussion, 33-34.
24. Passman MA, Moneta GL, Nehler MR, et al. Do normal early color-flow duplex surveillance examination results of infrainguinal vein grafts preclude the need for late graft revision?. *J Vasc Surg* 1995;22:476-481. discussion, 482-484.
25. Mills JL Sr, Wixon CL, James DC, Devine J, Westerband A, Hughes JD. The natural history of intermediate and critical vein graft stenosis: recommendations for continued surveillance or repair. *J Vasc Surg* 2001;33:273-278. discussion, 278-280.

chapter

7

Vascular Imaging and Radiation Safety

Marcelo Guimaraes, MD • Claudio Schönholz, MD • Renan Uflacker, MD • Walter Huda, PhD

Key Points

- Catheter angiography
  - Angiographic technique
  - Contrast media
  - Digital subtraction angiography
- Computed tomography angiography
  - Technical aspects of the MDCT angiography
  - Patient preparation
  - Scan acquisition
  - Post processing techniques
  - Maximum intensity projection (MIP)
  - Volume rendering (VR)
  - Multiplanar reconstruction (MPR)
  - Curved planar reconstruction (CPR)
  - Virtual angioscopy (VA)
  - CTA limitations
  - Contraindications for MDCT angiography
- Magnetic resonance angiography
  - Magnetic resonance angiography techniques
  - Phase-contrast magnetic resonance angiography
  - Time-of-flight magnetic resonance angiography
  - Three-dimensional half-fourier fast spin-echo magnetic resonance angiography
  - Balanced steady state free precession magnetic resonance angiography
  - Contrast-enhanced magnetic resonance angiography
  - Whole-body contrast-enhanced magnetic Resonance angiography
  - Patient preparation
  - Protocol and contrast media in CE-MRA
  - Specific sequences applications to the vascular anatomy
  - Synchronization of the contrast injection and acquisition in 3-D CE-MRA
  - MRA post-processing
- Clinical applications
  - Nonatherosclerotic vascular disease
  - Evaluation of peripheral artery stents
  - Lower extremities vascular occlusive disease
  - Thoracic and abdominal aorta
    - Aortic dissection
    - Aortic aneurysm
    - Aortic occlusive disease
  - Aneurysmal disease of the lower extremities
  - Pulmonary embolism
  - Carotid and supra-aortic arteries
  - Renal arteries
- Summary
- Radiation safety
  - X-rays and matter
  - Deterministic effects
  - Stochastic effects
  - Effective dose

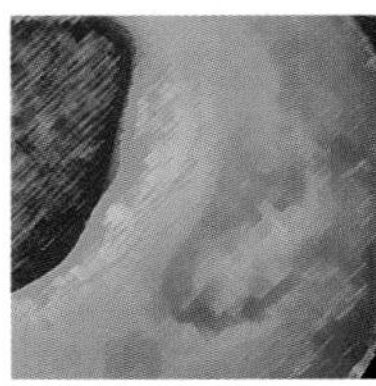

Peripheral vascular disease (PVD) accounts for 50,000 to 60,000 cases of percutaneous transluminal angioplasty and for about 100,000 cases of amputation annually in the United States. Proper treatment of the arterial disease requires a comprehensive assessment of the underlying vascular morphology because it is crucial to localize and gauge the severity of arterial lesions for further therapeutic decision making.

Digital subtraction angiography (DSA) has traditionally been used for anatomical assessment of PVD. DSA provides a precise roadmap for planning treatment, but because of its invasiveness, DSA is associated with a nondespicable morbidity risk.[1] As a result, catheter angiography is used less for diagnosis and more as an adjunct to endovascular procedures.

The noninvasive image techniques have many benefits, such as evaluation of the patient's vascular anatomy and its variations and treatment planning with much less risk to the patient inherent to the catheter angiography.

The development in the endovascular procedures has occurred in parallel with the availability of new and different noninvasive diagnostic vascular imaging applications. Doppler ultrasound, magnetic resonance angiography (MRA) and computed tomography angiography (CTA) are now among the tools of diagnostic algorithms for cardiovascular disease. They afford more widespread vascular screening, with subsequent early diagnosis and potential better prognosis. Noninvasive imaging techniques are increasingly being used for clinical decision making in patients with vasculites, arteriovenous malformations (AVMs), aneurysm, and dissections, as well as in suspected arterial occlusive disease. Most medical institutions have actually replaced catheter angiography for diagnostic purposes. For example, CTA is a well-established tool in assessing thoracic aortic aneurysm and abdominal aortic aneurysm (AAA) and ruling out the significant pulmonary embolism and pulmonary AVMs. Similarly, MRA is a great nonionizing radiation diagnostic tool for carotid and renal artery stenoses and assessing tool for potential kidney donors. The noninvasive vascular studies have revolutionized not only the diagnostic but also the comprehensive clinical management and treatment of PVD.[2]

The level, multiplicity, and severity of the vascular diseases, with arterial stenosis as a good example, may show significant variation that affects the final decision, including a more restricted and selective usage of the catheter angiography.[3] As the noninvasive imaging modalities have multiple applications, it is important to guarantee that the interpretations of these relatively new imaging techniques are reproducible and reliable.

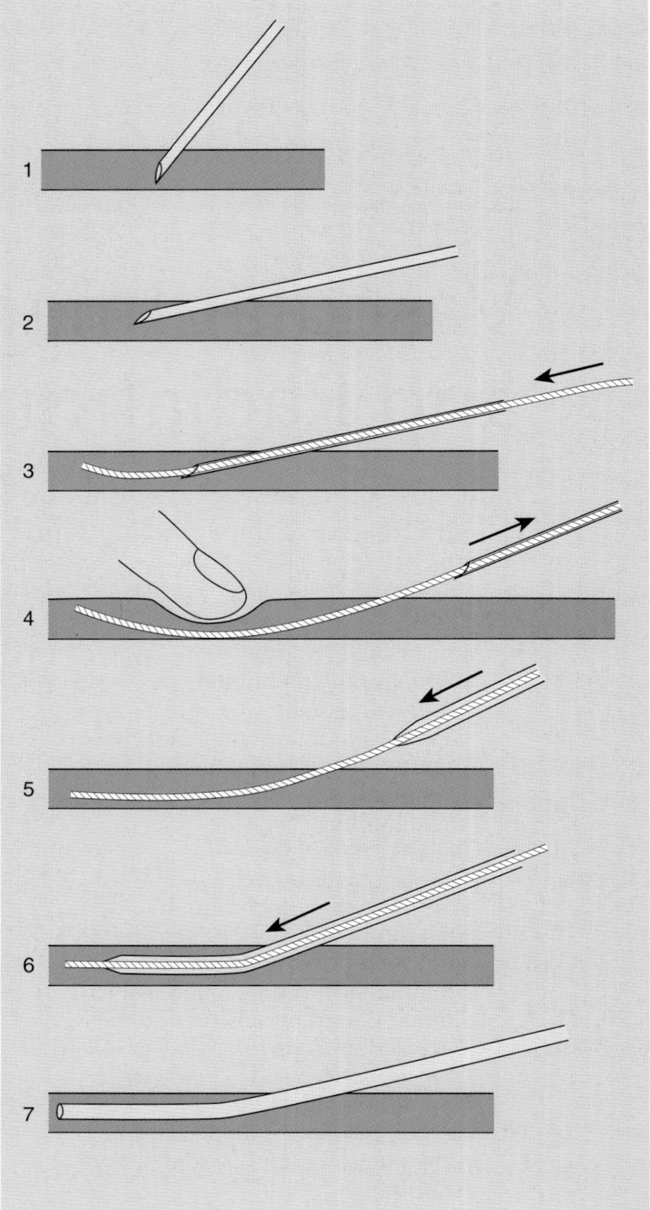

Figure 7-1. Seldinger technique. *(1)* Percutaneous vessel (artery or vein) puncture with a puncture needle, *(2)* backflow is observed through the needle, *(3)* a guide wire is advanced through the needle, *(4)* pressure is held over the puncture site while the needle is pulled out with the guide wire in place, *(5-6)* a diagnostic catheter or an introducer sheath may be advanced over the wire, and *(7)* the wire is removed and percutaneous intravascular access is obtained. (From Uflacker R. Wholley M. *Interventional radiology*. New York: McGraw Hill; 1991, 1.)

CATHETER ANGIOGRAPHY

The catheter angiography method of image provides vascular diagnosis with the highest resolution and accuracy. It is an invasive procedure requiring catheter placement in the area of interest of the vascular system, iodine-based contrast media injection, and ionizing radiation-based images. With simultaneous development of CTA and MRA diagnostic techniques, catheter angiography nowadays is mainly use in three situations: for diagnostic purposes when the vascular disease is still unclear after a noninvasive imaging study, in emergency situations when prompt endovascular or hybrid procedures are required, and as a guiding tool during elective endovascular procedures.

In 1953, the Norwegian physician Sven Ivan Seldinger described the technique principles of the percutaneous selective vascular catheterization (Figure 7-1).

Seldinger's innovative technique revolutionized catheter angiography because it allowed vascular access without surgical dissection and vessel exposure. The technique includes the following steps: vascular (artery or vein) percutaneous needle puncture, guide wire insertion, needle removal, and subsequent over-the-wire catheter intravascular placement. The development of thermoplastic and radiopaque catheters and excellent fluoroscopic equipment, associated with the dissemination of Seldinger's technique, were some important factors that paved the way for the development of the endovascular therapy.

Noninvasive imaging methods such as the Doppler ultrasound, CTA, and MRA have been widely used in the diagnosis of vascular diseases, with subsequent decrease in the number of catheter-based digital subtraction angiographies. Certainly this shift represents advancement in modern medical practice, with several advantages for the patients. However, the progressive reduction in the number of catheter-based angiographies may compromise the training of the future endovascular interventionists. The current "simulators" or the virtual training stations offer a promising "hands-on" opportunity to obtain adequate training, especially critical for procedures such as carotid artery stenting angioplasty. The main hands-on limitation is the lack of refined and gentle movements that real-life cases may require, resulting in a longer learning curve for appropriate hand skills.

Angiographic Technique

Before starting the procedure, every patient should be evaluated. The evaluation consists of obtaining an objective anamnesis to be aware of the patient's symptoms, a progression of the existing complaint (acute or chronic), comorbidities (e.g., diabetes mellitus or renal or hepatic insufficiency), prior surgeries, current medications, and history of drug allergy (e.g., previous exposure to iodine contrast). Physical examination should be focused to check the patient's vascular system according to the existing symptom, the potential vascular access (rule out local infection, presence of pulse), and the evidence of scar tissue related to prior surgical bypass and of chronic vascular disease such as skin trophic changes, lower extremities hair loss, positional redness, and skin temperature changes. Patients' blood pressure should be measured and, if necessary, controlled before any elective procedure to avoid complications. The blood pressure of bilateral upper extremities should be measured in case of brachial artery access or if the complaint is related to this vascular territory. Some essential precautions should be considered before the catheter angiogram. For insulin-dependent diabetes mellitus, the patient should take half of the usual dose when fasting starts. Blood glucose should be check before the procedure. In patients with renal and or hepatic insufficiency, it is important to check the dosage of medications used during the angiogram to avoid overdose and subsequent potential clinical complications, such as oversedation. Multiple myeloma and diabetic nephropathy patients have a higher chance of developing acute tubular necrosis and renal insufficiency when iodine-based contrast is used. Aggressive hydration should be taken into consideration if the patient can tolerate the volume (careful attention in dialysis and heart failure patients). Sickle cell disease and polycythemia vera patients have a higher risk of developing thromboembolic complications.

Contrast Media

The ideal contrast media is the one that presents excellent radiopacity, has easy blood solubility, is friendly to use, and causes no harm to the patient. The current iodine contrasts are close to achieving the ideal features to be used in the human body.

Table 7-1
Examples of Iodine Contrast Media and Their Osmolality

Agent Name	Brand Name	Osmolality*
Diatrizoato	Hypaque	1500-1700
Iotalamato	Convey	1500-1700
Iohexol	Ominpaque	600-700
Ioversol	Optiray	600-700
Ioxaglato	Hexabrix	560
Iodixanol	Visipaque	300

*Approximate osmolality in milliosmoles per kilogram of water.

There are two categories of iodine contrast agents: ionic and nonionic. The ionic contrast media agents have high solubility and low viscosity but have high osmolality. The higher osmolality in comparison to the blood is known to be the most important contributing factor to allergies and adverse reactions such as nausea and vomiting. On the other hand, the nonionic contrast media do not have electrical charge (cations free), so it is possible to reduce the osmolality of the contrast media. The main advantage is the increased safety profile, with the disadvantage of being more viscous. Table 7-1 shows examples of the most common iodine contrast media. Most allergic reactions to iodine contrast are mild and rare.

Nausea and pain represent the most common complaints. Most adverse reactions are related to contrast media osmolality, as the incidence of complications is higher when ionic contrast media are used (Table 7-2).

Nausea and vomiting are more common when the iodine contrast agent is administered intravenously than intraarterially. Apparently a central nervous system mechanism is responsible for the difference.[3]

The intravascular infusion of the contrast media may be performed manually or through a power injector. During the selective catheterizations, hand contrast injection may be performed, using a 10-ml syringe, to obtain a catheter angiography. It is a simple and safe method, as long as it was excluded the presence of air in the syringe. When the goal is to opacify multiple vessels simultaneously (e.g., celiac trunk angiogram) or a single large diameter vessel such as the aorta, power injectable injections are preferred because large volumes of contrast media and adequate injection flow are key elements for a diffuse and homogeneous opacification. Before connecting the diagnostic catheter into the power injector,

Table 7-2
Incidence of Adverse Reactions to Iodine Contrast Agents

Reaction	Incidence in Ionic Contrast	Incidence in Nonionic Contrast
Nausea	4.6%	1.0%
Vomiting	1.8%	0.4%
Itching	3.0%	0.5%
Urticaria	3.0%	0.5%
Sneezing	1.7%	0.2%
Dyspnea	0.2%	0.04%
Hypotension	0.1%	0.01%
Death	1:40,000	1:170,000

Table 7-3
Management of Mild Allergic Reactions

- First check the ABCs of the advanced cardiac life support: airway, breathing, circulation. Check the patient's airway. If the patient is capable of answering "no" to the question "Are you experiencing any difficulties in breathing or any sensation of tightness in your throat?," it is because there is no severe airway compromise. Administer oxygen using a nasal cannula or a venturi mask according to the oxygen saturation.
- Check the vital signs. Resuscitate with IV fluids if the patient experiences hypotension or if significant drop in the baseline blood pressure occurs. (Keep in mind that versed and fentanyl commonly used for conscious sedation also may cause a drop in blood pressure independent of the allergic reaction.)
- Double-check the patency of the existing venous access. If there is any difficulty, a second IV access must obtained immediately.
- Administer Benadryl, 50 mg IV, in bolus.
- Administer hydrocortisone, 100 mg IV, in bolus.
- For a mild bronchospasm:
    - Administer 0.5 ml (2.5 mg) of albuterol in 2.5 ml of normal saline using an inhalation nebulizer.
    - Administer 0.3 ml of epinephrine (1:1000) subcutaneously, repeating every 20 minutes as needed.

double-check whether the parameters have been set up correctly for that particular angiogram (total volume in milliliters, flow rate in cubic centimeters per second, and maximum injection pressure in pounds per square inch).

The pressure that every diagnostic catheter may tolerate is indicated on the catheter package label. If that level is not respected, catheter rupture may happen. The correct maximum injection pressure and flow rate are also important to prevent vascular dissection or to blow up a small vessel.

The major adverse reaction to iodine contrast is anaphylaxis contrast-induced nephropathy (CIN). Life-threatening anaphylaxis incidence related to contrast media is 1 in 40,000 to 170,000 procedures. The mild adverse reactions, such as urticaria and nasal congestion, are by far the most common, especially when ionic contrast media is used.

The treatment for severe adverse reactions to iodine contrast must be instituted immediately. As the airway obstruction is responsible for most reported deaths, material for endotracheal intubation should be promptly available in the angiography suite. The management of the mild allergic reactions and of the severe anaphylaxis is presented in Tables 7-3 and 7-4.[4]

Table 7-4
Management of Severe Allergic Reactions

- Call the "Code" team.
- Check the patient's airway as stated in Table 7-3. The goal is to keep the airway patent. Be ready to intubate or to perform cricothyroidotomy if needed.
- Double-check the IV access. In cases of severe hypotension, central IV access should be obtained.
- Administer 3-5 ml of epinephrine (1:10,000) IV or via endotracheal tube.
- Administer hydrocortisone, 500 mg IV, in bolus.
- Use aggressive fluid resuscitation with normal saline or lactated Ringer's solution.
- Start vasopressor IV if needed.
- Admit the patient to the intensive care unit.

Table 7-5
Prophylaxis for the Patients with History of Iodine Contrast Allergy

- Check the possibility of using a different diagnostic image method in case of a diagnostic arteriogram.
- Use nonionic contrast media.
- Give the following premedication IV (in bolus) before starting the procedure:
    - Benadryl, 50 mg
    - Hydrocortisone, 125 mg
    - Cimetidine, 300 mg

For those patients with a positive history of contrast allergy to contrast iodine, a detailed history of the episode should be obtained to rule out a true allergic reaction, as it is not uncommon that symptoms such as dizziness and headache to be misinterpreted as a contrast allergy. Once the history is confirmed, the procedure is canceled or the protocol medication for contrast allergy is administered before the beginning of the procedure (Table 7-5).

Since the CIN was identified in 1950s, a great body of knowledge has been built. However, a couple of key questions remain unclear. And although the anatomy of the pathology is clear, but the pathophysiology still needs to be better understood.[5]

How can the CIN be diagnosed? In general, an increase in the serum creatinine (sCr) level occurs in the first 24 to 48 hours after exposure to the contrast media, and the peak of the increased level may be reached in 72 to 96 hours. The patient may present oliguria and less often anuria. Usually, the sCr level drops to normal levels in 7 to 14 days. Nonetheless, today it is well known that the sCr level does not reflect the renal function or the glomerular filtration rate (GFR) accurately. As the sCr levels varies according to age, gender, race, and muscular mass, an isolated value of sCr of 1.2 mg/dl in a 20-year-old man can be completely normal. On the other hand, the same sCr level in an 80-year-old man may indicate marked GFR reduction. It is important to understand that no linear correlation exists between the GFR and sCr levels and their implications as markers of safety. For example, the kidney damage caused by CIN may be masked in patients with a normal sCr level before the diagnostic or interventional procedure. Of the total kidney parenchyma mass, 50% can be damaged without any alteration in the global renal function measured exclusively by the sCr, although the creatinine clearance is reduced in this case. Patients with an elevated baseline sCr level are at higher risk of developing CIN because they have a reduced renal functional reserve. Additional lost of 10% in the renal parenchyma may lead the patient to hemodialysis.[6]

According to this, large renal parenchymal damage may pass unnoticed after an endovascular intervention in patients with prior normal kidney function. The creatinine clearance is the best method to address such patients because it not only evaluates the relative risk of a single patient but also indicates the real effect of the contrast media in the kidney function. Although the creatinine clearance is the ideal exam, in real life it is recommended to check the creatinine level before major diagnostic or interventional angiographic procedures. For those patients with a sCr level higher than 1.5, diabetes mellitus, and dehydration, measurement of the creatinine clearance is recommended before the procedure.

Table 7-6
Risk Factors to the Development of Contrast-Induced Nephropathy

- Dehydration
- Diabetes mellitus
- Serum creatinine ≥1.5 mg/dl
- Chronic hypertension
- Cardiovascular disease
- Age >60 years
- Hyperuricemia
- Multiple myeloma
- High-osmolar contrast media
- Large volume of contrast in a short period
- Nephrotoxic medications

The CIN may occur in 15% to 25% of the patients, and the percentage can be higher in a diabetic patient with an existing deficit in the renal function (Table 7-6). Approximately 0.7% of these patients end up going for hemodialysis. The CIN has been considered the third cause of acute renal failure acquired in the hospital, and such incidence has increased from 5% to 6.4% in the last couple of years. The level of the preexisting renal function is the most important predicting factor in the development of contrast-induced acute renal failure. It is important to recognize that a decrease in kidney function after endovascular interventions may be partly or totally due to several events not related to the contrast use: nonsteroid antiinflammatory drugs, some antibiotics and chemotherapeutic agents, and some clinical scenarios, such as cardiac failure and after large surgical procedures. The risk of CIN can be estimated through predicting models that include elevated systolic blood pressure, need of vasopressors, severity of the cardiac failure, age older than 75 years, hematocrit level, amount of iodine contrast used, and sCr level.[5,6] Table 7-6 lists the risk factors for contrast-induced acute renal failure.[4]

Several therapeutic strategies can prevent CIN, including normal saline intravenously, hydration, N-acetylcysteine, aminophylline, fenoldopam, sodium bicarbonate, and endothelin antagonists. Intravenous hydration has been demonstrated to have the most consistent positive results; however, it is not clear which hydration regimen is the best. It seems to be wiser to orient the patient to have ideally oral or parenteral hydration for at least 12 hours before exposure to iodine contrast and for 24 hours afterward. Intravenous hydration associated to the restricted use of iodine contrast still is, independent of association with another preventive therapy, the most economic and best way to prevent the CIN. The current literature also advocates the potential benefit of sodium bicarbonate as a monotherapy in the reduction of CIN. A randomized clinical trial that compared hydration with sodium bicarbonate and hydration with sodium chlorate showed that the first method was more effective in the CIN prophylaxis.[7] On the other hand, N-acetylcysteine can possibly reduce the CIN through antioxidant effects and vasodilatation. After several studies with contradictory results, two relatively recent metaanalyses confirmed preventive benefits.[8,9] Nonetheless, the debate now is about the dose and route of administration, although it is clear that N-acetylcysteine is nontoxic. Marenzi et al.[10] showed that the intravenous administration of 1200 mg of N-acetylcysteine in bolus before the procedure followed by 1200 mg orally every 12 hours for 2 days was superior to the placebo group and to the usual regimen of 600 mg intravenously of N-acetylcysteine followed by the same dose orally every 12 hours for 2 days. The oral and intravenous N-acetylcysteine responses in the prevention on CIN were dose dependent and statistically significant.[11]

Part of the prevention strategy for CIN is the use of alternative contrast media such as carbon dioxide (CO_2) and gadolinium. CO_2 has been used as a contrast agent since 1914, when it was originally used in the visualization of intraabdominal organs. Following the development of DSA and safer CO_2 injection systems, CO_2 angiography became a feasible alternative. Some CO_2 features are that it is nontoxic, invisible, and highly compressible; has no viscosity and no allergy reaction or renal toxicity; and is 20 times more soluble than oxygen, quickly diluting into the blood. Instead of mixing with blood, as happens with iodine contrast, the CO_2 actually dislocates the blood to form a column of negative contrast. The CO_2 may be used in below-diaphragm arteriographies and in any venography, unless there is right-to-left intracardiac communication.[12]

The CO_2 injection can be performed manually and vigorously or through a closed bag system. Ideally, the hand injection can be done with 50- to 60-ml syringes for adequate contrast in relation to the surrounding tissues. Because it is invisible, the CO_2 syringe may easily be contaminated by other gases. It is critical to have a closed system for CO_2 hand injection. A CO_2 cylinder should be connected into the diagnostic catheter through connecting tubing, with a three-way stopcock interposing on the two. The large syringe should be filled passively to prevent air contamination. It is critical to push the column of fluid out of the diagnostic catheter with a small puff of CO_2; otherwise, when performing the forceful CO_2 injection, the fluid column will be injected quickly into the vessel, predisposing the patient to vessel wall damage as the compressed gas pressure is transferred to the column of fluid.

Avoiding CO_2 injection above the diaphragm or with the patient's head elevated is recommended due to the risk of CO_2 contrast injection into the cerebral circulation, which could cause cerebral toxicity, as demonstrated by an animal model study.[10]

In pending vascular territories, as in the iliac arteries, the CO_2 angiogram may hyperestimate the degree of stenosis, which can be resolved by either increasing the volume of the CO_2 injection or turning the area of interest up to have better filling of the vessel by the column of CO_2. Another drawback of the CO_2 angiography is the fragmentation of the CO_2 column, particularly in below-knee arteriograms, which can be resolved by advancing the diagnostic catheter as distally as possible toward the femoropopliteal transition or using "stacking" software in the angiography equipment. There is no maximum limit in the amount of CO_2 injection intravascularly, as long as less than 100 ml of CO_2 is injected every 2 minutes. The CO_2 is eliminated by the lungs after a quick dissolution in the blood.

Initially developed as a contrast material for magnetic resonance (MR), gadolinium has a superior safety profile compared to iodine contrast. Gadolinium may be used as an alternative contrast media for catheter angiography for those patients with documented iodine contrast allergy, but its used is limited in patients with decreased GFR, as further discussed, to avoid nephrogenic systemic fibrosis. In patients with normal kidney function, usually a total dose of 40 to 60 ml or 0.1 to 0.3 ml/kg can be safely used. Sometimes to achieve a good vascular opacification it is necessary to use higher dose of gadolinium, which can be nephrotoxic as well. The nephrotoxicity of gadolinium seems to be dose dependent.[13] Superior vascular opacification is obtained with the iodine contrast in a lower molecular dose because one benzene ring has three iodine-attenuating atoms, while the gadolinium quelate has only one attenuating atom. In an animal model study, gadolinium-based contrast agents were found to be more nephrotoxic than iodine-based contrast when equimolar doses were administered intraarterially.[14]

Digital Subtraction Angiography

Current angiography equipment is used for diagnostic and therapeutic procedures and offers several image applications. The most common ones in practice are DSA and native fluoroscopy (unsubtracted images). DSA is a computer-based digital image-processing technique by which an initial no-contrast mask image is electronically subtracted from subsequent serial images of an angiogram.

DSA includes special techniques such as stepping table DSA, bolus-chasing DSA, and three-dimensional (3D) rotational angiography. Only used in peripheral angiography, the stepping table involves table movement in a series of overlapping steps. A bolus of contrast injection is performed while the table is advanced when the vessels in that position are opacified. On average, five positions are required to cover the area from the abdominal aorta down to the feet. The more symmetrical the flow in the lower extremities, the better the result of the angiogram. The bolus-chasing DSA resembles and has the same application as the stepping table technique. The mask images are obtained approximately every 5 cm, and the table is then panned to keep up with the contrast bolus. The 3D rotational angiography requires rotation of the image intensifier or C-arm around the patient while masks are acquired, followed by repeated rotation while the contrast is injected. Postprocessing 3D reconstruction may be obtained in the workstation to provide an overview of the area of interest in addition to the rotational images. This technique is useful when multiple anticipated oblique projections are required, as in the angiographic evaluation of an internal iliac artery aneurysm or of a renal transplant artery stenosis.

There are several formats of diagnostic catheters (Figure 7-2) and guide wires with different applications. Some specific vessels require a special catheter to be safely catheterized, such as the vertebral catheter for the selective catheterization of the supraaortic vessels or the cobra catheter for the renal arteries catheterization. Using hand or power injection, iodine-based contrast is typically used to obtain images in DSA or in native (unsubtracted) fluoroscopy. Every vascular territory has a specific protocol for power injections that determine how much contrast needs to be injected (total volume) and the injection rates (in cubic centimeters per second; Table 7-7).

However, injection rates and image-acquisition programs should be tailored for the patient when indicated. Specific setup also exists in the angiography equipment for the most common clinical applications. These settings are related to the number of frames per second and the length of acquisition time during the DSA used for a particular study. For example, for a celiac trunk angiogram, three pulses each second is adequate and approximately 40 seconds of acquisition time is necessary to document opacification of the portal vein (venous phase). To control and ideally decrease the amount of exposure to radiation, the number of pulses per second may be chosen during fluoroscopy to have a balance between the best image resolution with the minimum patient and operator radiation exposure.

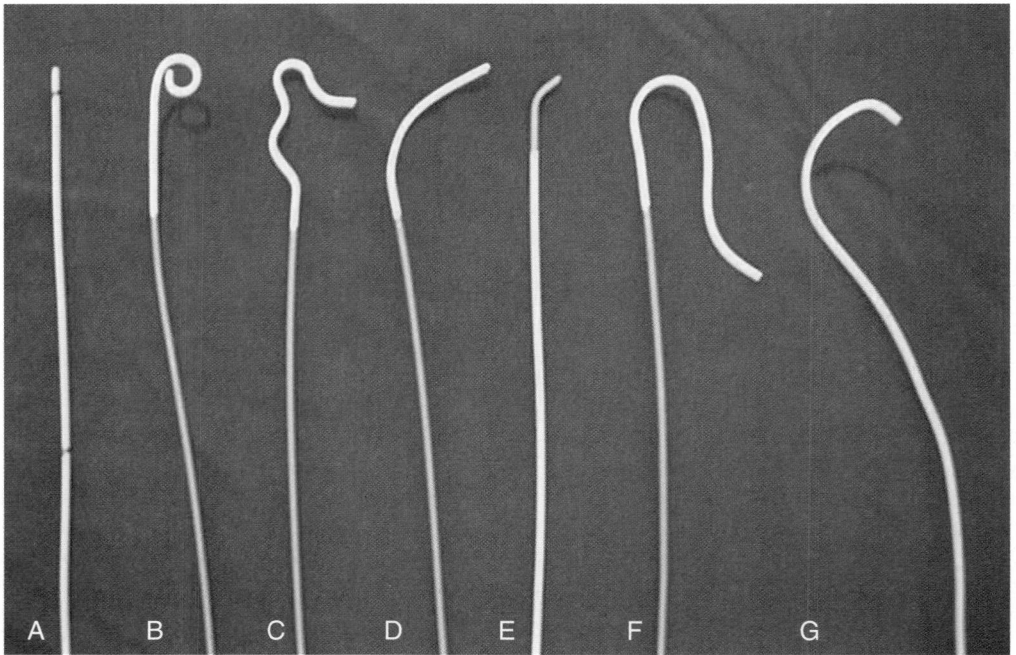

Figure 7-2. Examples of five French diagnostic catheters. High-flow catheters or catheters with side-holes: straight catheter with side-holes between the radiopaque markers (used for fibrinolytic therapy; **A**), pigtail **(B)**. Selective catheters or with end-hole orifice: Mickaelson **(C)**, multipurpose **(D)**, Kumpe **(E)**, Simmons **(F)**, Cobra **(G)**.

Table 7-7
Protocols for Peripheral and Visceral Arteriograms

Protocol	Total Volume of Contrast	Injection Rate of Contrast
Abdominal aortogram	30 ml	15 ml/sec
Thoracic aortogram	30 ml	15 ml/sec
Pelvic angiogram	20 ml	10 ml/sec
Unilateral lower extremities angiogram (iliac arteries)	10 ml	4 ml/sec
Selective renal transplant angiogram	8 ml	4 ml/sec
Renal angiogram	12 ml	4 ml/sec
Celiac angiogram	36 ml	6 ml/sec
Superior mesenteric angiogram	36 ml	6 ml/sec
Inferior mesenteric angiogram	18 ml	3 ml/sec
Hepatic angiogram	16 ml	4 ml/sec
Carotid arteries	9 ml	3 ml/sec
Vertebral arteries	8 ml	2 ml/sec
Hand angiogram (midbrachial artery)	9 ml	3 ml/sec

Most diagnostic and therapeutic procedures are done under intravenous conscious sedation (using midazolam and fentanyl) that, in general, provides adequate comfort to the patient during the procedure. However, there are situations in which no sedation should be administered, such as in carotid stenting when, ideally, the patient should be fully awake so that preservation of the cerebral function can be checked.

The incidence of complications during peripheral arteriogram is low; however, the incidence tends to increase with the duration of the procedure and if it is performed by some operator with lack of experience or poor training. Table 7-8 shows the incidence of the most common complications in arteriographic procedures.

COMPUTED TOMOGRAPHY ANGIOGRAPHY

The introduction of spiral computed tomography (SCT) in 1990 was the first of many improvements in diagnostic imaging. Compared to conventional computed tomography, SCT allowed faster acquisition of a large volume of data associated with improved longitudinal spatial resolution and decreased respiratory motion. In the beginning, CTA clinical applications only provided imaging of large vessels such as the thoracic and abdominal aortas, pulmonary vessels, and aortic branches such as the carotid and renal arteries.

Table 7-8
Complications of Angiography by Type and Incidence

Complications	Femoral (%)	Axillary (%)
Overall incidence	1.73	3.29
Death	0.03	0.09
Puncture site (total)	0.47	1.70
Arteriovenous fistula	0.01	0.02
Limb amputation	0.01	0.02
Pseudoaneurysm	0.05	0.22
Hemorrhage	0.26	0.68
Arterial occlusion	<0.20	<0.10
Contrast allergy		
Requiring hospitalization	0.10	
Fatal outcome	0.006	

Table 7-9
Main Clinical Applications of Computed Tomography Angiography

Thoracoabdominal aorta
Diagnosis of congenital and degenerative aortic diseases
Diagnosis of pulmonary embolism
Assessment of acute aortic injuries and dissections
Evaluation of visceral arteries (celiac, superior mesenteric, and renal arteries)
Preoperative planning and follow up
Tumor staging and surgical planning
Renal arteries
Assessment of anatomy for donor transplants
Diagnosis of renal artery stenosis in hypertensives or deteriorating renal function
Assessment of renal arteries after revascularization
Peripheral arterial system
Assessment of peripheral vascular disease
Assessment of bypass grafts
Carotid/intracranial circulation
Characterization of the atherosclerotic disease
Assessment of aortic arch vessels
Diagnosis of internal carotid artery stenosis
Preoperative planning of endovascular or surgical treatment of intracranial aneurysms and vascular malformations

The development of the helical technology in the late 1980s significantly reduced the acquisition time of one slice to approximately 1 second and eliminated the time interval between each image acquisition. This technology allowed the development of multidetector row computed tomography (MDCT), which was introduced in 1998. It started with the 4-detector row CT and in the last 10 years has quickly evolved to 16, 32, 64, and more recently 128 and 256 detectors. Before the MDCT technology, conventional CT and helical CT allowed only partial evaluation of the peripheral arteries. Currently, complete coverage of the lower extremity inflow and runoff arteries is possible with one acquisition using a single-contrast bolus. The considerably more rapid scanning times, improved z-axis resolution, and resulting thinner slice thicknesses achievable with 16- to 64-MDCT scanners mean that diagnostic angiography, for example, of the aortoiliac and peripheral runoff vasculature to the level of the foot is now a practical procedure at many centers. Additional benefits of 16- to 64-CTA compared with CTA performed using older CT technologies and with catheter angiography include a lower overall effective radiation dose and, given the rapid scanning times, the possibility of using less contrast agent.

True isotropic high spatial resolution of the entire acquired volume is now possible using the 64-MDCT scanner. The improvements in x-ray tube capacity and scan speed allow submillimeter acquisition of a large coverage without limitations. These developments made multidetector computed tomography angiography (MDCTA) an accurate alternative for the assessment of the peripheral arteries. Using standardized scanning and protocols, peripheral CTA is a robust, noninvasive technique for evaluating acute and chronic diseases of the central and peripheral arteries. In practice, CTA has replaced conventional catheter angiography in many diagnostic studies for PVD, especially in the evaluation of the carotid, supraaortic, and renal arteries and in the thoracic and abdominal aortas. The main clinical applications of CTA are summarized in the Table 7-9.

The procedure time and the amount of contrast media may be significantly decreased when MDCTA is performed compared with when catheter angiography is used. The comprehensive vascular evaluation permits not only the study of the vascular territory related to the patient's symptoms but also the best vascular access in case of indication for endovascular therapy or for a hybrid procedure. It allows planning of the whole procedure strategy: standard or alternative arterial access (femoral versus axillary, radial or brachial), the most appropriate devices (guide wires, diagnostic angiography catheters, guiding catheters), balloon and stent dimensions and type, and best technique (open, endovascular or hybrid revascularizations). Lesion morphology assessment plays a key role in most clinical decision making, especially for peripheral vascular interventions. In some clinical scenarios such as in carotid artery stenosis and in AAA, the device to be used can be chosen before the procedure by non-catheter-based angiography. In many situations, it permits identification of the lesion characteristics, such as calcification, ulceration, dissection, soft or hard plaque, thrombus, intimal hyperplasia, vessel inflow and outflow, and tortuosities (e.g., the aortic arch type 3 during the evaluation for possible carotid stenosis stenting). For example, the inclusion of the aortic arch is important during the evaluation of carotid arteries, and it is critical to include the common femoral arteries during the AAA workup with CTA. The additional information may anticipate potential associated abnormalities or simply variations of the anatomy that can be studied in detail. For open revascularizations, it may be important to choose the best access site, incision and dissection extensions and their location, clamping placement, etc. With the preprocedure vascular anatomy in mind, it allows adequate tailoring of the peripheral vascular intervention devices to the specific lesion or lesions to be treated and minimizes the amount of iodine-based contrast used and the length of the procedure. The ongoing development of MDCT scanners will further increase CTA capabilities. The volumetric data sets generated are suitable for 3D reconstructions. This process is becoming easier and faster with the advent of more powerful computer processors and software in commercially available workstations. Despite the rapid progress in MRA, the widespread use of MDCT scanners ensures the future of CTA. For patients with a history of stent placement for the treatment of PVD, CTA offers a great tool for patient surveillance, especially when an adequate ultrasound Doppler is not feasible (e.g., in the interposition of bowel gas) or when there is no definitive result. Unlike MRA, stents, pacemakers, and ferromagnetic aneurysm clips do not necessarily preclude CTA. Usually it does not have significant image artifacts generated by a ferromagnetic device as it does when the patient is submitted to an MRA. A recent systematic review of the literature described pooled sensitivity, specificity, and accuracy rates of 92%, 91%, and 91%, respectively, at all arterial levels; 92%, 94%, and 93%, respectively, at aortoiliac arteries; 96%, 85%, and 92%, respectively, at femoropopliteal arteries; and 91%, 85%, and 87%, respectively, at infrapopliteal arteries. A significant difference was found in the sensitivity of MDCTA in PAD between 4-slice MDCT and 16-slice MDCT scanners, between aortoiliac and femoropopliteal arterial segments, and between femoropopliteal and infrapopliteal arterial segments ($P < 0.05$). In comparison with conventional angiography, 16-MDCTA has shown 96% sensitivity and 97% specificity in the detection of hemodynamically significant stenosis in all aortoiliac and peripheral vascular segments.

The most recent progress in CT technology was seen through the development of the dual-source CT scan (Siemens), the 256-detector CT (Philips), and the "dynamic volume" CT scanner based on 320 slices (Toshiba). Presented in 2005, the dual-source scan consists of a dual x-ray tube and a dual array of 64-slice detectors. The dual sources increase the temporal resolution by reducing the rotation angle required to acquire a complete image, thus permitting cardiac studies without the use of heart rate–lowering medication, as well as permitting imaging of the heart in systole. The use of two x-ray units makes possible the use of dual energy imaging, which allows an estimation of the average atomic number in a voxel, as well as the total attenuation. This permits automatic differentiation of calcium (e.g., in bone or diseased arteries) from iodine (in contrast medium) or titanium (in stents), which might otherwise be impossible to differentiate. In 2007, the 256-slice CT scanner and the dynamic-volume CT scanner based on 320 slices were announced. The clinical capabilities of both technologies are under investigation, but they have demonstrated the potential to significantly reduce radiation exposure for patients.

Technical Aspects of MDCTA

MDCTA requires the synchronization of high-flow, intravenous, contrast medium injection with a fast volumetric acquisition timed to the arterial or venous phase. The scan acquisition, volume, concentration and speed of the contrast media administration, and image after processing and display are the most important technical components of MDCTA. The protocols and techniques have evolved from the single-detector row scanner to the MDCT scanners, minimizing the acquisition time and the radiation exposure, optimizing the amount of contrast use, simplifying the image display, and maximizing the capabilities of the scanners.

Patient Preparation

Before scanning preparations, just a few specifics are necessary for MDCTA of the aorta or of the peripheral arteries. Usually, the patient is placed comfortably in a supine position and the area of interest is kept still to avoid movement-related artifacts. Taking the legs as an example, the area of interest is stabilized with cushions around them and slightly strapped with adhesive tape distally. It is important that the patient does not wear metal zippers or buttons on clothing, since this can have a negative influence on the image quality, especially when using postprocessed images. The intravenous contrast material is typically administered through a cannula that is placed in the patient's antecubital vein. For neck, upper extremity, or upper chest studies, the contrast injection should be done either in the lower limbs or in the contralateral arm to the side of interest to decrease the streaking artifact from high-density contrast medium in the veins. When scanning the chest or the upper abdomen, both arms should be extended toward the patient's head to avoid image artifacts. Contrast material needs to be administered at body temperature to decrease the viscosity.

Table 7-10A
Computed Tomography Protocol—16-Slice Scanner*

Specific Anatomical Region	Aorta	Carotid	Liver or Pancreas	Renal
Kilovolts	120	120	120	120
Effective milliampere-seconds	200	200	200	200
Rotation time (seconds)	0.5	0.5	0.5	0.5
Detector collimation (millimeters)	0.75	0.75	0.75	0.75
Slice thickness (millimeters)	1.0	0.75	1.0	1.0
Feed or rotation (millimeters)	12	12	12	12
Reconstruction interval	0.7	0.3	0.7	0.7
IV contrast volume	140 ml Omnipaque 350	140 ml Omnipaque 350	140 ml Omnipaque 350	140 ml Omnipaque 350
Injection rate	4 ml/sec	4 ml/sec	4 ml/sec	4 ml/sec
Scan delay	Bolus tracking	20 seconds	Bolus tracking	Bolus tracking
3D, MIP, and MPR reconstructions	3D	3D or MIP	MIP	3D or MIP

*3D, three-dimensional; MIP, maximum intensity projection; MPR, multiplanar reconstruction.

Table 7-10B
Computed Tomography Protocol—64-Slice Scanner*

Specific Anatomical Region	Carotid	Liver or Pancreas	Renal	Pulmonary Embolism Study	Stent Graft
Kilovolts	120	120	120	120	120
Effective milliampere-seconds	159	279	288	220	276
Rotation time (seconds)	0.33	0.37	0.33	0.5	0.37
Detector collimation (millimeters)	0.6	0.6	0.6	0.6	0.6
Slice thickness (millimeters)	0.6	Arterial: 1.5 Venous: 3.0	Arterial: 1.5 Venous: 3.0	1.0	1.5
Pitch	1.2	0.75	0.65	0.7	0.75
Reconstruction interval	0.4	0.3-3.0	0.8- 3.0	0.5	0.8
IV contrast volume	140 ml Omnipaque 350	140 ml Omnipaque 350	140 ml Omnipaque 350	100 ml Omnipaque 350	140 ml Omnipaque 350
Injection rate	4 ml/sec	4 ml/sec	4 ml/sec	4 ml/sec	4 ml/sec
Scan delay (seconds)	Bolus tracking at 120 HU	Without: 0 Arterial: bolus tracking Venous: 35 Delay: 120	Arterial: bolus tracking Venous: 50	Bolus tracking at 120 HU	Bolus tracking
3D, MIP, or MPR reconstructions	3D or sagittal or coronal MPR	3D	3D	Sagittal or coronal MIP	3D or sagittal or coronal MPR

*3D, three-dimensional; HU, Hounsfield units; MIP, maximum intensity projection; MPR, multiplanar reconstruction.

Scan Acquisition

The main challenge for peripheral CTA is the great range of the vascular system that needs to be depicted. MDCTA should be performed, ideally, on a 16- to 128-detector scanner. The scan protocols are designed to provide comprehensive evaluations with high image quality and accurate disease depiction and characterization. To maximize exam efficiency and patient throughput, routine protocols are generally adequate for most patients. On the other hand, according to the patient's clinical situation, the protocol must be tailored for that particular individual. Scan protocol is perhaps the most undervalued and overlooked part of the examination. Making sure that the area of interest is covered and that the primary diagnostic question is answered are important actions to prevent a nondiagnostic test. The necessity of precontrast scans or delayed scans should be decided beforehand. Having established scanning protocols also ensures reproducibility and smooth workflow. Examples of the most common MDCT protocols used in our institution are in Table 7-10A and B.

As a general rule, the MDCTA protocol should allow only the use of negative oral contrast when gastric or bowel distention is required. No positive contrast should be taken orally. Potentially, the high-density contrast material (e.g., barium) may decrease the quality of the postprocessing images, with subsequent limitations for study interpretation. All MDCTA protocols should start with an anterior–posterior load dose scout view focused in the area of interest to check full coverage and the field-of-view extension (Figure 7-3). To optimize the scan, a lateral scout view should also be performed just before the upper or lower extremities MDCT angiogram. After an

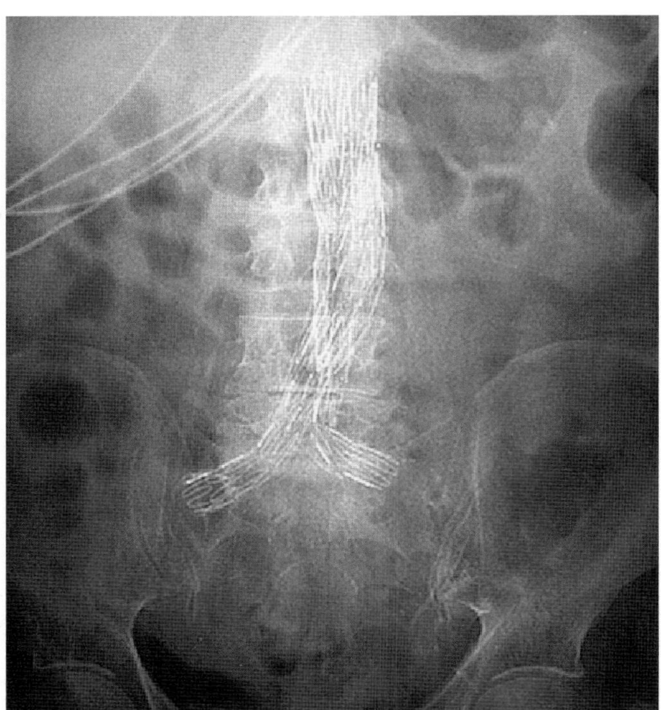

Figure 7-3. Computed tomography scout in anterior–posterior view. This first computed tomography acquisition is important for planning the field of view. It also may provide information about high-density structures such as the integrity prosthetic endografts.

initial scout image (120 kV, 100 mAs) is obtained, the scanning range is planned to encompass the entire vascular system of the area of interest. Image thickness may vary from 0.75 to 5.0 mm and depends on how small the vessels of interest are.

Initial noncontrasted CT scan images are not essential for all MDCTA examinations. However, depending on the vascular territory, it is wiser to obtain non-contrast-enhanced images as a baseline acquisition for further comparative analysis with the iodine contrast-enhanced acquisition. The non-contrast-enhanced images are helpful in the localization and extension of vascular calcifications, residual intravenous contrast, endovascular stents and stent grafts, aneurysm wall calcifications, foreign body, bone fragments due to trauma, surgical clips, surgical grafts, radiopaque embolic agents (glue, onyx, and ethiodol), and intramural hematoma or hemorrhage. Other benefits include deciding the field of coverage and deciding an appropriate site to place the cursor for contrast bolus tracking.

Following the non-contrast-enhanced images, an iodine-based nonionic contrast material is administered intravenously through an antecubital vein; a 20- to 22-gauge intravenous cannula is needed for the maximal flow rates of 5.0 to 3.0 ml/sec, respectively. This corresponds to an iodine administration rate of 1.0 to 1.4 g/sec using a contrast media concentration of approximately 320 to 350 mg I/ml. By increasing the iodine concentration to 400 mg I/ml, the iodine administration rate can be increased to 1.6 g/sec to increase the enhancement. Automatic power injection is required during the peripheral MDCTA to obtain a high and homogenous enhancement of the arterial tree and to synchronize the acquisition with the enhancement. The optimization of acquisition timing and contrast medium delivery is essential for vascular assessment and image after processing. The amount of contrast media depends on the scan duration and on the flow rate. The volume of contrast material ranges from 100 to 160 ml for a typical scan duration of 40 seconds. Based on the reported literature, the average values of contrast media volume, concentration, injection rate, and administration rate are 134 ml, 341 mg I/ml, 3.5 ml/sec, and 1.2 g/sec, respectively. Normally, attenuation values higher than 200 Hounsfield units (HU) in the arteries are considered suitable in MDCTA. However, to ensure the enhancement of all arteries, the injection duration should not be shorter than 30 seconds. In fast scan protocols, a delay time needs to be added to prevent outrunning of the contrast bolus. Appropriate timing optimizes contrast and allows either arteries or veins to be scanned. Scanning the abdominal aorta at 25 seconds after the start of the injection usually gives satisfactory images. In a healthy patient, empirical timing may suffice; however, time to peak enhancement varies, particularly in patients with cardiac compromise.

Two methods can be used to ensure correct timing. The first uses a series of static scans at a single level of interest, i.e., the aortic arch for cases of suspected dissection and the level of the renal arteries for assessment of AAAs. Then, 15 to 20 ml of contrast is injected at the anticipated injection rate and a scan is performed every 3 seconds, beginning 10 seconds after injection. A region of interest is then placed on the vessel, and the time to peak vascular enhancement is calculated.

The second method is semiautomated. A series of scans is performed at the start of contrast injection. Image acquisition is triggered when a preset enhancement threshold (attenuation of 100 HU above the baseline attenuation) is reached within a preselected region of interest. Visual assessment can be used to override the semiautomated software and commence scanning earlier.

Volumetric data acquisition is typically performed craniocaudally. In general, it is important to tailor contrast medium use in CTA depending on patient and investigation variables. The guiding principles are intravenous access, saline chase, injection rate, timing, and physiological factors. An appropriately sized antecubital vein is the most convenient. In view of the high flow rates needed, ensuring the cannula is not kinked due to the patient's position is important. The use of a saline chaser not only reduces the amount of contrast medium needed but also prevents streaking artifacts. The saline chaser can be used either after loading the contrast medium in a single barrel injector or by using one of the double-barrel injectors available. An optimum injection rate is important to achieve homogeneous enhancement of the small vessels. The contrast density level and synchronization of the contrast medium injection with image acquisition is critical. Nonionic 300 mg I/ml contrast is typically used, except in some institutions for cases of suspected pulmonary embolism or dissection of the thoracic aorta. In these instances, lower concentrations of contrast media may be used (150 to 240 mg/ml) because dense contrast medium may obscure low-density thrombus or an intimal flap.

As mentioned earlier, saline bolus chasers of 50 to 70 ml are employed to force the contrast through the tubing and the venous system to prolong the plateau phase of enhancement. A more homogenous enhancement can be achieved using a biphasic injection at a higher rate (5 to 6 ml/sec) at the beginning (during the first 5 seconds) of the injection and at a lower rate (3 ml/sec) for the remaining volume. In other words, an initial faster phase results in a peak in the corresponding curve

Table 7-11
Computed Tomography Angiography Scan Parameters*

Data Acquisition	Data Reconstruction
Tube current and voltage	Reconstruction algorithm
Pitch	Field of view
Gantry rotation speed	Slice thickness
Detector row width	Reconstruction interval
Cardiac gating	Half-scan reconstruction
Retrospective ECG gating	Multisector ECG reconstruction
Prospective ECG gating	

*ECG, electrocardiogram.

but with a more prolonged plateau. In clinical practice, a monophasic injection rate is often used because it is a simple method and it has resulted in adequate image quality with reproducible results that have less interpatient variation. Also important, the key physiological factors to be taken into consideration are body size, cardiac output, and the high concentration of contrast medium. Body size relates to proportionate blood volume. In general, we use 1.0 ml of contrast medium per kilogram of body weight. In patients with low cardiac output, the peak arterial enhancement is later. Hence, to achieve uniform enhancement, it is often useful to place the cursor for bolus tracking at the bottom of the aortic aneurysm, for example.

It is important to remember that mean contrast enhancement in patients with high cardiac output is actually less. With faster scanners, high-concentration contrast medium (more than 350 mg I/ml) is useful to achieve a high concentration of iodine in the vessels. It is possible to reduce both the injection rate and the total volume of contrast medium needed if high-concentration contrast medium is used.

According to the patient's clinical scenario, the acquisition of venous or delayed phases (or both) may be required and no supplementary contrast media may be necessary. The acquisition of delayed CTA images may be critical in situations such as ruling out the presence of stent graft endoleaks or of active bleeding. In some circumstances, cardiac gating is necessary to deal with motion artifacts, especially if the area of interest is close to the heart.

MDCTA scan parameters can be divided into those used for the data acquisition and those used for the data reconstruction (Table 7-11). Each MDCT scanner requires a specific protocol that needs to be tailored for the acquisition of images of a particular area. According to the number of detectors (or channels), it may have a specific competitive advantage. In other words, a carotid artery CTA in a 4-MDCT may require a different protocol than a 16-MDCT for the same images acquisition. Similarly, a 64-MDCT scanner may be ideal for some clinical applications, such as for coronary angiogram, when the 4-MDCT is definitely not. The breath-hold time, potential motion-induced artifacts, and administration of the contrast medium are directly correlated to the duration of the CT scan.

The collimation should be chosen to be as narrow as possible but to still allow a table speed of 30 mm/sec. The collimation depends on the number of detector rows and heat capacity. On a 4-MDCT, the collimation is limited to 4 × 2.5 mm, whereas the 16-MDCT and 64-MDCT allow a submillimeter collimation of 16 × 0.75 mm and 32 × 2 × 0.6 mm, respectively. Using the 16-MDCT in obese patients, the thin collimation protocol leads to unacceptable noise levels in the abdomen and pelvis because the tube is unable to deliver the necessary dose in this submillimeter configuration. To enable the tube to deliver a higher dose, a wider collimation (16 × 1.5 mm) with a reduced pitch factor of 0.7 is used to improve the image quality in obese patients. For the 64-MDCT scanner, there is no longer a tradeoff between resolution and scan speed; it allows, even in obese patients, a fast submillimeter scan protocol.

Post Processing Techniques

An MDCT angiographic study easily generates more than 1000 axial images. Postprocessing of these large-volume data sets is a challenge. Other core problems with these large data sets are image transfer rates on the system, hospital network, or both, as well as storage requirements both online and offline. These large data sets are also a challenge for radiologists or physicians who rely on film interpretation. The role of the postprocessing workstation is to optimize the diagnostic information to the end user. Ideally, the interpretation of the images should be done in a workstation environment. It provides the manipulation of the raw data using software that results in volumetric reconstructive images in grayscale or in colors. Initially, interpretation should be done on the axial source images. By displaying findings in a more familiar format, 3D reconstruction can help in difficult cases by revealing information present but not readily evident on axial images alone.

One result of the several new MDCT applications is the constantly evolving workstations. Not only do MDCT manufacturers have their own workstations, but numerous companies offer standalone workstations. Some picture archiving and communication system workstations also offer basic postprocessing functionality. An important aspect of workstation postprocessing is to understand the basics of various techniques. Commonly used techniques are maximum intensity projection (MIP), volume rendering (VR), multiplanar reconstruction (MPR), curved planar reconstruction, and virtual angioscopy. Usually, the transverse sections are reconstructed with a 2-mm slice thickness at an interval of 1 mm. The reconstructions are typically performed by one radiology technologist experienced in 3D postprocessing and segmentation techniques. Usually, segmentation is performed of both bone structures and vessel wall calcifications, resulting in images containing the contrast-enhanced vascular lumen without vessel wall calcifications and bones. Of these data sets, rotating VR images are generated using the commercially available software installed on the workstation. The final processed images may result in multiple angiogram-like images rotating more than 180 degrees for the area of interest.

Maximum Intensity Projection

Images can be displayed singly, as individual sections, or stacked, as a summary of several adjacent sections. A stacked display results in loss of detail but improved image contrast and decreased image noise. MIP (Figure 7-4) allows visualization of longer lengths of the arterial lumen and has proven more accurate for the detection of significant arterial stenosis than has multiplanar reformation or 3D VR reconstructions. A ray is projected along the data set in a user-selected direction, and the highest voxel value along the ray becomes the pixel value of a 2D MIP image. In other words, MIP views display the highest Hounsfield value voxel (contrast medium,

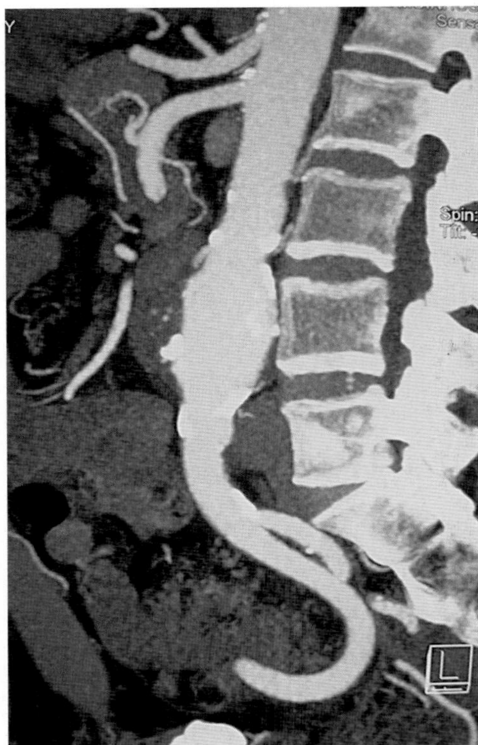

Figure 7-4. Abdominal computed tomography angiography in lateral view. Maximum intensity projection image shows an abdominal aorta with anterior wall thrombus. It also demonstrates a long aneurismal neck with favorable anatomical features for an endovascular stent graft repair.

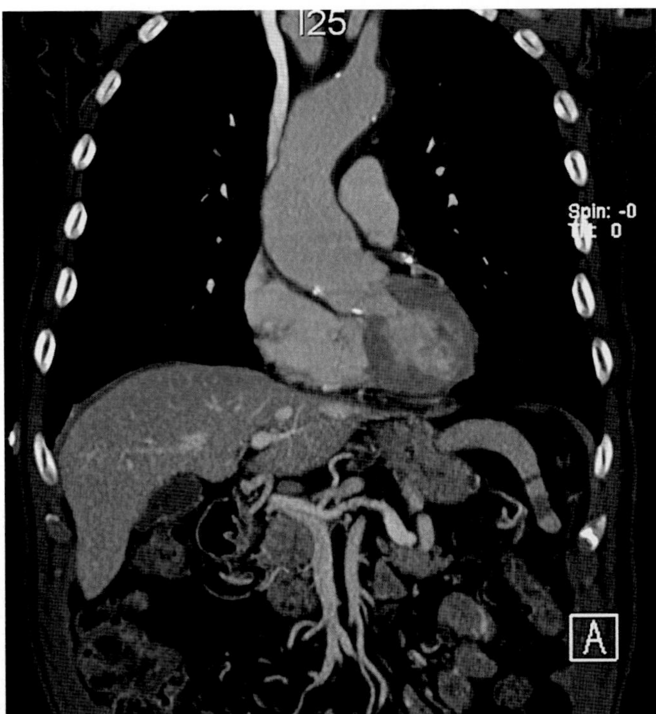

Figure 7-5. Coronal thoracic computed tomography angiography. Maximum intensity projection image shows in detail the ascending thoracic aortic aneurysm and its correlation with the surrounding anatomy.

calcium, bone) along any plane (Figure 7-5). MIP preserves relative attenuation values, and the resulting images are usually displayed with no surface shading or other devices to help the user appreciate the "depth" of the rendering (it lacks depth perception), making 3D relationships difficult to assess. This leads to difficulty in separating overlapping vessels in sites in which several vessels are opacified (e.g., pulmonary artery and thoracic aorta) and in identifying small intravascular hypodense lesions (e.g., thrombus and intimal flaps). If another high-density material lies along the ray through a vessel (such as calcification), the displayed pixel intensity only represents the calcification and contains no information from the intravascular contrast medium. This can lead to overestimation of stenosis, or it may obscure adjacent pathology. Also, normal vessels passing obliquely through a volume can have a "string of beads" appearance. Therefore, MIPs in more than one direction may be needed to evaluate a data set.

Volume Rendering

VR involves reconstruction of the entire volume of image data and display of the data from a selected viewer orientation. The contributions of each voxel along a line from the viewer's eye through the data set are summed, pixel by pixel, to obtain a single composite image. This is done repeatedly to determine each pixel value in the displayed image. VR algorithms are capable of revealing internal structures that would normally be hidden when using traditional surface rendering techniques (Figure 7-6). It also achieves a display that highlights tissues

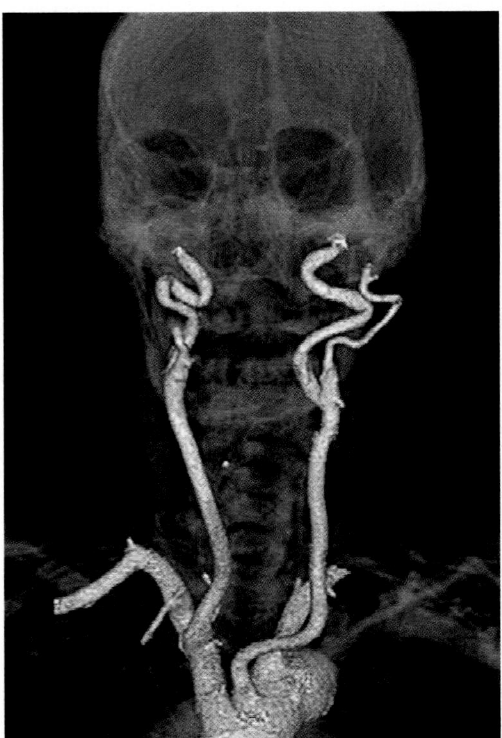

Figure 7-6. Aortic arch and carotid arteries multidetector row computed tomography angiogram. Colored volume rendering reconstruction using software available in workstations, showing the overlapping bone anatomy and the capability of having a 360-degree animation for full evaluation.

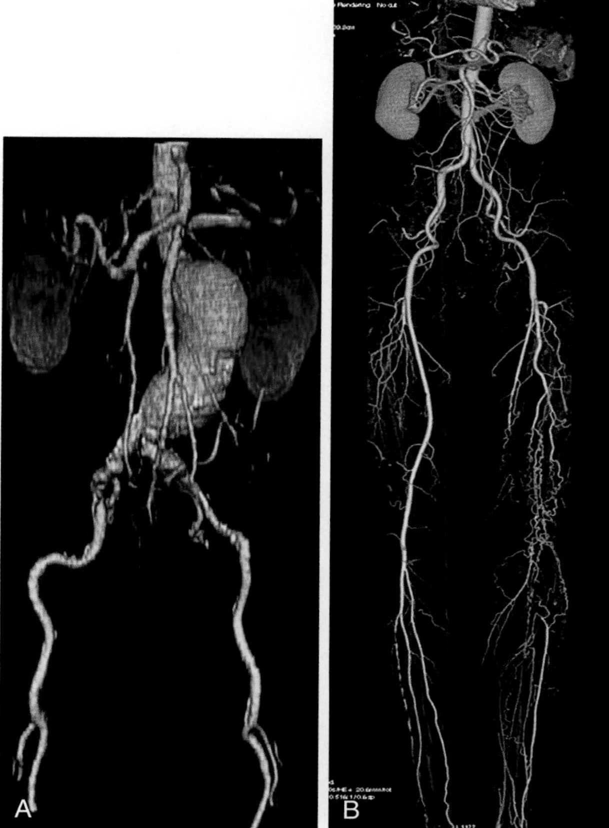

Figure 7-7. **A,** Abdominal aorta and pelvic multidetector row computed tomography (MDCT) angiogram. Colored volume rendering (VR) reconstruction using software available in workstations, providing information for the infrarenal AAA treatment strategy. **B,** Abdominal aorta and lower extremities MDCT angiogram. Colored VR shows superficial femoral artery occlusion associated with severe tibioperoneal disease on the left and two vessels' runoff on the right. Information provided is critical for the left lower-extremity revascularization strategy.

and relationships of interest. One of the biggest advantages of VR is perspective or depth information. Transfer functions are used to map properties such as opacity, brightness, color, and windowing to the voxel in the volume of interest, with all voxel in the volume potentially contributing to the final image. In real time, the displayed image can be cut and rotated, and transfer functions can be altered. It follows that this type of reconstruction needs more powerful processing computers. This technique is useful for detecting arterial anomalies, and it may be useful for surgical planning (Figure 7-7).

Multiplanar Reconstruction

MPR is useful for rapidly reviewing all information in coronal, sagittal, or oblique views. This technique is most often used to generate cross-sectional images, such as short-axis or long-axis views, of any small vessel or of any particular finding that was not clearly studied in single projection alone. The image plane can be chosen arbitrarily. A significant disadvantage is that the structure of interest should lie in one plane. However, an important advantage is the simultaneous parenchymal or surrounding tissues information, which is especially important in visceral CTA studies.

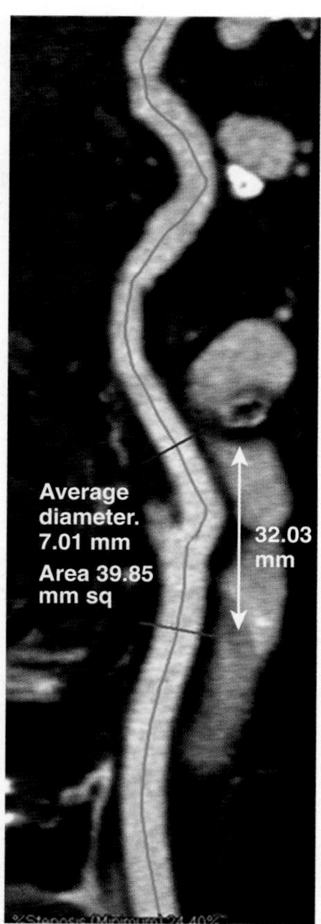

Figure 7-8. Carotid artery multidetector row computed tomography angiogram followed by curved planar reconstruction. Using workstation software, the vessel lumen is tracked along the segment of interest. This is an operator-dependent vascular analysis and allows measurements for therapeutic planning.

Curved Planar Reconstruction

This postprocessing algorithm allows the depiction of the entire course of a particular artery on a single image. The image plane is adjusted to follow the centerline of the vessel (Figure 7-8). The resultant display is most useful for depicting the lumen of an artery in a specific length. Curved planar reconstructions are useful to analyze individual vessels, especially heavily calcified ones. It is important to recognize that curved planar reconstruction is operator dependent, is a single-voxel-thick tomogram, and should be evaluated carefully.

Virtual Angioscopy

Specific software is applied to the MDCTA raw images in the workstation, and intraluminal images are generated as virtual angioscopy. After the VR reconstruction images are processed, it is possible to navigate thought the blood vessels and to evaluate the origin of branch vessels, calcified plaques, and focal or segmental stenosis correlations with the surrounding vascular branches and lumen of the stents (Figure 7-9).

CTA Limitations

The main disadvantages of MDCTA are the use of radiation, the use of potentially nephrotoxic iodinated contrast medium, the time-consuming 3D reconstruction techniques,

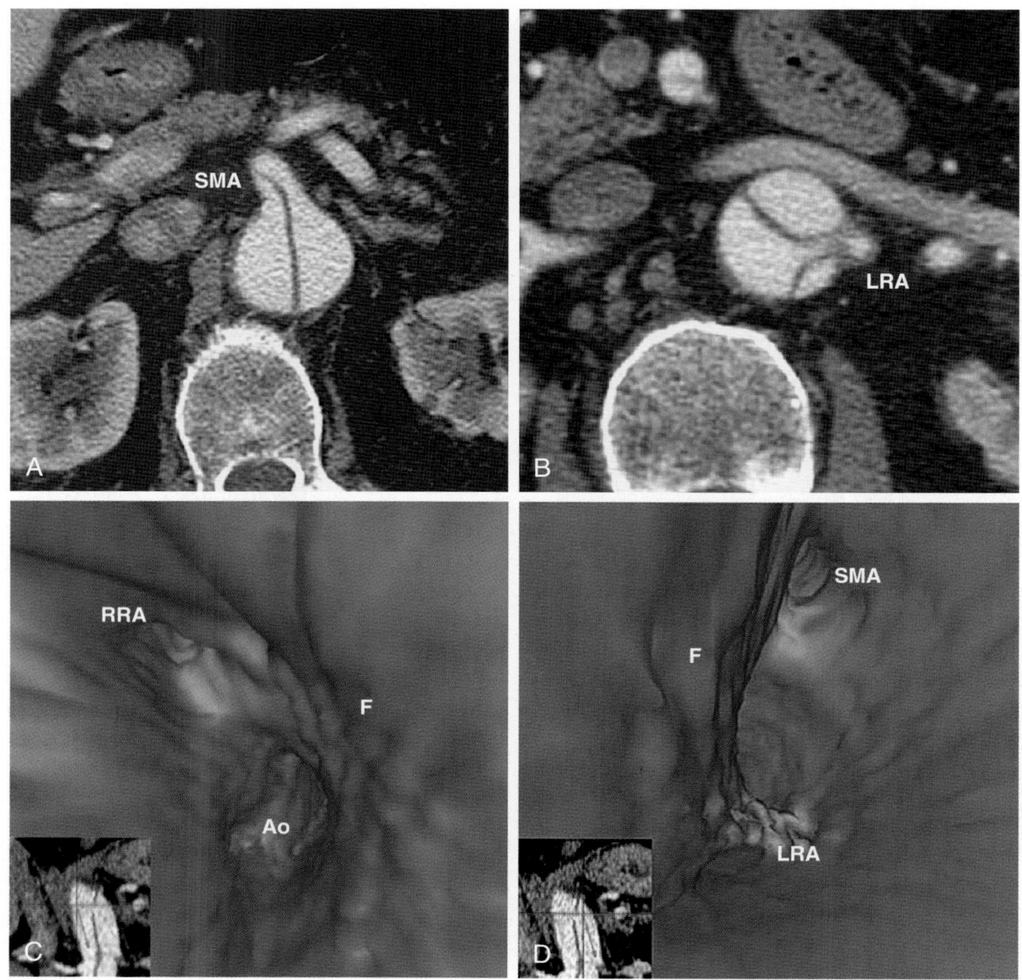

Figure 7-9. Abdominal aortic dissection involving the origin of the superior mesenteric artery (SMA) and the left renal artery (LRA). **A, B,** Axial computed tomography images showing the dissection. **C, D,** Virtual angioscopy views showing both lumens. RRA, right renal artery; Ao, aorta; F, dissection flap. (From Capuñay C, Carrascosa P, Martin López E, et al. Multidetector CT angiography and virtual angioscopy of the abdomen. *Abdom Imaging* 2009;34(1):81-93.)

and the difficulty in assessing the lumen stenosis of small arteries in the presence of vessel wall calcifications. Extensive arterial wall calcifications of the aorta and of the peripheral arteries are often seen in patients with vascular disease (Figure 7-10), and combined with a small vessel diameter, they may interfere with image interpretation, such as with the crural arteries. It is important to note that the apparent obscuration of the arterial lumen by vessel wall calcifications strongly depends on the window settings. Despite the impairment of vessel analysis in the presence of vessel wall calcifications, the possibility of localizing arterial wall calcifications that may have therapeutic relevance may be an advantage of MDCTA. Patients with metallic prosthetic grafts, such as knee replacement, may have significant image artifact that prevents adequate vessel evaluation.

Contraindications for MDCTA

Severe renal insufficiency, severe adverse reactions to iodinated contrast agent, and the need for an emergency intervention may limit CTA in some patients.

MAGNETIC RESONANCE ANGIOGRAPHY

MRA has evolved over the last decade, after several technical improvements and advances in scanner hardware and software, into a technique widely applied in clinical practice. Significantly better spatial resolution, speed, and reliability of the contrast-enhanced magnetic resonance)angiography (CE-MRA) led to high accuracy of this method, which is now comparable with that of CTA or even conventional catheter angiography in the aorta and its proximal main branches. Initially considered an experimental imaging modality, MRA is now widely implemented in noninvasive evaluation of PVD. The high accuracy, noninvasiveness, combination of morphological and functional information in a single examination, high spatial resolution, lack of ionizing radiation, and use of contrast agent with relatively small potential nephrotoxicity are the appealing features for broad acceptance of CE-MRA in initial diagnosis and repeated follow-up studies of patients with PVD.

Magnetic resonance imaging (MRI) is the result of digital representation based on the detection of radio-frequency

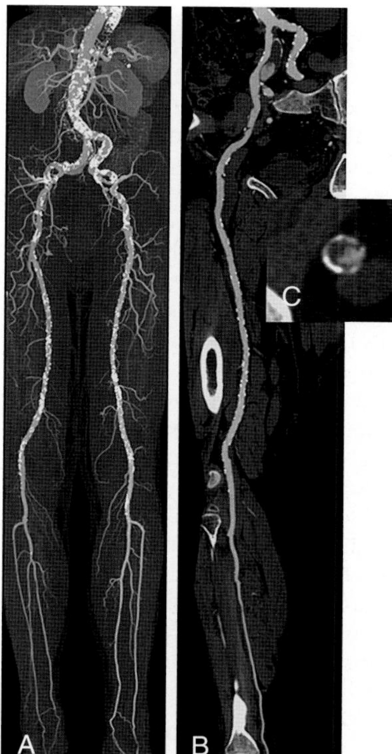

Figure 7-10. Abdominal aorta and lower extremities multidetector row computed tomography angiograms. **A,** Coronal maximum intensity projection (MIP) image shows severe and diffuse calcifications in the aorta, iliac, and superficial femoral arteries may lead to overestimation of stenosis. **B,** Coronal MIP image demonstrates moderate atherosclerotic disease in the superficial femoral artery. For a precise determination of the grade of vascular stenosis, the axial images must be carefully evaluated. **C,** In a situation like this, it is possible to underestimate the existing stenosis because of noncalcified plaque.

signals emitted by protons within a powerful magnetic field. Although all human body atoms are affected, the MR image is generated from the water hydrogen atoms, which are present in 70% of the human body. The T_1-weighted images represent the recovery of the "longitudinal magnetization" after the cessation of the radio-frequency waves in the exposed protons and are based on short echo times.

Table 7-12
Essential Magnetic Resonance (MR) Signal Features

- Solid organs, blood vessels, muscles, and fat tissue have different MR signals when they are normal, with pathology (tumor, bleeding, etc.) or exposed to contrast material. Usually, a bright signal follows contrast administration.
- Air and bone have a low signal.
- Blood flow is usually black (signal void), especially when the flow is fast and there is not enough time for the signal acquisition as it moves out of the field of view.
- The vessel wall inflammatory process has a high signal.
- Vascular calcifications are not visualized.
- There are different MR signals for different ages of the thrombus (static blood), but in general there are specific T_1- and T_2-weighted features for each age:
    - <24 hours: both T_1 and T_2 with an intermediate signal
    - 24-72 hours: both with low signals (dark)
    - 7-14 days: both with high signals (bright)

Table 7-13
Pros and Cons of the Most Used Magnetic Resonance Angiography (MRA) Sequences

Phase-Contrast MRA
(+) Velocity and direction of the blood flow
(–) Long volume imaging time, limited anatomical coverage

Time-of-Flight MRA
(+) Possible good distal lower leg and feet images
(–) Long imaging time, inherent artifact; slow flow and blood vessel course may cause artificial vascular occlusion and overestimation of the degree and length of stenoses
(–) Signal loss or artifacts due to:
1. Saturation bands that eliminate signal from retrograde flow
2. Slice misalignment due to patient motion between acquisitions
3. Ghosting artifacts due to vessel pulsatility and large variations in blood flow velocity during the cardiac cycle

Contrast-Enhanced MRA
(+) Fast volumetric image acquisition of large vascular territories
(+) Single breath-hold acquisition; slow or in-plane flow causes no vascular signal loss
(+) No need for tissue saturation
(+) Minimal background signal
(+) Invisible bones
(–) Importance of acquisition time, which is critical in unilateral, severe, proximal vascular disease in the lower extremities and essential for arterial or venous differentiation

The T_2-weighted images result from the necessary time for the disappearance of the "transverse magnetization" to take place during the deviation of the transversal axis, and the images are based on long echo times. MRI may be acquired directly in the plane of interest and has the capability to create multiple planes and large field-of-view images. This is a key competitive advantage over CTA, which requires processing techniques after scanning to generate multiple plane images.

Among several MRA techniques used to study the blood vessels, CE-MRA is the most popular because it permits vessel lumen visualization during the initial arterial passage of contrast material. In most MR sequences, the blood vessels and the organs usually become bright after the intravenous administration of contrast media. Different human body tissues have different MR signals on T_1- and T_2-weighted images. General MR features are basic knowledge to interpret the MR images correctly (Table 7-12).

MRA has replaced diagnostic catheter angiography and duplex ultrasonography in many institutions. In the last decade, MRA has evolved into a reliable noninvasive technique and has become solidly integrated in clinical practice for the investigation of several vascular diseases.

MRA Techniques

Several MRA techniques to evaluate the blood vessels have been described, including phase-contrast MRA, time-of-flight or inflow MRA, 3D half-Fourier fast spin-echo MRA, balanced steady-state free precession (bSSFP) MRA and CE-MRA. There are pros and cons for each MRA technique (Table 7-13); however, the CE-MRA or gadolinium-enhanced MRA technique is by far the most widely used.

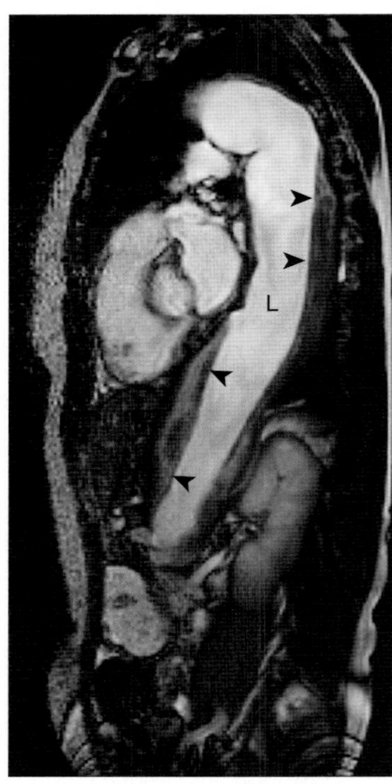

Figure 7-11. Mural thrombus *(arrowheads)* can easily be differentiated from the luminal blood (L). In addition, these images are useful as a localizer to plan subsequent high-resolution contrast-enhanced magnetic resonance angiography sequences (From Leiner T. Magnetic resonance angiography of abdominal and lower extremity vasculature. *Top Magn Reson Imaging* 2005;16(1):21-66).

Phase-Contrast MRA

In 1985, the first paper was published describing successful use of MRI to image arteries using the phase-contrast MRA technique.[17] It is a noninvasive evaluation of the peripheral vasculature, where a vessel-to-background contrast is generated by displaying the accumulated phase difference in transverse magnetization between moving protons in blood and stationary background tissues. Two data sets are acquired whereby polarity of the gradient lobes is shifted between successive acquisitions. As a result of the lack of net phase shift for stationary spins between acquisitions, a preferential image of the vascular tree is generated as their signal is suppressed after subtracting the two data sets. Besides the vascular anatomy evaluation, phase-contrast MRA allows a physiological evaluation because the flow can be quantified. However, the maximum blood flow velocity in the vessel of interest must be known to avoid artifacts.

Time-of-Flight MRA

In the time-of-flight MRA technique, the vessel-to-background contrast is generated by the inflow of fresh protons or unsaturated blood in a saturated background tissue slice. The inflowing unsaturated blood is seen in the imaged slice as an area of high signal intensity. Intravascular protons are also subject to saturation effects, which are proportional to the time protons reside in the imaging slice.[18] Their occurrence can be prevented by using systolic cardiac synchronization; however, it increases the imaging time even more. Depending on the blood flow velocity, imaging slice thickness, and flip angle, rapid extinction of the blood's longitudinal magnetization might occur, just as in the stationary tissues surrounding the arteries. Accelerated intravoxel phase dispersion occurs when the normal, laminar flow pattern in the artery becomes turbulent, as is the case distal to stenoses. This phenomenon also leads to signal loss on MRA images. Although intravoxel phase dispersion often leads to overestimation of degree and length of stenosis, in vitro studies have shown that the magnitude of the signal void directly correlates with the pressure gradient across a stenosis. Because arteries and veins are close to each other, it is necessary to suppress the signal from venous blood entering into the imaging slice. In time-of-flight MRA, this is done by placing concatenated saturation bands a few millimeters distal to the imaging slice. When arterial blood flow is in the craniocaudal direction and venous blood flow is in the opposite direction, the signal from veins is effectively suppressed. However, because the signal of all blood flowing from distal to proximal is suppressed, this may also lead to extinction of signal from retrograde arterial flow (arterial tortuosities). Clinically, this can lead to overestimation of occlusion length, as in the case of unilateral iliac artery occlusion or superficial femoral occlusion with retrograde flow.[19]

3D Half-Fourier Fast Spin-Echo MRA

A 3D flow-spoiled, half-Fourier fast spin-echo, echocardiography-triggered imaging technique has been described for non-CE-MRA of the peripheral vasculature.[20] The fresh-blood imaging technique permits the depiction of slow-flow vessels in T_2-weighted MR images and of fast-flow vessels by acquiring data during the slow-flow cardiac phase. In fast-flow vessels, the fresh-blood imaging technique, electrocardiogram-triggered 3D half-Fourier fast spin-echo MRI with short echo train spacing, shows both arteries and veins as bright blood in diastole-triggered images, whereas the technique shows dark-blood arteries and bright-blood veins in systole-triggered images. Subsequent subtraction of systole-trigged images from diastole-triggered images yields a selective arterial image.[21]

Balanced Steady-State Free Precession MRA

Other techniques that are increasingly being applied in the workup of patients with arterial disease are bSSFP MRI and MRA. Various acronyms are used to describe bSSFP pulse sequences; the most common terms are true fast imaging in steady-state free precession (TrueFISP; Siemens Medical Solutions), balanced fast field echo (bFFE; Philips Medical Systems), and fast imaging employing steady-state excitation (FIESTA, General Electric). The bSSFP sequences are characterized by a high signal-to-noise ratio and image contrast that is primarily determined by the T_2-to-T_1 ratio. The different T_2-to-T_1 ratios of blood and surrounding tissue allow for angiographic imaging with bSSFP. However, because of the bright fat signal, efficient fat saturation is necessary in cases in which arteries are surrounded by fat. Injection of gadolinium chelate contrast media can help further increase contrast between arteries and surrounding tissue. The bSSFP technique is useful for the quick differentiation of arterial lumen from thrombus in aneurysms (Figure 7-11) (1-second acquisition time), and it clearly demonstrates thoracoabdominal aortic aneurysm.[22]

Table 7-14
Limitations of Contrast-Enhanced Magnetic Resonance Angiography

- Claustrophobic patients may require sedation.
- Image compromise may occur with patient motion.
- The technique requires specific nonferromagnetic equipment (for monitoring, ventilation).
- There is a tendency toward stenosis overestimation.
- Signal loss may occur because of the following:
  - Heavy calcifications in small arteries (i.e., arteries below the knee)
  - Metal artifacts (surgical clips, vena cava filters, etc.)

Contrast-Enhanced MRA

The CE-MRA technique is the most popular MRA technique in the evaluation of patients with innumerous forms of arterial disease. It uses a gradient echo T_1-weighted sequence in association with the intravenous contrast media administration. The acquired 3D image is an arterial luminogram obtained during initial arterial passage of contrast material. The CE-MRA basically involves a balance among the desire for high spatial resolution and volumetric coverage (long image acquisition), the desire to avoid disturbing venous enhancement (short image acquisition), and high vessel-to-background contrast. Each sequence may take between 10 and 20 seconds, and the total CE-MRA examination can usually be completed within approximately 20 minutes, depending in the equipment used. Ideally, optimal image quality and the shortest possible imaging acquisition time are desired during the planning of 3D CE-MRA volumes. Initially, the volumetric field of view of the vascular territory to be studied is selected through an initial "scout" or "localizer" images. Scout scans are usually transverse, thick-slice, low-resolution time-of-flight scans.

Whole-Body CE-MRA

The minimum anatomical coverage for evaluation of PVD comprises aortic bifurcation to the ankles; however, because of the systemic nature of atherosclerosis, hypertension, renal, or cerebrovascular diseases often coexist. Thus, many clinicians desire evaluation of the whole-body arterial vasculature. The introduction of faster gradient MR systems, in addition to the implementation of the bolus chase technique and integrated table motion algorithms, has made a great contribution to overcoming the limitation of whole-body MR angiography imaging, which is now integrated into routine clinical practice in many centers throughout the world.[23]

Patient Preparation

It is critical to rule out any contraindication for the use of gadolinium (e.g., pregnancy) or to submit the patient to a magnetic field (e.g., some surgical clips).

Peripheral intravenous access is usually in one of the arms in the antecubital fossa. Claustrophobic patients usually require intravenous conscious sedation (midazolam) and monitoring (Table 7-14).

Once the patient is on the table, preparation starts with careful instructions not to move. Fixation of the area of interest is critical. Using the lower extremities runoff as an example, for a patient's comfort the feet should be fixed in no more than 20- to 30-degree plantar flexion and 20- to 30-degree exorotation.

Table 7-15
Strategies to Decrease the Disturbing Venous Enhancement

- Increase in acquisition speed (the most important one)
- Multielement surface coils and parallel imaging (multiple reception coils)
- Time-resolved acquisition strategy
- Use of venous compression
- Separate acquisition of the lower leg station (for lower extremities magnetic resonance angiography)

Nowadays, the venous enhancement in the lower extremities station is the most important problem standing in the way of universal acceptance of peripheral CE-MRA as an alternative for catheter angiography. This problem is particularly prevalent in patients with cellulites and AVMs in the context of diabetes mellitus (such patients also comprise a large subgroup of the patients with chronic critical ischemia). Taking the lower extremities arteries as an example, adequate depiction of the vascular territory is mandatory because they are often candidates for peripheral bypass surgery. In this scenario, the calves should be suspended by placing soft foam padding in the popliteal fossa, and a tourniquet or blood pressure cuff should be applied just above the knee to delay venous enhancement. Other strategies to avoid disturbing venous enhancement, which are useful for several vascular territories, are shown in Table 7-15.

Once contraindications are excluded (Table 7-16), it is important to rule out renal insufficiency through the patient's GFR, especially in patients with an inflammatory condition, which increases the risk of developing nephrogenic systemic fibrosis.[24]

Protocol and Contrast Media in CE-MRA

CE-MRA relies on synchronizing maximum T_1 shortening with acquisition of pre- and postcontrast injection. However, injection of gadolinium chelate only leads to transient T_1 shortening of the blood pool. The contrast agents quickly diffuse into the extracellular space following a briefly enhancement of the intravascular space. The intravascular half-life of commercially approved agents is about 90 seconds.[25] To decrease the T_1 of blood to values smaller than those of stationary surrounding tissues, enough contrast must be administered intravenously. To selectively depict the blood vessels, this means that the T_1 of blood must be reduced to a value well below that of fat (T_1 at 1.5 T is 270 milliseconds). The

Table 7-16
Contraindications for Magnetic Resonance Angiography

- Anaphylaxis
- Renal insufficiency (estimated glomerular filtration rate <60 ml/min for every 1.73 m^2)*
- Gadolinium during pregnancy
- Cardiac pacemaker
- Ferromagnetic cochlear prosthesis
- Poppen-Blaylock carotid clips
- Cerebral aneurysm clip (except titanium clips)

*Magnetic resonance angiography may be performed individually.

Table 7-17
Protocol for Gadolinium-Enhanced Magnetic Resonance Angiography

- Fast three-dimensional sequence (10-20 seconds)
- Image acquisition before and after IV bolus contrast injection
- Dose of 0.1 to 0.3 mmol/kg, usually between 15 to 45 ml for a 75-kg patient
- 1.5-3 mm slice thickness
- 1-2 mm reconstruction
- Acquisition plane according to the longer axis of the vessel

rate of contrast injection should be such that an arterial T_1 of about 50 milliseconds or less is achieved. In nearly all reported CE-MRA studies, conventional 0.5 M extracellular contrast agents were used. Typically, between 0.1 and 0.3 mmol/kg of contrast agents is injected (i.e., between 15 and 45 ml for a 75-kg patient), followed by a 15- to 30-ml saline injection to flush contrast from injection tubing and veins into the central venous and arterial circulations.

The lower extremities are usually imaged with 15 to 20 ml of contrast medium, and the aortoiliac and upper extremities arteries are imaged with 20 to 25 ml. When a time-resolved 2D test-bolus approach is used to image the lower extremities and pedal arteries first, usually around 5 to 7 ml of contrast is used, followed by a slightly larger saline flush volume to guarantee that the contrast agent is flushed from tubing and veins into the central circulation. Currently, there is no single preferred injection protocol (Table 7-17), although an empirical strategy that works well in clinical practice is that the contrast injection duration should be about 40% to 60% of the acquisition duration. The rationale for this strategy is twofold. First, due to contrast dilution at the leading and trailing edges of the bolus, as well as variable transit times through different portions of the pulmonary circulation, contrast bolus length increases in the body (usually with about 5 to 7 seconds).[26] Second, contrast that is injected after about half of the typical scan duration (10 to 20 seconds) does not arrive in the arterial bed of interest before k-space lines contributing to contrast enhancement in the image are acquired. The amount of contrast to be injected, the injection speed, and the amount of saline flush depend on other variables, such as the scan duration and technique used (i.e., single versus multiple injection). A publication from Boos et al. showed that increasing the amount of contrast injected and the saline flush volume increases bolus length and improves small vessel conspicuity but does not necessarily result in higher vessel-to-background contrast.[27]

The gadolinium-based contrast agents are commonly used to improve the visibility of internal structures when patients undergo MRI. Five types of gadolinium-based contrast agents have been approved by the Food and Drug Administration (FDA) for use in the United States: Magnevist (gadopentetate dimeglumine), Ominiscan (gadodiamide), OptiMARK (gadoversetamide), MultiHance (gadobenate dimeglumine), and Prohance (gadoteridol). The gadolinium atom is tightly bound to a small-molecular-weight linear chelate based on diethylenetriamine pentaacetic acid; it is toxic to the human body if used in isolation. It may be injected intravenously; it is excreted almost exclusively by the kidneys, providing a high signal (bright or white color) on T_1-weighted images; and it can be safely used in patients with iodine contrast allergy.

Gadolinium is contraindicated in patients with history of anaphylaxis (incidence of 1 in 20,000 exams) and in pregnancy. Potential teratogenicity has been demonstrated in an animal study.[28] Initially, it was advocated as a nonnephrotoxic contrast agent and was used as an alternative contrast media to iodine during catheter angiography in patients with renal function impairment.

Never identified before 1997, nephrogenic fibrosing dermopathy, more recently known as nephrogenic systemic fibrosis, is a disease of fibrosis of the skin and internal organs that occurs in patients with renal insufficiency that underwent to MRA studies with the administration of a gadolinium chelate contrast agent. Apparently a combination of factors, including altered kidney function, intense inflammatory burden, and exposure to gadolinium-based contrast agents (which can be found in tissue samples of nephrogenic systemic fibrosis), may play a role in the development of nephrogenic systemic fibrosis. It is particularly true for patients who have acute or chronic renal disease with a GFR lower than 30 ml/min for every 1.73 m^2. However, theoretical risks should be considered for patients with milder renal insufficiency.[29,30] Because chronic renal disease can manifest without causing symptoms and generally is underdiagnosed in the population,[31] a substantial number of patients who are referred for MRI may have undetected chronic renal disease. Determining the incidence of nephrogenic systemic fibrosis associated with the use of different gadolinium chelate contrast agents in large populations will lead to a better understanding of the pathogenesis of nephrogenic systemic fibrosis and to better management of all patients. Although evidence associates the development of nephrogenic systemic fibrosis in patients with renal failure with only some of the FDA-approved gadolinium-based MR contrast agents to date, prudence dictates that we apply our concern to all gadolinium-based MR contrast agents in this regard until more definitive information is forthcoming. A recent publication demonstrated that the incidence of nephrogenic systemic fibrosis at four medical universities of large patient populations was significantly lower ($P < 0.001$) at the two centers where gadopentetate dimeglumine was used compared with the incidence at the two centers where gadodiamide was used.[32]

The current recommendation is that the administration of gadolinium-containing agents should be avoided for all patients even with a mild level of renal insufficiency (estimated GFR of less than 60 ml/min for every 1.73 m^2), particularly if the patient is hospitalized with a proinflammatory condition. In many situations, an alternative imaging examination can help answer the clinical question without the use of a gadolinium-based agent. An unenhanced MRI technique as described earlier, MDCT without or with iodinated contrast material, Doppler ultrasonography, CO_2 catheter angiography, and conventional radiography, alone or combination, can provide answers to many clinical questions. If the patient is already undergoing dialysis, CT with an iodinated contrast agent may be a viable option. If the use of a gadolinium-based contrast agent is considered to be clinically indicated, the referring physician and the patient should be informed of the potential risks of developing nephrogenic systemic fibrosis and a detailed informed consent should be obtained. Lower doses of the contrast agent or the use of a contrast agent that is not implicated as strongly as gadodiamide could also be considered. In patients who are already undergoing renal replacement therapy, dialysis after exposure to gadolinium increases the clearance of the molecule.[33] It should be noted that no data demonstrate that either dialysis therapy after gadolinium or a lower dose of a gadolinium-based contrast agent reduces the incidence of nephrogenic systemic fibrosis. This is a debilitating and sometimes fatal disease. As it is a preventable disease, every effort should be made to screen and manage patients at risk of developing nephrogenic systemic fibrosis.

Specific Sequences Applied to the Vascular Anatomy

Even though CE-MRA is by far the most common sequence used nowadays, phase-contrast MRA and time-of-flight MRA sequences can be useful for the evaluation of high-flow vessels such as in the neck and pelvic, as well as the portal vein and the intracranial arteries (ICAs) and intracranial veins, especially the circle of Willis. Specific plane (2D technique) or volume (3D technique) images may be generated by both sequences. As discussed earlier, the potential stenosis overestimation and the differentiation between high-grade stenosis and vessel occlusion represent the main limitations of these techniques. The limitations are related to the turbulent or slow flow, where a stenosis promotes low or absent signal in the blood vessel, when a high-grade stenosis may be misrepresented as an occlusion (pseudoocclusion).

Thoracoabdominal aortic aneurysms require special attention because the flow may be markedly slower compared to the flow for patients without aneurysms. If insufficient delay time is observed between injection of contrast and imaging, incomplete opacification of the aneurysm results at the time of imaging. To avoid this problem, either a longer delay between injection and start of acquisition or a multiphasic acquisition should be used. The CE-MRA sequence surpassed the limitations related to turbulence or to slow flow, as it does not depend on the blood vessel flow. In general, even when the blood flow is decreased, this gadolinium-enhanced sequence may evaluate the vascular anatomy appropriately.

The 3D time-resolved imaging of contrast kinetics (TRICKS) technique combines appropriately, extending to 3D imaging, with several MRI elements permitting reconstruction of a series of 3D image sets having an effective temporal frame rate of one volume every 2 to 6 seconds.[34] Although this technique is capable of reducing venous contamination, the drawback is that to some extent it leads to a reduction in vessel-to-background contrast.[35]

Synchronization of the Contrast Injection and Acquisition in 3D CE-MRA

As with the CTA technique, there are two options for contrast injection and image acquisition synchronization. However, MRI is a slow imaging technique and the peak arterial enhancement time depends on several variables: injection rate and volume, amount and rate of saline flush, and cardiac output are the most important ones.[36]

The time of peak arterial enhancement has interpatient variation, which requires individualization of the technique to synchronize it with acquisition of the central area of interest to obtain a study of diagnostic quality. Also, the individual contrast arrival time must be taken into consideration to prevent ringing artifacts and suboptimal opacification of arteries in the field of view due to too-early acquisition and to prevent venous overlay.[37]

The first technique to obtain synchronization, for example, during an abdominal aorta MRA, is a 2D time-resolved test bolus in which the optimal scan delay time can be determined by measuring the arrival time of a small bolus (1 to 3 ml) of contrast medium in the infrarenal aorta, followed by 25 to 35 ml of saline injected at the same rate as the full contrast bolus will be injected later. A temporal resolution of about 1 to 2 seconds per image should be used. The scan delay should be chosen to coincide with the frame in which maximum enhancement is observed. Acquisition orientation of the timing bolus scan should be in the coronal or sagittal plane, as this provides not only the exact time at which enhancement commences but also the rate at which enhancement progresses along the 40 to 45 cm of the arterial tree in the field of view.

In contrast to the first technique described, there is real-time bolus (with injection of the total volume of contrast material) monitored by the operator through visual feedback or automatically detected by the scanner when the desired signal enhancement reaches the arterial territory of interest, and the 3D CE-MRA images are acquired. These so-called real-time bolus monitoring software packages have been introduced by all major MRI system vendors and are now considered the state of the art for CE-MRA; they include BolusTrak (Philips Medical Systems, Best, the Netherlands), CareBolus (Siemens Medical Solutions, Erlangen, Germany), and Fluoro Trigger (General Electric, Waukesha, Wisconsin).

MRA Resolution

DSA has an excellent in-plane spatial resolution of $0.3 \times 0.3\ mm^2$, which is already challenged by MDCTA with isotropic voxel sizes of approximately $0.7 \times 0.7 \times 0.7\ mm^3$. In contrast, the in-plane resolution of MRA has been on the order of $1.5 \times 1.5\ mm^2$, with slice thicknesses often exceeding 2 mm, thus hampering the depiction of fine anatomical structures and subtle pathological changes such as fibromuscular dysplasia (FMD). For example, for the detection and grading of renal artery stenosis (RAS), a recent multicenter study found poor sensitivities and specificities for MRA for which the authors blamed poor spatial resolution.[38] As various studies have proven that the area stenosis is more accurate than the traditionally used diameter stenosis, the acquired voxels should be isotropic to allow lossless reformatting (Figure 7-12).[39]

MRA Postprocessing

Dedicated MRA postprocessing work is critical to obtain good quality for imaging interpretation. Even if great images can be generated by the postprocessing tools, review of cross-sectional images remains an integral part of the MRA evaluation. Among the several postprocessing techniques are MIP (Figure 7-13), surface reconstruction (also called shaded surface display), and MPR. Newer reconstruction techniques commonly used are VR and virtual angioscopy. The most popular 3D MRA data display is MIP because it is operator independent, free of intensity thresholding, and fast.[40] Nowadays, most postprocessing workstations can generate and manipulate MIP images, where only voxels with the highest signal intensity are displayed, almost in real time. In the shaded surface display, the image information with signal intensity lower

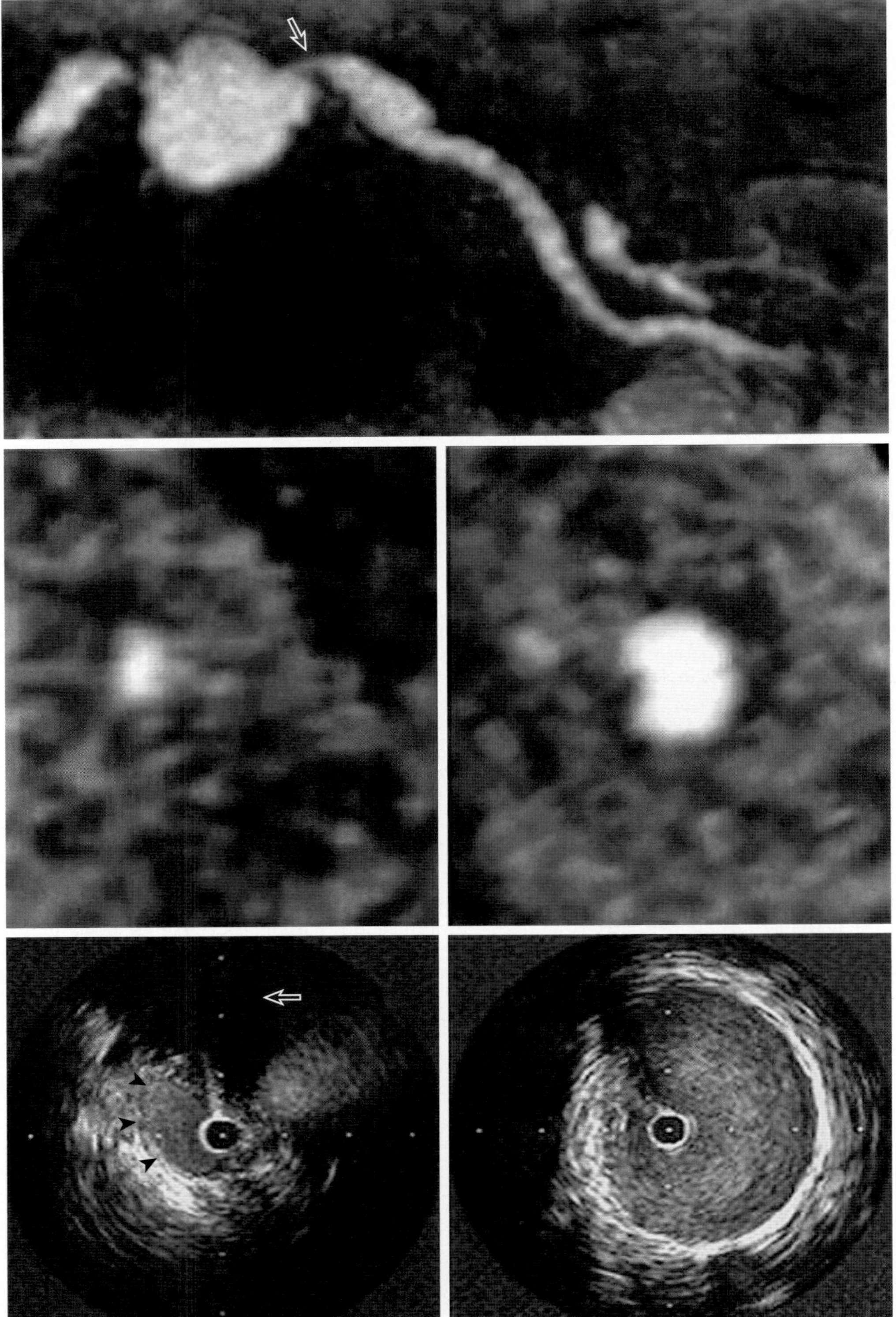

Figure 7-12. A thin, maximum intensity projection *(upper image)* of a proximal, high-grade renal artery stenosis *(arrow)*. The cross-sectional view *(lower image)* of the renal artery at the site of the stenosis with high-spatial-resolution magnetic resonance angiography (MRA; *upper row*) and intravascular ultrasound (IVUS; *lower row*) and distal of the stenosis *(right column)*. This example demonstrates the good correlation between area stenosis in MRA and IVUS. This feature of MRA and IVUS also enables the exact grading of eccentric stenoses, as in this case; grading is prone to errors when only the diameter stenosis is measured. (From Michaely HJ, Dietrich O, Nael K, et al. MRA of abdominal vessels: technical advances. *Eur Radiol* 2006;16:1637-1650.)

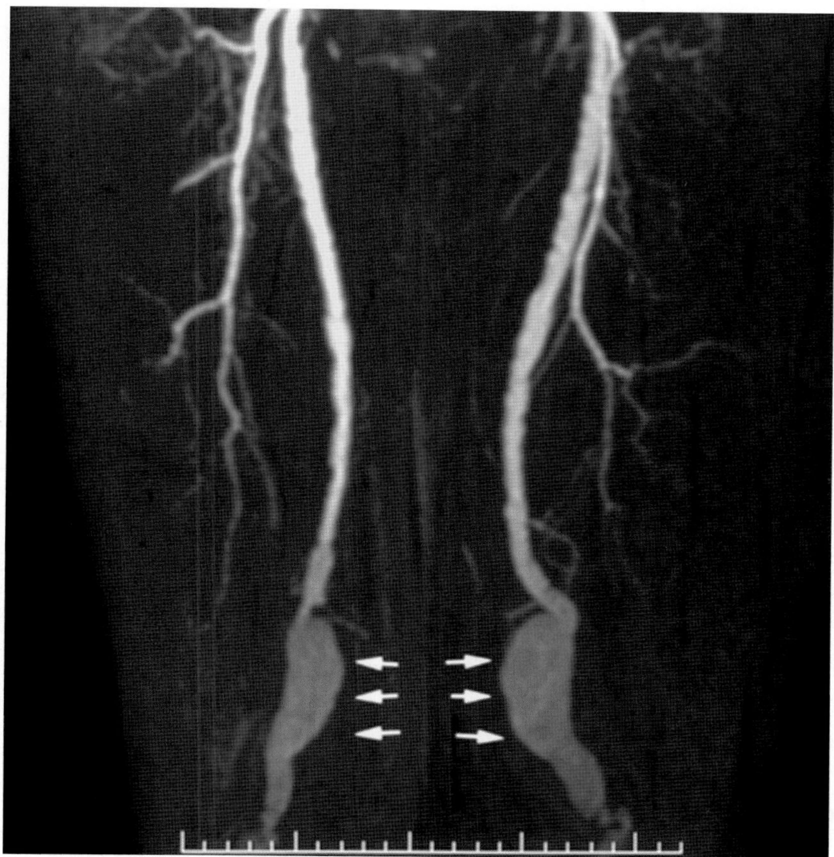

Figure 7-13. Coronal MIP image from contrast-enhanced lower extremities MRA show aneurysms of both popliteal arteries *(arrows)*. (From the RSNA Refresher Courses MR Imaging of Aortic and Peripheral Vascular Disease. Tatli S, Lipton MJ, Davison BD, et al. *Radiographics* 2003;23:S59-S78.)

than the predefined threshold in voxels is subtracted. The advantage is the depiction of complex anatomical relationships among large vessels. The misinterpretation of vascular pseudostenoses and occlusions may occur when the threshold is increased or when low signal intensity is seen in small artery stenosis. In other words, shaded surface display should be taken into consideration only when significant contrast occurs between the lumen of the vessel and the background.

The 3D CE-MRA data sets can be studied from multiple angles, which can be helpful in the eccentric stenoses evaluation. Digital subtraction is especially useful in increasing the contrast between the arteries and the background, which exacerbates the amount of gadolinium per voxel, providing lower signal-to-noise ratio. This has a particular advantage in the evaluation of small severely diseased arteries. Although not necessary for the larger vessels in the thorax, abdomen, and thigh, it may be useful in improving conspicuity of small branch vessels and collaterals.[41]

When multiple anatomical segments are studied with repeated injections of contrast medium, the residual venous enhancement from prior administration may obscure arterial detail in subsequent acquisitions if subtraction is not used.[42,43] According to a metaanalysis conducted by Hany et al.,[44] reviewing raw data (source images), in addition to viewing MIP images, increases the diagnostic accuracy remarkably, decreasing the chance of overprojection of structures with higher signal intensity (veins, subcutaneous fat, or bone marrow) and of wrong threshold data when shaded surface display or VR is used.[44,45] Original, thin-slice MRA images must be reviewed in multiple views (e.g., coronal, sagittal, and transverse) (Figure 7-14A and B), in association with the image reconstruction tools (MIP, shaded surface display, or VR) when there is a question of possible vascular occlusion stenosis. The grade of a vascular stenosis should be described in quantitative terms, which may be accomplished by generating a line profile across the vascular lumen and by plotting the range of signal intensities as a function of the position along the line.[46] Commercially available vascular tracking software may increase the accuracy that can be achieved by finding a center-lumen line with minimal user interaction and may allow for automatic extraction of luminal diameter and stenosis percentages.

CLINICAL APPLICATIONS

Both MRA and CTA are increasingly used for noninvasive vascular imaging. The Diagnostic Imaging in Patients with Peripheral Arterial Disease multicenter, randomized, controlled trial was designed to compare the costs and effects of Doppler ultrasound, MRA, and MDCTA as the initial imaging test in the diagnostic workup of patients with PVD.[47] Significantly higher confidence and less additional imaging were found for MRA and CTA compared with duplex ultrasonography. No statistically significant differences were found in improvement in functional patient outcomes and quality of life among the groups. The total costs were significantly higher

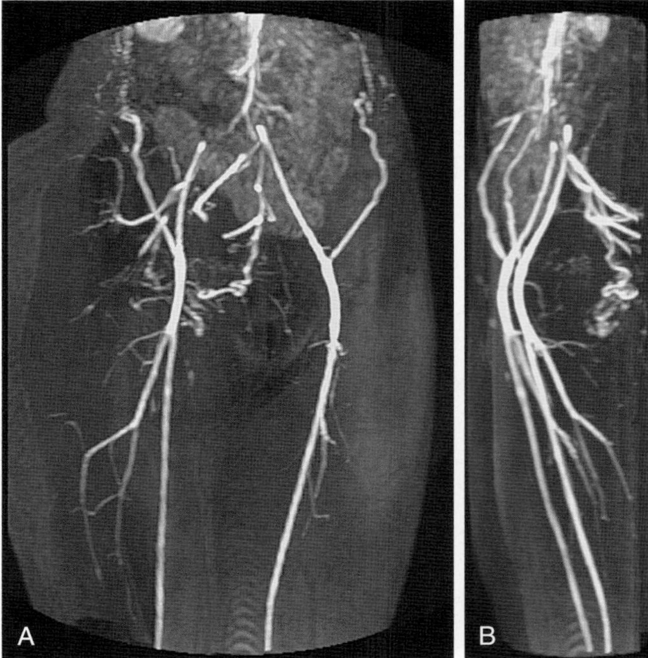

Figure 7-14. Contrast-enhanced magnetic resonance angiography images in right-anterior oblique and in lateral views. Bilateral occlusion of the common iliac arteries is shown.

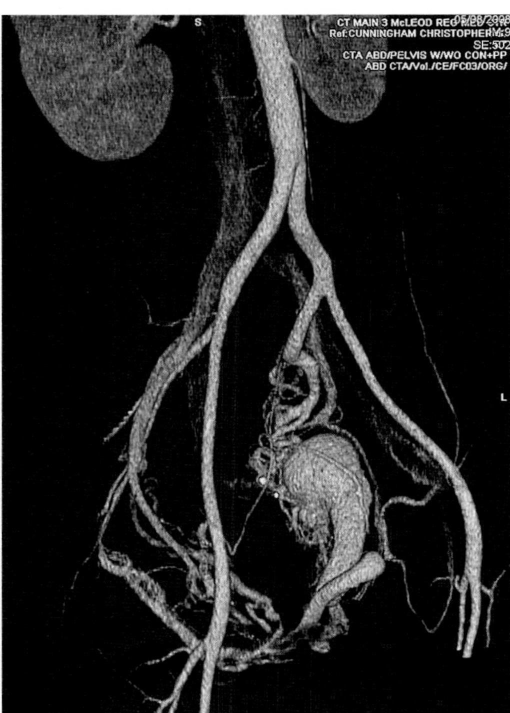

Figure 7-15. Right-anterior oblique three-dimensional reconstruction of a multidetector row computed tomography angiogram of a pelvis. Complex AVM associated with an enlarged drainage vein is demonstrated.

for MRA and duplex ultrasonography than for CTA. The imaging peripheral arterial disease study, a randomized, controlled trial comparing CE-MRA and MDCTA, was designed to evaluate the clinical utility, patient outcomes, and costs for initial imaging in the diagnostic workup of patients with PVD. Patients demonstrated no statistically significant difference in clinical utility and patient outcomes between both methods.[48] However, CTA provided a statistically significant reduction in the total diagnostic costs compared with MRA. At the time of the publication, the average cost for diagnostic imaging was €359 ($438) higher in the MRA group than in the MDCTA group (95% confidence interval: €209, €511 [$255, $623]; $P < 0.001$). Therapeutic costs were higher in the MRA group, but the difference was not significant. The therapeutic confidence for MDCTA was slightly higher than that for MRA, but both were comparable to the mean therapeutic confidence of 8.2 (in a scale from 0 to 10) for DSA that was observed in a previous study.[49] Probably because of the lower confidence in MRA, the physicians requested additional imaging more often in the MRA group than in the MDCTA group.

CTA more accurately depicts the extent and localization of disease, which results in better treatment and better patient outcomes. The results suggest that CTA has some advantages over MRA in the initial imaging evaluation of patients with PVD.[48]

Nonatherosclerotic Vascular Disease

Contrast-enhanced MDCTA and CE-MRA are increasingly used not only for noninvasive vascular imaging evaluation of atherosclerotic disease but also for assisting in the diagnosis and clinical management in various nonatherosclerotic vascular diseases, including vascular tumors (angiosarcoma), carotid body tumors, inflammatory diseases (e.g., Takayasu arteritis), AVMs (Figure 7-15), and arteriovenous fistulas. The initial minimally invasive angiographic evaluation may provide enough information to plan the clinical management or the procedure and to have a more objective therapeutic approach during the catheter angiography. Best arterial access, vessel size, number of vessels involved, surrounding tissues, collateral circulation (Figure 7-16), venous drainage, and potential vessel challenge anatomy (tortuosities) may be assessed. This information may anticipate complications and technical problems and may ultimately facilitate the performance of the surgical or endovascular procedure.

Evaluation of Peripheral Artery Stents

Generally, peripheral artery stents are larger and better evaluated under CTA than the small coronary artery stents, especially when specific MDCTA processing software is applied in the raw data. MIP (Figure 7-17), MPR, VR (Figure 7-18), and intrastent endoluminal reconstructions are useful for a comprehensive stent evaluation. The high-resolution MDCT scanner images usually correlate well with the catheter angiography findings. It is possible to study not only stent patency (to rule out intrastent restenosis or thrombosis) in several peripheral arteries but also stent fracture, crushing, kinking, adequate expansion, tine apposition, edge dissection, stent graft migration, and related endoleaks.

Lower Extremities Vascular Occlusive Disease

The diagnosis and planning of a therapeutic procedure for patients with advanced peripheral occlusive disease requires information about the location, degree, and length of the

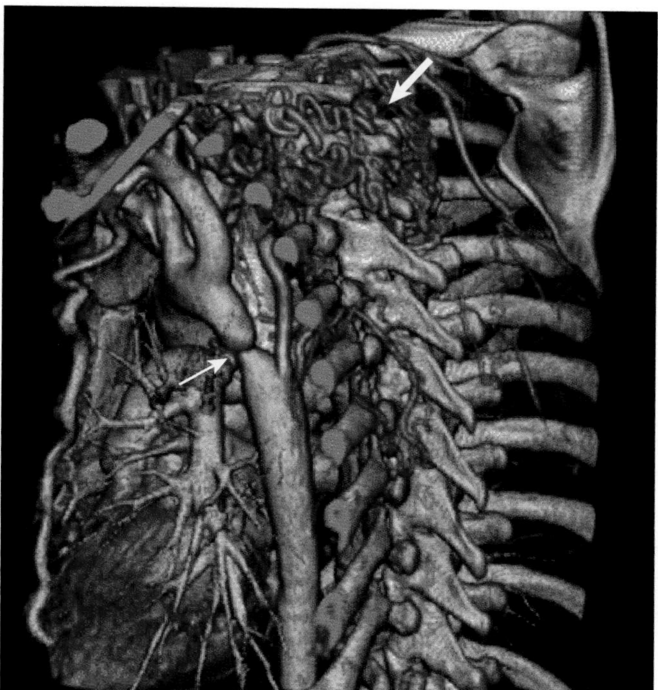

Figure 7-16. Colored volume rendering reconstruction of a thorax multidetector row computed tomography angiogram. Focal stenosis *(thin arrow)* is depicted that is consistent with aortic coarctation associated with well-developed collateral circulation *(thick arrow)*.

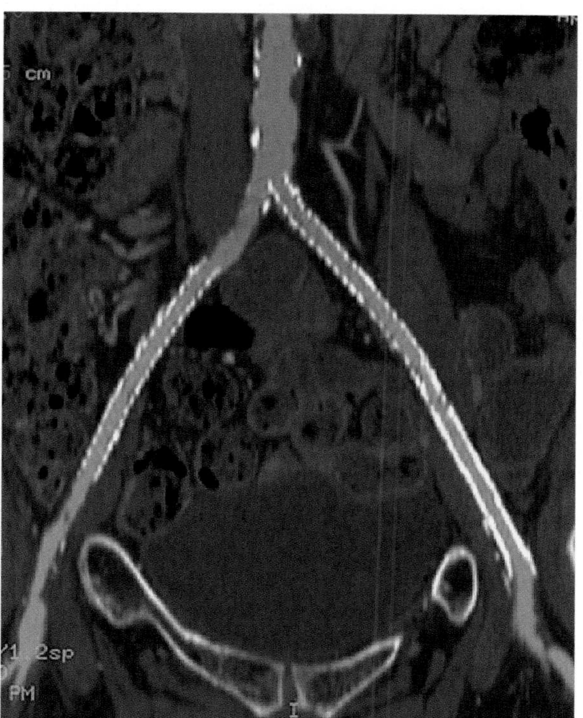

Figure 7-17. Maximum intensity projection reconstruction of a multidetector row computed tomography angiogram of the pelvis. Example is in a patient with previous stent placement to recanalize bilateral occlusions of the iliac arteries.

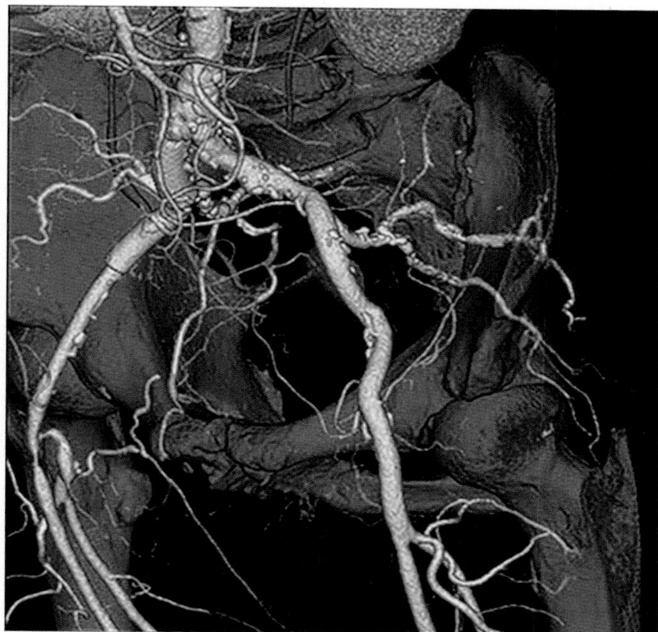

Figure 7-18. Colored volume rendering reconstruction of a multidetector row computed tomography angiogram for right iliac artery stent surveillance. Left-anterior oblique view demonstrates patency of the iliac artery stent and stenosis in the proximal superficial femoral artery.

lesion or lesions and the configuration of the inflow and runoff vessels. MDCTA and MRA are helpful in detecting hemodynamically significant occlusive lesions in peripheral arteries. Duplex ultrasonography evaluation of the arteries of an entire lower extremity is operator dependent and labor intensive and does not provide a roadmap equivalent to that provided by MR, CT, or catheter-based angiography. Thus, duplex ultrasonography would be expected to play only a supplementary role in evaluating restricted segments of lower extremity arteries. The great advantage of MDCTA is that it allows evaluation of all aortoiliac and lower extremity arteries in a single acquisition. The reported sensitivities and specificities of 4-MDCTA compared with DSA in detecting significant stenoses of the aortoiliac and lower extremity arteries are 91% to 99% for the sensitivities and 83% to 99% for the specificities, respectively.[53-55] With the introduction of the multidetector computer tomographers, especially with 64 channels, it becomes possible to evaluate larger vascular territories with a submillimeter slice thickness (approximately 0.6 mm) and high-resolution images with a short scanning time (Figure 7-7B).

A specific pitfall of MDCTA can occur when the timing of scanning does not coincide with the arrival of contrast material in the targeted lower extremity arteries, especially the infrapopliteal arteries. This discrepancy may cause misdiagnosis or overestimation of stenotic occlusion in calf arteries due to insufficient luminal enhancement in conditions such as low cardiac output or aortic aneurysm. The evaluation might be suboptimal due to limited spatial resolution or venous contamination as well.[54,56] This problem may be overcome by using CT scanners with 16 or more detector rows with submillimeter collimation.

When evaluating the peripheral vasculature, it is important to describe the morphological pattern of occlusive disease. Three distinct patterns of aortoiliac occlusive disease

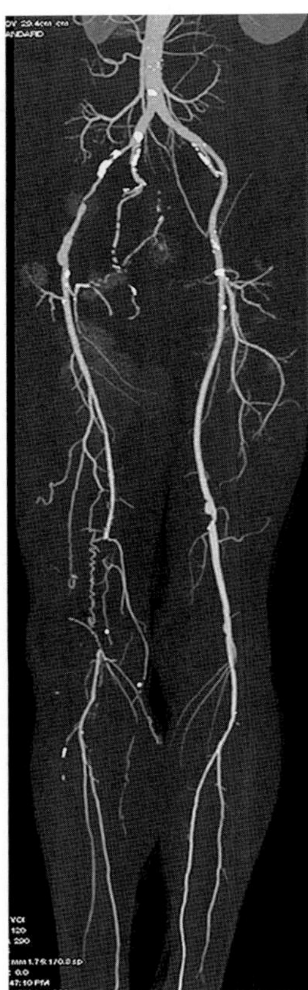

Figure 7-19. Contrast-enhanced magnetic resonance angiography showing the types of peripheral arterial occlusive disease. Type I: Disease limited to aorta and common iliac arteries. Type II: Disease limited to suprainguinal peripheral arteries. Type III: Central and peripheral arterial multilevel occlusive disease.

can be distinguished (Figure 7-19). The clinical significance lies in the distinction between types I and II and type III, as this latter group of patients has a much worse prognosis.[57,58] In the case of an aortic occlusion (LeRiche syndrome) or unilateral iliac artery occlusion, the site of distal reconstitution should be evaluated because this determines the type of revascularization. The easiest and most widely used method of measuring diameter reduction is to simply measure the maximum degree of luminal reduction on MIP images, analogous to how stenoses are measured on DSA images. A stenosis is generally considered to be "hemodynamically significant" when reduction of the luminal diameter exceeds 50%.

The key differentiation that must be made when evaluating the upper leg vasculature is whether there is a relatively short, focal stenosis or a complete occlusion over a long segment. The most common site of stenoses or occlusions is where the superficial femoral artery courses through the adductor (Hunter's) canal (Figure 7-20).

Patients with chronic occlusive disease are generally good candidates for imaging with CE-MRA. This is in contrast to patients with acute limb ischemia, who are experiencing a surgical emergency and for whom the decision to obtain an imaging test is based on the clinical status and presumed etiology of the occlusion. In the case of a suspected embolus or thrombosis, immediate surgical exploration is indicated, with possible catheter angiography on the surgical table. CE-MRA is an excellent modality to image the lower extremities, and it is possible to study from the abdominal aorta down to the toes in a single acquisition or simply evaluate selectively the femoropopliteal segment, for example. A surface coil such as the phased-array body coil or a dedicated peripheral vascular coil should be used to image the whole lower extremity vasculature whenever possible. In addition, the use of parallel imaging capable coils that cover multiple stations allow shortening of acquisition duration. Truly acquired slice thickness should not exceed 2.0 to 2.5 mm to prevent overestimation of stenosis severity. Subtraction of a nonenhanced "mask" scan helps increase vessel-to-background contrast but is not essential because the intravascular signal is usually much higher compared with that of subcutaneous fat. The reported sensitivities and specificities of CE-MRA compared with DSA in detecting significant stenoses of the aortoiliac and lower extremity arteries are 93% to 96% for the sensitivities and 90% to 95% for the specificities, respectively.[59,60] Relatively recent studies have demonstrated that MRA can have a sensitivity of up to 97% and a specificity of up to 100% for more than 50% stenosis in the femoropopliteal segment.[61-63]

In cases in which additional coverage is needed in the anteroposterior direction, for instance, in the presence of an AAA or a femorofemoral crossover bypass graft, or when LeRiche syndrome is suspected, the number of slices should be increased to cover all relevant anatomy.

In the infrapopliteal segment, exact lesion CTA assessment can be problematic due to small vessel diameters.[54] Although depiction of the infragenicular arterial system in patients with intermittent claudication is important, it is usually not the location of the lesions that causes symptoms or the target for invasive intervention, except in patients with diabetes mellitus.[64] This is opposed to the group of patients with chronic critical ischemia (i.e., rest pain, tissue loss, or both). The angiographic hallmarks of chronic critical ischemia are bilateral, multiple stenoses and occlusions at different levels in the peripheral arterial tree (type III occlusive disease). Patients with diabetes are a well-recognized subgroup with primarily distal atherosclerotic occlusive disease and preservation of normal inflow.

The diameter of the lower leg arteries gradually decreases from approximately 5 to 6 mm in the distal popliteal artery to about 2 to 3 mm in the foot. To reliably diagnose arterial occlusive disease, the spatial resolution should be $1.0 \times 1.0 \times 1.0$ mm^3 or better. On modern 1.5 T MR scanners equipped with state-of-the-art gradient systems, this resolution is certainly feasible. As yet, there is no standardized approach to MRA of the distal lower extremity. Below-knee MRA remains challenging, and deep venous opacification adjacent to the arteries can be a major problem resulting in suboptimal interpretation. Like MRA, MDCTA may face this problem, especially in diabetic patients or in below-knee cellulites (Figure 7-21). When needed, additional dedicated MRA and MDCTA imaging of calf arteries with a reduced field of view may be acquired for better evaluation (Figure 7-22). To obtain the best possible MRA image quality in the vascular territory below the knee, it is essential to understand that the goal is not so much to keep up with the arterial bolus but to acquire relevant image information before massive, deep venous enhancement. Exclusion of pedal arterial anatomy because of too-small imaging volume is a common mistake and can be avoided by meticulous review of localizer original partitions. Stenosis of the dorsalis pedis

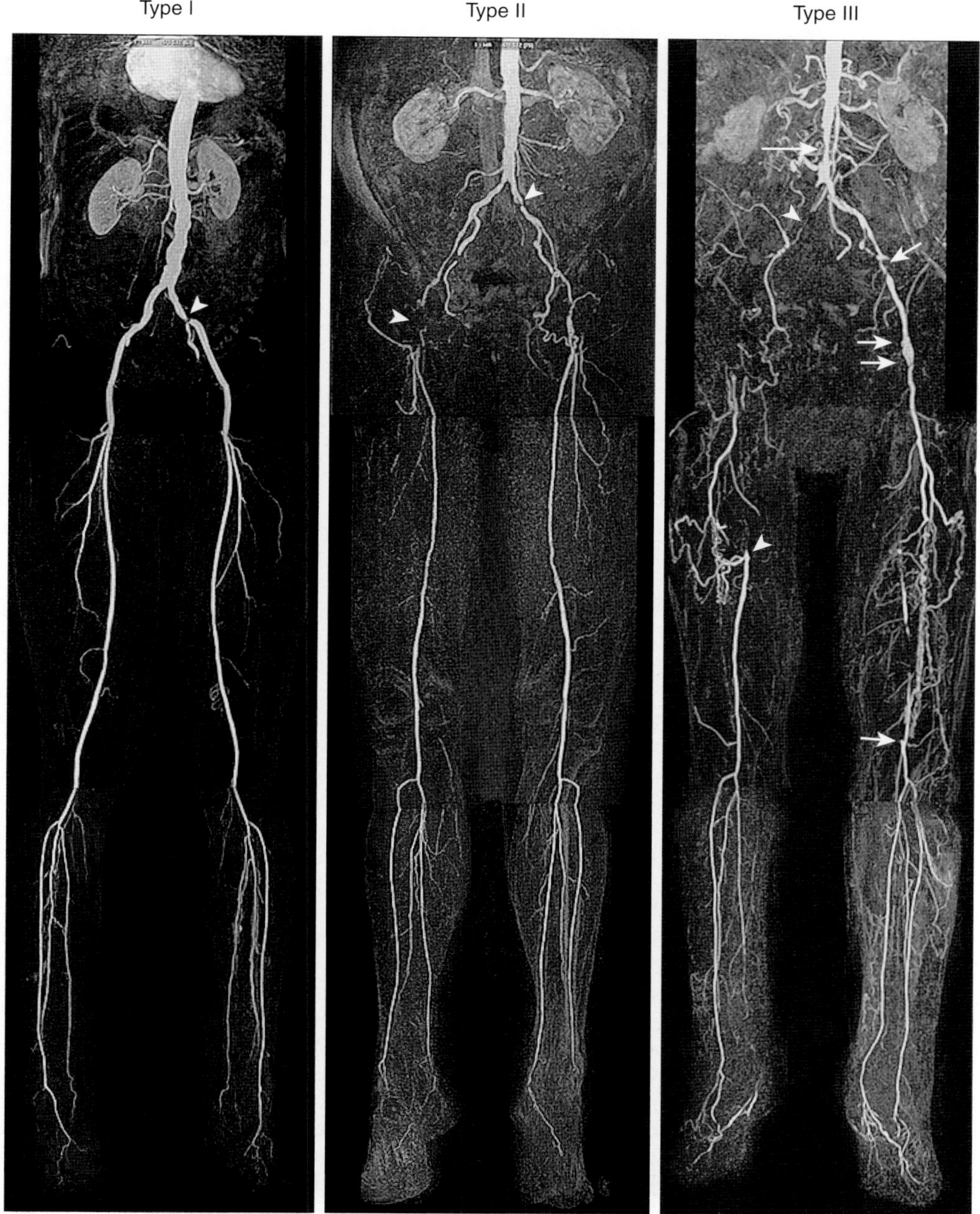

Figure 7-20. Coronal lower extremities multidetector row computed tomography angiography. Maximum intensity projection image shows high-grade stenosis in the right external iliac and occlusion of the distal right superficial femoral with reconstitution of the popliteal artery through collateral circulation. This study offers enough information for revascularization planning. (From Leiner TT. Magnetic resonance angiography of abdominal and lower extremity vasculature. *Top Magn Reson Imaging* 2005;16(1):21-66.)

artery can artifactually be induced by tight straps and when the foot is imaged in plantar flexion. The cause of this latter "Ballerina sign" artifact is compression of the dorsal pedal artery by the distal part of the retinaculum extensorum.[6]

Thoracic and Abdominal Aortas

MDCTA and MRA are great diagnostic tools during the investigation of possible aneurysms and dissection of the thoracic and abdominal aortas. With MDCTA and MRA, it is feasible to study the aorta from the aortic valve down to the bifurcation and the visceral branches, and the study may be extended to the toes if needed.

Aortic Dissection

Aortic dissection is the most common acute disease of the aorta, and it requires prompt diagnosis and management because it is potentially life threatening. Both MDCTA and MRA perform as well as transesophageal echo in the evaluation of dissection. Axial images best demonstrate the intimal flap because they have the highest resolution, and they should

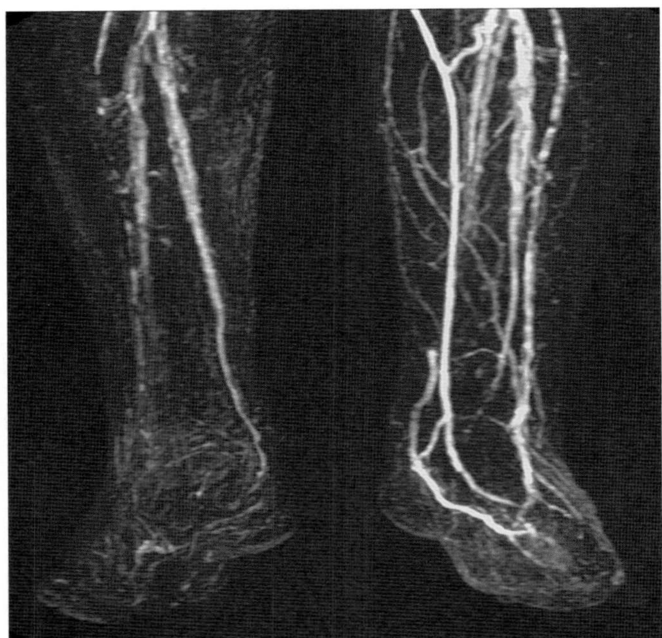

Figure 7-21. Below-knee magnetic resonance angiography (MRA). This type of MRA remains challenging because of the potential arterial and venous simultaneous demonstration, which can result in suboptimal interpretation.

be always compared to the findings in the 3D or MIP views. Potential problem exists when the dissection extends into a horizontally oriented vessel, but usually the current protocols for 16- to 128-MDCTA, with submillimeter slice thickness, and the MPR reconstruction may help in detection of subtle or difficult lesions. Confident diagnosis and correct classification of aortic dissection are based on the detection of an intimal flap in the aorta that separates the true and false lumens (Figure 7-23). The true and false lumens can be differentiated on the basis of signal intensity (for MRA) and contrast enhancement (for CTA), morphological features, the relationship between the lumens, and the appearance of thrombosis. Like MDCTA, CE-MRA shows the true lumen with higher signal intensity than the false lumen because of a higher concentration of contrast material during the arterial phase—a finding that is clearly depicted on MIP images. The true lumen is usually smaller than the false lumen and would be thin or flat from being pressed, appearing oval or semiround in the axial plane. The false lumen is expanded or large, appearing crescentic or semiround or winding around the true lumen in the axial plane (Figure 7-23). Regarding the relationship between the lumens, they may be parallel to each other, the false lumen may wind around the true lumen, or the true lumen may look like a ribbon floating in the false lumen. In relation to the appearance of thrombosis, the false lumen usually contains a degree of thrombus, especially at the retrograde end of the initial entry site, whereas the true lumen contains no thrombus in most cases.[65]

The manifestation of entry sites, especially the initial entry tear, is the greatest concern in clinical application, especially for planning endovascular treatment.[66] The initial entry can be clearly seen in the axial plane, but its 3D relationship to the surrounding anatomical structures cannot. In contrast, VR and MPR images can display both the initial entry and its 3D relationship to the neighboring arterial orifice.

The initial entry in Stanford type A dissection is usually located above the root of the ascending aorta (Figure 7-24), whereas that in type B dissection is usually located at the descending junction of the aortic arch. In the latter case, attention should be paid to the relationship between the entry and the left subclavian artery (Figure 7-25) because this relationship directly affects choice of therapy. Depiction of the initial entry and its relationship with the neighboring arterial orifice may be clearer on VR or MPR images than on DSA images, which greatly facilitates endovascular treatment by helping determine the correct projection direction for DSA. MIP or MPR images can help accurately measure the length and diameter of the proximal neck, the size of the initial entry, the diameters of various parts of the descending aorta, and the maximum diameter of the false lumen. In rare cases, the initial entry may be at the middle or lower segment of the descending aorta, the abdominal aorta, or even the renal artery. In most cases, the reentry site is at the iliac artery on the left side, the right side, or both. Occasionally, the reentry site can be at the abdominal aorta, descending aorta, renal artery, or celiac artery. Unlike the initial entry site, the reentry site is sometimes difficult to visualize clearly during the arterial phase because less contrast material is found in the false lumen, although it can be clearly seen during the venous phase.

Numerous studies evaluating the efficacy of CTA in diagnosing aortic dissection have demonstrated sensitivities of 90% to 100% but lower specificities ranging from 87% (lower than MRA or transesophageal echocardiography) to 100%.[67-70] However, these studies compared conventional CT, which has largely been supplanted by faster multidetector helical scanners. More recent study using MDCTA have reported sensitivities and specificities of 100%.[71] Complete aortogram in the newer generation MDCT (16 or more channels) scanners may be done in a single scan, a single breathhold. Following the non-contrast-enhanced CT examination, contrast-enhanced arterial and venous phases are performed to also rule out the presence of dissection, intramural hematoma, contrast extravasation, and penetrating parietal ulcer, which are part of the full image workup. The extension of the dissection into the aortic braches may be appreciated, as well as organ ischemia (Figure 7-26). Compared to MRA, MDCTA is faster and promptly available in most medical centers, which is important in avoiding compromise of the emergency care of unstable patients.

Another application of the MDCT is the posttreatment image follow-up of these patients. The exclusion of an aortic dissection by a stent graft or by a surgical graft, the presence of endoleak and of previously unseen points of communication between the false and the true lumens, and the dissection stabilizations or progression in a patient treated conservatively may be evaluated in detail. MRA is an excellent image method for the detection and assessment of aortic dissection, with a sensitivity of 98% and a specificity of 98%. An MRA examination of the aorta produces a 3D reconstruction of the aorta, allowing the identification of the intimal tear location, the involvement of branch vessels, and the location of any secondary tears. It can also detect and quantitate the degree of aortic insufficiency. MRA is a good alternative in patients with acute aortic dissection and who are hemodynamically stable (because the scan is relatively time consuming) and in the follow-up of patients with chronic aortic dissection. In addition, MRA clearly shows the presence of intramural hematoma

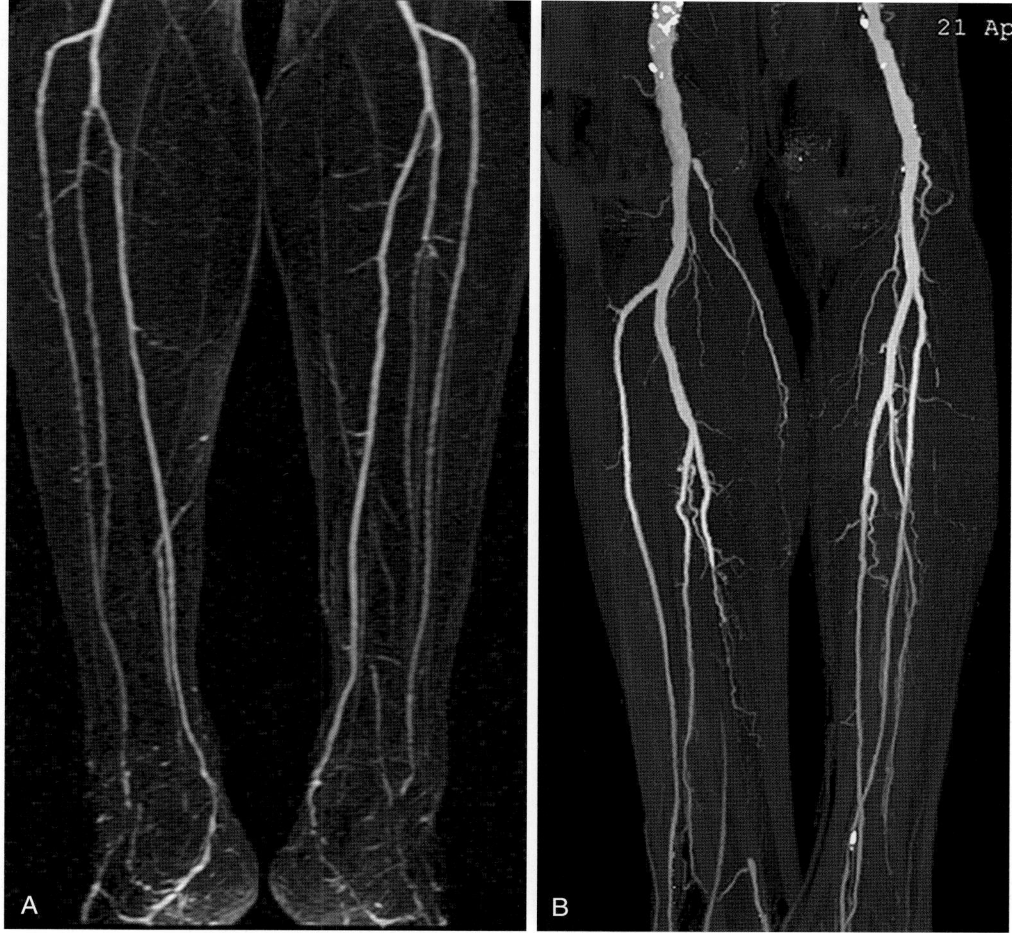

Figure 7-22. **A,** Dedicated magnetic resonance angiography demonstrates normal calf arteries with a reduced field of view. **B,** Dedicated multidetector row computed tomography angiogram in a reduced field of view shows calcifications in the popliteal arteries bilaterally and in the distal left anterior tibial artery, associated with occlusion of the posterior tibial artery at the midthird on the left.

and its progression, so it may also be useful in the follow-up of patients who underwent postaortic dissection surgical repair, as up to 15% and 25% of these patients will require a reoperation in 5 and 10 years, respectively.

Aortic Aneurysm

An aneurysm is defined as a focal enlargement of an artery to more than 1.5 times its normal diameter. For the aorta the general cutoff value is 3 cm, and for the iliac arteries it is 1.8 cm. Aneurysms are either "true," when intima, media, and adventitia are involved, or "false," if fewer than three layers are involved. False aneurysms are often associated with confined rupture of arterial vessel wall, either spontaneous or due to trauma. Morphologically, aneurysms are described as being fusiform or saccular, and they are often lined with thrombus. The most common aneurysms are of the nonspecific, degenerative type and are predominantly found in the infrarenal abdominal aorta and the iliac, femoral, and popliteal arteries.

CE-MRA imaging is an excellent modality for the workup and (postinterventional) follow-up of AAA. In dedicated medical centers, Doppler ultrasound can also be a suitable imaging modality for this purpose. However, in emergency cases, MDCTA is preferred. The workup of AAA demands a full morphological description of the AAA itself (exact location, diameter, presence of thrombus and calcifications) and the relationship to branch vessels and surrounding organs (Table 7-18).

AAA rupture risk increases with size[72]; however, when the aortic diameter is below 4 cm, rupture risk is close to zero.[73] When the diameter exceeds 5 cm, rupture risk rises to 3% to 15% per year.[74] The lower threshold for elective intervention is therefore when the diameter of the lumen, including any mural thrombus, exceeds 5.0 to 5.5 cm.[75,76] Facing a thoracic or abdominal aneurysm, it is essential to evaluate whether it has indication of treatment. If positive, it is important to study whether it is suitable for endovascular or surgical repair. In the case of an endovascular approach, preinterventional imaging is even more important because patient selection and sizing of the endograft depend on it (Figure 7-27).

MDCTA is ideal in the preoperative evaluation of thoracic and abdominal aneurysms because it is capable to show the location, extension, potential rupture, hematoma formation, involvement of the aortic braches, and relationships to the left subclavian artery and celiac trunk and to the renal and iliac arteries (Figure 7-28). MDCTA is also useful in the assessment of thoracic and abdominal aorta surgical repair and post–stent graft placement. MIP and VR images are favored in this scenario, as the metallic component of

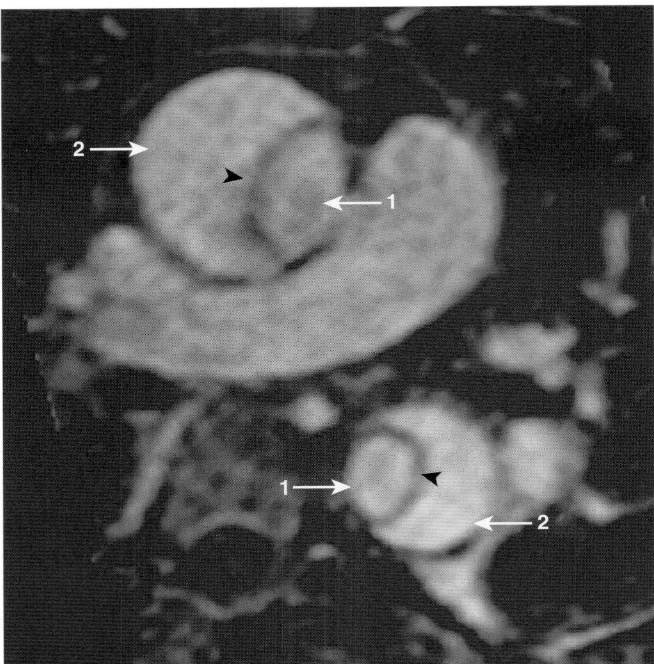

Figure 7-23. Axial image magnetic resonance angiography of the thoracic aorta. The image clearly shows a type A dissection. (From Liu Q, Ping Lu J, Wang F, et al. Three-dimensional contrast-enchanced MR angiography of aortic dissection: A pictorial essay. *RadioGraphics* 2007;27:1311-1321.)

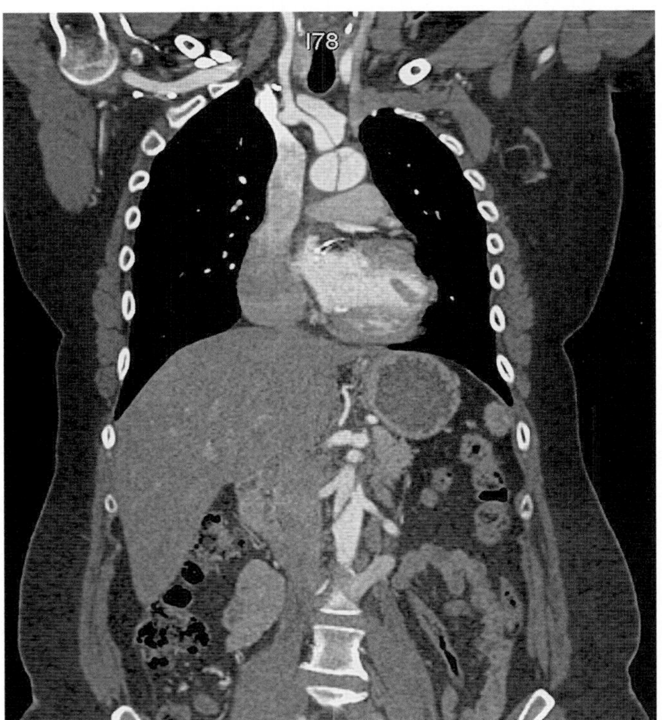

Figure 7-24. Coronal view of a multidetector row computed tomography angiogram maximum intensity projection reconstruction. This view depicts a type A dissection involving the supraaortic branches and extending into the thoracic aorta. The blood flow into right renal artery is coming from the false lumen and into left renal artery from the true lumen.

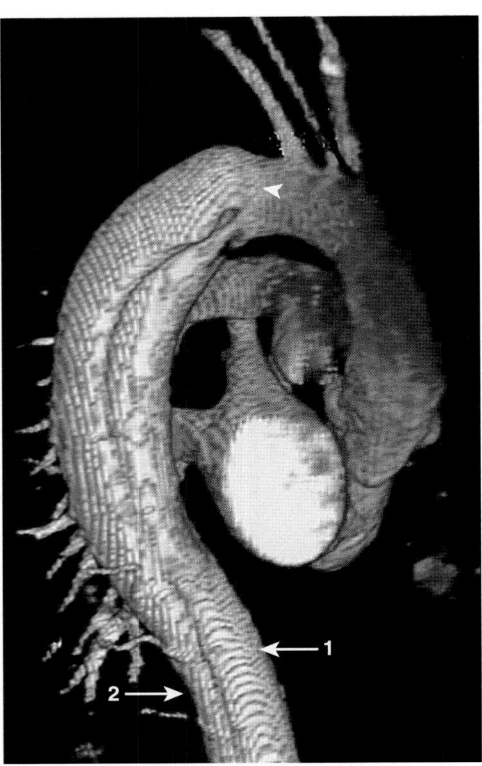

Figure 7-25. Posterior view of a magnetic resonance angiography volume rendering reconstruction of the thoracic aorta. This view demonstrates the dissection entry point distal to the left subclavian artery *(arrow head)* and the true *(1)* and false *(2)* lumens. (From Liu Q, Ping Lu J, Wang F, et al. Three-dimensional contrast-enchanced MR angiography of aortic dissection: A pictorial essay. *RadioGraphics* 2007; 27:1311-1321.)

the graft can be identified clearly (Figures 7-14A to B and 7-29). MDCTA adequately evaluates the stent graft position, the expansion and exclusion of the aneurysm sac, and the patency of the aortic branches and potential complications such as stent graft migration. Delayed images are also critical in the evaluation of endoleaks in the aneurismal sac after thoracic and abdominal stent graft placement. This is not an uncommon complication; it occurs in up to 20% of patients, and it refers to an incomplete exclusion of the aneurysm sac from the systemic circulation with leakage outside of the endoprosthesis.[77,78]

MRA with gadolinium is an excellent method of diagnostic image to evaluate the aorta. Using MIP and 3D reconstruction images, it is possible to study the aorta from multiple angles and planes. Aorta diameter, tortuosities, sometimes complex anatomy, atherosclerotic disease, original and proximal segments of its branches, aneurysm, and dissection can be identified accurately by MRA as well. Congenital abnormalities and coarctation of the aorta can also be evaluated. Presence of aortic wall disease, such as mycotic aneurysm and aortitis, are also studied because MR is capable of studying the wall of the aorta and clearly demonstrating whether an inflammatory process is going on. The bSSFP MRA is well suited to quickly determining the true size of aneurysms because of its ability to differentiate mural thrombus from patent lumen (Figure 7-11).

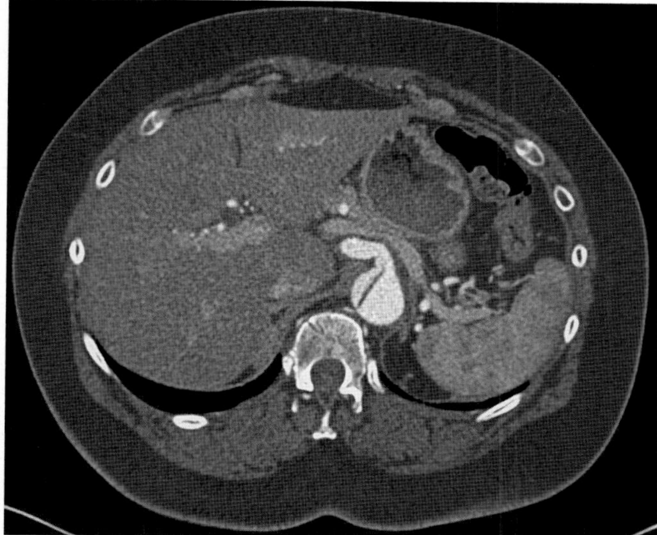

Figure 7-26. Axial image of multidetector row computed tomography aortogram. The image shows the extension of the dissection into the origin of the celiac trunk.

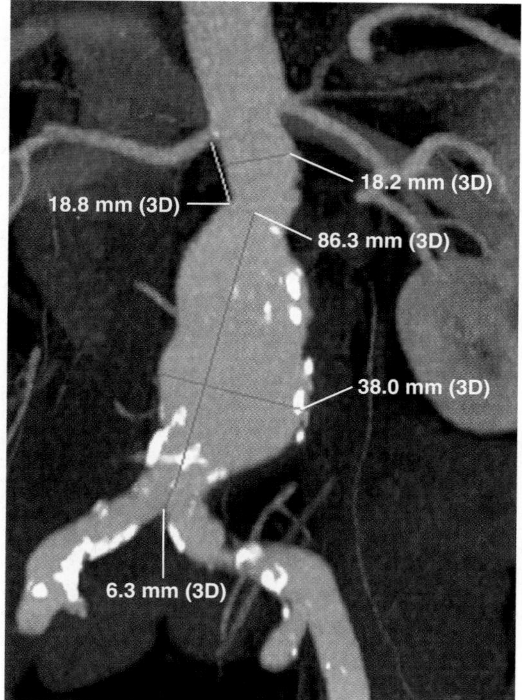

Figure 7-27. Coronal maximum intensity projection image of multidetector row computed tomography angiography of the abdominal aorta. The image shows some required measurements for the correct selection of the abdominal aortic aneurysm stent graft device. Multiple aneurismal change occurs in the ascending aorta.

MRA allows the evaluation of the entire aorta (thoracic and abdominal), which may be critical because one third of patients with thoracic aneurysm also have abdominal aneurysm (Figure 7-30). Aortic diameter measurements should always be performed on MPR, perpendicular to a center-lumen line through the vessel and including any mural thrombus. Although the CE-MRA MIP reconstruction only provides an aortic luminogram, the source images are well suited to determine the presence of thrombus. At present, it is not easy to assess the presence and extent of mural calcifications with MRI. For the evaluation of aortic aneurysms, it is important to obtain delayed 3D MRA images to rule out large aneurysm with slow filling, false lumen of an aneurismal dissection, and collateral circulation. The delayed images also allow the evaluation of the aortic wall and of the periaortic space. This is important for the differential diagnosis between aneurismal wall thrombus with slow flow and mycotic aneurysm, which is going to show

Table 7-18
Abdominal Aortic Aneurysm Features

- Length of normal infrarenal aorta
  - Above aneurysm: aortic neck length of at least 1.5 cm (when endovascular intervention is considered)
  - Below aneurysm: extension into iliac arteries
- Maximum diameter: aortic diameter of <3.0 cm is normal; iliac artery diameter of <1.8 cm is normal
- Relationship to renal arteries
  - Suprarenal: aneurysm extends above renal arteries
  - Juxtarenal: aneurysm begins within 1.0 cm of renal arteries
  - Infrarenal: >1.0 cm of normal aorta below main renal arteries
- Renal anatomy: presence of renal vein variants (e.g., retroaortic left renal vein) and kidney variants (e.g., horseshoe kidney)
- Presence of occlusive disease: calcifications, stenoses, and occlusion in aorta, iliac, and femoral arteries
- Patency of the inferior mesenteric artery (prominent artery may increase the risk of type II endoleaks)
- Inflammatory aortic wall process

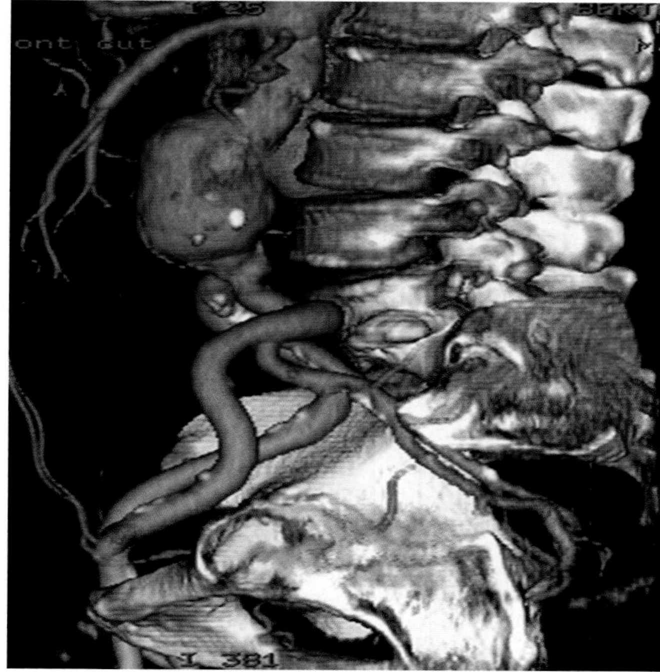

Figure 7-28. Lateral view of the volume rendering reconstruction image of an abdominal aortogram demonstrating a large infrarenal abdominal aorta.

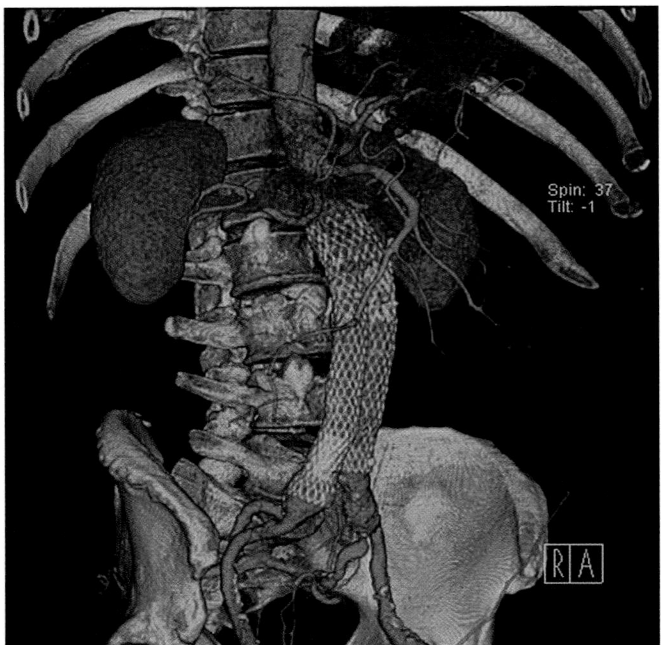

Figure 7-29. Control multidetector row computed tomography abdominal aortogram postinfrarenal abdominal aortic aneurysm stent graft repair. Colored volume rendering image shows patency and adequate stent graft position, with complete aneurysm sac exclusion.

periaortic-space gadolinium enhancement. The CE-MRA may be used in the follow-up of a patient who underwent open or endovascular repair of aortic aneurysms, and usually a period of at least 30 days is recommended to perform this study. Before this period, the inflammatory response to the endograft may mimic aortic infection. In general, even if the MRA follow-up may exclude hemodynamically significant stenosis (more than 50%) in nitinol, titanium, and Elgiloy (nonferromagnetic materials) stents, the potential image artifacts of MRA assure MDCTA as the method of choice for AAA patient surveillance after endovascular repair. The well-known stenosis-mimicking artifact of MRA after endograft placement is the loss of signal at the ends of the stent graft or complete loss of signal in the graft, depending on the composition of the graft material.

Aortic Occlusive Disease

The most common cause of aortic occlusive disease in Western countries is atherosclerosis. Other far less common causes are Takayasu disease, giant cells arteritis, and postradiation therapy. The MDCTA or MRA of the aorta offers a noninvasive evaluation of the level of the aortic occlusion, collateral circulation, and reconstitution of the distal branched and enough information for surgical planning (Figure 7-31).

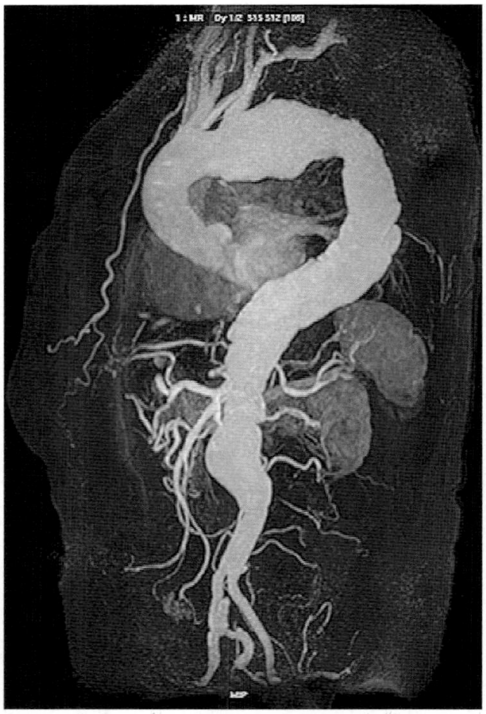

Figure 7-30. High-resolution left-anterior oblique image of magnetic resonance angiography maximum intensity projection reconstruction. The image demonstrates thoracoabdominal aortic aneurysm due to extensive atherosclerotic disease. (From Leiner TT. Magnetic resonance angiography of abdominal and lower extremity vasculature. *Top Magn Reson Imaging* 2005;16(1):21-66.)

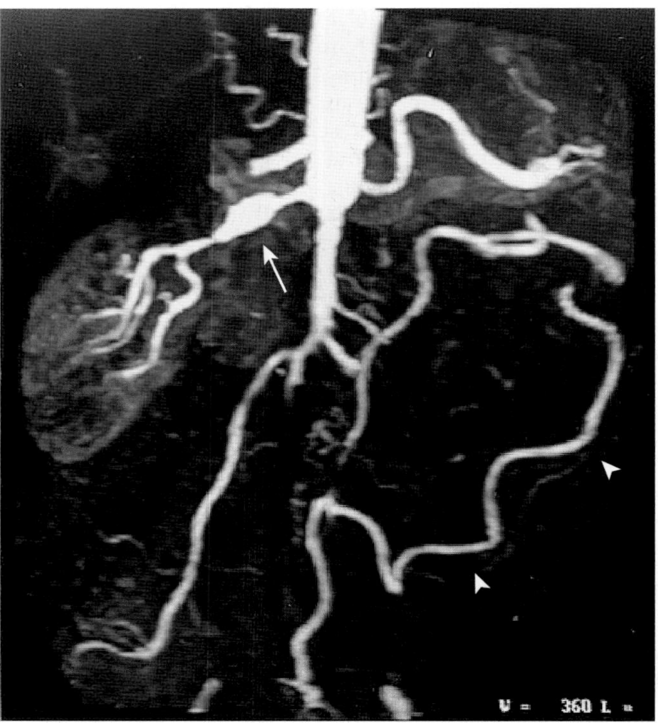

Figure 7-31. Multifocal vascular disease involving the aorta, mesenteric arteries, and renal arteries. Coronal maximum intensity projection image from an arterial-phase contrast-enhanced magnetic resonance angiography reveals occlusion of the abdominal aorta below the right renal artery origin. The left renal artery is not visualized, nor is the inferior mesenteric artery. Note the fusiform aneurysm of the proximal right renal artery *(arrow)* and the prominent collateral vessel supplying the left side of the colon *(arrowheads)*. (From Glockner JF. Three-dimensional gadolinium-enhanced MR angiography: Applications for abdominal imaging. *Radiographics* 2001;21:357-370.)

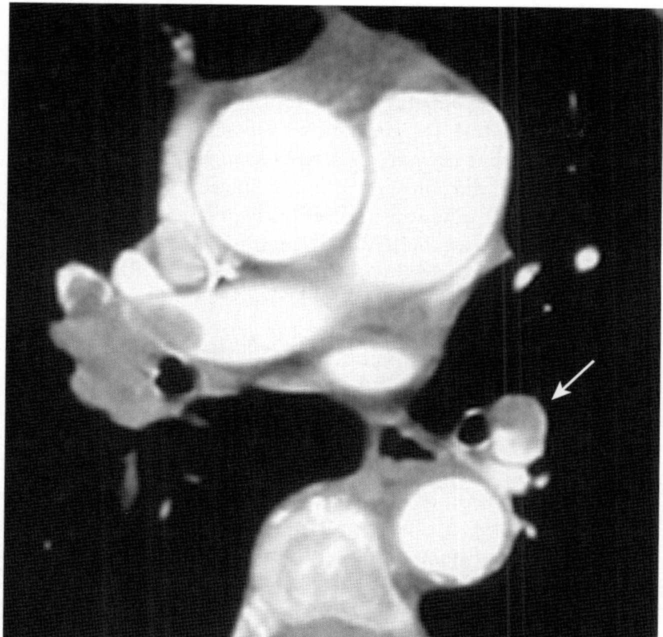

Figure 7-32. Axial image of multidetector row computed tomography pulmonary angiography. The image demonstrates massive right pulmonary artery embolism and a small thrombus in a peripheral pulmonary artery branch on the left *(arrow)*.

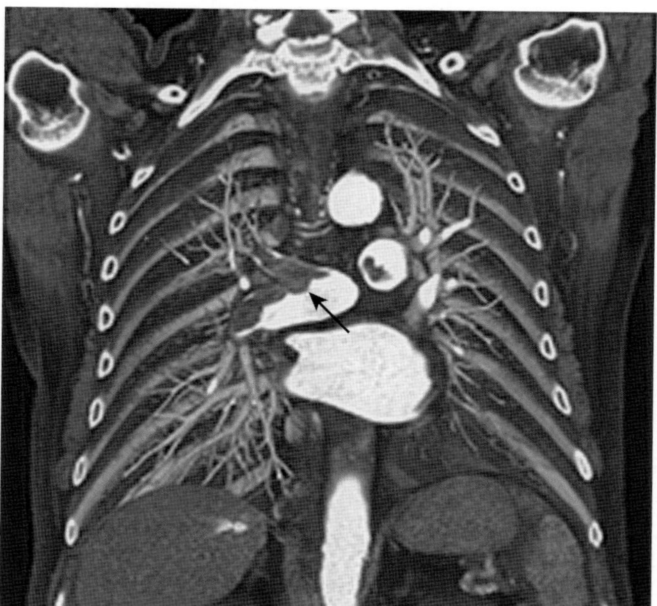

Figure 7-33. Coronal view of a chest multidetector row computed tomography angiogram. This view shows pulmonary embolism in the bifurcation of the main right pulmonary artery *(arrow)*.

As an alternative to CTA, phase contrast and TRICKS MR sequences can be performed to provide details about the flow lentification and retrograde flow in the primary or collateral arteries that may provide a pathway to the reconstitution of the distal circulation.[79]

Aneurysmal Disease of the Lower Extremities

Aneurysms in the lower extremity are clinically important because of the potential for limb-threatening complications. In addition, over 70% of patients with peripheral aneurysms have concomitant AAA[80] and it is therefore mandatory to image the abdominal aorta when a peripheral aneurysm is discovered. Peripheral aneurysms are predominantly found in the superficial femoral and popliteal arteries, and are of non-specific, postinterventional, or traumatic origin (see Figure 7-13). The popliteal artery is considered aneurysmal if its diameter exceeds 0.7 cm.[81] Similar to iliac artery aneurysms, popliteal aneurysms are bilateral in about half of all cases; carefully review of MRA source images reveals whether this is the case. Differential diagnostic possibilities such as a Baker's cyst (distention of the gastrocnemius-semimembranosus bursa with synovial fluid from the knee), cystic adventitial disease (multiple loculated cysts in the popliteal artery wall), or other soft-tissue tumors can also be investigated in the same imaging session. Aneurysms of the popliteal artery can be complicated by thrombosis, embolization, or rupture. The suspected presence of a peripheral arterial aneurysm necessitates bilateral imaging of the entire lower extremity vasculature, from the infrarenal aorta down to the pedal arch, to determine the optimal treatment strategy.

Pulmonary Embolism

CTA is widely used for the diagnosis of pulmonary emboli (PE), although ongoing debate relates to the precise place in the hierarchy of investigations for those patients with suspected PE. With the introduction of MDCT, CTA has been firmly established as the modality of choice for imaging the pulmonary arteries, particularly in the clinical scenario with suspected acute PE (Figures 7-32 and 7-33). The current resolution of MDCTA allows detection of PE to fourth order (segmental) vessels, covering the pulmonary artery tree with submillimeter slices in a 10-second breath-hold. The significance of PE in more distal vessels is uncertain.[82] If the MDCT angiogram is negative, it effectively rules out clinically significant PE. The examination is performed caudocranially to minimize respiratory motion artifact. Generally, 3-mm collimation and a pitch of 1.5 to 2 are used. Lower-density contrast medium (150 to 240 mg/ml) may be used to ensure that small emboli are not obscured. The sensitivity and specificity of CTA for central emboli have been reported as 91% and 78%, respectively. The MPR is used as a problem-solving tool for exclusion of PE when the axial images are inconclusive. Although the diagnosis or exclusion of acute pulmonary embolism is the most common and important application of pulmonary CTA, the ease of scan acquisition and the high spatial resolution of modern MDCT techniques make this test ideally suited for most congenital and acquired acute and chronic disorders of the pulmonary arteries and of the chest vessels (Figure 7-16).[83]

Initial studies have demonstrated that real-time MRA without the use of radiation or iodinated contrast material is comparable to angiography in the detection of PE.[84] In a study involving 207 combined MRI examinations for acute PE and deep vein thrombosis, perfusion MRI had a sensitivity ranging from 100% to 93% (subsegmental PE) and specificity ranging from 91% to 94%. Sensitivity of MRA was 81% and only 55%

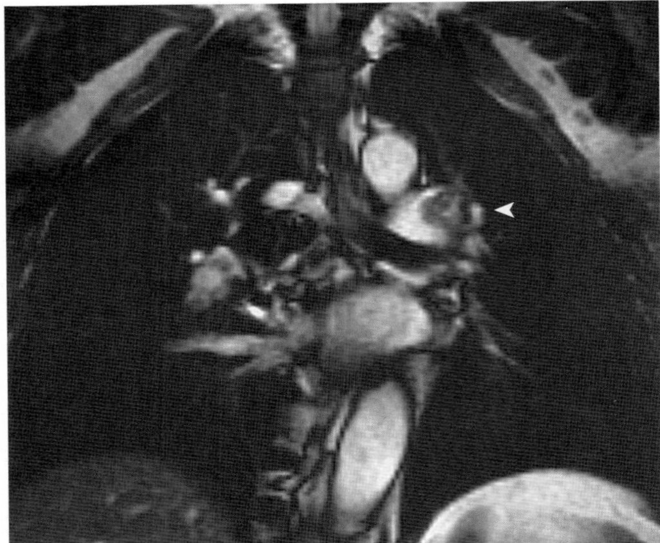

Figure 7-34. Large pulmonary embolism in the left pulmonary artery. The embolism is demonstrated in a real-time magnetic resonance image in coronal view *(arrow)*.

for subsegmental PE, and specificity ranged from 89% to 100%. Real-time MRI achieved a sensitivity of 89% and a specificity of 98%. Thus, perfusion MRI was the most sensitive technique, but MRA and real-time MRI were more specific. The combination of these techniques reached 100% sensitivity and 93% specificity for the diagnosis of PE.[85] Compared to fluoroscopic venography, MR venography may have sensitivity as high as 100% and specificity of 88% to 100% for deep vein thrombosis.[86] Other studies have shown that PE may be detected by using CE-MRA standard or gated spin-echo techniques, which have a sensitivity of 77% to 85% and a specificity of 96% to 100% for central or lobar emboli. MRI is inadequate for the diagnosis of subsegmental emboli. PE demonstrates increased signal intensity within the pulmonary artery. By obtaining a sequence of images, the signal that originated from slow blood flow may be distinguished from PE (Figure 7-34).[87]

Carotid and Supra-aortic Arteries

Accurate estimation of the degree of stenosis is crucial for optimizing the benefits from carotid artery surgery or stenting. Besides the symptoms, the indication of the carotid artery revascularization is based on the grade of stenosis and morphology of the plaque. Thus, precise quantification of stenosis of the ICAs is critical for patient clinical management and for interventional procedure, if indicated. DSA is the current gold standard; however, it carries a small but significant risk of complications (1.3%).[88] The noninvasive imaging modalities, such as Doppler ultrasound, MRA, and MDCTA, are reliable tools for detecting carotid artery stenosis.[89]

MRA and MDCTA modalities are superior to Doppler ultrasound in that they are relatively objective, are less operator dependent, and allow arterial evaluation from the aortic arch to the ICAs. The sensitivities and specificities of Doppler ultrasound, CTA, and MRA for detecting 70% to 99% stenosis of the ICA are compared with those of DSA in Table 7-19.

MDCTA may evaluate in a single breath-hold scan the entire intracranial, as well as extracranial, neurovascular system. In a recent study of 37 patients and 73 vessels, the reported sensitivity and specificity of the CTA for high-grade stenosis were 75% and 96%, respectively, and for moderate stenosis were 88% and 82%, respectively.[90] Furthermore, MDCT can assess the composition of the atherosclerotic plaque and the homodynamic of the brain circulation by using CT brain perfusion.[91,92] Another study demonstrated 100% agreement between CTA and DSA in cases of carotid stenosis higher than 70%. Overall, agreement between the two techniques was 89% using 2-mm collimation and a pitch of 1 (using only 100 ml of 270 mg/ml contrast). The overall agreement between Doppler ultrasound and DSA was 75%. While CTA outperformed Doppler ultrasound in this study, CTA and ultrasound showed no significant difference in identifying patients whose stenoses required surgery. This lack of significance most likely reflects the relatively small study population: only 28 patients and 56 arteries. The addition of VR and MIP images does not improve performance significantly.

Table 7-19
US, CT Angiography, and MR Angiography versus DSA in the Detection of 70%–99% Stenosis of the ICA

Modality	Sensitivity (%)	Specificity (%)
US	86 (84-89)*	87 (84-90)
CTA	85 (79-89)	93 (89-96)
MRA	95 (92-97)	90 (86-93)

*Numbers in parentheses indicate 95% confidence interval.

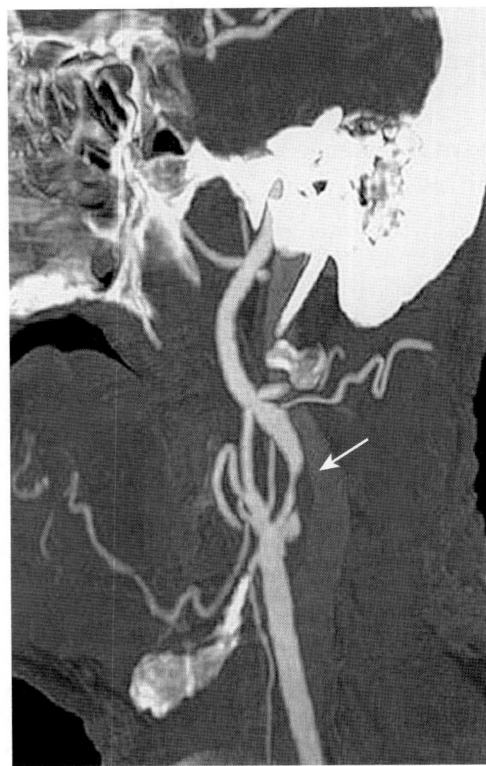

Figure 7-35. Multidetector row computed tomography angiogram of the neck. Sagittal maximum intensity projection reconstruction image shows intracranial artery stenosis caused by noncalcified, ulcerated plaque *(arrow)*.

Nevertheless, the exact role of MDCT in the management of carotid disease needs to be further defined. In addition, Doppler ultra sound plays an important role in the evaluation of carotid artery stenosis because it is by far the most common imaging modality in this setting and carotid endarterectomy is performed solely on the basis of Doppler ultrasound findings at many institutions.[93,94] On the other hand, Doppler ultrasound measurement of flow velocity in the ICA has a specific pitfall: if an ICA has significant stenosis, a compensatory increase in blood flow often occurs in the contralateral ICA to maintain intracranial blood flow. Thus, overestimation of stenosis may occur in ICAs with less than 70% stenosis that are contralateral to ICAs with greater than 70% stenosis or that are occluded.[95] Ideally, images of the aortic arch, neck, extracranial arteries, and ICAs should be obtained during the same study as part of an MDCTA protocol for stroke or transient ischemic attack with or without previous evidence of carotid artery stenosis. The high-resolution axial MDCTA images associated to the MIP reconstructions may provide some details about the carotid artery plaque, such as plaque ulceration (Figure 7-35). Compared to carotid MRA, MDCTA does have calcification-related artifacts. In heavily calcified carotid arteries, it may be difficult to quantify precisely the grade of stenosis (Figure 7-36).

Several methods exist for the carotid artery stenosis measurement: North American Symptomatic Carotid Endarterectomy Trial (NASCET) criteria, European Carotid Surgical Trial (ECST) criteria, and the carotid stenosis index. The NASCET criteria are the most popular, where the ICA stenosis was classified angiographically: % ICA stenosis = (1 − [narrowest ICA diameter/diameter normal distal cervical ICA]) × 100%. As with catheter angiography analysis, the grade of stenosis is stratified in mild (0% to 29%), moderate (30% to 69%), and high (70% to 99%) grades[96] (Figure 7-37).

During image evaluation of carotid atherosclerotic disease, not only the grade of stenosis but also the morphology of the plaque is important. The vulnerable plaque is defined as a plaque rich in lipids (lipid core) with a necrotic center and covered by a fine fibrotic layer, sometimes with evidence of superficial tearing.[97]

Catheter angiography still is the gold standard for diagnosing carotid artery stenosis (Figure 7-38), but with the association of the Doppler ultrasound and the MRA studies it is possible to exclude conventional angiography in the routine workup of patients under investigation for carotid artery disease. Carotid artery MRA is usually performed using a gadolinium-enhanced sequence, but the time-of-flight MRA sequence without gadolinium using 2D and 3D images can be useful when needed. Both sequences usually provide anatomical information similar to a catheter angiography (Figure 7-39), with the time-of-flight sequence having a higher chance of image artifacts.

CE-MRA has sensitivity of up to 100% and specificity of about 90% in the diagnosis of hemodynamically significant stenosis, and usually this MR sequence does not have flow artifacts. This is the ideal sequence because it provides great images to study the brain feeding vessels from the aortic arch up to the intracranial circulation, including the circle of Willis (Figure 7-40).

The high-resolution MRA images associated with VR reconstruction provide great information for the carotid artery

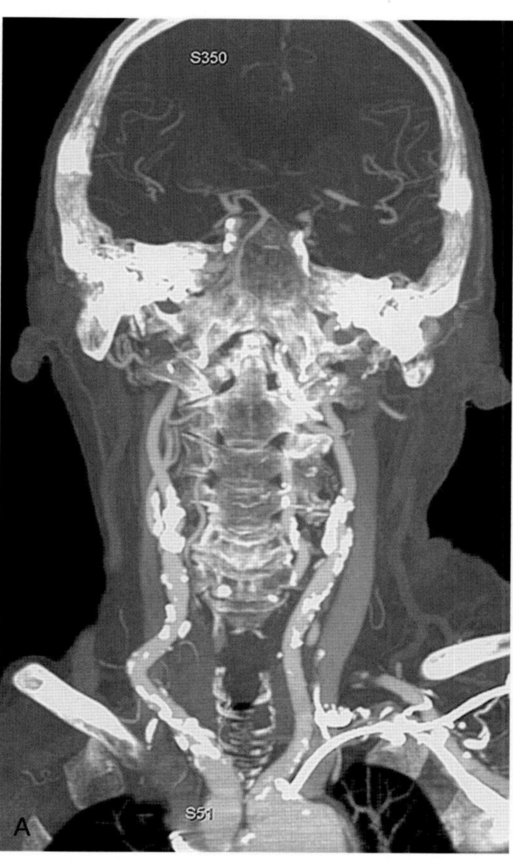

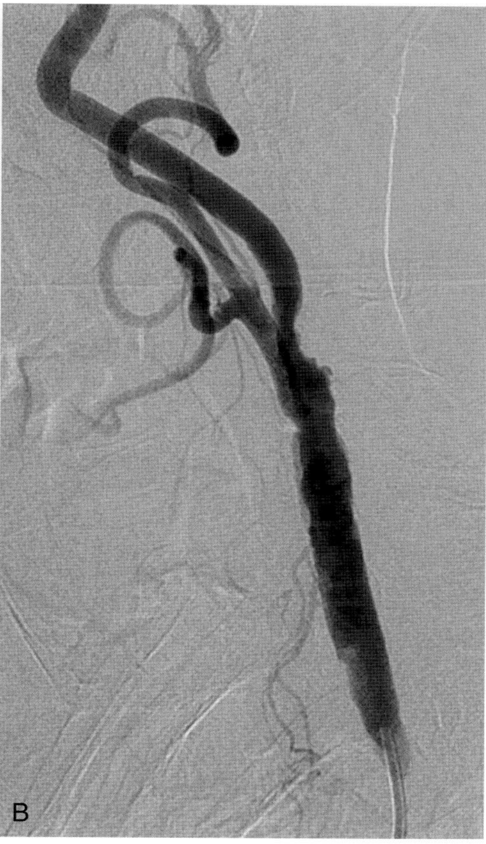

Figure 7-36. Patient with recent recurrent transient ischemic attacks. **A,** Multidetector row computed tomography angiogram of the upper thorax and neck. Coronal maximum intensity projection reconstruction shows heavily calcified plaques in both proximal intracranial arteries, which makes evaluation of the grade of stenosis difficult. **B,** Initial carotid artery surgery angiogram showing an intracranial artery stenosis associated with ulcerated plaque.

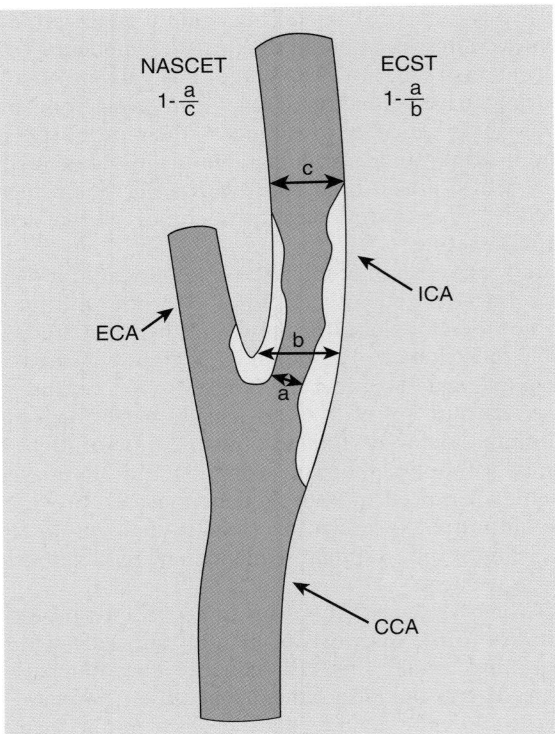

Figure 7-37. The percentage of diameter stenosis in an intracranial artery measured in the North American Symptomatic Carotid Endarterectomy Trial (NASCET) and the European Carotid Surgical Trial (ECST) criteria. The NASCET criteria use the formula 1 − (*a/c*), where *a* is the residual luminal diameter at the stenosis and *c* is the luminal diameter at a visible, disease-free point above the stenosis. The ECST criteria use the formula 1 − (*a/b*), where *b* is the estimated luminal diameter at the level of the lesion based on a visual impression of where the normal arterial wall was before development of the stenosis. CCA, common carotid artery; ECA, external carotid artery.

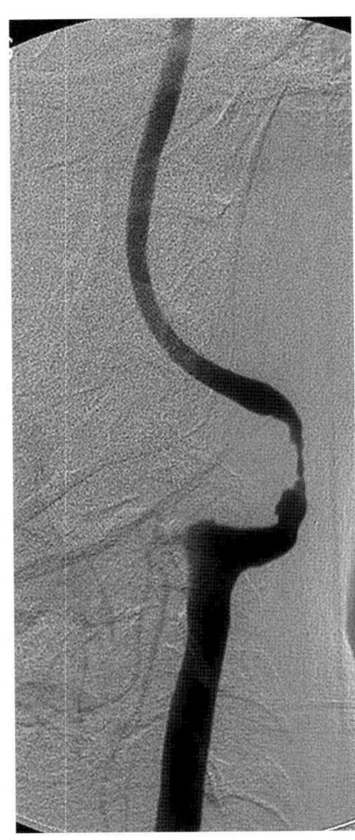

Figure 7-38. Lateral view of a left carotid artery digital subtraction angiography. This view demonstrates a 90% stenosis in the internal carotid artery associated with occlusion of the external carotid artery.

plaque morphology evaluation, with plaque ulceration analysis and better quantification of the carotid stenosis. Compared to carotid CTA, MRA does not have calcification-related artifacts, so it may demonstrate the true lumen (luminogram) of the carotid calcified stenosis.[98] To study the carotid plaque morphology, multiple MR sequences are required (base on T_1-weighted, T_2-weighted, time-of-flight, and protonic density sequences). With these sequences, it is possible to evaluate the plaque composition (lipid core, calcium, fibrotic layer, hemorrhage) because every component of the plaque has a specific MR signal.[97,99]

In general, the lipid core and the fibrous cap have similar signal intensity and they may be differentiated with the intravenous administration of gadolinium. The fibrous cap has gadolinium enhancement, and it is possible to characterize plaque thickness, contour, and presence of tearing (Figure 7-41).[100] The calcification presents with a low signal in all sequences. The hemorrhagic area has the signal intensity determined by the age of the bleeding. It can be acute, recent, or old. Acute usually has a high signal in T_1-weighted and time-of-flight sequences, recent can present with a high signal in T_1- or T_2-weighted and protonic density sequences, and the old hemorrhage typically has a low signal associated with poor border definition.

Renal Arteries

The two main indications for renal angiography are to image the renal anatomy of live donors and to identify possible RASs in cases of suspected renovascular hypertension or in some cases of deteriorating renal function. When imaging the renal anatomy of live donors (Figure 7-42), the importance is in detecting any anatomical variations, such as accessory arteries, early renal artery branching, or venous anomalies, as these affect the difficulty and risk of complications in an operation being conducted for altruistic reasons.[101] It has been reported that MDCTA with MIP reconstruction is faster and more accurate than MRA (Figure 7-43) and ultrasound in identification of accessory renal arteries.[103] MDCTA has an advantage over MRA in that it is more acceptable to patients (no claustrophobia, faster scan time) and misses fewer accessory renal arteries,[104] and the scan range should extend to the pelvic inlet to ensure identification of accessory arteries. Typical parameters are a 3-mm collimation, a pitch of 1.2 to 2, and 100 to 150 ml of contrast more than 3 ml/sec. The enhanced scout or topographic image demonstrates calcifications, and a delayed scout or topographic image after the CTA adequately depicts the collecting system and ureters and thus obviates the need for an intravenous urogram.

Although MDCTA involves radiation and a nephrotoxic contrast agent, it is an excellent screening tool of the renal arteries. Kidney donors, by nature, have good renal function where a single MDCT angiogram has a minimal negative effect when compared to potential complications inherent to a catheter angiogram. MDCTA should not be used when a

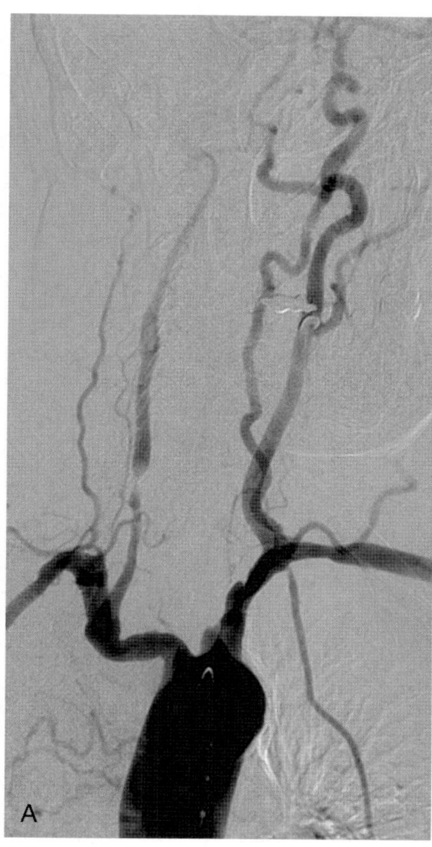

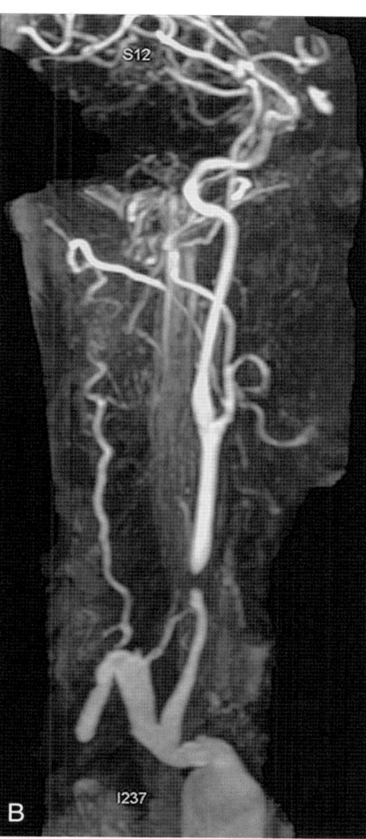

Figure 7-39. Carotid artery digital subtraction angiography and contrast-enhanced magnetic resonance angiography. The gadolinium-enhanced sequence shows great correlation of the anatomical findings between catheter angiography **(A)** and magnetic resonance angiography (MRA; **B**). The abnormalities observed in detail during catheter angiography are also demonstrated in a different oblique of the MRA study.

patient has poor renal function or an iodine allergy, although now there is also concern about the use of some MRA contrast agents and the risk of nephrogenic systemic fibrosis. It is also important to identify incidental renal pathology on the donor side, such as renal cyst or tumor. Studies looking at the sensitivity and specificity for the detection of accessory renal arteries using MDCTA have, using operative findings or DSA as the gold standard, showed sensitivity between 80% and 100% with specificity between 96% and 100%.[101,105,106] The sensitivity and specificity of the detection of early arterial branching was reported as 100% in one study, although the sensitivity in another study was only 89%, with a specificity of 100%.[105] Regarding venous anomalies, different studies showed a sensitivity of between 97% and 100%.[101,105,106]

RAS is the underlying cause of renovascular hypertension, which is the most frequent cause of secondary hypertension, with an estimated prevalence of 3% to 5% in the population of hypertensive patients.[108] Despite this low percentage, detection of RAS is important because it is a potentially curable cause of hypertension. In most cases, renovascular hypertension is caused by either atherosclerotic RAS or FMD. Atherosclerosis accounts for 70% to 90% of cases of RAS and usually involves the ostium and proximal third of the main renal artery.[108,109]

FMD is a collection of vascular diseases that affects the intima, media, and adventitia and is responsible for 10% to 30% of cases of RAS. Intraarterial DSA is traditionally regarded as the definitive test to diagnose the presence of RAS. However, both the invasive nature of DSA and the difficulty

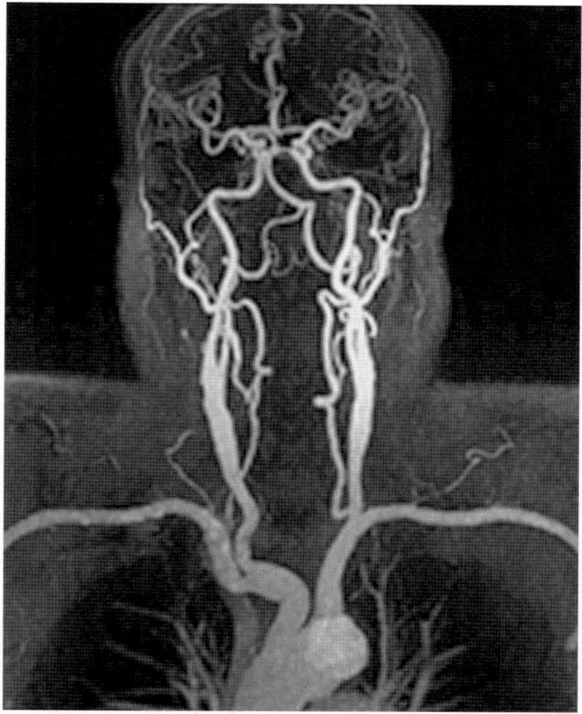

Figure 7-40. Contrast-enhanced magnetic resonance angiography protocol for carotid stenosis workup. The study includes the brain feeding vessels from the aortic arch up to the intracranial circulation, including the circle of Willis.

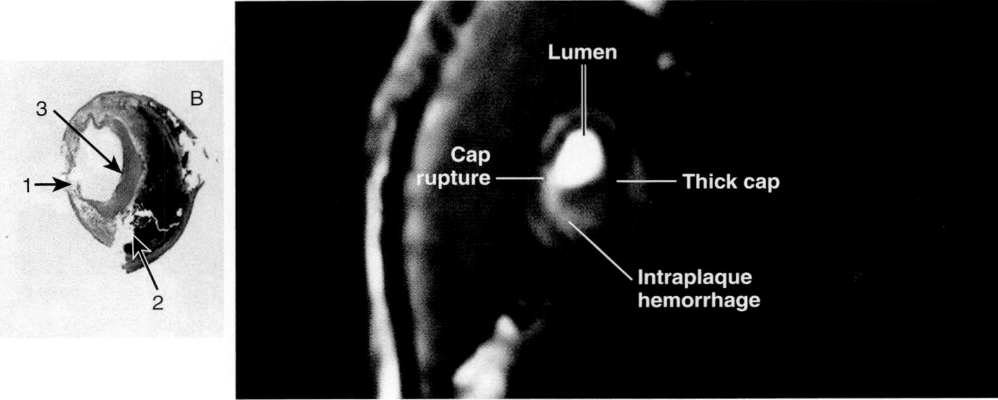

Figure 7-41. Example of plaque with fibrous cap rupture on gross section, histology (Masson's trichrome stain), and magnetic resonance imaging (MRI). On gross and histological sections, there is an area of cap rupture *(arrow 1)* next to a region where the fibrous cap is thick *(arrow 3)*. The cap rupture site corresponds to a region where a dark band is absent, and a hyperintense, bright region is seen adjacent to lumen on MRI. The hyperintense region in the plaque core on MRI corresponds to a region of recent intraplaque hemorrhage on gross and histological cross sections *(arrow 2)*. (From Huda W. *AJR Am J Roentgenol* 1997;169:1487-1488.)

in assessing the pathophysiological significance of stenotic lesions and substantial interobserver variation for the detection of RAS have encouraged the search for widely available noninvasive diagnostic tests. FMD may be detected as a single and focal stenosis in the middle third or in the distal portions of the renal artery, as multifocal stenosis ("string of pearls"), or as aneurysm formation (Figure 7-44). Little information exists about the use of MRA for diagnosis of FMD. Fain et al.[110] and Shetty et al.[111] have reported several instances in which they successfully detected angiographically confirmed FMD. Although overt cases of FMD can be diagnosed with CE-MRA, the general opinion is that CE-MRA is currently not able to detect FMD with high accuracy in the presence of only subtle anatomical changes.

The renal arteries arise ventrolaterally from the abdominal aorta and assume a dorsoinferolateral course until they enter the kidney at the renal hilum. About one third of the general population shows variations in number, location, and branching patterns of the renal arteries, with more than 30% of subjects having one or more accessory renal arteries.[6,38] This is clinically important because RAS in an accessory renal artery can, albeit rarely, also be responsible for renovascular hypertension.[112] There is no consensus on what constitutes a "significant" stenosis, but most authors use a reduction in luminal diameter of 50% as the cutoff point.[113] Precise knowledge of renal arterial anatomy is important because it determines the spatial resolution that any given imaging technique must be able to achieve to reliably differentiate a stenosed from a healthy vessel. At least three pixels are needed across

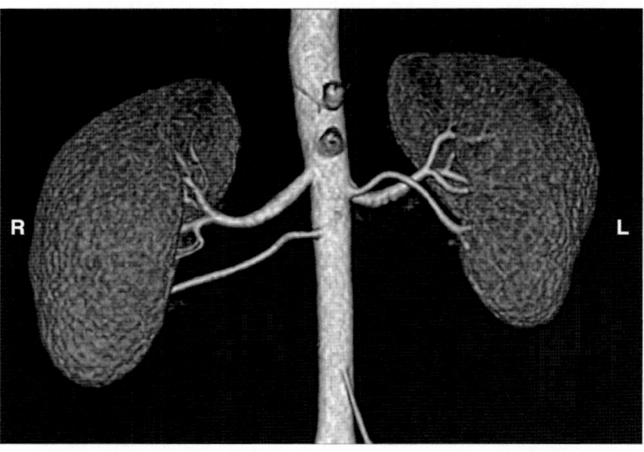

Figure 7-42. Volume rendering reconstruction of renal arteries multidetector row computed tomography angiography. Observe the presence of accessory renal arteries bilaterally, on the right inferiorly to the main right renal branch and on the left at the same level of the left main renal branch.

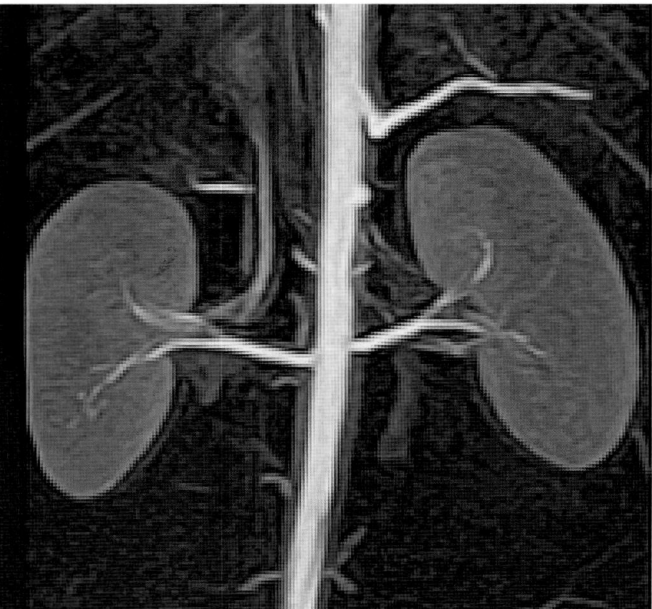

Figure 7-43. Contrast-enhanced magnetic resonance angiography. This is a good alternative to multidetector row computed tomography angiography for renal arteries and can be used as part of the renal live donor workup.

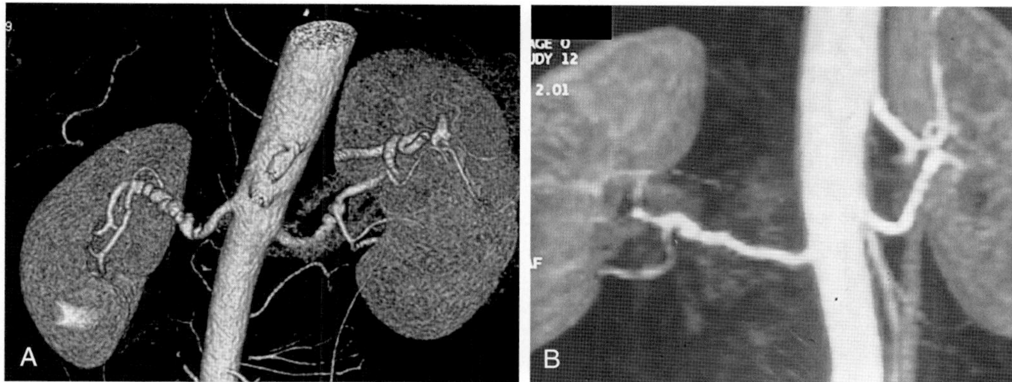

Figure 7-44. Fibromuscular dysplasia (FMD) in different patients with renovascular hypertension. **A,** Bilateral FMD is depicted in the volume rendering reconstruction of multidetector row computed tomography angiography. **B,** Bilateral FMD is poorly demonstrated in the maximum intensity projection reconstruction of contrast-enhanced magnetic resonance angiography. Note the superior resolution for the diagnosis of FMD in the computed tomography angiography study.

the lumen of an artery to quantify the degree of stenosis, with a maximum error of approximately 10%.[114] Taking into account the average diameter of 5 to 6 mm, the spatial resolution of any given imaging technique is ideally on the order of $1.0 \times 1.0 \times 1.0$ mm^3. In addition to the arterial supply, it is important to evaluate renal size, cortical thickness, and corticomedullary differentiation and to compare these parameters with the contralateral kidney.[115]

Doppler ultrasound can be used to look for RAS, although it has the disadvantages of requiring an expert user, relying on a reasonable patient body habitus, and being unreliable in detecting accessory renal arteries. Doppler ultrasound compared to DSA has a sensitivity of 75% and a specificity of 89.6% for RAS. Both MRA and MDCTA can be used to evaluate RAS as well (Figures 7-45 and 7-46). One study found no significant difference between the two, with sensitivities of 93% and 92% and specificities of 100% and 99%, respectively. Finally, this study showed higher patient acceptance for MDCTA. As the renal arteries run axially, scan protocol is particularly important. Sensitivity of 100% has been reported for stenoses greater than 50% using axial images associated with MPR and MIP reformats.[110] MDCTA is superior to catheter angiography in the measurement of eccentric RAS and in the differentiation of soft versus calcified plaques and ostial versus truncal stenoses. Nonatherosclerotic RAS, such as in arteritis or in FMD, may be demonstrated as well. A normal MDCT angiogram virtually excludes the presence of a stenosis, and it can be used for renal artery stenting surveillance to detect disease recurrence, as well as appropriate stent position and expansion (Figure 7-47).

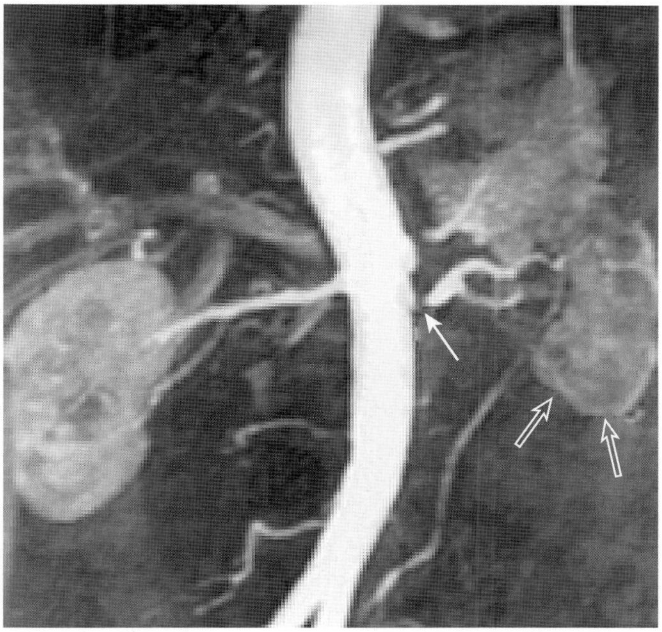

Figure 7-45. Coronal images obtained with multiphase three-dimensional contrast-enhanced magnetic resonance angiography. The images show the evolution of renal enhancement. Late arterial-phase image shows the stenosis *(solid arrow)* and delayed enhancement of the shrunken left kidney *(open arrows)*. (From Dong Q, Schoenberg S, Carlos RC, et al. Diagnosis of renal vascular disease with MR angiography. *Radiographics* 1999;19:1535-1554.)

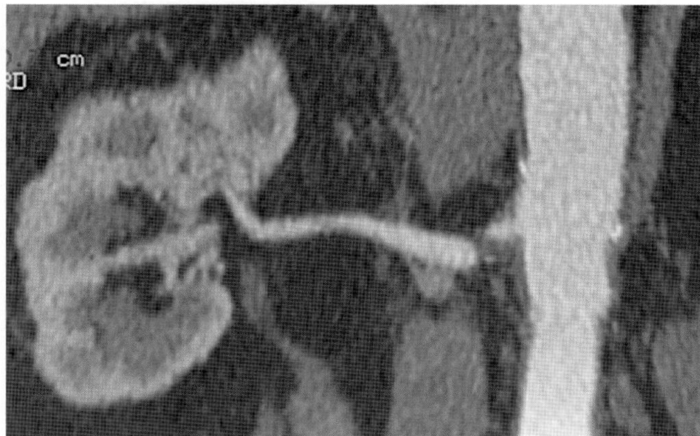

Figure 7-46. Maximum intensity projection reconstruction of a right renal multidetector row computed tomography angiogram. The reconstruction shows a proximal high-grade stenosis secondary to a noncalcified plaque.

Both nonenhanced and CE-MRA techniques have been used to investigate narrowing of the renal arteries. Currently, CE-MRA performed at a 1.5 T field strength, in a coronal plane, is the best MR technique for the detection of RAS.[116] Some authors advocate the use of phase-contrast MRA techniques to supplement the anatomical information obtained. For best results, a breath-hold during the acquisition is necessary that typically lasts about 15 to 20 seconds. Contrast medium is injected at 3.0 ml/sec, followed by a 25-ml saline flush. Using this approach, the abdominal aorta and renal arteries can be visualized with high accuracy (Figure 7-43). Arteries can usually be evaluated down to the proximal part of the segmental arteries. Distal segmental and interlobar branches cannot be evaluated reliably with this method. Another limitation is the risk of motion artifacts. A patient who is unable to sustain the breath-hold and the inherent linear caudocranial motion of the kidneys are potential contributing factors.[117] Both nonenhanced MRA (2D time-of-flight and phase-contrast) and CE-MRA techniques can be used for detection of RAS, and in a metaanalysis no significant differences were found among different MRA techniques.[114] Reported sensitivities and specificities for the detection of atherosclerotic RAS in these CE-MRA studies are uniformly above 90%.[111,118]

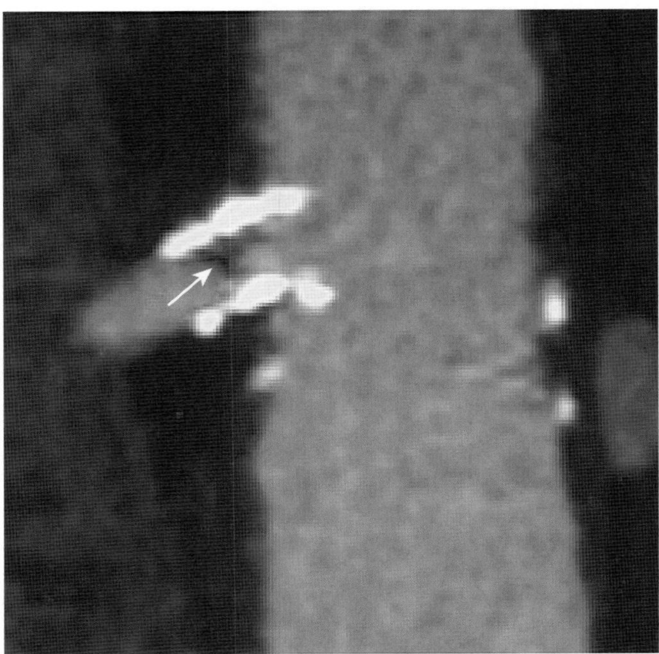

Figure 7-47. Patient with history of right renal artery stenting. Follow-up maximum intensity projection reconstruction of a multidetector row computed tomography angiogram follow-up shows intrastent restenosis *(arrow)*.

SUMMARY

Even if the catheter angiography is still considered the gold standard for the evaluation of PVD, diagnostic MDCTA of the aorta and of the peripheral arteries provides high-definition images not only of vascular structures but also of the vessel wall and of the adjacent anatomy. It can assist in the decision between conservative, conventional surgery and endovascular treatment and is an excellent tool for follow-up after revascularization procedures. The relatively recent introduction of MDCT scanners (16, 64, and 128 detectors) has resulted in shorter acquisition time, increased volume coverage, lower dose of contrast medium, and improved spatial resolution, with significant improvement of MDCTA for PVD.

CE-MRA has emerged as the MRA technique of choice for vascular imaging of the abdominal aorta, visceral branches, renal arteries, and lower extremities. Additional MRI sequences

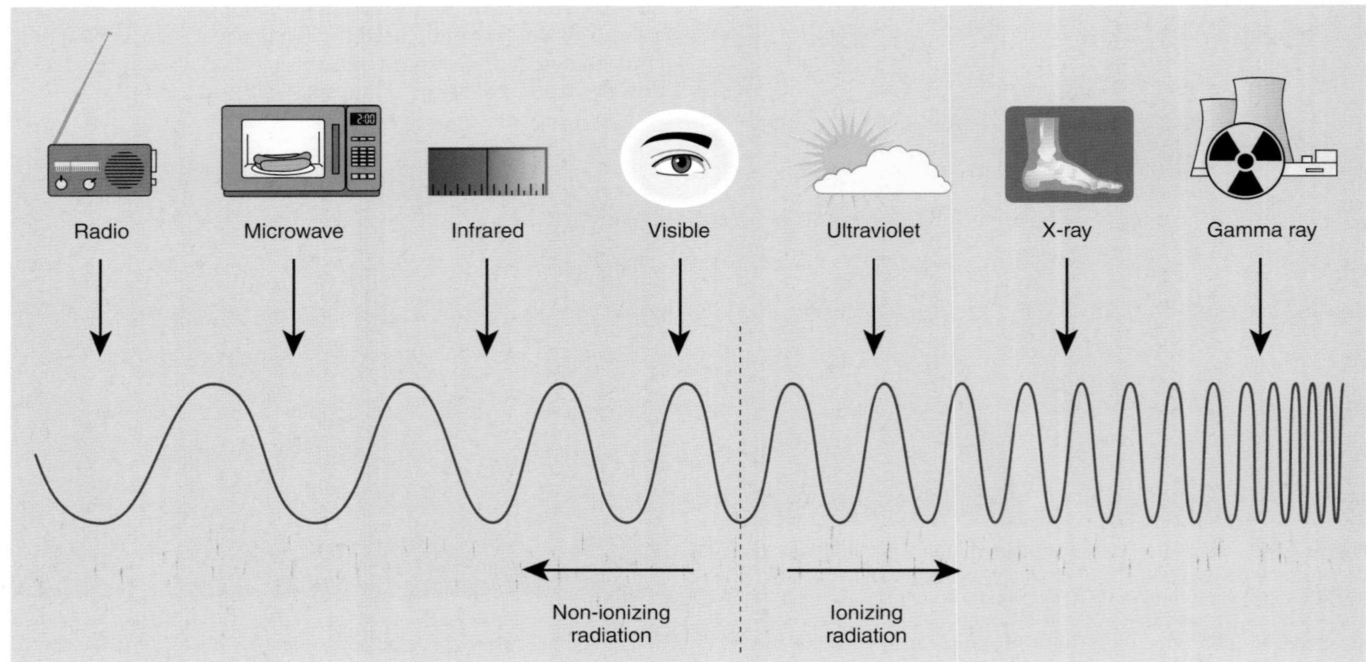

Figure 7-48. Electromagnetic spectrum showing that frequencies that exceed those of visible light are ionizing radiations.

also allow functional evaluation of vascular pathology. Ongoing technical improvements have significantly improved not only image quality but also speed, reliability, and ease of use, demonstrating high accuracy for the detection and characterization of several vascular diseases.

A decision as to which image test should be implemented in routine clinical practice must take into account the local expertise, availability of equipment, and considerations concerning ionizing radiation and renal insufficiency.

RADIATION SAFETY

X-Rays and Matter

X-rays are electromagnetic waves similar to visible light and radio waves, as depicted in Figure 7-48. Electromagnetic waves all travel at the speed of light (300 million m/sec) in a vacuum. Electromagnetic waves have a wavelength that is inversely proportional to frequency, so electromagnetic waves with a high frequency have a short wavelength, and vice versa. X-rays are produced in x-ray tubes when energetic electrons are stopped in a tungsten target. X-rays have a high frequency (i.e., short wavelength) and are considered by physicists to behave like discrete bundles of energy called photons. The photon energy is proportional to the frequency; Table 7-20 shows typical frequencies of various forms of electromagnetic radiation, together with the corresponding photon energies. X-rays have high photon energies that are approximately 100,000 times higher (see Table 7-20) than those of visible light.

X-rays interact with matter by transferring energy from x-rays to energetic electrons. These energetic electrons travel through the patient, losing part of their energy by knocking out outer-shell electrons. Atoms that lose electrons become positive ions, and x-rays are therefore deemed to be ionizing radiation. The important characteristic of x-ray photons is that they have sufficient energy to knock out atomic and molecular electrons. X-rays can break apart molecules; therefore, they are called ionizing radiations, as depicted in Figure 7-49. Visible light and lower-energy photons do not possess enough energy to eject electrons from atoms and are therefore nonionizing. When x-rays deposit energy in living cells, this energy can break apart molecules that may be biologically important (e.g., DNA), which can result in a cell being killed or undergoing a harmful modification.

The amount of energy deposited in an irradiated organ defines the absorbed dose to this organ. Absorbed dose *(D)* is the energy deposited (*E,* in joule) divided by the mass of the absorber (*M,* in kilograms); *D* is *E*/*M* and is measured in grays (Gy), with 1 Gy being equal to 1,000 mGy.[119] The absorbed dose to a specified tissue is used to predict the biological consequences to this tissue.[120] For patients undergoing multiple x-ray examinations, the cumulative dose to a given tissue is used to predict the likelihood of any harmful effects.

Deterministic Effects

Deterministic effects of ionizing radiation are related to cell killing. A deterministic radiation effect has a threshold dose below which the effect does not occur. When the threshold dose is exceeded, deterministic effects are possible. At doses just above the threshold dose, the effect occurs in the most radiosensitive individuals. However, at doses well above the threshold dose, the effect always occurs in all exposed patients, as depicted by the sigmoidal curve in Figure 7-50.

The most common deterministic effect in interventional radiology is skin damage.[121] The skin normally receives the highest dose where the x-ray beam enters the patient.[122] At skin doses that exceed about 2 Gy, transient erythema may occur in hours. Skin doses of about 6 Gy produce erythema 1 to 2 weeks following exposure. Skin doses that exceed 10 Gy can produce dry desquamation. Dry desquamation arises from the loss of clonogenic skin cells. Moist desquamation occurs at doses exceeding 15 Gy. Skin effects are reversible if the population of basal cells can recover. Table 7-21 provides a list of deterministic effects that can occur in patients subject to high doses of x-ray radiation.

In interventional radiology, the entrance (skin) of a patient may be irradiated continuously in fluoroscopy at a rate measured in milligrays per minute. In fluoroscopy, the total skin dose is obtained by multiplying this exposure rate by the total exposure time (in minutes). In addition, individual radiographic images may be obtained (e.g., during an arteriogram), with each image resulting in a patient skin dose that is measured in milligrays per image. In radiographic imaging, the total skin dose is obtained by multiplying the exposure per frame by the total number of acquired frames (i.e., images). One important factor that affects the skin dose in x-ray imaging is the patient thickness. Table 7-22 shows typical fluoroscopy and radiographic skin doses as a function of patient thickness. Operators need to be aware of the cumulative patient (skin) dose and take steps to minimize patient doses by keeping all exposures *as low as r*easonably *a*chievable (ALARA). It is important that valuable diagnostic medical information is not lost by using too little radiation and that the acquired image quality is sufficient to achieve a satisfactory level of diagnostic performance.[123]

The practical threshold dose for use in diagnostic radiology is 2 Gy. Below 2 Gy, clinically significant deterministic effects are most unlikely. Above 2 Gy, deterministic effects are possible, and the patient should be monitored for this possibility. As doses rise above 2 Gy, deterministic effects are increasingly likely to occur. Interventional radiology is one of the few areas in diagnostic imaging where deterministic effects are possible. When skin doses exceed 2 Gy, it is imperative that patients are advised of the possibility of deterministic effects and are monitored appropriately. Deterministic effects in interventional radiology are rare when procedures are performed by operators who are properly trained in dose and image quality issues. It has been estimated that fewer than 1 in 10,000 patients who undergo interventional radiology procedures by qualified personnel will suffer from a serious deterministic effect.

Stochastic Effects

Below the threshold dose for the induction of deterministic effects (i.e., less than 2 Gy), few cells are killed, and the deposition of ionizing x-ray energy is associated with cell transformation. A transformed cell may remain viable but have incurred some damage to biologically important molecules (e.g., DNA). Radiation risks at low doses are called stochastic because of their random nature, and they include carcinogenesis and the induction of genetic mutations. For stochastic radiation risks, the magnitude of the dose (in grays) determines

Table 7-20
Electromagnetic Radiation Frequencies and Their Photon Energies

Type of Electromagnetic Radiation	Frequency (Cycles Per Second)	Photon Energy (eV)
Radio waves (AM)	10^5	0.000000001
Television waves	10^8	0.000001
Microwaves	10^{10}	0.0001
Infrared	10^{13}	0.1
Visible light	10^{14}	1
Ultraviolet	10^{16}	100
X-rays	10^{19}	100,000

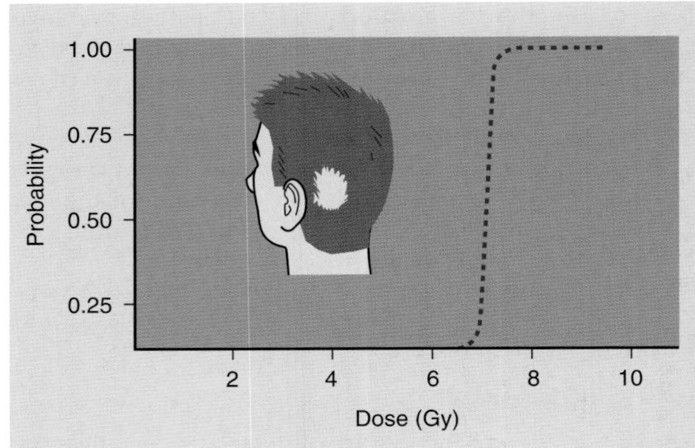

Figure 7-50. Probability of inducing epilation as a function of radiation dose, illustrating a threshold dose of about 7 Gy.

the probability of the effect but not the severity of the effect. Increasing the radiation dose to an organ increases the likelihood of inducing a cancer, but the type of cancer produced is independent of the radiation dose. In the 1950s, genetic effects were considered to be the most important; nowadays, cancer risk is of greatest concern. The organs that are most sensitive to radiation-induced cancer are the red bone marrow for the induction of leukemia and the (female) breast, lungs, stomach, and colon for induction of solid tumors. Moderately radiosensitive organs include the bladder, esophagus, liver, and thyroid.[124,125]

Radiation-induced cancers are no different from those that occur naturally and can only be identified in epidemiological studies. Performing such epidemiological studies is difficult, because the background incidence is high. In the United States, data shows that approximately 44% of the population will get cancer in their lifetime, and approximately 22% are expected to die from caner. Knowledge of cancer risks is obtained from epidemiological studies of groups exposed medically (Table 7-23), occupationally, or in the A-bomb exposure in Hiroshima and Nagasaki. It is important to note the long latent period between exposure to ionizing radiations and the appearance of radiation-induced cancers. For leukemia, the latent period is a few years, with a peak incidence about 8 years after the exposure occurred. For solid tumors, the latent period is measured in decades; radiation-induced cancers are still being observed in the survivors of the A-bomb attacks on Hiroshima and Nagasaki in 1945.

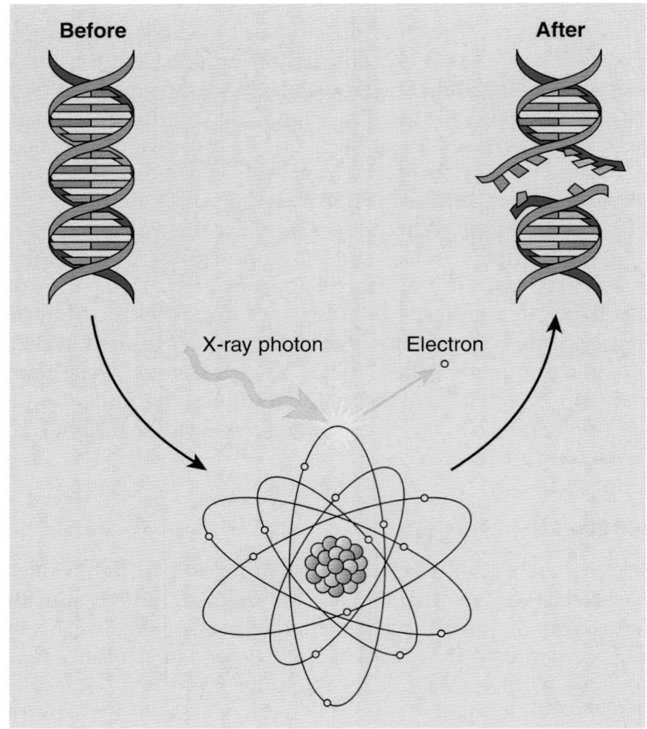

Figure 7-49. Effects of ionizing radiation on a DNA molecule showing that x-rays can knock out atomic electrons, and can thereby break apart a DNA molecule.

Radiological examinations generally produce a complex 3D pattern of energy distribution within the patient. In interventional radiological examinations, the directly irradiated skin receives the highest level of radiation dose, and if the dose exceeds a threshold dose, it may result in the induction of a deterministic effect. Directly irradiated organs and tissues deeper within the body receive lower levels of radiation

Table 7-21
Deterministic Effects of Ionizing Radiations and Approximate Threshold Doses

Deterministic Effect	Threshold Dose (Gy)	Comment
Epilation (temporary)	4	Hair color changes are likely (e.g., gray)
Epilation (permanent)	7	Onset of hair loss occurs about 10 days after exposure
Cataract (acute exposure)	2	Eye lens lack a mechanism for removal of damaged cells
Cataract (chronic exposure)	5	Interventional radiologists may risk getting x-ray-related cataracts
Sterility (male; acute exposure)	6	Fractionated exposure is *more* likely to cause sterility than acute exposure
Sterility (female; prepuberty)	12	Threshold dose for premenopausal women is much lower (i.e., about 2 Gy)

Table 7-22
Representative Skin Doses Associated with the Fluoroscopic and Radiographic Phases of Interventional Radiological Procedures

Imaging Mode	Patient Thickness—Soft-Tissue Equivalence (cm)	Entrance Skin Dose (mGy)
Fluoroscopy (1 minute exposure time)	18	10
	23	20
	28	40
Radiograph (single exposure)	18	1.5
	23	3
	28	6

Table 7-23
Patients Exposed to Medical Radiation that Subsequently Showed Excess Rates of Cancer

Medically Exposed Group of Patients	Excess Cancer
Ankylosing spondylitis	Leukemia
Acne and tonsillitis radiation treatment	Thyroid
Epilation for tinea capitis (ringworm)	Thyroid
Postpartum mastitis	Breast
Tuberculosis (multiple fluoroscopy exams)	Breast
Radium injections for tuberculosis and ankylosing spondylitis	Bone
Radiation therapy (adult and childhood)	Various

than the skin, and those tissues adjacent to the directly irradiated region receive much lower doses from scattered radiation. Radiation doses to distant tissues (e.g., more than 10 cm or so) are low and are normally negligible. As a result, most procedures in interventional radiology result in the irradiation of multiple organs and tissues. Dose descriptors of the stochastic patient radiation risk must therefore take into account all irradiated organs and tissues, as well as their relative radiosensitivity.

Effective Dose

The effective dose is a radiation dose descriptor commonly used in medical imaging that is directly related to the total stochastic risk in the exposed patient.[124] The effective dose is obtained by taking into account how much radiation is received by any individual organ, as well as the organ radiosensitivity. Effective doses are measured in sieverts (Sv), with 1 Sv being equal to 1,000 mSv. Effective doses are related to the whole-body risk associated with any given deposition of ionizing radiation in an individual. For nonuniform radiation, the effective dose is the equivalent uniform whole-body dose that results in the same radiation risk as a given nonuniform dose. A patient with an abdominal aortic stent may have an effective dose of 20 mSv, and this means that the patient's stochastic risk is the same as that arising from a uniform whole-body dose of 20 mGy.

The effective dose is the best single parameter for quantifying the total amount of radiation a patient receives during any radiological examination. The effective dose metric permits a direct comparison of all types of radiological examination that use ionizing radiation, including radiography, fluoroscopy, CT, and nuclear medicine. For example, an adult chest CT scan typically results in a patient effective dose of 5 mSv, whereas that for a chest radiographic examination is only 0.05 mSv. As a result, the chest CT examination is associated with a stochastic radiation risk that is 100 times larger than a conventional chest x-ray examination. Table 7-24 shows representative values of effective doses to adult patients undergoing diagnostic x-ray examinations of the head, abdomen, and heart.[126]

In interventional radiology, the patient dose depends on the complexity of the procedure, as well as the experience of the operator. Interventional radiology patient effective doses are among the highest encountered in diagnostic radiology. In 2006, it is estimated that 13 million interventional radiology procedures were performed in the United States, with an average patient effective dose of 8.6 mSv. Figure 7-51 shows that interventional radiology contributes to 2% of all radiological examinations but accounts for 12% of the average dose to the U.S. population from medical radiation. It is important to note that some procedures have much higher doses, with the average effective dose for a transjugular intrahepatic portosystemic shunt procedure being about 70 mSv.

Effective doses may also be compared with other benchmark radiation doses, such as background radiation from cosmic radiation, terrestrial radioactivity, and radionuclides incorporated in the body. In the United States, cosmic radiation, terrestrial radioactivity, and primordial radionuclides contribute an average dose to the whole U.S. population of approximately 1 mSv/year (Table 7-25).[127] A transcontinental U.S. flight results in a dose of approximately 0.03 mSv, and air crews receive an additional 5 mSv/year, assuming 1000 flying hours at 30,000 feet. Leadville, Colorado, has elevated levels of terrestrial radioactivity, which results in an additional dose of approximately 0.7 mSv/year. The biggest contribution to natural background is from domestic radon. Average annual doses from radon are about 2 mSv/year, but radon exposure levels vary widely. For example, radon levels in high-rise buildings are low, whereas radon levels can be high in poorly ventilated basements.

Table 7-24
Representative Patient Effective Dose in Diagnostic Radiology

Body Region	Type of Procedure	Effective Dose (mSv)
Head	Radiographic examination	0.1
	Head CT	2
Heart	Cardiac catheterization procedure (diagnostic)	7
	Cardiac angioplasty of radio-frequency ablation	15
	Cardiac CT	18
	Cardiac stress test (thallium-201)	40
Abdomen	Radiographic examination	0.7
	Abdominal CT (single phase)	8
	Barium enema	8
	Abdominal aorta angiography	12

CT, computed tomography.

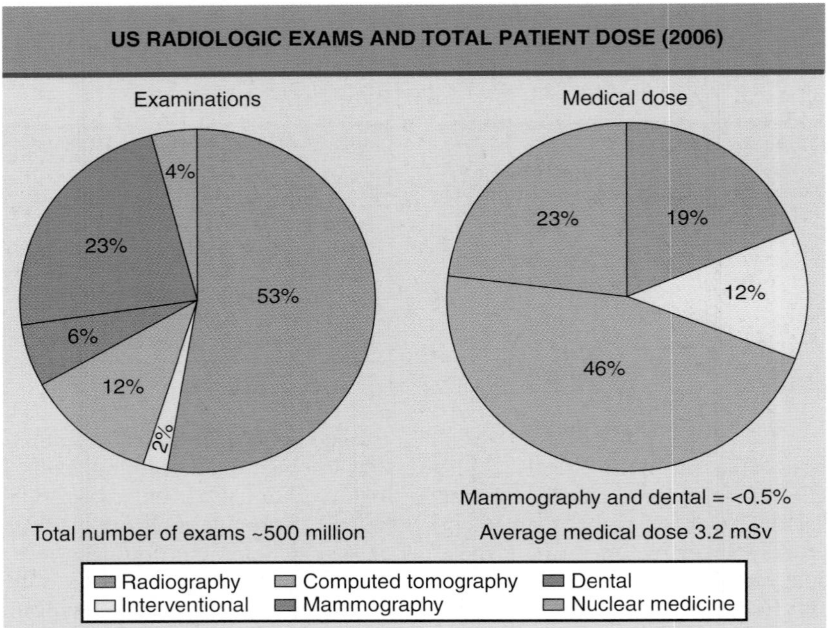

Figure 7-51. Diagnostic radiological exams performed in the United States in 2006 (500 million), and their contribution to the corresponding population medical dose from all diagnostic x-rays. The 2006 average patient dose (3.2 mSv) is a 600% increase over the value reported in 1980 (0.55 mSv), before the widespread clinical of computed tomography, nuclear medicine, and interventional radiology.

Table 7-25
Major Sources of Background Radiation Exposure to the U.S. Population

Source	Average Exposure (mSv/Year)	Comment
External	0.3	Radioactivity in soil (e.g., radium-226)
Internal	0.4	Primordial radionuclides (e.g., potassium-40)
Cosmic	0.3	Varies with altitude and latitude

References

1. Rutkow IM, Ernst CB. An analysis of vascular surgical manpower requirements and vascular surgical rates in the United States. *J Vasc Surg* 1986;3:74-83.
2. Martin EC. Transcatheter therapies in peripheral and noncoronary vascular disease: introduction. *Circulation* 1991;83:I1-I5.
3. Waugh JR, Sacharias N. Arteriographic complications in the DSA era. *Radiology* 1992;182:243-246.
4. Malden ES, Picus D, Vesely TM, Darcy MD, Hicks ME. Peripheral vascular disease: evaluation with stepping DSA and conventional screen-film angiography. *Radiology* 1994;191:149-153.
5. Picus D, Hicks ME, Darcy MD, Kleinhoffer MA. Comparison of nonsubtracted digital angiography and conventional screen-film angiography for the evaluation of patients with peripheral vascular disease. *J Vasc Interv Radiol* 1991;2:359-364.
6. Kaufman J, Michael L. *Vascular and interventional radiology: the requisites*. Philadelphia: Mosby; 2004.
7. Levy E, Viscoli CM, Horwitz RI. The effect of acute renal failure on mortality: a cohort analysis. *JAMA* 1996;275:1489-1494.
8. Pannu N, Wiebe N, Tonelli M, et al. Prophylaxis strategies for contrast-induced nephropathy. *JAMA* 2006;295:2765-2779.
9. Merten GJ, Burgess WP, Gray LV, et al. Prevention of contrast-induced nephropathy with sodium bicarbonate. *JAMA* 2004;291:2328-2334.
10. Marenzi G, Assanelli E, Marana I, et al. N-acetylcysteine and contrast-induced nephropathy in primary angioplasty. *N Engl J Med* 2006;354 (26):2773-2782.
11. Liu R, Nair D, Ix J, Moore DH, Bent S. N-acetylcysteine for the prevention of contrast-induced nephropathy: a systematic review and meta-analysis. *J Gen Intern Med* 2005;20(2):193-200.
12. Birck R, Krzossok S, Markowetz F, Schnulle P, van der Woude FJ, Braun C. Acetylcysteine for prevention of contrast nephropathy: meta-analysis. *Lancet* 2003;362 (9384):598-603.
13. Hawkins IF. Carbon dioxide digital subtraction arteriography. *AJR Am J Roentgenol* 1982;139(1):19-24.
14. Wilson AJ, Boxer MM. Neurotoxicity of angiographic carbon dioxide in the cerebral vasculature. *Invest Radiol* 2002;37 (10):542-551.
15. Deleted in proof.
16. Deleted in proof.
17. Wedeen VJ, Meuli RA, Edelman RR, et al. Projective imaging of pulsatile flow with magnetic resonance. *Science* 1985;230 (4728): 946-948.
18. Ho KY, Leiner T, de Haan MW, et al. Peripheral MR angiography. *Eur Radiol* 1999;9:1765-1774.
19. Mustert BR, Williams DM, Prince MR. In vitro model of arterial stenosis: correlation of MR signals dephasing and trans-stenotic pressure gradients. *Magn Reson Imaging* 1998;16:301-310.
20. Miyazaki M, Takai H, Sugiura S, et al. Peripheral MR angiography: separation of arteries from veins with flow-spoiled gradient pulses in electrocardiography-triggered three-dimensional half-Fourier fast spin-echo imaging. *Radiology* 2003;227:890-896.
21. Miyazaki M, Sugiura S, Tateishi F, et al. Non-contrast-enhanced MR angiography using 3D ECG-synchronized half-Fourier fast spin echo. *J Magn Reson Imaging* 2000;12:776-783.
22. Foo TK, Ho VB, Marcos HB, et al. MR angiography using steady-state free precession. *Magn Reson Med* 2002;48:699-706.
23. Nael K, Fenchel MC, Kramer U, Finn JP, Ruehm SG. Whole-body contrast-enhanced magnetic resonance angiography: new advances at 3.0 T. *Top Magn Reson Imaging* 2007;18(2):127-134.
24. Swaminathan S, Horn TD, Pellowski D, et al. Nephrogenic systemic fibrosis, gadolinium, and iron mobilization. *N Engl J Med* 2007;357 (7):720-722.
25. Schmiedl U, Moseley ME, Ogan MD, et al. Comparison of initial biodistribution patterns of Gd-DTPA and albumin-(Gd-DTPA) using rapid spin echo MR imaging. *J Comput Assist Tomogr* 1987;11:306-313.

26. Prince MR, Grist TM, Debatin JF. *3D Contrast MR angiography*. Berlin: Springer; 2003.
27. Boos M, Scheffler K, Haselhorst R, et al. Arterial first pass gadolinium-CM dynamics as a function of several intravenous saline flush and Gd volumes. *J Magn Reson Imaging* 2001;13:568-576.
28. Yip YP, Capriotti C, Talagala SL, Yip JW. Effects of MR exposure at 1.5 T on early embryonic development of the chick. *J Magn Reson Imaging* 1994;4:742-748.
29. U.S. Food and Drug Administration. Public health advisory: gadolinium-containing contrast agents for magnetic resonance imaging (MRI)—Omniscan, OptiMARK, Magnevist, ProHance, and MultiHance. Available at: http://www.fda.gov. Accessed November 19, 2007.
30. Thomsen HS. European Society of Urogenital Radiology (ESUR). ESUR guideline: gadolinium-based contrast media and nephrogenic systemic fibrosis. *Eur Radiol* 2007;17:2692-2696.
31. Levey AS, Coresh J, Balk E, et al. National kidney practice guidelines for chronic kidney disease: evaluation, classification and stratification. *Ann Intern Med* 2003;139:137-147.
32. Wertman B, Altun E, Martin D, et al. Risk of Nephrogenic Systemic fibrosis: evaluation of gadolinium chelate contrast agents at four American universities. *Radiology* 2008;248(3):799-806.
33. Okada S, Katagiri K, Kumazaki T, Yokoyama H. Safety of gadolinium contrast agent in hemodialysis patients. *Acta Radiologica* 2001;42:339.
34. Korosec FR, Frayne R, Grist TM, Mistretta CA. Time-resolved contrast-enhanced 3D MR angiography. *Magn Reson Med* 1996;36(3):345-351.
35. Hany TF, Debatin JF, Leung DA, et al. Evaluation of the aortoiliac and renal arteries: comparison of breath-hold, contrast-enhanced, three-dimensional MR angiography with conventional catheter angiography. *Radiology* 1997;204:357-362.
36. Prince MR. Contrast-enhanced MR angiography: theory and optimization. *Magn Reson Imaging Clin N Am* 1998;6:257-267.
37. Ho KY, Leiner T, van Engelshoven JM. MR angiography of run-off vessels. *Eur Radiol* 1999;9:1285-1289.
38. Vasbinder GB, Nelemans PJ, Kessels AG, et al. Accuracy of computed tomographic angiography and magnetic resonance angiography for diagnosing renal artery stenosis. *Ann Intern Med* 2004;141:674-682.
39. Schoenberg SO, Rieger J, Weber CH, et al. High-spatial-resolution MR angiography of renal arteries with integrated parallel acquisitions: comparison with digital subtraction angiography and U.S. *Radiology* 2005;235:687-698.
40. Huang Y, Webster CA, Wright GA. Analysis of subtraction methods in three-dimensional contrast-enhanced peripheral MR angiography. *J Magn Reson Imaging* 2002;15:541-550.
41. Ruehm SG, Nanz D, Baumann A, et al. 3D contrast-enhanced MR angiography of the run-off vessels: value of image subtraction. *J Magn Reson Imaging* 2001;13:402-411.
42. Rofsky NM, Morana G, Adelman MA, et al. Improved gadolinium-enhanced subtraction MR angiography of the femoropopliteal arteries: reintroduction of osseous anatomic landmarks. *AJR Am J Roentgenol* 1999;173:1009-1011.
43. Westenberg JJ, Wasser MN, van der Geest RJ, et al. Scan optimization of gadolinium contrast-enhanced three-dimensional MRA of peripheral arteries with multiple bolus injections and in vitro validation of stenosis quantification. *Magn Reson Imaging* 1999;17:47-57.
44. Hany TF, Schmidt M, Davis CP, et al. Diagnostic impact of four postprocessing techniques in evaluating contrast-enhanced three-dimensional MR angiography. *AJR Am J Roentgenol* 1998;170:907-912.
45. Nelemans PJ, Leiner T, de Vet HC, et al. Peripheral arterial disease: meta-analysis of the diagnostic performance of MR angiography. *Radiology* 2000;217:105-114.
46. Westenberg JJ, van der Geest RJ, Wasser MN, et al. Vessel diameter measurements in gadolinium contrast-enhanced three-dimensional MRA of peripheral arteries. *Magn Reson Imaging* 2000;18:13-22.
47. Ouwendijk R, de Vries M, Stijnen T, et al. Multicenter randomized controlled trial of the costs and effects of noninvasive diagnostic imaging in patients with peripheral arterial disease: The DIPAD trial. *AJR Am J Roentgenol* 2008;190:1349-1357.
48. Ouwendijk R, de Vries M, Pattynama P, et al. Imaging peripheral arterial disease: a randomized controlled trial comparing contrast-enhanced MR angiography and multi-detector row CT angiography. *Radiology* 2005;236:1094-1103.
49. Adriaensen ME, Kock MC, Stijnen T, et al. Peripheral arterial disease: therapeutic confidence of CT versus digital subtraction angiography and effects on additional imaging recommendations. *Radiology* 2004;233:385-391.
50. Deleted in proof.
51. Deleted in proof.
52. Deleted in proof.
53. Martin ML, Tay KH, Flak B, et al. Multidetector CT angiography of the aortoiliac system and lower extremities: a prospective comparison with digital subtraction angiography. *AJR Am J Roentgenol* 2003;180:1085-1091.
54. Portugaller HR, Schoellnast H, Hausegger KA, Tiesenhausen K, Amann W, Berghold A. Multi-slice spiral CT angiography in peripheral arterial occlusive disease: a valuable tool in detecting significant arterial lumen narrowing? *Eur Radiol* 2004;14:1681-1687.
55. Ofer A, Nitecki SS, Linn S, et al. Multidetector CT angiography of peripheral vascular disease: a prospective comparison with intra-arterial digital subtraction angiography. *AJR Am J Roentgenol* 2003;180:719-724.
56. Romano M, Mainenti PP, Imbriaco M. Multidetector row CT angiography of the abdominal aorta and lower extremities in patients with peripheral arterial occlusive disease: diagnostic accuracy and interobserver agreement. *Eur J Radiol* 2004;50:303-308.
57. Hertzer NR. The natural history of peripheral vascular disease: implications for its management. *Circulation* 1991;83:I12-I19.
58. Brewster DC. Direct reconstruction for aortoiliac occlusive disease. In Rutherford RB, ed. *Vascular surgery*. Philadelphia: WB Saunders; 2000: 943-972.
59. Loewe C, Schoder M, Rand T, et al. Peripheral vascular occlusive disease: evaluation with contrast-enhanced moving-bed MR angiography versus digital subtraction angiography in 106 patients. *AJR Am J Roentgenol* 2002;179:1013-1021.
60. Hentsch A, Aschauer MA, Balzer JO. Gadobutrol-enhanced moving-table magnetic resonance angiography in patients with peripheral vascular disease: a prospective, multi-centre blinded comparison with digital subtraction angiography. *Eur Radiol* 2003;13:2103-2114.
61. Binkert CA, Baker PD, Petersen BD, Szumowski J, Kaufman JA. Peripheral vascular disease: blinded study of dedicated calf MR angiography versus standard bolus-chase MR angiography and film hard-copy angiography. *Radiology* 2004;232(3):860-866.
62. Janka R, Fellner C, Wenkel E, Lang W, Bautz W, Fellner FA. Contrast-enhanced MR angiography of peripheral arteries including pedal vessels at 1.0 T: feasibility study with dedicated peripheral angiography coil. *Radiology* 2005;235(1):319-326.
63. Meissner OA, Rieger J, Weber C, et al. Critical limb ischemia: hybrid MR angiography compared with DSA. *Radiology* 2005;235(1): 308-318.
64. Menzoian JO, LaMorte WW, Paniszyn CC, et al. Symptomatology and anatomic patterns of peripheral vascular disease: differing impact of smoking and diabetes. *Ann Vasc Surg* 1989;3:224-228.
65. Cigarroa JE, Isselbacher EM, DeSanctis RW, Eagle KA. Diagnostic imaging in the evaluation of suspected aortic dissection: old standards and new directions. *N Engl J Med* 1993;328:35-43.
66. Nienaber CA, Fattori R, Lund G, et al. Nonsurgical reconstruction of thoracic aortic dissection by stent graft placement. *N Engl J Med* 1999;340:1539-1545.
67. Ballal RS, Nanda NC, Gatewood R, et al. Usefulness of transesophageal echocardiography in assessment of aortic dissection. *Circulation* 1991;84(5):1903-1914.
68. Laissy JP, Blanc F, Soyer P, et al. Thoracic aortic dissection: diagnosis with transesophageal echocardiography versus MR imaging. *Radiology* 1995;194(2):331-336.
69. Nienaber CA, von Kodolitsch Y, Nicolas V, et al. The diagnosis of thoracic aortic dissection by noninvasive imaging procedures. *N Engl J Med* 1993;328(1):1-9.
70. Sommer T, Fehske W, Holzknecht N, et al. Aortic dissection: a comparative study of diagnosis with spiral CT, multiplanar transesophageal echocardiography, and MR imaging. *Radiology* 1996;199(2): 347-352.
71. Yoshida S, Akiba H, Tamakawa M, et al. Thoracic involvement of type A aortic dissection and intramural hematoma: diagnostic accuracy–comparison of emergency helical CT and surgical findings. *Radiology* 2003;228(2):430-435.
72. Nevitt MP, Ballard DJ, Hallett Jr JW. Prognosis of abdominal aortic aneurysms: a population-based study. *N Engl J Med* 1989;321:1009-1014.
73. Ernst CB. Abdominal aortic aneurysm. *N Engl J Med* 1993;328: 1167-1172.
74. Reed WW, Hallett JW Jr., Damiano MA, et al. Learning from the last ultrasound: a population-based study of patients with abdominal aortic aneurysm. *Arch Intern Med* 1997;157:2064-2068.
75. Brewster DC, Cronenwett JL, Hallett JW Jr., et al. Guidelines for the treatment of abdominal aortic aneurysms: report of a subcommittee of the Joint Council of the American Association for Vascular Surgery and Society for Vascular Surgery. *J Vasc Surg* 2003;37:1106-1117.

76. Isselbacher EM. Thoracic and abdominal aortic aneurysms. *Circulation* 2005;111:816-828.
77. Moore WS, Rutherford RB. Transfemoral endovascular repair of abdominal aortic aneurysm: results of the North American EVT phase 1 trial—EVT investigators. *J Vasc Surg* 1996;23:543-553.
78. Baum RA, Stavropoulos SW, Fairman RM, et al. Endoleaks after endovascular repair of abdominal aortic aneurysms. *J Vasc Interv Radiol* 2003;14:1111-1117.
79. McGuigan EA, Sears ST, Corse WR, et al. MR angiography of the abdominal aorta. *Magn Reson Imaging Clin N Am* 2005;13:65-89.
80. Dent TL, Lindenauer SM, Ernst CB, et al. Multiple arteriosclerotic arterial aneurysms. *Arch Surg* 1972;105:338-344.
81. Wright LB, Matchett WJ, Cruz CP, et al. Popliteal artery disease: diagnosis and treatment. *Radiographics* 2004;24:467-479.
82. Goodman LR, Lipchik RJ, Kuzo RS, et al. Subsequent pulmonary embolism: risk after a negative helical CT pulmonary angiogram-prospective comparison with scintigraphy. *Radiology* 2000;215:535-542.
83. Schoepf U. Pulmonary artery CTA. *Tech Vasc Interv Radiol* 2006;9(4): 180-191.
84. Haage P, Piroth W, Krombach G, et al. Pulmonary embolism: comparison of angiography with spiral CT, MRA and real-time MR imaging. *Am J Respir Crit Care Med* 2003;167(5):729-734.
85. Kluge A, Mueller C, Strunk J, et al. Experience in 207 combined MRI examinations for acute pulmonary embolism and deep vein thrombosis. *AJR Am J Roentgenol* 2006;186:1686-1696.
86. Kluge A, Rominger M, Schönburg M, Bachmann G. Indirect MR venography: contrast media protocols, postprocessing and combination with MRI diagnostics for pulmonary embolism. *Rofo* 2004;176:976-984.
87. Oudkerk M, van Beek EJ, Wielopolski P, et al. Comparison of contrast-enhanced magnetic resonance angiography and conventional pulmonary angiography for the diagnosis of pulmonary embolism: a prospective study. *Lancet* 2002;359:1643-1647.
88. Willinsky RA, Taylor SM, TerBrugge K, et al. Neurologic complications of cerebral angiography: prospective analysis of 2899 procedures and review of the literature. *Radiology* 2003;227:522-528.
89. Long A, Lepoutre A, Corbillon E, Branchereau A. Critical review of non- or minimally invasive methods: duplex ultrasonography, MR, and CT angiography. *Eur J Vasc Endovasc Surg* 2002;24:43-52.
90. Silvennoinen HM, Ikonen S, Soinne L, et al. CT angiographic analysis of carotid artery stenosis: comparison of manual assessment, semiautomatic vessel analysis, and digital subtraction angiography. *AJNR Am J Neuroradiol* 2007;28:97-103.
91. de Wert TT, Outhouse M, Mitering E, et al. In vivo characterization and quantification of atherosclerotic carotid plaque components with MDCT and histopathological correlation. *Arterioscler Thromb Vascul Biol* 2006;26:2366-2372.
92. Wintermark M, Fischbein NJ, Smith WS, et al. Accuracy of dynamic perfusion CT with deconvolution in detecting acute hemispheric stroke. *AJNR Am J Neuroradiol* 2005;26:104-112.
93. Grant EG, Benson CB, Moneta GL, et al. Carotid artery stenosis: grayscale and Doppler U.S. diagnosis—Society of Radiologists in Ultrasound Consensus Conference. *Radiology* 2003;229:340-346.
94. Landwehr P, Schulte O, Voshage G. Ultrasound examination of carotid and vertebral arteries. *Eur Radiol* 2001;11:1521-1534.
95. van Everdingen KJ, van der Grond J, Kappelle LJ. Overestimation of a stenosis in the internal carotid artery by duplex sonography caused by an increase in volume flow. *J Vasc Surg* 1998;27:479-485.
96. Ota H, Takase K, Rikimaru H, et al. Quantitative vascular measurements in arterial occlusive disease. *Radiographics* 2005;25(5):1141-1158.
97. Ouhlous M, Flach HZ, de Weert TT, et al. Carotid plaque composition and cerebral infarction: MR imaging study. *AJNR Am J Neuroradiol* 2005;26(5):1044-1049.
98. Raggi P, Taylor A, Fayad Z, et al. Atherosclerotic plaque imaging: contemporary role in preventive cardiology. *Arch Intern Med* 2005;165(20):2345-2353.
99. Kampschulte A, Ferguson MS, Kerwin WS, et al. Differentiation of intraplaque versus juxtaluminal hemorrhage/thrombus in advanced human carotid atherosclerotic lesions by in vivo magnetic resonance imaging. *Circulation* 2004;110(20):3239-3244.
100. Hatsukami TS, Ross R, Polissar NL, Yuan C. Carotid plaque in vivo with high-resolution magnetic resonance imaging visualization of fibrous cap thickness and rupture in human atherosclerotic. *Circulation* 2000;102:959-964.
101. Laugharne M, Haslam E, Archer L, et al. Multidetector CT angiography in live donor renal transplantation: experience from 156 consecutive cases at a single centre. *Transpl Int* 2007;20:156-166.
102. Deleted in proof.
103. Rountas C, Vlychou M, Vassiou K, et al. Imaging modalities for renal artery stenosis in suspected renovascular hypertension: prospective intraindividual comparison of color Doppler U.S., CT angiography, GD-enhanced MR angiography, and digital substraction angiography. *Ren Fail* 2007;29:295-302.
104. Schlunt LB, Harper JD, Broome DR, et al. Improved detection of renal vascular anatomy using multidetector CT angiography: is 100% detection possible? *J Endourol* 2007;21:12-17.
105. Raman SS, Pojchamarnwiputh S, Muangsomboon K, et al. Utility of 16-MDCT angiography for comprehensive preoperative vascular evaluation of laparoscopic renal donors. *AJR Am J Roentgenol* 2006;186:1630-1638.
106. Kim T, Murakami T, Takahashi S, et al. Evaluation of renal arteries in living renal donors: comparison between MDCT angiography and gadolinium-enhanced 3D MR angiography. *Radiat Med* 2006;24: 617-624.
107. Deleted in proof.
108. Derkx FH, Schalekamp MA. Renal artery stenosis and hypertension. *Lancet* 1994;344:237-239.
109. Working Group on Renovascular Hypertension. Detection, evaluation, and treatment of renovascular hypertension: final report. *Arch Intern Med* 1987;147:820-829.
110. Fain SB, King BF, Breen JF, et al. High-spatial-resolution contrast-enhanced MR angiography of the renal arteries: a prospective comparison with digital subtraction angiography. *Radiology* 2001;218:481-490.
111. Shetty AN, Bis KG, Kirsch M, et al. Contrast-enhanced breath-hold three-dimensional magnetic resonance angiography in the evaluation of renal arteries: optimization of technique and pitfalls. *J Magn Reson Imaging* 2000;12:912-923.
112. Bude RO, Forauer AR, Caoili EM, et al. Is it necessary to study accessory arteries when screening the renal arteries for renovascular hypertension? *Radiology* 2003;226:411-416.
113. Vasbinder GB, Nelemans PJ, Kessels AG, et al. Diagnostic tests for renal artery stenosis in patients suspected of having renovascular hypertension: a meta-analysis. *Ann Intern Med* 2001;135:401-411.
114. Hoogeveen RM, Bakker CJ, Viergever MA. Limits to the accuracy of vessel diameter measurement in MR angiography. *J Magn Reson Imaging* 1998;8:1228-1235.
115. Safian RD, Textor SC. Renal-artery stenosis. *N Engl J Med* 2001;344: 431-442.
116. Schoenberg SO, Prince MR, Knopp MV, et al. Renal MR angiography. *Magn Reson Imaging Clin N Am* 1998;6:351-370.
117. Vasbinder GB, Maki JH, Nijenhuis RJ, et al. Motion of the distal renal artery during three-dimensional contrast-enhanced breath-hold MRA. *J Magn Reson Imaging* 2002;16:685-696.
118. Bakker J, Beek FJ, Beutler JJ, et al. Renal artery stenosis and accessory renal arteries: accuracy of detection and visualization with gadolinium-enhanced breath-hold MR angiography. *Radiology* 1998;207:497-504.
119. Huda W. Radiation dosimetry in diagnostic radiology. *AJR Am J Roentgenol* 1997;169:1487-1488.
120. Hall EJ, Giaccia AJ. *Radiobiology for the radiologist*. 6th ed, Philadelphia: Lippincott Williams & Wilkins; 2006.
121. Wagner LK, Eifel PJ, Geise RA. Potential biological effects following high x-ray dose interventional procedures. *J Vasc Inter Radiol* 1994;5: 71-84.
122. Gkanatsios NA, Huda W, Peters KR. Adult patient doses in interventional neuroradiology. *Med Phys* 2002;29:717-723.
123. U.S. Food and Drug Administration. Avoidance of serious x-ray induced skin injuries to patients during fluoroscopically-guided procedures (1994). Available at: http://www.fda.gov. Accessed March 30, 2009.
124. International Commission on Radiological Protection. 2008 recommendations of the International Commission on Radiological Protection. Publication 103. *Annals of the IRCP* 2007;37:204.
125. National Academy of Sciences Committee on the Biological Effects of Ionizing Radiation. Health effects of exposure to low levels of ionizing radiations: time for reassessment? Report VII. Washington, DC: BEIR; 2005.
126. United Nations Scientific Committee on the Effects of Atomic Radiation. *Sources and effects of ionizing radiation*. New York: UNSEAR; 2000.
127. National Council on Radiation Protection and Measurements. Exposure of the U.S. population from diagnostic medical radiation. Report 100. Washington, DC: NCRP; 1989.

II

Chronic Lower Extremity Ischemia

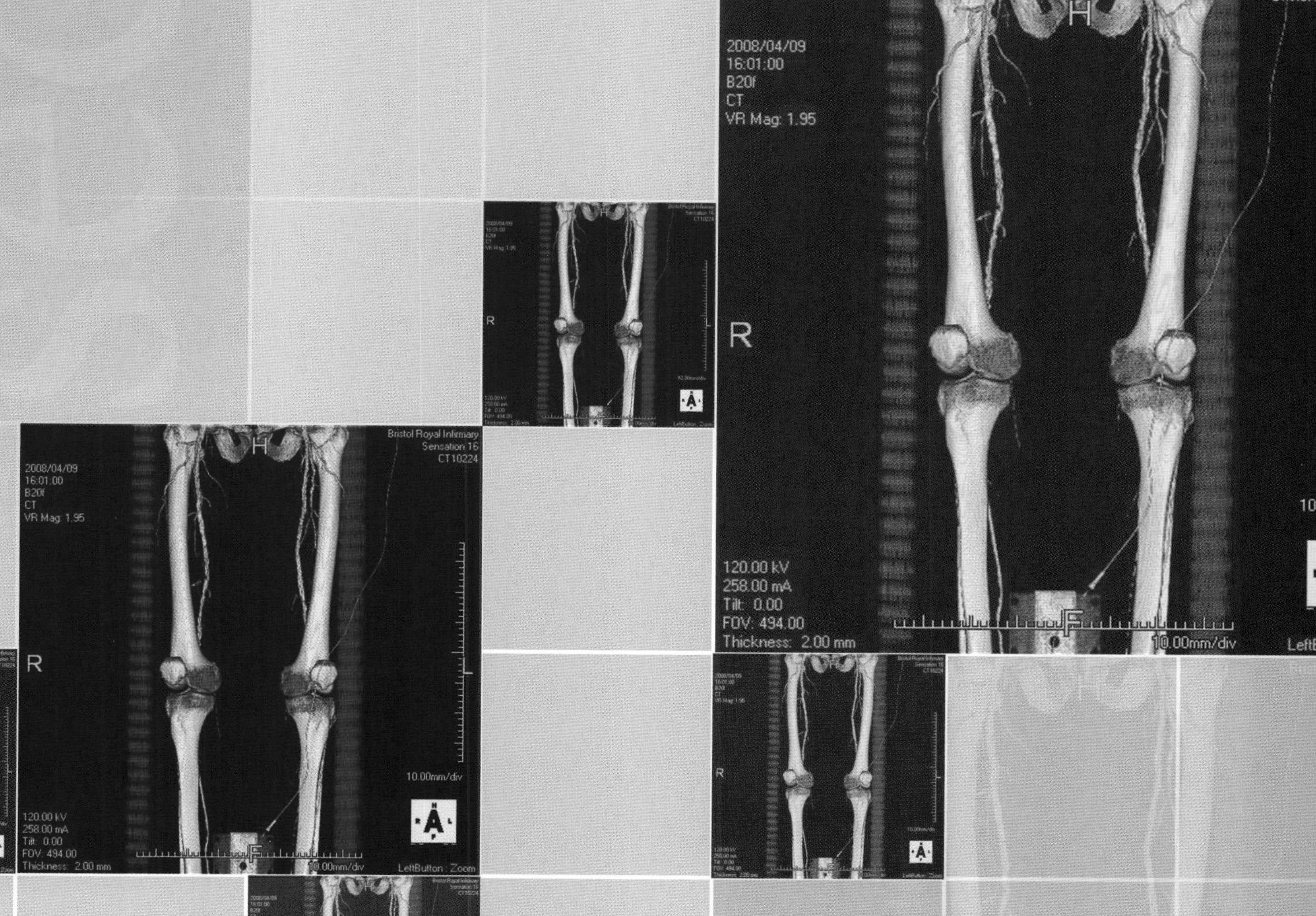

chapter

8

Natural History and Medical Management of Chronic Lower Extremity Ischemia

Frank C.T. Smith, BSc, MD, FRCS • Paritosh Sharma, MRCS • Constantinos Kyriakides, MD, FRCS

Key Points

- Peripheral arterial disease is common in the developed world, affecting approximately 14% to 20% of the adult population, with a ratio between symptomatic and asymptomatic individuals of 1:3 to 1:4.
- Chronic lower-extremity ischemia includes both intermittent claudication and more severe, critical limb ischemia (CLI).
- Approximately 25% of claudicants deteriorate in terms of clinical stage, most often in the first year after diagnosis.
- CLI affects between 500 and 1000 per 1 million population per year; 30% of patients with CLI undergo an amputation within the first year after diagnosis.
- The 5-year mortality for patients with CLI is 50% to 70%, 35% of these being cardiovascular deaths.
- Intermittent claudication is a manifestation of peripheral arterial disease, reflecting systemic atherosclerosis in which the coronary and cerebrovascular systems may also be involved.
- Treatment of chronic leg ischemia due to atherosclerotic disease should encompass secondary prevention for coronary and cerebrovascular events.
- Best medical treatment involves control of risk factors, including smoking cessation, supervised exercise, control of hyperlipidemia, hypertension, diabetes, and hyperhomocysteinemia.
- Aspirin, clopidogrel, statins, and angiotensin-converting enzyme inhibitors have established benefits in the prevention of secondary events.
- Naftidrofuryl and oxypentifylline have limited efficacy in improving walking capacity, but cilostazol has recently been shown to improve claudication distance and appears to have a beneficial effect on quality of life.

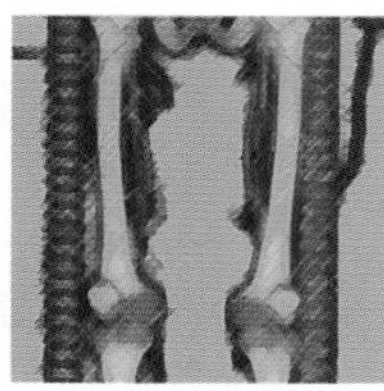

Chronic lower-extremity ischemia due to atherosclerotic arterial disease, encompassing intermittent claudication (IC) and the more severe critical limb ischemia (CLI), is a common cause of morbidity and mortality in Western populations (Figure 8-1). The incidence of chronic lower-extremity ischemia is likely to rise with the increasing elderly population. Patients are faced with disability affecting their legs and an increased likelihood of requiring an amputation, but more significantly, they are at an increased risk of morbidity and mortality due to cardiac and cerebrovascular ischemic events.

IC, defined as pain in the leg muscles following activity, is the earliest and most common presentation of chronic lower-extremity ischemia. Claudication pain is localized in the calf,

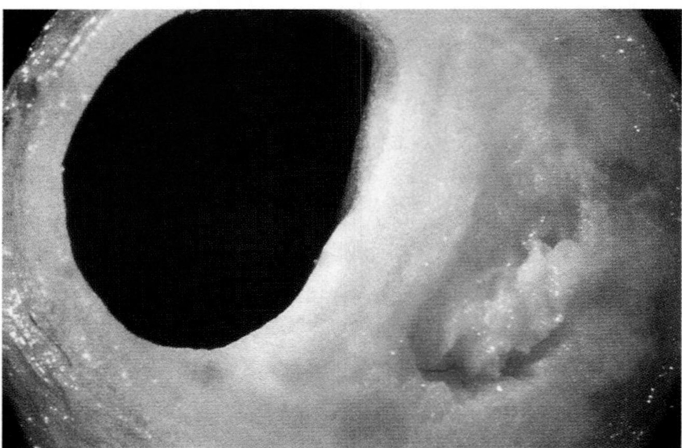

Figure 8-1. Arterial stenosis caused by an eccentric atherosclerotic plaque. Liquefaction occurs within the lipid core of the plaque, but the fibrous plaque cap remains intact. Stenosis or occlusion of the lower limb arteries is responsible for the symptom of intermittent claudication.

thigh, or buttock muscles, depending on the distribution of the arterial compromise. As the disease progresses in severity, patients develop pain at rest, particularly when the legs are elevated in bed at night. This pain is usually relieved by dependency. In contrast to IC, ischemic rest pain typically affects the foot. Severe tissue hypoperfusion then ensues, resulting in ischemic ulceration and gangrene. Significantly, CLI that includes rest pain and tissue loss is associated with an annual mortality rate of 20%.[1] The aim, therefore, is to develop management strategies that modify the progression of chronic lower-extremity ischemia and reduce the incidence of other adverse vascular events. These include risk factor identification, lifestyle modifications, pharmacotherapy, other forms of noninterventional treatment such as exercise rehabilitation and physiotherapy, and less commonly, percutaneous interventions and surgery.

ETIOLOGY

Atherosclerotic arterial disease is responsible for almost all lower limb arterial insufficiency and consequently CLI (Table 8-1). However, several rare conditions, listed here, tend to affect younger patients, and it is imperative that they are diagnosed early.

Persistent Sciatic Artery

The persistent sciatic artery is a congenital anomaly resulting from the lack of regression of the axial limb sciatic artery during early embryological development. The persisting axial artery continues to supply the limb while the iliofemoral segment remains underdeveloped. The persistent sciatic artery is prone to aneurysmal degeneration and can result in thrombosis or distal embolization.[2]

Thromboangiitis Obliterans: Buerger's Disease

Thromboangiitis obliterans, first described by Buerger in 1908, typically affects young Middle Eastern and Asian men usually between 20 and 40 years of age who are heavy smokers. It is characterized by segmental, thrombotic occlusions of the small- and medium-sized arteries, usually of the distal limbs. Patients typically present with rest pain and ischemic ulceration of the hands and toes. Buerger's disease has also been described as accelerated atherosclerosis.

Table 8-1
Causes of Lower Limb Arterial Occlusive Disease

Causes of Arterial Occlusive Lesions in the Lower Extremity
Atherosclerosis—occlusive or aneurysmal
Embolic disease
Trauma
Persistent sciatic artery
Thromboangiitis obliterans—Buerger's disease
Cystic adventitial disease
Fibromuscular dysplasia
Popliteal artery entrapment
Arteritis
Congenital and acquired coarctation of aorta
Primary vascular tumors

Cystic Adventitial Disease

Cystic adventitial disease is caused by a cystic abnormality of the adventitial layer of the arterial wall. The condition is common in young men between 20 and 50 years of age and typically affects the popliteal artery, although cases involving the iliac and femoral arteries have also been reported. The cysts are typically unilocular or multilocular with mucinous or gelatinous contents. These contents resemble that of a ganglion, and occasionally the cysts may be in communication with the synovium of an adjacent joint.[3]

Fibromuscular Dysplasia

Fibromuscular dysplasia is a condition of unknown etiology that typically affects the medium- to large-sized arteries in 20- to 50-year-old females. Although it primarily tends to affect the renal and carotid arteries, it can also involve the iliac and other arterial segments.

Popliteal Artery Entrapment Syndrome

Popliteal artery entrapment results from an aberrant relationship between the gastrocnemius muscle and the popliteal artery and commonly affects young athletes. The artery is compressed on flexing the knee joint and eventually, aneurysmal degeneration, distal embolization, and thrombosis occur.

DIAGNOSTIC CRITERIA

The Trans-Atlantic Inter-Society Consensus (TASC II) for the management of peripheral arterial disease (PAD) defines IC as muscle discomfort in the lower limb reproducibly produced by exercise and relieved by rest within 10 minutes.[4] Typical claudication symptoms occur in up to a third of patients with PAD and most commonly affect the calf but may also affect the thigh and the buttocks. However, it is important to note that typical claudication symptoms may not occur in patients with comorbidities that prevent sufficient activity to produce

Table 8-2
Classification of Peripheral Arterial Disease[5,6]

Fontaine Classification		Rutherford Classification	
Stage	Clinical	Grade	Clinical
I	Asymptomatic	0	Asymptomatic
IIa	Mild claudication	1	Mild claudication
IIb	Moderate to severe claudication	2	Moderate claudication
		3	Severe claudication
III	Ischemic rest pain	4	Ischemic rest pain
IV	Ulceration or gangrene	5	Minor tissue loss
		6	Major tissue loss

Table 8-3
Definitions of Critical Limb Ischemia

International Vascular Symposium Working Party Definition[7]
Severe rest pain requiring opiate analgesia for at least 4 weeks, and one of the following:
- Ankle pressure <40 mm Hg
- Ankle pressure <60 mm Hg in the presence of tissue necrosis or digital gangrene

Modified International Vascular Symposium Working Party Definition[8]
Severe rest pain requiring opiate analgesia for at least 4 weeks, and one of the following:
- Ankle pressure <40 mm Hg
- Tissue necrosis or digital gangrene

First European Working Group Definition[9]
Severe rest pain requiring opiate analgesia for at least 2 weeks, or both of the following:
- Ulceration or gangrene
- Ankle pressure <50 mm Hg

Second European Consensus Document[10]
- Persistently recurring ischemic pain requiring analgesia for more than 2 weeks and ankle systolic pressure <50 mm Hg and/or toe systolic pressure <30 mm Hg
- Alternatively, ulceration or gangrene of the foot or toes and ankle systolic pressure <50 mm Hg or toe systolic pressure <50 mm Hg

limb symptoms, such as severe lung disease, cardiac failure, and musculoskeletal disease.

A diagnosis of IC is usually established on history and examination, including measurement of the ankle–brachial index (ABI). A reduced ABI in symptomatic individuals confirms the diagnosis of hemodynamically significant occlusive disease, with a lower ABI corresponding to increased severity. The typical cutoff ABI for diagnosing PAD is 0.9 at rest. Falsely elevated ankle pressure readings may be obtained in diabetics and patients with renal disease who can have incompressible ankle arteries due to excessive calcification. Subjecting such symptomatic patients to additional diagnostic testing, including toe systolic pressures, pulse volume readings, transcutaneous oxygen measurements, and vascular imaging, may help confirm the diagnosis of PAD. Claudicants with isolated proximal disease may have a normal ABI at rest; however, with exercise, such lesions may become hemodynamically significant. Reduced postexercise ABI in these patients diagnoses PAD.

CLI is a manifestation of PAD that describes patients with typical chronic ischemic rest pain or with ischemic skin lesions through Fontaine stages III to IV or Rutherford categories 4 to 6 (Table 8-2).

The TASC II document recommends that the term CLI should only be used in relation to patients with chronic ischemic disease, defined by the presence of symptoms for more than 2 weeks.[4] The various definitions of CLI are summarized in Table 8-3.

Despite the multiplicity of definitions, the prevalence of CLI has been difficult to determine in population surveys. This is because CLI populations are difficult to study as large numbers of patients are lost to follow-up or die in longitudinal studies. In addition, it has not been possible to undertake accurate studies of the natural history of CLI because a significant majority of these patients require surgical intervention. Thus, most epidemiologic data for CLI populations relate to the group of patients with chronic lower-extremity ischemia. Nevertheless, detailed data can be obtained from hospital records as most patients with CLI are referred to hospital for treatment.

The terms "subcritical" and "critical" ischemia have been proposed to clarify subgroups within the CLI population.[11] Subcritical ischemia describes patients with rest pain and ankle pressure greater than 40 mm Hg, while critical ischemia has been used to describe patients with rest pain and tissue loss, ankle pressure below 40 mm Hg, or both. Important differences have been identified in these two groups with respect to outcomes. In the subcritical group, 27% of patients achieve limb survival without surgical intervention, compared to only 5% in the critically ischemic group, at 1 year. Evaluating cumulative graft patency at 1 year for surviving patients, 36% in the subcritical group benefited from conservative treatment, while 93% in the critically ischemic group needed surgery. For the critically ischemic group, intervention was virtually essential for limb viability. There was no evidence that the use of pharmacotherapy, sympathectomy, or spinal cord stimulation could improve limb salvage in this group.

There appears to be a group of patients with CLI, tissue loss and ankle pressure below 40 mm Hg in whom radiological or surgical intervention appears to be virtually imperative to save the limb. However, a less severely affected group exists with CLI, tissues intact, and ankle pressure above 40 mm Hg, in which limb loss does not appear to be inevitable and for which medical management may be effective.

A subgroup of PAD falls outside the definitions of both claudication and CLI. These patients have severe PAD but are asymptomatic either because of comorbidities that limit activity or because they are diabetics with peripheral neuropathy that reduces pain perception. Clinical assessment of these patients may reveal an ABI of 0.4 and absolute ankle pressures below 40 mm Hg. The term "chronic subclinical limb ischemia" has been used to describe this patient group, and it is important to identify these patients because they are thought to be vulnerable to progression to clinical CLI.[4,12]

PREVALENCE AND INCIDENCE

Several studies have looked at the prevalence of symptomatic and asymptomatic PAD in the same population and found that the ratio of the two is independent of age and is usually in the range of 1:3 to 1:4. These studies have also evaluated the prevalence of IC, and this appears to increase from 3% in patients aged 40% to 6% in those age 60 or older.[13-18] There have been some inconsistencies in the data obtained for the prevalence of symptomatic PAD. These have been attributed to varying methodologies, such as whether questionnaire surveys or ABI measurements were employed. Remember that while IC is the main symptom of PAD, the presence of this symptom does not always predict the presence of PAD. This is because symptoms are variable and may easily be confused with other causes of leg pain, such as spinal stenosis, arthritis, or venous disease.

Little direct information is available on the incidence of CLI; however, indirect evidence has been obtained from studies looking at progression of IC, population surveys on prevalence, and assumptions based on major amputation rates. Using these different methodologies, the incidence of CLI has been estimated to be 500 to 1000 new cases every year in a population of 1 million.[4,19-22]

A recent Swedish study evaluating prevalence found that 18% of the population suffered from PAD, with 0.5% having CLI.[23] These results are comparable to those reported by other population-based studies.[4,19-22]

RISK FACTORS

Several risk factors have been shown to be associated with the development and progression of chronic limb ischemia. In general, risk factors for the development of PAD can be divided into those that cannot be modified, such as age, and those that are modifiable, such as cigarette smoking, diabetes, dyslipidemia, and hypertension. Diabetes, smoking, dyslipidemia, increasing age, and a worsening ABI have also been suggested to be independent and probably additive risk factors associated with an increased incidence of CLI.[4,19]

Age

All large population-based studies have found that the incidence of both IC and CLI increases with age.[4,13-19]

Smoking

Smoking has been shown to be an independent risk factor for the development of PAD.[4,19] Smoking is considered to confer a two- to sixfold increase in the risk of developing PAD.[24] The association of smoking with PAD is thought to be stronger than its association with coronary artery disease. The severity of PAD appears directly proportional to the number of cigarettes smoked. Smoking cessation has been associated with a decline in the incidence of IC. The Edinburgh artery study found a relative risk of 3.7 to 3 for developing IC in smokers compared to ex-smokers.[18]

Diabetes

Diabetes mellitus is associated with a twofold increase in the risk of developing PAD.[4,19] This risk is directly proportional to the severity and duration of the diabetes. For every 1% increase in hemoglobin A1C, a corresponding 26% increase has been suggested in the risk of developing PAD.[25] PAD in diabetics is also more aggressive, with early involvement of large vessels and distal neuropathy. Diabetic patients suffer from sensory neuropathy and have a reduced resistance to infection that contributes to a five- to tenfold increase in the rate of major amputations compared to nondiabetics.[4,19,26-28]

Dyslipidemia

Elevated total serum cholesterol, low-density lipoprotein (LDL) cholesterol, decreased high-density lipoprotein (HDL), and hypertriglyceridemia have been associated with an increased risk of developing PAD.[4,19] This risk is thought to increase by 5% to 10% for every 10 mg/dl rise in total cholesterol.[29] The Framingham study found a doubling of the incidence of IC with a serum cholesterol greater than 7 mmol/L but suggested that the best predictor for PAD was the ratio of total to HDL cholesterol. It has also been suggested that smoking enhances the effects of hypercholesterolemia. Low serum HDL levels may also be related to smoking and reduced physical activity, although in the Edinburgh Artery Study the strong inverse relationship between HDL cholesterol and PAD was independent of smoking, other lipids, obesity, diabetes, and alcohol consumption.[30,31]

Evidence suggests that control of serum cholesterol and triglyceride levels decreases both the incidence and the progression of PAD.[32,33] Current guidelines recommend aggressive treatment of these patients with lipid-lowering drugs, as in patients with coronary artery disease.[34]

Hypertension

Hypertension is associated with an increased risk of developing PAD, although the association is considered to be weaker than for cerebrovascular and coronary disease. The risk is also less when compared to smoking and diabetes. The Framingham heart study found a 2.5-fold increase in the incidence of PAD in patients with hypertension, and this risk was proportional to the severity of the hypertension.[35]

Hyperhomocysteinemia

Increased homocysteine levels are detected in approximately 30% to 40% of patients with lower-extremity PAD. Hyperhomocysteinemia also appears to increase the risk of progression of PAD.[36] The association between hyperhomocysteinemia and PAD has also been suggested to be stronger than that for coronary artery disease.[4]

PROGNOSIS

Patients with PAD not only are at risk for progression of the disease but more significantly have been found to be susceptible to other cardiovascular events. The Reduction of Atherothrombosis for Continued Health registry that followed up patients with PAD, coronary artery disease, cerebrovascular disease, and subjects with more than 3 risk factors for atherothrombosis found PAD patients to have the highest cardiovascular mortality at 1-year follow-up.[37] Other studies have also found that these cardiovascular ischemic events are more common than any limb ischemic events[19,38]: there is a 20% to 60% increased risk of having a myocardial infarction, and the risk of having a stroke is increased by 40% in patients with PAD.[19,39-41]

The clinical course of PAD, as far as the leg is concerned, has been found to be surprisingly stable in most cases. All evidence gathered by large studies over the last 40 years has demonstrated that only a quarter of patients with IC will ever deteriorate significantly.[4] This stabilization has been attributed to the development of collaterals, metabolic adaptation of ischemic muscle, and the alteration of gait by the patient to favor nonischemic muscle groups.

A total of 25% of patients with IC deteriorate with time by the clinical stage, most in the first year after diagnosis (7% to 9%) compared to 2% to 3% per year thereafter.[4] Reviews suggest that only 1% to 3% of patients with IC need a major amputation over the next 5 years. In patients with IC, a worsening ABI is the best predictor for deterioration of PAD. The risk of progression to severe ischemia or limb loss for patients with low ankle pressures of 40 to 60 mm Hg is 8.5% per year.[4]

Studies suggest that approximately 60% to 90% of patients with CLI require some form of revascularization procedure, the rest undergoing a primary major amputation. It is therefore difficult to describe the natural history of the critically ischemic limb.

CLI is associated with a generally poor prognosis for patients. The TASC II document suggests that approximately 50% of patients with CLI undergo revascularization as primary treatment. At 1 year, only about 25% of these patients have resolution of their symptoms, 20% continue to have symptoms, 30% have undergone an amputation, and 25% are dead.[4] There have also been several studies on patients, with unreconstructable disease or for which attempts at reconstruction have failed, who have been managed with pharmacotherapy. The 6-month follow-up results from these studies indicate that approximately 40% of patients end up with an amputation and 20% die.[4] The mortality rates of patients who present with CLI have been reported in several large, single-center surgical series and vary from 40% to 70% over a 3- to 5-year follow-up.[42-44]

Management strategies for patients with PAD should therefore be developed, recognizing their cardiovascular burden, and especially those at risk of CLI, who should be identified early and treated actively.

TREATMENT FOR INTERMITTENT CLAUDICATION

The traditional goals of treatment for IC are to relieve the symptoms of pain on walking, to increase walking capacity, and to improve quality of life. However, recognition of the interrelationship of IC with other manifestations of cardiovascular disease means that intervention should be directed not only at improving focal symptoms but also at reducing the rate of coronary and cerebrovascular events. The recent TASC II and American College of Cardiology/American Heart Association (ACC/AHA) consensus documents have reviewed approaches to diagnosis and to the treatment of PAD, providing detailed discussion that places the use of appropriate medical and surgical therapeutic strategies in context.[4,19]

Control of risk factors for both claudication and other sequelae of cardiovascular disease is central to the medical management of claudication. There is sufficient evidence to argue for risk factor modification in all patients with PAD regardless of the severity of symptoms.[45] Beyond this, the decision to intervene for claudication depends on the individual's quality of life and on the extent to which the symptoms interfere with occupation and daily activities.

Objective evaluation of the impact of claudication on an individual patient is fraught with difficulties. The patient's assessment of their own walking distance, obtained when taking a medical history, is often unreliable. Patient and doctor may lack insight into the wide-ranging effects of the patient's symptoms on quality of life. IC has been shown to affect sleep, emotional behavior, and social interactions, in addition to mobility.[46]

Quality-of-life questionnaires such as the non-disease-specific Medical Outcomes Short Form–36 Questionnaire (SF-36) or the disease-specific Walking Impairment Questionnaire (WIQ) may help define functional, physical, and mental limitations but need to be interpreted cautiously, particularly with respect to the effect of concomitant medical conditions.

ASSESSMENT

Routine investigations include measurement of fasting blood glucose or hemoglobin A1C and lipid concentrations; a full blood cell count to exclude anemia, polycythemia, leukemia and thrombocythemia, urea, creatinine, and electrolytes for baseline assessment of renal function; and liver function tests before and during statin therapy. Thrombophilia screens and measurement of homocysteine levels should be performed selectively. An electrocardiogram should be taken. Many patients with claudication have a history of smoking, and a chest x-ray is advised to exclude an occult bronchial carcinoma.

An ABI of less than 0.9 at rest is useful in confirming the diagnosis of peripheral vascular disease and in helping distinguish this from nonvascular causes of leg pain, such as spinal stenosis (Figure 8-2). Patients with leg pain on walking who have an ABI of 0.91 to 1.30 should undergo an exercise test. Treadmill testing is helpful to define maximal walking distance (MWD) and pain-free walking distance (PFWD) but may not adequately simulate the patient's normal walking pace. In a patient with an ABI of more than 0.9, a decrease by more than 20% postexercise is indicative of arterial disease.

Patients with an ABI of more than 1.0 but with symptoms of claudication may have incompressible arteries. This clinical picture often occurs in diabetic patients due to calf vessel calcification. Other useful investigations in this situation include Doppler assessment of toe pressures, the "pole test,"[47]

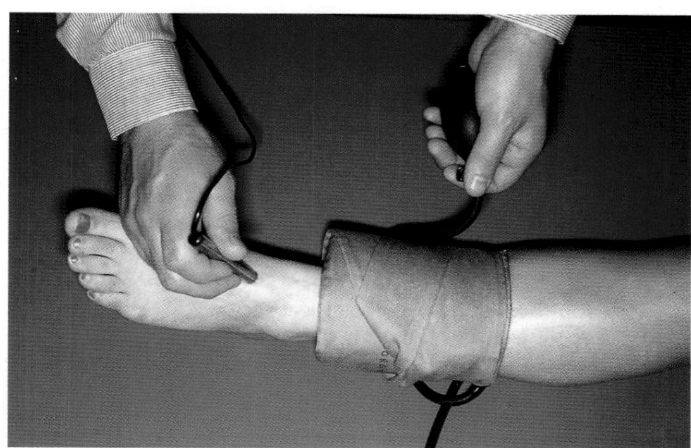

Figure 8-2. Continuous wave Doppler measurement of ankle pressures is the primary investigation in assessment for intermittent claudication. Measurement of postexercise pressures may increase the diagnostic sensitivity of the test.

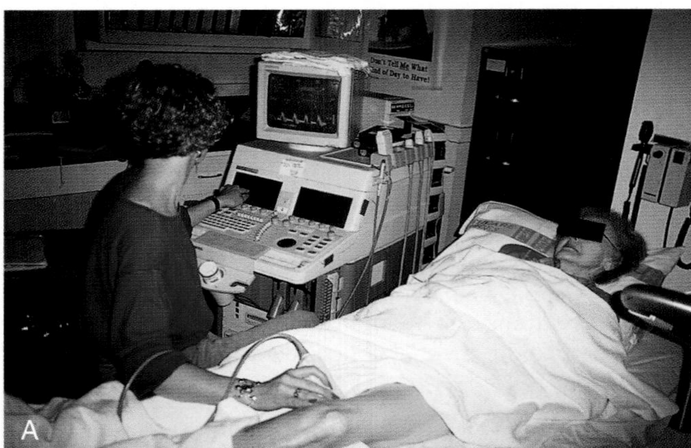

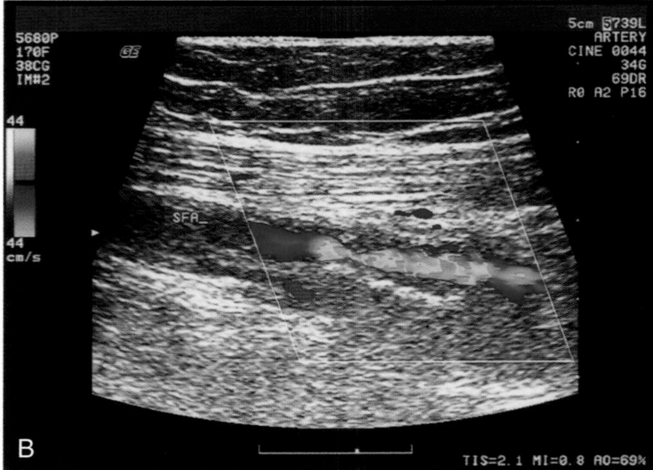

Figure 8-3. **A,** Noninvasive duplex Doppler assessment of the lower limb arteries provides both morphological and hemodynamic information about the nature of vessel disease. **B,** B-mode color-flow duplex ultrasound showing a tight stenosis in the superficial femoral artery of a claudicant. Turbulent blood flow in the vicinity of the stenosis is indicated by the change of color from blue to orange. Spectral analysis demonstrated a sixfold increase in blood flow velocity through the stenotic region.

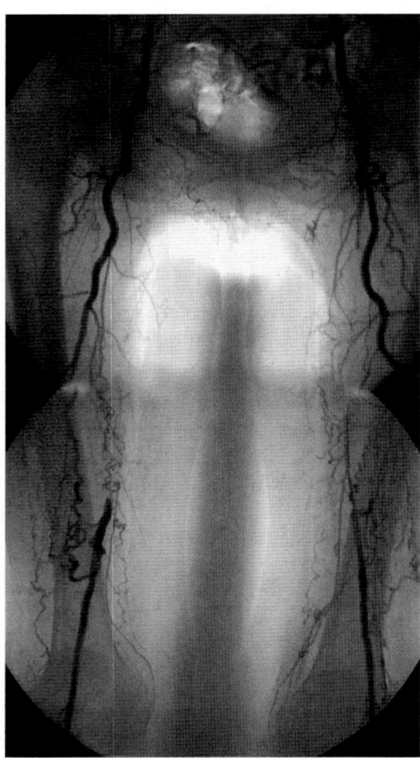

Figure 8-4. Digital subtraction angiography demonstrating bilateral superficial femoral artery occlusions, with development of extensive collateral circulations, in a patient with calf claudication in both legs.

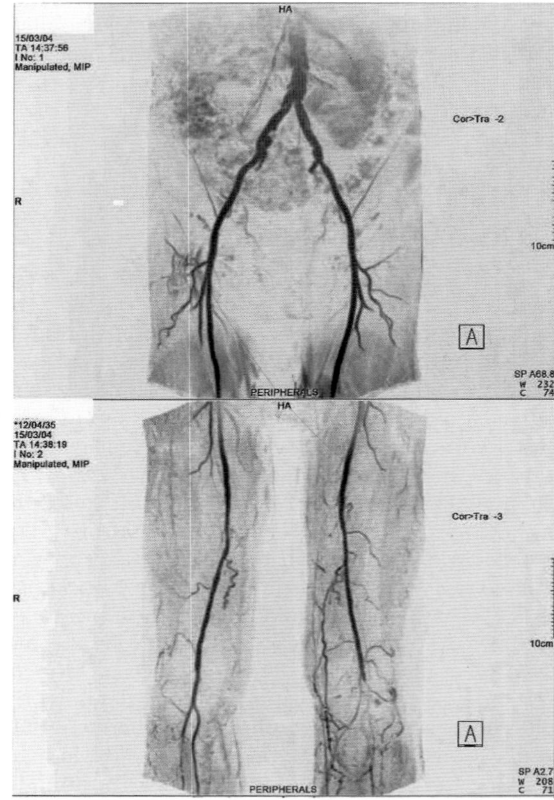

Figure 8-5. Magnetic resonance angiography demonstrating bilateral iliac artery disease and left above-knee popliteal artery occlusion with extensive collateral vessel development.

Doppler measurement of ankle pressures on leg elevation, and duplex ultrasound assessment of iliac, superficial femoral, and calf vessels (Figure 8-3).

At this time, duplex imaging or digital subtraction angiography are the investigations of choice when intervention by angioplasty or surgery is to be considered (Figure 8-4). However, magnetic resonance angiography (MRA; Figure 8-5) is a valuable noninvasive adjunctive investigation for localizing stenotic or occlusive peripheral vascular disease. Advantages of MRA include its safety and ability to provide rapid, high-resolution, three-dimensional (3D) imaging of the entire abdomen, pelvis, and legs simultaneously. MRA is useful for treatment planning before intervention and in assessing the suitability of lesions for an endovascular approach. Preprocedural MRA may minimize use of iodinated contrast material and exposure to radiation.

Multidetector computed tomography angiography (MDCTA; Figure 8-6) is also being widely adopted for initial diagnostic evaluation and treatment planning of PAD. The rapid evolution of technology, the deployment of fast

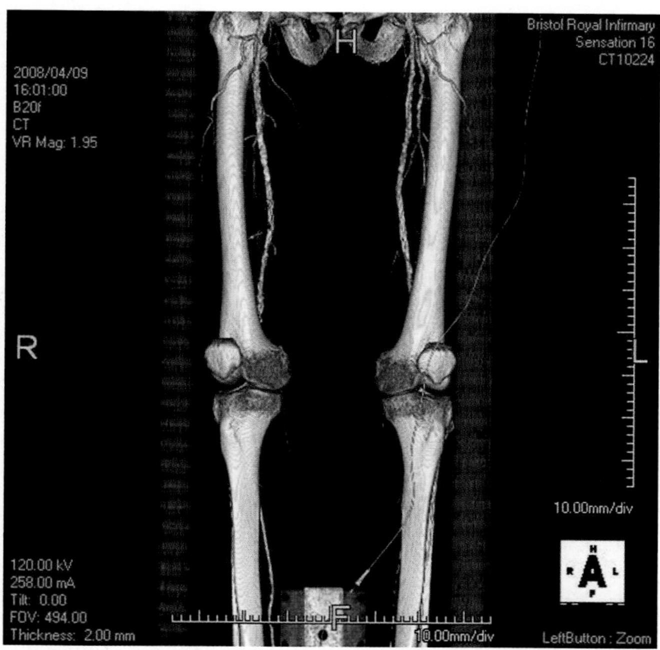

Figure 8-6. Contrast computed tomography angiography demonstrating diffuse, nonocclusive, stenotic right superficial femoral artery disease.

MDCTA multislice systems in the community, the familiarity with computed tomography technology, and ease of use are some factors driving its popularity. Multislice MDCTA enables fast imaging of the entire lower extremity and abdomen in one breath-hold at submillimeter isotropic voxel resolution. Although there are few prospectively designed studies with MDCTA, emerging data suggest that the sensitivity, specificity, and accuracy of this technique may rival invasive angiography.[48,49]

MODIFICATION OF RISK FACTORS

Hyperlipidemia

Alterations in lipid metabolism are a major risk factor for all forms of atherosclerosis. Evidence from several large epidemiological studies demonstrates that elevated serum total cholesterol and LDL cholesterol levels, and decreased HDL cholesterol levels, are significantly associated with cardiovascular mortality.[50,51] The role of elevated triglyceride levels has been debated, and it has been suggested that a strong association between triglyceride and cholesterol levels may account for the apparent effect of triglycerides. However, recent studies have shown conclusively that elevated triglyceride levels are also a strong and independent predictor of both ischemic heart disease and PAD.

Specific lipid fractions appear to be important in determining the extent and progression of atherosclerosis. Elevated total cholesterol, LDL cholesterol, triglycerides, and lipoprotein A levels are independent risk factors for PAD.[52,53] Increases in HDL cholesterol and apolipoprotein A1 confer protection.[53] For every increase of 10 mg/dl in total cholesterol, the risk of PAD rises by approximately 10%. Increases in lipoprotein Ap126 a levels appear to increase the risk of coronary disease twofold, and similar results have been noted in patients with PAD. Critical levels are 30 mg/dl or greater. Apolipoprotein B, a large protein contained within LDL particles, has also been associated with development of PAD. Higher levels of apolipoprotein B have been found in patients with peripheral vascular disease than in controls, and there appear to be differences in the apolipoprotein B gene locus between these groups.[54]

A metaanalysis of seven randomized, controlled trials of lipid-lowering therapy in patients with PAD found inconsistencies in outcome with respect to changes in ABI and walking distances.[55] In these trials, 698 patients were treated with various lipid-lowering therapies, including diet, probucol, cholecystyramine, and nicotinic acid, for intervals of 4 months to 3 years. The difference in mortality of 0.7% in treated patients versus 2.9% in controls did not achieve statistical significance. However, lipid-lowering therapy was effective in reducing disease progression as assessed by angiography and the severity of claudication symptoms.

Attempts to reduce lipid levels by diet alone achieved reductions of only 5% to 10%, and several of the drugs employed in the previously noted studies had considerable side effects. In the Cholesterol Lowering Atherosclerosis Study,[56] 188 men with both coronary disease and PAD were randomized to colestipol plus niacin or placebo, after initial diet control. The treated group had regression or stabilization of femoral atherosclerosis compared to the control group. In the St. Thomas' Trial,[57] 25 patients were treated with diet, cholecystyramine, nicotinic acid, or clofibrate for a mean of 19 months with an apparent beneficial effect on femoral atherosclerosis.

Probucol is a drug that reduces LDL and cholesterol HDL concentrations. The Probucol Qualitative Regression Swedish Trial[58] studied 303 patients with PAD who were treated by diet and cholecystyramine and then by either probucol or placebo for 3 years. No significant beneficial effect of probucol treatment was demonstrated on either femoral atherosclerosis or ABI. In the Program on the Surgical Control of the Hyperlipidemias Trial,[59] ileal bypass was used to lower lipid concentrations and patients were followed for 10 years. This trial evaluated specific lower limb clinical endpoints. At 5 years, the relative risk of an abnormal ABI in the treated group was 0.6, the 95% confidence interval was 0.4 to 0.9, absolute risk reduction was 15%, and $P < 0.01$; the risk of claudication or limb-threatening ischemia was 0.7, the 95% confidence interval was 0.2 to 0.9, absolute risk reduction was 7%, and $P < 0.01$ compared to the control group.

Statins

Statins are 3-hydroxy-3-methylglutaryl–coenzyme A reductase inhibitors and effectively reduce serum cholesterol (Figure 8-7). However, they also have valuable ancillary effects on endothelial function, including plaque stabilization and antithrombogenic properties, and reduce plasma fibrinogen levels (Table 8-4).

The statins differ with respect to cytochrome P450 metabolism and drug interactions, but all may cause rhabdomyolysis. Statins should be used cautiously in patients with liver disease. Baseline and follow-up liver function tests should be performed within 1 to 3 months of starting treatment and thereafter every 6 months for 1 year.

Five major randomized, controlled trials have shown a reduction in total mortality and major coronary events by lowering levels of serum cholesterol with statin therapy in patients with or without a history of cardiac disease.

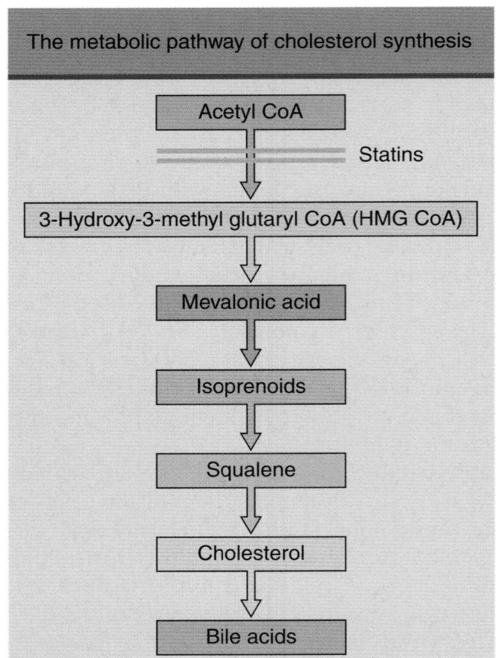

Figure 8-7. The metabolic pathway of cholesterol synthesis. Blockade by statins, 3-hydroxy-3-methylglutaryl–coenzyme A reductase inhibitors, occurs at the first, rate-limiting step.

A metaanalysis of these studies demonstrated mean reductions of total and LDL cholesterol of 20% and 28%, respectively, and of triglycerides by 13%, as well as a 5% HDL–cholesterol increase.[60] In the Long-Term Intervention with Pravastatin in Ischaemic Disease Study,[61] subgroup analysis of 905 out of 9014 patients with coronary heart disease and claudication showed a significant reduction in myocardial and cerebrovascular events in patients treated with pravastatin. In the Heart Protection Study,[62] 6748 patients with a total cholesterol level greater than 135 mg/dl were randomized to receive simvastatin or placebo. Risk of heart attack, stroke, and leg revascularization in patients with PAD was reduced by 25% at the 5-year follow-up. Average reductions of total cholesterol of 2 mmol/L and of LDL cholesterol of 1.5 mmol/L were achieved.

The main reason for using these drugs to date, therefore, has been to reduce cardiovascular events. However, specifically with respect to PAD, results from the 4S Scandinavian Simvastatin Survival Study[63] suggested that the incidence of new or worsening IC was reduced by 38% after 3 years in patients on statin therapy versus placebo (relative risk, 0.62; 95% confidence interval, 0.44 to 0.88; absolute risk reduction, 1.3%). A prospective trial demonstrated that atorvastatin increased the distance walked to the onset of claudication but did not increase MWD.[64] Two other single-center trials have suggested a similar benefit with respect to time to claudication onset in patients treated with simvastatin.[65,66]

Table 8-4
Nonlipid Lowering Effects of Statins

- Inhibition of vascular smooth muscle cell proliferation and migration
- Improved endothelial function and vasomotion
- Reduced oxygen free radical production by activated macrophages
- Reduced low-density lipoprotein oxidation
- Reduced platelet aggregability
- Increased fibrinolysis
- Reduced fasting insulin concentrations

In a study that investigated the effect of plasma apheresis to reduce serum lipoprotein a concentration, 42 patients were randomized to receive simvastatin alone or simvastatin plus apheresis.[67] Follow-up was continued for 2 years. The peripheral arterial endpoints included assessment of femoral and tibial artery atherosclerotic disease by duplex ultrasonography. An increase occurred in the number of hemodynamically significant stenoses in patients treated with simvastatin alone, compared to a decrease in the number of stenoses in patients who also had apheresis ($P = 0.002$). Although apheresis has little practical scope as a routine therapy, these results achieved statistical significance and provide further evidence for the implication of lipoprotein A in peripheral atherogenesis.

In summary, lipid-lowering therapy benefits patients with PAD who often have concomitant coronary and cerebrovascular disease. Revision of the National Cholesterol Education Program Adult Treatment Panel III guidelines recommends that patients with PAD and an LDL cholesterol level of 100 mg/dl or greater be treated with a statin. The recommended LDL cholesterol goal is less than 100 mg/dl, but when the risk is very high an LDL cholesterol goal of less than 70 mg/dl is a therapeutic option. Patients with very high cholesterol concentrations, greater than 8 mmol/L, may be suffering from a familial hyperlipidemia and should be referred to a specialist lipid clinic for advice, since these patients may benefit from combination therapy.

Hyperhomocysteinemia

High serum homocysteine levels are an independent risk factor for development of PAD.[68] Hyperhomocysteinemia may be related to an autosomal recessive inborn error of metabolism or due to nutritional, physiological, or pathological factors, including dietary folate deficiency and alterations in vitamin B_{12} metabolism. Patients with hyperhomocysteinemia and symptomatic PAD have a fourfold risk of vascular mortality and morbidity compared to patients with a normal level.[69] Approximately one third of patients with PAD have elevated serum homocysteine levels[70]; for every 5 μmol/L rise in fasting homocysteine levels, there is an increase in relative risk of atherosclerotic disease of about 35% for men and 42% for women.

The mechanism of action of homocysteine is not fully elucidated but is thought to involve facilitation of oxidation of LDL cholesterol. Homocysteine is implicated in generation of oxygen free radicals resulting in endothelial dysfunction with impaired nitric oxide generation and proliferation of smooth muscle cells, leading to acceleration of the process of atherosclerosis. It may also be implicated in blood hypercoagulability.

Homocysteine synthesis and metabolism are outlined in Figure 8-8. High serum homocysteine levels can be lowered by dietary supplementation with B_{12} and B_6 vitamins and folate. However, no randomized clinical trials have shown that lowering serum homocysteine concentrations results in an improvement in claudication. These areas are being explored.

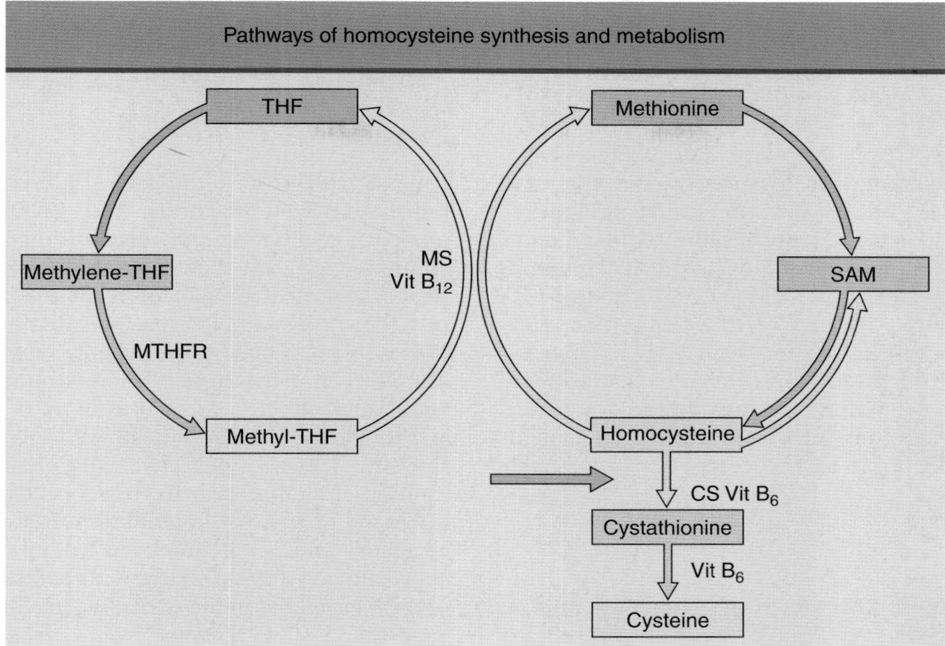

Figure 8-8. Pathways of homocysteine synthesis and metabolism and the involvement of vitamins B_6, B_{12}, and folate. The block arrow indicates the site of deficiency of the enzyme cystathionine synthase, which occurs in homocystinuria, as a result of an autosomal recessive inborn error of metabolism. CS, cystathionine synthase; MS, methionine synthase; MTHFR, methylene tetrahydrofolate reductase; SAM, S-adenosyl methionine; THF, tetrahydrofolate.

Diabetes Mellitus

Lower limb arterial disease is a well-recognized complication of diabetes mellitus and may result from both macrovascular and microvascular disease. The incidence of claudication and low ABI is two- to sixfold higher in diabetic patients than in the age-matched population. Intensive control of blood glucose is well established in the treatment of microvascular complications of diabetes, but its role in prevention of macrovascular sequelae is less well defined.

In the U.K. Prospective Diabetes Study 3867, type II diabetic patients were randomized to "intensive" versus "usual care."[71] Intensive therapy involved treatment with sulphonylureas or insulin, and conventional care was achieved with diet therapy. Intensive care resulted in the reduction of diabetes-related myocardial infarction ($P = 0.05$) and other diabetes-related endpoints. The major part of this reduction was directly attributable to a reduction in microvascular-related complications. Risks of amputation, however, were not altered by intensive diabetic control.

In another important study, the Diabetes Control and Complications Trial,[72] 1441 patients with type I diabetes were treated by intensive or conventional insulin therapy. A lower incidence of cardiovascular events was seen in the intensively treated patients, which did not quite achieve statistical significance ($P = 0.08$). However, a negligible difference appeared in outcome with respect to peripheral vascular disease. These results suggest that good diabetic control in patients with type I and type II diabetes may not be sufficient to improve the outcome of associated peripheral vascular disease. The cornerstone of PAD management, therefore, is to attempt good diabetic control, but in conjunction with aggressive management of other risk factors such as diet, provision of adequate exercise, and control of smoking and blood pressure.

Current recommendations from the ACC/AHA guidelines advise the following:[34a]

> Proper foot care, including use of appropriate footwear, chiropody/podiatric medicine, daily foot inspection, skin cleansing, and use of topical moisturizing creams, should be encouraged and skin lesions and ulcerations should be addressed urgently in all diabetic patients with lower-extremity PAD. Treatment of diabetes in individuals with lower-extremity PAD, by administration of glucose control therapies to reduce the hemoglobin A1C to less than 7%, can be effective to reduce microvascular complications and potentially improve cardiovascular outcomes.

Hypertension

Hypertension has a strong association with the presence of PAD, the risk of claudication being increased up to threefold in hypertensive patients.[35] Treatment of hypertension may reduce cardiovascular deaths by 14% and the stroke rate by 38%, with a reduction in peripheral vascular events of 26%. However, there are few data to suggest that treatment alters either the progress of peripheral atherosclerosis or the symptoms of IC.

Early studies suggested that treatment of hypertensive patients with β-adrenergic antagonists aggravated the symptoms of claudication. These reports have been superceded by a metaanalysis of 11 randomized, controlled trials in which no detrimental effect of the drugs on walking distance or symptoms of claudication in patients with PAD was demonstrated.[73] The current view is that beta-blockers are safe to administer to patients with mild to moderate PAD; however, if symptoms deteriorate after administration, then other appropriate antihypertensive medication, for instance, the calcium antagonist nifedipine, should be prescribed.

Angiotensin-converting enzyme (ACE) inhibitors may have a valuable cardioprotective role in patients with PAD. In large studies, ACE inhibitors such as ramipril have been shown to reduce death from vascular causes, nonfatal myocardial infarcts, and strokes in hypertensive patients. The Heart Outcomes Prevention Evaluation study randomized patients with coronary artery disease, cerebrovascular disease, PAD, diabetes, or a combination of these to the ACE inhibitor ramipril or placebo. The study included 4051 patients with PAD. Ramipril reduced the risk of myocardial infarction, stroke, or vascular death in patients with PAD by approximately 25%, a level of efficacy comparable to that achieved in the entire study population.[74] It is therefore recommended that ACE inhibitors be considered as treatment for patients with lower-extremity PAD to reduce the risk of adverse cardiovascular events.

Smoking

Epidemiological studies have shown that a lifetime of cigarette smoking approximately doubles the risk of morbidity and mortality from ischemic heart disease, compared to not smoking.[75] The risk is related to the amount and duration of smoking. Stopping smoking rapidly reduces this risk, although it may take 20 years, if ever, before the risk is reversed. Heavy smokers are three times more likely to develop IC than nonsmokers, and the risks of developing CLI or requiring amputation are three- to fivefold higher among patients with PAD who continue to smoke. Patients with PAD should therefore be encouraged and helped to stop smoking and to prevent restarting.

The value and application of effective antismoking strategies has largely been neglected in everyday clinical practice. Unfortunately, long-term quit rates for behavioral interventions alone are poor, with only 15% to 30% of patients remaining abstinent after 1 year of treatment. However, there is good evidence that nicotine replacement therapy (NRT)[76] and oral bupropion[77] may improve the rates in motivated patients by two- to threefold at 1 year.

Cigarette smoking has two deleterious components: nicotine, which is addictive but plays no significant role in atherogenesis, and tar and other chemicals such as oxidizing agents, which exert powerful damaging atherogenic and carcinogenic effects and impair lung function (Figure 8-9). The strategy with NRT is to encourage patients to stop smoking abruptly. This precipitates nicotine withdrawal symptoms, which are alleviated by NRT via transdermal or sublingual routes, or by nasal inhalation. The oral bioavailability of nicotine is low. Transdermal and sublingual administration of NRT may be combined to achieve the required plasma levels to relieve symptoms of nicotine withdrawal, including agitation, sleep disturbance, and sympathetic nervous effects. NRT is then gradually reduced over 2 to 3 months.

Bupropion is an antidepressant licensed for use as part of a smoking cessation program. In recent clinical trials, it has been demonstrated to be at least as effective as NRT in promoting smoking cessation, although combined therapy has been shown to be more effective than either treatment alone.[77,78]

Although the rationale for smoking cessation is still poorly understood and randomly applied by physicians, the cost effectiveness of this intervention in patients with PAD compares favorably with other medical treatments, such as statins and ACE inhibitors.

Exercise

Patients with IC have diminished exercise performance and impaired overall functional and physical capacities. Peak oxygen consumption measured during treadmill testing is approximately half that of normal subjects and equivalent to that reported for patients with significant heart failure. Impairment in walking capacity is detrimental to other normal everyday functions and quality of life. Improvement of mobility per se, therefore, is an important goal for the patient with claudication.

Providing patients with advice to walk more has been shown to be largely ineffective, but formal supervised exercise training programs seem to have a beneficial effect. A recent Cochrane review of 10 randomized trials of exercise therapy estimated an overall improvement in walking distance of approximately 150%.[79] Exercise was supervised in all but one of these trials, and in the remaining trial evidence of unsupervised exercise was obtained from exercise log books and by providing patients with pedometers.

A meta analysis of 21 exercise training programs showed that by training for at least 6 months, by walking to near-maximum pain tolerance, a significant improvement in PFWD and MWD was achieved.[80] However, similar dramatic improvements have also been reported in trials that used shorter periods of exercise, from 1 to 3 months, with symptomatic improvement persisting beyond the period of supervision.

The reduction in cardiac risk is an added benefit of supervised exercise programs. Physical inactivity is an independent risk factor for atherosclerosis, and exercise has been shown to reduce blood pressure and to improve lipid profile and glucose metabolism in a healthy population. Furthermore, exercise rehabilitation reduces the risk of cardiovascular death after myocardial infarction by about 25%.

Exercise intensity, the rate at which work is performed, must be taken into consideration when designing an exercise program for the individual patient. It is important that the exercise intensity for aerobic work falls within the specific physiological capabilities the individual and is sufficiently strenuous to produce a training response.

Various mechanisms may produce the beneficial effects achieved by exercise training. Training is not associated with a substantial increase in blood flow to the legs, and the changes that do occur fail to predict clinical responses. Improved cardiovascular fitness is a nonspecific benefit of exercise; indeed, even upper limb training is effective in improving claudication. Some benefits are probably due to improved oxygen extraction by leg muscles. Alterations in muscle metabolism may also be implicated. Furthermore, training results in improvements in gait and walking efficiency.

Continued participation is an essential component of exercise therapy; thus, both initial and subsequent intensities of the training programs must be acceptable to the patient, who needs to remain motivated. The time of day at which a patient exercises may affect compliance. Individuals who exercise regularly at the same time of day experience psychological benefits at that time of day and are more likely to continue to comply with an exercise program.

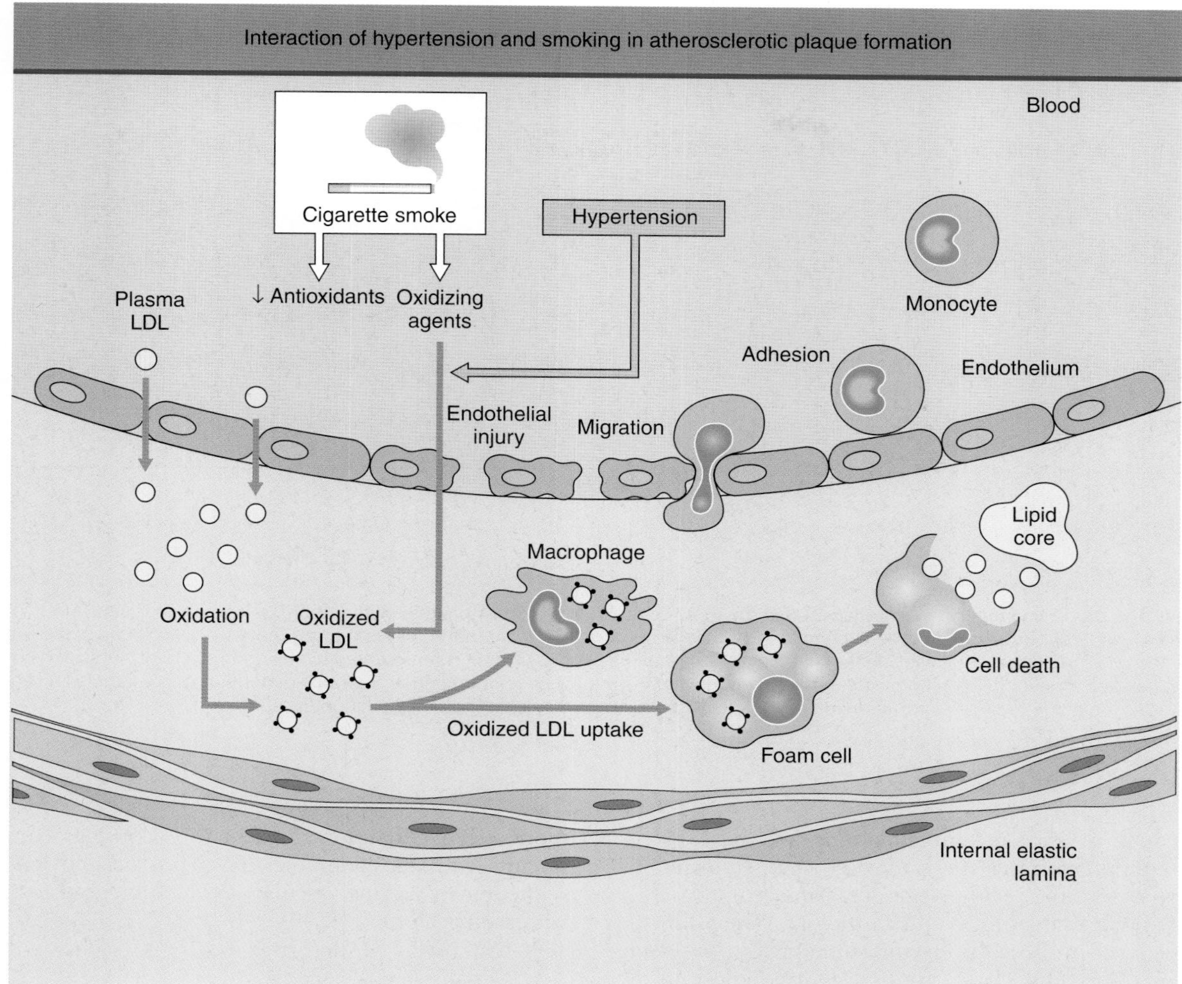

Figure 8-9. Interaction of hypertension and smoking in atherosclerotic plaque formation. Monocytes adhere to the vascular endothelium and migrate to the intima. Low-density lipoprotein (LDL) also enters the intima, where it becomes oxidized and is taken up by monocytes to become foam cells. Foam cell death caused by apoptosis, or due to necrosis induced by lipid peroxides, releases lipid, which is incorporated into the lipid core. Cigarette smoke contains oxidizing species whose passage across the endothelium is facilitated in the presence of hypertension. These oxidizing agents and the decreased levels of antioxidants found in smokers promote oxidation of LDL, speeding up the process of atherogenesis.

Two trials comparing exercise therapy with angioplasty for claudication produced conflicting data. In a study from Oxford, exercise was found to be more effective than angioplasty at 1-year follow-up, but this advantage was lost at 70 months, when only one third of patients still undertook exercise.[81] In the other trial from Edinburgh, a benefit from angioplasty seen at 6 months was lost after 2 years.[82] Both trials, however, had a relatively small number of patients, and larger, multicenter randomized trials of supervised exercise therapy versus angioplasty in patients with claudication are awaited.

Despite its efficacy, exercise therapy has various limitations. Supervised exercise is not readily available, and unsupervised exercise remains the mainstay of conservative treatment. Currently in the United Kingdom, referral to a supervised exercise program is available to only 27% of vascular surgeons.[83] Moreover, in the United States, exercise training programs are not covered by medical insurance, hindering their widespread use.

Current ACC/AHA recommendations are that a program of supervised exercise training should be initial treatment for patients with IC. Supervised exercise training should occur for a minimum of 30 to 45 minutes, on a treadmill, at least three times per week for a minimum of 12 weeks.

Exercise therapy appears to be cheaper and safer than surgery or angioplasty, but the optimum duration, intensity, and cost effectiveness of exercise programs still have to be determined.

DRUG THERAPY

Unequivocal evidence now supports the value of antiplatelet agents in providing secondary protection against cardiovascular events in patients with PAD. No drug, however, has yet proven effective enough for the symptoms of claudication to gain widespread acceptance or universal usage, although various drugs have been advocated for this purpose. Evidence for use of these drugs has been reviewed extensively in the recent ACC/AHA 2005 Guidelines for the Management of Patients with Peripheral Arterial Disease and the Inter-Society Consensus for the Management of Peripheral Arterial Disease TASC II 2007 documents.[4]

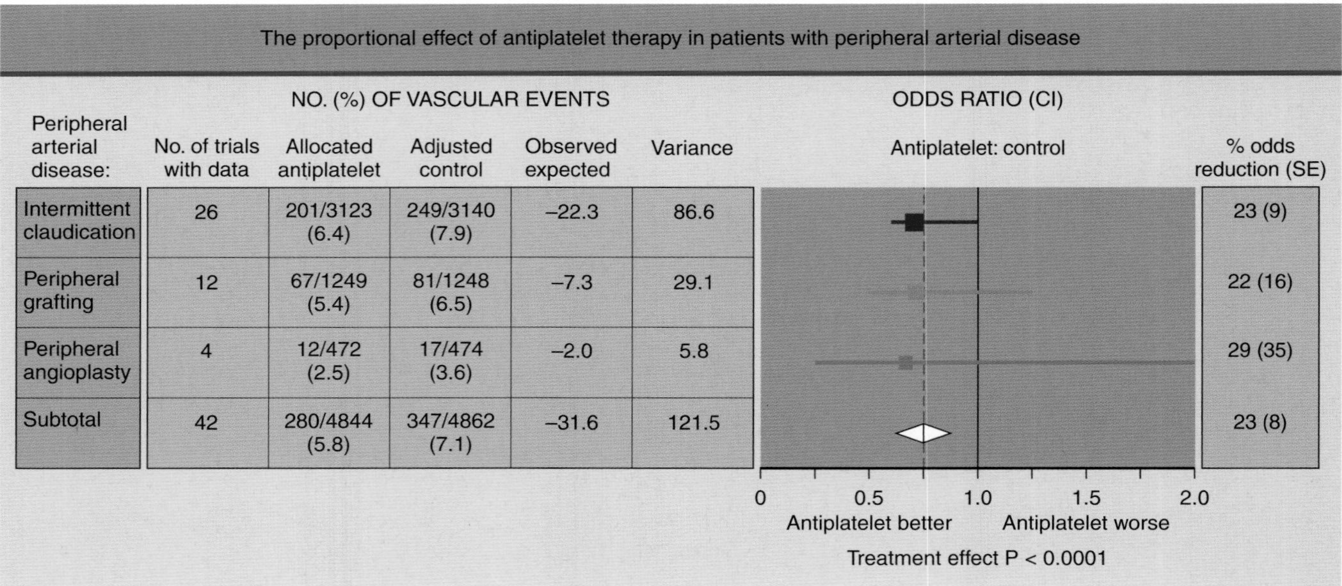

The proportional effect of antiplatelet therapy in patients with peripheral arterial disease

Peripheral arterial disease:	No. of trials with data	NO. (%) OF VASCULAR EVENTS Allocated antiplatelet	Adjusted control	Observed expected	Variance	% odds reduction (SE)
Intermittent claudication	26	201/3123 (6.4)	249/3140 (7.9)	−22.3	86.6	23 (9)
Peripheral grafting	12	67/1249 (5.4)	81/1248 (6.5)	−7.3	29.1	22 (16)
Peripheral angioplasty	4	12/472 (2.5)	17/474 (3.6)	−2.0	5.8	29 (35)
Subtotal	42	280/4844 (5.8)	347/4862 (7.1)	−31.6	121.5	23 (8)

Figure 8-10. The proportional effect of antiplatelet therapy in 42 trials involving 9214 patients with peripheral arterial disease (PAD). The stratified ratio of odds of an event in treatment groups compared to that in control groups is plotted for each group of trials (*square*), together with its 99% confidence interval (*horizontal line*). Metaanalysis of the results for all categories of PAD is represented by the *open diamond*. Adjusted control totals were calculated after converting any unevenly randomized trials to even ones by counting control groups more than once. Other statistical calculations were based on actual numbers from individual trials. (Data from Antithrombotic Trialists' Collaboration *BMJ* 2002;324:71-86.)

The contents and recommendations of these documents present consensus views, devised and endorsed by international societies, with representations from vascular surgery, radiology, angiology, and cardiology. The following drugs have been proposed as having some proven but small benefits in improving claudication distance: naftidrofuryl, oxypentifylline, cilostazol, and buflomedil.

Antiplatelet Therapy

Aspirin

In patients with systemic cardiovascular disease, including those with PAD, current evidence suggests that antiplatelet drugs confer significant benefit, principally in terms of secondary prevention of vascular events.

In a recent metaanalysis of updated data from the Antithrombotic Trialists' Collaboration involving 9214 patients with PAD treated with antiplatelet agents in 42 trials, a proportional reduction of 23% was found in serious vascular events (P = 0.004; Figure 8-10).[84] Similar benefits were observed among patients with IC and those undergoing peripheral bypass surgery or peripheral angioplasty.

Aspirin is the most comprehensively investigated antiplatelet drug. Within a few days of beginning 75 mg of aspirin daily, platelet cyclooxygenase-mediated production of thromboxane A_2 is virtually eliminated, producing an antithrombotic effect. In the Physicians Health Study,[85] a primary prevention trial, aspirin was found to reduce the subsequent need for arterial surgery. Aspirin has also been shown to reduce vascular graft occlusion rates in patients with PAD who have previously undergone arterial bypass surgery.[86]

High doses of aspirin, 500 to 1500 mg, which carry greater potential risk of gastrointestinal side effects, appear to be no more effective than low doses of 75 to 150 mg. Combination therapy with dipyridamole may be associated with further reduction in serious vascular events compared to treatment with aspirin alone.

Ticlopidine and Clopidogrel

These drugs are both thienopyridines that inhibit platelet adenosine diphosphate–induced aggregation and activation. The effect of these agents is complementary to aspirin, which inhibits thromboxane-dependent activation. In patients with PAD, ticlopidine has been shown to reduce the risks of fatal and nonfatal myocardial infarction and stroke. However, the beneficial effects of ticlopidine were partially negated by the substantial risk of thrombocytopenia, neutropenia, and thrombotic thrombocytopenic purpura. These significant side effects occur in 1 in 2000 to 4000 patients, and treatment therefore necessitates scrupulous hematological monitoring.

Clopidogrel is a second-generation thienopyridine with fewer side effects than ticlopidine. The platelet inhibitory effects of clopidogrel and aspirin are illustrated in Figure 8-11. Evidence for the benefit of clopidogrel was principally derived from the Clopidogrel versus Aspirin in Patients at Risk of Ischemic Events Trial.[87] This was a large, randomized, controlled trial conducted in 16 countries comparing the benefits of 75 mg of clopidogrel per day with aspirin at 375 mg per day. More than 19,000 patients participated in the trial. Primary outcome measures in this study had a composite endpoint, including myocardial infarction, fatal or nonfatal ischemic stroke, or other vascular death. Overall risk reduction was 8.7% ($P < 0.05$) in favor of clopidogrel compared to aspirin.

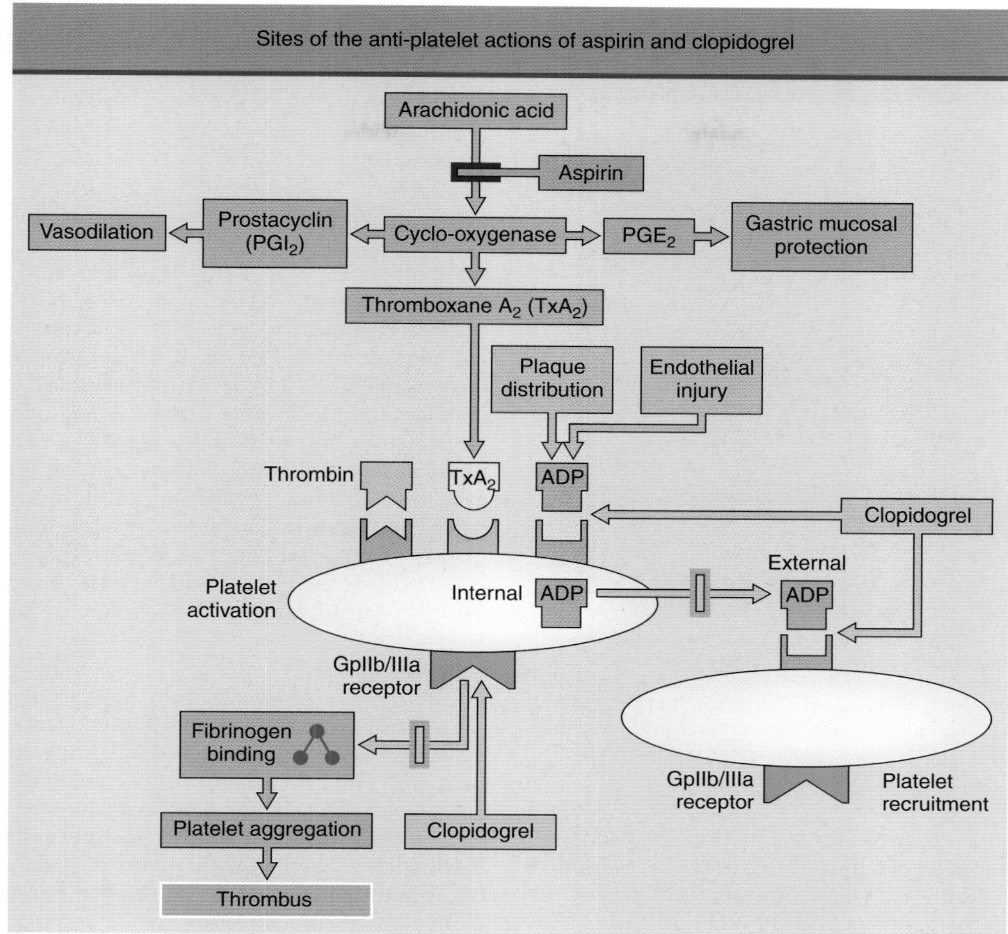

Figure 8-11. Sites of the antiplatelet actions of aspirin and clopidogrel.

In this study, 6452 patients had either a history of claudication, with previous peripheral bypass surgery, or claudication, with an APBI of 0.85 or less. Subgroup analysis of these patients with moderate PAD showed an overall 23.8% risk reduction on treatment with clopidogrel, with an average event rate per year for aspirin of 4.86% versus clopidogrel at 3.7% ($P = 0.0028$; Figure 8-12). Patients taking clopidogrel had a higher incidence of rash, diarrhea, and pruritus than those taking aspirin but a lower incidence of gastrointestinal bleeding. An overlap in confidence intervals that went from negligible benefit to a 20% further reduction in vascular events in favor of clopidogrel in this trial means that the true size of any difference between aspirin and clopidogrel could not be reliably estimated.

Interest in combination therapy has been stimulated by the results of another large trial, the Clopidogrel in Unstable Angina to Prevent Recurrent Ischemic Events Study,[88] which suggested improved outcome when clopidogrel was used with aspirin in patients with acute coronary syndrome. To date, however, no evidence supports the efficacy of combined aspirin and clopidogrel treatment versus a single antiplatelet agent in patients with lower-extremity PAD.

In summary, current evidence suggests that aspirin, at a dose of 75 to 325 mg daily, is a safe and effective antiplatelet regimen in PAD, unless patients have a definite contraindication to aspirin. Clopidogrel, at 75 mg daily, is an appropriate alternative. The value of combination therapy still has to be vindicated.

Cilostazol

Cilostazol is a phosphodiesterase type 3 inhibitor that increases cellular levels of cyclic adenosine monophosphate. It acts to inhibit platelet aggregation and thrombus formation but also reduces vascular smooth muscle cell proliferation and has a direct effect as a vasodilator. Vasodilator-type drugs generally reduce systemic blood pressure, leading to a reduction in lower limb perfusion pressure. They may also result in a steal of blood from ischemic regions in which blood vessels are already maximally dilated; thus, the rationale for treatment with vasodilators has been questioned in claudication. The mechanisms by which cilostazol exerts its beneficial effects in claudication, therefore, have not been fully elucidated.

Cilostazol is metabolized by hepatic routes involving the 3A4, 2C19, and 1A2 isoforms of cytochrome P450. Because of this, drugs-inhibiting cytochrome P450 may increase its serum levels. Various side effects have been described, principally due to the vasodilatory properties of the drug. These include headaches and gastrointestinal disturbances.

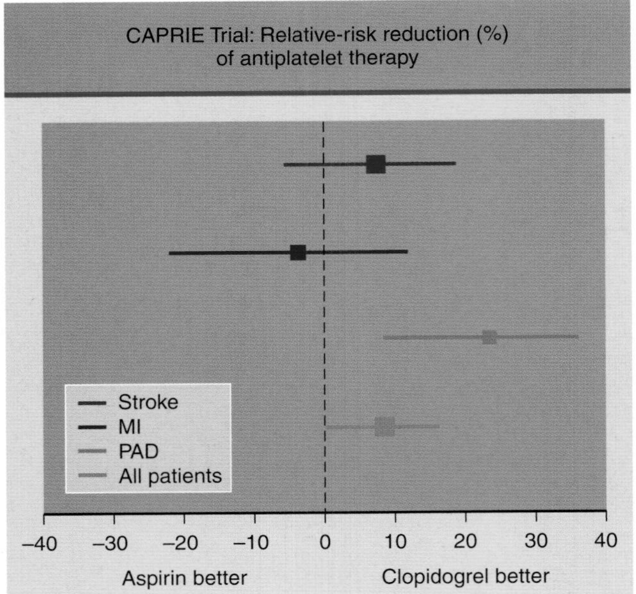

Figure 8-12. Relative risk reduction and 95% confidence intervals, by disease subgroups, in patients with vascular disease who were treated with aspirin or clopidogrel in the Clopidogrel versus Aspirin in Patients at Risk of Ischemic Events Trial. MI, myocardial infarction; PAD, peripheral arterial disease. (Data from Clopidogrel versus Aspirin in Patients at Risk of Ischemic Events Steering Committee. *Lancet* 1996;348:1329-1339.)

The drug was first approved for use by the U.S. Food and Drug Administration in claudicants in 1999. In four randomized, placebo-controlled trials, cilostazol at a dose of 50 to 100 mg twice daily increased both PFWD and MWD.[89-92] Importantly, cilostazol also improved physical function and quality of life, as assessed by the SF-36 questionnaire.[90-92] Other beneficial endpoints were increases in ABI and raised serum HDL cholesterol concentrations. This drug, therefore, has promise for the treatment of claudication, although the U.S. Food and Drug Administration has warned that cilostazol should not be used in patients with heart failure.

Picotamide

Picotamide is an antiplatelet drug that inhibits thromboxane A_2 synthase, blocking thromboxane A_2 receptors. In a major trial involving 2304 patients with PAD, a reduction of fatal and nonfatal ischemic events by 19% was achieved in the treatment group compared to controls.[93] However, this failed to achieve statistical significance.

Naftidrofuryl

Naftidrofuryl has been available in Europe, but not in the United States, for the treatment of claudication for several decades. It has a local anesthetic action and acts at tissue level, improving oxygenation, increasing adenosine triphosphate levels, and reducing lactic acid, thus potentially attenuating symptoms of claudication. Mechanisms of action may include antagonism of 5-hydroxytryptamine.

In a review of nine double-blind placebo-controlled trials, a placebo response was seen in all studies, producing a mean improvement in PFWD by approximately 25%[94] A further improvement of approximately 30% was seen in patients treated with naftidrofuryl after 3 to 6 months. These results were supported in two metaanalyses. However, MWD was not improved. Naftidrofuryl may lead to a slight symptomatic improvement in patients with moderate claudication, but no evidence supports any long-term benefit in disease outcome.

Oxypentifylline

Oxypentifylline is a methyl-xanthine derivative that exerts its effects by reducing blood viscosity. It increases red blood cell deformability, reduces plasma fibrinogen levels, and has antiplatelet effects. Results of studies investigating the use of oxypentifylline as a treatment for claudication have provided conflicting evidence and were bedeviled by variable methodology. Early controlled trials suggested a benefit over placebo in increasing initial and absolute claudication distance. However, metaanalyses of randomized, double-blind, controlled trials subsequently concluded that the limited amount and quality of reported data precluded reliable estimates of efficacy and that there is insufficient data to support widespread use of oxypentifylline.[95,96]

Buflomedil

Buflomedil is an agent with α-1 and -2 adrenolytic effects. It decreases vasoconstriction and has some antiplatelet effects, increases red cell deformability, and has a weak calcium antagonist effect. It has been available for the treatment of claudication in some countries for more than 12 years. Two small trials involving 127 patients have shown some benefit on absolute walking distance in claudicants for buflomedil, compared to placebo. However, a recent Cochrane review suggested that these studies were undermined by publication bias and found little overall evidence for efficacy of buflomedil in claudication.[97]

Antioxidants and Chelation Therapy

Oxidative injury is implicated in the pathogenesis of PAD, and patients have diminished antioxidant capacity. Antioxidant vitamins C and E have been employed to reduce or attenuate this oxidative damage. However, little evidence points to efficacy in this role in PAD.

Chelation therapy involves the use of repeated ethylenediaminetetraacetic acid injections, administered twice weekly by intravenous injection, and concurrent treatment with vitamins, trace elements, and iron supplements. It has been suggested that this technique reduces the calcium content of atherosclerotic plaques, lowering LDL oxidation and facilitating activity of hydroxyl radical scavengers. Platelet adhesion is also diminished, and chelation therapy appears to attenuate reperfusion injury. However, observed benefits of chelation therapy in randomized, controlled trials, to date, are likely to have been due to powerful placebo responses. Overall, trials have demonstrated no significant changes in PFWD or MWD.

Inositol Nicotinate

This drug is licensed in the United Kingdom for the treatment of claudication. Its mechanism of action is thought to involve vasodilation of skin blood vessels, fibrinolysis, and lipid lowering. It may also have a role in inhibition of oxidative metabolism in anoxic tissues. In randomized, controlled trials, no significant benefits were demonstrated for patients with PAD.

Cinnarizine

Cinnarizine is an antagonist to the endogenous vasoconstrictor substances 5-hydroxytryptamine, angiotensin, and noradrenaline. It may also exert a beneficial effect on blood rheology. Current studies evaluating cinnarizine have not employed standard methods of assessment, and it is not possible to conclude whether this drug is beneficial in PAD at this time.

Levocarnitine and Propionyl Levocarnitine

Various metabolic derangements occur in the skeletal muscle of patients with PAD. These anomalies include impairment of mitochondrial activity with accumulation of acyl carnitines, which are intermediates of oxidative metabolism. Diminished exercise performance is proportional to the accumulation of these metabolites. Both levocarnitine and propionyl levocarnitine have been used to treat these deleterious effects, the latter having a greater benefit. In a limited number of randomized trials, propionyl levocarnitine improved MWD by 54% to 73% and PFWD, compared to placebo, with beneficial effects on quality of life. However, larger phase III trials are still awaited, and at present propionyl-L-carnitine is not licensed for the treatment of PAD.

Prostaglandins

Prostaglandin E1 and stable PGI_2 prostacyclin derivatives such as iloprost and beraprost have been used extensively in the treatment of rest pain in critical ischemia, and in Raynaud's disease. However, few trials have critically investigated the efficacy of these compounds in claudicants. One disadvantage is that they are metabolized rapidly and until recently have had to be administered parenterally. Side effects are associated with their vasodilatory properties and include headaches, nausea, and facial flushing. In recent trials with oral analogues such as beraprost, positive but statistically insignificant effects on MWD and quality of life were found. These results were associated with a reduction in cardiovascular events. The results of larger-scale trials are awaited.

Angiogenic Growth Factors

Angiogenic growth factors, including vascular endothelial growth factor, basic fibroblast growth factor (bFGF), and hypoxia-inducible factor-1, have been proposed as possible therapeutic interventions for treatment of symptomatic PAD. The rationale is that these drugs have been shown to promote collateral blood vessel formation and to increase limb blood flow in experimental models of hindlimb ischemia.[98,99]

Angiogenic growth factors have been administered as recombinant proteins or via gene transfer with naked plasmid DNA, or adenoviral vectors encoding the angiogenic growth factor.[100,101] In a small, phase 1, double-blind, placebo-controlled study, administration of bFGF via the femoral artery on 1 or 2 consecutive days increased calf blood flow at both 1 month and 6 months later.[102] In a randomized, placebo-controlled study, intraarterial administration of recombinant fibroblast growth factor-2, a single dose of 30 μg/kg increased peak walking time after 90 days by 19%, although its administration on two occasions 30 days apart did not improve peak walking time compared with placebo.[103]

Adverse effects have been reported. One study that involved the intravenous administration of bFGF to patients with claudication was terminated prematurely when 4 of 16 subjects who received bFGF developed proteinuria.[104] A larger, double-blind, randomized, placebo-controlled trial of intramuscular administration of vascular endothelial growth factor isoform 121 in 105 patients with claudication failed to demonstrate any clinical efficacy but did provoke limb edema.[105] At the present time, therefore, it is premature to recommend angiogenic growth factors for the treatment of IC.

Immune Modulation

Recently, a small, randomized trial suggested that claudicants may improve MWD when treated with autologous blood subjected to thermal, ultraviolet, and oxidative stresses.[106] This pilot study was carried out to investigate evidence gathered from anecdotal reports, and larger-scale trials are awaited.

SUMMARY

PAD is just one component of systemic atherosclerosis. IC, one of the most common symptoms of PAD, results in impaired functional capacity and loss of quality of life. To date, clinical trials in PAD have not received the emphasis accorded to ischemic heart disease and cerebrovascular disease. Despite this shortcoming, evidence exists that patients with PAD should be considered for secondary-prevention strategies in the same way as patients with coronary disease.

Antiplatelet agents reduce the risk of both fatal and nonfatal cardiovascular events. Aspirin should be considered for all patients with PAD, with clopidogrel as an effective alternative therapy. Control of hyperlipidemia with statins and of hypertension with ACE inhibitors also confers secondary protective effects. Smoking cessation and participation in a supervised exercise program are conservative measures that improve functional capacity and have other cardiovascular benefits. Various drugs, including naftidrofuryl and oxypentifylline, have been shown to have limited efficacy in improving walking capacity, but more recently cilostazol has shown promise, not only improving PFWD and MWD but also enhancing quality of life. Other therapeutic avenues are still under investigation.

References

1. Ouriel K. Peripheral arterial disease. *Lancet* 2001;358:1257-1264.
2. Jung AY, Lee W, Chung JW, et al. Role of computed tomographic angiography in the detection and comprehensive evaluation of persistent sciatic artery. *J Vasc Surg* 2005;42:678-683.
3. Sharma P, Padhiar N, Kyriakides C. Popliteal cystic adventitial disease causing intermittent claudication in a young athlete: a case report. *South Med J* 2008;101(11):1154-1156.
4. Norgren L, Hiatt WR, Dormandy JA, et al. Intersociety consensus for the management of peripheral arterial disease TASC II. *Eur J Vasc Endovasc Surg* 2007;33:S1-S75.
5. Fontaine R, Kim M, Kieny P. Die chirurgische behandling der peripheren durch-blutungsstorungen. *Helv Chir Acta* 1954;21:499.

6. Ad Hoc Committee on Reporting Standards. Suggested standards for reports dealing with lower extremity ischaemia. *J Vasc Surg* 1986;4:80-94.
7. Bell PRF, Charlesworth D, De Palma PG. The definition of critical ischemia of the limb: Working Party of the International Vascular Symposium Editorial. *Br J Surg* 1982;69:S2.
8. Tyrrell MR, Wolfe JH. Critical leg ischaemia: an appraisal of clinical definitions. Joint Vascular Research Group. *Br J Surg* 1993;80:177-180.
9. European consensus on critical limb ischemia. *Lancet* 1989;1:737-738.
10. Second European consensus document on chronic critical limb ischemia. *Circulation* 1991;84(4 Suppl):IV1-IV26.
11. Wolfe JH, Wyatt MG. Critical and subcritical ischaemia. *Eur J Vasc Endovasc Surg* 1997;13:578-582.
12. White JV, Rutherford RB, Ryjewski C. Chronic subcritical limb ischemia: a poorly recognised stage of chronic limb ischaemia. *Semin Vasc Surg* 2007;20:62-67.
13. Meijer WT, Hoes AW, Rutgers D, et al. Peripheral arterial disease in the elderly: the Rotterdam study. *Arterioscler Thromb Vasc Biol* 1998;18: 185-192.
14. Criqui MH, Fronek A, Barrett-Connor E, et al. The prevalence of peripheral arterial disease in a defined population. *Circulation* 1985;713: 510-551.
15. Hiatt WR, Hoag S, Hamman RF. Effect of diagnostic criteria on the prevalence of peripheral arterial disease: the San Luis Valley Diabetes Study. *Circulation* 1995;915:1472-1479.
16. Selvin E, Erlinger TP. Prevalence of and risk factors for peripheral arterial disease in the United States: results from the National Health and Nutrition Examination Survey, 1999-2000. *Circulation* 2004;1106: 738-743.
17. Hirsch A, Criqui M, Treat-Jacobson D, et al. Peripheral arterial disease detection, awareness, and treatment in primary care. *JAMA* 2001;28611: 1317-1324.
18. Fowkes FG, Housley E, Cawood EH, et al. Edinburgh Artery Study: prevalence of asymptomatic and symptomatic peripheral arterial disease in the general population. *Int J Epidemiol* 1991;20:384-392.
19. Hirsch AT, Haskal ZJ, Hertzer NR, et al. ACC/AHA 2005 guidelines for the management of patients with peripheral arterial disease lower extremity, renal, mesenteric, and abdominal aortic: a collaborative report from the American Association for Vascular Surgery/Society for Vascular Surgery, Society for Cardiovascular Angiography and Interventions, Society for Vascular Medicine and Biology, Society of Interventional Radiology, and the ACC/AHA Task Force on Practice Guidelines Writing Committee to Develop Guidelines for the Management of Patients with Peripheral Arterial Disease. *J Am Coll Cardiol* 2006;47:1-192.
20. Dormandy J, Heeck L, Vig S. Predicting which patients will develop chronic critical leg ischemia. *Semin Vasc Surg* 1999;122:138-141.
21. Novo S, Coppola G, Millio G. Critical limb ischemia: definition and natural history. *Curr Drug Targets Cardiovasc Haematol Disord* 2004;43:219-225.
22. Wolfe J. Defining the outcome of critical limb ischaemia: a one-year prospective study. *Br J Surg* 1986;73:321.
23. Sigvant B, Wiberg-Hedman K, Bergqvist D, et al. A population-based study of peripheral arterial disease prevalence with special focus on critical limb ischemia and sex differences. *J Vasc Surg* 2007;45:1185-1191.
24. Kannel WB, Shurtleff D. The Framingham study: cigarettes and the development of intermittent claudication. *Geriatrics* 1973;28:61-68.
25. Selvin E, Marinopoulos S, Birkenblit G, et al. Meta-analysis: glycosylated haemoglobin and cardiovascular disease in diabetes mellitus. *Ann Intern Med* 2004;1416:421-431.
26. McDaniel MD, Cronenwett JL. Basic data related to the natural history of intermittent claudication. *Ann Vasc Surg* 1989;3:273-277.
27. Dormandy JA, Murray GD. The fate of the claudicants: a prospective study of 1969 claudicants. *Eur J Vasc Surg* 1991;5:131-133.
28. Most RS, Sinnock P. The epidemiology of lower extremity amputations in diabetic individuals. *Diabetes Care* 1983;6:87-91.
29. Senti M, Nouges X, Pedro-Botet J, et al. Lipoprotein profile in men with peripheral vascular disease: role of intermediate density lipoproteins and apoprotein E phenotypes. *Circulation* 1992;851:30-36.
30. Fowkes FG, Housley E, Riemersma RA, et al. Smoking, lipids, glucose intolerance, and blood pressure as risk factors for peripheral atherosclerosis compared with ischemic heart disease: the Edinburgh Artery Study. *Am J Epidemiol* 1992;135:331-340.
31. Murabito JM, Evans JC, Nieto K, et al. Prevalence and clinical correlates of peripheral arterial disease in the Framingham offspring study. *Am Heart J* 2002;143:961-965.
32. Tilly-Kiesi M. The effect of lovastatin treatment on low-density lipoprotein hydrated density distribution and composition in patients with intermittent claudication and primary hypercholesterolaemia. *Metabolism* 1991;40:623-628.
33. Khan F, Litchfield SJ, Stonebridge PA, Belch JJ. Lipid-lowering and skin vascular responses in patients with hypercholesterolaemia and peripheral arterial obstructive disease. *Vasc Med* 1999;4:233-238.
34. Expert Panel on Detection, Evaluation and Treatment of High Blood Cholesterol in Adults. Executive summary of the third report of the National Cholesterol Education Program (NCEP) Expert Panel on Detection, Evaluation, And Treatment of High Blood Cholesterol in Adults: adult treatment panel III. *JAMA* 2001;285:2486-2497.
35. Kannel WB, McGee DL. Update on some epidemiologic features of intermittent claudication: the Framingham study. *J Am Geriatric Soc* 1985;33:13-18.
36. Taylor LM Jr., Moneta GL, Sexton GJ, et al. Prospective blinded study of the relationship between plasma homocysteine and progression of symptomatic peripheral arterial disease. *J Vasc Surg* 1999;29:8-19.
37. Steg PG, Bhatt DL, Wilson PW, et al. One-year cardiovascular event rates in outpatients with atherothrombosis. *JAMA* 2007;297:1197-1206.
38. Weitz JI, Byrne J, Clagett GP, et al. Diagnosis and treatment of chronic arterial insufficiency of the lower extremities: a critical review. *Circulation* 1996;94:3026-3049. erratum, Circulation 2000;102:1074.
39. Smith GD, Shipley MJ, Rose G. Intermittent claudication, heart disease risk factors, and mortality: the Whitehall Study. *Circulation* 1990;82:1925-1931.
40. Leng GC, Lee AJ, Fowkes FG, et al. Incidence, natural history and cardiovascular events in symptomatic and asymptomatic peripheral arterial disease in the general population. *Int J Epidemiol* 1996; 25:1172-1181.
41. Criqui MH, Langer RD, Fronek A, et al. Mortality over a period of 10 years in patients with peripheral arterial disease. *N Engl J Med* 1992;326:381-386.
42. Ouriel K, Fiore WM, Geary IE. Limb-threatening ischemia in the medically compromised patient: amputation or revascularization? *Surgery* 1988;104:667-672.
43. Veith FJ, Gupta SK, Samson RH, et al. Progress in limb salvage by reconstructive arterial surgery combined with new or improved adjunctive procedures. *Ann Surg* 1981;194:386-401.
44. Hickey NC, Thomson IA, Shearman CP, Simms MH. Aggressive arterial reconstruction for critical lower limb ischaemia. *Br J Surg* 1991;78:1476-1478.
45. Hiatt WR. Medical treatment of peripheral arterial disease and claudication. *N Engl J Med* 2001;34421:1608-1621.
46. Khaira HS, Hanger R, Shearman CP. Quality of life in patients with intermittent claudication. *Eur J Vasc Endovasc Surg* 1996;12:65-69.
47. Smith FCT, Shearman CP, Simms MH, Gwynn BR. Falsely elevated ankle pressures in severe leg ischaemia: the Pole Test—an alternative approach. *Eur J Vasc Surg* 1994;8:408-412.
48. Jakobs TF, Wintersperger BJ, Becker CR. MDCT-imaging of peripheral arterial disease. *Semin Ultrasound CT MR* 2004;252:145-155.
49. Ota H, Takase K, Igarashi K, et al. MDCT compared with on angiography for assessment of lower extremity arterial occlusive disease: importance of reviewing cross-sectional images. *AJR Am J Roentgenol* 2004;1821:201-209.
50. Martin MJ, Hulley SB, Browner WS, et al. Serum cholesterol, blood pressure, and mortality: implications from a cohort of 361,662 men. *Lancet* 1986;2:933-936.
51. Gordon DJ, Probstfield JL, Garrison RJ, et al. High-density lipoprotein cholesterol and cardiovascular disease: four prospective American studies. *Circulation* 1989;79:8-15.
52. Murabito JM, D'Agostino RB, Silbershatz H, Wilson WF. Intermittent claudication: a risk profile from the Framingham heart study. *Circulation* 1997;96:44-49.
53. Johansson J, Egberg N, Hohnsson H, Carlson LA. Serum lipoproteins and haemostatic function in intermittent claudication. *Arterioscler Thromb* 1993;13:1441-1448.
54. Monsalve MV, Young R, Jobsis J, et al. DNA polymorphism of the gene for apolipoprotein B in patients with peripheral arterial disease. *Atherosclerosis* 1988;70:123-129.
55. Leng GC, Price JF, Jepson RG. Lipid-lowering for lower limb atherosclerosis. *Cochrane Database Syst Rev* 2000;2. CD000123.
56. Blankenhorn DH, Azen SP, Crawford DW, et al. Effects of colestipol–niacin therapy on human femoral atherosclerosis. *Circulation* 1991;83: 438-447.

57. Lewis B. Randomised controlled trial of the treatment of hyperlipidaemia on progression of atherosclerosis. *Acta Med Scand Suppl* 1985;701: 53-57.
58. Walldius G, Erikson U, Olsson AG, et al. The effect of probucol on femoral atherosclerosis: the Probucol Quantitative Regression Swedish Trial (PQRST). *Am J Cardiol* 1994;74:875-883.
59. Buchwald H, Bourdages HR, Campos CT, et al. Impact of cholesterol reduction on peripheral arterial disease in the Program on the Surgical Control of the Hyperlipidemias (POSCH). *Surgery* 1996;120:672-679.
60. LaRosa JC, He J, Vupputuri S. Effect of statins on risk of coronary disease: a meta-analysis of randomized controlled trials. *JAMA* 1999;282:2340-2346.
61. Long-term Intervention with Pravastatin in Ischaemic Disease Study Group. Prevention of cardiovascular events and death with pravastatin in patients with coronary heart disease and a broad range of initial cholesterol levels. *N Engl J Med* 1998;339:1349-1357.
62. MRC/BHF Heart Protection Study of cholesterol-lowering therapy and of antioxidant vitamin supplementation in a wide range of patients at increased risk of coronary heart disease death: early safety and efficacy experience. *Eur Heart J* 1999;2010:725-741.
63. Pedersen TR, Olsson AG, Faergeman O, et al. The effect of simvastatin on ischaemic signs and symptoms in the Scandinavian Simvastatin Survival Study 4S. *Am J Cardiol* 1998;81:333-335.
64. Mohler ER 3rd, Hiatt WR, Creager MA. Cholesterol reduction with atorvastatin improves walking distance in patients with peripheral arterial disease. *Circulation* 2003;108:1481-1486.
65. Aronow WS, Nayak D, Woodworth S, et al. Effect of simvastatin versus placebo on treadmill exercise time until the onset of intermittent claudication in older patients with peripheral arterial disease at six months and at one year after treatment. *Am J Cardiol* 2003;92: 711-712.
66. Mondillo S, Ballo P, Barbati R, et al. Effects of simvastatin on walking performance and symptoms of intermittent claudication in hypercholesterolemic patients with peripheral vascular disease. *Am J Med* 2003;114:359-364.
67. Kroon AA, van Asten WN, Stalenhoef AF. Effect of apheresis of low-density lipoprotein on peripheral vascular disease in hypercholesterolaemic patients with coronary artery disease. *Ann Intern Med* 1996; 125:945-954.
68. Aronow WS, Ahn C. Association between plasma homocysteine and peripheral vascular disease in older persons. *Coron Artery Dis* 1998;9:49-50.
69. Cheng SW, Ting AC, Wong J. Fasting total plasma homocysteine and atherosclerotic peripheral vascular disease. *Ann Vasc Surg* 1997;11: 217-223.
70. van der Berg M, Boers GH. Homocysteinuria: what about mild hyperhomocysteinaemia? *Postgrad Med J* 1996;72:513-518.
71. UK Prospective Diabetes Study Group. Intensive blood–glucose control with sulphonylureas or insulin compared with conventional treatment and risk of complications in patients with type 2 diabetes: UKPDS 33. *Lancet* 1998;352:837-953. Erratum, *Lancet* 1999;354:602.
72. Effect of intensive diabetes management on macrovascular events and risk factors in the Diabetes Control and Complications Trial. *Am J Cardiol* 1995;75:894-903.
73. Radack K, Deck C. β-Adrenergic blocker therapy does not worsen intermittent claudication in subjects with peripheral arterial disease: a meta-analysis of randomised controlled trials. *Arch Intern Med* 1991;151:1769-1776.
74. Yusuf S, Sleight P, Pogue J, et al. Effects of an angiotensin-converting enzyme inhibitor, ramipril, on cardiovascular events in high-risk patients: the Heart Outcomes Prevention Evaluation Study Investigators. *N Engl J Med* 2000;342:145-153. Errata, *N Engl J Med* 2000;342:1376; N Engl J Med 2000;342:748.
75. Doll R, Peto R, Wheatley K, et al. Mortality in relation to smoking: 40 years' observations on male British doctors. *BMJ* 1994;309: 901-911.
76. Joseph AM, Norman SM, Ferry LH, et al. The safety of transdermal nicotine as an aid to smoking cessation in patients with cardiac disease. *N Engl J Med* 1996;335:1793-1798.
77. Jorenby DE, Leischow SJ, Nides MA, et al. A controlled trial of sustained-release bupropion, a nicotine patch, or both for smoking cessation. *N Engl J Med* 1999;340:685-691.
78. Tonstad S, Farsang C, Klaene G, et al. Bupropion SR for smoking cessation in smokers with cardiovascular disease: a multicentre, randomised study. *Eur Heart J* 2003;2410:946-955.
79. Leng GC, Fowler B, Ernst E. Exercise for intermittent claudication. *Cochrane Database Syst Rev* 2000;2. CD000990.
80. Garner AW, Poehlman ET. Exercise rehabilitation programs for the treatment of claudication pain. *JAMA* 1995;274:975-980.
81. Perkins JMT, Collin JC, Morris PJM. Angioplasty versus exercise for stable claudication: long-term results of a prospective randomised trial. *Br J Surg* 1995;82:557-558.
82. Whyman MR, Fowkes FGR, Kerracher E, et al. A randomised controlled trial of percutaneous balloon angioplasty PTA versus observation for intermittent claudication. *Eur J Vasc Endovasc Surg* 1996;12:167-172.
83. Stewart AHR, Lamont PM. Exercise for intermittent claudication. *BMJ* 2001;323:703-704.
84. Antithrombotic Trialists' Collaboration. Collaborative meta-analysis of randomised trials of anti-platelet therapy for prevention of death, myocardial infarction, and stroke in high risk patients. *BMJ* 2002;324: 71-86.
85. Goldhaber SZ, Manson JE, Stampfer MJ, et al. Low-dose aspirin and subsequent peripheral arterial surgery in the Physicians' Health Study. *Lancet* 1992;340:143-145.
86. Collaborative overview of randomised trials of anti-platelet therapy. II. Maintenance of vascular graft patency by anti-platelet therapy. *BMJ* 1994;308:159-168.
87. Clopidogrel versus Aspirin in Patients at Risk of Ischemic Events Steering Committee. A randomised, blinded trial of clopidogrel versus aspirin in patients at risk of ischaemic events. *Lancet* 1996;348: 1329-1339.
88. Clopidogrel in Unstable Angina to Prevent Recurrent Ischemic Events Study Investigators. Effects of clopidogrel in addition to aspirin in patients with non-ST segment elevation acute coronary syndromes. *N Engl J Med* 2001;345:494-502.
89. Dawson DL, Cutler BS, Hiatt WR, et al. A comparison of cilostazol and pentoxifylline for treating intermittent claudication. *Am J Med* 2000;109:523-530.
90. Dawson DL, Cutler BS, Meissner MH, Strandness DEJ. Cilostazol has beneficial effects in treatment of intermittent claudication: results from a multicenter, randomised, prospective, double-blind trial. *Circulation* 1998;98:678-686.
91. Money SR, Herd JA, Isaacsohn JL, et al. Effect of cilostazol on walking distances in patients with intermittent claudication caused by peripheral vascular disease. *J Vasc Surg* 1998;27:267-274.
92. Beebe HG, Dawson DL, Cutler BS, et al. A new pharmacological treatment for intermittent claudication: results of a randomised multicenter trial. *Arch Intern Med* 1999;159:2041-2050.
93. Balsano F, Violi F. Effect of picotamide on the clinical progression of peripheral vascular disease: a double-blind placebo-controlled study. *Circulation* 1993;87:1563-1569.
94. Diagnosis and management of peripheral arterial disease. Guideline 89. *Scottish Intercollegiate Guidelines Network* 2006;Section, p14.
95. Hood SC, Moher D, Barber GG. Management of intermittent claudication with pentoxifylline: meta-analysis of randomised controlled trials. *CMAJ* 1996;155:1053-1059.
96. Girolami B, Bernardi E, Prins MH, et al. Treatment of intermittent claudication with physical training, smoking cessation, pentoxifylline, or nafronyl: a meta-analysis. *Arch Intern Med* 1999;159:337-345.
97. de Backer TL, Bogaert M, Vander Stichele R. Buflomedil for intermittent claudication. *Cochrane Database Syst Rev* 2008;1. CD000988. Update of *Cochrane Database Syst Rev* 2007;4:CD000988.
98. Yang HT, Deschenes MR, Ogilvie RW, et al. Basic fibroblast growth factor increases collateral blood flow in rats with femoral arterial ligation. *Circ Res* 1996;79:62-69.
99. Takeshita S, Zheng LP, Brogi E, et al. Therapeutic angiogenesis: a single intraarterial bolus of vascular endothelial growth factor augments revascularization in a rabbit ischemic hind limb model. *J Clin Invest* 1994;93:662-670.
100. Tsurumi Y, Takeshita S, Chen D, et al. Direct intramuscular gene transfer of naked DNA encoding vascular endothelial growth factor augments collateral development and tissue perfusion. *Circulation* 1996;94:3281-3290.
101. Ohara N, Koyama H, Miyata T, et al. Adenovirus-mediated ex vivo gene transfer of basic fibroblast growth factor promotes collateral development in a rabbit model of hind limb ischemia. *Gene Ther* 2001;8: 837-845.
102. Lazarous DF, Unger EF, Epstein SE, et al. Basic fibroblast growth factor in patients with intermittent claudication: results of a phase I trial. *J Am Coll Cardiol* 2000;36:1239-1244.

103. Lederman RJ, Mendelsohn FO, Anderson RD, et al. Therapeutic angiogenesis with recombinant fibroblast growth factor-2 for intermittent claudication the TRAFFIC study: a randomised trial. *Lancet* 2002;359:2053-2058.
104. Cooper LT Jr., Hiatt WR, Creager MA, et al. Proteinuria in a placebo-controlled study of basic fibroblast growth factor for intermittent claudication. *Vasc Med* 2001;6:235-239.
105. Rajagopalan S, Mohler ER 3rd, Lederman RJ, et al. Regional angiogenesis with vascular endothelial growth factor in peripheral arterial disease: a phase II randomized, double-blind, controlled study of adenoviral delivery of vascular endothelial growth factor 121 in patients with disabling intermittent claudication. *Circulation* 2003;108:1933-1938.
106. McGrath C, Robb R, Lucas A, et al. A randomised, double-blind, placebo-controlled study to investigate the efficacy of immune modulation therapy in the treatment of patents suffering from peripheral arterial occlusive disease with intermittent claudication. *Eur J Vasc Endovasc Surg* 2002;23:381-387.

chapter 9a

Endovascular Treatment of Lower Extremity Arterial Occlusive Disease: Interventional Treatment for Aortoiliac Disease

Dierk Vorwerk, MD

Key Points

- The Fontaine and Rutherford classifications offer clinically useful categorizations of patients with intermittent claudication (IC).
- IC may cause significant disability in the activities of daily living (lifestyle limitation) in some individuals but is unlikely to result in critical limb ischemia.
- Aortoiliac occlusive disease is generally more amenable to percutaneous intervention than is femoropopliteal occlusive disease.
- Lesion length, composition (calcification, thrombus), and morphology (concentric, eccentric) influence outcome of percutaneous intervention. Trans-Atlantic Inter-Society Consensus (TASC) classification should be used to guide determination of the appropriateness of percutaneous intervention.
- Balloon angioplasty with or without stenting is the best initial therapy for most TASC-A and TASC-B iliac lesions. Kissing balloon or stenting techniques are extremely useful for aortoiliac bifurcation lesions.

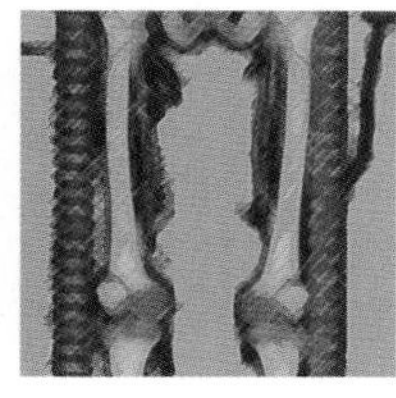

While iliac artery interventions are classical procedures, interventions in the infrarenal aorta are relatively rare. Patients with iliac artery stenoses and occlusions count for about one third of all patients with peripheral occlusive disease, but about two thirds of them are candidates for percutaneous treatment. Aortoiliac lesions usually lead to limited walking distance but—as a single lesion—rarely cause limb-threatening ischemia. An exception is the blue toe syndrome that may be caused by emboli also caused by aortic or iliac plaques.

In contrast, patients with limb-threatening ischemia may also show iliac or femoral lesions, in combination with lesions involving the lower leg arteries and small arteries of the foot. In such instances, however, treatment of the iliac and femoral arteries does not differ technically from treatment of claudicants.

OVERVIEW AND CLINICAL INDICATIONS FOR TREATMENT

It has generally been suggested that a surgical approach to peripheral vascular disease requires major clinical symptoms such as rest pain, nonhealing ulceration, or at least, severe claudication. Using the European Fontaine classification, an advanced IIb or III stage is therefore accepted as requisite for invasive surgical management.

Endovascular treatment, however, is associated with low morbidity, an even lower mortality, and satisfactory patient outcomes. Thus, it is fair to reconsider why an endovascular approach should be reserved only for those with severe clinical symptoms. Furthermore, occlusive arterial disease tends to occur earlier in life, because of changed smoking and dietary habits among the population, and may affect individuals still in the active phases of a professional life.

On the other hand, intermittent claudication is not likely to worsen over time and only about 5% of claudicants ever develop critical limb ischemia if no important comorbid factors such as diabetes are present. In light of this benign natural history, any proposed intervention should be associated with minimal risk and provide acceptable durability.

PROBLEMS OF CLASSIFICATION

Classification of intermittent claudication is difficult without the application of standardized methods. Patients are unreliable in defining their true walking distance, which may also be limited by their general physical abilities, coexisting angina pectoris, and individual circumstances of living. Precise definition of walking distance requires a standardized treadmill test.

In the Fontaine classification, stage IIa defines a walking distance of more than 200 m and IIb one of less than 200 m.

The Rutherford system distinguishes among categories 1 (mild claudication), 2 (moderate), and 3 (severe). Comparing both systems, Fontaine stage IIa is equivalent to Rutherford category 1, while Fontaine stage IIb includes both Rutherford categories 2 and 3.[1] Nevertheless, while both systems offer an objective framework to provide guidelines for treatment and are useful tools for scientific reporting, they may not reflect the degree of disability in an individual patient.

LIFESTYLE-LIMITING CLAUDICATION

Intermittent claudication may affect a patient's life in various degrees and result in different levels of activity limitation. It is obvious that a patient with coexisting major angina pectoris or severe emphysema may not experience major disability even from severe peripheral arterial disease since the coexisting diseases limit that patient's walking capacity. An 85-year-old patient with significantly limited physical abilities may therefore be less affected by peripheral arterial disease than a young and active patient of 45 years. However, in an amputee, even mild claudication in the remaining leg may cause major restrictions of lifestyle since the patient fully depends on the remaining limb. People living in a flat area may not have major problems compared with those living in a mountainous region or on the seventh floor of an inner-city apartment block with no access to a lift. A younger individual used to an active sports life will hardly accept mild claudication since it is preventing that person from pursuing activities that are important to the lifestyle.

Therefore, in each patient, the individual circumstances of living should be taken into account before determining whether invasive therapy is indicated. Lifestyle-limiting claudication is an appropriate term, and lifestyle alteration should be considered when evaluating a patient for potential interventional therapy.

COMPARISON OF ENDOVASCULAR AND SURGICAL TREATMENT

Endovascular therapy is perceived to be a less invasive form of therapy associated with good technical success and fair overall patency. For percutaneous transluminal angioplasty (PTA) of iliac lesions (data derived from five publications totaling 1264 procedures), an average complication rate of 3.6%, an initial success rate of 95%, and a 5-year patency rate of 61% have been reported.[1] The results of iliac stenting for stenoses (analysis of nine publications including 1365 patients) are somewhat better, with 99% technical success and 72% 5-year patency. The weighted average complication rate was 6.3%.[1]

Surgery offers a limb-based 5-year patency of 91% for aortobifemoral bypasses; weighted average mortality was 3.3%. For femoropopliteal reconstruction, an average 5-year patency of 80% for vein bypasses and 65% to 75% for expanded polytetrafluoroethylene (EPTFE) bypasses has been reported. Combined mortality and amputation risk was calculated to be about 2.2% for aortobifemoral reconstructions and 1.4% for femoropopliteal reconstructions.[1]

The clinician must consider that life expectancy of patients with intermittent claudication is limited compared with a nonclaudicant control group. Mortality rates after 5, 10, and 15 years are approximately 30%, 50%, and 70%, respectively, although most patients will not die from peripheral vascular causes but rather from cardiac, cerebral, or nonvascular causes.[1]

Despite better clinical outcome for surgery, therefore, recommendation 37 of the TASC guidelines proposes that surgery should be used as a treatment for intermittent claudication only when other forms of medical therapy have been recommended but have either failed or been rejected for good reasons.[1] Furthermore, there should be a high benefit-to-risk ratio for the proposed operation.[1] This is difficult to achieve in patients with mild to moderate claudication. Thus, endovascular therapy appears to be the method of choice, if interventional therapy is required, in this subgroup of patients with mild–moderate intermittent claudication.

LESION LOCATION

Claudication is mainly related to lesions in the aortoiliac or the femoropopliteal segments. It is less likely the result of infrapopliteal lesions, and there is general agreement that treatment below the knee should be strictly limited to patients with critical limb ischemia, i.e., stage III and IV (Fontaine) or category 4 to 6 (Rutherford).

In the aortoiliac segment, a major proportion of lesions are amenable to percutaneous treatment with an acceptable outcome. In the femoropopliteal segment, overall success and long-term efficacy of percutaneous treatment is less and the lesion type becomes a more important determinant of success.

Thus, the location of a lesion and its type must be taken into consideration before treatment is recommended. While most aortoiliac lesions are approachable with endovascular therapy, this is not generally true for femoropopliteal lesions. In addition, the risk of treatment is related to the lesion type and location and requires careful consideration before embarking upon an endovascular approach.

LESION MORPHOLOGY

Lesion morphology influences the technical success rate, long-term results, and risk of treatment. The TASC 2000 document therefore introduced a classification system to categorize lesions with regard to their appropriateness for either percutaneous treatment or surgery:

- Focal type A lesions, which are ideal for percutaneous approach
- Type B lesions, in which the percutaneous approach is still the preferred technique
- Type C lesions, for which the surgical approach should be preferred
- Type D lesions, for which surgery is the option of choice

The TASC classification supersedes older classifications since it takes into account all available and published techniques, including stent technology, which offer a much wider variety of treatment and an effective tool to deal with current acute complications of PTA, such as occluding dissection or vascular rupture.

If we consider percutaneous therapy as the preferred method to deal with those patients presenting with mild or moderate claudication, treatment might be offered to those presenting with type A or B lesions but should be discussed in depth with patients with type C lesions, since the risk and the potential benefit of treatment are adversely affected by the underlying morphology (Figure 9a-1).

For iliac lesions, single stenoses up to 3 cm in length both in the common iliac artery (CIA) and in the external iliac artery (EIA) are classified as type A lesions, while single stenoses of 3 to 10 cm (not involving the common femoral artery, or CFA), tandem stenoses not longer than 5 cm each, and unilateral occlusions of the CIA are classified as type B lesions. Bilateral long stenoses (5 to 10 cm in length), unilateral EIA occlusions not extending into the CFA, and unilateral EIA stenoses extending into the CFA are classified as type C. More advanced lesions are classified as type D.

Based on this system of classification, many iliac lesions meet the criteria for types A and B, opening a potentially growing field for endovascular procedures if applied to mild and moderate claudicants. My experience suggests that percutaneous treatment may be appropriate in selected type C lesions, particularly for EIA occlusions not extending into the CFA. However, published data are lacking to support widespread adoption of this approach.

TASC 2007 has modified the classification of iliac arterial lesions to some extent. Type A now includes all types of unilateral or bilateral stenoses of the CIA and short stenoses below 3 cm of the EIA, both unilaterally or bilaterally. Type B now also includes short stenoses of the infrarenal aorta, as well as unilateral occlusions of the EIA. TASC type C (2007) includes bilateral stenoses of 3 to 10 cm of the EIA, unilateral stenosis of the EIA extending into the CFA, and unilateral occlusion of the EIA involving the orifice of the internal iliac artery or the CFA, calcified occlusions of the EIA, and bilateral stenoses of the EIA of 3 to 10 cm in length. Finally, type D now includes diffuse stenoses of the iliac axis, including the CFA, long occlusions of the iliac axis, bilateral occlusions of the EIA, extensive disease involving both iliac arteries and the infrarenal aorta, chronic Leriche syndrome, and patients who suffer from an infrarenal aortic aneurysm that requires treatment.

Some of these changes reflect the clinical situation and appear rational and logical. Some are still difficult to understand and will not meet the day-to-day setting in interventional radiology suites. The impact of the changed classification on my patients seemed rather small.

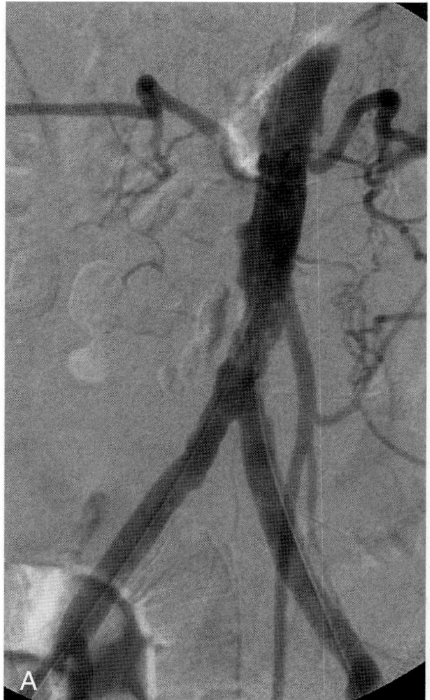

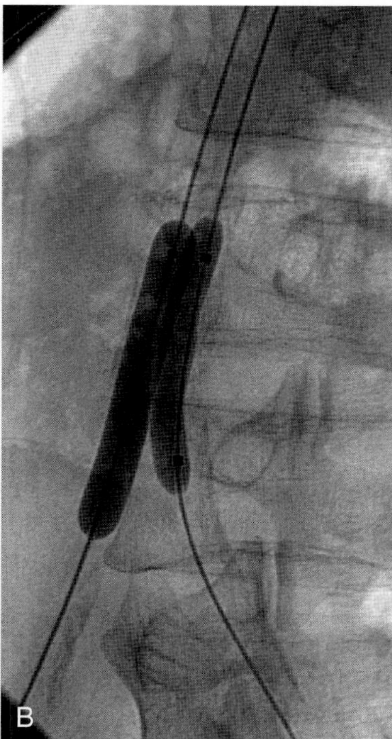

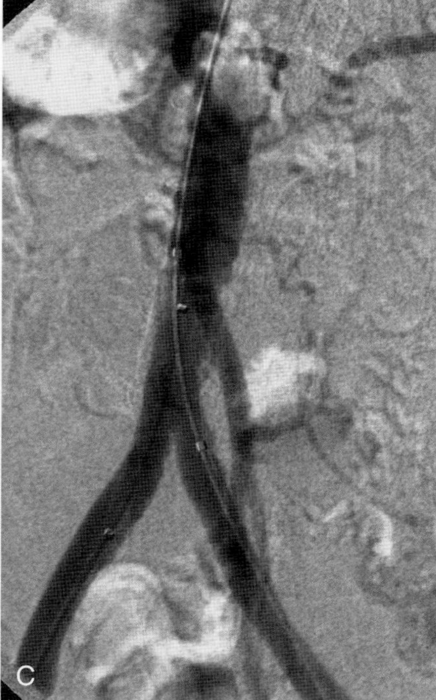

Figure 9a-1. Percutaneous transluminal angioplasty (PTA) of aortic stenosis in a 46-year-old male patient presenting with bilateral upper thigh claudication with symmetrical onset of symptoms after a walking distance of 250 m. **A,** Irregular calcific stenosis of infrarenal aorta; angiographically of moderate severity. **B,** Bilateral 7-mm kissing balloons in place. **C,** After PTA, improved diameter of the aortic lumen. Patient became asymptomatic.

MULTILEVEL DISEASE

Sometimes only mild symptoms may be caused by multilevel disease, i.e., an iliac stenosis and a well-collateralized femoropopliteal lesion. There is some chance that intervention solely for the iliac stenosis may be sufficient to improve the clinical situation. Multilevel disease does not necessarily preclude endovascular treatment in such patients.

ADJUVANT FORMS OF TREATMENT

It is widely accepted that smoking cessation and a well-conducted physical exercise program should precede any type of interventional treatment of intermittent claudication. The reality, however, is that in many institutions it is difficult to develop an infrastructure that provides state-of-the-art physical exercise in claudicants. As far as smoking is concerned, a major difference lies between willing and doing.

Moreover, even with state-of-the-art exercise, a young patient may not recover completely from claudication in all activities, including sports. The process will be longer and may compromise the patient's abilities in professional life. Therefore, it might be worth considering, especially for the subgroup of young and active patients, whether they should be vigorously treated with the axiom of physical exercise first or whether invasive treatment might be offered earlier in their course.

DECISION MAKING

The decision regarding invasive treatment should be based on the individual circumstances in each patient presenting with claudication. Age, social life, physical abilities, and professional situation require consideration, and simple administration of rigid classification systems should be avoided. Under some circumstances, patients with mild-to-moderate claudication might become candidates for invasive treatment. Because of its low morbidity and mortality, endovascular therapy should be considered as the method of choice unless precluded by morphological or other factors. The type of percutaneous treatment, however, depends on the morphological features of each particular lesion.

TECHNICAL OPTIONS OF TREATMENT

Percutaneous Transluminal Angioplasty

The basic endoluminal technique remains PTA. Over the years, balloon catheter technology has improved markedly. Various options are available, ranging from noncompliant balloons holding the determined diameter to semicompliant balloons that allow pressure-guided adaptation of the definitive balloon diameter to the actual vessel diameter and high-pressure balloons withstanding pressure up to 20 atm as rated burst pressure, which might be exceeded by up to 50% (i.e., 30 atm). The introduction diameter has been reduced to 6F introducer systems, or with smaller guide wires, down to 4F introducer sheath compatibility. Inflation and deflation times have become shorter, and a smooth profile is maintained even after deflation. These improvements certainly contribute to the safety and ease of performance of the procedure; their influence on outcome, however, is difficult to determine.

Technical success of PTA is usually determined by angiographic appearance of the lesion after PTA, improved flow and pulse, and hemodynamic parameters such as pressure gradients across the lesion, particularly in iliac artery lesions.

Endovascular Stents

The introduction of stent technology into the peripheral arterial arena has led to an enormous improvement in treatment, particularly with respect to iliac artery lesions. Since the late 1980s, stent implantation has rapidly increased.

In principle, two types of stents are available:

- Balloon-expandable stents
- Self-expanding stents

Balloon-expandable stents are mounted on a balloon catheter and are passively enlarged to a desired diameter at the site of implantation by dilation of the balloon. Newer balloon-expandable stents are precrimped onto the balloon, permitting easy deployment. Older, hand-crimped stents are more difficult to employ in curved vessels and pose a risk of dislodgment from the balloon. Hand-crimping, however, allows use of a single type of stent for several vessel diameters, which is advantageous from an inventory standpoint. Balloon-expandable stents are usually short, are made from stainless steel, and are preferred for well-circumscribed lesions. They are advantageous if precise placement is required.

Self-expanding stents open actively after being released from a dedicated delivery system. The self-expanding character depends either on the braiding structure (Wallstent—Boston Scientific, Watertown, Massachusetts—made from stainless steel) or on the type of alloy (nitinol). Most modern types of stents are made from nitinol, with different geometries of the stent structure. The Wallstent may be withdrawn even after partial deployment, which provides an additional safety feature in delicate situations, such as lesions near the iliac artery orifice. Although they are self-expanding, nitinol stents should not be moved after opening. Nitinol stents are less radiopaque compared with stainless steel, and visibility is enhanced by markers on the stent or the delivery system. Wallstents shorten considerably, while nitinol stents do not. Self-expanding stents come in various lengths up to 80 mm and are of particular advantage in curved vessels, long lesions, and arterial occlusions. A recent innovation is the development of self-expanding stents that are deliverable through 6F introducer sheaths.

Especially in femoral arteries, neointimal overgrowth leading to significant restenosis is an unsolved problem. Therefore, drug-eluting stents that might help reduce neointimal growth are being evaluated. Sirolimus (rapamycin) and taxol are the agents under investigation and are released for use in the coronary circulation. Some experimental work has been done on radiating stents, but logistical problems and long-term sequelae with pronounced stenosis at the stent ends have prevented broad clinical application. Afterloading therapy is difficult to perform for logistic reasons, and dedicated catheters are no longer on the market.

Stent Grafts

Stent grafts play a limited role in the treatment of peripheral obstructive disease. Stent grafts are stent bodies carrying a full jacket coating around their surface. While in bare stents only a small percentage of the vessel surface is covered by foreign material, in stent grafts there is a total coverage. Two coatings are clinically available: Dacron and EPTFE. Animal experiments have shown that Dacron tends to stimulate a more pronounced neointimal growth compared with bare stents,[2] while EPTFE seems not to lead to a stimulated neointimal growth.[3] Again, the carrying stent might be balloon-expandable nonmounted stent grafts (Jomed Stent Graft, now Abbott, Brussels, Belgium), premounted stent grafts (Advanta V12, Atrium Mijdrecht, the Netherlands), which are already crimped onto balloon or self-expanding (Wallgraft, Boston Scientific; Hemobahn, Gore, Flagstaff, Arizona), Fluency stent grafts (Bard Inc., Karlsruhe, Germany). Stent grafts, especially in diameters larger than 8 mm, require larger 9F to 11F introducer systems. In the iliac segment, stent grafts are predominantly used to treat aneurysmal or pseudoaneurysmal disease or rare cases of rupture, perforation, or arteriovenous fistulas.

Atherectomy

Atherectomy catheters were introduced for the treatment of peripheral disease in the early 1990s. The most widely used device was a peripheral directed catheter—the Simpson atherectomy catheter (Guidant, Brussels, Belgium). This device consists of a collecting chamber with a lateral opening and a rotating blade. An eccentric balloon presses the open chamber against the plaque while the rotating blade is advanced. The plaque material is cut and stored within the chamber. Then the balloon is deflated and the catheter is removed. The device was especially helpful in removing markedly eccentric and calcified plaques. Another indication was removal of neointimal tissue from self-expanding stents. In a population of patients, however, results after atherectomy did not show an improvement in patency compared with PTA alone. The device is no longer available.

As an alternative, an atherectomy device, the fox-hollow atherectomy system (EV3, Plymouth, Minnesota), has been introduced in which an eccentrically shaped catheter comes into contact with the arterial wall where an oscillating round blade cuts into the plaque. The debris is collected in a distal chamber, which is cleared after removing the catheter.

Atherectomy in iliac arteries is less effectively used, because the mismatch between the catheter size and the larger vascular lumen prevents a highly efficient recanalization diameter.

ACCESS

Usually the access to an iliac arterial lesion is most easily performed using retrograde transfemoral access either via the ipsilateral femoral groin or via a contralateral approach. Ideally, the CFA below the inguinal ligament is used as an entry zone to the artery. An ipsilateral approach is easily performed in case a femoral pulse is still palpable. Sometimes, however, there is no or a weak pulse present but the artery may palpated as a stringlike structure or, during fluoroscopy, calcifications delineate the assumed course of the femoral artery. Alternatively, ultrasound- or Doppler-guided puncture may be performed.

Crossover access to an iliac lesion is recommended if a lesion is close to the potential ipsilateral entry point into the femoral artery or the ipsilateral femoral artery is small. Also, in obese patients crossover access may be a good choice. A crossover approach is problematic in lesions that are close to the aortic bifurcation because sometimes wire passage is difficult or placement of balloons and stents may be complicated. Then an ispilateral approach is preferable.

As an alternative, a transbrachial approach may be used by placing a long 90 to 100 cm 6F sheath from above to allow proper periprocedural imaging. Via this access, both iliac accesses are easily reachable but a long instrument with working lengths of 120 to 135 cm should be used. This approach may be used if an access to the ipsilateral groin is not possible (recent femoral cutdown, planned surgery in the near future, large groin hematoma, florid infection, etc.) And a crossover approach is not recommendable due to the proximal location of the lesion.

Increasingly, hybrid interventions are performed that combine an open approach to the groin (femoropopliteal bypass or crossover femoral bypass) with an interventional procedure in the iliac axis. These procedures may be performed in the operating procedure room but also in specially designated angio suites offering operating procedure conditions like laminar airflow. Also, a percutaneous intervention may precede surgery and the patient may be transported to the operation theater with a sheath in place.

In complex lesions and maneuvers, sometimes bilateral femoral access is unavoidable, such as aortic bifurcational lesions, kissing balloon techniques, or iliac occlusions difficult to pass.

The availability of closure devices facilitates bleeding control at the entry site. They are quite easily and safely applicable in retrograde femoral artery access. Although closure devices are helpful in reducing the time needed for an intervention, allowing the patient to get up quite early, after around 4 hours, and offer the chance to perform more interventions on an outpatient basis, they have created their own complications, such as femoral artery occlusion, infected groin hematomas, distal embolization, arterial laceration, or plaque removal. They have to be handled with care, and patients with narrow arteries, large plaques, or calcifications of the femoral artery may not be ideal candidates for the use of these systems.

TREATMENT OPTIONS RELATIVE TO LESION LOCATION AND MORPHOLOGY

Aortoiliac Arteries

The aorta and the iliac arteries have long been a primary field for percutaneous intervention. The ease of access to the lesion, the relatively large diameter of the target vessels, and the comparably benign outcome even of major complications contribute to the wide acceptance of percutaneous interventions for lesions in the aortoiliac system. Over the years, indications have broadened and now include treatment not only of focal stenoses but also of occlusive and aneurysmal disease. The introduction of vascular stents was particularly helpful in overcoming technical problems and as a tool to treat major technical complications that otherwise would have required open surgical repair.

Aorta

While the suprarenal abdominal aorta is rarely a target for percutaneous treatment, disease in the infrarenal segment may lend itself to PTA or related treatment. In more than 90% of cases, the cause of infrarenal aortic obstruction is atherosclerosis.[4] Clinically, solitary infrarenal aortic stenosis proximal to the

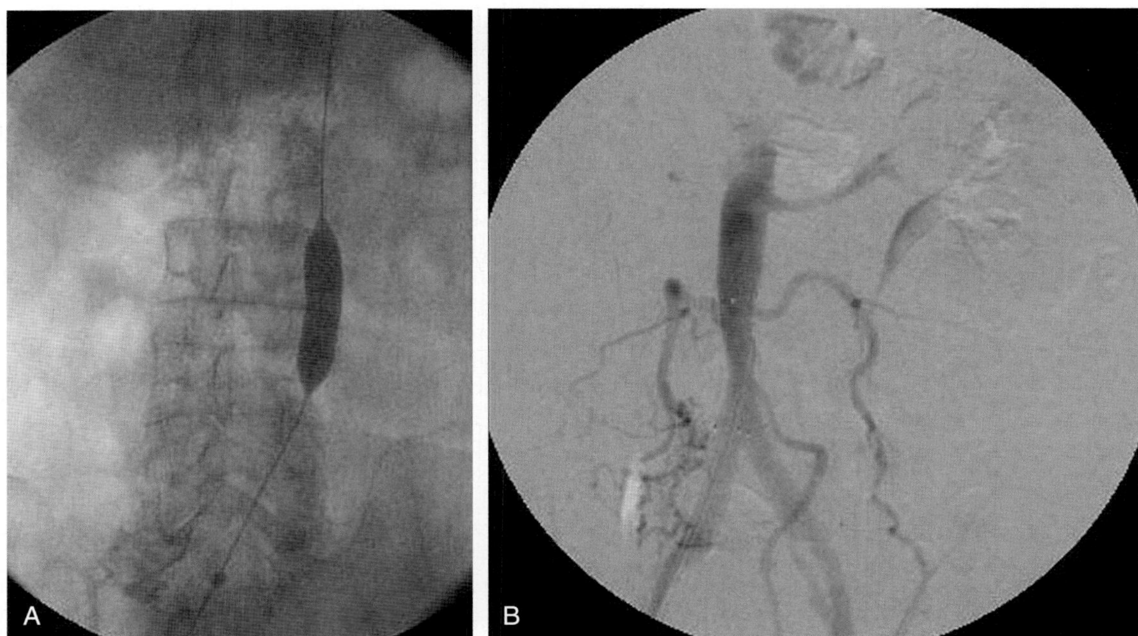

Figure 9a-2. Aortic stent placement. **A,** Tight stenosis of the infrarenal segment of the abdominal aorta with considerable residual stenosis after percutaneous transluminal angioplasty. **B,** After stent placement, only mild residual stenosis but otherwise sufficient patency. Patient became asymptomatic after treatment.

aortic bifurcation is rare, but a stenosis of both the distal aortic segment and the common iliac arteries is more common. This may be complicated by an acute or subacute thrombosis of the aortic bifurcation. Small distal aortic caliber, especially in female patients, may be a predisposing factor. Atherosclerotic stenosis above the orifice of the inferior mesenteric artery is rare.[4]

Embolic occlusion of the distal aorta (saddle embolus) is much less common but may occur in patients with mitral valve disease. Other rare causes of aortic obstruction are fibromuscular dysplasia, Takayasu's arteritis, and retroperitoneal fibrosis.

The typical age of patients with aortic obstruction ranges from 40 to 70 years. With respect to aortic occlusions, 55% are located at the level of the aortic bifurcation, 8% involve the entire infrarenal segment, and 37% involve aortic segments alone.[4] Collateral pathways are manifold via lumbar, epigastric, and mesenteric arteries.

Clinical symptoms of chronic aortic obstruction are bilateral claudication, predominantly with upper thigh symptoms, buttock pain, and erectile dysfunction in males. Symptoms must be differentiated from those of spinal stenosis. In occlusions, acute bilateral ischemia is present if no preexisting stenotic process has promoted earlier development of collateral pathways. Aortic aneurysmal disease is increasingly becoming a field of interest for endovascular therapy, and such may be applied to selected patients with associated atherosclerotic occlusive disease. Endovascular treatment of aneurysms, however, is beyond the scope of this chapter.

INDICATIONS FOR PERCUTANEOUS TREATMENT

Indications for percutaneous versus surgical treatment largely depend on the location, extent, chronology (acute versus chronic), and morphology of the responsible lesion.

Accepted indications for PTA alone (Figures 9a-1 and 9a-2) are concentric segmental stenosis and short-segment aortic bifurcation stenosis. Balloon angioplasty may be followed by stent insertion in cases of either insufficient luminal gain or occurrence of significant dissection after PTA.

PTA is relatively contraindicated if a complete calcified ring is present at the site of obstruction, as aortic rupture has been occasionally reported under such circumstances.[5] Because of the law of Laplace, the aorta is theoretically more easily prone to rupture than smaller-diameter vessels such as the iliac artery. In such instances, primary placement of a stent graft might be considered.

Long-segment diffuse disease of both the aorta and the iliac arteries is considered a contraindication to endovascular therapy; surgical aortobifemoral bypass grafts are generally a better choice (Figure 9a-3).

Focal bifurcational aortic stenosis is treatable by PTA using a simultaneous "kissing balloon" technique to dilate the distal aortic segment and both iliac orifices. Stent implantation has been increasingly used to achieve a stable postangioplasty widening by use of kissing stents in the distal aorta and both iliac arteries. In the case of distal aortic occlusion, few reports exist on remodeling the distal aortic segment or the aortic bifurcation by use of metallic stents.[6,7] In such difficult situations, use of advanced interventional techniques is certainly an advantage over simple balloon angioplasty.

Technical Aspects

No major differences exist between the aortic and the iliac segment concerning techniques of lesion passage or traversal of occluded segments, whether they are located purely in the aorta or also involve the iliac segment. This is also true for balloon dilation, which does not differ significantly from angioplasty

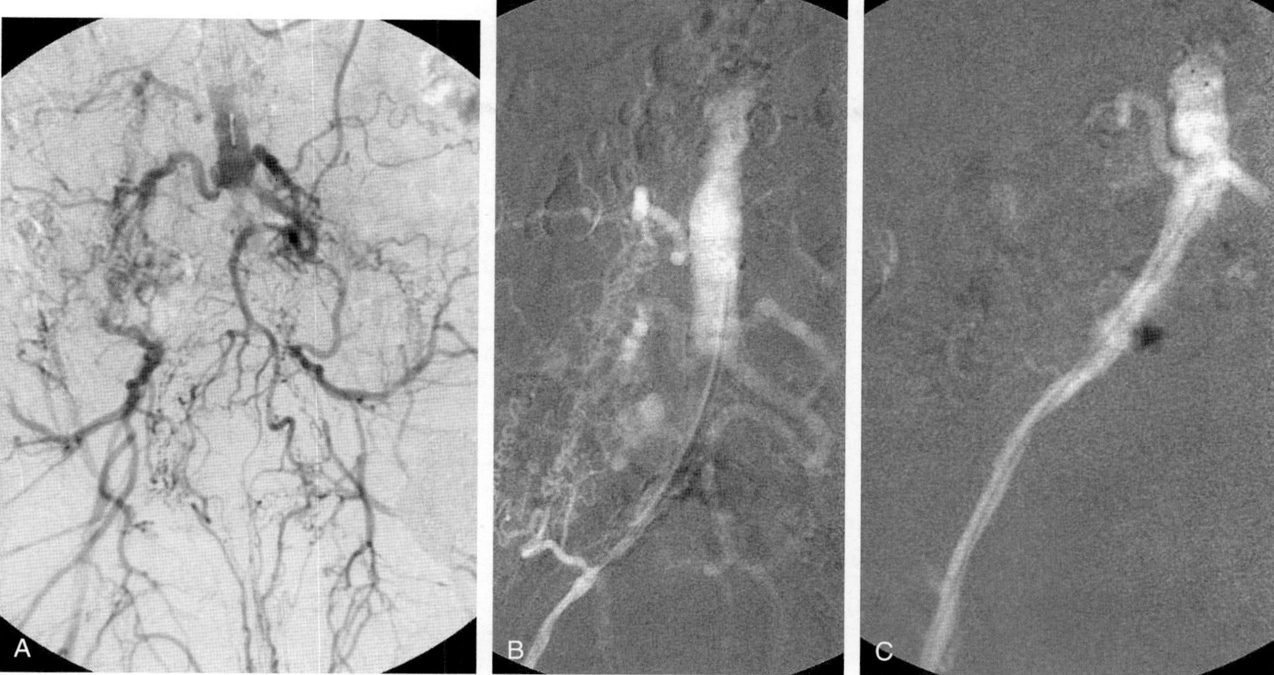

Figure 9a-3. Recanalization of a chronic Leriche syndrome. A 68-year-old obese patient presented with acute rupture of his right Achilles' tendon. He had suffered from bilateral claudication for a couple of years. To improve healing after surgery, recanalization of the right iliac axis was performed. **A,** Chronic Leriche syndrome with extensive collaterals. **B,** Passage of guide wire and catheter through occlusion. **C,** After placement of three stents starting with 14 mm diameter down to 8 mm, recanalization of the iliac axis was achieved.

elsewhere. The relatively large diameter of the aortic lumen, however, presents certain technical issues.

Kissing or Double Balloon Technique

Until recently, a major difficulty was the lack of suitable balloons of sufficient (16 to 20 mm) diameter. Thus, a double or triple balloon technique was recommended to open the aortic stenosis to a sufficiently large diameter. With two or three kissing balloons that are inserted by a bifemoral or by an additional transbrachial approach, respectively, and are inflated simultaneously, the aortic lumen can be widened to its original diameter. The kissing technique is still recommended for dilation of bilateral stenosis of the aortoiliac bifurcation and allows remodeling of the aortic bifurcation.

Single Balloon Technique

Recently, large-diameter balloons from 16 to 25 mm have become available (Boston Scientific, Cordis), permitting the use of a single balloon technique by a unifemoral approach. With these balloons, it is strictly necessary to locate the balloon entirely within the aortic lumen, not overriding the bifurcation, to avoid overdilation and rupture of the proximal iliac segment.

Stent insertion into the infrarenal aortic segment follows the same rules as elsewhere. Use of a stent of appropriate size, at least 14 to 16 mm, is necessary to avoid undersizing. The largest stent diameter can be achieved by use of the balloon-expandable Palmaz XXL stent (Johnson and Johnson) that can be mounted on a large balloon and inflated up to 25 mm in diameter.

Single Stent Technique

In lesions without involvement of the aortic bifurcation, a single stent can be implanted with no specific technical requirements. The stent type depends on the experience and preference of the interventionalist. Depending on the length of the stent and the location of the lesion, stent placement across the orifice of the inferior mesenteric artery may be unavoidable. A typical diameter is 12 to 16 mm in self-expanding stents.

However, if the lesion ends close to the bifurcation, placement of a single stent, especially of the balloon-expandable variety, may become difficult without overdilation of an iliac orifice. Under those circumstances, use of a self-expanding stent may be advantageous, while the aortic bifurcation is protected by a crossover catheter inserted from a contralateral approach. An alternative technique for distal aortic lesions or bifurcational lesions is use of the kissing stents.

Kissing Stent Technique

Analogous to the kissing balloon method, stents of preferably identical diameter and length are placed in kissing fashion within the distal aorta with their distal ends extending into the common iliac arteries. Often, the stents tend to meet the opposite aortic wall. Thus, instead of being shaped in a kissing fashion, they cross each other, forming a mirror-sided artificial iliac orifice.

Few reports of this technique have been made, and some questions remain open. Especially in stenotic lesions, it is not yet known whether there are potential sequelae from using two open stents that remain partly nonendothelialized in their aortic portion, possibly causing embolic disease or an increased tendency for thrombosis. It is unclear whether covered stents would be advantageous in such cases.

If a kissing stent technique is applied, it is mandatory that the proximal ends of both stents parallel meticulously side by side to avoid a situation in which one stent compromises inflow into the other. Consequently, use of noncompressible, balloon-expandable stents such as the Palmaz stent may be helpful.

Results

Aortic PTA has an excellent reported outcome compared with PTA at other sites. A primary success rate of 95% and a cumulative patency of 98% after 1 year and 80% after 5 years have been compiled from different series.[8]

Only anecdotal reports of stent placement for aortic stenosis have been made. Long et al.[9] reported two cases with successful stenting in Leriche syndrome. Dietrich[10] reported on six cases with chronic aortic occlusion that underwent thrombolysis and stenting by use of Palmaz stents. Long-term results are not available.

Complications

Complications that may occur after aortic dilation do not differ from those in other vascular provinces; however, they can have greater potential clinical impact. While severe dissection, recollapse, or residual stenoses are simply treatable by additional stent implantation, aortic rupture, although reported rarely, is potentially life-threatening and therefore may require immediate surgery. To control bleeding, a large occlusion latex balloon (Boston Scientific) should be positioned just below the renal arteries or covering the site of rupture and left inflated until the patient is prepared for surgical repair. To avoid this complication, computed tomography is recommended before the intervention to exclude complete or near-complete circular calcification of the aortic wall, which is said to be a risk factor for rupture. A covered stent graft may be placed across the site of rupture percutaneously; however, this method, to date, has only been reported for iliac arterial rupture and may risk occlusion of major collaterals and the inferior mesenteric artery.

Distal embolization develops in less than 1% of cases.[8] Subacute complications include thrombosis. This has not been reported for pure aortic dilation or stenting but is a risk in remodeling techniques of the aortic bifurcation. Thrombosis may be predisposed by adjacent aortic disease with plaques hanging over the stent orifice, thus causing inflow obstruction, or by adjacent outflow problems. If a technical reason has caused stent or post-PTA thrombosis, surgery is a reasonable option; if not, thrombolysis may be tried. Because of their large diameter, reobstruction of aortic stents occurs rarely but they may undergo repeat balloon dilation similar to iliac stents. In kissing stents, obstruction may be caused by neointimal hyperplasia; such lesions are treatable by reballooning, atherectomy, or placement of a second stent.

TREATMENT OF ILIAC OCCLUSIVE DISEASE

Iliac occlusive disease accounts for approximately one third of symptomatic lower-extremity occlusive arterial lesions, while two thirds are located infrainguinally. PTA lends itself to the treatment of many iliac artery lesions, and technical as well as clinical results are satisfying (Figure 9a-4).

Clinically, intermittent claudication starting in the upper thigh, together with lower limb claudication, is the leading symptom of iliac arterial disease. Erectile dysfunction may also be present. In isolated iliac lesions, critical ischemia is rare if not associated with additional infrainguinal disease. Rarely, blue toe syndrome might be present if cholesterol embolization has occurred from an ulcerated plaque in the iliac axis.

Weakened femoral pulses and reduced ankle–arm index are simple clinical signs that can indicate iliac obstruction, which can be verified by direct or poststenotic color-coded or duplex studies. For planning of a percutaneous intervention, magnetic resonance or conventional angiography is still most helpful.

Stent placement for stenotic iliac lesions should be performed if the angioplasty result is suboptimal (Figure 9a-5) as defined angiographically or by direct measurement of major pressure gradients. Since follow-up data are now available showing that iliac stent placement is relatively safe, a liberal approach is justified, although primary stenting of stenoses is not generally recommended because of socioeconomic constraints and potential follow-up problems. Furthermore, primary stenting is not superior to successful PTA alone.[10] Thus,

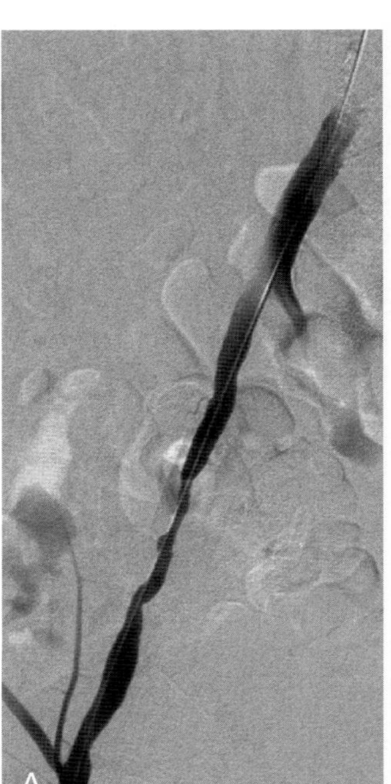

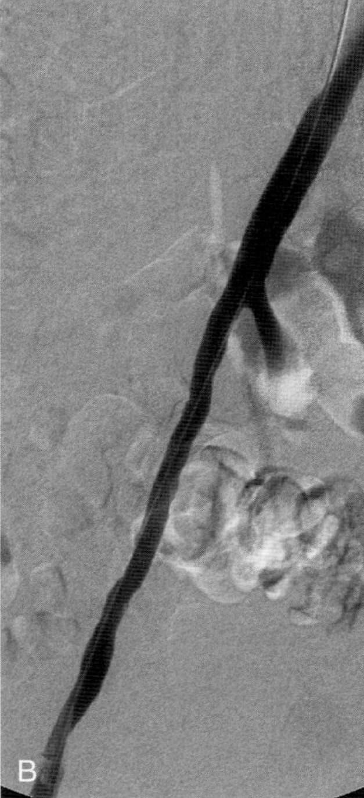

Figure 9a-4. Iliac percutaneous transluminal angioplasty (PTA) without stent. **A,** Eccentric long-segment stenosis of the right external iliac artery. Usually, these lesions tend to show dissections after PTA. **B,** After PTA with a 6-mm balloon of 40 mm length, smooth appearance of the treated lesion without dissection.

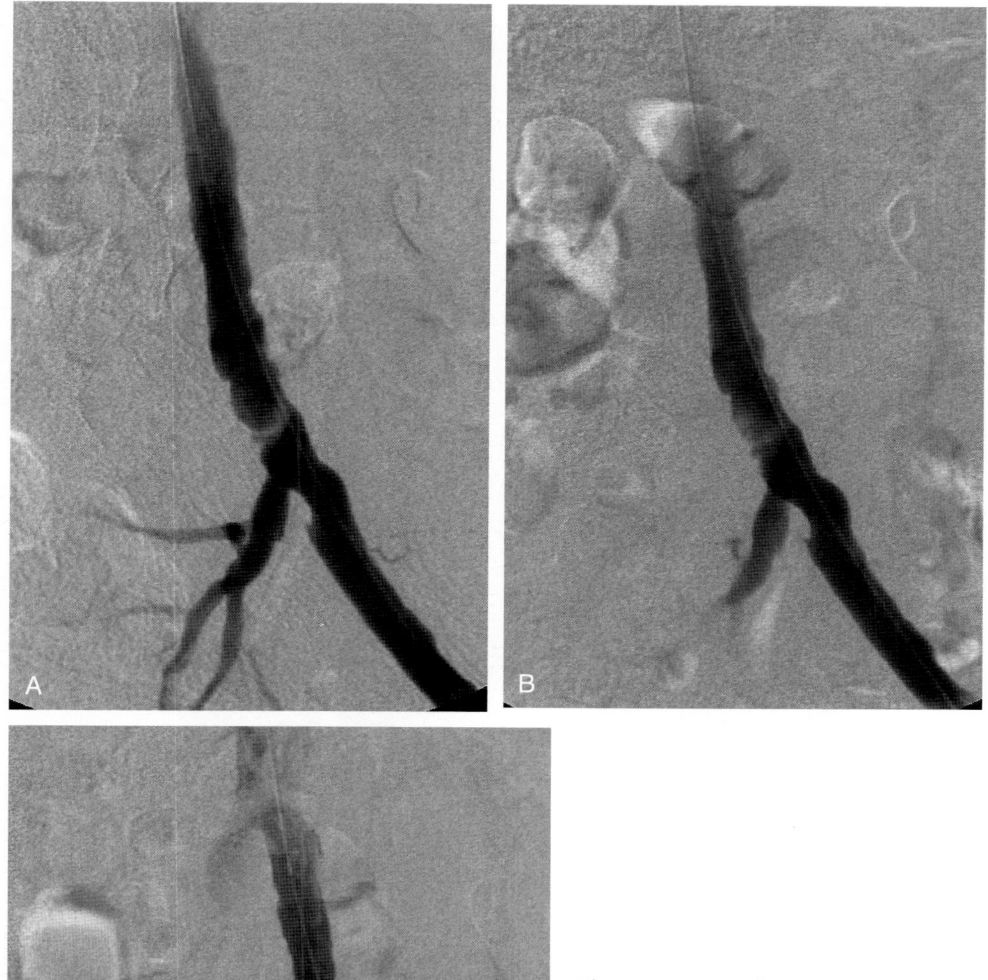

Figure 9a-5. Very short eccentric stenosis of distal common iliac artery *(left)* undergoing secondary stenting. **A,** Lesion before percutaneous transluminal angioplasty (PTA). **B,** After PTA, no major improvement has been achieved. **C,** After implantation of a self-expanding nitinol stent, the lumen is widely patent.

stenting is only performed for PTA failure (Figure 9a-5) or when technical requirements compromise success of simple PTA, such as for iliac occlusions (Figure 9a-6). As previously outlined, endovascular treatment is most appropriate for TASC type A and B lesions.

Iliac Artery Stenoses

Although PTA has proven to be an effective procedure in the treatment of iliac stenoses, the indication for stent placement should be restricted to lesions that are not primarily amenable to PTA alone. An inadequate postangioplasty result has been suggested as a general indication for stent placement, although the term remains ill defined. Residual pressure gradients are certainly a useful way to assess the angioplasty result,[11] but it is still unclear what the borderline gradient ultimately requiring additional intervention is. Moreover, the decision should not be made without reference to both morphological criteria and visibly reduced flow.

Long-segment stenoses with an irregular surface, aneurysmal formation, or markedly ulcerated plaques may be included in the group of complex lesions (Figure 9a-1).

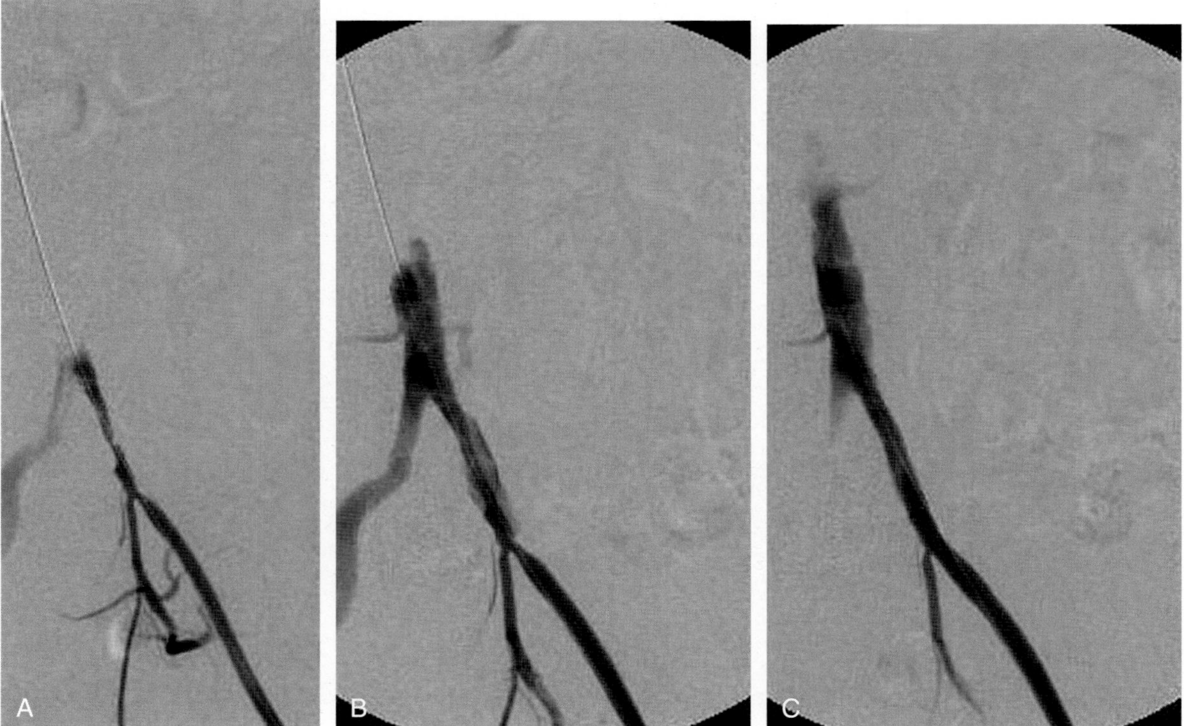

Figure 9a-6. Iliac artery dissection. **A,** Tight stenosis of distal common iliac artery and proximal external iliac artery. **B,** After PTA, there is severe dissection of the distal common iliac artery and minor dissection of the proximal internal iliac artery. **C,** After implantation of a self-expanding stent overriding the orifice of the internal iliac artery, the vessel is fully remodeled.

Eccentric stenoses and ostial lesions with extension to the aortic bifurcation are known not to respond well to balloon angioplasty alone. A stenotic lesion may respond well to initial balloon inflation but may collapse after balloon deflation, a process termed elastic recoil.

Such complications of PTA are treatable by stent placement (Figure 9a-5). This includes not only intramural hematoma but also flow-obstructing dissection complicating PTA, which may be an acute indication for stent placement to maintain the vascular lumen, obviating emergency surgery.

Iliac restenosis after previous PTA does not generally require stent placement as no proof exists that stenting prevents restenosis under those circumstances. However, stenting may be considered from a technical point of view in cases in which the result of balloon angioplasty remains compromised.

Internal Iliac Artery Stenoses

Indications to treat stenoses of the internal iliac or hypogastric artery are usually rare. In most cases, a network of collaterals is sufficient to feed the gluteal arteries from lumbar, contralateral iliac, or femoral pathways. However, in single cases a tight stenosis of the internal iliac artery and absence of sufficient collateralization may lead to severe and treatment-resistant buttock claudications. In these cases, angioplasty with and without stenting may be indicated.

Access to the internal iliac artery may be via a contralateral or an ipsilateral approach.

No established long-term data or larger series on this type of lesions exists that may give information about technical success, durability of treatment, or long-term success.

Iliac Artery Occlusions

Percutaneous treatment of selected iliac occlusions is technically feasible. In cases of acute thrombosis, thrombolysis is an alternative to surgical thrombectomy and might precede PTA of an underlying lesion. Mechanical thrombectomy via percutaneous access is still in its infancy and cannot be recommended as a routine approach since potential risks such as downward or crossover embolization are possible and no data are yet available to determine the overall complications of such a method.

In chronic occlusions with an occlusion time exceeding 3 months, balloon angioplasty alone, thrombolysis with subsequent balloon angioplasty and elective stenting, or mechanical passage of the occlusion followed by primary stent implantation have been described as alternative techniques (Figure 9a-7).

Metallic stents—and self-expandable endoprostheses, in particular—offer a new concept of percutaneous revascularization in chronic iliac occlusion, which my colleague and I believe is a primary indication.[12] Self-expandable stents are used to cover the occluding thrombotic material, thereby preventing peripheral dislodgment, a well-known complication of percutaneous recanalization of occlusions.

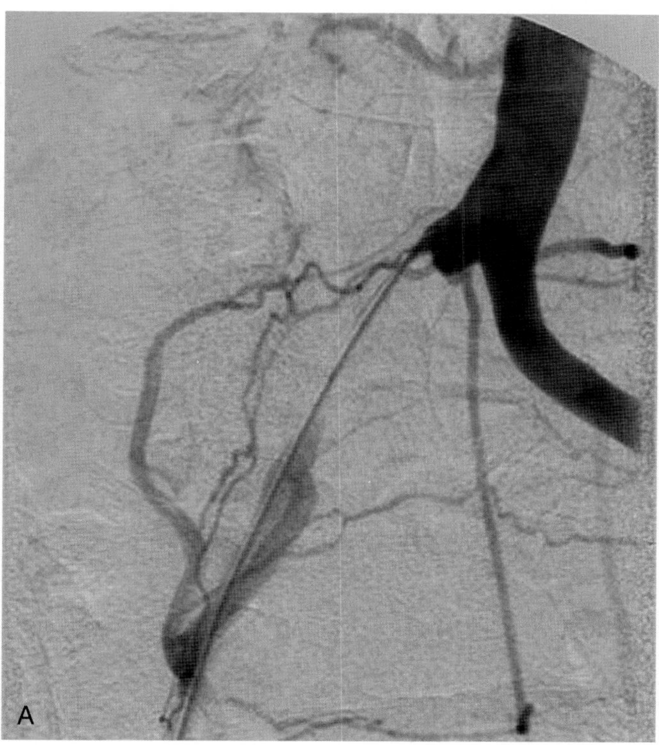

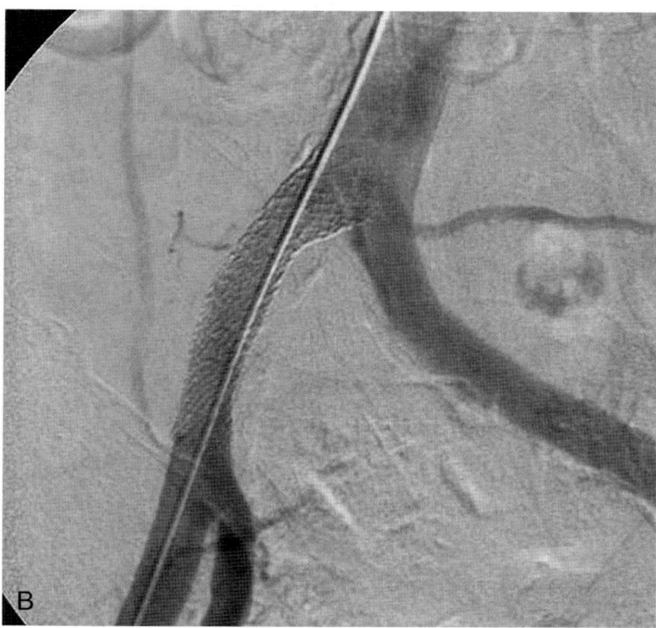

Figure 9a-7. Chronic iliac artery occlusion. **A,** After guide wire traversal of the occluded segment, primary stenting is performed. **B,** After placement of a self-expanding nitinol stent and subsequent percutaneous transluminal angioplasty, the segment is recanalized.

The indication for use of a metallic stent is almost always a technical one. Type and morphology of the lesion, technical outcome of PTA, and complicated situations are important criteria for use of stenting.

TECHNICAL CONSIDERATIONS IN THE ILIAC ARTERIES

Percutaneous Transluminal Angioplasty

Iliac artery PTA is relatively simple to perform. A retrograde transfemoral approach affords the easiest access to such stenotic lesions. Crossover dilation may be performed in special indications such as double-sided stenoses in case both lesions should be dilated in one session or in case an external iliac stenosis extends far down into the CFA. After careful traversal of the diseased segment, a suitable balloon is placed across the lesion and dilation is performed either manually or by using a pressure-monitoring gauge (Figure 9a-4). Balloon size may be selected either by film measuring or in digital subtraction angiography images by use of graduated catheters that allow fairly exact measurement of the vessel size.

By leaving the wire in place across the lesion and using backflush angiography through a previously inserted sheath or by reinserting an angiographic catheter and using downhill angiography, the postdilation result can be imaged. Backflush angiography was previously thought to be associated with a risk of retrograde dissection. However, with use of digital subtraction angiography, this is an extremely rare event and sequelae are limited as long as the guide wire is left in place.

There is wide agreement that both hemodynamic relevance of a lesion and post-PTA success can be accurately monitored by measuring the pressure gradient across the lesion. However, some dispute concerns criteria for success. A systolic pressure gradient of 10 mm Hg and less after peripheral drug-induced vasodilation is accepted by most authors to indicate successful PTA even if the morphological result is not perfect. Some authors use a mean pressure gradient of 10 mm Hg.

No data support anticoagulation following PTA of simple iliac lesions. I regularly keep my patients on full heparinization (500 to 1000 IU/hour) for 12 to 24 hours and recommend lifetime acetylsalicylic acid (aspirin) medication (100 mg/day).

Stent Implantation

If balloon angioplasty fails by either morphological or hemodynamic criteria, stent implantation can be considered. Technique depends on the type of stent employed. Most clinical series show similar results with various stents. Length and location of the lesion, experience of the investigator, and availability of appropriate size are important factors that may lead to preference of one or another type.

Precise placement is mandatory to avoid major complications, especially in cases where the stent must be placed close to the aortic bifurcation. While self-expanding Wallstents can be corrected during placement to a limited extent, balloon-expandable stents and self-expanding nitinol stents cannot undergo correction of their localization once inflation of the balloon has been started (Figure 9a-5).

Chronic iliac artery occlusions are primary indications for stent placement. I avoid predilation and place the stent directly into the occluded segment (Figure 9a-6). After stenting, careful balloon dilation is performed to avoid dislodgment of occluding material.

Atherectomy

Directional atherectomy does not play a major role in the treatment of iliac arterial disease. This is because the ratio of introduction and working diameter in most atherectomy systems is relatively low, which requires a considerably large puncture to achieve atherectomy of larger iliac diameters from 8 to 12 mm. The Simpson atherectomy catheter, the most widely used atherectomy system, requires an 11F sheath to sufficiently treat iliac lesions. Atherectomy may play an important role in the recanalization of stent reobstruction to debulk stents from reobstructing neointimal tissue.

Stent Reobstruction

Directional atherectomy and repeat PTA are both applicable to cases of in-stent restenosis. If PTA is used, a balloon size in accordance with the outer diameter of the placed stent is recommended to maximally compress the neointima, especially if occurring within a self-expanding stent that does not allow overexpansion. If a balloon-expandable stent has been used, slight overdilation of the stent is recommended to gain a larger diameter despite the presence of neointimal tissue. Some authors prefer atherectomy to debulk the stent. This is nicely achievable in smaller stents such as in the femorals but may require large instruments of 11F in iliac stents.

The treatment of stent occlusion is more difficult. Early acute occlusions are mainly due to technical problems, and it is mandatory to address these problems to maintain long-term success. Recent thrombosis should be treated by thrombolysis followed by PTA, additional stent placement, or both as required.

Late occlusion is mainly due to obstructing neointima within or adjacent to the stent. Little published experience relates to treatment of complete stent occlusion at a chronic stage. Thrombolysis, atherectomy, and mechanical aspiration followed by balloon angioplasty are possible techniques. A relatively easy method is the use of the stent-in-stent technique. Following traversal of the occluded stent, a stent is placed within the occluded segment, bridging it at both ends. The new stent is then carefully dilated, with a tendency to use an underdilation of 1 to 2 mm to avoid distal embolization.

RESULTS

Percutaneous Transluminal Angioplasty

For aortoiliac PTA, Becker and co-workers compiled data showing an average technical success of 92%, a 2-year patency of 81% (range 65% to 93%), and a 5-year-patency of 72% (range 50% to 87%) from available references in the literature, including 2679 procedures.[13] Gardiner and colleagues described a total complication rate of 4.5% and a major complication rate requiring surgery of 2.7% in 224 iliac procedures.[14] More recently, Tegtmeyer et al. reported on a single-center series of 200 patients, with a technical success of PTA of 88%, a total complication rate of 10.5%, and a major complication rate of 6.5%.[15] Follow-up results reported a 2-year patency of 90% and a 5-year patency of 85% among patients whose initial treatment was successful. Secondary patency was 99% and 92% after 2 and 5 years, respectively.

Improvement of these results seems difficult to achieve. The type of lesions that are treated, however, influences the technical results. The inclusion of eccentric lesions, calcified or ulcerated plaques, dissections, or iliac occlusions has a major impact on the technical outcome, and presumably on the long-term outcome, of iliac PTA. Stenting may be beneficial in such difficult cases and to treat complications of simple PTA.[13,16]

Stent Implantation

Stents are effective in the treatment of iliac artery stenoses. Use of the Wallstent placement in 118 patients with aortoiliac stenoses[16] with a mean length of the stenosed segment of 3 ± 2 cm was reported. Morphologically, 85 lesions were eccentric, 73 lesions showed major calcifications, and 52 lesions had irregular margins.

A total of 142 stents were placed, with a mean of 1.2 ± 0.5 stents per patient. Mean stented segment length was 4 ± 2 cm. Clinical stage improved in 112 patients; 89 patients improved by two or more stages (Fontaine classification). Mean ankle–arm index significantly improved to 0.92 ± 0.17. The primary cumulative patency was 97% after 6 months, 95% after 1 year, and 88% after 2 years; 4-year patency was 82%. Secondary or assisted patency was 97% after 6 months, 96% after 1 year, 93% after 2 years, and 91% at 4 years.

Chronic Iliac Occlusions

My colleagues and I also reported our experience with the treatment of 103 chronic iliac occlusions.[17] Mean length of the occluded segment was 5.1 ± 3.1 cm. In 44 patients, the occlusion was less than 5 cm (Society of Cardiovascular and Interventional Radiology class III); in 59 patients, it was more than 5 cm (Society of Cardiovascular and Interventional Radiology class IV).[10] The lesion included the orifice of the CIA in 48 patients and the orifice of the EIA in 41 patients. The lesion extended into the CFA in two patients. Mean ankle–arm index at rest was 0.48 ± 0.2 before treatment. The mean angiographic follow-up period was 26 ± 18 months, and the mean clinical follow-up interval was 29 ± 17 months.

A total of 154 stents were placed, with a mean of 1.6 ± 0.7 stents per patient. Mean stented segment length was 6.1 ± 3.3 cm. Arterial flow was successfully reestablished in 101 patients.

In two patients, the stent entered the aorta subintimally, thus leading to a compression of the stent entrance. In both patients, further intervention was abandoned to avoid arterial rupture and, despite heparinization, the new channel thrombosed within 24 hours. Thus, technical success of remodeling the vascular lumen was 98% (101 of 103 patients). Clinical stage improved in 99 patients. Mean ankle–arm index improved to 0.89 ± 0.19. Primary patency was 92% after 6 months, 87% after 1 year, 83% after 2 years, and 78% at 3 years. Secondary or assisted patency was 95% after 6 months, 94% after 1 year, and 90% after 2 years. The 3- and 4-year patencies were each 88%.

For iliac stent placement, larger series with follow-up data are now available for four specific types of vascular endoprostheses: the Strecker stent, the Palmaz stent, the Wallstent, and various types of nitinol self-expanding stents.[6,18] Device types differ with respect to stent design, radial expansile force, and surface geometry, all of which may theoretically influence respective long-term results.[19]

A multicenter study of the Palmaz stent including 486 patients revealed a technical success rate of 99% and a complication rate of 10%, with major complications reported in 4.7%. Clinical follow-up patency was 90% at 1 year and 84% at 2 years.[18]

The Dutch Iliac Stent Trial[21] did not reveal a difference between primary stenting and selective stenting in the case of insufficient hemodynamic outcome after PTA.

Selective stent placement was done in 59 of the 136 patients (43%) with PTA first. The mean follow-up was 9.3 months (range 3 to 24). Initial hemodynamic success and complication rates were 119 of 149 limbs (81%) and 6 of 143 limbs (4%; primary stenting) versus 103 of 126 limbs (82%) and 10 of 136 limbs (7%; selective stenting), respectively. Quality of life improved significantly after intervention ($p < 0.05$), but no difference was found between the groups during follow-up. The 2-year cumulative patency rates were similar at 71% versus 70%, respectively, as were reintervention rates at 7% versus 4%, respectively. The conclusion was that primary stenting did not gain a benefit and PTA first is a good option.

Now, the long-term data of the Dutch Iliac Stent Trial with a follow-up of 5 to 8 years are available.[22] Patients who underwent PTA and selective stent placement had better improvement of symptoms than did patients treated with primary stent placement, whereas ABI, iliac patency, and score for quality of life for nine survey dimensions did not support a difference between treatment groups.

Also, with the Strecker stent, which is no longer available, Strecker and co-workers reported a technical success of 100% in 116 patients with iliac lesions who underwent implantation of a Strecker tantalum stent, with patencies of 95% at 1 and 2 years.[6] Long et al. reported on iliac implantation of Strecker stents in 64 patients.[20] The technical success rate was 98%; the complication rate was 12%, but the rate of major complications was only 3.1%. Restenosis occurred in 10 cases, and reocclusion in 8.[20]

With respect to published data on the use of various metallic stents in the iliac arterial system, no obvious difference is shown between such regarding technical success and midterm patency.

Other Stents

At present, clinical results mainly with small series are available for a couple of nitinol self-expanding stents. Hausegger et al. reported the first clinical results with the Cragg stent, which showed a high technical success.[23] Starck et al. presented follow-up data on 203 patients with the memotherm stent and reported technical success of 98%. They used the stent in the iliac (44%) and femoropopliteal region (52%) and claimed to have achieved a better outcome than with the Strecker stent.[24] These preliminary data, however, are uncontrolled and nonrandomized.

As some types of stents disappear from availability and other become available, randomized comparison data are missing, as well as randomized studies of types of stents for the iliac arteries. However, whatever type of stent was used, results are similar for the iliac artery and successful. Although on a randomized basis no clear benefit of primary stenting has been shown, use of stents in iliac arteries has become quite liberal.

Atherectomy

Data are scarce for iliac atherectomy using the Simpson directional atherectomy catheter. A technical success rate of 85% and a 3-year patency ranging from 57% to 84% have been reported.[8] Maynar et al. preferentially used the system to treat the EIA, which is more accessible to atherectomy because of its smaller diameter; 18-month patency was 87%.[25]

Reobstruction in Stents

In cases of reobstruction, percutaneous reintervention is often feasible. My colleagues and I analyzed our results of such in 26 instances.[26] Percutaneous reintervention was effective in all 10 cases of stent stenosis. For stent occlusion, the technical success rate was 88% (14 of 16 cases). Embolization was the major complication of reintervention, occurring in 2 of 26 cases. Patency after treatment of stent stenosis was 87% after 1 year, compared with a stent occlusion patency of 57%. Recurrent stent obstruction occurred in 8 of 24 (33%) initially successful reinterventions.

For some authors, atherectomy is the method of choice for treatment of in-stent stenosis and occlusion. Available data are insufficient to compare techniques of reintervention.

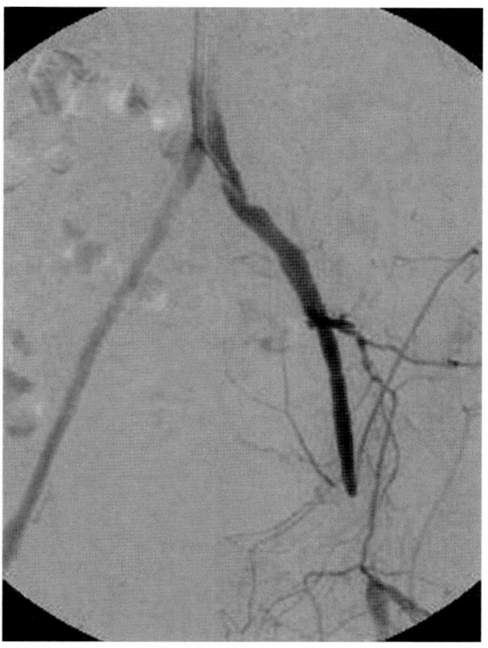

Figure 9a-8. Occlusion of common femoral artery due to a closure device. **A,** Patient experienced subacute ischemia of his left leg 1 day after iliac artery angioplasty and stenting. **B,** Angiography shows patent iliac segment but complete occlusion of the common femoral artery due to thrombosis onto a closure device (angioseal 6F), which was used to seal the access point.

Complications

Iliac artery PTA is relatively safe. The overall complication rate after iliac PTA has been reported to be 8.1%, with major complications in 2.7% and major complications requiring surgery in 1.2%. The most common complications are related to access problems such as hematoma (2.9%) and pseudoaneurysm (0.5%), acute occlusion (1.9%), embolization (1.6%), and arterial rupture (0.2%). Mortality is very low, with a mean of 0.2%.[8]

Stenting is useful not only to improve the technical results of iliac PTA but also to deal with specific complications such as acute occlusion. Use of stents, however, has expanded the application of percutaneous techniques to cases that otherwise would have required open surgery.

After stenting, the rate of complications in iliac arteries is relatively small. Using the Wallstent to treat iliac stenoses, a complication rate of 6.8% has been reported, with major complications—including subacute stent thrombosis—occurring in 3.4%.[16] For iliac occlusions, complications occurred in 11.7%. An additional surgical or percutaneous reintervention became necessary in six patients; thus, the major complication rate was 5.8%. The latter included arterial emboli, which was the most common type of complication in chronic arterial occlusions.[17]

In our series, my colleagues and I found that stent reobstruction occurred in 7.6% of stenoses and 17.5% of occlusions. Stent reobstruction was due to stenosis in 44% and occlusions in 56%.[26]

As generally in percutaneous interventions but especially after introduction of closure systems, access problems may occur. These may be due to local thrombosis, plaque disruption, or dissection of the CFA (Figure 9a-8). Although closure systems are usually safe and do not create more complications than manual compression, occlusion of the CFA is a particular problem.

CONCLUSIONS

Percutaneous recanalization with angioplasty and stent placement is widely accepted as the method of choice for most iliac and aortic lesions due to its low morbidity and complication rate. Differentiated therapy decision should include clinical image, morphological factors, and technical outcome to achieve best possible results.

References

1. Trans-Atlantic Inter-Society Consensus Working Group. Management of peripheral arterial disease (PAD). *J Vasc Surg* 2000;31:S1-S296.
2. Schurmann K, Vorwerk D, Uppenkamp R, et al. Iliac arteries: plain and heparin-coated Dacron-covered stent-grafts compared with noncovered metal stents—an experimental study. *Radiology* 1997;203:55-63.
3. Cejna M, Virmani R, Jones R, et al. Biocompatibility and performance of the Wallstent and several covered stents in a sheep iliac artery model. *J Vasc Interv Radiol* 2001;12:351-358.
4. Vollmar J. *Rekonstruktive chirurgie der arterien.* Stuttgart: Thieme; 1996: 207-214.
5. Berger T, Sörensen R, Konrad J. Aortic rupture: a complication of transluminal angioplasty. *Am J Roentgenol* 1986;146:373-374.
6. Strecker E, Hogan B, Liermann D, et al. Iliac and femoropopliteal vascular occlusive disease treated with flexible tantalum stents. *Cardiovasc Intervent Radiol* 1993;16:158-164.
7. Dietrich EB, Santiago O, Gustafson G. Preliminary observation on the use of the Palmaz stent in the distal portion of the abdominal aorta. *Am Heart J* 1993;125:490-500.
8. Rholl K, van Breda A. Percutaneous intervention for aortoiliac disease. In: Strandness E, van Breda A, eds. *Vascular diseases.* New York: Churchill Livingstone; 1994:433-466.
9. Long A, Gaux J, Raynaud AC, et al. Infrarenal aortic stents: initial clinical experience and angiographic follow-up. *Cardiovasc Intervent Radiol* 1994;16:203-208.
10. Dietrich EB. Endovascular techniques for abdominal aortic occlusions. *Int Angiol* 1993;12:270-280.
11. Tetteroo E, Haaring C, Van den Graaf Y, et al. Intraarterial pressure gradients after randomized angioplasty or stenting of iliac arterial lesions. *Cardiovasc Intervent Radiol* 1996;19:411-417.
12. Vorwerk D, Guenther RW. Mechanical revascularization of occluded iliac arteries with use of self-expandable endoprostheses. *Radiology* 1990;175:411-415.
13. Becker G, Katzen B, Dake M. Noncoronary angioplasty. *Radiology* 1989;170:921-940.
14. Gardiner G, Meyerovitz M, Stokes K, et al. Complications of transluminal angioplasty. *Radiology* 1986;159:201-208.
15. Tegtmeyer C, Hardwell G, Selby B, et al. Results and complications of angioplasty in aortoiliac disease. *Circulation* 1991;83:I53-I60.
16. Vorwerk D, Günther RW, Schürmann K, Wendt G. Aortic and iliac stenoses: follow-up results of stent placement after insufficient balloon angioplasty in 118 cases. *Radiology* 1996;198:45-48.
17. Vorwerk D, Guenther R, Schürmann K, et al. Primary stent placement for chronic iliac artery occlusions: follow-up results in 103 patients. *Radiology* 1995;194:745-749.
18. Palmaz JC, Labored J, Rivera F, Encarnacion C, Lutz J, Moss J. Stenting of the iliac arteries with the Palmaz stent: experience from a multicenter trial. *Cardiovasc Intervent Radiol* 1992;15:291-297.
19. Schatz R. A view of vascular stents. *Circulation* 1989;79:445-447.
20. Long A, Sapoval M, Beyssen B, et al. Strecker stent implantation in iliac arteries: patencies and predictive factors for long-term success. *Radiology* 1995;194:739-744.
21. Tetteroo E, Van der Graaf Y, Bosch JL, et al. Randomised comparison of primary stent placement versus primary angioplasty followed by selective stent placement in patients with iliac-artery occlusive disease. Dutch Iliac Stent Trial Study Group. *Lancet* 1998;351(9110):1153-1159.
22. Klein WM, Van der Graaf Y, Seegers J, et al. Dutch Iliac Stent Trial: long-term results in patients randomized for primary or selective stent placement. *Radiology* 2006;238(2):734-744.
23. Hausegger KA, Lafer M, Lammer J, et al. Iliac artery stenting: clinical experience with a nitinol prototype stent (Cragg stent). *Cardiovasc Intervent Radiol* 1993;16(Suppl):S25 (abstract).
24. Starck E, Dukiet C, Heinz C, Vierhauser S. Clinical experience with a new self-expanding nitinol stent. *Cardiovasc Intervent Radiol* 1995;18(Suppl):S72 (abstract).
25. Maynar M, Reyes R, Cabrera P. Percutaneous atherectomy of iliac arteries. *Semin Intervent Radiol* 1988;5:253-255.
26. Vorwerk D, Günther RW, Schürmann K, Wendt G. Percutaneous treatment of late obstruction in iliac arterial stents. *Radiology* 1995;197: 479-484.

chapter 9b

Endovascular Treatment of Lower Extremity Arterial Occlusive Disease: Femoropopliteal and Tibial Interventions

Bruce H. Gray, DO

Key Points

- Patients with critical limb ischemia (CLI) often have multilevel disease, systemic atherosclerosis, and a shorter life expectancy.
- Endovascular techniques have been used more often as first-line therapy to treat CLI because of technological improvements in wires, balloons, stents, and other devices.
- Percutaneous transluminal angioplasty (PTA) remains the mainstay of revascularization whenever possible, despite the availability of atherectomy, laser, cryoplasty, and cutting and scoring balloons.
- Nitinol self-expanding stents improve clinical durability for superficial femoral artery lesions.
- Tibial angioplasty is technically feasible and best reserved for patients with CLI.
- Antiplatelet (long-term) and anticoagulation (periprocedurally) agents are important to the success of the endovascular procedure.
- After revascularization, risk factors should be maximally treated.

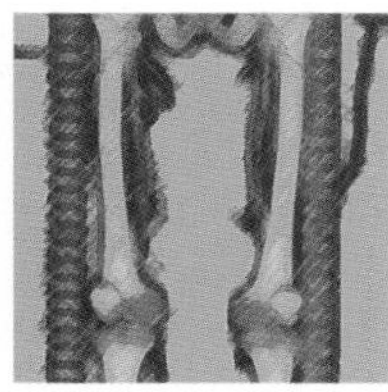

The treatment of infrainguinal arterial disease is the most controversial and perhaps one of the most evolutionary areas of vascular medicine. Several recent advances in our understanding of infrainguinal disease have modified patient care. The Bypass versus Angioplasty in Severe Ischaemia of the Leg (BASIL) Trial provides data regarding endovascular versus surgical treatment.[1] Other studies focusing on nontraditional endpoints, such as quality of life, functional status, and maintenance of independent living, challenge our emphasis on traditional endpoints of patency, limb salvage, or mortality.[2-5] And the development of devices and tools that increase the technical success of endovascular therapies has enabled clinicians to treat complex and longer lesions successfully. The vascular workforce has also changed, with many more vascular specialists being able to offer treatment than ever before.

Patients with critical limb ischemia (CLI) most often have infrainguinal atherosclerotic disease. Multilevel involvement (aortoiliac, femoropopliteal, tibial, or a combination of these) is the rule in CLI patients, whereas single-level disease is related to claudication. The BASIL Trial challenged the traditional surgical view that patients with CLI should be treated with bypass surgery. The main conclusions of this randomized trial, which compared a balloon angioplasty (percutaneous transluminal angioplasty first, or PTA-first) to a bypass surgery first treatment strategy (BS-first), showed PTA-first to be the most cost effective. However, the BS-first group showed greater patency beyond 2 years of follow-up. Even though the trial was well conducted and the conclusions are acceptable, practitioners can use these data as evidence to support either a PTA-first or a surgery-first strategy.

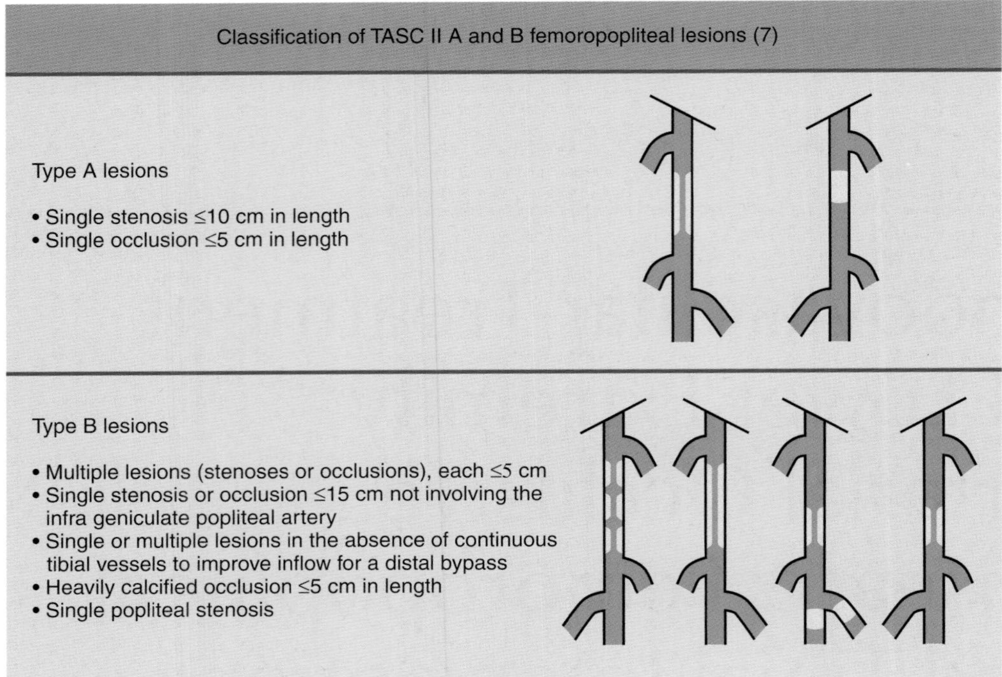

Classification of TASC II A and B femoropopliteal lesions (7)
Type A lesions
• Single stenosis ≤10 cm in length
• Single occlusion ≤5 cm in length
Type B lesions
• Multiple lesions (stenoses or occlusions), each ≤5 cm
• Single stenosis or occlusion ≤15 cm not involving the infra geniculate popliteal artery
• Single or multiple lesions in the absence of continuous tibial vessels to improve inflow for a distal bypass
• Heavily calcified occlusion ≤5 cm in length
• Single popliteal stenosis

Figure 9b-1. Classification of Trans-Atlantic Inter-Society Consensus II A and B femoropopliteal lesions.

The advanced disease present in CLI patients is representative of a systemic disease burden that leads to significant physical morbidity and mortality. The preferred treatment strategy must also minimize social, psychological, and functional burden of the disease. Endovascular treatments result in shorter hospital stays, less need for nursing home or assisted-living environments, and less functional disability, providing further incentive to consider a PTA-first strategy.

The Trans-Atlantic Inter-Society Consensus (TASC I and II) documents attempt to determine a treatment preference for femoropopliteal disease based on lesion severity (Figures 9b-1 and 9b-2).[6,7] Simple lesions (TASC-A) should be treated with an endovascular approach, and TASC-D lesions should be treated with a surgery-first approach based on available evidence. The TASC-B and TASC-C lesions represent the middle of the spectrum, and treatment bias toward PTA-first for TASC-B and surgery-first for TASC-C lesions. Significant differences exist between the first (published 2000) and second (published 2007) consensus documents as to lesion severity. As an example, shorter superficial femoral artery (SFA) lesions are defined in TASC II as less than 15 cm in length rather than 5 to 10 cm as in TASC I.

With these consensus documents and position papers, the treatment strategy must be individualized to the specific patient, with endovascular therapy viewed as complimentary rather than competitive to traditional open surgery (bypass, endarterectomy). Important factors to consider include the anatomical level of disease (TASC classification), the degree of ischemia at presentation (e.g., claudication, rest pain, or gangrene), the functional status (e.g., ambulatory, homebound, or bedridden), comorbidities (e.g., obesity, heart disease, or age), and technical factors (e.g., bypass target or integrity of autologous vein). This chapter explores the use of endovascular therapies for patients with femoropopliteal and tibial disease.

GENERAL CONCEPTS

Initial Evaluation and Anatomical Assessment

Individualized Treatment Plan

It is important before formulating a revascularization plan to distinguish between significant and nonsignificant lesions. Noninvasive studies (pulse volume recordings, segmental pressures) provide functional information and important clues as to the hemodynamic significance of lesions. They quantify the hemodynamic significance of collateralization and establish a baseline for comparative purposes. Segmental pressures across the iliac, femoral, tibial, and toe should be measured. Segmental pressure gradients *at rest* of 10 mm Hg are sometimes significant, a 20-mm Hg gradient is usually significant, and gradients more than 30 mm Hg are always significant.[8] A patient with a resting ankle–brachial index of 0.4 has a 10-mm Hg pressure drop across the iliac segment, a 50-mm Hg drop across the SFA or popliteal, and a 20-mm Hg drop across the tibial, which requires correction of at least the SFA component. In contrast, a drop of 60 mm Hg across the iliac, with a 20-mm Hg drop through the SFA and tibial, implies that the iliac lesion is most significant and should be initially treated. This is a grade A recommendation according to the American College of Cardiology/American Heart Association consensus document.[9] Then, with an inadequate clinical response, correction of the infrainguinal lesion would be necessary. Resolving these gradients and improving the corresponding PVR waveform can predict successful revascularization. Failure to correct the "functionally important" lesion results in poor outcomes.[10]

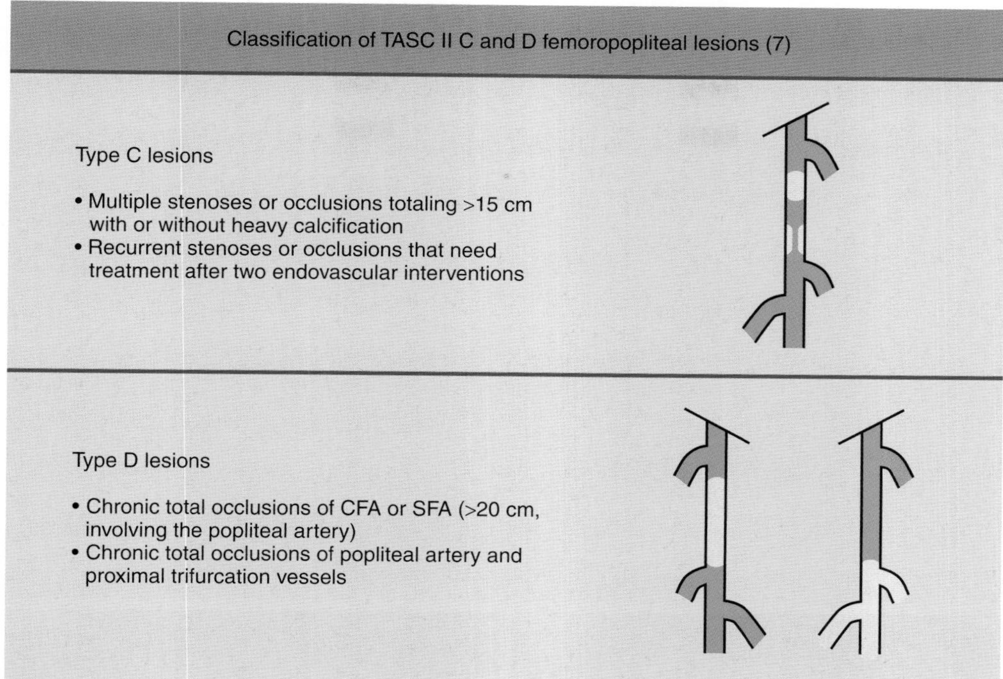

Figure 9b-2. Classification of Trans-Atlantic Inter-Society Consensus II C and D femoropopliteal lesions.

Intraarterial pressure gradients are an essential component to procedural success and are complimentary to the preprocedural noninvasive studies. Intraarterial gradients are usually higher than gradients obtained noninvasively. Superficial femoral and popliteal lesions induce large gradients and are more difficult to resolve with endovascular techniques. An 80-mm Hg gradient across the SFA can be reduced to 20 mm Hg, which may be acceptable. How these pressures are measured is critical. A gradient is induced by 4- or 5-French (Fr) catheters when placed across a lesion, whereas pressure wires (0.014 inches) do not, and can be used to even assess tibial artery lesions (Figure 9b-3). The utility of pharmacologically induced vasodilation (fractional flow reserve) with nitroglycerin or papaverine has been incompletely studied in the infrainguinal territory but may provide additional diagnostic information when assessing the clinical significance of a lesion.

Duplex ultrasound provides excellent information about patients with single-level disease but falters with multilevel disease.[11,12] A limitation is imaging obese patients, but for the rest duplex Doppler can be an excellent initial screening test in many CLI patients in experienced hands. Magnetic resonance angiography, computed tomography angiography, and duplex ultrasound have been used with increasing frequency to evaluate disease before revascularization therapy. The quality and resolution of these modalities have improved, supplementing diagnostic angiography.

Despite these advances in diagnostic imaging, digital subtraction arteriography provides the detail necessary for revascularization. Arteriography with posterior–anterior, lateral, and oblique projections can identify most lesions (Figure 9b-4). Contralateral oblique projections unmask proximal external iliac artery lesions from internal iliac artery overlap. Ipsilateral oblique projections of the femoral arteries uncover proximal SFA and profunda lesions. Lateral projections of the popliteal artery may be necessary in patients with orthopedic knee prostheses or in patients with nonatherosclerotic diseases. Lateral foot films identify the dorsalis pedis and plantar arch vessels best. Patients with extensive disease can be difficult to image when only injecting from a pigtail catheter in the aorta. Selective catheter placement at each infrainguinal level can provide better anatomical information (Figure 9b-5).

Selection of Procedure

Understanding the natural history of the disease in the context of the patient's history and physical examination is essential for proper treatment. Not all patients with CLI could or should undergo revascularization. Those with extensive necrosis or infectious gangrene or who are nonambulatory may be best served with primary amputation. Ambulatory patients with long arterial occlusions and heavily calcified arteries (usually diabetics) who have adequate autologous venous conduit and are expected to live for more than 2 years are best served with bypass surgery. Many CLI patients are poor surgical candidates because of medical comorbidities, compromised bypass target, and poor venous conduit; such patients would be best-treated endovascularly. These treatments are not mutually exclusive and should be viewed as complimentary.

Hybrid procedures that take into account the advantages of both surgery and endovascular therapy should be considered. The most common would be angioplasty and stenting of an iliac lesion before bypass of a long SFA occlusion. Some have used tibial angioplasty to improve the runoff after placement of a femoral bypass, which was limited by the length of usable autologous vein. Others have used angioplasty and stenting of the SFA before popliteal–tibial bypass.[13]

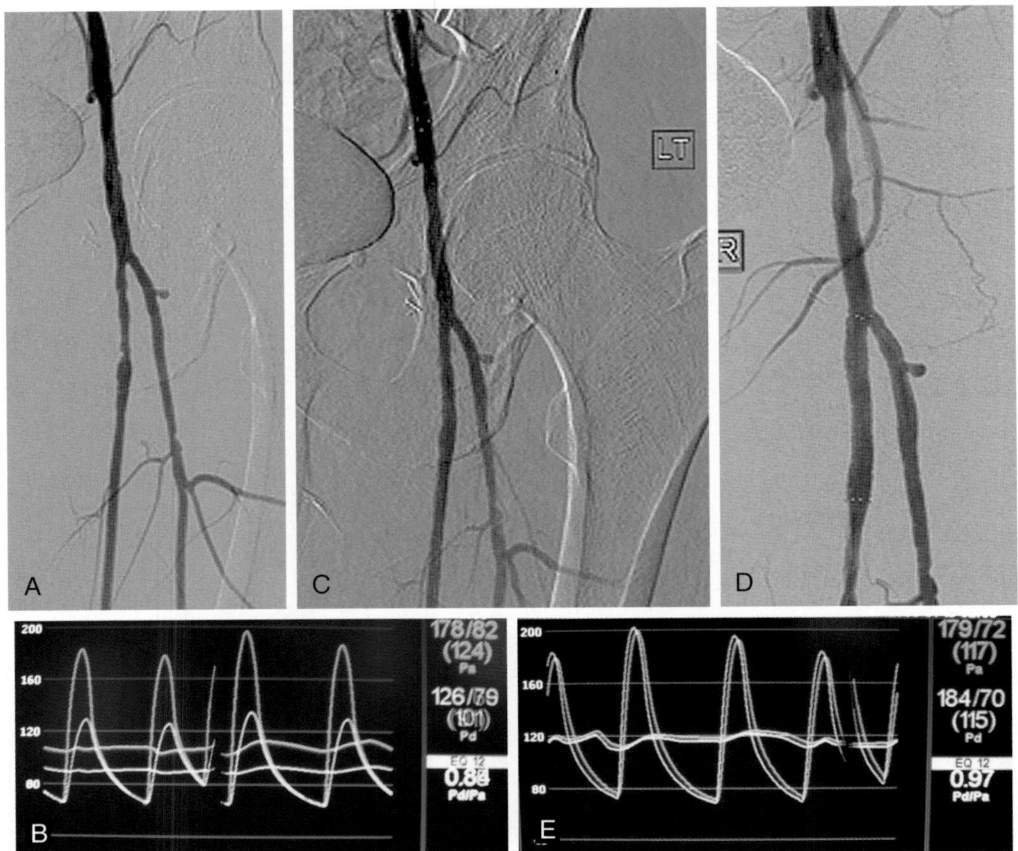

Figure 9b-3. **A,** Arteriogram demonstrating a Trans-Atlantic Inter-Society Consensus II A lesion of the proximal left superficial femoral artery. **B,** Corresponding pressure gradient across the lesion using an 0.014-inch pressure wire did not significantly change from baseline after percutaneous transluminal angioplasty **(C)** but did so after stenting **(D, E),** with corresponding pressure wire pictures.

Percutaneous Access Site

Potential percutaneous access sites include the radial, brachial, axillary, femoral, popliteal, and pedal arteries. The common femoral artery (CFA) is the most convenient, safest, and easiest access site for most diagnostic and therapeutic procedures. It can be accessed in an antegrade and/or a retrograde direction. The contralateral CFA is usually the best site for the initial diagnostic study. From this site, therapeutic intervention on the contralateral distal common iliac, external iliac, common femoral, profunda femoral, and SFA can be done. Ipsilateral, antegrade CFA access can be used for middle to distal SFA, popliteal, and tibial intervention. These distal lesions can also be done from the contralateral side, but catheter manipulation is much simpler with the antegrade approach.[14] Retrograde popliteal artery approach is excellent for proximal SFA occlusions with or without involvement of the CFA (Figure 9b-6).[15] Retrograde pedal artery access enables traversal of proximal tibial occlusions when the antegrade approach is unsuccessful.[16]

Percutaneous needle entry into the artery should be a single-stick, anterior wall puncture only. The Seldinger technique (anterior through posterior wall) should be avoided since arterial closure devices can only close a single anterior wall arteriotomy. Arterial puncture high in the CFA may predispose the patient to retroperitoneal bleeding, whereas low punctures at the level of the SFA have a higher incidence

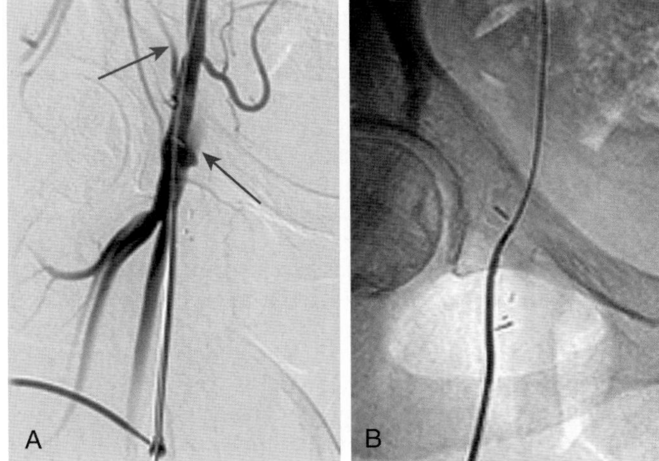

Figure 9b-4. Percutaneous access into aortobifemoral bypass by using a right anterior oblique projection **(A)** and a curved catheter to direct the wire anterior and medially **(B)** into the bypass graft rather than into the native external iliac artery.

of arteriovenous fistula, hematoma, and pseudoaneurysm formation. Occasionally, unplanned use of a fibrinolytic agent is necessary and a single wall puncture reduces groin complications associated with its use. Arterial puncture of a pulseless artery can be challenging. Helpful alternatives

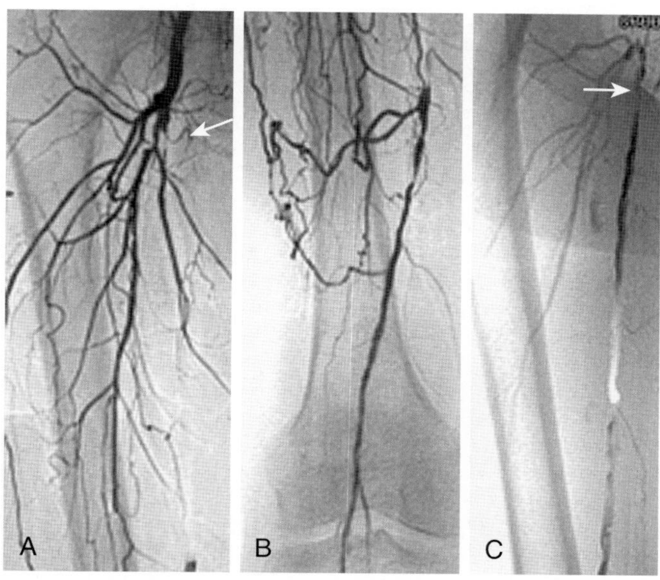

Figure 9b-5. A, B, Arteriogram of the right leg, which at first appears to be a long superficial femoral artery (SFA) occlusion with diffuse disease in the popliteal artery. **C,** On selective injection of the SFA, the area of severe stenosis is short *(arrow)*. Selective injections can alter treatment options.

include puncturing under fluoroscopy into the CFA 1 cm superior and medial to the lowest portion of the femoral head, using a Doppler "Smart" needle to locate the artery, puncturing calcification of the CFA seen fluoroscopically, or injecting contrast from a remote site and puncturing the contrast column while road mapping.

Wires

Many wires (entry wires, support or exchange wires, small vessel wires, glide wires) are available for therapeutic interventions. Improvements in wire technology have expanded the treatment of occlusions, particularly in smaller arteries (i.e., coronary and tibial). Stainless steel core wires maintain high pushability but deform easily. Nitinol-shaped metal alloys improve on the flexibility and shape retention easily lost in conventional wires.[17] Initial entry wires (0.035 inches) usually have a slight J shape that reforms as the wire passes through the needle into the artery. This wire design rarely passes subintimally, avoiding iatrogenic dissection. Exchange wires are long and sturdy and are important for coaxial catheter exchanges to reduce the risk of losing wire access. Support wires improve the trackability and deliverability of balloon catheters and stents but are poor in crossing lesions. Wires with slippery coatings (hydrophilic wires) facilitate traversal of occlusions and should not be used through entry needles since the coating can be sheared. After crossing a lesion with a hydrophilic wire, the clinician should exchange the wire for a support wire to avoid inadvertent loss of wire access. Small-caliber wires (0.014 to 0.018 inches) enable access into tibial vessels with small-vessel balloons, lasers, and stents. Wire characteristics that must be considered are size (0.010 to 0.038 inches), coating (bare or hydrophilic), length (35 to 300 cm), base metal construction (stainless steel, nitinol), and tip construction (coating, stiffness, shapeability, transition length).

Sheaths, Guides, and Catheters

Sheaths provide stable arterial access, minimize blood loss, and improve catheter manipulation. Sheaths are sized according to their inner diameter, with the outer sheath diameter ranging from 1.6 to 2.7 Fr, depending on the brand. Guiding catheters are sized according to the outer diameter. In practical terms, the inner diameter (working diameter) of an 8-Fr guiding catheter would be equivalent to a 6-Fr sheath. Most diagnostic and simple angioplasty procedures can be done through a 4- or 5-Fr sheath. Balloon-expandable and self-expanding stents require a 5- to 6-Fr sheath or 7- to 8-Fr guide. Long, flexible sheaths are needed for contralateral work. These sheaths are radially supported to minimize kinking when placed over the aortic bifurcation. Thin, smooth-walled sheaths produce a smaller arteriotomy and are preferred when access is from the upper extremity.

Pigtail catheters are the mainstay for diagnostic aortography and can be used to cross over the bifurcation by hooking the end of the catheter. When hooking the pigtail catheter on the aortic bifurcation is not possible, preshaped selective catheters can be used. Some catheters have a slippery hydrophilic coating that improves trackability. Trackability enables a catheter to advance through tortuous anatomy without pulling the wire out of position. The combination of hydrophilic-coated wires and catheters enables traversal of almost any lesion. Catheters can also have markers for measuring, radiopaque tips for better visibility, and tapering ends for improved crossability.

Reentry catheters are used to return to the arterial lumen from the subintimal space, distal to an occlusion. This avoids further distal extension of the subintimal plane, which could jeopardize important collaterals. Reentry is made with a curved needle extruded back into the lumen through which a 0.014-inch guide wire is passed. Orientation of this needle extrusion is performed with biplane imaging when using the Outback catheter (Cordis, Miami, Florida; Figure 9b-7) or with intravascular ultrasound guidance with the Pioneer catheter (Medtronic, Minneapolis, Minnesota; Figure 9b-8). Once the wire is safely into the distal lumen, then endovascular treatment can be completed.

The Crosser system (FlowCardia, Sunnyvale, California) uses vibration (20,000 cycles/sec) at the tip of a c atheter to "jackhammer" through an occlusion. The wire has received 510(k) clearance for use in the United States. The Patriot trial, which consisted of 40 peripheral arterial disease patients with occlusions showed success in most cases after traditional guide wire failure.[18] The Frontrunner catheter (Cordis) can be used to tease open the artery while it is gently advanced through an occlusion (Figure 9b-9).

Balloons

Balloon angioplasty causes a controlled injury to the vessel wall, producing localized dissection, plaque fracture, and medial or adventitial layer stretching. Dissections are usually nonflow limiting and are anticipated with concentric plaques. Eccentric plaque is more resistant, with expansion of the free wall accounting for improved luminal diameter. Stretching or disruption of the internal elastic lamina predisposes the patient to intimal hyperplasia.[19] Balloons differ in diameter, length, material strength, compliance, shaft size, shoulders, profile, and coaxial versus monorail design.

Noncompliant balloons assume their intended diameter even at high pressures. Compliant balloons are prone to

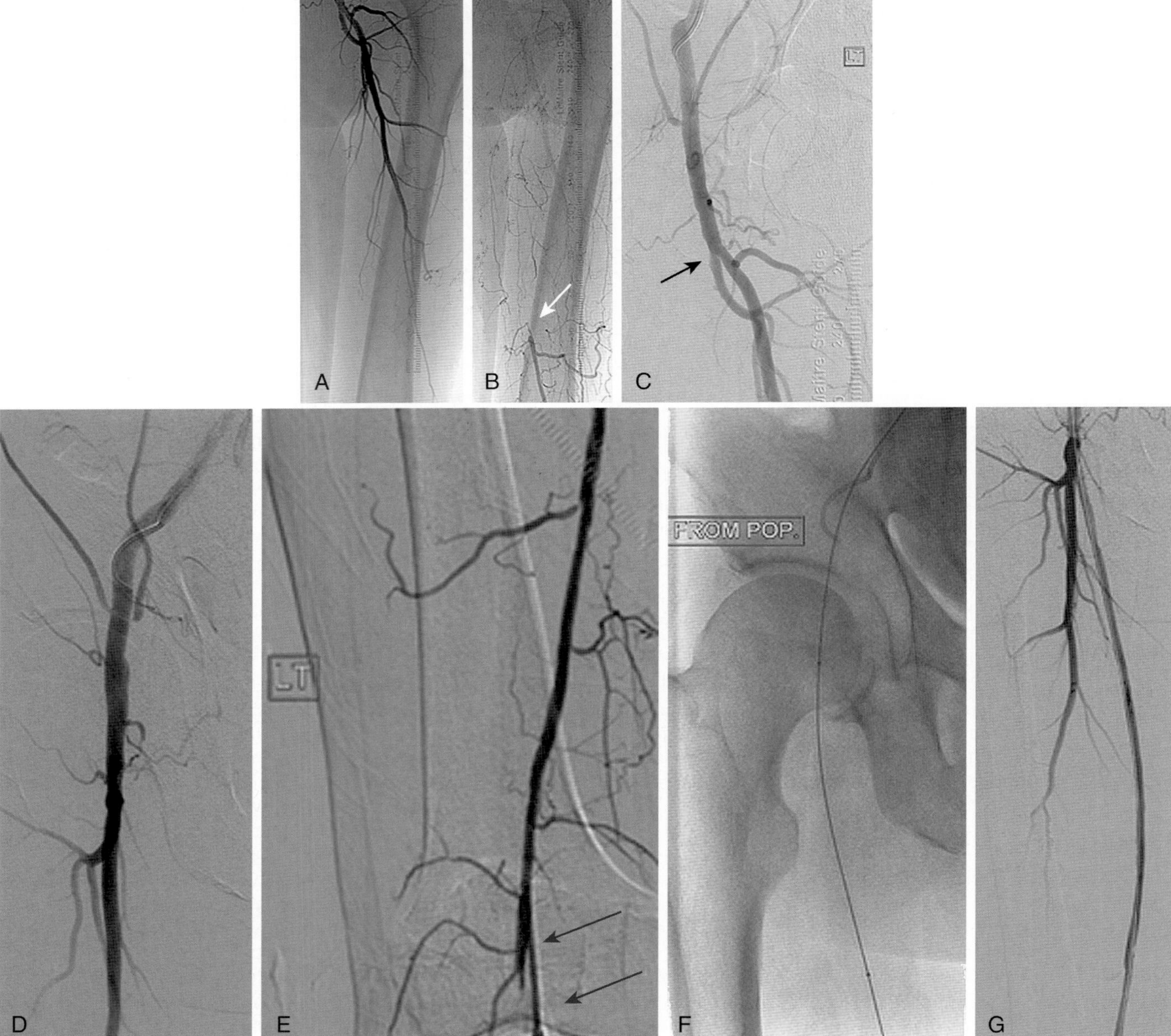

Figure 9b-6. Arteriogram showing left superficial femoral artery (SFA) occlusion **(A)** with late fill of the proximal popliteal artery **(B)** and no identifiable stump of the proximal SFA on a left anterior oblique projection **(C).** The patient is in a prone position **(D)** for retrograde popliteal access (**E;** *red arrow* highlights the sheath), wire traversal of the lesion **(F),** and completion after percutaneous transluminal angioplasty **(G).**

overstretching in areas of less plaque and do not exert equal forces with balloon expansion. Some balloons are considered noncompliant at low pressures and then become compliant or semicompliant at higher pressures. This enables the operator to alter the final balloon size by adjusting the balloon pressure.

Most balloons are made of polypropylene, polyethylene, or nylon. Nylon is noncompliant and puncture resistant, and it works well for stent delivery and postdilating. Compliant balloons should not be used for stent deployment. Smaller-profile balloons improve crossability. Upon deflation, balloons do not rewrap to their predilation diameter, so distal lesions should be crossed and dilated first, followed by more proximal lesions. Monorail designs or "rapid-exchange" technology has been extrapolated from coronary technology and applied in the periphery. These monorail systems allow the use of shorter wires, speeding up catheter exchange at the expense of pushability. Balloon inflation times vary according to operator preference. Maintaining the inflated balloon for 3 to 30 minutes reduces the incidence of dissection and stent use but does not improve the long-term patency of PTA compared to shorter inflation times.[20,21]

Pharmacotherapies

Adjunctive medications for endovascular procedures include antiplatelet therapy, anticoagulant therapy, and fibrinolytic therapy.

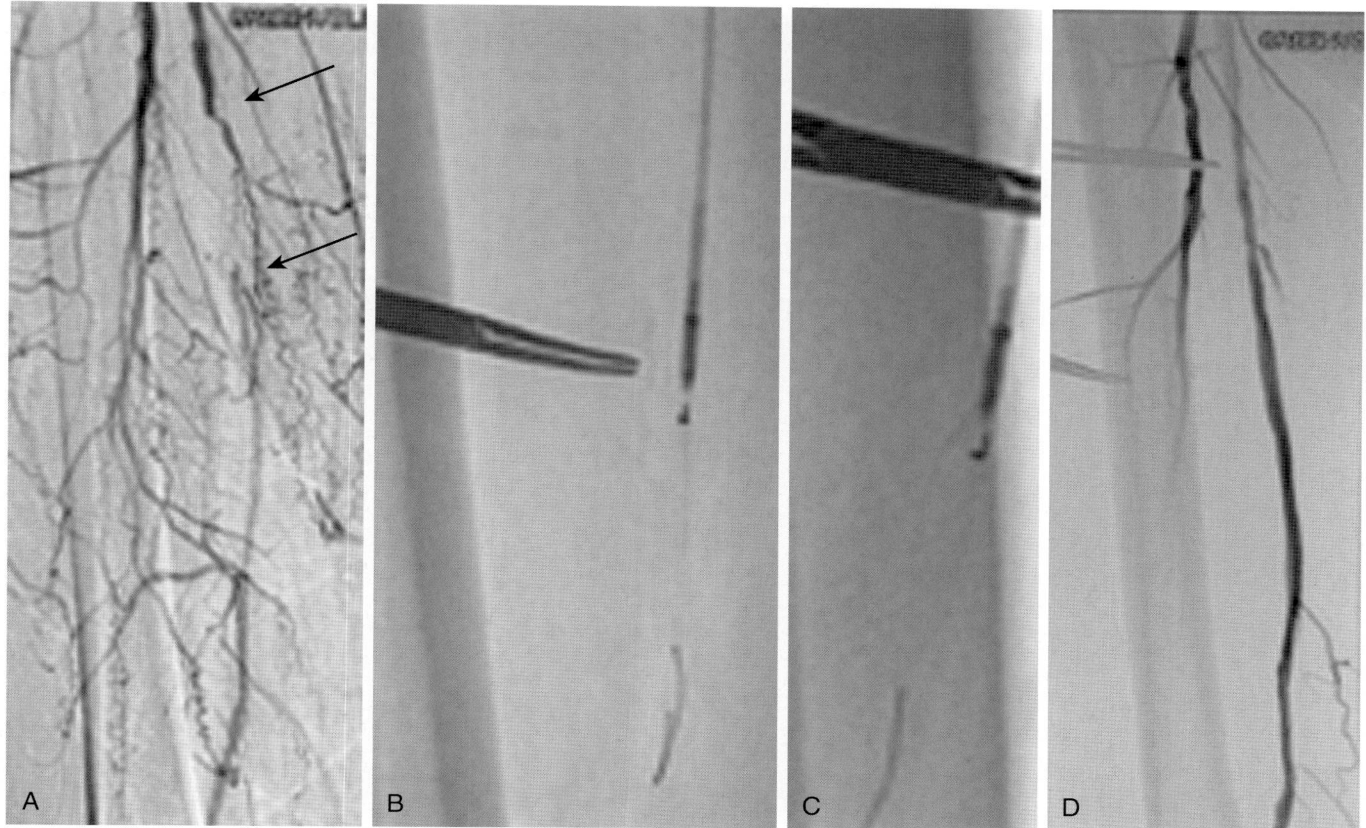

Figure 9b-7. **A,** Arteriogram of a Trans-Atlantic Inter-Society Consensus II B occlusion or stenosis with large collateral *(arrow)* at the proximal occlusion. **B,** Initial wire traversal was subintimal, so an Outback catheter was advanced over a 0.014-inch wire. **C,** The wire was then retracted into the catheter so that the reentry needle could be directed via the "L" and "T" markers toward the lumen. **D,** The wire was then advanced into the true lumen via the reentry needle, followed by percutaneous transluminal angioplasty.

Antiplatelet Agents

All patients with peripheral arterial disease should receive long-term antiplatelet therapy, and it should be started before the procedure. Antiplatelet agents including aspirin, ticlopidine, clopidogrel, prasugrel, dipyridamole, and picotamide have shown a statistically significant reduction in cardiovascular events.[22,23] No high-level evidence shows that these agents improve patency after PTA and stenting. Aspirin has the most rapid onset of action, within minutes, and peak action of less than 30 minutes. It produces about 20% platelet inhibition, and its effects last 5 to 7 days. It is the most cost-effective antiplatelet agent, with effective dosing at 81 to 325 mg/day.[22]

Ticlopidine and clopidogrel provide additive antiplatelet inhibition to aspirin, up to 40%. This translates into a reduction of serious adverse events by 9% over aspirin alone.[24] Clopidogrel takes 5 days to reach peak activity, with the daily dose of 75 mg. Loading doses of 300 to 900 mg reduce this to hours.[25] The risk of significant neutropenia is higher with ticlopidine, so clopidogrel is preferred. Long-term use of clopidogrel in all peripheral arterial disease patients can be justified; however, cost may be the limiting factor.[23,26] Dipyridamole combined with aspirin produced no greater effect on vascular risk reduction than did aspirin alone.[22] Picotamide, a thromboxane synthase inhibitor that is only available in Europe, is comparable to aspirin in reducing the risk of a cardiovascular event.[22]

Oral glycoprotein IIb and IIIa agents have not been superior to aspirin alone in several clinical studies involving cardiovascular patients.[23] Intravenous glycoprotein IIb and IIIa agents for peripheral intervention have been rarely used. These agents at full dose suppress platelet activity by more than 80% and substantially reduce the risk of acute arterial closure at the time of intervention. These agents—abciximab (ReoPro, Centocor, Malvern, Pennsylvania), eptifibatide (Integrilin, Schering-Plough, San Francisco, California), and tirofiban hydrochloride, (Aggrastat, Merck, Whitehouse Station, New Jersey)—escalate bleeding risk at the catheter entry site over unfractionated heparin (UFH).[27] Abciximab, an antibody, binds noncompetitively to the IIb or IIIa receptor site with high affinity. The drug therefore has a short plasma half-life but a prolonged receptor blockade. The drug dosing is unchanged by renal insufficiency, and its effects can be reversed with platelet infusion. The latter two drugs have low molecular weight, bind competitively to the IIb or IIIa receptor, and have a longer plasma half-life. They are excreted in the urine, and dosing must be adjusted in patients with renal insufficiency. Their effects cannot be reversed with platelet transfusions, but they resolve with time. The cost–benefit ratio has not been studied in CLI interventions. Intravenous IIb or IIIa inhibitors can be considered for long SFA, popliteal, or tibial revascularization that have a high risk of acute closure. The strategy to use a full-dose IIb or IIIa inhibitor with a reduced-dose (one-half to one-quarter) fibrinolytic has shown promise for subacute thromboses.[28] Combination therapy has not reduced the lytic infusion time over monotherapy, so further safety data are required to support widespread use.

Anticoagulant Therapy

Anticoagulation should be used routinely for peripheral interventions. Standard bolus doses of UFH (60 to 80 U/kg) can elevate the activated clotting time (ACT) above 250 seconds and is given after catheter insertion. This range minimizes the risk of pericatheter or sheath thrombosis and allows for prolonged balloon inflation times. The heparin half-life of 60 to 90 minutes, coupled with its low cost and low allergic risk, make it the ideal anticoagulant. Newer agents such as low-molecular-weight heparin, bivalirudin (Angiomax), or recombinant hirudin (Refludin) can be helpful, particularly in patients sensitive to UFH. Bivalirudin, a direct thrombin inhibitor, has a shorter half-life and less platelet activation but costs 10 to 20 times more than UFH. Refludin, another direct

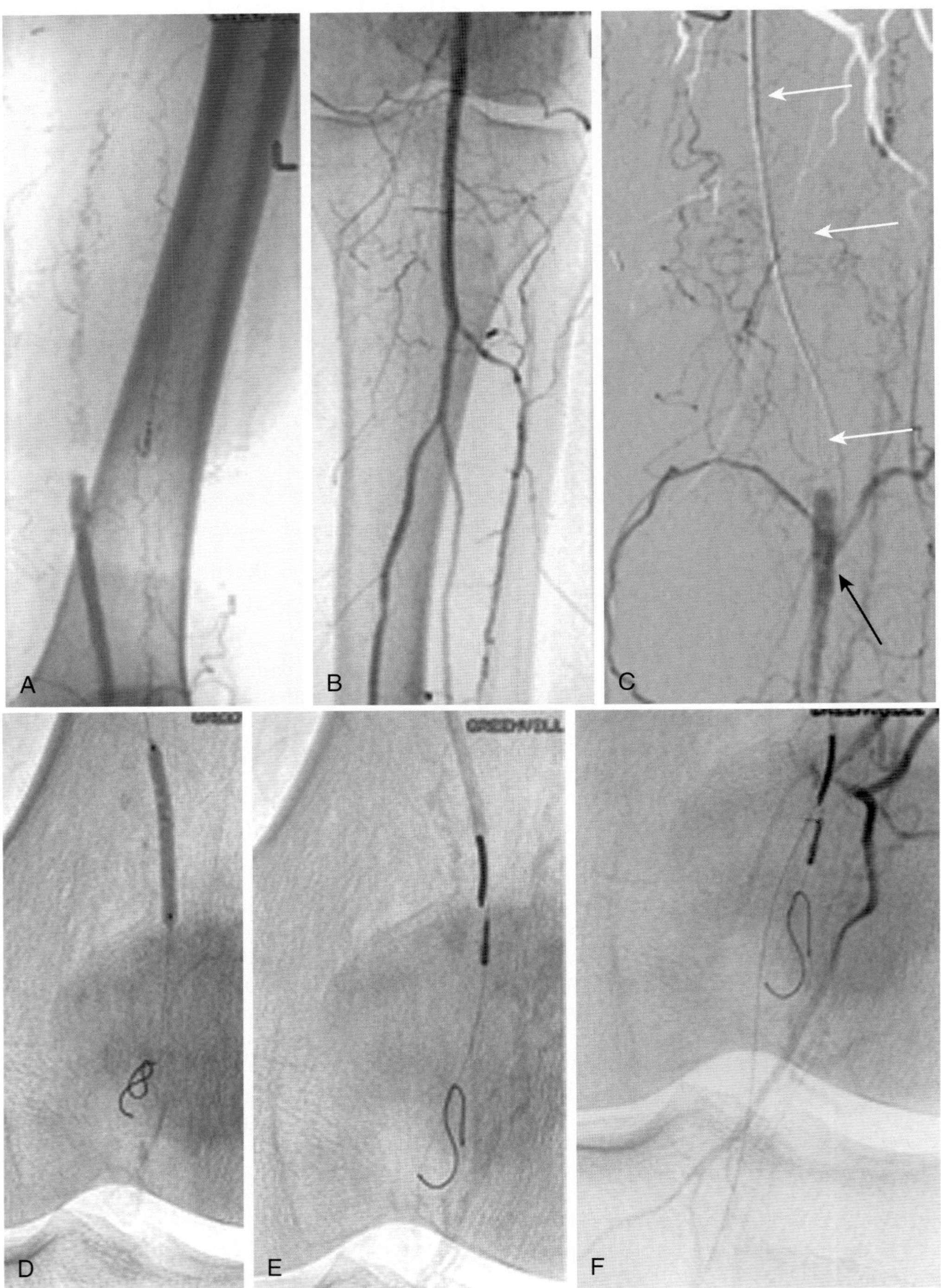

Figure 9b-8. A, B, Arteriogram demonstrating a Trans-Atlantic Inter-Society Consensus II D occlusion of the left superficial femoral artery with excellent runoff. **C,** Subintimal (SI) traversal to the proximal popliteal artery with a catheter. **D,** A small balloon is used to expand the SI space to deliver the Pioneer reentry catheter **(E)**. **F,** This is followed by needle reentry into the true lumen with a 0.014-inch wire.

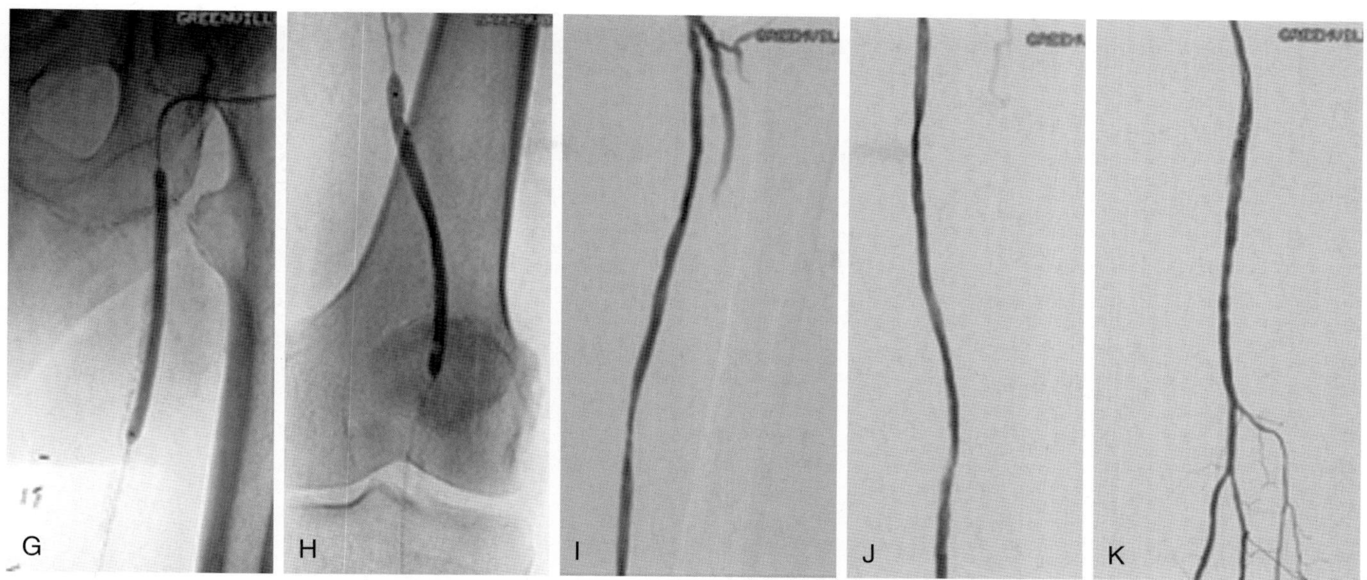

Figure 9b-8—cont'd, Percutaneous transluminal angioplasty **(G, H)** and stent grafting **(I** to **K)** follow.

thrombin inhibitor, can be used in patients allergic to heparin. This drug provides better thrombus penetration than UFH and may compliment fibrinolysis.

Fibrinolytic Therapy

Fibrinolytic therapy (streptokinase, urokinase, tissue plasminogen activator, recombinant plasminogen activator, tenecteplase, staphylokinase) has been used clinically for patients with acute arterial occlusion and for the pretreatment of chronic lesions.[28-34] Chemical clearance of the main artery and small resistance vessels without further endothelial trauma can simplify treatment of the underlying lesion. Efficacy is limited by the age of the thrombus, drug delivery, and lack of flow through the occlusion. Systemic infusions are ineffective, requiring intrathrombus catheter delivery. Other concerns of fibrinolytic therapy include a higher bleeding complication rate, drug expense, and prolonged ischemia time.[29,30] The feared complication of intracranial hemorrhage occurs in up to 2.9% of intraarterial catheter infusions and is associated with at least 78% mortality.[31] Specific risk factors for intracranial hemorrhage include recent cerebrovascular accident or transient ischemic attack (within 2 to 6 months), intracranial neoplasm, uncontrolled hypertension, or concomitant warfarin therapy. In these patients, fibrinolytic therapy should be avoided. The concomitant use of anticoagulation may contribute to bleeding risk; however, the safety margin produced with a less-than-full dose (activated partial thromboplastin time 1.5 to 2 times control) of heparin is unknown.[30]

Urokinase was used extensively in the United States until removal from the market in 1998. It was reintroduced in 2002. Typical doses range from 240,000 down to 60,000 U/hr and are infused from 4 to 36 hours.[28,29,31] The dose is usually tapered to the lower range after 4 hours and after reestablishing flow with the higher dose. Urokinase directly activates plasminogen, is less antigenic, and is a lower bleeding risk with greater efficacy compared to streptokinase. Streptokinase is of historical interest only and should no longer be used because of the antibody formation, which can induce allergic reactions.

Tissue plasminogen activator has been used extensively for peripheral arterial thromboses.[32,33] Weight-based doses have varied from 0.025 to 0.1 mg/kg/hr. Alternatively, non-weight-based doses of 0.25 to 10 mg/hr have been used. When given at 2 mg/hr, the fibrinogen level stays above 65% of baseline in 84% of patients, rarely dropping below 50%.[32] The fibrinolytic response can be quite rapid (6 hours or less) when fixed doses above 5 mg/hr are used.[33] The risk of intracranial hemorrhage with this drug appears to be higher than with traditional urokinase infusions.[31] Total dose limitation to 0.9 mg/kg or 100 mg does not eliminate this risk even though the drug is infused slowly and continuously. Current practice is to use 1 or 2 mg/hr (fixed dose) limited to 24 hours.

Retavase, a direct plasminogen activator, appears to be safe and effective for arterial occlusions.[34] Empirical dosing with the drug has been 0.5 or 1.0 U/hr. This drug has a longer half-life (18 minutes) than tissue plasminogen activator (4 to 5 minutes). The bleeding risks associated with an overnight infusion (0.5 U/hr) in 81 acute limb ischemia patients showed a major complication rate of 4.9% and a minor complication rate of 12.3%.[35] Some authors have used heparin quite sparingly with Retavase (100 to 500 U/hr).[34,35]

Exit Strategies

Arterial closure devices have influenced endovascular intervention. These devices promote prompt hemostasis, enabling early ambulation and avoidance of anticoagulation interruption.[36] Since arterial closure devices provide access site control, reservation lessens toward use of larger sheath sizes and

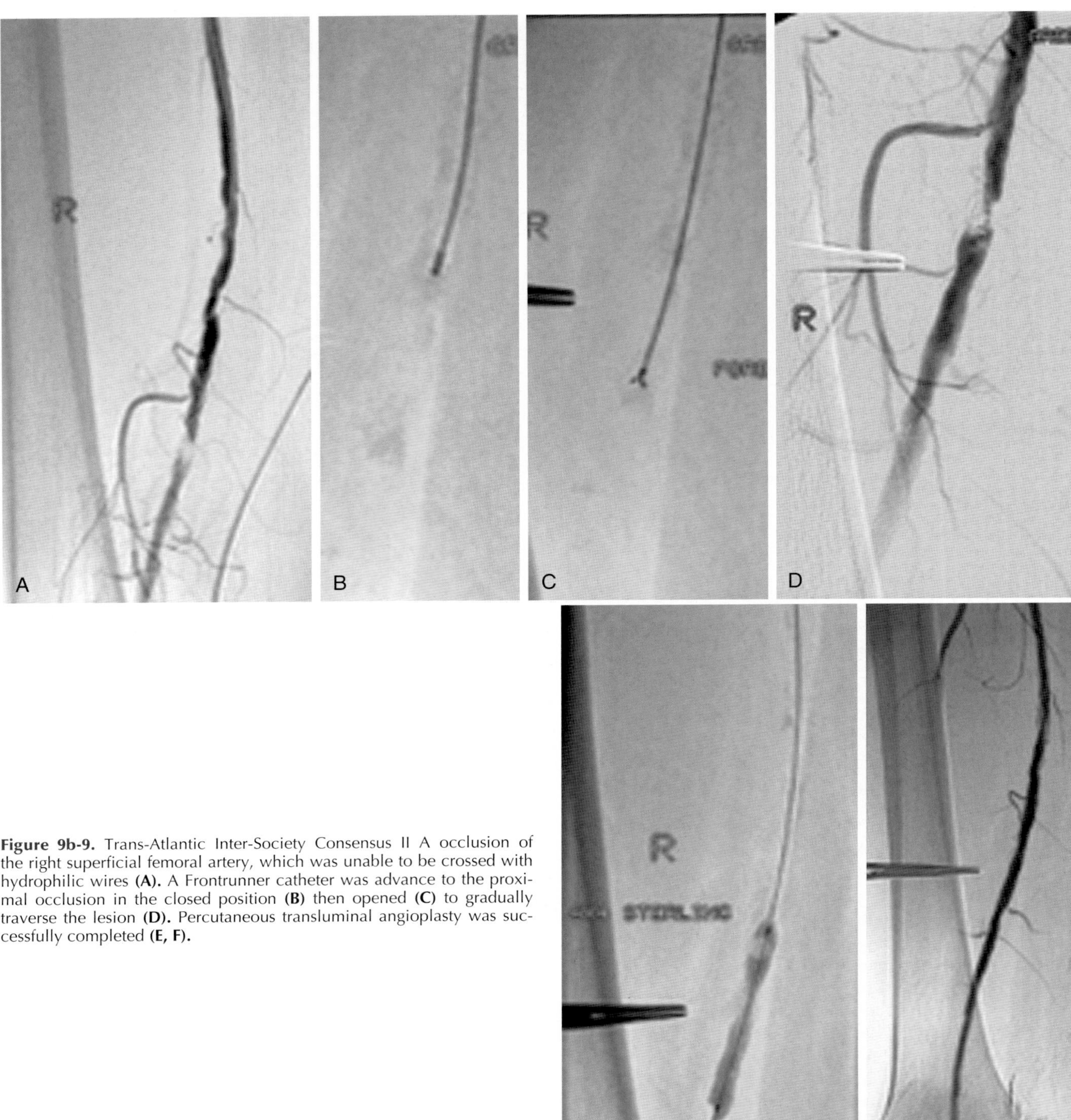

Figure 9b-9. Trans-Atlantic Inter-Society Consensus II A occlusion of the right superficial femoral artery, which was unable to be crossed with hydrophilic wires **(A).** A Frontrunner catheter was advance to the proximal occlusion in the closed position **(B)** then opened **(C)** to gradually traverse the lesion **(D).** Percutaneous transluminal angioplasty was successfully completed **(E, F).**

multiple or remote access sites. Some devices close the arteriotomy with suture (Perclose) or a collagen–disc sandwich (Angioseal). Others expedite the clotting process with extraarterial collagen (Vasoseal) or thrombin (Duett). Routine use can be justified by early ambulation and prompt discharge. Those patients who remain bedfast postprocedure for 4 to 6 hours do well with manual compression. The incidence of major access site complications does not lessen with closure devices. Major complications before closure devices of hematoma and pseudoaneurysm have been replaced with infection, acute closure of the access site and limb.[36] A learning curve relates to using each device and requires the development of tactile feel good

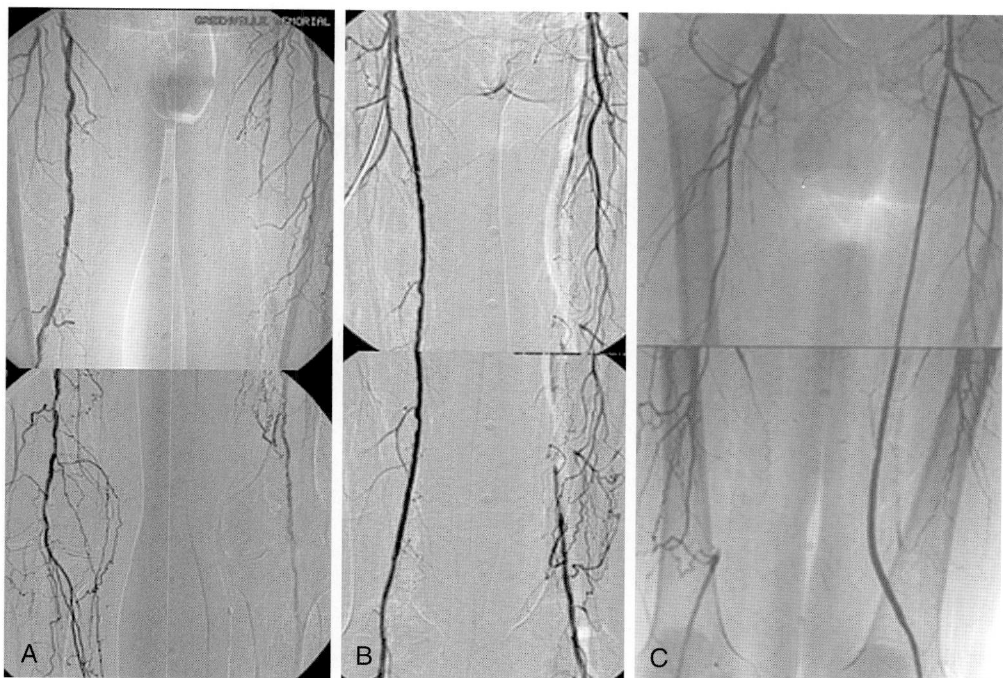

Figure 9b-10. **A,** Arteriogram demonstrating the plaque-dominant left superficial femoral artery (SFA) occlusion as based on the appearance of the patent contralateral SFA. **B,** A similar occlusion with less plaque and more thrombus. **C,** A thrombus-dominant occlusion.

results. There is no additional risk in peripheral arterial disease patients when using arterial closure devices.[37,38]

REVASCULARIZATION OPTIONS FOR FEMOROPOPLITEAL DISEASE

Femoropopliteal disease is more common than iliac disease and is the most common site of peripheral arterial involvement.[39,40] The atherosclerotic plaque can involve the entire 30-cm artery or it can be focal and discrete, illustrating the heterogeneity of lesions. Stenoses of the SFA are typically short, with 79% less than 5 cm, whereas occlusions are rarely less than 5 cm (9%).[41] In situ thrombosis converts atherosclerotic stenoses into occlusions. Often, the anatomy of the contralateral limb may provide a comparative basis as to the extent of atherosclerotic plaque since disease is often symmetrical (Figure 9b-10). This distinction is pivotal for endovascular intervention since the procedure can be modified to specifically treat thrombus, plaque, or both.

Endovascular techniques spare the autologous saphenous vein, can be done with local anesthesia, and minimize in-patient hospitalization and the need for outpatient extracare facilities. PTA carries a lower procedural risk than surgery with less durability. Early failure of PTA merely leaves the patient with unresolved limb ischemia without precluding surgical options. It rarely increases the risk of limb loss above the heightened risk associated with the disease condition. Late failure does not necessarily result in a return of the patient's original symptoms since clinical benefit outpaces patency.[42]

In CLI patients, direct flow into the foot needs to be established, so tibial intervention may also be necessary (Figure 9b-11). Concomitant treatment of tibial disease may also increase the durability of SFA angioplasty.[43] Early failure of PTA is predicted on the length of the lesion, while runoff integrity predicts long-term success.

Intimal or Subintimal Traversal Technique

Irrespective of stenosis or occlusion, high initial technical success rates can be achieved with current technology for short lesions. The use of hydrophilic wires allows the traversal of any occlusion. The wire shape and resistance as it traverses the lesion, coupled with the contour of the balloon on inflation, distinguishes an intimal from subintimal traversal (Figure 9b-7). Intimal traversal uses the tip of the wire to steer through the occlusion. Thus, the balloon has a "waist" at the site of atherosclerotic plaque (Figure 9b-9). Subintimal traversal pushes a loop of the wire under the plaque proximally and reenters the true lumen distal to the plaque. This balloon is smooth in contour on inflation, without the "waist" of the plaque (Figure 9b-8). Subintimal traversal, even unintentional, occurs commonly when crossing occlusions. Therefore, the subintimal technique is not as dependent on the length of the lesion as on the presence of a normal artery proximal and distal to the occlusion. The fibrous cap at the proximal end of an occlusion can be difficult to penetrate with a guide wire. The stiffness of the wire tip becomes an important variable since the wire stiffness needs to be greater than the force needed to penetrate the cap or else it will slip into the subintimal space. Wires with penetrating forces of 12 to 20 cm have been produced (Conquest or Conquest Pro [Confianza], Asahi Intec, Seto, Japan) that enable luminal traversal of difficult peripheral occlusions.[44]

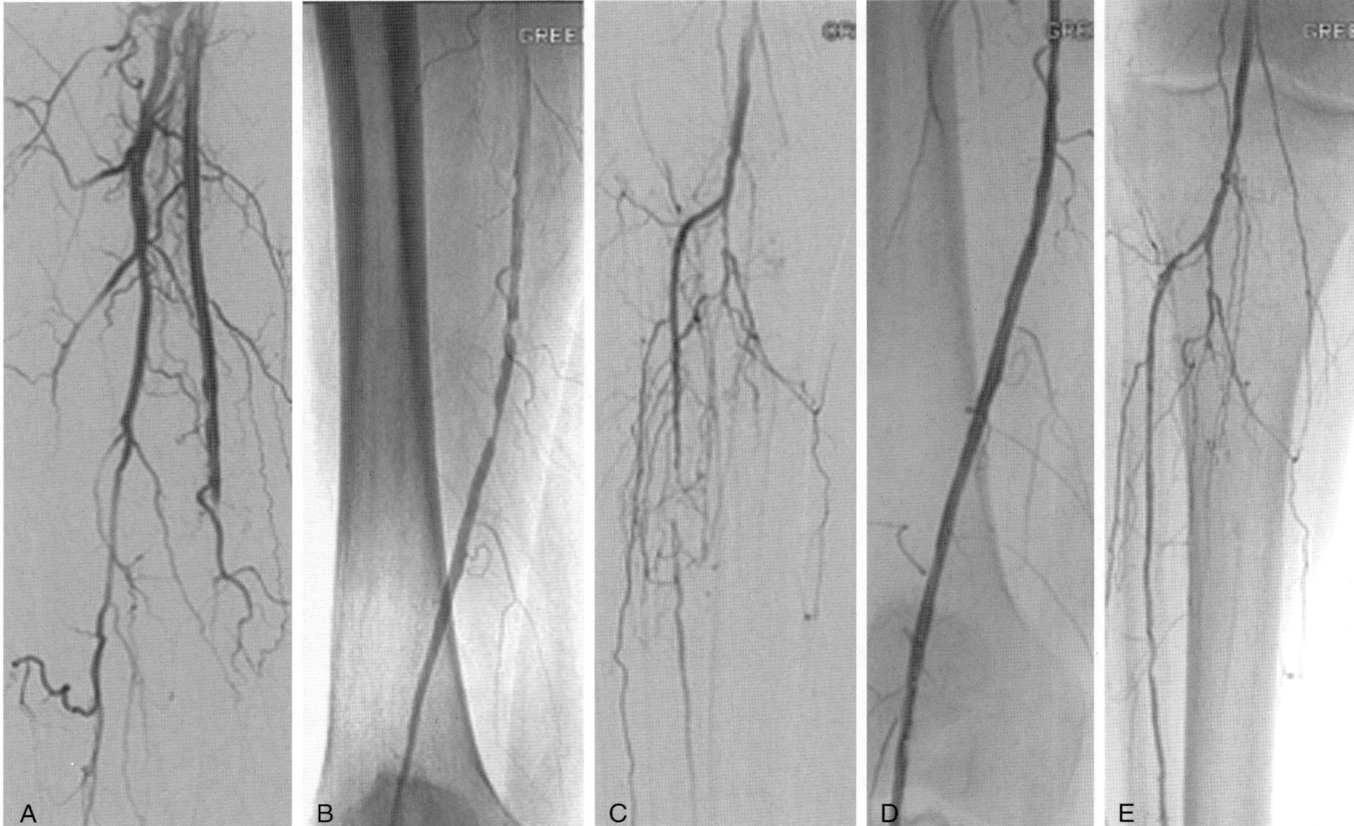

Figure 9b-11. Arteriographic example of a patient with critical limb ischemia and a right superficial femoral artery (SFA) occlusion **(A)** with reconstitution **(B)** and all tibial arteries occluded **(C).** SFA after percutaneous transluminal angioplasty (PTA) **(D)** and tibial PTA **(E).** Treatment of the tibial lesion is required to reestablish direct flow to the foot (Graziani class 6).

Standard PTA

Most femoropopliteal studies are composed of patients with claudication rather than CLI. In general, PTA of lesions less than 5 cm in length has a patency of 59% to 93% at 1 year.[45-49] SFA patency is also influenced by the quality of the runoff. Patency was 78% at 3 years after PTA in lesions less than 5 cm when two to three tibial vessels were patent versus 25% when zero to one tibial vessel was patent, emphasizing the importance of patent tibial vessels.[43] In a population of CLI patients, Jeans et al. noted that occlusions (31%) had a lower patency rate than stenoses (61%) at 5 years when the initial technical success rate was included.[45] Analysis after exclusion of these initial technical failures showed that the durability was unchanged by the presence of an occlusion.

Blair et al. conducted a retrospective study comparing PTA with bypass surgery in CLI patients.[46] Clinical improvement was seen in 72% (39 of 44) of PTA patients, with limb salvage of 78%. Bypass surgery patency was 68% at 2 years, with limb salvage of 90%. Hemodynamic benefit was better with bypass surgery, but limb salvage rates were not statistically different. Reintervention rates were higher with PTA as compared to bypass surgery. This study supports the contention that, despite late restenosis of the PTA-treated patients, the clinical impact on limb salvage is not substantially different. Lofberg et al. studied 92 CLI patients who underwent femoropopliteal PTA. The technical success rate was 88%, with primary patency of 32% for lesions less than 5 cm. Limb salvage was 86% and survival only 51% at 5 years.[47] Jamsen et al. reported on 100 consecutive CLI patients treated with femoropopliteal PTA.[48] Lifelong follow-up of each patient revealed that 32 patients underwent repeat PTA, 11 surgical revascularization, and 51 (37 major) amputations. Limb salvage was 65%, 60%, and 60% while survival rates were 41%, 26%, and 16% at 3, 5, and 8 years, respectively. This high mortality rate, secondary to cardiovascular causes, makes endovascular therapy appealing for TASC-A, TASC-B, and TASC-C lesions, even if secondary procedures are necessary.

Unsuccessful PTA occurs secondary to heavily calcified eccentric stenoses, extensive dissection, acute thrombosis, perforation, atheroemboli, or significant residual stenosis (Figure 9b-12). Acute closure due to dissection, thrombosis, or both can occur in 4% to 7%[49] (Figure 9b-13). An important endpoint after intervention is the reestablishment of brisk pedal pulses. This physical examination finding corresponds to improved ankle–brachial indices and volume flow. The restenosis rate at 12 months is better (24% versus 64%) when the 24-hour postinterventional ankle–brachial index is greater than 0.9.[50] Restenosis or recoil occurs within 3 months of the procedure and is not intimal hyperplasia. Restenosis within the first year is usually due to intimal hyperplasia and recoil. Restenosis occurs in 35% to 50% of noniliac peripheral arterial angioplasties within the first year.[51]

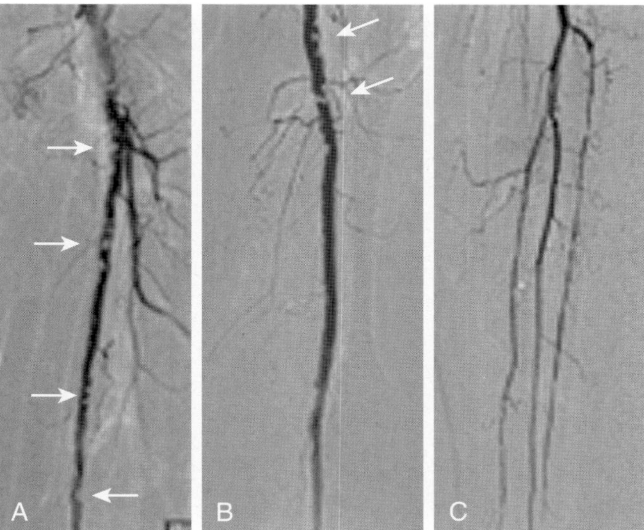

Figure 9b-12. Disease in a patient with ischemic ulceration. Note the focal areas of hard calcified atherosclerosis in the superficial femoral artery **(A)** and popliteal artery **(B)** with diffuse tibial lesions **(C)**. This popcorn-like plaque *(arrows)* does not fracture or compress well with percutaneous transluminal angioplasty. Stents also conform poorly in these types of lesions (Graziani class 1).

Long-Segment SFA PTA

Patients with CLI are often found to have long-segment occlusions of the SFA (TASC-D lesions). A study summarized the patency results after SFA intervention from the control arms (PTA-alone) of three device trials.[51] The primary patency of the 116 patients with a mean lesion length of 8.7 ± 3.1 cm (4 to 15 cm in length) was 28% at 12 months. They used a duplex ultrasound endpoint with a peak systolic velocity of more than 2.0 to define restenosis. Patency was adversely affected by lesion length, with an adverse event rate of 6.0%. They further summarized the randomized, controlled studies in the literature and found a combined 12-month primary patency rate of 37% in 191 patients treated with PTA for SFA lesions of an 8.9 cm mean length. Standalone PTA for long SFA lesions has a high incidence of restenosis and in general carries a primary patency estimate rate of 33% at 1 year.[52]

Bolia and Bell advocate intentional subintimal angioplasty for these lesions. They report an initial technical success of 80% in 200 patients (mean lesion length 11.5 cm, range 2 to 37 cm).[53] Life table analysis excluding technical failures revealed primary patency rates of 71% and 58% at 1 and 3 years, respectively. There were 2 major (1%) and 13 minor (6.5%) complications, with a 30-day mortality rate of 1.5%. These results are impressive; however, this technique may not be unique to this study. Unintentional subintimal traversal of SFA occlusions is common; thus, any study that includes the treatment of long SFA occlusions probably includes this technique.

Cryoplasty or Cold Balloon PTA

In an attempt to improve on the restenosis rate of plain balloon angioplasty, cryoplasty has been used. It involves the cooling of a balloon to −10° C using liquid nitrous oxide for inflation. The PolarCath (Boston Scientific, Natick, Massachusetts) is available in sizes to treat any infrainguinal artery. The proposed advantages of "cryo" are improved plaque modification, less elastic recoil, and induction of smooth muscle apoptosis, all of which could limit dissection and lower restenosis.[54] Comparative trials have not been done to substantiate these potential advantages. Cryo costs at least three times more, takes more time in inflate and deflate, and has less dilating force than conventional balloons. Until comparative data are available, the disadvantages outweigh the advantages.

Drug-Coated Balloon PTA

New data are emerging on the combination of balloon angioplasty and local delivery of an antirestenotic drug (i.e., sirolimus or paclitaxel).[55] Tepe et al. reported their experience with the local delivery of paclitaxel (3 ug/cm^2) at the site of SFA angioplasty in 154 patients. The mean lesion length was 7.4 cm, and the patients were followed with arteriography at 6 months and then duplex ultrasound at 12 and 24 months. The study design also included a group treated with uncoated balloon angioplasty (control group) and a group treated with uncoated balloon angioplasty with paclitaxol mixed in the contrast medium at a dose of 17.1 mg per 100 ml of contrast. The results showed a markedly improved patency rate when the drug was delivered locally and a significant reduction in target lesion revascularization at 24 months. If these data are consistent and reproducible, the treatment of SFA disease will be greatly affected. It will relegate stenting to recurrent lesions, make atherectomy a historical technique, and cause an industrywide frenzy for the next best antiproliferative drug.

Atherectomy

Atherectomy—rotational, directional, or ablational (laser)—catheters are designed to remove plaque. This debulking strategy, used as a standalone procedure or concomitantly with PTA, has not improved the results of PTA alone for infrainguinal intervention.[53,56-58]

Directional atherectomy (i.e., Simpson Atherocath, DVI, Redwood, California) consists of a circular cutting blade that excises plaque when pressed against the diseased side of the arterial wall with an inflated balloon on the backside of the catheter. The retained tissue samples are removed, debulking the lesion, and can be evaluated histologically. The depth of cutting with this device is difficult to control, often debulking to the media, which increases the risk of intimal hyperplasia. Restenosis rates at 6 months range to 65%.[56] This technique is more time consuming than PTA, requires a larger sheath, cannot remove heavily calcified plaque, and must be done ipsilateral to the lesion. These disadvantages have limited the use of atherectomy to removal of eccentric short focal lesions or retained valve cusps.

The SilverHawk plaque excision system (eV3, Minneapolis, Minnesota) is a newer generation of the DVI catheter. This catheter reportedly reduces the barotrauma of the earlier-generation device by eliminating the eccentric balloon. The rotational cutting blade is exposed to the wall of the artery on activation and advancement of the catheter. A ribbon of plaque is collected in the nose cone of the catheter. Multiple passes in various planes or quadrants lead to luminal enlargement. At least seven sizes are available for use in the SFA, popliteal, and tibial arteries. Several collection nose cones are

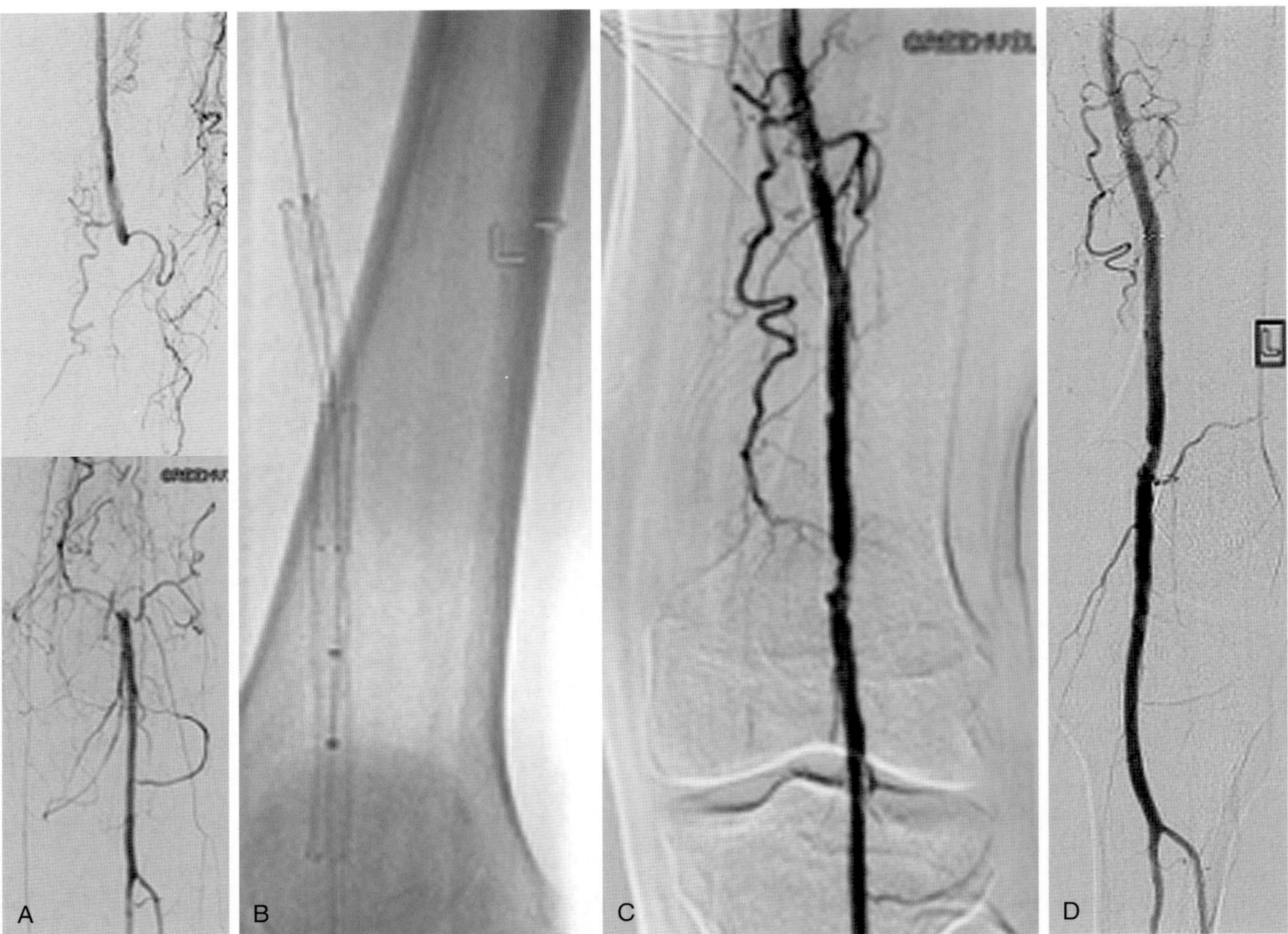

Figure 9b-13. **A, B,** A 76-year-old with occlusion of stents in the proximal left popliteal artery. **C,** Treated with Possis thrombectomy with some residual thrombus. **D,** Four hours of thrombolytic therapy showed complete resolution with residual stenosis in the midpopliteal segment.

also available for extra tissue collection and easier cleanout through flushing.

Raj et al. evaluated the SilverHawk in 25 consecutive patients with de novo stenotic SFA lesions.[57] Intravascular ultrasound was performed before and after atherectomy. Plaque was characterized, and overall plaque burden was quantified. Overall, an 11% decrease was found in plaque burden, from 64% to 53%, and a 6.3% increase was seen in luminal diameter. This catheter is unable to detect the depth of atherectomy and has a potential for perforation with overly aggressive use (Figure 9b-14). Further modifications may incorporate imaging to minimize this risk. Primary and secondary patency rates at 18 months were 49% to 73% and 79% to 89%, respectively, in 84 SFA claudication patients. De novo lesions fared better than restenotic lesions.[58] A limb salvage rate of 87% at 6 months was noted in 69 patients with CLI using the SilverHawk device.[59] Distal embolization is also a concern with atherectomy, leading some to advocate the concomitant use of embolic protection devices.[60] Comparative trials have not been performed to show the real advantage over PTA.

The Transluminal Extraction Catheter (TEC; Interventional Technologies, San Diego, California), and Rotablator (Heart Technologies, Redmond, Washington) are examples of rotational atherectomy devices. A sharp cutting blade (TEC) or diamond-studded metal tip (Rotablator) spins rapidly, shaving atheroma from the vessel wall as it passes over a guide wire. The TEC device aspirates the debris, while the Rotablator sends it distally. The new channel is only as large as the catheter itself, requiring ancillary PTA. Of initially successful procedures, 30% to 40% fail within the first 6 months, limiting the enthusiasm for debulking.[57] A newer-generation TEC-type catheter is the Pathway Medical PV (Pathway Medical Technologies, Redmond, Washington), which uses rotating scraping blades with ports between that allow flushing and aspiration during activation. And the new version of the Rotablator is the Orbital Atherectomy System (Cardiovascular Systems, St. Paul, Minnesota). This places the diamond-tipped burr in an off-center wire channel so that rotation causes a wider orbital path. Conceptually, this can lead to a larger lumen, greater flow, and improved patency. Data are forthcoming to determine the efficacy and safety of each device. The use of these atherectomy catheters will probably be in the infrapopliteal arteries and not in the SFA.

Laser-assisted angioplasty has had resurgence since technical improvements of pulsed (rather than continuous) light, use in a saline medium, and slow, gradual progression through

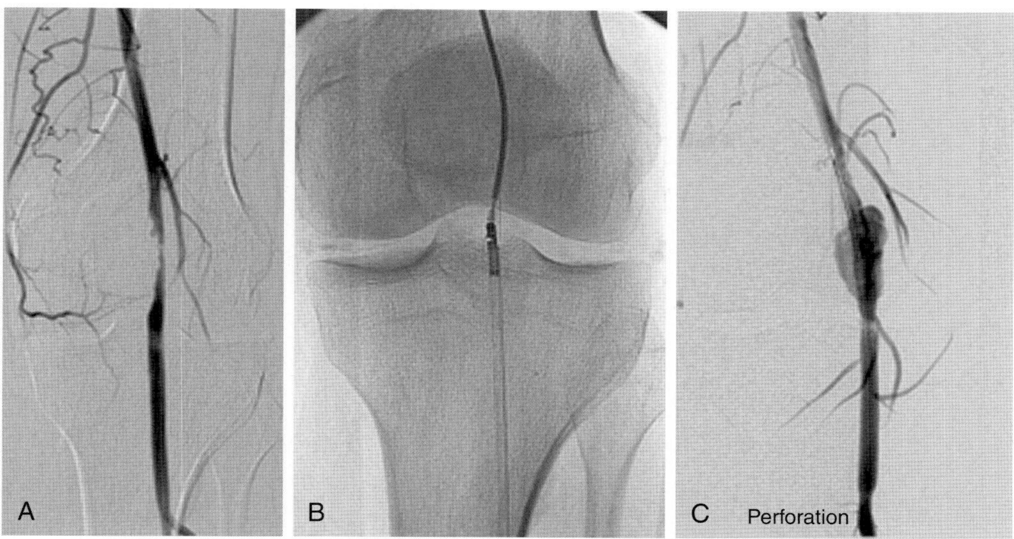

Figure 9b-14. **A,** Arteriogram of left popliteal artery stenosis (Trans-Atlantic Inter-Society Consensus II A lesion). **B,** SilverHawk directional atherectomy catheter. **C,** Perforation of popliteal artery after the third pass.

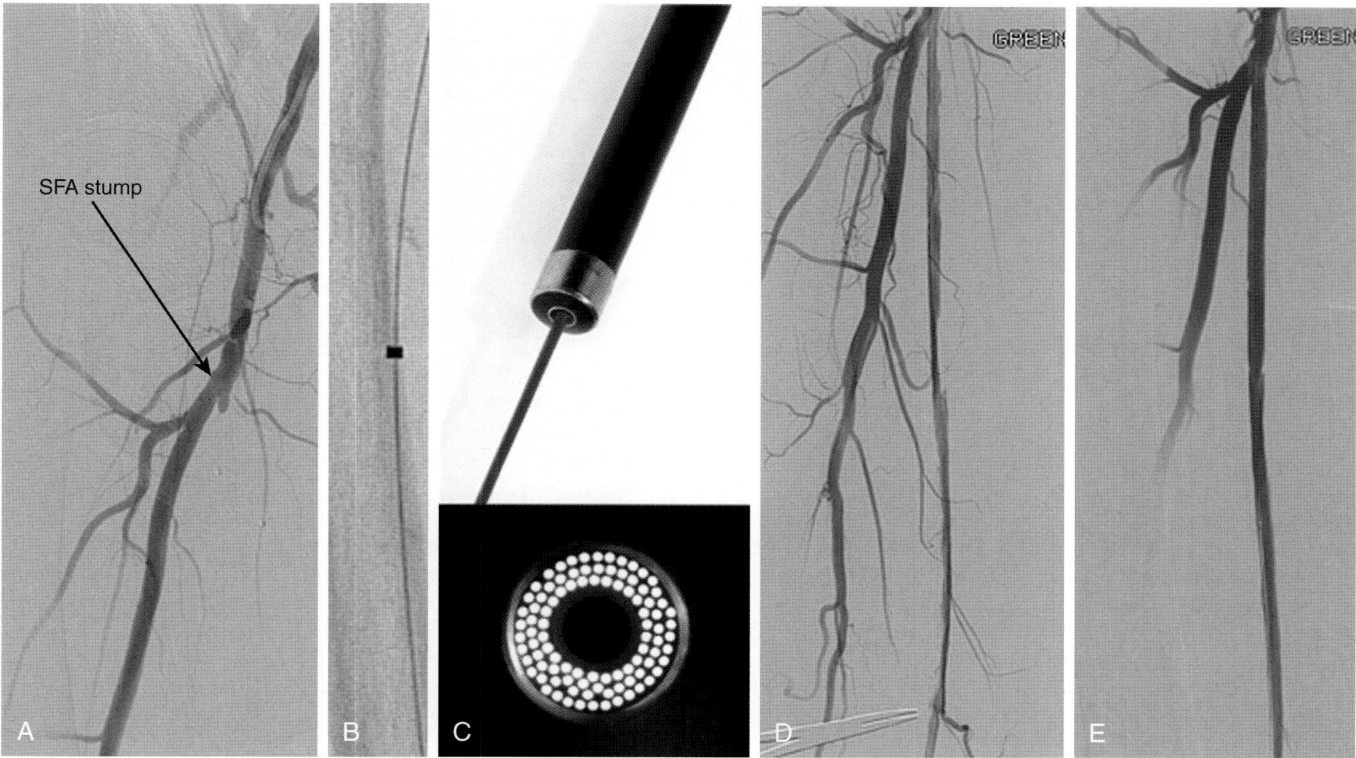

Figure 9b-15. Arteriogram of a long superficial femoral artery occlusion **(A).** After Excimer laser **(B, C)** atherectomy, a nice channel is produced **(D),** as it also is after percutaneous transluminal angioplasty without stenting **(E).**

the lesion. The use of pulsed light allows the heat to dissipate, minimizing thermal injury seen with earlier-generation lasers. The laser procedure is performed with continuous saline infusion. This limits dissections caused by acoustic trauma induced in a contrast or blood-filled medium. Excimer-laser (308 nm) light resolves chronic thrombus and some plaque without producing thermal injury. PTA after laser therapy can produce an excellent channel without a stent (Figure 9b-15). Laser-assisted angioplasty was performed in 411 patients with SFA occlusions averaging 19.5 cm in length.[61] The initial technical success rate was 83% from the contralateral approach, but the rate improved to 93% when a second access site (ipsilateral or popliteal) was used. The primary, primary-assisted, and secondary patency rates were 33%, 65%, and 75%, respectively. Stents were used in only 7.3% of patients. Restenosis usually occurred in a focal area, predictably at the site of greatest plaque burden.

Table 9b-1
Results of Three Randomized Superficial Femoral Artery Nitinol Stent Trials*

	Study Name		
Variable	**Schillinger[69]**	**FAST[68]**	**RESILIENT[70]**
Type	SC, R, Pros	MC, R, Pros	MC, R, Pros
Stent	Guidant Absolute	Bard Luminexx	Edwards LifeStent
Ischemia	Claudication	Claudication	Claudication
Number of patients	104	244	206
PTA	53	121	72
Stent	51	123	134
Mean lesion length			
PTA	127 mm	46 mm	<150 mm
Stent	132 mm	44 mm	<150 mm
Procedural success			
PTA	68%	79%	72%
Stent	93%	95%	86%
Restenosis rate (12/24 months)			
PTA	63%/74%	39%/NA	62%/NA
Stent	37%/49%	32%/NA	20%/NA
Conclusion	PS > SS	PS = SS	PS > SS

*MC, multicenter; NA, not applicable; Pros, prospective; PS, primary stenting; PTA, percutaneous transluminal angioplasty; R, randomized; SC, single center; SS, secondary stenting.

Repeat PTA or PTA with spot stenting was used for secondary intervention, producing high secondary patency rates. Acute reocclusion, perforation, distal thrombosis, or embolization occurred in only 7.1% of patients. This study highlights the benefit of laser assistance to simplify long occlusions by removing coexistent thrombus before PTA. Secondary procedures are common but lead to reasonable results in these long lesions.

The evidence to date, mostly single-center observational studies, does not support the routine use of atherectomy or any debulking strategy, like laser, for SFA lesions. Niche uses may include lesions at bifurcations, retained valve cusps in bypass grafts, or areas in which a no-stent strategy (i.e., popliteal artery) is preferred.

Bare Metal Stents

Both balloon-expandable and self-expanding stents have been used in the SFA. Balloon-expandable stents can be deformed from trauma or external compression, making self-expanding stents preferred.[62] Stents can be placed at the time of successful angioplasty (direct or primary stenting) or with failed angioplasty (secondary stenting). Three randomized trials in patients with short femoropopliteal lesions have shown no improvement in long-term success after primary nonnitinol stent placement as compared to PTA alone. Two small trials randomized PTA with PTA and balloon-expandable stents. They showed a 1-year PTA patency of 63% to 85% compared to 62% to 63% with stenting.[63,64] The largest randomized PTA versus PTA–stent trial using the Vascucoil (Intratherapeutics, Minnesota), consisted of 267 patients with 368 lesions. The mean lesion length was 3.5 cm with randomization to standalone PTA or PTA plus stent. Acute angiographic success rates were 94% with PTA and 98% with PTA plus stent. Restenosis rates at 9 months were 43% with PTA versus 46% with PTA plus stent. The complication rates were higher in the PTA (8.4%) group as compared to the stent group (1.5%).[65] Based on these data, the U.S. Food and Drug Administration approved the use of these stents for failed angioplasty (secondary stenting). There was no statistical difference to advocate the use of primary stenting for short-segment SFA lesions. Cost-effectiveness analysis also suggests that these favorable lesions should be treated with PTA initially.[66,67]

Three trials have since been published that provide randomization data between PTA and PTA with stenting using contemporary nitinol stents. The Femoral Artery Stenting Trial (FAST Trial), Schillinger SFA stent trial, and the Resilient Trial were conducted in a prospective, randomized protocol[68-70] (Table 9b-1). The FAST trial did not show benefit of stenting at a 12-month follow-up. This study used the Bard Luminexx stent that has been shown in the Femoral Stenting in Obstructions trial to have a high fracture rate.[71] The Schillinger and Resilient trials showed benefit to primary stenting at 12 and 24 months using the Dynalink/Absolute and Edwards Lifestent NT, respectively. Both of these stents have been less prone to fracture. In general, sustained benefit to primary stenting has been shown in longer rather than shorter lesions and in patients with claudication rather than CLI. Quality of life and improved functional capacity have also been favorably affected with primary stenting.[68-70]

Stent fracture is more common in longer stented segments (more than 80 mm), in areas of stent overlap, and in arterial segments subjected to more longitudinal, bending, and torsional forces, such as the popliteal artery (Figures 9b-16 and 9b-17). Stent fracture is based on the ability of the stent to handle axial compression. Stiffer stents fracture more easily when placed in the SFA.[71] Fracture is associated with restenosis, which may or may not be hemodynamically significant. The currently available nitinol stents used in the SFA are open cell design. The radial force generated by the stent counteracts the elastic recoil of the artery to maintain luminal diameter. Each has a relatively similar radial force, which is considered 5 to 10 times less than balloon-expandable stents. The dilating force of a balloon is exponentially greater than a self-expanding stent.

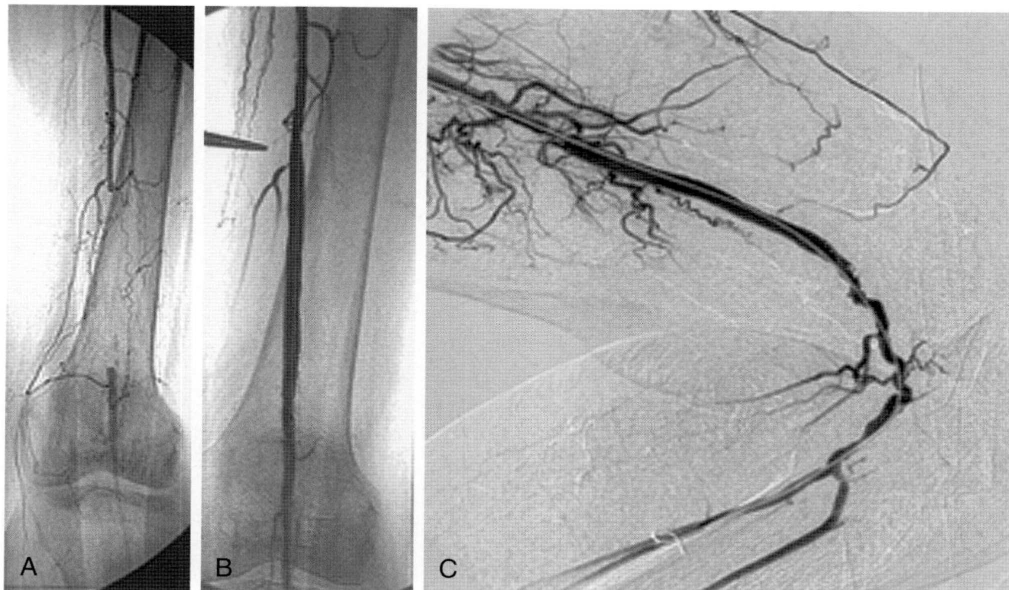

Figure 9b-16. Arteriogram of a left popliteal artery occlusion (Trans-Atlantic Inter-Society Consensus II B). Treated with percutaneous transluminal angioplasty **(A)** and stenting **(B).** Note the severe kinking in the unstented distal popliteal artery with the knee bent to 120 degrees **(C).**

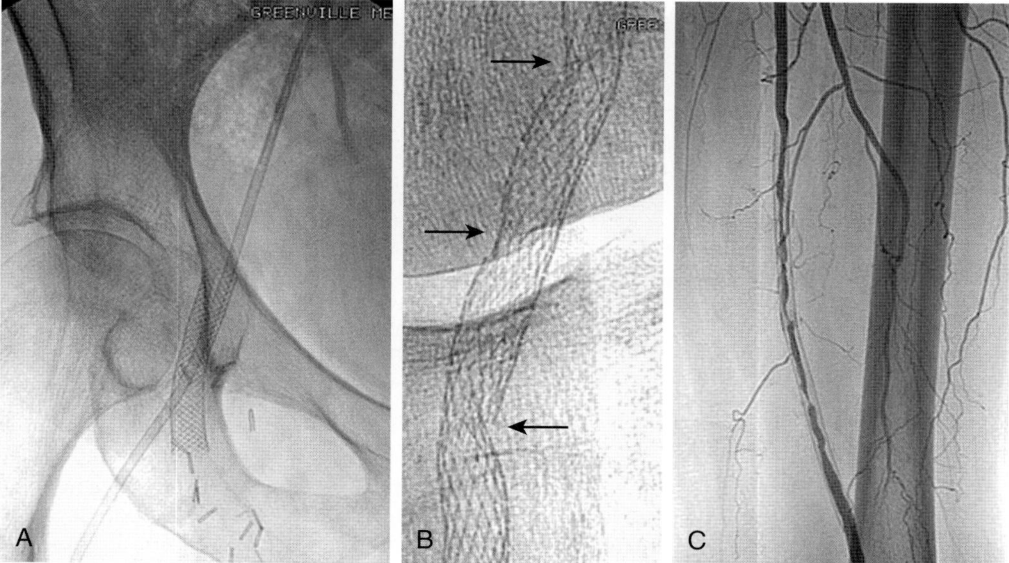

Figure 9b-17. The downside of arterial stents as demonstrated on this fluoroscopic image of a Wallstent in the right common femoral artery (CFA). **A,** The artery was then accessed percutaneously with sheath insertion. Stent placement in the CFA should be reserved for patients unable to undergo open endarterectomy. **B,** Multiple stent fractures *(arrows)* in the right popliteal artery. **C,** Diffuse in-stent restenosis in the left superficial femoral artery.

Flow dynamics through the infrainguinal arteries is different from the larger, more proximal arteries. The diseased segments are longer and resistance to flow is greater, which may increase the thrombosis risk after intervention. Early reports suggested the risk of acute stent thrombosis was as high as 25%, but as antiplatelet agents became more routine and were administered before and/or immediately afterward, the need for full anticoagulation (warfarin) was unnecessary to prevent acute thrombosis. The replacement of Wallstent with nitinol stents, which conform to the arterial wall better, may contribute to the lower risk.[72,73] Embolic protection devices may be helpful when acute thrombus is present with underlying atherosclerotic plaque (Figure 9b-18).

Since the restenosis rate is substantial, routine noninvasive laboratory testing should be performed. This is particularly true during the first year. I suggest routine duplex ultrasound surveillance every 3 months for the first year and then twice yearly thereafter. The definition of restenosis on duplex ultrasound varies. Most studies use a ratio (peak systolic velocity ratio between the stenotic segment and the normal proximal segment) of more than 2.0 to define restenosis.[51] Not all patients with restenosis have symptoms or require reintervention.

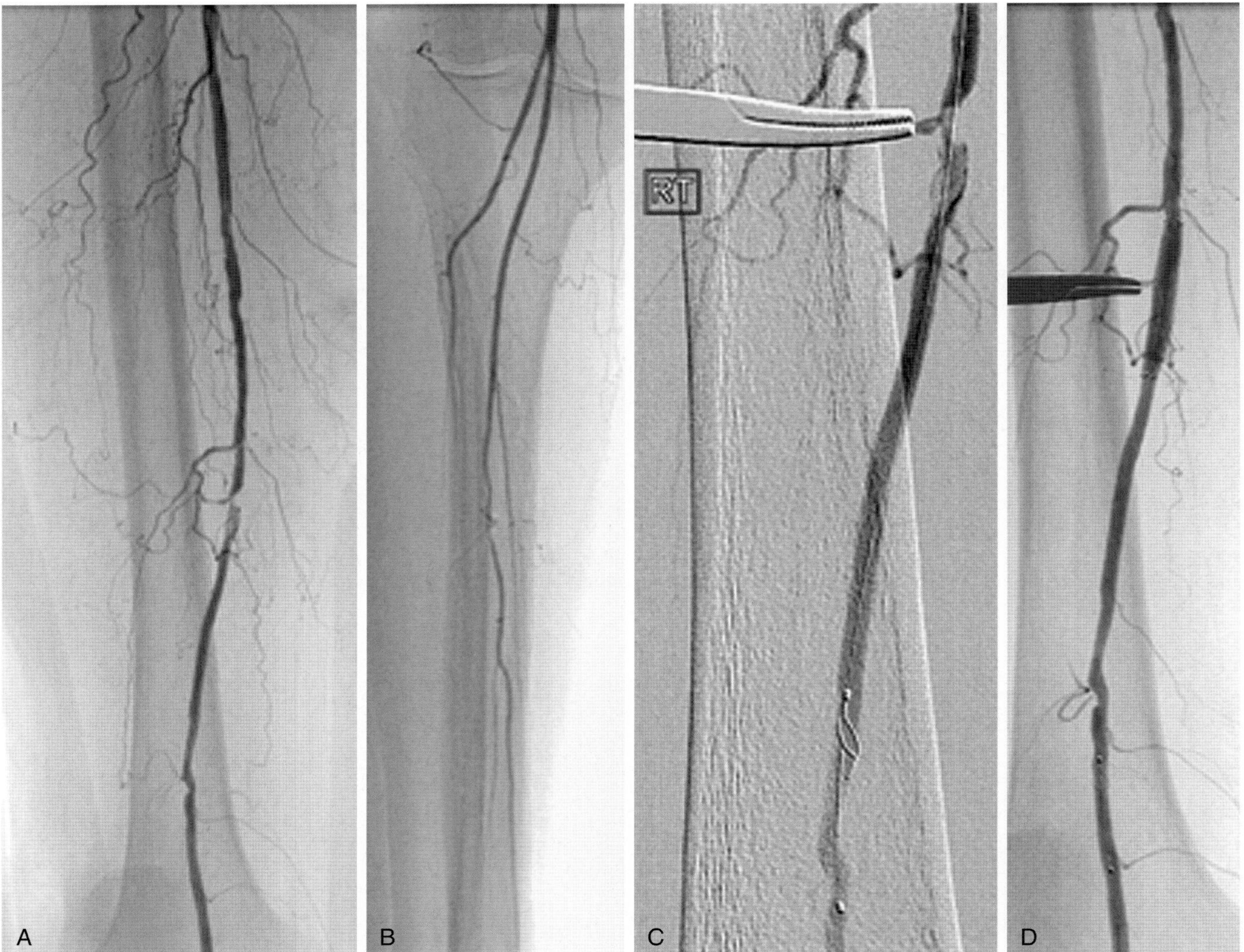

Figure 9b-18. Arteriogram of the right leg in a patient with acute change in her claudication. **A,** She was known to have a distal right superficial femoral artery stenosis, which appears to have thrombosed. **B,** Slow flow in the tibial arteries was noted, with a high takeoff of the anterior tibial artery. **C,** Embolic protection device was placed. **D,** Stenting with postdilation followed.

Drug-Eluting Stents

Drug-eluting stents (DESs) used to treat SFA disease have not met the same positive result of coronary DES. The Sirolimus Coated Cordis Smart Nitinol Self-Expandable Stent for the Treatment of SFA Disease (SIROCCO) trials used an equivalent drug dosage to that used in coronary stents (90 ug/cm^2). SIROCCO I randomized 36 SFA patients with lesions up to 20 cm in length and SIROCCO II randomized 57 patients with lesions up to 14.5 cm to either DES or the bare Smart stent. Overall, a nonsignificant trend was seen toward less in-stent restenosis in the DES group. The early benefit was lost by the 18-month follow-up duplex ultrasound. This trial also brought to light the issue of stent fracture, which occurred in six stents in SIROCCO I. The significance of fracture has been debated, but clearly patients with fracture are more likely to experience subclinical or clinical restenosis or occlusion.[74-76]

The Zilver PTX Stent Platform (Cook Medical, Bloomington, Indiana) is currently investigating polymer-free paclitaxol on Zilver stents for SFA lesions less than 14 cm in length. The dose is 3 μg/mm^2. The initial phase studied 60 patients and noted a 90% patency rate at 9 months as determined by duplex ultrasound. These encouraging results are being studied in a 420-patient cohort using a 12-month primary endpoint of event-free survival. Secondary endpoints will be 6- and 12-month patency.

The use of DES for SFA disease is investigational, and further study is warranted to determine the patients who may benefit, the proper dosage of drug, and the potential downside of treatment.

Covered Stents

Stent

Grafts have been used in the femoropopliteal distribution. Early devices such as the Dacron-covered nitinol stent (Cragg EndoPro System 1) were plagued by acute thrombosis in 17%, postimplantation pain and fever in 40%, and late failure in 83%.[77] The Hemobahn (Viabahn) polytetrafluoroethylene

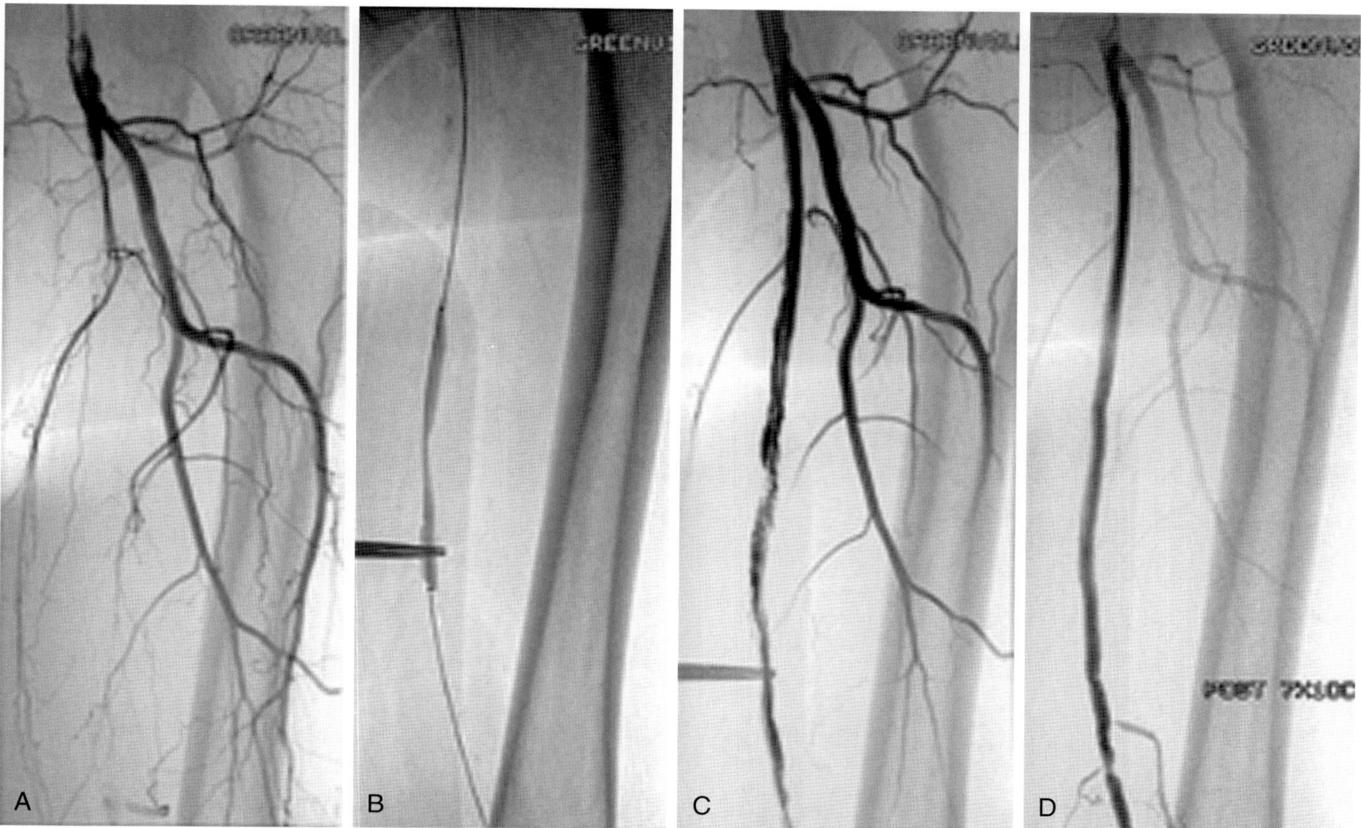

Figure 9b-19. Long superficial femoral artery occlusion **(A)** treated with percutaneous transluminal angioplasty **(B, C)** followed by Viabahn stent grafting **(D)**.

(PTFE) or nitinol stent graft has fewer thrombotic events, fewer postimplantation symptoms, and better patency rates, although these complications are not rare.[78,79] Primary and secondary patency rates at 4 years were 55% and 79%, respectively, in a study of 87 limbs in 76 patients. Lesion length did not affect patency, but smaller luminal diameter (less than 4.5 mm) was the strongest negative predictor. The stent prevents negative remodeling and may offer a distinct advantage over bare-stenting long SFA lesions. The Viabahn handles the axial compression forces of the SFA well, minimizing fracture and mechanical failure risk. Edge stenosis occurs in 13.6% of limbs, so Saxon et al suggest extending the Viabahn into larger disease-free segments of the artery.[80]

Despite the lower thrombogenicity of PTFE compared to Dacron, Fischer et al. noted a significant thrombotic risk as he studied 60 limbs (mean lesion length 10.7 cm). The 30-day risk of thrombosis was 10%; risk was 24% at 1 year and increased to 37% at 5 years after Viabahn placement. Nonideal candidates included patients with heavy SFA calcification in which the postdilation diameter is less than 6 mm, patients with entire SFA occlusions, and those patients who were noncompliant with aspirin therapy in follow-up.[81] Recent approval of heparin-coated PTFE Viabahn stent grafts may improve on this thrombotic tendency. Heparin is covalently bonded to the graft and has been shown to improve patency in PTFE bypass grafts. Despite the chronic exposure of the patient to heparin, no significant cases of heparin-induced thrombocytopenia have been reported. No comparative data are available to date.

Viabahn Stent

Grafts carry the highest patency in the literature for long SFA lesions treated with endovascular techniques. However, the cost of these devices is significant. A recent single-center trial randomized patients to an above-prosthetic bypass graft compared to the Viabahn device.[82] They were equivalent in patency with less morbidity in the Viabahn group, suggesting an expanded role for endovascular intervention in long SFA lesions using this device. These devices should not be oversized by more than 5% to 10% to avoid infolding and possible graft collapse.[83] Aggressive postimplantation angioplasty may minimize this risk. Angiographically, the results of stent grafting diffuse SFA disease are quite appealing (Figure 9b-19).

Brachytherapy

Endovascular brachytherapy treatment after PTA to prevent restenosis has shown mixed results to date. The need for γ-radiation over β-radiation, lack of an adequate centering catheter, coordination of radiation delivery outside of an angiography suite, and lack of convincing randomized trials (both coronary and peripheral) have lessened the enthusiasm for this technology. The Pediatric Amblyopia Risk Investigational Study used an iridium-192 γ-radiation source with a prescribed dose of 14 Gy in 40 patients with SFA lesions averaging almost 10 cm in length.[84] The angiographic restenosis rate at 6 months was 17%, and the clinical restenosis rate at 12 months was 13%. Brachytherapy has also been used after

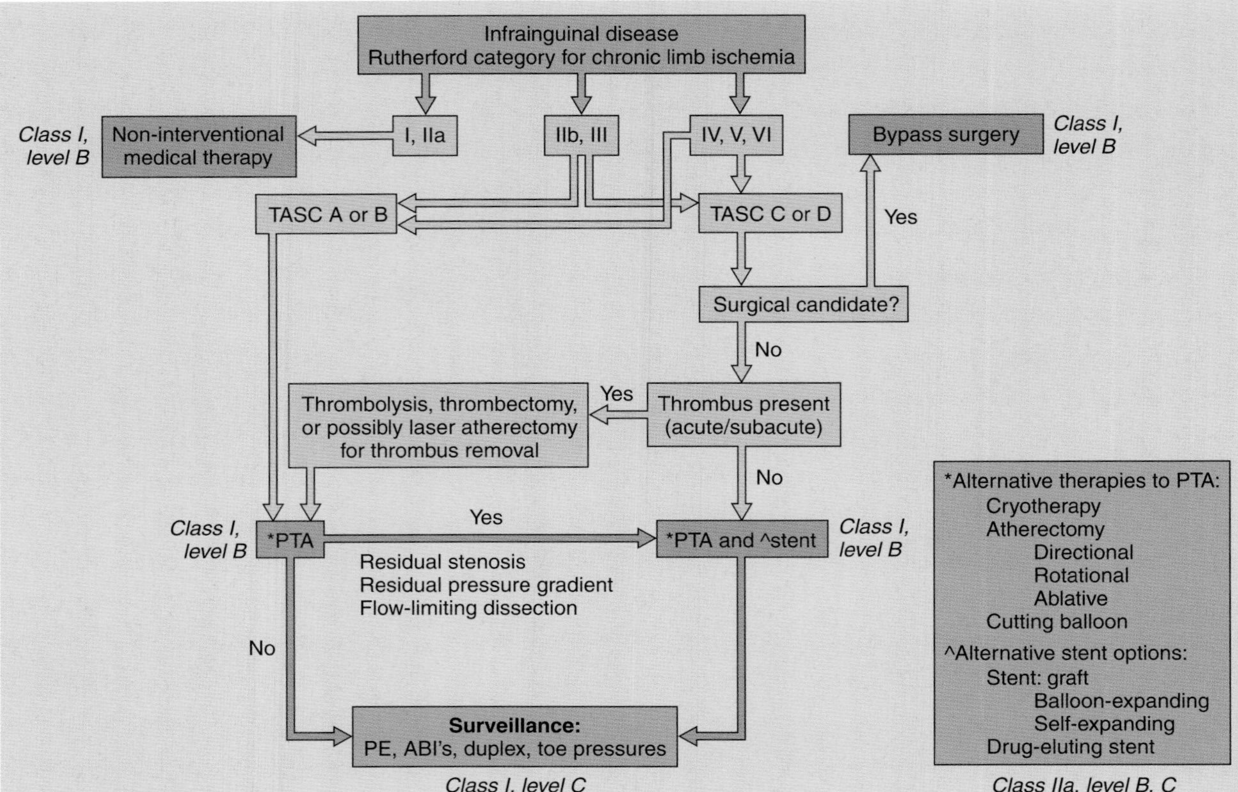

Figure 9b-20. Simplified treatment algorithm of symptomatic infrainguinal peripheral arterial disease, assuming concomitant aortoiliac disease has been treated and the patient is an acceptable candidate for revascularization.

stenting in a small study of 33 patients, with an average lesion length of 12 cm and a stent length of 17 cm.[85] At 6 months, 70% (23 of 33 arteries) were considered patent. Of the 10 early failures, 7 had sudden thrombotic occlusion and were treated with fibrinolysis. Only 4 of the 33 arteries (12%) had in-stent restenosis due to intimal hyperplasia.

Summary of SFA and Popliteal Artery Intervention

Patients with symptomatic infrainguinal disease should be considered for endovascular therapy. The lesions should be classified according to the TASC II document and treated accordingly. Angioplasty remains the mainstay treatment, with stenting primarily for longer lesions and secondarily for shorter lesions. Debulking strategies have not improved outcomes and should be reserved for special cases. Restenosis remains the Achilles' heel of intervention despite aggressive pharmacological cotherapy. Frequent follow-up with noninvasive studies is warranted to maintain acceptable primary-assisted and secondary patency rates (Figure 9b-20).[86]

TIBIAL ARTERY INTERVENTION

Typically, patients with CLI have multilevel disease. The mortality of this population is predicated on the extent of cardiovascular disease. Also, a worsening ankle–brachial index, an elevated serum creatinine, and the presence of renal artery stenosis negatively correlate with prognosis.

About 8% of patients have hemodynamically significant lesions involving the iliac, femoral, and tibial arteries. Of these, 60% present with femoral and tibial disease and 32% have isolated tibial disease.[87] The incidence of diabetes is 60% to 70% in the general CLI population and serves as a reference to the studied population. The TASC II document provides a grading scheme for the femoropopliteal segment but falls short of classifying multilevel disease in CLI patients. Graziani et al. proposed an arteriographic classification system based on concomitant SFA and tibial disease.[88] They used seven categories (Figure 9b-21). The seven classes of disease show a progressive involvement with a corresponding drop in the baseline transcutaneous oxygen level.

Patient Selection for Tibial Intervention

The general rule for revascularization in patients with CLI is to reestablish direct pulsatile flow to the foot via at least one tibial artery. So, those patients with ischemic rest pain, ulceration, or gangrene (Rutherford categories 4, 5, and 6, respectively) and with disease that prevents direct pulsatile flow to the foot should be considered candidates for revascularization. Those with extensive necrosis requiring amputation, bedridden patients with gangrene, or those with a short life expectancy secondary to comorbid conditions should undergo primary amputation. The selection of an open bypass procedure versus an endovascular procedure involves the balance of patient risk, presence of autologous vein, expected durability of the endovascular procedure, experience of the operator or team, and to a lesser degree, preference of the patient.

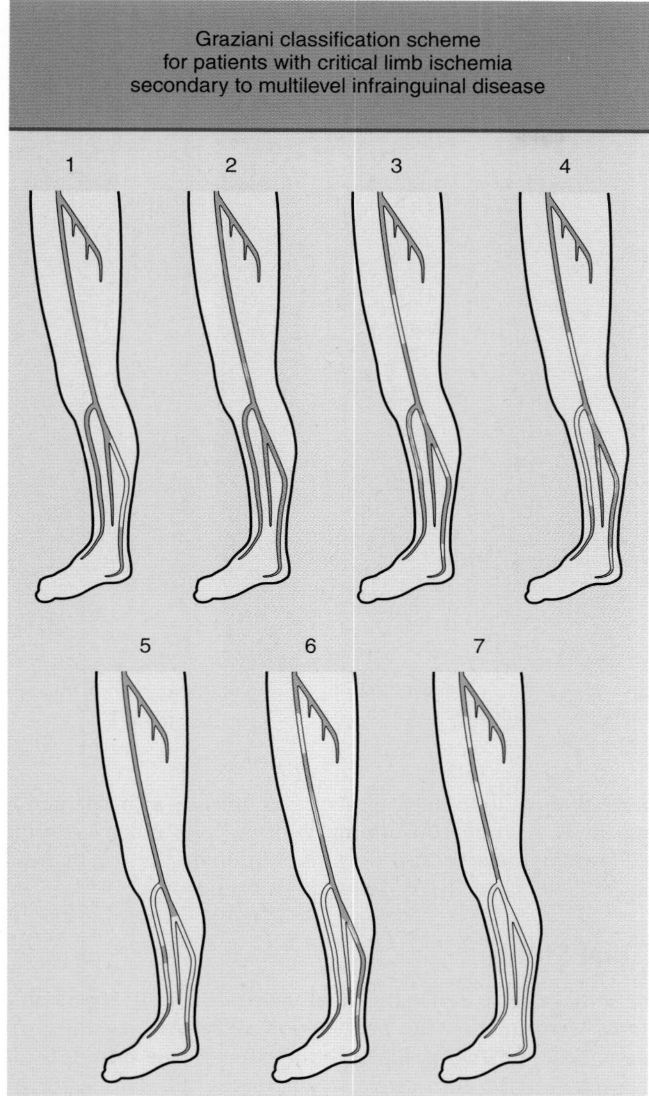

Figure 9b-21. Graziani classification scheme for patients with critical limb ischemia secondary to multilevel disease. (From Graziani L, et al. *Eur J Vasc Endovasc Surg* 2007;33:453-460.)

The accurate arterial assessment using noninvasive vascular testing can be challenging in patients with arterial calcification and multilevel disease. Segmental pressure measurements can miss moderate stenoses in the iliac segment, cannot discriminate arterial stenosis from occlusion, and can provide falsely elevated readings in calcified arteries. Pulse volume recordings are limited by concomitant disease since severe proximal disease affects the assessment of distal vascular beds. Toe pressure measurements using a small plethysmographic flow sensor help establish distal systolic pressure in patients with noncompressible tibial arteries. The toe pressure is normally 30 mm Hg less than the ankle pressure and can be used to predict healing potential and to serially follow the quality of the circulation.[7] Transcutaneous oxygen monitoring can also be performed serially and used to indirectly assess for healing potential (ideal $TcPO_2$ more than 50).

Treatment Approach and Anatomical Principles

The treatment of hemodynamically significant lesions in the largest inflow vessels should take preference over the smaller, more distal lesions. Often, suprainguinal lesions can be treated at a separate session and ischemia can be reevaluated. Persistent ischemia would then require the additional treatment of the outflow vessels. These infrainguinal lesions can then be treated to reestablish direct flow to the foot. Superficial femoral and popliteal lesions are usually treated simultaneously with tibial lesions. Not all tibial lesions need to be treated, and selecting the tibial artery with the best distal reconstitution should be the target of choice. The complexity of the lesion also dictates treatment since a stenosis, even in a less dominant artery, may take precedence over a long occlusion in a dominant one. Multiple tibial arteries can be treated (if acceptable risk) when feasible to maximize direct flow to the foot.

The access site of choice should minimize aortoiliac angles and tortuosity, be a relatively disease-free puncture site, be close to the treatment site, and be able to handle sheath diameter to minimize disruption of flow before, during, and after treatment. Consequently, using an antegrade approach to the CFA would allow the best access for most tibial interventions. Obesity, groin scar, or infection may force use of the contralateral CFA or a remote site (popliteal, pedal) for arterial entry. Antegrade access site closure can be performed with various devices and minimizes the need for extrinsic compression of the access site after intervention.

Treatment Options

Patients with CLI and multilevel disease are often treated with multiple techniques and devices. This makes analysis of any one particular technique or device problematic. Studies describing the impact of one modality are not representative of the treatment necessary to fix multilevel disease. Many studies fail to report patency rates and merely use amputation-free survival to demonstrate efficacy. Furthermore, randomized, comparative, device, or technical trials are lacking. This leaves the interventionalist with a need to "try" everything and make a personal assessment.

PTA can be performed with a plain, cutting, scoring, or cryoplasty balloon and remains the most commonly used technique for infrapopliteal lesions. Faglia et al. reported on 84% of 1191 diabetic patients with CLI who were treated with plain balloon PTA and provisional stenting. Over a median follow-up of 23 months, the amputation rate was only 1.7%. The clinical recurrence rate was 11.3%, with a 5-year cumulative patency rate of 88%. Of the original patients, 157 were treated with bypass surgery (13.2%), with an 8.3% major amputation rate. That left 47 patients without revascularization, of which 34% underwent major amputation.[87]

The cutting balloon (Boston Scientific, Natick, Massachusetts) consists of surgical microtomes mounted on the balloon. The blades mounted on the outside of the balloon focus the dilating force in four quadrants, causing more controlled trauma to the artery, which creates less dissection and plaque disruption. The cutting balloon can dilate recalcitrant lesions such as calcified stenoses, ostial lesions, bypass graft stenosis, and in-stent restenosis.[89] These lesions are commonly seen in diabetics with tibial artery calcification. Ansel et al. reported

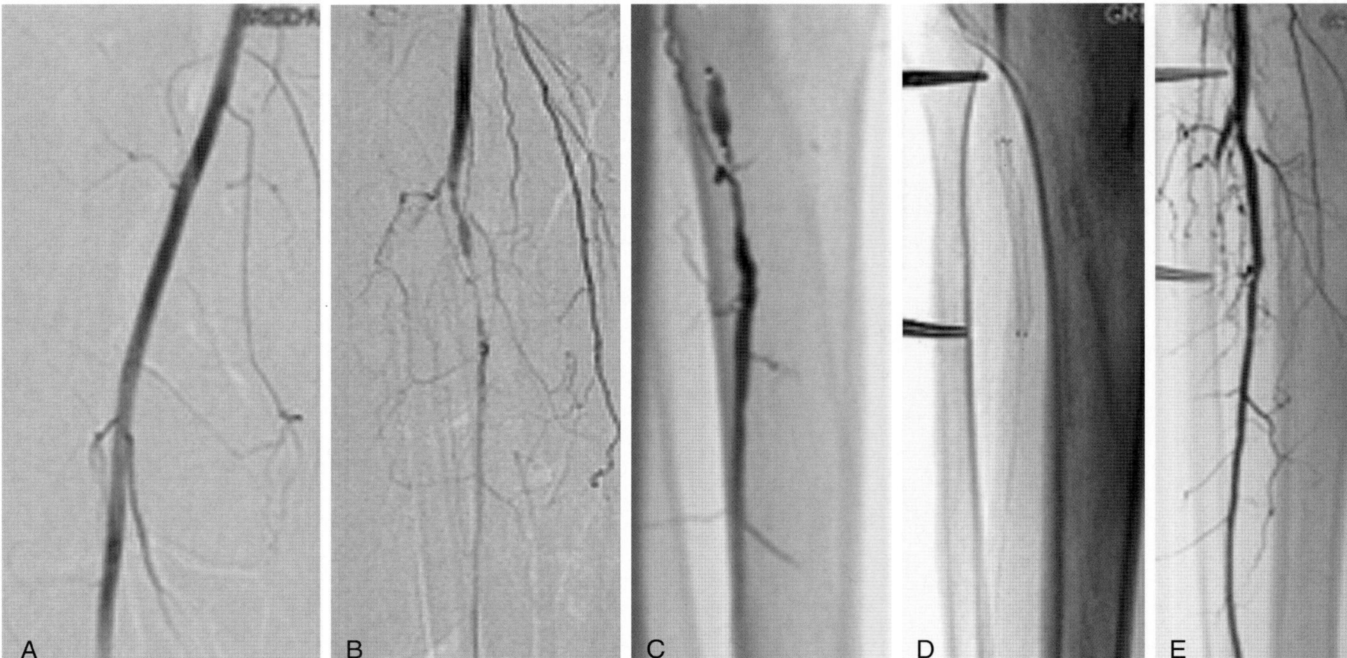

Figure 9b-22. Arteriogram. **A, B,** Arteriogram of isolated peroneal artery with stenosis with normal inflow. **C,** Selective arteriogram of stenosis. **D,** Treated with cutting balloon percutaneous transluminal angioplasty and stenting. **E,** Completion.

a 1-year limb salvage rate of 85.9% in 73 symptomatic patients treated with the cutting balloon. The need for adjunctive tibial artery stenting was 20%.[90] The crossing profile of this balloon is greater than plain balloon, and predilation is sometimes necessary to deliver the cutting balloon.

The AngioSculpt (Angioscore, Freemont, California) consists of a balloon with nitinol blades organized in a spiral configuration. The blade configuration may allow for easier lesion traversal than the cutting balloon. Scheinert et al. reported the use in tibial arteries. The technical success rate was high, with only 6 of 56 patients requiring stenting for dissection or residual stenosis. Most patients had CLI (90.5%), with a mean lesion length of 33.9 ± 42.2 mm. Patency rates were not reported.[91]

The PolarCath (Boston Scientific) uses nitrous oxide to inflate a balloon. This cools the balloon to −10° C, which conceptually minimizes dissection, arterial trauma, and the need for adjunctive stenting. Using a computerized inflation control unit, the nitrous oxide inflates the balloon to 8 atm of pressure. Deflation is via syringe aspiration. This process is completed within several minutes. The crossing profile of this balloon is greater than that of a regular balloon, but it can be used from a contralateral approach. The balloon has been studied in the Below-the-Knee Chill study. The study followed 106 patients with tibial lesions, mean lesion length of 4 cm, with a procedural success rate of 97%. They were followed for 12 months, with a limb salvage rate of 85%.[92]

Interest has been renewed in debulking tibial lesions with atherectomy with the development of the Excimer Laser, SilverHawk, Pathway Medical, and Orbital Atherectomy Systems. Each modality was described earlier. The data for the use of atherectomy for tibial disease is scant, nonrandomized, and limited to technical success and amputation-free survival. Considering the facts that atherectomy costs 4 to 12 times more than balloon angioplasty, is technically more demanding, is more time consuming, is often followed by routine balloon angioplasty, and does not eliminate the use or need of stents, it is hard to recommend its routine use.[93]

Tibial Stents

Stents have been used in the tibial arteries. Balloon-expandable stents were initially the only option since the crossing profile and diameter of self-expanding stents were nonideal for these 2.5- to 3.5-mm arteries. Scheinert et al. compared the use of sirolimus-eluting versus bare metal stents in 60 consecutive patients with infrapopliteal lesions. At 6 months follow-up, the mean degree of in-stent restenosis determined angiographically was 1.8% ± 4.8% in the sirolimus patients ($n = 27$) versus 53.0% ± 40.9% in the bare metal stent patients ($n = 26$).[94] This preliminary study suggests that DES technology may be beneficial and that balloon-expandable stents may be an acceptable alternative. A 4-Fr self-expanding nitinol stent (Xpert, Abbott Vascular, Redwood City, California) has been evaluated in 35 patients and had a arteriographic primary patency rate of 82% at 6 months[95] (Figure 9b-22). Bosiers et al. studied this same stent in 47 CLI patients and report a 12-month arteriographic primary patency rate of 76.3%.[96] These intriguing initial results will no doubt lead to further use of stents in the tibial arteries. At present, the use of provisional stenting should be limited to patients with CLI.

SUMMARY

Increasing evidence points to the effectiveness of endovascular therapy for patients with CLI. Patients who are at high risk for loss of life or limb have the most to gain with low-risk revascularization procedures. These procedures are not exclusive of traditional surgical treatment and should be viewed as complimentary. Technological advances in balloons, stents (bare, covered, coated), and pharmacotherapies allow application to a wider variety of clinical and anatomical problems. The aortoiliac component of multilevel disease should be treated initially. Patients with tissue loss require reestablishment of direct flow to the foot, which usually involves SFA and tibial revascularization. Endovascular strategies for SFA occlusions should start by removing the coexistent thrombus before treating the underlying atherosclerotic plaque. Covered or coated stents may prove useful, providing long-term benefit. After successful revascularization, close surveillance is required while maintaining a low threshold for reintervention (Figure 9b-20).

References

1. Adam DJ, Beard JD, Cleveland T, et al. Bypass versus Angioplasty in Severe Ischaemia of the Leg (BASIL): multicentre, randomized controlled trial. *Lancet* 2005;366:1925-1934.
2. Deutschmann HA, Schoellnast H, Temmel W, et al. Endoluminal therapy in patients with peripheral arterial disease: prospective assessment of quality of life in 190 patients. *AJR Am J Roentgenol* 2007;188: 169-175.
3. Nylaende M, Abdelnoor M, Stranden E, et al. The Oslo Balloon Angioplasty versus Conservative Treatment study (OBACT): the 2-years results of a single centre, prospective, randomized study in patients with intermittent claudication. *Eur J Vasc Endovasc Surg* 2007;33:3-12.
4. Golledge J, Askew C, Leicht A, et al. Outcome assessment for intermittent claudication. *Eur J Vasc Endovasc Surg* 2006;31:44-45.
5. Taylor SM, Kalbaugh CA, Blackhurst DW, et al. A comparison of percutaneous transluminal angioplasty versus amputation for critical limb ischemia in patients unsuitable for open surgery. *J Vasc Surg* 2007;45:304-310.
6. Trans-Atlantic Inter-Society Consensus Working Group. Management of peripheral arterial disease (PAD). *J Vasc Surg* 2000;31(1 Pt 2): S1-S296.
7. Norgren L, Hiatt WR, Dormandy JA, et al. Inter-Society Consensus for the management of peripheral arterial disease (TASC II). *J Vasc Surg* 2007;45(Suppl S):S5-S67.
8. Barretto S, Ballman KV, Rooke TW, Kullo IJ. Early-onset peripheral arterial occlusive disease: clinical features and determinants of disease severity and location. *Vasc Med* 2003;8:95-100.
9. Hirsch AT, Haskal ZJ, Hertzer NR, et al. ACC/AHA 2005 practice guidelines for the management of patients with peripheral arterial disease (lower extremity, renal, mesenteric, and abdominal aortic): a collaborative report from the American Association for Vascular Surgery/Society for Vascular Surgery, Society for Cardiovascular Angiography and Interventions, Society for Vascular Medicine and Biology, Society of Interventional Radiology, and the ACC/AHA Task Force on Practice Guidelines (Writing Committee to Develop Guidelines for the Management of Patients with Peripheral Arterial Disease); endorsed by the American Association of Cardiovascular and Pulmonary Rehabilitation, National Heart, Lung, and Blood Institute; Society for Vascular Nursing; Trans-Atlantic Inter-Society Consensus; and Vascular Disease Foundation. *Circulation* 2006;113:e463-e654.
10. Krajewski LP, Olin JW. Atherosclerosis of the aorta and lower-extremity arteries. In: Young JR, Olin JW, Bartholomew JR, eds. Peripheral vascular diseases. 2nd ed. St. Louis: Mosby; 1996:215-216.
11. Bandyk DF, Chauvapun JP. Duplex ultrasound surveillance can be worthwhile after arterial intervention. *Perspect Vasc Surg Endovasc Ther* 2007;19:354-359.
12. Roth SM, Bandyk DF. Duplex imaging of lower extremity bypasses, angioplasties, and stents. *Semin Vasc Surg* 1999;12:275-284.
13. Cotroneo AR, Iezzi R, Marano G, et al. Hybrid therapy in patients with complex peripheral multifocal steno-obstructive vascular disease: two-year results. *Cardiovasc Intervent Radiol* 2007;30:355-361.
14. Biondi-Zoccai GG, Agostoni P, Sangiorgi G, et al. Mastering the antegrade femoral artery access in patients with symptomatic lower limb ischemia: learning curve, complications, and technical tips and tricks. *Catheter Cardiovasc Interv* 2006;68:835-842.
15. Saha S, Gibson M, Magee TR, et al. Early results of retrograde transpopliteal angioplasty of iliofemoral lesions. *Cardiovasc Intervent Radiol* 2001;24:378-382.
16. Ansel GM, George BS, Botti CF Jr, et al. Infrapopliteal endovascular techniques: indications, techniques, and results. *Curr Interv Cardiol Rep* 2001;3:100-108.
17. Sutuo Y, Yamauchi K, Suzuki M, et al. High maneuverability guidewire with functionally graded properties using new superelastic alloys. *Minim Invasive Ther Allied Technol* 2006;15:204-208.
18. Melzi G, Cosgrove J, Biondi-Zoccai GL, et al. A novel approach to chronic total occlusions: the Crosser system. *Catheter Cardiovasc Interv* 2006;68:29-35.
19. Barth KH, Virmani R, Froelich J, et al. Paired comparison of vascular wall reactions to Palmaz stents, Strecker tantalum stents, and Wallstents in canine iliac and femoral arteries. *Circulation* 1996;93:2161-2169.
20. Zorger N, Manke C, Lenhart M, et al. Peripheral arterial balloon angioplasty: effect of short versus long balloon inflation times on the morphologic results. *J Vasc Intervent Radiol* 2002;13:355-360.
21. Soder H, Manninen HI, Rasanen HT, et al. Failure of prolonged dilation to improve long-term patency of femoropopliteal artery angioplasty: results of a prospective trial. *J Vasc Intervent Radiol* 2002;13:361-370.
22. Antithrombotic Trialists' Collaboration. Collaborative meta-analysis of randomized trials of antiplatelet therapy for prevention of death, myocardial infarction, and stroke in high risk patients. *Br Med J* 2002;324: 71-86.
23. Agnelli G. Rationale for the use of platelet aggregation inhibitors in PAD patients. *Vasc Med* 2001;6(Suppl 1):13-15.
24. CAPRIE Steering Committee. A randomized, blinded, trial of clopidogrel versus aspirin in patients at risk of ischaemic events (CAPRIE). *Lancet* 1996;348:1329-1339.
25. Lotrionte M, Biondi-Zoccai GG, Agostoni P, et al. Meta-analysis appraising high clopidogrel loading in patients undergoing percutaneous coronary intervention. *Am J Cardiol* 2007;100:1199-1206.
26. Steinhubl SR, Badimon JJ, Bhatt DL, et al. Clinical evidence for anti-inflammatory effects of antiplatelet therapy in patients with atherothrombotic disease. *Vasc Med* 2007;12:113-122.
27. Shlansky-Goldberg R. Combination therapy in peripheral vascular disease: the rationale of using both thrombolytic and antiplatelet drugs. *J Am Coll Surg* 2002;194(Suppl 1):S103-S113.
28. Duda SH, Banz K, Ouriel K, et al. Cost-effectiveness analysis of treatment of subacute peripheral artery occlusions with thrombolysis with and without adjunctive abciximab. *J Vasc Interv Radiol* 2001;21:S70.
29. Ouriel K, Vieth F, Sasahara AA. A comparison of recombinant urokinase with vascular surgery as initial treatment for acute arterial occlusion of the legs: Thrombolysis of Peripheral Arterial Surgery (TOPAS) Investigators. *N Engl J Med* 1998;338:1105-1111.
30. Weaver F, Toms C. The practical implications of recent trials comparing thrombolytic therapy with surgery for lower extremity ischemia. *Semin Vasc Surg* 1997;10:49-54.
31. Ouriel K, Gray BH, Clair DG, et al. Complications associated with the use of urokinase and recombinant tissue plasminogen activator for catheter-directed peripheral arterial and venous thrombolysis. *J Vasc Interv Radiol* 2000;11(3):295-298.
32. Earnshaw JJ, Comerota A. Towards international consensus in peripheral arterial thrombolysis. *Br J Surg* 1997;84:1332-1333.
33. Braithwaite BD, Birch PA, Poskitt KR. Accelerated thrombolysis with high dose bolus t-PA extends the role of peripheral thrombolysis but may increase the risks. *Clin Radiol* 1995;50:747-750.
34. Martin U, Kaufmann B, Neugebauer G. Current clinical use of reteplase for thrombolysis: a pharmacokinetic–pharmacodynamic perspective. *Clin Pharmacokinet* 1999;36:265-276.
35. Hanover TM, Kalbaugh CA, Gray BH, et al. Safety and efficacy of reteplase for the treatment of acute arterial occlusion: complexity of underlying lesion predicts outcome. *Ann Vasc Surg* 2005;19:817-822.
36. Koreny M, Riedmuller E, Nidfardjam M, et al. Arterial puncture closing devices compared with standard manual compression after cardiac catheterization: systematic review and meta-analysis. *JAMA* 2004;291:350-357.
37. Mackrell P, Kalbaugh CL, Langan EM 3rd, et al. Can the Perclose suture–mediated closure system be used safely in patients undergoing diagnostic and therapeutic angiography to treat chronic lower extremity ischemia? *J Vasc Surg* 2003;38:1305-1308.
38. Gray BH, Miller R, Langan EM 3rd, et al. The utility of StarClose arterial closure device in patients with peripheral arterial disease. *Ann Vasc Surg* 2008; Sep 20[Epub ahead of print].

39. Hertzer NR. The natural history of peripheral vascular disease: implications for its management. *Circulation* 1991;83(Suppl 1):I12-I19.
40. McDaniel MD, Cronenwett JL. Basic data related to the natural history of intermittent claudication. *Ann Vasc Surg* 1989;3:273-277.
41. Juergens JL, Barker NW, Hines EA Jr. Arteriosclerosis obliterans: review of 520 cases with special reference to pathogenic and prognostic factors. *Circulation* 1960;21:188-195.
42. Gray BH, Sullivan TM, Childs MB, et al. High incidence of restenosis/reocclusion of stents in the percutaneous treatment of long-segment superficial femoral artery disease after suboptimal angioplasty. *J Vasc Surg* 1997;25:74-83.
43. Desgrandes P, Boufi M, Lapeyre M, et al. Subintimal angioplasty: feasible and durable. *Eur J Vasc Endovasc Surg* 2004;28:138-141.
44. Mitsudo K. The how and why of chronic total occlusions. I. How to treat CTOs. *EuroIntervention* 2006;2:375-381.
45. Jeans WD, Amstrong S, Cole SE, et al. Fate of patients undergoing transluminal angioplasty for lower-limb ischemia. *Radiology* 1990;177:559-564.
46. Blair JM, Gewertz BL, Moosa H, et al. Percutaneous transluminal angioplasty versus surgery for limb-threatening ischemia. *J Vasc Surg* 1989;9:698.
47. Lofberg AM, Kavacagil S, Hellberg A, et al. Percutaneous transluminal angioplasty of the femoropopliteal arteries in limbs with chronic critical ischemia. *J Vasc Surg* 2001;34:114-121.
48. Jamsen T, Manninen H, Tulla H, et al. The final outcome of primary infrainguinal percutaneous transluminal angioplasty in 100 consecutive patients with chronic critical limb ischemia. *J Vasc Interv Radiol* 2002;13:455-463.
49. Gardiner GA Jr, Meyerovitz MF, Harrington DP, et al. Dissection complicating angioplasty. *AJR Am J Roentgenol* 1985;145:627-631.
50. Krepel VM, van Andel GJ, van Erp WF, et al. Percutaneous transluminal angioplasty of the femoropopliteal artery: initial and long-term results. *Radiology* 1985;156:325-328.
51. Johnston KW, Rae M, Hogg-Johnston SA, et al. Five-year results of a prospective study of percutaneous transluminal angioplasty. *Ann Surg* 1987;206:403-413.
52. Rocha-Singh KJ, Jaff MR, Crabtree TR, et al. Performance goals and endpoint assessments for clinical trials of femoropopliteal bare nitinol stents in patients with symptomatic peripheral arterial disease. *Catheter Cardiovasc Interv* 2007;69:910-919.
53. Bolia A, Bell PRF. Femoropopliteal and crural artery recanalization using subintimal angioplasty. *Semin Vasc Surg* 1995;8:253-264.
54. Rogers JH, Laird JR. Overview of new technologies for lower extremity revascularization. *Circulation* 2007;116:2072-2085.
55. Tepe G, Zeller T, Albrecht T, et al. Local delivery of paclitaxel to inhibit restenosis during angioplasty of the leg. *N Engl J Med* 2008;358:689-699.
56. Ahn SS, Auth DC, Marcus DR, et al. Removal of focal atheromatous lesions by angioscopically guided high-speed rotary atherectomy: preliminary experimental observations. *J Vasc Surg* 1988;7:292-300.
57. Rai P, Costa MA, Hu P, et al. Mechanism of lumen enlargement by SilverHawk atherectomy device in SFA and popliteal lesions: An IVUS study. *Am J Cardiol* 2006:98:S234-S240.
58. Zeller T, Rastan A, Sixt S, et al. Long-term results after directional atherectomy of femoropopliteal lesions. *J Am Coll Cardiol* 2006;48:1573-1578.
59. Kandarzi DE, Kiesz RS, Allie D, et al. Procedural and clinical outcomes with catheter-based plaque excision in critical limb ischemia. *J Endovasc Ther* 2006;13:12-22.
60. Lam RC, Shah S, Faries PL, et al. Incidence and clinical significance of distal embolization during percutaneous interventions involving the superficial femoral artery. *J Vasc Surg* 2007;46:1155-1159.
61. Scheinert D, Laird JR Jr, Schroder M, et al. Excimer laser-assisted recanalization of long, chronic superficial femoral artery occlusions. *J Endovasc Ther* 2001;8:156-166.
62. Rosenfield K, Schainfeld R, Pieczek A, et al. Restenosis of endovascular stents from stent compression. *J Am Coll Cardiol* 1997;29:328-338.
63. Cejna M, Thurnher S, Illiasch H, et al. PTA versus Palmaz stent placement in femoropopliteal artery obstructions: a multicenter prospective randomized study. *J Vasc Interv Radiol* 2001;12:23-31.
64. Vroegingeweij D, Vos LD, Tielbeek AV, et al. Balloon angioplasty combined with primary stenting versus balloon angioplasty alone in femoropopliteal obstructions: a comparative randomized study. *Cardiovasc Intervent Radiol* 1997;20:420-425.
65. Greenberg D, Rosenfield K, Garcia LA, et al. In-hospital costs of self-expanding nitinol stent implantation versus balloon angioplasty in the femoropopliteal artery (the VascuCoil Trial). *J Vasc Interv Radiol* 2004;10:1065-1069.
66. Muradin GS, Myriam Hunink MG. Cost and patency rate targets for the development of endovascular devices to treat femoropopliteal arterial disease. *Radiology* 2001;218:464-469.
67. Hunink MGM, Wong JB, Donaldson MC, et al. Revascularization for femoropopliteal disease: a decision and cost-effectiveness analysis. *JAMA* 1995;274:165-171.
68. Krankenberg H, Schluter M, Steinkamp HJ, et al. Nitinol stent implantation versus percutaneous transluminal angioplasty in superficial femoral artery lesions up to 10 cm in length: the Femoral Artery Stenting Trial (FAST). *Circulation* 2007;116:285-292.
69. Schillinger M, Sabeti S, Dick P, et al. Sustained benefit at 2 years of primary femoropopliteal stenting compared with balloon angioplasty with optional stenting. *Circulation* 2007;115:2745-2749.
70. Katzen B. Resilient trial. *Presented at the International Symposium on Endovascular Therapy meeting,* Jan 22, Miami: Florida; 2008.
71. Scheinert D, Scheinert S, Sax J, et al. Prevalence and clinical impact of stent fractures after femoropopliteal stenting. *J Am Coll Cardiol* 2005;45:312-315.
72. Do-dai-Do, Triller J, Walpoth BH, et al. A comparison study of self-expandable stents versus balloon angioplasty alone in femoropopliteal artery occlusions. *Cardiovasc Intervent Radiol* 1992;15:306-312.
73. White GH, Liew SCC, Waugh SC, et al. Early outcome and intermediate follow-up of vascular stents in the femoral and popliteal arteries without long-term anticoagulation. *J Vasc Surg* 1995;21:270-281.
74. Duda SH, Pusich B, Richter G, et al. Sirolimus-eluting versus bare nitinol stent for obstructive superficial femoral artery disease: six month results. *Circulation* 2002;106:1505-1509.
75. Duda SH, Bosiers M, Lammer J, et al. Sirolimus-eluting versus bare nitinol stent for obstructive superficial femoral artery disease: the SIROCCO II trial. *J Vasc Interv Radiol* 2005;16:331-338.
76. Duda SH, Bosiers M, Lammer J, et al. Drug-eluting and bare nitinol stents for the treatment of atherosclerotic lesions in the superficial femoral artery: long-term results from the SIROCCO trial. *J Endovasc Ther* 2006;13:701-710.
77. Rousseau HP, Raillat CR, Joffre FG, et al. Treatment of femoropopliteal stenosis by means of self-expandable endoprostheses: midterm results. *Radiology* 1989;172:961-964.
78. Alimi YS, Hakam Z, Hartung O, et al. Efficacy of Viabahn in the treatment of severe superficial femoral artery lesions: which factors influence long-term patency? *Eur J Vasc Endovasc Surg* 2008;35:346-352.
79. Jahnke T, Andresen R, Muller-Hulsbeck S, et al. Hemobahn stent-grafts for treatment of femoropopliteal arterial obstructions: midterm results of a prospective trial. *J Vasc Interv Radiol* 2003;14:41-51.
80. Saxon RR, Coffman JM, Gooding JM, Ponec DJ. Long-term patency and clinical outcome of the Viabahn stent-graft for femoropopliteal artery obstructions. *J Vasc Interv Radiol* 2007;18:1341-1350.
81. Fischer M, Schwabe C, Schulte KL. Value of the Hemobahn/Viabahn endoprosthesis in the treatment of long chronic lesions of the superficial femoral artery: 6 years of experience. *J Endovasc Ther* 2006;13:281-290.
82. Kadora J, Hohmann S, Garrett W, et al. Randomized comparison of percutaneous Viabahn stent grafts vs. prosthetic femoral–popliteal bypass in the treatment of superficial femoral arterial occlusive disease. *J Vasc Surg* 2007;45:10-16.
83. Ranson ME, Adelman MA, Cayne NS, et al. Total Viabahn endoprosthesis collapse. *J Vasc Surg* 2008;47:454-456.
84. Waksman R, Laird JR, Jurkovitz CT, et al. Intravascular radiation therapy after balloon angioplasty of narrowed femoropopliteal arteries to prevent restenosis: results of the PARIS feasibility clinical trial. *J Vasc Interv Radiol* 2001;12:915-921.
85. Wolfram RM, Pokrajac B, Ahmadi R, et al. Endovascular brachytherapy for prophylaxis against restenosis after long-segment femoropopliteal placement of stents: initial results. *Radiology* 2001;220:724-729.
86. Gray BH, Ramee S, Kandarpa K, et al. Lower extremity revascularization: state of the art. *Circulation* 2008;118(Suppl 1):S35-S39.
87. Faglia E, Dalla Paola L, Clerici G, et al. Peripheral angioplasty as the first-choice revascularization procedure in diabetic patients with critical limb ischemia: prospective study of 993 consecutive patients hospitalized and followed between 1999 and 2003. *Eur J Vasc Endovasc Surg* 2005;29:620-627.
88. Graziani L, Silvestro V, Bertone E, et al. Vascular involvement in diabetic subjects with ischemic foot ulcer: a new morphologic categorization of disease severity. *Eur J Vasc Endovasc Surg* 2007;33:453-460.
89. Engelke C, Morgan RA, Belli AM. Cutting balloon percutaneous transluminal angioplasty for salvage of lower limb arterial bypass grafts: feasibility. *Radiology* 2002;223:106-114.

90. Ansel GM, Sample NS, Botti CF, et al. Cutting balloon angioplasty of the popliteal and infrapopliteal vessels for symptomatic limb ischemia. *Catheter Cardiovasc Interv* 2004;61:1-4.
91. Scheinert D, Peeters P, Bosiers M, et al. Results of the multicenter first-in-man study of a novel scoring balloon catheter for the treatment of intra-popliteal peripheral arterial disease. *Catheter Cardiovasc Interv* 2007;70:1034-1039.
92. Das T, McNamara T, Gray BH, et al. Cryoplasty therapy for limb salvage in patients with critical limb ischemia. *J Endovasc Ther* 2007;14:753-762.
93. White CJ, Gray WA. Endovascular therapies for peripheral arterial disease: an evidence-based review. *Circulation* 2007;116:2203-2215.
94. Scheinert D, Ulrich M, Scheinert S, et al. Comparison of sirolimus-eluting vs. bare-metal stents for the treatment of infrapopliteal obstructions. *EuroIntervention* 2006;2:169-174.
95. Kickuth R, Keo HH, Triller J, et al. Initial clinical experience with the 4-F self-expanding Xpert stent system for infrapopliteal treatment of patients with severe claudication and critical limb ischemia. *J Vasc Interv Radiol* 2007;18:703-708.
96. Bosiers M, Deloose K, Verbist J, et al. Nitinol stenting for treatment of "below-the-knee" critical limb ischemia: 1-year angiographic outcome after Xpert stent implantation. *J Cardiovasc Surg (Torino)* 2007;48:455-461.

chapter

10a

Surgical Intervention for Lower Extremity Arterial Occlusive Disease: Aortoiliac Revascularization Operations

Amy B. Reed, MD • Magruder C. Donaldson, MD

Key Points

- Aortoiliac occlusive disease (AIOD) has a profound effect on peripheral perfusion, and its correction is correspondingly beneficial.
- Precise imaging allows classification of occlusive lesions using Trans-Atlantic Inter-Society Consensus definitions to assist with rational choice among multiple endovascular and open modalities for most effective revascularization option.
- Long-term patency of aortobifemoral bypass is 85% to 90% at 5 years and 70% to 75% at 10 years. Aortobifemoral bypass is the most durable therapy for diffuse long-segment AIOD.
- Extraanatomical axillobifemoral grafting is useful in selected high-risk patients requiring operation for bilateral diffuse AIOD due to medical comorbidities or anatomical considerations ("hostile abdomen," sepsis, etc.).
- Iliac endarterectomy, iliofemoral bypass, and femorofemoral bypass are useful approaches to patients with predominantly unilateral iliac occlusive disease not amenable to angioplasty.

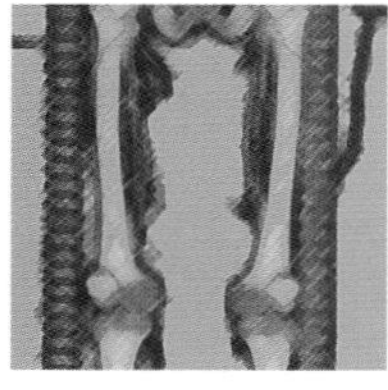

Clinically significant aortoiliac arterial occlusive disease occurs almost entirely based on longstanding chronic atherosclerosis. Although the disease is present throughout the aorta and both iliac arteries, distinct patterns of disease have been recognized among patients presenting with symptoms. Among these is so-called coral reef atherosclerosis, in which heavy, calcific circumferential plaque is present adjacent to the visceral and renal portion of the abdominal aorta. Focal high-grade stenosis may occur midaorta and more commonly in a "pantaloon" distribution straddling the aortic bifurcation and extending into the proximal common iliac arteries. Another common pattern involves a predominance of disease at the iliac bifurcation or bifurcations. Degrees of occlusive disease range from total infrarenal aortic and bilateral iliac occlusion to diffuse aortoiliac stenoses. AIOD is often combined with disease below the inguinal ligament, adding to the overall impact on the lower extremities. Nonatherosclerotic diseases occur occasionally, including fibromuscular dysplasia (most commonly in the external iliac arteries), hypoplasia of the aorta, coarctation of the abdominal aorta, and arterial dissection.

Clinical symptoms result most typically from chronic arterial insufficiency after years of gradual disease progression. Patients with combined segment disease involving both aortoiliac and infrainguinal arteries are more severely affected. On rare occasions, acute peripheral ischemia results from embolization of fragments of plaque and thrombus arising from the aortoiliac segment. Although in cases with diffuse disease it is impossible to prove the origin of such events, a focal ulcerated area may be detectable in the aorta or iliac artery proximal to the involved limb. Acute thrombosis of the aorta is unusual but most commonly results from a "saddle" embolus to the aortic or iliac bifurcation that is cardiac in origin (macroembolization).

Preventive and supportive measures are fundamental to management of all patients with vascular disease. Revascularization is appropriate when aortoiliac occlusion contributes to critical limb ischemia or disability. A wide array of alternatives is available for revascularization, often combining modalities to obtain the best results with the least morbidity. Endovascular techniques have been successfully employed in the aortoiliac segments for more than 25 years and are described in detail in Chapters 9a and 9b. Well-established open surgical options remain valuable in selective situations in the modern era using either direct arterial reconstruction or extraanatomical bypass. This chapter reviews diagnosis, surgical indications, perioperative management, technique, and results of these options.

EVALUATION

Clinical Presentation

The history and physical examination are usually sufficient to establish the diagnosis of peripheral arterial disease (PAD). The signs and symptoms depend on the location, extent, and acuity of the occlusive process (Figure 10a-1A).[1] Among claudicants, 25% have disease confined to the aortoiliac segment and 65% have more diffuse disease, both above and below the inguinal ligament, involving either the superficial femoral artery or the distal vessels. Focal AIOD limited to the distal abdominal aorta and common iliac arteries occurs in only a small number of patients and, in the absence of concomitant distal disease, rarely produces limb-threatening symptoms.[2,3] This focal pattern is most commonly identified among relatively young female smokers. The typical presentation is bilateral claudication involving the calves and the proximal musculature of the thigh, hip, or buttocks. Affected men may present with the characteristic triad of Leriche syndrome—bilateral claudication, impotence, and diminished or absent femoral pulses—caused by extensive disease in the aortoiliac segments. Except in relatively rare instances of acute aortic occlusion or distal embolization from the aortoiliac vessels, patients with critical ischemia have chronic combined segment occlusive disease affecting vessels below the inguinal ligament. These patients are older, are more likely to be male, and have a higher prevalence of diabetes, hypertension, and associated cerebrovascular and coronary atherosclerosis than claudicants.[4-6]

Among general findings, the vascular examination documents bilateral brachial blood pressure; cardiac rhythm; abdominal findings such as bruit or aneurysm; femoral, popliteal, and pedal pulses; and status of the feet. Abdominal or groin bruit or reduced or absent femoral pulses signify the presence of aortoiliac disease. Absence of peripheral pulses under these circumstances does not necessarily imply the presence of infrainguinal disease. Neuropathy and dependent rubor of the toes or forefoot imply borderline compensation for severe resting ischemia. Necrosis, ulceration, and infection involving the toes or foot are other signs of diffuse multisegment occlusive disease.

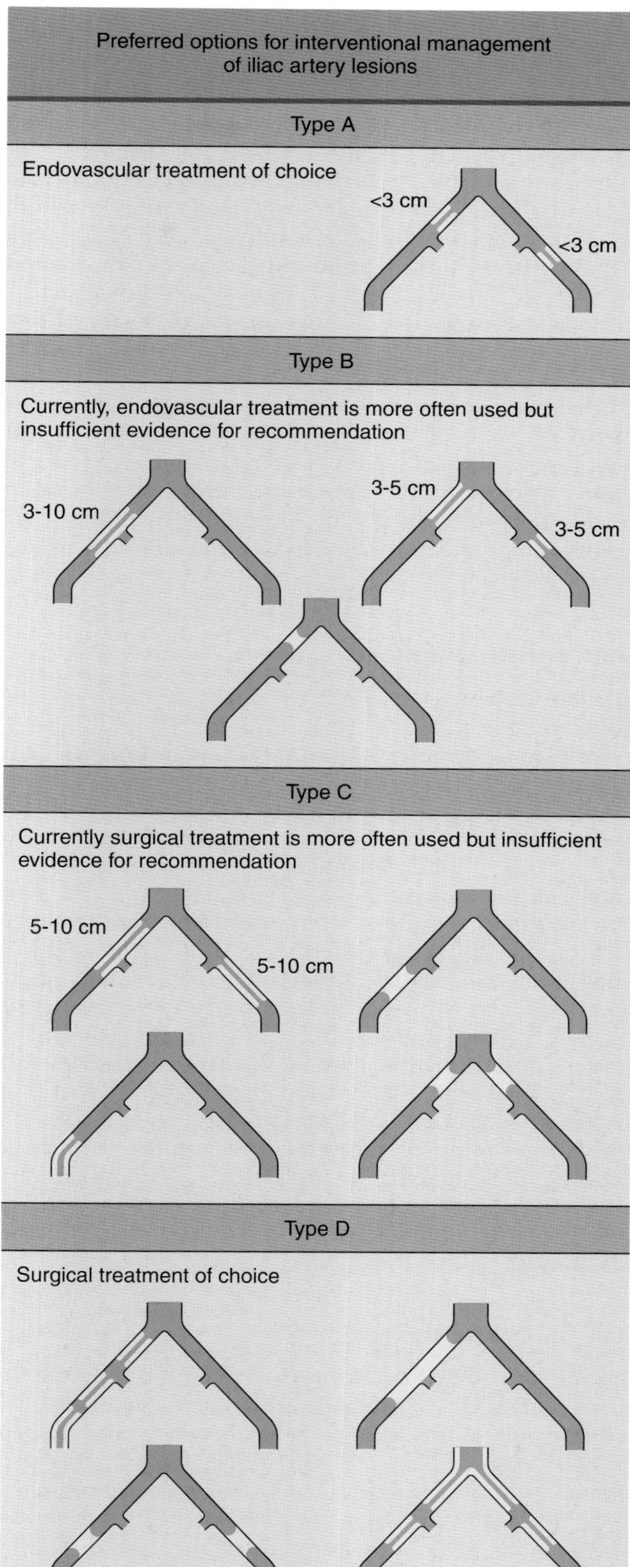

Figure 10a-1. Preferred options for interventional management of iliac artery lesions. (Adapted from Trans-Atlantic Inter-Society Consensus II Working Group. *J Vasc Surg* 2007;45[Suppl]:S5-S67.)

Physiological Assessment

Noninvasive laboratory evaluation by means of segmental limb pressures and pulse volume recordings is a useful adjunct to clinical assessment, especially when physical findings are equivocal or the history is atypical. The laboratory is especially valuable in clarifying the functional importance of vascular disease in patients with claudication symptoms and concomitant confounding conditions such as degenerative joint disease of the hip and spinal stenosis. For example, vasculogenic claudication can be difficult to distinguish from neurogenic claudication or other musculoskeletal pain syndromes, even though in most instances vascular claudication is relieved by standing after walking while pain caused by other etiologies is relieved only by sitting or lying down. Selective functional assessment of such complex patients using a physiological treadmill exercise study is a valuable adjunct to more routine studies performed at rest. Vascular laboratory data objectively confirm disease presence and severity and provide a baseline from which to follow the disease for progression.

Anatomical Diagnosis

Detailed evaluation of PAD by direct vascular imaging studies is indicated only when symptoms are sufficiently severe to warrant intervention. Magnetic resonance angiography (MRA), computed tomography angiography, or abdominal aortography with bilateral lower-extremity runoff is used to provide hard-copy images for interventional planning. Gadolinium-enhanced MRA is available in most centers and is increasingly used for diagnostic and planning purposes, despite concern regarding rare instances of chronic subcutaneous sclerosis possibly associated with gadolinium. Computed tomography angiography using rapid sequence, thin-slice image acquisition is also available, although it requires a bolus of intravenous iodinated contrast. Interpretation may be difficult in patients with heavy arterial wall calcification. Percutaneous aortography allows selective study of various vascular segments and affords the option of subtraction techniques to increase accuracy. This modality is increasingly available in various interventional settings and is often combined in one encounter with either endovascular or open surgical revascularization.

Risk Assessment

The presence of PAD is a strong marker for future cardiovascular events such as myocardial infarction (Figure 10a-2).[7] Results from several studies have shown 5- and 10-year mortality rates of 30% and 50%, respectively, among such patients, with most deaths due to cardiovascular complications.[1] A classic study from the Cleveland Clinic evaluated 1000 patients (381 with lower extremity ischemia) with coronary arteriography before elective vascular surgery and found normal coronary arteries in only 10%.[8] Of these patients, 28% had severe triple-vessel coronary disease or worse. Cardiology consultation is important before open surgical therapy, and most patients should be placed on beta-blockers and statins preoperatively. Ultrasound screening for coincident carotid disease is appropriate in patients

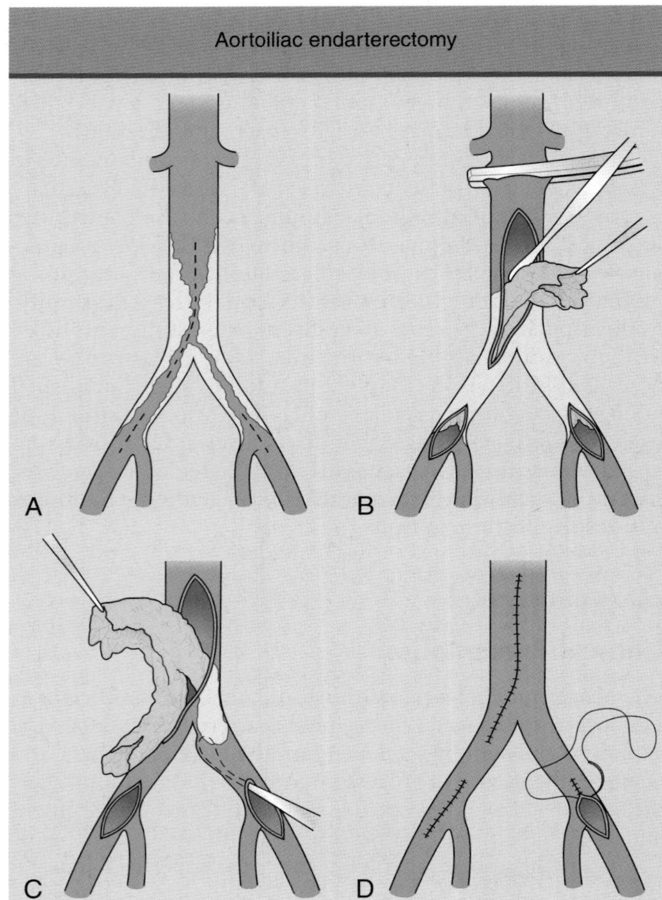

Figure 10a-2. Aortoiliac endarterectomy. Method of aortoiliac endarterectomy using longitudinal aortotomy and distal common iliac arterotomies to gain access to disease localized to the distal aorta and proximal common iliac arteries, with primary closure. (Adapted from Brewster DC. Direct reconstruction for aortoiliac occlusive disease. In: Rutherford RB, ed. *Vascular surgery*. 6th ed. Philadelphia: Elsevier/Saunders; 2005:1114.)

with chronic atherosclerosis. Smoking is common among patients who present with aortoiliac disease, and chest radiographs and assessment of secondary chronic obstructive pulmonary disease are appropriate. Presence and degree of diabetes, renal dysfunction, and coagulopathy should be assessed. Anatomical features such as obesity, previous abdominal surgery or vascular surgery, radiation, and infection need consideration during planning. Anomalies such as retroaortic left renal vein, duplicated inferior vena cava, or horseshoe kidney may affect choice of approach. The patient's sexual function should be considered, with implications for surgical planning.

TREATMENT

Risk factor modification, exercise, and appropriate pharmacotherapy should be recommended in all patients with PAD, particularly before embarking on surgical intervention.[1] Intervention should be limited to those patients who are truly disabled by claudication or those who develop signs or symptoms of resting ischemia and are judged acceptable risks for intervention. Patients with critical ischemia caused by either acute or chronic occlusive processes should generally receive supportive measures and expeditious evaluation followed by intervention unless deemed unduly hazardous. Once intervention is indicated based on patient symptoms and findings, a rational system to assist with the choice between endovascular and open surgical approach is useful. At present, many surgeons employ the system advocated by the TransAtlantic Inter-Society Consensus (TASC) Working Group. It divides lower extremity occlusive disease into aortoiliac and infrainguinal locations, categorizing the lesions according to preferred treatment options (Figure 10a-1).[1] Patients with short-segment iliac artery lesions (TASC-A) are treated preferentially with endovascular techniques. Longer stenotic segments of the aortoiliac segments or short common iliac or external iliac occlusions (TASC-B) are effectively treated with endovascular therapy. Surgical treatment is recommended for good-risk patients with TASC-C lesions, although endovascular techniques may also be effective. Open surgical revascularization is recommended for most patients with TASC-D lesions consisting of long or multisegment AIOD.

OPERATIVE SURGERY

Direct pharmacological management of vulnerable myocardium and preliminary cardiac intervention for selected patients have improved surgical morbidity and mortality rates for revascularization of the aortoiliac arteries. For example, a 30-day operative mortality rate for bypass or endarterectomy using an abdominal approach has been reduced to less than 2% in many centers.[9-13] With acceptably low morbidity and excellent long-term patency rates, use of open vascular reconstruction is appropriate in selected patients with symptomatic AIOD.

Aortoiliac Thromboembolectomy

Thromboembolectomy is indicated when clinical circumstances are highly suggestive of acute embolic occlusion of the aorta or iliac arteries. Preoperative arterial imaging is not mandatory, although it may be obtained if it can be done without undue delay. In many such circumstances, little underlying disease occurs in the aortoiliac segments and expeditious clot removal can be expected using simple balloon catheters. In principle, relatively simple bilateral femoral artery exposure allows thorough and prompt restitution of inflow, access for angiographic study of inflow and outflow vessels, and optional thromboembolectomy or revascularization of the distal vessels. If proximal thromboembolectomy is incomplete or underlying disease is uncovered, femoral access facilitates nearly all endovascular and surgical bypass options for consolidating inflow.

When embolization is suspected, the patient should be anticoagulated with intravenous heparin before surgery. Regional spinal or epidural anesthesia is therefore best avoided, and the procedure is started with local anesthesia and sedation, being prepared for conversion to general anesthesia as appropriate. The patient is placed on a fluoroscopy table. Both groins, the affected leg or legs, and the abdomen are prepped and draped, and access to the axillary artery on one side is considered to facilitate the option of axillofemoral bypass if necessary. If physical findings and history suggest unilateral iliac artery occlusion, a femoral incision is made on that side; if both femoral artery pulses are absent, bilateral incisions are made. The distal external iliac, entire common femoral, and proximal profunda femoris and superficial femoral arteries are exposed. The vessels should be carefully assessed for plaque burden to determine the possible need for endarterectomy and patch angioplasty if severe. Additional heparin is administered if necessary to allow full anticoagulation (activated clotting time of more than 240). If the arteries are minimally diseased, a transverse arteriotomy is made over the distal common femoral artery. If the occlusive disease is more extensive, a longitudinal arteriotomy may be preferable at the outset, although a transverse incision can be converted if necessary. Placement of elastic vessel loops facilitates multiple passages of the thromboembolectomy balloon catheter while minimizing blood loss and trauma to the vessel. A 5-French balloon thromboembolectomy catheter is used for initial passage retrograde into the aortoiliac segments. The catheter is advanced carefully, stopping if firm resistance is encountered. Placement of a curve in the end of the catheter facilitates passage beyond an area of tortuosity. In cases of unilateral iliac occlusion, thrombus flush with the common iliac artery origin is susceptible to dislodgement and embolization down the contralateral limb. In cases of bilateral iliac or aortoiliac occlusion, thromboembolectomy is performed sequentially on both sides, with temporary vascular occlusion on the side opposite to balloon passage.

In most instances, copious thrombus is extracted and the catheter is passed repeatedly until no further clot is returned and the inflow is pulsatile and vigorous. Ideally, the retrieved specimen has a meniscus at the proximal end, signifying the interface of the thrombus with liquid blood at the top of the occlusion and the likelihood that the thromboembolectomy is complete. The specimen should be sent to pathology for examination since, on rare occasions, tumor embolus can be found. A 4-French thromboembolectomy catheter should be passed distally into the profunda and superficial femoral arteries to be certain that there is no distal thrombus, after which dilute heparin solution is instilled into these vessels.

If there is poor inflow or questionable outflow after these maneuvers, fluoroscopic angiography is performed to identify the cause. Recalcitrant clot or fixed disease affecting the inflow is managed with further mechanical thrombectomy maneuvers and endovascular interventions such as balloon angioplasty or stenting. If residual disease in the external iliac cannot be corrected, a unilateral iliofemoral bypass can be performed. If one iliac is patent and free of hemodynamically significant disease, a femorofemoral bypass can be performed to correct residual unilateral iliac occlusion on the contralateral side. If satisfactory inflow cannot be obtained from either iliac system, axillobifemoral bypass may be the best available option. Direct reconstruction such as aortobifemoral bypass is generally neither necessary nor appropriate in such acute circumstances. The outflow should be imaged with fluoroscopy unless the thromboembolectomy catheter has passed without difficulty to at least 50 cm down the superficial femoral and 20 cm down the profunda. Residual outflow disease can most often be observed, expecting restoration of inflow to the profunda, the superficial femoral, or both to resolve threat to the limb. Nonvisualization of outflow vessels in the thigh or failure to visualize reconstituted vessels below the knee may compel further percutaneous or open surgery.

The femoral arteriotomy sites are closed with monofilament suture, either in running fashion or with a series of interrupted sutures if the artery is small or diseased, taking care to incorporate all layers of the artery. If concern exists about flap, dissection, or stenosis due to local plaque burden, endarterectomy and patch angioplasty should be performed. The lower extremities are examined before removal of drapes, using Doppler to insonate distal arteries and palpation to assess muscle compartment tension. Adjunctive peripheral bypass and fasciotomy should always be considered.

Restoration of baseline or improved perfusion can be expected in most patients after thromboembolectomy for acute occlusion. Patients have a high prevalence of underlying cardiac disease; since more than 90% of peripheral emboli arise from the heart, recurrence is possible. Accordingly, anticoagulation should be continued for at least the early postoperative period unless contraindicated. Postoperative cardiac monitoring is routine, and a complete cardiac evaluation should be carried out to clarify the need for antiarrhythmic therapy and long-term anticoagulation before hospital discharge.

Aortoiliac Endarterectomy

First performed in the early 1950s,[14] aortoiliac endarterectomy is still an appropriate choice of treatment for candidates selected from the 5% to 10% of patients with disease limited to the distal aorta and common iliac arteries. Since diffuse disease is so much more common, many surgeons lack experience with endarterectomy and may prefer not to use the method for this reason. Patients most likely to be candidates include early-middle-aged females with occlusive disease of the middle and distal abdominal aorta, with limited extension into the proximal common iliac arteries. Patients who present with atheroembolization from disrupted focal aortoiliac plaque may be best treated by endarterectomy to avoid risk of further embolization from catheter manipulation during catheter-based therapy. The principal benefit of aortoiliac endarterectomy is avoidance of prosthetic grafts and attendant possible complications of infection. The procedure may be less appealing for males because of concern over interference with the nervi erigentes coursing over the aortic bifurcation and proximal common iliac arteries. The main contraindication to endarterectomy is the existence of a degenerated or aneurysmal arterial wall.

A midline abdominal incision allows good exposure of the aorta as described for aortobifemoral bypass. When the iliac arteries are involved, the retroperitoneal incision is extended down both common iliacs, leaving the tissue at and between the iliac origins undissected if possible to preserve the periaortic nervi erigentes, which course lateral to the aorta and cross over the aortic bifurcation. The proximal external and internal iliac arteries are dissected out for clamping. Clamps are applied to the aorta at the level of the renal arteries and at the proximal internal and external iliac arteries, with bulldog clamps for lumbars and the inferior mesenteric artery. A longitudinal incision is made in the aorta at or above the target plaque and carried down to the aortic bifurcation. The endarterectomy plane is begun in the deep media, pushing the aortic wall away from the plaque. The plaque is transected below the level of the proximal aortic clamp. The distal endpoint is exposed by transverse or longitudinal counterincisions in the common iliac arteries, just proximal to the iliac bifurcation (Figure 10a-2). If the plaque does not taper to a satisfactory endpoint, it is sharply divided and mattress stitches are placed to tack it down. After irrigation with heparinized saline, backbleeding, and forward flushing, the aortotomy is closed with a continuous monofilament suture. The iliac incisions are closed primarily or using a patch, depending on arterial diameter and surgeon's preference.

Early complications specific to aortoiliac endarterectomy include limb ischemia related to embolization or dissection at the distal endpoint and hemorrhage from excessive thinning of an endarterectomized artery, most common when there is heavy plaque calcification. Over time, aneurysmal dilatation of the endarterectomized segment and progressive atherosclerotic disease may necessitate reoperation. In carefully selected patients, the 5-year patency rate after aortoiliac endarterectomy is 80% to 90%.[15,16]

Aortobifemoral Bypass Graft

Aortoiliac bypass is occasionally appropriate, using the common iliac bifurcation or external iliac arteries for the distal anastomosis. This procedure would be reasonable for a patient with proximal aortoiliac disease and normal external iliac arteries and would be preferable to aortobifemoral bypass in such patients if the groins were inhospitable for one reason or another. In most patients, disease involves the external iliac arteries to some extent, and placement of the graft proximal to the groin leaves the patient vulnerable to progression of disease in the external iliac, with a relatively arduous revision necessary in the event of graft failure. Since it has become clear that tunneling a prosthetic graft across the hip joint to the groin does not cause graft failure due to kinking, aortobifemoral bypass has become the preferred procedure for most patients with diffuse infrarenal aortoiliac disease.

Aortobifemoral bypass surgery commences with bilateral groin incisions to expose both common femoral arteries, taking care to control lymphatic tissue to minimize the possibility of postoperative lymph leak with associated wound complications and infection. The posterior aspect of the inguinal ligament is divided over most of the distal external iliac artery to facilitate tunneling of the graft, taking care to avoid injury to the deep circumflex iliac vein (the "vein of woe") crossing the external iliac artery just beneath the ligament. Dissection is carried distally to the common femoral artery bifurcation. If preoperative arteriography or intraoperative palpation reveals superficial femoral artery occlusion, the profunda femoris artery should be mobilized past any proximal disease, to the level of the medial and lateral femoral circumflex branches, to expose a more normal distal segment of the artery for possible profundaplasty at the time of construction of the distal anastomosis.

The infrarenal abdominal aorta may be exposed by various approaches, including left subcostal retroperitoneal and midline transperitoneal incisions. Using either approach, the proximal abdominal aorta is mobilized just below the renal arteries at the level of the left renal vein. Dissection proceeds distally, keeping to the right side of the anterior surface of the aorta to protect the inferior mesenteric artery to allow for possible reimplantation in the event of inadequate collateral flow to the left colon at the conclusion of surgery. The distal aorta is sufficiently mobilized for clamping at a level appropriate for the graft configuration chosen. A gentle atraumatic technique is necessary to avoid atheroembolization during dissection.

After completion of the femoral and aortic exposures, retroperitoneal tunnels are created from the aortic bifurcation to the groin to allow passage of the graft limbs. Gentle blunt dissection is carried out with both index fingers simultaneously, taking care to remain directly anterior to the common and external iliac arteries, posterior to the ureters, and anterior to the deep circumflex iliac vein. Passage of the graft posterior to the ureters is an important detail that minimizes the potential of ureteral compression and hydronephrosis.

Once the dissection and tunneling are complete, the patient is systemically heparinized and the aorta is cross-clamped infrarenally. The proximal anastomosis is constructed in an end-to-end or end-to-side configuration. A good deal of controversy remains as to the proper configuration of the aortobifemoral bypass graft.[12,17-20] Some authors believe that the end-to-end technique reduces the incidence of late aortoduodenal fistula because the graft does not project as anteriorly as it does after end-to-side anastomosis,[12,21,22] while others have not demonstrated any difference in complication or late patency rates between end-to-end and end-to-side grafts.[17-20] The end-to-end technique is best suited for patients who will not suffer any further hemodynamic compromise to the bowel and pelvic arterial beds from interruption of forward flow in the aorta, such as those with complete aortic occlusion below the renal arteries and those with patent external iliac arteries capable of retrograde flow from the groin into the internal iliacs. End-to-end anastomosis is mandatory in patients with aneurysmal disease of the infrarenal aorta. The end-to-side technique (Figure 10a-3) is reserved for those patients who have a patent and enlarged inferior mesenteric artery, a low-lying accessory renal artery arising from the distal aorta or proximal iliac artery, diffuse occlusive disease confined mainly to the external iliac arteries with an intact distal aorta and common iliac system, or reconstituted pelvic circulation via collateral arteries that might otherwise be lost in an end-to-end anastomosis. The end-to-end proximal anastomotic technique (Figure 10a-4) requires transection of the aorta between two clamps below the renal arteries, allowing for localized thromboendarterectomy of the proximal aortic stump under direct visualization if necessary. A segment of aorta is usually resected, and the distal aorta is either oversewn or stapled (Figure 10a-5). Construction of an end-to-side anastomosis involves placement of a longitudinal aortotomy as proximal as possible below the renals after clamping in a relatively less diseased section of aorta. Although a partially occluding Satinsky clamp may be used when disease is minimal, in most instances two clamps are best to facilitate exposure and selective flushing from each end of the aorta (Figure 10a-6). Care must be taken to remove all loose thrombus and debris from the excluded aortic segment between the occluding clamps.

Laparoscopic aortic surgery is a minimally invasive approach offering the potential for reducing some of the morbidity associated with open surgery. Dion performed the first laparoscopic aortobifemoral bypass in 1995 using a gasless technique.[23] He later improved on the technique through the use of carbon dioxide pneumoperitoneum, which aided

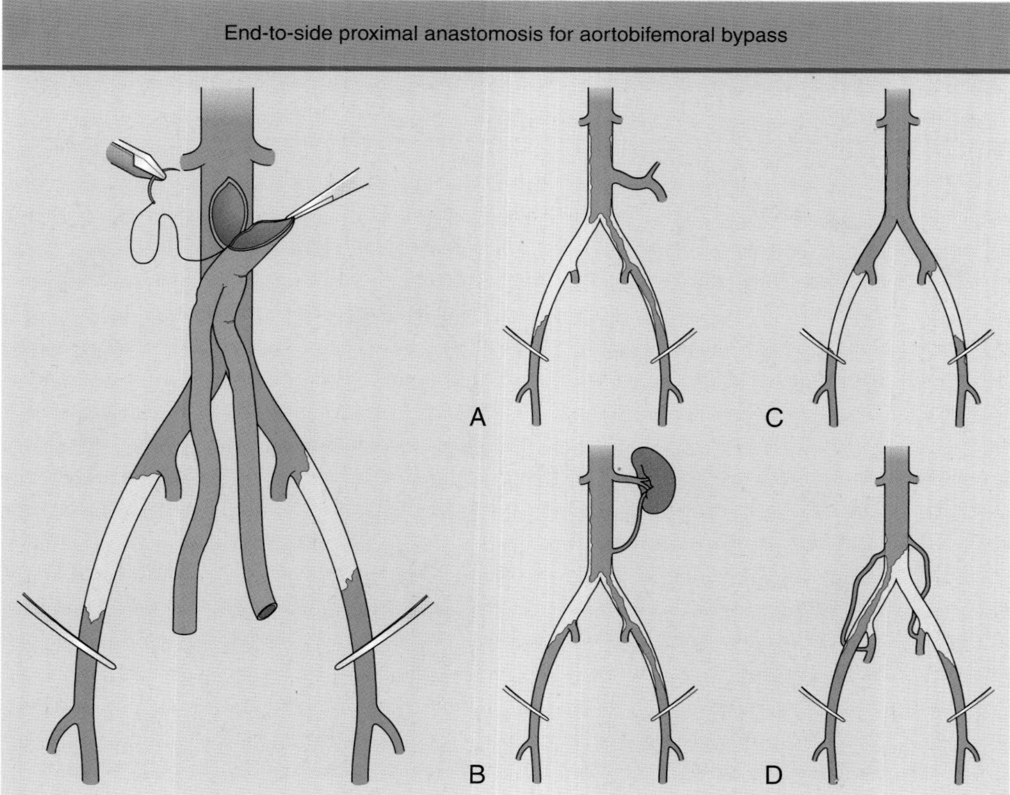

Figure 10a-3. End-to-side proximal anastomosis for aortobifemoral bypass. Pattern of aortoiliac occlusive disease appropriate for end-to-side proximal anastomosis of aortobifemoral bypass graft to preserve antegrade flow into important vascular beds. (Adapted from Brewster DC. Direct reconstruction for aortoiliac occlusive disease. In: Rutherford RB, ed. *Vascular surgery*. 6th ed. Philadelphia: Elsevier/Saunders; 2005:1116.)

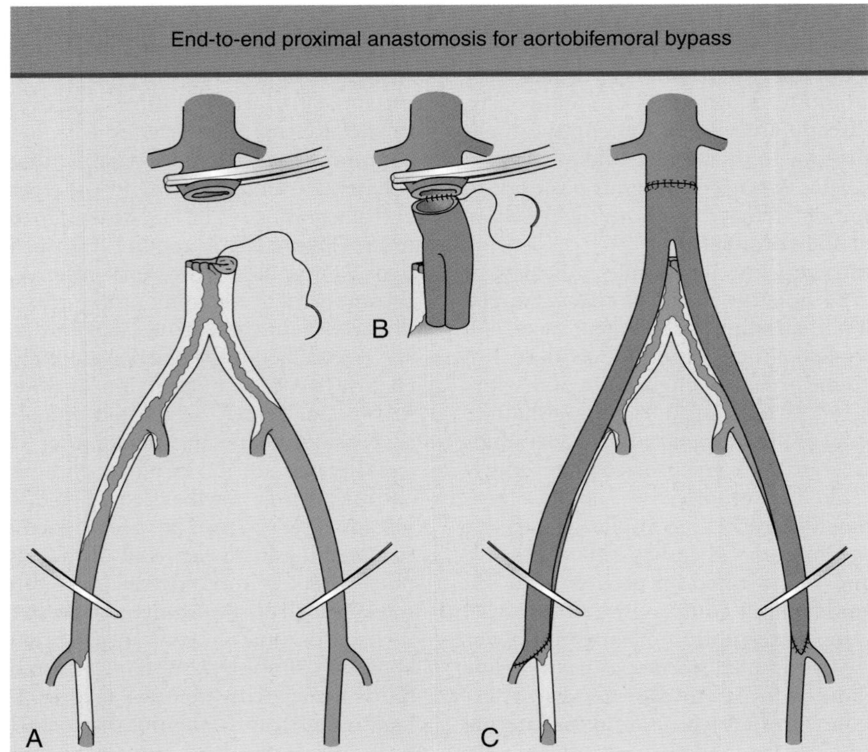

Figure 10a-4. End-to-end proximal anastomosis for aortobifemoral bypass. Pattern of aortoiliac occlusive disease appropriate for end-to-end proximal anastomosis of aortobifemoral bypass graft in which retrograde flow from femoral arteries supplies internal iliac arterial beds after occlusion of distal aorta. (Adapted from Brewster DC. Direct reconstruction for aortoiliac occlusive disease. In: Rutherford RB, ed. *Vascular surgery*. 6th ed. Philadelphia: Elsevier/Saunders; 2005:1115.)

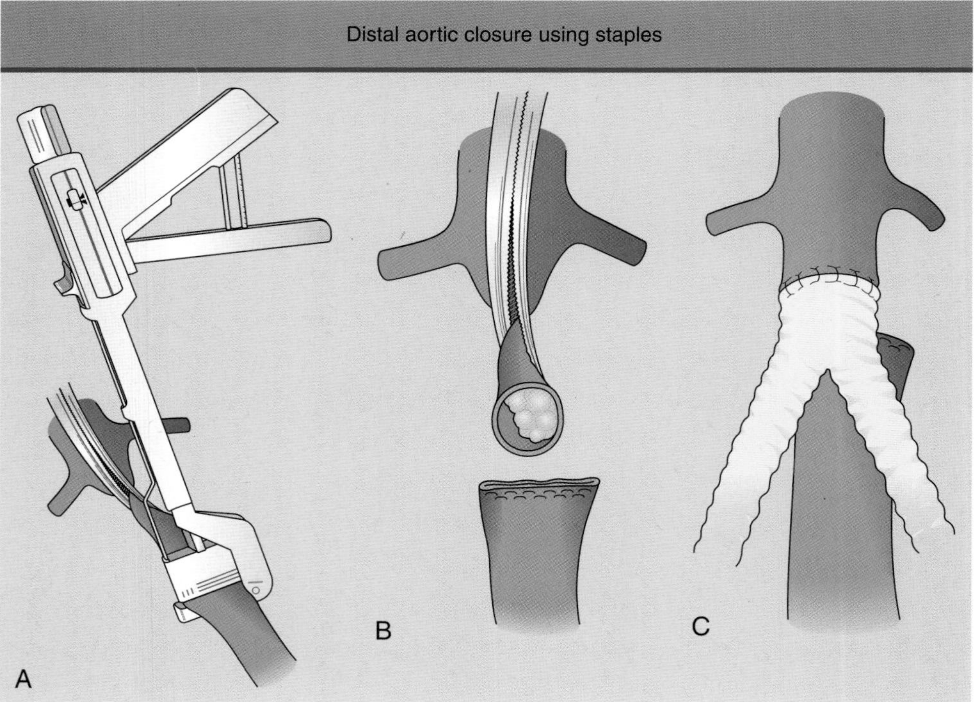

Figure 10a-5. Distal aortic closure using staples. The distal aorta may be conveniently closed using staples in aortas relatively free of calcium in patients undergoing aortobifemoral bypass with end-to-end proximal anastomosis. (Adapted from Belkin M, Whittemore AD, Donaldson MC, Mannick JA. Aortoiliac occlusive disease. In: Moore WS, ed. *Vascular surgery: a comprehensive review*. 6th ed. Philadelphia: WB Saunders; 2002:512.)

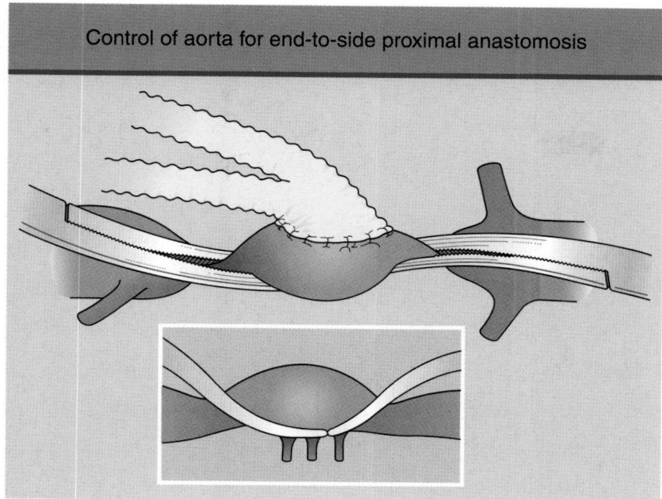

Figure 10a-6. Control of aorta for end-to-side proximal anastomosis. Method of clamping proximal aorta to allow occlusion and selective flushing of proximal and distal aorta, occlusion of lumbar arteries, and adequate exposure for local aortic thromboendarterectomy. (Adapted from Belkin M, Whittemore AD, Donaldson MC, Mannick JA. Aortoiliac occlusive disease. In: Moore WS, ed. *Vascular surgery: a comprehensive review.* 6th ed. Philadelphia: WB Saunders; 2002:513.)

exposure of the retroperitoneum. Since 1995, several technical aspects of trocar placement and set up have been standardized (Figures 10a-7 through 10a-9).[24] This approach is discussed in detail in Chapter 32.

The femoral anastomotic configuration depends on the degree of femoropopliteal occlusive disease. If the superficial femoral artery is occluded, the profunda femoris will be the predominant runoff for the graft limb. If obvious disease is at the profunda orifice, the common femoral arteriotomy should be extended down onto the first portion of the profunda femoris, where the toe of the graft limb serve as a patch profundaplasty (Figure 10a-10). If the status of the profunda orifice is unclear from preoperative imaging and palpation, the initial common femoral arteriotomy may be kept short and extended onto the profunda only if a 3.5- or 4.0-mm dilator cannot be easily passed into the profunda. Orificial or proximal profunda disease may be treated by endarterectomy, but care must be taken to avoid leaving a distal flap. Usually, endarterectomy is unnecessary and it is sufficient to simply open the profunda by patching with the hood of the bypass graft.

No evidence conclusively establishes superiority of one prosthetic graft material over another, and the choice can be made based on handling characteristics and the surgeon's preference. Dacron prostheses, optionally coated with either collagen or albumin, obviate the need for preclotting and are preferred by many surgeons because of absence of bleeding at suture holes, flexibility, and ease of manipulation. Others prefer expanded polytetrafluoroethylene (PTFE) for many of the same reasons. Regardless of which prosthetic graft is used, it is important to select the appropriate size based on the corresponding diameter of the patient's common femoral arteries. A 16 × 8 mm bifurcated prosthesis is appropriate for most patients, with smaller grafts commonly used in females and larger ones in patients with an element of arteriomegaly or ectasia.

With proper patient selection, preparation, and technical execution, 30-day postoperative mortality following aortoiliac

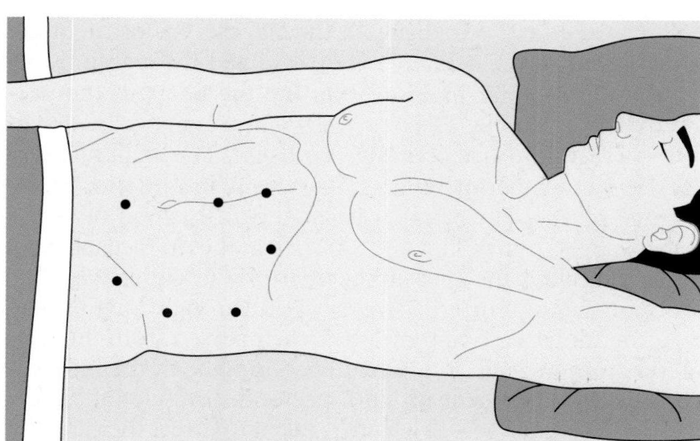

Figure 10a-7. Position of patient for laparoscopic aortobifemoral bypass with left hip elevated. (Adapted from Barbera L, Mumme A, Metin S, Volker Z, Kemen M. *J Vasc Surg* 1998;28:136-142.)

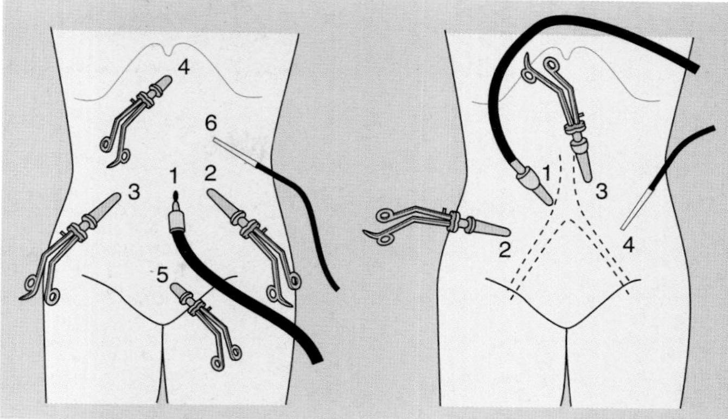

Figure 10a-8. Position of trocars for laparoscopic procedures on the infrarenal aorta. (Adapted from Barbera L, Mumme A, Metin S, Volker Z, Kemen M. *J Vasc Surg* 1998;28:136-142.)

Access site	Trocar diameter (mm)	Instruments
1	12.5	Laparoscope
2	12.5	Needle driver, scissor
3	12.5	Atraumatic grasper
4	10	Proximal clamp
5	10	Distal clamp
6	5	Grasper, suction device

Figure 10a-9. Standard access sites and instruments for laparoscopic aortic surgery. (Adapted from Barbera L, Mumme A, Metin S, Volker Z, Kemen M. *J Vasc Surg* 1998;28:136-142.)

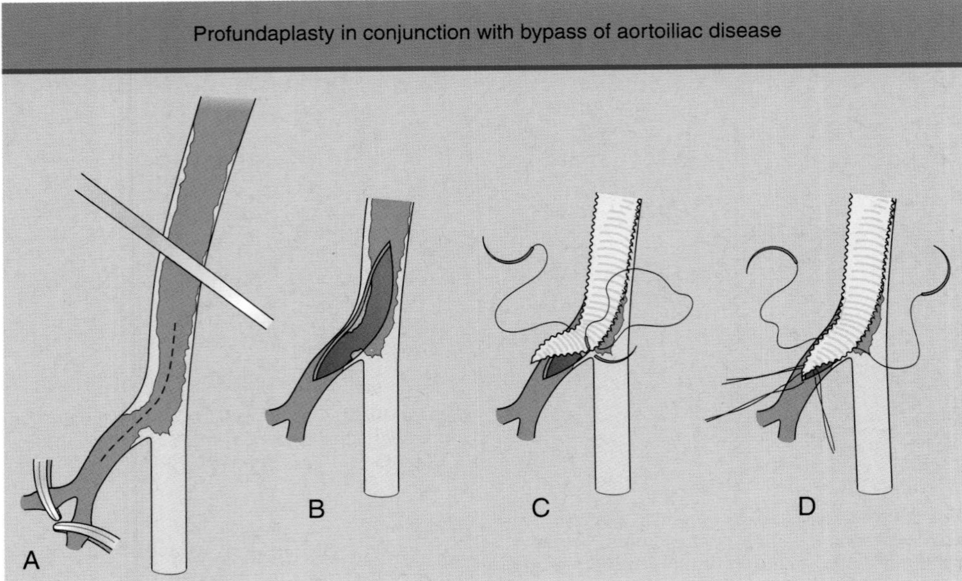

Figure 10a-10. Profundaplasty in conjunction with bypass of aortoiliac disease. The distal anastomosis of a prosthetic inflow graft should include angioplasty over significant proximal disease in the profunda femoris artery when present. (Adapted from Brewster DC. Direct reconstruction for aortoiliac occlusive disease. In: Rutherford RB, ed. *Vascular surgery*. 6th ed. Philadelphia: Elsevier/Saunders; 2005:1117.)

and aortofemoral reconstruction should not exceed 2%. No more than a small minority of additional patients should experience combined early morbidity specific to aortobifemoral bypass grafting, including the following:

- Renal dysfunction caused by hemodynamic instability, atheroembolism, renal artery occlusion, or ureteral injury
- Colon ischemia due to interruption of inflow or collaterals to the bed of the inferior mesenteric artery
- Lower extremity ischemia due to inflow occlusion or to embolism of thrombus or atheromatous debris
- Retrograde ejaculation due to injury of the nervi erigentes or interruption of the pelvic circulation

Long-term aortobifemoral bypass graft patency is excellent, with cumulative patency rates of 85% to 90% at 5 years and 70% to 75% at 10 years.[25,26] Younger patients with premature atherosclerosis and patients with small aortas, who are often female, have been shown to have inferior patency rates compared with the overall group of patients.[13]

Axillofemoral Bypass Graft

Extraanatomical bypass with axillofemoral grafting is used in patients with symptomatic aortoiliac disease who are deemed high risk for a major abdominal surgical procedure or who have a hostile abdomen due to prior irradiation, surgery, sepsis, or gastrointestinal stomas. Since few patients who meet these criteria are likely to complain solely of intermittent claudication, axillofemoral reconstructions are most commonly used for patients with critical ischemia. Unilateral axillofemoral (axillounifemoral) bypass is rarely used electively but is appropriate as a temporizing measure for aortic graft sepsis when the contralateral groin is infected or for temporary retrograde perfusion of the aorta during repair of a thoracoabdominal aneurysm. Because patency rates for axillofemoral grafts with distal anastomoses to both femoral arteries (axillobifemoral bypass) are significantly superior to the axillounifemoral configuration, partly due to increased flow through the common axillary graft limb, the axillobifemoral option is preferred for most situations when feasible.[27,28]

Construction of the axillobifemoral bypass begins by assessment of the blood pressure in each arm to select the optimal site for the proximal anastomosis. If pressures are equivalent, it is preferable to base the inflow on the right axillary artery because the innominate-right subclavian artery is less likely to develop hemodynamically significant occlusive disease than the left subclavian artery. Routine preoperative arteriography or other imaging has been recommended before axillofemoral bypass because of evidence of significant inflow disease in 25% of patients undetected by noninvasive testing in 75%.[29,30]

The patient is positioned supine with the donor arm supported on a narrow arm board and with slight flexion at the elbow in a "hand–in–pants pocket" configuration. This posture relaxes the pectoralis muscles to facilitate tunneling and axillary artery exposure beneath the clavicle. Exposure of the first portion of the axillary artery is gained through a transverse infraclavicular incision, splitting the fibers of the pectoralis major muscle. The pectoralis minor may be divided, if necessary, to improve operative exposure. The axillary artery lies deep and superior to the axillary vein and inferior to the brachial plexus. The artery is isolated by dissection toward a palpable pulse or by following a branch of the thoracoacromial trunk, reflecting the vein either inferiorly or superiorly. The common femoral arteries are exposed through longitudinal groin incisions. A long tunneler is then passed from the ipsilateral groin incision in a subcutaneous plane in the midaxillary line and then beneath both pectoralis muscles along the chest wall (Figure 10a-11). Care is taken to direct the tunneler medial to the anterior iliac spine and to remain superficial to the costal margin. Grafts tunneled too far anterior to the midaxillary line are prone to kinking.[31] Use of a long tunneler

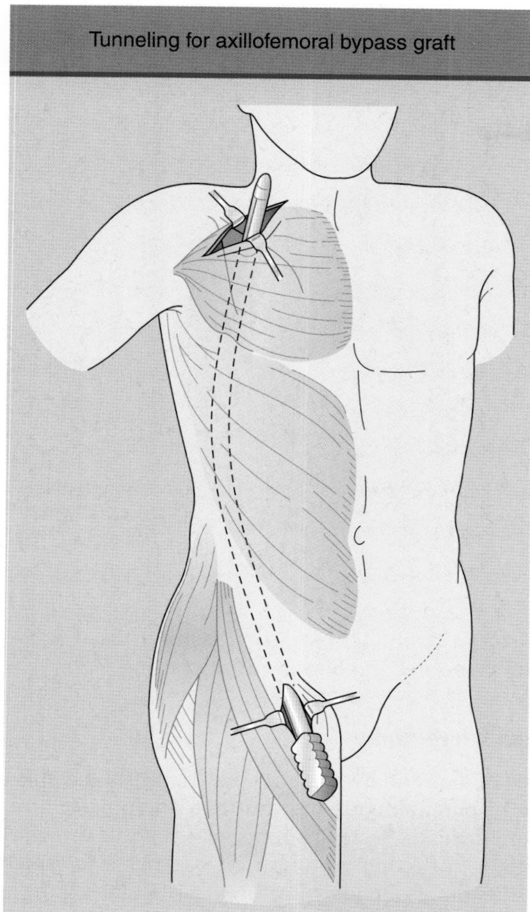

Figure 10a-11. Tunneling for axillofemoral bypass graft. A long tunneling instrument is used to create space for the graft in a subcutaneous plane, anterior to the iliac spine; in the midaxillary line; and under the pectoralis muscles on the chest wall, toward the proximal axillary artery. (Adapted from Taylor LM, Landry GJ, Moneta GL, Porter JM. Axillobifemoral bypass. In: Nyhus LM, Baker RJ, Fischer JE, eds. *Mastery of surgery*. 3rd ed. Boston: Little, Brown; 1997:2040.)

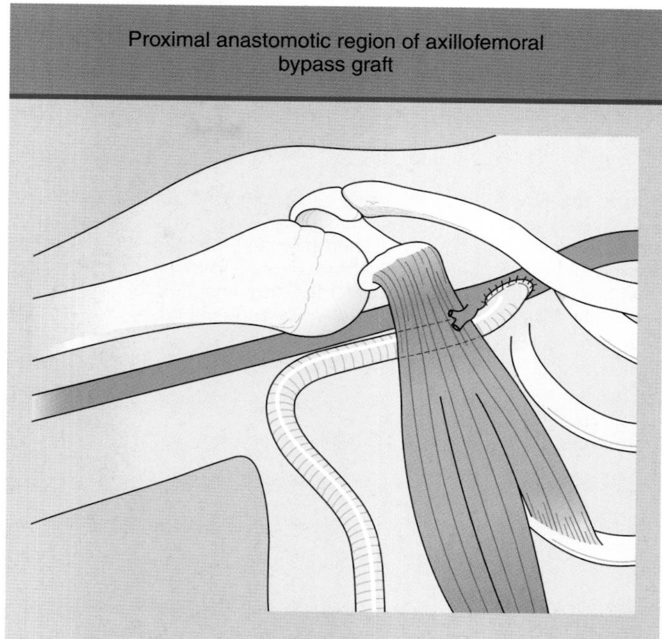

Figure 10a-12. Proximal anastomotic region of axillofemoral bypass graft. The graft is connected to the anterior–inferior surface of the proximal axillary artery adjacent to the chest wall, with oblique course along the artery under the pectoralis muscles and some laxity (exaggerated in figure for emphasis) to avoid undue tension at the anastomosis when the arm is elevated. (Adapted from Taylor LM, Landry GJ, Moneta GL, Porter JM. Axillobifemoral bypass. In: Nyhus LM, Baker RJ, Fischer JE, eds. *Mastery of surgery*. 3rd ed. Boston: Little, Brown; 1997:2040.)

avoids the need for a counter incision along the course of the graft and eliminates a potential source of wound complications. A femorofemoral tunnel is then created in a gentle inverted C shape in the subcutaneous plane on the fascia of the external oblique and anterior rectus sheath. Dacron and PTFE grafts have been used with equally good results, usually in an 8-mm diameter with optional external supporting rings to minimize the risk of graft compression. The graft may be passed through the long tunnel before or after the proximal anastomosis is constructed.

Once the patient is systemically heparinized, clamps are applied as proximally as possible on the axillary artery. The anastomosis is created proximal to the pectoralis minor muscle. An arteriotomy is made on the anterior–inferior aspect of the artery to allow gentle angulation of the anastomosis into the subcutaneous plane. Traumatic disruption of the axillary anastomosis has been reported with excessive arm abduction either because the graft was pulled down to the groin too tightly[32] or because the axillary arterial anastomosis was performed at too acute (less than 75 degrees) of an angle (Figure 10a-12). The graft is flushed and clamped at its origin to allow reperfusion of the arm while the ipsilateral femoral anastomosis is constructed. The graft is copiously flushed again just before final closure of the distal suture line and establishment of flow into the leg.

Several configurations have been advocated for the femorofemoral portion of the bypass, although no conclusive evidence favors one over another. Grafts are available with a preattached femoral sidearm, in which case the graft must be carefully positioned in the tunnels before creation of the axillary anastomosis to assure optimal alignment of the sidearm. Most surgeons prefer to construct the sidearm by excising a window on the medial aspect of the axillofemoral limb using one of several alternative configurations: (1) a “lazy S” shape, involving an anastomosis just below the anterior iliac spine; (2) an “inverted C” shape, with the anastomosis in the groin, just above or into the hood of the distal axillofemoral anastomosis; or even (3) dividing the distal external iliac artery and performing an end-to-end anastomosis between the femorofemoral prosthetic and the divided external iliac artery (Figure 10a-13). Configurations that eliminate the short arm of the graft system connected to the ipsilateral femoral artery may be preferred in situations when the runoff below the ipsilateral femoral artery is severely compromised, creating reduced flow in the short limb.

Early complications specific to axillofemoral bypass include injury to the axillary artery, axillary vein, and brachial plexus, in addition to inadvertent entry into the peritoneal or pleural cavity with the tunneler. Axillary anastomotic disruption and perigraft seroma are also occasionally associated with axillofemoral grafting.

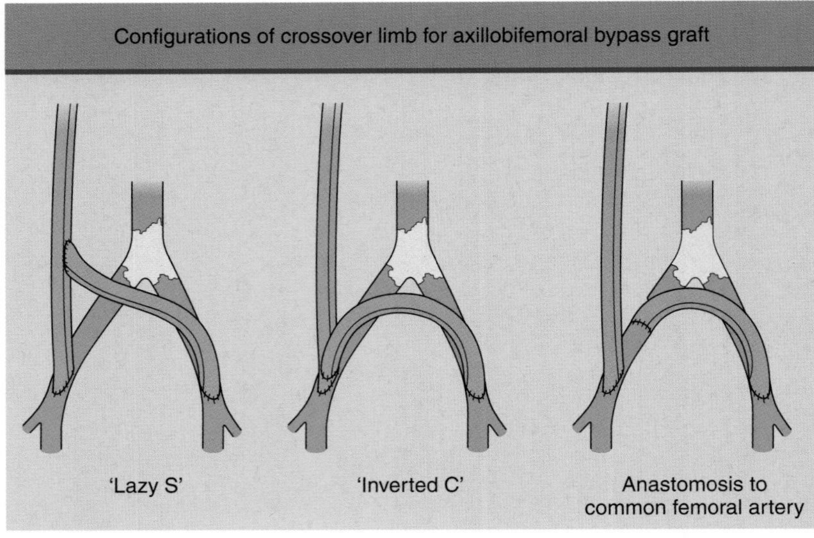

Figure 10a-13. Configurations of crossover limb for axillobifemoral bypass graft. Configurations that minimize low flow in the ipsilateral short femoral limb may be preferable when there is compromised runoff from the short limb. (Adapted from Schneider JR. Extra-anatomic bypass. In: Rutherford RB, ed. *Vascular surgery*. 6th ed. Philadelphia: Elsevier/Saunders; 2005:1143.)

Patency rates for axillofemoral bypass are strongly influenced by the operative indications, the graft configuration, and the status of the runoff vessels. When the procedure is performed for aortic sepsis following aortic aneurysm resection in the bifemoral configuration with patent superficial femoral artery runoff, 5-year primary patency rates may approach 90%. On the other hand, when performed for occlusive disease in the unilateral configuration with an occluded superficial femoral artery in the recipient groin, the long-term primary patency rate may be expected to be much lower. Circumstances between these relative extremes can be expected to yield intermediate patency results. Choice of supported or unsupported Dacron versus PTFE graft material has no clear patency advantage.[29,33] Secondary patency is substantially higher than primary patency, rewarding efforts to disobliterate and revise grafts when necessary.[34]

Isolated Iliac Occlusive Disease

Isolated iliac disease is relatively uncommon, as disease tends to affect both the aorta and the iliac arteries. Standard aortobifemoral bypass is the most definitive approach in good-risk younger patients, thus obviating any possible progression of disease in the less involved arteries over time. When the infrarenal aorta does not have significant disease and at least one common iliac artery is uninvolved, iliac disease may be successfully addressed independently of the aorta.[12,35] Since it can be assumed that atherosclerosis will eventually compromise the source of iliac inflow, this approach is most appealing among patients with minimal inflow disease at the outset and in whom longevity may be limited by age or concurrent illness.[36,37]

In addition to axillofemoral bypass, iliofemoral endarterectomy and iliofemoral or iliobifemoral bypass are options applicable to patients with suitable anatomy and excessive comorbidity for major abdominal surgery. Femorofemoral bypass is an excellent option, with good long-term success for patients with hemodynamically intact contralateral iliofemoral inflow to the groin. If necessary, mild-to-moderate iliac inflow disease may be corrected using endovascular techniques to allow subsequent surgical bypass based on the improved inflow to the groin. This strategy has been used successfully for femorofemoral and femorodistal grafting.[37,38]

Iliac Endarterectomy

The role of iliac endarterectomy has diminished with increasing use of percutaneous transluminal angioplasty and stenting. Nonetheless, selected patients with suitable short-segment involvement of either common or external iliac vessels have durable results after endarterectomy, particularly if the arteries are relatively large in caliber. This approach should not be used if there is aneurysmal change. Using the semiclosed technique without patching, endarterectomy obviates the need for prosthetic material and is thus an option when infection is a consideration. For patients with localized unilateral common iliac or external iliac occlusive disease, a retroperitoneal approach to the iliac fossa provides good access.[39,40] The common, internal, and external iliac artery are exposed through a "kidney transplant" incision. Once proximal and distal control are achieved, techniques similar to those described earlier for aortoiliac endarterectomy disease may be used. A semiclosed approach may be employed via transverse arteriotomies with a ring endarterectomy loop to remove the core of disease, followed by transverse closure without the need for patch angioplasty. In smaller arteries, or when the disease ends adjacent to the iliac bifurcation, longitudinal arteriotomies may be used to facilitate exposure of the distal endpoint, in which case closure is performed with a patch angioplasty of vein or prosthetic material. Less commonly, a single arteriotomy may afford adequate exposure to handle focal plaque. Concomitant common femoral endarterectomy, profundaplasty, or ipsilateral distal bypass may be combined with iliac endarterectomy in patients with unilateral multilevel disease.[39,41]

Iliofemoral Bypass

When the disease has caused occlusion of the external iliac artery but has largely spared the distal aorta and ipsilateral common iliac artery, the common iliac may serve well as the site of inflow for bypass to the ipsilateral femoral artery, with an adjunctive cross-limb to the contralateral femoral artery if necessary.[37] Although axillofemoral bypass and femorofemoral bypass may be equally applicable in similar situations, iliofemoral grafts may be preferable because of generally more favorable long-term success. The iliobifemoral option may be chosen for patients with favorable ipsilateral anatomy and severe contralateral iliac disease who are felt to be high risk for aortobifemoral bypass. Alternatively, the unilateral iliofemoral bypass is a good choice for relatively healthy and active individuals with unilateral disease in whom a durable, strictly ipsilateral solution is desired. Occasionally, the unilateral graft is helpful if there is good reason to avoid the contralateral groin, such as sepsis or previous surgery. Presence of heavy calcification in the donor iliac artery on preoperative imaging makes this method less attractive because of potential difficulties in clamping and sewing the artery.

Exposure of the common iliac artery is obtained with a retroperitoneal incision extending obliquely from the anterior axillary line near the tip of the eleventh rib to 2 to 3 cm below the umbilicus. The external and internal oblique muscles are divided. The medial extent of the incision may be terminated at the lateral edge of the rectus or with partial rectus incision in patients with wide costal margins. The transversus abdominus muscle is split in the line of its fibers, and a preperitoneal plane is developed and retracted medially. Use of a mechanical retractor system is of great help in gaining and maintaining adequate exposure of the deeper structures, particularly in relatively obese patients. The ureter is carefully mobilized away from the common iliac artery. The external and internal iliac artery origins are mobilized sufficiently for later control with loops or clamps. The common iliac artery should be mobilized to its origin and the exposure extended to include the proximal contralateral iliac artery and distal aorta if there is heavy calcification and no favorable place for clamping. After exposing the common femoral artery through a longitudinal groin incision, a tunnel is created under the inguinal ligament anterior to the external iliac artery and under the ureter if it has been mobilized distal to the common iliac artery.

Proximal control of the common iliac artery is easily obtained with a clamp if the vessel is soft and generally free of disease. If there is circumferential or partially circumferential calcification, however, clamping may be difficult or may create a dissection or injury sufficient to compromise the anastomosis. Under these circumstances, it may be preferable to make use of a 5- or 6-mm occluding balloon, passed through the graft and into the artery via a stab wound, to provide atraumatic inflow occlusion (Figure 10a-14). Most commonly, an 8-mm prosthesis is an appropriate graft choice, constructing the proximal anastomosis using a continuous "parachute" technique without tying down the heel and toe of the graft to provide better visualization deep in the wound. If an additional graft limb is planned to the contralateral side, a cross-limb may be attached to the graft in the retroperitoneum and passed across preperitoneally and under the contralateral inguinal ligament to the femoral artery. Alternatively and generally more easily, a femorofemoral bypass is constructed from the region of the ipsilateral femoral anastomosis across to the other femoral artery via the subcutaneous plane (Figure 10a-15).

Although iliofemoral bypass was originally most commonly performed among patients judged unfit for transabdominal

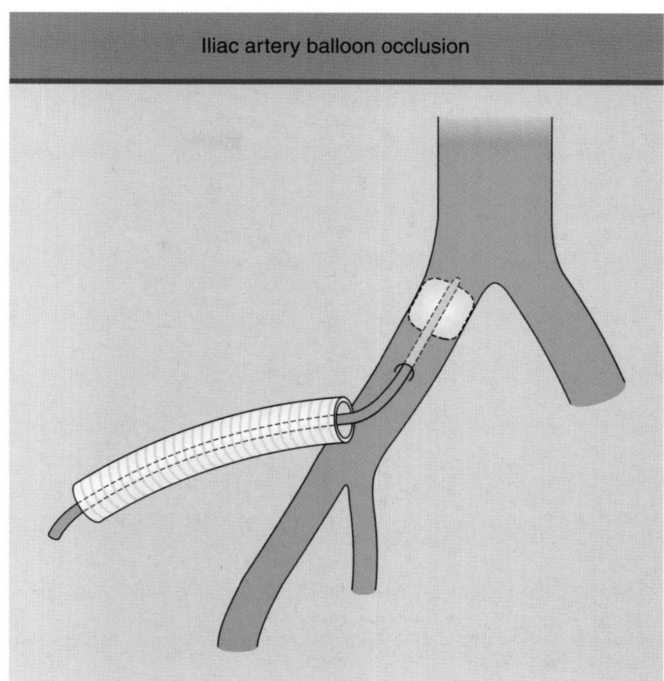

Figure 10a-14. Iliac artery balloon occlusion. Method for balloon occlusion of a calcified common iliac artery during iliofemoral bypass grafting. The prosthetic graft is loaded on the balloon before insertion and inflation for control of inflow and then tailored to be sewn end-to-side into the arterotomy created by enlarging the iliac puncture using Potts scissors. Proximal iliac or distal aortic exposure should be adequate to control inflow as backup in the event of balloon failure.

surgery, long-term patency rates have proven sufficient to allow indications to be extended to all patients with anatomically appropriate disease patterns.[37,42] Cumulative 5-year patency rates in the range of 80% are typical.[43] When applied for unilateral external iliac occlusion, patency rates for iliofemoral and femorofemoral bypass are equivalent in some reports,[44,45] but others demonstrate a small patency advantage for iliofemoral bypass, perhaps related to its antegrade configuration.[37,46-48] Other important advantages include avoidance of morbidity related to a second groin incision and placement of the graft deep within the pelvis, where it is less susceptible to external compression or kinking.

Iliofemoral Bypass via Obturator Foramen

Restoration of flow to the lower extremity may be problematic if the femoral triangle is unsuitable for anastomosis or routing of a graft conduit. Such circumstances occur in the patients with groin sepsis, malignancy, radiation injury, or trauma. Routing of a graft from a clean abdominal or pelvic source through the obturator foramen into the posteromedial thigh or popliteal space avoids wound morbidity from poor healing, infection, and hemorrhage.[49,50]

The procedure requires thorough preoperative imaging to establish the status of the iliac, superficial femoral, and popliteal arteries. The patient is prepared for abdominal and lower extremity exposure under general or high regional anesthesia. If the groin is infected or open, it is carefully prepped out to exclude contamination of the sterile operative field. In most

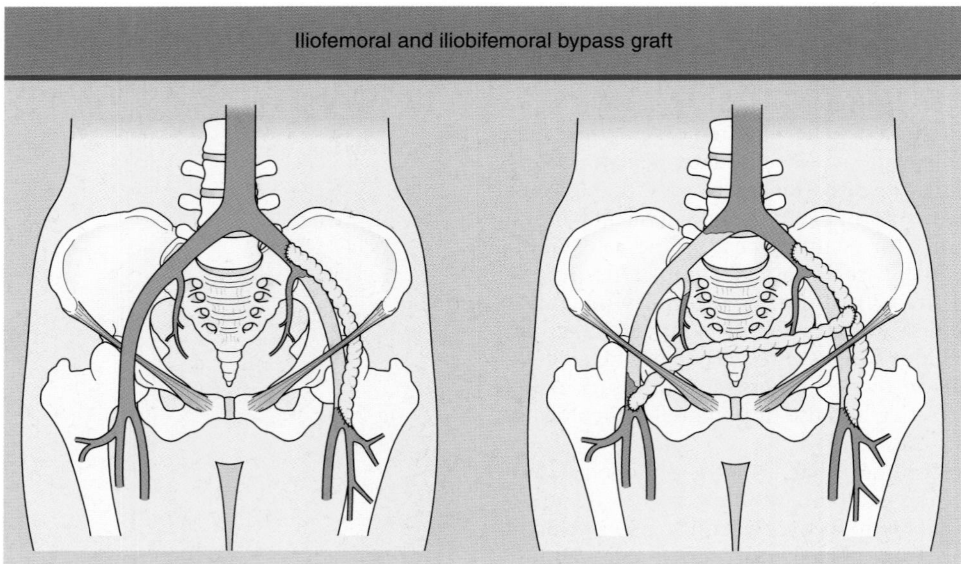

Figure 10a-15. Iliofemoral and iliobifemoral bypass graft. Configurations of retroperitoneal iliofemoral bypass for unilateral external iliac occlusion *(left)* and iliobifemoral bypass for bilateral iliac occlusions with common iliac artery sparing *(right)*. (Adapted from Belkin M, Whittemore AD, Donaldson MC, Mannick JA. Aortoiliac occlusive disease. In: Moore WS, ed. *Vascular surgery: a comprehensive review.* 6th ed. Philadelphia: WB Saunders; 2002:516.)

instances, the common iliac artery is the inflow vessel and the middle or distal superficial femoral or proximal popliteal artery is the recipient outflow vessel for the bypass graft. Either saphenous vein or prosthetic conduit may be chosen. Exposure of the iliac artery is performed through an oblique muscle splitting incision in the flank as described earlier. The pelvic peritoneum is reflected medially sufficiently to feel and then visualize the obturator foramen inferior to the symphysis pubis. The obturator artery and nerve penetrate the internal and external obturator muscles through an anteromedial canal, which can be palpated with the fingertip (Figure 10a-16). The membrane is carefully incised at this location to allow the fingertip to be pushed through into the upper thigh. A counterincision is made over the distal medial thigh through which the adductor magnus muscle is retracted to allow exposure of the distal superficial femoral or proximal popliteal artery. Blunt dissection allows tunneling back to the fingertip opening in the obturator foramen. An umbilical tape is passed from pelvis to leg through the foramen using a long aortic clamp.

After systemic heparinization, the distal anastomosis is created and the graft is flushed and clamped just above the anastomosis. The graft is carefully oriented and passed retrograde into the pelvis through the obturator foramen. The proximal anastomosis is then created using techniques described earlier. After flushing and completion, flow is established. Gentle palpation of the graft as it exits the pelvis assures absence of kinking or extrinsic compression. A completion arteriogram assures satisfactory flow and technique (Figure 10a-17). If resection of the femoral artery is indicated because of threat of hemorrhage due to infection, the external iliac artery may be oversewn proximally and distally within the pelvis, divided and the distal end tucked under a soft-tissue closure to exclude subsequent retrograde pelvic contamination. Wounds are closed in layers and left under sterile dressings with adhesive protection during any subsequent manipulations in the groin. When femoral artery resection is planned, presence of a functioning obturator bypass graft through clean tissue planes allows direct excision of the femoral artery and oversewing of the adjacent vessels with monofilament suture through the groin.

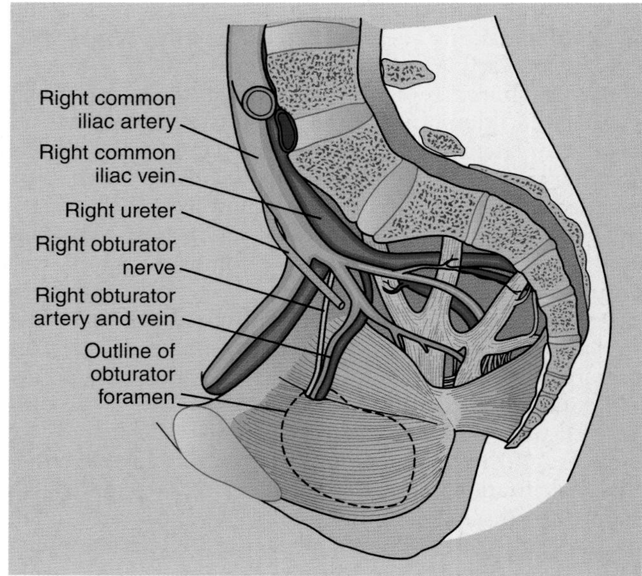

Figure 10a-16. Anatomy of the obturator foramen from within the pelvis, indicating the location of the canal through which the obturator artery, vein, and nerve penetrate the internal and external obturator musculofascial layers. (Adapted from Schneider JR. Extra-anatomic bypass. In: Rutherford RB, ed. *Vascular surgery.* 6th ed. Philadelphia: Elsevier/Saunders; 2005:1148.)

Although rarely necessary, the obturator bypass is a valuable method for managing difficult and challenging problems affecting the groin.[51-53] It has proven highly successful given adequate inflow and outflow, careful technique, and management of the adjacent groin issue. Hazards include prosthetic

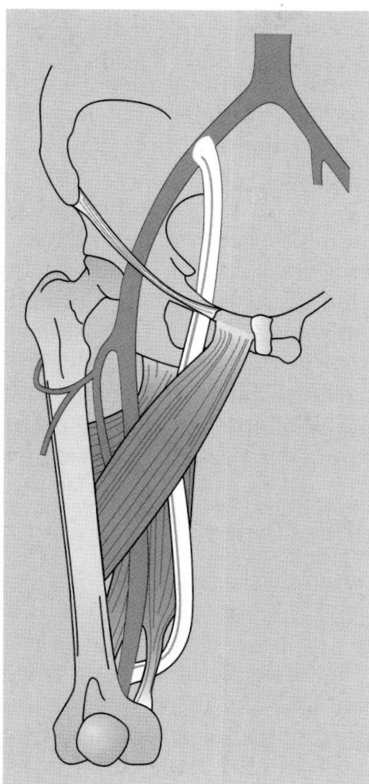

Figure 10a-17. Configuration of obturator bypass using prosthetic material from the iliac to popliteal arteries. (Adapted from Schneider JR. Extra-anatomic bypass. In: Rutherford RB, ed. *Vascular surgery.* 6th ed. Philadelphia: Elsevier/Saunders; 2005:1148.)

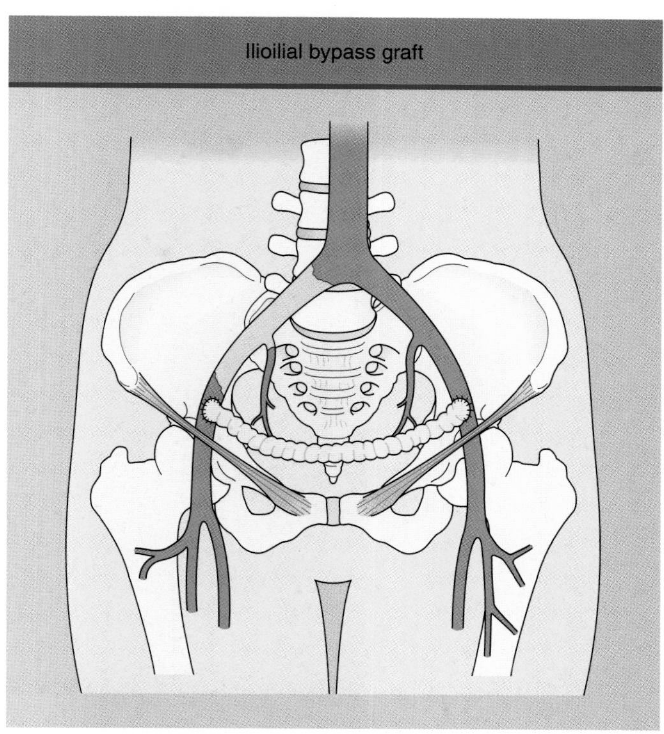

Figure 10a-18. Ilioiliac bypass graft. Configuration for graft crossing in preperitoneal plane from normal donor iliac artery to contralateral external iliac artery. (Adapted from Belkin M, Whittemore AD, Donaldson MC, Mannick JA. Aortoiliac occlusive disease. In: Moore WS, ed. *Vascular surgery: a comprehensive review.* 6th ed. Philadelphia: WB Saunders; 2002:516.)

graft contamination, hemorrhage from injury to the obturator vessels during tunneling, and kinking or twisting of the graft.

Ilioiliac Bypass

Under unusual circumstances, it may be advantageous to construct a bypass between a donor iliac and the contralateral iliac artery. This option is particularly appealing in patients who have had previous femoral artery procedures on either the donor or the recipient side or who have another compelling reason, such as sepsis, for avoiding one or the other groin. Another reason to avoid groin incisions might be a preference to preserve the groin for later distal bypass work. As for femorofemoral bypass, the donor iliac must be free of significant disease. The recipient-side anatomy consists of the relatively unusual pattern of common iliac occlusion with a virtually normal external iliac artery (Figure 10a-18). The external iliac arteries are exposed through an extraperitoneal plane via curvilinear oblique incisions parallel to and above the inguinal ligament. The prosthetic graft is tunneled through the preperitoneal plane via the space of Retzius, thus allowing deeper placement and better protection of the graft than is possible with femorofemoral bypass. The graft must be carefully routed past the bladder to avoid injury.

In a small series of patients undergoing ilioiliac bypass,[54] the cumulative patency rate was 96% at 4 years, demonstrating this technique to be an excellent option for selected patients with unilateral occlusive disease limited to the common iliac artery.

Femorofemoral Bypass

Patients whose occlusive disease is confined to one iliac artery, with the aorta and contralateral iliac system free of hemodynamically significant disease, may be candidates for femorofemoral bypass. Typical candidates include patients in whom unilateral iliac lesions are not amenable to percutaneous therapy and in whom direct aortobifemoral bypass is judged unduly arduous or unnecessary. It is critical that the donor iliac artery is assessed before performing femorofemoral bypass. Presence of a normal femoral pulse on physical examination is a reassuring sign that should be followed by imaging using duplex ultrasound, MRA, or contrast angiography to be certain no anatomical lesion creates more than a 50% diameter stenosis. If a lesion of questionable significance exists, hemodynamic assessment at preoperative angiography or early during surgery establishes its importance. Resting femoral artery pressure sampled through a needle or catheter should be no more than 10 mm Hg below the simultaneous pressure measured via a catheter in the radial artery or via a brachial cuff. The most precise assessment is obtained by advancing an end-hole catheter retrograde into the abdominal aorta and measuring pressure continuously as the catheter is pulled back through the lesion in question. Any pressure gradient is abnormal under these circumstances, and equivocal findings can be clarified by use of reactive hyperemia after thigh cuff occlusion or more readily by intraarterial injection of a vasodilator such as papaverine. A 15% or greater drop in the femoral pressure with these maneuvers is consistent with

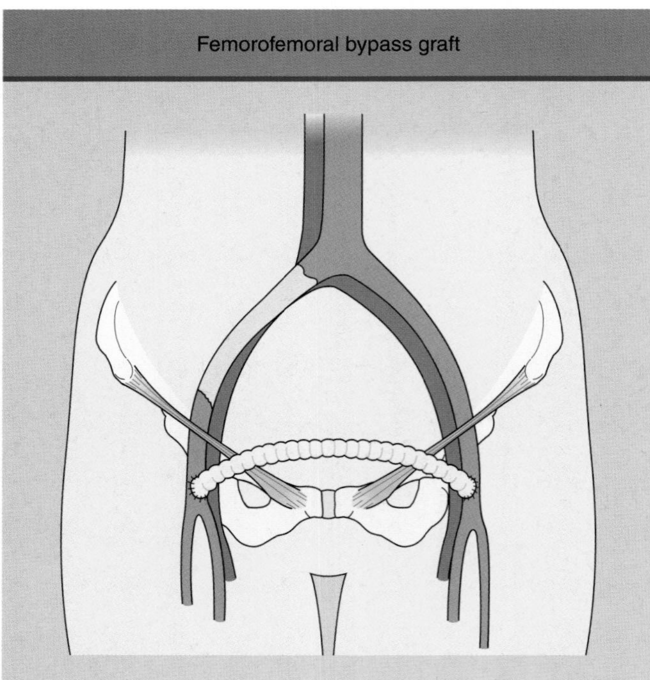

Figure 10a-19. Femorofemoral bypass graft. Configuration of the femorofemoral bypass with graft in a deep subcutaneous plane above the pubic rim in a simple inverted U pattern. To minimize kinking, the ends of the graft should approach the groins more parallel to the common femoral arteries than shown in figure. (Adapted from Belkin M, Whittemore AD, Donaldson MC, Mannick JA. Aortoiliac occlusive disease. In: Moore WS, ed. *Vascular surgery: a comprehensive review.* 6th ed. Philadelphia: WB Saunders; 2002:516.)

the presence of significant inflow disease.[55] If a hemodynamically significant focal lesion is identified, it can be corrected by balloon angioplasty or stent. Inflow thus corrected has been found to be reliable when used for femorofemoral and femorodistal grafts.[37,38]

Femorofemoral bypass is particularly applicable to high-risk patients as it can be performed under regional or even local anesthesia. The lower abdomen and upper thighs should be included in the sterile field to allow access to the external iliac arteries, as well as the superficial and deep femoral arteries. Both common femoral arteries are exposed through longitudinal groin incisions. The incisions are connected via a subcutaneous suprapubic tunnel created by blunt dissection just anterior to the deep fascia. A gentle inverted U configuration is constructed well above the pubic rim to avoid compression (Figure 10a-19). The ends of the graft should approach the anastomotic regions without undue tension and parallel to the femoral arteries, with the arteriotomies usually angled obliquely toward the profunda femoris artery, to avoid kinking of the graft and to facilitate profundaplasty if necessary. Prosthetic grafts of the surgeon's choice are equally suitable, usually 8 mm in diameter. Care must be taken to close the wounds without residual dead space but to accommodate the graft as it transits from the deep tissue under the femoral sheath into the subcutaneous plane.

Reported primary patency rates of femorofemoral bypass are highly variable and range from 50% to 90% at 5 years, perhaps reflecting differences in patient selection criteria.[56] For example, under ideal circumstances with virtually normal iliofemoral artery inflow and patent superficial femoral artery outflow, primary patency may exceed 90%, compared with 50% when the superficial femoral artery is occluded. With close surveillance, reported secondary patency rates may exceed 90% at 4 years.[48] In patients with a patent superficial femoral artery, femorofemoral bypass patency rates can be expected to be similar to those for aortobifemoral bypass.[35] Hemodynamically, addition of the contralateral lower extremity to the runoff below the donor iliac artery results in increased volume and velocity of blood flow through the donor iliac system. This may result in significant dilatation of the donor iliac artery over time.[57] If the donor iliac artery is hemodynamically normal, it is capable of providing adequate flow to both limbs without creating a "steal" phenomenon, which becomes a clinically important issue only if the donor iliac is stenotic.[58]

Internal Iliac Artery Bypass

Internal iliac artery revascularization is generally reserved for patients with symptoms of gluteal claudication or vasculogenic impotence and for selected patients undergoing endovascular repair of bilateral iliac artery aneurysms.[59-61] The ipsilateral external iliac and the hypogastric artery of interest are dissected free from their surrounding structures, generally through an extraperitoneal plane using a curvilinear, transplant incision several centimeters proximal to the inguinal ligament. A 6- or 8-mm prosthetic graft is then sewn end to side to the anteromedial aspect of the external iliac artery. The graft is tunneled cephalad and medial. An end-to-side anastomosis constructed in a continuous "parachute" technique facilitates exposure as the distal anastomosis is constructed along the inferomedial aspect of the hypogastric artery.

CONCLUSIONS

Surgical intervention for lower extremity arterial occlusive disease should be offered to treat severe symptoms only after nonoperative and endovascular management has failed or been rejected for appropriate reasons. If surgery is undertaken, it should have a high benefit-to-risk ratio with realistic expectations regarding functional outcome goals. The surgeon must take into account the natural history data regarding expected patient survival and limb amputation rates in this patient population. Procedural morbidity and mortality must be carefully considered for each patient within the context of the surgeon's own institution, despite excellent statistics in the literature. Once intervention has been chosen, surgery should be used with catheter-based techniques to achieve the best possible result with the least attendant cost and morbidity.

References

1. Trans-Atlantic Inter-Society Consensus II Working Group. Inter-Society consensus for the management of peripheral arterial disease (TASC II). *J Vasc Surg* 2007;45(Suppl):S5-S67.
2. McDaniel MD, Cronenwett JL. Basic data related to the natural history of intermittent claudication. *Ann Vasc Surg* 1989;3:273-277.
3. Brewster DC, Darling RC. Optimal methods of aortoiliac reconstruction. *Surgery* 1978;84:739-748.
4. Staple T. The solitary aortoiliac lesion. *Surgery* 1968;64:569.
5. Moore W, Cafferata HT, Hall AD, Blaisdell FW. In defense of grafts across the inguinal ligament. *Ann Surg* 1968;168:207.
6. Mozersky DJ, Sumner DS, Strandness DE. Long-term results of reconstructive aortoiliac surgery. *Am J Surg* 1972;123:503-509.

7. Criqui MH, Langer RD, Fronek A, et al. Mortality over a period of 10 years in patients with peripheral arterial disease. *N Engl J Med* 1992;326:381-386.
8. Hertzer NR, Beven EG, Young JR, et al. Coronary artery disease in peripheral vascular patients: a classification of 1000 coronary angiograms and results of surgical management. *Ann Surg* 1984;199:223-233.
9. Whittemore A, Donaldson MC, Mannick JA, et al. Aortoiliac occlusive disease. *Philadelphia: WB Saunders* 1998:483-494.
10. Valentine RJ, Hansen ME, Myers SI, et al. The influence of sex and aortic size on late patency after aortofemoral revascularization in young adults. *J Vasc Surg* 1995;21:296-305, discussion, 305-306.
11. Crawford ES, Bomberger RA, Glaeser DH, et al. Aortoiliac occlusive disease: factors influencing survival and function following reconstructive operation over a twenty-five-year period. *Surgery* 1981;90:1055-1067.
12. Brewster DC. Current controversies in the management of aortoiliac occlusive disease. *J Vasc Surg* 1997;25:365-379.
13. Reed AB, Conte MS, Donaldson MC, et al. The impact of patient age and aortic size on the results of aortobifemoral bypass grafting. *J Vasc Surg* 2003;37:1219-1225.
14. Wylie E. Thromboendarterectomy for arteriosclerotic thrombus of major arteries. *Surgery* 1952;32:275-292.
15. Inahara T. Evaluation of endarterectomy for aortoiliac and aortoiliofemoral occlusive disease. *Arch Surg* 1975;110:1458-1464.
16. van den Akker PJ, van Schilfgaarde R, Brand R, et al. Long-term results of prosthetic and non-prosthetic reconstruction for obstructive aorto-iliac disease. *Eur J Vasc Surg* 1992;6:53-61.
17. Mikati A, Marache P, Watel A, et al. End-to-side aortoprosthetic anastomoses: long-term computed tomography assessment. *Ann Vasc Surg* 1990;4:584-591.
18. Rutherford RB, Jones DN, Martin MS, et al. Serial hemodynamic assessment of aortobifemoral bypass. *J Vasc Surg* 1986;4:428-435.
19. Ameli FM, Stein M, Aro L, et al. End-to-end versus end-to-side proximal anastomosis in aortobifemoral bypass surgery: does it matter? *Can J Surg* 1991;34:243-246.
20. Melliere D, Labastie J, Becquemin JP, et al. Proximal anastomosis in aortobifemoral bypass: end-to-end or end-to-side? *J Cardiovasc Surg (Torino)* 1990;31:77-80.
21. Robbs JV, Wylie EJ. Factors contributing to recurrent lower limb ischemia following bypass surgery for aortoiliac occlusive disease, and their management. *Ann Surg* 1981;193:346-352.
22. Sanders RJ, Kempczinski RF, Hammond W, DiClementi D. The significance of graft diameter. *Surgery* 1980;88:856-866.
23. Dion YM, Gaillard F, Demalsy JC, Gracia CR. Experimental laparoscopic aortobifemoral bypass for occlusive disease. *Can J Surg* 1996;39: 451-455.
24. Barbera L, Mumme A, Metin S, et al. Operative results and outcome of twenty-four totally laparoscopic vascular procedures for aortoiliac occlusive disease. *J Vasc Surg* 1998;28:136-142.
25. Hertzer NM, Bena JF, Karafa MT. A personal experience with direct reconstruction and extra-anatomic bypass for aortoiliofemoral occlusive disease. *J Vasc Surg* 2007;45:527-535.
26. de Vries SO, Hunink MGM. Results of aortic bifurcation grafts for aortoiliac occlusive disease: a meta-analysis. *J Vasc Surg* 1997;26:558-569.
27. van den Dungen JJ, Boontje AH, Kropveld A. Unilateral iliofemoral occlusive disease: long-term results of the semi-closed endarterectomy with the ring-stripper. *J Vasc Surg* 1991;14:673-677.
28. Ascer E, Veith FJ, Gupta SK, et al. Comparison of axillounifemoral and axillobifemoral bypass operations. *Surgery* 1985;97:169-175.
29. Schneider JR. Extra-anatomic bypass. In: Rutherford RB, ed. Vascular surgery. 6th ed. Philadelphia: Elsevier; 2005:1141-1147.
30. Calligaro KD, Veith FJ, Gupta SK, et al. Unsuspected inflow disease in candidates for axillofemoral bypass operations: a prospective study. *J Vasc Surg* 1990;11:832-837.
31. Mannick JA, Williams LE, Nabseth DC. The late results of axillofemoral grafts. *Surgery* 1970;68:1038-1043.
32. Taylor Jr LM, Park TC, Edwards JM, et al. Acute disruption of polytetrafluoroethylene grafts adjacent to axillary anastomoses: a complication of axillofemoral grafting. *J Vasc Surg* 1994;20:520-526.
33. Johnson WC, Lee KK. Comparative evaluation of externally supported Dacron and polytetrafluoroethylene prosthetic bypasses for femorofemoral and axillofemoral arterial reconstructions: Veterans Affairs Cooperative Study No. 141. *J Vasc Surg* 1999;30:1077-1083.
34. Schneider JR, Golan JF. The role of extraanatomic bypass in the management of bilateral aortoiliac occlusive disease. *Semin Vasc Surg* 1994;7: 35-44.
35. Piotrowski JJ, Pearce WH, Jones DN, et al. Aortobifemoral bypass: the operation of choice for unilateral iliac occlusion? *J Vasc Surg* 1988;8: 211-218.
36. Brener BJ, Brief DK, Alpert J. Femorofemoral bypass: a twenty-five year experience. In: Yao JST and Pearce WH, eds. *Long-term results in vascular surgery.* Norwalk, Conn: Appleton & Lange;1993:385-393. Mosby; 2001:405-406.
37. Kalman PG, Hosang M, Johnston KW, Walker PM. Unilateral iliac disease: the role of iliofemoral bypass. *J Vasc Surg* 1987;6:139-143.
38. Brewster DC, Cambria RP, Darling RC, et al. Long-term results of combined iliac balloon angioplasty and distal surgical revascularization. *Ann Surg* 1989;210:324-330.
39. Taylor Jr LM, Freimanis IE, Edwards JM, Porter JM. Extraperitoneal iliac endarterectomy in the treatment of multilevel lower extremity arterial occlusive disease. *Am J Surg* 1986;152:34-39.
40. Vitale GF, Inahara T. Extraperitoneal endarterectomy for iliofemoral occlusive disease. *J Vasc Surg* 1990;12:409-413.
41. Brewster DC, Veith FJ. Combined aortoiliac and femoropopliteal occlusive disease. In: Veith FJ, Hobson RW 2nd, Williams RA, eds. Vascular surgery: principles and practice. 2nd ed. New York: McGraw-Hill; 1994: 459-472.
42. Cham C, Myers KA, Scott DF, et al. Extraperitoneal unilateral iliac artery bypass for chronic lower limb ischaemia. *Aust NZ J Surg* 1988;58: 859-863.
43. Darling 3rd RC, Leather RP, Chang BB, et al. Is the iliac artery a suitable inflow conduit for iliofemoral occlusive disease: an analysis of 514 aortoiliac reconstructions. *J Vasc Surg* 1993;17:15-19.
44. Lorenzi G, Domanin M, Costanini A, et al. Role of bypass, endarterectomy, extra-anatomic bypass and endovascular surgery in unilateral iliac occlusive disease: a review of 1257 cases. *Cardiovasc Surg* 1994;2:370-373.
45. Hanafy M, McLoughlin GA. Comparison of iliofemoral and femorofemoral crossover bypass in the treatment of unilateral iliac arterial occlusive disease. *Br J Surg* 1991;78:1001-1002.
46. Sidawy AN, Menzoian JO, Cantelmo NL, LoGerfo FW. Retroperitoneal inflow procedures for iliac occlusive vascular disease. *Arch Surg* 1985;120:794-796.
47. Kalman PG, Hosang M, Johnston KW, Walker PM. The current role for femorofemoral bypass. *J Vasc Surg* 1987;6:71-76.
48. Ricco J-B, Probst H. Long-term results of a multicenter randomized study on direct versus crossover bypass for unilateral iliac artery occlusive disease. *J Vasc Surg* 2008;47:45-54.
49. Shaw RS, Baue AE. Management of sepsis complicating arterial reconstructive surgery. *Surgery* 1963;53:75-86.
50. Sautner T, Niederle B, Herbst F, et al. The value of obturator canal by pass: a review. *Arch Surg* 1994;129:718-722.
51. Patel A, Taylor SM, Langan EM III, et al. Obturator bypass: a classic approach for the treatment of contemporary groin infection. *Am Surg* 2002;68:653-659.
52. Nevelsteen A, Mees U, Deleersnijder J, Suy R. Obturator bypass: a sixteen-year experience with 55 cases. *Ann Vasc Surg* 1987;1:558-563.
53. Pearce WH, Ricco JB, Yao JST, et al. Modified technique of obturator bypass in failed or infected grafts. *Ann Surg* 1983;197:344-347.
54. Couch NP, Clowes AW, Whittemore AD, et al. The iliac-origin arterial graft: a useful alternative for iliac occlusive disease. *Surgery* 1985;97: 83-87.
55. Flanigan DP, Ryan TJ, Williams LR, et al. Aortofemoral or femoropopliteal revascularization? A prospective evaluation of the papaverine test. *J Vasc Surg* 1984;1:215-223.
56. Criado E, Farber MA. Femorofemoral bypass: appropriate application based on factors affecting outcome. *Semin Vasc Surg* 1997;10: 34-41.
57. da Gama AD. The fate of the donor artery in extraanatomic revascularization. *J Vasc Surg* 1988;8:106-111.
58. Donor limb vascular events following femoro-femoral bypass surgery: a Veterans Affairs Cooperative Study. *Arch Surg* 1991;126:681-685.
59. Flanigan DP, Sobinsky KR, Schuler JJ, et al. Internal iliac artery revascularization in the treatment of vasculogenic impotence. *Arch Surg* 1985;120:271-274.
60. Seagraves A, Rutherford RB. Isolated hypogastric artery revascularization after previous bypass for aortoiliac occlusive disease. *J Vasc Surg* 1987;5:472-474.
61. Utikal P, Kocher M, Bachleda P, et al. Femoral–internal iliac bypass in aortoiliac aneurysm endovascular repair. *Biomed Pap Med Fac Univ Palacky Olomouc Czech Repub* 2004;148:91-93.

chapter 10b

Surgical Intervention for Lower Extremity Arterial Occlusive Disease: Femoropopliteal and Tibial Interventions

Nick J.M. London, MD, FRCS, FRCP

Key Points

- The optimal management of a patient with chronic lower limb ischemia (CLLI) often requires a combination of endovascular and open surgical techniques.
- Preoperative independent mobility best predicts postoperative status after infrainguinal bypass for CLLI.
- Patients with CLLI have a profoundly reduced quality of life that is immediately improved by successful treatment of CLLI.
- Primary amputation is more expensive than bypass for CLLI.
- Autologous vein is the conduit of choice for infrainguinal bypass.
- Poor runoff status and lack of continuity of calf vessels with the plantar arch are significant risk factors for graft occlusion.
- No patient should be denied an attempted reconstruction based on results of preoperative arteriography alone.
- The results of infrainguinal in situ and reverse vein bypass are similar.
- Between 15% and 25% of infrainguinal vein bypass grafts are technically flawed or harbor intrinsic defects, and some form of postreconstruction quality control is essential.
- All patients with CLLI should be prescribed an antiplatelet agent. The addition of warfarin to an antiplatelet agent carries a considerable risk of major hemorrhage and therefore should only be used in patients with "high risk" grafts.
- Evidence favors duplex surveillance of vein grafts, whereas no evidence supports duplex surveillance of prosthetic grafts.

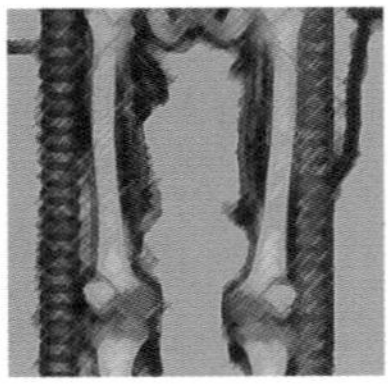

Chronic lower limb ischemia (CLLI) is nearly always the result of arterial obstruction due to atherosclerosis. Although other rare causes lead to arterial obstruction, such as distal embolization in the blue toe syndrome, these conditions are not discussed here. Similarly, this chapter does not discuss the relative role of endovascular techniques and surgery because this depends on local facilities and expertise. Chronic critical lower limb ischemia usually results from multilevel disease. Increasingly, it is possible to treat one level of disease by percutaneous transluminal angioplasty (PTA) while another component is best managed surgically. This combined approach can take the form of PTA in the angiography suite before surgery or an "on-table" angioplasty can be performed at the same time as the surgical procedure.

Although at one time lumbar sympathectomy was used for the treatment of CLLI, in modern vascular surgical practice, operative lumbar sympathectomy has little of a role to play. However, for the rare patient in whom it is not possible to treat CLLI by either endovascular or surgical methods, a chemical lumbar sympathectomy may provide useful analgesia. Therefore, the techniques of lumbar sympathectomy are not discussed here, nor is the as-yet-unproven technique of distal venous arterialization.[1]

PATIENT SELECTION

A detailed social history is essential for the optimal management of the patient with CLLI. In particular, it is vital that the clinician assesses the functional status of the threatened limb. Thus, the bedbound patient using an ischemic leg to transfer to and from a wheelchair or from a wheelchair to a toilet poses a different management issue to the bedbound patient who never uses the leg. The clinician should also clarify whether a dying leg reflects a dying patient or is an isolated event in an otherwise reasonably fit patient. The general condition of the patient may be so poor and the chances of survival so limited by comorbidity that it is appropriate simply to make the patient comfortable. A reasonably fit patient may have lost so much tissue in the foot that any attempt to save it is futile. Similarly, patients who have developed fixed flexion contractions of the knee and the hip may be best managed by primary amputation. These management issues involve complex, individualized decision making and are best made in consultation with the patient, the patient's relatives, and the rehabilitation team looking after the patient.

Preoperative independence and mobility have been shown to best predict postoperative status after infrainguinal bypass for CLLI.[2,3] Thus, only 4% of survivors who are not living independently before surgery achieve independent living 6 months postoperatively. Therefore, it would seem that there is little point in undertaking extensive revascularization in the hope of achieving independence for a patient already requiring care in a nursing home. Conversely, 99% of survivors who live independently before developing the need for limb salvage surgery remain independent 6 months after surgery. Certainly, age itself should not be considered a contraindication to surgery, and several studies report benefit in patients over the age of 80.[4]

IMPACT OF SURGERY ON QUALITY OF LIFE IN PATIENTS WITH CLLI

It has been shown, using the Nottingham Health Profile, that compared to a normal control population patients with CLLI have a profoundly reduced quality of life.[5] Studies that have looked at the impact of successful surgical revascularization on quality of life have uniformly shown that a patent graft following infrainguinal arterial reconstruction for CLLI results in an immediate and lasting improvement in health-related quality of life. Conversely, symptomatic graft occlusion leads to a reduction in quality of life. Amputation results in a striking deterioration in physical function, particularly after failed secondary revascularization. A successful patent graft particularly improves the domains of physical functioning, social functioning, role physical, and pain.[6-9]

ECONOMICS AND COST EFFECTIVENESS

The precise costs of procedures vary among countries and among institutions within countries. Also, the cost of health care is continually increasing; therefore, comparison of costs quoted by studies performed in different eras is not possible. For these reasons, this section focuses on the comparative cost of various approaches. Several studies, from both Europe and North America,[10-12] have shown that the overall costs 1 year after intervention are between 1.5 and 2 times greater for primary amputation than for femorodistal grafting. These studies have included in the costs of femorodistal grafting the costs of graft failure and secondary amputation. The main reason that primary amputation costs more is the community costs in the first year after amputation. In general, two to three times as many patients who undergo successful primary reconstruction are able to return home compared to those who undergo amputation. A study from Finland by Luther[11] has shown that among patients undergoing amputation the total costs for those already in an institution are one sixth of those required by patients who return home after amputation. This substantial difference results from the longer hospital stay, longer survival, and home care of the group not institutionalized before amputation. Interestingly, a study from Sheffield by Singh et al.[13] has shown no significant difference over 1 year in the cost of managing a patient with CLLI by angioplasty or of surgical reconstruction. This is because the major costs in both groups were related to the length of in-patient stay, which was similar in the two groups. Presumably, this reflects that the length of hospital stay is related more to the state of the foot and social factors than to the intervention received.

FACTORS AFFECTING OUTCOME

Several studies have investigated the factors influencing graft patency, limb salvage, and mortality rate after lower limb bypass procedures for CLLI. Although most surgeons would attempt a bypass procedure in the presence of one or two adverse risk factors, the presence of numerous adverse risk factors may influence the decision to attempt a bypass. In addition, knowledge of the risk factors discussed here is important with respect to informed consent and counseling the patient about the risks and likely outcome of bypass surgery.

Gender

The literature concerning the effect of gender on outcome after infrainguinal bypass is contradictory. Thus, some authors identify female gender as an adverse risk factor with respect to long-term survival[14] and graft patency,[14,15] whereas others do not.[16,17] There does, however, seem to be a consensus that the combination of female gender and diabetes significantly reduces 3-year postoperative survival, graft patency, and limb salvage.[14,16]

Age

With increasing age, several important risk factors become more prevalent. These include diabetes, female gender, and cardiac risk factors. A multivariate analysis,[16] which took account of these confounding factors, found no independent effect of age on operative mortality, graft patency, leg salvage, or survival. A more recent multivariate analysis found that infrainguinal bypass grafts were 2.2 times more likely to occlude in patients less than 50 years of age compared to those over the age of 70.[18] Certainly, age itself should not be a contraindication to infrainguinal bypass surgery.

Diabetes

Disagreement surrounds the influence of diabetes on the patency of infrainguinal bypass grafts. Some authors conclude that diabetes has no effect[17,19] or even improves outcome,[18] while others conclude that diabetes adversely affects outcome.[15,16,20] One of the reasons for these differences may be the nature of the analyses performed. Thus, some authors who have found diabetes to be a risk factor for graft occlusion in univariate analysis have found that this disappears on multivariate analysis.[14,16] This suggests that, although diabetic patients are more likely to have risk factors for graft occlusion than nondiabetics, diabetes itself is not a significant risk factor. Contrary to previous studies,[14,16] a recent paper from Hamdan et al.[21] reported that diabetes is not associated with an increased postoperative mortality after vascular surgery. Diabetic patients do, however, have markedly reduced long-term survival compared to nondiabetics.[14,16,21]

Renal Failure

There seems little doubt that patients with chronic renal failure who require lower limb revascularization have a high perioperative mortality,[22] spend more time in a hospital,[23] have a reduced graft patency,[24] and have a poor long-term survival rate.[25] However, evidence also indicates that, provided autologous vein is used, acceptable graft patencies can be achieved.[25] Certainly, it would seem that for hemodialysis-dependent patients the use of prosthetic material is not worthwhile.[25]

Smoking

Although some authors[24,26] have reported that smoking significantly reduces late graft patency, somewhat surprisingly others have not found this association.[15,18] This is probably because smoking history is not a true reflection of smoking activity. However, in view of the overall health benefits of smoking cessation, all patients who smoke should be encouraged to desist.

GRAFT MATERIAL

Vein versus Prosthetic

Although prosthetic materials can achieve acceptable results for below-knee bypass grafts,[27] there is no doubt that the best results below the knee are obtained with autologous vein.[18,27,28] It is clear from prospective randomized trials that autologous vein is also superior to prosthetic grafts in the above-knee position.[29,30] For example, a study from Boston[29] randomized 752 patients to receive autologous vein, polytetrafluoroethylene (PTFE), or human umbilical vein. In patients with critical ischemia, the 5-year patency of saphenous vein was 68% compared to 52% and 37% for human umbilical vein and PTFE, respectively. It has been shown that below-knee composite vein-prosthetic grafts have poor patency rates[31] and offer no advantage over prosthetic grafts alone.[32] Thus, for grafts both above- and below-knee, autologous vein is undoubtedly the conduit of choice.

Radial Artery

In patients with no vein or insufficient available vein, often in the setting of redo surgery, the radial artery is one option to consider. This can be used to replace a segment of diseased vein or extend a vein graft further distally.[33] Although few cases have been reported, the principle seems a good one and is worth consideration in patients who have exhausted their own vein.

Source of Vein

Although there are descriptions of the use of cold-stored vein allografts and cryopreserved vein or arterial allografts, the reported patency rates are poor.[34] The options for autogenous vein are ipsilateral long and/or short saphenous veins, ipsilateral femoral–popliteal vein (FPV), contralateral saphenous veins, or arm veins. Any of these veins can be joined or spliced together to produce vein of adequate total length. No doubt, the first choice is ipsilateral long saphenous vein. However, the ipsilateral long saphenous vein is only available in approximately 45% of cases.[35] The ipsilateral short saphenous vein is a good alternative that can often be used without the need to join it to other vein.[36]

The use of the FPV as an infrainguinal bypass conduit was introduced by Schulman et al. in 1981[37] and has subsequently been used by others.[38,39] While there seems no doubt that it provides excellent patency rates,[37,38] harvesting the vein is more difficult than saphenous vein and 20% to 30% of patients are troubled by postoperative limb swelling.[39] Compartment syndrome may also develop after FPV harvest.

Although some surgeons routinely use long saphenous vein from the contralateral leg,[40] others are reluctant to do so because of the chance that the patient may require contralateral lower limb bypass at a future date. It has been reported that at 2 years after surgery for CLLI 20% of patients have developed critical ischemia in the contralateral limb[41] and that by 5 years 30% of patients will have required intervention for contralateral CLLI.[42] Multivariate analysis has shown that diabetes, coronary artery disease, an ankle–brachial index less than 0.7, and age less than 70 years are all significant independent predictors of the need for contralateral intervention.[42] Although, based on these data it would seem unwise to use the contralateral long saphenous vein in patients less than 70 years of age and in diabetics, Chew et al.[40] have routinely used the contralateral long saphenous vein when required without compromising the contralateral leg, even in diabetics. Robin et al.[43] report that the only contraindication to using the contralateral long saphenous vein is the presence of trophic changes in the contralateral leg at the time of surgery.

Kakkar[44] suggested the use of arm vein for lower limb bypass grafting in 1969, and since then several authors have described its use.[45,46] The incidence of diseased veins in the arm is as high as 63%,[46] considerably higher than the value of 12% for the long saphenous vein.[47,48] Many of these abnormalities are thought to result from previous phlebotomy, intravenous cannulation, or both, and this explains why the incidence of disease in the more accessible forearm cephalic vein is 49% while in the less accessible basilic vein it is only 12%.[46] It has been reported[45] that the patency of composite arm vein is significantly less than that of single-length arm vein (29% versus 52% at 5 years). However, Marcaccio et al.[46] found that if angioscopy was used to detect and "upgrade" diseased arm veins the patency of composite vein grafts was no different from single-length grafts. This would seem to imply that providing the surgeon is technically proficient, composite arm vein grafts are acceptable when the conjoined vein segments are disease free. Certainly, composite vein grafts are preferable to prosthetic grafts[49] and are preferable to single-length long saphenous vein that contains sclerotic or diseased areas.[50]

VEIN DIAMETER AND QUALITY

Diameter

Most vascular surgeons believe that the size and quality of the venous conduit are the most important determinants of long-term patency of infrainguinal bypass grafts. Disagreement concerns the minimum usable vein diameter. Thus, whereas Shah et al.[17] consider 4 mm to be the minimum, Wengerter et al.[51] demonstrated increasing graft patency with graft diameters ranging from 3 to 4 mm. Sumner[52] has shown, based on theoretical considerations, that long vein grafts with diameters less than 3 mm produce unacceptably high pressure gradients. Varty et al.[50] concluded that vein grafts with a diameter less than 3 mm are at increased risk of developing stenoses, and Ishii et al.[53] found markedly reduced patency rates in grafts with a diameter of less than 3 mm. Based on the available data, it would appear preferable to use vein with a diameter greater than 3 mm.

Quality

Vein quality can be assessed either macroscopically or microscopically. Although the latter may be of importance with respect to the development of vein graft stenosis, it is primarily of research interest.[54] The macroscopic vein appearance is crucially important to the practicing vascular surgeon[55] because it profoundly influences both early and late graft patency.[48,55] Thus, Panetta et al.[48] found that 63 of 513 (12%) infrainguinal vein bypasses contained abnormalities such as thick walls, postphlebitic occlusions, postphlebitic stenoses, calcification, or varicosities. Preoperative duplex was able to identify 62% of these macroscopically abnormal veins. The remaining abnormalities were detected intraoperatively (vide infra).

SITE OF DISTAL ANASTOMOSIS, RUNOFF, AND PLANTAR ARCH STATUS

Although it has been shown that the patency of above-knee bypass grafts is better than below-knee grafts, it has also been shown that the patencies of below-knee vein grafts that are anastomosed to tibial vessels are as good as those placed onto the below-knee popliteal artery itself.[56] Many studies conclude that poor runoff is an independent risk factor for graft failure,[20,53,57,58] and it has been shown that lack of continuity of the calf vessels with the plantar arch[57,59,60] is a significant risk factor for graft occlusion. It has been suggested that grafts to the peroneal artery do not do as well as grafts to the anterior or posterior tibial arteries.[61] However, a substantial literature contradicts this view,[17,62] and the most important factor is that the artery chosen for the distal anastomosis is disease free distally and is in continuity with the pedal arch.

GENERAL CONSIDERATIONS BEFORE SURGERY

A substantial body of evidence now indicates that patients with peripheral vascular disease should be prescribed an antiplatelet agent such as aspirin or clopidogrel and that this agent should be continued in the perioperative period.[63,64] Recent studies have shown that patients already receiving beta-blockers or statins before surgery should continue them.[65] Only patients needing heart rate control, blood pressure control, or both in the perioperative period should start treatment with beta-blockers. The need for vigilance with respect to the medical management of patients with CLLI has been highlighted by a Danish study showing that only the minority of patients with CLLI are receiving adequate risk factor management.[66] All patients who smoke should be encouraged to stop.

Although intraoperative anticoagulation with intravenous heparin has been widely believed to provide adequate protection against thromboembolic phenomena, it has been shown[67] that 18% of patients undergoing lower limb vascular reconstruction without specific deep vein thrombosis (DVT) prophylaxis develop postoperative DVT. A randomized, controlled trial comparing low-molecular-weight heparin with unfractionated heparin for the prevention of postoperative DVT in patients undergoing femorodistal bypass reported that the postoperative DVT rate was 3.4%, with no significant difference between the two heparin types.[68] These studies, taken in conjunction with the general literature on DVT prophylaxis, suggest that patients undergoing lower limb revascularization should receive DVT prophylaxis.

With respect to antibiotic prophylaxis, it is recommended that antibiotic prophylaxis be used in the context of clean operations whenever intravascular prosthetic material is inserted or if deep infection would pose a catastrophic risk. Thus, although vascular procedures are usually clean, they often qualify for prophylaxis. The agent used for prophylaxis should be active against staphylococci, and although no evidence supports a prolonged course of antibiotic prophylaxis in vascular patients, most surgeons continue prophylaxis for at least 24 hours and longer in patients with indwelling central venous or arterial lines.[69]

PREOPERATIVE IMAGING

Imaging of the arterial tree has already been covered in Chapters 6 and 7. This section therefore addresses specific issues that are pertinent to lower limb bypass grafting. The two most important aspects of preoperative imaging are the identification of arterial runoff vessels and the determination of the availability and suitability of vein that can be used as a bypass conduit.

Imaging of the Arterial System

It is advantageous to initially image the arterial tree by noninvasive techniques. This approach allows the surgeon to assess the potential role of endovascular therapy, and if PTA is chosen, a noninvasive arterial map facilitates an endovascular approach. In addition, it is easier to have an informed discussion with the patient about the available treatment options if the surgeon has a noninvasive arterial map at hand.[70] The three most commonly used noninvasive techniques for imaging the arterial tree are color duplex scanning, multidetector computed tomography (CT), and magnetic resonance imaging (MRI) angiography.[70-72] The choice depends on local facilities and expertise. Duplex scanning has the advantages that it can be performed as part of a single visit assessment and that it provides both an anatomical and a hemodynamic

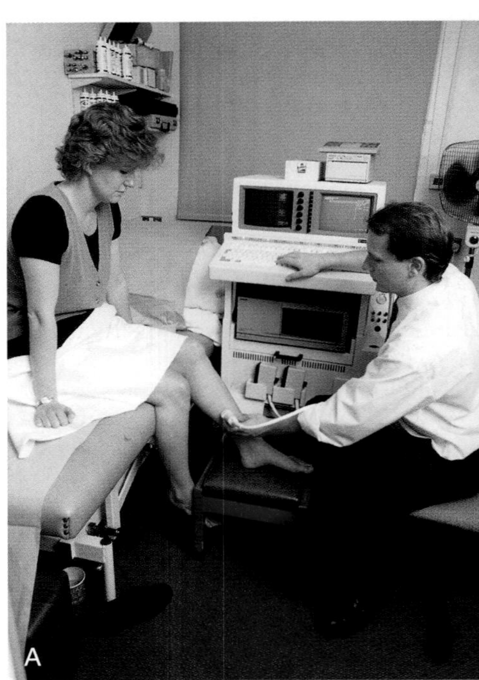

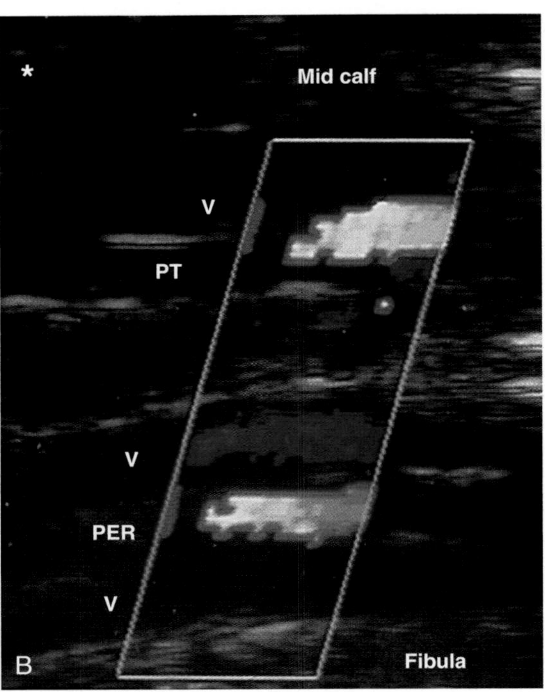

Figure 10b-1. Duplex scanning. **A,** The tibial vessels are best scanned with the leg dependent. **B,** This scan shows the peroneal (PER) and posterior tibial (PT) arteries and associated veins (V) at midcalf level.

map (Figure 10b-1). It is also cheaper than CT or MRI angiography. The major disadvantage of color duplex scanning is that it is operator dependent. Duplex scanning, CT, and MRI angiography may demonstrate distal vessels not seen on digital subtraction angiography (DSA).[70-73] Several studies have shown that it is safe to proceed to lower limb arterial reconstruction based solely on the results of duplex scanning.[70,74]

One of the major disadvantages of intraarterial DSA is that in the face of severe proximal arterial obstruction it may fail to show patent distal vessels revealed by intraoperative arteriography. An additional approach that can prove useful is dependent Doppler[75,76] (Figure 10b-2). This technique allows the accurate detection of calf vessels that have continuity with the pedal arch.

Several authors have developed "runoff scores" based on preoperative angiography, Doppler, or a combination of these modalities.[59,60] Most of these scoring systems have a low positive predictive value and a high negative predictive value for amputation (e.g., 50% and 97%, respectively).[60] This means that these systems are better at predicting patency rather than occlusion and most surgeons would therefore not deny a patient the chance of vessel exploration with intraoperative prereconstruction arteriography solely on the basis of an unfavorable score.

Imaging of the Venous System

It has been shown by several authors that preoperative duplex scanning of the superficial veins of the legs and arms can identify veins that are not visible clinically, can size veins (Figure 10b-3), and can detect veins with macroscopic disease caused by postphlebitic sclerosis (Figure 10b-4), calcification or varicosities.[48,77,78] If a vascular technologist marks the site of the chosen vein with a skin marker, this greatly aids exposure of the vein and reduces the likelihood of undermining skin flaps that may then become necrotic.

ANESTHETIC CONSIDERATIONS

Lower limb bypass surgery can be performed under general anesthesia, epidural anesthesia, or local infiltration anesthesia.[75,79] The choice often is determined by the precise nature of the planned surgery and the cardiorespiratory status of the patient. Although consensus is growing that those patients undergoing major vascular surgery who receive combined general and epidural anesthesia with postoperative epidural anesthesia have significantly lower cardiac morbidity than those receiving general anesthesia alone,[80] not all studies support this view.[81-83] It has been reported that epidural anesthesia after lower limb vascular reconstruction reduces platelet hyperaggregability[84] and is accompanied by less inhibition of fibrinolysis[85] compared to general anesthesia. It has also been shown that epidural anesthesia significantly decreases peripheral vascular resistance and increases graft blood flow in femorodistal grafts.[86] However, a significant difference has not been convincingly shown in the graft thrombosis rate between patients undergoing lower limb vascular reconstruction who receive epidural anesthesia and those who receive general anesthesia.[83,86] Therefore, the choice between general anesthesia and epidural anesthesia should be based on traditional anesthetic considerations.

Among the potential risks of epidural anesthesia is epidural hematoma, particularly in patients who receive large doses of anticoagulants or fibrinolytic agents. Effective epidural anesthesia may provide such adequate pain relief that graft thrombosis is not immediately recognized, and temperature differences between the limbs may be incorrectly ascribed to

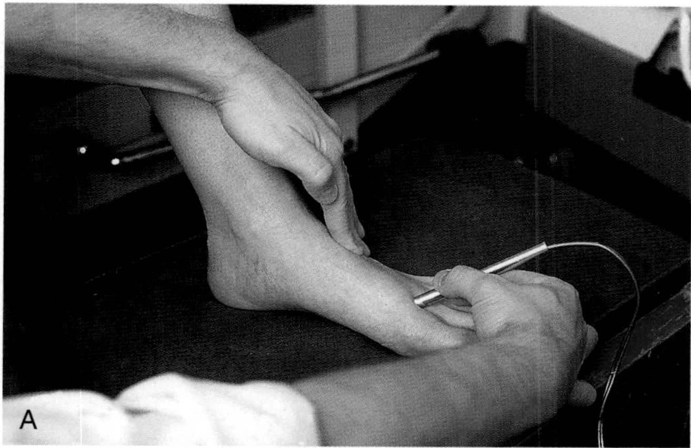

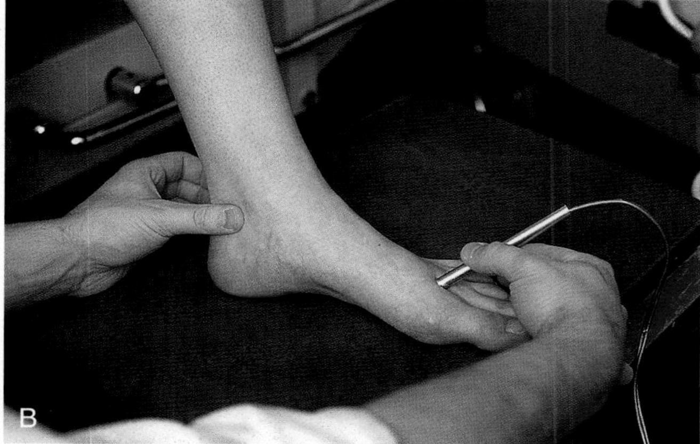

Figure 10b-2. Dependent Doppler. The leg is placed in a dependent position, and a Doppler signal is obtained in the first web space over the area of the deep plantar artery. Individual calf vessels are then compressed in turn at the ankle joint (**A,** the dorsalis pedis; **B,** the posterior tibial artery). If only one calf vessel communicates with the pedal arch, then the Doppler signal is obliterated. If more than one tibial vessel is in continuity with the arch, compression results in attenuation of the pedal arch signal. The vessel that gives the greatest attenuation is defined as the major inflow vessel to the arch.

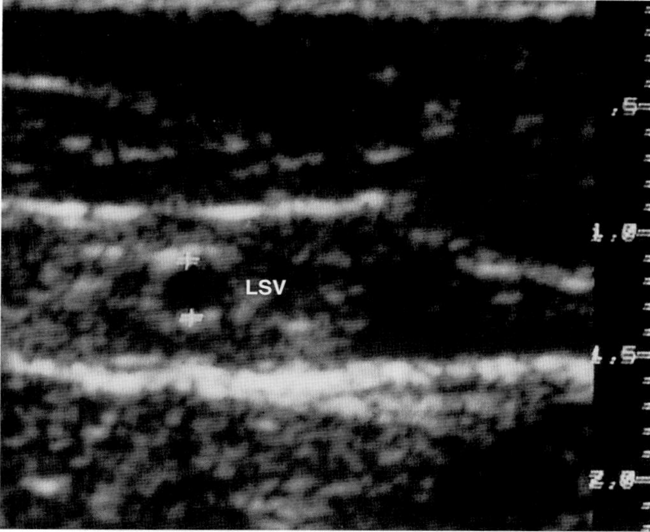

Figure 10b-3. Small saphenous vein. Even with venous occlusion, this long saphenous vein (LSV) will not dilate beyond 2 mm and is therefore not suitable for use as a bypass conduit.

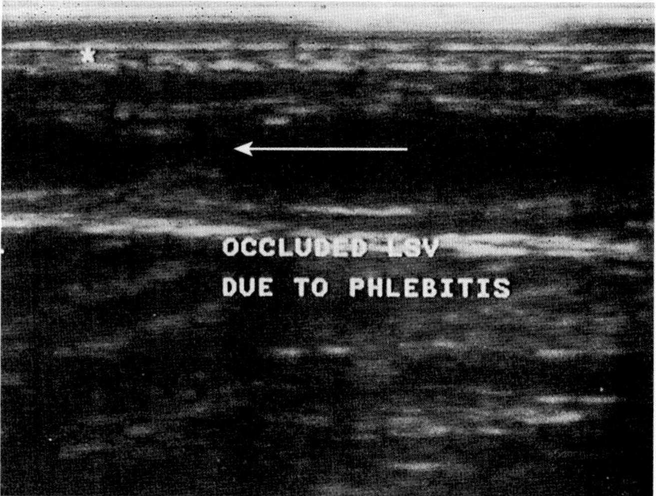

Figure 10b-4. Postphlebitic occlusion. This long saphenous vein has been occluded *(arrow)* by previous phlebitis.

epidural anesthesia. An additional anesthetic consideration is that if the patient is to undergo arterial reconstruction using arm vein it is important to ensure that the anesthetist does not cannulate the arm vein chosen as a bypass conduit.

SURGICAL STRATEGY

Precise surgical strategy depends on the distribution of obstructive arterial disease, the cardiorespiratory status of the patient, the nature and extent of any previous abdominal or lower limb procedures, and the availability and location of autogenous vein. One of the intellectual challenges facing the surgeon is to "tailor the procedure" to the patient. Thus, the operative strategy needs to take into account the length of available autogenous vein and the potential inflow and outflow sites. While it is not sensible to compromise the principles of unimpaired inflow and outflow sites, for the patient with limited autogenous vein it may be possible to move the inflow site more distally using PTA of proximal disease before or during surgery[87] or to move the outflow site more proximally using on-table PTA of distal disease.[88] Finally, in patients with CLLI and a major tissue defect, a combined approach between plastic and vascular surgeons using free flap transfers can produce excellent long-term results.[89] Broadly, surgical treatments can be divided into profundoplasty or endarterectomy or infrainguinal bypass. Sometimes a combination of approaches is required.

Profundoplasty and Endarterectomy

Profundoplasty

Although profundoplasty is most commonly performed as an adjunct to an inflow procedure such as aortobifemoral bypass,[90] it may have a role as an isolated procedure in selected patients with CLLI.[91,92] Profundoplasty may be a good option in patients with a superficial femoral artery occlusion and a concomitant significant stenosis (more than 50%) or occlusion of the origin of the profunda femoris artery who also lack autogenous vein for a bypass. Criteria for successful outcome after isolated profundoplasty include the presence of well-developed distal profunda femoris artery collaterals and patent tibial vessels. Cumulative 3-year limb salvage rates of 83%[91] and 76%[92] have been reported. Kalman et al.[92] noted that the best results were obtained in those with two or three patent tibial arteries.

Endarterectomy

Although no longer commonly performed, it should not be forgotten that iliofemoral endarterectomy is a technique that may still have a role in the patient with critical ischemia. A recent series from France reported 5- and 10-year actuarial limb salvages of 98% and 90%, respectively.[93] An alternative to open endarterectomy is endarterectomy through a single arteriotomy using a ring cutter.[94] Although described and used predominantly in the superficial femoral artery segment, the technique has also been used with success in the iliac arteries.[94]

Infrainguinal Bypass

Before discussing detailed operative techniques, it is necessary to consider general operative strategies and planning for infrainguinal bypass procedures.

General Considerations

There is no doubt that femorodistal reconstruction can be demanding of a surgeon's time, technical skills, and patience. There is also no doubt that a successful outcome requires meticulous attention to detail, gentle tissue handling, and unwillingness to accept technical imperfection. With this in mind, these procedures should be performed in an environment that is not time constrained. It is also invaluable to have at least two experienced surgeons, particularly if vein needs to be harvested from several sites. Many surgeons find loupe magnification greatly facilitates these procedures, in particular the distal anastomosis. Intraoperative assessment and quality control are facilitated by an operating theater that is equipped with either mobile or static DSA equipment. Finally, it is well established that surgeon-determined judgmental or technical error accounts for most graft failures in the first month after surgery,[95] and it cannot be stressed enough that it is highly preferable to spend time and effort getting these procedures right the first time. Early graft thrombosis not only poses a difficult challenge for the surgeon but also markedly decreases secondary graft patency[20,96] and increases the morbidity and mortality of these procedures.

Choice and Use of Bypass Material

As discussed earlier, the preferred bypass conduit is autogenous vein.

The importance of using good-quality vein cannot be overstressed, and it is preferable to use composite vein grafts composed of good-quality vein than to use a single length of poor-quality vein that contains diseased segments. Composite vein-prosthetic grafts offer no advantage over prosthetic grafts alone; the alternative to autogenous vein is therefore a prosthetic graft.

Reversed Vein versus In Situ Vein

Since first described by Kunlin in 1949,[97] reversed saphenous vein has been the most commonly used method for autogenous vein bypass. The in situ technique was first described in 1965[98] and became increasingly popular in the early 1970s with the development of a valve stripper that could be inserted through the open end of the greater saphenous vein.[99] The major proposed theoretical advantage of the in situ technique is that it keeps the vasa vasorum intact and thereby preserves the endothelial lining. However, it has been shown that the valve stripper causes extensive endothelial and smooth muscle damage, which is more severe in the case of in situ vein than that of reversed vein.[100] Several prospective randomized studies[101-105] and a large retrospective comparative review[106] have concluded that the incidence of vein graft stenosis and the long-term patency of reversed and in situ grafts are remarkably similar. Thus, the decision concerning in situ or reversed vein should be made on an individual patient basis and not in the belief that either technique provides superior long-term patency.

One of the major disadvantages of the in situ technique is that the use of an ipsilateral long saphenous vein is mandatory and this is not available in between 30% and 40% of limbs.[17,104] It has been suggested that one potential advantage of the in situ technique is that it allows the use of smaller-caliber vein because it allows a better match to the recipient distal artery.[107] However, small veins have been shown to perform badly for both the in situ and the reversed technique,[101-105] and as discussed earlier, it would not seem sensible to use a vein less than 3 mm in diameter. One of the advantages of the in situ technique is that in the event of graft thrombosis it is relatively easy to unblock the graft because the valves have been lysed. Unblocking a reversed vein graft with intact valves can be more difficult.

Angioscopy of Bypass Vein

Angioscopy has been used both for the detection of unsuspected venous disease[108] and for the minimally invasive preparation of in situ vein grafts.[109] Sales et al.[108] used angioscopy to examine 32 long saphenous veins before their use as bypass conduits and found a significantly better 1-year patency in an angioscopically normal compared to an abnormal group (70% versus 14%). More recently, Thorne et al.[110] used angioscopy to inspect roughly one third of in situ vein bypasses before the formation of the distal anastomosis. Interestingly, angioscopy detected partially occluding thrombus in 16% of veins but itself damaged the vein in 9% of cases. Although the 1-year primary patency was significantly better in those bypasses that had undergone angioscopy, the secondary patency rate achieved was no different. It is also interesting to note that this study was hampered by angioscope breakage and that a major problem with angioscopy is the delicate nature of the equipment and the costs of its repair or replacement.

Angioscopically assisted in situ vein bypass became popular in the early 1990s, with the angioscope used to assist valve lysis and aid vein branch identification and occlusion. It was hoped that angioscopy would reduce operative morbidity, shorten hospital stays, and improve graft patency. A prospective study by Clair et al.[109] in 1994 randomized 59 patients and concluded that angioscopically assisted in situ bypass conferred no benefit in terms of operative morbidity, hospital stay, or graft patency. A more recent multicenter study[111] randomized 273 patients undergoing in situ vein bypass to an angioscopically assisted or a conventional procedure. The angioscopic group underwent angioscopically guided valvulotomy and side branch occlusion using an angioscopic side branch occlusion system. The 3-year primary patency, secondary patency, and limb salvage rates were similar. However, small veins (less than 3 mm diameter) in the angioscope group fared badly with a 1-year graft thrombosis rate of 15%. Wound complications, length of hospital stay, and overall costs were less in the angioscope group. It would appear, therefore, that angioscopically assisted in situ bypass does have advantages, provided that the vein is more than 3 mm in diameter. For smaller veins, instrumentation damage to the vein and subsequent graft thrombosis would appear to outweigh the potential benefits.

Prosthetic Grafts

If it is not possible to use autologous vein, prosthetic grafts are an alternative. Controversy surrounds the role of prosthetic infrainguinal grafts to a single calf vessel, and many surgeons would not use a prosthetic graft in this context. Careful patient selection is crucial, and it should be borne in mind that the most important determinants of short- and long-term patency are the state of the runoff, the completeness of the plantar arch, and the degree of continuity between the two.[57,112] The choice of graft material lies between PTFE and Dacron. Although most surgeons prefer PTFE, little clinical evidence indicates it is better than Dacron. A randomized trial[112] comparing PTFE with gelatin-sealed Dacron for femoropopliteal bypass found no difference in 3-year primary patency (52% versus 47%), and a randomized trial[113] comparing PTFE with heparin-bonded Dacron found that, although the latter had a significantly superior 3-year patency (55% versus 42%), there was no difference at 5 years. It should be noted that in both studies most bypasses were to the above-knee popliteal artery. Although observational studies have been made of heparin-bonded PTFE grafts,[114,115] no randomized trials compare them with standard PTFE. A prospective multicenter, randomized trial[116] compared carbon-impregnated PTFE with standard PTFE and found no difference in patency at 3 years (43% versus 38%).

It has been shown in a prospective randomized study that the patency of below-knee PTFE grafts is improved by the addition of a vein cuff at the distal anastomosis.[117] This study did not include patients with bypass grafts to single calf vessels. However, it would seem reasonable to extrapolate the results and to use a vein cuff in such situations. A prospective randomized study demonstrated that the addition of a distal arteriovenous fistula to a vein cuff does not improve the patency of PTFE grafts to infrapopliteal vessels.[118]

Selection of Inflow Site

The inflow for infrainguinal bypass grafts has traditionally been based on the common femoral artery. However, no reason exists that more distal arteries cannot serve as inflow sites, provided that that no significant proximal arterial obstruction occurs. The potential advantages of these distal origin grafts include the increased likelihood of using autogenous vein and the reduced surgical morbidity and recovery time. Ballotta et al.[119] have shown in a prospective randomized study that the patency rates of vein grafts originating below the common femoral artery (distal superficial femoral artery, popliteal artery, or tibioperoneal trunk) are the same as for those arising from the common femoral artery. Distal origin grafts may be particularly useful in diabetic patients because of the typical diabetic pattern of infrapopliteal disease with relative sparing of inflow vessels above the knee.

If doubt exists about the suitability of a possible inflow site at the time of surgery, intraarterial pressure measurements at rest and after papaverine can be helpful.[120] The principle is to compare the intraarterial pressure at the proposed inflow site with brachial or radial arterial pressure. The inflow artery is punctured by a needle connected to a pressure transducer; the brachial or radial artery is also punctured, and the pressure difference noted. A resting pressure difference of more than 10 mm Hg is significant. The inflow artery–brachial pressure ratio is recorded, papaverine (30 mg) is injected into the inflow artery, and the percentage fall in the ratio measured. A fall of 15% after papaverine is considered significant.[120]

Isolated Popliteal Segment

The most commonly used definition of an isolated popliteal segment is a distally occluded popliteal artery without direct runoff or with runoff into a single infrapopliteal artery that is patent for a distance of less than 5 cm.[121,122] Although it would seem unlikely that a graft to an isolated popliteal segment remains patent for long, the published results are surprisingly good. In a prospective randomized study of patients with an isolated popliteal artery segment, Darke et al.[123] found that the 1-year patency of bypasses to the isolated segment were not significantly different from those randomized to a reconstituted distal vessel lower in the calf (79% versus 70%). The conduit used in most patients in this study was in situ vein.

Kram et al.[121] reported a 10-year experience of 217 femoropopliteal bypasses to isolated popliteal artery segments. Most of these procedures (98%) were for critical ischemia, and most of the bypass conduits (85%) were PTFE. Although the 5-year secondary patency for the saphenous vein group was significantly higher than for the PTFE group (74% versus 56%), the 5-year limb salvage rates were the same (78%). Other authors have also reported reasonable limb salvage results using PTFE grafts to an isolated popliteal segment.[122,124,125] Therefore, it would appear that, in patients with an isolated popliteal artery segment who only have a short length of autogenous vein, a bypass to the isolated segment is a good option. If no autogenous vein is available, then a PTFE bypass to an isolated popliteal artery segment is reasonable.

Prereconstruction Intraoperative Arteriography

The underlying principles of prereconstruction intraoperative angiography are to identify distal vessels that may not have been revealed by preoperative investigations and to be certain that the site chosen for the distal anastomosis is appropriate. Some surgeons[75] do not perform preoperative angiography in the presence of a normal femoral pulse and instead always perform prereconstruction intraoperative angiography. Most surgeons use prereconstruction intraoperative arteriography selectively, depending on the results of preoperative imaging. The technique most commonly used is to study the preoperative investigations and then expose the most proximal site that provides visualization of the predicted distal bypass target artery. The vessel is then cannulated with a small-gauge butterfly needle, and 10 to 20 ml of an ionic contrast medium is manually injected under x-ray screening.

Postreconstruction Quality Control

Although numerous techniques have been used to provide quality control for femorodistal bypass grafting, the three most commonly used are angioscopy,[126,127] postreconstruction arteriography,[126,127] and duplex scanning.[128] Comparisons of angioscopy with arteriography have shown that angioscopy is better at detecting abnormalities within the conduit[126,127] but that angioscopy can miss abnormalities beyond the distal anastomosis. Miller et al.[127] prospectively randomized 293 patients undergoing infrainguinal bypass grafts to angioscopy or completion arteriography. Although more abnormalities were detected by angioscopy than by arteriography, this did not result in improved 1-month patency rates in the angioscopy group.

Gilbertson et al.[129] compared duplex with arteriography and angioscopy in a series of 20 in situ vein grafts. The results of this study suggest that angioscopy may be of particular value for in situ vein grafts because it is particularly good at detecting residual competent valves or unligated tributaries. A recent report from Johnson et al.[128] has described the use of papaverine-augmented intraoperative completion duplex scans to provide quality control for infrainguinal bypass procedures. A 15% intraoperative revision rate was seen, and a normal intraoperative duplex scan on initial imaging or after revision was associated with a 30-day graft thrombosis rate of only 0.2%.

It is pertinent to note that, regardless of the quality control technique used, the overall intraoperative graft revision rate is high (15% to 25%) in most studies. The important points are that some form of quality control is essential and that the technique used depends on local facilities and expertise.

Use of a Tourniquet

The use of tourniquets in infrainguinal bypass surgery was first described by Bernhard et al.[130] in 1980. Since then, several other authors have described their use. Distal vascular control during femorodistal reconstruction can be awkward. Vascular clamps, silastic slings, intraluminal flow arresters, and intraluminal balloons are commonly used methods of obtaining vascular control. These techniques may not work well in the presence of calcified vessels, may cause intimal flaps, and can clutter the operative field and reduce visibility and access. Proponents of the tourniquet technique argue that many of these technical problems are reduced and suggest that the reduced intimal trauma produced by tourniquets may improve both short- and long-term patency rates.[131] The latter point has not, however, been proven. The technique most commonly used is to obtain proximal vessel control in the normal way with clamps or slings, expose (but not mobilize) the distal vessels, tunnel the graft if necessary, heparinize the patient, exsanguinate the leg, apply the tourniquet at midthigh level, and then perform the distal anastomosis.[132]

OPERATIVE TECHNIQUES

Profundaplasty

A vertical groin incision is made over the common femoral artery and is carried approximately 5 cm proximal to the inguinal crease. The length of profunda femoris artery that needs to be exposed determines the distal extent of the incision. The common femoral artery and its branches are then exposed, as is the superficial femoral artery for 4 to 5 cm from its origin. This allows the superficial femoral artery to be mobilized, which then facilitates dissection of the profunda femoris artery. The origin of the profunda femoris artery from the posterior aspect of the common femoral artery is identified, and the dissection then continues down the anterior surface of the artery. At this point, the surgeon has to be aware that several large veins cross anterior to the profunda femoris artery, including the lateral circumflex femoral vein. These veins need to be carefully ligated and divided (Figure 10b-5). The length of the extent of dissection down the profunda femoris artery depends on the distal extent of disease within the artery. This is best ascertained by palpation. The dissection down the profunda femoris artery should continue to the first set of branches beyond the disease so that distal control can be obtained.

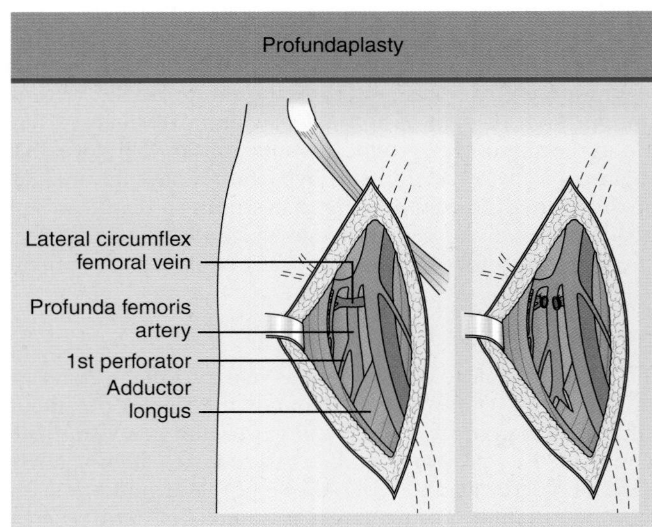

Figure 10b-5. Profundaplasty. Several large veins cross anterior to the profunda femoris artery, including the lateral circumflex femoral vein. These veins need to be carefully ligated and divided to expose the profunda femoris artery.

In patients who have had previous groin surgery and vascular repair, an alternative approach is to expose the midportion of the profunda femoris artery through an anterior thigh incision. The sartorius muscle is retracted laterally to expose the superficial femoral vessels, which are then retracted medially (Figure 10b-6). The fascia deep to the superficial artery is incised to expose the profunda femoris vessels between the first and second perforator branches.

Once the dissection has been completed, 5000 units of heparin are given intravenously and the vessels are controlled by whatever means the surgeon prefers. A vertical incision is made in the anterior aspect of the common femoral artery, which then continues down the anterior wall of the profunda femoris for 1 cm or more beyond the transition between abnormal and normal artery. Thromboendarterectomy is carried out as far as the transition zone, at which point it may be necessary to place tacking sutures (Figure 10b-7A and B). The arteriotomy is then closed with a patch (Figure 10b-7C) that can be formed from a segment of adjacent occluded superficial femoral artery, from saphenous vein (preferably a major branch of the long saphenous vein rather than the long saphenous vein itself), or a prosthetic patch. The latter should only be used if

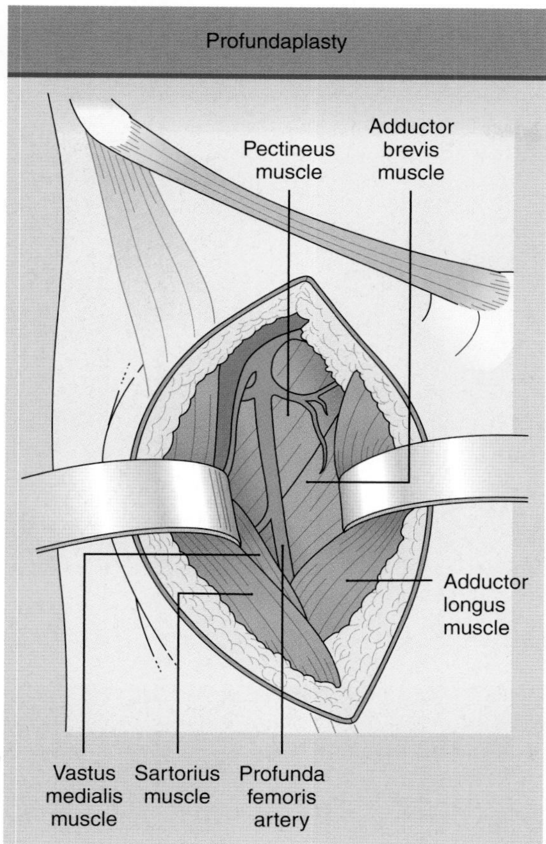

Figure 10b-6. Profundaplasty. The midportion of the profunda femoris artery is exposed by lateral retraction of the sartorius muscle and medial retraction of the superficial femoral vessels.

no vein is used. The patch is tailored and sutured in such a way that it produces a gradually tapering lumen.

Infrainguinal Bypass

The patient should be prepared for surgery as previously described (vide supra). This should usually include subcutaneous heparin DVT prophylaxis, prophylactic antibiotics, and preoperative duplex marking of the vein that is intended for use. In the case of arm vein, it is important to ensure that the anesthetist does not use the intended vein for intravenous access. If arm vein is to be used, the arms should be abducted and placed on arm boards. The patient usually lies supine unless a posterior approach is intended, in which case the patient is placed prone. Exposure of many lower limb vessels is facilitated if the knee is flexed, and it is useful to have a heavy sandbag that can be placed under the sole of the foot to hold the leg in a flexed position.

Vessel Exposure

Common Femoral, Profunda Femoris, and Superficial Femoral Artery

If just the common femoral artery or the origin of the profunda femoris or superficial femoral artery needs to be exposed, then the preferred incision is an oblique incision placed above and parallel to the groin crease (Figure 10b-8). This is because, compared to vertical groin incisions, the wound infection rate is significantly reduced.[133] If, however, it is necessary to dissect some distance down the profunda femoris or superficial femoral artery, then a vertical incision is the preferred choice. The common femoral artery is exposed from the level of the inguinal ligament to its bifurcation, the proximal superficial femoral artery and profunda femoris artery are mobilized, and control is obtained. If it is necessary to expose the distal profunda, the technique described earlier for profundaplasty is followed. It is straightforward to follow the superficial femoral artery down the thigh by extending the vertical incision and dissecting the superficial femoral artery out of the loose areolar tissue surrounding it.

Above-Knee Popliteal Artery

The above-knee popliteal artery is exposed through a medial thigh incision (Figure 10b-8) to expose the sartorius muscle, which is then retracted posterolaterally. The underlying deep fascia is incised over the adductor canal, and the popliteal artery is dissected free of accompanying structures as it lies posterior to the femur. The artery is then mobilized as far as necessary distally. This is best determined by palpation. Flexion of the knee facilitates distal dissection.

Below-Knee Popliteal Artery

The below-knee popliteal artery is exposed through a medial calf incision posterior to the medial femoral condyle (Figure 10b-8), extending distally medial to the tibial crest. Care should be taken not to damage the underlying saphenous vein, which should be carefully mobilized. The deep muscular fascia is incised, and the medial head of gastrocnemius is reflected posterolaterally to expose the popliteal artery. The distal popliteal artery is mobilized from the popliteal vein, which usually lies medially. Great care should be taken to avoid damage to surrounding veins. By following the dissection distally, the tibioperoneal trunk can be exposed, as can the origin of the anterior tibial artery.

Anterior Tibial Artery

The anterior tibial artery can be exposed at its origin as it leaves the below-knee popliteal artery, as described earlier. More commonly, however, the anterior tibial artery is approached through a longitudinal incision over the anterior compartment of the leg (Figures 10b-8 and 10b-9) and is exposed by reflection of the anterior tibial muscle anteromedially and the digital extensor muscles laterally. The vessels are found lying on the interosseous membrane close to the tibia.

Posterior Tibial Artery

The proximal posterior tibial artery is best isolated by continued dissection down the tibioperoneal trunk, as described earlier. The midposterior tibial artery is exposed through a medial calf incision (Figures 10b-8 and 10b-9). The distal posterior tibial artery is exposed through an incision just posterior to the medial malleolus (Figure 10b-8), and its medial and lateral plantar branches are exposed by extension of the incision on to the medial surface of the foot.

Peroneal Artery

The proximal peroneal artery can be exposed by continuation of dissection down the tibioperoneal trunk, as described earlier. Several techniques are available for exposure of the

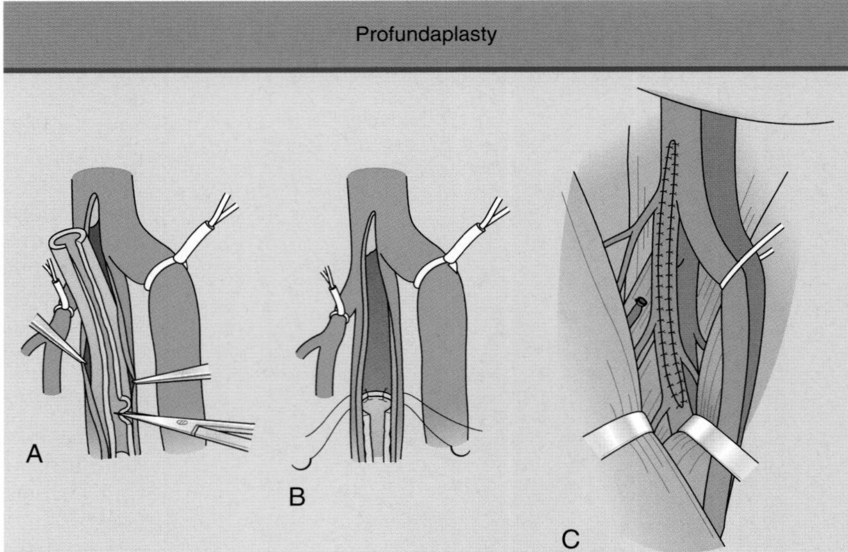

Figure 10b-7. Profundaplasty. **A,** Endarterectomy of profunda femoris artery. **B,** After completion of the endarterectomy, the distal intimal flap is tacked down. **C,** The arteriotomy is closed with a patch.

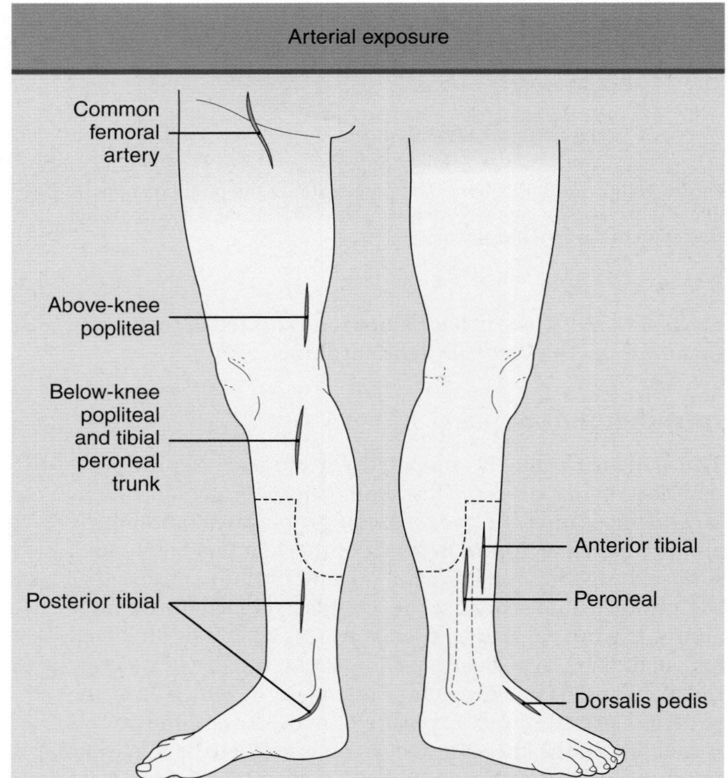

Figure 10b-8. Arterial exposure. Sites of incisions for exposure of major lower limb arteries.

distal peroneal artery. One technique involves placing a longitudinal incision over the distal fibula (Figures 10b-8 and 10b-10), mobilizing the long peroneal muscle from the fibula and reflecting it posteriorally, along with the flexor hallucis longus. A 10-cm length of fibula is then resected, and the peroneal artery and its accompanying veins are located just deep to a thin layer of fascia lying on the surface of the posterior tibial muscle. This lateral approach can be followed by postoperative pain and distal lower-extremity edema; an alternative is a posterior approach to the peroneal artery (Figure 10b-11). This approach is particularly useful when the inflow source is the popliteal artery and the conduit to be used is lesser

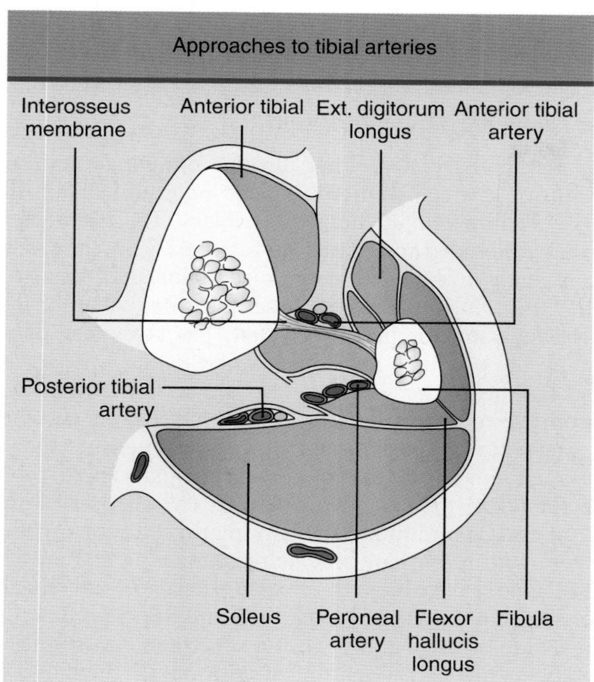

Figure 10b-9. Approaches to tibial arteries. Anatomical approaches to the anterior tibial, peroneal, and posterior tibial arteries in the midcalf.

saphenous vein. The patient is placed prone on the operating table, and a longitudinal incision is made in the midline at the level of the proposed anastomosis to the peroneal artery. The midperoneal artery is exposed by splitting the muscle fibers of the gastrocnemius and soleus muscles. This can be facilitated with the use of a handheld intraoperative pencil Doppler. The distal peroneal artery is readily isolated by medial displacement of the lateral body of the gastrocnemius and soleus muscles, followed by incision of the deep investing fascia in lateral to tendo calcaneus. The flexor hallucis longus muscle is retracted laterally, and the fibula is palpated as a landmark running immediately lateral to the artery.[134] Up to 15 cm of the vessel can be exposed before it bifurcates into anterolateral and posteromedial collateral branches running to the anterior and posterior tibial arteries, respectively.

Dorsalis Pedis Artery

This vessel is easily exposed through a longitudinal incision on the dorsum of the foot just lateral to the extensor hallucis longus tendon (Figure 10b-9). It is important to provide a wide skin bridge between the arterial incision and that required for exposure and subsequent mobilization of the distal saphenous vein.

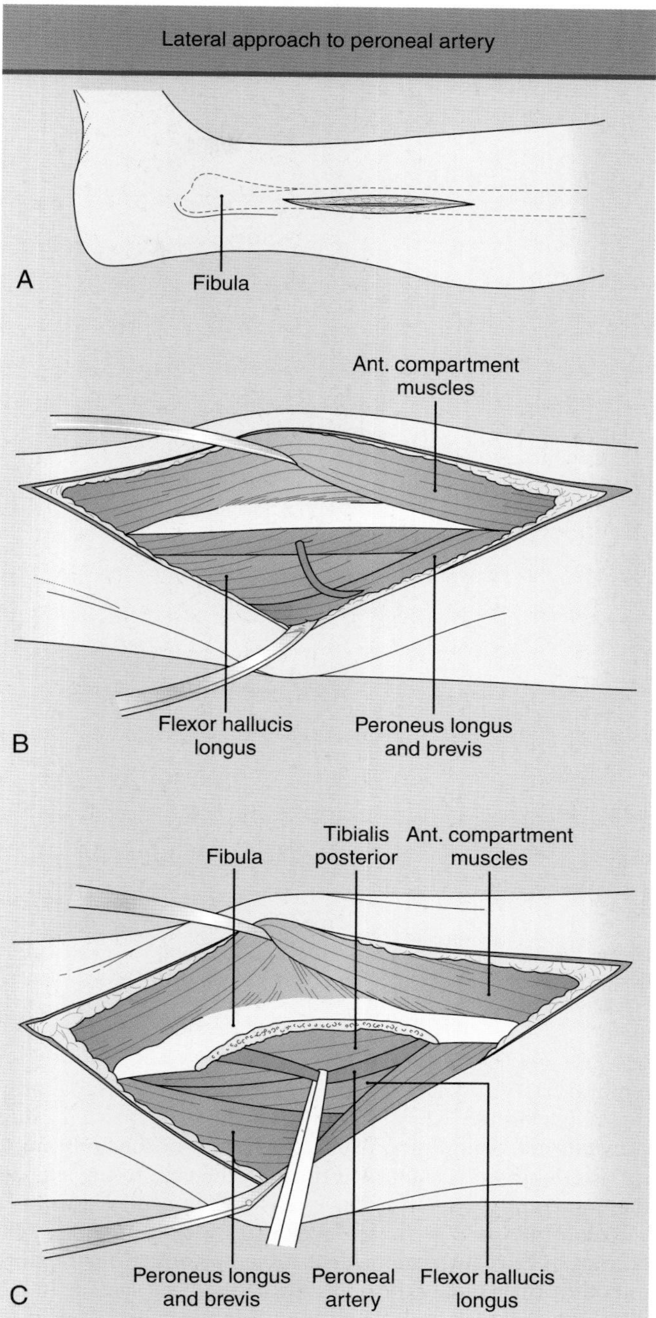

Figure 10b-10. Lateral approach to peroneal artery. The fibula is exposed and a 10-cm length is resected to reveal the peroneal artery and vein lying beneath it.

In Situ Bypass

In situ bypass can be performed by exposing the entire length of the long saphenous vein or, if an angioscope is used to identify vein tributaries, multiple small incisions are used. As described earlier, a further extension of the use of the angioscope is occlusion of patent tributaries with small metal coils. Although there is little doubt that these angioscopic approaches are appealing, a significant learning curve exists and operative times can be significantly prolonged. The in situ method requires that the proximal anastomosis be initially constructed after transection of the saphenofemoral junction and closure of the common femoral venotomy. The proximal anastomosis is usually located in the distal common femoral artery, but the precise site is dictated by the level of the saphenofemoral junction. It is usual to mobilize a segment of proximal saphenous vein and to excise the cusps of the first venous value under direct vision. Once control of the relevant inflow arteries has been obtained, an arteriotomy is made in the distal common

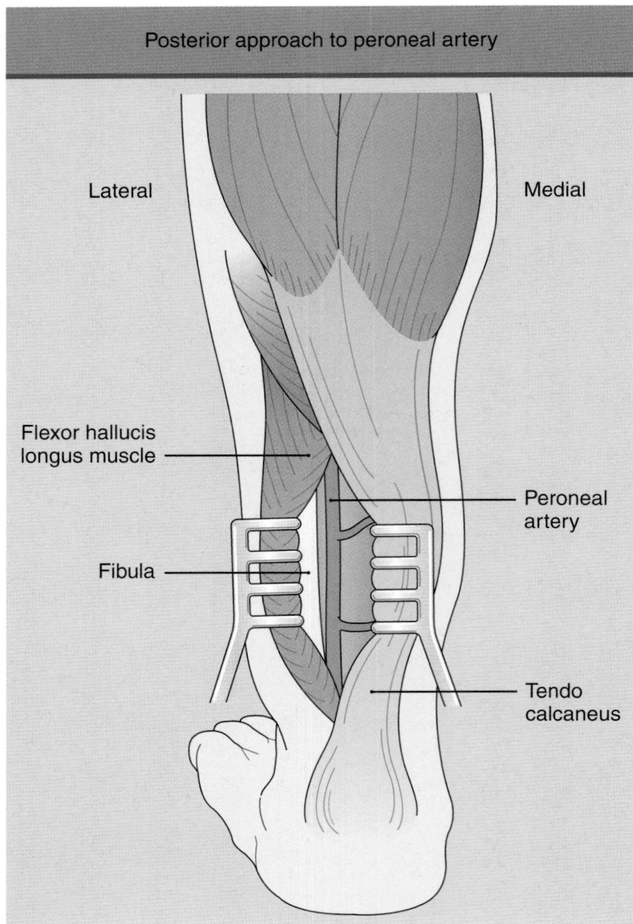

Figure 10b-11. Posterior approach to peroneal artery. The tendo calcaneus is retracted medially and flexor hallucis longus is retracted laterally to expose the peroneal artery.

femoral artery and, if necessary, a preliminary endarterectomy can be performed. The anastomosis is then constructed using conventional techniques. After completion of the anastomosis, arterial flow is established through the vein to the level of the first competent valve. Valve lysis is then achieved using a valvulotome, such as those developed by Hall or Mills. The efficacy of valve lysis can be determined by observing the flow out of the open end of the graft. An arteriotomy is made in the distal target vessel, and the anastomosis is performed using a fine monofilament suture. Some surgeons like to perform the distal anastomosis with a fine catheter in the distal artery to reduce the chance of technical error.

Nonreversed Saphenous Vein

If the ipsilateral long saphenous vein is not available and it is felt that the practical advantages of the in situ technique, such as a better size match between the artery and the vein at the proximal and distal anastomoses is desirable, then an alternative approach described by Beard et al.[135] may be used. In this approach, the vein is harvested from its bed and the proximal valve is then excised under direct vision. The proximal anastomosis is completed, and the valves are lysed as described for the in situ bypass operation. The graft may then be tunneled if necessary and the distal anastomosis performed.

Reversed Long Saphenous Vein

Vein may be harvested either through one long continuous incision or through numerous short longitudinal skin incisions with intervening cutaneous bridges. The tributaries of the vein are divided and ligated, and after excision, the reversed vein is gently flushed with heparinized saline and then stored in the flush solution until use. Either the proximal or the distal anastomosis may be performed first. The advantage of performing the proximal anastomosis first is that it is easier to detect kinking of the vein. The vein is then tunneled using an appropriate tunneling device down to the relevant distal target artery. It is important after tunneling to ensure that the vein is not kinked and that there is an adequate length of vein with the leg in the extended position. The chances of kinking can also be minimized by marking the anterior surface of the vein with methylene blue before tunneling and ensuring that the marks remain on the anterior surface of the vein after tunneling. Although it is usual to tunnel the vein down the medial side of the leg, it is entirely acceptable to tunnel the vein subcutaneously along the anterior lateral thigh and calf to the anterior tibial artery if necessary.

Pedal Bypass

A recent metaanalysis has shown that, with careful patient selection, excellent results can be achieved with bypass to the foot.[136] This approach is of particular value in patients with diabetes. Ouriel[137] has described a posterior approach when the inflow vessel is the popliteal artery. The patient is placed in a prone position, and the short saphenous vein is used as the bypass conduit. The popliteal artery is exposed through a posterior midline short saphenous vein harvest incision that is placed between the two heads of the gastrocnemius muscle (Figure 10b-12). The proximal 10 cm of the soleus muscle can then be divided to expose the proximal portion of the crural vessels. Only the first 2 cm of the anterior tibial artery can be exposed, but this can be extended by dividing the interosseous membrane. The exposure of the peroneal and posterior tibial arteries is shown in Figures 10b-11 and 10b-13, respectively. The anterior tibial artery is exposed through the standard anterior lateral incision by externally rotating the leg to bring the cleft between the anterior tibial and the extensor hallucis longus muscles into an accessible view. If the anterior tibial artery is the target vessel, the vein can be tunneled from the posterior fossa to the anterior tibial artery through the interosseous membrane.

Optimizing the Use of Autogenous Vein

Several techniques can be used to optimize the use of autogenous vein. These are shown diagrammatically in Figures 10b-14 to 10b-16.

Prosthetic Bypass

As discussed earlier, if a prosthetic bypass is to be used with a distal anastomosis to the below-knee popliteal artery or more distally, a vein cuff should be used. Three types of vein cuff are commonly used. These are illustrated in Figure 10b-17.

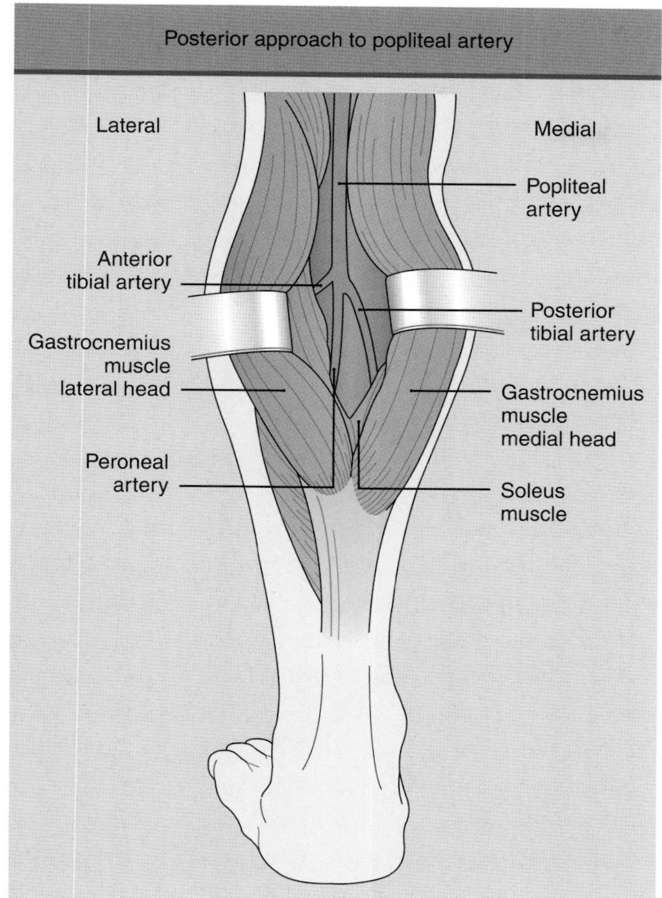

Figure 10b-12. Posterior approach to popliteal artery. The two heads of the gastrocnemius muscle are separated, and the proximal soleus muscle is divided to reveal the proximal tibial vessels.

INTRAOPERATIVE CONSIDERATIONS

Although several small studies have examined the effect of intraoperative iloprost on graft patency, the largest study is from the Iloprost Bypass International Study Group.[138] This prospective, multicenter, placebo-controlled study randomized 517 bypass grafts (424 vein, 92 prosthetic) to receive either intravenous iloprost or placebo intraoperatively followed by daily 6-hour infusions for the first three postoperative days. All patients had critical ischemia, and in 97.5% of cases the distal anastomosis was distal to the below-knee popliteal artery. Iloprost had no effect on 1-year primary patency or limb salvage in either the prosthetic or the vein group.

POSTOPERATIVE CONSIDERATIONS

Antiplatelet Agents

Numerous relatively small trials have suggested that aspirin improves the patency of infrainguinal bypass grafts, in particular of prosthetic grafts.[139] Although this finding is of interest, its relevance to clinical practice has been diminished because all patients with peripheral vascular disease should be on an antiplatelet agent anyway because of their cardioprotective and cerebroprotective effects.[140] It has also been shown

Posterior approach to the posterior tibial artery

Lateral

Medial

Posterior tibial artery

Flexor digitorum longus muscle

Tendo calcaneus

Figure 10b-13. Posterior approach to the posterior tibial artery. The tendo calcaneus is retracted laterally and the flexor digitorum longus muscle medially to reveal the posterior tibial artery.

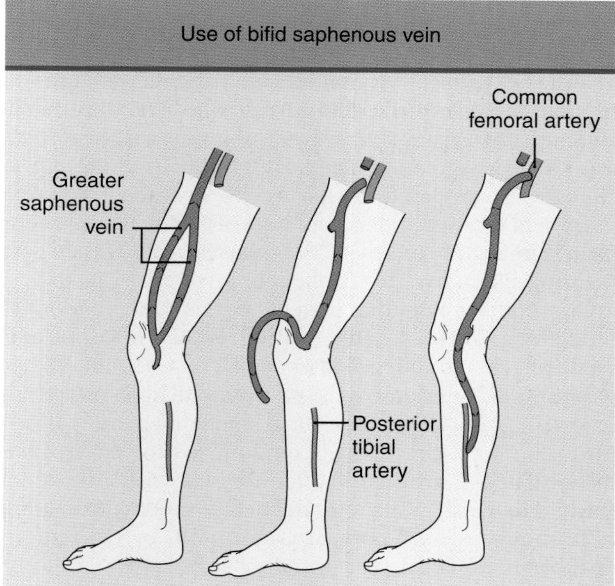

Figure 10b-14. Use of bifid saphenous vein. One proximal end of the bifid vein is divided and rotated to become the distal end of the graft. The proximal half of the graft is kept in situ, and the valves are lysed with a valvulotome. The distal rotated segment is reversed; therefore, valve lysis is not necessary.

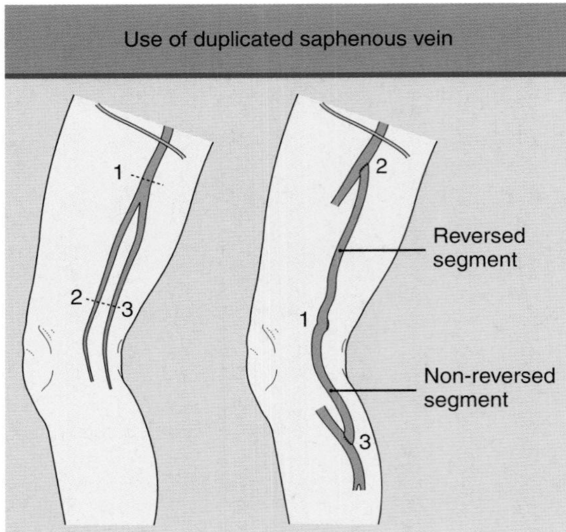

Figure 10b-15. Use of duplicated saphenous vein. Both branches of the saphenous vein are mobilized, and the trunk with the largest diameter is reversed and used for the proximal part of the graft. The smaller branch is used as a distal nonreversed segment, and its valves are lysed. The excised bifurcation zone is sutured.

that these agents should be continued in the perioperative period.[63] If patients are intolerant of aspirin, then clopidogrel is an alternative.[141]

Anticoagulants

Only one long-term placebo-controlled study has assessed the effect of anticoagulation on long-term infrainguinal bypass patency.[142] This study randomized 130 patients undergoing infrainguinal vein bypass to phenprocoumon or placebo and reported a significant improvement in graft patency limb salvage and patient survival in the phenprocoumon group. The Dutch Bypass Oral Anticoagulants or Aspirin Study randomized patients undergoing infrainguinal bypass to aspirin or oral anticoagulants.[143] A total of 2690 patients were randomized, and analysis of the data revealed no overall difference between the two groups. However, subgroup analysis revealed that oral anticoagulation significantly improved the patency of vein grafts compared to aspirin with a relative risk of graft occlusion of 0.69 (confidence interval of 0.64 to 0.88), whereas aspirin significantly increased the chances of a prosthetic graft remaining patent by 1.26 (confidence interval of 1.03 to 1.55). It is important to note that patients in this study randomized to oral anticoagulation had a relative risk of a major bleeding episode of 1.96 (confidence interval of 1.42 to 2.71).

Sarac et al.[144] randomized 56 patients with high-risk infrainguinal vein grafts to receive aspirin alone or a combination of aspirin plus warfarin. Patients randomized to warfarin were anticoagulated immediately after surgery with intravenous heparin. High-risk grafts were defined as those with a suboptimal venous conduit, poor arterial runoff, or redo infrainguinal bypasses. The 3-year primary patency was significantly higher in the warfarin plus aspirin group (74% versus 51%), as was the 3-year limb salvage (81% versus 31%). However, this improved outcome was gained at the expense of significantly more postoperative wound hematomas in the warfarin plus aspirin group (32% versus 3.7%). One quarter of the

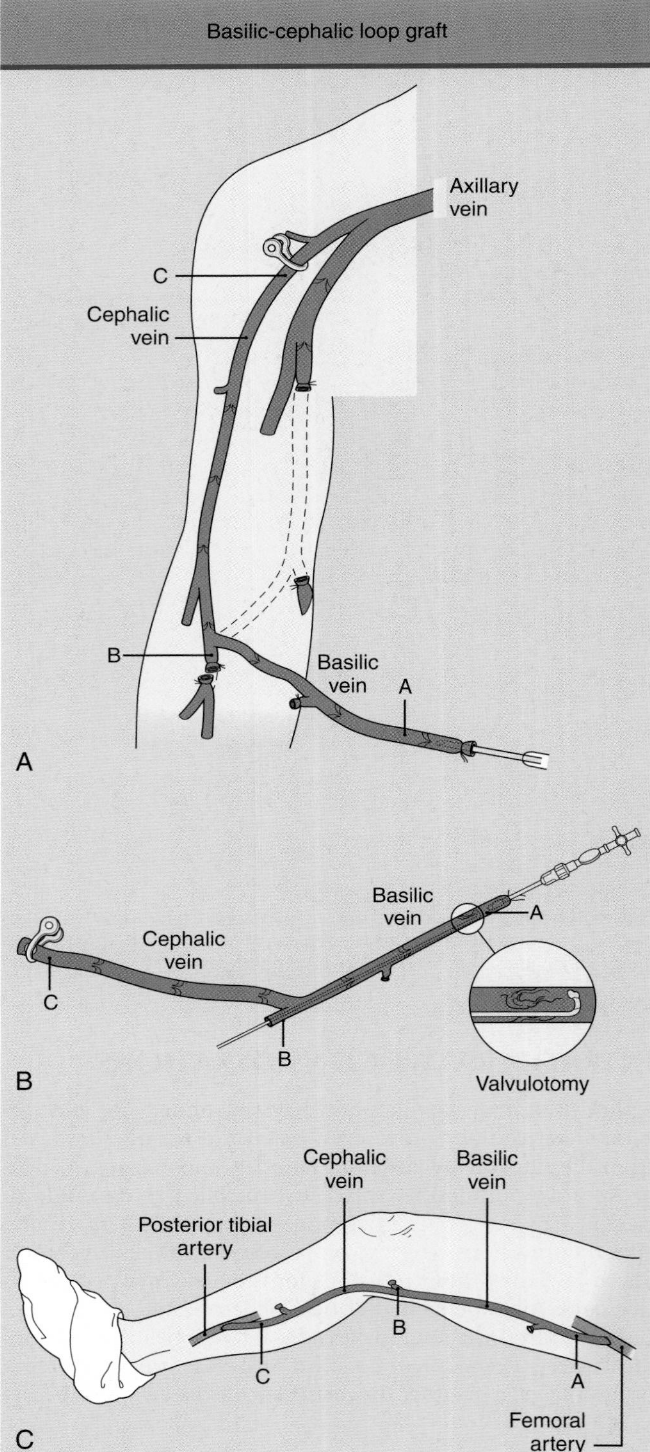

Figure 10b-16. Basilic–cephalic loop graft. The basilic and cephalic veins are mobilized **(A)** and the valves of the distended basilic vein are lysed **(B).** The proximal basilic vein is then placed in "nonreversed" orientation **(C),** while the distal cephalic segment is used in the reversed orientation. (Modified from LoGerfo FW, Paniszyn CW, Menzoian J. A new arm vein graft for distal by bypass. *J Vasc Surg* 1987;5:889-89.)

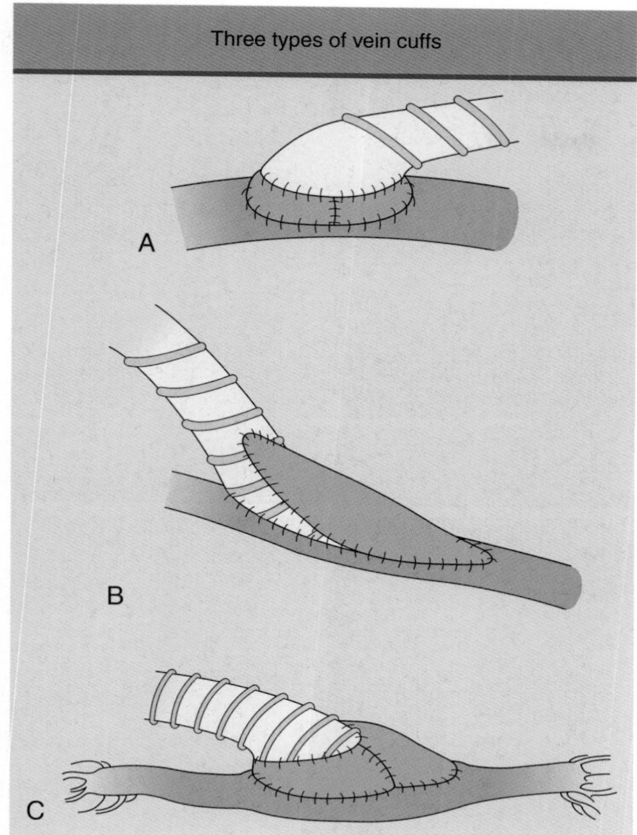

Figure 10b-17. Three types of vein cuffs: Miller collar (A), Taylor patch (B), and St. Mary's boot (C).

wound hematomas in the warfarin plus aspirin group required operative evacuation.

Johnson et al.[145] reported the results of a Veterans Affairs Cooperative Study that included 665 patients with infrainguinal bypasses who were randomized to aspirin alone or aspirin plus warfarin. The addition of warfarin to aspirin had no effect on vein bypass patency but did reduce the risk of prosthetic bypass occlusion by a factor of 0.62 (confidence interval of 0.42 to 0.92). Twice as many major hemorrhagic events occurred in those taking warfarin, and the risk of death was increased by a factor of 1.41 (confidence interval of 1.09 to 1.84). There seems no doubt from the preceding studies in patients with peripheral vascular disease that combining an anticoagulant with aspirin carries significant risks. It had been shown in a randomized, placebo-controlled trial[146] that the addition of low-molecular-weight heparin (dalteparin, 5000 IU daily) to aspirin for the first 3 months after lower limb bypass surgery does not improve vein or prosthetic graft patency.

All patients with peripheral vascular disease should be on an antiplatelet agent for its cardioprotective and cerebroprotective effects, which means that the decision to be made in the case of the patient with an infrainguinal bypass graft is whether to add an anticoagulant to the antiplatelet agent. Current evidence suggests that for prosthetic grafts and "high risk" vein grafts there may be some benefit in terms of graft patency. However, this improved patency is gained at the expense of roughly double the risk of a major hemorrhage compared to taking aspirin alone. Therefore, a reasonable approach is to use anticoagulants selectively and only anticoagulate patients with "high risk" vein or prosthetic grafts, provided that the patient does not have a raised baseline risk of a hemorrhagic event.

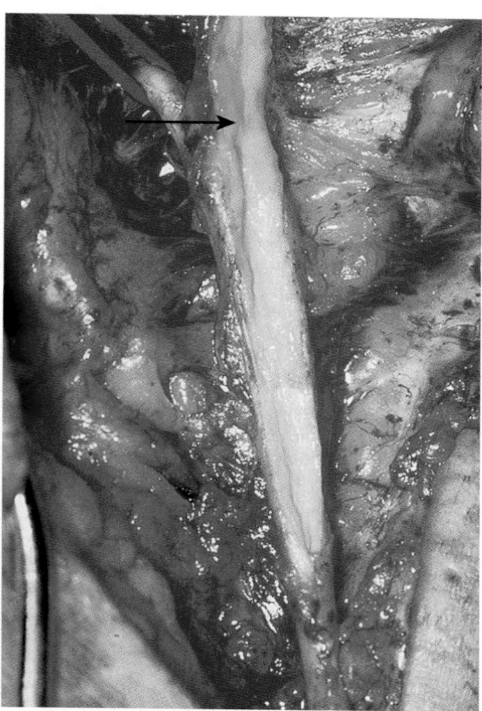

Figure 10b-18. Vein graft stenosis. Operative photograph of a vein graft stenosis *(arrow)*.

GRAFT SURVEILLANCE

The principle behind a graft surveillance program is to detect failing grafts before they occlude. Graft occlusion during the first postoperative month most commonly results from technical error or poor runoff. After 1 month, the commonest cause of graft occlusion is intimal hyperplasia causing a localized graft stenosis (Figures 10b-18 and 10b-19). Up to 30% of vein grafts develop a patency-threatening stenosis in the first two postoperative years. Color duplex scanning can detect stenoses (Figure 10b-20), and the criterion most commonly used is the peak systolic velocity ratio across the stenosis. Stenoses with a peak systolic velocity ratio of more than 3.0 require treatment.[147] The treatment options are surgical vein patch angioplasty or PTA.[148,149] It has been reported that lesions involving anastomoses are better treated surgically whereas focal midgraft lesions do equally well with surgery or PTA (Figure 10b-21).

Although color duplex scanning can detect graft stenoses, controversy surrounds the effectiveness of graft surveillance programs. Lundell et al.[150] randomized patients with infrainguinal vein grafts to intensive duplex surveillance or not and found that intensive surveillance significantly improved secondary patency at 3 years (82% versus 56%). Ihlberg et al.[151] also randomized patients to duplex surveillance or not and were not able to show any benefit from duplex surveillance. However, only 60% of patients randomized to duplex surveillance actually received a duplex scan and 8% of patients

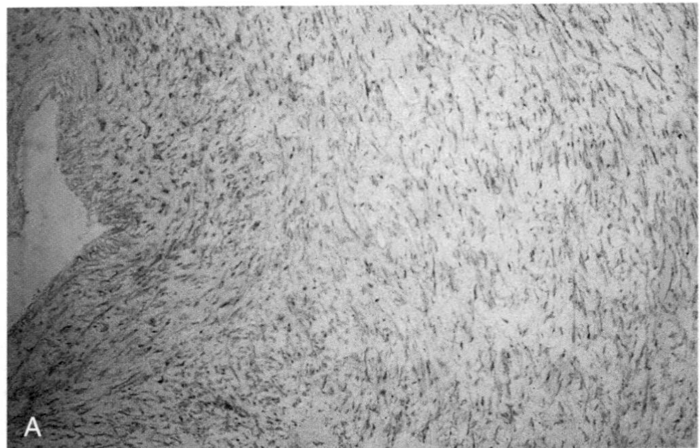

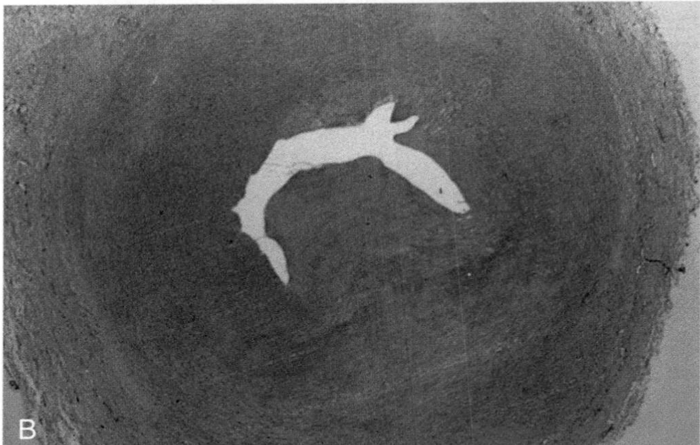

Figure 10b-19. Histology of vein graft stenosis. Photomicrograph of a vein graft stenosis stained with antismooth muscle actin **(A)** and Alcian blue or periodic acid–Schiff **(B).** The former stains smooth muscle cells red, and the latter stains matrix mucopolysaccharides blue. It can be seen that the intimal hyperplastic lesion contains large numbers of smooth muscle cells that are producing copious extracellular matrix.

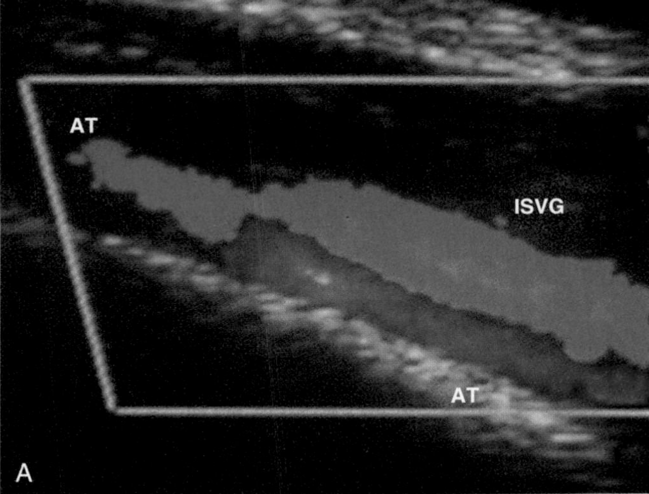

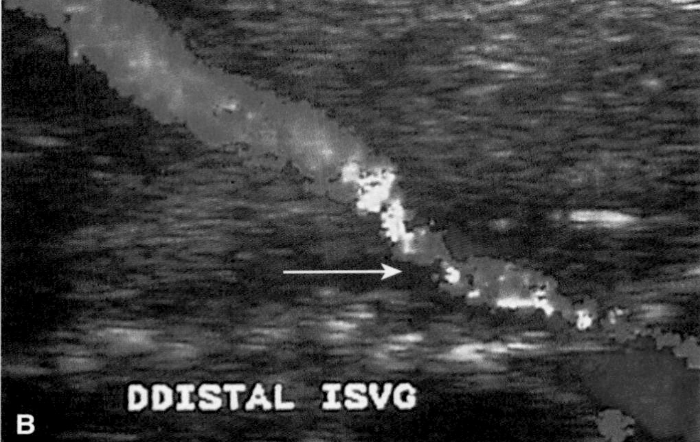

Figure 10b-20. Duplex scanning. **A,** A normal in situ vein graft (ISVG) is seen joining the anterior tibial artery (AT). **B,** In the distal portion of this in situ vein graft is a flow disturbance *(arrow)* that was causing a peak systolic velocity ratio of 4.5 across the stenosis.

in the nonsurveillance group underwent duplex surveillance at the request of their surgeon. The results of this study are therefore difficult to interpret. Visser et al.[152] examined the cost effectiveness of vein graft duplex surveillance and concluded that in patients with CLLI it is highly effective and leads to a reduction in major amputation and consequently in cost. More recently, in a prospective randomized trial, Davies et al.[153] found that duplex surveillance did not improve vein graft patency. Therefore, although the role of vein graft surveillance is still controversial, there is agreement that surveillance of prosthetic grafts is not worthwhile.[150,154,155]

MANAGEMENT OF GRAFT THROMBOSIS

Early graft thrombosis within 30 days of surgery can result from technical error, poor inflow, poor outflow, or hypotension in the immediate postoperative period. In addition, a small number of grafts, particularly prosthetic grafts, occlude in the immediate postoperative period for no identifiable reason. Graft failure between 1 month and 2 years usually results from intimal hyperplasia. After 2 years, progression of atherosclerosis in either inflow or outflow arteries becomes increasingly important. Early graft thrombosis often results in acute critical ischemia, requiring immediate reoperation, whereas late graft thrombosis more often results in the return of preoperative symptoms. Although in the latter situation immediate surgery to save the leg is unnecessary, the longer a graft remains thrombosed, particularly a vein graft, the more difficult it is to unblock. An underlying principle behind the management of all thrombosed grafts is the need to ascertain and correct the cause or causes of the graft failure. It is particularly helpful in this respect if the surgeon performing the original procedure records in the operation note any areas of concern or likely causes of graft failure. Most surgeons would consider revised thrombosed grafts as "high risk" and in the absence of contraindications anticoagulate the patient.

EARLY GRAFT THROMBOSIS

Early graft thrombosis often results in severe acute ischemia and requires an immediate reoperation. The return to theater should not be delayed by arteriography, because this can be performed on table. It is, however, invaluable to request a vascular technologist to search for and mark any usable vein in the contralateral leg or arms. However, this should not significantly delay the return to theater. If for any reason the return to theater is unavoidably delayed, the surgeon

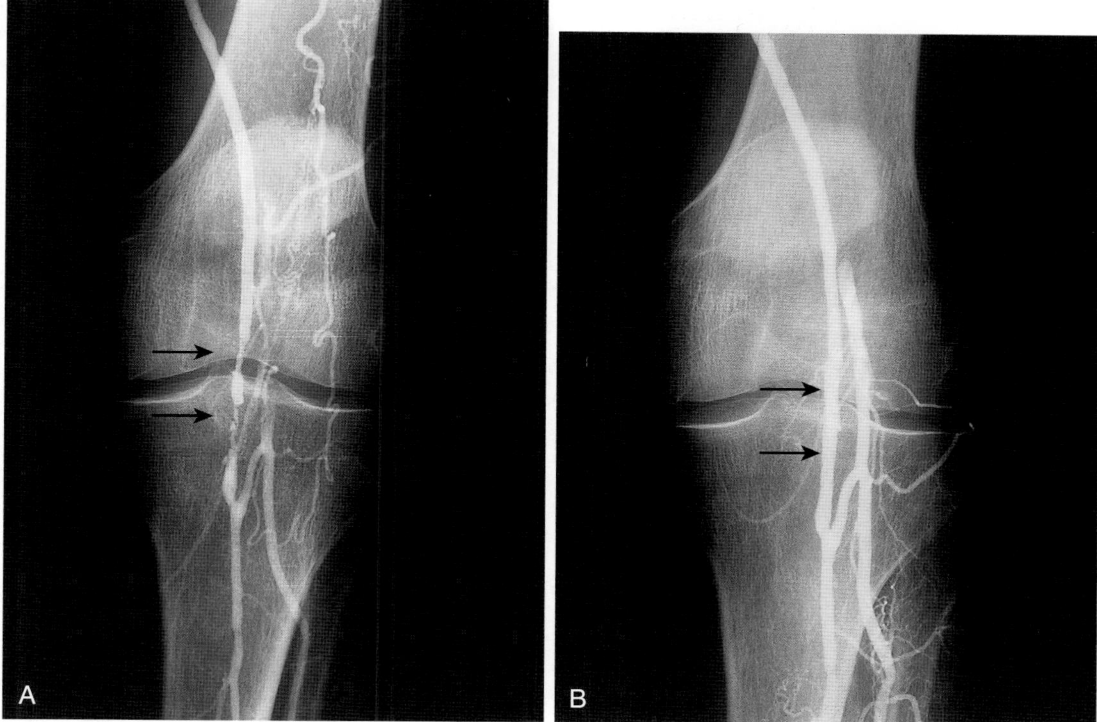

Figure 10b-21. Percutaneous transluminal angioplasty of vein graft stenoses. Two stenoses *(arrows)* in vein graft to below-knee popliteal artery before **(A)** and after **(B)** angioplasty.

may have to consider performing a fasciotomy. Finally, these reoperative procedures are particularly demanding and are greatly aided by the assistance of a "fresh" experienced vascular surgeon.

Vein Grafts

The distal incision is reopened, and after anticoagulation with intravenous heparin, a linear venotomy is made in the hood of the graft. Any visible clot is removed with fine forceps and a balloon catheter is passed distally. An on-table arteriogram is then performed to examine the state of the runoff vessels. If fresh clot occurs in the vessels, this can be resolved by direct infusion of tissue plasminogen activator (5 to 10 mg in 50 ml of saline infused over 20 minutes) into the vessels. If there is longstanding runoff disease, this can be dealt with by either extension of the bypass or on-table PTA. The choice of approach depends on factors such as the availability of additional autogenous vein and the nature of the distal disease. Although thrombus in the body of the graft sometimes can be removed using a balloon catheter passed up from the distal venotomy, it is often necessary to expose the proximal anastomosis and remove thrombus through a proximal venotomy. Reversed vein grafts can be particularly troublesome because of intact valves obstructing the passage of balloon catheters. The technique described by Pit and Lawson[156] is particularly useful in this respect (Figure 10b-22).

If a cause for the graft thrombosis can be identified and corrected using the original vein graft, then a completion arteriogram including the full length of the graft should be performed to ensure that indeed no problems remain. If the vein graft itself cannot be unblocked or is an inadequate conduit, then every effort should be made to replace it with alternative autogenous vein, including if necessary composite vein. If no additional autogenous vein can be found, the decision regarding the use of a prosthetic graft is based on the state of the runoff, the completeness of the plantar arch, and the degree of continuity between the two.[57,112] If a prosthetic graft is used, it has to be accepted that the risk of infection is increased in the circumstance of an often-prolonged revision procedure occurring soon after the primary operation.

If the previously described techniques do not demonstrate a cause for graft failure, a final investigation once graft flow has been established is to measure the pressure (vide supra) in the inflow artery. If pressure measurements reveal an inflow problem, then this is best dealt with by on-table PTA. Sometimes no cause for the early failure of a vein graft can be found, and even in this circumstance simple thrombectomy can result in long-term patency.

Prosthetic Grafts

The surgical principles underlying the management of the early thrombosis of a prosthetic graft are the same as those for a vein graft. However, the graft itself is usually easier to unblock than a vein graft, and it is more common to not find an identifiable cause of graft failure. If a below-knee prosthetic graft has not had a vein cuff placed at the distal anastomosis, then one should be inserted. If no cause for graft failure can be found, in theory one approach is to replace the prosthetic with autologous vein, However, in practice most surgeons would only use a prosthetic graft for the primary procedure if vein was not available. Therefore, it is unlikely that vein will be available.

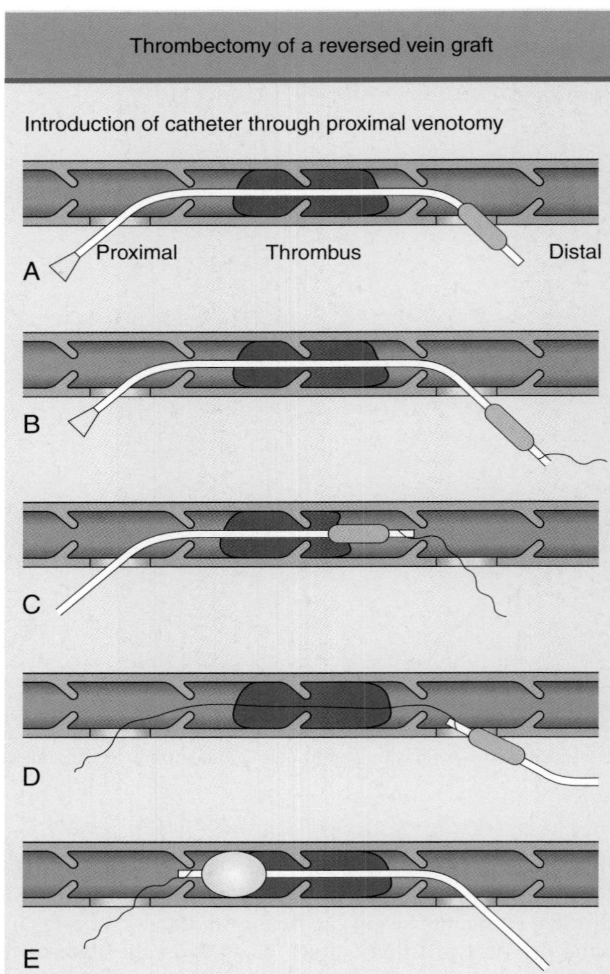

Figure 10b-22. Thrombectomy of a reversed vein graft. Thrombectomy of a reversed vein graft using a Fogarty balloon catheter is impeded by the presence of valves. **A,** The graft is opened with small proximal and distal incisions, and a Fogarty catheter is introduced through the proximal incision. **B,** A thread is attached to the catheter tip. **C,** This is then pulled through the graft and out of the proximal incision. **D,** The distal thread is now attached to the catheter tip, which is then pulled up through the valves against the flow direction. **E,** The catheter balloon is then inflated and thrombectomy proceeds. Steps **D** and **E** can be repeated as required. (Adapted from Pit MJ, Lawson JA. *Eur J Vasc Surg* 1993;7:452-453.)

LATE GRAFT THROMBOSIS

Late graft thrombosis does not usually lead to acute ischemia and in some cases may not lead to a recurrence of the patient's preoperative symptoms. The first course of action therefore may be a risk–benefit discussion with the patient concerning the need for and potential benefits of reintervention. If reintervention is required, then the arterial system of the affected limb should be investigated by duplex scanning. If this reveals disease that is amenable to PTA, then this is an excellent solution to the problem. However, this option is rarely available since the original bypass procedure was performed because the original arterial disease was not suitable for PTA. If further surgery is required, the patient should have all remaining leg and arm veins mapped so that the surgeon can assess the available options. If vein mapping reveals sufficient length to replace the thrombosed graft, then this is the best option. If sufficient vein is not available, then the options depend on the type of graft that has thrombosed.

Vein Grafts

Vein grafts that have been thrombosed for more than 48 hours are usually impossible to unblock using surgical techniques. One approach to the problem, which can be used for up to 14 days after graft thrombosis, is thrombolysis. Initial enthusiasm for the use of thrombolysis in thrombosed vein grafts has been tempered by the risks of hemorrhagic complications and poor long-term patencies.[157,158] Thus, although the rate for successful thrombolysis of thrombosed vein grafts can be as high as 77%,[157] up to 25% of patients suffer a serious hemorrhage and up to 67% require an adjunctive radiological or surgical procedure.[158] Therefore, it would seem that thrombolysis is best viewed as a technique to open a thrombosed vein graft before a radiological or surgical procedure to correct the underlying cause of the graft failure. In view of the risks of thrombolysis, it is probably best reserved for those occasions when there is not enough autogenous vein to replace a thrombosed vein graft.

Prosthetic Grafts

Unlike vein grafts, it is usually possible to unblock prosthetic grafts using conventional surgical techniques. Conversely, the results of thrombolysis of occluded prosthetic grafts are poor.[158] If autogenous vein is not available, then one approach is surgical graft thrombectomy combined with on-table thrombolysis in an attempt to rid the distal runoff vessels of thrombus. The nature of any corrective procedure is determined by the findings of on-table arteriography. Chronic runoff vessel disease can be dealt with either by on-table PTA or by a distal extension of the prosthetic bypass. Distal or proximal anastomotic intimal hyperplasia is best managed by patch angioplasty using vein.

A PERSONAL VIEW

The preceding sections have summarized the evidence for several approaches to the management of CLLI. In this section I summarize my own approach to management of the patient with CLLI, not in the belief that my own approach is necessarily the best but because it at least gives one approach to the problem. My initial investigation of the patient with CLLI is always a color duplex scan of the lower limb arterial tree. Based on this scan, I then decide whether a PTA is possible. If a PTA is technically feasible, I discuss the pros and cons of such an approach with the patient, including the complication rate. If a PTA looks unlikely to be technically possible or successful, I then request a scan of the patient's lower limb veins and, if necessary, arm vein. If no autogenous vein is available, this would make me more likely to request an attempted angioplasty in a borderline case, whereas if autogenous is available, I would proceed to surgery. I routinely perform a dependent Doppler examination to confirm that the proposed target distal vessel is in continuity with the pedal arch. I would never proceed to a primary amputation in a patient in whom I was intending to salvage the leg without intraoperative prereconstruction arteriography.

I routinely use subcutaneous low-molecular-weight heparin thromboprophylaxis and at least three doses of antibiotic prophylaxis. I try to tailor the operative plan to the individual patient. In particular, it is often possible to use autogenous by being creative about inflow and outflow sites, including, if required, preoperative and intraoperative PTA. I would use contralateral long saphenous vein or arm vein or composite autologous vein rather than use a prosthetic graft. I always request preoperative duplex marking of the intended venous conduit to detect diseased segments and to minimize undermining skin flaps. I routinely use loupe magnification. Although I only rarely request preoperative arteriography, as discussed earlier I routinely perform prereconstruction arteriography, the site of which is dictated by a preoperative duplex scan. I favor a reversed vein technique because I find that valve lysis in small veins can be difficult and because I like to tunnel the vein deep to thigh or calf wounds that, if they become infected, may threaten an underlying in situ vein graft. I routinely perform completion arteriography in the expectation that approximately 20% of grafts will harbor a technical error that requires correction. I would only use a prosthetic graft if the patient had excellent runoff that was in continuity with the plantar arch. If I use a prosthetic graft, I always use a vein cuff when the outflow is below the knee. I always enter vein grafts into a surveillance program but never do so with prosthetic grafts.

References

1. Lu XW, Idu MM, Ubbink DT, Legemate DA. Meta-analysis of the clinical effectiveness of venous arterialization for salvage of critically ischaemic limbs. *Eur J Vasc Endovasc Surg* 2006;31:493-499.
2. Abou-Zamzam AM, Lee RW, Moneta GL, et al. Functional outcome after infrainguinal bypass for limb salvage. *J Vasc Surg* 1997;25: 287-295.
3. Taylor SM, Kalbaugh CA, Blackhurst DW, et al. Determinants of functional outcome after revascularization for critical limb ischemia: an analysis of 1000 consecutive vascular interventions. *J Vasc Surg* 2006;44:747-756.
4. Eskelinin E, Luther M, Eskelinen A, Lepentalo M. Infrapopliteal bypass reduces amputation incidence in elderly patients: a population-based study. *Eur J Vasc Endovasc Surg* 2003;26:65-68.
5. Klevsgard R, Hallberg IR, Risberg B, Thomsen MB. Quality of life associated with varying degrees of chronic lower limb ischaemia: comparison with a healthy sample. *Eur J Vasc Endovasc Surg* 1999;17:319-325.
6. Kukkonen T, Junnila J, Aittola V, Makinen K. Functional outcome of distal bypasses for lower limb ischemia. *Eur J Vasc Endovasc Surg* 2006:258-261.
7. Tangelder MJD, McDonnell J, Van Busschbach JJ, et al. Quality of life after infrainguinal bypass grafting surgery. *J Vasc Surg* 2002;29:913-919.
8. Nguyen LL, Moneta GL, Conte MS, et al. Prospective multicenter study of quality of life before and after lower extremity vein bypass in 1404 patients with critical ischaemia. *J Vasc Surg* 2006;44:977-984.
9. Holtzman J, Caldwell M, Walvatne C, Kane R. Long-term functional status and quality of life after lower extremity revascularization. *J Vasc Surg* 1999;29:395-402.
10. Johnson BF, Evans L, Drury R, et al. Surgery for limb threatening ischaemia: a reappraisal of the costs and benefits. *Eur J Vasc Endovasc Surg* 1995;9:181-188.
11. Luther M. Surgical treatment for chronic critical leg ischaemia: a 5 year follow-up of socioeconomic outcome. *Eur J Vasc Endovasc Surg* 1997;13:452-459.
12. Cheshire NJ, Wolfe JH, Noone MA, et al. The economics of femorocrural reconstruction for critical leg ischemia with and without autologous vein. *J Vasc Surg* 1992;15:167-174.
13. Singh S, Evans L, Datta D, et al. The costs of managing lower limb-threatening ischaemia. *Eur J Vasc Endovasc Surg* 1996;12:359-362.
14. Magnant JG, Cronenwett JL, Walsh DB, et al. Surgical treatment of infrainguinal arterial occlusive disease in women. *J Vasc Surg* 1993;17:67-76.
15. Enzler MA, Ruoss M, Seifert B, Berger M. The influence of gender on the outcome of arterial procedures in the lower extremity. *Eur J Vasc Endovasc Surg* 1996;11:446-452.
16. Luther M, Lepantalo M. Femorotibial reconstructions for chronic critical leg ischaemia: influence on outcome by diabetes, gender and age. *Eur J Vasc Endovasc Surg* 1997;13:569-577.
17. Shah DM, Darling RC III, Chang BB, et al. Long-term results of in situ saphenous vein bypass: analysis of 2058 cases. *Ann Surg* 1995;222: 438-446.
18. Singh N, Sidawy AN, DeZee KJ, et al. Factors associated with early failure of infrainguinal lower extremity bypass. *J Vasc Surg* 2008:556-561.
19. Tordoir JH, van der Plas JP, Jacobs MJ, Kitslaar PJ. Factors determining the outcome of crural and pedal revascularisation for critical limb ischaemia. *Eur J Vasc Surg* 1993;7:82-86.
20. Olojugba DH, McCarthy MJ, Reid A, et al. Infrainguinal revascularisation in the era of vein-graft surveillance: do clinical factors influence long-term outcome? *Eur J Vasc Endovasc Surg* 1999;17:121-128.
21. Hamdan AD, Saltzberg SS, Sheahan M, et al. Lack of association of diabetes with increased postoperative mortality and cardiac morbidity. *Arch Surg* 2002;137:417-421.
22. Peltonen S, Biancari F, Lindgren L, et al. Outcome of infrainguinal bypass surgery for critical leg ischaemia in patients with chronic renal failure. *Eur J Vasc Endovasc Surg* 1998;15:122-127.
23. Nguyen LL, Lipsitz SR, Bandyk DF, et al. Resource utilisation in the treatment of critical ischemia: the effect of tissue loss, comorbidities, and graft-related events. *J Vasc Surg* 2006:971-976.
24. Giswold ME, Landry GJ, Sexton GJ, et al. Modifiable patient factors are associated with reverse vein graft occlusion in the era of duplex scan surveillance. *J Vasc Surg* 2003;37:47-53.
25. Meyerson SL, Skelly CL, Curi MA, et al. Long-term results justify autogenous infrainguinal bypass grafting in patients with end-stage renal failure. *J Vasc Surg* 2001;34:27-33.
26. Willigendael EM, Teijink JAW, Bartelink M-L, et al. Smoking and the patency of lower extremity bypass grafts: a meta-analysis. *J Vasc Surg* 2005;42:67-74.
27. Sayers RD, Raptis S, Berce M, Miller JH. Long-term results of femorotibial bypass with vein or polytetrafluoroethylene. *Br J Surg* 1998;85: 934-938.
28. Pereira CE, Albers M, Romiti M, et al. Meta-analysis of femoropopliteal bypass grafts for lower extremity arterial insufficiency. *J Vasc Surg* 2006;44:510-517.
29. Johnson WC, Lee KK. A comparative evaluation of polytetrafluoroethylene, umbilical vein, and saphenous vein bypass grafts for femoral–popliteal above-knee revascularization: a prospective randomized Department of Veterans Affairs Cooperative Study. *J Vasc Surg* 2000;32:268-277.
30. Klinkert P, Schepers A, Burger DHC, et al. Vein versus polytetrafluoroethylene in above-knee femoropopliteal bypass grafting: five-year results of a randomized controlled trial. *J Vasc Surg* 2003;37:149-155.
31. Neufang A, Espinola-Klein C, Dorweiler B, et al. Infrapopliteal composite bypass with autologous vein and second generation glutaraldehyde stabilized human umbilical vein (HUV) for critical ischaemia. *Eur J Vasc Endovasc Surg* 2007;34:583-589.
32. Fichelle JM, Marzelle J, Colacchio G, et al. Infrapopliteal polytetrafluoroethylene and composite bypass: factors influencing patency. *Ann Vasc Surg* 1995;9:187-196.
33. Leshnower BG, Leshnower LE, Leshnower AC. Adjunctive uses of the radial artery for emergency infrapopliteal bypass in patients presenting with acute limb-threatening ischemia. *Vasc Endovasc Surg* 2007;41: 348-351.
34. Albers M, Romiti M, Pereira CAB, Wulkan M. Meta-analysis of allograft bypass grafting to infrapopliteal arteries. *Eur J Vasc Endovasc Surg* 2004;28:462-472.
35. Donaldson MC, Whittemore AD, Mannick JA. Further experience with an all-autogenous tissue policy for infrainguinal reconstruction. *J Vasc Surg* 1993;18:41-48.
36. Chang BB, Paty PS, Shah DM, Leather RP. The lesser saphenous vein: an underappreciated source of autogenous vein. *J Vasc Surg* 1992;15: 152-156.
37. Schulman ML, Badhey MR, Yatco R. Superficial femoral–popliteal veins and reversed saphenous veins as primary femoropopliteal bypass grafts: a randomized comparative study. *J Vasc Surg* 1987;6:1-10.
38. Sladen JG, Reid JD, Maxwell TM, Downs AR. Superficial femoral vein: a useful autogenous harvest site. *J Vasc Surg* 1994;20:947-952.
39. Wells JK, Hagino RT, Bargmann KM, et al. Venous morbidity after superficial femoral–popliteal vein harvest. *J Vasc Surg* 1999;29:282-289.

40. Chew DK, Owens CD, Belkin M, et al. Bypass in the absence of ipsilateral greater saphenous vein: safety and superiority of the contralateral greater saphenous vein. *J Vasc Surg* 2002;35:1085-1092.
41. de Vries SO, Donaldson MC, Hunink MG. Contralateral symptoms after unilateral intervention for peripheral occlusive disease. *J Vasc Surg* 1998;27:414-421.
42. Tarry WC, Walsh DB, Birkmeyer NJ, et al. Fate of the contralateral leg after infrainguinal bypass. *J Vasc Surg* 1998;27:1039-1047.
43. Robin C, Lermusiaux P, Bleuet F, Martinez R. Distal bypass for limb salvage: should the contralateral great saphenous vein be harvested? *Ann Vasc Surg* 2006;20:761-766.
44. Kakkar VV. The cephalic vein as a peripheral vascular graft. *Surg Gynecol Obstet* 1969;128:551-556.
45. Londrey GL, Bosher LP, Brown PW, et al. Infrainguinal reconstruction with arm vein, lesser saphenous vein, and remnants of greater saphenous vein: a report of 257 cases. *J Vasc Surg* 1994;20:451-456.
46. Marcaccio EJ, Miller A, Tannenbaum GA, et al. Angioscopically directed interventions improve arm vein bypass grafts. *J Vasc Surg* 1993;17:994-1002.
47. Miller A, Stonebridge PA, Jepsen SJ, et al. Continued experience with intraoperative angioscopy for monitoring infrainguinal bypass grafting. *Surgery* 1991;109:286-293.
48. Panetta TF, Marin ML, Veith FJ, et al. Unsuspected preexisting saphenous vein disease: an unrecognized cause of vein bypass failure. *J Vasc Surg* 1992;15:102-110.
49. Kreienberg PB, Darling RC III, Chang BB, et al. Early results of a prospective randomized trial of spliced vein versus polytetrafluoroethylene graft with a distal vein cuff for limb-threatening ischemia. *J Vasc Surg* 2002;35:299-306.
50. Varty K, London NJ, Brennan JA, et al. Infragenicular in situ vein bypass graft occlusion: a multivariate risk factor analysis. *Eur J Vasc Surg* 1993;7:567-571.
51. Wengerter KR, Veith FJ, Gupta SK, et al. Influence of vein size (diameter) on infrapopliteal reversed vein graft patency. *J Vasc Surg* 1990;11:525-531.
52. Sumner DS. Haemodynamics and rheology of vascular disease: applications to diagnosis and treatment. In: Haimovici H, ed. *Haimovici's vascular surgery.* Cambridge: Cambridge-Blackwell Science; 1996:104-123.
53. Ishii T, Gossage JA, Dourado R, et al. Minimum internal diameter of the greater saphenous vein is an important determinant of successful femorodistal bypass grafting that is independent of the quality of the runoff. *Vascular* 2004;12:225-232.
54. Marin ML, Veith FJ, Panetta TF, et al. Saphenous vein biopsy: a predictor of vein graft failure. *J Vasc Surg* 1993;18:407-114.
55. Stansby G. Vein quality in vascular surgery. *Lancet* 1998;351:1001-1002.
56. Shah DM, Paty PS, Leather RP, et al. Optimal outcome after tibial arterial bypass. *Surg Gynecol Obstet* 1993;177:283-287.
57. Schweiger H, Klein P, Lang W. Tibial bypass grafting for limb salvage with ringed polytetrafluoroethylene prostheses: results of primary and secondary procedures. *J Vasc Surg* 1993;18:867-874.
58. Copeland GP, Edwards P, Wilcox A, et al. GORA: a scoring system for the quantification of risk of graft occlusion. *Ann R Coll Surg Engl* 1994;76:132-135.
59. Scott DJ, Horrocks EH, Kinsella D, Horrocks M. Preoperative assessment of the pedal arch using pulse generated runoff and subsequent femorodistal outcome. *Eur J Vasc Surg* 1994;8:20-25.
60. Alback A, Biancari F, Saarinen O, Lepantalo M. Prediction of the immediate outcome of femoropopliteal saphenous vein bypass by angiographic runoff score. *Eur J Vasc Endovasc Surg* 1998;15:220-224.
61. Elliott BM, Robison JG, Brothers TE, Cross MA. Limitations of peroneal artery bypass grafting for limb salvage. *J Vasc Surg* 1993;18:881-888.
62. Bergamini TM, George Jr. SM, Massey HT, et al. Pedal or peroneal bypass: which is better when both are patent? *J Vasc Surg* 1994;20: 347-355.
63. Neilipovitz DT, Bryson GL, Nichol G. The effect of perioperative aspirin therapy in peripheral vascular surgery: a decision analysis. *Anesth Analg* 2001;93:573-580.
64. Sonksen J, Gray R, Hickman PJ. Safer non-cardiac surgery for patients with coronary artery disease. *Br Med J* 1998;317:1400-1401.
65. Bolsin S, Colson M, Conroy M. Beta-blockers and statins in non-cardiac surgery. *BMJ* 2007;334:1283-1284.
66. Bismuth J, Klitfod L, Sillesen H. The lack of cardiovascular risk factor management in patients with critical limb ischaemia. *Eur J Vasc Endovasc Surg* 2001;21:143-146.
67. Hollyoak M, Woodruff P, Muller M, et al. Deep venous thrombosis in postoperative vascular surgical patients: a frequent finding without prophylaxis. *J Vasc Surg* 2001;34:656-660.
68. Farkas JC, Chapuis C, Coombe S, et al. A randomised controlled trial of a low-molecular-weight heparin (Enoxaparin) to prevent deep-vein thrombosis in patients undergoing vascular surgery. *Eur J Vasc Surg* 1993;7:554-560.
69. Mangram AJ, Horan TC, Pearson ML, Silver LC, Jarvis WR. Guideline for prevention of surgical site infection, 1999: Centers for Disease Control and Prevention (CDC) Hospital Infection Control Practices Advisory Committee. *Am J Infect Control* 1999;27:97-132.
70. Pemberton M, Nydahl S, Hartshorne T, et al. Can lower limb vascular reconstruction be based on colour duplex imaging alone? *Eur J Vasc Endovasc Surg* 1996;12:452-454.
71. Collins C, Burch J, Cranny G, et al. Duplex ultrasonography, magnetic resonance angiography, and computed tomographic angiography for diagnosis and assessment of symptomatic, lower limb peripheral arterial disease: systematic review. *BMJ* 2007;334:1257-1261.
72. Ouwendijk R, de Vries M, Pattynama PMT, et al. Imaging peripheral arterial disease: a randomised controlled trial comparing contrast-enhanced MR angiography and multi-detector row CT angiography. *Radiology* 2005;236:1094-1103.
73. Dorweiler B, Neufang A, Kreitner K-F, et al. Magnetic resonance angiography unmasks reliable target vessels for pedal bypass grafting in patients with diabetes mellitus. *J Vasc Surg* 2002;35:766-772.
74. Avenarius JK, Breek JC, Lohle PNM, et al. The additional value of angiography after colour-coded duplex on decision making in patients with critical limb ischaemia: a prospective study. *Eur J Vasc Endovasc Surg* 2002;23:393-397.
75. Hickey NC, Thomson IA, Shearman CP, Simms MH. Aggressive arterial reconstruction for critical lower limb ischaemia. *Br J Surg* 1991;78: 1476-1478.
76. McCarthy MJ, Nydahl S, Hartshorne T, et al. Colour-coded duplex imaging and dependent Doppler ultrasonography in the assessment of cruropedal vessels. *Br J Surg* 1999;86:33-37.
77. Leopold PW, Shandall A, Kupinkski AM, et al. Role of B-mode venous mapping in infrainguinal in situ vein–arterial bypasses. *Br J Surg* 1989;76:305-307.
78. Bagi P, Schroeder T, Sillesen H, Lorentzen JE. Real time B-mode mapping of the greater saphenous vein. *Eur J Vasc Surg* 1989;3:103-105.
79. Barkmeier LD, Hood DB, Sumner DS, et al. Local anesthesia for infrainguinal arterial reconstruction. *Am J Surg* 1997;174:202-204.
80. Buggy DJ, Smith GS. Epidural anaesthesia and analgesia: better outcome after major surgery? *Br Med J* 1999;319:530-531.
81. Rivers SP, Scher LA, Sheehan E, Veith FJ. Epidural versus general anesthesia for infrainguinal arterial reconstruction. *J Vasc Surg* 1991;14: 764-768.
82. Christopherson R, Beattie C, Frank SM, et al. Perioperative morbidity in patients randomized to epidural or general anesthesia for lower extremity vascular surgery: Perioperative Ischemia Randomized Anesthesia Trial Study Group. *Anesthesiology* 1993;79:422-434.
83. Pierce ET, Pomposelli Jr FB, Stanley GD, et al. Anesthesia type does not influence early graft patency or limb salvage rates of lower extremity arterial bypass. *J Vasc Surg* 1997;25:226-232.
84. Naesh O, Haljamae H, Hindberg I, et al. Epidural anaesthesia prolonged into the postoperative period prevents stress response and platelet hyperaggregability after peripheral vascular surgery. *Eur J Vasc Surg* 1994;8:395-400.
85. Rosenfeld BA, Beattie C, Christopherson R, et al. The effects of different anesthetic regimens on fibrinolysis and the development of postoperative arterial thrombosis: Perioperative Ischemia Randomized Anesthesia Trial Study Group. *Anesthesiology* 1993;79:435-443.
86. Hickey NC, Wilkes MP, Howes D, et al. The effect of epidural anaesthesia on peripheral resistance and graft flow following femorodistal reconstruction. *Eur J Vasc Endovasc Surg* 1995;9:93-96.
87. Brewster DC, Cambria RP, Darling RC, et al. Long-term results of combined iliac balloon angioplasty and distal surgical revascularization. *Ann Surg* 1989;210:324-331.
88. Gross GM, Johnson RC, Roberts RM, et al. Results of peripheral endovascular procedures in the operating room. *J Vasc Surg* 1996;24:353-362.
89. Tukiainen E, Kallio M, Lepantalo M. Advanced leg salvage of the critically ischaemic leg with major tissue loss by vascular and plastic surgeon teamwork: long-term outcome. *Ann Surg* 2006;244:949-958.
90. Edwards WH, Jenkins JM, Mulherin Jr JL, et al. Extended profundoplasty to minimize pelvic and distal tissue loss. *Ann Surg* 1990;211:694-702.
91. Hansen AK, Bille S, Nielsen PH, Egeblad K. Profundaplasty as the only reconstructive procedure in patients with severe ischemia of the lower extremity. *Surg Gynecol Obstet* 1990;171:47-50.

92. Kalman PG, Johnston KW, Walker PM. The current role of isolated profundaplasty. *J Cardiovasc Surg (Torino)* 1990;31:107-111.
93. Radoux JM, Maiza D, Coffin O. Long-term outcome of 121 iliofemoral endarterectomy procedures. *Ann Vasc Surg* 2001;15:163-170.
94. Ho GH, Moll FL, Hedeman Joosten PP, et al. Endovascular remote endarterectomy in femoropopliteal occlusive disease: one-year clinical experience with the ring strip cutter device. *Eur J Vasc Endovasc Surg* 1996;12:105-112.
95. Donaldson MC, Mannick JA, Whittemore AD. Causes of primary graft failure after in situ saphenous vein bypass grafting. *J Vasc Surg* 1992;15:113-118.
96. Belkin M, Donaldson MC, Whittemore AD, et al. Observations on the use of thrombolytic agents for thrombotic occlusion of infrainguinal vein grafts. *J Vasc Surg* 1990;11:289-294.
97. Kunlin J. Le traitement de l'arterite obliterante par la greffe veineuse. *Arch Mal Coeur Vaiss* 1949;42:371-372.
98. May AG, DeWeese JA, Rob CG. Arterialized in situ saphenous vein. *Arch Surg* 1965;91:743-750.
99. Skagseth E, Hall KV. In situ vein bypass: experiences with new vein valve strippers. *Scand J Thorac Cardiovasc Surg* 1973;7:53-58.
100. Sayers RD, Watt PA, Muller S, et al. Structural and functional smooth muscle injury after surgical preparation of reversed and non-reversed (in situ) saphenous vein bypass grafts. *Br J Surg* 1991;78:1256-1258.
101. Harris PL, How TV, Jones DR. Prospectively randomized clinical trial to compare in situ and reversed saphenous vein grafts for femoropopliteal bypass. *Br J Surg* 1987;74:252-255.
102. Harris PL, Veith FJ, Shanik GD, et al. Prospective randomized comparison of in situ and reversed infrapopliteal vein grafts. *Br J Surg* 1993;80:173-176.
103. Moody AP, Edwards PR, Harris PL. In situ versus reversed femoropopliteal vein grafts: long-term follow-up of a prospective, randomized trial. *Br J Surg* 1992;79:750-752.
104. Wengerter KR, Veith FJ, Gupta SK, et al. Prospective randomized multicenter comparison of in situ and reversed vein infrapopliteal bypasses. *J Vasc Surg* 1991;13:189-197.
105. Watelet J, Soury P, Menard JF, et al. Femoropopliteal bypass: in situ or reversed vein grafts? Ten-year results of a randomized prospective study. *Ann Vasc Surg* 1997;11:510-519.
106. Lawson JA, Tangelder MJ, Algra A, Eikelboom BC. The myth of the in situ graft: superiority in infrainguinal bypass surgery?. *Eur J Vasc Endovasc Surg* 1999;18:149-157.
107. Leather RP, Shah DM, Chang BB, Kaufman JL. Resurrection of the in situ saphenous vein bypass. 1000 cases later. *Ann Surg* 1988;208:435-442.
108. Sales CM, Goldsmith J, Veith FJ. Prospective study of the value of prebypass saphenous vein angioscopy. *Am J Surg* 1995;170:106-108.
109. Clair DG, Golden MA, Mannick JA, et al. Randomized prospective study of angioscopically assisted in situ saphenous vein grafting. *J Vasc Surg* 1994;19:992-999.
110. Thorne J, Danielsson G, Danielsson P, et al. Intraoperative angioscopy may improve the outcome of in situ saphenous vein bypass grafting: a prospective study. *J Vasc Surg* 2002;35:759-765.
111. Rosenthal D, Arous EJ, Friedman SG, et al. Endovascular-assisted versus conventional in situ saphenous vein bypass grafting: cumulative patency, limb salvage, and cost results in a 39-month multicenter study. *J Vasc Surg* 2000;31:60-68.
112. Robinson BI, Fletcher JP, Tomlinson P, et al. A prospective randomized multicentre comparison of expanded polytetrafluoroethylene and gelatin-sealed knitted Dacron grafts for femoropopliteal bypass. *Cardiovasc Surg* 1999;7:214-218.
113. Devine C, McCollum C. Heparin-bonded Dacron or polytetrafluoroethylene for femoropopliteal bypass: five-year results of a prospective randomized multicenter clinical trial. *J Vasc Surg* 2004;40:924-931.
114. Dorigo W, Di Carlo F, Troisi N, et al. Lower limb revascularization with a new bioactive prosthetic graft: early and late results. *Ann Vasc Surg* 2008;22:79-87.
115. Peeters P, Verbist J, Deloose K, Bosiers M. Results with heparin bonded polytetrafluoroethylene grafts for femorodistal bypasses. *J Cardiovasc Surg* 2006:407-413.
116. Kapfer X, Meichelboeck W. Groegler F-M. Comparison of carbon-impregnated and standard PTFE prostheses in extra-anatomical anterior tibial artery bypass: a prospective randomized multicenter study. *Eur J Vasc Endovasc Surg* 2006;32:155-168.
117. Griffiths GD, Nagy J, Black D, Stone PC. Randomized clinical trial of distal anastomotic interposition vein cuff in infrainguinal polytetrafluoroethylene bypass grafting. *Br J Surg* 2004;91:560-562.
118. Laurila K, Lepantalo M, Teittinen K, et al. Does an adjuvant AV fistula improve the patency of a femorocrural PTFE bypass with distal vein cuff in critical ischaemia? A prospective randomised multicentre trial. *Eur J Vasc Endovasc Surg* 2004;27:180-185.
119. Ballotta E, Renon L, De Rossi A, et al. Prospective randomized study on reversed saphenous vein infrapopliteal bypass to treat limb-threatening ischemia: common femoral artery versus superficial femoral or popliteal and tibial arteries as inflow. *J Vasc Surg* 2004;40:732-740.
120. Flanigan DP, Williams LR, Schwartz JA, et al. Hemodynamic evaluation of the aortoiliac system based on pharmacologic vasodilatation. *Surgery* 1983;93:709-714.
121. Kram HB, Gupta SK, Veith FJ, et al. Late results of two hundred seventeen femoropopliteal bypasses to isolated popliteal artery segments. *J Vasc Surg* 1991;14:386-390.
122. Karacagil S, Almgren B, Bowald S, Eriksson I. Bypass grafting to the popliteal artery in limbs with occluded crural arteries. *Am J Surg* 1991;162:19-23.
123. Darke S, Lamont P, Chant A, et al. Femoropopliteal versus femorodistal bypass grafting for limb salvage in patients with an "isolated" popliteal segment. *Eur J Vasc Surg* 1989;3:203-207.
124. Loh A, Chester JF, Taylor RS. PTFE bypass grafting to isolated popliteal segments in critical limb ischaemia. *Eur J Vasc Surg* 1993;7:26-30.
125. Samson RH, Showalter DP, Yunis JP. Isolated femoropopliteal bypass graft for limb salvage after failed tibial reconstruction: a viable alternative to amputation. *J Vasc Surg* 1999;29:409-412.
126. Woelfle KD, Kugelmann U, Bruijnen H, et al. Intraoperative imaging techniques in infrainguinal arterial bypass grafting: completion angiography versus vascular endoscopy. *Eur J Vasc Surg* 1994;8:556-561.
127. Miller A, Marcaccio EJ, Tannenbaum GA, et al. Comparison of angioscopy and angiography for monitoring infrainguinal bypass vein grafts: results of a prospective randomized trial. *J Vasc Surg* 1993;17:382-396.
128. Johnson BL, Bandyk DF, Back MR, et al. Intraoperative duplex monitoring of infrainguinal vein bypass procedures. *J Vasc Surg* 2000;31:678-690.
129. Gilbertson JJ, Walsh DB, Zwolak RM, et al. A blinded comparison of angiography, angioscopy, and duplex scanning in the intraoperative evaluation of in situ saphenous vein bypass grafts. *J Vasc Surg* 1992;15:121-127.
130. Bernhard VM, Boren CH, Towne JB. Pneumatic tourniquet as a substitute for vascular clamps in distal bypass surgery. *Surgery* 1980;87:709-713.
131. Ciervo A, Dardik H, Qin F, et al. The tourniquet revisited as an adjunct to lower limb revascularization. *J Vasc Surg* 2000;31:436-442.
132. Eyers P, Ashley S, Scott DJ. Tourniquets in arterial bypass surgery. *Eur J Vasc Endovasc Surg* 2000;20:113-117.
133. Chester JF, Butler CM, Taylor RS. Vascular reconstruction at the groin: oblique or vertical incisions? *Ann R Coll Surg Engl* 1992;74:112-114.
134. Mukherjee D. Posterior approach to the peroneal artery. *J Vasc Surg* 1994;19:174-178.
135. Beard JD, Wyatt M, Scott DJ, et al. The non-reversed vein femoro-distal bypass graft: a modification of the standard in situ technique. *Eur J Vasc Surg* 1989;3:55-60.
136. Albers M, Romiti M, Brochado-Neto FC, et al. Meta-analysis of popliteal-to-distal vein bypass grafts for critical ischaemia. *J Vasc Surg* 2006;43:498-503.
137. Ouriel K. The posterior approach to popliteal–crural bypass. *J Vasc Surg* 1994;19:74-79.
138. Iloprost Bypass International Study Group. Effects of perioperative iloprost on patency of femorodistal bypass grafts. *Eur J Vasc Endovasc Surg* 1996;12:363-371.
139. Watson HR, Belcher G, Horrocks M. Adjuvant medical therapy in peripheral bypass surgery. *Br J Surg* 1999;86:981-991.
140. Antiplatelet Trialists' Collaboration. Collaborative overview of randomised trials of antiplatelet therapy. I. Prevention of death, myocardial infarction, and stroke by prolonged antiplatelet therapy in various categories of patients. *BMJ* 1994;308:81-106.
141. CAPRIE Steering Committee. A randomised, blinded, trial of clopidogrel versus aspirin in patients at risk of ischaemic events (CAPRIE). *Lancet* 1996;348:1329-1339.
142. Kretschmer G, Herbst F, Prager M, et al. A decade of oral anticoagulant treatment to maintain autologous vein grafts for femoropopliteal atherosclerosis. *Arch Surg* 1992;127:1112-1115.
143. Dutch Bypass Oral Anticoagulants or Aspirin Study Group. Efficacy of oral anticoagulants compared with aspirin after infrainguinal bypass surgery: a randomised trial. *Lancet* 2000;355:346-351.

144. Sarac TP, Huber TS, Back MR, et al. Warfarin improves the outcome of infrainguinal vein bypass grafting at high risk for failure. *J Vasc Surg* 1998;28:446-457.
145. Johnson WC, Williford WO. Department of Veterans Affairs Cooperative Study. Benefits, morbidity, and mortality associated with long-term administration of oral anticoagulant therapy to patients with peripheral arterial bypass procedures: a prospective randomized study. *J Vasc Surg* 2002;35:413-421.
146. Jivegard L, Drott C, Gelin J, et al. Effect of three months of low molecular weight heparin (dalteparin) treatment after bypass surgery for lower limb ischaemia: a randomised placebo-controlled double blind multicentre trial. *Eur J Vasc Endovasc Surg* 2005;29:190-198.
147. Olojugba DH, McCarthy MJ, Naylor AR, et al. At what peak velocity ratio value should duplex-detected infrainguinal vein graft stenoses be revised? *Eur J Vasc Endovasc Surg* 1998;15:258-260.
148. Hagino RT, Sheehan MK, Jung I, et al. Target lesion characteristics in failing vein grafts predict the success of endovascular and open revision. *J Vasc Surg* 2007;46:1167-1172.
149. Berceli SA, Hevelone ND, Lipsitz SR, et al. Surgical and endovascular revision of infrainguinal vein bypass grafts: analysis of midterm outcomes from the PREVENT III trial. *J Vasc Surg* 2007;46:1173-1179.
150. Lundell A, Lindblad B, Bergqvist D, Hansen F. Femoropopliteal–crural graft patency is improved by an intensive surveillance program: a prospective randomized study. *J Vasc Surg* 1995;21:26-33.
151. Ihlberg L, Luther M, Tierala E, Lepantalo M. The utility of duplex scanning in infrainguinal vein graft surveillance: results from a randomised controlled study. *Eur J Vasc Endovasc Surg* 1998;16:19-27.
152. Visser K, Idu MM, Buth J, et al. Duplex scan surveillance during the first year after infrainguinal autologous vein bypass grafting surgery: costs and clinical outcomes compared with other surveillance programs. *J Vasc Surg* 2001;33:123-130.
153. Davies AH, Hawdon AJ, Sydes MR, Thompson SG. Is duplex surveillance of value after leg vein bypass grafting? Principal results of the vein graft surveillance randomised trial (VGST). *Circulation* 1985-1991;2005;(112).
154. Dunlop P, Sayers RD, Naylor AR, et al. The effect of a surveillance programme on the patency of synthetic infrainguinal bypass grafts. *Eur J Vasc Endovasc Surg* 1996;11:441-445.
155. Lalak NJ, Hanel KC, Hunt J, Morgan A. Duplex scan surveillance of infrainguinal prosthetic bypass grafts. *J Vasc Surg* 1994;20:637-641.
156. Pit MJ, Lawson JA. A simple technique for thrombectomy of a reversed saphenous vein arterial bypass graft. *Eur J Vasc Surg* 1993;7:452-453.
157. Nehler MR, Mueller RJ, McLafferty RB, et al. Outcome of catheter-directed thrombolysis for lower extremity arterial bypass occlusion. *J Vasc Surg* 2003;37:72-78.
158. Conrad MF, Shepard AD, Rubinfield IS, et al. Long-term results of catheter-directed thrombolysis to treat infrainguinal bypass graft occlusion: the urokinase era. *J Vasc Surg* 2003;37:1009-1016.

chapter 11

Diabetic Foot Problems

Jeffrey A. Kalish, MD • Frank B. Pomposelli Jr, MD

Key Points

- In patients with diabetes mellitus, neuropathy and ischemia promote the development of foot ulcers, pressure necrosis, nonhealing wounds, and secondary infection.
- Soft-tissue infection is usually polymicrobial, often involves tendon or bone, and can cause extensive destruction.
- Treatment of complications of infection, neuropathy, or both often requires surgery; if circulation is inadequate, it must be corrected; otherwise, measures to treat infection, neuropathy, or both will fail.
- The concept of "small vessel disease" is erroneous and has no place in the diagnosis or management of foot ischemia, which is due to atherosclerosis.
- Atherosclerosis in the ischemic diabetic foot usually involves the tibial or peroneal arteries but usually spares the foot arteries.
- In the treatment of foot ischemia, a carefully planned approach, including prompt control of infection when present, and an extreme distal arterial reconstruction to maximize foot perfusion (often to the foot arteries) should lead to rates of limb salvage in diabetic patients that equal or exceed those achieved in the nondiabetic patient population.
- Minimally invasive endovascular interventions can be performed in diabetic patients to restore circulation for limb salvage, and current studies are comparing the outcomes to traditional bypass surgery.

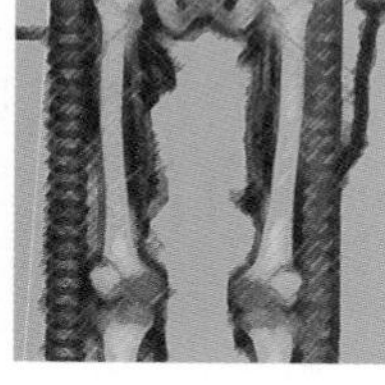

Problems related to the foot still remain the most common cause for hospitalization for patients with diabetes mellitus.[1,2] Approximately 15% of the nearly 21 million people in the United States with diabetes mellitus will be hospitalized for a foot problem at least once during their lifetime. The annual health-care cost for this problem alone exceeds $1.5 billion.[3] The pathological combination of neuropathy and ischemia sets the stage for foot ulcers, pressure necrosis, and nonhealing wounds. The resultant loss of continuity of the "skin envelope" often leads to destructive polymicrobial infection and further tissue loss. A vicious cycle is created, which explains the high risk of gangrene and amputation that stems from an initially minor insult (Figure 11-1). In the United States, patients with diabetes account for approximately 60% of nontraumatic limb amputations annually, even though they comprise only 7% of the population.[4]

For the physicians involved in the care of these patients, understanding the interaction of the etiological triad of neuropathy, infection, and ischemia is critical to achieving successful foot salvage. The following sections separately discuss neuropathy, infection, and ischemia, but it is important to understand that they seldom work in isolation and must be evaluated and treated simultaneously in a successful treatment plan.

NEUROPATHY

Neuropathy is a common complication of diabetes mellitus and is one of the hallmark pathological conditions associated with this disease, along with retinopathy and nephropathy.

Pathophysiology

Diabetic neuropathy is a polyneuropathy, affecting the autonomic and the somatic nervous system and leading to a complex and polymorphous group of disorders.

The pathogenesis of diabetic neuropathy is not fully understood. Possible explanations are based on theories of alterations in the nerves supplying blood vessels (vasa nervorum) or abnormalities in metabolism. The vascular theory is based on observations of thickening of the nutrient vessels, which may occlude with progression, resulting in ischemic injury to the nerve. A more popular theory for the pathogenesis of neuropathy is the increased activity of the polyol (sorbitol) pathway.[5] Accumulation of sorbitol has been demonstrated in aortic intima and media. Excess sorbitol may produce toxic effects, resulting in demyelination and impaired velocity of peripheral

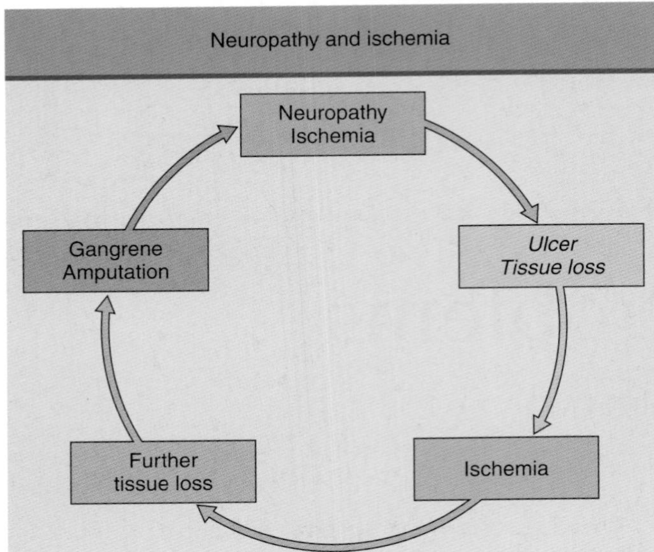

Figure 11-1. Neuropathy and ischemia. The presence of neuropathy and ischemia sets the stage for the development of ulcers (neuroischemic ulcers) and tissue loss. If ischemia is not corrected with appropriate arterial reconstruction, tissue loss will occur and will lead to gangrene and amputation.

nerve conduction. These pathological findings have been reported in human diabetic neuropathy.[6] Several studies suggest a decrease in neurotrophic factors may be important for the development of diabetic neuropathy.[7,8] As with microangiopathic complications of retinopathy and nephropathy, the severity of neuropathy is related to the duration of diabetes.

Neuropathy involving the autonomic system may lead to a shunting away of the blood through arteriovenous connections in the microcirculation.[9] This leads to decreased tissue perfusion, even in the presence of normal arterial supply. Recent work has demonstrated that oxygen saturation is reduced in the skin of diabetic patients, and this impairment is accentuated in the presence of neuropathy.[10] The second interaction between neuropathy and perfusion involves the nociceptive reflex. When a (peripheral) sensory fiber is stimulated, the signal travels to the central nerve cell body and the spinal cord and then to other axon branches (axon reflex). This reflex releases substance P from the nerve, which triggers mast cells to release histamine resulting in a "wheal and flare." This response to a noxious stimulus is greatly attenuated in patients with diabetes and may even precede clinically apparent neuropathy.[11] The absence of this reflex may contribute to the blunted neuroinflammatory response in diabetics, which helps explain the typical underestimation of the severity of a diabetic foot infection.[12] Last, autonomic neuropathy causes the skin to become dry through loss of sweat and oil gland function. This dry skin exhibits markedly increased susceptibility to skin breakdown and fissures, thus creating a portal of entry for bacteria.

Motor neuropathy decreases the neural stimulation of the intrinsic muscles of the foot; leads to atrophy and wasting of these muscles, which are important in maintaining digital stability at the metatarsophalangeal joint level; and increases tonus of the long flexors. With intrinsic muscle wasting, the metatarsal bones are fixed and the toes are drawn up in a "claw" position (Figure 11-2). The resultant deformity creates abnormal pressure points beneath the metatarsal heads and over the dorsum and the tip of the toes, which may lead to ulcers.

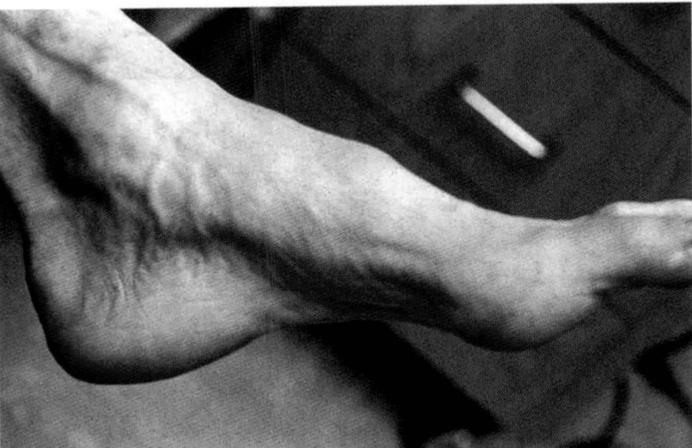

Figure 11-2. The "claw" position. Motor neuropathy causes loss of normal balance between flexor and extensor muscles through decreased neural stimulation, causing atrophy of the intrinsic muscles of the foot. The plantar arch is exaggerated, and the toes are fixed in a claw position.

Sensory neuropathy affects the small-diameter pain and temperature fibers first, and susceptibility to injury is increased because these patients are less sensitive to pressure-related trauma or other usually minor skin abrasions. High-pressure penetrating injuries, low-pressure repetitive stress from walking or standing (especially in a foot deformed by neuropathy), and thermal injury may go unrecognized due to this loss of pain sensation and can lead to ulcers, necrosis, and tissue loss.[13]

Joints can also be affected by neuropathy. Neuropathic arthropathy (Charcot foot) is a relatively painless, progressive, and degenerative arthropathy of single or multiple joints. In patients with diabetes, the areas primarily affected are the joints of the foot and the ankle (Figure 11-3). In the presence of severe sensory neuropathy, proprioception is lost and the joints of the foot are subjected to extreme ranges of motion without "warning." This leads to capsular and ligamentous stretching, joint laxity, distension, and subluxation—without any discomfort for the patient. As weight bearing continues and instability increases, the dislocated articular surfaces grind on adjacent bone and may result in osteochondral fragmentation and joint fractures. These osteoporotic areas are more susceptible to trauma, and a vicious cycle of continued bony destruction is created. The unfortunate result is collapse of the normal architecture of the foot and severe foot deformity. During the period of joint destruction, a natural hyperemic response occurs, and this hyperemia is often mistaken for infection.

Clinical Presentation

On inspection, the neuropathic foot often has a characteristic appearance. The toes may be "clawed." The skin is usually dry and may be cracked due to the loss of sweating and oil secretion (autonomic neuropathy). Heavy, thick callus, which may ulcerate over time, is often evident at points of increased

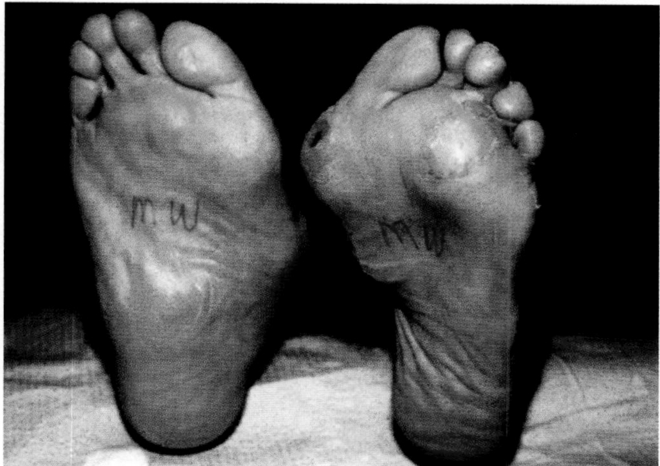

Figure 11-3. Neuropathic arthropathy (Charcot foot). Severe foot deformity and collapse of the normal architecture of the foot leads to abnormal bony prominences ("rocker bottom" deformity). These prominences are common causes of ulceration.

pressure and weight bearing. Atrophy of small muscles of the foot may or may not be apparent. Color and temperature changes can range from hyperemic and warm in a patient with an acute Charcot fracture to pale and cool in a patient with concomitant ischemia and neuropathy. In addition, in the presence of arteriovenous shunting, an ischemic foot may appear pink and relatively warm even with significant loss of arterial perfusion.

In individuals with a Charcot foot, collapse of the arch, a "rocker bottom" deformity (Figure 11-3), or other severe abnormalities may be seen. Crepitus is a common finding with acute fractures, most notably on passive range of motion of involved joints or excessive subluxation.

The loss of pinprick sensation is the most distinguishing physical finding with neuropathy. Loss of soft touch sensation tends to be preserved even in moderate to severe neuropathy, and ankle reflexes are almost always absent in older patients. Testing for vibration sense can be useful in detecting the younger patient at risk for developing clinically significant neuropathy later in life.

Diagnosis

The presence of neuropathy can usually be determined with a careful history and physical examination. Loss of pinprick sensation can be determined by the use of a Semms-Weinstein monofilament (Figure 11-4). In multiple prospective studies, this instrument has identified patients at risk for foot ulceration with a sensitivity ranging from 66% to 91% and a specificity ranging from 34% to 86%.[14] A simple and inexpensive test for vibratory sensation involves the use of a tuning fork, although it is less predictive of ulceration than the Semms-Weinstein monofilament. A more expensive version is a biothesiometer, another handheld device that assesses vibration perception threshold. Occasionally, nerve conduction or electromyelographic studies may be helpful, but these are not essential and are not widely available. Plain film radiographs are helpful in the diagnosis of Charcot disease, foreign bodies, and infection; the osteoarthropathy takes on the appearance of a severely destructive form of degenerative arthritis.

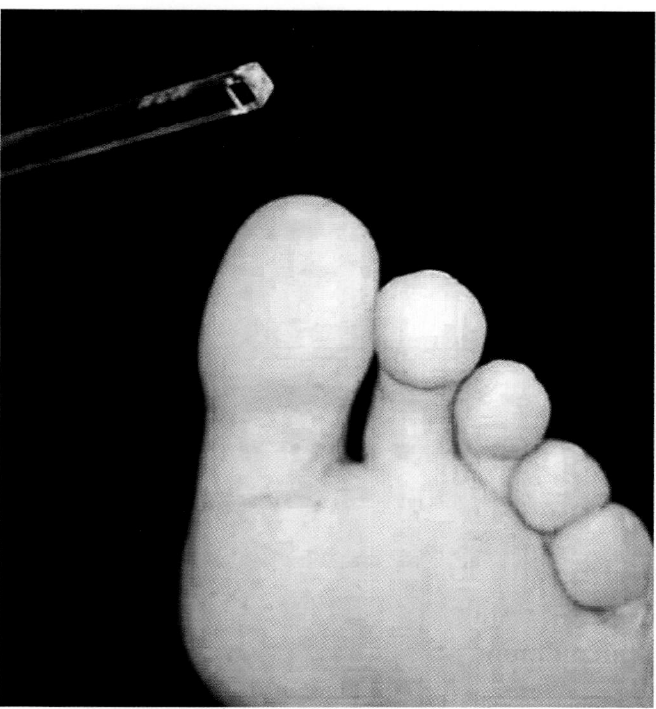

Figure 11-4. Assessment of loss of pinprick sensation using Semms-Weinstein filaments. The monofilament should be applied firmly to create a bend.

Computed tomography and magnetic resonance imaging scans may be required, especially when planning foot reconstructive surgery. Computerized methods to demonstrate points of high pressure under the sole have been developed. With pedobarography, specially designed sensors can be embedded within the insoles of the patient's shoes, and pressures under the soles of both feet can be recorded while the patient is standing upright or during walking (Figure 11-5). Increased forces exerted on different areas of the sole can be visualized and analyzed both before and after treatment.[15]

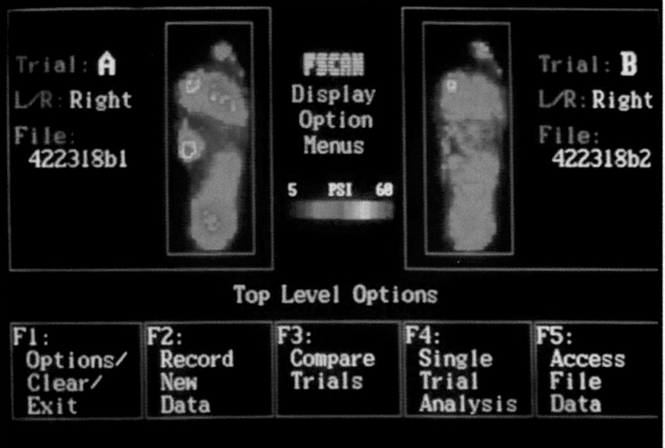

Figure 11-5. Pedobarography. Points of high pressure under the sole are recorded by sensors embedded within the insoles of the patient's shoes. Increased forces exerted on the midfoot *(left)* and over the first metatarsal head can be visualized and analyzed before and after treatment.

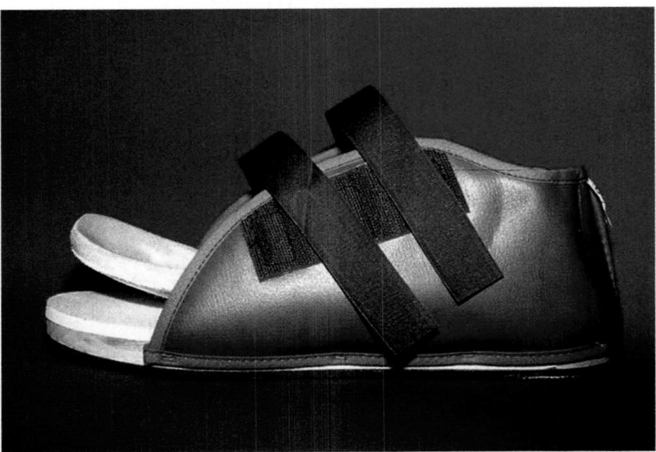

Figure 11-6. Management of diabetic neuropathy. To relieve any pressure from healing ulcers, shoes are replaced by a stiff-soled healing sandal until the ulcer has closed. A custom-molded orthotic protects the foot during weight bearing.

Management

The first step in the treatment of any type of neuropathic complication is restriction of weight bearing of the involved extremity. Patients with ulcers complicated by limb-threatening infections (described later), as well as noncompliant patients, require hospitalization and bed rest. Treatment of associated infection or ischemia must be undertaken simultaneously.

For uncomplicated neuropathic ulcers, topical therapy and non–weight bearing often heal the ulcer, and a trial of outpatient care is warranted. Patients should be instructed not to soak or bathe the foot. Topical dressings should be aimed at maintaining a moist environment with saline impregnated gauze, topical antibiotic ointments, or similar agents. Weight bearing can be limited by the use of a walker, crutches, or a wheelchair. The ulcer should be protected from excessive pressure by placement of an accommodative pad around the lesion to distribute the pressure around the ulcer to surrounding tissues. Heavy callus around the edges of the lesion should be trimmed away to reduce peak plantar pressure, and shoes should be replaced with a stiff-soled "healing sandal" (Figure 11-6) until the ulcer has closed. Only after wound healing is achieved should weight bearing be reinstituted back to baseline levels, and consultation with a physical therapist should be obtained when necessary. In addition, custom-molded orthotics and extradepth shoes, running shoes, or custom-molded shoes, in the case of severe foot deformity, are prescribed to prevent future recurrence.[16]

Patient education about the dangers of neuropathy, along with proper shoes and regular podiatric care, are essential preventive measures. Patients should be advised to call their health-care providers early and often because of their increased susceptibility to infection and ulceration in the hopes that vigilance will prevent dreaded limb-threatening complications. When conservative measures fail, however, surgical therapy to correct underlying bony deformities or mechanical derangements may be indicated.

In the presence of both ischemia and neuropathy, arterial revascularization is critically important to bring maximal circulation to the foot to allow healing (as described later).

In the management of the Charcot foot, the goals are to protect the affected extremity, prevent further collapse and deformity, and protect the opposite foot. The first step of treatment is an extended period of non–weight bearing (3 to 6 months) and cast or splint immobilization to promote eventual healing of the joint. In the initial phase of treatment, hospitalization may be required to provide adequate treatment of potentially infected ulcers and to reduce swelling of the affected foot. The duration of immobilization is determined by the anatomic location of the fracture, as well as evidence of fracture healing by clinical examination and foot x-rays. As with the management of any foot ulcer, the use of accommodative footwear is essential to long-term management. Surgery is rarely indicated, and a stabilizing procedure is done most safely after a quiescent stage of the disease has been reached. Amputation is reserved for those rare patients with severe uncorrectable deformities, with chronic ulcers plagued by such extensive osteomyelitis that the foot is unsalvageable, or after failed open reconstructions.

INFECTION

The infected foot is the most common cause for hospitalization of the patient with diabetes, accounting for more in-hospital days than any other complication of diabetes.[1]

Pathophysiology

Sensory neuropathy results in sensory loss to pain and pressure and results in unrecognized trauma and ulcers. Autonomic neuropathy leads to loss of sweating and oil secretion, causing cracks and fissures. Both are causes of skin breakdown and create a portal of entry for various types of bacteria, many of which naturally colonize the skin and soft tissues. The signs of infection are often diminished due to the reduced neurogenic inflammatory response.

Metabolic State and Arterial Insufficiency

Hyperglycemia causes a relatively immune-compromised state in which patients are more prone to numerous types of infection.[17] Resulting proteinuria leads to loss of albumin, which affects tissue nutrition. Furthermore, infection increases metabolic rate and a subsequent elevation of the oxygen demand in local tissues. In the ischemic foot, the inability to meet this increased oxygen requirement due to the infection may accelerate and exacerbate tissue necrosis. Without adequate restoration of blood flow, measures to treat infection fail and may even lead to a more proximal anatomical amputation level.

Classification or Microbiology

Non-limb-threatening infections are characterized by superficial ulcers with local signs of infection (e.g., cellulitis), no bone or joint involvement, limited or absent systemic signs of infection, and no evidence of severe limb ischemia. In collected microbiological specimens, the most prevalent pathogens are aerobic gram-positive cocci, usually *Staphylococcus aureus,* coagulase-negative staphylococci, or β-hemolytic streptococci. Gram-negative bacilli and anaerobes are occasionally present but not common in these infections.

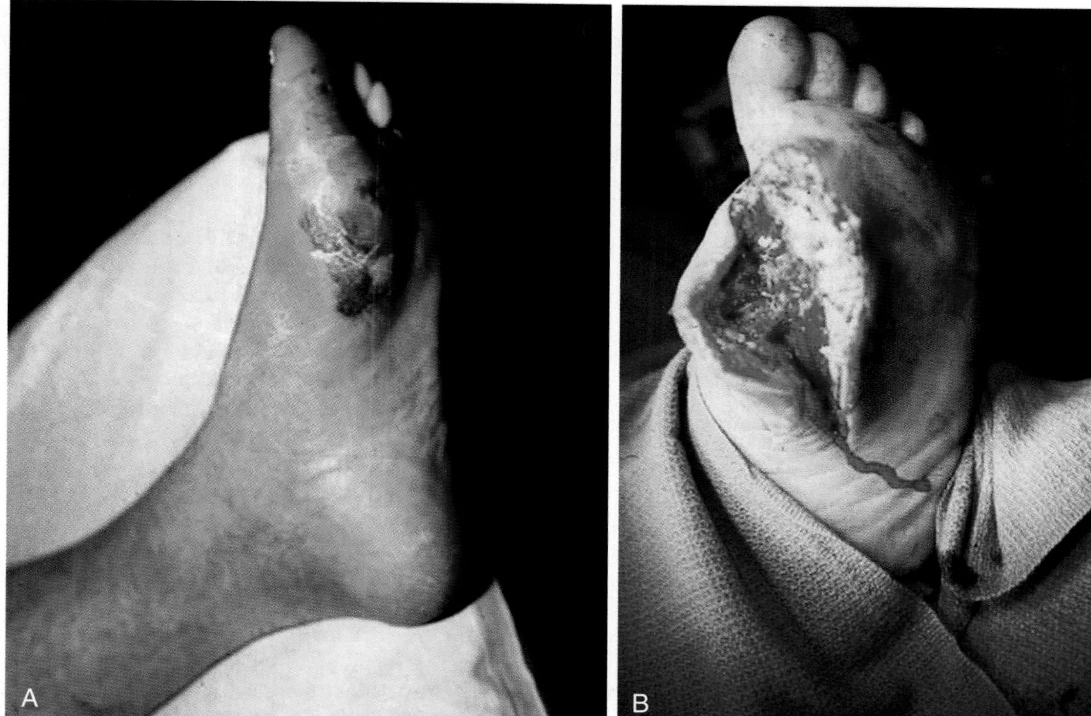

Figure 11-7. Deep space infection of the forefoot caused by ulceration of the plantar surface over the first metatarsal head. **A,** Note the diffuse swelling, erythema, and subcuticular hemorrhage. The drainage from the ulcer had a foul odor, and the patient was febrile and hyperglycemic. **B,** Extensive necrosis of the underlying fascia and septic arthritis of the metatarsophalangeal joint was seen at surgery. An open first-ray amputation was performed.

Limb-threatening infections are classified as deep ulcers involving tendon, bone, or joint or any infection with associated tissue necrosis (wet gangrene) or severe ischemia (Figure 11-7). Cellulitis is common, and lymphangitis may be present. Systemic signs may be present, but hyperglycemia may be the only manifestation of an underlying infection. Because bacteremia and septic shock can occur, such infections can become life threatening as well. Collected microbiological specimens usually reveal polymicrobial flora consisting of gram-positive organisms (staphylococci, streptococci, enterococci), gram-negative organisms (*Escherichia coli,* proteus), and anaerobes (peptostreptococci, bacteroides, clostridia; Table 11-1). More chronic infections or those previously treated with antibiotics may have additional "opportunistic" species (enterobacter, pseudomonas, yeast). The presence of anaerobes should always be suspected in any ulcer with foul-smelling drainage or when there is a deep space abscess.

Osteomyelitis

Soft-tissue ulceration and infection of the ischemic and neuropathic diabetic foot can lead to osteomyelitis, septic arthritis, or both. Most cases of osteomyelitis in diabetic patients originate from penetrating ulcers at pressure points beneath the metatarsal heads (Figure 11-8). Extension of osteomyelitis into the joint space can cause loss of the subchondral bone plate and joint space narrowing associated with septic arthritis. Spontaneous fracture, subluxation, and dislocation of the bones and joints may follow.

Clinical Presentation and Diagnosis

Since many patients with diabetes have a blunted neurogenic inflammatory response, typical inflammatory signs of infection may be absent or diminished (e.g., erythema, rubor, cellulitis, or tenderness). In addition, the usual systemic manifestations of infection (e.g., fever, tachycardia, or elevated white blood cell count) are often absent[17,18]; therefore, these patients require extreme vigilance so that providers do not overlook life-threatening conditions. Unexplained hyperglycemia should prompt an aggressive search for a source of infection because the elevated glucose may be the only sign of impending problems.

Careful palpation of the foot for areas of tenderness or fluctuance is an important approach to detect undrained abscesses in deeper tissue planes. All ulcers must be carefully inspected and probed, and superficial eschar unroofed, to look for potential deep space abscesses that are not readily apparent by visual inspection alone. The use of a sterile metallic probe to explore the ulcer not only determines the ulcer depth and extent but may also determine the involvement of bony structures. Grayson et al. revealed that if this sterile probe hits bone, then osteomyelitis can be diagnosed with a sensitivity of 66%, a specificity of 85%, and a positive predictive value of 89%.[19]

Plain radiographs of the foot should be obtained in every patient with suspected foot infection. It is the first step to determining the presence of a foreign body, gas, osteolysis, or joint effusion, as well as to assess anatomy for surgical planning. Further evaluation with a bone scan or tagged white blood cell scan should be reserved for cases in which the metal

Table 11-1
Pathogens detected in microbiologic specimens from patients with moderate/severe (limb-threatening) diabetic foot infections.

Pathogens	Patients (%) with pathogens isolated
Monomicrobial	16
Polymicrobial	80
Staphylococcus aureus	56
Coagulase-negative staphylococci	13
Streptococci	36
Enterococci	29
Klebsiella sp.	5
Proteus sp.	7
Other gram-negatives	6-44
Pseudomonas aeruginosa	7
Anaerobes	42
Fungi	3

Modified from Grayson ML. Diabetic foot infections: antimicrobial therapy. *Infect Dis Clin North Am* 1995;9:143-161.

probe test is equivocal, when an abscess or multifocal disease is suspected, or in patients with neuropathic osteoarthropathy, i.e., Charcot foot (because the associated bony changes and inflammatory response can be misinterpreted as osteomyelitis). A bone scan may be positive 24 hours after the onset of osteomyelitis, and a three-phase bone scan can be useful in distinguishing osteomyelitis from cellulitis. Magnetic resonance imaging has shown to be a highly sensitive diagnostic tool (up to 100%) but is only about 80% specific since osteomyelitis and fracture may have similar appearances.[20]

Management

Antibiotic Therapy

Patients with limb-threatening infections require immediate hospitalization, immobilization, and intravenous antibiotics. Cultures from the depths of the ulcer should be sent to the microbiology laboratory; wound swabs are unreliable and should not be performed. Establishment of high serum concentrations of antibiotics is essential when local host factors such as reduced arterial supply, edema, devitalized tissue, and altered tissue pH might impede delivery or impair efficacy of the drug or drugs at the site of infection. Pending culture and sensitivity data, empirical broad antibiotic therapy should be initiated to cover the presumed polymicrobial infections usually seen in patients with diabetes (i.e., gram-positive, gram-negative, and anaerobic organisms).[1,21] Empirical antibiotic regimens are dictated by institutional preferences, local resistance patterns, availability, and cost. Numerous trials of antibiotic therapy have been conducted to evaluate different regimens.[22-24] The Study of Infections in Diabetic Feet Comparing Efficacy, Safety, and Tolerability of Ertapenem versus Piperacillin-Tazobactam is the largest and most recent randomized, multicenter study evaluating antibiotics regimens in moderate-to-severe diabetic foot infections.[25] This trial found no difference in eradication rates, clinical outcomes, and adverse events between once-daily ertapenem and four-times-daily piperacillin/tazobactam. The investigators were permitted to add vancomycin to the regimen as needed for methicillin-resistant *S. aureus* or enterococcus.

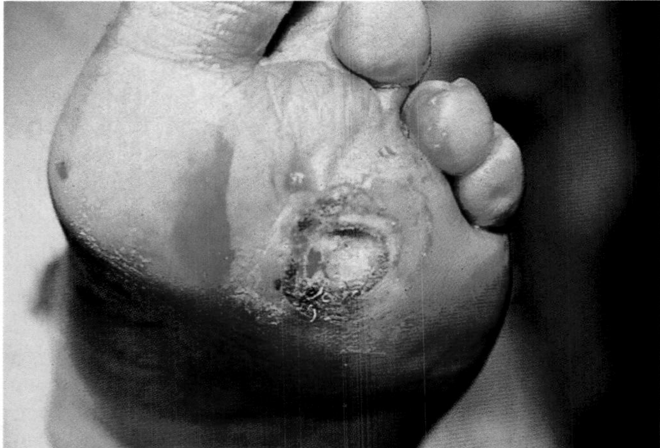

Figure 11-8. Penetrating ulcer located at a pressure point over the fourth metatarsal head, with resulting deep space abscess and osteomyelitis.

The antibiotic protocol in our tertiary-care center has undergone many changes over the last 20 years. Currently, a combination of vancomycin, ciprofloxacin, and metronidazole is our empirical "first line" choice. Given the increasing prevalence of methicillin-resistant *S. aureus* in hospital-acquired infections, as well as in community isolates, empirical therapy with vancomycin is warranted.[26] Major advantages of fluoroquinolones are their potent activity against both gram-positive and gram-negative organisms, the high tissue concentrations obtained with oral administration, and the safety in penicillin-allergic patients. Metronidazole is added to cover anaerobic bacteria against which levofloxacin has no activity.[27] Once culture results become available, antibiotics should be appropriately tailored to prevent development of resistance. Mild infections usually require only 7 to 10 days of antibiotic therapy, whereas moderate and severe infections may require up to 3 weeks of treatment.[28]

Incision and Drainage

Patients with diabetes and foot infections do not tolerate undrained pus or devitalized infected tissue. Patients with abscess formation, septic arthritis, necrotizing fasciitis, etc., must undergo prompt incision, drainage, and debridement, including partial open toe, ray, or forefoot amputation as dictated by findings at operation.[29] The incision should be fashioned longitudinally such that each respective superficial layer is opened further than the corresponding deeper layer so that no pus can accumulate in a hidden space. Tendon sheaths should be probed as proximally as possible and excised if infected. Despite fears to the contrary, long and extensive drainage incisions heal when infection is controlled and foot circulation is adequate. Wounds should be packed open with saline-moistened gauze, and dressings should be changed two to three times a day. The moist gauze allows faster healing, causes less scarring, promotes autolytic debridement (from macrophages), and promotes angiogenesis; subsequent removal of the dried gauze allows mechanical debridement. Wounds should be examined daily, and additional bedside or operative debridement should be repeated as needed.

Numerous adjunctive modalities exist for wound care, such as topical growth factors, synthetic skin grafts, electrical stimulation, hyperbaric oxygen chambers, and vacuum-assisted closure. Each has its own merits, but economic constraints and patient compliance should be kept in mind when comparing these to the well-established modality of simple gauze dressings. A recent randomized trial revealed the efficacy of the vacuum-assisted closure (negative pressure wound therapy) compared to standard moist gauze dressings. In diabetic patients with partial foot amputations and adequate perfusion, vacuum-assisted closure therapy resulted in a higher proportion of healed wounds, faster healing rates, and potentially fewer reamputations than standard care.[30] Overall, health-care providers must always remember that any new wound care modalities are simply adjuncts to frequent clinical examinations and local wound care.

Traditional therapy for osteomyelitis was accepted as 4 to 6 weeks of intravenous antibiotics,[31] but recent studies have documented a recurrence rate greater than 30% using this modality alone.[32] As a result, our standard practice involves surgical debridement of infected bone with an adequate margin, followed by a shorter duration antibiotic course. We believe that an aggressive and early surgical approach to pedal osteomyelitis shortens healing times, decreases the need for long-term antibiotic therapy, limits the emergence of resistant bacteria, and reduces both inpatient and outpatient economic costs. In our experience, long-term antibiotic therapy without excision of infected bone is rarely successful in these patients.

ISCHEMIA

The management of ischemic complications of the diabetic foot has changed dramatically in the last two decades. The results of open lower-extremity arterial reconstruction remain outstanding, but less invasive endovascular options are becoming more widely available and potentially applicable to this patient population. Unfortunately, inappropriate pessimism persists regarding such aggressive interventions, leading to many needless and avoidable amputations. Our experience suggests that neither the basic treatment principles applied nor the outcomes expected for patients with lower extremity ischemia should significantly differ based on whether or not they suffer from diabetes.

Pathophysiology

The most important principle in treating foot ischemia in patients with diabetes is the recognition that the cause of their presenting symptoms is macrovascular occlusion of the leg arteries due to atherosclerosis. For many decades, clinicians incorrectly assumed that the ischemic complications in diabetic patients were due to microvascular occlusion of arterioles—so-called small vessel disease. The idea originated from a single histological study by Goldenberg and coworkers who microscopically evaluated amputated limb specimens from diabetic patients. They observed a periodic acid–Schiff–positive material occluding the arterioles and named this process "arteriolosclerosis."[33] A subsequent prospective study[34] of amputation specimens from diabetic and nondiabetic patients, however, demonstrated no histological evidence of a specific arteriolar occlusive lesion associated with diabetes. Current literature supports the notion that diabetic patients typically suffer from tibial and peroneal arterial occlusive disease with relative sparing of the foot arteries, especially the dorsalis pedis and its branches, and ischemia results from both atherosclerotic macrovascular disease and microcirculatory dysfunction.[35]

In the minds of many clinicians and their patients, the concept of small vessel disease has resulted in a pessimistic attitude toward treatment of ischemia in diabetic patients that all too often leads to unnecessary limb amputation without any attempt at arterial reconstruction. This attitude and approach is antiquated, is inappropriate, and must be discouraged. In fact, the results of lower extremity bypass grafting in diabetic patients are equal or even superior to results in nondiabetic patients.[36] In our opinion, rejection of the small vessel theory alone and adoption of evidence-based guidelines could probably decrease the fortyfold increase of major limb amputation diabetic that patients face during their lifetime compared to nondiabetic counterparts.

Atherosclerosis in the diabetic patient is histologically similar to that of nondiabetic patients, but there are clinically relevant differences. The likelihood of cardiovascular mortality is higher, generalized atherosclerosis is more prevalent (coronary,[37,38] cerebrovascular, and peripheral vascular[39]), and atherosclerosis progresses more rapidly in diabetic patients. In those patients presenting with an ischemic lower extremity, gangrene and tissue loss are more likely to be present compared to nondiabetics. Diabetic patients with coronary atherosclerosis and significant polyneuropathy are more likely to develop "silent ischemia," or the absence of typical angina and other symptoms of myocardial infarction.[40]

These findings imply that arterial reconstruction in diabetic patients should be associated with a higher risk of a perioperative myocardial infarction, death, or both. In fact, both Eagle et al.[41] and Lee et al.[42] identified diabetes as an independent risk factor for adverse cardiac events in patients undergoing major vascular surgery. In our experience, however, this has not been the case. For diabetic patients undergoing lower extremity arterial reconstruction, the in-hospital mortality rate was 1%; long-term graft patency, limb salvage, and patient survival rates were comparable or better than nondiabetic patients treated over the same period.[36] In a larger study reviewing the outcomes of more than 6000 arterial reconstructive procedures, perioperative mortality rates were no different for patients with or without diabetes.[43] In fact, preoperative cardiac evaluation did not predict or improve postoperative morbidity, mortality, or 36-month survival in asymptomatic, diabetic patients undergoing elective lower-extremity arterial reconstruction.[44]

From a surgical perspective, the most important difference in lower extremity atherosclerosis in the patient with diabetes is the anatomical location or distribution of the arterial lesions.[35] Diabetic patients typically have significant occlusive disease in the crural arteries, while arteries of the foot are spared (Figure 11-9). This "tibial artery disease" requires a different approach to arterial reconstruction and presents special challenges for the surgeon.

Patient Selection Criteria

Even in the absence of palpable foot pulses, no surgical intervention is warranted for diabetic patients without symptoms or signs of lower extremity occlusive disease. For patients who do require surgery, several factors must be taken into consideration, and additional decisions need to be made

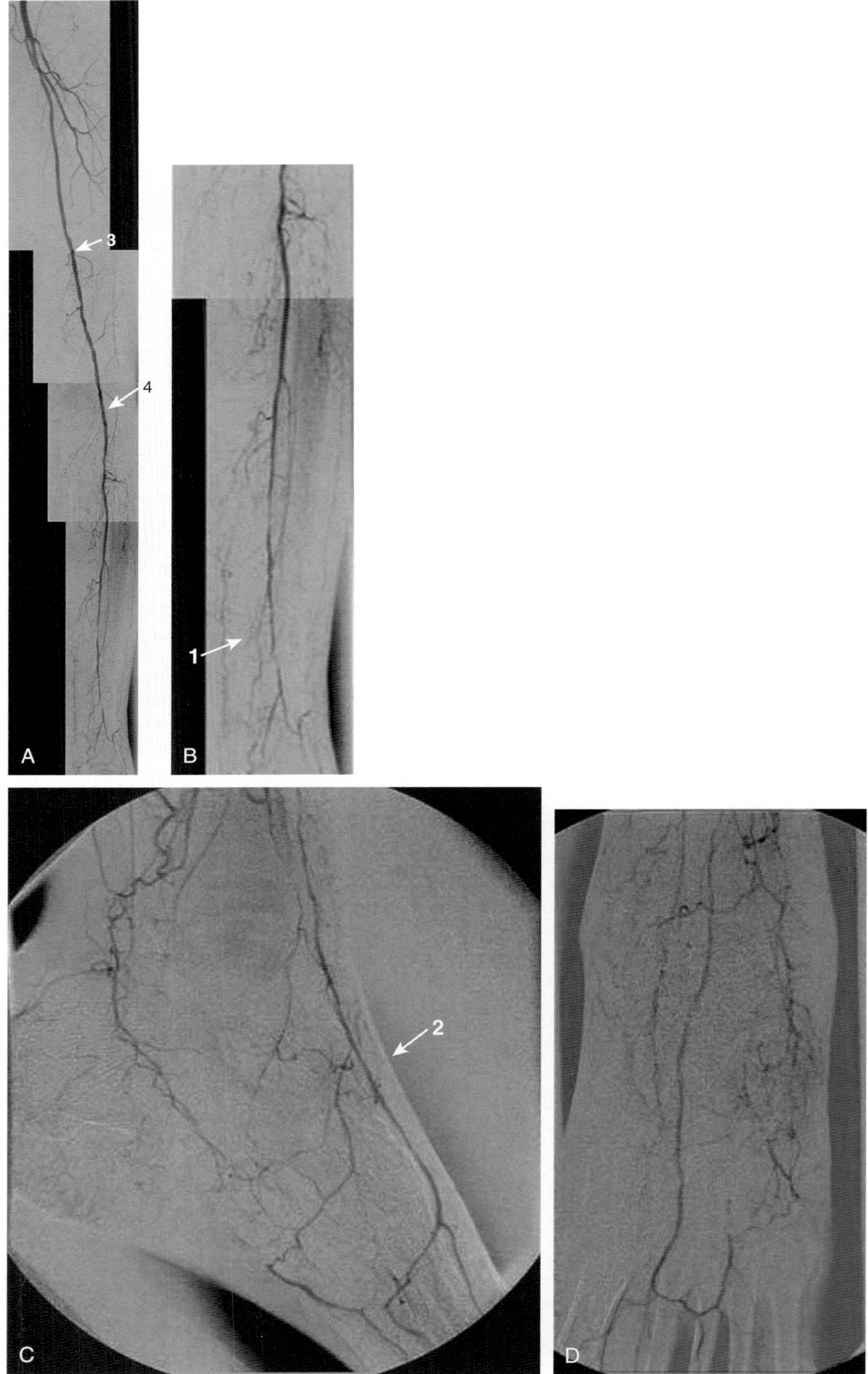

Figure 11-9. Location of the arteriosclerotic lesions in diabetic patients. The most significant lesions are found at the crural level distal to the knee joint. The foot arteries are usually spared, especially the dorsalis pedis artery. *(1)* Peroneal artery. *(2)* Dorsalis pedis artery. *(3)* Superficial femoral artery. *(4)* Popliteal artery.

regarding the use of traditional surgical reconstruction versus less invasive endovascular interventions. Certain patients may not be appropriate candidates for arterial reconstruction based on their overall health status. Elderly patients with severe dementia, other organic brain syndromes, or both who are nonambulatory or bedridden or who have severe flexion contractures of the knee, hip, or both have no prospect of rehabilitation and are inappropriate candidates for traditional vascular procedures. Age alone, however, is not a contraindication for arterial reconstruction. Our results with arterial reconstruction in those patients 80 years of age or older showed similar graft patency, limb salvage, and perioperative mortality rates compared to younger patients. Moreover, two important quality-of-life outcomes—the ability to ambulate and the ability to return to living at home—were analyzed. One year after surgery, more than 80% were still ambulatory and residing in their homes.[45]

Patients with terminal cancer with short life expectancy or similar lethal comorbidities do poorly with open revascularization and are probably better served by endovascular intervention or primary amputation. Patients with an unsalvageable foot due to extensive necrosis from ischemia, or ischemia and infection, also require primary amputation.

Patients with salvageable ischemic foot lesions and concomitant active infection need to have the infection brought under control before vascular surgical intervention (as described earlier). In addition to instituting broad-spectrum antibiotics, options include open debridement and drainage or partial foot amputation. A short delay (usually less than 5 days) before revascularization to control active infection is justified; however, waiting longer than necessary to "sterilize wounds" is inappropriate and may result in further necrosis, tissue loss, or lost opportunity to save the foot. During this intervening period, contrast arteriography and other preoperative evaluations (e.g., cardiac or pulmonary testing) can be performed as necessary. Once cellulitis, lymphangitis, and edema have improved or resolved, especially in any areas of expected incisions for bypass, bypass can be undertaken without further delay.

Patients with limb ischemia and signs and symptoms of coronary artery disease require medical stabilization of their cardiac disease (and rarely a coronary artery intervention) before lower extremity arterial reconstruction. Virtually, patients with diabetes and lower extremity ischemia have occult coronary artery disease,[46] so the value of routine screening tests for occult coronary ischemia remains unclear. Quantifying the degree of coronary disease with dipyridamole–thallium imaging testing has occasionally been useful to stratify patients at excessive risk for cardiac morbidity and mortality; however, most patients with severely abnormal scans usually have obvious clinical signs or symptoms as well.[47] At our institution, preoperative cardiac stress testing did not predict or improve postoperative morbidity, mortality, or 36-month survival in asymptomatic, diabetic patients undergoing elective lower-extremity arterial reconstruction.[44] As a result, we rely mostly on the patient's clinical presentation and electrocardiography in determining when further evaluation is needed and use imaging studies selectively in patients with unclear or atypical symptoms. Furthermore, numerous recent studies have addressed the issue of preoperative coronary revascularization in patients undergoing noncardiac vascular surgery (Coronary Artery Revascularization Prophylaxis and Dutch Echocardiographic Cardiac Risk Evaluation Applying Stress Echocardiography trials), and the results have shown that medical optimization is equivalent to coronary revascularization with regards to myocardial infarction, in-hospital mortality, and long-term mortality.[48,49]

Our perioperative routine involves the following tactics: (1) ensuring patients are placed on the optimal and appropriate pharmacological regimens, including beta-blockers, aspirin, and statins; (2) frequent use of invasive perioperative cardiac monitoring, including pulmonary arterial catheters or intraoperative transesophageal echocardiograms in highly selected patients; (3) specialized anesthesia teams dedicated to treating patients with ischemic heart disease; and (4) postoperative monitoring in cardiovascular care units with specially trained nurses. We believe that these modalities have significantly reduced the perioperative cardiac morbidity and mortality in our patients.

The presence of renal failure presents special challenges. If acute renal failure occurs, most commonly following contrast arteriography, surgery is delayed until renal function is stabilized or has returned to baseline. Affected patients have transient elevations of serum creatinine levels without other symptoms, and they rarely become anuric or require hemodialysis. Patients with dialysis-dependent end-stage renal disease can safely undergo arterial reconstruction with reasonable initial graft patency rates. However, gangrene and tissue loss are often present, and the healing response is poor even with restoration of arterial blood flow. Studies have demonstrated that graft patency and limb salvage in these patients are lower compared to in patients without renal failure and that some even require amputation with a patent bypass graft.[50,51] Moreover, long-term survival in our experience has been exceedingly poor for this group[52]; therefore, careful patient selection is extremely important to determine which patients should have arterial reconstructive surgery versus primary amputation.

Vascular Evaluation and Diagnostic Studies

Patients requiring surgical intervention for lower extremity arterial insufficiency usually present with severely disabling intermittent claudication or signs and symptoms of limb-threatening ischemia. A complete vascular examination is imperative in any patient reporting symptoms consistent with claudication or rest pain, and the examination findings may correlate with the reported location of the patient's symptoms. Femoral pulses may be absent with aortoiliac disease, popliteal pulses absent with superficial femoral artery disease, and distal foot pulses absent with tibioperoneal disease. Nocturnal muscle cramping is a common complaint but is not a typical symptom of vascular disease and should not be mistaken for intermittent claudication.

Studies of the natural history of intermittent claudication have demonstrated that progression to limb-threatening ischemia in patients presenting with claudication is uncommon.[53] In fact, multiple studies show amputation rates of 1% to 7% from 5 to 10 years after a diagnosis is made and rates of only 10% after 10 years or more.[54] Most patients with intermittent claudication never require surgical intervention; thus, conservative options (i.e., exercise regimens, smoking cessation programs, and risk factor reduction for atherosclerosis)[55] and pharmacological therapy (cilostazol)[56]

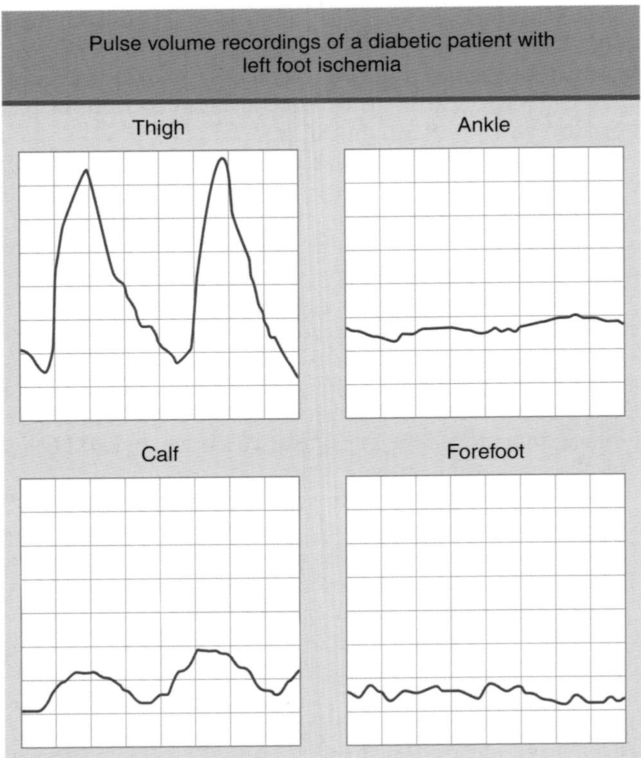

Figure 11-10. Pulse volume recordings of a diabetic patient with left foot ischemia. The severely abnormal calf waveform suggests popliteal artery occlusion and flat waveforms at the ankle and forefoot level are consistent with additional tibial arterial occlusive disease.

may be all that are required for many of these patients. Traditional surgical or endovascular interventions for claudication are reserved for patients presenting with a limited functional capacity and those who are unable to work due to their symptoms. However, distal bypass procedures to the pedal or tarsal vessels are reserved for foot or limb salvage.

Most patients with diabetes who require revascularization have limb-threatening ischemia manifested by a nonhealing ulcer with or without associated gangrene or infection. Some patients are referred after a minor surgical procedure when the foot fails to heal due to ischemia. Patients with limb-threatening ischemia can also present with ischemic rest pain with or without associated tissue loss. Ischemic rest pain typically occurs in the distal forefoot, particularly the toes. It is exacerbated by recumbence and relieved by dependency of the involved extremity. It is imperative, albeit difficult, to distinguish rest pain from painful diabetic neuropathy, which may also be subjectively worse at night. Neuropathic patients may present without rest pain despite severe ischemia due to complete loss of sensation. In those cases in which the etiology of the patient's foot pain is unclear, noninvasive vascular laboratory studies are particularly useful. Patients with severe ischemia usually have ankle brachial indices of less than 0.4. Many diabetic patients, however, have artificially elevated ankle pressures due to calcification of the arterial wall.[57] Therefore, pulse volume recordings are useful since they are unaffected by arterial wall calcification (Figure 11-10). Some centers have found toe pressures[57] and transcutaneous oxygen measurements[58] to be useful in diabetic patients. Following surgery, the same noninvasive testing can quantify the degree of improvement in distal circulation. Furthermore, postoperative duplex ultrasonography of vein grafts has been useful in detecting areas of stenosis due to intimal hyperplasia, which can be corrected before the occurrence of graft thrombosis.[59]

On the other hand, noninvasive testing adds little information to the evaluation of a patient with obvious signs of foot ischemia and the absence of a palpable posterior tibial artery, dorsalis pedis artery, or both. In these patients, contrast arteriography should be performed as the first diagnostic (and potentially therapeutic) test.

Arteriography

Ultimately, the decision to perform a tibial or pedal bypass is based on a carefully performed arteriogram. The outflow target artery should be relatively free of occlusive disease and demonstrate unimpeded arterial flow into the arteries of the foot. In general, the most proximal artery distal to the occlusion meeting these two criteria is chosen. Because of the propensity for diabetic patients to have occlusive lesions in the tibial arteries, it is essential that arteriograms incorporate the complete infrapopliteal circulation, including the foot vessels. It is our preference to exclusively use intraarterial digital subtraction arteriography to evaluate the lower extremity arterial circulation. Patients with mild to moderate renal insufficiency (a glomerular filtration rate, or GFR, less than 60 ml/min/1.73 m^2) receive preprocedure and postprocedure hydration with a sodium bicarbonate intravenous fluid, while those with moderate to severe renal insufficiency (GFR less than 35 ml/min/1.73 m^2) follow the same hydration protocol in addition to taking an oral mucomyst regimen. Isoosmolar Visipaque contrast is used for all patients with GFR less than 60 ml/min for every 1.73 m^2 due to its decreased likelihood of causing contrast-induced nephropathy in these patients.[60] Although magnetic resonance arteriography had been used more often during the past decade to plan arterial reconstructions in patients with more marginal renal function,[61] recent reports about nephrogenic systemic fibrosis[62] have shifted clinical practice back to conventional arteriography. Moreover, we have found that conventional digital subtraction arteriography continues to provide the best-quality images and the risk of contrast-induced nephropathy can be minimized by adhering to a strict protocol, as listed earlier.

Management

Arterial Reconstruction

One of the most important developments in vascular surgery has been the demonstration that autogenous saphenous vein gives the best short- and long-term results for distal bypass. In a large multicenter, prospective, randomized trial, 6-year graft patency of saphenous vein grafts was consistently better than that of prosthetic grafts in the above- and below-knee positions.[63]

For more than five decades, the standard conduit for lower extremity revascularization has been the reversed greater saphenous vein.[64] An inherent problem with reversing the vein, which is necessary to overcome the impediment to flow from the valves, is a size discrepancy that results between the

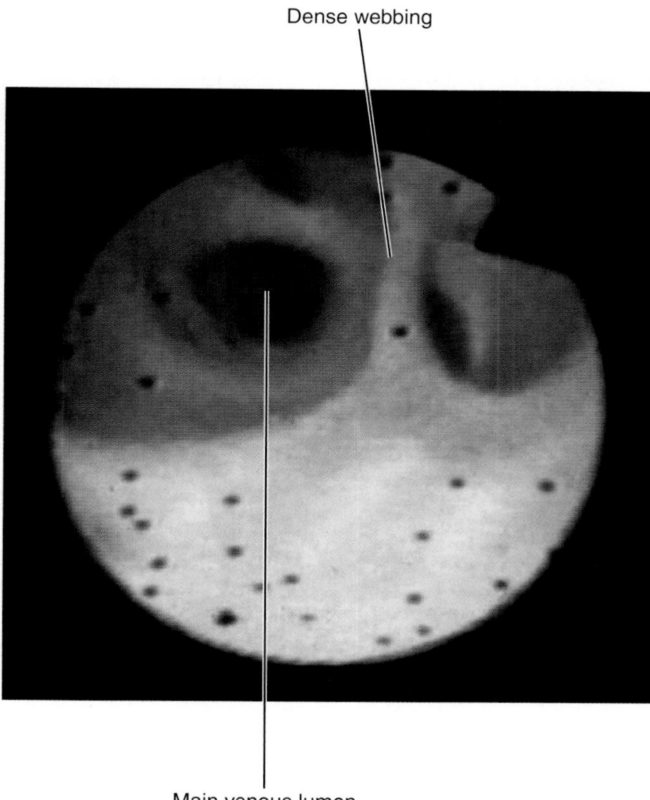

Figure 11-11. Angioscopy of the lumen of arm vein, demonstrating dense "webbing." These lesions occur as a result of previous venipunctures. Segments of vein with these findings are not suitable for use as bypass conduits.

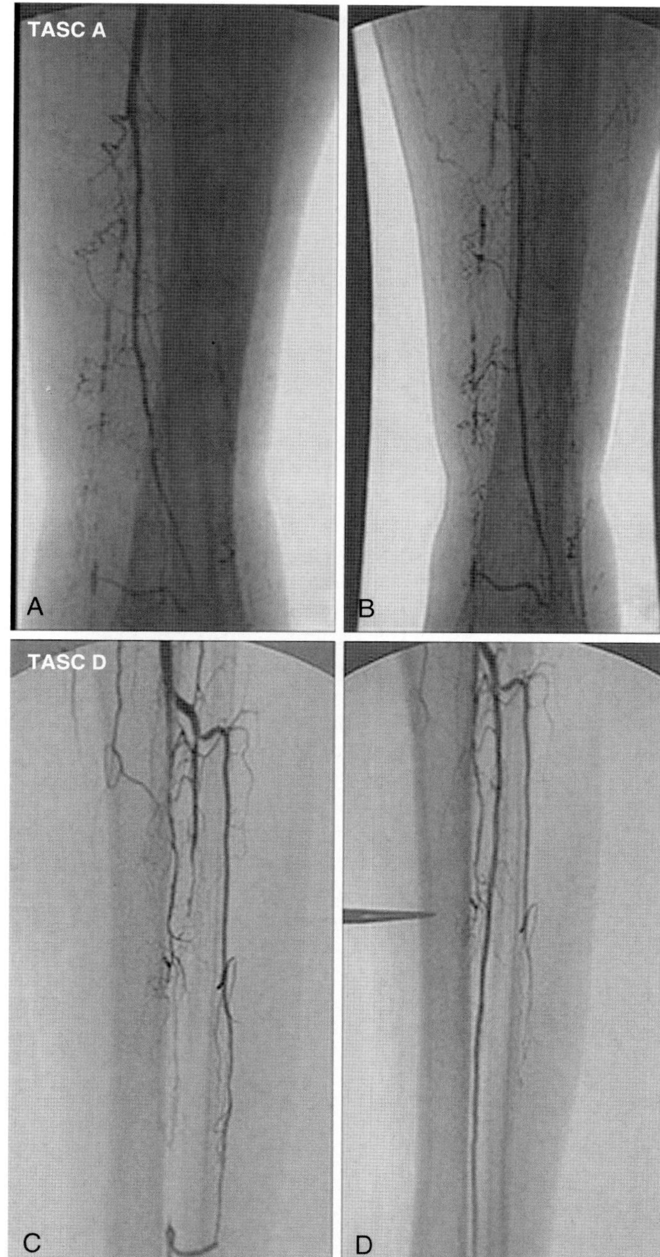

Figure 11-12. Trans-Atlantic Inter-Society Consensus A and D tibial lesions. These lesions are typical of diabetic patients before **(A, C)** and after **(B, D)** endovascular intervention with balloon angioplasty.

arteries and veins when they are connected. Methods were developed early on to render the valves incompetent and allow use of nonreversed or in situ vein, but the first widely accepted technique was described in the late 1970s by Leather et al.,[65] who incorporated a modified Mills valvulotome to cut the valves atraumatically and quickly. Although many believed that the in situ bypass was biologically superior to the reversed saphenous vein graft, evidence to support this concept is lacking.[66] Similarly, when in situ bypasses are compared to reversed saphenous vein grafts, no apparent superiority is evident.[67,68]

In the 1980s, the first series of bypass grafts with originating from the popliteal artery was reported,[69] with reported results equivalent to arterial reconstructions taking inflow from the common femoral artery.[70,71] In patients with diabetes, the superficial femoral artery is often spared from significant occlusive disease, thus allowing the popliteal artery to be used as inflow for the distal vein graft. Doing so shortens the operative procedure and avoids potentially troublesome wound complications in the groin. Short vein grafts also benefit patients with a limited quantity of adequate saphenous vein. Our experience with extreme distal bypasses has shown that popliteal inflow is possible in about 60% of diabetic patients undergoing lower extremity vascular reconstruction.[68]

When the greater saphenous vein is unavailable due to previous harvesting or vein stripping, alternative sources of conduits must be used, such as contralateral saphenous vein, arm vein, or lesser saphenous vein. Our experience has demonstrated, that in patients lacking ipsilateral saphenous vein, the likelihood of requiring another vascular reconstruction in the contralateral extremity approaches 40% at 3 years following the first operation.[72] Therefore, because we prefer not to harvest the contralateral saphenous vein, our next conduit of choice has been arm vein. Our results with arm vein grafts continue to improve with the use of angioscopy to identify and exclude vein segments with strictures or webs induced by previous venipuncture and thrombosis (Figure 11-11).[73] Creation of composite grafts made of various segments of arm vein, including the cephalic–basilic vein loop graft,[74] can provide sufficient length to reach from the groin to the midcalf or foot vessels, thus reducing our use of prosthetic conduits. Our results with arm vein grafts are inferior to those with de novo reconstructions done with saphenous vein but significantly better than those reported with prosthetic conduits.[75]

Each operation must be individualized based on the patient's available venous conduit and arterial anatomy, as demonstrated in the preoperative arteriogram. Our experience has demonstrated that in 10% of cases a foot artery usually the dorsalis pedis artery is the only suitable outflow vessel. In an additional 15% of patients, the dorsalis pedis artery appears to be the best target vessel in comparison to other patent but diseased tibial vessels. As a result, we began performing bypasses to the dorsalis pedis artery in the early 1980s. In one of the most comprehensive studies to date regarding dorsalis pedis revascularization in diabetic patients, we reported results from more than 1000 bypasses spanning a decade.[76] Primary patency, secondary patency, and limb salvage rates were 56.8%, 62.7%, and 78.2% at 5 years and 37.7%, 41.7%, and 57.7% at 10 years, respectively. Patient survival was 48.6% and 23.8% at 5 and 10 years, respectively, and perioperative mortality was only 0.9%. The popliteal artery was the source of inflow in 53.2% of the patients. Moreover, even in the presence of foot infection, pedal bypass can be performed safely as long as invasive sepsis is controlled before surgery.[77] Although pedal artery bypass represents the most "extreme" type of distal arterial reconstruction, it is almost always possible, particularly when the surgeon is flexible in terms of venous conduit and location of proximal anastomosis.

Distal arterial reconstruction presents special technical challenges to the vascular surgeon and requires meticulous attention to detail. The distal target arteries can be small (1 to 2 mm in diameter) and are often severely calcified. Despite these challenges, the incorporation of dorsalis pedis artery bypass into the treatment algorithm of the diabetic foot has resulted in a significant decline in all amputations performed for ischemia.[78]

Endovascular Intervention

Although surgical reconstruction is the current gold standard for diabetic foot revascularization, an avalanche of technology has allowed endovascular interventions to become integrated into the management strategies employed by vascular surgeons and interventionalists. Research has definitively shown that balloon angioplasty and stenting are well suited to focal, short-segment iliac stenoses or occlusions, which exist in 10% to 20% of patients with diabetes.[79] Not only can this intervention be performed easily in the same setting as the preoperative diagnostic arteriogram, but this procedure improves inflow for potential distal bypass grafts at a markedly lower morbidity and mortality rate compared to aortic level and extraanatomical bypass procedures.

With regard to outflow bypass procedures, the morbidity of open surgery can be quite significant and not simply limited to local wound complications or myocardial infarctions. Readmissions to the hospital, reoperations, slow time to healing, and time spent in rehabilitation must be factored into the risk–benefit analysis.[80] In fact, the ideal outcome (patent graft, healed wound, no additional operations in a fully ambulatory patient who can sustain independent living) may only be obtainable 14% to 22% of the time,[81] so functional outcomes must be considered in this patient population as well. When factoring in the potential pitfalls accompanying traditional surgical approaches to limb salvage, as well as the overall poor health and life expectancy of patients with peripheral vascular disease, less invasive endovascular therapy can represent an attractive alternative.

Unfortunately, the literature supporting endovascular interventions consists mainly of individual case series and retrospective reviews and does not compare with the research describing traditional open bypasses. The Trans-Atlantic Inter-Society Consensus Working Group initially stratified femoropopliteal and tibial lesions in 2000[79] and made recommendations for therapy based on lesion type (stenosis versus occlusion), location, and length. Figure 11-12 shows examples of typical tibial lesions in diabetic patients and their results after balloon angioplasty. The best and most recent scientific attempt to compare open and endovascular interventions was the Bypass versus Angioplasty in Severe Ischemia of the Leg Trial.[82] Although only 42% of the patients in this trial were known to have diabetes, the level of ischemia was comparable to the typical disease patterns seen in this patient population. Over a 5-year period, 452 patients with severe limb ischemia (rest pain, ulceration, gangrene) from infrainguinal disease were randomized to either a bypass surgery–first or a balloon angioplasty–first strategy. Perioperative (30-day) morbidity was higher with surgery; all-cause mortality trended higher with surgery for the first 6 months but then trended lower for the next 6 months; amputation-free survival was similar in both groups. Hospital costs were higher with surgery over the first 12 months, while reinterventions were more common with angioplasty. Longer-term post hoc analysis revealed that after 2 years surgery seemed to be associated with a reduced risk of future amputation, death, or both. Overall, the trialists concluded that, although the strategies are roughly equivalent at medium-term follow-up with regard to mortality and amputation-free survival, angioplasty should be used first for patients with significant comorbidities and with a life expectancy of less than 1 to 2 years. Longer follow-up from this trial will continue to provide more statistically guided information in the years to come.

SUMMARY

This chapter reviewed the principles of evaluation, diagnosis, and treatment of arterial disease patients with diabetes and lower extremity ischemia. Rejecting the small vessel disease hypothesis and acknowledging the true location of atherosclerotic disease in diabetic patients is crucial to the institution of proper treatment. Ultimate success with limb salvage hinges on a thorough understanding of the complex interplay of neuropathy, infection, and ischemia. A carefully planned approach, including prompt control of infection, high-quality arteriography with lateral foot views, and extreme distal arterial reconstruction or endovascular intervention to maximize foot perfusion, should lead to rates of limb salvage in diabetic patients that equal or exceed those achieved in the nondiabetics.

References

1. Gibbons GW, Eliopoulos GM. Infection of the diabetic foot. In: Kozak GP, Campbell DR, Frykberg RG, et al., eds. *Management of diabetic foot problems.* 2nd ed. Philadelphia: WB Saunders; 1984:121-130.
2. Edmonds ME. The diabetic foot: pathophysiology and treatment. *Clin Endocrinol Metab* 1986;15(4):889-916.

3. Grunfeld C. Diabetic foot ulcers: etiology, treatment, and prevention. *Adv Intern Med* 1992;37:103-132.
4. National Institute of Diabetes and Digestive and Kidney Diseases. National Diabetes Statistics fact sheet: general information and national estimates on diabetes in the United States, 2005. Available at: http://diabetes.niddk.nih.gov/dm/pubs/statistics/index.htm. Accessed April 16, 2008.
5. Kozak GP, Giurini JM. Diabetic neuropathies: lower extremities. In: Kozak GP, Campbell D, Frykberg R, et al., eds. *Management of diabetic foot problems.* 2nd ed. Philadelphia: WB Saunders; 1995:43-52.
6. Gabbay KH. The sorbitol pathway and the complications of diabetes. *N Engl J Med* 1973;288(16):831-836.
7. Apfel SC. Introduction to diabetic neuropathy. *Am J Med* 1999; 107(2B):1S.
8. Ishii DN. Implication of insulin-like growth factors in the pathogenesis of diabetic neuropathy. *Brain Res Brain Res Rev* 1995;20(1):47-67.
9. Boulton AJ, Scarpello JH, Ward JD. Venous oxygenation in the diabetic neuropathic foot: evidence of arteriovenous shunting? *Diabetologia* 1982;22(1):6-8.
10. Greenman RL, Panasyuk S, Wang X, et al. Early changes in the skin microcirculation and muscle metabolism of the diabetic foot. *Lancet* 2005;366(9498):1711-1717.
11. Walmsley D, Wiles PG. Early loss of neurogenic inflammation in the human diabetic foot. *Clin Sci (Lond)* 1991;80(6):605-610.
12. Parkhouse N, Le Quesne PM. Impaired neurogenic vascular response in patients with diabetes and neuropathic foot lesions. *N Engl J Med* 1988;318:1306-1309.
13. Kosiak M. Etiology and pathology of ischemic ulcers. *Arch Phys Med Rehabil* 1959;40:62-69.
14. Singh N, Armstrong DG, Lipsky BA. Preventing foot ulcers in patients with diabetes. *JAMA* 2005;293(2):217-228.
15. Lobmann R, Kayser R, Kasten G, et al. Effects of preventative footwear on foot pressure as determined by pedobarography in diabetic patients: a prospective study. *Diabet Med* 2001;18(4):314-319.
16. Tyrrell W. Orthotic intervention in patients with diabetic foot ulceration. *J Wound Care* 1999;8(10):530-532.
17. Tan JS, Anderson JL, Watanakunakorn C, et al. Neutrophil dysfunction in diabetes mellitus. *J Lab Clin Med* 1975;85(1):26-33.
18. Bagdade JD, Root RK, Bulger RJ. Impaired leukocyte function in patients with poorly controlled diabetes. *Diabetes* 1974;23:9-15.
19. Grayson ML, Gibbons GW, Balogh K, et al. Probing to bone in infected pedal ulcers: a clinical sign of underlying osteomyelitis in diabetic patients. *JAMA* 1995;273(9):721-723.
20. Marcus CD, Ladam-Marcus VJ, Leone J, et al. MR imaging of osteomyelitis and neuropathic osteoarthropathy in the feet of diabetics. *Radiographics* 1996;16(6):1337-1348.
21. Grayson ML, Gibbons GW, Habershaw GM, et al. Use of ampicillin/sulbactam versus imipenem/cilastatin in the treatment of limb-threatening foot infections in diabetic patients. *Clin Infect Dis* 1994;18(5): 683-693.
22. Lipsky BA, Itani K, Norden C. Linezolid Diabetic Foot Infections Study Group. Treating foot infections in diabetic patients: a randomized, multicenter, open-label trial of linezolid versus ampicillin-sulbactam/amoxicillin-clavulanate. *Clin Infect Dis* 2004;38(1):17-24.
23. Harkless L, Boghossian J, Pollak R, et al. An open-label, randomized study comparing efficacy and safety of intravenous piperacillin/tazobactam and ampicillin/sulbactam for infected diabetic foot ulcers. *Surg Infect (Larchmt)* 2005;6(1):27-40.
24. Lipsky BA, Stoutenburgh U. Daptomycin for treating infected diabetic foot ulcers: evidence from a randomized, controlled trial comparing daptomycin with vancomycin or semi-synthetic penicillins for complicated skin and skin-structure infections. *J Antimicrob Chemother* 2005;55(2):240-245.
25. Lipsky BA, Armstrong DG, Citron DM, et al. Ertapenem versus piperacillin/tazobactam for diabetic foot infections (SIDESTEP): prospective, randomised, controlled, double-blinded, multicentre trial. *Lancet* 2005;366(9498):1695-1703.
26. Lipsky BA. Empirical therapy for diabetic foot infections: are there clinical clues to guide antibiotic selection? *Clin Microbiol Infect* 2007;13(4): 351-353.
27. Ellison MJ. Vancomycin, metronidazole, and tetracyclines. *Clin Podiatr Med Surg* 1992;9(2):425-442.
28. Lipsky BA, Berendt AR, Deery HG, et al. Diagnosis and treatment of diabetic foot infections. *Clin Infect Dis* 2004;39(7):885-910.
29. Gibbons GW. The diabetic foot: amputations and drainage of infection. *J Vasc Surg* 1987;5(5):791-793.
30. Armstrong DG, Lavery LA, Diabetic Foot Study Consortium. Negative pressure wound therapy after partial diabetic foot amputation: a multicentre, randomised controlled trial. *Lancet* 2005;366(9498):1704-1710.
31. Bamberger DM, Daus GP, Gerding DN. Osteomyelitis in the feet of diabetic patients: long-term results, prognostic factors, and the role of antimicrobial and surgical therapy. *Am J Med* 1987;83:653-660.
32. Tice AD, Hoaglund PA, Shoultz DA. Outcomes of osteomyelitis among patients treated with outpatient parenteral antimicrobial therapy. *Am J Med* 2003;114:723-728.
33. Goldenberg SG, Alex M, Joshi RA, et al. Nonatheromatous peripheral vascular disease of the lower extremity in diabetes mellitus. *Diabetes* 1959;8:261-273.
34. Strandness DE, Priest RE, Gibbons GW. Combined clinical and pathological study of diabetic and nondiabetic peripheral arterial disease. *Diabetes* 1964;13:366-372.
35. LoGerfo FW, Coffman JD. Current concepts: vascular and microvascular disease of the foot in diabetes—implications for foot care. *N Engl J Med* 1984;311(25):1615-1619.
36. Akbari CM, Pomposelli FB Jr, Gibbons GW, et al. Lower extremity revascularization in diabetes: late observations. *Arch Surg* 2000;135(4): 452-456.
37. Kannel WB, McGee DL. Diabetes and cardiovascular disease: the Framingham study. *JAMA* 1979;241(19):2035-2038.
38. Smith JW, Marcus FI, Serokman R. Prognosis of patients with diabetes mellitus after acute myocardial infarction. *Am J Cardiol* 1984;54(7): 718-721.
39. Petersen CM, Kaufman J, Jovanovic L. Influence of diabetes on vascular disease and its complications. In: Moore WS, ed. *Vascular surgery: a comprehensive review.* 5th ed. Philadelphia: WB Saunders; 1998: 146-167.
40. Zarich S, Waxman S, Freeman RT, et al. Effect of autonomic nervous system dysfunction on the circadian pattern of myocardial ischemia in diabetes mellitus. *J Am Coll Cardiol* 1994;24(4):956-962.
41. Eagle KA, Coley CM, Newell JB, et al. Combining clinical and thallium data optimizes preoperative assessment of cardiac risk before major vascular surgery. *Ann Intern Med* 1989;110(11):859-866.
42. Lee TH, Marcantonio ER, Mangione CM, et al. Derivation and prospective validation of a simple index for prediction of cardiac risk of major noncardiac surgery. *Circulation* 1999;100(10):1043-1049.
43. Hamdan AD, Saltzberg SS, Sheahan M, et al. Lack of association of diabetes with increased postoperative mortality and cardiac morbidity: results of 6565 major vascular operations. *Arch Surg* 2002;137(4):417-421.
44. Monahan TS, Shrikhande GV, Pomposelli FB, et al. Preoperative cardiac evaluation does not improve or predict perioperative or late survival in asymptomatic diabetic patients undergoing elective infrainguinal arterial reconstruction. *J Vasc Surg* 2005;41(1):38-45.
45. Pomposelli FB Jr., Arora S, Gibbons GW, et al. Lower extremity arterial reconstruction in the very elderly: successful outcome preserves not only the limb but also residential status and ambulatory function. *J Vasc Surg* 1998;28(2):215-225.
46. Nesto RW. Screening for asymptomatic coronary artery disease in diabetes. *Diabetes Care* 1999;22(9):1393-1395.
47. Zarich SW, Cohen MC, Lane SE, et al. Routine perioperative dipyridamole 201 T_1 imaging in diabetic patients undergoing vascular surgery. *Diabetes Care* 1996;19(4):355-360.
48. McFalls EO, Ward HB, Moritz TE, et al. Coronary–artery revascularization before elective major vascular surgery. *N Engl J Med* 2004;351(27): 2795-2804.
49. Poldermans D, Schouten O, Vidakovic R, et al. A clinical randomized trial to evaluate the safety of a noninvasive approach in high-risk patients undergoing major vascular surgery: the DECREASE-V Pilot Study. *J Am Coll Cardiol* 2007;49(17):1763-1769.
50. Korn P, Hoenig SJ, Skillman JJ, et al. Is lower extremity revascularization worthwhile in patients with end-stage renal disease? *Surgery* 2000;128(3):472-479.
51. Johnson BL, Glickman MH, Bandyk DF, et al. Failure of foot salvage in patients with end-stage renal disease after surgical revascularization. *J Vasc Surg* 1995;22(3):280-286.
52. Ramdev P, Rayan SS, Sheahan M, et al. A decade experience with infrainguinal revascularization in a dialysis-dependent patient population. *J Vasc Surg* 2002;36(5):969-974.
53. Dormandy J, Heeck L, Vig S. The natural history of claudication: risk to life and limb. *Semin Vasc Surg* 1999;12(2):123-137.
54. Muluk SC, Muluk VS, Kelley ME, et al. Outcome events in patients with claudication: a 15 year study in 2777 patients. *J Vasc Surg* 2001;33: 251-257.

55. Hertzer NR. The natural history of peripheral vascular disease: implications for its management. *Circulation* 1991;83(2 Suppl):I12-I19.
56. Thompson PD, Zimet R, Forbes WP, Zhang P. Meta-analysis of results from eight randomized, placebo-controlled trials on the effect of cilostazol on patients with intermittent claudication. *Am J Cardiol* 2002;90: 1314-1319.
57. Weitz JI, Byrne J, Clagett GP, et al. Diagnosis and treatment of chronic arterial insufficiency of the lower extremities: a critical review. *Circulation* 1996;94(11): 3026-3049; erratum, *Circulation* 2000;102(9):1074.
58. Hauser CJ, Klein SR, Mehringer CM, et al. Superiority of transcutaneous oximetry in noninvasive vascular diagnosis in patients with diabetes. *Arch Surg* 1984;119(6):690-694.
59. Bandyk DF, Seabrook GR, Moldenhauer P, et al. Hemodynamics of vein graft stenosis. *J Vasc Surg* 1988;8(6):688-695.
60. Jo SH, Youn TJ, Koo BK, et al. Renal toxicity evaluation and comparison between Visipaque (iodixanol) and Hexabrix (ioxaglate) in patients with renal insufficiency undergoing coronary angiography: the RECOVER study—a randomized controlled trial. *J Am Coll Cardiol* 2006;48(5): 924-930.
61. Carpenter JP, Baum RA, Holland GA, et al. Peripheral vascular surgery with magnetic resonance angiography as the sole preoperative imaging modality. *J Vasc Surg* 1994;20(6):861-869: discussion, 869-871.
62. Shabana WM, Cohan RH, Ellis JH, et al. Nephrogenic systemic fibrosis: a report of 29 cases. *AJR Am J Roentgenol* 2008;190(3):736-741.
63. Veith FJ, Gupta SK, Ascer E, et al. Six-year prospective multicenter randomized comparison of autologous saphenous vein and expanded polytetrafluoroethylene grafts in infrainguinal arterial reconstructions. *J Vasc Surg* 1986;3(1):104-114.
64. Kunlin J. Le traitment de làrterite obliterante par la greffe veinuse. *Arch Mal Coeur Vaiss* 1949;42:371.
65. Leather RP, Powers SR, Karmody AM. A reappraisal of the in situ saphenous vein arterial bypass: its use in limb salvage. *Surgery* 1979;86(3): 453-461.
66. Cambria RP, Megerman J, Brewster DC, et al. The evolution of morphologic and biomechanical changes in reversed and in situ vein grafts. *Ann Surg* 1987;205(2):167-174.
67. Taylor LM Jr., Edwards JM, Porter JM. Present status of reversed vein bypass grafting: five-year results of a modern series. *J Vasc Surg* 1990;11(2):193-206.
68. Pomposelli FB Jr., Jepsen SJ, Gibbons GW, et al. A flexible approach to infrapopliteal vein grafts in patients with diabetes mellitus. *Arch Surg* 1991;126(6):724-729.
69. Ascer E, Veith FJ, Gupta SK, et al. Short vein grafts: a superior option for arterial reconstructions to poor or compromised outflow tracts? *J Vasc Surg* 1988;7(2):370-378.
70. Cantelmo NL, Snow JR, Menzoian JO, et al. Successful vein bypass in patients with an ischemic limb and a palpable popliteal pulse. *Arch Surg* 1986;121(2):217-220.
71. Stonebridge PA, Tsoukas AI, Pomposelli FB Jr, et al. Popliteal-to-distal bypass grafts for limb salvage in diabetics. *Eur J Vasc Surg* 1991;5(3): 265-269.
72. Holzenbein TJ, Pomposelli FB Jr., Miller A, et al. Results of a policy with arm veins used as the first alternative to an unavailable ipsilateral greater saphenous vein for infrainguinal bypass. *J Vasc Surg* 1996;23(1):130-140.
73. Stonebridge PA, Miller A, Tsoukas A, et al. Angioscopy of arm vein infrainguinal bypass grafts. *Ann Vasc Surg* 1991;5(2):170-175.
74. Balshi JD, Cantelmo NL, Menzoian JO, et al. The use of arm veins for infrainguinal bypass in end-stage peripheral vascular disease. *Arch Surg* 1989;124(9):1078-1081.
75. Faries PL, Arora S, Pomposelli FB Jr., et al. The use of arm vein in lower-extremity revascularization: results of 520 procedures performed in eight years. *J Vasc Surg* 2000;31(1 Pt 1):50-59.
76. Pomposelli FB, Kansal N, Hamdan AD, et al. A decade of experience with dorsalis pedis artery bypass: analysis of outcome in more than 1000 cases. *J Vasc Surg* 2003;37:307-315.
77. Tannenbaum GA, Pomposelli FB Jr., Marcaccio EJ, et al. Safety of vein bypass grafting to the dorsal pedal artery in diabetic patients with foot infections. *J Vasc Surg* 1992;15(6):982-990.
78. LoGerfo FW, Gibbons GW, Pomposelli FB Jr., et al. Trends in the care of the diabetic foot. Expanded role of arterial reconstruction. *Arch Surg* 1992;127(5):617-621.
79. Dormandy JA, Rutherford RB. Management of peripheral arterial disease (PAD): TASC Working Group. *J Vasc Surg* 2000;31:S1-S296.
80. Goshima KR, Mills JL, Hughes JD. A new look at outcomes after infrainguinal bypass surgery: traditional reporting standards systematically underestimate the expenditure of effort required to attain limb salvage. *J Vasc Surg* 2004;39:330-335.
81. Nicoloff AD, Taylor LM, McLafferty RB, et al. Patient recovery after infrainguinal bypass grafting for limb salvage. *J Vasc Surg* 1998;27: 256-263.
82. Adam DJ, Beard JD, Cleveland T, et al. BASIL Trial Participants. Bypass versus Angioplasty in Severe Ischaemia of the Leg (BASIL): multicentre, randomised controlled trial. *Lancet* 2005;366(9501):1925-1934.

chapter 12

Amputation

Kenneth R. Woodburn, MB ChB, MD FRCSG (Gen) •
Benjamin Lindsey, MB BS, FRCSE

Key Points

- Only a small percentage of patients with chronic intermittent claudication progress to develop critical limb ischemia that requires amputation.
- Preoperative epidural analgesia reduces postoperative stump pain but not the rate of phantom limb pain.
- Complex quantitative measures of skin perfusion add little to the judgment of an experienced clinician when determining amputation level and remain research tools.
- The likelihood of walking on a prosthesis is much higher if the knee joint is preserved, i.e., following amputation below the knee.
- No evidence exists for an optimal surgical technique when performing below-knee amputation; all have consistently lower healing rates than above-knee amputation.
- Major limb amputation carries a mortality of 6% to 13%, reflecting the comorbidities of this patient population rather than the magnitude of the operation.
- Rehabilitation following amputation requires teamwork, with the anesthetists, physiotherapists, and occupational therapists all playing roles.

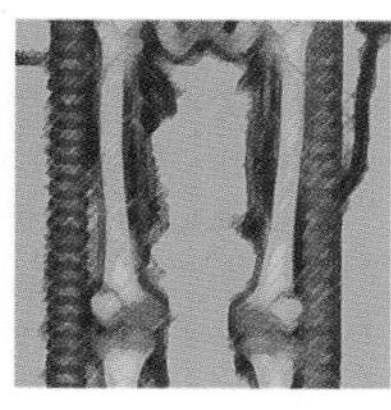

Although considered by many to be the fate of the patient with peripheral arterial disease, the rate of amputation in patients with intermittent claudication is reported to be around 1.6% per annum,[1] with historical studies indicating that fewer than 10% of claudicants require major limb amputation within 10 years of diagnosis.[2]

The global incidence of lower limb amputation is highest in northern America and northern Europe, while Japan and southern Europe have some of the lowest rates.[3-5] Peripheral vascular disease has been cited as the etiology in 70% of amputees referred to the U.K. prosthetics services in 2001 and 2002.[6] Diabetes mellitus, smoking, and a reduced ankle–brachial index are the major risk factors for amputation.[7] Some studies have suggested that an aggressive approach to vascular surgical reconstruction reduces the incidence of major amputation,[8,9] while others have failed to show improved limb salvage rates with increasing surgical activity.[10] The average life expectancy of an amputee is 4 years, reflecting the systemic nature of atherosclerosis.[11] These data highlight the importance of decision making when managing patients with critical limb ischemia (CLI). Amputation for vascular disease is often regarded as the manifestation of failed vascular reconstruction and may be the reason patients reach the end of the line, physiologically and mentally drained at the end of a series of failed interventions.

In conjunction with their patient, experienced clinicians should strive to identify when revascularization, amputation with a view to full ambulatory rehabilitation, palliative amputation, or medical palliation is appropriate and in the patient's best interests. Amputation should be seen as a positive procedure, one preserving life, often ending chronic pain and sepsis, and offering the opportunity to regain independent mobility. The procedure itself needs to be led by a senior surgeon rather than delegated to an unsupervised inexperienced junior, the outcome of which has been shown to be inferior.[12]

Getting it right the first time requires the clinician to have a thorough understanding of the general principles of amputation. These include preoperative planning, a technically meticulous procedure, and a multidisciplinary team approach to recovery and rehabilitation. The rationale and data supporting the many components of this approach are discussed in this chapter, optimizing patient recovery and return to an acceptable quality of life.

Table 12-1
Indications for Extremity Amputation in Peripheral Arterial Disease

Dead
Nonviable tissue
Dry gangrene
Wet gangrene
"Fixed" mottling in an acutely ischemic limb
Deadly
Spreading infection and compromising survival
Diabetic neuropathic tissue
Necrotizing fasciitis
Chronic ulceration
Disabling
Nonfunction or limited recovery of function
Traumatic
Postrevascularization
Intractable pain
Chronic irreversible ischemia
Chronic ulceration
Nonhealing wounds
Diabetic neuroischemic tissue

INDICATIONS FOR MINOR AND MAJOR AMPUTATION, INCLUDING CLINICAL COURSE OF AMPUTATION

The indications for the amputation of tissue in patients with peripheral arterial disease are summarized in Table 12-1. Minor amputation is usually undertaken for localized tissue destruction, where the removal of infected or necrotic tissue leaves an acceptable wound-healing environment with a vascularity that favors healing. Failing that, the blood supply can be improved by angioplasty or bypass to achieve healing. Major limb amputation is indicated if a limb is dead, deadly, or disabling. An experienced clinician is familiar with the three distinct disease patterns described here, tailoring management to the age and comorbidities of the individual. However, these patterns are not mutually exclusive, and many patients who are being considered for amputation have a mixture of features.

Small Vessel Disease

Small vessel disease leading to major limb amputation rarely exists in isolation. While vasospastic conditions such as frostbite and secondary Raynaud's disease may lead to digital necrosis (Figure 12-1), local amputation of necrotic tissue can be undertaken with a high chance of success. It is usually reserved for pain relief or when previously dry gangrene becomes secondarily infected (wet gangrene). More commonly, and typically in the diabetic patient, small vessel disease coexists with atherosclerotic disease in the larger vessels, as well as other systemic and local complications that render successful tissue healing unlikely. Therefore, diabetic patients are usually advised to retain nonviable digits as long as the gangrene remains dry. The moment they exhibit signs of wet gangrene or spreading cellulitis, the leg becomes deadly and major limb amputation becomes necessary to prevent fatal decline. Sadly, revascularization is rarely an option in these individuals because blood flow at the ankle is reasonable and the problem lies at the microvascular level, often in combination with a peripheral neuropathy. Diabetic patients also suffer extensive comorbidity and are often dialysis-dependent. In some instances, these diabetic patients present acutely and are unstable, with systemic sepsis arising from deep tissue infection in a compromised extremity, when an emergency amputation becomes a lifesaving operation.

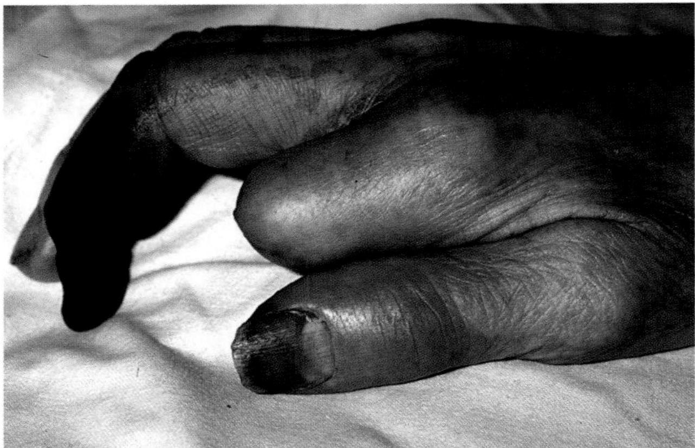

Figure 12-1. Digital gangrene following microvascular occlusion. Note prior healed digital amputation.

Large Vessel Disease

Despite adequate risk factor management and appropriate attempts at revascularization, a small proportion of patients with intermittent claudication go on to develop CLI.[13] The annual incidence of this group is rising,[1] partly due to an aging population, as well as the increasing prevalence of insulin resistance in the young.[14] This latter group is challenging to manage, and the choice of treatment is based on a detailed consideration of individual circumstances, coupled with informed discussion among health-care professionals, the patient, and the family or caregivers. The value of multidisciplinary input into the decision-making process for these patients cannot be overemphasized.

Advocates of an aggressive revascularization policy for CLI cite benefits of a reduced operative mortality,[15,16] economic advantage,[17] and improved quality of life.[18,19] A definitive study in which patients with CLI are randomized to reconstruction or primary amputation has never been carried out and would be difficult to conduct ethically. Such a study would take away the bias of appropriate medical selection that inevitably skews the data quoted previously.[15-22] Clear evidence of the superiority of limb salvage over amputation is therefore not available, and decision-making continues to be subjective in these patients.

In some patients with CLI, primary amputation may be preferable to distal revascularization; survival rates have been reported following major amputation that are considerably better[21] than those following limb salvage surgery.[23] Studies of quality of life incorporate a mobility score that inevitably favors the limb salvage group. When the mobility score is excluded, quality of life for both amputees and patients with limb salvage is comparable in terms of social isolation, pain, lethargy, or sleep disturbance.[22] Other studies have suggested that restricted mobility alone does not prevent independent living.[20]

While most patients with macrovascular disease being considered for major limb amputation have a long history of previous symptomatic arterial disease, increasing longevity leads to a higher rate of asymptomatic peripheral arterial disease.[24] Increasingly, these patients present for the first time with an acutely ischemic leg precipitated by hypotension, the result of a cardiac event or the dehydration that accompanies an illness such as gastroenteritis. A large percentage of these patients have a nonsalvageable leg, and it is a challenge to treat every patient optimally.

Trauma

The vascular, orthopedic, and plastic surgical literature contains many examples of valiant limb salvage marathons necessitated by trauma. Prolonged unsuccessful attempts are costly, carry high morbidity, and are sometimes lethal. The Mangled Extremity Severity Score[25] is one of the most thoroughly validated classification systems developed to help clinicians decide whether a concerted effort to salvage a limb is likely to succeed in both military and civilian settings.[26-28] Mangled Extremity Severity Scores comprise the extent of soft tissue and skeletal injury, the severity and duration of ischemia, and circulatory shock, as well as age. A value of greater than 7 suggests that early amputation offers the best outcome, while values below this indicate that salvage attempts may deliver acceptable functional results. The recent escalation of global military conflict has sadly confirmed the value of applying this scoring system.[29,30]

INFLUENCE OF PREVIOUS SURGICAL REVASCULARIZATION

The need for major amputation may follow one or several failed revascularization procedures, exposing the patient to increasing and cumulative risk. Predictably, younger patients with more aggressive disease fare less well,[31,32] and this is strongly related to smoking status. Some studies have suggested that the price of seeking revascularization is that the level of amputation may be compromised.[33] Conversely, careful case selection has given rise to several large reports on surgical bypass for claudication, reporting minimal limb loss over 5 years,[34-36] and no convincing evidence shows that prior revascularization compromises a later amputation, should that be required.

The lack of an easily palpable femoral pulse has been associated with failure of a transtibial amputation to heal.[37] Furthermore, healing of a transfemoral amputation may also be compromised, although it is usually achieved at this level even in the absence of a femoral pulse. The advantages to mobility conferred by preservation of the knee joint[38,39] mandate every effort to improve inflow by iliac angioplasty or stenting or, less commonly, by a surgical inflow procedure.

PREOPERATIVE PREPARATION AND PATIENT OPTIMIZATION

Disabling Limbs

Some patients needing amputation have a disabling leg with stable critical ischemia or possibly a previously salvaged but useless leg. There is time for these patients to have adequate preparation and counseling, to be discharged home with appropriate analgesia, and to return for routine surgery once they have accepted that an amputation is right choice for them. They can embark on an amputation care pathway, agreed upon and managed by a multidisciplinary team, which has been shown to optimize rehabilitation.[40] Ideally, psychological, occupational, and physiotherapy assessment are completed, along with the required home modifications, before the operation is done. Patients are directed to think about their impending amputation as a gateway to freedom and should be taught exercises that maintain muscle strength, as well as limit flexion deformity at the knee. Anesthetic optimization, including an epidural placed 24 hours in advance of surgery, is also possible, which may reduce the rate of phantom limb pain (described later).

Dead and Deadly

A dead leg that is cold and mottled, with fixed skin staining, needs a quicker approach. There is still often time for a full and frank discussion with the patient and their relatives. This takes into consideration the patient's existing quality of life and should limit the number of patients for whom a major amputation is endured in the closing few days of life. These are often frail and elderly patients with an acute ischemic event that is secondary to cardiogenic or hypovolemic shock. If the decision is made to proceed to major amputation, then there is still time for optimization of cardiac and respiratory function, correction of clotting, and even placement of a preoperative epidural catheter.

Sepsis in an ischemic leg is deadly because it can spread rapidly, especially in a diabetic patient. This constitutes an emergency, and by definition, resuscitation should take place in parallel with the surgery. Fundamental principles of treatment include preoperative intravenous antibiotics followed by adequate drainage of pus and removal of all nonviable tissue. When sepsis and tissue loss extend above the forefoot, a definitive transtibial amputation may be carried out with planned delayed closure of the wound in 5 to 7 days.[41] Alternatively, a guillotine procedure can be undertaken to allow resolution of sepsis before proceeding to definitive stump formation later. This two-stage approach has been shown to reduce stump infection, as well as the need for revision, without increased mortality in some series[42] but not in others.[43] A guillotine amputation can be managed using a vacuum-assisted closure device.

A temporizing strategy for when a patient is too unstable for any surgery has been reviewed by Hunsaker et al.[44]: Cryoanesthesia is used to cool the gangrenous limb by either immersing it in dry ice or using a cryoamputation boot. With the addition of a tourniquet, systemic toxicity is reduced until the patient is stable enough to withstand amputation; this is then associated with reduced postoperative mortality.[45-47]

ADJUVANT THERAPY

Acute CLI caused by thromboembolism is usually treated by Fogarty balloon catheter embolectomy.[48] Surgical thromboembolectomy may be detrimental for acute in situ thrombosis where the arteries are diseased. Percutaneous thrombolysis may help differentiate between these two etiologies; failure of lysis can identify patients with extensive runoff disease for whom primary amputation is the best treatment.[49]

Many medical treatments have been explored in patients with unreconstructable chronic CLI. These include intravenously administered prostanoids, such as iloprost or prostaglandin E1, which are vasodilators that improve microcirculation at the endothelial level.[50] Individual tolerance to prostanoids is variable, and side effects can include drastic hypotension, flushing, and severe headache. In acute ischemia, prostanoids have been shown to reduce the rate of primary amputation, as well as death, in a placebo-controlled study.[31] A metaanalysis suggested that the benefit can last for at least 6 months.[51]

Lumbar sympathectomy and dorsal column stimulation can help reduce pain in chronic CLI and in appropriately selected patients may postpone major limb amputation, at least until tissue necrosis supervenes.

OPERATIVE MANAGEMENT

Principles Applying to All Levels of Amputation

Optimization of the outcome of any amputation, major or minor, is governed by adherence to several general principles. Amputations undertaken for ischemia generally should not include the use of a tourniquet. Occasionally, in a patient with distal disease and normal proximal arteries undergoing transtibial amputation, significant blood loss may be anticipated and a tourniquet is indicated. This allows accurate and timely identification of blood vessels and limits blood loss.[52,53] Antibiotics should be administered according to the protocol described later. Patients undergoing amputation are particularly at risk for deep vein thrombosis[54,55] and should receive daily fractionated heparin or low-molecular-weight heparin throughout their hospital admission, particularly since thromboembolic deterrent stockings cannot normally be used on the contralateral leg.

Surgery aims to achieve complete removal of diseased, necrotic, or infected tissue. Damage to healthy marginal tissue can be reduced by the avoidance of unnecessary cautery and instrumentation with forceps. Separation of skin and subcutaneous fat from the underlying fascia should be limited, and muscle is cut firmly and cleanly with a blade, not electrocautery. Bone is better sectioned and contoured with a power saw than with a handsaw. A rasp is used to smooth the surface of the bone, and the bone dust is washed away with saline to prevent heterotopic calcification. Nerves are cut on the stretch so that they retract into the stump, limiting localized hematoma and neuroma formation. It is preferable to separate and ligate vessels individually; large patent arteries and veins should be transfixed using absorbable sutures. If suction drainage is required, it should not be sutured to the skin so that it can be removed after 24 hours without disturbing the dressing. No evidence exists that routine wound drainage reduces the rates of wound hematoma or other complications. Muscles are either firmly sutured to one another over the ends of the bone or directly to the bone through predrilled holes. This stabilization prevents deformation of the stump during muscle contraction.

Periodically opposing the edges of the marginal fascia together, while fashioning the muscle flaps, informs the surgeon of the anticipated stump shape, as well as ensuring that the skin may finally be closed without tension. Skin can be closed either using continuous nonabsorbable or absorbable sutures or using interrupted staples or nonabsorbable stitch. No evidence supports one of these as an optimal method. Adhesive paper strips are an acceptable adjunct. The definitive stump dressing is discussed later.

Selection of Amputation Level

Local minor amputation of any number of toes, releasing undrained sepsis, and removing necrotic tissue should halt tissue destruction and leave the patient with a useful foot. When three or four toes need to be removed, it may be better to remove all five, resulting in a transmetatarsal forefoot amputation. This avoids having a single protruding digit exposed to trauma that may restart the cycle of infection and necrosis. Digital, ray, and transmetatarsal amputations may all be left open to heal by secondary intention, and this has been greatly improved by the principle of vacuum-assisted closure.[32,56]

Many patients needing a transmetatarsal amputation also require a revascularization procedure to ensure robust healing.[57] If this is not successful, then half need revision to transtibial amputation.[58] Transmetatarsal amputation preserves foot function, avoids the need for tendon transfers, and allows walking to return to normal with little more than an ankle-high lace-up boot containing a filler. Therefore, it has been advocated as preferable to a single first-ray amputation because of the superior loading dynamic of the foot.[59]

More proximal unconventional ankle amputations include Lisfranc's forefoot disarticulation at the level of the tarsal–metatarsal joints and Chopart's disarticulation at the talonavicular and calcaneocuboid joints. These procedures are generally the domain of the specialist orthopedic ankle surgeon and are not recommended for CLI unless carried out by a vascular surgeon with particular expertise.[60] In patients with a patent posterior tibial artery and an intact heel, a Syme's amputation has been reported to serve these exacting requirements well.[61,62]

For most patients who need a major limb amputation, the choice is between operation below, through, or above the knee. The more proximal the amputation, the higher the chance of healing; the more distal, the better the chance of walking on a prosthesis. If a major amputation is indicated in immobile or wheelchair-bound individuals, then transfemoral amputation is better since it has a significantly higher healing rate than transtibial amputation.[20] In patients able to sit out in a chair, a through-knee amputation may afford more core stability and a lower center of gravity without increasing the rate of nonhealing.[63,64]

While patients may well be fitted with prosthesis after above-knee amputation, mobilization on an artificial limb is more reliable following a transtibial amputation, when excellent healing and subsequent functional results are possible.[65,66] This should encourage the restoration of a good pulse at the groin, knowing that without one healing rates are less than 25%.[37] Patients with a fixed flexion deformity at the knee of 15 degrees (that cannot be improved by physiotherapy) will never mobilize after transtibial amputation as they cannot use the prosthesis, and those with 45 degrees of flexion will not achieve stump healing due to pressure necrosis of stump skin. These patients should only be offered a transfemoral amputation.

Many techniques have been investigated to help improve the clinician's judgment about the most distal level at which healing is likely after amputation. The severity of the arterial disease on angiography and the presence of rest pain, tissue loss, or both are, not surprisingly, associated with poor healing after transtibial amputation.[67] Conversely, a palpable popliteal pulse almost guarantees healing of a transtibial amputation.[68] The predictive value of ankle–brachial index for healing after transtibial amputation is described in some studies but refuted by others.[69]

Transcutaneous oxygen measurements can predict amputation wound healing, but with variable accuracy.[37,68,69] A range of predictive values has been suggested: oxygen tension below 20 mm Hg seems to predict stump failure, whereas above 40 mm Hg predicts healing.[70-74] Other more complex and specialist techniques include radioisotope washout[72,75] or laser Doppler fluximetry, which have both been used to predict amputation healing. The actual cutoff values used, however, varied among centers,[76,77] which suggests that the methods are better suited to use in the research laboratory than as clinical tools. Similar techniques have been used to investigate transmetatarsal amputation healing, without conclusive results.[78]

Skin temperature at the site of amputation can be valuable,[69,79] along with the ratio of temperatures measured at the front and back of the calf when considering a long posterior flap[80]; other measurements are less clear.[81]

Despite the application of these techniques, the transtibial amputation failure rate remains 15% to 25%. The clinical judgment of an experienced surgeon based on the apparent vascularity of skin and muscle at operation remains one of the most reliable predictors of healing.[38,73]

Anesthetic Techniques

The anesthetic technique can influence wound healing, as well as survival, but needs to be modified according to the general state of the patient and the urgency of the procedure. The 30-day mortality rates after transtibial and transfemoral amputation have been reported to be 6.3% and 13.3%, respectively,[82] the leading cause of death being cardiac complications.[73] Previous coronary artery bypass grafting triples the likelihood of surviving a major amputation.[71]

Dialysis-dependent patients should be managed with advice from their renal physicians; ideally, the patient should have surgery shortly after dialysis. The preceding factors, as well as the presence of respiratory disease or clotting dysfunction, dictate whether a regional or general anesthetic technique can be used. In patients with acute ischemia, it may be worth stopping a heparin infusion for a few hours so that an epidural can be sited. Finally, the more distal minor amputations can be carried out with a local anesthetic ankle block, particularly since many patients also have a diabetic sensory neuropathy.

Most operations can be carried out under epidural anesthetic, supplemented by sedation or light general anesthesia. Placement of the epidural catheter at least 24 hours before the amputation has been suggested to reduce the subsequent rate of phantom limb pain, as has the insertion of a perineural sheath catheter for local anesthetic infusion at the time of surgery. This debate will influence the anesthetic technique used and is discussed later.

Antibiotics

Historically, antibiotic prophylaxis was employed to prevent clostridial infection or gas gangrene, usually with penicillin and metronidazole. Local hospital microbiology policy dictates which agent or agents should be used and for how long.[34,83] Good evidence shows that a short course of antibiotic prophylaxis reduces the rate of amputation stump breakdown. More recently, colonization with methicillin-resistant *Staphylococcus aureus* (MRSA) has been shown to affect the outcome of major limb amputation adversely.[72] Most units have a local policy for antibiotic use that takes into account the prevalence of MRSA in their community. In the United Kingdom, all patients are now screened for MRSA on hospital admission. In those colonized, eradication is attempted before surgery.

TECHNIQUES OF MAJOR LIMB AMPUTATIONS

The general vascular surgical principles have already been described; the specific technical issues pertaining to each technique follow.

Transfemoral Amputation

The indications for an above-knee amputation include doubtful prospect of healing at the transtibial level, low likelihood of mobilization, and fixed flexion deformity at the knee.

The placement of equal anterior and posterior cutaneous flaps is dictated by the level of proposed femoral section; this should be kept as long as possible, while leaving space to incorporate both muscle flap coverage (myoplasty) and the knee joint mechanism of a prosthetic limb.

In practical terms, the femur is sectioned about 12 cm from the knee joint and the skin flaps are based on a circumferential skin incision centered 2 to 3 cm distal to this. Suturing of the lateral and medial muscle groups over the sectioned femur may be stabilized by the additional drilling of holes near the end of the bone. The quadriceps and hamstring muscles are then sutured to each other, forming the second muscle layer over the bone. A robust myoplasty and myodesis technique affords good stump shape, reduced pain, and a balanced action of flexors and extensors, which improves proprioception and function.[84-87]

Transtibial Amputation

For almost 30 years, two common techniques have been used for performing a transtibial amputation: the long posterior flap or the skew flap. The long posterior flap method was described by Burgess et al. and is popular in the United States.[88] It requires the skin quality on the posterior calf to be good enough to cover the gastrocnemius muscle flap on which the technique is based. Although a good pad of muscle is used to cover the end of the sectioned tibia, the suture line in the skin and fascia lie directly over the sectioned edge of the tibia. This may lead to wound breakdown following minimal trauma, which can delay limb fitting. Also "dog ears" at each end of the suture line can be difficult to avoid using this technique.

The skew flap was designed in 1982[89] and displaces the skin incision away from the anterior tibia. This, along with better

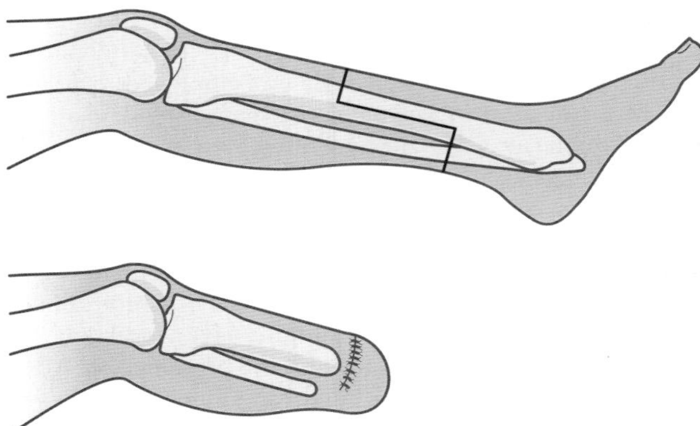

Figure 12-2. Skin incision and closure for long posterior flap (Burgess type) below-knee amputation. (Adapted from Rutherford 6th ed.:2466, Figure 172.5A.)

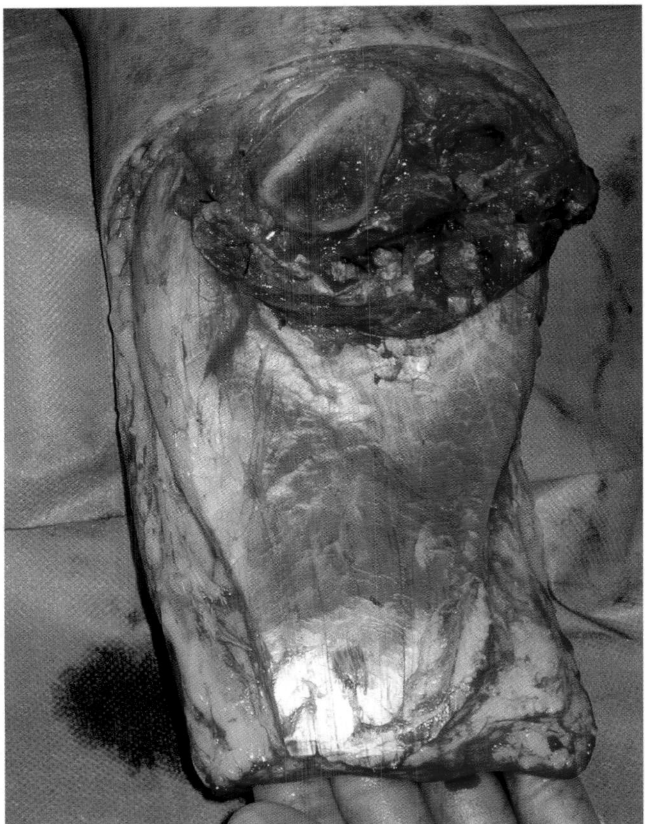

Figure 12-3. The appearance of the completed posterior flap following cleavage in the plane between gastrocnemius and soleus.

blood supply of the shorter flaps,[90] may be the reason for better healing than after the Burgess technique in some series,[91] although a recent randomized study showed equivalent outcomes for both methods.[92]

Long Posterior Flap Transtibial Amputation

After positioning the patient according to the operating surgeon's preference, a proximal skin incision is made at a point one handbreadth (10 cm) below the tibial tuberosity. The incision should include almost two thirds of the calf circumference at this level. The long posterior flap then extends from the medial and lateral ends of this transverse incision along the length of the limb for a distance at least half the length of the transverse incision. At this point, a posterior transverse incision completes the flap, which can be trimmed to exact length later in the procedure (Figure 12-2).

These incisions are then deepened through subcutaneous tissue and deep fascia, ligating bleeding points as required. At the level of tibial transection, the muscles of the anterior compartment are divided transversely, the anterior tibial vessels are ligated, the nerve is transected, and the interosseous membrane is incised. After cleaning the fibula proximally for 1 to 2 cm, it is divided at a level 2 cm above the planned level of tibial transaction. The tibia is then divided with a power saw at the originally identified level. Thereafter, the deep muscles of the calf are divided transversely, the vessels are ligated, the nerves are divided, and the plane between gastrocnemius and soleus is developed until soleus can be excised along with the limb; gastrocnemius is divided transversely at the distal extent of the posterior flap. This leaves a long posterior flap consisting solely of gastrocnemius muscle, along with overlying skin and subcutaneous tissue (Figure 12-3). The tendinous portion of gastrocnemius is then sutured to the anterior tibial periosteum, and the muscle length is reduced as required to ensure apposition without tissue tension or undue redundancy. The skin is then closed to complete the procedure (Figure 12-4).

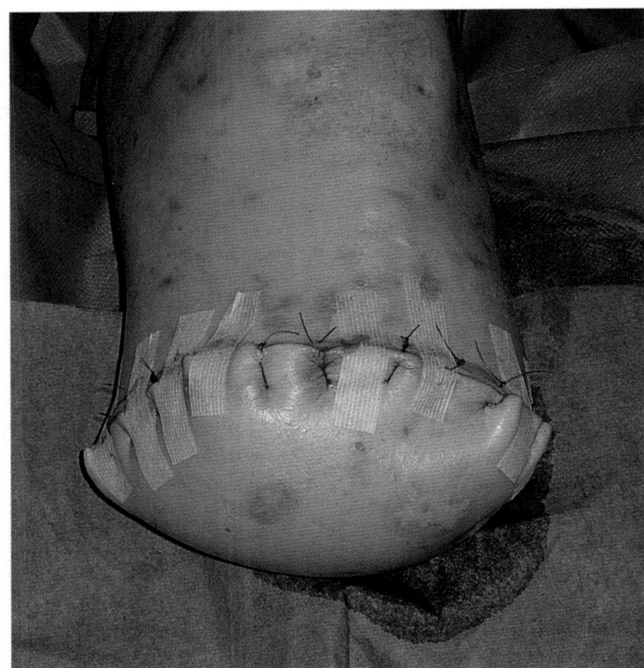

Figure 12-4. Appearance of a newly completed left transtibial amputation stump.

Skew Flap Transtibial Amputation

This procedure again uses a flap of gastrocnemius muscle but with the creation of anteromedial and posterolateral fasciocutaneous flaps based on the cutaneous blood supply of the lower limb. Flaps are again marked at a level one handbreadth below the tibial tuberosity, and the circumference of the calf is measured at this point. The base for each fasciocutaneous flap is determined as half of this circumference.

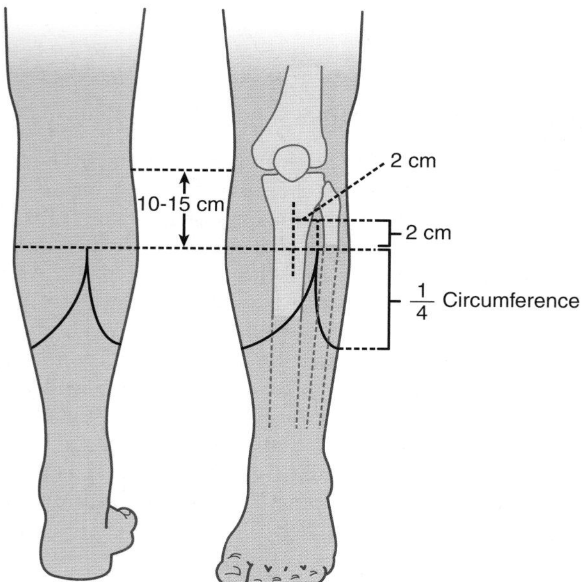

Figure 12-5. Skin incisions for the skew flap transtibial amputation. (Adapted from Rutherford 6th ed. :2466, Figure 172.5B.)

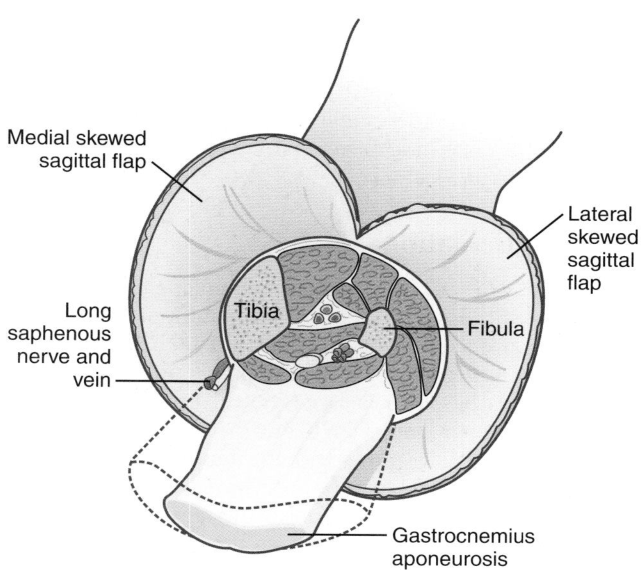

Figure 12-6. Diagrammatic representation of skew flaps. The procedure is completed by placing the gastrocnemius flap obliquely over the bone ends and suturing it to the anterior periosteum and deep fascia. (Adapted from Rutherford 6th ed. :2468, Figure 172.7A.)

The anterior junction of the flaps lies over the anterior muscle compartment 2.5 cm from the tibial crest, the posterior junction being at a point 180 degrees around the calf. The midpoint of the base of each flap is marked and used as the center of the semicircular cutaneous flap (Figure 12-5). At the anterior junction of the two flaps, a proximal incision is made to facilitate access to the line of bone section.

On incision, the fasciocutaneous flaps can be reflected proximally to enable the operation to continue as described for the long posterior flap. The gastrocnemius tendon and fascia is cut approximately 5 cm longer than the skin flap and can be trimmed and brought obliquely forward to be sutured to the anterior tibial periosteum (Figure 12-6). Skin can be approximated with either suture or adhesive paper strips or preferably with both.

Through-Knee Amputation

The rationale for amputation at this level is both a functional and a practical extension of the transfemoral amputation. While it does not preclude the fitting of a prosthesis,[26] the intention is to provide a longer lever and retained muscle fixation. The former gives better core stability for the nonambulant amputee when transferring and sitting; the latter avoids late flexion contracture at the knee or hip following transtibial or transfemoral amputation, respectively. Through-knee amputation is a good option in a patient who already has an above-knee amputation on the other side since it improves balance and stability.

Disarticulation of the knee joint is particularly suited to medically high-risk patients because it may be undertaken swiftly with minimal blood loss. The technique is based on generous equal medial and lateral flaps that are closed in the midline over the patella, which in turn has been taken off its tibial insertion and sutured to the hamstrings and cruciate ligaments posteriorly. The Gritti-Stokes amputation is a modification of this method, where the end of the femur is sectioned by removing the condyles with a power saw. The back of the patella is is also shaved flat after it is removed from its tibial insertion, and it is then hinged over the flat end of the femur, which has been cut with a posterior facing 30-degree slant. The opposing bone surfaces are fixed with the aid of holes drilled in the periosteum and heavy suture material, and the patella is covered by a long anterior skin flap. The Gritti-Stokes method has a good record of healing, with less of a synovial fluid leak than simple disarticulation. Comparison of the two techniques suggested the Gritti-Stokes method to be better.[93]

Transmetatarsal Amputation

Wet gangrene, necrosis, osteomyelitis, or ulceration of one or more digits is dealt with by amputation through the base of the proximal phalanx. The incision is fashioned to allow healthy skin to overlap the bone, healing by secondary intention. More proximal disease requires amputation at the level of the metatarsal neck, along with a wedge containing all nonviable or infected soft tissue. The first and fifth transmetatarsal amputations are undertaken using a racquet handle incision, the handle being the incision that allows access to and division of the metatarsal shaft. Preservation of the base of the fifth metatarsal ensures that peroneus brevis can still carry out foot eversion.

Any combination of digital and transmetatarsal amputations may be undertaken as long as the blood supply to the foot is adequate; however, if only one or two isolated and exposed digits remain, it may be better to employ a transmetatarsal amputation, for which far better mobility is achieved than after a more proximal amputation. Up to half of transmetatarsal amputations undertaken for forefoot ischemia require conversion to a transtibial amputation.[58]

The skin incision on the dorsum of the foot joins the first and fifth midmetatarsal points before passing distal along the lateral borders of their shafts and being joined in an arc just behind the sulcus of the toes on the plantar surface. Once the metatarsal shafts have been sectioned, the plantar flap is bought up over the defect and closed without tension, resulting in a moccasin appearance of the forefoot. When advanced sepsis occurs in the toes, guillotine amputation may be performed and the resulting defect may be healed with a vacuum-assisted closure device.

Hip Disarticulation

Predictably, when undertaken for ischemia, gangrene, or an infected nonhealing transfemoral amputation, the hip disarticulation procedure is associated with high mortality and accounts for fewer than 1% of all major amputations.[94] In summary, it is based on a large gluteal myocutaneous flap running posteriorly from 3 cm below the pubic tubercle to the anterior superior iliac spine. Once the femoral, sciatic, gluteal, and obturator neurovascular bundles have been suture-ligated individually—with the exception of the nerves, which are all divided on the stretch—the muscles are sectioned, the hip is disarticulated, and the gluteal fascia is sutured to the inguinal ligament. A hip spica is used to obliterate the space between the flap and the pelvis.

POSTOPERATIVE CARE

The use of a perioperative epidural catheter has been shown to reduce postoperative stump pain.[95] Moderate elevation can reduce postoperative swelling, and regular conventional analgesia is prescribed. Neuromodulation with carbamazepine and amitriptyline has been superseded by gabapentin.[96] The rehabilitation process ideally starts before the amputation, and it should continue seamlessly early in the postoperative phase.

Phantom Limb Pain

Pain at the site of an amputation stump is entirely predictable; it only requires investigation if it persists, at which point investigation may be required to detect a deep infection or neuroma. The sensation of pain in the absent limb is termed phantom pain, and it is debilitating in 25% of the patients affected. The literature is divided as to whether it diminishes with time.[97,98] Sometimes, the symptoms are restricted to phantom sensation alone, which is not usually problematic and indeed may aid rehabilitation.[5] The mechanisms of phantom pain are unclear. The obvious explanation is that inappropriate afferent signals arise from stump nerves leading to spinal sensitization. A more intriguing explanation is that a mismatch occurs between the sensation of the limb being present and the opposing visual feedback. This causes cortical jarring, which can be treated with mirror therapy. This emerging therapy has been described anecdotally by Ramachandran.[99]

There appears to be a correlation between severity and location of preamputation pain and postoperative phantom limb pain[98] that has led clinicians to attempt to limit the former. An obvious strategy that has been reported in two small studies is to site an epidural 24 to 72 hours before amputation.[100,101] The benefits that were reported in the first small studies could not be reproduced in a large Danish, double-blind, randomized trial.[102] The use of perineural infusion of bupivucaine via a catheter placed alongside the major nerve bundle at the time of surgery may reduce postoperative stump pain[95] but not phantom pain.[103]

Rigid Stump Dressings

The application of a rigid plaster of Paris dressing to the transtibial amputation stump is claimed to reduce stump swelling, pain, contracture, and exposure to trauma.[88] This rigid stump dressing is applied in the operating theater and can be left undisturbed for up to 14 days (Figure 12-7).[104] Some evidence indicates that its use may shorten the time to first limb fitting[105] as it offers protection from trauma and assists in shaping the stump (Figure 12-8). Previous randomized trials comparing rigid postoperative dressings with standard soft dressings have shown a trend toward advantage for the rigid dressing that did not reach statistical significance[106,107] for both earlier healing and limb fitting. Nawijn et al. concluded that evidence supports the practice of rigid stump dressings, although larger trials are needed.[108]

Mobilization and Rehabilitation

In fitter patients, with adequate analgesia, and with an appropriate stump dressing, mobilization can begin on the first postoperative day. This includes bed mobility and joint exercises, as well as strengthening of the upper limbs and remaining leg. The potential for rehabilitation on a prosthesis becomes evident by about a week. Early mobilization can minimize complications and improve rehabilitation, an extreme example of which is the immediate application of a prosthetic device on the operating table.[109] Once the skin has healed, a firm stump stocking is applied to help reduce edema and shrink the stump into a shape ready for limb fitting. Morale can be boosted significantly by using early walking aids such as the pneumatic postamputation mobility aid. This prosthesis is attached via a one-size-fits-all socket comprising an adjustable pneumatic cuff. Once mobile, amputees may begin physiotherapy to relearn the postural reflexes and balance needed to achieve energy-efficient walking. Vascular amputees generally have their first limb fitting consultation from 6 to 8 weeks after

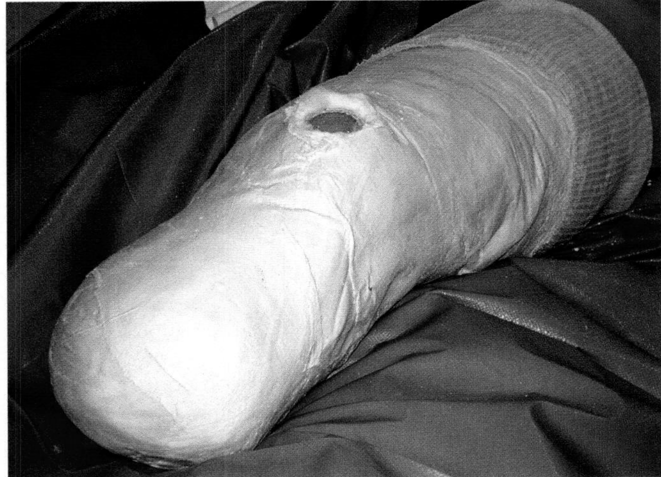

Figure 12-7. A rigid stump dressing applied to the transtibial amputation stump shown in Figure 12-4.

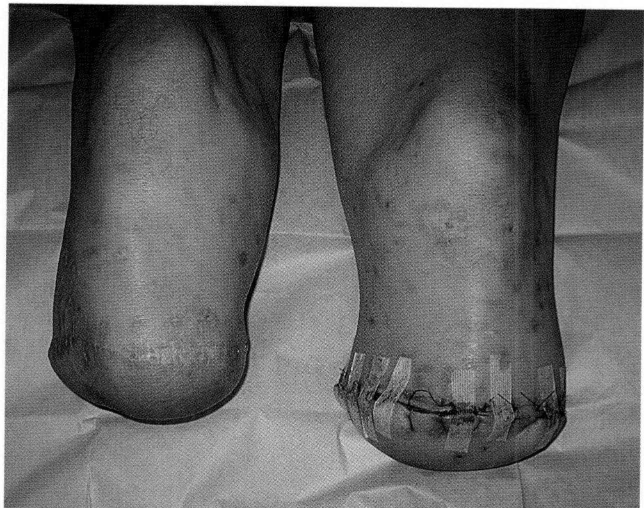

Figure 12-8. Appearance of the stump 10 days postoperatively, on removal of the rigid stump dressing. This is the same stump shown in Figure 12-4, and this figure clearly illustrates the early reduction in stump volume and the beneficial molding of the stump shape achieved by the rigid dressing. The healed right transtibial amputation was performed 8 months previously.

amputation. Developments in material science and technology, combined with a modular design, have led to prostheses that are lighter, are quicker to manufacture, and may be tailored to individual requirements. In younger amputees, this has led to some remarkable results.[110-112]

PSYCHOLOGICAL SUPPORT

Some management decisions surrounding limb salvage and amputation are not always straightforward. This may cause the patient to be unclear of what to expect, and fear of the unknown provokes anxiety. This can be minimized by giving the patient realistic expectations as the clinical picture unfolds. The emergence of a multidisciplinary care pathway has helped this tremendously, ensuring opportunity for preoperative and postoperative discussion with the rehabilitation team.[112] An opportunity to meet with other amputees before the surgery and at different stages of rehabilitation is also helpful.

OUTCOMES AND SURVIVAL

Both early and contemporary series demonstrate consistent and unchanged outcomes over the last 30 years.[20,113,114] This highly morbid group has a 30-day mortality of 10% and a 1-year survival rate of only 60% to 80%. Three-year survival rates following transtibial and transfemoral amputation are reported to be around 57% and 39%, respectively, with a more proximal amputation being associated with a poorer prognosis.[82] Morbidity is also high, with 35% of transmetatarsal, 15% of transtibial, and 6% of transfemoral amputations requiring conversion to a higher level within 2 years. Of patients undergoing major amputation, 15% require a major contralateral amputation, also within 2 years.[114]

In a study from the United Kingdom, it was reported that approximately equal numbers of transtibial and transfemoral amputation operations were performed; 17% of the patients died during the same hospital admission, and a further 25% were not suitable for rehabilitation. Of the 68% referred for limb fitting and rehabilitation, one fifth had died by 2 years. At this time, only 17% of the patients the original study cohort could walk around their own home, only one third of whom were confident enough to venture outside on their prosthesis.[115]

SUMMARY

Major limb amputation is a high-risk procedure, and a palliative option may be chosen in selected patients. For patients in whom surgery is appropriate, a planned multidisciplinary team approach is required, with an emphasis on good communication, medical optimization, and technically exacting surgery to achieve the appropriate quality of life to which all amputees are entitled.

References

1. Dormandy JA, Murray GD. The fate of the claudicant: a prospective study of 1969 claudicants. *Eur J Vasc Surg* 1991;5:131-133.
2. Bloor K. Natural history of atherosclerosis of the lower extremities. *Ann R Coll Surg Engl* 1961;28:36-52.
3. Global Lower Extremity Amputation Study Group. Epidemiology of lower extremity amputation in centres in Europe, North America and East Asia. *Br J Surg* 2000;87:328-337.
4. Hirsch AT, Treat-Jacobson D, Lando HA, et al. The role of tobacco cessation, antiplatelet and lipid-lowering therapies in the treatment of peripheral arterial disease. *Vasc Med* 1997;2:243-251.
5. McDermott MM, Feinglass J, Slavensky R, et al. The ankle–brachial index as a predictor of survival in patients with peripheral vascular disease. *J Gen Intern Med* 1994;9:445-449.
6. Information and Statistics Division. *Amputee Statistical Database for the United Kingdom 2001-02. Edinburgh: National Health Service Scotland* 2003:2008.
7. Beckman JA, Creager MA, Libby P. Diabetes and atherosclerosis: epidemiology, pathophysiology, and management. *JAMA* 2002;287:2570-2581.
8. Gutteridge B, Torrie P, Galland B. Trends in arterial reconstruction, angioplasty and amputation. *Health Trends* 1994;26:88-91.
9. Ebskov LB, Schroeder TV, Holstein PE. Epidemiology of leg amputation: the influence of vascular surgery. *Br J Surg* 1994;81:1600-1603.
10. Westcoast Vascular Surgeons Study Group. Variations of rates of vascular surgical procedures for chronic critical limb ischemia and lower limb amputation rates in western Swedish counties. *Eur J Vasc Endovasc Surg* 1997;14:310-314.
11. Stewart CPU, Jain AS, Ogden SA. Lower limb amputee survival. *Prosthet Orthot Int* 1992:11-198.
12. Carrington AL, Abbott CA, Griffiths J, et al. Peripheral vascular and nerve function associated with lower limb amputation in people with and without diabetes. *Clin Sci (Lond)* 2001;101:261-266.
13. McDaniel MD, Cronenwett JL. Basic data related to the natural history of intermittent claudication. *Ann Vasc Surg* 1989;3:273-277.
14. Houghton AD, Taylor PR, Thurlow S, et al. Success rates for rehabilitation of vascular amputees: implications for preoperative assessment and amputation level. *Br J Surg* 1992;79:753-755.
15. Hobson RW, Lynch TG, Jamil Z, et al. Results of revascularization and amputation in severe lower extremity ischemia: a five-year clinical experience. *J Vasc Surg* 1985;2:174-185.
16. Taylor LM Jr, Hamre D, Dalman RL, et al. Limb salvage vs amputation for critical ischemia: the role of vascular surgery. *Arch Surg* 1991;126:1251-1257.
17. Wolfe JH, Tyrrell MR. Justifying arterial reconstruction to crural vessels: even with a prosthetic graft. *Br J Surg* 1991;78:897-899.
18. Johnson BF, Singh S, Evans L, et al. A prospective study of the effect of limb-threatening ischemia and its surgical treatment on the quality of life. *Eur J Vasc Endovasc Surg* 1997;13:306-314.
19. Thompson MM, Sayers RD, Reid A, et al. Quality of life following infragenicular bypass and lower limb amputation. *Eur J Vasc Endovasc Surg* 1995;9:310-313.

20. Nehler MR, Coll JR, Hiatt WR, et al. Functional outcome in a contemporary series of major lower extremity amputations. *J Vasc Surg* 2003;38:7-14.
21. Pell J, Stonebridge P. Association between age and survival following major amputation: the Scottish Vascular Audit Group. *Eur J Vasc Endovasc Surg* 1999;17:166-169.
22. Pell JP, Donnan PT, Fowkes FG, et al. Quality of life following lower limb amputation for peripheral arterial disease. *Eur J Vasc Surg* 1993;7:448-451.
23. Abou-Zamzam Jr AM, Lee RW, Moneta GL, et al. Functional outcome after infrainguinal bypass for limb salvage. *J Vasc Surg* 1997;25:287-295.
24. Barnes RW, Thornhill B, Nix L, et al. Prediction of amputation wound healing: roles of Doppler ultrasound and digit photoplethysmography. *Arch Surg* 1981;116:80-83.
25. Johansen K, Daines M, Howey T, et al. Objective criteria accurately predict amputation following lower extremity trauma. *J Trauma* 1990;30:568-572.
26. Helfet DL, Howey T, Sanders R, et al. Limb salvage versus amputation: preliminary results of the Mangled Extremity Severity Score. *Clin Orthop Relat Res* 1990:80-86.
27. Slauterbeck JR, Britton C, Moneim MS, et al. Mangled Extremity Severity Score: an accurate guide to treatment of the severely injured upper extremity. *J Orthop Trauma* 1994;8:282-285.
28. Sharma S, Devgan A, Marya KM, et al. Critical evaluation of Mangled Extremity Severity scoring system in Indian patients. *Injury* 2003;34:493-496.
29. Rush Jr RM, Kjorstad R, Starnes BW, et al. Application of the Mangled Extremity Severity Score in a combat setting. *Mil Med* 2007;172:777-781.
30. Starnes BW, Beekley AC, Sebesta JA, et al. Extremity vascular injuries on the battlefield: tips for surgeons deploying to war. *J Trauma* 2006;60:432-442.
31. McCready RA, Vincent AE, Schwartz RW, et al. Atherosclerosis in the young: a virulent disease. *Surgery* 1984;96:863-869.
32. Valentine RJ, Jackson MR, Modrall JG, et al. The progressive nature of peripheral arterial disease in young adults: a prospective analysis of white men referred to a vascular surgery service. *J Vasc Surg* 1999;30:436-444.
33. Stirnemann P, Walpoth B, Wursten HU, et al. Influence of failed arterial reconstruction on the outcome of major limb amputation. *Surgery* 1992;111:363-368.
34. Byrne J, Darling RC III, Chang BB, et al. Infrainguinal arterial reconstruction for claudication: is it worth the risk? An analysis of 409 procedures. *J Vasc Surg* 1999;29:259-267.
35. Donaldson MC, Mannick JA. Femoropopliteal bypass grafting for intermittent claudication: is pessimism warranted? *Arch Surg* 1980;115:724-727.
36. Kent KC, Donaldson MC, Attinger CE, et al. Femoropopliteal reconstruction for claudication: the risk to life and limb. *Arch Surg* 1988;123:1196-1198.
37. O'Dwyer KJ, Edwards MH. The association between lowest palpable pulse and wound healing in below knee amputations. *Ann R Coll Surg Engl* 1985;67:232-234.
38. Harris JP, Page S, Englund R, et al. Is the outlook for the vascular amputee improved by striving to preserve the knee? *J Cardiovasc Surg (Torino)* 1988;29:741-745.
39. Carmona GA, Lacraz A, Assal M. Walking activity in prosthesis-bearing lower-limb amputees. *Rev Chir Orthop Reparatrice Appar Mot* 2007;93:109-115.
40. Conte MS, Belkin M, Donaldson MC, et al. Femorotibial bypass for claudication: do results justify an aggressive approach? *J Vasc Surg* 1995;21:873-880.
41. Kernek CB, Rozzi WB. Simplified two-stage below-knee amputation for unsalvageable diabetic foot infections. *Clin Orthop Relat Res* 1990:251-256.
42. Desai Y, Robbs JV, Keenan JP. Staged below-knee amputations for septic peripheral lesions due to ischemia. *Br J Surg* 1986;73:392-394.
43. Fisher Jr DF, Clagett GP, Fry RE, et al. One-stage versus two-stage amputation for wet gangrene of the lower extremity: a randomized study. *J Vasc Surg* 1988;8:428-433.
44. Hunsaker RH, Schwartz JA, Keagy BA, et al. Dry ice cryoamputation: a twelve-year experience. *J Vasc Surg* 1985;2:812-816.
45. Brinker MR, Timberlake GA, Goff JM, et al. Below-knee physiologic cryoanesthesia in the critically ill patient. *J Vasc Surg* 1988;7:433-438.
46. Bunt TJ. Physiologic amputation: preliminary cryoamputation of the gangrenous extremity. *AORN J* 1991;54:1220-1224.
47. Winburn GB, Wood MC, Hawkins ML, et al. Current role of cryoamputation. *Am J Surg* 1991;162:647-650.
48. Ray SA, Buckenham TM, Belli AM, et al. The predictive value of laser Doppler fluxmetry and transcutaneous oximetry for clinical outcome in patients undergoing revascularization for severe leg ischemia. *Eur J Vasc Endovasc Surg* 1997;13:54-59.
49. Marty B, Wicky S, Ris HB, et al. Success of thrombolysis as a predictor of outcome in acute thrombosis of popliteal aneurysms. *J Vasc Surg* 2002;35:487-493.
50. Bunt TJ, Manship LL, Bynoe RP, et al. Lower extremity amputation for peripheral vascular disease: a low-risk operation. *Am Surg* 1984;50:581-584.
51. Toursarkissian B, Shireman PK, Harrison A, et al. Major lower-extremity amputation: contemporary experience in a single Veterans Affairs institution. *Am Surg* 2002;68:606-610.
52. Taylor SM, Kalbaugh CA, Blackhurst DW, et al. Preoperative clinical factors predict postoperative functional outcomes after major lower limb amputation: an analysis of 553 consecutive patients. *J Vasc Surg* 2005;42:227-235.
53. Hertzer NR, Bena JF, Karafa MT. A personal experience with the influence of diabetes and other factors on the outcome of infrainguinal bypass grafts for occlusive disease. *J Vasc Surg* 2007;46:271-279.
54. Fletcher JP, Batiste P. Incidence of deep vein thrombosis following vascular surgery. *Int Angiol* 1997;16:65-68.
55. Yeager RA, Moneta GL, Edwards JM, et al. Deep vein thrombosis associated with lower extremity amputation. *J Vasc Surg* 1995;22:612-615.
56. Taylor SM, Kalbaugh CA, Blackhurst DW, et al. Determinants of functional outcome after revascularization for critical limb ischemia: an analysis of 1000 consecutive vascular interventions. *J Vasc Surg* 2006;44:747-755.
57. La Fontaine J, Reyzelman A, Rothenberg G, et al. The role of revascularization in transmetatarsal amputations. *J Am Podiatr Med Assoc* 2001;91:533-535.
58. Thomas SR, Perkins JM, Magee TR, et al. Transmetatarsal amputation: an 8-year experience. *Ann R Coll Surg Engl* 2001;83:164-166.
59. Funk C, Young G. Subtotal pedal amputations: biomechanical and intraoperative considerations. *J Am Podiatr Med Assoc* 2001;91:6-12.
60. Gregg RO. Bypass or amputation? Concomitant review of bypass arterial grafting and major amputations. *Am J Surg* 1985;149:397-402.
61. Hudson JR, Yu GV, Marzano R, et al. Syme's amputation: surgical technique, prosthetic considerations, and case reports. *J Am Podiatr Med Assoc* 2002;92:232-246.
62. Weaver FA, Modrall JG, Baek S, et al. Syme amputation: results in patients with severe forefoot ischemia. *Cardiovasc Surg* 1996;4:81-86.
63. Faber DC, Fielding LP. Gritti-Stokes (through-knee) amputation: should it be reintroduced? *South Med J* 2001;94:997-1001.
64. Hagberg E, Berlin OK, Renstrom P. Function after through-knee compared with below-knee and above-knee amputation. *Prosthet Orthot Int* 1992;16:168-173.
65. Chiodo CP, Stroud CC. Optimal surgical preparation of the residual limb for prosthetic fitting in below-knee amputations. *Foot Ankle Clin* 2001;6:253-264.
66. Smith DG, Fergason JR. Transtibial amputations. *Clin Orthop Relat Res* 1999:108-115.
67. Yip VS, Teo NB, Johnstone R, et al. An analysis of risk factors associated with failure of below knee amputations. *World J Surg* 2006;30:1081-1087.
68. Ballard JL, Eke CC, Bunt TJ, et al. A prospective evaluation of transcutaneous oxygen measurements in the management of diabetic foot problems. *J Vasc Surg* 1995;22:485-490.
69. Wagner WH, Keagy BA, Kotb MM, et al. Noninvasive determination of healing of major lower extremity amputation: the continued role of clinical judgment. *J Vasc Surg* 1988;8:703-710.
70. Dormandy J, Belcher G, Broos P, et al. Prospective study of 713 below-knee amputations for ischemia and the effect of a prostacyclin analogue on healing: Hawaii Study Group. *Br J Surg* 1994;81:33-37.
71. Stone PA, Flaherty SK, Aburahma AF, et al. Factors affecting perioperative mortality and wound-related complications following major lower extremity amputations. *Ann Vasc Surg* 2006;20:209-216.
72. Harris JP, McLaughlin AF, Quinn RJ, et al. Skin blood flow measurement with xenon-133 to predict healing of lower extremity amputations. *Aust NZ J Surg* 1986;56:413-415.
73. Keagy BA, Schwartz JA, Kotb M, et al. Lower extremity amputation: the control series. *J Vasc Surg* 1986;4:321-326.
74. McCollum PT, Spence VA, Walker WF. Amputation for peripheral vascular disease: the case for level selection. *Br J Surg* 1988;75:1193-1195.
75. Avci S, Musdal Y. Skin blood flow level and stump healing in ischemic amputations. *Orthopedics* 2000;23:33-36.

76. Adera HM, James K, Castronuovo Jr JJ, et al. Prediction of amputation wound healing with skin perfusion pressure. *J Vasc Surg* 1995;21: 823-828.
77. Dwars BJ, van den Broek TA, Rauwerda JA, et al. Criteria for reliable selection of the lowest level of amputation in peripheral vascular disease. *J Vasc Surg* 1992;15:536-542.
78. Sanders LJ. Transmetatarsal and midfoot amputations. *Clin Podiatr Med Surg* 1997;14:741-762.
79. Spence VA, Walker WF, Troup IM, et al. Amputation of the ischemic limb: selection of the optimum site by thermography. *Angiology* 1981;32:155-169.
80. Stoner HB, Taylor L, Marcuson RW. The value of skin temperature measurements in forecasting the healing of a below-knee amputation for end-stage ischemia of the leg in peripheral vascular disease. *Eur J Vasc Surg* 1989;3:355-361.
81. Burnham SJ, Wagner WH, Keagy BA, et al. Objective measurement of limb perfusion by dermal fluorometry: a criterion for healing of below-knee amputation. *Arch Surg* 1990;125:104-106.
82. Feinglass J, Pearce WH, Martin GJ, et al. Postoperative and late survival outcomes after major amputation: findings from the Department of Veterans Affairs National Surgical Quality Improvement Program. *Surgery* 2001;130:21-29.
83. Oral Iloprost in Severe Leg Ischaemia Study Group. Two randomized and placebo-controlled studies of an oral prostacyclin analogue (iloprost) in severe leg ischemia. *Eur J Vasc Endovasc Surg* 2000;20: 358-362.
84. Konduru S, Jain AS. Trans-femoral amputation in elderly dysvascular patients: reliable results with a technique of myodesis. *Prosthet Orthot Int* 2007;31:45-50.
85. Gottschalk F. Transfemoral amputation: biomechanics and surgery. *Clin Orthop Relat Res* 1999:15-22.
86. Chadwick SJ, Lewis JD. Above-knee amputation. *Ann R Coll Surg Engl* 1991;73:152-154.
87. Pinzur M. Current concepts: amputation surgery in peripheral vascular disease. *Instruct Course Lect* 1997;46:501-509.
88. Burgess EM, Romano RL, Zettl JH, et al. Amputations of the leg for peripheral vascular insufficiency. *J Bone Joint Surg Am* 1971;53: 874-890.
89. Robinson KP, Hoile R, Coddington T. Skew flap myoplastic below-knee amputation: a preliminary report. *Br J Surg* 1982;69:554-557.
90. Johnson WC, Watkins MT, Hamilton J, et al. Transcutaneous partial oxygen pressure changes following skew flap and Burgess-type below-knee amputations. *Arch Surg* 1997;132:261-263.
91. Harrison JD, Southworth S, Callum KG. Experience with the "skew flap" below-knee amputation. *Br J Surg* 1987;74:930-931.
92. Ruckley CV, Stonebridge PA, Prescott RJ. Skew flap versus long posterior flap in below-knee amputations: multicenter trial. *J Vasc Surg* 1991;13:423-427.
93. Campbell WB, Morris PJ. A prospective randomized comparison of healing in Gritti-Stokes and through-knee amputations. *Ann R Coll Surg Engl* 1987;69:1-4.
94. Sugarbaker PH, Chretien PB. A surgical technique for hip disarticulation. *Surgery* 1981;90:546-553.
95. Pinzur MS, Garla PG, Pluth T, et al. Continuous postoperative infusion of a regional anesthetic after an amputation of the lower extremity: a randomized clinical trial. *J Bone Joint Surg Am* 1996;78:1501-1505.
96. Katsamouris A, Brewster DC, Megerman J, et al. Transcutaneous oxygen tension in selection of amputation level. *Am J Surg* 1984;147: 510-517.
97. Bianchi C, Montalvo V, Ou HW, et al. Pharmacologic risk factor treatment of peripheral arterial disease is lacking and requires vascular surgeon participation. *Ann Vasc Surg* 2007;21:163-166.
98. Jensen TS, Krebs B, Nielsen J, et al. Immediate and long-term phantom limb pain in amputees: incidence, clinical characteristics and relationship to pre-amputation limb pain. *Pain* 1985;21:267-278.
99. Dwyer AJ, Paul R, Mam MK, et al. Modified skew-flap below-knee amputation. *Am J Orthop* 2007;36:123-126.
100. Bach S, Noreng MF, Tjellden NU. Phantom limb pain in amputees during the first 12 months following limb amputation, after preoperative lumbar epidural blockade. *Pain* 1988;33:297-301.
101. Jahangiri M, Jayatunga AP, Bradley JW, et al. Prevention of phantom pain after major lower limb amputation by epidural infusion of diamorphine, clonidine and bupivacaine. *Ann R Coll Surg Engl* 1994;76:324-326.
102. Nikolajsen L, Staehelin JT. Phantom limb pain. *Curr Rev Pain* 2000;4:166-170.
103. Lambert A, Dashfield A, Cosgrove C, et al. Randomized prospective study comparing preoperative epidural and intraoperative perineural analgesia for the prevention of postoperative stump and phantom limb pain following major amputation. *Reg Anesth Pain Med* 2001;26: 316-321.
104. Mars M, McKune A, Robbs JV. A comparison of laser Doppler fluxmetry and transcutaneous oxygen pressure measurement in the dysvascular patient requiring amputation. *Eur J Vasc Endovasc Surg* 1998;16:53-58.
105. Mooney V, Harvey Jr JP, McBride E, et al. Comparison of postoperative stump management: plaster vs. soft dressings. *J Bone Joint Surg Am* 1971;53:241-249.
106. Deutsch A, English RD, Vermeer TC, et al. Removable rigid dressings versus soft dressings: a randomized, controlled study with dysvascular, trans-tibial amputees. *Prosthet Orthot Int* 2005;29:193-200.
107. Woodburn KR, Sockalingham S, Gilmore H, et al. A randomized trial of rigid stump dressing following trans-tibial amputation for peripheral arterial insufficiency. *Prosthet Orthot Int* 2004;28:22-27.
108. Nawijn SE, van der LH, Emmelot CH, et al. Stump management after transtibial amputation: a systematic review. *Prosthet Orthot Int* 2005;29:13-26.
109. Berlemont M, Weber R, Wilson SE. Ten years of experience with the immediate application of prosthetic devices to amputees of the lower extremities on the operating table. *Prosthet Orthot Int* 1969;3: 8-18.
110. Buckley JG. Biomechanical adaptations of transtibial amputee sprinting in athletes using dedicated prostheses. *Clin Biomech (Bristol, Avon)* 2000;15:352-358.
111. Osterman H. The process of amputation and rehabilitation. *Clin Podiatr Med Surg* 1997;14:585-597.
112. Tang PCY, Ravji K, Key JJ, et al. Let them walk. I. Current prosthesis options for leg and foot amputees. *J Am Coll Surg* 2008;206:548-560.
113. Rush DS, Huston CC, Bivins BA, et al. Operative and late mortality rates of above-knee and below-knee amputations. *Am Surg* 1981;47: 36-39.
114. Stone PA, Flaherty SK, Hayes JD, et al. Lower extremity amputation: a contemporary series. *WV Med J* 2007;103:14-18.
115. Dormandy J, Heeck L, Vig S. Major amputations: clinical patterns and predictors. *Semin Vasc Surg* 1999;12:154-161.

Section

III

Acute Limb Ischemia

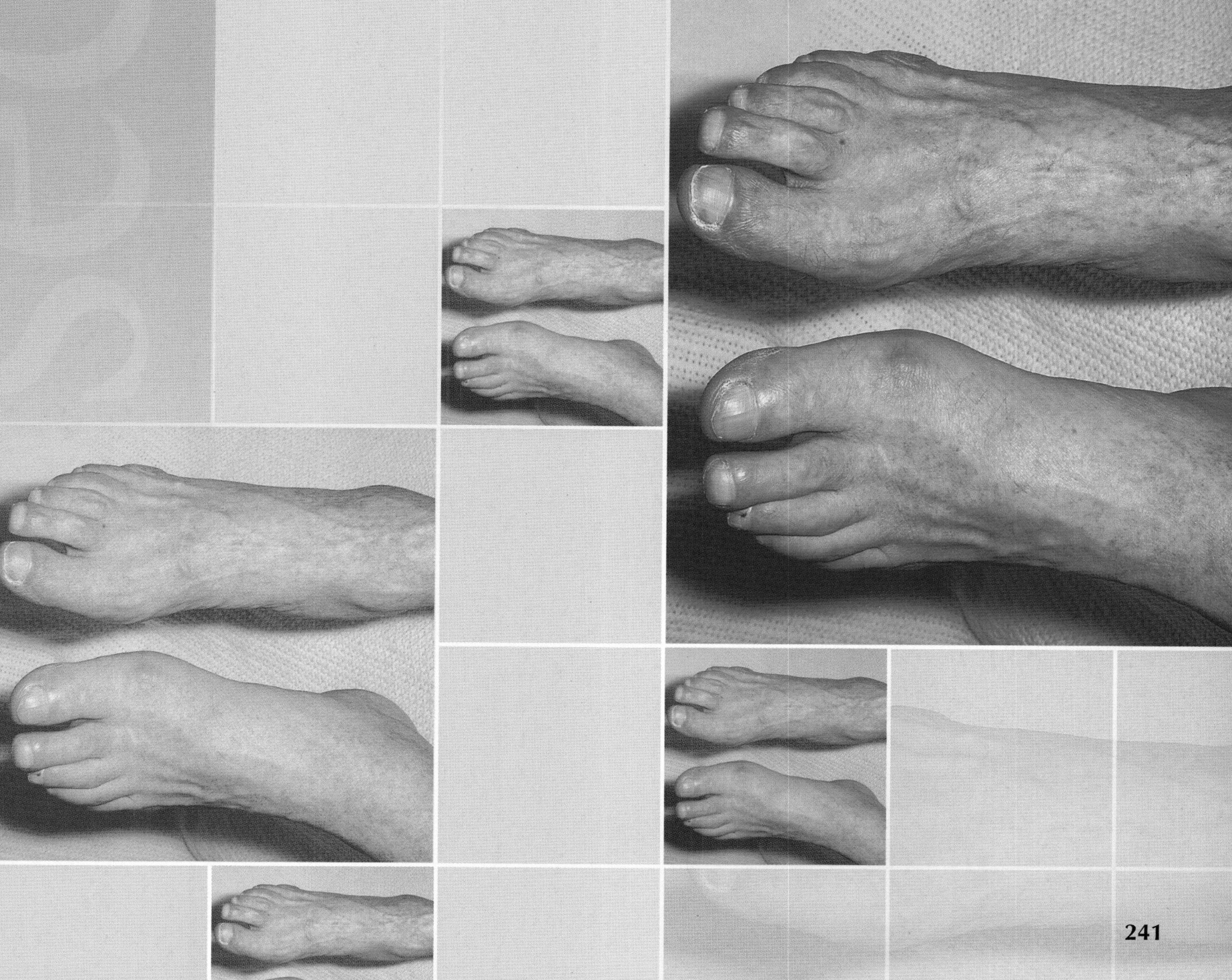

chapter 13

Etiology and Natural History: Diagnosis and Evaluation

John Byrne, MCh FRCSI (Gen)

Key Points

Acute Leg Ischemia

- The incidence of acute leg ischemia is 14 per 100,000 population per year, accounting for 12% of operations in the average vascular unit.
- Acute arterial thrombosis accounts for more episodes of acute leg ischemia than acute emboli.
- With increasing use of endovascular therapy, iatrogenesis is a growing cause of acute leg ischemia.
- Angiography is being replaced by duplex imaging for documenting arterial anatomy, but assessing limb viability and gauging urgency of intervention remain clinical.
- Acute arterial thrombosis carries a greater risk of limb loss; acute arterial embolism carries a greater risk of death.
- Life expectancy for patients with acute leg ischemia is similar to many cancers: only 17% to 44% are still alive at 5 years.
- In the absence of intervention for acute ischemia, two thirds of patients come to immediate amputation. Thrombosis (versus embolism), total ischemia time, advanced age, and omission of postoperative anticoagulation predict a greater chance of amputation.

Acute Arm Ischemia

- Acute arm ischemia accounts for one fifth of limb ischemia (2.4 cases per 100,000 population per year) but has a better prognosis than leg ischemia for both life and limb.
- Arm ischemia is due to embolism in 90% of patients, usually associated with atrial fibrillation. Conservative management is associated with a significant rate of limb dysfunction.

In General

- Vascular specialists have better limb salvage rates than do general surgeons and are increasingly in a position to offer both endovascular and open surgical options.

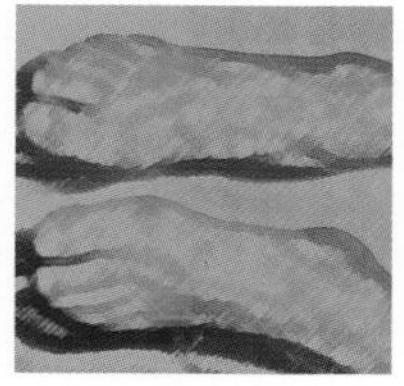

The management of acute arm and leg ischemia is often demanding. The need for urgent intervention is usually clear. However, clinical decisions can be difficult in anesthetized patients or at the extremes of age in nonverbal patients. With acute limb ischemia, the surgeon must restore blood flow quickly, so preoperative testing must be used judiciously. Increasingly, vascular specialists can offer both endovascular and open surgical options, sometimes in the same operating room. Initial symptoms may improve in some patients with anticoagulation, and gauging the urgency of revascularization requires careful judgment. Those who have unsuccessful outcomes for acute ischemia are more likely to end up with an above-knee amputation than are chronically ischemic patients with a failed reconstruction.[1] Not all acutely ischemic limbs are salvageable. Primary amputation can be both appropriate and lifesaving. Rarely, profound limb ischemia may be a manifestation of terminal illness and palliation, rather than aggressive attempts at limb salvage, may be the best approach.

Thromboembolic events still account for more than 90% of cases of acute limb ischemia. The remainder are due to trauma or are iatrogenic. Acute limb ischemia is often taxing, and surgeons may need to employ their full armamentarium, from simple embolectomy to complex extraanatomic and tibial bypass.

Despite the nihilism and frustration that sometimes attends management of acute limb ischemia, attempts at limb salvage are worthwhile and satisfying. Limb salvage can be achieved in up to 80% of patients.[2] Initial diagnosis and clinical evaluation are crucial for good outcomes.

ACUTE LEG ISCHEMIA

Diagnostic Criteria

Clinical Evaluation

Acute limb ischemia was redefined by the Trans-Atlantic Inter-Society Consensus (TASC II) Working Group in 2007 as "any sudden decrease in limb perfusion causing a potential threat to limb viability."[3] The emphasis is on threat to limb survival. It excludes sudden changes in limb perfusion that do not endanger the limb, such as acute onset claudication. No reliable biochemical or radiological markers of limb viability exist. Initial assessment of the "threatened limb," therefore, is clinical.

History (Three P's)

Pain

Pain is usually the first symptom. With embolus or trauma, the pain is acute; with in situ arterial thrombosis, the onset is more insidious. Once established, however, the pain is severe. It requires opiates but can be resistant to narcotic analgesia. The patient complains of diffuse pain throughout the entire affected limb—a distinguishing point from the rest pain of chronic ischemia, which is limited to the forefoot. In the neonate with acute ischemia due to iatrogenic intervention, or the elderly confused patient, no history may be forthcoming.

Pain accompanies leg ischemia, with one exception: in acute aortic thrombosis with profound leg ischemia, the first symptom may be paralysis and not pain. This has led to patients being referred incorrectly to a neurologist or internist. Batz and Brückner[4] reported that 84% of patients with acute aortic occlusion presented with paralysis. Only 14% had pain, and 55% had already been referred to a neurologist.

Paresthesia

Paresthesia, when present, is a clear indication of deteriorating neurological function and is a sign of progressive ischemia. Proprioception and light sensation are conveyed by small myelinated fibers and are lost early in acute ischemia. Larger sensory nerves convey temperature, pain, and pressure, and these are maintained unless ischemia is prolonged.

Paralysis

Paralysis is an ominous symptom. It is also a misnomer. It should be termed "loss of motor function," as it reflects ischemic myopathy rather than nerve hypoperfusion. Loss of function of the intrinsic muscles of the foot occurs first (patients cannot flex and extend toes). Absent foot dorsiflexion and plantar flexion indicate loss of function of the extensor and flexor muscles of the lower leg. If ischemia continues, patients develop calf tenderness due to swelling of the gastrocnemius and soleus muscles, although the anterior compartment muscles can also be affected. This indicates muscle infarction. In patients with paralysis or muscle tenderness, there is no place for expectant management with anticoagulants. These patients need urgent restoration of blood flow. Passive movement of the ankle may show the foot to be unyielding and "fixed" due to degeneration of the muscle fibers, leading to loss of elasticity. After 8 hours of absolute ischemia, skeletal muscle becomes rigid and contracted (muscle rigor) indicating an unsalvageable limb.

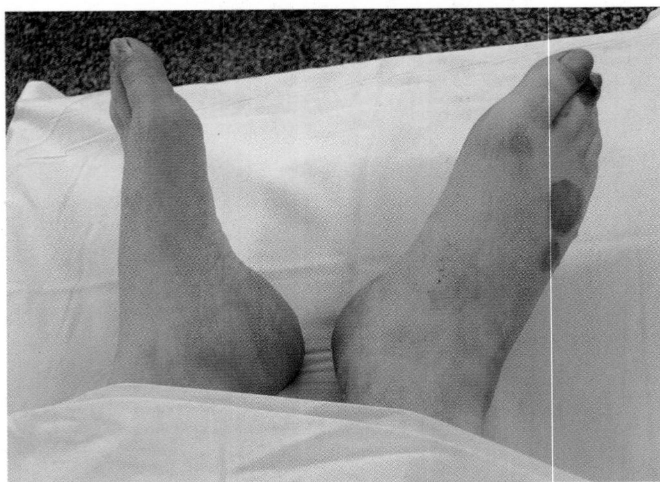

Figure 13-1. Waxy white appearance of a profoundly ischemic right leg before above-knee amputation.

Clinical Examination (Three P's)

Pallor

Pallor indicates obstruction of a major arterial trunk to the leg. In the absence of collateral circulation, this produces a marble white, waxy leg with absent capillary refill and collapsed veins or "venous guttering" (Figure 13-1). The leg may even appear cadaveric. In arterial thrombosis, initial pallor may be followed by gradual improvement, with return of skin perfusion and capillary refill, over 6 to 12 hours due to opening of preformed collaterals. Capillary refill on blanching the skin indicates that the leg is still retrievable, even if the foot is mottled and cyanosed. However, fixed mottling and fixed staining (cyanosed or purple areas of skin that fail to blanch on pressure) indicate that the capillaries have thrombosed and ruptured. Such limbs are unsalvageable. Fixed staining may also be seen in synergistic gangrene, especially gas gangrene. These patients often are septic, and the relative warmth of the affected leg and the finding of crepitus are important differentiating clinical signs.

Pulselessness

Pulselessness is the absolute prerequisite of acute ischemia. In the presence of a full set of peripheral pulses, arterial ischemia can be excluded and other diagnoses for acute foot pain and cyanosis should be entertained, such as blue toe syndrome

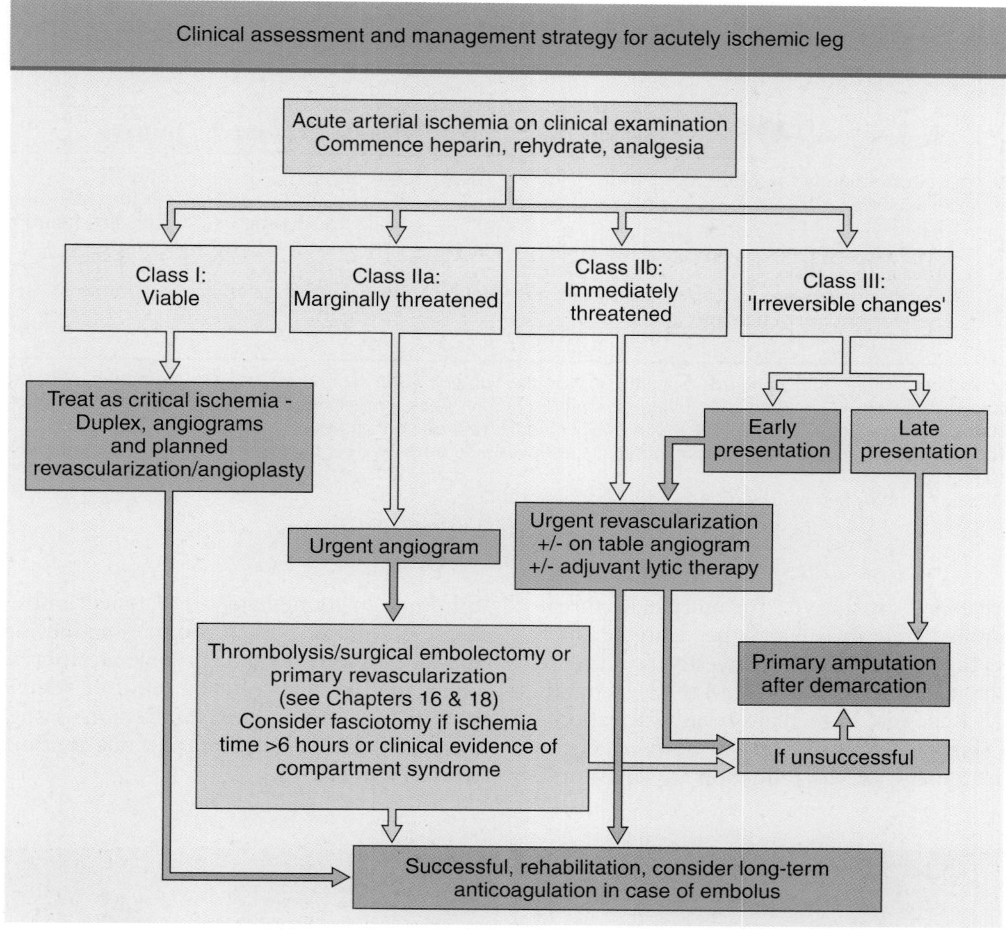

Figure 13-2. Clinical assessment and management strategy for an acutely ischemic leg.

(atheroemboli lodging in the digital arteries) or venous gangrene (often a paraneoplastic syndrome). An intact set of pulses in the contralateral leg suggests an embolic process in the affected one; absent pulses in the contralateral leg indicate underlying peripheral arterial disease and point to in situ thrombosis. The discovery of a popliteal artery aneurysm in either leg suggests popliteal aneurysm thrombosis as the cause of acute ischemia.

Perishing Cold

Perishing cold is easy to elicit, especially when compared to the other leg. However, in an acute aortic occlusion, both legs will be equally cold. Correlating the extent of coolness with the level of an arterial occlusion is difficult, but if the buttock and thigh are cold and cyanosed, an aortoiliac occlusion is likely.

Leg Viability: How Quickly Is Intervention Needed on Clinical Grounds?

Most patients present within 2 weeks of the acute event and with a spectrum of leg ischemia. While the diagnosis can be made quickly when the preceding signs and symptoms are present, assessing viability can be difficult and requires good judgment. Most vascular surgeons prefer to operate in the daytime, with all support systems in place. However, knowing which patients need to go to the operating room immediately is not just intuitive or the result of years of accumulated wisdom—clinical pointers help (Figure 13-2).

Systematic Approach

In response to the need for uniform reporting standards, a scoring system was derived by the Society for Vascular Surgery/International Society for Cardiovascular Surgery (SVS/ISCVS; Table 13-1). It was initially devised in 1986[5] and modified in 1997.[6] It requires clinical assessment of motor and sensory function in the limb and the use of a handheld Doppler probe. While not tested prospectively in a clinical setting, it at least offers guidance. Inevitably, a small number of patients do not fit comfortably into any category.

Viable

The viable category usually includes patients with acute-on-chronic arterial thrombosis. The onset is sudden, but sensation is preserved and normal motor function is present. The leg is noticeably cooler. Doppler examination detects both arterial and venous signals. Patients in this group require no immediate intervention and can be anticoagulated while investigations are organized (Figure 13-3A).

Table 13-1
SVS/ISCVS Criteria for Limb Viability* †

Category	Description/Prognosis	Findings		Doppler Signals	
		Sensory Loss	Muscle Weakness	Arterial	Venous
I. Viable	Not immediately threatened	None	None	Audible	Audible
II. Threatened					
a. Marginally	Salvageable if promptly treated	Minimal or none	None	(Often) inaudible	Audible
b. Immediately	Salvageable with immediate revascularization	More than toes; often rest pain	Mild, moderate	(Usually) inaudible	Audible
III. Irreversible	Major tissue loss or permanent nerve damage inevitable	Profound, anesthetic	Profound, paralysis (rigor)	Inaudible	Inaudible

From the Ad Hoc Committee on Reporting Standards, Society for Vascular Surgery/North American Chapter, International Society for Cardiovascular Surgery. Suggested standards for reports dealing with lower extremity ischemia. *J Vasc Surg* 1986;4:80-94. Rutherford RB, Baker JD, Ernst C, et al. Recommended standards for reports dealing with lower extremity ischemia: revised version. *J Vasc Surg* 1997;26(3):517-538.
*SVS/ISCVS, Society of Vascular Surgery/International Society for Cardiovascular Surgery; TEE, transesophageal echocardiography; TTE, transthoracic echocardiography.
†Clinical categories of acute limb ischemia (based on SVS/ISCVS classification).

Threatened

All legs in the threatened category (A for marginally threatened and B for immediately threatened) need urgent intervention. However, there is still time for investigation in level IIA ischemia, as long as close surveillance of the leg is maintained. In level IIB ischemia, immediate revascularization is needed. Reduced skin sensation is found in both categories. In marginally threatened legs, the reduction in sensation is minimal; in immediately threatened limbs, the reduction is more profound. Loss of motor function indicates an immediately threatened limb. In general, arterial Doppler signals are inaudible in threatened legs but venous signals are still present. Of course, this subdivision is slightly artificial. In practice, patients present as part of a continuous clinical spectrum (Figure 13-3B).

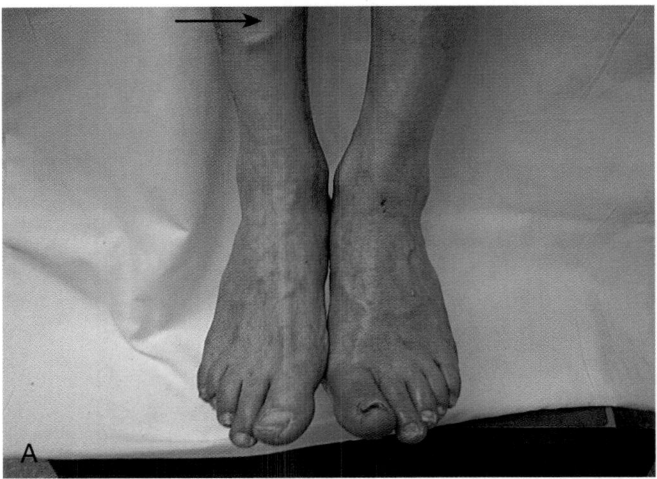

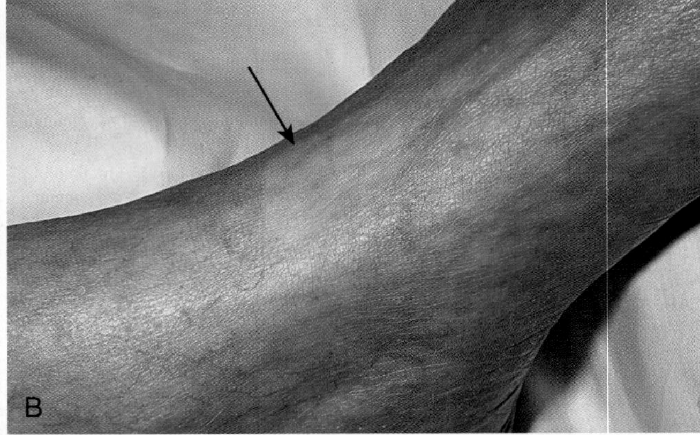

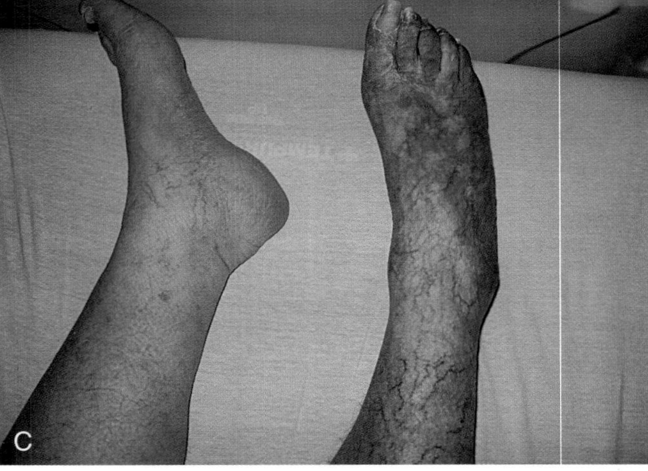

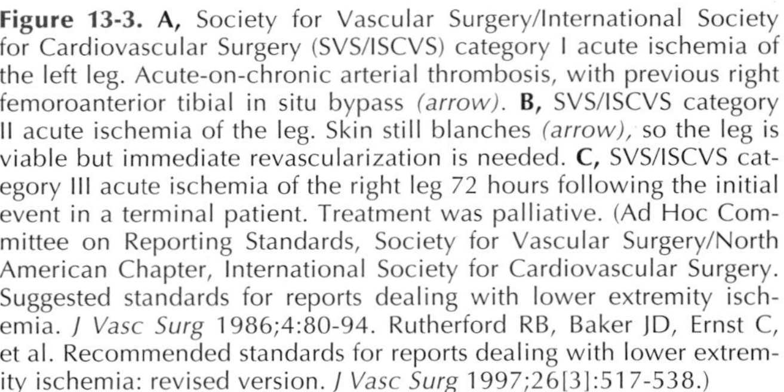

Figure 13-3. A, Society for Vascular Surgery/International Society for Cardiovascular Surgery (SVS/ISCVS) category I acute ischemia of the left leg. Acute-on-chronic arterial thrombosis, with previous right femoroanterior tibial in situ bypass *(arrow)*. **B,** SVS/ISCVS category II acute ischemia of the leg. Skin still blanches *(arrow)*, so the leg is viable but immediate revascularization is needed. **C,** SVS/ISCVS category III acute ischemia of the right leg 72 hours following the initial event in a terminal patient. Treatment was palliative. (Ad Hoc Committee on Reporting Standards, Society for Vascular Surgery/North American Chapter, International Society for Cardiovascular Surgery. Suggested standards for reports dealing with lower extremity ischemia. *J Vasc Surg* 1986;4:80-94. Rutherford RB, Baker JD, Ernst C, et al. Recommended standards for reports dealing with lower extremity ischemia: revised version. *J Vasc Surg* 1997;26[3]:517-538.)

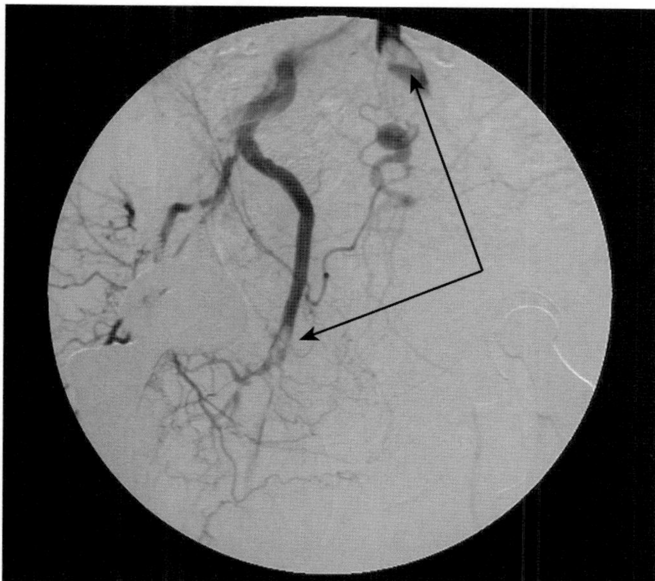

Figure 13-4. Bilateral arterial emboli *(arrows)* affecting the left common iliac and right common femoral arteries. Note normal vessels and classic meniscus signs on both sides. Emboli are often multiple and can cause bilateral ischemia.

Irreversible

A cold cyanosed limb with fixed staining and calf muscle rigor is clearly unsalvageable. Sensory loss is profound, and Doppler examination fails to elicit either arterial or venous signals (especially in the popliteal vein). Such patients are usually systemically unwell and may require expeditious amputation to save their life (Figure 13-3C).

Pragmatic Approach

In many centers, a more practical approach is often employed. Patients with acute onset symptoms with normal or reduced sensation and normal motor function are anticoagulated, and imaging is arranged. Patients with absent sensation and decreased motor function undergo emergency surgery. Evidence shows that such an approach is employed widely. In a 1998 survey,[7] Swedish surgeons ranked loss of motor function as the most important indicator of the need for immediate surgery. Doppler signals, as suggested by the SVS/ISCVS classification, were ranked very low. Emergency revascularization, as opposed to heparinization and scheduled angiography, was needed in approximately 30% of patients with an acutely ischemic leg.[8]

Regardless of the approach used initially to evaluate an acutely ischemic leg, if treatment is to be delayed, the impaired leg must be monitored closely. A leg that appears "viable" in the evening can easily be "irreversible" by morning.

Angiography: When Is It Required?

In patients with acute leg ischemia, traditional teaching is that investigations should not delay revascularization. However, preoperative imaging can reduce operating time, and angiography is entirely appropriate for patients with viable or marginally threatened legs (category I and IIA ischemia). However, many patients with acute leg ischemia present outside the working schedule of most vascular technologists or radiology technicians. On-table angiograms are an alternative, and with the increasing sophistication of vascular operating rooms, the quality of these images match those of the interventional radiology suite. However, in many hospitals, this is still not the case and the quality of images obtained in the operating room is often poor. In patients with renal insufficiency or dye allergies, carbon dioxide can give reasonable pictures. Gadolinium is no longer used in the United States for patients with renal impairment due to the risk of nephrogenic systemic fibrosis.[9]

In Albany, New York, a low threshold exists for obtaining angiograms, partly because most surgeons perform their own studies. Providing angiography does not delay surgery by a substantial amount; it allows for a more focused and directed approach to revascularization (Figure 13-4) and reduces time spent exploring occluded arteries. It also allows treatment of inflow lesion before embarking on emergency distal bypass, for example.

Other Imaging Modalities

Duplex imaging is a noninvasive alternative that gives similar information to angiography in expert hands. Many vascular specialists have prompt access to a vascular laboratory or are gaining expertise themselves, such that an anatomical diagnosis can be obtained quickly using duplex, even at the patient's bedside.[10]

In addition, magnetic resonance angiography and in particular computed tomography angiography are becoming more widely available for assessment of the acutely ischemic leg. Despite advances in both modalities, they still fall short of catheter angiography, in particular since they do not allow simultaneous endovascular therapy.

The Role of Routine Echocardiography and Thrombophilia Screening

In a patient with an acutely ischemic leg who has been treated successfully, the question is, what precipitated the problem? This often prompts a reflex ordering of an echocardiogram and a thrombophilia screen (activated protein C resistance, factor V Leiden, homocysteine levels, antithrombin III, protein C, protein S, lupus anticoagulant, and anticardiolipin antibodies). However, how often do they actually alter management?

Echocardiography

Following embolectomy, many patients are referred for transthoracic echocardiography (TTE) as part of the hunt for the source of the embolus. The yield for this test is variably reported between 5% and 56%.[11,12] Many surgeons think that even 5% is an overestimate, and TTE has such a low return for good reasons. The left atrial appendage is the most common source of cardiac thrombus, but it is poorly visualized by TTE. The maximum resolution of TTE is 2 mm, which means that small vegetations on the valve leaflets are not visible. TTE alters management of patients with acute leg ischemia less than 5% of the time. Transesophageal echocardiography (TEE), although more invasive, readily demonstrates the left atrium and ascending aorta with good resolution. It also detects very low flow prethrombotic areas (spontaneous echocontrast). In the setting of peripheral arterial embolism, it is significantly better than TTE imaging in detecting cardiac lesions.[13] However, it is difficult to prove conclusively that any defect detected is the source of the embolus. If TTE is negative (95% of patients), only an additional 0% to 4% of patients

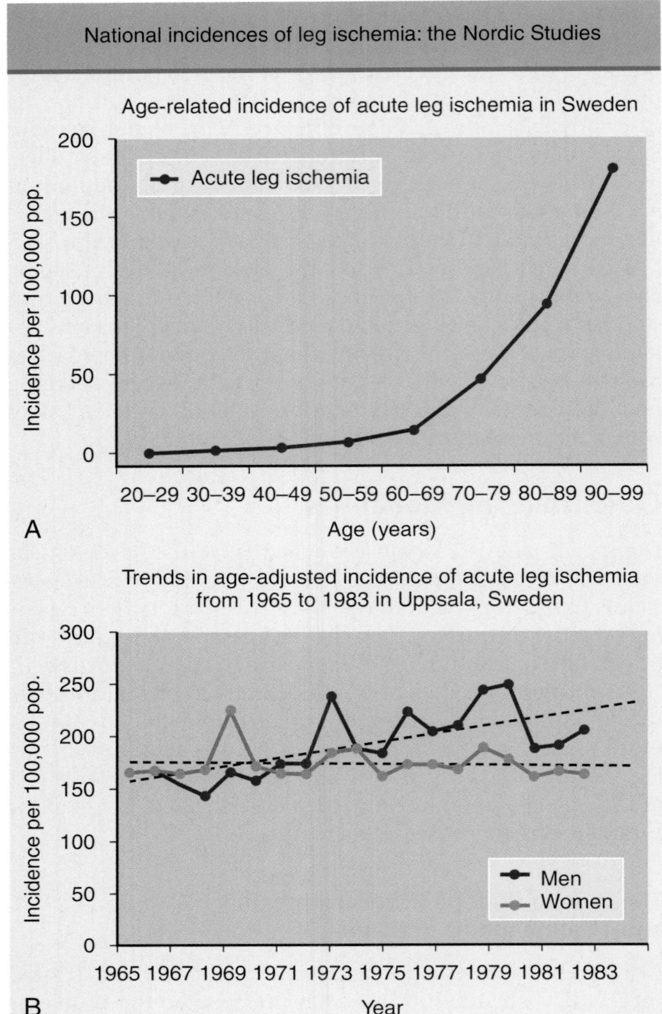

Figure 13-5. National incidences of leg ischemia: the Nordic studies. **A,** Age-related incidence of acute leg ischemia in Sweden. **B,** Trends in age-adjusted incidence of acute leg ischemia from 1965 to 1983 in Uppsala, Sweden. (**A,** Dryjski M, Swedenborg J. Acute ischemia of the extremities in a metropolitan area during one year. *J Cardiovasc Surg [Torino]* 1984;25[6]:518-522. **B,** Ljungman C, Adami HO, Bergqvist D, et al. Risk factors for early lower limb loss after embolectomy for acute arterial occlusion: a population-based case-control study. *Br J Surg* 1991;78[12]:1482-1485.)

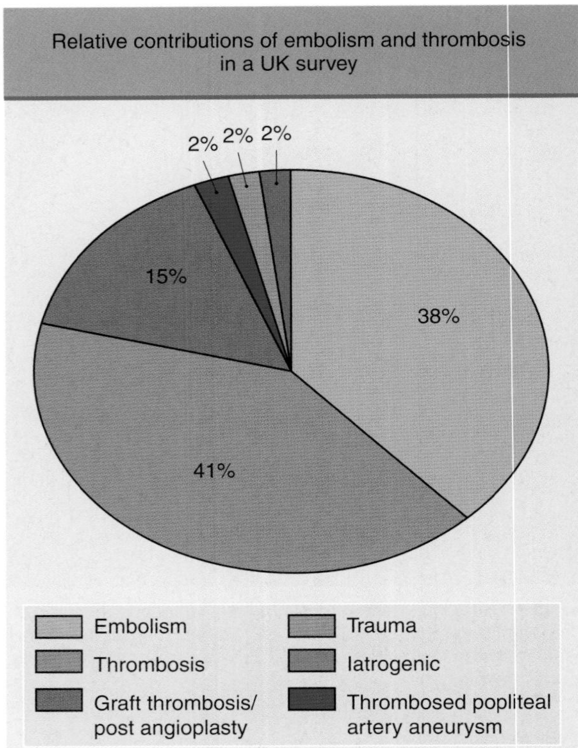

Figure 13-6. Relative contributions of embolism and thrombosis in a UK survey. (Davies B, Braithwaite BD, Birch PA, et al. Acute leg ischaemia in Gloucestershire. *Br J Surg* 1997;84[4]:504-508.)

have their management altered by subsequent TEE.[12] While TTE should not be abandoned, especially in today's litigious environment, where it might be regarded as the standard of care, the limitations of the investigation are clear.

Thrombophilia Screening

Most patients are placed on lifelong warfarin following an episode of acute limb ischemia, with good reason in the case of peripheral arterial emboli, making a diagnostic workup irrelevant. Scant evidence in the literature supports routine thrombophilia screening in patients with acute leg ischemia. The TASC II report[3] in 2007 recommended that a thrombophilia screen (anticardiolipin and antiplatelet factor IV antibodies) and measurement of homocysteine levels be performed in young patients with acute arterial thrombosis or in those with a strong family history of thrombotic events and no predisposing cause for thrombosis. Contemporary literature goes further and dismisses any link between inherited thrombophilias or homocysteine levels and arterial thrombosis.[13-15]

Prevalence and Incidence

National Incidences of Leg Ischemia

The Nordic Studies

Much of the early epidemiological data on acute leg ischemia came from Sweden (Figure 13-5). In 1984, Dryjski and Swedenborg[16] estimated the crude incidence of acute leg ischemia in greater Stockholm (population 1.5 million) to be 9 per 100,000, with a peak incidence of 180 per 100,000 in patients over 90. Subsequently, Ljungman et al.[17] analyzed temporal trends in acute ischemia over a 19-year interval (1965 to 1983) in Uppsala (population 1.3 million). They demonstrated an annual increase of 2.7% to 3.9% over the study interval. Some of this might be expected in an aging population; however, even when age adjusted, a 2.7% annual increase occurred in men.[18] More contemporary data are needed to see whether this trend has continued or the incidence has peaked. The Swedish vascular registry (Swedvasc) was established in 1987. In 1998, it reported an average national incidence of acute leg ischemia of 13 per 100,000 population.[19] The Finnish vascular registry (Finnvasc) covers a population of 5 million. While no incidence figures are available, the committee identified 509 cases of acute ischemia over 23 months.[20]

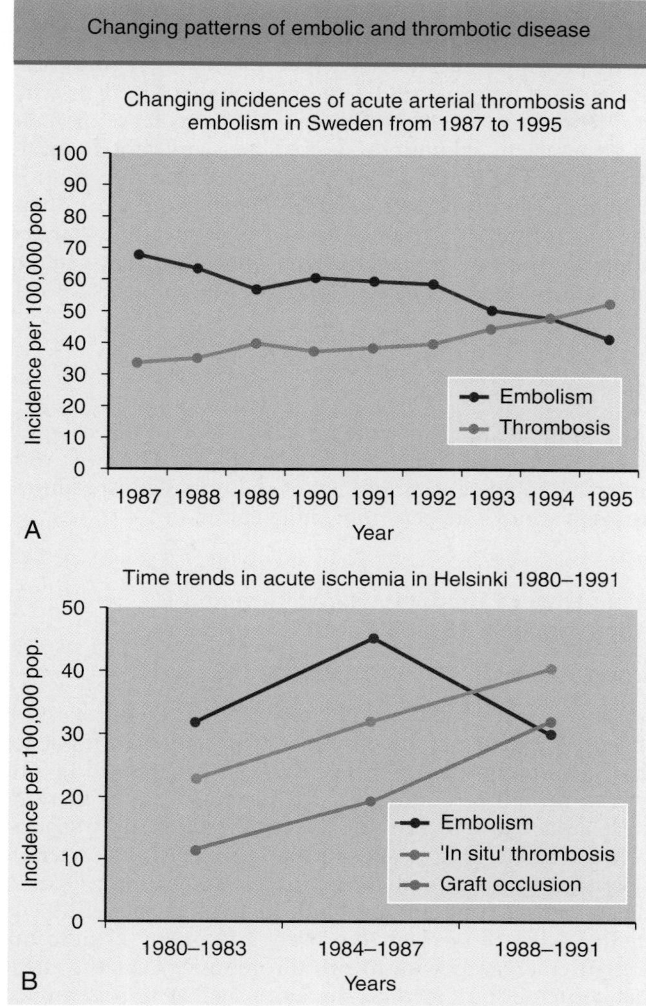

Figure 13-7. Changing patterns of embolic and thrombotic disease. **A,** Changing incidences of acute arterial thrombosis and embolism in Sweden from 1987 to 1995. **B,** Time trends in acute ischemia in Helsinki from 1980 to 1991. (**A,** Bergqvist D, Tröeng T, Elfstrom J, et al. Auditing surgical outcome: ten years with the Swedish vascular registry, Swedvasc. *Eur J Surg* 1998;164[S7]:3-32. **B,** Luther M, Alback A. Acute leg ischemia: a case for the junior surgeon? *Ann Chir Gynaecol* 1995;84:373-378.)

The British Studies

In 1989, Clason et al.[21] reported that the incidence of acute leg ischemia in southeast Scotland was 3.7 per 100,000 population. This was based on a survey of patients referred to the regional specialist unit in Edinburgh. The Gloucestershire study in 1997 proposed a definition of acute limb ischemia as "sudden deterioration in the circulation of a previously symptom-free leg at rest"[22] (Figure 13-6). This definition is remarkably close to the one subsequently adopted by the TASC group in 2000. The incidence of acute leg ischemia was estimated for the county of Gloucestershire (population 540,000) for a single year (1994) using hospital charts, general practice records, and death certificates. The incidence was 14 per 100,000 population. When thrombosed vascular grafts were included, the incidence in Gloucestershire rose to 16 per 100,000.

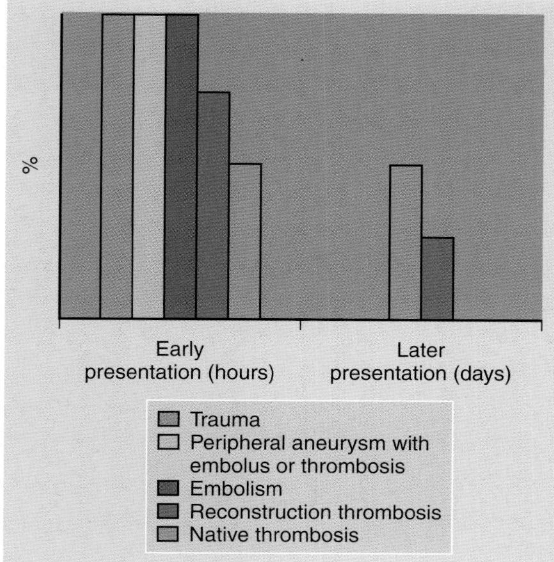

Figure 13-8. Time to presentation in relation to etiology. (Adapted from Norgren L, Hiatt WR, Dormandy JA, et al.; TASC II Working Group. Inter-society consensus for the management of peripheral arterial disease [TASC II]. *J Vasc Surg* 2007;45[Suppl]:S5-S67.)

Acute versus Chronic Ischemia

Acute leg ischemia is less common than chronic ischemia. From data supplied by national vascular registers, acute leg ischemia accounts for 11.9% of operations undertaken by vascular surgeons. Chronic ischemia, by comparison, comprises 40.2% of vascular reconstructions. This would reflect the experience of many vascular surgeons.[23]

Changing Patterns of Embolic and Thrombotic Disease

The relative incidences of acute arterial thrombosis and embolism have altered over the past decades (Figure 13-7). Previously, acute arterial embolus was the commonest cause of limb ischemia; now it is in situ thrombosis. Arterial emboli have declined for several reasons: the disappearance of rheumatic fever, aggressive surgical management of rheumatic valve lesions, and use of systemic anticoagulation for atrial fibrillation. At the same time, the at-risk population for arterial thrombosis has increased with the aging of most Western populations. Data from single centers suggest that embolic disease is now responsible for as few as 9% of episodes of acute leg ischemia.[24] However, population data show the change has been more gradual. Data from Sweden[19] covering 1987 to 1995 show the incidence of embolism has declined from 65% to 43% (Figure 13-7A). A survey of British vascular surgeons in 1998 showed less dramatic differences (in situ thrombosis at 44%, embolus at 40%, and graft occlusion at 16%).[25]

Timing of Presentation

As pointed out in the TASC II document,[3] the timing of presentation is related to the severity of ischemia and access to health care (Figure 13-8). Patients with trauma present early, as might be expected. Patients with acute arterial emboli and

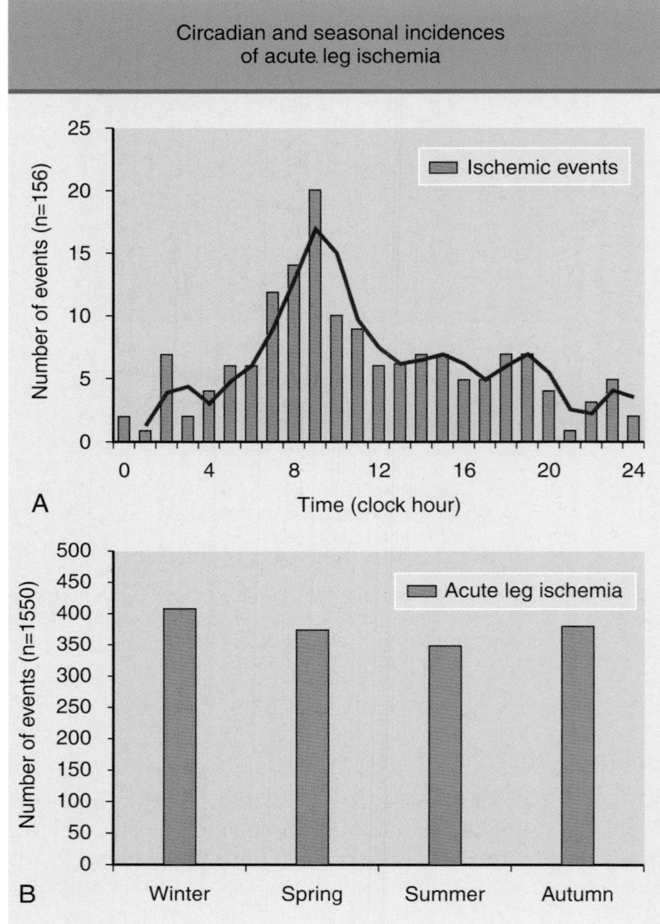

Figure 13-9. Circadian **(A)** and seasonal **(B)** incidences of acute leg ischemia. (**A,** Manfredini R, Gallerani M, Portaluppi F, et al. Circadian variation in the onset of acute critical limb ischemia. *Thromb Res* 1998;92[4]:163-169. **B,** Kuukasjärvi P, Salenius JP, Lepäntalo M, et al.; Finnvasc Study Group. Weekly and seasonal variation of hospital admissions and outcome in patients with acute lower limb ischaemia treated by surgical and endovascular means. *Int Angiol* 2000;19[4]:354-357.)

thrombosed popliteal artery aneurysms also are similar early presenters due to the severity of ischemia and the lack of collaterals. Patients with an occluded prosthetic graft also tend to present early, quite often with profound ischemia due to extension of thrombus into the native arteries. Late presenters usually include patients with in situ thrombosis or those with an occluded vein bypass graft or an occluded stent.

Circadian and Seasonal Incidences

Evidence is accumulating for a circadian pattern to cardiovascular events (Figure 13-9).[26] Transient myocardial ischemia has a diurnal peak, usually within 1 to 2 hours of awakening. Neural and hormonal factors also follow a diurnal variation, as do vasoconstrictors such as norepinephrine and renin. Fibrinogen and factor VIII also have a morning peak, and plasma fibrinolytic activity has a morning trough. Analysis of the circadian incidence of acute leg ischemia has shown that it, too, has a morning peak, with a large cluster of events around 9 AM.[27] Interestingly, paroxysmal atrial fibrillation also has a morning peak.

While a circadian variation in acute leg ischemia is plausible, seasonal variations in the incidence of cardiovascular events are more questionable. In 1983, it was reported the incidence of brachial and femoral emboli peaked in winter.[28] However, a review of the monthly incidence of acute leg ischemia in Edinburgh showed no significant monthly variation.[29] The Finnvasc study group revisited the question in 2000 in a study of 1550 patients.[30] They found that admissions for acute leg ischemia peaked in winter but that the difference was not significant. They concluded that patients with acute limb ischemia seek help in a nonuniform seasonal pattern.

Etiology

The common causes of acute leg ischemia have not changed over the past decade (Figures 13-10 and 13-11). However, with increasing sophistication and use of endovascular procedures, iatrogenic causes are becoming more common.

Acute Lower Extremity Arterial Thrombosis (Approximately 50% of Cases)

Atherosclerosis

Peripheral arterial disease is clearly the commonest cause of acute leg ischemia. It comprises most patients with acute arterial thrombosis. Atherosclerosis can progress to in situ arterial thrombosis and acute leg ischemia due to increasing plaque burden, intraplaque hemorrhage, or transient hypotension leading to clot formation in diseased arteries. The risk for patients with intermittent claudication progressing to critical ischemia and limb loss has been well documented.[3] It is less clear, however, how many claudicants present emergently with in situ thrombosis. Also, the effect that contemporary medical therapies such as statins, angiotensin-converting enzyme inhibitors and antiplatelet agents, have had in reducing such events has not been studied in detail. Most vascular surgeons would probably agree that, among their own population of medically managed patients with claudication, the number who present with acute leg ischemia is low. Anecdotally, most acute in situ thrombosis seems to occur in patients with undiagnosed peripheral arterial disease.

Popliteal Artery Disease

Acute popliteal artery occlusion can be particularly difficult to manage. In elderly men, thrombosed popliteal artery aneurysms account for 10% of acute arterial occlusions. Up to 50% of these patients also have a contralateral popliteal aneurysm.[31] Amputation rates can be high, even with aggressive thrombolytic and surgical management. Popliteal artery entrapment syndrome is caused by compression of a healthy popliteal artery by an anomalous medial head of gastrocnemius muscle. It ought to be considered in an otherwise fit and healthy man younger than 40 years with severe acute ischemia due to popliteal artery thrombosis. Often, a history of claudication exists, but occasionally it presents acutely. It is bilateral in 25% of cases. Cystic adventitial disease of the popliteal artery is much less common but can cause popliteal artery compression; patients usually present with claudication, not acute ischemia.

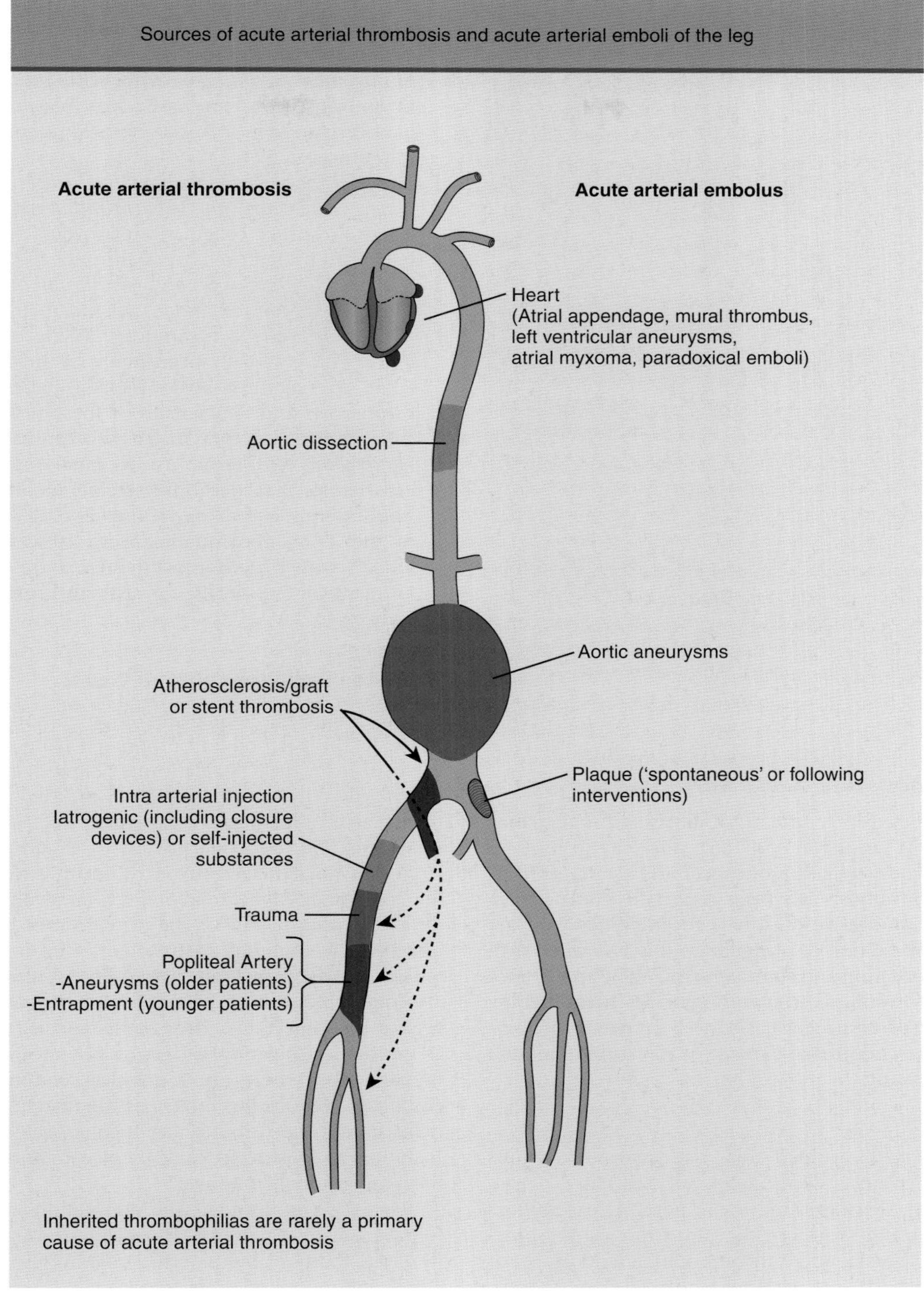

Figure 13-10. Sources of acute arterial thrombosis **(A)** and acute arterial emboli **(B)** of the leg.

Aortic Dissection and Intraarterial Injection

Other conditions that predispose patients to thrombosis are aortic dissection and intraarterial injection of narcotics by intravenous drug users. Aortic dissection ought to be considered in any patient who complains of severe chest pain before developing acute ischemia. Lower limb vessels are involved in 10% of patients, and rarely acute leg ischemia may be the first presentation of acute aortic dissection. It usually predicts a poor outcome, as the visceral branches of the aorta are also likely to be involved.[32]

Intravascular injection of narcotics causes intense vasospasm of the entire artery and is a significant source of acute ischemia in young people in Western countries.

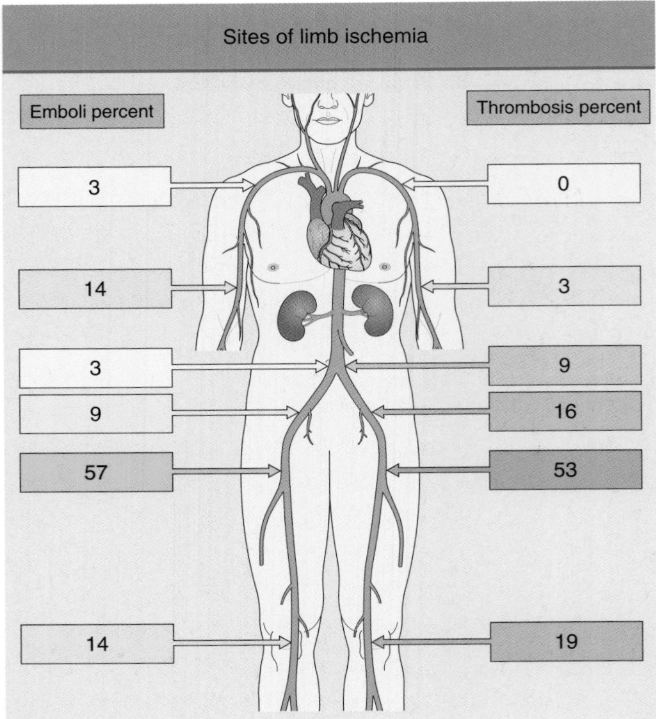

Figure 13-11. Sites of limb ischemia. (Adapted from Dryjski).[54]

Arterial Thrombosis and Malignancy

The association between venous thrombosis and malignancy was recognized by Trousseau[33] in 1861, allegedly in himself. Less common is the association of cancer and arterial thrombosis. Arterial thrombosis has been reported in association with lung, breast, and gastrointestinal cancers. When it occurs as the initial manifestation of malignancy, it is associated with a high risk of amputation and short survival.[34] The appearance of acute arterial thrombosis after commencing chemotherapy with cisplatin-based treatment is also well known to oncologists, due either to endothelial damage or elevation of plasma von Willebrand factor.[35]

Thrombophilia

Hypercoagulable states are particular risk factors for venous thrombosis. In certain circumstances, such as failed bypass grafts or occluded stents, they may be important contributors to arterial thrombosis. However, they are a rare cause of primary acute leg ischemia, and a thrombophilia workup is not indicated for most patients with acute arterial insufficiency. Nonetheless, they warrant consideration.

1. *Factor V Leiden mutation.* Activated protein C resistance is present in 12% of whites. In 90% of cases, activated protein C resistance is attributable to a mutation in the factor V gene (factor V Leiden). It predicts early graft thrombosis and is found in 35% of patients under 51 years with leg ischemia.[36]
2. *Antiphospholipid antibody syndrome.* The presence of lupus anticoagulants and anticardiolipin antibodies characterizes this syndrome. Up to 30% of patients with the syndrome suffer venous thrombosis during their lives. Peripheral arterial reconstructions in patients with antiphospholipid antibody syndrome are 5.6 times more likely to fail.
3. *Endogenous fibrinolytic system.* These defects also seem important. In young patients with unexplained arterial thrombosis, deficient tissue-type plasminogen activator has been found in 45% and elevated plasminogen activator inhibitor-1 in 59%.
4. *Hyperfibrinogenemia, elevated Von Willebrand factor, "sticky platelet syndrome," and heparin-induced thrombocytopenia.* These are other coagulation disorders that predispose a patient to premature arterial thrombosis.
5. *Protein C, protein S, and antithrombin III deficiencies.* These are all natural anticoagulants; their lack predisposes patients to venous thrombosis. While often touted, few reports have actually been made of these defects causing acute arterial thrombosis. Usually, patients with arterial thrombosis and deficiencies of these proteins have other significant risk factors, such as severe atherosclerosis.
6. *Hyperhomocysteinemia.* An accepted risk factor for atherosclerosis is hyperhomocysteinemia. It was previously implicated in acute arterial thrombosis.[37] This is reflected in the TASC recommendations. However, today, individuals with hyperhomocysteinemia are believed to have an identical risk profile for arterial thrombosis as normal subjects.[15]

Acute Leg Embolism (40% of Cases)

Approximately three quarters of leg emboli originate in the heart. In the past, emboli originated from rheumatic aortic valves or from atrial fibrillation as a consequence of rheumatic mitral valve disease. Now, emboli mostly arise from clot in the left atrial appendage of patients with atrial fibrillation due to atherosclerotic coronary artery disease or, less commonly, from clot on damaged myocardium due to recent myocardial ischemia. Myocardial infarction results in an area of dyskinesia that promotes the formation of mural thrombus. Thrombus is found at postmortem in up to 40% of patients with acute myocardial infarction. Ventricular aneurysms may also develop and become a source for recurrent emboli. Of course, emboli can arise from other cardiac pathologies such as mechanical heart valves, bacterial endocarditis, and atrial myxoma, but these are much less common. Paradoxical embolism (venous thrombus passing through a cardiac septal defect) is also a possibility, although it is seldom encountered. It should be considered in a patient with both venous thrombosis and arterial embolism.

Regardless of etiology, the destination of cardiac emboli follows a distinct pattern: the leg is most often affected (50% to 60%), followed by the arm (15% to 20%), brain (15% to 20%), and mesenteric vessels (5%).

The remaining leg emboli (approximately 25%) arise from extracardiac sources. Of these, atherosclerotic plaques account for two thirds and aneurysms (usually abdominal aortic aneurysm) account for most of the remainder. In some cases, emboli from atherosclerotic plaques are the consequence of an endovascular procedure.

Preventing arterial emboli, naturally, should be the goal. Atrial fibrillation is the biggest single contributor. Adequate prophylactic anticoagulation should prevent emboli in patients with atrial fibrillation. However, in 2006, a study in the United Kingdom showed that two thirds of patients with acute arterial emboli and atrial fibrillation presenting to their unit were not on anticoagulants.[11,37] Of course, just taking the medication is not enough; it is clear that tight control of anticoagulation is also important as those with good international normalized ratio control have a significantly lower number of thromboembolic events compared to those with poor control.[38]

Iatrogenic Trauma (5% of Cases)

As the number of percutaneous and endoluminal vascular procedures increases, the risk of vascular injury has also risen.[39,40] Iatrogenic arterial trauma now accounts for one third of acute arterial injuries, mainly to the femoral artery. The risk of acute ischemia in diagnostic angiography is low at 0.10% to 0.15%. For diagnostic studies, a low-profile catheter such as a 4 French (Fr) or 5 Fr is used, which is tolerated well by most patients. When therapeutic intervention is required, 6-Fr systems or larger are used and the incidence of complications rises to 1% to 2%, although for femoral catheterization, bleeding, or pseudoaneurysm formation is more common than ischemia. For endovascular repair of abdominal aortic aneurysms, the size of the sheath used is typically 12 Fr or 18 Fr, and delivery sheaths for thoracic aneurysms are up to 21 Fr, sometimes requiring access through the iliac arteries. Acute leg ischemia complicates almost 3% of endovascular repairs of abdominal aortic aneurysms, either intraoperatively or following surgery as a result of graft limb occlusion.[41]

With the use of larger sheaths and catheters, many interventionalists now liberally use "closure" devices to ensure hemostasis and reduce recovery time. The most commonly used devices are the PerClose and StarClose devices (Abbott Vascular, Redwood City, California) and the Angio-Seal (St. Jude Medical, Minnetonka, Minnesota). Although effective, ischemic complications have been reported with all three due to intraluminal deployment.[42-44] For the consulting vascular surgeon, it is important to be aware of this possibility when reviewing a patient with leg ischemia following a catheter intervention.

Acute leg ischemia is well recognized in patients undergoing cardiac surgery. In one large series covering 7620 procedures, the overall incidence of acute leg ischemia was 0.85%, most (86%) due to injury during intraaortic balloon pump insertion. Overall, 27% of aortic balloon pumps are associated with leg ischemia.[45] Fortunately, most episodes of leg ischemia will respond to simple withdrawal of the device.

Military and Civilian Trauma (5% of Cases)

Motor vehicle accidents account for most blunt arterial injuries. The mechanism of injury is bony fracture or dislocation in three quarters of cases. Less commonly, injury is due to traction or contusion. Approximately two thirds of cases have complete disruption of the artery; in one third, intimal or medial tears are found. Motorcycle accidents are associated with a disproportionately high incidence of arterial disruption. Increasingly, gunshot injuries are featuring in civilian trauma.

The superficial femoral artery is the most commonly injured arterial segment in modern conflicts, where leg trauma is twice as common as arm injury. Up to 40% of cases also have a major venous injury that increases the risk of amputation. A quarter also have a major bony injury. As with nontraumatic ischemia, total ischemia time correlates with the risk of amputation: 22% if treated within 12 hours, 93% if the delay is greater than 12 hours. The most recent data on acute leg ischemia due to trauma in combat comes from the U.S. Army experience in Iraq. Most vascular injuries were to the lower extremity, and the superficial femoral artery was by far the most often injured artery requiring repair.[46]

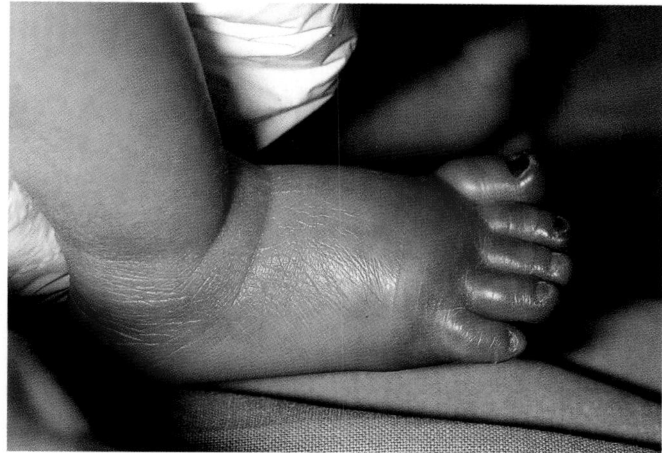

Figure 13-12. Neonate with acute ischemia due to iatrogenic intervention.

Acute Leg Ischemia in Children (Rare)

Advances in neonatal care have increased the need for vascular access for intravenous therapy and continuous arterial pressure monitoring. With increasing use comes the possibility of complications. In centers with large neonatal units, the first physician consulted when signs of acute leg ischemia develop in a preterm infant is often the on-call vascular surgeon. Usually umbilical artery catheterization is the cause (Figure 13-12). These children are at the opposite end of the spectrum from the standard vascular patient, sometimes as young as 28 weeks gestation and usually weighing less than 5 kg. Presentation is usually with cyanosis of their toes or, in extreme conditions, cyanosis extending to the lower abdomen. Diagnosis is made based on clinical examination, absent Doppler signals, and ultrasound examination.[47]

Differential Diagnosis

Vasospastic disorders are rarely a cause of acute ischemia, as the history is usually longstanding. The initial appearances of a patient with an exacerbation of Raynaud's syndrome or acrocyanosis may be deceptive (Figure 13-13). A duplex scan provides objective confirmation of the integrity of the vessels. Similarly, arteritis seldom causes acute ischemia. Takayasu's disease rarely affects the legs, and Buerger's disease presents as chronic, not acute, ischemia. Phlegmasia cerula dolens (Figure 13-14) and the rarer entity, phlegmasia alba dolens, are extreme manifestations of extensive deep venous thrombosis. The affected foot may be cool and cyanosed with "fixed staining." The leg may also be swollen, making pulse examination difficult. Awareness of the condition and duplex examination usually resolve any doubts. Congestive cardiac failure with a low cardiac index and decreased peripheral perfusion may confuse the unwary. Palpable pulses confirm viability of

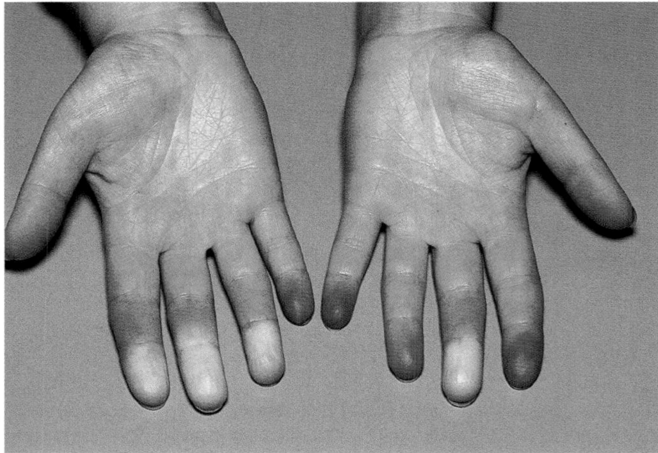

Figure 13-13. Not acute hand ischemia: severe Raynaud's disease.

the limb. Rarely, a vascular specialist is asked to see patients in an intensive care setting with thrombotic complications of meningococcal septicemia (Figure 13-15).

Prognosis

Natural History of Acute Leg Ischemia

Understandably, few contemporary studies have been done on the natural history of untreated acute leg ischemia. In 1948, Warren and Linton[48] described 24 patients with acute arterial emboli seen at the Massachusetts General Hospital from 1937 to 1946. The amputation rate was high: 17 per 24 (71%). They also described an additional 32 legs in which "conservative therapy" was employed. This consisted of lumbar sympathectomy, papaverine, and a special boot to apply intermittent compression. A small number of patients also received heparin. In this group, the amputation rate was 38%. A subsequent review of unoperated patients in the same institution from 1937 to 1953 with lower limb emboli showed an in-hospital mortality of 33% to 58%, with aortoiliac occlusions associated with a particularly high mortality.[49] In 1950, Haimovici[50] reported the outcome of 300 patients with acute leg ischemia. A 13% mortality rate occurred, and 27% developed gangrene. Of course, these data do not include the morbidity experienced by patients who survived without amputation: the number with rest pain or nonhealing wounds must have been substantial. To place this in context, contemporary operative mortality rates for acute leg ischemia are less than 10%, with limb salvage rates of more than 80% in most published series.

Life Expectancy of a Patient with Acute Leg Ischemia

Acute leg ischemia is a marker for reduced life expectancy (Figure 13-16). Data from Portland, Oregon,[24] showed 15% of their patients had died by 1 month and 49% were dead within 3 years of presentation. Swedish figures[18] for 1965 to 1983 showed 4-year survival rates of 33% to 43%. Aune and Trippestad[51] in 1998 looked specifically at 5-year survival rates in Norwegian patients with acute leg ischemia and compared them with expected survival rates in the general population (Figure 13-16). However, other factors also affect survival after treatment of acute leg ischemia. Patients with acute arterial emboli have shorter life expectancies than those presenting with acute arterial thrombosis. Predictably, age at presentation and poor cardiac function are associated with higher mortality.

Embolism versus Thrombosis

The 5-year survival rate for patients treated for an acute arterial embolus in population studies is 17%, significantly lower than the expected survival rate of 62%.[51] More patients with acute arterial thrombosis live to 5 years, but the 44% survival rate is still less than the expected 74% for matched controls in the population. Explanations commonly advanced for the discrepancy between survival after embolism and thrombosis are the older age profile of patients with embolic disease and the greater incidence of cardiac disease, given that 75% of embolic lesion are cardiac in origin, and usually the consequence of coronary artery disease.

Heart Disease and Acute Leg Ischemia

Patients with acute leg ischemia and New York Heart Association class 3 to 4 disease (angina or dyspnea with usual activity or at rest) have a mortality rate six times higher than those with class 1 to 2 disease (no symptoms or only on severe exertion).[52] Jivegård et al.[53] examined patients with acute leg ischemia due to presumed embolic disease and found a 60% mortality rate within 10 days in patients with a cardiac index less than 1.7 l/min m^2. Data from the Finnish national vascular

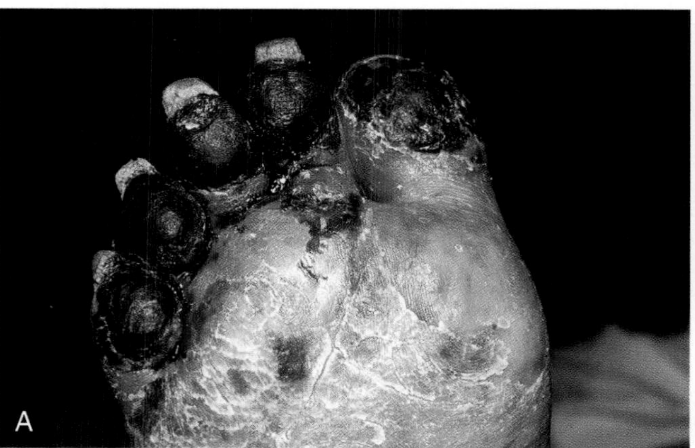

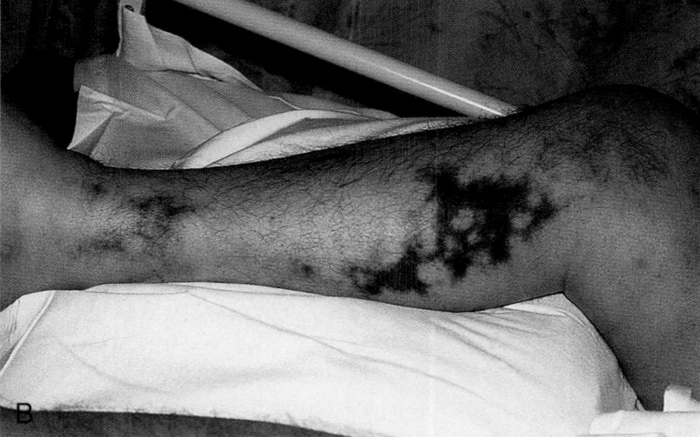

Figure 13-14. Venous gangrene in a 56-year-old man with an occult primary malignancy.

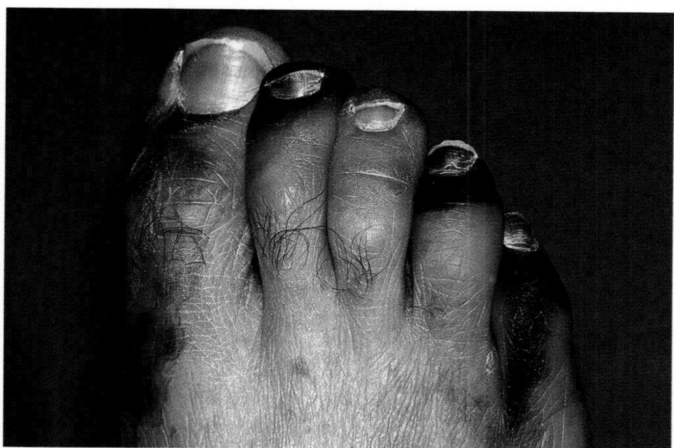

Figure 13-15. Meningococcal septicemia.

database in 1994 also confirmed that cardiac and pulmonary disease adversely affected survival.[20]

Age

Not unexpectedly, age affects survival; older patients fare worse than the young. Dryjski and Swedenborg[54] showed that patients over 80 years with acute arterial thrombosis had a 50% mortality compared to 5% in those under 60. Population studies from Sweden in 1996[55] showed 5-year survival rates of 31% in patients with acute ischemia older than 80 years, compared to 86% in those younger than 50 years.

Prognosis for the Limb in a Patient with Acute Leg Ischemia

As a rule, patients with acute arterial embolism are more likely to die; those with acute arterial thrombosis are more likely to require amputation (Figure 13-17). The higher limb salvage rates after embolization reflect the relative ease of balloon embolectomy versus the technical challenges of tibial bypass, for example, especially in the emergency setting.

Embolism versus Thrombosis

Cambria and Abbott[56] reported the outcome of patients with acute leg ischemia. Limb salvage rates were significantly lower in patients with acute arterial thrombosis than in those with embolism (63% versus 81%). Reports that are more contemporary support this. Data from the Finnvasc registry[20] in 1994 also reported higher amputation rates after thrombosis when compared to embolus (26% versus 10%). The Swedish vascular registry analyzed outcomes in 1189 patients and confirmed the risk of amputation in thrombosis to be twice that of embolic disease.[17]

Early versus Late Presentation

In 1998, the Swedvasc database showed that patients who present with established leg ischemia fare worse than those presenting early. The risk of amputation in patients with symptoms for more than 25 hours is four times greater (odds ratio, 4.3) than those with symptoms for less than 6 hours.[19] This seems self-evident. After all, muscle fiber function can hardly improve with prolonged ischemia time. In 2004, however, the report of the National Audit of Thrombolysis for Acute Leg Ischemia (NATALI) investigators showed that a shorter duration of leg

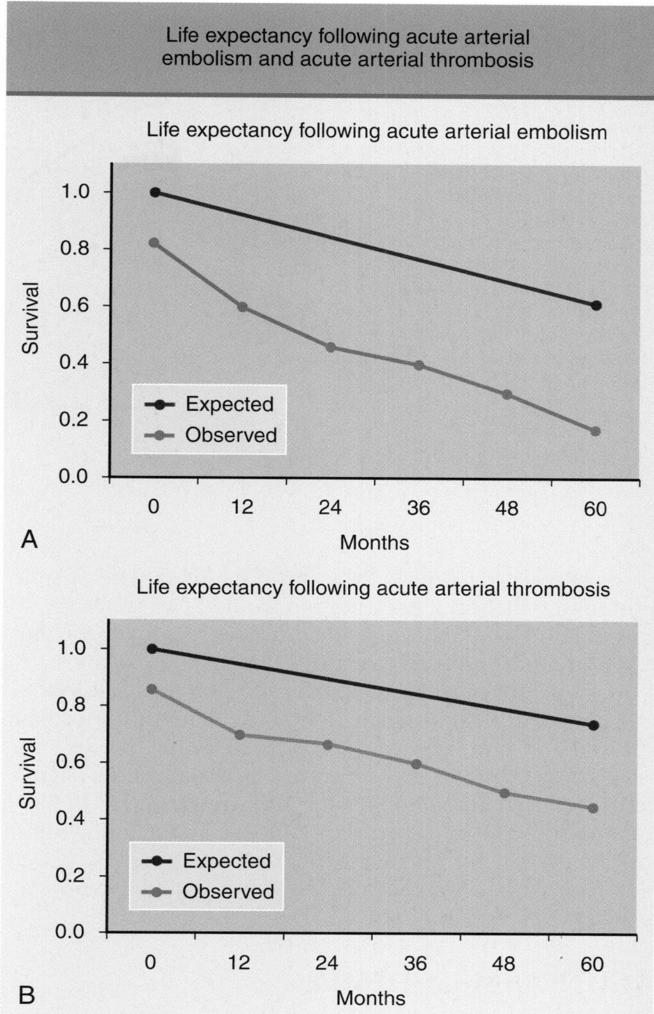

Figure 13-16. Life expectancy following acute arterial embolism **(A)** and acute arterial thrombosis **(B).** (Aune S, Trippestad A. Operative mortality and long-term survival of patients operated on for acute lower limb ischaemia. *Eur J Vasc Endovasc Surg* 1998;15[2]:143-146.)

ischemia before treatment meant a higher risk of amputation and death.[2] The reason is probably referral bias. The NATALI group was only selecting patients undergoing thrombolysis, not those who were brought directly to the operating room for revascularization or primary amputation or those assigned to conservative management. Patients with a shorter duration of ischemia at time of presentation were probably those with more severe disease, unlikely to benefit from lytic therapy.

Systemic Factors Influencing Limb Salvage

Some predictors of limb loss may not be so obvious. The Thrombolysis or Peripheral Arterial Surgery Trial[57] prospectively collected data on 544 patients with acute leg ischemia from 113 centers worldwide. Univariate analysis of the data showed eight factors predicted the likelihood of being alive with a viable limb at 1 year (amputation-free survival). Patients at higher risk were nonwhite, age less than 65 years, body weight less than 160 pounds (72 kg), history of malignancy, neurological or cardiac disease, mottled skin at presentation, and ischemic pain at rest. Most of these factors are

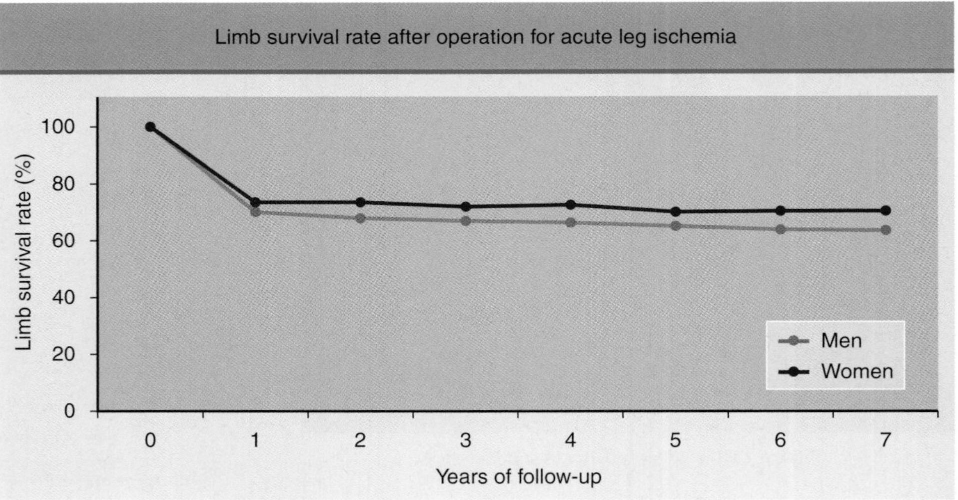

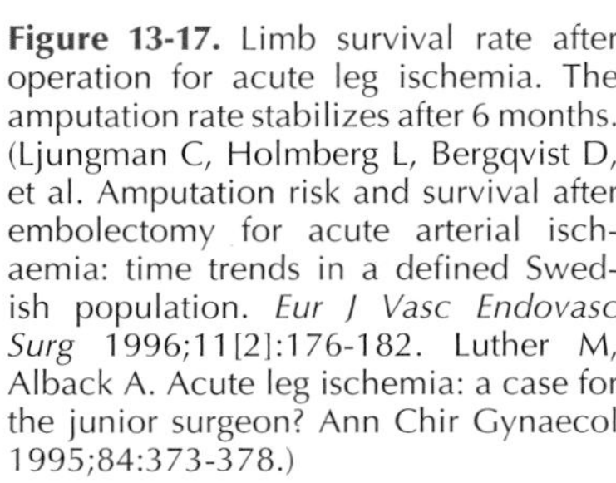
Figure 13-17. Limb survival rate after operation for acute leg ischemia. The amputation rate stabilizes after 6 months. (Ljungman C, Holmberg L, Bergqvist D, et al. Amputation risk and survival after embolectomy for acute arterial ischaemia: time trends in a defined Swedish population. *Eur J Vasc Endovasc Surg* 1996;11[2]:176-182. Luther M, Alback A. Acute leg ischemia: a case for the junior surgeon? Ann Chir Gynaecol 1995;84:373-378.)

predictable, as patients with severe systemic disease or more profound ischemia at presentation would be expected to fare worse. However, race, age, and body mass as prognostic indicators are more difficult to explain.

Postoperative management may affect limb salvage. Abbott emphasized the importance of anticoagulation in improving survival and limb salvage rates.[56] In 1998, the Swedish registry confirmed that postoperative anticoagulation significantly reduced amputation rates (odds ratio, 0.3).[19] In 2000, Campbell et al.[58] reported the results at 2-year follow-up of 287 British patients with acute leg ischemia. Patients who were warfarinized had significantly less chance of recurrent acute ischemia (7% versus 17%).

ACUTE ARM ISCHEMIA

Acute arm ischemia is uncommon but has a better prognosis than leg ischemia. It is usually not immediately limb threatening due to the rich network of collateral vessels supplying the arm. However, the consequences of a poor outcome can be devastating. Conservative therapy suffices in some but can leave others with debilitating forearm claudication. Whether or not to operate in a patient with a viable arm at time of presentation remains contentious.

Diagnostic Criteria

Acute arm ischemia can be divided into three categories: acute embolic events, iatrogenic trauma, and uncommon conditions.

Clinical Evaluation: History and Examination

In nontraumatic arm ischemia, patients present with a history of acute onset of coldness in the hand, often exacerbated by use. Often they also give a history of transient pain and paresthesia. Objectively, the hand feels cooler than the healthy limb and appears noticeably paler (Figure 13-18). Motor function is preserved, although initially the hand may be a little weaker than normal. Examination confirms absent radial, ulnar, brachial, or axillary pulses, depending on the level of occlusion. Usually within 24 hours of instigating heparin, the hand is appreciably "pinker" and movement is restored. "Mottling" of the arm or hand is rare in embolic disease. Using the SVS/ISCVS system,[6] most cases are class I or IIA ischemia.

In trauma, however, pain and paresthesia are often present from the outset, with marked pallor and loss of motor function. Pulses are absent distal to the injury. All these injuries are class IIB or III ischemia. Urgent surgical revascularization is needed.

Angiography: When Is It Required?

The situation with regard to angiography is different in acute arm ischemia. Most patients have a viable limb at presentation, and the overwhelming majority (more than 90%) have a simple embolus amenable to embolectomy. In practice, many patients are successfully managed on clinical grounds alone. For example, in a patient with arm ischemia and atrial fibrillation, brachial embolectomy under local anesthesia is highly effective. In these patients, angiography is obviously superfluous. While the odds in acute arm ischemia highly favor a diagnosis of acute arterial embolus, in a minority of patients, the clinical picture is less clear and diagnostic imaging is needed. Patients with acute ischemia and previous axillary or subclavian artery surgery (e.g., axillofemoral, carotid–subclavian bypass) should undergo duplex imaging and angiography.

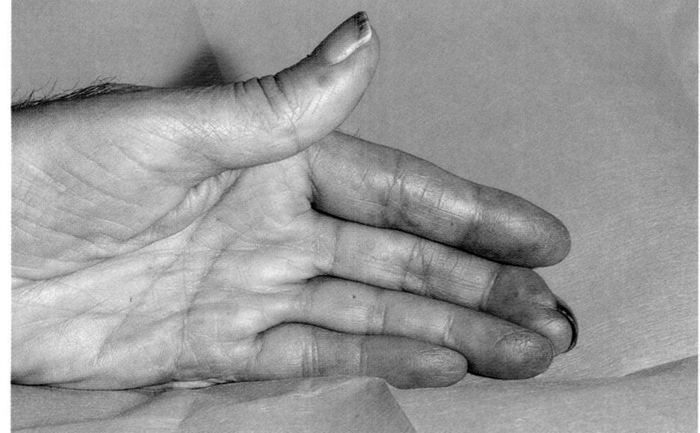
Figure 13-18. Acutely ischemic left hand due to brachial artery embolus.

A history compatible with thoracic outlet syndrome, clinical evidence of a subclavian artery aneurysm, or suspicion of in situ thrombosis also mandate investigation. Persistent digital microemboli (blue finger syndrome) or isolated digital ischemia are also clear indications.

Few authors have looked specifically at the place of diagnostic imaging. However, a review of 251 patients with acute arm ischemia in 2001 from Munich suggested that angiograms are needed in as few as 4% of patients.[59] Based on their experience, the authors stated that diagnostic angiograms are only indicated in the absence of a carotid pulse or in patients with generalized atherosclerosis and a long occlusion.

Other Imaging Modalities

Magnetic resonance angiography and computed tomography angiography probably have less of a role here than in leg ischemia, although Duplex examination again can prove useful. The arguments for and against echocardiography are identical to those in acute leg ischemia. Most patients are warfarinized empirically following successful brachial embolectomy. Therefore, using the criteria for leg ischemia, it is possible to rationalize the use of TTE and TEE.

Incidence

Acute arm ischemia accounts for one fifth of all episodes of acute limb ischemia. There seems to be a female-to-male preponderance in all series of approximately 2:1. Patients with acute arm ischemia are also slightly older than those with acute leg ischemia (67 years versus 62 years). Most published series include only those patients who have surgery. In reality, between 9% and 30% of patients seen by vascular specialists are managed conservatively as they either are unfit for surgery or have minimal symptoms. In Dryjski and Swedenborg's survey[16] of acute limb ischemia in Stockholm, the incidence of acute arm ischemia was 1.13 per 100,000 population. Most current estimates would suggest an incidence of 1.2 to 3.5 per 100,000 population.

Causes of Acute Arm Ischemia

In contrast to acute leg ischemia, nearly all cases of acute arm ischemia are due to emboli (Figure 13-19). In situ thrombosis is a rare entity. Complications of dialysis access procedures may also comprise a few presentations.

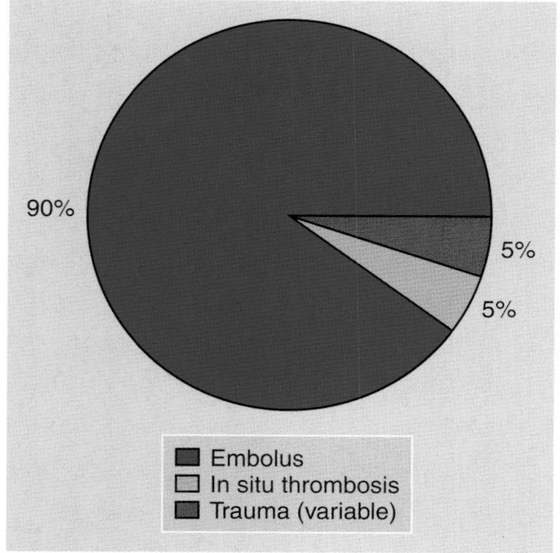

Figure 13-19. Etiology of acute arterial ischemia of the arm.

Embolus (90% of Cases)

As with acute leg ischemia, at least 75% of arm emboli come from the heart (Figure 13-20). Most are due to atrial fibrillation. The remainder are due to recent myocardial infarction, ventricular aneurysms, atrial myxomas, and paradoxical emboli. In most of these patients, clinical examination and basic investigations, including a 12-lead electrocardiogram, point to the cause of the embolus.

The remaining emboli are extracardiac (13%) or of indeterminant origin (12%). The extracardiac arm emboli usually arise in the aorta, brachiocephalic arteries, or subclavian arteries. They can be due to atherosclerotic plaque embolization (atheroemboli) or extrinsic compression due to fibrous bands or cervical ribs. Subclavian artery aneurysms are rare but can be a source of embolic material. Even rarer causes are malignant emboli and fibromuscular dysplasia.

As with leg emboli, arm emboli follow a distinct pattern of embolization, regardless of source. In most cases, they conveniently lodge in the brachial artery (60%). The next most common site is the axillary artery (26%). A slightly greater frequency of emboli occurs in the right arm, possibly due to the brachiocephalic artery being closer to the heart.

Thrombosis (5% of Cases)

In situ thrombosis of the arm is rare. Approximately 5% of community episodes of acute arm ischemia are due to thrombosis. Eyers and Earnshaw[60] suggest that the more proximal the occlusion, the more likely it is to be thrombosis. As with acute leg ischemia, patients who are initially misdiagnosed and subjected to inappropriate embolectomy fare worse. The most common predisposing cause is atherosclerotic plaques, although thoracic outlet syndrome, aneurysms, and arteritis are also implicated. Less common causes include hypercoagulable conditions, malignancy (Trousseau syndrome), and radiotherapy injury.

Military and Civilian Trauma (2.5% of Cases)

Acute arm ischemia in civilian practice is mostly due to blunt rather than penetrating injury. Outcome and limb function, however, usually depend on the extent of associated nerve injuries. Blunt shoulder injury resulting in damage to the axillary and subclavian arteries is almost always associated with brachial plexus disruption. Disruption of the brachial artery is associated with major nerve injury in half of cases.[61,62] Endovascular therapy has a role in the management of such injuries, but contemporary data suggest only about half of patients are suitable for such management.[63]

In the Iraqi conflict, the incidence of arm trauma has been well documented.[64] The brachial artery is the most often injured (58%). The remaining injuries were equally divided between the subclavian–axillary artery and the territory distal to the elbow. However, early limb loss was 10% reflecting significant soft-tissue loss and associated nerve and bone injuries.

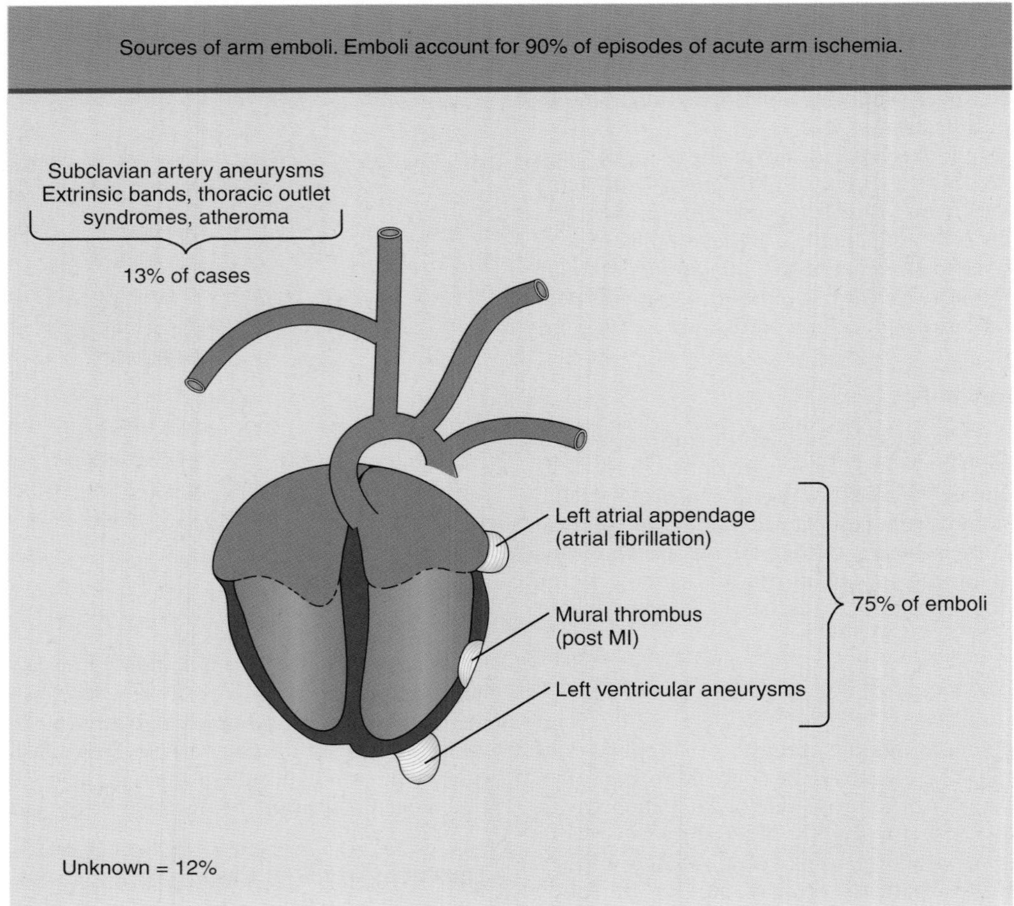

Figure 13-20. Sources of arm emboli. Emboli account for 90% of episodes of acute arm ischemia.

Iatrogenic Injuries (2.5% of Cases)

While not the first option, occasionally arterial access for angiography can only be obtained via the brachial artery. However, if a 6-Fr sheath is needed in this relatively small-diameter brachial artery, the risk of thrombosis and dissection is greater than in the femoral artery. In many patients in whom hand ischemia develops during brachial catheterization, complete reversal of symptoms occurs upon termination of the procedure. For those who still have evidence of ischemia, however, surgical exploration is mandatory and is usually done under local anesthesia.

The rising incidence of diabetes in most Western countries has led to a corresponding rise in the number of patients in whom vascular access is required for hemodialysis.[65,66] As reconstructions become more complex, these patients are increasingly coming under the care of vascular surgeons. An unfortunate consequence of the growing number of upper-arm fistulas is that the incidence of dialysis-associated steal syndrome (DASS) is increasing as well. DASS is less common after Cimino or radiocephalic fistula procedures,[67] but it occurs in 6% to 8% of patients who undergo upper-arm brachial artery–based fistula or graft procedures.[68,69] DASS may present in either an acute form (characterized by severe rest pain and obvious ischemia developing within 24 hours) or a chronic form (characterized by symptoms and signs developing several weeks or even months after the original operation), each of which is managed differently. In cases of acute ischemia, the fistula is ligated to restore flow down the native arteries. In cases of chronic ischemia, the aim is to preserve the fistula and avoid ligation, usually by distal revascularization–interval ligation. Accidental intraarterial injection may rarely be responsible (Figure 13-21).

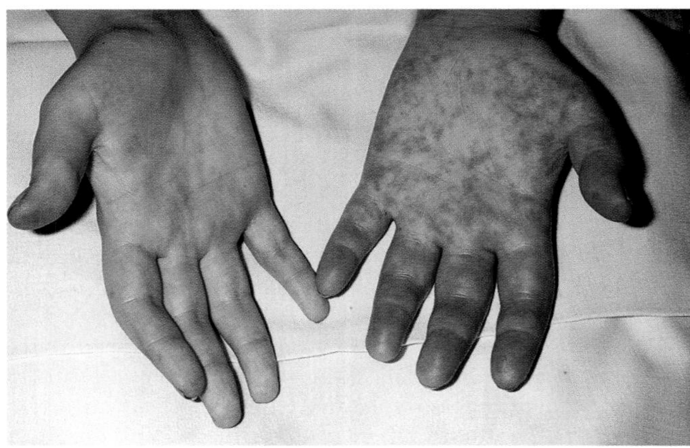

Figure 13-21. Acute ischemia of the left hand due to intraarterial injection of narcotics.

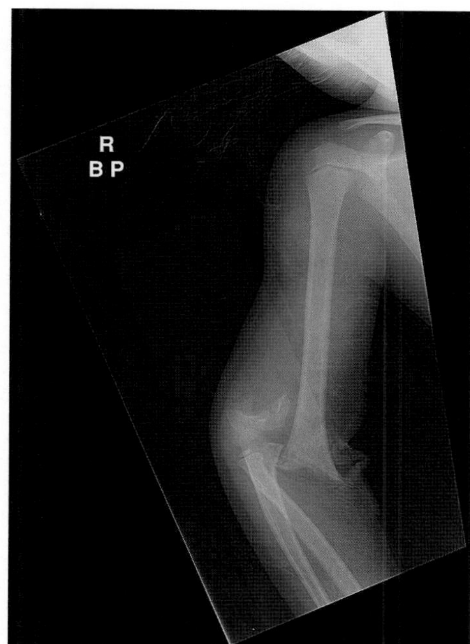

Figure 13-22. Supracondylar fracture of right humerus in a 5-year-old girl resulting in a brachial artery injury.

Acute Arm Ischemia in Children (Rare)

Acute nontraumatic arm ischemia in the very young is rare. Isolated reports have appeared of acute ischemia due to axillary catheterization in neonates, but thankfully, this is a rare event. However, most vascular surgeons encounter acute ischemia in older children, usually due to a supracondylar fracture of the humerus resulting in brachial artery injury (Figure 13-22). This occurs usually between the ages of 5 and 8, more often in girls than boys, and more often affecting the left arm than the right.[70] It occurs in 14% of children with Gartland grade III supracondylar fractures (complete displacement of distal humerus either posteromedially or posterolaterally). Three quarters of children regain their radial pulse following reduction of the fracture; the rest are left with a "pink pulseless hand"[71] or rarely a pale pulseless hand. Doppler examination reveals a monophasic or absent signal over the radial artery. Volkmann's ischemic contracture is the most feared complication in this situation. These injuries are often managed by brachial artery exploration by a vascular surgeon. However, the largest contemporary series in the literature comes from plastic surgeons with an expertise in microsurgery.[72]

Prognosis

Natural History

In contrast to leg ischemia, untreated nontraumatic acute arm ischemia is relatively benign. All natural history series predate the development of the Fogarty embolectomy catheter in 1963. Warren and Linton[48] reported the Massachusetts General Hospital experience in 1948 of 14 patients who received no treatment. In all cases the arm survived, but no information was provided about subsequent function. Abbott et al.[73] analyzed all nonoperated patients with arm ischemia presenting to a single center from 1937 to 1953. He showed an in-hospital mortality rate of 17%. By 1980, mortality rates for acute arm ischemia had fallen to 6%.

Mortality Rates and Long-Term Survival

Perioperative survival rates are good in patients with acute arm ischemia. However, acute nontraumatic arm ischemia is a marker of reduced long-term survival. Hernandez-Richter et al.[59] quote a 5-year survival rate for patients of 56% following brachial embolectomy. When specifically compared to outcomes for patients with acute leg ischemia, patients with acute arm ischemia fare better. Stonebridge et al.[74] reported that patients with arm ischemia had a 5% in-hospital mortality rate, versus 30% for leg ischemia. While patients with arm ischemia were older and had a similar incidence of cardiac dysrhythmias, they had significantly fewer cardiopulmonary symptoms.

Arm Function and Recurrent Embolization

The reported operative mortality rate after brachial embolectomy is 5.5% to 19.2%. Following successful brachial embolectomy, 95% to 98% of patients are symptom free, with as few as 2% reporting long-term arm claudication.

Conservatively managed patients are probably underrepresented in the literature. In the few reported series, assessment of symptoms and disability tends to be inconsistent. However, in a series of 95 patients reported in 1964, 32% were left with abnormal function of the arm. In 1977, Savelyev et al.[75] reported that 75% of patients managed conservatively had a poor functional outcome. More recently, Galbraith and colleagues[76] confirmed that 50% of their conservatively managed patients had persistent forearm claudication.

Recurrent embolization was reported in 11% of patients managed in Edinburgh, despite full anticoagulation.[74] All had ongoing atrial fibrillation. Recurrent emboli are also more likely when the underlying cause was acute myocardial ischemia. In patients who are not anticoagulated, the outlook is worse, with up to 33% experiencing recurrent emboli. As might be expected, recurrent embolization is associated with a higher mortality rate.

SUMMARY

Acute limb ischemia remains a major problem for the vascular specialist. Most patients are elderly, and many have significant comorbidities. The incidence of acute limb ischemia is slowly increasing. This reflects the aging population and increased prevalence of peripheral vascular disease. Accordingly, the commonest cause of leg ischemia is now acute arterial thrombosis. Embolic disease is still the main cause of nontraumatic arm ischemia.

Improvements in limb salvage rates have been dramatic since the 1950s. However, even with improved limb salvage techniques, only 70% of patients leave the hospital with an intact limb. Of the remaining 30%, half die and half require a major amputation. Only 10% to 15% of these amputees regain any degree of independent activity. Early, appropriate intervention can save life and limb. Compelling evidence shows that outcomes are better when these patients are treated by a vascular specialist. Approximately 30% of those admitted with acute leg ischemia require immediate surgical revascularization, either bypass or embolectomy. Where the diagnosis of embolus can confidently be made, embolectomy is immediately effective. The other patients ought to have diagnostic imaging, unless they are unfit for further intervention. The roles of magnetic resonance angiography and computed tomography angiography remain uncertain, and with best intentions, ancillary investigations are probably overused. Ultimately, assessment remains clinical and early treatment is the best guarantee of an optimal outcome.

References

1. Campbell WB, Marriott S, Eve R, et al. Amputation for acute ischaemia is associated with increased comorbidity and higher amputation level. *Cardiovasc Surg* 2003;11(2):121-123.
2. Earnshaw JJ, Whitman B, Foy C. National Audit of Thrombolysis for Acute Leg Ischemia (NATALI): clinical factors associated with early outcome. *J Vasc Surg* 2004;39(5):1018-1025.
3. Norgren L, Hiatt WR, Dormandy JA, et al. TASC II Working Group. Inter-society consensus for the management of peripheral arterial disease (TASC II). *J Vasc Surg* 2007;45(Suppl):S5-S67.
4. Batz W, Brückner R. Symptoms and therapy of aortic bifurcation embolism. *Chirurg* 1985;56(3):166-169.
5. Ad Hoc Committee on Reporting Standards. Society for Vascular Surgery/North American Chapter, International Society for Cardiovascular Surgery. Suggested standards for reports dealing with lower extremity ischemia. *J Vasc Surg* 1986;4:80-94.
6. Rutherford RB, Baker JD, Ernst C, et al. Recommended standards for reports dealing with lower extremity ischemia: revised version. *J Vasc Surg* 1997;26(3):517-538.
7. Jivegård L, Wingren U. Management of acute limb ischaemia over two decades: the Swedish experience. *Eur J Vasc Endovasc Surg* 1999;18(2): 93-95.
8. Jivegärd L, Bergqvist D, Holm J. When is urgent revascularization unnecessary for acute lower limb ischaemia? *Eur J Vasc Endovasc Surg* 1995;9(4):448-453.
9. U.S. Food and Drug Administration. Information for healthcare professionals: gadolinium-based contrast agents for magnetic resonance imaging (marketed as Magnevist, MultiHance, Omniscan, OptiMARK, ProHance). Available at: http://www.fda.gov/cder/drug/InfoSheets/HCP/gcca_200705.htm. Accessed 2008.
10. Boström A, Ljungman C, Hellberg A, et al. Duplex scanning as the sole preoperative imaging method for infrainguinal arterial surgery. *Eur J Vasc Endovasc Surg* 2002;23(2):140-145.
11. Gossage JA, Ali T, Chambers J, Burnand KG. Peripheral arterial embolism: prevalence, outcome, and the role of echocardiography in management. *Vasc Endovascular Surg* 2006;40(4):280-286.
12. Egeblad H, Andersen K, Hartiala J, et al. Role of echocardiography in systemic arterial embolism: a review with recommendations. *Scand Cardiovasc J* 1998;32(6):323-342.
13. Linnemann B, Schindewolf M, Zgouras D, et al. Are patients with thrombophilia and previous thromboembolism at higher risk to arterial thrombosis? *Thromb Res* 2008;121(6):743-750.
14. de Moerloose Boehlen F. Inherited thrombophilia in arterial disease: a selective view. *Semin Hematol* 2007;44(2):106-113.
15. Lijfering WM, Coppens M, van der Poel MH, et al. The risk of venous and arterial thrombosis in hyperhomocysteinaemia is low and mainly depends on concomitant thrombophilic defects. *Thromb Haemost* 2007;98(2):457-463.
16. Dryjski M, Swedenborg J. Acute ischemia of the extremities in a metropolitan area during one year. *J Cardiovasc Surg (Torino)* 1984;25(6):518-522.
17. Ljungman C, Adami HO, Bergqvist D, et al. Risk factors for early lower limb loss after embolectomy for acute arterial occlusion: a population-based case-control study. *Br J Surg* 1991;78(12):1482-1485.
18. Ljungman C, Adami HO, Bergqvist D, et al. Time trends in incidence rates of acute, non-traumatic extremity ischaemia: a population-based study during a 19-year period. *Br J Surg* 1991;78(7):857-860.
19. Bergqvist D, Tröeng T, Elfstrom J, et al. Auditing surgical outcome: ten years with the Swedish vascular registry, Swedvasc. *Eur J Surg* 1998;164(S7):3-32.
20. Kuukasjärvi P, Salenius JP. Perioperative outcome of acute lower limb ischaemia on the basis of the national vascular registry: the Finnvasc Study Group. *Eur J Vasc Surg* 1994;8(5):578-583.
21. Clason AE, Stonebridge PA, Duncan AJ, et al. Acute ischaemia of the lower limb: the effect of centralizing vascular surgical services on morbidity and mortality. *Br J Surg* 1989;76(6):592-593.
22. Davies B, Braithwaite BD, Birch PA, et al. Acute leg ischaemia in Gloucestershire. *Br J Surg* 1997;84(4):504-508.
23. Salenius JP, Lepäntalo M, Ylönen K, Luther M. Treatment of peripheral vascular diseases: basic data from the nationwide vascular registry Finnvasc. *Ann Chir Gynaecol* 1993;82(4):235-240.
24. Yeager RA, Moneta GL, Taylor LM Jr, et al. Surgical management of severe acute lower extremity ischemia. *J Vasc Surg* 1992;15(2):385-391.
25. Campbell WB, Ridler BM, Szymanska TH. Current management of acute leg ischaemia: results of an audit by the Vascular Surgical Society of Great Britain and Ireland. *Br J Surg* 1998;85(11):1498-1503.
26. Maemura K, Layne MD, Watanabe M, et al. Molecular mechanisms of morning onset of myocardial infarction. *Ann NY Acad Sci* 2001;947:398-402.
27. Manfredini R, Gallerani M, Portaluppi F, et al. Circadian variation in the onset of acute critical limb ischemia. *Thromb Res* 1998;92(4):163-169.
28. Clark CV. Seasonal variation in incidence of brachial and femoral emboli. *Br Med J (Clin Res Ed)* 1983;287(6399):1109.
29. John TG, Stonebridge PA. Seasonal variation in operations for ruptured abdominal aortic aneurysm and acute lower limb ischaemia. *J R Coll Surg Edinb* 1993;38(3):161-162.
30. Kuukasjärvi P, Salenius JP, Lepäntalo M, et al. Finnvasc Study Group. Weekly and seasonal variation of hospital admissions and outcome in patients with acute lower limb ischaemia treated by surgical and endovascular means. *Int Angiol* 2000;19(4):354-357.
31. Hamish M, Lockwood A, Cosgrove C, et al. Management of popliteal artery aneurysms. *Aust NZ J Surg* 2006;76(10):912-915.
32. Henke PK, Williams DM, Upchurch GR Jr, et al. Acute limb ischemia associated with type B aortic dissection: clinical relevance and therapy. *Surgery* 2006;140(4):532-539.
33. Trousseau A. *Clinique médicale de l'Hôtel-Dieu de Paris. Vol 2.* Paris: JB Baillière; 1861.
34. Javid M, Magee TR, Galland RB. Arterial thrombosis associated with malignant disease. *Eur J Vasc Endovasc Surg* 2008;35(1):84-87.
35. Grenader T, Shavit L, Ospovat I, et al. Aortic occlusion in patients treated with cisplatin-based chemotherapy. *Mt Sinai J Med* 2006;73(5): 810-812.
36. Deitcher SR, Carman TL, Sheikh MA, Gomes M. Hypercoagulable syndromes: evaluation and management strategies for acute limb ischemia (review). *Semin Vasc Surg* 2001;14(2):74-85.
37. Kottke-Marchant K, Green R, Jacobsen DW, et al. High plasma homocysteine: a risk factor for arterial and venous thrombosis in patients with normal anticoagulation profiles. *Clin Appl Thromb Hemost* 1997;34:329-344.
38. Parkash R, Wee V, Gardner MJ, et al. The impact of warfarin use on clinical outcomes in atrial fibrillation: a population-based study. *Can J Cardiol* 2007;23(6):457-461.
39. Rudström H, Bergqvist D, Ogren M, Björk M. Iatrogenic vascular injuries in Sweden. *Eur J Vasc Endovasc Surg* 2008;35(2):129-130.
40. Giswold ME, Landry GJ, Taylor LM, Moneta GL. Iatrogenic arterial injury is an increasingly important cause of arterial trauma. *Am J Surg* 2004;187(5):590-592.
41. Cochennec F, Becquemin JP, Desgranges P, et al. *Eur J Vasc Endovasc Surg* 2007;34(1):59-65.
42. Derham C, Davies JF, Shahbazi R, Homer-Vanniasinkam S. Iatrogenic limb ischemia caused by angiography closure devices. *Vasc Endovascular Surg* 2006-2007;40(6):492-494.
43. Wille J, Vos JA, Overtoom TT, et al. Acute leg ischemia: the dark side of a percutaneous femoral artery closure device. *Ann Vasc Surg* 2006;20(2):278-281.
44. Stock U, Flach P, Gross M, et al. Intravascular misplacement of an extravascular closure system: StarClose. *J Interv Cardiol* 2006;19(2):170-172.
45. Allen RC, Schneider J, Longenecker L, et al. Acute lower extremity ischemia after cardiac surgery. *Am J Surg* 1993;166(2):124-129.
46. Fox CJ, Gillespie DL, O'Donnell SD, et al. Contemporary management of wartime vascular trauma. *J Vasc Surg* 2005;41(4):638-644.
47. Chaikof EL, Dodson TF, Salam AA, et al. Acute arterial thrombosis in the very young. *J Vasc Surg* 1992;16(3):428-435.
48. Warren R, Linton RR. The treatment of arterial embolism. *N Engl J Med* 1948;238:421-429.

49. Warren R, Linton RR, Scannell JG. Arterial embolism: recent progress. *Ann Surg* 1954;(I)40: 311-317.
50. Haimovici H. Peripheral arterial embolism: a study of 330 unselected cases of embolism of the extremities. *Angiology* 1950;1:20-45.
51. Aune S, Trippestad A. Operative mortality and long-term survival of patients operated on for acute lower limb ischaemia. *Eur J Vasc Endovasc Surg* 1998;15(2):143-146.
52. Dregelid EB, Stangeland LB, Eide GE, Trippestad A. Characteristics of patients operated on because of suspected arterial embolism: a multivariate analysis. *Surgery* 1988;104(3):530-536.
53. Jivegård L, Arfvidsson B, Frid I, et al. Cardiac output in patients with acute lower limb ischaemia of presumed embolic origin: a predictor of severity and outcome? *Eur J Vasc Surg* 1990;4(4):401-407.
54. Dryjski M, Swedenborg J. Acute nontraumatic extremity ischaemia in Sweden: a one-year survey. *Acta Chir Scand* 1985;151(4):333-339.
55. Ljungman C, Holmberg L, Bergqvist D, et al. Amputation risk and survival after embolectomy for acute arterial ischaemia: time trends in a defined Swedish population. *Eur J Vasc Endovasc Surg* 1996;11(2): 176-182.
56. Cambria RP, Abbott WM. Acute arterial thrombosis of the lower extremity: its natural history contrasted arterial embolism. *Arch Surg* 1984;119:784-787.
57. Ouriel K, Veith FJ. Acute lower limb ischemia: determinants of outcome. *Surgery* 1998;124:3336-3341.
58. Campbell WB, Ridler BM, Szymanska TH. Two-year follow-up after acute thromboembolic limb ischemia: the importance of anticoagulation. *Eur J Vasc Endovasc Surg* 2000;19:169-173.
59. Hernandez-Richter T, Angele MK, Helmberger T, et al. Acute ischemia of the upper extremity: long-term results following thrombembolectomy with the Fogarty catheter. *Langenbecks Arch Surg* 2001;386(4):261-266.
60. Eyers P, Earnshaw JJ. Acute non-traumatic arm ischaemia. *Br J Surg* 1998;85(10):1340-1346.
61. Shaw AD, Milne AA, Christie J, et al. Vascular trauma of the upper limb and associated nerve injuries. *Injury* 1995;26(8):515-518.
62. Joshi V, Harding GE, Bottoni DA, et al. Determination of functional outcome following upper extremity arterial trauma. *Vasc Endovascular Surg* 2007;41(2):111-114.
63. Danetz JS, Cassano AD, Stoner MC, et al. Feasibility of endovascular repair in penetrating axillosubclavian injuries: a retrospective review. *J Vasc Surg* 2005;41(2):246-254.
64. Clouse WD, Rasmussen TE, Perlstein J, et al. Upper extremity vascular injury: a current in-theater wartime report from Operation Iraqi Freedom. *Ann Vasc Surg* 2006;20(4):429-434.
65. National Center for Health Statistics. *Health, United States, 2005, with chartbook on trends in the health of Americans.* Hyattsville, Maryland: National Center for Health Statistics; 2005:255.
66. U.S. Renal Data System. *USRDS 2005 annual data report: atlas of end-stage renal disease in the United States.* Bethesda, Maryland: National Institutes of Health, National Institute of Diabetes and Digestive and Kidney Diseases; 2005.
67. van Hoek F, Scheltinga MR, Kouwenberg I, et al. Steal in hemodialysis patients depends on type of vascular access. *Eur J Vasc Endovasc Surg* 2006;32(6):710-717.
68. Revanur VK, Jardine AG, Hamilton DH, Jindal RM. Outcome for arteriovenous fistula at the elbow for haemodialysis. *Clin Transplant* 2000;14 (4 Pt 1):318-322.
69. Wolford HY, Hsu J, Rhodes JM, et al. Outcome after autogenous brachial–basilic upper arm transpositions in the post–National Kidney Foundation Dialysis Outcomes Quality Initiative era. *J Vasc Surg* 2005;42(5):951-956.
70. Baratz M, Micucci C, Sangimino M. Pediatric supracondylar humerus fractures. *Hand Clin* 2006;22(1):69-75.
71. Ruch DS, Seal CN, Koman LA, Smith BP. The pink pulseless hand. *J South Orthop Assoc* 2002;11(3):174-178.
72. Noaman HH. Microsurgical reconstruction of brachial artery injuries in displaced supracondylar fracture humerus in children. *Microsurgery* 2006;26(7):498-505.
73. Abbott WM, Maloney RD, McCabe CC, et al. Arterial embolism: a 44 year perspective. *Am J Surg* 1982;143(4):460-464.
74. Stonebridge PA, Clason AE, Duncan AJ, et al. Acute ischaemia of the upper limb compared with acute lower limb ischaemia: a 5-year review. *Br J Surg* 1989;76(5):515-516.
75. Savelyev VS, Zatevakhin II, Stepanov NV. Artery embolism of the upper limbs. *Surgery* 1977;81(4):367-375.
76. Galbraith K, Collin J, Morris PJ, Wood RF. Recent experience with arterial embolism of the limbs in a vascular unit. *Ann R Coll Surg Engl* 1985;67(1):30-33.

chapter

14

Management of Acute Limb Ischemia

Jonathan D. Beard, FRCS, ChM, Med • Jonothan J. Earnshaw, DM, FRCS

Key Points

- The practical management of acute leg ischemia remains a challenge, as it involves one of the most complex decision pathways in vascular surgery.
- Treatment should be based on the severity of the ischemia rather than the underlying cause.
- A successful outcome depends on collaboration between an experienced vascular radiologist and a vascular surgeon (or a dedicated vascular specialist) with access to, and the ability to use, the full range of therapeutic techniques that may be required.
- A patient with a threatened limb who presents to a hospital without adequate vascular staffing or imaging capability should be transferred to the nearest vascular center without delay.
- Catheter angiography, computed tomography angiography, magnetic resonance angiography, or duplex ultrasound imaging should be obtained in all patients with a threatened limb, but the target of treatment within 6 hours should not be compromised.
- If a catheter angiogram is performed, the catheter must not be removed until a decision has been made about the treatment pathway (percutaneous or surgical).
- The role of conventional balloon catheter embolectomy is diminishing due to the decreasing incidence of cardiac embolism, increasing incidence of peripheral arterial disease, and proliferation of new endovascular techniques.
- Despite several large trials, the precise role of each treatment modality remains unclear.

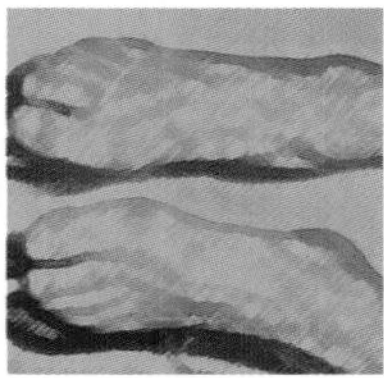

The revised (2007) Trans-Atlantic Inter-Society Consensus (TASC) defines acute limb ischemia (ALI) as any sudden decrease in limb perfusion causing a potential threat to limb viability.[1] Although the incidence of ALI seems to be increasing, the role of conventional balloon catheter embolectomy is diminishing. The reasons for this include the following:

- Increasing availability of percutaneous techniques such as thrombolysis, aspiration thrombectomy, and mechanical thrombectomy
- Decreasing frequency of cardiac embolism due to the falling incidence of rheumatic heart disease and greater use of oral anticoagulation for patients with atrial fibrillation
- Increasing use of antiplatelet and thrombolytic agents after myocardial events resulting in a reduction in cardiac embolism from mural thrombus
- More thrombosis due to the increasing incidence of peripheral arterial disease (PAD) and bypass grafting

Patients with cardiac embolism may also suffer from PAD, as atherosclerosis is often systemic. This increases the difficulty in establishing the cause of the ischemia (see Chapter 13). The presence of underlying PAD can prevent successful embolectomy, even if the cause is embolic.

The implication of all these changes is that "blind" embolectomy by a trainee surgeon is no longer acceptable as a treatment for ALI. The management of ALI can involve one of the most complex decision pathways in vascular surgery. A successful outcome depends on collaboration between an experienced vascular radiologist and a vascular surgeon (or a dedicated vascular specialist) with access to, and the ability to use, the full range of imaging and interventional techniques that may be required. Outcomes seem better when decisions about treatment are made based on the severity of the ischemia, rather than the cause.

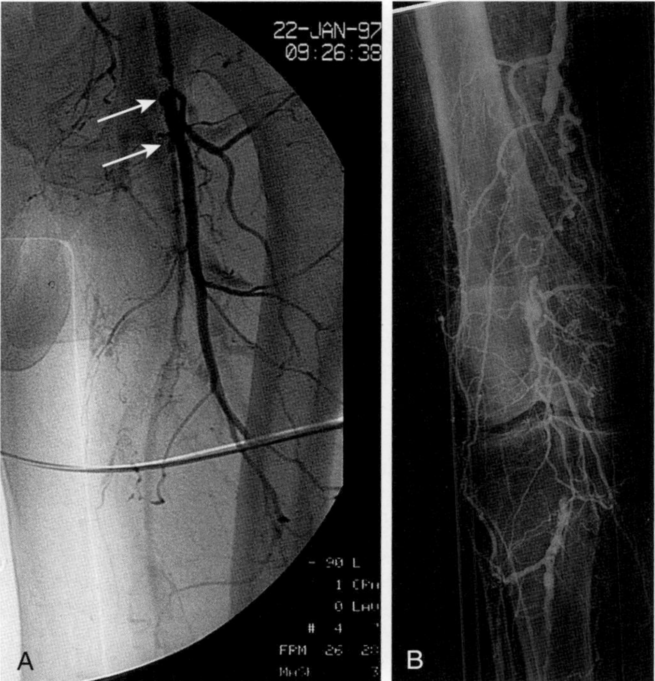

Figure 14-1. **A,** Angiogram of a typical embolus lodged at the bifurcation of the common femoral artery (CFA; *arrows*) with poor filling of the superficial femoral artery (SFA) below this. **B,** Contrast this appearance with a typical thrombosis of the popliteal artery. The extensive collaterals suggest a preexisting stenosis.

SEVERITY OF ISCHEMIA

The severity of leg ischemia is often defined according to Society for Vascular Surgery/International Society for Cardiovascular Surgery criteria.[2] This classification is more useful for reporting results than for planning treatment. TASC defines three categories of ALI based on the severity of ischemia[1] as this, rather than the underlying cause, determines the care pathway; these categories are described here.

Viable Leg

In this category, there is an acute onset of a painful, cold leg, but no neurological deficit is found and an audible arterial Doppler signal is heard at the ankle. The cause is often acute thrombosis of an atherosclerotic artery or previous bypass graft. There may be a history of progressive claudication before the acute event. Such patients can be treated with anticoagulation while awaiting urgent arteriography or duplex ultrasound imaging. Thromboembolectomy is unlikely to successfully treat thrombosis of a stenosed artery or graft. The therapeutic alternatives in these patients are surgical reconstruction, percutaneous thrombolysis with a view to endovascular intervention, or careful observation to see whether leg perfusion improves as collaterals open. This last option allows an acute thrombosis to mature, which reduces the risk of embolization if endovascular intervention is subsequently required.

Threatened Leg

Patients with a threatened leg have loss of sensation and variable loss of motor function and there are no audible arterial Doppler signal in the pedal vessels. These patients require emergency intervention, especially if the calf muscles are tender. An acute white leg with no prior history of claudication, normal contralateral pulses, and atrial fibrillation makes embolism the likely cause, but in many cases it is difficult to differentiate between embolism and thrombosis (Figure 14-1). Some debate focuses on whether preoperative imaging provides beneficial information or wastes valuable time. When the femoral pulse is absent, imaging helps exclude alternative diagnoses, such as dissection, and plan inflow surgery or stenting. Patients without motor loss can also be treated with accelerated thrombolysis if a suitable lesion is found, while percutaneous aspiration embolectomy and mechanical thrombectomy are now alternatives to conventional balloon catheter thromboembolectomy. Therefore, good reasons exist for all such patients to undergo arteriography or duplex ultrasound, but the target of treatment within 6 hours should not be compromised. If a conventional catheter arteriogram is undertaken, the catheter should not be removed until a decision on the treatment pathway (percutaneous or surgical) has been agreed. Otherwise, the puncture site may bleed if thrombolysis is performed subsequently. A patient with a threatened leg who presents to a hospital that lacks adequate vascular staffing or imaging capability should be transferred to the nearest vascular center without delay.

Dead Leg (Irreversible Ischemia)

In this category, acute ischemia has become irreversible, with complete neurological deficit, tense muscles due to rigor mortis, and fixed skin staining due to capillary breakdown. Attempts at revascularization risk causing death from renal and cardiac toxicity due to reperfusion syndrome. Such patients require resuscitation and emergency amputation if they are to survive, but the prognosis is often poor. Terminal care may be the kindest option for moribund patients with severe comorbidity.[3]

Thrombosed Popliteal Aneurysm

The presence of an easily palpable contralateral popliteal pulse, or an ipsilateral popliteal mass, raises the possibility of a thrombosed popliteal aneurysm (Figure 14-2). Duplex ultrasound imaging confirms the diagnosis. The bulk of thrombus within the aneurysm restricts the use of thrombolysis because of the high risk of massive distal embolization,[4] slow clearance, and large amount of residual thrombus after recanalization. If thrombolysis does have a role to play, then it is to open runoff vessels for distal bypass grafting. This is achieved by placing a catheter through the popliteal artery into a tibial vessel and then lysing it until a distal vessel becomes patent for bypass. Alternatively, surgical exploration may be performed, with intraoperative angiography and thrombolysis to clear the runoff, before exclusion bypass.[5]

Ischemic Arm

ALI of the arm is usually embolic in origin, as PAD of the upper limb is rare. The same TASC classification system for severity of ischemia can be used, but most patients with features sufficiently severe to warrant intervention can proceed to balloon catheter thromboembolectomy without an arteriogram. The

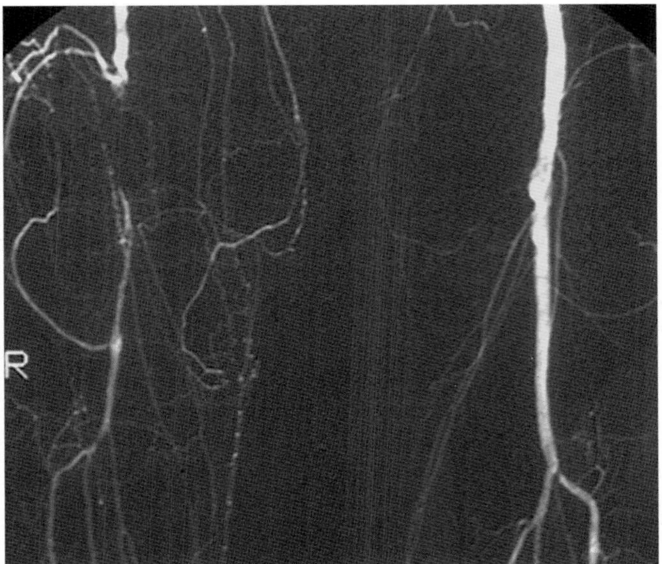

Figure 14-2. Angiogram showing occlusion of a right popliteal aneurysm. The ectatic left popliteal artery provides a clue to the diagnosis. A duplex scan confirmed thrombosis of a 3-cm popliteal aneurysm.

exception is when subclavian artery pathology is suspected. This includes an absent subclavian pulse (due to dissection or thrombosis) or a prominent subclavian pulse (due to an underlying cervical rib or subclavian artery aneurysm). Some surgeons advise conservative treatment with heparin anticoagulation and operation only if the arm does not improve. A risk is that a patient will be left with neurological symptoms and forearm claudication if a threatened limb is left untreated. Therefore, conservative treatment requires careful monitoring and immediate intervention should deterioration occur.[6]

GENERAL MANAGEMENT

Treatment is associated with a high mortality rate of up to 30% because ALI patients are often in poor general health and suffer from associated cardiovascular disease (Table 14-1). Blood should be taken for full blood count, coagulation profile, urea, electrolytes, and glucose. An electrocardiogram and chest radiograph should be requested, a urethral catheter inserted, and cardiac monitoring and pulse oximetry commenced. The patient should be given 24% oxygen by face mask, as some experimental evidence indicates its benefit.[7] Further oxygen therapy is titrated based on the results of blood gas analysis.

Dehydration is common and is best treated with an intravenous infusion of 5% dextrose. A central venous line should be inserted if any suggestion is found of cardiac impairment, and appropriate treatment of cardiac failure, arrhythmia, or both should occur with diuretics, antiarrythmics, or both. An adequate diuresis also reduces the risk of renal impairment due to contrast toxicity. Morphine is usually required for pain relief and is best given by an intravenous pump. Intramuscular analgesia should be avoided because of the risk of bleeding if thrombolysis is used. Intravenous unfractionated heparin (5000 U) should be usually be given immediately, followed by continuous heparin infusion to maintain an activated partial thromboplastin time ratio of more than 2. The aim is to restrict propagation of thrombus and reduce the risk of further embolization (if this is the cause) as some evidence shows that heparinization improves the prognosis.[8] Anticoagulation may, however, prevent the use of epidural anesthesia if surgical intervention is required. Many patients are not fit for general anesthesia, and an epidural provides excellent postoperative analgesia. Heparin may be withheld temporarily if surgery under epidural is contemplated.[2]

Table 14-1
Early (In-Hospital or 30-Day) Rates of Amputation and Death in Selected Series of Patients with Recent Peripheral Arterial Occlusion, Treated with Primary Open Surgical Intervention

Study*	Year	Amputation Rate	Mortality Rate
Blaisdell et al.[8]	1978	25%	30%
Jivegård et al.[56]	1988	—	20%
Rochester[52]	1994	14%	18%
STILE[57]	1994	5%	6%
TOPAS[58]	1998	2%	5%

*STILE, Surgery or Thrombolysis for the Ischemic Lower Extremity; TOPAS, Thrombolysis or Peripheral Arterial Surgery.

SELECTION OF TREATMENT

The question of whether thrombolysis is better than surgery for ALI has been addressed by large randomized studies such as the Surgery or Thrombolysis for the Ischemic Lower Extremity (STILE) and the Thrombolysis or Peripheral Arterial Surgery (TOPAS) trials. Like all new therapies, thrombolysis was initially adopted with great enthusiasm, followed by increasing caution. The results of these trials are discussed later, but the precise role of each of the treatment modalities and their relationship to each other remain open questions. Many patients with ALI require a combination of thrombolysis followed by conventional surgery: thrombolysis may reveal a chronic occlusion that requires a surgical bypass.

The diagnosis of acute leg ischemia is normally a clinical one. Handheld Doppler can help assess the severity of ischemia. Vascular imaging is rarely necessary to confirm the diagnosis. The aims of such imaging are to establish the site and extent of the arterial occlusion and to determine whether it is embolic or thrombotic in nature. Transfemoral catheter angiography is the conventional method of imaging. Advantages are found in using noninvasive methods such as duplex ultrasound, computed tomography angiography (CTA), or magnetic resonance angiography (MRA), all of which are becoming increasingly available. Many vascular surgeons are also becoming competent in the use of duplex ultrasound, and both duplex and MRA have the advantage of avoiding the nephrotoxicity associated with iodinated contrast media. The identification of runoff vessels can be difficult in patients with acute leg ischemia because the distal vessels may not opacify due to the severity of ischemia even though they are patent. If intraarterial angiography is used, the number of arterial punctures should be minimized (ultrasound-guided arterial access is quite useful) and a small sheath and catheter should be used to reduce the risk of subsequent bleeding. The catheter must not be removed until a decision on the treatment pathway (percutaneous or surgical) has been agreed upon.

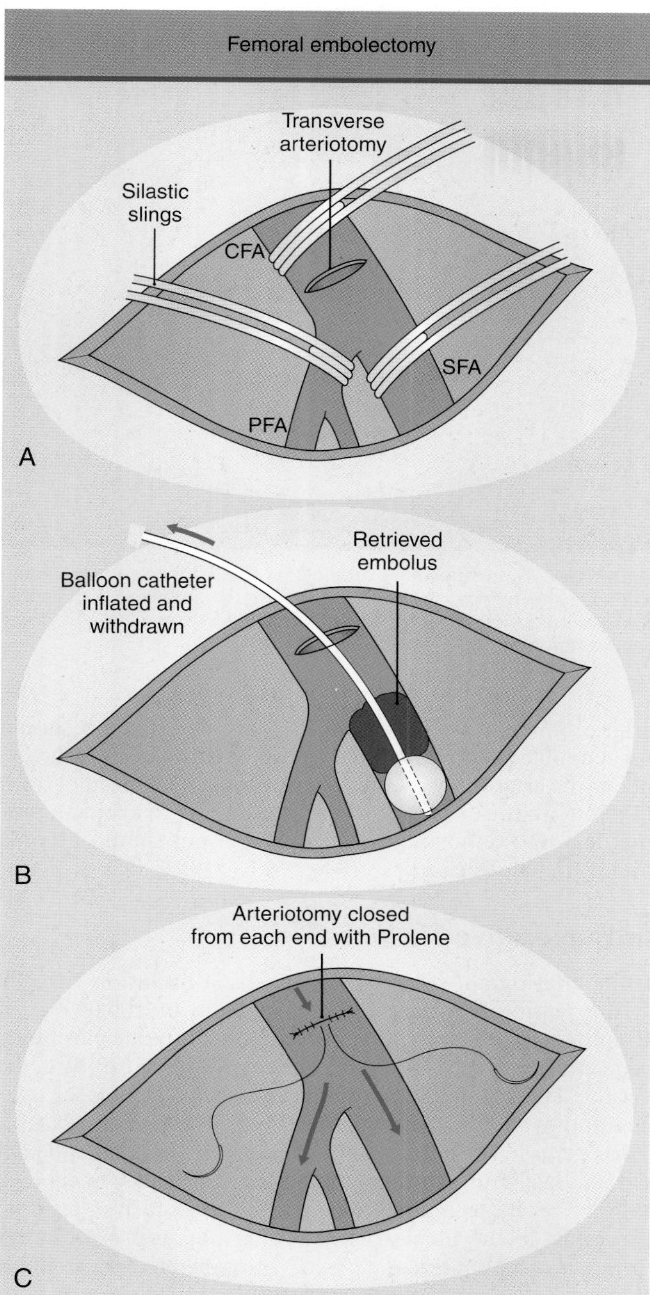

Figure 14-3. Femoral embolectomy. **A,** Via an oblique groin incision, a transverse arteriotomy is made in a soft portion of the common femoral artery (CFA) after control of the bifurcation with slings. **B,** The thromboembolus is retrieved by gentle inflation and withdrawal of the balloon catheter. **C,** The arteriotomy is closed with 4/0 Prolene from each end, after flushing with heparinized saline. PFA, profunda femoris artery; SFA, superficial femoral artery.

SURGICAL MANAGEMENT

With the increasing age of the population, underlying atherosclerosis often complicates ischemia, even if the cause is primarily embolic. Consequently, complex secondary procedures may well be necessary if initial balloon catheter thromboembolectomy fails. Operation under local anesthesia may be preferred in a slim patient with a clear-cut embolus and high cardiac risk, but although wound analgesia can be achieved, the embolectomy and arteriography remain painful. Pain during embolectomy and arteriography can be abolished by intraarterial injection of a small volume of plain 1% lidocaine (lignocaine).[9] An anesthetist should always be present during surgery (even when done under local anesthetic) to monitor the electrocardiogram and oxygen saturation, administer sedation or analgesia, and convert to general anesthesia, if required. Obesity, confusion, and the likelihood of additional procedures seem good reasons for general or epidural anesthesia.

Femoral Artery Exploration

Femoral embolectomy remains the standard surgical treatment for lower limb–threatening ALI. Both the groin and the entire leg should be prepared to permit surgical access and intraoperative angiography. The lower abdomen should also be prepared if any doubt exists about the inflow. The foot is placed in a sterile transparent bag for easy inspection. The common femoral artery bifurcation is exposed via an oblique groin incision, which reduces wound-healing problems, and the vessels are controlled with silastic slings (Figure 14-3). It is important to take care not to damage the great saphenous vein and its lateral tributary. The former may be required for a bypass graft, and the latter can be used to patch the arteriotomy if the femoral artery is severely diseased. Clamps should be avoided initially because they may fragment thrombus that may otherwise be removed intact. A transverse arteriotomy is made in the common femoral artery proximal to the bifurcation, avoiding any obvious plaque. A transverse arteriotomy is easier to close without narrowing, and it can be converted to a diamond shape for proximal anastomosis if a bypass is required. Any thrombus at the bifurcation can be removed by gentle suction or forceps and momentary release of the sling. A balloon embolectomy catheter is then used to retrieve any proximal or distal thrombus. Before use, the stilette should be removed from the catheter and the balloon inflated with air to test integrity and volume required. Air is preferred to saline since it is compressible and therefore arterial wall damage is less likely.

Inflow

If pulsatile inflow is not present, then a 5-French (Fr) or 6-Fr balloon catheter is passed proximally up the iliac artery into the aorta, inflated, and withdrawn. Pressure should be applied to the contralateral femoral artery during this procedure to prevent contralateral embolization. A saddle embolus of the aortic bifurcation can usually be retrieved by bilateral femoral embolectomy, withdrawing both balloons simultaneously to prevent the saddle embolus from moving from side to side. If the catheter cannot be passed up the iliac artery, then the surgeon should try to shape the tip into a "J." If this does not work, a guide wire may be passed under fluoroscopic control. If good inflow cannot be achieved, then a femorofemoral or axillofemoral bypass is required.

Runoff

Next, a 3-Fr or 4-Fr balloon catheter is passed as far distally as possible down both the profunda and the superficial femoral arteries. Force should not be used if resistance is met, as dissection or perforation may result. The balloon should be inflated

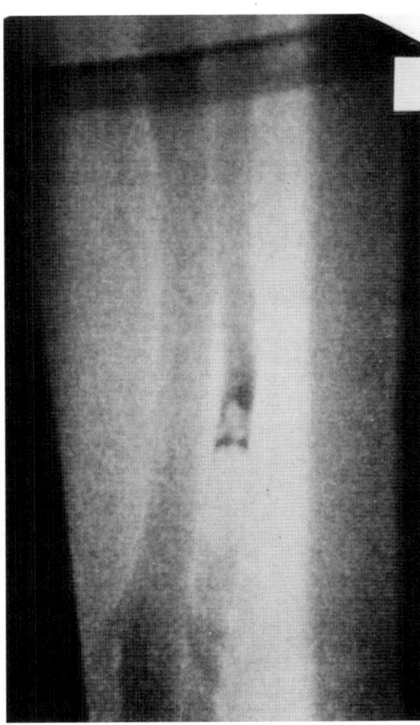

Figure 14-4. Balloon catheter embolectomy using the "negative contrast" method. The artery is filled with contrast, and the air-filled balloon is withdrawn under fluoroscopic control. The embolus and balloon show up clearly against the contrast-filled artery.

only as the catheter is withdrawn, and the amount of inflation should be adjusted to avoid excessive intimal friction. The procedure is repeated until no more thromboembolic material can be retrieved. Conventional embolectomy is performed blindly, and the surgeon has no control over the direction of the catheter past the popliteal trifurcation.[10] Use of an end-hole balloon catheter permits selective catheterization of the tibial arteries, over a guide wire, under fluoroscopic control. Use of a guide wire also reduces the risk of an intimal dissection. It is better to fill the artery with contrast and the balloon with air, which can then be seen fluoroscopically as a negative image (Figure 14-4). Filling the balloon with contrast makes inflation and deflation difficult due to the viscosity of the contrast.

Completion Arteriography

A completion arteriogram should always be performed because persistent thrombus may be present even if the catheter passes to the foot.[11] Backbleeding is of no prognostic value as it may arise from established proximal collaterals. Most operating theaters now have excellent fluoroscopic units capable of high-quality arteriography. If a C-arm image intensifier is not available, the surgeon can use a film cassette wrapped in a towel under the leg, centered on the knee. Fifty milliliters of contrast medium infused rapidly down the superficial femoral artery (SFA) via a Tibbs cannula or umbilical catheter, with a silastic snugger to prevent backflow, provides good images of the distal vessels. If the SFA is chronically occluded, contrast can be infused down the profunda femoris artery to image the distal runoff. The contrast should be flushed with copious amounts of heparin saline, and if no thrombus is present, the

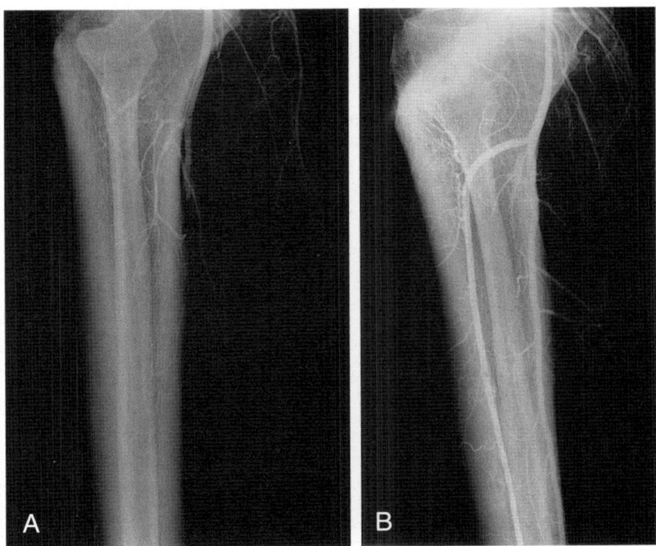

Figure 14-5. A, Intraoperative arteriogram after balloon catheter embolectomy, showing persistent occlusion of the popliteal trifurcation. **B,** A short infusion of 10 mg of r-tPA resulted in complete lysis of the residual thrombus.

arteriotomy is closed with 5/0 Prolene. The surgeon should use a double needle suture cut in two, starting from each corner of the arteriotomy, remembering to pass the needles from in to out on the distal side of the arteriotomy to avoid an intimal flap. On removing the clamps, the foot should become pink with palpable pulses.

Intraoperative Thrombolysis

If the arteriogram shows persistent distal occlusion (usually at the popliteal trifurcation), an infusion of 100,000 U of streptokinase (SK) or 10 mg of recombinant tissue plasminogen activator (r-tPA) in 60 ml of heparin saline can be given via the Tibbs cannula or umbilical catheter in boluses over 30 minutes and the arteriogram can be repeated (Figure 14-5). This results in complete lysis in about a third of cases and partial lysis facilitating further embolectomy or bypass in another third.[12-14] The technique may also be used to lyse residual thrombus in the tibial arteries during popliteal exploration or repair of a popliteal aneurysm.[5] Intraoperative thrombolysis seems effective because the lack of blood flow ensures a high concentration of lytic agent despite the low dose, which reduces the problem of systemic bleeding complications. If an underlying stenosis of the SFA is revealed, on-table balloon angioplasty may be attempted (Figure 14-6). Thrombolysis may also be continued postoperatively in patients with no "reflow" after thromboembolectomy. Law et al.[15] used 58,000 U/hr of urokinase and achieved limb salvage in 7 of 12 patients. The angiographic appearance of blushing or tufting due to extravasation of contrast from the muscle capillaries is a bad prognostic sign as it indicates muscle necrosis.

Popliteal Exploration

Persistent distal occlusion requires exploration of the below-knee popliteal artery. A skin incision is made on the medial side of the knee, extending down from the femoral condyle,

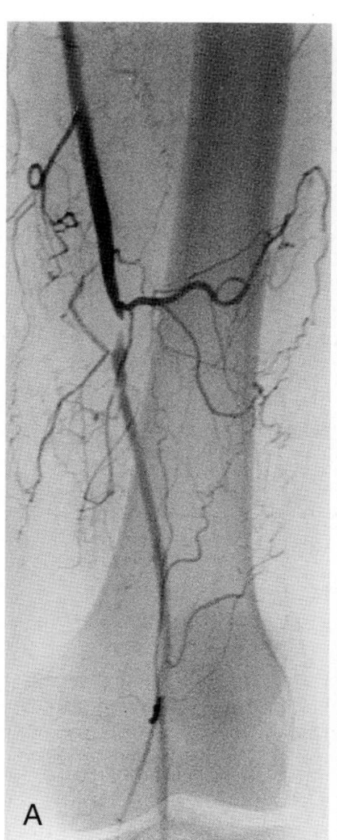

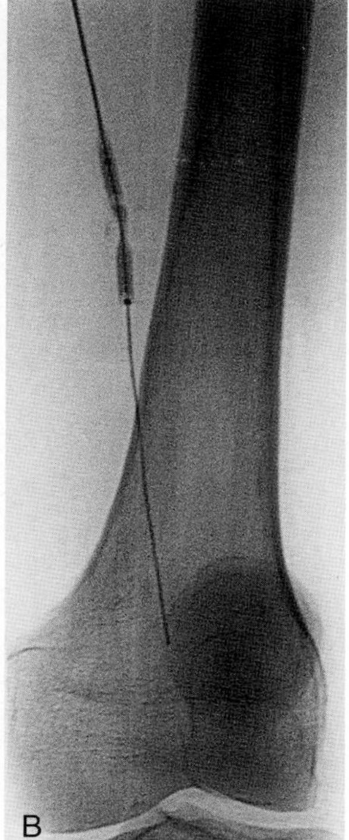

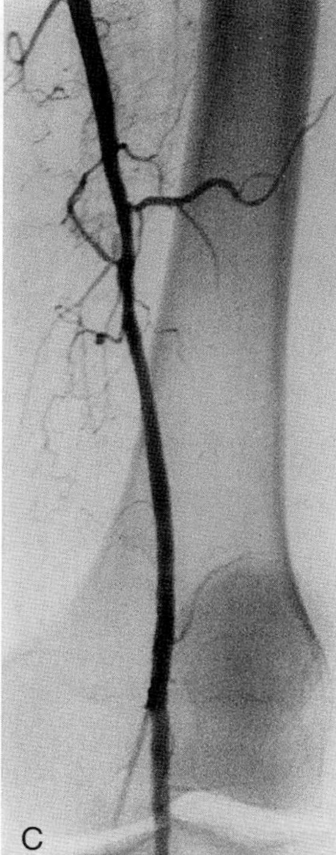

Figure 14-6. A, Intraoperative angiogram after balloon catheter embolectomy and lysis showing an underlying severe stenosis of the distal superficial femoral artery. **B, C,** This was successfully treated by intraoperative balloon angioplasty.

making sure to preserve the long saphenous vein. The origins of the anterior tibial artery, tibioperoneal trunk, posterior tibial artery, and peroneal artery should be controlled with slings. Access often requires extensive dissection and division of the anterior tibial vein, which crosses in front of the trifurcation (Figure 14-7). If the popliteal artery is disease free, a transverse arteriotomy may be used, but this is rarely the case. A longitudinal arteriotomy is usually the best option, as it can be extended into the tibioperoneal trunk, if required. Selective embolectomy of each tibial artery is performed with a 2-Fr or 3-Fr catheter. Thrombus lodged at the adductor hiatus may also be successfully retrieved in retrograde fashion via a popliteal embolectomy if the femoral approach fails. Persistent occlusion of the SFA, popliteal artery, or both requires a femoropopliteal–distal bypass graft. A longitudinal popliteal arteriotomy should be repaired with a vein patch. The fascial layer should not be closed, and if any suggestion of muscle tension occurs, the skin incision should also be left open.

Tibial Embolectomy

Tibial embolectomy should be considered if embolectomy, intraoperative thrombolysis, or both via the popliteal artery fail because of distal mature thrombus or atheroembolism (trash foot). The anterior and posterior tibial arteries are exposed at the ankle level via short, vertical incisions. A 2-Fr embolectomy catheter is passed up to the popliteal level and down into the foot via a small transverse arteriotomy.[16,17] It is important to take care not to split the arteriotomy when withdrawing the balloon. Simms performed tibial embolectomy in 22 of 233 surgical procedures for ALI. Overall limb salvage was only 50% at 6 months, but six of seven trashed feet were salvaged (unpublished data). Wyffels et al. employed an adjuvant intraoperative infusion of urokinase during 16 tibial embolectomies in 12 legs and continued the infusion postoperatively in 14 arteries that did not lyse after the intraoperative bolus.[18] Four patients required concomitant bypass grafting, and four required transfusion for bleeding.

Upper Limb Embolectomy

Upper limb embolectomy is usually performed via the brachial approach. This can normally be done under local anesthesia, but the same requirements regarding monitoring and the presence of an anesthetist apply.[6] The entire arm, axilla, and supraclavicular fossa should be prepared, and the arm should be placed on a board with the hand in a transparent bowel bag. Surgical exposure is via a lazy "S" incision swinging laterally over the bicipital aponeurosis to end in the midline, over the bifurcation of the brachial artery (Figure 14-8). The medial cutaneous nerve of the forearm and cubital veins should be preserved if possible. Damage to the nerve results in an irritating paresthesia, and the vein is a useful conduit or patch. Additional local anesthetic may result in a temporary median nerve palsy, which should be anticipated. The brachial artery and the origins of the radial and ulnar arteries are controlled with silastic slings, and clamps should be avoided if possible. A transverse arteriotomy is made proximal to the bifurcation, and a 3-Fr or 4-Fr embolectomy catheter is passed up the brachial artery if pulsatile inflow is not present. The runoff is then cleared with a 2-Fr or 3-Fr embolectomy guided selectively down the radial and ulnar arteries in turn. The arteriotomy is closed using interrupted 6/0 Prolene. Hematoma formation is common, so it is wise to apply a well-padded crepe bandage, after carefully checking that the radial pulse is present.

Failed brachial embolectomy is rare, as the runoff vessels are accessible, but occasionally distal embolectomy is required via the radial artery at the wrist. Failure to establish

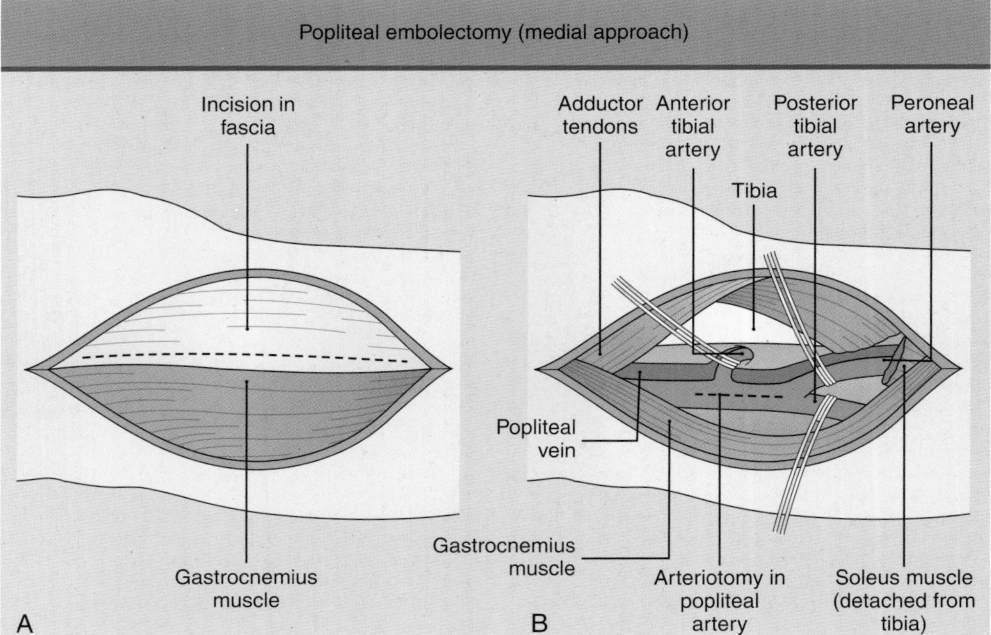

Figure 14-7. Popliteal embolectomy. **A,** The medial incision extends down from the femoral condyle and is deepened by incising the fascia anterior to gastrocnemius. **B,** Division of the proximal attachment of the soleus to the back of the tibia and one of the tibial veins is required to completely expose the popliteal trifurcation. The arteriotomy must cross the origin of the anterior tibial artery and requires closure with a vein patch.

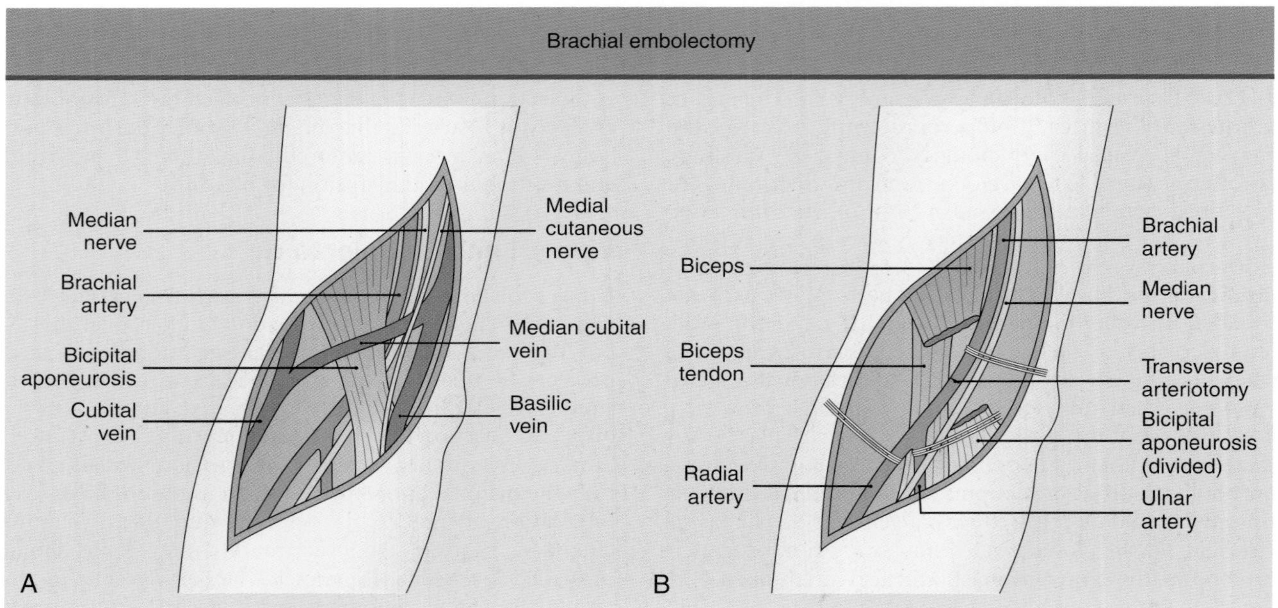

Figure 14-8. Brachial embolectomy. **A,** The brachial bifurcation is exposed via a lazy "S" incision, swinging laterally over the bicipital aponeurosis to end in the midline. The bifurcation is controlled with slings after division of the bicipital aponeurosis, taking care to protect the median nerve. **B,** A 120-degree transverse arteriotomy should be made proximal to the bifurcation and then closed with 6/0 interrupted Prolene sutures.

inflow should raise the possibility of a subclavian aneurysm or chronic proximal disease. This is why the subclavian pulse should be palpated and a preoperative arteriogram or duplex scan requested if a proximal aneurysm or occlusion is suspected. Sometimes a larger embolus lodged in the axillary or subclavian artery cannot be retrieved via the smaller caliber brachial artery. This requires retrieval via an axillary or supraclavicular approach. A proximal subclavian artery occlusion is best treated by intraoperative stenting via the brachial arteriotomy, with placement guided by a transfemoral catheter positioned in the aortic arch. A cervical rib causing arterial compression or aneurysm formation requires excision. Following removal of the rib, enough redundant length of subclavian artery often permits excision of the damaged or aneurysmal segment and end-to-end repair, without the need for interposition grafting.

Fasciotomy

Revascularization of ischemic muscle can result in considerable swelling within the fascial compartments of the leg. This compartment syndrome leads to further muscle and nerve

Table 14-2
Properties of the Components of the Fibrinolytic System*

Component	Molecular Weight	Plasma $t_{1/2}$	Properties
Streptokinase	48,000	16 minutes, then 90 minutes	Complexes with plasmin or plasminogen to gain activity
Urokinase	32,000/54,000	14 minutes	Direct plasminogen activator
r-Urokinase	32,000	7 minutes	Similar in most respects to natural urokinase
r-Prourokinase	49,000	7 minutes	Little intrinsic activity, converted to urokinase
r-tPA	68,000	3.5 minutes	Exhibits great degree of fibrin activity and specificity
TNK-tPA	65,000	15 minutes	Modified tPA with a longer half-life
Reteplase	39,000	14 minutes	Truncated tPA with a longer half-life
Plasminogen	88,000	2.2 days	Binds to fibrin, converted to active plasmin
Plasmin	88,000	0.1 seconds	Serine protease that cleaves fibrin
α_2-Antiplasmin	70,000	3 days	Inactivates free plasmin
PAI-1	52,000	Unknown	Inactivates the plasminogen activators

*PAI-1, plasminogen activator inhibitor-1; r-tPA, recombinant tissue plasminogen activator; TNK-tPA, tenecteplase; tPA, tissue plasminogen activator.

damage if not relieved. All muscle compartments should be decompressed via full-length skin and fascial incisions from knee to ankle if any muscle tenseness is present, or when ischemia has been prolonged (see Chapter 15 for more details).[19]

FURTHER MANAGEMENT

The operating surgeon should document the pulse status of the limb at the end of the operation. The surgeon should also decide whether reintervention is worthwhile if it becomes clear that reperfusion is inadequate. The wounds, pulse status, color, and capillary refilling of the extremity should be documented hourly. Wound hematomas are common because of anticoagulation[20] and are best drained unless small.

Revascularization of an ischemic limb results in a sudden venous return of blood with low pH and a high potassium concentration. The anesthetist must be prepared to correct these, as hypotension and arrhythmias may occur. Reperfusion of a large mass of ischemic tissue results in a systemic inflammatory reaction caused by neutrophil activation. This may cause multiple organ dysfunction, including renal and pulmonary failure (see Chapter 18). Initial reperfusion with a hypertonic perfusate containing antioxidants, combined with venous drainage, reduces this systemic injury.[21] Renal function may be further impaired by myoglobinuria. This can be avoided by maintaining a good diuresis, but it is important to beware of pushing a patient with poor cardiac reserve into heart failure. Established renal failure requires hemofiltration, dialysis, or both. Careful monitoring on a high-dependency unit is beneficial for all patients with significant comorbidity. Inotropes may be required for cardiac or renal support.

Following embolectomy, anticoagulation with unfractionated heparin and then coumadin (warfarin) is continued as this reduces the risk of recurrent embolism, especially if atrial fibrillation is present.[20,22,23] A search for a proximal source should be undertaken in patients with clear-cut embolism who do not have atrial fibrillation. This includes an abdominal ultrasound scan to exclude an aneurysm, a 24-hour electrocardiogram to exclude paroxysmal arrhythmias, and an echocardiogram to exclude cardiac thrombus or valvular pathology. Little evidence exists regarding the role of anticoagulation in patients without atrial fibrillation.[24] For many patients, an individual decision needs to be made, based on the risks of warfarinization and the state of the distal circulation. Where contraindications exist to warfarin therapy, some clinicians use dual antiplatelet therapy (e.g., aspirin with clopidogrel) as an alternative. Anticoagulation with low-molecular-weight heparin is a reasonable alternative to unfractionated heparin after 24 hours or so. It is inadvisable to use it around the time of surgery because of the long half-life and difficulty in monitoring and reversal.

THROMBOLYTIC AGENTS

Pharmacology

All available thrombolytic agents in clinical use are plasminogen activators (Table 14-2). As such, they do not directly degrade fibrinogen. Rather, they are trypsin-like serine proteases that have high specific activity directed at the cleavage of a single peptide bond in the plasminogen zymogen, converting it to plasmin. Plasmin is the active molecule that cleaves fibrin polymer to cause the dissolution of thrombus. The importance of plasminogen was first noted in 1941, when it was found that clots formed with highly purified fibrinogen and thrombin were not lysed by streptococcal fibrinolysin unless a small amount of human serum (plasminogen) was added. Recognizing this direct role of plasminogen, early investigators attempted to dissolve occluding thrombi with the administration of exogenous plasmin. Free plasmin, however, was ineffective as a thrombolytic agent as it is extremely unstable at physiological pH. Effective thrombolysis can only be achieved when fibrin-bound plasminogen is converted to its active form, plasmin, at the site of the thrombus.

Thrombolytic agents can be classified by their pharmacological actions: those that are "fibrin specific" (bind to fibrin but not fibrinogen) versus those that are nonspecific and those that have a great degree of "fibrin affinity" (bind avidly to fibrin) versus those that do not (Table 14-3). They can also be divided into groups based on the origin of the parent compound. It is most efficient to divide the agents into three groups: the SK compounds, the urokinase compounds, and the tPAs.

Table 14-3
Properties of the Thrombolytic Agents

Agent*	Fibrin Specificity	Fibrin Affinity
Streptokinase	Low	Low
Urokinase	Low	Low
tPA	High	High
TNK-tPA	Very high	High
Reteplase	High	Low

*TNK-tPA, tenecteplase; tPA, tissue plasminogen activator.

Streptokinase Compounds

SK, originating from the streptococcus bacteria, was the first thrombolytic agent to be described.[25] SK is a 50-kDa molecule with a biphasic half-life comprising a rapid $t_{1/2}$ of 16 minutes and a second, slower $t_{1/2}$ of 90 minutes. Whereas the initial half-life is accounted for by the formation of a complex between the molecule and the SK antibodies, the second half-life represents the actual biological elimination of the protein. SK differs from other thrombolytic agents with respect to plasminogen binding. Whereas other agents directly convert plasminogen to plasmin, SK must form a complex with a plasmin or plasminogen molecule to gain activity. Only then can this SK–plasmin or plasminogen complex activate a second plasminogen molecule to form active plasmin; thus, two plasminogen molecules are used in SK-mediated plasmin generation.

SK has significant antigenic potential. Preformed antibodies exist to a certain extent in all patients who have been infected with the streptococcus bacterium. Similarly, patients with exposure to SK may have high antibody titers on repeat exposure. These neutralizing antibodies inactivate exogenously administered SK. SK antibodies may be overwhelmed through the use of a large initial bolus of SK. Some investigators have recommended measurement of antibody titers before beginning SK therapy, gauging the loading dose on the basis of this titer.[26] While SK administration may be complicated by allergic reactions such as urticaria, pyrexia, periorbital edema, and bronchospasm, the major untoward effect associated with SK is hemorrhage, although this is no different from bleeding associated with any thrombolytic agent.

Urokinase Compounds

The fibrinolytic potential of human urine was first described by Macfarlane and Pinot in 1947.[27] The active molecule was extracted, isolated, and named "urokinase" in 1952.[28] This urokinase-type plasminogen activator is a serine protease composed of two polypeptide chains, occurring in low-molecular-weight (32 kDa) and high-molecular-weight (54 kDa) forms. The high-molecular-weight form predominates in urokinase isolated from urine, while the low-molecular-weight form is found in urokinase obtained from tissue culture of kidney cells. Unlike SK, urokinase directly activates plasminogen to form plasmin; prior binding to plasminogen or plasmin is not necessary for activity. Also in contrast to SK, preformed antibodies to urokinase are not observed. The agent is nonantigenic, and untoward reactions of fever or hypotension are rare. Most urokinase is now of tissue-culture origin, manufactured from human neonatal kidney cells, or manufactured from recombinant techniques using a murine hybridoma cell line (recombinant urokinase).

Tissue Plasminogen Activators

tPA is a naturally occurring fibrinolytic agent produced by endothelial cells and intimately involved in the balance between intravascular thrombogenesis and thrombolysis.[29] Natural tPA is a single-chain (527 amino acid) serine protease with a molecular weight of approximately 65 kDa. Plasmin hydrolyzes the Arg275–Ile276 peptide bond, converting the single-chain molecule into a two-chain moiety. In contrast to most serine proteases (e.g., urokinase), the single-chain form of tPA has significant activity. tPA has potential benefits over other thrombolytic agents. The agent exhibits significant fibrin specificity. In plasma, the agent is associated with little plasminogen activation. At the site of the thrombus, however, the binding of tPA and plasminogen to the fibrin surface induces a conformational change in both molecules, greatly facilitating the conversion of plasminogen to plasmin and dissolution of the clot. tPA also manifests the property of fibrin affinity; that is, it binds strongly to fibrin.

r-tPA was produced in the 1980s after molecular cloning techniques were used to express human tPA DNA. In an effort to lengthen the duration of bioavailability of tPA, the molecule has been systematically bioengineered. Tenecteplase (TNK-tPA) is a novel molecule with a greater half-life and fibrin specificity. The longer half-life of TNK-tPA allowed successful administration as a single bolus for acute myocardial infarction, in contrast to the requirement for an infusion with r-tPA. In addition, TNK-tPA manifests greater fibrin specificity than r-tPA, resulting in less fibrinogen depletion. In studies of acute coronary occlusion, TNK-tPA performed at least as well as r-tPA, concurrent with greater ease of administration.[30]

The r-tPA reteplase is similar to tenecteplase. Reteplase has a longer half-life than r-tPA, potentially enabling bolus injection versus prolonged infusion. The fibrin affinity of reteplase was only 30% of that exhibited with tPA, similar to urokinase. The decrease in fibrin affinity was hypothesized to reduce the incidence of distant bleeding complications in a manner similar to that of SK over r-tPA in the Global Use of Strategies to Open Occluded Coronary Arteries (GUSTO) Trial.[31] Reteplase has demonstrated some benefit over r-tPA in the GUSTO III Study for acute myocardial infarction.[32]

Comparison of Thrombolytic Agents

Few well-designed clinical comparisons have been made of various thrombolytic agents in acute limb ischemia. Various in vitro studies and retrospective clinical trials exist, most pointing to improved efficacy and safety of urokinase and r-tPA over SK.[33,34] In an analysis of data collected in a prospective, single institution registry at the Cleveland Clinic Foundation, urokinase demonstrated a diminished rate of bleeding complications when compared with r-tPA.[35] Efficacy was not evaluated in this trial.

Two prospective, randomized comparisons have been made of urokinase and r-tPA, neither of which was blinded. Meyerovitz and associates from the Brigham and Women's

Hospital randomized 32 patients with peripheral arterial or bypass graft occlusions of less than 90 days' duration to r-tPA (10-mg bolus, 5 mg/hr to a maximum of 24 hours) or urokinase (60,000-IU bolus, 4000 IU/min for 2 hours, 2000 IU/min for 2 hours, then 1000 IU/min to a maximum of 24 hours' total administration).[36] Significantly greater systemic fibrinogen degradation occurred in the r-tPA group ($p = 0.01$), indicating that the fibrin specificity of r-tPA was lost at this dose. r-tPA achieved more rapid initial thrombolysis, but efficacy was identical in the two groups by 24 hours. The tradeoff to more rapid thrombolysis was a trend toward a higher rate of bleeding complications in the r-tPA-treated patients ($p = 0.39$).

The second randomized comparison of urokinase and r-tPA was the STILE Trial, a three-armed multicenter comparison of urokinase (250,000-IU bolus, 4000 IU/min for 4 hours, then 2000 IU/min for up to 36 hours), r-tPA (0.05 to 0.1 mg/kg/hr for up to 12 hours), and primary operation.[37] One intracranial hemorrhage occurred in the urokinase group (0.9%), and two happened in the r-tPA group (1.5%, no significant difference). Although actual rates of overall bleeding complications and efficacy were not reported for the two thrombolytic groups, the authors remarked that no significant differences were detected in any of the outcome variables. In a subsequent "reanalysis" of the data, reported in 1999, the frequency of complete clot lysis was similar with urokinase and r-tPA at the time of the early arteriographic study.[38] This recent information suggests that the rate of thrombolysis may be similar, in contrast to the popularly held view that r-tPA is a more rapidly acting agent.

INTRAARTERIAL THROMBOLYSIS

Every vascular interventionalist who undertakes intraarterial thrombolysis has a personal preference regarding thrombolytic agent and method. Each uses a subtly different technique, but the following schedule emphasizes the important components of an episode of intraarterial thrombolysis.[39]

Catheter Insertion

Once the diagnosis is confirmed, an infusion catheter needs to be inserted within the arterial obstruction. The occlusion is usually approached from the contralateral groin if it is above the inguinal ligament or in the proximal SFA, using the diagnostic catheter puncture site if possible. The approach is from the ipsilateral groin for distal femoropopliteal occlusions and often requires a second puncture. An introducer sheath facilitates catheter changes during progression of thrombolysis but does leave a larger puncture site for later hemostasis. The infusion catheter should be inserted 7 cm into the thrombus. The catheter size used is usually 3 Fr or 4 Fr, with a single end hole. Catheters with multiple side holes can be used, provided that all side holes are situated within the thrombus. A mistake made when thrombolysis was in its infancy was to position the catheter proximal to the thrombus, with resulting poor outcomes. If a guide wire is used to place the infusion catheter, this can also be used to probe the arterial occlusion. The ability to cross the occlusion with a guide wire (guide wire traversal test) is an excellent predictor of successful thrombolysis. If the thrombus is impenetrable, the arterial occlusion is likely chronic. Occasionally, infusion of the lytic agent just proximal to a chronic occlusion softens it sufficiently for a catheter to be inserted.

Low-Dose Infusion

Conventionally, 0.5 to 1 mg of tPA, or its equivalent, are infused per hour. A reasonable volume of fluid should be infused so that a steady concentration of lytic drug is maintained (5 to 10 ml of fluid per hour). Concomitant heparin is used by some to prevent pericatheter thrombosis. Other maneuvers that speed the duration of lysis include lacing and debulking. Lacing the entire length of the thrombus with lytic drug can speed up the process. Debulking using aspiration embolectomy can also accelerate thrombolysis (as described later). Once the infusion is running, sequential angiography is performed. Usually, an initial angiogram after 4 hours confirms the position of the catheter and commencement of lysis; after this, angiography should be performed at least every 12 hours until the occlusion is lysed (Figure 14-9). The infusion is stopped if no clot lysis occurs between two 12-hour angiograms or if complications ensue. If the occlusion is long, it often is necessary to advance the infusion catheter as the occlusion is gradually lysed. Some experienced practitioners feel it is better to lyse the occlusion from distal to proximal by sequentially withdrawing the catheter to try to prevent distal embolization. Often, successful thrombolysis uncovers a significant arterial stenosis. Angioplasty may be performed at any stage during the lytic process; some radiologists perform it as early as possible, as soon as a stenosis is identified. Angioplasty should certainly not be left until days after a successful procedure, as rethrombosis is highly likely. The fundamental principle of intraarterial thrombolysis is to establish forward flow as soon as possible.

Systemic heparin is often administered before and after thrombolysis to counteract the associated prothrombotic tendency, although some data from trials of the thrombolytic treatment of acute stroke suggest that heparin may increase hemorrhagic complications. An alternative is concurrent administration of low-dose heparin (200 U/hr) via the proximal arterial sheath while delivering the thrombolytic agent via an end-hole catheter to an occlusion below the inguinal ligament.

Accelerated Methods of Thrombolysis

Conventional low-dose intraarterial thrombolysis takes between 18 and 30 hours to clear most arterial occlusions. This may be too long for a patient with a threatened leg, who may have established muscle and skin damage at this stage. Several techniques speed the duration of lysis, either by using special catheters or by varying the lytic schedules. Pulse spray thrombolysis uses an infusion catheter with multiple side holes shaped as slits (Figure 14-10). A special infusion pump is attached to the catheter, and this delivers small pulses of lytic agent throughout the thrombus as a fine spray. This technique partially macerates the occlusion and delivers drug throughout its whole length. The technique speeds thrombolysis, and good results have been published.[40,41] However, the equipment required is expensive.

Various methods of altering lytic infusions have been tested. One that has been investigated in a randomized, controlled trial is high-dose bolus lysis.[42] Three 5-mg boluses

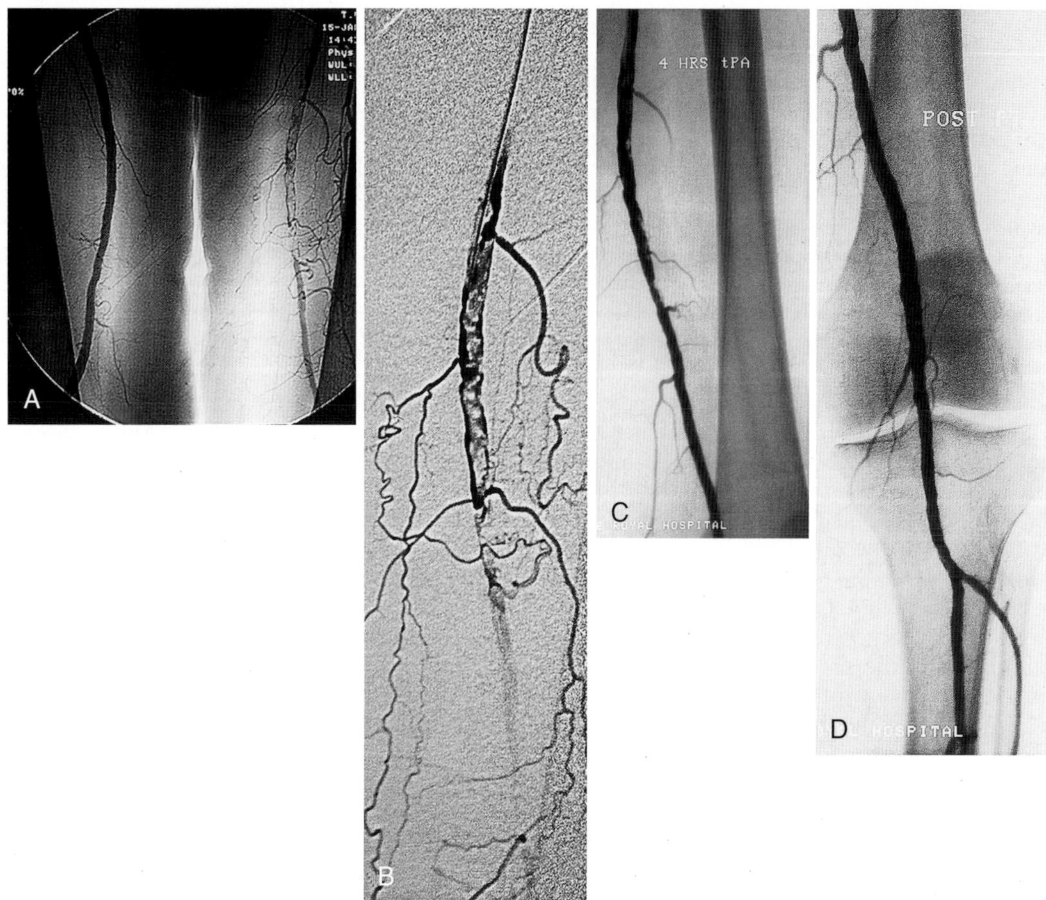

Figure 14-9. Low-dose intraarterial thrombolysis. A, Superficial femoral artery (SFA) thrombosis of 14 days' duration. B, Thrombogram after catheter insertion. C, After 4-hour lysis with tPA at 0.5 mg/hr, the SFA was patent but with a midpoint stenosis. D, Good result after angioplasty.

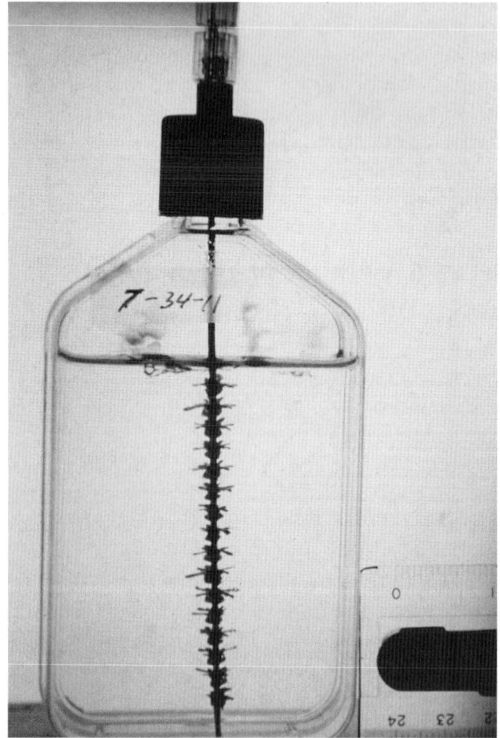

Figure 14-10. Pulse spray lysis catheter in a gelatin bottle. Note the multiple side holes.

of tPA are given over 30 minutes, laced into the full length of the occlusion. If this approach results in no angiographic improvement, lysis is abandoned and the patient is taken for surgery. This is termed the trial of lysis. If after 30 minutes some dissolution of the thrombus has occurred, an infusion of 3.5 mg of tPA per hour is continued for the next 4 hours. Most patients have complete or partial thrombolysis by the end of the 4 hours. If not, treatment can be continued, but the dose is usually reduced to 0.5 to 1 mg/hr. The median duration of lysis using this technique is reduced from 24 to 7 hours (Figure 14-11).

The use of accelerated thrombolysis means that patients with a threatened limb and a partial neurological deficit can be treated by endovascular means. No specific clinical advantage has been seen, and none of the trials has shown improved results with accelerated thrombolysis over conventional techniques in equivalent patients. In patients with a viable leg and no neurosensory deficit, vascular specialists are free to choose the technique they prefer, and an individual decision is acceptable.

Aspiration Embolectomy

The principle of aspiration embolectomy is to remove small fragments of clot percutaneously.[43] The easiest way of doing this is to use a 5-Fr or 7-Fr catheter with the tapered end removed (modified Van Andel predilator). This is passed into

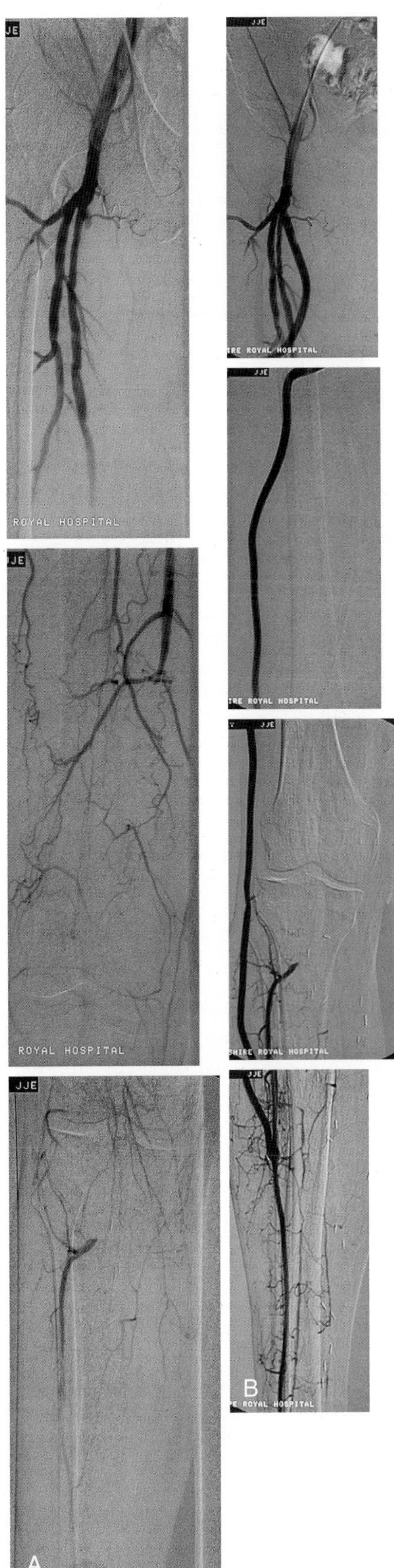

Figure 14-11. Composite angiograms showing occluded femoropopliteal polytetrafluoroethylene graft **(A)** treated successfully with high-dose bolus tPA within 4 hours **(B).**

the occlusion and pulled back through it. A 50-ml syringe is attached to the end of the catheter and aspirated when it is withdrawn through the occlusion. The aspirated clot is collected, and angiography is used to confirm forward flow. Manufacturers have created sets containing all equipment needed to perform this technique (Cook Single-Handed Aspiration Set, Cook, United Kingdom). The results in selected patients with small emboli are good. Adjuvant thrombolysis is often required if larger occlusions are treated. The technique is useful when distal embolization occurs during endovascular therapy. It has obvious advantages over conventional surgical embolectomy.

Percutaneous Mechanical Thrombectomy

The aim with percutaneous mechanical thrombectomy is to break up thrombus within the vessel and aspirate it percutaneously. All available percutaneous mechanical thrombectomy devices are relatively expensive single-use items and are only recommended in fresh occlusions less than 14 days old. There are several principles. The Amplatz Thrombectomy device (Microvena) uses an air-driven impeller rotating at 100,000 to 150,000 rpm to create a vortex that attracts and then macerates thrombus into tiny fragments, which disperse into the circulation. The Arrow-Trerotola device has a four-wire basket spinning at 3000 rpm. Both devices have little steerability, tend to embolize distally because there is no mechanism for aspirating debris, and cause hemolysis (which is only rarely clinically significant). More popular are the devices that use high-pressure saline jets to create a vacuum (Venturi principle) so that thrombus is aspirated into a maceration chamber and then removed through a separate channel. This technique has the hazard that a significant volume of blood can be lost during aspiration of a long occlusion. Current devices include the Hydrolyser (Cordis), Oasis (Boston Scientific), and Angiojet (Possis). The Ekos Catheter uses high-frequency, low-energy ultrasound to loosen the fibrin, thus making it more accessible to thrombolytic drugs. The Acolysis catheter uses low-frequency, high-energy ultrasound to directly lyse clot. It is proposed that it be used alone or as an adjunct to pharmacological thrombolysis. The Resolution 360 wire vibrates a titanium wire at 20 kHz to create microbubbles and clot dissolution without drugs.

Although the U.S. Food and Drug Administration has approved eight percutaneous mechanical thrombectomy devices for use in occluded hemodialysis grafts, only the Angiojet is licensed for use in peripheral arterial occlusions. All of these devices have the advantage of immediacy but in general are used mainly in patients with stable acute ischemia. No comparative trials have been done with surgery, or more importantly with thrombolysis. It is often necessary to supplement thrombectomy with further thrombolysis. Large puncture wounds are needed in the groin, and hematoma formation is common. Significant arterial damage is also an occasional complication. However, results comparable with other treatments have been reported in selected patients.[44,45]

Further Management

Patients should be monitored in a suitable area. Ideally, a ward staffed by specialist vascular nurses or a high-dependency unit should be employed. Clinicians who feel that lysis should only be performed in a high-dependency unit run the risk that this procedure will not be able to be carried out unless such a bed is available. Vital signs should be assessed regularly, and arterial puncture sites should be monitored carefully for signs of bleeding. The perfusion status of the leg should be monitored hourly. Dehydration should be avoided with intravenous fluids to maintain a good diuresis. Patients can receive oral fluids, but it is best to avoid giving them food, just in case urgent surgery becomes necessary. Supplemental oxygen is beneficial.[7] Intraarterial thrombolysis can be uncomfortable, and analgesia is important. If oral analgesia is not adequate, intravenous opiate infusion is better than intramuscular injections, which run the risk of bruising. The most efficient way of caring for patients undergoing intraarterial thrombolysis is to use a care pathway that contains reminders of all of these items. Regular hematological monitoring does not seem to improve outcome or reduce the risk of bleeding complications. The only coagulation factor that predicts bleeding complications is a low plasma fibrinogen level. The activated partial thromboplastin time should also be monitored carefully if heparin has been administered.

Once successful thrombolysis has been achieved, the infusion catheter should be removed as soon as possible. Groin puncture sites need firm pressure, often for 20 to 30 minutes. Pressure should not occlude the artery, as this can cause rethrombosis. Arterial closure devices (e.g., Perclose) can be useful in this situation.[46] A rebound risk of hypercoagulability occurs after thrombolysis, and patients should be anticoagulated with heparin for at least 48 hours. The role of prolonged anticoagulation is as controversial here as after embolectomy. Some vascular surgeons anticoagulate patients with sodium warfarin for long periods. Others feel that antiplatelet medication alone is satisfactory in those who have high flow through a vessel treated with angioplasty and good runoff. Duplex ultrasound imaging postprocedure is advisable, particularly if the cause of occlusion has not been found.

Minimizing the Risks of Intraarterial Thrombolysis

Many vascular surgeons and radiologists believe that intraarterial thrombolysis is a particularly dangerous undertaking. However, if managed carefully, the risks of intraarterial thrombolysis need be no greater than those of major surgery. Thrombolysis driven by protocol and using care pathways helps optimize the results and minimize the risks.[47]

Bleeding is the most common complication and can be severe in up to 10% of patients. Minor puncture site bleeding is more common and can be seen in up to half of the procedures (Figure 14-12). Usually, simple pressure over the groin, possibly with a sandbag, can keep oozing under control. If a significant groin hematoma occurs, or signs of major blood loss or shock appear, thrombolysis needs to be stopped. Resuscitation and blood transfusion then need to be given. Considerable retroperitoneal bleeding is possible and occurs particularly after high antegrade arterial puncture. Computed tomography or ultrasound imaging is occasionally needed to make the diagnosis. If the risk to life becomes greater than the risk to the leg, it may be necessary to reverse the bleeding tendency caused by thrombolysis. Clotting factors can be given, although cryoprecipitate is the most useful infusion to restore levels of fibrinogen that have been degraded by the lytic agents. Antifibrinolytic drugs such as tranexamic acid may have a role. All fibrinolytic drugs cause abnormalities of coagulation, particularly if therapy is prolonged.

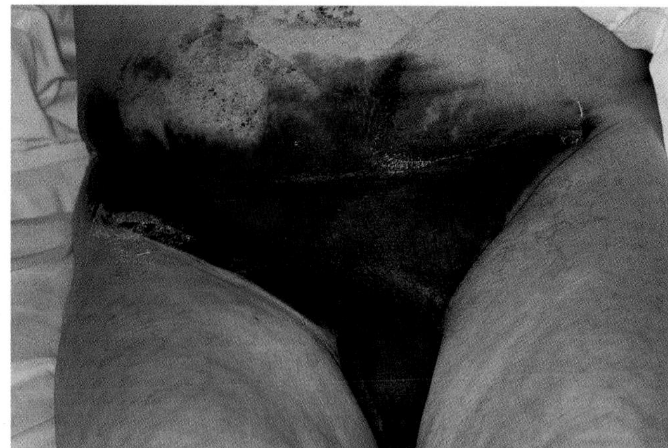

Figure 14-12. Extensive groin hematoma after successful intraarterial thrombolysis.

Stroke is the most feared complication of intraarterial thrombolysis, occurring in approximately 2% of procedures. In fact, only 50% of the strokes are hemorrhagic; the other 50% are thrombotic due to the nature of the high-risk patient group being treated. If a stroke occurs during thrombolysis, urgent brain computed tomography is required. If the stroke is hemorrhagic, thrombolysis should clearly be stopped; the dilemma is whether or not to continue thrombolysis in a patient who has a thrombotic occlusion. The incidence of stroke during thrombolysis means that pretreatment consent is an important part of counseling.

Distal embolization occurs in up to 10% of patients due to the breakup of thrombus during lysis. In most patients, continued infusion clears the small distal occlusions. If the foot does not improve after 4 hours of continued thrombolysis, surgical embolectomy is required to retrieve the distal thrombus. The highest risk of distal embolization is during the thrombolysis of an acutely thrombosed popliteal aneurysm.[4] Rethrombosis is rare after properly conducted thrombolysis. If it occurs, the reason is usually that the thrombolysis was inadequate or that an underlying cause was not corrected.

EVIDENCE FOR THROMBOLYTIC THERAPY

The British Thrombolysis Study Group has collected information on more than 1000 episodes of peripheral arterial thrombolysis.[48] Their overall results show an amputation-free survival rate of 75% at 30 days, a mortality rate of 12.5%, and an amputation with survival rate of 12.5%. A multivariate analysis was performed to evaluate factors that affected outcome. Amputation-free survival was improved in patients taking warfarin before the episode and was poorer in diabetic patients, those who had threatened legs with a neurological deficit, and those with a short duration of ischemia. Other factors that adversely affected mortality and amputation rates included female gender, a history of ischemic heart disease, and an occlusion due to embolism. In general, amputation rates were higher in patients with a thrombosis and mortality

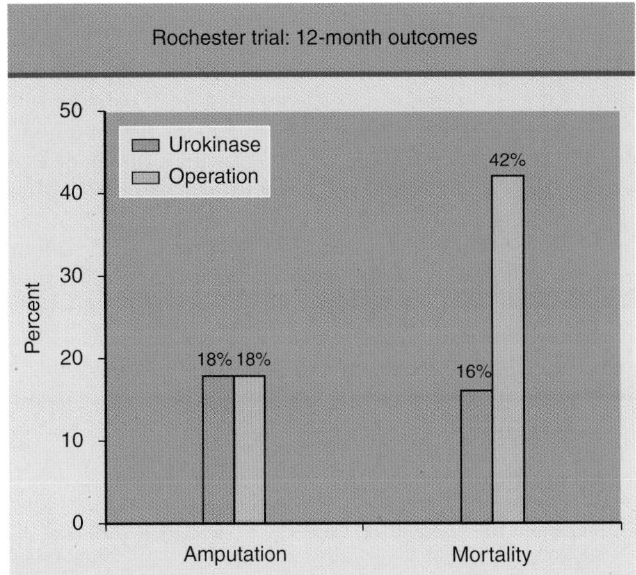

Figure 14-13. Rochester trial: 12-month outcomes. The rate of amputation was identical in the two treatment groups in the Rochester trial, but the mortality rate was significantly lower in patients assigned to thrombolytic therapy.

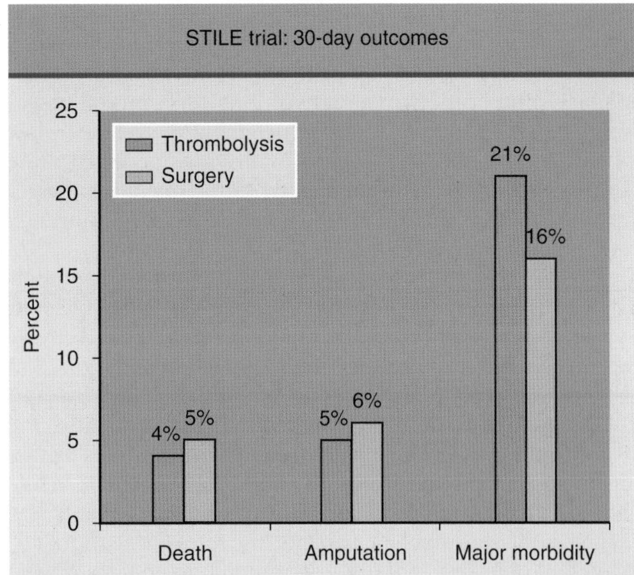

Figure 14-14. Surgery or Thrombolysis for the Ischemic Lower Extremity Trial: 30-day outcomes. Note that the rates of death and amputation are similar.

rates were higher in patients with embolism. Amputation rates and mortality were not insubstantial when patients with acute claudication were treated with thrombolysis, and this is no longer recommended.[49] Physiological scoring systems can help predict mortality after thrombolysis.[50]

Three well-controlled, randomized comparisons have been made of thrombolytic therapy versus primary operation in patients with recent peripheral arterial occlusion. From the start, the clinician must realize that thrombolytic therapy alone is seldom sufficient therapy. Successful pharmacological dissolution of thrombus must be followed by definitive therapy to address the underlying lesion that caused the occlusion. When no such lesion can be found, the risk of early rethrombosis is unacceptably high.[51] As testimony to this caveat, Sullivan et al. observed postthrombolysis 2-year patency rates of 79% in bypass grafts with a flow-limiting lesion identified and corrected by angioplasty or surgery versus only 9.8% in patients without such lesions.[51]

The first study of thrombolysis versus surgery, the Rochester series, compared urokinase to primary operation in 114 patients presenting with what has subsequently been called hyperacute ischemia.[52] Enrolled patients in this trial all had severely threatened limbs (Rutherford class IIB) with a mean symptom duration of approximately 2 days. This was a single-center trial funded by the Thrombolysis and Thrombosis Program Project National Institutes of Health grant at the University of Rochester, Rochester, New York. After 12 months of follow-up, 84% of patients randomized to urokinase were alive, compared to only 58% of patients randomized to primary operation (Figure 14-13). By contrast, the rate

Table 14-4
Results of the TOPAS Trial, Demonstrating Similar Mortality Rates and Amputation-Free Survival Rates after Thrombolysis or Surgery

	Native Artery Occlusions (n = 242)			Bypass Graft Occlusions (n = 302)		
Intervention	Urokinase (n = 122)	Surgery (n = 120)	p Value	Urokinase (n = 150)	Surgery (n = 152)	p Value
Complete dissolution of clot on final angiogram	67/112 (60%)	NA*	—	100/134 (75%)	NA	—
Increase in ankle–brachial index†	0.44 ± 0.04	0.52 ± 0.04	0.15‡	0.48 ± 0.03	0.50 ± 0.03	0.76‡
Mortality (%):						
6 months	20.8	15.9	0.33§	12.1	9.4	0.45§
1 year	24.6	19.6	0.36§	16.2	15.0	0.77§
Amputation-free survival (%):						
6 months	67.6	76.1	0.15§	75.2	73.9	0.79§
1 year	61.2	71.4	0.10§	68.2	68.8	0.91§

*NA, not applicable.
†Mean ± standard error.
‡The p value was based on one-way analysis of variance.
§The p value was based on Kaplan–Meier analysis.

of limb salvage was identical at 80%. A closer inspection of the raw data revealed that the defining variable for mortality differences was the development of perioperative cardiopulmonary complications. The rate of long-term mortality was high when such complications occurred but was relatively low when they did not. That such complications occurred more commonly in patients taken directly to the operating theater was the only explanation for the greater long-term mortality rate in the operative group.

The second prospective, randomized analysis of thrombolysis versus surgery was the STILE Trial.[37] Genentech (South San Francisco, California), the manufacturer of the Activase brand of r-tPA, funded the study. At its termination, 393 patients were randomized to one of three treatment groups: r-tPA, urokinase, or primary operation. Subsequently, the two thrombolytic groups were combined for purposes of data analysis when the outcome was found to be similar. While the rate of the composite endpoint of untoward events was higher in the thrombolytic patients, the rates of the more relevant and objective endpoints of amputation and death were equivalent (Figure 14-14). Articles then appeared in the literature comprising subgroup analyses of the STILE data, one relating to native artery occlusions[53] and one to bypass graft occlusions.[54] Thrombolysis appeared to be more effective in patients with graft occlusions. The rate of major amputation was higher in native arterial occlusions treated with thrombolysis (10% thrombolysis versus 0% surgery at 1 year, $p = 0.0024$). By contrast, amputation was lower in patients with acute graft occlusions treated with thrombolysis ($p = 0.026$). These data suggest that thrombolysis may be of greatest benefit in patients with acute bypass graft occlusions of less than 14 days' duration.

The third and final randomized comparison of thrombolysis and surgery was the TOPAS Trial, funded by Abbott Laboratories (Abbott Park, Illinois). Following completion of a preliminary dose-ranging trial in 213 patients,[55] 544 patients were randomized to a recombinant form of urokinase or primary operative intervention. After a mean follow-up of 1 year, the rate of amputation-free survival was identical in the two treatment groups: 68.2% and 68.8% in the urokinase and surgical patients, respectively (Table 14-4). While this trial failed to document improvement in survival or limb salvage with thrombolysis, 31.5% of the thrombolytic patients were alive without amputation with nothing more than a percutaneous procedure after 6 months of follow-up. After 1 year, this number had decreased only slightly, with 25.7% alive without amputation and with only percutaneous interventions. Thus, the original goal of the TOPAS Trial, to generate data on which regulatory approval of recombinant urokinase would be based, was not achieved. Nevertheless, the findings confirmed that acute leg ischemia could be managed with catheter-directed thrombolysis, achieving similar amputation and mortality rates but avoiding the need for an open surgical procedure in a significant percentage of patients.

SUMMARY

The practical management of ALI remains a challenge, as it involves one of the most complex decision pathways in vascular surgery. A successful outcome depends on collaboration between an experienced vascular radiologist and a vascular surgeon (or a dedicated vascular specialist) with access to, and the ability to use, the full range of imaging and interventional techniques that may be required. Treatment should be based on the severity of the ischemia rather than the underlying cause. An arteriogram should be obtained in all patients with a threatened limb, but the target of treatment within 6 hours should not be compromised. A patient with a threatened leg who presents to a hospital without adequate vascular staffing or imaging capability should be transferred to the nearest vascular center without delay. The role of conventional balloon catheter embolectomy is diminishing, due to the proliferation of new percutaneous techniques and the decreasing incidence of cardiac embolism. However, the precise role of each treatment modality remains unclear, and the choice should be made on an individual basis for each patient.

References

1. Rutherford RB, Flanigan DP, Gupta SK, et al. Suggested standards for reports dealing with lower extremity ischemia. *J Vasc Surg* 1986;4:80-94.
2. Norgren L, Hiatt WR, Dormandy JA, et al. Inter-society consensus for the management of peripheral arterial disease. *Eur J Vasc Endovasc Surg* 2007;33:S1-S75.
3. Campbell WB. Non-intervention and palliative care in vascular patients. *Br J Surg* 2000;87:1601-1602.
4. Galland RB, Earnshaw JJ, Baird RN, et al. Acute limb deterioration during intra-arterial thrombolysis. *Br J Surg* 1993;80:1118-1120.
5. Thompson JF, Beard J, Scott DJA, Earnshaw JJ. Intraoperative thrombolysis in the management of thrombosed popliteal aneurysm. *Br J Surg* 1993;80:858-859.
6. Eyers P, Earnshaw JJ. Acute non-traumatic arm ischaemia. *Br J Surg* 1998;85:1340-1346.
7. Berridge DC, Hopkinson BR, Makin GS. Acute lower limb arterial ischaemia: a role for continuous oxygen inhalation. *Br J Surg* 1980;76:1021-1023.
8. Blaisdell FW, Steele M, Allen RE. Management of lower extremity arterial ischaemia due to embolism and thrombosis. *Surgery* 1978;84:822-834.
9. Campbell WB, Ballard PK. Intra-arterial lignocaine in embolectomy. *Br J Surg* 1996;83:244.
10. Gwynn BR, Shearman CP, Simms MH. The anatomical basis for the route taken by Fogarty catheters in the lower leg. *Eur J Vasc Surg* 1987;1:129-132.
11. Bosma HW, Jorning PJG. Intraoperative arteriography in arterial embolectomy. *Eur J Vasc Surg* 1990;4:469-472.
12. Beard JD, Nyamekye I, Earnshaw JJ, et al. Intraoperative streptokinase: a useful adjunct to balloon catheter embolectomy. *Br J Surg* 1993;80:21-24.
13. Knaus J, Ris HB, Do D, Stirnemann P. Intraoperative catheter thrombolysis as an adjunct to surgical revascularization for infrainguinal limb threatening ischaemia. *Eur J Vasc Surg* 1993;7:507-512.
14. Quinones-Baldrich WJ, Baker D, Busuttil RW, et al. Intraoperative infusion of lytic drugs for thrombotic complications of revascularization. *J Vasc Surg* 1989;10:408-417.
15. Law MM, Gelabert HA, Colburn MD, et al. Continuous postoperative intra-arterial urokinase infusion in the treatment of no reflow following revascularization of the acutely ischaemic limb. *Ann Vasc Surg* 1994;8:66-73.
16. Youkey JR, Clagett GP, Cabellon Jr S, et al. Thromboembolectomy of arteries explored at the ankle. *Ann Surg* 1984;199:367-371.
17. Wyffels PL, DeBord JR. Increased limb salvage with distal tibial–peroneal artery thrombectomy–embolectomy in acute lower limb ischaemia. *Am J Surg* 1990;56:468-475.
18. Wyffels PL, DeBord JR, Marshall JS, et al. Increased limb salvage with intraoperative and postoperative ankle level urokinase infusion in the treatment of no reflow following revascularisation of the acutely ischaemic limb. *Ann Vasc Surg* 1994;8:66-73.
19. Ernst CB. Fasciotomy in perspective. *J Vasc Surg* 1989;9:829-830.
20. Hammarsten J, Holm J, Shersten T. Positive and negative effects of anticoagulant treatment during and after arterial embolectomy. *J Cardiovasc Surg* 1978;19:373-379.
21. Walker PM, Romaschim AD, Davis S, Piovesan J. Lower limb ischemia: phase 1 results of salvage perfusion. *J Surg Res* 1999;84:193-198.

22. Ljungman C, Adami H-O, Bergqvist D, et al. Risk factors for early lower limb loss after embolectomy for acute arterial occlusion: a population-based case-control study. *Br J Surg* 1991;78:1482-1485.
23. Campbell WB, Ridler BM, Szymanska TH. Two year follow-up after acute thromboembolic leg ischaemia: the importance of anticoagulation. *Eur J Vasc Endovasc Surg* 2000;19:169-173.
24. Connolly SJ. Anticoagulation for patients with atrial fibrillation and risk factors for stroke. *BMJ* 2000;320:1219-1220.
25. Tillett WS. Garner RL The fibrinolytic activity of hemolytic streptococci. *J Exp Med* 1933;58:485-502.
26. Jostring H, Barth U, Naidu R. Changes of antistreptokinase titer following long-term streptokinase therapy. In: Martin M, Schoop W, Hirsh J, eds. *New concepts of streptokinase dosimetry*. Vienna: Hans Huber; 1978;110.
27. Macfarlane RG, Pinot JJ. Fibrinolytic activity of normal urine. *Nature* 1947;159:779.
28. Sobel GW, Mohler SR, Jones NW, et al. Urokinase: an activator of plasma fibrinolysin extracted from urine. *Am J Physiol* 1952;171:768-769.
29. Hoylaerts M, Rijken DC, Lijnen HR, Collen D. Kinetics of the activation of plasminogen by human tissue plasminogen activator: role of fibrin. *J Biol Chem* 1982;257:2912.
30. Cannon CP, Gibson CM, McCabe CH, et al. TNK-tissue plasminogen activator compared with front-loaded alteplase in acute myocardial infarction: results of the TIMI 10B trial. Thrombolysis in Myocardial Infarction (TIMI) 10B investigators. *Circulation* 1998;98:2805-2814.
31. Global Use of Strategies to Open Occluded Coronary Arteries Investigators. An international randomized trial comparing four thrombolytic therapies for acute myocardial infarction. *N Engl J Med* 1993;329: 673-682.
32. Anonymous. A comparison of reteplase with alteplase for acute myocardial infarction: the Global Use of Strategies to Open Occluded Coronary Arteries (GUSTO III) investigators. *N Engl J Med* 1997;337:1118-1123.
33. van Breda A, Robison JC, Feldman L, et al. Local thrombolysis in the treatment of arterial graft occlusions. *J Vasc Surg* 1984;1:103-112.
34. Ouriel K, Welch EL, Shortell CK, et al. Comparison of streptokinase, urokinase, and recombinant tissue plasminogen activator in an in vitro model of venous thrombolysis. *J Vasc Surg* 1995;22:593-597.
35. Ouriel K, Gray BH, Clair DG, Olin JW. Complications associated with the use of urokinase and recombinant tissue plasminogen activator for catheter-directed peripheral arterial and venous thrombolysis. *J Vasc Intervent Radiol* 2000;11:295-298.
36. Meyerovitz M, Goldhaber SZ, Reagan K, et al. Recombinant tissue-type plasminogen activator versus urokinase in peripheral arterial and graft occlusions: a randomized trial. *Radiology* 1990;175:75-78.
37. Anonymous. Results of a prospective randomized trial evaluating surgery versus thrombolysis for ischemia of the lower extremity: the STILE Trial. *Ann Surg* 1994;220:251-266.
38. Comerota AJ. A re-analysis of the STILE data. Presented at the Montefiore Symposium, 1999, New York, New York.
39. Ouriel K. Current status of thrombolysis for peripheral arterial occlusive disease. *Ann Vasc Surg* 2002;16:797-804.
40. Yusuf SW, Whitaker SC, Gregson RHS, et al. Prospective randomized comparative study of pulse spray and conventional local thrombolysis. *Eur J Vasc Endovasc Surg* 1995;10:136-141.
41. Armon MP, Yusuf SW, Whitaker SC, et al. Results of 100 cases of pulse spray thrombolysis for acute and subacute leg ischaemia. *Br J Surg* 1997;84:47-50.
42. Braithwaite BD, Buckenham TM, Galland RB, et al. Prospective randomized trial of high-dose bolus versus low dose tissue plasminogen activator infusion in the management of acute limb ischaemia. *Br J Surg* 1997;84:646-650.
43. Cleveland TJ, Cumberland DC, Gaines PA. Percutaneous aspiration thromboembolectomy to manage the embolic complications of angioplasty and as an adjunct to thrombolysis. *Clin Radiol* 1994;49:549-552.
44. Kasirajan K, Haskal ZJ, Ouriel K. The use of mechanical thrombectomy devices in the management of acute peripheral arterial occlusive disease. *J Vasc Interv Radiol* 2001;12:405-411.
45. Morgan R. Belli A-M. Percutaneous thrombectomy: a review. *Eur Radiol* 2001;12:205-217.
46. Starnes BW, O'Donnell SD, Gillespie DL, et al. Percutaneous arterial closure in peripheral vascular disease: a prospective randomized evaluation of the Perclose device. *J Vasc Surg* 2003;38(2):263-271.
47. Whitman B, Parkin D, Earnshaw JJ. Management of acute leg ischaemia. In: Beard JD, Murray S, eds. *Pathways of care in vascular surgery*. Worcester, United Kingdom: TFM Publishing; 2002:99-105.
48. Earnshaw JJ, Whitman B, Foy C. On behalf of the Thrombolysis Study Group. National Audit of Thrombolysis for Acute Leg Ischaemia (NATALI) database: final clinical analysis. *Br J Surg* 2003;90:A504-A505.
49. Braithwaite BD, Tomlinson MA, Walker SR, et al. Peripheral thrombolysis for acute onset claudication. *Br J Surg* 1999;86:800-804.
50. Neary B, Whitman B, Foy C, et al. Value of POSSUM physiology scoring to assess outcome after intra-arterial thrombolysis for acute leg ischaemia. *Br J Surg* 2001;88:1344-1345.
51. Sullivan KL, Gardiner GAJ, Kandarpa K, et al. Efficacy of thrombolysis in infrainguinal bypass grafts. *Circulation* 1991;83(2 Suppl):I99-I105.
52. Ouriel K, Shortell CK, DeWeese JA, et al. A comparison of thrombolytic therapy with operative revascularization in the initial treatment of acute peripheral arterial ischemia. *J Vasc Surg* 1994;19:1021-1030.
53. Weaver FA, Comerota AJ, Youngblood M, et al. Surgical revascularization versus thrombolysis for nonembolic lower extremity native artery occlusions: results of a prospective randomized trial: The STILE investigators—Surgery versus Thrombolysis for Ischemia of the Lower Extremity. *J Vasc Surg* 1996;24:513-521.
54. Comerota AJ, Weaver FA, Hosking JD, et al. Results of a prospective, randomized trial of surgery versus thrombolysis for occluded lower extremity bypass grafts. *Am J Surg* 1996;172:105-112.
55. Ouriel K, Veith FJ, Sasahara AA. Thrombolysis or peripheral arterial surgery: phase I results. TOPAS investigators. *J Vasc Surg* 1996;23:64-73.
56. Jivegård L, Holm J, Scherstén T. Acute limb ischemia due to arterial embolism or thrombosis: influence of limb ischemia versus pre-existing cardiac disease on postoperative mortality rate. *J Cardiovasc Surg* 1988;29:32-36.
57. Anonymous. Results of a prospective randomized trial evaluating surgery versus thrombolysis for ischemia of the lower extremity. The STILE trial. *Ann Surg* 1994;220:251-266.
58. Ouriel K, Veith FJ, Sasahara AA. A comparison of recombinant urokinase with vascular surgery as initial treatment for acute arterial occlusion of the legs. *N Engl J Med* 1998;338:1105-1111.

chapter 15

Metabolic and Systemic Consequences of Acute Limb Ischemia

Frank Padberg Jr, MD • Walter N Durán, PhD

Key Points

- The severe consequences of acute limb ischemia are considered in three broad categories: ischemia, reperfusion, and local effects (compartment syndrome).

Ischemia

- Tissue and organ tolerance for ischemia is highly variable. The duration and extent of ischemia are major factors affecting outcome.
- Prompt restoration of blood flow remains the most effective intervention to minimize the deleterious effects of ischemia–reperfusion injury.
- Innovative experimental approaches developed to ameliorate the adverse effects of reperfusion have yet to translate into clinical practice.

Reperfusion

- Revascularization produces both local and systemic effects from release of toxic metabolites and stimulation of inflammatory mediators.

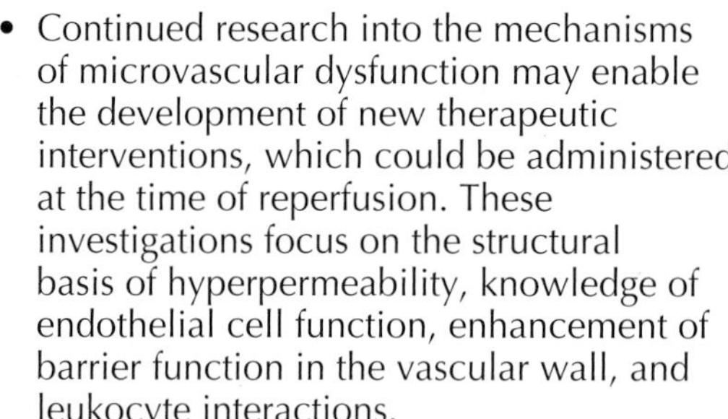

- Continued research into the mechanisms of microvascular dysfunction may enable the development of new therapeutic interventions, which could be administered at the time of reperfusion. These investigations focus on the structural basis of hyperpermeability, knowledge of endothelial cell function, enhancement of barrier function in the vascular wall, and leukocyte interactions.

Local Effects

- A diffuse increase in microvascular permeability produces the clinical finding of tissue edema. Reperfusion edema constrained by a restrictive fascial envelope results in compartmental hypertension.
- Compartment syndrome remains primarily a clinical diagnosis; however, measurement of compartment pressures may resolve an indistinct clinical presentation.
- Prompt, thorough fasciotomy decompresses compartmental hypertension.

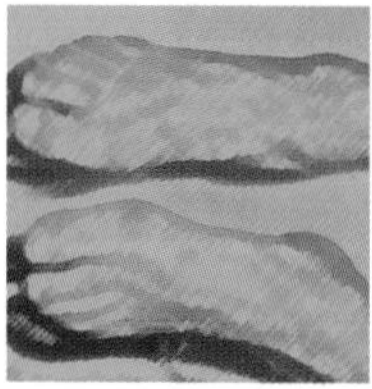

Acute limb ischemia may result from arterial trauma, arterial occlusion, thrombosis of a previous reconstruction, or thromboemboli. The magnitude of acute ischemic injury increases proportionally with the duration of ischemia and the mass of tissue affected. The mechanism of injury in reperfusion involves a series of events including inadequate oxygen delivery, reduction in cellular energy stores, accumulation of noxious metabolites, and oxygen-derived free radical injury.[1] The release of toxic metabolic products into the systemic circulation causes remote organ cellular dysfunction, increases in microvascular permeability, and produces tissue edema. Increased permeability to macromolecules is one of the earliest signs of dysfunction in skeletal muscle. Intravital microscopy techniques indicate that a significant increase in macromolecular transport occurs during the reperfusion phase.[2] The cellular alterations produced by ischemia are exaggerated by reperfusion. In addition, reperfusion causes new injury due to complex interactions between the newly reintroduced molecular oxygen and the cellular metabolic state set up by ischemia.

Significant secondary complications such as tissue necrosis, neuromuscular dysfunction, amputation, sepsis, multisystem

Table 15-1
SVS/ISCVS Criteria for Limb Viability. Clinical Categories of Acute Limb Ischemia (Based on SVS/ISCVS Classifcation)

Category	Description/Prognosis	Sensory Loss	Muscle Weakness	Arterial	Venous
I. Viable	Not immediately threatened	None	None	Audible	Audible
II. Threatened					
a. Marginally	Salvageable if promptly treated	Minimal or none	None	(Often) inaudible	Audible
b. Immediately	Salvageable with immediate revascularization	More than toes; often associated with rest pain	Mild, moderate	(Usually) inaudible	Audible
III. Irreversible	Major tissue loss or permanent nerve damage inevitable	Profound, anesthetic (rigor)	Profound, paralysis	Inaudible	Inaudible

organ failure, and death may follow acute arterial ischemia–reperfusion (IR) of skeletal muscle.[3-5] When the increase in permeability occurs within a restricted space, progressive swelling may obstruct venous return, capillary perfusion, and finally arterial flow. The combined effect produces ischemic injury to the tissues within that space. This condition, known as compartment syndrome, may be amenable to interventions including mechanical decompression by fasciotomy or pharmacotherapy designed to prevent or reduce tissue edema.

CLINICAL SIGNIFICANCE

The morbidity and mortality associated with acute limb ischemia are significant. The mortality rate for acute limb ischemia is 9% to 25%.[5,6] The major amputation rate is 13% to 25%. Factors reported to be associated with reduced risk of mortality are patient age less than 63 years, heparin administration, and percutaneous transluminal angioplasty. Increased risk of mortality has been associated with embolectomy, amputation, and fasciotomy.[6] In one large review, approximately 10% of the amputations were performed as the primary procedure for limbs deemed nonsalvagable. In one small series of patients with severe, bilateral limb ischemia and paralysis from acute aortic occlusion, mortality was 63% with amputation and paraplegia present in two of the three survivors.[4]

Patients presenting with acute limb ischemia are classified into three basic categories corresponding to recommendations for management.[5,7] The three categories of ischemia—viable, threatened, and irreversible—are in turn based on the clinical findings of sensory loss (none to extensive), muscle weakness (none to paralysis, rigor), and presence (or absence) of a pedal Doppler signal (Table 15-1).[5,7]

Effective management of acute limb ischemia and its sequelae may require fasciotomy. A contemporary study based on the U.S. National Inpatient Sample reported fasciotomy in 4.3% of limbs coded for acute embolism and thrombosis of the lower extremities. Fasciotomy was more common (25%) in a concomitant, retrospective experience at an academic institution. Those requiring fasciotomy were also at greater risk of amputation and death, presumably reflecting more advanced ischemia.[6]

ETIOLOGY

Ischemia followed by restoration of blood flow precipitates increases in permeability and local edema. The duration of ischemia can often be assessed accurately after trauma but is often less clear after an episode of arterial thromboembolism.[4,8] Combined arteriovenous injuries are more likely to result in tissue edema, especially when associated with venous occlusion. Coexistent hypotension exacerbates the IR injury.

Edema due to reperfusion of an ischemic extremity may develop several hours following revascularization; therefore, monitoring for compartmental hypertension should be a routine part of the careful postoperative evaluation.

It may be difficult to distinguish isolated compartment syndrome from acute limb ischemia. Clinical situations in which acute compartmental hypertension may mimic acute arterial ischemia are noted in Table 15-2. The most common nonarterial cause is fracture with secondary hemorrhage within a compartment. Other examples include prolonged compression of a muscular part, which may result from positioning for protracted surgery or prolonged immobilization

Table 15-2
Causes of Compartment Syndromes

Decreased compartment volume	Closure of fascial defects Application of excessive traction
Increased compartment content	Bleeding Major vascular coagulation disorder Increased capillary filtration Bites–Reptiles or insects Ischemia–reperfusion Trauma Intraarterial drug injection Cold Orthopedic injury Increased capillary pressure Acute venous obstruction Diminished serum osmolarity Nephrotic syndrome Other causes Infusion infiltration Pressure transfusion Muscular hypertrophy Popliteal cyst
Externally applied pressure	Tight casts, dressings, or splints Increased pressure on the limb due to prolonged immobilization during long surgical procedures or after recreational drug use

after recreational drug use.[8-12] A dressing or a cast that is too tight can cause external pressure. Crush injury and constriction from a circumferential burn eschar can be devastating.[3] Less common causes of compartment syndrome include massive soft-tissue swelling following the bite of a poisonous snake or insect due to release of toxins, unintentional extravascular infusion of intravenous fluids or medications, and iatrogenic compartment syndrome resulting from prolonged application of an extremity tourniquet or military antishock trousers.[13] Other unusual causes include phlegmasia cerulea dolens, malfunctioning pneumatic venous compression boots, and intraaortic balloon counterpulsation devices.[14-16] Complications related to intraarterial drug injections include diffuse arterial injury and acute ischemia from ligation of the infected arterial pseudoaneurysm.[10] Common clinical situations involving arterial compromise and associated compartmental hypertension include thromboembolism, occlusion of arterial reconstructions, primary arterial thrombosis, thrombosis of an aneurysm, arterial injuries, and high-velocity injuries with extensive soft-tissue damage.[4,6,8,17-19]

PATHOPHYSIOLOGY

The clinical components of acute limb ischemia may be considered in three broad categories: ischemia, reperfusion with its potential systemic effects, and local tissue hypertension. Some tissues are more susceptible than are others.

Ischemia

The magnitude of the ischemic insult is directly related to the duration and mass of ischemic tissue, as well as the severity of hypoperfusion. Skeletal muscle can tolerate complete ischemia for 4 to 6 hours, after which the injury becomes irreversible. Studies performed in our laboratory using canine models demonstrated that 6 hours of complete ischemia consistently produced skeletal muscle necrosis. This was verified in whole-limb preparations with both tourniquet and multiple ligation–induced ischemia and with isolated gracilis muscle preparations.[20,21] Following clinical episodes of arterial embolization in humans, mortality and amputation rates increase when the ischemia is prolonged for greater than 6 hours.[22] When ischemia is prolonged, the microvasculature loses its integrity and massive increases in permeability may accompany restoration of arterial perfusion. Systemic hypotension in the presence of acute limb ischemia amplifies the ischemia reperfusion injury response in the affected tissues. Ischemia, along with reperfusion injury to these tissues, may result in permanent impairment of function, amputation, or death.

Reperfusion

The reperfusion phase following ischemia is complex and may produce both local metabolic abnormalities and a systemic inflammatory response due to the release and activation of toxic metabolic products. Hemodynamically, reperfusion is characterized by diffuse hyperemic flow to the entire extremity.[21] Clinically important consequences include the development of acidosis, hyperkalemia, renal failure, acute respiratory insufficiency, arrhythmias, and neuromotor dysfunction. Acidosis and hyperkalemia result from the washout of accumulated byproducts of anaerobic metabolism. The factors responsible for the development of IR injury are the toxic metabolites of molecular oxygen such as superoxide radicals and hydroxyl radicals. The electronic configurations of these free radicals are highly unstable, and they react with other molecules to stabilize rapidly; however, in so doing, they cause structural and functional changes in cell membranes and organelles, resulting in their disruption. Many of these reactions result in the further release of free radicals, which, by themselves, are capable of propagating this process.[23]

Specific Tissues: Organs

Studies suggest that the fundamental mechanisms of reperfusion injury are similar in many organs, including the gastrointestinal tract, skin, heart, kidneys, and brain. Remote organ injury, including lungs, kidneys, heart, gastrointestinal tract, and brain, as a consequence of IR is a major cause of morbidity and even death from multiorgan failure.

Vulnerability to ischemia and reperfusion injury is variable and depends on the organ, the tissue, and the clinical situation. The brain, kidneys, and bowel are more susceptible to ischemia reperfusion injury than are the extremities. The duration of ischemia that can be tolerated by an organ is also variable; it is as short as 3 to 4 minutes for the brain and as much as 40 to 60 minutes for the kidneys.

With respect to the extremities, the most sensitive tissues are the sensory and motor nerves, followed by skeletal muscle, skin, and bone, which is why a neurosensory deficit is often the earliest clinical finding, preceding muscular dysfunction. Bourne and Rorabeck have shown that muscle blood flow and peroneal nerve conduction velocities decreased proportionately to the duration and magnitude of tissue hypertension.[24] Peroneal nerve conduction was lost with 30 minutes of complete arterial ischemia.

Local Tissue Hypertension

Increased microvascular permeability promotes local edema. Arteriolar and capillary flows are the most sensitive to changes in compartment pressures. Subcutaneous tissues tolerate uncontrolled edema reasonably well, but when the edema is contained within a fascial compartment, the pressure soon exceeds the intraluminal pressure of the venules, resulting in regional venous obstruction. Compartment syndrome has been described as a clinical condition in which increased pressure within a fascial compartment compromises the circulation and function of the tissues within that space.[11]

Ashton measured critical, closing pressures in the capillaries and found they were 21 and 33 mm Hg in the leg and the arm, respectively.[25] Depending on the situation, compartmental pressures as low as 20 to 40 mm Hg may result in compromised arterial inflow and tissue ischemia. Significant nerve damage has been reported when pressures of 30 to 40 mm Hg were present for 6 to 12 hours.[12] Early mechanical decompression by fasciotomy is believed to be effective in minimizing the secondary local complications of compartment syndrome.

DIAGNOSIS AND MANAGEMENT

Ischemia

Clinical recognition of the severity of acute limb ischemia is critical to successful management since timely revascularization is the most effective means of minimizing the deleterious effects of injury. Immediate limb viability is not usually in question when ankle brachial indices or absolute ankle pressures can be obtained (Society for Vascular Surgery/International Society for Cardiovascular Surgery category I); these measurements quantitate the degree of arterial insufficiency and can be repeated as needed. The threatened limb, characterized by minimal sensory loss and absence of muscle weakness (category IIA), is salvageable with prompt revascularization. Associated ischemic pain at rest with mild to moderate muscle weakness (category IIB) requires immediate intervention. An anesthetic extremity with muscular paralysis and absence of a pedal Doppler signal is indicative of profound ischemia.[5,7,10] Depending on the severity of these findings and the duration of ischemia, such limbs may have sustained irreversible ischemia[5]; the presence of profound limb anesthesia and muscle rigor suggests irreversible ischemia (category III), and such patients should not be revascularized. The morbidity and mortality of acute limb ischemia are increased when ischemia has persisted for more than 6 hours, fasciotomy is required, or amputation is performed.[5,6,22]

Early recognition of the extent of ischemia is the first step, followed by expeditious revascularization. Immediate administration of heparin is beneficial, but thrombolysis has not been proven superior to surgical intervention.[5,8] Diagnostic arteriography is advantageous when the clinical evaluation suggests a problem proximal to the inguinal ligament or the clavicle but is often unnecessary in traumatic extremity injuries. When time is short or prolonged transport is needed, temporary bypass using an appropriately sized carotid shunt is a valuable tool for diminishing the ischemia. This is most useful in battlefield or trauma surgery.

Reperfusion

Reperfusion after successful revascularization releases toxic metabolites that have accumulated during the ischemia. The reperfusion syndrome is characterized by acidosis, hyperkalemia, myoglobinuria, renal failure, and refractory dysrhythmias.[26,27] The presence of myoglobin in the urine is signaled by a dark, reddish color; the urine is dipstick positive for hemoglobin, but no red cells are present on microscopy or pigmented granular casts are noted in the sediment. Urine myoglobin of more than 20 mg/dl is predictive of acute renal failure.[5] Creatinine phosphokinase is a marker of ischemic muscle injury; half of those patients with creatinine phosphokinase greater than 5000 U/L also develop acute renal failure.[5] Replacement of intravascular volume helps avoid renal hypoperfusion and increases parenchymal and tubular flow; in addition, administration of intravenous mannitol and alkalinization of the urine can minimize precipitation of myoglobin in the renal tubules.[3] Acidosis and hyperkalemia contribute to myocardial irritability; specific antiarrhythmic therapy to reduce these sequelae may be supplemented by infusion of dextrose, insulin, and fluids. Pharmacotherapy aimed at prevention and treatment of reperfusion-induced injury continues to be actively investigated. Additional management options include restricted flow restoration, outflow washout, preperfusion agents, and leukocyte depletion.[28-32] However, none of these modalities has yet been shown to have clinical utility.

Local Tissue Hypertension

The clinical diagnosis of compartmental hypertension may be quite subtle, since it is normally suggested by various nonspecific clinical findings. As a result, heightened suspicion and good clinical judgment play large roles in formulating therapy; objective measurement of intracompartmental pressures may help determine the need for surgical intervention in patients with inconclusive findings. The clinical findings of compartmental hypertension are often subtle and delayed in onset. Pain is an early complaint and is often remarkable because it seems to be out of proportion with the physical findings; however, its absence may be falsely reassuring in a patient with spinal cord injury or an altered level of consciousness. Severe tenderness, paresthesia, paresis, and pain on passive stretch are signs of compartment syndrome. Unfortunately, all of these findings are nonspecific. On palpation, the compartment may feel tense and sometimes even boardlike. Neurological findings such as hypoesthesia, paresthesia, decreased motor function, or a combination of these, especially if progressive, are strongly suggestive of compartment syndrome. The earliest abnormality is often numbness in the dorsal web space between the first and the second toes; sensory innervation of this anatomical site is distributed through the lateral anterior tibial nerve, a branch of the deep peroneal nerve that exits the anterior compartment. However, in the trauma setting, these deficits must be differentiated from those due to direct nerve injury, highlighting the importance of an adequate baseline neurological examination. Loss of pulses or diminution of arterial Doppler signals constitutes a late sign of compartmental hypertension and indicates pathological elevation of compartmental pressures in the absence of arterial injury. Changes in venous Doppler signals in the affected extremity have been suggested as an early marker since normal venous pressure is rapidly exceeded as compartmental hypertension progresses; however, this observation requires further clinical corroboration and the technique has not been widely adopted.

Ulmer applied probability theory to articles on compartment syndrome to evaluate the reliability of clinical diagnosis. The four findings evaluated were pain, paresthesias, paresis, and pain on passive stretch. In general, the sensitivity of clinical findings for the diagnosis of compartment syndrome of the leg is low (13% to 19%).[33] The positive predictive value of the clinical examination was 11% to 15%, and the specificity and negative predictive value were both 97% to 98%. These findings suggest that the clinical features of compartment syndrome of the lower leg are more useful by their absence in excluding the diagnosis than by their presence in confirming the diagnosis. The probability of compartment syndrome with one clinical finding was approximately 25% but increased to 93% in the presence of three clinical findings.[33]

When an at-risk patient complains of pain that is clinically suspicious of compartment syndrome, the first step should be to remove all circumferential dressings. If a plaster cast is present, it may be split and removed or a window may be cut for additional evaluation. If the clinical findings are convincing, complete fasciotomy should be considered. However, if

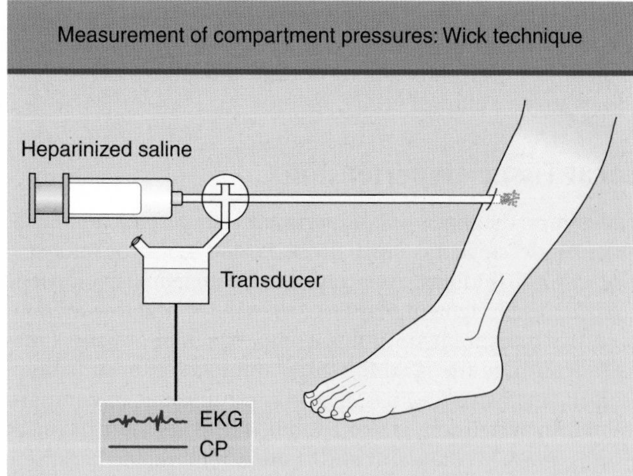

Figure 15-1. Measurement of compartment pressures: wick technique. Continuous monitoring of tissue pressures can be maintained for as long as necessary. This may be helpful in the patient who has an evolving clinical course and whose examination is equivocal.

the diagnosis remains uncertain, determination of compartment pressures may be of value.

COMPARTMENTAL DECOMPRESSION

Measurement of Compartment Pressures

Whenever it is impossible to assess sensorimotor function (i.e., in patients with altered level of consciousness or spinal cord injury and in children), measurement of compartment pressures is one of the few methods available to establish or exclude the diagnosis of compartment syndrome. Feliciano et al. recommended that compartment pressure measurements be considered routinely in the susceptible patient.[34] Reperfusion edema may develop insidiously and may not be evident immediately. Continuous or repeated pressure measurements may be required, in conjunction with repeated clinical evaluations, when fasciotomy is not performed at the initial procedure. Several catheters have been used for measurement of intracompartmental pressures. Wick or slit catheters (Figure 15-1) are equally efficacious for continuous monitoring of compartment pressures. The Stryker needle (intracompartmental pressure monitoring system, Stryker Surgical, Kalamazoo, Michigan; Figure 15-2A) is a portable instrument that allows single-puncture measurement of compartment pressure at the bedside and is currently the most popular method in the North America. However, no special instrument is required for measuring compartment pressure in the operative or critical care setting. A standard intravascular transducer system can be used for one-time determination of tissue pressure; when flushed between measurements, the same needle and transducer may be used to probe multiple fascial compartments (Figure 15-2B). A decrease in tissue pressure following decompression may also be documented.

Indications for Fasciotomy

Fasciotomy should be performed whenever firm clinical evidence exists of compartment syndrome. However, since the clinical findings are often nonspecific, compartment pressure measurements should be considered in equivocal cases to aid in clinical decision making. In the final analysis, the decision to proceed with fasciotomy remains controversial and must be based on clinical judgment and experience.

Based on experimental work, decompressive fasciotomy is recommended when intracompartmental pressure exceeds 30 to 45 mm Hg. Unfortunately, no specific threshold pressure exists at which compartment syndrome occurs. Matsen et al. demonstrated uniform damage when tissue pressures have exceeded these values,[35] but compartment syndrome can occur at pressures as low as 20 to 30 mm Hg. The duration of the compartmental hypertension, the systemic hemodynamics of the patient, and the presence or absence of coexisting

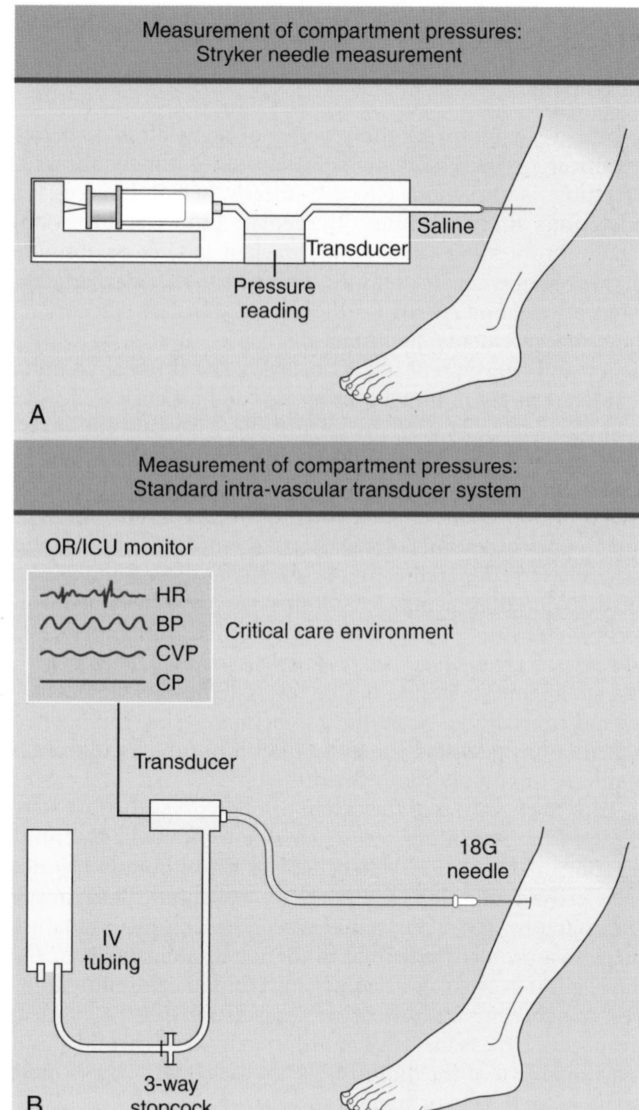

Figure 15-2. Measurement of compartment pressures. **A,** The Stryker is a portable instrument that allows single-puncture measurement of compartment pressures at the bedside. **B,** The standard intravascular transducer system may be used to determine tissue pressures at a given time, and the same needle may be used to probe multiple fascial compartments.

peripheral vascular disease are among the factors that may lower the threshold for performing decompressive fasciotomy.

Heppenstall et al. emphasized the concept of compartmental perfusion pressure (CPP), defined as the mean systemic arterial pressure minus the compartmental pressure.[36] An increasing compartmental pressure with coexistent systemic hypotension can rapidly reduce the CPP to zero. Compartment syndrome is seen often when the difference between the mean arterial pressure and the pressure in the involved compartment is less than 40 mm Hg; blood flow ceases when the CPP is 25 mm Hg or less.[37]

COMMON LOCATIONS AND MANAGEMENT

The forearm and the lower leg are the usual locations for compartment syndrome. However, the alert clinician is aware of its occurrence at less common sites such as the hand or the foot or even less commonly the shoulder, the upper arm, the buttock, or the thigh. These unusual sites are more typically involved when there has been prolonged inadvertent compression of muscle groups, such as when an unattended subject remains collapsed after a stroke or drug overdose. The compression is relieved when the affected extremity is moved and reperfusion commences. Compartment syndrome may be more common in the forearm and leg because the musculature is constrained by firm, well-defined fascial boundaries in a relatively limited anatomical space.

Operative Treatment

Mechanical decompression of established compartmental hypertension is achieved by the release of skin and fascia by incision. When a tense firm fascia is incised in the limb with compartmental hypertension, muscles bulge into the operative field, change color from pale to dusky to bright red, and become soft and pliable.

LOWER EXTREMITY

Compartment syndrome may involve all four compartments of the leg. The anterior tibial compartment is most likely to be involved (Figure 15-3A) but significant damage is most common in the deep posterior compartment (Figure 15-3B).[12] The likelihood of compartment syndrome is increased after combined arterial and venous injury, as opposed to isolated arterial or venous injury. Once recognized, immediate fasciotomy is indicated for decompression of the muscle compartment to prevent tissue necrosis and irreversible loss of neuromuscular function.

Anatomical Considerations

A major nerve traverses each of the four compartments of the leg (Figure 15-4), the identification of which is important in localizing symptoms. Knowledge of their anatomical course is useful in performing successful uncomplicated fasciotomy. The deep peroneal nerve arises from the common peroneal nerve and traverses the anterior compartment to exit as the anterior tibial nerve. It carries sensory innervation to the dorsum of the foot in the first web space and motor fibers to the forefoot extensors. The superficial peroneal nerve also arises from

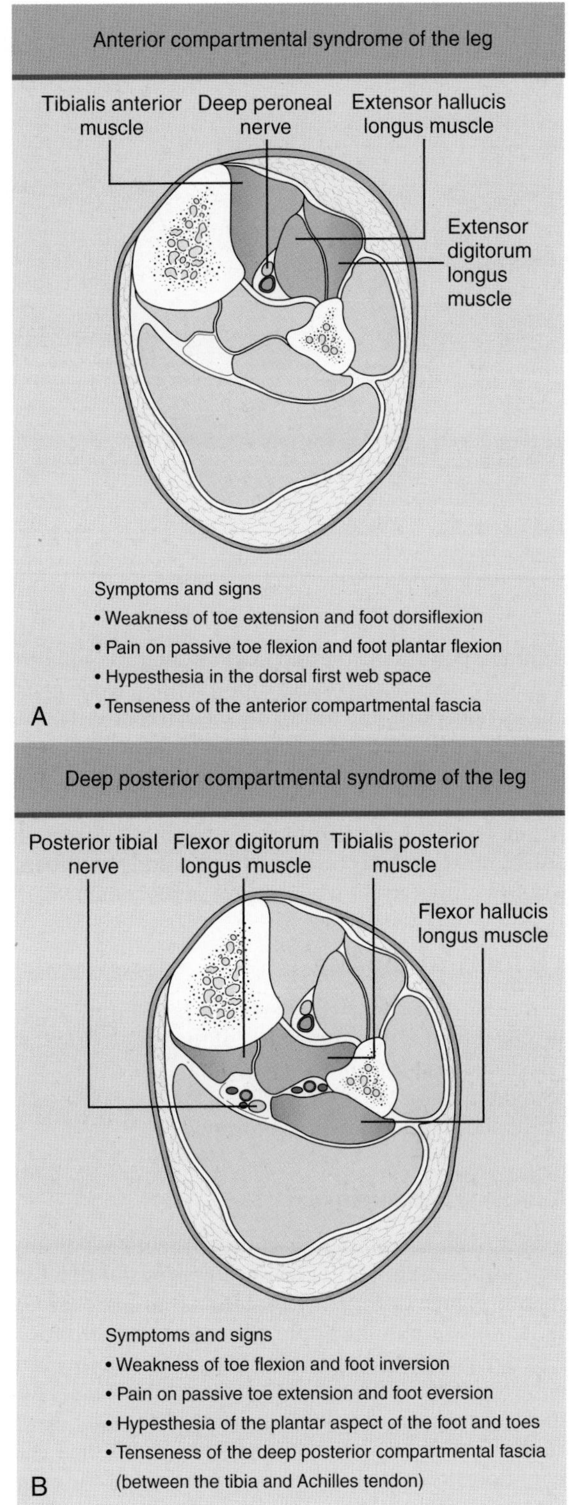

Figure 15-3. Compartmental syndromes of the leg. **A,** Anterior compartmental syndrome of the leg. The anterior compartment contains the deep peroneal nerve (DPN), along with three muscles: tibialis anterior (TA), extensor hallucis longus (EHL), and extensor digitorum longus (EDL). **B,** Deep posterior compartmental syndrome of the leg. The deep posterior compartment contains the posterior tibial nerve (PTN), as well as three muscles: tibialis posterior (TP), flexor hallucis longus (FHL), and flexor digitorum longus (FDL).

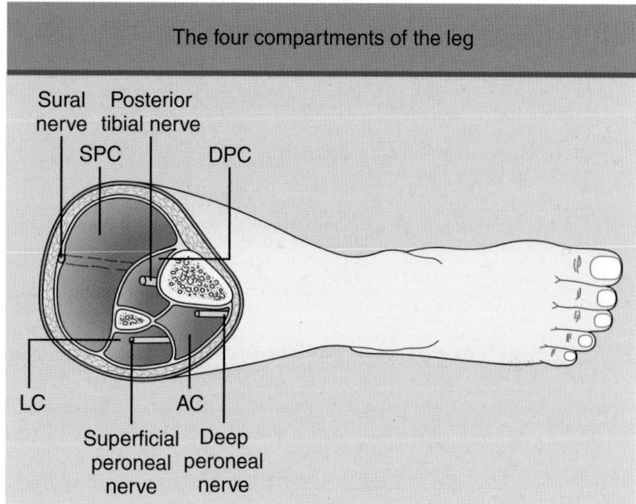

Figure 15-4. The four compartments of the leg. Anterior compartment (AC), lateral compartment (LC), superficial posterior compartment (SPC), and deep posterior compartment (DPC).

the common peroneal nerve and exits the lateral compartment midleg; it provides sensory innervation to the medial great toe and the second, third, and fourth dorsal web spaces. This nerve is identified during fasciotomy to prevent injury. The posterior tibial nerve forms the nerve of the deep posterior compartment and is responsible for plantar sensation and toe flexion. The superficial posterior compartment contains the gastrocnemius and soleus muscles and is traversed by the sural nerve that provides sensory input to the lateral aspect of the foot.

Fasciotomy of the Leg

Three techniques of four-compartment fasciotomy are commonly discussed for decompression of the leg:

- Dual-incision fasciotomy
- Single-incision fasciotomy
- Lateral or fibulectomy fasciotomy

Dual-Incision Fasciotomy

We prefer dual-incision, four-compartment fasciotomy to ensure complete skin and fascial decompression of all compartments (Figure 15-5). The temptation is to spare the length of the skin incision in the hope of avoiding the need for subsequent skin grafting; however, inadequate fasciotomy is most often the result of inadequate skin or fascial incisions. The initial incision includes skin and subcutaneous tissue down to the fascia. The lateral and anterior fasciotomy is then started in the midportion of the leg over the junction of the anterior and lateral compartments, with particular attention paid to the identification and preservation of the superficial peroneal nerve that exits the fascia at the level of the midleg. The fascia is incised from the extensor retinaculum at the ankle to just below the fibular head using a long, blunt-tipped scissor. The medial fasciotomy begins in the middle third of the leg. The saphenous vein is retracted anteriorly, and the superficial posterior compartment is incised. The deep posterior compartment is opened posteromedially, where the superficial posterior muscles form the Achilles' tendon and the avascular plane of the posterior intermuscular septum is incised.

Single-Incision Fasciotomy

Single-incision four-compartment fasciotomy begins laterally over the posterior fibular border from just below the fibular head to 4 cm above the malleolus (Figure 15-6). Anterior and posterior skin flaps are raised, and longitudinal incisions are made in the anterior, lateral, and superficial posterior compartments. Retracting the muscles of the lateral compartment anteriorly, the attachment of the soleus to the posterior fibula aids identification and incision of the deep posterior compartment. Care must be taken to avoid injury to the peroneal and posterior tibial neurovascular bundles, which are located adjacent and medial to the fibula. Some authors have expressed difficulty with this approach when severe disruption of tissue planes occurs. In addition, tibial fracture management is difficult through this incision.

Fibulectomy Fasciotomy

Fibulectomy fasciotomy achieves decompression of the posterior and anterior compartments through fibulectomy via the periosteal bed. Fibulectomy must not include the fibular head or the distal 8 cm of the fibula to minimize deformity and to maintain stability of the ankle. Removal of the fibula requires considerably more dissection than the other methods and destabilizes the limb if the tibia is fractured. In addition, free tissue transfer techniques based on the fibula are no longer available after its excision. Since equivalent decompression is achieved with the single- and dual-incision techniques, this procedure has not gained widespread acceptance.

Fasciotomy of the Thigh and Buttock

Thigh and gluteal compartment syndromes are rare and seldom recognized. They occur most commonly in individuals with altered mental status who remain in one position for an extended period following drug or alcohol use. The physiology and manifestations are similar to those seen in the more common and readily recognized compartment syndromes of the lower leg. Diagnosis is often delayed, resulting in significant morbidity and possible mortality. The mainstay of treatment consists of fasciotomy and debridement.

Decompression of the anterior and posterior compartments of the thigh may be accomplished with full-length incisions. The gluteus is easily decompressed through longitudinal cutaneous incisions. Individual epimysial envelopes may also require separate incisions for decompression.

UPPER EXTREMITY

Fasciotomy of the Upper Extremity

Compartment syndromes in the upper extremity are uncommon and difficult to diagnose. Intracompartmental pressure measurements may help confirm the diagnosis. In addition to acute disruption of arterial flow, compartment syndrome in the upper extremities should be suspected in patients with supracondylar fracture, fractures of the forearm, brachial artery puncture, subfascial intravenous infiltrations, crush injuries, extremity replantations, and gunshot wounds. The deep volar compartment of the forearm is most vulnerable as it is supplied by the anterior interosseous artery, which has no significant collateral flow.

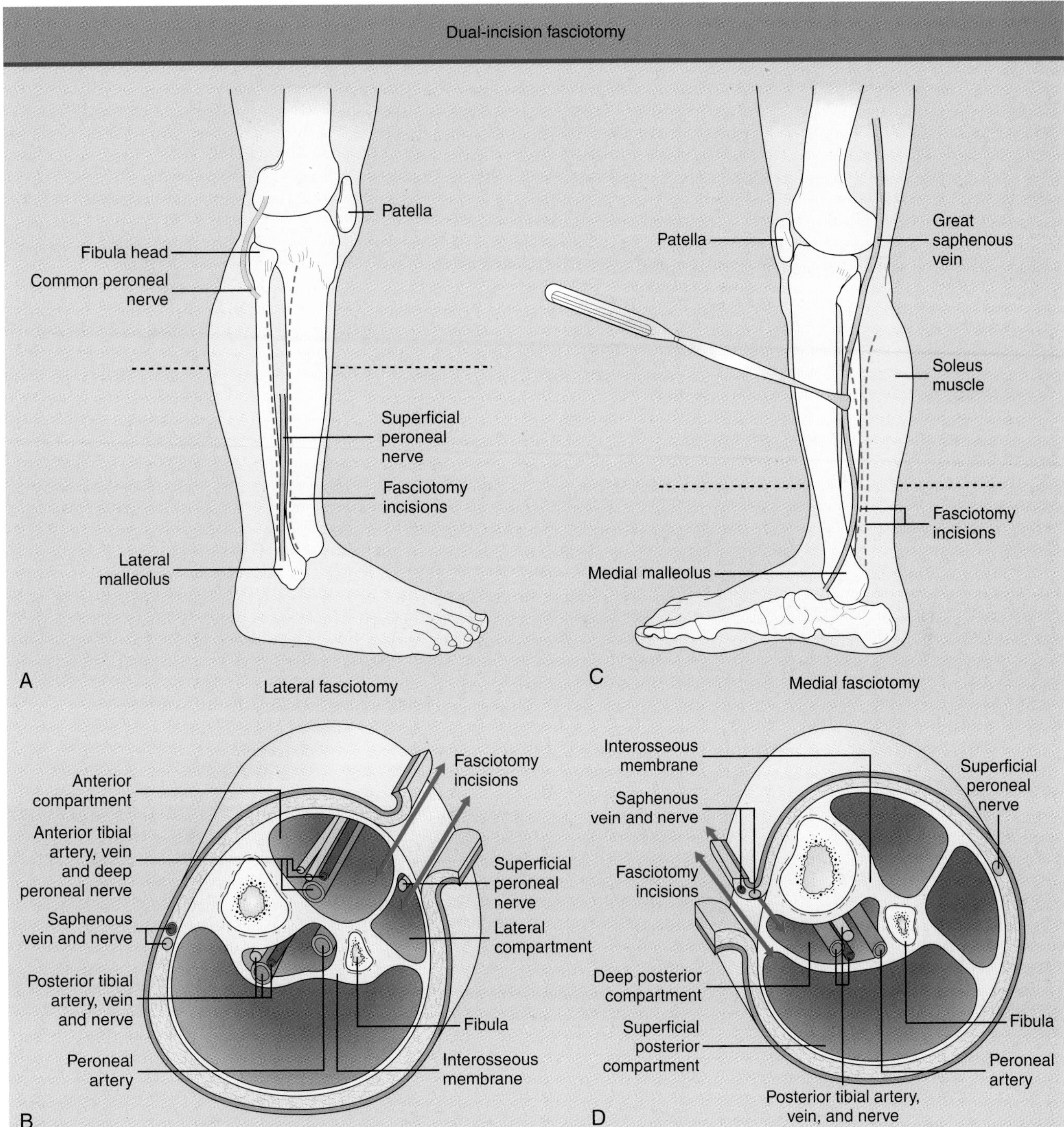

Figure 15-5. Dual-incision fasciotomy. The longitudinal incisions are illustrated in the top figures **(A, C)**; the level of the cross-sections **(B, D)** are indicated with a dotted horizontal line. **A, B,** The anterior and lateral compartments are decompressed by longitudinal fascial incisions beneath a lateral skin incision. The superficial peroneal nerve exits the fascia close to the skin incision. **C, D,** The superficial and deep posterior compartments are decompressed through longitudinal incisions on the medial aspect of the leg. The greater saphenous vein and nerve are preserved and retracted anteriorly.

Technique of Fasciotomy

Fasciotomy is performed through the incisions outlined in Figure 15-7. Typically, a dorsal incision and a volar incision are required to decompress the forearm. A curvilinear volar incision allows release of the flexor compartment. The course of the incision may be altered to accommodate preexisting traumatic wounds. In the forearm, the muscles at risk are predominantly located on the volar aspect. Decompressive fasciotomy should relieve the median ulnar and radial nerves and the thumb and finger muscles (Figure 15-8). Although volar release is usually sufficient, dorsal incisions may also be needed. Intraoperative compartmental pressure measurement may be valuable in determining the need for a dorsal incision. A longitudinal incision provides release to the extensor compartment. In severe cases, the deep intramuscular fascia

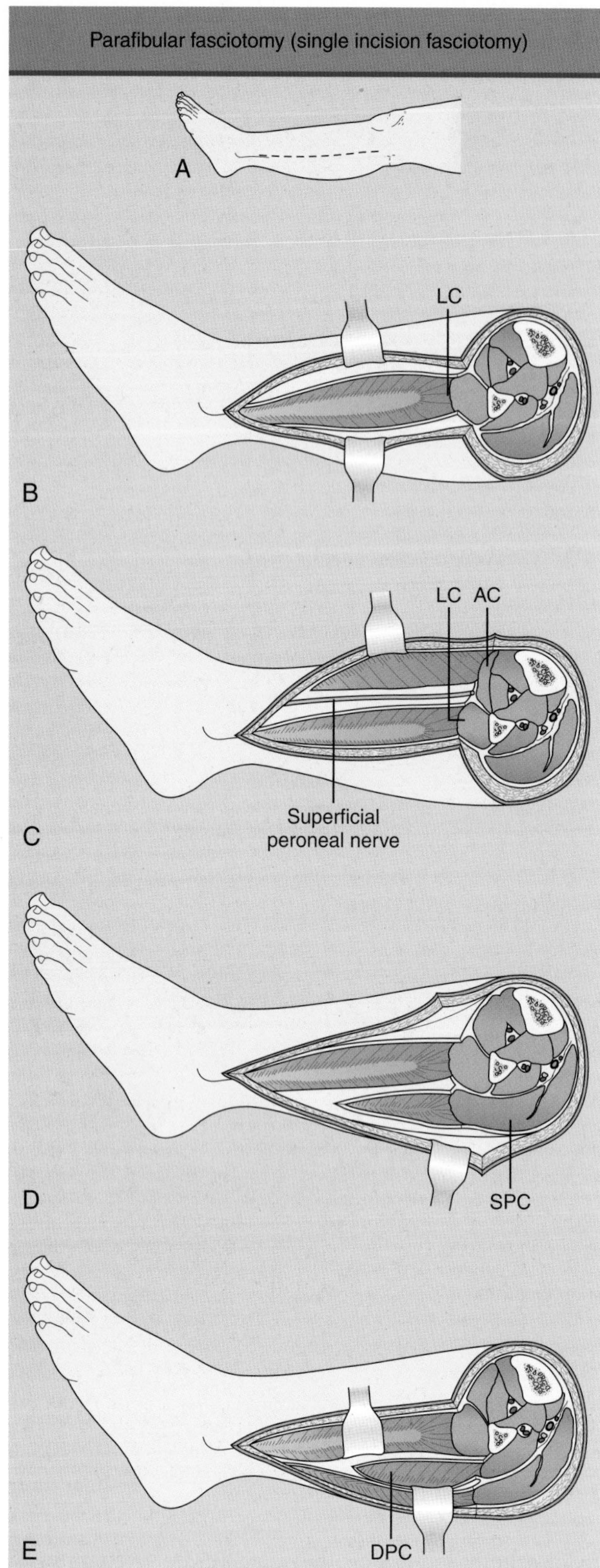

Figure 15-6. Parafibular fasciotomy (single-incision fasciotomy). **A,** The skin incision runs along the fibula. **B,** The lateral compartment (LC) lies just under the skin. **C,** The anterior compartment (AC) is exposed by retracting the anterior skin flap. **D,** The superficial posterior compartment (SPC) is exposed by retracting the posterior skin flap. **E,** The deep posterior compartment (DPC) is exposed by retracting the lateral compartment anteriorly and the superficial posterior compartment posteriorly and then dividing the fibular attachments of the soleus.

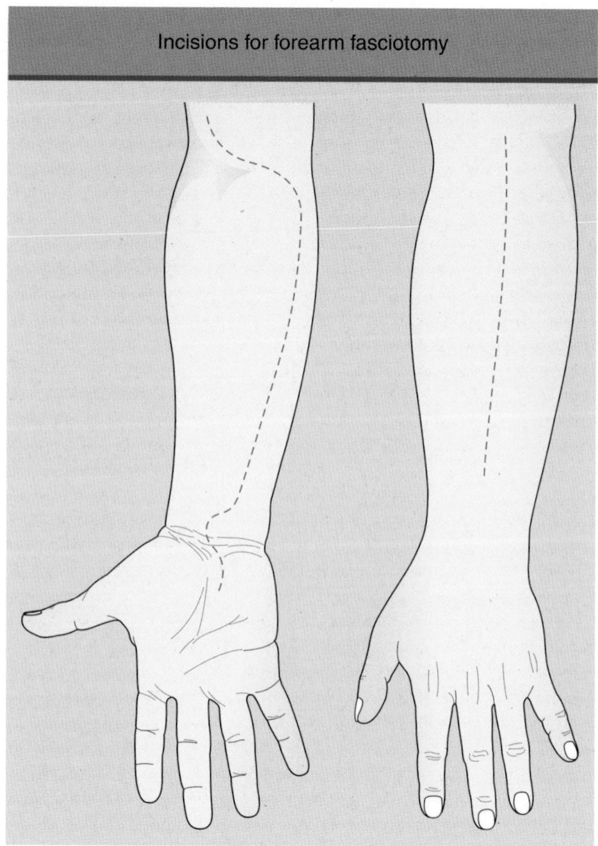

Figure 15-7. Incisions for forearm fasciotomy.

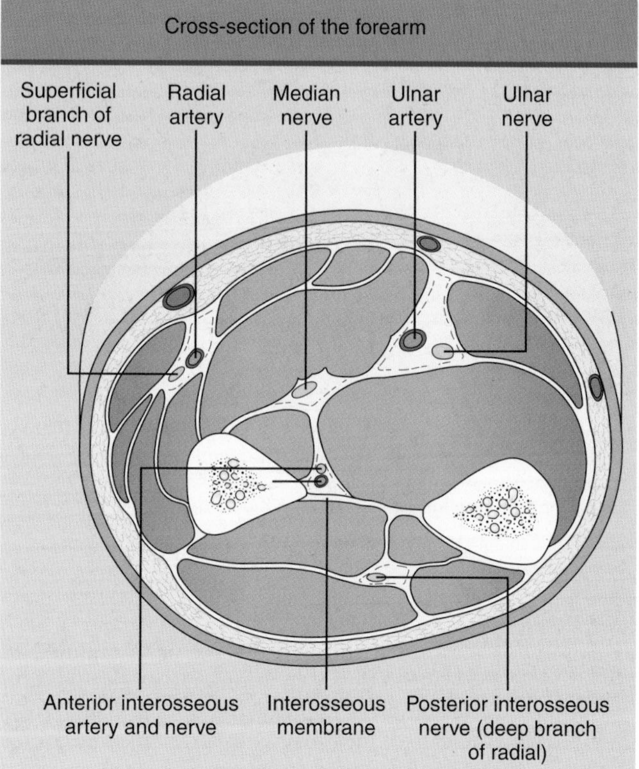

Figure 15-8. Cross-section of the forearm.

enveloping the flexor digitorum superficialis, the flexor digitorum profundus, and the flexor pollicis longus may have to be opened as well. The thick transcarpal ligament is divided distally to perform a carpal tunnel release. The proximal incision should release the lacertus fibrosus to decompress the median nerve at the elbow.

CONTRAINDICATIONS TO REVASCULARIZATION AND COMPLICATIONS

In cases of prolonged and advanced ischemia, tissue necrosis may have already occurred and revascularization may be contraindicated. Ascertaining the extent of preexisting tissue damage is one of the most difficult decisions for the surgeon, especially in moribund patients with acute ischemia, who can neither provide a history nor cooperate with the clinical examination. For the patient with a painful, immobile, insensate extremity, functional recovery may be limited by neuropathic pain, weakness, contracture, and loss of protective sensation. Reperfusion following reconstruction, fasciotomy, or both may result in the release of toxic metabolites into the systemic circulation, resulting in myoglobinuric renal failure, systemic inflammatory response syndrome, sepsis, shock, multisystem organ failure, and death. All of these effects are exaggerated in a patient with concomitant hypotension.

The decision to proceed with revascularization and fasciotomy rather than primary amputation is based primarily on the severity of the clinical findings, the duration of ischemia, and the muscle mass involved in the ischemic insult. If the duration of profound limb ischemia is more than 6 to 12 hours, the likelihood of tissue salvage becomes small and the risk of complications following revascularization increases significantly. However, systemic effects of IR are less pronounced when less tissue has been subjected to the ischemic insult. Thus, time is not the sole determinant in the decision-making process. The experienced clinician must individualize therapy according to the specific circumstances of each patient.

Fasciotomy incisions may create new issues related to wound healing in a patient with preexisting chronic peripheral vascular disease. Thus, comorbidies predispose the patient to additional complications such as conversion of closed to open fractures, osteomyelitis, delayed wound closure, wound sepsis, bleeding, and cosmetic deformity. Reasons for perceived failure of fasciotomy may relate to associated profound ischemia, delay in fascial decompression, incomplete fasciotomy, and errors in technique. Following successful revascularization, most patients experience few problems with wound healing; however, additional operations for split thickness skin grafts or closure by direct suture may be required.

MECHANISMS OF MICROVASCULAR DYSFUNCTION AFTER IR

Increased Microvascular Permeability

The microcirculation represents the first barrier in IR injury in all tissues and may be a useful target for therapeutic interventions. Increased permeability to macromolecules, stimulated adhesion and emigration of leukocytes, and no-reflow phenomenon are characteristic responses of ischemic microvessels. One of the key concepts of the structural basis of increased microvascular permeability relates to widening of the intercellular gap junctions due to endothelial cell contraction.[38] The postcapillary venules are the main site of hyperpermeability induced by inflammatory mediators as studied by electron and fluorescence microscopy.[39] These microvessels are also responsible for the permeability alterations in IR.

The signaling pathways for inflammatory agents that cause hyperpermeability involve the activation of protein kinase C, activation of nitric oxide (NO) synthetase, and synthesis of NO.[40-45] Reports are consistent with the hypothesis that endothelial NO synthetase activity and release of NO result in activation of soluble guanyl cyclase and synthesis of guanosine 3′,5′-cyclic monophosphate.[46] Guanosine 3′,5′-cyclic monophosphate activates the mitogen-activated protein kinases p42/44, which are important in the regulation of baseline, as well as agonist-induced, permeability.[47] The final step in the sequence of molecular modifications appears to involve proteins located at the cell junctional–cytoskeletal complex. Studies performed mainly in tissue culture have identified vascular endothelial–cadherin and β-catenins as possible key molecules. Phosphorylation induced by mitogen-activated protein kinase and disorganization of the vascular endothelial–cadherin may result in structural changes in the cellular cytoskeleton and hyperpermeability.[48]

Hyperpermeability, a hallmark of inflammation, is among the important initial events in the microvascular response to IR. Knowledge of the dynamics of this fundamental process and the development of adequate therapies has focused on investigating how to prevent the onset and the maintenance of the elevated permeability. Thus, we have learned much about how to counteract or inhibit the action of specific agents that elevate permeability. Less effort has been devoted to understanding the mechanisms that normally enhance the barrier properties of the microvascular wall, knowledge that once acquired might be applied to prevent or terminate excessive increases in microvascular permeability.

Endothelial Cell and Vascular Wall Interactions

The xanthine oxidase–containing microvascular endothelial cells, along with the neutrophils, are the most probable sources of oxygen-derived free radicals. Ischemia activates a calcium-dependent protease that catalyzes the conversion of xanthine dehydrogenase to its oxidase form. As ischemia continues, adenosine triphosphate is degraded to hypoxanthine, which is then converted to uric acid by xanthine oxidase with the production of superoxide anion. Superoxide dismutase converts superoxide anion to hydrogen peroxide, which in the presence of ferric ion produces the hydroxyl radical, a highly toxic oxidant. Support for the role of oxygen-derived free radicals in the microvascular dysfunction associated with IR[1,29] comes from the observed efficacy of free radical scavengers in the reduction of the indices of IR-induced microvascular dysfunction to about half of their unopposed values.

NO, derived from L-arginine, is produced by vascular and perivascular cells and has been implicated in IR-induced microvascular dysfunction. It may serve as an antiadhesive substance to protect the endothelium against leukocyte adherence.[49] In addition, the uncoupling of NO and formation of peroxynitrite ($ONOO^-$), a powerful reactive oxygen metabolite, leads to formation of hydroxyl radicals.[50] Peroxynitrite, the reaction product of superoxide and NO, is potentially more harmful than either superoxide or hydroxyl radical due to its longer half-life.

Endothelial cells are involved in the control of blood flow, microvascular permeability, vessel contractility, angiogenesis, coagulation, leukocyte traffic, and immunity. These endothelial functions are exquisitely modulated by endogenous and exogenous factors. Deviations from the normal balance because of a deficiency or an excess of the regulatory factors may lead to pathological states. Thus, a better understanding of the endothelial pathophysiological mechanisms involved in IR may provide opportunities for successful clinical interventions. Most research on IR and inflammation has focused on prevention of hyperpermeability and on modulation or control of proinflammatory agents that increase basal permeability. Much less attention has been given to elements that would normally contribute to the maintenance of the integrity of the microvascular wall and that would enhance its barrier properties. Based on the premise that knowing how hyperpermeability signals are terminated is just as important as understanding how they are generated, it seems important to foster advances in signaling processes that are aimed at maintaining the barrier properties of the microvascular wall and should contribute to inactivation of the inflammatory increase in permeability and return the barrier properties of the microvascular wall to baseline levels after IR.

Recent advances in cell research have provided a solid framework to consider cyclic adenosine monophosphate (cAMP) as an important second messenger in regulating and promoting cell adhesion and, by extension, the integrity of the microvascular barrier. cAMP is produced by adenyl cyclases and is a pleiotropic-signaling second messenger. The classical view has been that most, if not all, actions of cAMP proceed by activation of protein kinase A and are terminated by phosphodiesterase 4–catalyzed degradation. This view has been significantly changed since the recent discovery of Epac, an exchange protein activated by cAMP,[51] which is a guanine nucleotide exchange factor and responds with specificity to activation by cAMP.[52]

Specific stimulation of Epac–Rap1 enhances the endothelial barrier properties in human umbilical vein endothelial cells,[53,54] a process involving formation and tightening of cell junctions through vascular endothelial–cadherin.[55] Prostacyclin and forskolin, which enhance cAMP production, induced cortical actin rearrangement in a Rap1-dependent manner and decreased permeability in human umbilical vein endothelial cells.[54] These findings provide a subcellular explanation for a report that iloprost, a prostacyclin analogue, reduced the impact of IR on hyperpermeability in striated muscle.[56,57]

Current management of acute limb ischemia is based on the restoration of blood flow to the ischemic extremity as rapidly as possible to reduce the degree of ischemic injury. Superimposed on this algorithm is the use of pharmacological agents and nonpharmacological methods for reducing IR injury. These algorithms respond to the double jeopardy facing the vascular surgeon—namely, that unattended ischemia leads to necrosis, making prompt restoration of blood flow a must, but reperfusion compounds the problem, and its consequences (including compartment syndrome) may interfere significantly with survival of the organ and the patient. Studies advancing knowledge of the mechanisms that maintain the vascular wall barrier properties will be clinically relevant as they contribute an approach that will allow vascular surgeons to implement a directed and timed enhancement of the barrier properties of the microvascular wall.

LEUKOCYTES

After a period of controversial reports, it now seems established that hyperpermeability in response to an inflammatory challenge is regulated by endothelial cells, mainly through endothelial NO synthase.[41,44,58] Endothelial NO synthetase–modulated processes are orchestrated in synchrony with cell contraction and junctional reorganization induced by polymorphonuclear leukocytes.[59-61] Support for the involvement of leukocytes in IR comes from experiments in which either the animal or the experimental muscle has been rendered leukopenic by radiation, chemical, or physical means.[62,63] Leukopenia decreases the impact of IR on changes in microvascular permeability by reducing the increase in transport of macromolecules from a sevenfold down to a twofold increase compared to that obtained in the untreated ischemic muscle.[62,64] nicotinamide adenine dinucleotide phosphate (reduced form) oxidase (NADPH oxidase), within the leukocytes, converts cytoplasmic NADPH to nicotinamide adenine dinucleotide phosphate (oxidized form), resulting in the formation of superoxide anion and hydrogen peroxide, with subsequent release of hydroxyl radicals. Leukocytes also possess myeloperoxidase, an enzyme that catalyzes a reaction between hydrogen peroxide and chloride to form hypochlorous acid, a powerful oxidant. Levels of myeloperoxidase have been found to remain constant during ischemia and to increase at 15 minutes and 1 hour of reperfusion.[65] In addition, activated neutrophils release elastase, collagenase, and cathepsin G, substances that are able to degrade microvascular basement membrane and lead to increases in permeability and cellular dysfunction.

OTHER CHEMICAL MEDIATORS AND SIGNALING MOLECULES

Calcium ions modulate the activity of leukocytes, as well as the contractile properties of endothelial cells, and play an important role in the pathophysiology of skeletal muscle IR injury and associated microvascular injury.[65] Thromboxane A_2 has been implicated in causing microvascular alterations in the lung following reperfusion of ischemic canine hindleg.[63]

Platelet-activating factor is a vasoconstrictor, a strong promoter of microvascular permeability, and a powerful neutrophil chemoattractant.[66] The possibility that hydrogen peroxide may be the stimulus for platelet-activating factor synthesis in IR is indirectly supported by experiments in which human recombinant superoxide dismutase administered intravenously caused a 30% decrease in neutrophil adherence.[67]

PREVENTIVE STRATEGIES

What can be done to protect organs and tissues from the effects of ischemia and reperfusion injury? Early operation and revascularization decrease ischemic time, temporary bypass shunts maintain tissue perfusion, and oxygenation and tissue cooling may be used to decrease metabolic demands.

In elective ischemic events such as transplantation, tissue preservation can be enhanced by preischemic interventions. However, with acute limb ischemia, additional opportunities only present themselves during management of the reperfusion phase. Hypothermic and controlled reperfusion can reduce edema and necrosis.[68] The clinical applicability of biochemical interventions designed to reduce reperfusion-induced injury in end organs remains unproven. Much experimental work has been done to study pharmacological intervention for the prevention and treatment of reperfusion-induced injury. The potential beneficial effects of substances such as verapamil, mannitol, prostacyclin, monoclonal antibodies, superoxide dismutase, hetastarch high-molecular-weight carbohydrates, and heparin continue to be investigated. Many of these agents have demonstrated benefit in experimental studies that have not translated into clinical advantages.

Because leukocyte–endothelium interactions play an important role in bringing about IR damage,[63,69] these cells and their biochemical processes are considered possible targets for therapeutic interventions. A major aim is to minimize adhesion of leukocytes to microvascular endothelium.[70] Similarly, receptor antagonists to platelet-activating factor, administered just before reperfusion, effectively inhibit the ability of the phospholipid to recruit leukocytes to the injured area and abrogate their adhesion to the microvascular wall.[70] Reduction or elimination of leukocyte adhesion to endothelium may inhibit the oxidative stress that leads to parenchymal and cellular dysfunction.

Restriction of calcium in reperfusion, either by using entry blockers (such as verapamil)[64] or by administration of low calcium–modified solutions, may also be a useful way to decrease damage in reperfused muscle and to restore contractile function.[68]

Monoclonal antibodies directed against adhesion molecules on endothelium, leukocytes, or both also provide effective protection against immediate IR damage.[69] Clinical application of monoclonal antibodies awaits improvement in their design that will avoid rendering these critically ill patients immunodeficient for a significant interval after treatment. These monoclonal antibodies, and specific receptor-blocking agents, work effectively when administered immediately before reperfusion and offer the possibility for development of therapeutic approaches applicable at the time of revascularization.

SUMMARY

Ischemic tissue injury is the primary cause of morbidity and mortality from acute interruption of arterial blood flow. However, the main component of this injury occurs during reperfusion. Early recognition of the severity of limb ischemia with prompt restoration of blood flow is an obvious method for reducing the duration of ischemia. However, intervention at the time of reperfusion offers a broad additional opportunity since treatment is initiated when tissue perfusion is restored. The cascade of events that occurs after successful revascularization of an ischemic limb may be amenable to innovative interventions. Current investigations are targeted at understanding these cellular mechanisms and interactions to develop new therapeutic measures to diminish the detrimental metabolic and systemic consequences of ischemia and reperfusion. Research directed toward alteration of endothelial function includes reducing permeability, enhancing barrier properties, and discouraging leukocyte adherence to the endothelium.

Since IR injury cannot be well controlled, the alert physician must remain ever vigilant when faced with the common clinical settings in which compartmental hypertension is known to occur. The incidence may be much higher than reported because some of its late sequelae, including joint stiffness, claw toes, and equinus deformities, may be quite subtle. The diagnosis of compartment syndrome is not always straightforward. However, in clinical practice, its recognition is often delayed and fasciotomy is performed too late. Clinicians are advised to err on the side of early fasciotomy to avoid significant and permanent morbidity. Measurement of compartment pressures may be useful in equivocal cases or in sedated or neurologically impaired patients who are difficult to assess clinically. No substitutes exist for experience and sound clinical judgment.

References

1. Korthuis RJ, Granger DN, Townsley MI, Taylor AE. The role of oxygen-derived free radicals in ischemia-induced increases in canine skeletal muscle vascular permeability. *Circ Res* 1985;57:599-609.
2. Durán WN, Dillon PK. Effects of ischemia-reperfusion injury on microvascular permeability in skeletal muscle. *Microcirc Endothelium Lymphatics* 1989;5:223-239.
3. Odeh M. Role of reperfusion induced injury in the pathogenesis of the crush syndrome. *N Engl J Med* 1991;324:1417-1422.
4. Meagher AP, Lord RSA, Hill DA. Acute aortic occlusion presenting with lower limb paralysis. *J Cardiovasc Surg* 1991;32:643-647.
5. Norgren L, Hiatt WR, Dormandy JA, et al. Inter-society consensus for the management of peripheral arterial disease (TASC II). *J Vasc Surg* 2007;45:S5A-S67A. on behalf of the Trans-Atlantic Inter-Society Consensus II working group.
6. Eliason JL, Wainess RM, Proctor MC, et al. A national and single institutional experience in the contemporary treatment of acute lower extremity ischemia. *Ann Surg* 2003;238:382-390.
7. Rutherford RB, Baker JD, Ernst C, et al. Recommended standards for reports dealing with lower extremity ischemia: revised version. *J Vasc Surg* 1997;26:517-538.
8. Blaisdell W, Steele M, Allen RE. Management of acute lower extremity arterial ischemia due to embolism and thrombosis. *Surgery* 1978;84:822-834.
9. Yeager RA, Hobson RW II, Padberg FT, et al. Vascular complications related to drug abuse. *J Trauma* 1986;27:305-308.
10. Padberg FT, Hobson RW, Lee BC, et al. Femoral pseudoaneurysm from drugs of abuse: ligation or reconstruction? *J Vasc Surg* 1992;15:642-648.
11. Matsen FA III, Mubarak SJ, Rorabeck CH. A practical approach to compartment syndromes. In: *Instructional courses lectures.* vol. 32, Rosemont, IL: Academy of American Orthopedic Surgeons; 1983:88-113.
12. Mubarak SJ, Hargens A. *Compartment syndromes and Volkmann's contracture.* Philadelphia: Saunders; 1981.
13. Perry MO. Compartment syndromes and reperfusion injury. *Surg Clin North Am* 1988;68:853-864.
14. Patman RD, Thompson JE, Persson AV. Use and technique of fasciotomy as an adjunct to limb salvage. *South Med J* 1973;66:1108-1116.
15. Werbel GB, Shybut GT. Acute compartment syndrome caused by a malfunctioning pneumatic compression pump. *J Bone Joint Surg* 1986;68A:1445-1446.
16. Glenville B, Crockett JR, Bennett JG. Compartment syndrome and intraaortic balloon. *Thorac Cardiovasc Surg* 1986;24:292-294.
17. Yeager RA, Hobsons RW II, Lynch TG, et al. Popliteal and infrapopliteal arterial injuries: differential management and amputation rates. *Am Surg* 1983;50:155-158.
18. Lim LT, Michuda MS, Flanigan DP, et al. Popliteal artery trauma: 31 cases without amputation. *Arch Surg* 1980;115:1307-1313.
19. Wagner WH, Calkins ER, Weaver FA, et al. Blunt popliteal artery trauma: one hundred consecutive injuries. *J Vasc Surg* 1988;7:737-748.
20. Franco CD, RW11 Hobson, Padberg FT, et al. Hemodynamic changes during canine hindlimb reperfusion: comparison of thigh tourniquet and multiple ligation models. *Curr Surg* 1987;44:34-37.

21. Padberg FT, Franco CD, Kerr JC, et al. Acute ischemia reperfusion injury in the canine hindlimb. *J Cardiovasc Surg* 1989;30:925-931.
22. Kendrick J, Thompson BW, Read RC, et al. Arterial embolectomy in the leg: results in a referral hospital. *Am J Surg* 1981;142:739-742.
23. Bulkley GB. The role of oxygen free radicals in human disease processes. *Surgery* 1983;94:407-411.
24. Bourne RB, Rorabeck CH. Compartment syndromes of the lower leg. *Clin Orthop Relat Res* 1989;240:97-104.
25. Ashton H. Critical closing pressures in human vascular beds. *Clin Sci* 1962;22:79-87.
26. Haimovici H. Metabolic complications of acute arterial occlusions. *J Cardiovasc Surg* 1979;20:349-357.
27. Presta M, Ragnotti G. Quantification of damage to striated muscle after normothermic or hypothermic ischemia. *Clin Chem* 1981;27:297-302.
28. Wright JG, Belkin M, Hobson RW II. Hypothermia and controlled reperfusion, two nonpharmacologic methods which diminish ischemia reperfusion injury in skeletal muscle. *Microcirc Endothelium Lymphatics* 1989;53:315-334.
29. Walker PM, Lindsay TF, Labbe A, et al. Salvage of skeletal muscle with free radical scavengers. *J Vasc Surg* 1987;5:68-75.
30. Keller MP, Hoch JR, Silver D. Urokinase and mannitol modification of skeletal muscle ischemia reperfusion injury. *Surg Forum* 1991;42:330-332.
31. Blebea J, Kerr J, Hobson RW II. Effect of oxygen free radical scavengers on skeletal muscle ischemia and reperfusion injury. *Curr Surg* 1987;44:396-398.
32. Buchbinder D, Karmody A, Leather RD, et al. Hypertonic mannitol, its use in the prevention of revascularization syndrome after acute arterial ischemia. *Arch Surg* 1981;116:414-421.
33. Ulmer T. The clinical diagnosis of compartment syndrome of the lower leg: are clinical findings predictive of the disorder? *J Orthop Trauma* 2002;16(8):572-577.
34. Feliciano DV, Cruse PA, Spjint Patrinly V, et al. Fasciotomy after trauma to the extremities. *Am J Surg* 1988;156:533-536.
35. Matsen FA III, Winquist RA, Krugmire RB. Diagnosis and management of compartment syndrome. *J Bone Joint Surg* 1980;62A:286-291.
36. Heppenstall RB, Balderston R, Goodwin C. Pathophysiologic effects distal to a tourniquet in the dog. *J Trauma* 1979;19(4):234-238.
37. Hartsock LA, O'Farrell D, Seaber AV, Urbaniak JR. Effect of increased compartment pressure on the microcirculation of skeletal muscle. *Microsurgery* 1998;18(2):67-71.
38. Suval WD, Durán WN, Boric MP, et al. Microvascular transport and endothelial cell alterations precede skeletal muscle damage in ischemia–reperfusion injury. *Am J Surg* 1987;154:211-218.
39. Gawlowski DM, Ritter AB, Durán WN. Reproducibility of microvascular permeability responses to successive topical applications of bradykinin in the hamster cheek pouch. *Microvasc Res* 1982;24:354-363.
40. Hood JD, Meninger CJ, Ziche M, et al. VEGF upregulates ecNOS message protein, and NO production in human endothelial cells. *Am J Physiol* 1998;274:H1054-H1058.
41. Huang Q, Yuan Y. Interaction of PKC and NOS in signal transduction of microvascular hyperpermeability. *Am J Physiol* 1997;273:H2442-H2452.
42. Kobayashi K, Kim D, Hobson RW, et al. Platelet activating factor modulates microvascular transport by stimulation of protein kinase C. *Am J Physiol* 1994;266:H1214-H1220.
43. Mayhan WG. Role of nitric oxide in modulating permeability of the hamster cheek pouch in response to adenosine 5′-diphosphate and bradykinin. *Inflammation* 1992;16:295-305.
44. Ramirez MM, Quardt SM, Kim D, et al. Platelet activating factor modulates microvascular permeability through nitric oxide synthesis. *Microvasc Res* 1995;50:223-234.
45. Ramirez MM, Kim D, Durán WN. Protein kinase C modulates microvascular permeability through nitric oxide synthase. *Am J Physiol* 1996;271:H1702-H1705.
46. He P, Zeng M, Curry FE. cGMP modulates basal and activated microvessel permeability independently of [Ca 2+]i. *Am J Physiol* 1998;274:H1865-H1874.
47. Varma S, Breslin JW, Lal BK, et al. p42/44 MAPK regulates baseline permeability and cGMP-induced hyperpermeability in endothelial cells. *Microvasc Res* 2002;63:172-178.
48. Kevil CG, Payne DK, Mire E, Alexander JS. Vascular permeability factor/vascular endothelial cell growth factor–mediated permeability occurs through disorganization of endothelial junctional proteins. *J Biol Chem* 1998;273:15099-15103.
49. Kubes P, Granger DN. Nitric oxide modulates microvascular permeability. *Am J Physiol* 1992;262:H611-H615.
50. Beckman JS, Beckman TW, Chen J, et al. Apparent hydroxyl radical production by peroxynitrite: implications for endothelial cell injury from nitric oxide and superoxide. *Proc Nat Acad Sci USA* 1990;87:1620-1624.
51. de Rooij J, Zwartkruis FJ, Verheijen MH, et al. Epac is a Rap1 guanine-nucleotide-exchange factor directly activated by cyclic AMP. *Nature* 1998;396:474-477.
52. Christensen AE, Selheim F, de Rooij J, et al. cAMP analog mapping of Epac1 and cAMP kinase: discriminating analogs demonstrate that Epac and cAMP kinase act synergistically to promote PC-12 cell neurite extension. *J Biol Chem* 2003;278:35394-35402.
53. Cullere X, Shaw SK, Andersson L, et al. Regulation of vascular endothelial barrier function by Epac, a cAMP-activated exchange factor for Rap GTPase. *Blood* 1950-1955;2005(105).
54. Fukuhara S, Sakurai A, Sano H, et al. Cyclic AMP potentiates vascular endothelial cadherin–mediated cell–cell contact to enhance endothelial barrier function through an Epac–Rap1 signaling pathway. *Mol Cell Biol* 2005;25:136-146.
55. Kooistra MR, Corada M, Dejana E, Bos JL. Epac1 regulates integrity of endothelial cell junctions through VE–cadherin. *FEBS Lett* 2005;579:4966-4972.
56. Blebea J, Cambria RA, Defouw D, et al. Iloprost attenuates the increased permeability in skeletal muscle after ischemia and reperfusion. *J Vasc Surg* 1990;12:657-666.
57. Belkin M, Wright JG, Hobson RW II. Iloprost infusion decreases skeletal muscle injury after ischemia reperfusion. *J Vasc Surg* 1990;11:77-83.
58. Hatakeyama T, Pappas PJ, Hobson RW II, et al. Endothelial nitric oxide synthase regulates microvascular hyperpermeability in vivo. *J Physiol* 2006;574:275-281.
59. Breslin JW, Sun H, Xu W, et al. Involvement of ROCK-mediated endothelial tension development in neutrophil-stimulated microvascular leakage. *Am J Physiol Heart Circ Physiol* 2006;290:H741-H750.
60. Yuan SY, Wu MH, Ustinova EE, et al. Myosin light chain phosphorylation in neutrophil-stimulated coronary microvascular leakage. *Circ Res* 2002;90:1214-1221.
61. Yuan Y, Huang Q, Wu HM. Myosin light chain phosphorylation: modulation of basal and agonist-stimulated venular permeability. *Am J Physiol* 1997;272:H1437-H1443.
62. Breitbart GB, Dillon PK, Suval WD, et al. Leukopenia reduces microvascular clearance of macromolecules in ischemia reperfusion injury. *Curr Surg* 1990;47:8-12.
63. Belkin M, Lamorte WL, Hobson RW, et al. The role of leukocytes in the pathophysiology of skeletal muscle ischemic injury. *J Vasc Surg* 1989;10:14-19.
64. Klausmer JM, Paterson IS, Valeri CR, et al. Limb ischemia induced increase in permeability is mediated by leukocytes and leukotrienes. *Ann Surg* 1988;208:755-760.
65. Smith JK, Grisham GB, Granger DN, et al. Free radical defence mechanisms and neutrophils infiltration in postischemic skeletal muscle. *Am J Physiol* 1989;256:H789-H793.
66. Durán WN, Dillon PK. Acute microcirculatory effects of platelet activating factor. *J Lipid Mediat* 1990;2:S215-S227.
67. Kubes P, Suzuki M, Granger DN. modulation of PAF-induced leukocyte adherence and increased microvascular permeability. *Am J Physiol* 1990;259:G859-G869.
68. Beyersdorf F, Matheis G, Kruger S, et al. Avoiding reperfusion injury after limb revascularization: experimental observations and recommendations for clinical application. *J Vasc Surg* 1989;9:757-766.
69. Ferrante RJ, RW11 Hobson, Miyasaka M, et al. Inhibition of white blood cell adhesion at reperfusion decreases tissue damage in postischemic striated muscle. *J Vasc Surg* 1996;24:187-193.
70. Milazzo VJ, Sabido F, Hobson RW II, et al. Platelet activating factor blockade inhibits leukocyte adhesion to endothelium in ischemia reperfusion. *Surg Forum* 1992;43:376-378.

section

IV

Upper Extremity Problems

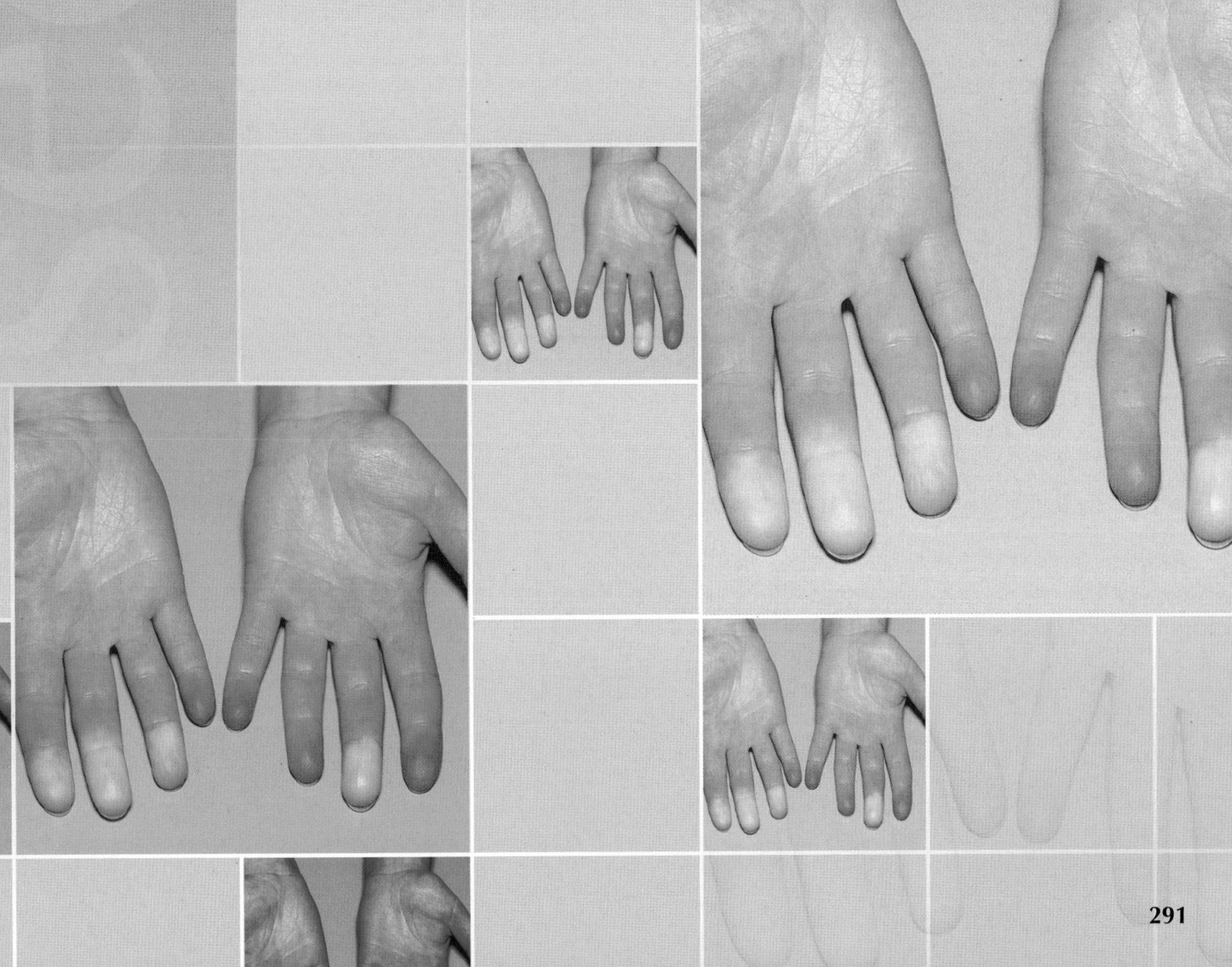

chapter

16

Upper Extremity Ischemia: Aortic Arch

Jeffrey M. Rhodes, MD • Kenneth J. Cherry Jr, MD • Michael D. Dake, MD

Key Points

- Aortic arch branch disease is defined as disease of the innominate, subclavian, or common carotid arteries resulting in flow-limiting stenosis or embolization to the brain, upper extremities, or both.
- Etiology of these lesions is most often atherosclerotic. However, large vessel arteritis must also be considered in the differential diagnosis.
- Short-segment extraanatomical reconstructions (subclavian-to-carotid grafting) are safe and durable reconstructions for isolated proximal lesions.
- Carotid–subclavian transposition should be used where technically feasible due to superior long-term patency compared to carotid–subclavian bypass grafting for isolated subclavian pathology.
- Direct transsternal reconstructions are necessary when multiple vessels are involved and are superior to extraanatomical bypasses in this situation.
- Endovascular reconstructions, when technically feasible, have a low morbidity and good midterm patency rates.

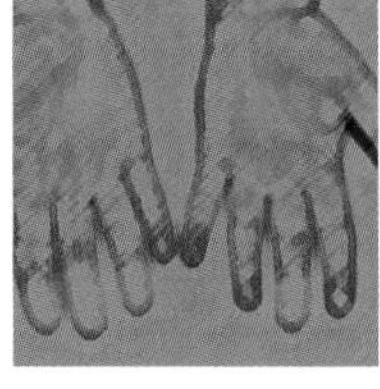

While carotid bifurcation disease is often encountered by the vascular surgeon, the need to treat the more proximal disease of the great vessels is uncommon in practice. Despite this, the vascular specialist must always consider the possibility of proximal disease when approaching patients with neurological or upper extremity symptoms.

Throughout the 1960s, reports emerged regarding the treatment of occlusive lesions of the great vessels. Crawford at al.[1] reported their experience with both extraanatomical and direct transsternal repairs. Although they demonstrated the technical feasibility of both approaches, they also demonstrated a significant difference in mortality between the two. As their experience increased, they shifted from 100% transsternal repairs to approximately 20% by the end of the decade. Their preferred alternative became short-segment extraanatomical reconstructions such as carotid–subclavian bypasses, but they still advocated direct repairs for multiple lesions and when adequate inflow was a concern. In attempts to find a revascularization option with less morbidity than transsternal repairs, some investigators pursued remote extraanatomical repairs such as axilloaxillary[2] or femoral-to-axillary bypasses. Contemporary surgical series have demonstrated decreased morbidity and mortality for each type of revascularization, with excellent long-term patency for both direct transsternal repairs and short-segment extraanatomical bypasses.[3-5] Even remote extraanatomical reconstructions can produce excellent long-term results.[6] However, some authors have reported a significantly decreased midterm patency, making extraanatomical reconstructions more controversial.[7] When considering open surgical approaches only, short-segment extraanatomical bypasses are the preferred reconstruction. However, if multiple vessels are involved, a direct transsternal repair is best, saving the remote extraanatomical bypasses for those patients who are prohibitive operative risks.

With the emergence of endovascular therapies, the debate now centers less on the ideal surgical approach than on whether endovascular or "conventional" surgical approaches should be used as primary therapy for great vessel occlusive disease.[8,9] While endovascular therapy does not have the four decades of experience of surgical revascularization, promising midterm data are emerging that support strong consideration of this approach when technically feasible. Similar to treating lower extremity occlusive disease, a combination of

Table 16-1
Anatomical Distribution of Disease in Takayasu's Arteritis*

	Degree of Stenosis	
	≥50%	100%
	No. (%)	No. (%)
Innominate artery	10 (77)	5 (38)
Right common carotid artery	9 (69)	4 (31)
Left common carotid artery	8 (62)	4 (31)
Right subclavian artery	8 (62)	5 (38)
Left subclavian artery	12 (92)	10 (77)

*Distribution of hemodynamically significant (>50%) stenoses and complete (100%) occlusions in 13 patients with symptomatic great vessel disease from Takayasu's arteritis.

endovascular correction of the inflow lesion and either subsequent or simultaneous repair of the "outflow" lesion may be warranted. This chapter discusses the etiology and clinical presentation of aortic arch branch vessel disease, the indications for therapy, and the outcomes of various surgical and endovascular approaches.

ANATOMY AND PATHOLOGY

Occlusive lesions of the great vessels are predominately atherosclerotic. In surgical series of direct transsternal revascularization, the incidence of atherosclerotic lesions has been reported to be 69% to 100%.[4,10] Takayasu's arteritis is the next most common in the United States, with the Mayo Clinic series reporting a 22% incidence in patients requiring surgery.[4] Secondary arteritis from radiation is also seen occasionally and can represent a formidable clinical challenge.

Since the pathological features of atherosclerotic vascular disease were discussed in Chapter 2, we focus on those vasculitic changes specific to the great vessels. The etiology of Takayasu's arteritis remains unclear but is likely multifactorial. The arterial inflammation is an immune-mediated response with a genetic predisposition. Infectious agents have been implicated by some as the triggering event, but these findings are inconsistent.[11] Initial histopathological changes consist of plasma cells and lymphocytes within the adventitia and media. Giant cells can form within the media, and elastic fibers can be identified within these lesions. After degradation of the media elastic fibers, it becomes fibrotic. This fibrosis results in the long, tapered stenosis of the affected vessels. The intimal injury and subsequent proliferation or thickening results from damage in the vaso vasorum. This intimal damage contributes to development of atherosclerosis that can cause significant stenoses and occlusions years after quiescence of the inflammatory stage.[11]

The anatomical distribution of disease in Takayasu's arteritis varies depending on the ethnicity, location, or both of the study population. Japanese populations have a higher incidence of isolated supraaortic and aortic arch involvement. The distribution of disease in the United States is not well defined. Table 16-1 demonstrates the frequency with which each vessel may be involved, highlighting the diffuse nature of this disease.

Atherosclerosis often affects multiple arteries. Contemporary surgical series of transsternal repairs have documented multiple great vessel involvement in 70% to 80% of patients.[4,5,10,12] When considering all reconstructions of the innominate, common carotid, or subclavian arteries, Crawford and colleagues reported only a 24% incidence of multiple vessel involvement.[1] The discrepancy may be due to the inclusion of isolated subclavian lesions that underwent carotid–subclavian bypass. Perhaps the more important question is, What is the likely distribution of disease in a patient who presents with neurological symptoms? Debakey et al.[13] reported on 942 consecutive patients with neurological symptoms, all of whom underwent arteriography. Extracranial stenoses were identified in 41% of patients. Not surprisingly, the most common location of occlusive disease in this symptomatic population was the carotid bifurcation (64% of lesions), although 67% of patients were noted to have multiple vessels involved. The vertebral arteries accounted for 19% of lesions, the subclavians accounted for 8%, and the common carotids and the innominate arteries accounted for 3.6% each.

Hass et al.[14] reported the anatomical results of the joint study of extracranial arterial occlusion. Nearly 5000 patients were included in this prospective registry of patients presenting with neurological symptoms. Figure 16-1 summarizes the frequency with which a given artery was involved, including

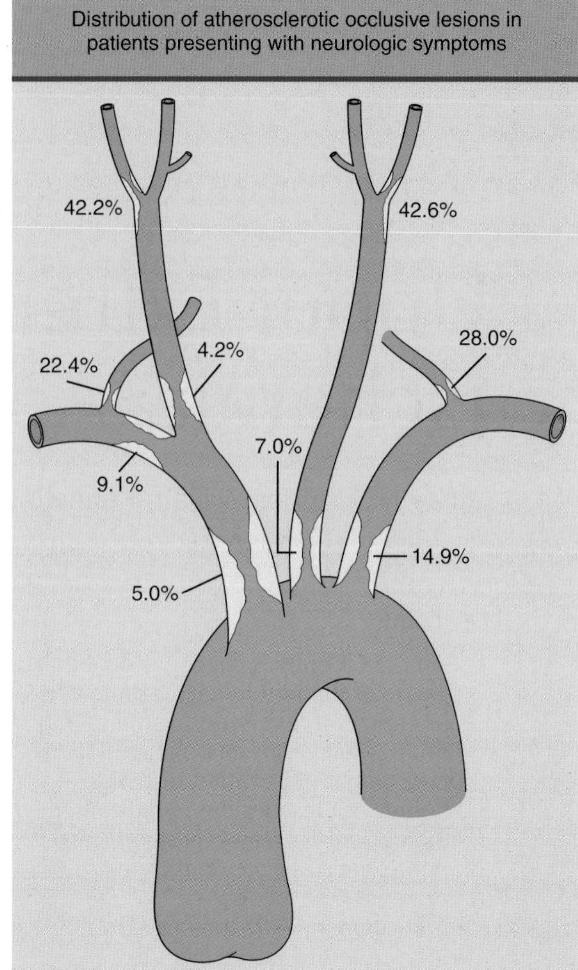

Figure 16-1. Distribution of atherosclerotic occlusive lesions in patients presenting with neurological symptoms. (Adapted from Hass WK, Fields WS, North RR, et al. *JAMA* 1968;203:159-166.)

both stenosis and occlusions, on a per patient basis. Strikingly similar to Debakey's series, 67.3% of patients had multiple vessels involved. No identifiable lesion was seen in 19% of patients, and surgically inaccessible lesions alone were seen in 6%. Again, despite the carotid bifurcation being the most common lesion, proximal great vessel disease must be considered in every patient.

PATHOPHYSIOLOGY

As for occlusive lesions at the carotid bifurcation, the morbidity from great vessel occlusive disease can result from thromboembolic events to either the brain or the upper extremity. In addition, given the frequency of multiple vessel involvement, low-flow states resulting in global ischemic symptoms or vertebrobasilar insufficiency play a significant role in the pathophysiology. This is particularly true for patients with Takayasu's arteritis. Such patients in the Mayo Clinic series had a 70% incidence of global ischemic symptoms due to flow-limiting lesions.[4] In addition, 54% had upper extremity claudication from innominate or subclavian stenoses. Despite the smooth tapering lesions seen with Takayasu's arteritis, embolic events also occur. Of these patients, 31% had neurological events due to emboli, half of whom also had microemboli to the digits.

The pathophysiology of atherosclerotic lesions is different given the potentially irregular nature of the luminal surface. For those lesions requiring surgical intervention, it is twice as likely that an embolic event is the cause of the presenting symptom. In the atherosclerotic (atherosclerosis obliterans, ASO) patients from the same Mayo Clinic series,[4] 63% had embolic events, 53% causing neurological symptoms and 10% causing pure upper extremity symptoms, with 5% of patients having both territories affected.

CLINICAL PRESENTATION

The clinical scenario of a patient presenting with symptomatic great vessel disease varies based on the type of lesion, the location and extent of those lesions, and most importantly, the underlying pathology, which affects not only the presentation but also the long-term outcome.

The typical patient with Takayasu's arteritis is female. Initial presentation is before the age of 40.[11] However, the age at which the patient seeks intervention for vascular complaints has been reported in two series to range from 18 to 58 years.[4,15] During the early phases of the disease, complaints can be nonspecific, including fever, malaise, and myalgia. Some patients complain of limb claudication or pain overlying an involved artery. Hypertension and its sequelae are the most common presentation.[11] Hypertension can be from renal artery stenosis, aortic coarctation, or carotid involvement with alteration in the usual baroreflex. Neurological symptoms related to the hypertension can include headache, visual changes, stroke, or even encephalopathy. As the disease advances and the subclavian, innominate, and carotid arteries develop progressive diameter reduction, low-flow symptoms can emerge. Lightheadedness, dizziness, photophobia, visual disturbances, and clinical subclavian steal syndrome can all occur. Upper extremity claudication without clinical steal remains more common than true symptomatic steal.

Most patients with Takayasu's arteritis have signs of significant vascular involvement on initial presentation. The classical description is of pulselessness of one or both upper extremities. Early in the course of disease, there may only be discrepancies in blood pressures between the arms or between the arms and the lower extremities. Subclavian or carotid bruits can often be heard, as well as intraabdominal bruits. Carotid pulses may also be blunted or absent. In the presence of significant subclavian disease, the hands can be pale with sluggish capillary refill. In the case of embolic lesions, splinter hemorrhages may occur. Rarely, embolization may even occur to the lateral chest wall, causing ulceration. These physical examination findings are not specific for Takayasu's arteritis; they apply to atherosclerotic patients as well.

Some differences between ASO patients and those with Takayasu's arteritis were discussed in the Pathophysiology section. Specifically, ASO patients are more likely to have lesions that result in embolic events. The typical neurological symptoms that result from emboli include hemispherical events referable most often to the anterior circulation and amaurosis fugax. The other major area of difference is the demographics and associated comorbidities. Comparing the risk factors of ASO and Takayasu's patients from the Mayo Clinic series,[4] the mean age was significantly older for the ASO group (59 ± 10 years versus 40 ± 11 years, $p < 0.001$) and all Takayasu's patients were female compared with 66% in the ASO group ($p < 0.05$). When comparing other variables, including history of previous transient ischemic attack or cerebrovascular accident, diabetes, hypertension, tobacco use, hyperlipidemia, known coronary artery disease, renal insufficiency, or previous symptomatic lower extremity peripheral vascular disease, the only significant difference was history of tobacco use. Tobacco abuse was almost uniform in the ASO patients, with 95% reporting a significant or ongoing use of tobacco. The Takayasu's group still had a high rate of tobacco use (69%), but this was significantly less than for ASO patients ($p = 0.02$). The risk factors are almost identical to those identified by Berguer and colleagues,[12] including age, female predominance, and tobacco use.

Patients with radiation-induced stenosis of the carotid arteries and great vessels can present with both embolic and low-flow signs and symptoms.[16] The duration from therapeutic irradiation to development of symptomatic arterial disease is usually a decade, but this is variable and may be within years or several decades later.[17,18] The radiation injury predisposes to atherosclerotic changes in the vessels, often in locations not typical of uncomplicated atherosclerosis. Despite the relatively common use of radiation therapy in the treatment of malignancy, it is relatively rare that these patients develop significant lesions that require revascularization. The presenting symptoms are often global ischemia from a low-flow state since multiple vessels are often involved. Vertebrobasilar and upper extremity symptoms have also been reported.[16,17]

Regardless of the etiology of occlusive disease, a phenomenon often talked about is the subclavian steal syndrome. True subclavian steal syndrome occurs when a proximal subclavian stenosis or occlusion is present. During upper extremity activity, blood flows retrograde down the vertebral to supply the arm and results in compromised cerebral perfusion. Although the radiographic finding of subclavian steal is common, the clinical syndrome is rare.[19] Of 168 patients identified with true radiographic subclavian steal in the joint study of extracranial arterial occlusion, none were reported to have worsening symptoms with arm use and 80% had significant lesions in other vessels, which likely contributed to the vertebrobasilar or low-flow-state symptoms.[20] The radiographic finding is more important as a marker for proximal disease than for its clinical relevance.

Taking into consideration that patients rarely present to the vascular specialist's office with a pathological and anatomical diagnosis in hand, the questions when seeing these patients are as follows:

1. What is the lesion responsible for the symptom?
2. What is the cause of that lesion?
3. What are the risks of correcting that lesion?

The clinician must always be aware of the possibility that the cause of the presenting neurological symptom may not be the carotid bifurcation lesion seen on duplex ultrasound. This is especially true if the severity of that lesion does not correspond to the given symptom. Based on history and physical examination findings, the clinician must consider further imaging or investigation. A female patient with a history of heavy tobacco use who presents at a relatively young age (fifth or sixth decade of life) constitutes a subgroup that has an increased risk of proximal great vessel disease. This is true regardless of the etiology of the lesion. While not an indication in itself to image the great vessels, a low threshold should exist in this population. Physical examination findings of a proximal bruit or discrepancies in blood pressures also warrant further investigation of the great vessels.

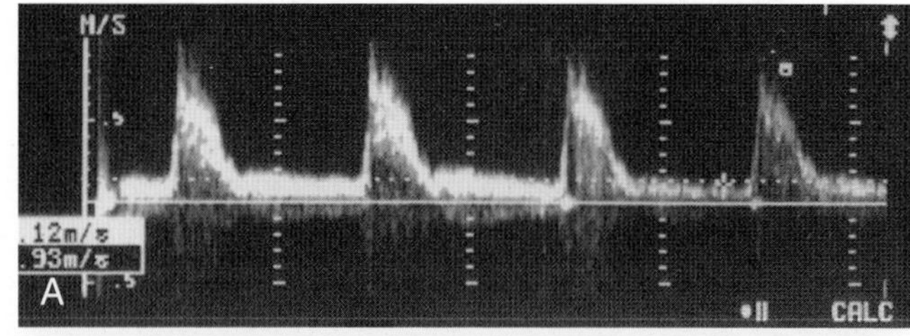

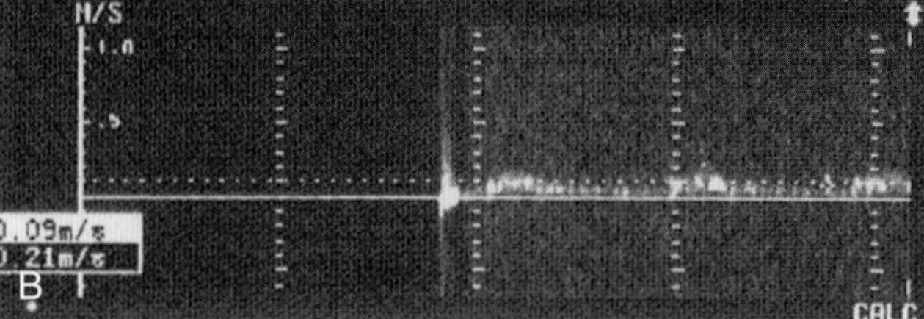

Figure 16-2. Spectral analysis of the left **(A)** and right **(B)** common carotid arteries. The left has mild diffuse stenotic (16% to 49%) disease. The right spectral waveform is altered by a significant (more than 50%) stenosis of the innominate artery that cannot be directly visualized in this patient.

DIAGNOSTIC TECHNIQUES

Although the proximal extent of the carotid and subclavian arteries cannot be directly visualized using duplex ultrasound, significant information can be gained from this imaging modality. Rarely, the origin of the right common carotid artery and even a portion of the innominate artery can be seen directly in slender individuals. Usually, the presence of proximal carotid or innominate disease is inferred from the Doppler waveform characteristics in the common carotid artery. The normal waveform has a sharp systolic upstroke, is triphasic, and has a clear spectral window. In the presence of hemodynamically significant proximal disease, the waveform may be blunted, may be monophasic, and may have spectral broadening consistent with turbulent flow (Figure 16-2). Other findings on duplex scan indicating more proximal disease include abnormal subclavian flow similar to the changes mentioned for the common carotid; retrograde vertebral flow, indicating a flow-limiting proximal subclavian stenosis; or discrepancy of 10 mm Hg or greater in upper extremity blood pressure measurements.

Although it is now common practice to intervene in carotid bifurcation disease based on duplex ultrasound findings alone, initial criticism of this approach was that significant proximal disease would be missed. Akers et al.[21] examined 1000 consecutive arch angiograms to determine whether this added to patient management over noninvasive testing alone. These studies were not compared directly with duplex ultrasound studies, and it appears that asymptomatic patients were included. A 10.5% incidence of proximal disease occurred, but most was vertebral artery occlusive disease. When excluding the vertebral arteries, 1.8% of patients had significant proximal lesions. The authors concluded that routine arteriography is not necessary except when a significant discrepancy occurs in upper extremity blood pressures or if noninvasive testing does not find a lesion that adequately accounts for the patient's symptoms. To better define the role of duplex ultrasound for the diagnosis of aortic arch branch vessel disease, McLaren et al.[22] examined a series of 650 consecutive carotid duplex scans that all underwent confirmatory arteriography. Using the criteria mentioned earlier, they accurately predicted the presence of 27 proximal lesions (4%). Only one lesion was missed by duplex. This yielded a sensitivity and a specificity of 96% and 100%, respectively. More importantly, the positive and negative predictive values were 100% and 99%, respectively. The authors stressed that 50% of the proximal lesions identified did require surgical intervention, highlighting the importance of recognizing these lesions. These findings were confirmed in a prospective manner by Kadwa and colleagues,[23] who examined 129 patients undergoing carotid endarterectomy. They found a 14.5% incidence of proximal disease, half involving either the innominate or the common carotid artery and half involving the subclavians. All proximal lesions could be predicted by a combination of pulse and blood pressure abnormalities, presence of bruits, and duplex findings. Of these patients, 37% required surgical correction of these additional lesions.

The gold-standard examination to delineate the extent and location of great vessel pathology remains arch aortography with four-vessel runoff. With present digital subtraction techniques, the contrast load has decreased, as has the time to complete the study. A typical study can now be performed with 100 ml or less of contrast. Figure 16-3 demonstrates a standard arch aortogram in a patient with atherosclerotic occlusive disease (Figure 16-3A) and in a patient with Takayasu's arteritis (Figure 16-3B). The criticisms of intraarterial contrast studies have been their invasive nature, the risk of stroke from catheter manipulations, the nephrotoxicity of the contrast agents, and the possibility of missing irregular lesions due to inability to visualize them through the column of contrast. Although gadolinium can be used as an alternative agent to decrease renal toxicity, the image quality may be suboptimal.

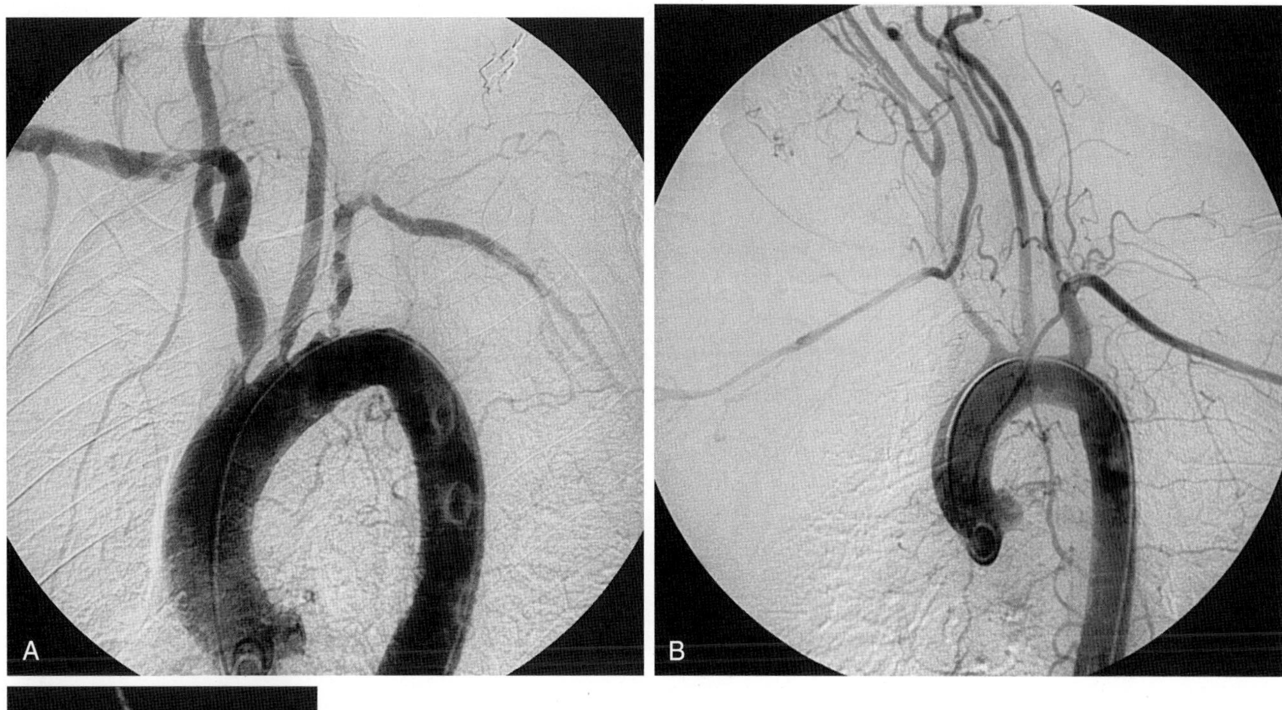

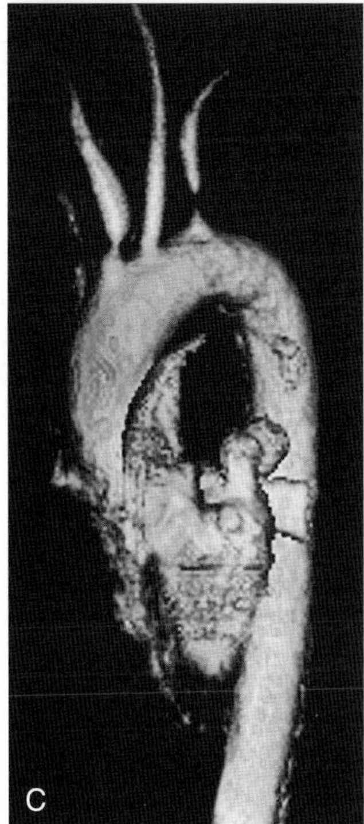

Figure 16-3. Standard arch aortogram in a patient with atherosclerotic occlusive disease **(A)** and in a patient with Takayasu's arteritis **(B)**. Magnetic resonance angiography of atherosclerotic disease involving innominate and left common carotid arteries **(C)**.

The Asymptomatic Carotid Atherosclerosis Study identified the risk of stroke in asymptomatic patients undergoing angiography to be 1.2%.[24] A contemporary series by Johnston and associates compared the risk of neurological complications in patients undergoing cerebral angiography—50% of whom were symptomatic—at a university medical center versus at a community hospital practice.[25] They found no difference in cerebrovascular risk between the two settings. The overall risk of stroke and transient ischemic attack was 0.5% and 0.4%, respectively.

Although conventional arteriography is associated with a low risk, it is not risk free. The desire of both the patient and the physician to find a less invasive means of imaging the aortic arch and its branches has led to further developments in both computed tomography angiography and magnetic resonance angiography (MRA; Figure 16-3C). Much of the data published on MRA centers on cervical carotid disease. The American Heart Association published a summary on use of MRA imaging and, for carotid artery disease, stated that it should be used in conjunction with duplex ultrasound, reserving conventional angiography for discrepant results.[26] In a review of 11 studies comparing MRA with conventional angiography in a total of nearly 700 patients, the median sensitivity was 93% (range 86% to 100%) and the median specificity was 88%

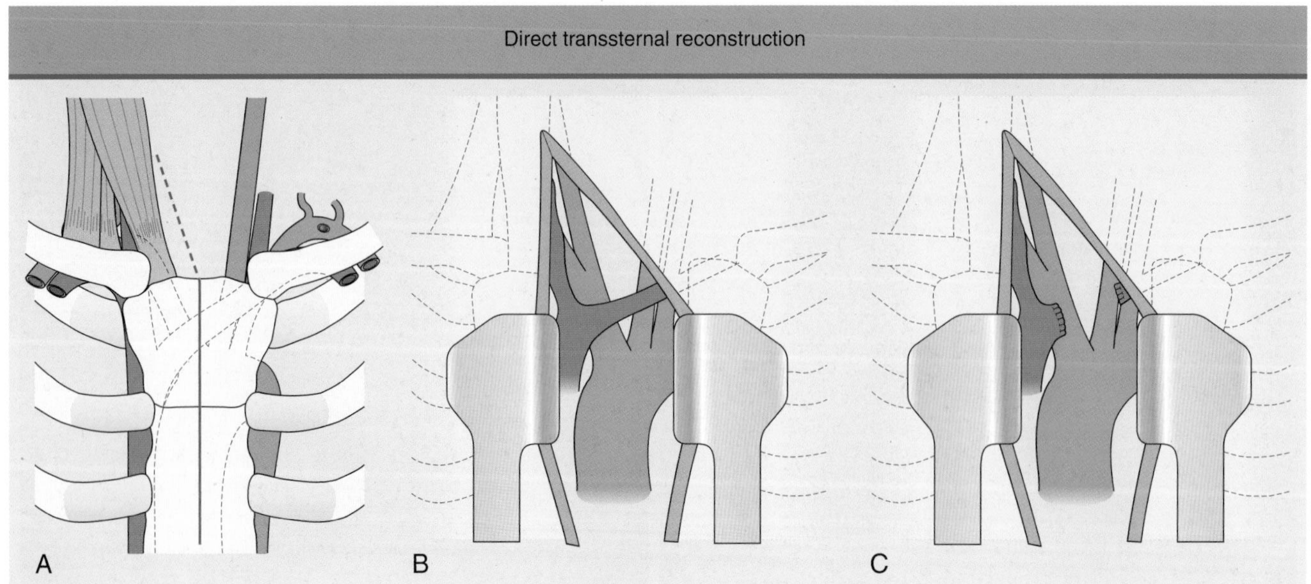

Figure 16-4. Direct transsternal reconstruction. **A, B,** Initial exposure of the ascending aorta and its branches by a transsternal approach. **C,** The left brachiocephalic vein can be divided and oversewn to facilitate exposure.

(range 75% to 98%), making it a reasonable adjunct to duplex ultrasound for cervical carotid artery disease.[26]

The criticism that duplex ultrasound first received—the possibility of missing more proximal lesions—is now directed toward MRA. Carpenter et al.[27] prospectively studied MRA for aortic arch occlusive disease, all patients having both MRAs and conventional angiograms performed. The sensitivity of MRA was only 73% (specificity, 89% to 98%), leading the authors to conclude that although a normal study excludes significant disease the technology was not yet to the point at which MRA could replace conventional angiography. Prince et al.[28] summarized their experience with thoracic aortic MRA for various aortic and nonaortic pathologies. A subset of 19 patients was analyzed who had occlusive disease of major aortic branches. This included not only great vessel disease (excluding vertebrals) but also mesenteric and renal disease. Despite these limitations, the sensitivity and the specificity at detecting a hemodynamically significant stenosis was promising, at 90% and 96%, respectively. As the technology and techniques for both obtaining and analyzing data are improved, MRA is likely to become accurate enough to replace conventional arteriography of the aortic arch and its branches.

Proponents of MRA also point out that, in regards to plaque morphology and ulceration, MRA may be more sensitive than conventional angiography, which can obscure the details of a lesion by the column of contrast.[26] Randoux et al.[29] confirmed this finding for carotid bifurcation lesions, but no data exist for aortic branch vessel pathology. The other aspect of their study was the validation of computed tomography angiography in the evaluation of the cervical carotid artery. This technique can also be used to image the aortic arch and branch vessels.

In summary, the radiographic evaluation of a patient suspected of having symptomatic carotid bifurcation or great vessel occlusive disease should begin with duplex ultrasonography. If the study does not demonstrate a lesion that is clearly responsible for the symptom or is suggestive of a proximal stenosis, further imaging of the aortic arch and great vessels should be performed. If clinical suspicion for significant proximal disease is low, an MRA or a computed tomography angiogram beginning at the level of the aorta should be obtained. A normal study excludes significant pathology. If suspicion of a lesion that will require intervention is high, a conventional intraarterial angiogram is recommended, especially if a percutaneous intervention at the time of angiography is being considered. However, using computed tomography angiography or MRA before intervention could be helpful in guiding an endovascular intervention. Recent concerns about the safety of gadolinium as a magnetic resonance contrast agent in patients with a glomerular filtration rate of less than 30 ml/min, resulting in potential nephrogenic systemic fibrosis, have decreased its utility in this subgroup.[30]

MANAGEMENT AND PROGNOSIS

Direct transsternal reconstruction for aortic branch vessel occlusive disease has been the gold standard for patients with disease affecting multiple vessels. For isolated disease of the common carotid or subclavian arteries, short-segment extraanatomical bypasses (subclavian–carotid bypass) are the surgical treatment of choice. When comparing the results of remote extraanatomical bypasses and endovascular approaches, it is important to compare treatments of similar lesions to understand which therapy is best. In this section, we discuss both the technical aspects of each of the therapies and data regarding both complications and long-term success.

Direct transsternal repair is performed through a median sternotomy, with extension of the incision to the right neck if needed (Figure 16-4A and B). Alternatively, a ministernotomy to the third intercostal space can be performed with transection of the sternum at that level.[31] The left brachiocephalic vein is fully mobilized; if necessary, this can be divided and oversewn to facilitate exposure and allow proper lie of the graft without significant long-term sequelae to the left upper extremity (Figure 16-4C).[4] Separate cervical incisions are made if the target vessels are the carotid bifurcations. Extending the

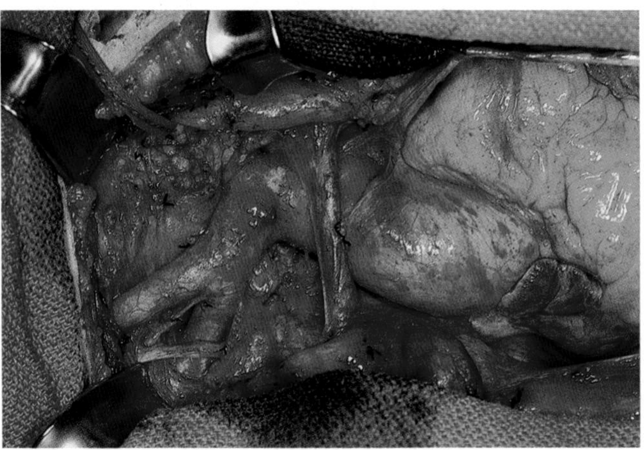

Figure 16-5. Intraoperative photograph of the transsternal approach to the ascending aorta and innominate bifurcation. The brachiocephalic vein was left intact.

sternal incision into the right neck can facilitate exposure of the innominate and proximal right subclavian and common carotid arteries (Figure 16-5). The proximal anastomosis is placed as far laterally on the ascending aorta as possible (Figure 16-6). This allows a smooth lie of the graft and keeps the bulk in the anterior mediastinum to a minimum, preventing encroachment onto the graft after closure of the chest. We prefer the use of knitted 7-, 8-, or 10-mm polyester grafts, with additional sidearms placed as needed (Figures 16-6B and 16-7). Some authors prefer the use of bifurcated grafts (Figure 16-6D), but again, care must be taken to avoid excessive mediastinal contents that could kink or impinge on the graft. Resectioning of the diseased innominate artery is one way to provide additional space for a graft.

When planning revascularization, arteries that have complete proximal occlusions are grafted first to maximize cerebral blood flow during each stage of the procedure. If available, electroencephalographic monitoring can be helpful, but the need for shunt placement is uncommon (less than 10%) and

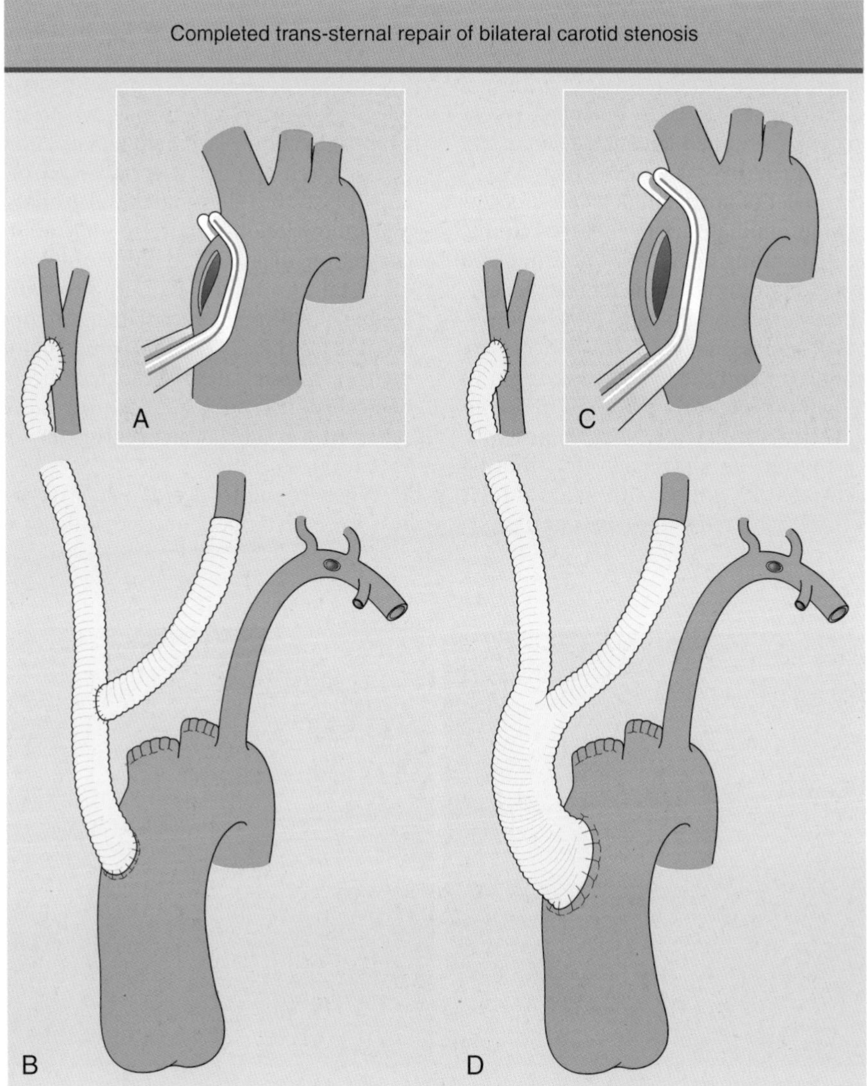

Figure 16-6. Completed transsternal repair of bilateral carotid stenosis using an 8-mm polyester graft with a sidearm that was added **(A, B)** or using a bifurcated graft **(C, D).**

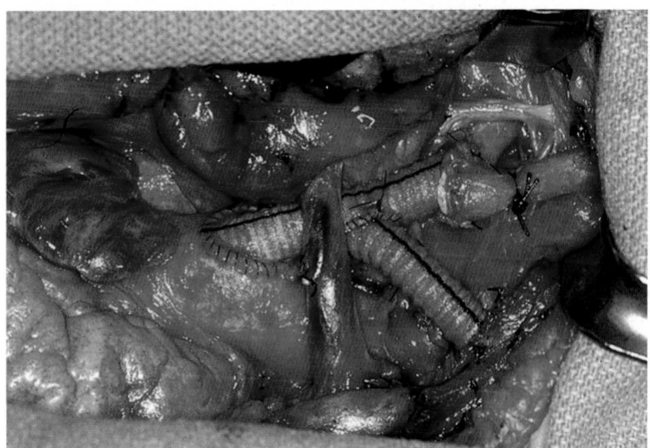

Figure 16-7. Intraoperative photograph of a completed aortoinnominate and left common carotid bypass using an 8-mm polyester graft to the innominate bifurcation, with a single sidearm added that goes to the left common carotid artery (not pictured), in a patient with Takayasu's arteritis.

often the decision to place a shunt is based on the preoperative clinical scenario (Figure 16-8).[4] Although the Texas Heart Group has favored reconstruction of all occluded vessels, we have found that the left subclavian can be dealt with in a staged fashion if necessary (Figure 16-9). In our most recent series, none of the 16 patients who had left subclavian artery occlusions required a subsequent bypass.

The other procedural aspect of aortic branch vessel occlusive disease is the utility of innominate artery endarterectomy. This is technically more demanding than bypass grafting, and patients must have proper anatomy to allow its use. Specifically, the aorta at the innominate origin must not have significant calcification. Also, approximately 1 cm is necessary between the innominate origin and the left carotid origin to allow proper clamping without compromising perfusion to both hemispheres (Figure 16-10). Extensive experience with this technique by the group at the University of California at San Francisco demonstrated its utility, with patency rates equal to or better than those achieved with bypass grafting.[32] It is particularly useful when simultaneous coronary artery bypass grafting will be necessary, since the ascending aorta can be left free for the proximal vein grafts.

When feasible, short-segment cervical reconstructions (subclavian–carotid bypasses or carotid–subclavian transposition) are performed for disease isolated to a single vessel (Figure 16-11). Synthetic conduits, 8-mm knitted polyester, are preferred over vein grafts in this location. Remote, nonanatomical bypass grafts can also be performed in patients who are at a prohibitive risk for transsternal repairs and are not candidates for short-segment cervical bypasses because of involvement of the usual inflow vessel. These reconstructions include axilloaxillary bypasses, carotid–carotid bypasses (with either pretracheal or retroesophageal tunneling), and femoral–axillary bypasses (Figures 16-12 and 16-13). Synthetic materials, often externally supported, are used for these reconstructions.

Endovascular therapy for aortic branch vessel occlusive disease has been reported for atherosclerotic lesions, radiation-induced stenoses, and Takayasu's and giant cell arteritis.[33,34] Percutaneous approach can be from the ipsilateral brachial–axillary artery or from either femoral approach. The use of cerebral protection devices during the treatment of common carotid origin or innominate lesions may be beneficial for symptomatic embolic lesions, but a device specifically for this purpose does not presently exist and the use of internal carotid artery filters may not afford sufficient guide wire support to allow placement and accurate deployment of stents across often-angulated great vessel origins.[35] Intraoperative angioplasty and stenting may also allow correction of a proximal inflow lesion via a retrograde approach during operative correction of a carotid bifurcation lesion, with the benefit of distal carotid control to prevent embolization (Figure 16-14).[36] Although recanalizing a completely occluded segment is technically feasible using angioplasty and stent placement, a higher rate of both technical failure and restenosis or occlusion is seen.[37] Technical success rates of 100% was achieved for subclavian stenoses in one series compared to 65% for occlusions.[38]

When trying to decide which revascularization option is best for a given patient, the clinician must consider the risk

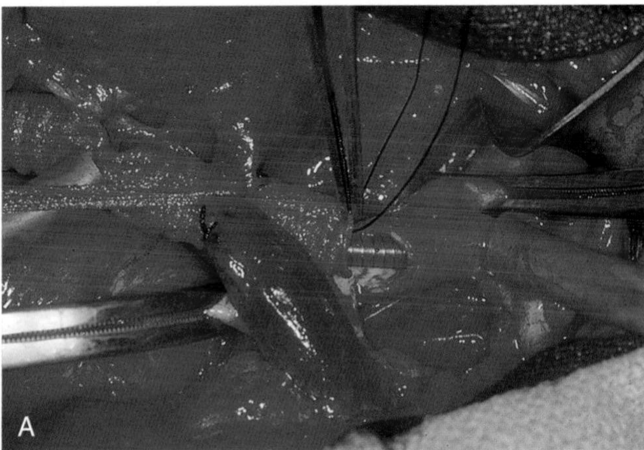

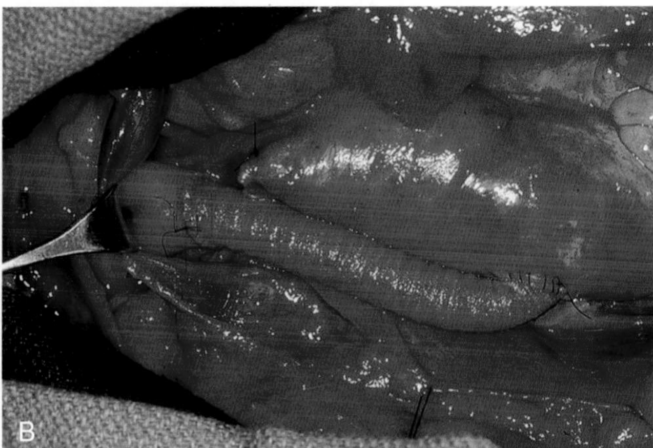

Figure 16-8. Shunt placement. **A,** Intraoperative photograph of an aortoinnominate bypass using a shunt for cerebral protection. Note that this is secured into the graft and common carotid arteries with Rummel tourniquets and the right subclavian artery is clamped. **B,** Completed repair after shunt removal.

of the given procedure and the long-term benefits of that procedure. When comparing various approaches, it is also important to compare treatment of similar lesions, similar extent of disease, and similar pathologies. These comparisons also need to be among contemporary series when available. No prospective comparison exists among the various surgical approaches, nor are there any data regarding direct, prospective comparisons of open versus endovascular options. Farina et al.[39] assessed carotid–subclavian bypass versus percutaneous transluminal angioplasty (PTA) without stenting for proximal stenoses of less than 4 cm length in a retrospective cohort fashion. Patients with innominate or common carotid disease were excluded, as were those with complete occlusions. In this group of 36 patients, no difference occurred in the incidence of immediate complications between the two procedures; however, 5-year primary patency data favored surgical reconstruction (87% versus 54%). The authors concluded that PTA should be reserved for elderly patients or those who have prohibitive medical comorbidities for surgery. Whether the addition of stents to the PTA arm would have improved patency is unclear.

The remainder of the data on revascularization of aortic branch vessel disease comes from individual series. Tables 16-2 and 16-3 summarize available contemporary data over the past decade for surgical and endovascular repairs. Although direct comparisons can be made for the initial outcomes and complications, it is more difficult to compare long-term outcomes since those data are incomplete for endovascular therapies. Few life-table data exist for endovascular repairs, and the use of "long-term" often applies to follow-up periods of less than 2 years.

Direct, transsternal repair carries with it the highest morbidity and mortality of all approaches discussed because of the scope of the operative procedure and the extent of disease. The overall neurological event rate is 6%, with a perioperative death rate of 5% (Table 16-2, upper panel). Risk factors identified for poor early outcomes have included the presence of a hypercoagulable state (or thrombophilia) and renal insufficiency.[4] Although identifying hypercoagulable patients preoperatively would likely improve these results, screening of all patients undergoing great vessel repair would not be cost effective. We advocate screening only those patients who have a history of multiple graft thromboses, regardless of the location of those grafts. This approach is relevant whether considering a direct, extraanatomical, or endovascular repair. In addition, any patient who experiences an acute graft, endarterectomy, or PTA site or stent thrombosis should be evaluated. Renal insufficiency should be considered a significant risk factor for poor initial outcome, and these patients may benefit from minimizing the complexity or invasiveness of the procedure. Unfortunately, the extent of disease is more likely to be the determinant of which approach is necessary. The etiology of disease (ASO, Takayasu's arteritis, or radiation-induced arteritis) is not a predictor of initial outcomes.

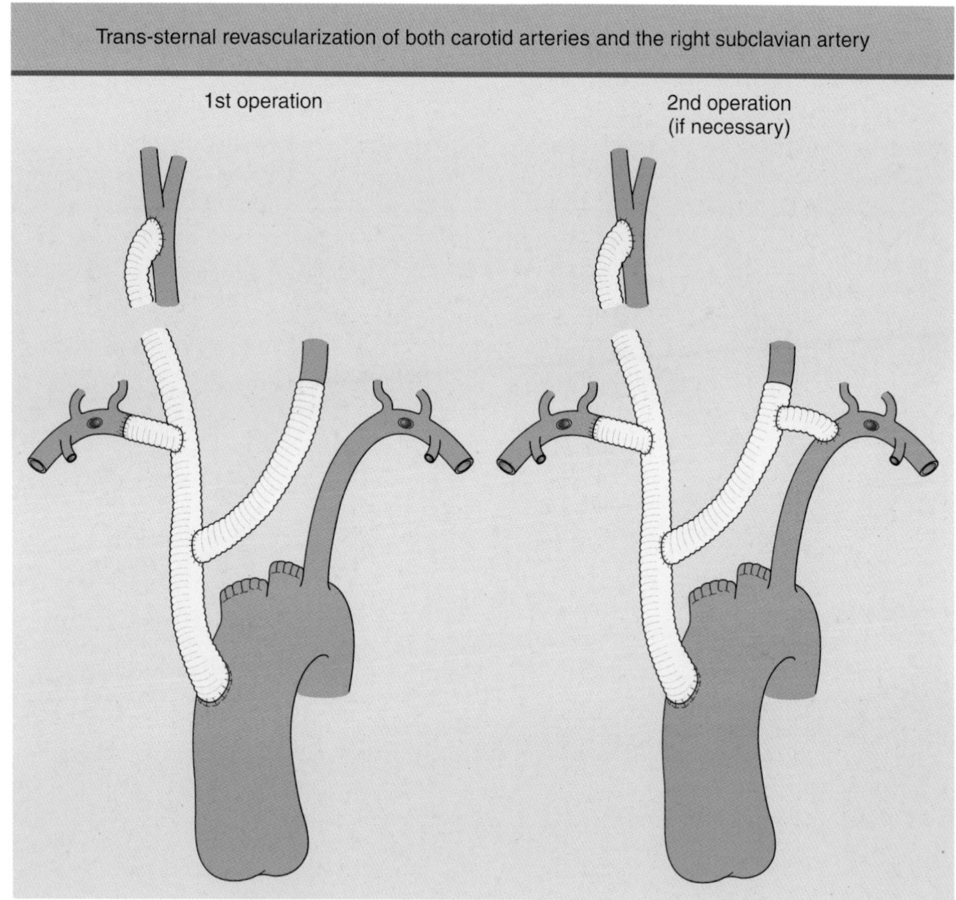

Figure 16-9. Transsternal revascularization of both carotid arteries and the right subclavian artery. Revascularization of the left subclavian artery can be performed later but is rarely necessary.

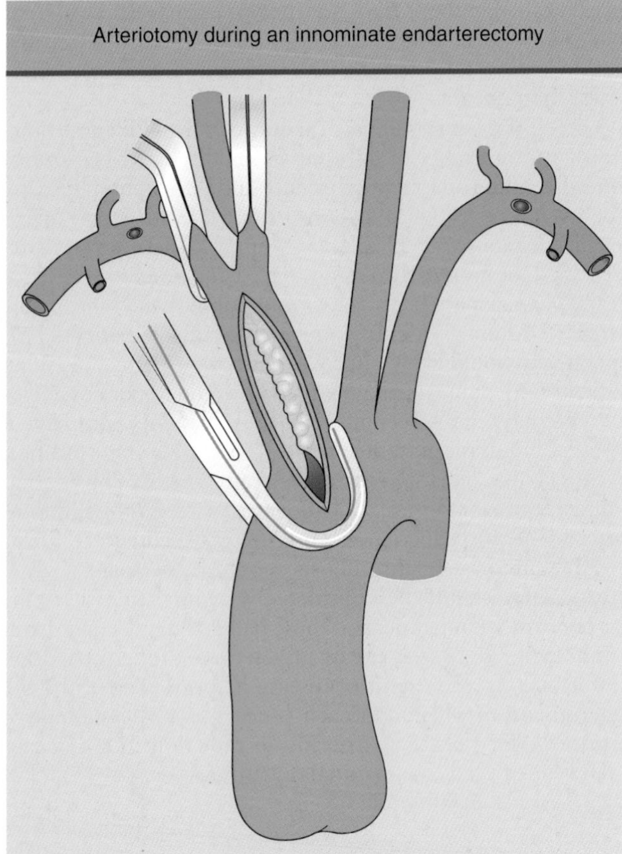

Figure 16-10. Arteriotomy during an innominate endarterectomy. Note that the arteriotomy is carried onto the aorta as needed and that the proximal clamp is placed to allow adequate flow to the left common carotid artery.

The higher rate of perioperative complications influenced Crawford et al. to shift from a universal transsternal approach for all patients to short extraanatomical bypasses in 80%.[1] The contemporary perioperative neurological event rate for short-segment extraanatomical (subclavian–carotid and carotid–subclavian) bypass grafting is 1.4%, with a death rate of 0.7% (Table 16-2). It is also a durable repair, with 5-year patency rates in the high-80% to mid-90% range and excellent stroke-free survival rates. This is the open revascularization approach of choice when the anatomy is suitable. Several authors prefer a subclavian–carotid transposition when technically feasible. This too has a low risk of perioperative neurological events (1.3%, Table 16-2), although the death rate was higher in analysis. Most of these reports are a bit older and the deaths were isolated to one series; however, the patency was uniformly excellent when this reconstruction is used.

The most recent report from the Texas Heart Institute reviewed the results in 154 consecutive patients undergoing with innominate artery disease either alone or with other great vessel disease.[5] Transternal repair was done in 72%, and 28% underwent extrathoracic repair. The strength of this series is its consecutive nature; however, selection bias was likely introduced given the nonrandomized nature of it. The perioperative death rates were similar (2.7% versus 2.3%), and the extrathoracic reconstructions actually had a trend toward higher perioperative neurological events (2.7% transsternal versus 6.8% extrathoracic). The authors postulated that this was related to clamping both sides of the cerebral circulation. The 10-year survival rate was similar in both groups at just under 70%; however, 10-year freedom from graft failure strongly favored transthoracic repair (94% versus 60%).

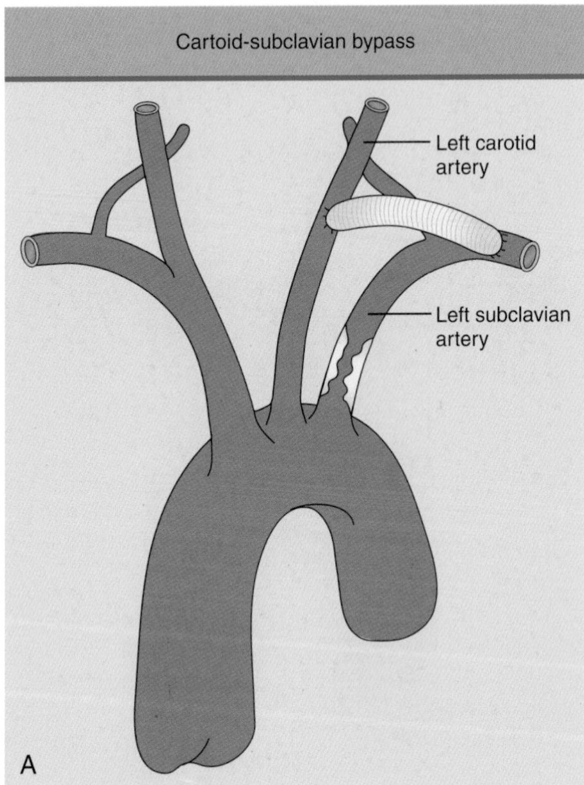

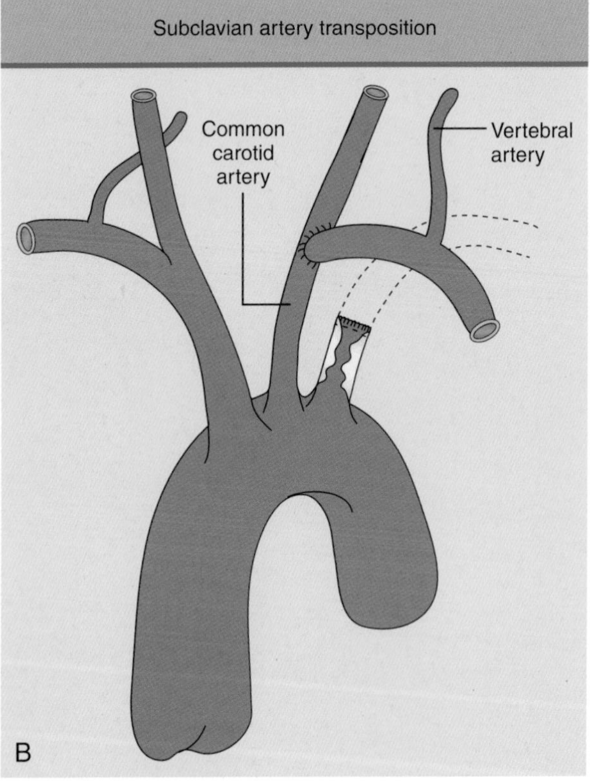

Figure 16-11. Short segment extraanatomical carotid–subclavian bypass **(A)** and subclavian to carotid transposition **(B)**.

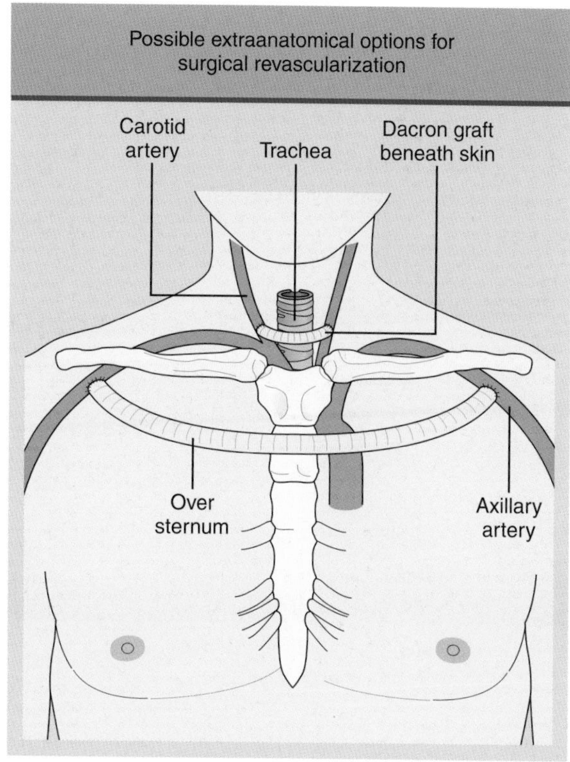

Figure 16-12. Possible extraanatomical options for surgical revascularization. Both an axilloaxillary artery bypass and a pretracheal carotid–carotid bypass are depicted.

Some authors have advocated remote extraanatomical approaches, such as axilloaxillary bypass, when a suitable ipsilateral inflow vessel is not available. Although the recent reported series often included significant numbers of patients with pure upper extremity symptoms, the axilloaxillary bypass has low stroke and death rates of 0% and 1.3%, respectively (Table 16-2, lower panel). Patency has also been acceptable, from 87% to 90% at 5 years. However, not all series share these patency rates. Schanzer et al.[51] reported a 5-year primary patency rate of 72%, and Brewster et al.[7] and Salam et al.[44] reported a 50%-plus occlusion rate. The other theoretic disadvantage of this approach is the course of the graft, which traverses the sternum, making future procedures through a median sternotomy potentially problematic. Despite these concerns, axilloaxillary bypass grafting is a reasonable option for the patient who is a prohibitive operative risk for a transsternal repair, who is not a candidate for subclavian–carotid grafting because of anatomical considerations, and for whom an endovascular solution is not possible.

Much of the available data on endovascular therapy for aortic branch vessel occlusive disease are from individual series, with follow-up data expressed as patency during a mean follow-up period rather than by life-table analysis. This makes direct comparisons with the contemporary surgical literature problematic. In addition, the claim of having long-term follow-up data when the mean follow-up period is often less than 2 years is inadequate. Acknowledging these limitations, meaningful comparisons can be made on complication rates, and trends for patency can be noted. An example of how

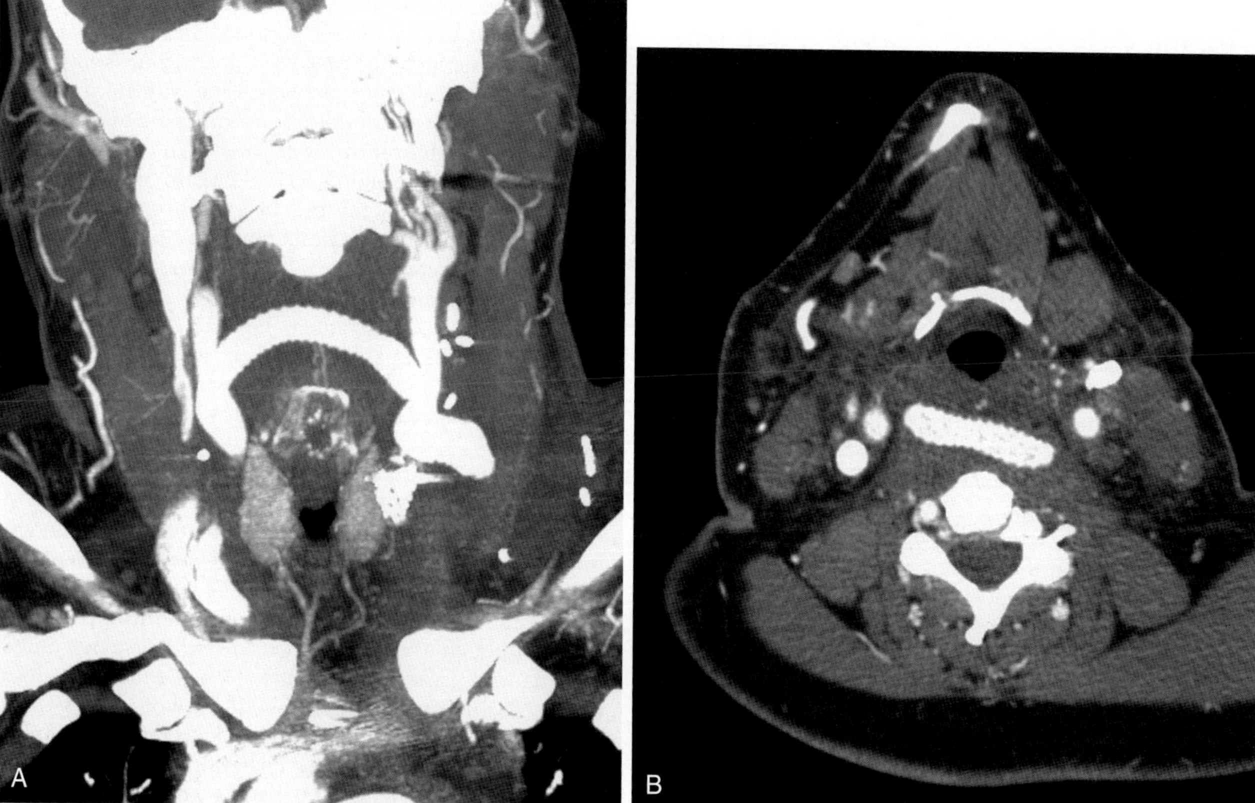

Figure 16-13. Computed tomography angiogram of a retroesophageal carotid–carotid bypass performed with ringed polytetrafluoroethylene in coronal **(A)** and cross-sectional **(B)** views.

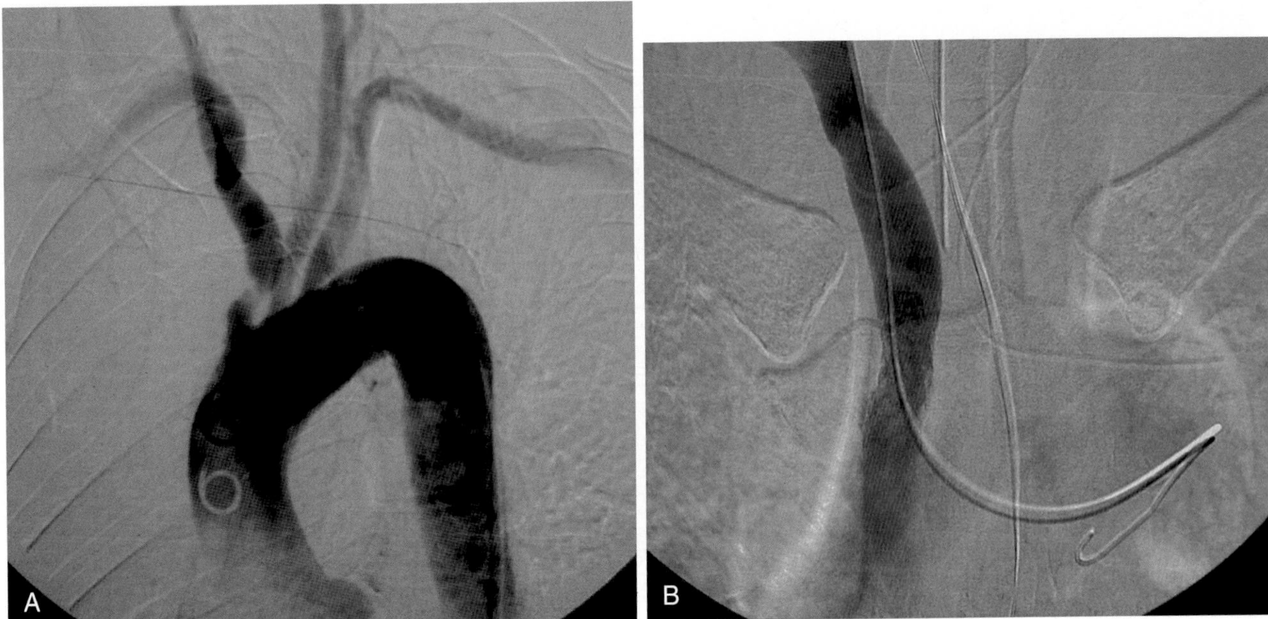

Figure 16-14. Innominate artery stenosis **(A)** treated with stent placement from the carotid approach **(B)**.

patency data can be misleading is seen in Farina et al.'s study,[39] where they did report 5-year life-table patency rates. The raw value for patency of subclavian PTA was 78% at a mean of 40 months; however, the 5-year patency by life-table analysis was only 54%.

The technical success and complication data for endovascular therapy versus open surgical techniques are directly comparable. For isolated subclavian lesions, technical success was achieved in 93% of cases (Table 16-3, upper panel). Those series with a higher rate of total occlusions tended to have a lower technical success rate, often due to an inability to cross the lesion. Data regarding the routine use of stents are not clear. Presently, no definitive data support one approach over the other. Significant complications with endovascular therapy were rare or nonexistent. When they occurred, they were most often related to the access site. The mortality rate was 0.7%, comparable to that seen with carotid–subclavian bypass grafting. No neurological events were reported, thus comparing favorably with carotid–subclavian grafting, which had a 1.4% stroke rate.

The durability of endovascular repair of proximal subclavian lesions remains less clear. In distinction to Farina et al.'s series,[39] Selby et al.[53] reported a 97% 5-year life-table patency in 32 nonoccluded lesions treated with PTA alone. The aggregate patency of subclavian PTA with or without stenting at a mean of 27 months was 84% based on raw data. Based on limited life-table data, the patency at 4 to 5 years appears to be 70% to 80% (Table 16-3). While the life-table patency appears less compared to short-segment bypasses, endovascular therapy is a reasonable first choice for isolated proximal stenotic subclavian lesions. This may prohibit the option of a subclavian–carotid transposition, however. The endovascular treatment of total occlusions remains controversial.

When examining the results of endovascular treatment of the innominate and common carotid arteries, it is not surprising that the complication rates increase compared to subclavian intervention (Table 16-3, lower panel). The neurological event rate in this group was 2.1%, with a mortality of 0.7%, but remains significantly lower than transthoracic repairs (6% neurological events, 5% mortality). Most innominate or common carotid stenting series were performed simultaneously with ipsilateral carotid endarterectomy, raising the question of which portion of the procedure was responsible for the neurological event. van Hattum et al. reported their results with percutaneous treatment of isolated innominate artery lesions in 30 patients over a 10-year period.[64] Stenting was reserved for residual stenosis and was used in two thirds of patients. Their neurological event rate was 3.1% with no mortalities. The tradeoff in lower complications compared to open repairs appears to be significantly lower patency in this series, with a primary patency rate of only 50% at 2 years. Since the authors used life-table analysis, this may be a truer comparison for the surgical series than the conglomerate of raw numbers obtained from the other reported series. Nonetheless, an endovascular approach is certainly attractive based on the safety profile. Close follow-up is warranted, however, given the limited available data. In a patient who is at increased surgical risk due to medical comorbidities, endovascular therapy should be strongly considered as first-line therapy based on these limited data.

Numerous reports have been made of endovascular treatment for Takayasu's arteritis involving the aortic branch vessels. Tyagi et al.[65] directly compared the results of PTA alone for symptomatic subclavian artery stenosis in patients with either Takayasu's arteritis or ASO. The lesions included were stenoses less than 6 cm in length and occlusions less than 2 cm. Although a trend occurred toward worse outcomes in patients with Takayasu's arteritis (19% restenosis versus 5% in ASO at a mean of 43 months), it did not reach statistical significance. All lesions were amenable to repeat angioplasty, and one required an additional dilatation. Other workers have reported the use of stents for patients with Takayasu's disease, but no data exist other than short-term follow-up to determine whether this is superior to PTA alone.[15,33]

Table 16-2

Results of Contemporary Surgical Series for Repair of Aortic Arch Branch Lesions by Direct Transsternal Repair, Short-Segment Extraanatomical Bypass Grafting (Subclavian–Carotid and Carotid–Subclavian Bypass), and Remote Extraanatomical Bypass (Axilloaxillary Bypass)*

Authors	No.	CVA/TIA No. (%)	Death No. (%)	Primary Patency (5 Years)	Secondary Patency (5 Years)	Stroke-Free Survival (5 Years)	Survival (5 Years)
Transsternal Surgical Repairs							
Kieffer et al.[10]	148	8 (5)	8 (5)	98%	99%	89%	78%
Berguer et al.[12]	100	10 (10)	8 (8)	94%	97%	87%	73%
Rhodes et al.[4]	58	4 (7)	2 (3)	80%	91%	86%	88%
Azakie et al.[32]	94	6 (6)	3 (3)	—	—	—	85%
Takach et al.[5]	113	3 (3)	3 (3)	94%†	—	87%†	69%†
Total	513	31 (6)	24 (5)	NA	NA	NA	NA
Short-Segment Extraanatomical Bypass							
Authors	**No.**	**CVA/TIA No.(%)**	**Death No.(%)**	**Primary Patency (5 Years)**	**Secondary Patency (5 Years)**	**Stroke-Free Survival (5 Years)**	**Survival (5 Years)**
Law et al.[3]	60	2 (3.3)	1 (1.7)	88%	—	86%	84%
Aburahma et al.[40]	51	0	0	96%	98%	82%	86%
Perler and Williams[41]	31	1 (3.2)	0	92%	—	71%	88%
Synn et al.[42]	32	0	0	77%	—	74% (87% CVA free)	—
Vitti et al.[43]	124	0	1 (0.8)	94%	—	90%	83%
Farina et al.[39]	15	0	0	87%	100%	100%	—
Salam et al.[44]	28	0	0	77%	—	—	—
Cinar et al.[45]	66	1 (1.5)	1 (1.5)	83%	—	—	93%
Paty et al.[46]	10	0	0	100%	100%	—	—
Total	417	6 (14)	3 (0.7)	NA	NA	NA	NA
Subclavian–Carotid Transposition							
Authors	**No.**	**CVA/TIA No. (%)**	**Death No. (%)**	**Primary Patency (5 Years)**	**Secondary Patency (5 Years)**	**Stroke-Free Survival (5 Years)**	**Survival (5 Years)**
Salam et al.[44]	6	0	0	100%	—	—	—
Schardey et al.[47]	108	2 (1.9)	0	100%	100%	—	82%
Cina et al.[48]	23	0	0	100%	—	—	—
Edwards et al.[49]	178	2	5	100%‡	—	—	—
Total	315	4 (1.3)	5 (1.6)	NA	NA	NA	NA
Axilloaxillary Bypass							
Authors	**No.**	**CVA/TIA No. (%)**	**Death No. (%)**	**Primary Patency (5 Years)**	**Secondary Patency (5 Years)**	**Stroke-Free Survival (5 Years)**	**Survival (5 Years)**
Mingoli et al.[6]	61	0	1 (1.6)	87%	88%	98%	93%
Rosenthal et al.[50]	32	0	0	90%	—	—	92%
Schanzer et al.[51]	33	0	1 (3.0)	72%	—	—	—
Weiner et al.[52]	19	0	0	89%	—	—	—
Salam et al.[44]	7	0	0	46%	—	—	—
Total	152	0	2 (1.3)	NA	NA	NA	NA

*CVA, cerebrovascular accident; NA, not applicable; TIA, transient ischemic attack.
†10-year life-table data.
‡Not life-table data.

Use of PTA with or without stenting has appeal in those patients who have postirradiation stenosis, given the risk of graft infection and wound-healing difficulties encountered with direct repairs.[4] The data on endovascular repair of these lesions are limited. Melliere et al.[66] reported a group of six patients who had angioplasty of carotid, subclavian, iliac, or femoral vessels. Four of six were successful, but data were lacking on follow-up. Given the poor results with surgical therapy in this population, despite minimal available data, PTA with or without stenting should be considered where feasible.

SUMMARY

Aortic arch branch disease is a relatively uncommon cause of significant neurovascular symptoms in the general population. Although the true incidence is unknown, duplex ultrasound

Table 16-3
Results of Endovascular Therapy for Subclavian Stenoses and for Innominate and Common Carotid Lesions*

Endovascular Treatment of Subclavian Artery Stenoses

Authors	No.	Death No. (%)	Occlusion No. (%)	Stents No. (%)	Technical Success No. (%)	Primary Patency†	Follow-up (Months)
Duber et al.[37]	8	0	8 (100)	0	7 (88)	38%	17
Selby et al.[53]	29	0	0	0	32 (100)‡	97%	36
Marques et al.[54]	31	1 (3)	6 (19)	4 (13)	31 (100)	97%	37
Sullivan et al.[55]	66	—	10 (15)	62 (100)§	62 (94)	89%	13
Queral and Criado[56]	12	0	5 (42)	10 (100)§	10 (83)	66%	27
Hebrang et al.[57]	52	0	9 (17)	0	45 (87)	79%	29
Farina et al.[39]	21	0	0	0	21 (91) ‖	78%	40
Schillinger et al.[58]	109	0	27 (25)	26 (24)	93 (85)	79% at 4 years¶	46
de Vries et al.[38]	110	1 (0.9)	20 (18)	59 (54)	102 (93)	89% at 4 years¶	34
Aburahma et al.[59]	121	1 (0.8)	25 (21)	119 (98)	119 (98)	70% at 5 years¶	41
Total	559	3 (0.6)	110 (20)	280 (50)	522 (93)	84%	27

Endovascular Treatment of Innominate and Common Carotid Stenoses

Authors	No.	CVA/TIA No. (%)	Death No. (%)	Occlusion No. (%)	Stents No. (%)	Technical Success No. (%)	Primary Patency	Follow-Up (Months)
Ruebben et al.[60]	8	0	0	0	8 (100)	8 (100)	100%	17
Sullivan et al.[55]	21	2 (9.5)	1 (4.8)	0	21 (100)	20 (95)	—	—
Queral and Criado[56]	14	0	0	3 (21)	14 (100)	14 (100)	93%	27
Lutz et al.[61]	5	0	0	—	5 (100)	5 (100)	80%	19
Grego et al.[62]	16	0	0	—	14 (88)	14 (88)	88%	—
Allie et al.[63]	34	0	0	—	34 (100)	34 (100)	91%	34
Payne et al.[36]	12	0	0	0	3 (25)	12 (100)	92%	30
Vanhattum et al.[64]	30	1 (3.3)	0	5 (17)	20 (67)	25 (83)	50%¶	24
Total	140	3 (2.1)	1 (0.7)	8 (9.4)	119 (85)	132 (94)	92%	29

*CVA, cerebrovascular accident; TIA, transient ischemic attack.
†Based on intent to treat.
‡32 lesions treated in 29 patients.
§All lesions able to be crossed were stented.
‖23 lesions in 21 patients.
¶Life-table analysis.

and angiographic studies suggest the incidence of significant proximal lesions to be about 2% to 4% in a symptomatic population.[21,22] Symptoms can be related to emboli from these lesions or from low-flow states when multiple vessels are involved. Low-flow symptoms include presyncope and other vertebrobasilar complaints. In addition, 50% of patients have isolated or concomitant upper extremity symptoms.[4]

The etiology of occlusive disease of the great vessels is most often atherosclerosis, with Takayasu's arteritis accounting for one fifth of patients in contemporary surgical series.[4] Radiation arteritis is an uncommon cause but often difficult to deal with due to high delayed wound-healing and high infection rates. Diagnostic imaging should include a duplex ultrasound, and any suggestion of a more proximal lesion on this or by physical examination (i.e., proximal noncardiac bruit or blood pressure discrepancy) warrants further imaging. Intra-arterial angiography remains the gold standard for definitive imaging but MRA or computed tomography angiography is an acceptable alternative, especially if the suspicion for proximal disease is low.

Surgical options to treat these lesions include direct transsternal repairs, including endarterectomy, or bypass grafting originating from the ascending aorta. Isolated stenoses of the subclavian or carotid origins can be treated with short-segment extraanatomical bypasses (carotid–subclavian bypass). Remote extraanatomical bypasses (axilloaxillary bypass) are reserved for those patients who represent a high surgical risk. PTA and stenting is gaining popularity as first-line therapy for proximal lesions because of its low morbidity and rare mortality, both of which compare favorably with surgical therapies. The long-term patency of these endovascular approaches remains unclear; midterm results are promising, although they still appear inferior to those achieved with surgical repairs. If restenosis occurs, these lesions can often be re-treated by endovascular means with good assisted primary patency and have even been described in treating recurrent stenoses at surgical bypass sites.[67] As stent and cerebral protection technology evolves, the already promising results of endovascular therapy are likely to improve further.

References

1. Crawford ES, Debakey ME, Morris GC, Howell JF. Surgical treatment of occlusion of the innominate, common carotid, and subclavian arteries: a 10-year experience. *Surgery* 1969;65:17-31.
2. Myers WO, Lawton BR, Sautter RD. Axillo-axillary bypass graft. *JAMA* 1971;217:826.
3. Law MM, Colburn MD, Moore WS, et al. Carotid–subclavian bypass for brachiocephalic occlusive disease: choice of conduit and long-term follow-up. *Stroke* 1995;26:1565-1571.

4. Rhodes JM, Cherry KJ, Clark RC, et al. Aortic-origin reconstruction of the great vessels: risk factors for early and late complications. *J Vasc Surg* 2000;31:260-269.
5. Takach TJ, Reul GJ, Cooley DA, et al. Brachiocephalic reconstruction I: operative and long-term results for complex disease. *J Vasc Surg* 2005;42:47-54.
6. Mingoli A, Sapienza P, Feldhaus RJ, et al. Long-term results and outcomes of crossover axilloaxillary bypass grafting: a 24-year experience. *J Vasc Surg* 1999;29:894-901.
7. Brewster DC, Moncure AC, Darling C, et al. Innominate artery lesions: problems encountered and lessons learned. *J Vasc Surg* 1985;2:99-112.
8. Hadjipetrou P, Cox S, Piemonte T, Eisenhauer A. Percutaneous revascularization of atherosclerotic obstruction of aortic arch vessels. *J Am Coll Cardiol* 1999;33:1238-1245.
9. Woo EY, Fairman RM, Velazquez OC, et al. Endovascular therapy of symptomatic innominate–subclavian arterial occlusive lesions. *Vasc Endovasc Surg* 2006;40:27-33.
10. Kieffer E, Sabatier J, Koskas F, Bahnini A. Atherosclerotic innominate artery occlusive disease: early and long-term results of surgical reconstruction. *J Vasc Surg* 1995;21:326-337.
11. Sharma BK, Jain S. Takayasu's arteritis. In: Ball GV, Bridges SL, eds. *Vasculitis*. New York: Oxford University Press; 2002:278-289.
12. Berguer R, Morasch MD, Kline RA. Transthoracic repair of innominate and common carotid artery disease: immediate and long-term outcome for 100 consecutive surgical reconstructions. *J Vasc Surg* 1998;27:34-42.
13. Debakey ME, Crawford ES, Morris GC, Cooley DA. Surgical consideration of occlusive disease of the innominate, carotid, subclavian, and vertebral arteries. *Ann Surg* 1961;154:698-725.
14. Hass WK, Fields WS, North RR, et al. Joint study of extracranial arterial occlusions. II. Arteriography, techniques, sites, and complications. *JAMA* 1968;203:159-166.
15. Bali HK, Jain S, Jain A, Sharma BK. Stent supported angioplasty in Takayasu arteritis. *Int J Cardiol* 1998;66S:S213-S217.
16. Hassen-Khodja R, Kieffer E. Radiotherapy-induced supra-aortic trunk disease: early and long-term results of surgical and endovascular reconstruction. *J Vasc Surg* 2004;40:254-261.
17. Andros G, Schneider PA, Harris RW, et al. Management of arterial occlusive disease following radiation therapy. *Cardiovasc Surg* 1996;4:135-142.
18. Phillips GR, Peer RM, Upson JF, et al. Late complications of revascularization for radiation-induced arterial disease. *J Vasc Surg* 1992;16: 921-925.
19. Gosselin C, Walker PM. Subclavian steal syndrome: existence, clinical features, diagnosis and management. *Semin Vasc Surg* 1996;9:93-97.
20. Fields WS, Lemak NA. Joint study of extracranial arterial occlusion. VII. Subclavian steal: a review of 168 cases. *JAMA* 1972;222:1139-1143.
21. Akers DL, Markowitz IA, Kerstein MD. The value of aortic arch study in the evaluation of cerebrovascular insufficiency. *Am J Surg* 1987;154: 230-232.
22. McLaren JT, Donaghue CC, Drezner AD. Accuracy of carotid duplex examination to predict proximal and intrathoracic lesions. *Am J Surg* 1996;172:149-150.
23. Kadwa AM, Robbs JV, Abdool-Carrim AT. Aortic arch angiography prior to carotid endarterectomy: is its continued use justified? *Eur J Vasc Endovasc Surg* 1997;13:527-530.
24. Executive Committee for Asymptomatic Carotid Atherosclerosis Study. Endarterectomy for asymptomatic carotid artery stenosis. *JAMA* 1995;273:1421-1428.
25. Johnston DCC, Chapman K, Goldstein LB. Low rate of complications of cerebral angiography in routine clinical practice. *Neurology* 2001;57: 2012-2014.
26. Yucel EK, Anderson CM, Edelman RR, et al. Magnetic resonance angiography: update on applications for extracranial arteries. *Circulation* 1999;100:2284-2301.
27. Carpenter JP, Holland GA, Golden MA, et al. Magnetic resonance angiography of the aortic arch. *J Vasc Surg* 1997;25:145-151.
28. Prince MR, Narasimham DL, Jacoby WT, et al. Three-dimensional gadolinium-enhanced MR angiography of the thoracic aorta. *AJR Am J Roentgenol* 1996;166:1387-1397.
29. Randoux B, Marro B, Koskas F, et al. Carotid artery stenosis: prospective comparison of CT, three-dimensional gadolinium enhanced MR, and conventional angiography. *Radiology* 2001;220:179-185.
30. U.S. Food and Drug Administration Alert. Gadolinium-based contrast agents for magnetic resonance imaging: information for healthcare professionals. Available at: http://www.fda.gov. Accessed May 23, 2007.
31. Sakopoulos AG, Ballard JL, Gundry SR. Minimally invasive approach for aortic arch branch vessel reconstruction. *J Vasc Surg* 2000;31:200-202.
32. Azakie A, McElhinney DB, Hagashima R, et al. Innominate artery reconstruction: over 3 decades of experience. *Ann Vasc Surg* 1998;228: 402-410.
33. Sharma BK, Jain S, Bali HK, et al. A follow-up study of balloon angioplasty and de novo stenting in Takayasu's arteritis. *Int J Cardiol* 2000;75: S147-S152.
34. Amann-Vesti BR, Koppensteiner R, Rainoni L, et al. Immediate and long-term outcome of upper extremity balloon angioplasty in giant cell arteritis. *J Endovac Ther* 2003;10:371-375.
35. Criado FJ, Abul-Khoudoud O. Interventional techniques to facilitate supraaortic angioplasty and stenting. *Vasc Endovasc Surg* 2006;40: 141-147.
36. Payne DA, Hayes PD, Bolia A, et al. Cerebral protection during open retrograde angioplasty/stenting of common carotid and innominate artery stenoses. *Br J Surg* 2006;93:187-190.
37. Duber C, Klose KJ, Kopp H, Schmiedt W. Percutaneous transluminal angioplasty for occlusion of the subclavian artery: short and long-term results. *Cardiovasc Intervent Radiol* 1992;15:205-210.
38. de Vries JPPM, Jager LC, van den Berg JC, et al. Durability of percutaneous transluminal angioplasty for obstructive lesions of proximal subclavian artery: long-term results. *J Vasc Surg* 2005;41:19-23.
39. Farina C, Mingoli A, Schultz RD, et al. Percutaneous transluminal angioplasty versus surgery for subclavian artery occlusive disease. *Am J Surg* 1989;158:511-514.
40. Aburahma AF, Robinson PA, Jennings TG. Carotid–subclavian bypass grafting with polytetrafluoroethylene grafts for symptomatic subclavian artery stenosis or occlusion: a 20-year experience. *J Vasc Surg* 2000;32:411-419.
41. Perler BA, Williams GM. Carotid–subclavian bypass: a decade of experience. *J Vasc Surg* 1990;12:716-723.
42. Synn AY, Chalmers RTA, Sharp WJ, et al. Is there a conduit of preference for a bypass between the carotid and subclavian arteries? *Am J Surg* 1993;166:157-162.
43. Vitti MJ, Thompson BW, Read RC, et al. Carotid–subclavian bypass: a twenty-two year experience. *J Vasc Surg* 1994;20:411-418.
44. Salam TA, Lumsden AB, Smith RB. Subclavian artery revascularization: a decade of experience with extrathoracic bypass procedures. *J Surg Res* 1994;56:387-392.
45. Cinar B, Enc Y, Kosem M, et al. Carotid–subclavian bypass in occlusive disease of subclavian artery: more important today than before. *Tohoku J Exp Med* 2004;204:53-62.
46. Paty PSK, Mehta M, Darling C, et al. Surgical treatment of coronary subclavian steal syndrome with carotid subclavian bypass. *Ann Vasc Surg* 2003;17:22-26.
47. Schardey HM, Meyer G, Rau HG, et al. Subclavian carotid transposition: an analysis of a clinical series and a review of the literature. *Eur J Vasc Endovasc Surg* 1996;12:431-436.
48. Cina CS, Safar HA, Lagana A, et al. Subclavian carotid transposition and bypass grafting: consecutive cohort study and systematic review. *J Vasc Surg* 200;35:422-429.
49. Edwards WH, Tapper SS, Edwards WH, et al. Subclavian revascularization: a quarter century experience. *Ann Surg* 1994;219:673-678.
50. Rosenthal D, Ellison RG, Clark MD, et al. Axilloaxillary bypass: is it worthwhile? *J Cardiovasc Surg* 1988;29:191-1195.
51. Schanzer H, Chung-Loy H, Kotok M, et al. Evaluation of axillo-axillary artery bypass for the treatment of subclavian or innominate artery occlusive disease. *J Cardiovasc Surg* 1987;28:258-261.
52. Weiner RI, Deterling RA, Sentissi J, O'Donnell TF. Subclavian artery insufficiency: treatment with axilloaxillary bypass. *Arch Surg* 1987: 876-880.
53. Selby JB, Matsumoto AH, Tegtmeyer CJ, et al. Balloon angioplasty above the aortic arch: immediate and long-term results. *AJR Am J Roentgenol* 1993;160:631-635.
54. Marques KMJ, Ernst SMPG, Mast EG, et al. Percutaneous transluminal angioplasty of the left subclavian artery to prevent or treat the coronary–subclavian steal syndrome. *Am J Cardiol* 1996;78:687-690.
55. Sullivan TM, Gray BH, Bacharach JM, et al. Angioplasty and primary stenting of the subclavian, innominate, and common carotid arteries in 83 patients. *J Vasc Surg* 1998;28:1059-1065.
56. Queral LA, Criado FJ. The treatment of focal aortic arch branch lesions with Palmaz stents. *J Vasc Surg* 1996;23:368-375.
57. Hebrang A, Maskovic J, Tomac B. Percutaneous transluminal angioplasty of the subclavian arteries: long-term results in 52 patients. *AJR Am J Roentgenol* 1991;156:1091-1094.

58. Schillinger M, Haumer M, Schillinger S, et al. Outcome of conservative versus interventional treatment of subclavian artery stenosis. *J Endovasc Ther* 2002;9:139-146.
59. Aburahma AF, Bates MC, Stone PA, et al. Angioplasty and stenting versus carotid–subclavian bypass for the treatment of isolated subclavian artery disease. *J Endovasc Ther* 2007;14:698-704.
60. Ruebben A, Tettoni S, Muratore P, et al. Feasibility of intraoperative balloon angioplasty and additional stent placement of isolated stenosis of the brachiocephalic trunk. *J Thorac Cardiovasc Surg* 1998;115:1316-1320.
61. Lutz HJ, Do DD, Schroth G, et al. Hybrid therapy of symptomatic stenosis of the innominate artery. *Eur J Vasc Endovasc Surg* 2002;24:184-185.
62. Grego F, Frigatti P, Lepidi S, et al. Synchronous carotid endarterectomy and retrograde endovascular treatment of brachiocephalic or common carotid artery stenosis. *Eur J Vasc Endovasc Surg* 2003;26:392-395.
63. Allie DE, Hebert CJ, Lirtzman MD, et al. Intraoperative innominate and common carotid intervention combined with carotid endarterectomy: a "true" endovascular surgical approach. *J Endovasc Ther* 2004;11:258-262.
64. van Hattum ES, de Vries JPPM, Lalezarif, et al. Angioplasty with or without stent placement in the brachiocephalic artery: feasible and durable? A retrospective cohort study. *J Vasc Interv Radiol* 2007;18:1088-1093.
65. Tyagi S, Verma PK, Gambhir DS, et al. Early and long-term results of subclavian angioplasty in aortitis (Takayasu disease): comparison with atherosclerosis. *Cardiovasc Intervent Radiol* 1998;21:218-224.
66. Melliere D, Becquemin JP, Berrahal D, et al. Management of radiation-induced occlusive arterial disease: a reassessment. *J Cardiovasc Surg* 1997;38:261-269.
67. Anzuini A, Chiesa R, Vivekananthan K, et al. Endovascular stenting for stenoses in surgically reconstructed brachiocephalic bypass grafts: immediate and midterm outcomes. *J Endovasc Ther* 2004;11:263-268.

chapter 17

Upper Extremity Ischemia: Small Artery Occlusive Disease

James M. Edwards, MD

Supported in whole or in part by grant M01 RR000334 to the Oregon Clinical Translational Research Institute, National Institutes of Health, Bethesda, Maryland.

Key Points

- Raynaud's syndrome is defined as episodic digital ischemia in response to cold or emotional stress.
- Most patients have normal digits between attacks.
- Raynaud's syndrome may be due to fixed obstruction or episodic vasospasm.
- Raynaud's syndrome is associated with autoimmune diseases.
- Evaluation by the vascular laboratory is useful.
- Initial therapy consists of cold avoidance.
- Medication therapy comprises calcium channel blockers and angiotensin-converting enzyme inhibitors.
- Tissue loss is rare and is best treated conservatively.
- Most patients do not develop progressive hand ischemia.

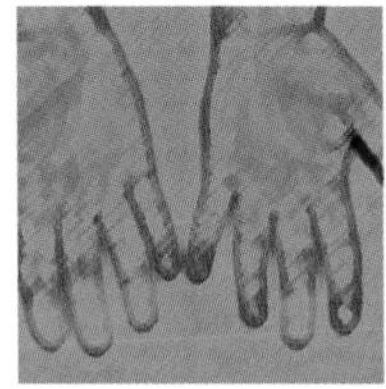

Upper extremity ischemia accounts for less than 5% of patients presenting to a vascular surgeon for evaluation of limb ischemia, with the vast majority of patients in most practices presenting with leg ischemia secondary to atherosclerosis.

Patients with upper extremity occlusive disease usually present with Raynaud's syndrome. Raynaud's syndrome is intermittent digital ischemia occurring in response to cold or emotional stress. Most patients describe tricolor changes, with the fingers initially turning white, then blue or purple, and finally red after rewarming. The physiological sequence responsible for these color changes is as follows: the initial pallor is caused by digital ischemia; the cyanosis occurs when blood initially returns to the digit and becomes deoxygenated; and the rubor on rewarming occurs as the result of reactive hyperemia. There are a subgroup of Raynaud's patients that do not have the classical tricolor changes, including a small group of patients who have no color changes. These patients appear to be otherwise indistinguishable from those patients with color changes. In most patients, the digits are normal between attacks.

Raynaud's syndrome may be due to an intrinsic abnormality in the digital blood vessels, sympathetic nervous system, or thermoregulatory system or may be secondary to an associated disease, as discussed later in this chapter. Patients with intrinsic abnormalities often have a lifelong history of Raynaud's syndrome and may be regarded as otherwise-normal individuals who are hypersensitive to cold. The traditional division of Raynaud's patients was into *Raynaud's phenomenon* and *Raynaud's disease,* where phenomenon refers to patients with a diagnosed associated disease and disease refers to those with episodic digital ischemia in the absence of a diagnosed associated disease.[1] This classification was described long before modern serological testing was available, and while still widely used, has two significant limitations.[2,3] First, the most common associated diseases, the connective tissue diseases, may not become clinically apparent until years after the Raynaud's syndrome is diagnosed, meaning patients may be shifted from one group to another without a change in clinical condition. Second, this division does not address the underlying digital artery pathology that may be present. Since the presence or absence of arterial pathology or associated disease is the primary and perhaps only objective data available on patients with Raynaud's syndrome, it seems better to group Raynaud's patients based on these two factors. By categorizing all patients with either fixed or episodic digital ischemia as having Raynaud's syndrome and then subcategorizing patients (according to the presence or absence of associated disease and the presence or absence of arterial occlusive disease), the treating physician is better able to determine the natural history that a particular patient may anticipate.

This chapter discusses the pathophysiology and classification of Raynaud's syndrome, the mechanisms of vasospasm thought to be important in Raynaud's syndrome, the variety of connective tissue disorders and small vessel diseases that may be associated with Raynaud's syndrome, and a clinical approach to patients who present with Raynaud's syndrome.

PATHOPHYSIOLOGY

The pathophysiological mechanism or mechanisms underlying Raynaud's syndrome remain unknown despite more than a century of study.[4,5] Multiple abnormalities including those of the sympathetic nervous system,[6,7] digital blood vessels, altered sensitivities, numbers of α-adrenoceptors[8,9] and β-adrenoceptors,[10] and vasoactive peptides, including calcitonin gene-related peptide[11-13] and endothelin,[14-17] have been hypothesized over the last century to explain Raynaud's syndrome. Evidence also suggests it is a combination of both local factors[18] and alterations in the function of the sympathetic nervous system.[19] The recognized physiology of blood vessel contraction and relaxation is becomingly increasingly complex, and it is increasingly clear that the pathophysiological mechanisms responsible for Raynaud's syndrome are varied, probably overlap, and likely differ from patient to patient.

While no way exists of determining the exact pathophysiological mechanism or mechanisms of vasospasm in a given patient, experience indicates that patients with Raynaud's syndrome can easily be separated into groups by looking at objective characteristics. As noted earlier, patients may easily be divided into four groups based on the presence or absence of arterial obstructive disease and the presence or absence of an associated disease. Division of patients into groups based on the presence or absence of arterial obstructive disease results in two groups—vasospastic and obstructive. These groups have symptoms based on significantly different pathophysiological mechanisms.

Patients with vasospastic Raynaud's syndrome have normal digital artery pressure at rest. Because of cold or emotional stress, these patients experience an abnormally forceful contraction of digital artery smooth muscle leading to palmar and digital artery closure. This results in profound, albeit temporary, digital ischemia and pallor. The pathophysiological mechanism responsible for this abnormally forceful contraction is not known and may vary among patients or even vasospastic episodes. Upon rewarming or relief of stress, the vasoconstriction ceases and the digits return to normal.

Patients with obstructive Raynaud's syndrome have palmar and digital artery occlusive disease, proximal obstruction of the large arteries of the upper extremity, or a combination of the two that results in decreased resting digital blood pressure. These patients usually have relatively normal-appearing fingers at rest but may also have symptomatic digital ischemia or tissue loss under nonstressed conditions. With cold or emotional stress, a normal (or possibly abnormal) vasoconstrictive response of the digital artery smooth muscle is able to overcome the decreased intraluminal distending pressure and cause arterial closure with subsequent symptoms. With this mechanism, hypothesizing an abnormally forceful vasoconstrictive response in these patients is unnecessary, but overlap is likely among mechanisms such that several patients experience both an abnormally forceful contractile response and a palmar or digital artery obstructive disease.

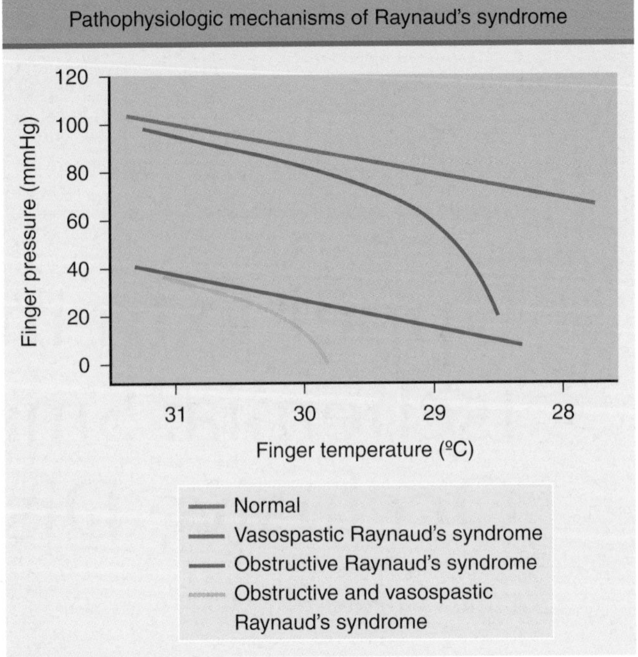

Figure 17-1. Pathophysiological mechanisms of Raynaud's syndrome. Finger blood pressure response to digital cooling in normals decreases gradually with decreasing finger temperature. Finger blood pressure response to digital cooling in patients with obstructive disease also decreases gradually with decreasing temperature, but it reaches zero. Finger blood pressure response to digital cooling in patients with either vasospastic disease alone or both obstructive and vasospastic disease decreases gradually until a critical temperature is reached, at which time it decreases rapidly to zero.

The two pathophysiological mechanisms are shown diagrammatically in Figure 17-1. The vasospastic patient has a normal digital pressure at room temperature that falls rapidly after a critical temperature is reached. The obstructive group starts at a lower initial digital pressure, and the hypothermia-induced pressure decline parallels that of normal individuals until arterial closure occurs. If a patient with obstruction also has a vasospastic component, the resulting curve is a combination of the two.

A few diseases, including the autoimmune connective tissue diseases, Buerger's disease, and hypersensitivity angiitis, have a predilection for damaging the small vessels of the extremities, primarily the fingers and to a lesser extent the toes. The reason these diseases have a predilection for damaging distal extremity vessels is not known, but thermally sensitive antigen–antibody reaction with immune complex deposition has been postulated. Not surprisingly, the digits are the coolest part of the body, and this finding may explain why the process primarily occurs in the digits. In the next section, I briefly present the clinical and laboratory features of the small vessel arteriopathies encountered most often.

Raynaud's syndrome has been described with several pharmacological agents. Beta-blockers, particularly propranolol, are perhaps the most widely named prescription drugs, but little evidence supports a causal link. The initiation or discontinuation of estrogens, with or without progesterone, have been linked with both the onset and the cessation of Raynaud's syndrome. Various chemotherapeutic agents, particularly bleomycin, have the rare side effect of digital necrosis.[20] Nicotine and caffeine have also been implicated in Raynaud's syndrome, but at typical use levels they may aggravate the preexisting disease but not cause it.

COMMON SMALL VESSEL ARTERIOPATHIES

Scleroderma

The most common connective tissue disease in patients with Raynaud's syndrome is scleroderma. Scleroderma (progressive systemic sclerosis) is a generalized disorder of connective tissue, the microvasculature, and the small arteries.[21] The name scleroderma is derived from the Greek for "hard skin." Scleroderma has a female-to-male ratio of about 3:1, and the incidence is approximately 10 per 1 million population per year in the United States. An estimated 50,000 patients in the United States have scleroderma. Cutaneous involvement in scleroderma is almost universal. The clinical course of scleroderma is characterized by progressive scarring and small vessel occlusions in the skin, gastrointestinal tract, kidneys, lungs, and heart. Raynaud's syndrome is present in 80% to 97% of patients with scleroderma. The syndrome usually begins as the vasospastic type and progress to the obstructive type over time in a subgroup of patients. It is the most commonly associated condition in the Oregon Health and Science University experience in patients with digital ulceration.[22]

Scleroderma patients may be divided into those who present with involvement of primarily the skin of the hands, forearms, and face (limited involvement group) and those who present with diffuse cutaneous and visceral involvement (diffuse involvement). Members of the first group, which represents about half of the total, often present with finger swelling and longstanding Raynaud's syndrome. Perhaps because of the usual delay in presentation to a physician, these patients in the limited involvement group are older than those in the diffuse involvement group. The limited involvement group appears to have a relatively benign course with prolonged survival in comparison to the diffuse involvement group. This limited cutaneous involvement syndrome has been termed the CREST (for calcinosis, Raynaud's syndrome, esophageal dysmotility, sclerodactyly, and telangiectasias), although many patients with limited involvement do not manifest all these features.

Patients in the diffuse involvement group tend to be younger and usually present soon after development of symptoms of generalized skin involvement or arthritis. The skin involvement often is most severe in the upper arms and the trunk and is progressive. Renal involvement is common in this group.

Patients with scleroderma may also be divided into subgroups based on the presence or absence of various antibodies. Patients with limited involvement often have a positive anticentromere antibody, while those patients with diffuse involvement are more likely to have antibodies to topoisomerase I (anti-Scl-70).

While the pathophysiological mechanisms of scleroderma are still being elucidated, the damage seen in scleroderma is likely mediated through cytotoxic antibodies to the endothelium.[23,24] Histopathological features of scleroderma include a vasculitis of the small arteries with fibrinoid necrosis and concentric thickening of the intima with deposition of layers of mucopolysaccharides. The cellular infiltrates seen on histopathology are composed of T cells. Capillary abnormalities may be seen in patients with scleroderma using nailfold microscopy.[25] These abnormalities include giant capillary loops and capillary dropout. On electron microscopy, these capillaries have thickened basement membranes and endothelial damage.[26]

Systemic Lupus Erythematosus

While systemic lupus erythematosus (SLE) occurs most often in young females, approximately 10% of patients are male and cases of SLE have been reported in all age groups.[27] The pathophysiology of SLE remains unknown, and the damage to the affected organs appears caused primarily by immune complex deposition. Abnormalities in apoptosis have also been postulated in SLE.[28] The diagnosis of SLE is made primarily clinically since the available laboratory tests in patients with SLE, such as the antinuclear antibody, while quite sensitive, are not specific.[29] The clinical criteria include fevers, arthralgias, skin rash, Raynaud's syndrome, and nephritis.

The pathological lesions of SLE typically involve small arteries and capillaries and occur throughout the vascular system. The lesions in the small arteries are characterized by necrosis of all or part of the vessel wall, fibroblastic hyperplasia of the intima or media, and occlusive fibrin deposits. Raynaud's syndrome is one of the most common clinical manifestations of SLE, with as many as 80% of patients reporting this symptom. In most patients, this is a nuisance condition, but a small number develop significant digital arteriopathy with resulting digital artery occlusion, digital ischemia, and in the extreme digital ulceration and gangrene.[30]

Rheumatoid Arthritis

Rheumatoid arthritis is a chronic inflammatory joint disease. Patients with rheumatoid arthritis have a progressive and inflammatory synovitis with resulting destruction of the articular cartilage, the joint, and the surrounding structures. The etiology of rheumatoid arthritis is unknown, but it likely results from immune-mediated damage. Most patients have the HLA-DRW-4 allele, and it has been theorized that this marks a genetic predisposition that, in response to an unknown stimulus such as infection, leads to immune complex deposition and inflammation. The diagnosis is based on clinical and laboratory findings, the most important of which is the presence of rheumatoid factor, an immunoglobulin M. Rheumatoid factor is present in most patients with rheumatoid arthritis, and almost all patients with extraarticular involvement have rheumatoid factor.

While rheumatoid arthritis invariably involves the joints, a subgroup of patients has extraarticular involvement of the skin, eyes, lungs, spleen, and arteries.[31] Several types of vasculitis have been described in patients with rheumatoid arthritis, the most severe of which is termed rheumatoid vasculitis, a systemic process involving both arteries and veins.[32]

The pathological lesions found in rheumatoid vasculitis include intimal proliferation with vessel occlusion, medial necrosis, and obliterative fibrosis.[33] The clinical manifestations of vasculitis include Raynaud's syndrome with or without digital gangrene, polyneuropathy, purpura, cutaneous gangrene and ulceration, and rarely involvement of the systemic arteries, including the coronary and visceral arteries. The diagnosis of rheumatoid vasculitis is made by biopsy, as well as clinical and laboratory findings.

Sjögren's Syndrome

Sjögren's syndrome is characterized by dry eyes and a dry mouth (keratoconjunctivitis sicca and xerostomia). Sjögren's syndrome may be primary, or it may be secondary to another connective tissue disease, including scleroderma, rheumatoid arthritis, or SLE.[34] The diagnosis of Sjögren's syndrome is made primarily on clinical grounds and may be confirmed by buccal salivary gland biopsy.

Sjögren's syndrome may be associated with a small vessel arteriopathy, which may be divided into acute necrotizing, leukocytoclastic, and lymphocytic vasculitis.[35] The necrotizing form involves small- and medium-sized arteries, while the others involve capillaries and venules. The vasculitic lesions usually appear several years after diagnosis and may involve the fingers with resulting ulceration. The diagnosis of vasculitis in Sjögren's syndrome requires biopsy.

Mixed and Undifferentiated Connective Tissue Disease

Mixed connective tissue disease (MCTD) and undifferentiated connective tissue disease (UCTD) are terms used to describe a group of disease states that are clearly autoimmune diseases but do not fall into a named disease category. Patients with UCTD have Raynaud's syndrome, isolated keratoconjunctivitis sicca, unexplained polyarthritis, and at least three other criteria from a list consisting of Raynaud's syndrome, myalgias, rash, pleuritis, pericarditis, and six other items.[36] While this is a diagnosis of exclusion, it represents a sufficiently large subset of patients with connective tissue disease in that it is a widely accepted diagnostic condition. MCTD clinically presents as an overlap syndrome with features of two or more connective tissue disease, such as SLE, rheumatoid arthritis, or scleroderma.[37] Patients characteristically have high titers of antibodies to an extractable nuclear antigen, which consists of ribonucleic acid and protein. Patients with both MCTD and UCTD may have a diffuse vasculitis, and in my experience, these two groups account for a small but significant proportion of patients with severe digital ischemia and digital ulceration.

Buerger's Disease

Buerger's disease (thromboangiitis obliterans) describes a clinical syndrome characterized by the occurrence of segmental thrombotic occlusions of the small- and medium-sized arteries.[38,39] The lower extremities are most often involved, but upper extremity involvement with resulting Raynaud's syndrome and digital ischemia occurs in as many as 50% of these patients. Ischemic digital ulcerations are common. Buerger's disease classically occurs in young male smokers and is often associated with both migratory thrombophlebitis and Raynaud's syndrome. The diagnostic criteria include age less than 45 years, tobacco abuse, exclusion of other diseases with similar clinical findings, normal arteries proximal to the popliteal or brachial arteries, and documentation by objective means of digital arterial occlusion.[40] Buerger's disease has also been reported after prolonged marijuana use.[41]

The pathological lesion of Buerger's disease, in the acute stage, is one of neutrophilic inflammation with preservation of the internal elastic lamina.[42] In contrast, disruption of the internal elastic lamina occurs in most immune arteritides and in atherosclerosis. Other distinguishing features include preservation of the arterial wall and lack of vascular wall calcification, aneurysms, and atheroma. Lesions eventually develop a predominance of mononuclear cells and occasional giant cells. Late lesions are characterized by intense perivascular fibrosis.

The natural history of Buerger's disease is one of progression of disease with major lower extremity amputation in 20% to 30% of patients. Interestingly, life expectancy does not appear to be shortened, probably reflecting the typical absence of significant cardiac, cerebral, and visceral vessel disease in these patients. The cornerstone of treatment of Buerger's disease is cessation of smoking. With this, most lesions heal with simple conservative therapy.

Vibration Arterial Injury

The finding of Raynaud's syndrome after long-term use of vibrating tools was first reported about a century ago.[43,44] The patients in the initial group were stonecutters, but since that time similar groups of patients have been described in various occupations, including welders or grinders in shipyards, timber fellers, and most recently windshield replacement technicians in the auto-glass industry.[45] This condition has been termed vibration white finger. The pathophysiological mechanism of vibration white finger is not known, but clearly kinetic energy imparted to the small vessels and nerves of the hand by vibrating tools with power in certain frequency bands is harmful. This appears to be a cumulative trauma disorder in that the damage accumulates over time without healing between exposures. Early on, these patients have vasospastic Raynaud's syndrome, but in the late stage, usually after decades of vibrating tool use, digital artery occlusive disease is seen.[46,47]

Hypersensitivity Angiitis

The term hypersensitivity angiitis describes a group of patients who fit an unusual but similar disease process. These patients present with the acute onset of significant digital ischemia, usually with ischemic ulceration, but have no demonstrable underlying abnormality, such as a connective tissue disease or embolic source.[48] My colleagues and I have hypothesized that these patients have digital artery occlusions occurring on the basis of immune-mediated arterial wall injury, although we have no objective evidence to support this hypothesis. We have noted that the palmar and digital arterial injury and occlusion in these patients appears to be a one-time event quite unlike the ongoing small vessel arteriopathic injury seen in patients with connective tissue diseases. In our experience, patients with hypersensitivity angiitis do not have further episodes of digital ischemia and their clinical course has been one of progressive improvement.

Fibromuscular Disease

The presence of fibromuscular disease involving the forearm arteries and the palmar and digital arteries has been described but is extremely uncommon.[49] This small group of patients often presents with significant finger ischemia because of arterial embolization and occlusion. My colleagues and I have postulated that the condition known as hypothenar hammer syndrome, in which patients have the acute onset of hand ischemia after using the heel of their hand as a hammer, is actually due to acute trauma to a preexisting fibromuscular disease lesion.[50] This is based on most of these patients having an abnormal palmar artery on the opposite (nontraumatized) side; in addition, the pathological appearance of resected aneurysms is consistent with fibromuscular disease.

Malignancy

Raynaud's syndrome has been reported in association with several malignancies.[51-53] While the mechanism of the digital artery occlusions in these patients is unknown, it appears related to tumor-based immunological processes, probably including both small vessel arteritis and immune complex deposition and possibly including cryoglobulins. Spontaneous improvement with treatment of the tumor has been reported.

Frostbite

Freeze injury of the small vessels of the digits results in Raynaud's syndrome. Mild frostbite usually results in vasospastic Raynaud's syndrome, while significant freezing injury may result in occlusive disease of the digital arteries.

CLINICAL PRESENTATION AND EVALUATION

The usual clinical presentation of Raynaud's syndrome in a primary care setting is that of a young female with finger color changes in response to cold or emotional stress, although in our tertiary referral center my colleagues and I often see patients of all ages who present with a spectrum of digital ischemia. This spectrum includes patients presenting with only nuisance symptoms and those presenting with severe acute or chronic digital ischemia, including the presence of digital gangrene or ulceration. All patients undergo a complete history and physical examination, with specific attention to signs and symptoms of underlying connective tissue diseases. Special attention is paid to determining a threshold for cold sensitivity. By asking patients whether they experience Raynaud's attacks in response to various cold stimuli, the threshold temperature can be simply estimated (cold, wet winter days at 10° C, cool fall nights at 15° C, air-conditioned buildings at 20° C). The basic evaluation consists of the clinical laboratory tests and noninvasive vascular laboratory tests shown in Table 17-1. If this initial battery of tests is nondiagnostic and the patients have significant obstructive disease (by vascular laboratory criteria) or digital ulceration, further testing to determine the presence of a hypercoagulable state is conducted. This screening battery consists of antithrombin III, protein C, and protein S levels, tests for the presence of anticardiolipin and antiphospholipid (lupus inhibitor) antibodies, Lp(a) levels in patients with hyperlipidemia, and tests for familial hypercoagulable states such as factor V Leyden.

Table 17-1
Evaluation of Raynaud's Syndrome

Vascular Laboratory
Finger pressures
Finger photoplethysmographic waveforms
Cold challenge test
Basic Clinical Laboratory
Complete blood count
Erythrocyte sedimentation rate
Antinuclear antibodies
Rheumatoid factor
Additional Tests in Select Cases
Hypercoagulable screening
Protein C
Protein S
Antithrombin III
Lupus anticoagulant
Anticardiolipin and antiphospholipid antibodies
Lipoprotein A
Factor V Leyden
Thyroid panel

The noninvasive vascular laboratory provides the information needed to differentiate patients with baseline arterial obstruction from those with normal resting digital pressures. Furthermore, the performance of both upper extremity arterial examination and finger pressures allows the differentiation of large artery disease (abnormal upper extremity examination) from small artery disease (normal upper extremity examination, abnormal lower extremity examination). It is important to record finger temperature when performing finger pressure measurement, as most patients with cold hands have abnormal finger pressures. Ensuring normal finger temperature precludes the false positive of obstructive Raynaud's syndrome. Multiple noninvasive vascular laboratory tests have been suggested for the objective and quantitative diagnosis of the cold-induced vasospasm seen in Raynaud's syndrome, all of which have a cold challenge component. Clinically an objective test is not necessary since treatment of Raynaud's syndrome is not curative but only for symptomatic benefit and no evidence shows that severity of cold sensitivity correlates with outcome. However, for both research and compensation, an objective, qualitative test for the severity of cold sensitivity in Raynaud's syndrome is essential. The most basic test for cold sensitivity is finger temperature recovery after ice-water immersion. Normal individuals have recovery of digital temperatures to preimmersion levels in 5 minutes. The sensitivity of the finding of prolonged temperature recovery after ice-water immersion is near 100%, but the specificity is only about 50% with many otherwise-normal individuals testing positive. A diagrammatic representation of normal and abnormal temperature recovery after ice-water immersion is shown in Figure 17-2.

Numerous cold challenge tests have been used by the many researchers in the field of Raynaud's. In the past, my colleagues and I relied on the ischemic digital hypothermic challenge test as described by Nielsen and Lassen, which has the highest

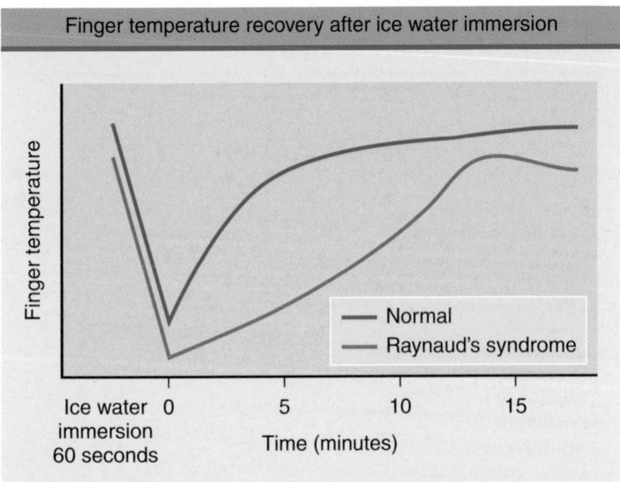

Figure 17-2. Finger temperature recovery after ice-water immersion. A normal response to ice-water immersion is recovery to baseline temperature in less than 5 minutes. In an abnormal response, finger temperature recovery takes more than 5 minutes.

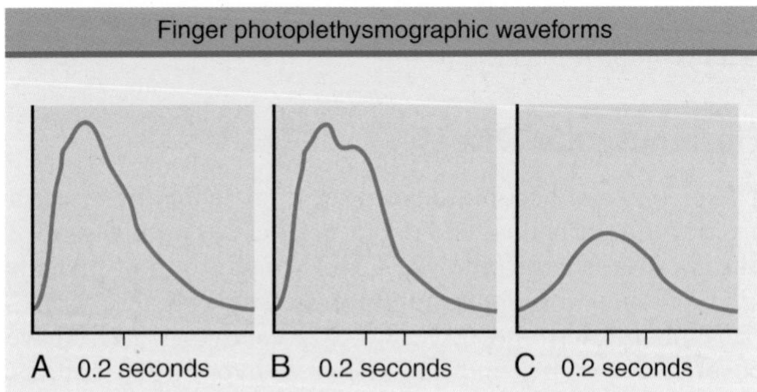

Figure 17-3. Finger photoplethysmographic (PPG) waveforms. **A,** Normal PPG waveform. **B,** "Peaked pulse" pattern often seen in vasospastic Raynaud's syndrome. **C,** Obstructive pattern.

sensitivity and specificity for the diagnosis of Raynaud's syndrome.[54,55] However, the machine that used to perform this test is no longer manufactured or maintained. Therefore, we do not perform cold challenge testing or recommend a specific test; instead, we rely on clinical history. Perhaps the most promising test described in the literature is cold finger lactate content before and after cold challenge testing (cold finger fingertip lacticemy).[56] In a recent paper, this has been shown to demonstrate the response to therapy in patients with either no associated disease or scleroderma.[57] Since this test involves analysis of lactate levels in blood obtained from a finger stick, the general usefulness outside of the research realm remains unknown.

Three digital photoplethysmography patterns are often observed in patients with Raynaud's syndrome (Figure 17-3). The first is a normal pulsatile pattern with a sharp upstroke, which is normal. Patients with vasospastic Raynaud's syndrome may have a "peaked pulse," with the addition of a second, smaller peak just after the peak upstroke apparently related to increased arterial resistance or elasticity.[58] Patients with obstructive Raynaud's syndrome have dampened waveforms with a slower upstroke (greater than 0.2 seconds). It is important to remember that photoplethysmography waveforms are qualitative, not quantitative, and that the height of the wave is not important, just the shape and upstroke time. In addition, both normal patients and those with vasospastic Raynaud's syndrome have digital blood pressures within 20 mm Hg of brachial pressure, while patients with obstructive Raynaud's syndrome have digital blood pressures below this level.

We reserve arteriography for those patients with unexplained digital artery occlusions in an asymmetrical distribution (e.g., several digits on one hand only) to rule out a surgically correctable proximal lesion. Thus, a patient with diffuse occlusions of all fingers of both hands and a high-titer antinuclear antibody would not have arteriography, while a patient with the acute onset of ischemia of two fingers of one hand would have arteriography recommended, as well as echocardiography. When ordering and performing arteriography, the entire upper extremity circulation from the aortic arch to the fingertips, including magnification hand arteriography, should be visualized. In addition, both upper extremities should be imaged. The presence of significant occlusive disease bilaterally, which may be seen even with unilateral symptoms, is an indication of a systemic disease state rather than an embolic source. An example of hand arteriography in a patient with multiple digital and palmar arterial occlusions is shown in Figure 17-4. Magnetic resonance arteriography performed with the proper sequences and reconstructed by skilled individuals may provide the necessary diagnostic information.[59]

TREATMENT

Most patients with Raynaud's syndrome are best managed by cold and tobacco avoidance without the need for medication. In addition, if the patient has recently started medications such as beta-blockers and has noted a worsening of symptoms, alternatives to the medication should be sought. Patients should be instructed to limit their caffeine and nicotine intake for a period to determine whether this ameliorates their symptoms.

Several medications have been shown to be beneficial in the treatment of Raynaud's syndrome in randomized trials. The most effective drug treatment to date has been the calcium channel blocker nifedipine.[60,61] The administration of 30 mg of the extended release formulation relieves or improves the symptoms in about half the patients with vasospastic Raynaud's syndrome. Losartan, an angiotensin-converting enzyme-2 inhibitor, has been demonstrated to be effective in patients with Raynaud's syndrome in randomized trials, although in my experience the results are not as dramatic as those seen with nifedipine.[62,63] Fluoxetine, a selective serotonin uptake inhibitor, has also been shown in a double-blind, randomized, controlled trial.[64] Other drugs that have a modest clinical benefit and have been used in the treatment of Raynaud's syndrome include prazosin,[65] sildenafil,[66] reserpine, cilostazol,[67] captopril,[68] guanethidine, niacin, ω-3 fatty acids, and dibenzyline. Bosentan, an endothelin receptor blocker, appears to particularly beneficial in patients with scleroderma.[69]

Unfortunately, the results in patients with obstructive Raynaud's syndrome are less satisfying. Since this group of patients probably does not have abnormal contraction of the digital arteries in response to cold, pharmacological intervention is predictably less effective. About 20% to 30% of patients do not tolerate nifedipine because of headache, ankle swelling, or a diffuse feeling of lassitude. Thus, drug therapy of

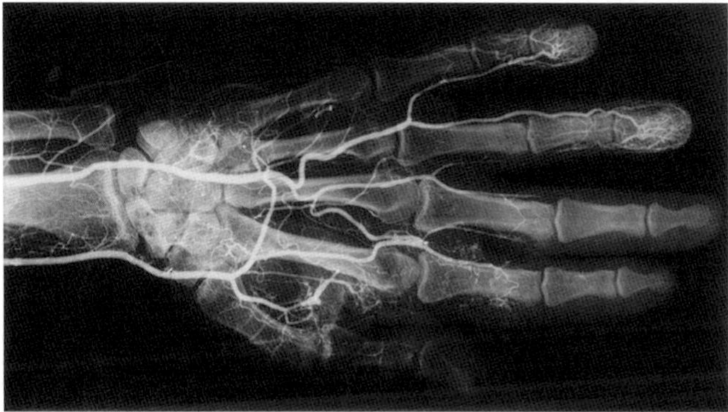

Figure 17-4. Arteriography from a patient with obstructive Raynaud's syndrome.

Raynaud's syndrome appears effective in about half of the small number of Raynaud's syndrome patients requiring drug therapy.

Thoracic sympathectomy has been used both for the treatment of digital artery vasospasm and as an adjunct for healing of digital ischemic ulceration. As a treatment for vasospasm, thoracic sympathectomy is usually initially successful, but the symptoms of vasospasm invariably return rapidly, usually within 3 to 6 months. My colleagues and I have performed thoracic sympathectomy for hyperhidrosis in patients with concomitant Raynaud's syndrome and have noted a lifelong cessation of sweating but the rapid recurrence of Raynaud's attacks. The underlying pathophysiological basis for this differential remains unknown but probably relates to incomplete sympathectomy. Thoracic sympathectomy as an adjunctive measure for the treatment of digital ulceration is unproven. Our results without sympathectomy in 100 patients with digital ulceration are as good or better than those reported with sympathectomy.[70,71] Patients with digital ulceration have obstructed digital arteries and are most likely already maximally vasodilated; thus, it appears sympathectomy is unlikely to improve blood flow. While sympathectomy is now often performed via a thoracoscopic approach, little evidence exists that sympathectomy via this approach is any more effective than sympathectomy via thoracotomy.[72]

Other treatments that have been reported for the treatment of severe Raynaud's syndrome include spinal cord simulation,[73] biofeedback,[54] and periarterial digital sympathectomy.[74] None have been shown to be effective in well-designed controlled trials.

My current recommendation for patients with severe digital ischemia and ulceration is local cleansing and debridement, with simple soap and water washing, and antibiotics as needed. Medical therapy with nifedipine or losartan is also used if tolerated but without proven benefit for ulcer healing. Resectional debridement of the ulcers is often needed, including local resection of protruding phalangeal bone tips, but major amputations to the metacarpal–phalangeal joint are rarely required. My colleagues and I no longer perform thoracic sympathectomy for digital ulceration. With this regime, our ulcer healing rates without recurrence are approximately 90%, although the time to healing is often many months. Patients who present with ulceration or gangrene during the cold months of the year, particularly in northern latitudes, may not heal until the onset of warmer weather in the spring and summer. Figure 17-5 demonstrates healing of a significant digital ulcer with this treatment regime. To date, ulcer recurrences have been limited to those patients with connective tissue disease who have ongoing digital artery damage from an associated small vessel arteriopathy. Treatment of diseases causing the small vessel arteriopathy is beyond the scope of this chapter. While controlling the associated disease does not have any curative effect on the digital arteries, the arrest or attenuation of the vasculitis associated with many of these diseases may prevent progression of digital ischemia in this patient group.

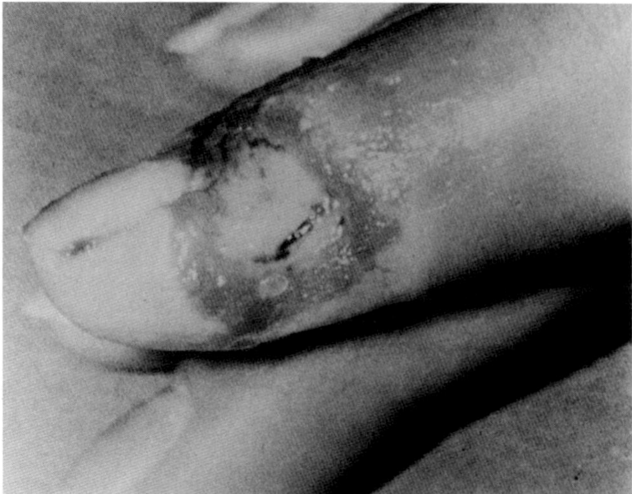

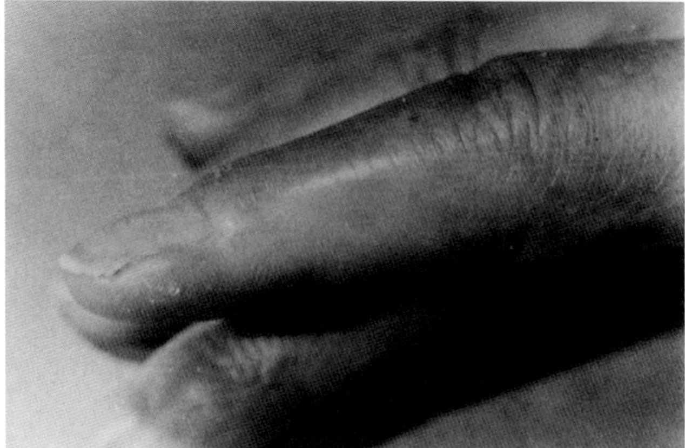

Figure 17-5. Healing of a significant digital ulcer.

PROGNOSIS

Since Allen and Brown's pivotal publications in 1932 dividing patients with Raynaud's syndrome into Raynaud's disease and Raynaud's phenomenon (based on the presence or absence of an associated disease), a great deal of interest has focused on the incidence and the subsequent development of associated diseases in patients presenting with Raynaud's syndrome.[1,2,75-77] Oregon Health and Science University has had a clinic devoted to Raynaud's syndrome patients for more than 30 years and has enrolled more than 1300 patients. All of these patients have been prospectively evaluated with several serological, radiological, and noninvasive vascular laboratory tests both to evaluate the Raynaud's syndrome and to detect the presence of an associated disease process.

In a review of this experience, patients were divided into four groups based on the presence or absence of upper extremity occlusive disease or associated systemic disease.[22] Patients without evidence of occlusive disease or an associated disease had a low incidence of progression to developing an associated disease, similar to that seen in the general population (2% in 10 years). Patients with occlusive disease without evidence of an associated disease were unlikely to develop evidence of an associated disease (8.5% in 10 years) but had a 48% risk of ulcer occurrence. Patients with an associated disease but without evidence of occlusive disease had a moderate risk of developing ulcers (15.5% at 10 years) or occlusive disease. Patients with both occlusive disease and an associated disease were the most likely to develop new or recurrent ulcers (56%). Amputation was uncommon in all groups. Curiously, patients appeared to have their most severe symptoms at the time of presentation. Only about 50% of patients presenting with digital ulceration had recurrent ulcers.

The experience with the subgroup of patients who presented with severe finger ischemia and ischemic digital ulceration has also been reviewed.[30,78] Severe digital ischemia with ulceration is limited to patients with small vessel occlusions caused by various diseases, most often the digital arteriopathy of connective tissue disease. In 100 patients with ischemic finger ulceration, 54% had a connective tissue disease, most often scleroderma, and the remainder had various other conditions, including Buerger's disease, hypersensitivity angiitis, and atherosclerosis. All patients with recurrent ulceration in the series suffered from a connective tissue disease.

SUMMARY

Raynaud's syndrome is a condition characterized by episodic digital ischemia in response to cold or emotional stress. In most patients, it is a nuisance condition that can be treated by cold and tobacco avoidance. A few patients have symptoms that require treatment with vasodilators, and an even smaller number of patients, all of whom have palmar and digital artery obstruction, have ischemic digital ulceration.

The small vessel arteriopathies are a common cause of digital arterial damage that may result in severe digital ischemia and in some cases digital ulceration. The diagnosis of the underlying disease is made based on clinical and laboratory findings. Regardless of the underlying disease process, satisfactory healing of digital ulceration from small vessel arteriopathies can be expected with conservative therapy, although recurrence can be expected in approximately 50% of patients if the underlying disease process is ongoing.

References

1. Allen E, Brown G. Raynaud's disease: a critical review of minimal requisites for diagnosis. *Am J Med Sci* 1932;83:187-200.
2. Priollet P, Vayssairat M, Housset E. How to classify Raynaud's phenomenon: long-term follow-up study of 73 cases. *Am J Med* 1987;83:494-498.
3. Weiner ES, Hildebrandt S, Senécal JL, et al. Prognostic significance of anticentromere antibodies and anti-topoisomerase I antibodies in Raynaud's disease: a prospective study. *Arthritis Rheum* 1991;34:68-77.
4. Raynaud M. *On local asphyxia and symmetrical gangrene of the extremities: in selected monographs.* London: New Sydenham Society; 1888.
5. Lewis T, Pickering G. Observations upon maladies in which the blood supply to the digits ceases intermittently or permanently and upon bilateral gangrene of the digits: observations relevant to so-called "Raynaud's disease." *Clin Sci* 1934;1:327-366.
6. de Takats G, Fowler EF. The neurogenic factor in Raynaud's phenomenon. *Surgery* 1962;51:9-18.
7. Ekenvall L, Lindblad LE. Is vibration white finger a primary sympathetic nerve injury? *Br J Ind Med* 1986;43:702-706.
8. Edwards JM, Phinney ES, Taylor LM Jr, Keenan EJ, Porter JM. α_2-Adrenergic receptor levels in obstructive and spastic Raynaud's syndrome. *J Vasc Surg* 1987;5:38-45.
9. Freedman RR, Subhash SC, Desai N, Wenig P, Mayes M. Increased α-adrenergic responsiveness in idiopathic Raynaud's disease. *Arthritis Rheum* 1989;32:61-65.
10. Brotzu G, Susanna F, Roberto M, Palmina P. Beta-blockers: a new therapeutic approach to Raynaud's disease. *Microvasc Res* 1987;33:283-288.
11. Terenghi G, Bunker CB, Liu YF, et al. Image analysis quantification of the peptide-immunoreactive nerves in the skin of patients with Raynaud's phenomenon and systemic sclerosis. *J Path* 1991;164:245-252.
12. Bunker CB, Goldsmith PC, Leslie TA, et al. Calcitonin gene-related peptide, endothelin-1, the cutaneous microvasculature and Raynaud's phenomenon. *Br J Derm* 1996;134(3):399-406.
13. Cooke JM, Marshall JM. Mechanisms of Raynaud's disease. *Vasc Med* 2005;10:293-307.
14. Cimminiello C, Milani M, Uberti T, et al. Endothelin, vasoconstriction, and endothelial damage in Raynaud's phenomenon. *Lancet* 1991;Jan 12:114-115.
15. Zamora MR, O'Brien RF, Rutherford RB, Weil JV. Serum endothelin-1 concentrations and cold provocation in primary Raynaud's phenomenon. *Lancet* 1990;Nov 10:1144-1147.
16. Freedman RR, Girgis R, Mayes MD. Abnormal responses to endothelial agonists in Raynaud's phenomenon and scleroderma. *J Rheumatol* 2001;28(1):119-121.
17. Mayes MD. Endothelin and endothelin receptor antagonists in systemic rheumatic disease. *Arthritis Rheum* 2003;48(5):1190-1199.
18. Lewis T, Landis EM. Observations upon the vascular mechanism in acrocyanosis. *Heart* 1930;15:229-246.
19. de Trafford JC, Roberts VC. Thermal entrainment. In: Cooke E, Nicolaides A, Porter J, eds. *Raynaud's syndrome.* London: Med-Orion Publishing; 1991:111-123.
20. Hladunewich M, Sawka C, Fam A, Franssen E. Raynaud's phenomenon and digital gangrene as a consequence of treatment for Kaposi's sarcoma. *J Rheumatol* 1997;24(12):2371-2375.
21. Johnson SR, Feldman BM, Hawker GA. Classification criteria for systemic sclerosis subsets. *J Rheumatol* 2007;34(9):1855-1863.
22. Landry GJ, Edwards JM, McLafferty RB, et al. Long-term outcome of Raynaud's syndrome in a prospectively analyzed patient cohort. *J Vasc Surg* 1996;23:76-86.
23. Kahaleh MB, Sherer GK, Leroy ED. Endothelial injury in scleroderma. *J Exp Med* 1979;149:1326-1335.
24. Silveri F, De Angelis R, Poggi A, et al. Relative roles of endothelial cell damage and platelet activation in primary Raynaud's phenomenon (RP) and RP secondary to systemic sclerosis. *Scand J Rheumatol* 2001;30(5):290-296.
25. Mariq HR, Spencer-Green G, Leroy EC. Skin capillary abnormalities as indicators of organ involvement in scleroderma (systemic sclerosis), Raynaud's syndrome and dermatomyositis. *Am J Med* 1976;61: 862-870.
26. Fleischmajer R, Perlish JS, Shaw KV, et al. Skin capillary changes in early systemic sclerosis. *Arch Dermatol* 1976;112:1553-1557.
27. Grishman E, Spiera H. Vasculitis in connective tissue disease, including hypocomplementemic vasculitis. In: Churg A, Churg J, eds. *Systemic vasculitides.* Igaku-Shoin: New York; 1991:273-292.
28. Gordon C, Salmon M. Update on systemic lupus erythematosus: autoantibodies and apoptosis. *Clin Med* 2001;1(1):10-14.
29. Tan EM, Cohen AS, Fries JF, et al. The 1982 revised criteria for the classification of systemic lupus erythematosus. *Arthritis Rheum* 1982;25: 1271-1277.
30. Mills JL, Friedman EI, Taylor LM Jr, Porter JM. Upper extremity ischemia caused by small artery disease. *Ann Surg* 1987;206:521-528.
31. Ragan C, Farrington E. The clinical features of rheumatoid arthritis. *JAMA* 1967;181:663-667.
32. Panush RS, Katz P, Longlry S, et al. Rheumatoid vasculitis: survival and associated risk factors. *Medicine* 1986;65:365-375.
33. Bywaters EGL. Peripheral vascular obstruction in rheumatoid arthritis and its relationship to other vascular disorders. *Ann Rheum Dis* 1957;16:84-103.
34. Talal N. Sjögren's syndrome and connective tissue diseases associated with other immunologic disorders. In: McCarty DJ, ed. *Arthritis and allied conditions.* 11th ed. William and Wilkins; Philadelphia. 1987:1197-1213.

35. Tsokos M, Lazarou SA, Moutsopoulos HM. Vasculitis in Sjögren's syndrome: histologic classification and clinical presentation. *Am J Clin Pathol* 1987;88:26-31.
36. Alarcon GS, Williams GV, Singer JZ, et al. Early undifferentiated connective tissue disease. I. Early clinical manifestation in a large cohort of patients with undifferentiated connective tissue diseases compared to cohorts of well established connective tissue disease. *J Rheumatol* 1991;18:1332-1339.
37. Sharp GC, Irwin WS, Tan ES, et al. Mixed connective tissue disease: an apparently distinct rheumatic disease syndrome associated with a specific antibody to an extractable nuclear antigen (ENA). *Am J Med* 1972;52: 149-159.
38. Mills JL, Porter JM. Buerger's disease (thromboangiitis obliterans). *Ann Vasc Surg* 1992;5:570-572.
39. Puechal X, Fiessinger JN. Thromboangiitis obliterans or Buerger's disease: challenges for the rheumatologist. *Rheumatology* 2007;46(2): 192-199.
40. Mills JL, Taylor LM Jr, Porter JM. Buerger's disease in the modern era. *Am J Surg* 1987;154:123-129.
41. Schneider HJ, Jha S, Burnand KG. Progressive arteritis associated with cannabis use. *Eur J Vasc Endovasc Surg* 1999;18(4):366-367.
42. Shionoya S, Ban I, Nakata Y, et al. Diagnosis, pathology, and treatment of Buerger's disease. *Surgery* 1974;75:695-700.
43. Loriga G. Pneumatic tools: occupation and health. *Boll Inspett Lav* 1911;2:35.
44. Hamilton A. A study of spastic anemia in the hands of stonecutters: effect of the air hammer on the hands of the stonecutters. *US Bureau Labor Stat Bull* 1918;236:53-66.
45. McLafferty RB, Edwards JM, Ferris BL, et al. Raynaud's syndrome in workers who use vibrating pneumatic air knives. *J Vasc Surg* 1999;30: 1-7.
46. Schatz IJ. Occlusive disease on the hand due to occupational trauma. *N Engl J Med* 1963;268:281-284.
47. Cherniack M, Brammer AJ, Lundstrom R, et al. The Hand–Arm Vibration International Consortium (HAVIC): prospective studies on the relationship between power tool exposure and health effects. *J Occup Environ Med* 2007;49:289-301.
48. Baur GM, Porter JM, Bardana EJ Jr, et al. Rapid onset of hand ischemia of unknown etiology. *Ann Surg* 1977;186:184-189.
49. Edwards JM, Antonius JI, Porter JM. Critical hand ischemia caused by forearm fibromuscular dysplasia. *J Vasc Surg* 1985;2:459-463.
50. Ferris BL, Taylor LM Jr, Oyama K, et al. Hypothenar hammer syndrome: proposed etiology. *J Vasc Surg* 2000;31:104-113.
51. Friedman SA, Bienenstock H, Richter IH. Malignancy and arteriopathy. *Angiology* 1969;20:136-143.
52. Vayssairat M, Fiessinger JN, Bordet F, Housset E. Rapports entre necroses digitales du membre superieur et affections malignes. *Nouv Presse Med* 1978;7:1279-1282.
53. Taylor LM Jr, Hauty MG, Edwards JM, Porter JM. Digital ischemia as a manifestation of malignancy. *Ann Surg* 1987;206:62-68.
54. Nielsen SL, Lassen NA. Measurement of digital blood pressure after local cooling. *J Appl Physiol* 1977;43:907-910.
55. Gates KH, Tyburczy JA, Zupan T, et al. The noninvasive quantification of digital vasospasm. *Bruit* 1984;8:34-37.
56. Pucinelli MLC, Fontenelle SMA, Andrade LEC. Determination of fingertip lacticemy before and after cold stimulus in patients with primary Raynaud's phenomenon and systemic sclerosis. *J Rheumatol* 2002;29:1401-1403.
57. Fontenelle SMA, Kayser C, Pucinelli MLC, Andrade LEC. Cold stimulus fingertip lacticemy test: an effective method to monitor acute therapeutic intervention on primary Raynaud's phenomenon and systemic sclerosis. *Rheumatology* 2008;47:80-83.
58. Sumner DS, Strandness DE Jr. An abnormal finger pulse associated with cold sensitivity. *Ann Surg* 1972;175:294.
59. Walcher J, Strecker R, Goldacker S, et al. High resolution 3 Tesla contrast-enhanced MR angiography of the hands in Raynaud's disease. *Clin Rhematol* 2007;26:587-589.
60. Kiowski W, Erne P, Buhler FR. Use of nifedipine in hypertension and Raynaud's phenomenon. *Cardiovasc Drug Ther* 1994;5(Suppl):935-940.
61. Anonymous. Comparison of sustained-release nifedipine and temperature biofeedback for treatment of primary Raynaud phenomenon: results from a randomized clinical trial with 1-year follow-up. *Arch Int Med* 2000;160(8):1101-1108.
62. Dziadzio M, Denton CP, Smith R, et al. Losartan therapy for Raynaud's phenomenon and scleroderma: clinical and biochemical findings in a fifteen-week, randomized, parallel-group, controlled trial. *Arthritis Rheum* 1999;42(12):2646-2655.
63. Wood HM, Ernst ME. Renin–angiotensin system mediators and Raynaud's phenomenon. *Ann Pharmacother* 2006(40):1998-2002.
64. Coleiro B, Marshall SE, Denton CP, et al. Treatment of Raynaud's phenomenon with the selective serotonin reuptake inhibitor fluoxetine. *Rheumatology* 2001;40(9):1038-1043.
65. Harding SE, Tingey PC, Pope J, Fenlon D, Furst D, Shea B, Silman A, Thompson A, Wells GA. Prazosin for Raynaud's phenomenon in progressive systemic sclerosis. *Cochrane Database of Systematic Reviews* 1998, Issue 2. Art. No.: CD000956. DOI: 10.1002/14651858.CD000956.
66. Fries R, Shariat K, von Wilmowsky H, Bohm M. Sildenafil in the treatment of Raynaud's phenomenon resistant to vasodilatory therapy. *Circulation* 2005;112:2980-2985.
67. Rajagopalan S, Pfenninger D, Somers E, et al. Effects of cilostazol in patients with Raynaud's syndrome. *Am J Cardiol* 2003;92(11): 1310-1315.
68. Aikimbaev KS, Oguz M, Ozbek S, et al. Comparative assessment of the effects of vasodilators on peripheral vascular reactivity in patients with systemic scleroderma and Raynaud's phenomenon: color Doppler flow imaging study. *Angiology* 1996;47(5):475-480.
69. Hettema ME, Zhang D, Bootsma H, Kallenberg CG. Bosentan therapy for patients with severe Raynaud's phenomenon in systemic sclerosis. *Ann Rheum Dis* 2007;66:1398-1399.
70. Machleder HI, Wheeler E, Barber WF. Treatment of upper extremity ischemia by cervico-dorsal sympathectomy. *Vasc Surg* 1979;13:399-404.
71. Dale WA. Occlusive arterial lesions of the wrist and hand. *J Tenn Med Assoc* 1964;57:402-406.
72. Maga P, Kuzdzal J, Nizankowski R, et al. Long-term effects of thoracic sympathectomy on microcirculation in the hands of patients with primary Raynaud disease. *J Thor Cardiovasc Surg* 2007;133(6):1428-1433.
73. Neuhauser B, Perkmann R, Klingler PJ, et al. Clinical and objective data on spinal cord stimulation for the treatment of severe Raynaud's phenomenon. *Am Surg* 2001;67(11):1096-1097.
74. McCall TE, Petersen DP, Wong LB. The use of digital artery sympathectomy as a salvage procedure for severe ischemia of Raynaud's disease and phenomenon. *J Hand Surg Am* 1999;24:173-177.
75. Harper F, Mariq H, Turner R, et al. A prospective study of Raynaud phenomenon and early connective tissue disease. *Am J Med* 1982;72: 883-888.
76. Kallenberg C, Wouda A, The T. Systemic involvement and immunologic findings in patients presenting with Raynaud's phenomenon. *Am J Med* 1980;69:675-680.
77. Velayos E, Roginson H, Porciuncula F, Masi A. Clinical correlation analysis of 137 patients with Raynaud's phenomenon. *Am J Med Sci* 1970;262:347-356.
78. McLafferty RB, Edwards JM, Taylor LM Jr, Porter JM. Diagnosis and long-term clinical outcome in patients diagnosed with hand ischemia. *J Vasc Surg* 1995;22:361-369.

chapter

18

Thoracic Outlet Syndrome

David Rigberg, MD • Julie Freischlag, MD

Key Points

- The thoracic outlet is a limited space through which numerous important structures must traverse (subclavian artery and vein and brachial plexus).
- The form of thoracic outlet syndrome (TOS) depends on the structure compressed: nerve (neurogenic), venous (axillosubclavian thrombosis), or arterial.
- Neurogenic is the most common form, and it generates considerable controversy regarding both its diagnosis and its treatment.
- Usually, excision of the first rib decompresses the thoracic outlet, regardless of the form of TOS.
- The presentation of the vascular forms can be dramatic. Neurogenic TOS presents with pain and paresthesias that can be a diagnostic challenge.
- History and physical examination are the cornerstones of diagnosis. Ancillary testing is helpful mostly for excluding other conditions.
- Arteriography and venography play important roles in the arterial and venous forms.
- Treatment is conservative for most patients (physical therapy), but a significant number have symptoms that persist. Surgical decompression is warranted in these cases.
- Both the transaxillary and the supraclavicular approaches to first-rib excision are used, and each approach has benefits and limitations.
- Well-performed clinical outcomes studies are needed to objectively assess the results of first-rib resection in these patients.

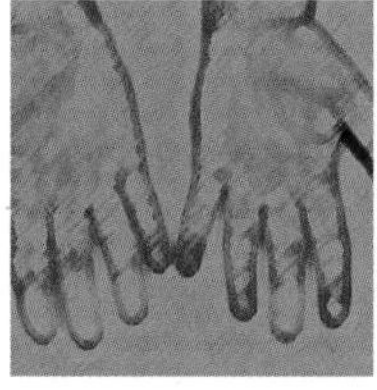

Thoracic outlet syndrome (TOS) describes a spectrum of symptoms and signs related to the passage of key anatomical structures through a narrow aperture on their way to the distal upper extremity. This syndrome is manifest in three main forms based on the tissues damaged: neurogenic, venous, and arterial. Considerable controversy surrounds the diagnosis, and some would even argue the existence of the most common, neurogenic form. The objective findings in the other two variants preclude this discussion. Nonetheless, a large patient population continues to present with the constellation of symptoms, and the vascular surgeon should be able to recognize and treat the various forms of this disorder.

Several early anatomists, most notably Galen described the presence of cervical ribs, and this structure was considered the key etiological agent as physicians first gained an appreciation for compressive symptoms of the thoracic outlet. In 1821, Sir Astley Cooper related this structure to the development of ischemic fingers secondary to subclavian artery compression. Twenty years later, Gruber published what is still considered the definitive classification of cervical ribs. In 1861, Coote demonstrated the development of a subclavian artery aneurysm in a patient with a cervical rib. He then went on to resect the rib via a supraclavicular approach. Both Mayo and Halsted published on subclavian aneurysms related to TOS, with Mayo describing a first-rib exostosis as the cause. Mention should be made at this point of the work of Paget and Schroetter who, in 1875, simultaneously published their findings of axillosubclavian venous thrombosis in what has become known as the Paget-Schroetter syndrome.

By the early twentieth century, physicians were looking to the cervical rib not only as a cause of vascular conditions but for neurogenic symptoms as well. Keene in 1907 presented his series of TOS patients, most of whom had neurogenic complaints. About the same time, however, Branwell published descriptions of TOS patients who had neither cervical ribs nor any identifiable first-rib anomalies. As early as 1910, Murphy was performing excision of normal first ribs

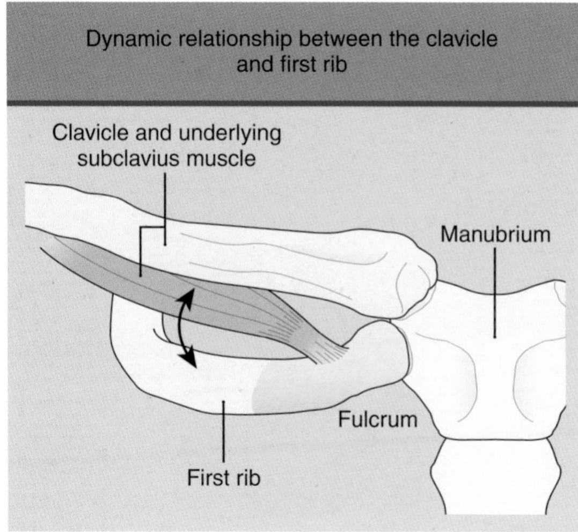

Figure 18-1. Dynamic relationship between the clavicle and the first rib. Note the potential for impingement of structures with movement of the arm.

for what had become known as cervical rib syndrome. Law's descriptions of ligamentous attachments to cervical rib, followed by Adson and Coffey's publications in 1927 on dividing the anterior scalene muscle, helped shift the focus off the cervical rib. The scalenus anticus syndrome, described in the late 1930s by both Naffziger and DeBakey, was treated for a time by scalenectomy. This operation, which involved dividing the muscle in the neck, did not prove to be particularly effective and even when successful had a high rate of recurrence.

In the early 1950s, following work by Telford and Stopford describing the bony confines provided by the normal first rib, attention had shifted so that compression between the clavicle and the first rib was considered the culprit. This was termed the costoclavicular syndrome and led briefly to the use of claviculectomy, described by Rosati and Lord, as the treatment of choice. Because it is disfiguring, the operation was usually performed bilaterally to maintain symmetry. It was not particularly effective and soon fell out of favor.

The major shift to the modern conception of TOS occurred in 1956 with Peet et al.'s coining of the term TOS and his description of a therapeutic exercise program, essentially the first physical therapy for TOS.[1] The term was used again by Standeven and Rob 2 years later and encompassed all previous "anatomical" names used for this set of symptoms. This also coincided with the therapeutic focus shifting to the first rib, and in 1962 Clagett presented his high thoracoplasty for first-rib resection, an operation requiring the division of the trapezius and rhomboid muscles.[2] Roos in 1966 described what has become for many the modern treatment of choice for TOS, the transaxillary first-rib resection.[3] This operation was fashioned after the transaxillary sympathectomy, and first-rib resection by this route offered reasonable exposure and minimal morbidity, especially when compared to previously employed techniques. Gol's infraclavicular approach was described a year later but required a large, cosmetically displeasing scar and was often a difficult exposure. This operation never gained widespread use.

ANATOMY

The limited space and numerous important structures that must traverse the neck and chest areas on their way to the upper arm make the thoracic outlet an area like no other in the body. Although any number of anatomical anomalies can predispose a patient to or directly cause compression to the neural, venous, or arterial structures within its confines, the normal anatomy itself leaves little room for stress positioning.

Definitions may vary from author to author, but it is generally accepted that the thoracic outlet is the area from the edge of the first rib extending medially to the upper mediastinum and superiorly to the fifth cervical nerve. The clavicle and subclavius muscles can be pictured as forming a roof, while the superior surface of the first rib forms the floor. Machleder's description of the thoracic outlet as a triangle with its apex pointed toward the manubrium is helpful in visualizing the three-dimensional orientation of the structures, as well as the dynamic changes that can lead to injury.[4] In this model, the clavicle and its underlying subclavius muscle and tendon form the superior limb, while the base is the first thoracic rib. The point at which these two structures "overlap" medially can be pictured as the fulcrum of a pair of scissors that open and closes as the arm moves, potentially causing compression of the thoracic outlet contents (Figure 18-1).

Although most TOS symptoms are related to nerve compression, almost any structure that travels through the thoracic outlet can be involved (Figure 18-2). Moving medially to laterally, the clinician first encounters the exiting of the subclavian vein, usually positioned adjacent to the region where the first rib and clavicular head fuse to form a fibrocartilaginous joint with the manubrium. Immediately lateral to the vein is the anterior scalene muscle, which inserts onto a prominence on the first rib. Lateral to this site is the subclavian artery so that the anterior scalene muscle lies between the subclavian artery and the vein, with the artery deep, lateral, and somewhat cephalad. The brachial plexus is the next structure encountered. The C4 to C6 roots are superiorly oriented, and the C7 to T1 roots inferior. As shall

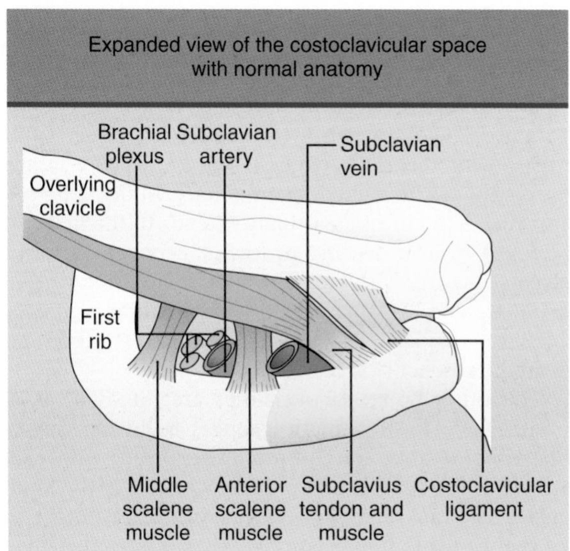

Figure 18-2. Expanded view of the costoclavicular space with normal anatomy.

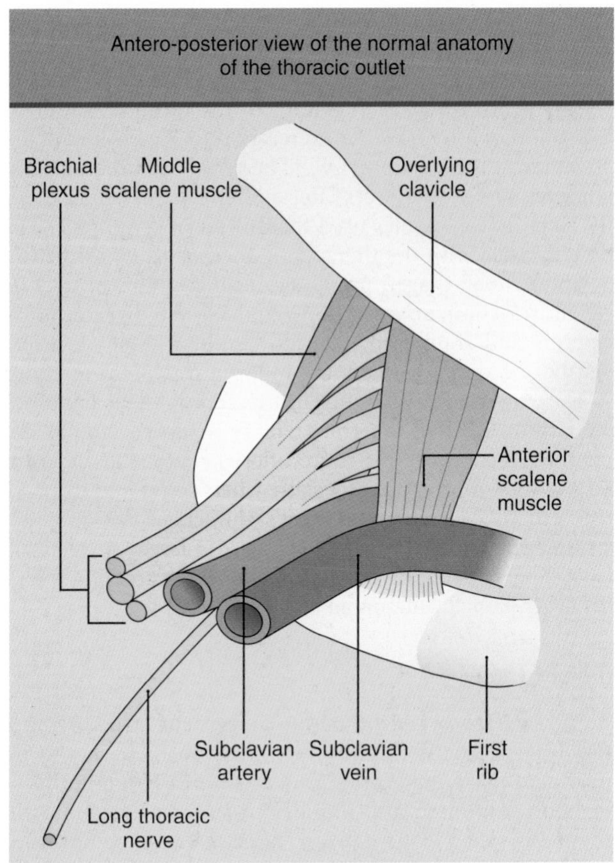

Figure 18-3. Anteroposterior view of the normal anatomy of the thoracic outlet. Note the course of the long thoracic nerve and the potential for injury to the nerve during operations in this area.

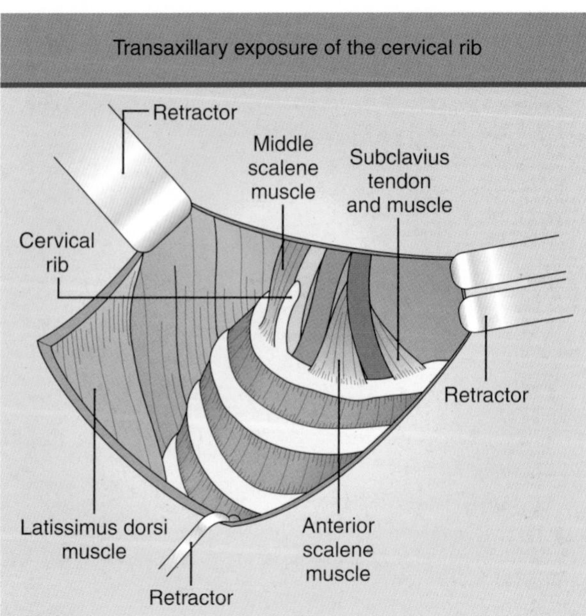

Figure 18-4. Transaxillary exposure of the cervical rib. Note the impingement on the brachial plexus, as well as the cervical rib's origin from the first rib. The middle scalene muscle is displaced laterally and is intimately associated with the cervical rib.

be seen, this arrangement has important implications for the symptom constellation in neurogenic TOS. Posterior and lateral to the plexus, generally a rather broad attachment of the middle scalene to the first rib is found. This is an area of particular importance during operative decompression of the thoracic outlet, for here the long thoracic nerve can be inadvertently injured as it travels to the serratus anterior muscle (Figure 18-3).

Other structures encountered in the thoracic outlet include the phrenic and dorsal scapular nerves, the stellate ganglion, the thoracic duct, and the cupola of the lung. The phrenic nerve lies between the prescalene fat pad and the anterior scalene muscle. Compression of this structure does not generally occur, but it can be injured during supraclavicular approaches and must be left intact while the underlying scalene muscle is dissected. The dorsal scapular nerve comes off the brachial plexus on its way to innervate the medially inserting muscles of the scapula (rhomboids and levator scapulae). It is usually neither involved nor encountered. The stellate ganglion is found along the sympathetic chain. This structure can be involved in compression, and occasionally a cervicothoracic sympathectomy is part of the treatment plan for TOS. The thoracic duct may be encountered if a left supraclavicular approach is undertaken, and care must be taken not to injure it or to ligate it if injury occurs. Finally, the clinician must watch for pleural injury in any approach to TOS and be prepared to evacuate pneumothoraces when indicated.

PATHOPHYSIOLOGY

Once the normal anatomy of the thoracic outlet is appreciated, it becomes clear that any structure that intrudes into or limits the flexibility of this region predisposes the nerves, arterial structures, and venous structures to compression. Although specific anatomical configurations favor the development of each form of TOS, they are not entirely specific, and considerable overlap can occur. In addition to the obvious gross consequences of injury to the contents of the thoracic outlet, histological and biochemical changes are observed in the involved tissues. These stress the uniqueness of the outlet's configuration and offer objective support to the chronicity of many of these injuries.

The cervical rib is the most obvious bony abnormality contributing to TOS, and autopsy studies indicate that roughly 0.5% of the population have this structure (Figures 18-4 and 18-5).[5] Series from the United States generally report 10% of TOS patients with cervical ribs, although others have reported up to 65%. The European literature reports closer to 25%. The reason for this discrepancy is not known. Cervical ribs can be completely formed or rudimentary. In the latter case, a compressive band of tissue usually extends to the first rib. As they project from transverse processes, cervical ribs displace involved structures forward. The subclavian artery is particularly vulnerable to damage in this configuration, and some authors feel that arterial changes secondary to TOS rarely occur in the absence of a cervical rib.

Several other bony abnormalities are found in association with TOS. Posttraumatic changes following clavicular or first-rib fractures are commonly reported, with callous formation at the clavicle and pseudoarthroses of the first rib. Elongated C7 transverse processes are also occasionally seen. These changes can often be appreciated radiographically.

Most TOS cases are associated with some form of soft-tissue anomaly. Work by Juvonen, Raymond and others led to

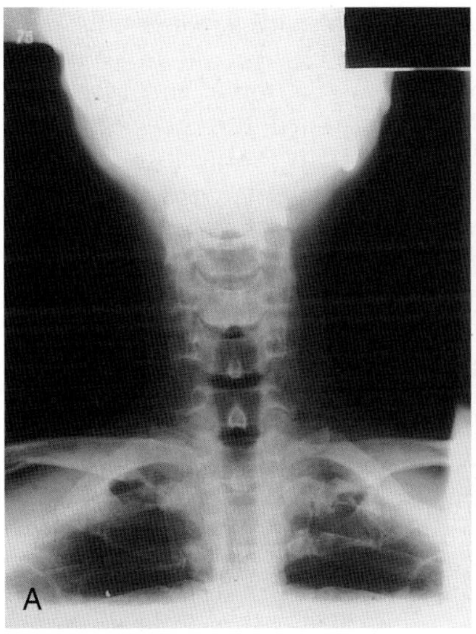

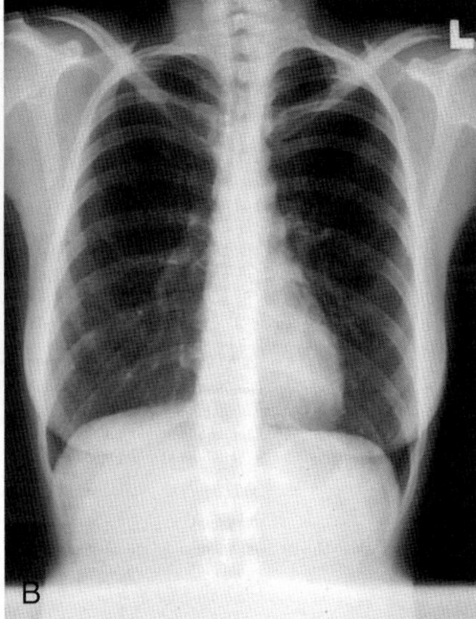

Figure 18-5. Bilateral cervical ribs in a patient with symptoms of neurogenic thoracic outlet syndrome in neutral position **(A)** and with arms partially abducted **(B).**

Table 18-1
Roos Classification System of Anatomical Variations in Anatomical Pathology of Thoracic Outlet Syndrome

Type I	Incomplete cervical rib; band beneath T1 root attached to first rib
Type II	Abortive cervical rib with band to first rib
Type III	Accessory muscle between neck and tubercle of first rib; separates T1 nerve and the subclavian artery
Type IV	Large middle scalene compressing T1 nerve root; pins nerve to the vertebral body (ulnar symptoms)
Type V	Scalenus minimus muscle attaching to the first rib behind the scalene tubercle
Type VI	Scalenus minimus muscle attaching to the endothoracic fascia covering the cupola of lung
Type VII	Band extending from the middle scalene to the costal cartilage or sternum
Type VIII	Band from middle scalene under the subclavian vein; associated with Paget-Schroetter syndrome
Type IX	Web filling the inner curve of the first rib
Type X	Double band from cervical rib attaching to the cupola with a band to the costocartilage or sternum

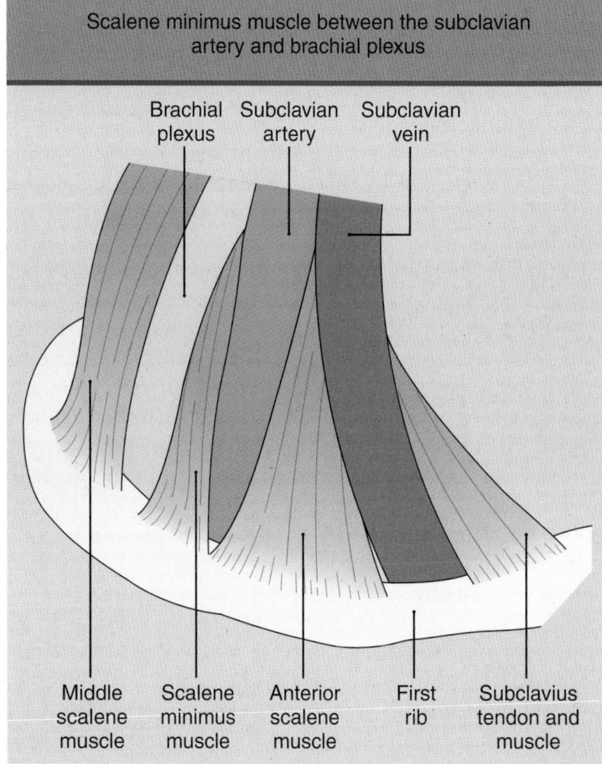

Figure 18-6. Scalene minimus muscle between the subclavian artery and the brachial plexus. This is a type V Roos deformity.

appreciation of the multiple forms occurring. However, the classification system of Roos is the most thorough, with 10 distinct anomalies with several subtypes observed intraoperatively[6] (Table 18-1 and Figure 18-6).

As would be expected, these anomalies often occur in association with one another and do not tend to be symmetrical. Several other muscular anomalies exist, mostly involving thickened muscle branches encompassing nerves, for example, slips of anterior scalene between the C5 and the C7 nerve roots or even a bulky muscle anteriorly displacing the nerves. Reports have been made of these muscle fibers becoming incorporated into the epineurium of these nerves as well. One particularly interesting configuration is when a fibrous band stretches over the proximal C5 nerve. Muscular spasm of the neck and shoulder can then lead to direct compression, with upper cord symptoms.

In addition to these anatomical arrangements, hypertrophy of the normal musculature or tendons has been implicated in TOS. For example, some authors report a link between Paget-Schroetter syndrome and subclavius tendon hypertrophy, particularly in the presence of an enlarged insertion tubercle (Figure 18-7). Others have implicated a role for the pectoralis minor muscle. Another scenario is the weight lifter,

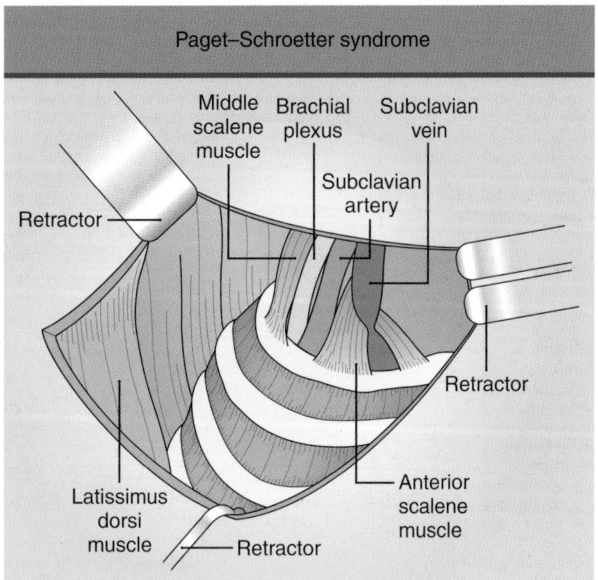

Figure 18-7. Paget-Schroetter syndrome. Transaxillary exposure of the thoracic outlet demonstrating a subclavian vein compressed by subclavius and anterior scalene muscles. These are originating from first-rib exostosis. This is one of several configurations that can be associated with Paget-Schroetter syndrome.

often a young man, with hypertrophied scalene musculature. Anatomical studies have documented the compression of the subclavian vein by this muscle into the costoclavicular notch. This has clear implications for axillosubclavian vein thrombosis.

Trauma is generally implicated in the pathogenesis of neurogenic TOS, particularly localized to the neck and shoulder. Hyperextension, or whiplash injuries, occurs in this patient population with some frequency. Neurogenic TOS can also be seen with repetitive motion–type injuries. In Sanders et al.'s review of operative TOS patients, 86% had a history of trauma.[7] This is considerably higher than many other reports, but it stresses the role that trauma can play in the disorder. Chronic trauma, such as that associated with poor posture, has also been implicated. This is termed the pectoralis minor syndrome, and the symptoms can be reproduced with an external compression of the pectoralis musculature.[8]

In a large series of patients, Machleder determined the etiology for operative cases of TOS when approached via a transaxillary incision.[9] Interestingly, no anatomical defect was visualized in 34%. This stands in contrast to other studies in which defects were almost always found. Cervical ribs were found in 8.5%, 10% had a scalenus minimus muscle, 19.5% had a defect in the subclavius tendon or its insertion, 43% had a developmental or insertional defect in the scalene musculature, and 7.5% had anatomical configurations whose developmental history was unclear.

As mentioned previously, histological and biochemical changes in the tissues are involved with TOS. Work by Sanders et al.[10] demonstrated inflammation surrounding compressed nerve trunks. This inflammation could cause direct irritation of the nerve trunks or set up a perineural inflammatory process leading to vasospasm in the vasa nervorum. Histological changes in both the mesoneurium and the endoneurium of involved nerves have been described, and the local formation of edema and adhesions is often observed.

On the molecular level, several reports have noted the transition from type 2 to type 1 muscle fibers in TOS. Sanders and others have published on this topic, and Machleder et al.'s studies clearly demonstrated this phenomenon.[11] Briefly, most skeletal muscle fibers are the quick-reacting type 2 fibers that have reactivity with phosphorylase and myosin ATPase. The slower, type 1 fibers have an increased oxidative capacity and a pronounced, slow, tonic, contractile pattern. Immunohistochemical analysis shows greater numbers of type 1 fibers in the anterior scalene muscle of TOS patients than in any other kind of tissue. The signaling required for this transition is not completely understood, but it does provide a molecular backdrop to the gross changes seen in TOS. Recent studies of TOS and bone mineral density have failed to show a difference between such measurements in the forearm in TOS patients and those in controls.[12]

PRESENTATION

Neurogenic TOS

Patients can present with the symptoms of neurogenic TOS at any age, although the usual case is a young to middle-aged adult with no other major health issues. When confronted by the pediatric or younger teenage patient with purely neurogenic symptoms, most authors recommend a period of waiting to see whether growth allows the symptoms to abate. Recent data from our institution suggest that earlier intervention may be appropriate in selected adolescents.[13] Eighteen such patients underwent treatment (age range from 13 to 19), with all eventually returning to their full preoperative activities. However, the need for reintervention was notably higher than in adult patients.[13] Care must be taken when evaluating extremely young patients, as the presentation may be unusual, including reports of cervical rib fractures causing symptoms.[14]

The neurogenic symptoms generally can range in severity from nuisance to severely debilitating pain. Motor effects are seen, and although gross dysfunction of the upper extremity is unusual, a degree of weakness is not. This occasionally manifests as a decrease in grip strength. Gilliat et al.'s description of classic neurogenic TOS with muscle wasting in the hand is not common.[15]

The pain may originate anywhere in the upper extremity, but the most common site is the back of the shoulder. The suprascapular portion of the trapezius may be involved. From the shoulder, pain can spread up the ipsilateral extremity, along the back and neck, or even up the face. This situation can lead to hemicranial headaches that can be labeled migraines.

Pain involving the arm can be focused to a particular nerve distribution or generalized. When localized, ulnar symptoms tend to be the most common, leading to difficulties with the ring and small fingers. Many authors report that these "lower plexus" (C8 to T1) symptoms are more common than "upper" (C5 to C7) manifestations.

Patients may report pain at rest that is not relieved by positioning. However, the typical patient reports that stress positioning exacerbates symptoms. This is particularly the case with work-related situations. People who must perform tasks with elevated arms or hold their arms in other awkward positions note they are no longer able to perform these tasks. Examples include waitresses, mechanics, and truck drivers. With prolonged stress positioning, patients may report finger discoloration, coolness of the extremity, or even swelling.

Driving an automobile can be difficult, with the concomitant numbness and tingling in the fingers.

Patients often report that their symptom complex started following a traumatic event. These can be chronic, repetitive-type injuries such as seen with pitchers and other athletes. Direct injury to the chest wall or shoulder can also precipitate symptoms, particularly if associated with a clavicular fracture or an acromioclavicular joint dislocation. Whiplash-type injuries are also associated with TOS. Even a relatively minor injury can "unmask" the syndrome in a previously asymptomatic individual.

Given all of these symptoms, a review of several series reveals that the most common finding is some form of paresthesia, which occurs in more than 90% of patients. This is followed by upper limb pain, which is reported almost as often. The incidence of suprascapular pain is roughly 80%. Headache complaints vary widely in reported series, although some studies report them in as many as 65% of patients.[16]

Two unusual presenting symptoms should be mentioned. First, ipsilateral hyperhidrosis can occur, and the proximity of the sympathetic chain to the other involved structures explains this phenomenon. The hyperhidrosis of TOS always occurs in association with other complaints.

Second, a pseudo-angina has been described in which TOS presents with symptoms consistent with coronary artery disease.[17] Interestingly, many of these patients do not have the usual upper extremity symptoms with their initial presentation, leading to delay in diagnosis. The more common symptoms often occur as time goes by, leading to the correct diagnosis.

Paget-Schroetter Syndrome

Paget-Schroetter syndrome (axillosubclavian vein thrombosis or "effort" thrombosis) usually presents suddenly in a previously healthy patient with no symptoms of neurogenic TOS. Typically, the patient is a young athlete or worker with a component to the sport or job that requires prolonged or repetitive stressful positioning of the arm. Examples include baseball players, swimmers, weight lifters, volleyball players, and mechanics. This presentation is dramatic compared to neurogenic TOS, and patients usually seek medical attention immediately.

The involved extremity often has a degree of discoloration, from rubor to cyanosis. The redness may be confused with the erythema of an infection, leading to a delay in diagnosis. Physical examination may reveal the presence of dilated collateral veins around the shoulder and upper arm. The remainder of the physical examination is normal at this point.

If the condition is left untreated, the swelling will resolve over the course of days or weeks. Patients will note that they return to their normal state at rest but that they are unable to use their arm for any period, particularly in a stressed (abducted, externally rotated) position. The collateral channels that develop and allow the swelling to abate are rarely adequate to accommodate the increased venous return that occurs with activity.

An alternate presentation is in association with an acute traumatic injury. Typically, the patient has an injury to the shoulder area. After a few days pass, some degree of ipsilateral arm swelling occurs. The natural history of these two variants is the same, reflecting that the injury most likely contributed to compression in the thoracic outlet so that the thrombosis associated with injury is really the same insult seen in "spontaneous" thrombosis.

As mentioned previously, symptoms of neurogenic TOS are not usually associated with Paget-Schroetter syndrome. Although not common, ipsilateral sympathetic hyperactivity is not rare in this setting.

Arterial Complications

Because subclavian artery compression can lead to several injuries, its presentation is the most varied of the three forms of TOS. Damage to the subclavian artery itself can lead to anywhere from a small stenosis to aneurysm formation or complete occlusion. Each of these can then have its own sequelae secondary to embolization or thrombosis or the extremely rare rupture of a subclavian aneurysm.

Patients are commonly misdiagnosed with collagen vascular disease because of the cold sensitivity, Raynaud's phenomena, and other symptoms. These patients may go on to have frank ischemic conditions of the hands, with paronychial ulcers or fingertip gangrene. If the subclavian artery is completely occluded, patients may present with early fatigue of the involved side. This can be in the form of crampy pain with exercise and has led to the term arm claudication.

As with Paget-Schroetter syndrome, arterial TOS is not usually accompanied by symptoms of the neurogenic form. This probably contributes to the difficulty in making this diagnosis.

DIAGNOSIS

It is important to point out from the outset that no generally accepted battery of tests must be performed to confirm the presence of TOS. Most surgeons routinely dealing with the disorder require at a minimum a physical examination consistent with the symptoms, cervical films to rule out disc disease, and a chest radiograph to visualize any bony abnormalities. Various other tests may be applied in different clinical situations or when the diagnosis is not clear. Different specialists also can have differing approaches to the diagnosis, and the need for invasive or expensive tests is an area of considerable debate.

History and Physical Examination

An extensive history should be taken from the patient, including any injuries and the patient's occupation. Activities that worsen and improve the discomfort or other symptoms should be ascertained. In conjunction with a good history, most cases of TOS are diagnosed on the basis of physical examination. In addition, the physical examination plays an important role in ruling out other causes of a patient's symptoms. A thorough examination should focus not only on the site of complaints but also on other areas commonly involved in neurological conditions. This includes the general appearance of the patient and other signs of symptom impact. Note should be made of symmetry of the muscle groups of the shoulders and upper extremities. Serratus anterior atrophy is occasionally present with TOS, as demonstrated by a winged scapula. Although cervical symptoms are common with TOS, limited cervical range of motion is not and should not be excessive tenderness over the vertebral bodies. The presence of either of these suggests an alternate diagnosis. Deep-tendon reflexes, grip strength, and pulses should be routinely assessed. Palmar hyperhidrosis should be noted if present. Machleder points out that, even in neurogenic TOS, changes in pulses can sometimes be readily detected. Specific provocative neurological maneuvers, such as downward compression of the head to rule out cervical disc disease, can be used when necessary. After this general neurological assessment, tests more specific for the presence of thoracic outlet compression can be undertaken.

Patients with TOS generally do not have obvious muscle atrophy; rather, they have nearly normal gross baseline sensory and motor exams. However, useful information can still be obtained if the clinician uses an organized approach. Initial palpation of the structures of the chest wall, cervical area, and shoulder can be useful before undertaking provocative testing. The region overlying the anterior scalene muscle is often exquisitely tender in the face of brachial plexus entrapment or irritation. In addition, percussion of the clavicle can reproduce pains and paresthesias in TOS patients. These simple maneuvers should be performed before more complex maneuvering of the patient, which may cloud later findings.

The most used TOS test is probably the elevated arm stress test (EAST), which was originally described by Roos and Owens in 1966 as a means for eliciting upper extremity claudication and neurological symptoms.[18] In the test, patients are asked to completely elevate the shoulders and arms (hold-up position) and then to repeatedly clench and unclench their hands (Figure 18-8). This positioning is designed to constrict the costoclavicular space and by many reports will bring on weakness and paresthesias in the ulnar and median nerve distributions in patients with TOS within 3 minutes. Its proponents argue that it is specific for TOS and that the time of onset of symptoms correlates with the severity of TOS. In addition, it is felt by many that the test is good for reproducing the symptoms that patients suffer while using their upper extremities at work. Attention should also be made to the color of the hands during the EAST, as one may become pale and ischemic if arterial compromise in involved.

This test is not without its detractors. Although anecdotally reported to have excellent specificity, a study from 1985 found a positive test in more than 80% of patients with carpal tunnel syndrome,[19] and an earlier study by this same group found a positive EAST is almost all healthy patients, although the researchers did note that the positive tests occurred earlier in patients with TOS. In addition, some question the anatomical basis for the test, particularly how clenching and unclenching of the hand can lead to stress of the brachial plexus.[20]

Closely related to the EAST is the abduction and external rotation test (Figure 18-9). The arm is abducted, rotated, and held in that position. This test works by a similar mechanism and likewise produces the weakness and numbness seen with EAST in a similar distribution, namely, the C8 to T1 fibers supplying the median and ulnar nerves. In addition, the examiner can sometimes detect a bruit below the lateral portion of the clavicle that is attributable to partial compression of the axillary artery. Both of these tests appear particularly suited to work-related and repetitive motion–associated TOS.[21]

Several variants and positional tests can be used, each with its own benefits and shortcomings. The "military brace" position can often reproduce TOS symptoms in patients with the disorder. The shoulders are braced backward and downward, effectively causing a narrowing of the thoracic outlet. Symptoms arise within 2 minutes in a susceptible patient. The upper limb tension test uses graduated tension to test for irritation of the brachial plexus by extending the forearm with the shoulder abducted and externally rotated. Other tests include the timed Morley and Eden studies.

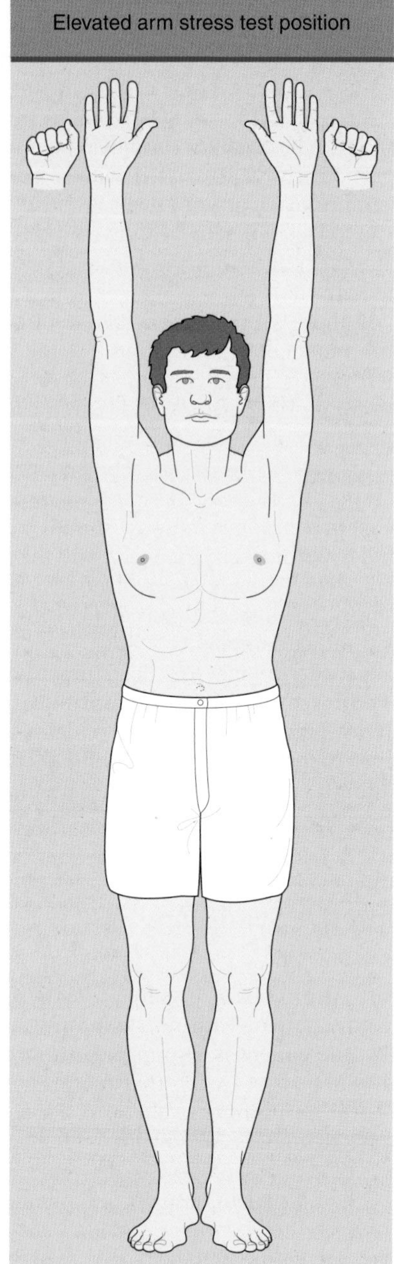

Figure 18-8. Elevated arm stress test position. The fists are repeatedly clenched and unclenched, usually for 3 minutes, or less if the symptoms start earlier. The costoclavicular space is narrowed via this maneuver (see Figure 18-1).

Additional information can be gained by adding pulse examination to the preceding tests. The original Adson's test consisted of assessment of the radial pulse following rotation of the neck to the contralateral side and deep inspiration (Figure 18-10). Adson's sign is the subsequent loss of the radial pulse. This test is notoriously nonsensitive and has been

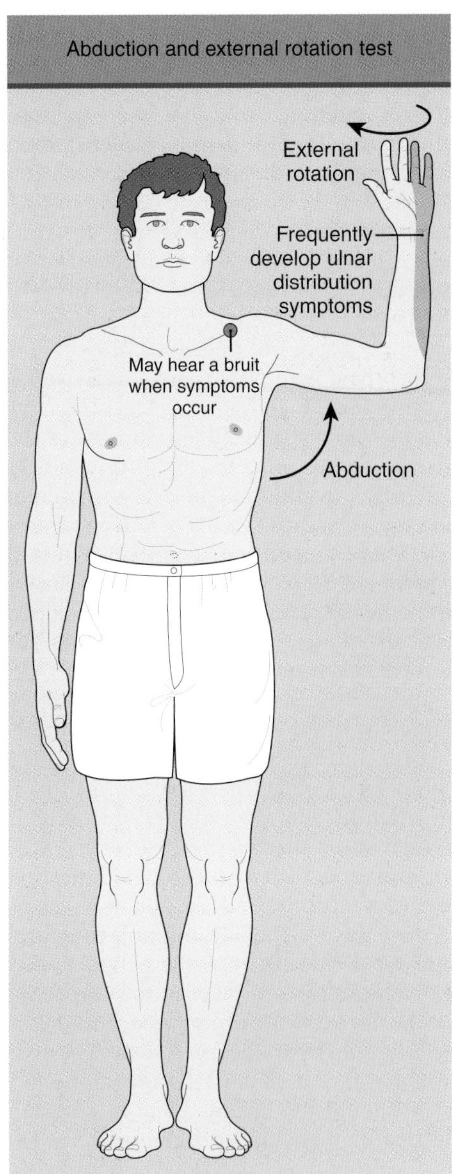

Figure 18-9. Abduction and external rotation test. The patient may be asked to clench and unclench the fist. A bruit is sometimes heard over the lateral aspect of the clavicle (axillary artery).

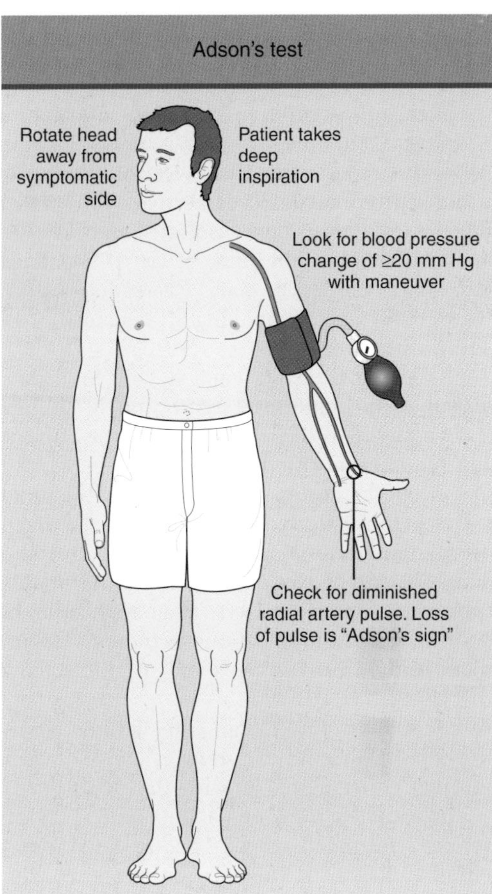

Figure 18-10. Adson's test. This test is notoriously insensitive, with only about 3% of patients with thoracic outlet syndrome demonstrating loss of the radial pulse. Changes in blood pressure can add to the sensitivity, but this test is rarely helpful.

reported to be positive in less than 3% of TOS patients.[22] In 1945, Wright described the hyperabduction position, which is also of little clinical utility given its positive result in most healthy individuals. However, measurements that quantify blood pressure are more sensitive, and a drop of 20 mm Hg after movement from neutral position or the same pressure difference from one extremity to the other is often present in TOS. These tests are facilitated by using the Doppler probe. Additional positioning tests can be used with simultaneous pulse assessment, including both the costoclavicular and the anticus maneuvers. Of note, the cutaneous color changes associated with stress positioning do not correlate well with the presence of TOS.[23] None of these aforementioned tests are pathognomonic, but the presence of one or more of them can help support the diagnosis of TOS. Combined with the proper history, other disorders can be effectively ruled out and other tests can be avoided.

Objective Testing

The cervical spine film and chest radiograph are the most important objective studies needed in making the diagnosis of TOS. Clearly, cervical disease must be excluded as a cause of neurological symptoms, and the bony abnormalities of TOS (cervical ribs, elongated C7 transverse processes, fractures with exostosis or callous formation) can be appreciated on plane chest films. Magnetic resonance imaging is often used in the workup for TOS. Certainly, a sizable number of these patients undergo magnetic resonance imaging in their evaluation or other neurological etiologies to explain their symptoms. Current protocols include measurement of the interscalene triangle and the costoclavicular space, as well as the thickness of the various muscles and any obvious neural of vascular compression.[24] Provocative maneuvers can increase the utility of these studies.[25] Nonetheless, a recent review of available evidence suggests that magnetic resonance imaging is not particularly useful in this setting.[26] Computed tomography has also been used to assess for TOS. The exact role for this study has not been determined, but it does appear that provocative maneuvers are beneficial in revealing the anatomical abnormalities.[27]

The use of objective neurodiagnostic tests for TOS has met with some success, although it continues to be an area of considerable controversy. Perhaps the main criticism of these tests is that they only tend to be positive in patients with advanced disease, in whom history and physical examination should be sufficient. Thus, no less an authority than Roos suggests they offer "little definitive diagnostic information" and that the clinician "still must rely on careful history and physical."[28] All of this reflects that most electrophysiological tests evaluate larger myelinated nerve fibers, not the smaller fibers whose injury mediates the pain associated with TOS. A recent study by Franklin et al. found that, of 158 TOS patients, only 7.6% had abnormalities in their electrodiagnostic tests.[16] Nonetheless, they can aid in making the diagnosis of TOS and in excluding other conditions.

Neurophysiological testing came to the forefront in the early 1960s, but the anatomical constraints of attempting to measure changes across the brachial plexus have always made its application in this position difficult. After Jebsen published the results of conduction velocity testing for the ulnar nerve in 1968, Urschel investigated its potential in the diagnosis of TOS. Hongladhom subsequently applied F-wave studies to the field in 1976, and Glover did the same with somatosensory evoked potentials (SSEPs) in 1981. Their application has continued to evolve, and modifications in these techniques have led to them being more sensitive and specific when applied to TOS.

Nerve conduction studies can offer limited information in the workup of TOS and can show evidence of carpal tunnel syndrome, either alone or with the double-crush syndrome; approximately 20% of patients with TOS can have carpal tunnel syndrome as well. Conduction studies do not offer definitive diagnostic information as specifically relates to TOS. To measure velocities usefully, the nerve must be stimulated proximal to the potential point of injury. For compression at the thoracic outlet, this could mean stimulation at the roots, a site not conducive to easy testing. Several authors have described their experience using ulnar conduction velocity from Erb's point (above the clavicle and lateral to the insertion of the sternocleidomastoid muscle) to the elbow to assess TOS, but this technique has been criticized.[19] However, if severe disease with concomitant axonal damage occurs, changes in ulnar action potentials can be demonstrated. A reasonable approach to conduction studies includes sensory testing of the median and ulnar nerves at the wrist to screen for carpal tunnel syndrome and TOS, respectively. The addition of motor nerve conduction velocities can be considered if additional information is needed to rule out carpal tunnel syndrome or ulnar entrapment neuropathy. However, no specific motor pathways for demonstrating TOS have been determined.

Electromyography (EMG) is also capable of showing objective data supporting the diagnosis of TOS, although this is again in a setting of advanced disease. This study can demonstrate spontaneous firing of acutely denervated muscle fibers (positive sharp waves, fibrillation potentials), but this is not the usual clinical situation for TOS. Rather, after reinnervation, prolonged and irregular potentials are seen. Because this is a reflection of previous denervation injury, many of these patients have atrophy of the involved muscle groups, and EMG can confirm that the lower trunk of the brachial plexus was injured. However, in patients without evidence of atrophy, this test is not likely to reveal these findings. This is supported by studies showing that standard EMG tests are negative in 62% of TOS patients.[29] However, these tests can be used to examine the paraspinal muscles, which can be important in ruling out radiculopathy as the cause of the patient's symptoms.

EMG has an additional role that bears mentioning, that of an adjunct to needle placement for scalene block. This test has utility as a predictor of surgical outcome for neurogenic TOS, with relaxation of the anterior scalene muscle approximating the decompression achieved with first-rib resection or scalenectomy. Inadvertent needle placement can confuse the results of this test or cause injury, particularly to the brachial plexus itself or even the sympathetic ganglia at that level. Patients are given a series of injections of either lidocaine or saline, and then pain with provocative maneuvers is assessed (generally using EAST). Jordan and Machleder reported on 122 patients in whom this technique was used and found a 90% positive predictive value for correlation with the clinical diagnosis of TOS.[30] In addition, for patients undergoing first-rib resection for TOS, those with a positive scalene block had a greater chance of a good outcome (94%) than those with a negative preoperative scalene block (50%). This test can be positive with other disorders, particularly radiculopathies, but is another useful adjunct to not only diagnosis of TOS but also likelihood of surgical benefit.

F-wave studies are an attractive concept for evaluating TOS because they allow distal propagation of the stimulus back to the spinal cord, thus crossing the brachial plexus and obviating the need for proximal nerve access. In this technique, nerve stimulation at the wrist leads not only to an immediate action potential in the affected muscle groups but also to this proximal propagation, with a concomitant reflection from the cord leading to a secondary action potential. This returning potential is the F wave. Generally, multiple trails are recorded, and the shortest period between the percutaneous stimulus and the secondary response is taken as the latency. This period is delayed if the nerve fibers are damaged, and this can be seen with TOS. Additional parameters can be assessed, but it is not clear whether these add any relevant information to TOS evaluations. It should also be noted that these tests tend to be poorly tolerated by many patients and it is prudent to avoid their use unless other tests have proved unrewarding and further diagnostic information is required.

Somatosensory evoked potentials (SSEPs) can play a role in the workup of TOS. Since 1979, when Siivola et al. showed that multiple position recordings could be used to help locate peripheral nerve deficits related to the brachial plexus, the technique has been refined and applied to TOS.[31] Currently, assessment of the ulnar and median nerves can be used for evidence of their compression at the thoracic outlet. These studies, when abnormal, tend to show lower plexus injury (ulnar) with normal median function. This is seen primarily as a blunting of the Erb's point peak (Figure 18-11).[32] Several studies have documented abnormal SSEPs with TOS. Machleder and colleagues showed that 74% of their patients carrying a clinical diagnosis of TOS had abnormal evoked responses. Furthermore, when these patients were studied following operative decompression of their thoracic outlets, more than 90% had correlation between improved symptoms and normalization of their SSEPs.[33] Other series have shown 45% to 70% of patients with TOS demonstrating corresponding changes in their SSEPs. Increases of the sensitivity of these tests can be achieved with provocative maneuvers, such as arm positioning, although these maneuvers can also cause SE changes in

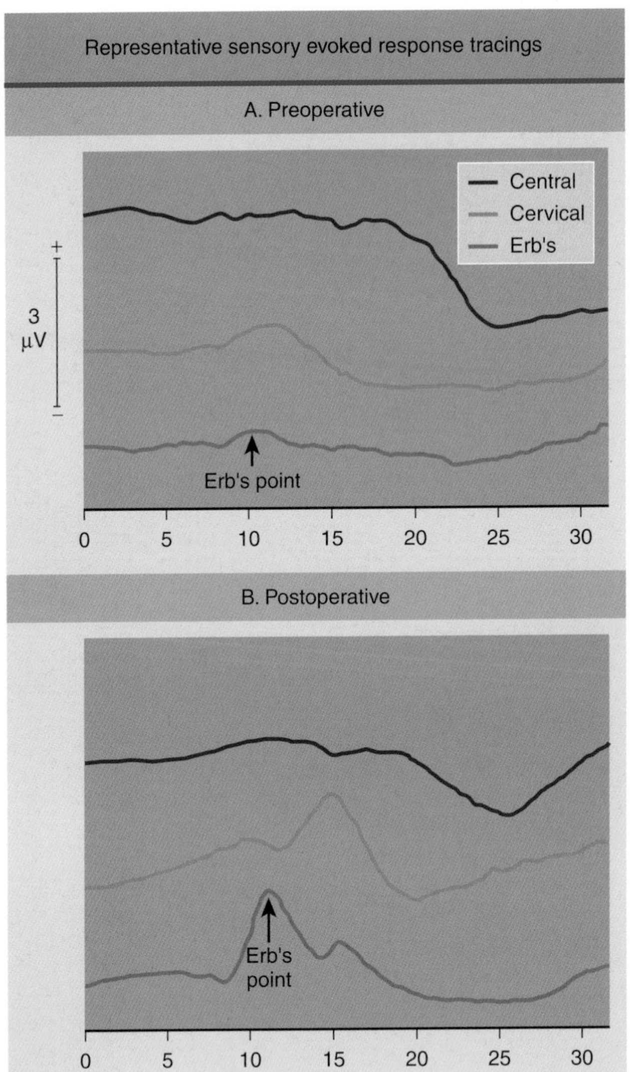

Figure 18-11. Representative sensory-evoked response tracings, preoperatively **(A)** and postoperatively **(B).** The improved amplitude at Erb's point, recorded over the brachial plexus, is often seen when preoperative blunting is present. This tracing is from a patient with lower (ulnar) symptoms.

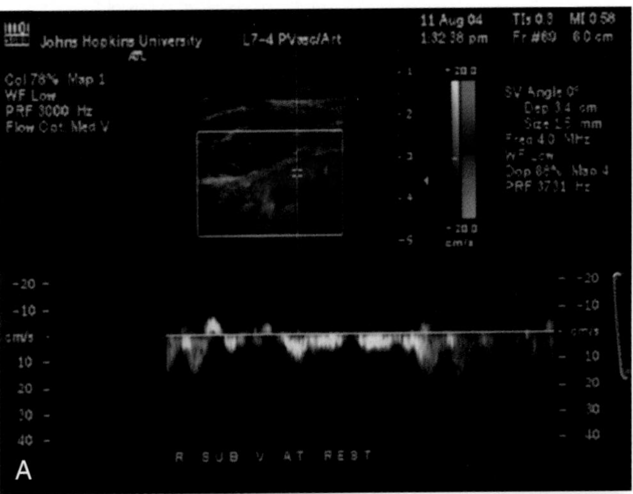

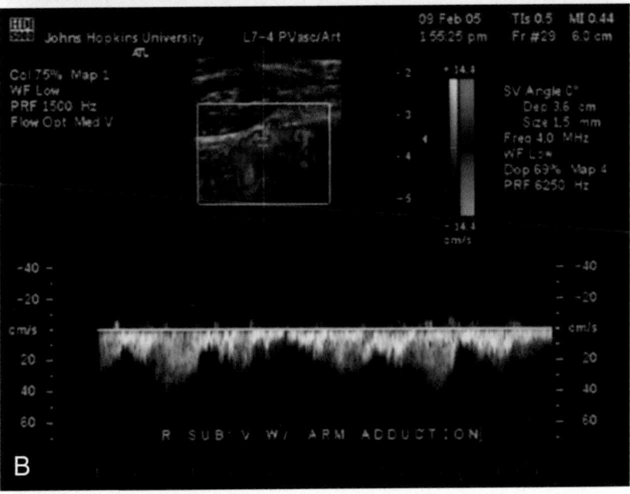

Figures 18-12. Duplex evaluation of the right subclavian vein in a patient with intermittent arm swelling and Paget-Schroetter syndrome. The vein is patent with normal arm positioning **(A)** but partially compressed in a stressed (abduction and external rotation) position **(B).**

patients with no clinical evidence of TOS. As with other forms of TOS testing, most patients with abnormal SSEPs also have an abnormal physical examination and other electrophysiological examination. As with these other tests, SSEPs can be used to diagnose other processes causing the patient's symptoms.

Paget-Schroetter Syndrome

In the TOS patient who presents with upper extremity swelling, the diagnosis of axillosubclavian vein thrombosis is suggested by the physical examination and history. Assessment of the venous system is usually initiated with noninvasive duplex ultrasonography. Provocative positioning, such as external rotation and abduction, can increase the sensitivity of these tests. Other authors describe a two-position technique, with the arms fully adducted and then abducted 90 degrees (Figure 18-12). Magnetic resonance venography can also be useful in evaluating these patients, particularly gadolinium-enhanced images. Again, provocative positioning can document compression of the axillosubclavian veins, particularly when studying the side contralateral to an occlusion.

Most patients go on to have a diagnostic venogram, which is the gold standard for thrombosis in this position (Figure 18-13). In the acute setting, this is usually followed by the administration of lytic therapy. Although this test confirms the diagnosis of thrombosis, the occasional patient needs further clarification as to its cause. Neurogenic symptoms are usually not present, and the clinician must often rely on the exclusion of other causes in this situation.

Arterial Disease

As discussed in the previous section, several symptoms and signs can be a consequence of arterial involvement in TOS. Physical examination can reveal a pulsatile mass in the supraclavicular fossa, but this is not a consistent finding. Clearly, the diagnostic algorithm is not straightforward. Patients may initially be worked up with digital plethysmography or upper extremity duplex examination. These may be abnormal depending on the lesion, and arteriography is almost always required in this setting. When arterial compression

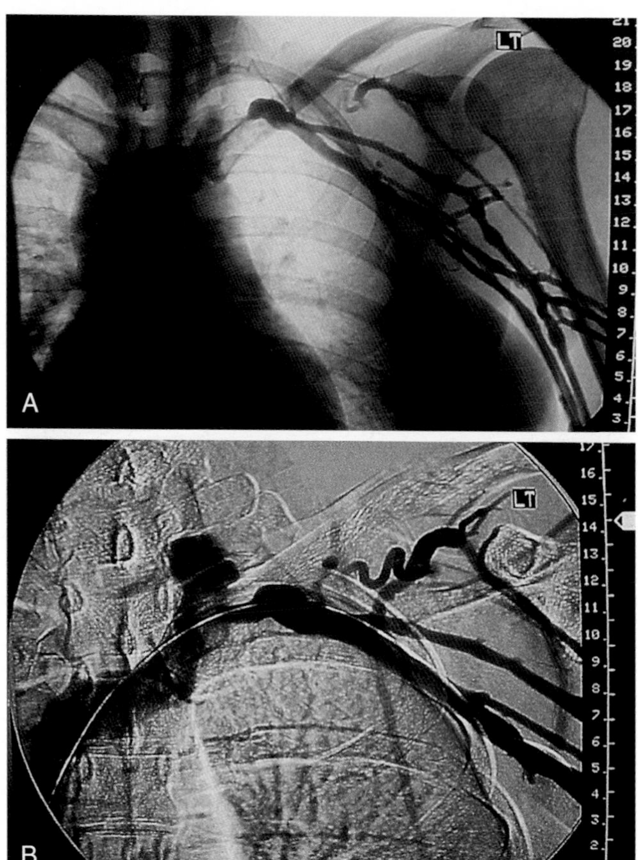

Figure 18-13. Venography and Paget-Schroetter syndrome. **A,** Pretreatment venogram from a patient with axillosubclavian thrombosis (Paget-Schroetter syndrome). This patient underwent thrombolysis, and a venogram **(B)** was obtained. This therapy was followed by transaxillary first-rib resection.

is suspected, attention should first be toward an arch study to include the subclavian and axillary arteries more distally. Often, arterial compression can be better visualized if the arm is abducted 90 degrees, and most studies are obtained with the arms in neutral and abducted positions (Figure 18-14). When distal embolization is suggested, the angiography should encompass the target sites, often requiring studies of the hand on the affected side.

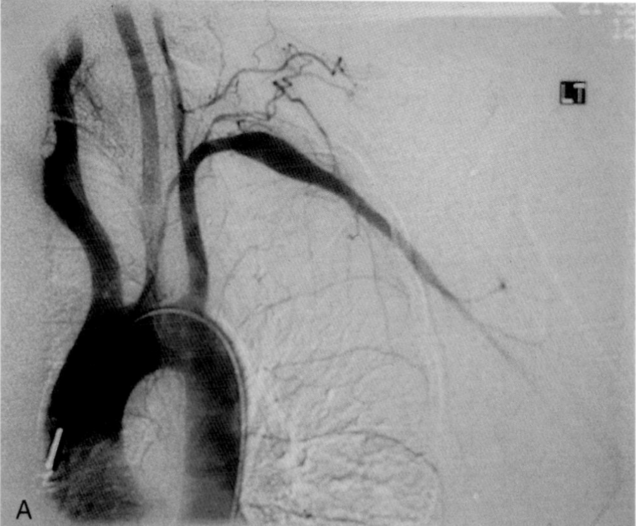

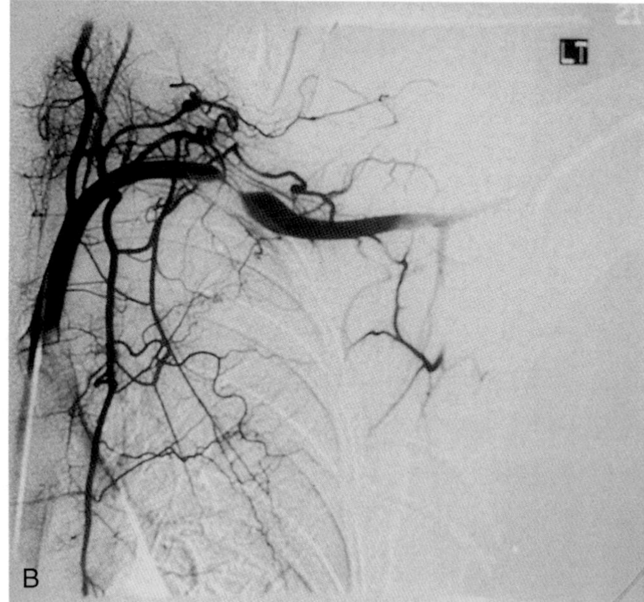

Figure 18-14. Arteriograms showing arterial changes in thoracic outlet syndrome. **A,** A subclavian aneurysm at the site of the thoracic outlet is shown. **B,** When the arm is abducted into a stressed position, a tight stenosis proximal to the area of dilatation is revealed.

TREATMENT

Most patients with neurogenic TOS go undiagnosed and thus receive no therapy. This reflects the range of severity inherent in the spectrum of symptoms associated with TOS. For those who seek medical intervention, most clearly have substantial improvement without operation. Although the numbers are controversial and depend on the modalities used to make the diagnosis, more than 95% of patients avoid operation. Considerable debate currently surrounds neurogenic TOS surgery, with several groups reporting no long-term benefit from operation versus physical therapy. Nonetheless, most surgeons with considerable experience with neurogenic TOS report good surgical results with properly selected patients.

Before embarking on a treatment plan for a patient with a secure diagnosis of TOS, it is important to consider the variant of the syndrome being addressed. This discussion starts with the neurogenic form, which we have already noted is the most common. Differences in treatments for the other forms are considered at the end of this section.

Neurogenic TOS

For many TOS surgeons, their referral patterns are such that patients have already undertaken unsuccessful conservative therapy before seeking further consultation. It is important for surgeons to be aware of this selection bias. It is also important to have an algorithm for conservative treatment so that the correct patients are selected for operation. Recent reports suggest that a minimum of 6 weeks of physical therapy is required before its effects can be evaluated. It is also key that the correct program is used, as it has been recognized that inappropriate physical therapy can worsen TOS symptoms. In general, these programs are designed to relax muscle groups

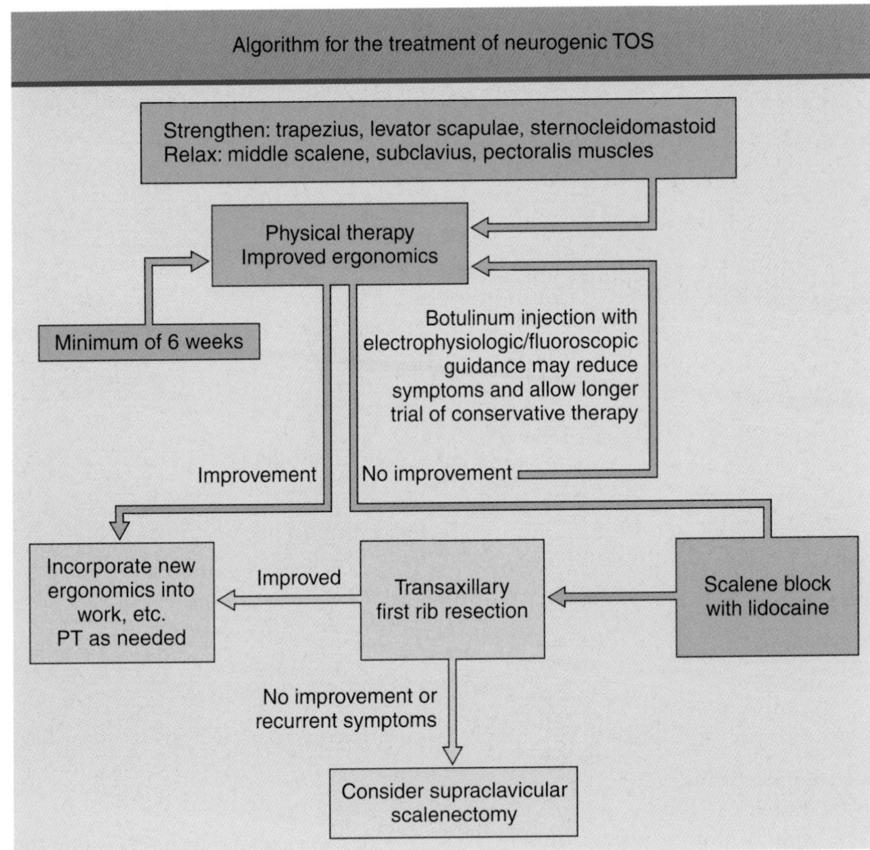

Figure 18-15. Algorithm for the treatment of neurogenic thoracic outlet syndrome. Some surgeons prefer a supraclavicular scalenectomy as the initial route of intervention. This can be done with or without first-rib resection.

that tighten the thoracic outlet while conditioning those that open it. Aligne and Barral thus described a program in which the trapezius, levator scapulae, and sternocleidomastoid muscles are strengthened and the middle scalene, subclavius, and pectoralis muscles are relaxed.[34] These goals can be met via many protocols, usually with a combination of supervised and at-home exercises.

Other nonsurgical interventions are available. Following the concept of diagnostic scalene blocks, attempts have been made at therapeutic blockade of the scalene muscles. Steroid injection has not been successful, and early attempts at using botulinum toxin were complicated by dysphagia in as many as 20% of attempts. However, recent work by Jordan and colleagues demonstrated that electrophysiological and fluoroscopic guidance of needle placement decreased the incidence of dysphagia and relieved symptoms for a mean duration of 88 days.[35] This technique may prove to be a useful tool either in relieving symptoms in the preoperative period or in allowing the patient to tolerate an extended period of physical therapy or other adjustments, such as in their ergonomics at work. Recent work has shown that the combination of EMG and ultrasound works as well as EMG and fluoroscopy.[36]

When a symptomatic patient who has sought treatment fails to improve with physical therapy, surgical intervention is warranted. For most TOS surgeons, the initial operative treatment is transaxillary first-rib resection (Figure 18-15). The patient is placed in the lateral decubitus position, with the head neutral. No paralytic agents are used. Various devices are available for elevation of the arm on the operative side, all of which should be used for easy lowering of the extremity intermittently throughout the case to allow periods of increased arterial inflow and decreased tension on stretched nerves. The incision is placed between the pectoralis major and the latissimus dorsi in the lower aspect of the axilla. Dissection is carried out, with care taken to identify intercostal brachial cutaneous nerves. These structures should be avoided and preserved when possible, but it is preferable to sacrifice them rather than to leave them injured and to subject the patient to possible causalgic pain. Care must be taken in the region of the posterior scalene muscle to identify the long thoracic nerve, as injury with resulting winged scapula has been reported when this structure aberrantly passes closer to the midaxillary line.

After the connective tissue over the thoracic outlet is opened using blunt techniques with a peanut, the subclavian vein and artery, anterior scalene muscle, and lower trunk of the brachial plexus can be identified and cleared (Figure 18-16). The anterior scalene muscle is now carefully separated from the subclavian vessels, and its attachment to the first rib can be divided. The subclavius tendon is also divided. Before the rib can be removed, further attachments between it and the middle scalene and first intercostal muscle must be released, with particular care taken not to injure the T1 nerve. A right-angled rib shear is next positioned posteriorly over the first rib so that it approaches the transverse process of T1. Anteriorly, the rib is divided almost at the level of the costal cartilage. Considerable care must be taken following removal of the rib to smooth the posterior stump and thus to prevent any subsequent T1 injury. At this point, any further anomalies (fibromuscular bands, scalenus minimus muscles) encountered should be resected. Cervical ribs are resected in

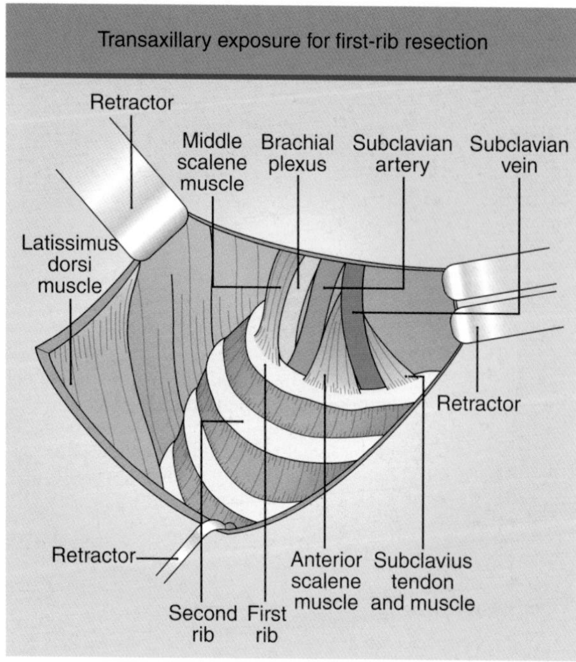

Figure 18-16. Transaxillary exposure for first-rib resection.

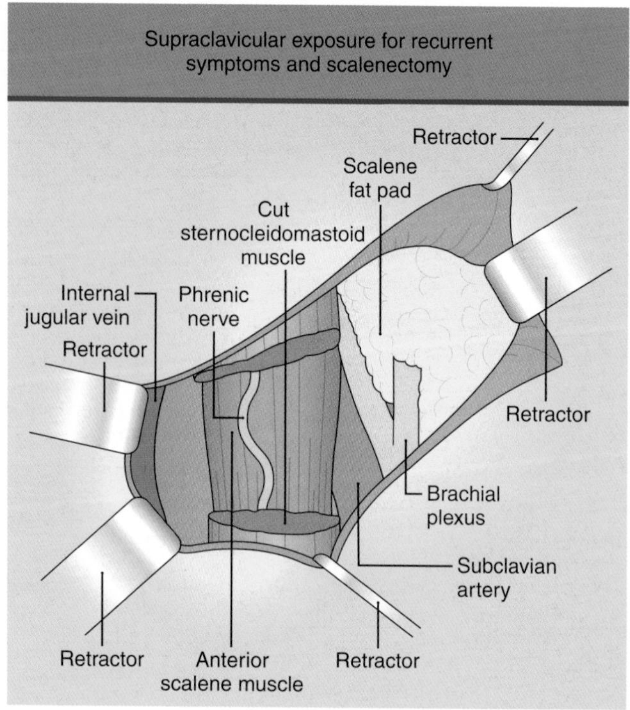

Figure 18-17. Supraclavicular exposure for recurrent symptoms and scalenectomy.

a similar fashion to the first rib, requiring division of their attachments to the middle scalene and intercostal muscles.

Before closure, irrigation is placed into the wound and inspection is made for a pleural leak. In the presence of a leak, a small chest tube can be used for pleural drainage. This can usually be removed the following day. A postoperative chest radiograph is obtained. Most patients are discharged home on postoperative day 1 or 2. Careful follow-up and physical therapy are also employed in the early postoperative period.

Supraclavicular Scalenectomy

Three situations occur in which scalenectomy is considered for TOS. First, when the patient's symptoms are particularly suggestive of upper brachial plexus involvement (as opposed to the more common lower plexus), as has been described by Roos, it is reasonable to use an approach in which these nerves can be more directly decompressed. Second, for patients who have undergone transaxillary operation but now have upper plexus symptoms, the operation can be employed. Third, some surgeons feel that the supraclavicular approach is as effective as the transaxillary operation and that it is safer. Thus, they use this approach routinely. The first rib can also be resected as a component of this procedure, although some argue that it cannot be done with the same margins as the transaxillary approach.

As with the transaxillary approach, no paralytics are used so that nerve function can be assessed intraoperatively. The patient is placed in the semi-Fowler position, with the head turned from the operative side. An incision is placed two fingerbreadths above the clavicle, extending from the external jugular vein to the sternocleidomastoid muscle. This muscle is subsequently mobilized medially, while the omohyoid muscle must usually be transected. The scalene fat pad is carefully divided, taking care to avoid the underlying phrenic nerve. This structure must be protected throughout the course of the operation (Figure 18-17). Underlying the nerve is the anterior scalene muscle. This is divided inferiorly at its insertion on the first rib. Usually, adhesions are found between the muscle and the subclavian artery and brachial plexus components that also must be freed, and the origin end of the muscle is divided medially to expose the C5 to C7 roots. The area between the C7 root and the subclavian artery is next cleaned, including the division of a subclavius minimus muscle if present. At this point, the five roots should be completely cleared and tested using a nerve stimulator, although several authors have noted that is often difficult to assess the T1 nerve root in this manner.

If the operation is to include first-rib resection, the middle scalene muscle must be divided. The rib is divided posteriorly, and a finger is used to dissect it from the pleura while elevating the divided end. The subclavian artery must be freed from the anterior portion of the rib before it is divided. It can then be carefully extracted.

Irrigation is placed in the wound to assess for pleural leak. If present, the soft, closed suction drain can be positioned so that the tip drains the pleural space. Otherwise, the drain can be placed to drain the wound. Postoperative chest radiograph is obtained, and the patient is usually discharged home within 1 or 2 days.

Mention should be made here of thoracoscopic first-rib resection. This procedure has not gained widespread acceptance, as some question the benefits versus the transaxillary approach. Nonetheless, it is offered at several centers, and it remains to be seen what place this operation will play in the treatment of TOS.[37]

Paget-Schroetter Syndrome

Unlike the elective nature of neurogenic TOS therapies, venous occlusion at the thoracic outlet should be treated expeditiously. Although this disease was once treated with anticoagulation and arm elevation, therapeutic protocols now stress the importance of dissolving the clot, maintaining patency of the axillosubclavian veins, and correcting any anatomical abnormalities contributing to the thrombosis. Once the diagnosis has been established, the patient should be taken for catheter-directed fibrinolysis of the clot. Streptokinase, urokinase, and tissue plasminogen activator have all been used in the past, and the agent employed is institution dependent. A recent trial by Gelabert et al. compares tissue plasminogen activator and urokinase in this setting and suggests that the drugs' profiles are similar.[38] In addition to the clot-directed therapy, patients are heparinized and then placed on oral coumadin. Work by Perler and Mitchell, later supported by that of Machleder and Kunkel, demonstrated that a period of 1 to 3 months of anticoagulation allowed for intimal healing of the damaged vein before the patient was taken for definitive surgery in the form of first-rib resection.[39-41] Following surgery, the vein is again assessed. If residual stricture exists, the patient undergoes further catheter-based treatment.

The preceding protocol and variants of it have been widely adopted at centers treating Paget-Schroetter syndrome. However, in attempts to decrease the period of disability between the initial lysis and the definitive operation, some authors have advocated first-rib resection during the initial hospitalization. The University of California–Los Angeles (UCLA) group recently reported a series of patients treated in this fashion and noted no increased morbidity compared to those patients with delayed operation.[42] In particular, none of the theoretical concerns for bleeding following thrombolytic instillation were observed, nor were there particular technical problems secondary to the inflammation associated with the venous thrombosis. Although no randomized prospective trial has yet to compare these two protocols, several centers likely will adopt a policy of early surgical intervention.

Recent data from Johns Hopkins addresses the question of treating chronically occluded veins in this setting.[42a] Even for patients with documented symptoms and occlusions for an average of 6 months before treatment was performed, good outcomes were attained. The protocol currently in use for such patients involves surgical decompression followed by long-term anticoagulation. Lysis of the chronically occluded vein is not performed. Intermediate results (average 7 months follow-up) shows that the veins recanalize. Longer-term follow-up and greater numbers of patients are needed to validate this approach, but it does show potential for members of this difficult cohort who are not treated early for their occlusion.

We should mention complicated venous injuries in the setting of TOS. Angioplasty for residual stricture appears to work quite well in this setting following correction of the anatomical problems. Stenting has not been particularly useful, however. Meier et al. reported on the high incidence of stent deformity in the setting of TOS, even after first-rib resection.[43] Nonetheless, some authors continue to use stents for postoperative venous strictures. Finally, cases exist in which the vein is so severely damaged that the only operative repair that can be performed is a jugular–subclavian bypass. This is only indicated if the patient has continued symptoms of venous hypertension, and it is rarely performed.

For patients with thrombus that resists thrombolysis, a component of chronic disease is common. Machleder and colleagues observed that these patients might have intermittent periods of clot propagation for which their collaterals are not adequate to compensate. It is during these times that "acute" swelling occurs. It is not clear what the ideal treatment is in this situation. If the patient has resolution of the acute symptoms, observation with anticoagulation is a reasonable option. For symptomatic patients, some surgical or endovascular procedure tailored to the particular problem is warranted.

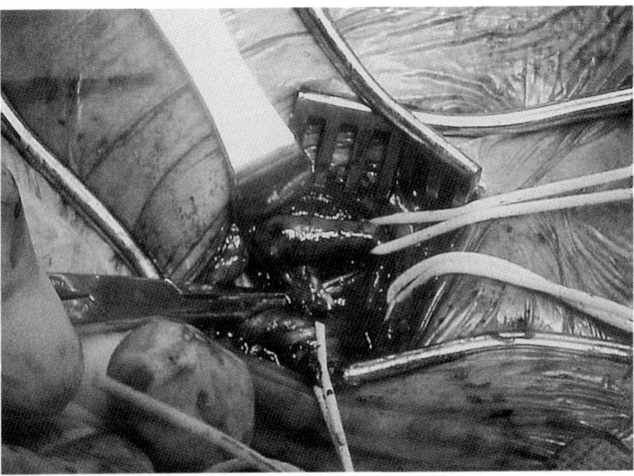

Figure 18-18. Supraclavicular exposure of a subclavian artery aneurysm and cervical rib. Vessel loops are around the artery, and the right angle clamp is partially elevating the cervical rib.

Arterial Disease

As previously discussed, several arterial problems can arise from thoracic outlet obstruction, although they are uncommon. Clearly, the urgency of intervention depends on the severity of the problem, with ischemia dictating an expeditious approach. For most, transaxillary first-rib resection followed by arterial repair remains the treatment of choice. If there is a cervical rib, it needs to be removed as well. The area of arterial involvement is usually the retroscalene subclavian to prepectoral region of the axillary artery. If treating a patient with emboli, catheter-based thrombolysis is usually necessary before addressing their source.

Aneurysms secondary to TOS usually are treated no differently than such lesions when due to atherosclerosis, namely, resection and graft reconstruction. This holds true for axillosubclavian poststenotic dilatation and obstruction. These operations are described elsewhere in this text, so only a few points are made about them here. Standard approaches are used, with a high anterior thoracotomy for proximal lesions on the left and median sternotomy for the right. For more distal lesions, various clavicular incisions may be used (Figures 18-18 and 18-19). Graft material is a matter of surgeon's preference, but it is clear that synthetic material, vein, and arterial grafts have all been used with success in this position. Postoperative anticoagulation is not usually indicated, and patients tend to do well if the thoracic outlet is adequately decompressed and the vessel is no longer subjected to trauma.

An additional consideration in these patients is the presence of reflex sympathetic dystrophy, causalgia, or other autonomic dysfunction. Cervicodorsal or cervicothoracic sympathectomy is offered to these patients and can often be performed at the time of the arterial repair by standard approaches.

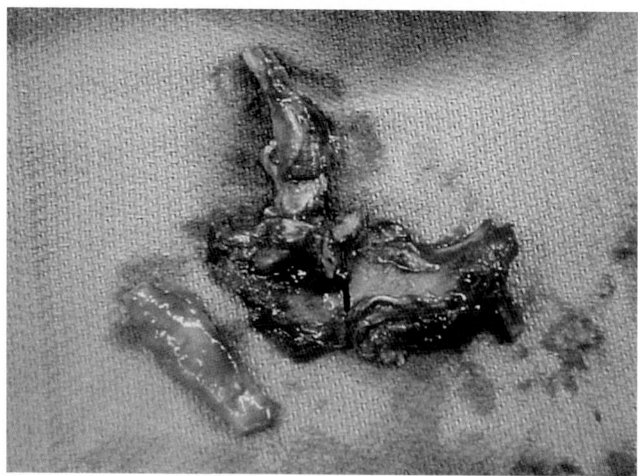

Figure 18-19. Specimen from first-rib resection and repair of subclavian artery aneurysm. This lesion was approached via the supraclavicular route. The aneurysm, cervical rib, and first rib are shown.

Alternatively, this operation can be done at a separate setting via a thoracoscopic route if its need is not clear. It should also be noted that these same symptoms can occur in patients with primary neurogenic TOS if the sympathetics in the inferior trunk of the brachial plexus are involved. These patients can also be treated by sympathectomy if needed.

Finally, patients with arterial consequences of TOS can have diverse complications. Machleder reported an embolizing aneurysm of the posterior humeral circumflex artery necessitating aneurysm excision and cephalic vein bypass of the distal common and posterior humeral circumflex artery to the anterior humeral circumflex artery.[44] Clearly, the variety of problems arising from arterial involvement in TOS leads to the most varied presentations and concomitantly to the most varied therapies.

Treatment for Recurrent TOS

Recurrence of TOS following operative intervention is not uncommon. Published series have reported rates as low 2.2%, but most are in the range of 15% to 20%.[45-48] Defining recurrence in this situation is often difficult, because it is not always clear that the patient's symptoms ever improved. These tend to be similar to the original complaints, with paresthesias of the hand and pain of the neck and shoulder the most common manifestations. The etiology of recurrence is usually not clear, although postoperative scarring is considered one of the main culprits. Several studies have looked at the implications of a long posterior stump to the first rib, but little correlation is found with return of symptoms. Other reported etiologies include middle scalene reattachment, calcified rib masses, and missed cervical ribs or cervical rib stumps. Some have drawn a distinction between a spontaneous recurrence attributable to scar and a recurrence secondary to a traumatic insult. In the latter situation, the patient again tends to have the original symptoms, even though the thoracic outlet has already been decompressed. A whiplash-type injury often occurs in this scenario.

The workup for recurrence is essentially the same as for untreated disease. Special emphasis should be placed on ruling out other causes, as a percentage of patients failing treatment will have done so on the basis of a faulty diagnosis. Iatrogenic injury to the plexus, carpal tunnel syndrome, tendonitis, cervical arthritis, or spine injury must be sought before treatment for the recurrence is started. A conservative plan is initially undertaken, although the overwhelmingly positive response seen with physical therapy in TOS patients who avoid the original operation is not reproduced here. If conservative methods fail, reoperation is considered, although it should be noted that only a 50% improvement rate is quoted for these patients.

Although clinical practices vary, many surgeons have adopted an algorithm for reoperation. If the original operation was via a transaxillary approach, a supraclavicular approach is taken. Care is taken to identify any remaining first rib and to resect it all the way to the transverse process. If the patient's original operation did not include first-rib resection, it is removed now. Most surgeons also add some form of neurolysis to the reoperation, whereby the scar around the nerves is carefully removed. Some surgeons remove the middle scalene during the course of reexploration. If the supraclavicular approach was already used, the transaxillary is used for the second operation. Again, care is taken to remove the entire first rib, any remaining attachments, and scar. Neurolysis can be performed via this route, with some advocating it over the supraclavicular route, particularly when ulnar symptoms predominate.

Several methods have been tried to prevent the formation of scar tissue and adhesions following thoracic outlet decompression, particularly in the face of reoperation. After clearing the nerve roots, they are usually covered with the overlying adipose tissue, although the benefit of this technique has never been documented. Similarly, care is taken to replace the scalene fat pad, but this does not appear to influence the formation of scar. Attempts to control scarring with the administration of exogenous agents, including steroids, have also been disappointing. Sheets of polytetrafluoroethylene have been used to cover the nerves, but this technique has been abandoned by most and probably leads to additional scar formation. The use of hyaluronic acid gels showed some promise several years ago, but it is not clear whether these products are particularly helpful and they are not approved by the U.S. Food and Drug Administration for this use.

Complications

Any structure encountered in the dissection for first-rib resection is a potential site of injury. The catastrophic complications of brachial plexus injury, subclavian artery, and subclavian vein injury occur rarely. Concern about brachial plexus injury dates back to the early days of first-rib resection. Particularly in the neurology literature, this has been a controversial topic. For several years, only a few case reports were made of plexus injuries. However, Dale in 1982 published the results of a survey of thoracic surgeons performing first-rib resections and discovered 273 injuries, 19% of which were permanent.[49] While this study certainly suggested underreporting of this complication, reports of plexus injuries remained low, although not the almost negligible rate that had been accepted.

What is most notable about the publications that followed is that no mention is made of the incidence of this injury. Wilbourn in 1988 reported on eight patients with plexus injuries from the Cleveland Clinic. They underwent first-rib resection sometime between 1974 and 1983, but total number of procedures performed is not given.[50] Likewise, Horowitz reported on four cases of plexus injury, but no figures are given regarding the number of procedures performed from which these patients were taken.[51] The same can be said of the four cases reported by Cherington et al. in 1986.[52] In several large, recent surgical series, most notably that of Roos, the incidence of such injuries is very low (0% to 2%). In the UCLA experience, there have been no such injuries. It is fair to say that plexus injuries certainly do occur but that the risk of the injury must be weighed against the possible benefits of the procedure.

Another issue regarding plexus injuries is that of retraction. It is more than likely that most neurological injuries were related to stretching of the perineurium with resultant ischemia. During the transaxillary approach, a considerable amount of stretch is applied to the arm, and most surgeons relieve the traction intermittently to allow blood flow. This was not necessarily the case when an assistant was retracting. Specialized retraction systems, such as the Machleder retractor, allow for periods of extremity relaxation with easy repositioning to continue the procedure.

The incidence of major arterial or venous injury during first-rib resection is also difficult to determine. Clearly, these injuries can and do occur, and they demand immediate attention. In a review of 2445 cases, Roos reported only 3 instances of major injuries of this nature (0.12%).[53] In all 3 cases, the patients had full recovery. Delayed bleeding, usually from a small subclavian branch or intercostals artery, is also seen. Roos reported 7 cases of delayed bleeding in the same series (0.2%). The patients also had complete recovery. In Green et al.'s review of 136 patients, there were no major vascular injuries.[54] UCLA reported one such injury in its series over 10 years of operations.

We recently completed a review of in-hospital injuries to the brachial plexus and major blood vessels during first-rib resection.[55] This study was performed using the nationwide inpatient sample database and revealed a 0.6% incidence of brachial plexus injury and a 1.74% incidence of vascular injury.

Injuries to other nerves occur, particularly the long thoracic. Roos reported a 0.12% incidence, with two of the patients having complete recoveries and one lost to follow-up. In Sharp et al.'s series of 36 patients, there was 1 such injury.[56] Most of these tend to be temporary, but permanent winged scapula can occur. Phrenic injuries are not common and are more associated with the anterior approach, particularly with reoperative cases. Most of these injuries result in temporary, subclinical diaphragmatic paralysis, although complete division with permanent injury is possible.

The most common nerve injury is not a true complication but a byproduct of the operation: division of intercostals brachial cutaneous branches leading to cutaneous numbness. This occurs to some extent in most patients, not unlike that which occurs with axillary dissection for other disease states. It is usually well tolerated and resolves.

Reports of patients with postoperative causalgia or other pains are also difficult to place into clinical perspective. In most series, they are unusual. Significant causalgia is usually attributed to brachial plexus injury and thus should parallel the incidence of that injury. In the Washington state workers' compensation study, 6% of patients were reported to have causalgia, and 13% had "other pains." It is not clear what these represented. Green's series of 136 cases had 3 patients with some form of postoperative vasospasm. Finally, postoperative Horner's syndrome occurs in between 0.5% and 2% of patients in most series. In almost all reported cases, it is self-limited.

Entry into the pleural space occurs in as many as 30% of cases. This is usually recognized and easily evacuated at the time of operation without the need for a chest tube. The highest reported incidence of postoperative pneumothorax is 5%.

As mentioned previously, reports note injuries to all structures encountered during first-rib resection. Thus, supraclavicular approaches can lead to thoracic duct or even recurrent laryngeal nerve injury, although these injuries are rare. The risk of complications is increased with reoperative surgery. Many structures tend to be adherent in a particular pattern during these procedures, for example, the subclavian artery to the anterior scalene muscle. Care must be taken in these cases to identify all structures adequately.

PROGNOSIS

For most patients diagnosed with TOS, the prognosis is excellent, with improvement in symptoms following physical therapy or other adjustments in their working postures or activities. However, for the patients with more debilitating symptoms that require surgical intervention, the long-term prognosis is not clear. In addition, it is difficult to objectively study the outcomes following surgery for neurogenic TOS. With regards to functional outcomes, a small series of patients with neurogenic and venous TOS demonstrated an improvement in the disability of arm shoulder and hand instrument scores, a validated means of assessing upper extremity function.[57] However, larger controlled series are still lacking. We are currently collecting these data at our centers.

Several series have recurrence rates between 15 and 20% following first-rib resection by either the transaxillary or the supraclavicular route. Sanders reported a similar range and noted that most of these occur within 2 years of the initial operation.[59] In this same study, it was reported that the subjectively determined immediate postoperative success rate of 84% decreased to 59% at 2 years, 69% at 5 years, and as low as 41% at the 10- to 15-year interval using life-table analysis. Reoperation for these patients resulted in improvement so that at the 5- to 10-year interval 86% of patients still were reporting subjective benefits from their procedures. Patients with symptoms that were persistent, rather than recurrent, also tended to worse following reoperation.

A study by Sharp et al. focused on patients' ability to return to work following TOS surgery, noting that 80% of the patients in their study were able to do so and that 85% of the patients subjectively described their outcomes as good to excellent.[56] As was noted previously, employment and disability issues complicate outcomes in TOS. In Franklin's Washington state workers' compensation study, 40% of postoperative TOS patients were still not working 2 years after their operations; this percentage was actually worse at 5 years (44%).[16] Interestingly, the conservatively treated patients in this study did better in these regards, although this was a retrospective study in which the cohorts were not particularly well matched. Numerous other studies have shown worse outcomes when the patients have work or legal issues related to their TOS.[58]

Other factors predicting outcome following TOS surgery have been studied. Trauma as the event precipitating TOS is associated with poor outcomes in several series but not in others.[54,59] In addition, preoperative depression has been linked to worse outcome. In a report by Axelrod et al., those patients with preoperative depression were more likely to have continued functional and vocational disability following operation.[60] This study combined preoperative and postoperative interviews, psychological evaluations, and patient examinations, with an overall 67% subjectively reported "good or average" outcome. At an average of 47 months follow-up, 64% of patients were satisfied with their outcomes and 69% reported they would undergo operation again if faced with the same symptoms. At that time, 18% of the patients considered themselves disabled.

In one of the largest series of TOS patients, Roos reported that in 1844 transaxillary first-rib resections, 90% of patients were able to return to performing tasks they had been unable to perform preoperatively. In addition, 97% said that they would recommend rib resection to other patients with symptoms from TOS. A 5% recurrence was seen, which was better than the 19% seen with scalenectomy (although this was without rib resection). Green also reported higher recurrence following an anterior approach, although other authors have reported that the two approaches yielded equivalent recurrence rates.

The prognosis for untreated axillosubclavian venous thrombosis was one of progressive disability. Even after the institution of immobilization and anticoagulation, a study in 1970 revealed that 75% of patients had poor outcomes.[61] Following modern treatment protocols, most patients are able to resume normal activities, which is of particular importance in this group of predominantly young and otherwise healthy patients. The most important factor is the time to treatment following thrombosis, with most treatment failures occurring in the face of delays. As far as long-term results, Feugier et al. reported that all treated patients were asymptomatic at an average follow-up of 45 months.[62] If treated expeditiously, with complete recanalization of the vein and removal of the compressive rib, long-term sequelae are uncommon.[62] However, if this cannot be accomplished, repeated venous problems occur and can lead to debilitating situations.

A recent series evaluated outcomes in competitive athletes with axillosubclavian thrombosis.[63] In the series, 32 such patients underwent treatment, including lysis and decompression, and all patients eventually returned to full premorbid activities at an average interval of 3.5 months from operation to resumption of sports. Early operation correlated with a shorter postoperative convalescence.

The prognosis for patients with arterial involvement in TOS is highly variable, depending on the pattern of disease. Again, if the compressive element of the process is adequately dealt with, the issue becomes the arterial repair itself. The data for subclavian artery repairs can be found elsewhere but are generally good. Likewise, the outcomes from the rarely required sympathectomy parallel those for reflex-sympathetic dystrophy when performed in appropriately selected patients.

SUMMARY

Neurogenic TOS is a controversial diagnosis, and despite more than a century of treatment plans, acceptance of the diagnosis—or for that matter, the treatment—is still not universal in many cases. At the center of the controversy is the lack of objective tests for the most commonly diagnosed neurogenic form of the syndrome. Although physical maneuvers and data from scalene blocks can certainly support the diagnosis, it remains a clinical diagnosis in the absence of vascular involvement.

Likewise, assessing the outcomes of intervention for the neurogenic form is difficult and an area of debate. Studies have shown conflicting results, with patients reporting dissatisfaction with their first-rib resection but the willingness to undergo the operation again if the same symptoms were to develop contralaterally. Although an oversimplification, most surgical series reflect fairly high patient satisfaction, while reviews by other specialists tend to be less positive.

It is clear that outcome data will be of great value in this debate. First-rib surgery is mostly patient driven. Many of these patients have dealt with their symptoms for prolonged periods with no relief. They are more than willing to undergo surgery because nothing else has worked. Quality-of-life data from these patients will help surgeons decide to what extent interventions are actually helping improve the upper extremity function for these patients, as well the role surgeons can play in relieving their symptoms.

References

1. Peet RM, Hendricksen JD, Anderson TP, et al. Thoracic outlet syndrome: evaluation of the therapeutic exercise program. *Mayo Clin Proc* 1956;31:281-287.
2. Clagett OT. Presidential address: research and prosearch. *J Thorac Cardiovasc Surg* 1962;44:153-166.
3. Roos DB. Transaxillary approach for first rib resection to relieve thoracic outlet compression syndrome. *Ann Surg* 1966;163:354.
4. Machleder HI. *Vascular disorders of the upper extremity*. 3rd ed. Mt. Kisco, New York: Futura Press; 1999.
5. Roos DB. Historical perspectives and anatomic considerations: thoracic outlet syndrome. *Semin Thor Cardiovasc Surg* 1996;8:183-189.
6. Roos DB. Congenital anomalies associated with thoracic outlet syndrome: anatomy, symptoms, diagnosis and treatment. *Am J Surg* 1976;132: 771-778.
7. Sanders RJ, Haug CE, Pearce WH, et al. Recurrent thoracic outlet syndrome. *J Vasc Surg* 1990;12:390-400.
8. Nakada T, Knight RT, Mani RL. Intermittent venous claudication of the upper extremity: the pectoralis minor syndrome. *Ann Neurol* 1982;11: 433-434.
9. Machleder HI. Thoracic outlet syndromes: new concepts from a century of discovery. *Cardiovasc Surg* 1994;2:137-145.
10. Sanders RJ, Jackson CGR, Baushero N, et al. Scalene muscle abnormalities in traumatic thoracic outlet syndrome. *Am J Surg* 1990;159:231-236.
11. Machleder HI, Moll F, Verity A. The anterior scalene muscle in thoracic outlet compression syndrome. *Arch Surg* 1986;121:1141-1144.
12. Kaymak B, Ozçakar L, Inanici F, et al. Forearm bone mineral density measurements in thoracic outlet syndrome. *Rheumatol Int* 2008;28(9):891-893. [Epub 2008 Jan 30].
13. Rigberg DA, Gelabert HA. The management of thoracic outlet syndrome in teenaged patients. Ann Vasc Surg (in press).
14. Martins RS, Siqueira MG. Cervical rib fracture: an unusual etiology of thoracic outlet syndrome in a child. *Pediatr Neurosurg* 2007;43(4): 293-296.
15. Gilliat RW, LeQuesne PM, Logue V, et al. Wasting of the hand associated with a cervical rib or band. *J Neurol Neurosurg Psychiatry* 1970;33: 615-624.
16. Franklin GM, Fulton-Kehoe D, Bradley C, et al. Outcome of surgery for thoracic outlet syndrome in Washington state workers' compensation. *Neurology* 2000;54:1252-1257.
17. Urschel Jr HC, Razzuk MA, Hyland JW, et al. Thoracic outlet syndrome masquerading as coronary artery disease. *Ann Thorac Surg* 1973;16:239-248.
18. Roos DB, Owens JC. Thoracic outlet syndrome. *Arch Surg* 1966;93: 71-74.

19. Costigan DA, Wilbourn AJ. The elevated arm stress test: specificity in the diagnosis of thoracic outlet syndrome. *Neurology* 1985;35(Suppl 1): 74-75.
20. Wilbourn AJ. Thoracic outlet syndrome is overdiagnosed. *Muscle Nerve* 1999;22:130-136.
21. Toomingas A, Nilsson T, Hagberg M, et al. Predictive aspects of the abduction external rotation test among male industrial and office workers. *Am J Ind Med* 1999;35:32-42.
22. Roos DB. The place for scalenectomy and first-rib resection in thoracic outlet syndrome. *Surgery* 1982;92:1077-1085.
23. Abe M, Katsuaki I, Nishida J. Diagnosis, treatment and complications of thoracic outlet syndrome. *J Orthop Sci* 1999;4:66-69.
24. Demondion X, Bacqueville E, Paul C, et al. Thoracic outlet: assessment with MR imaging in asymptomatic and symptomatic populations. *Radiology* 2003;227(2):461-468.
25. Demirbag D, Unlu E, Ozdemir F, et al. The relationship between magnetic resonance imaging findings and postural maneuver and physical examination tests in patients with thoracic outlet syndrome: results of a double-blind, controlled study. *Arch Phys Med Rehabil* 2007;88(7): 844-851.
26. Estilaei SK, Byl NN. An evidence-based review of magnetic resonance angiography for diagnosing arterial thoracic outlet syndrome: review. *J Hand Ther* 2006;19(4):410-420; quiz, 420.
27. Hasanadka R, Towne JB, Seabrook GR, et al. Computed tomography angiography to evaluate thoracic outlet neurovascular compression. *Vasc Endovascular Surg* 2007;41(4):316-321.
28. Roos DB. Thoracic outlet syndrome is underdiagnosed. *Muscle Nerve* 1999;12:260-264.
29. Smith T, Trojaborg W. The diagnosis of thoracic outlet syndrome: value of sensory and motor conduction studies and quantitative electromyography. *Arch Neurol* 1987:1161-1163.
30. Jordan SE, Machleder HI. Diagnosis of thoracic outlet syndrome using electrophysiologically guided anterior scalene blocks. *Ann Vasc Surg* 1998;12:260-264.
31. Siivola J, Myllyla VV, Sulg I, et al. Brachial plexus and radicular neurography in relation to cortical evoked responses. *J Neurol Neurosurg Psychiatry* 1979;42:1151-1158.
32. Siivola J, Sulg I, Pokela R. Somatosensory evoked responses as a diagnostic aid in thoracic outlet syndrome (a preoperative study). *Acta Chir Scand* 1982;148:647-652.
33. Machleder HI, Mill F, Nuwer M, et al. Somatosensory evoked potentials in the assessment of thoracic outlet compression syndrome. *J Vasc Surg* 1987;6:177-184.
34. Aligne C, Barral X. Rehabilitation of patients with thoracic outlet syndrome. *Ann Vasc Surg* 1992;6:381-389.
35. Jordan SE, Ahn SS, Freischlag JA. Selective botulinum chemodenervation of the scalene muscles for treatment of neurogenic thoracic outlet syndrome. *Ann Vasc Surg* 2000;14:365-369.
36. Jordan SE, Ahn SS, Gelabert HA. Combining ultrasonography and electromyography for botulinum chemodenervation treatment of thoracic outlet syndrome: comparison with fluoroscopy and electromyography guidance. *Pain Physician* 2007;10(4):541-546.
37. Ohtsuka T, Wolf RK, Dunsker SB. Port-access first-rib resection. *Surg Endosc* 1999;13:940-942.
38. Gelabert HA, Jimenez JC, Rigberg DA. Comparison of retavase and urokinase for management of spontaneous subclavian vein thrombosis. *Ann Vasc Surg* 2007;21(2):149-154.
39. Perler BA, Mitchell SE. Percutaneous transluminal angioplasty and transaxillary first rib resection. A multidisciplinary approach to the thoracic outlet syndrome. *Am Surg* 1986;52:485-488.
40. Machleder HI. Evaluation of a new treatment strategy for Paget-Schroetter syndrome: spontaneous thrombosis of the axillary–subclavian vein. *J Vasc Surg* 1993;17:305-317.
41. Kunkel JM, Machleder HI. Treatment of Paget-Scroetter syndrome: a staged, multidisciplinary approach. *Arch Surg* 1989;124:1153-1158.
42. Angle N, Gelabert HA, Farooq MM, et al. Safety and efficacy of early surgical decompression of the thoracic outlet for Paget-Schroetter syndrome. *Ann Vasc Surg* 2001;15:37-42.
42a. de León R, Chang DC, Busse C, Call D, Freischlag JA. First rib resection and scalenectomy for chronically occluded subclavian veins: what does it really do? *Ann Vasc Surg* 2008;22(3):395-401.
43. Meier GH, Pollak JS, Rosenblatt M, et al. Initial experience with venous stents in exertional axillary–subclavian vein thrombosis. *J Vasc Surg* 1996;24:974-983.
44. Machleder HI. *Vascular disorders of the upper extremity*. 3rd ed. Armonk, New York: Futura Publishing; 1998;217–218.
45. Lindgren KA, Leino E, Lepantalo M, et al. Recurrent thoracic outlet syndrome after first rib resection. *Arch Phy Med Rehabil* 1991;72:208-210.
46. Roos DB. Recurrent thoracic outlet syndrome after first rib resection. *Acta Chir Belg* 1980;79:363-372.
47. Sessions RT. Recurrent thoracic outlet syndrome: causes and treatment. *South Med J* 1982;75:1453-1461.
48. Sanders RJ, Monsour JW, Gerber FG, et al. Scalenectomy versus first rib resection for treatment of the thoracic outlet syndrome. *Surgery* 1979;85:109-121.
49. Dale WA. Thoracic outlet compression syndrome. *Arch Surg* 1982;164: 149-153.
50. Wilbourn AJ. Thoracic outlet syndrome surgery causing severe brachial plexopathy. *Muscle Nerve* 1988;11:66-74.
51. Horowitz SH. Brachial plexus injuries with causalgia resulting from transaxillary rib resection. *Arch Surg* 1985;120:1189-1191.
52. Cherington M, Happer I, Machanic B, et al. Surgery for thoracic outlet syndrome may be hazardous to your health. *Muscle Nerve* 1986;9:632-634.
53. Roos DB. Thoracic outlet nerve compression. In: Rutherford; RB, ed. *Vascular surgery*. 3rd ed. Philadelphia: WB Saunders; 1989:858-875.
54. Green RM, McNamara J, Ouriel K. Long-term follow-up after thoracic outlet decompression: an analysis of factors determining outcome. *J Vasc Surg* 1991;14:739-746.
55. Chang DC, Lidor AO, Matsen SL, Freischlag JA. Reported in-hospital complications following rib resections for neurogenic thoracic outlet syndrome. *Ann Vasc Surg* 2007;21(5):564-570.
56. Sharp WJ, Nowak LR, Zamani T, et al. Long-term follow-up and patient satisfaction after surgery for thoracic outlet syndrome. *Ann Vasc Surg* 2001;15:32-36.
57. Cordobes-Gual J, Lozano-Vilardell P, Torreguitart-Mirada N, et al. Prospective study of the functional recovery after surgery for thoracic outlet syndrome. *Eur J Vasc Endovasc Surg* 2008;35(1):79-83.
58. Lepantalo M, Lindgren KA, Leino E, et al. Long-term outcome after resection of the first rib for thoracic outlet syndrome. *Br J Surg* 1989;76: 1255-1256.
59. Sanders RJ, Pearce WH. The treatment of thoracic outlet syndrome: a comparison of different operations. *J Vasc Surg* 1989;10:626-632.
60. Axelrod DA, Proctor MC, Geisser ME, et al. Outcomes after surgery for thoracic outlet syndrome. *J Vasc Surg* 2001;33:1220-1225.
61. Tilney ML, Griffiths HJ, Edwards EA. Natural history of major venous thrombosis of the upper extremity. *Arch Surg* 1970;101:792-796.
62. Feugier P, Aleksic I, Salari R, et al. Long-term results of venous revascularization for Paget-Scroetter syndrome in athletes. *Ann Vasc Surg* 2001;15:212-218.
63. Melby SJ, Vedantham S, Narra VR, et al. Comprehensive surgical management of the competitive athlete with effort thrombosis of the subclavian vein (Paget-Schroetter syndrome). *J Vasc Surg* 2008;47(4):809-820. [Epub 2008 Feb 14].

section

V

Mesenteric Vascular Disease

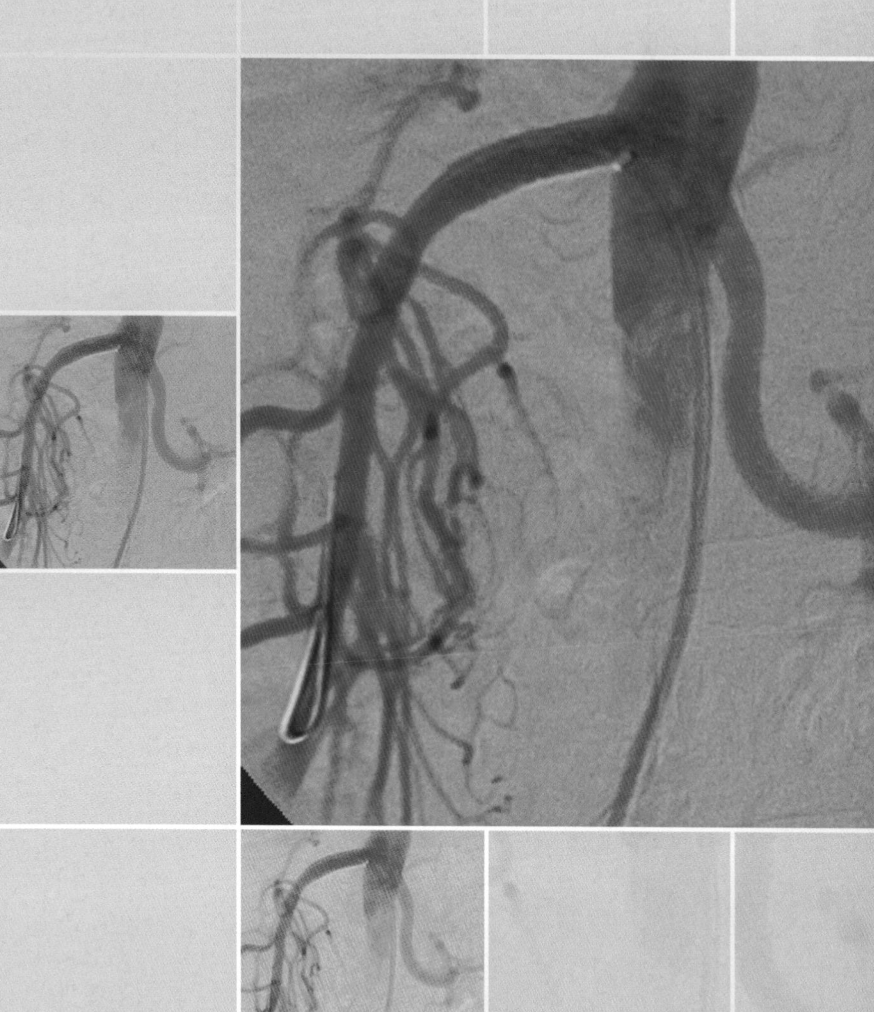

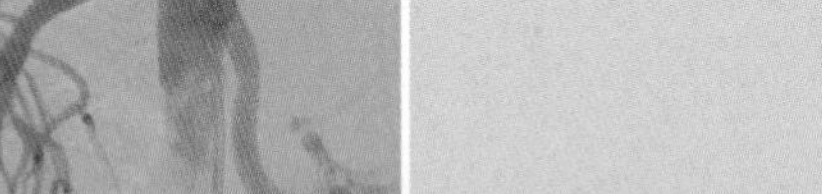

chapter 19

Acute and Chronic Mesenteric Ischemia

Thomas C. Bower, MD • Gustavo S. Oderich, MD

Key Points

Acute Mesenteric Ischemia

- Etiology
- Clinical presentation
- Diagnosis
- Treatment
- Results

Chronic Mesenteric Ischemia

- Prevalence and natural history
- Clinical presentation
- Diagnosis
- Percutaneous treatment
- Superior mesenteric artery versus celiac stenting
- Results
- Surgical treatment
- Bypass grafting
- Endarterectomy
- Postoperative management
- Outcomes

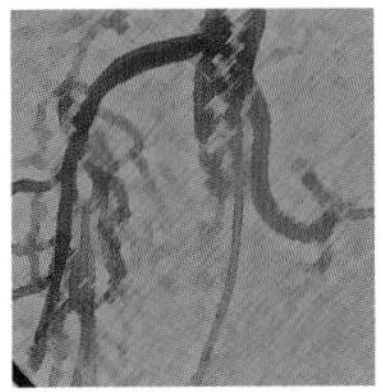

The diagnosis and management of patients with acute mesenteric arterial ischemia (AMAI) or chronic mesenteric arterial ischemia (CMAI) is challenging. Surgical results for patients treated with CMAI have improved, but there has been little advance in the early diagnosis and treatment of patients with AMAI. Endovascular therapy has emerged as an option in patients with CMAI.

This chapter reviews the classification, etiology, clinical presentation, diagnosis, and treatment for patients with AMAI and CMAI. The management of patients with nonocclusive mesenteric ischemia is not discussed. Much of the information in this chapter is based on our experience, as well as selected comparative data from the literature.

ACUTE MESENTERIC ISCHEMIA

The etiology of AMAI is primarily due to arterial obstruction.[1-3] Emboli usually originate in the heart but may come from proximal aortic aneurysms or atherosclerotic lesions.[1-2] Typically, the proximal small bowel is spared but the remainder of the small intestine and proximal colon are ischemic because the embolus occludes the superior mesenteric artery (SMA) a few centimeters beyond its origin, sparing the proximal branches.[1]

Acute thrombosis of the SMA is often secondary to an underlying proximal atherosclerotic lesion.[1] Dissections, aneurysms, and vasculitis are rare causes. Most of the small bowel and colon are ischemic in various proportions depending on the status of the collateral circulation.[1]

Clinical Presentation and Diagnosis

Most patients are in the sixth or seventh decade of life.[1-2,4] The patients have a history of severe abdominal pain out of proportion to their physical examination findings. From a recent review at our institution by Park et al., 55 of 58 patients (95%) had abdominal pain for a median of 24 hours before presentation to the hospital.[2] The other three patients presented in extremis with acidosis and shock. Nausea and diarrhea occurred in 30% to 40% of patients, and blood per rectum happened in only 16%.[2]

No laboratory abnormality is 100% specific for AMAI. Leukocytosis, lactic acidosis, seromuscular enzyme levels, and phosphate abnormalities are the most common findings but are noted late in the course of the acute episode.[3]

In the 10-year review by Park et al., AMAI occurred more often in women than men.[2] The mean age of patients was 67 years, but AMAI was seen over a wide age range. Mesenteric artery thrombosis occurred in 64% of patients, embolism in 28%, and nonocclusive mesenteric ischemia in the remaining 8%. Atherosclerosis in other vascular beds was common, regardless of etiology. Patients with embolic occlusion of the SMA were older than those with thrombosis and had atrial fibrillation or ventricular arrhythmias more often. Patients with SMA thrombosis were usually female, and more than half had a history of chronic abdominal pain and weight loss consistent with CMAI.[2]

Diagnosis

The key in diagnosis is a high index of clinical suspicion.[1-18] In many cases, because of the nonspecific nature of the pain, computed tomography (CT) is the first study performed. Whether CT is performed with standard axial images or with an angiographic format (CTA), diagnosis can be made on the basis of this study alone.[2,19-20] In our experience, approximately 60% of patients with AMAI had CT scan abnormalities, including dilatation, thickening of the bowel, pneumatosis intestinalis, and filling defects in the proximal SMA.[2]

Embolic occlusion of the SMA appears as an abrupt cutoff or meniscus sign several centimeters beyond the origin of the artery. The middle colic artery is often spared, and delayed images show refilling of the distal SMA branches. The SMA may not fill with contrast in patients with in situ thrombosis. In patients with acute or chronic symptoms, the celiac artery, inferior mesenteric artery (IMA), or internal iliac artery may be stenotic, but intestinal collaterals may be well developed (e.g., meandering mesenteric artery). The SMA trunk beyond the occlusion may be seen if delayed images are done, but it is difficult to image the distal arcades.[1,21]

Treatment

AMAI is a surgical emergency. Patients with abdominal pain or other risk factors suggestive of AMAI should undergo arteriography or CTA before operation if there is no evidence of peritonitis or shock. Patients with rebound tenderness, abdominal rigidity, severe acidosis, or shock should undergo immediate operation.[1-2]

Since the mortality rate for patients treated operatively for AMAI is high, select patients may be candidates for other therapies.[1-20] Thrombolysis followed by balloon angioplasty or stent placement of the stenotic artery at the time of arteriography is a reasonable option if diagnosis is made early, the patient is hemodynamically stable, there are no signs of peritonitis, and the thrombus burden is small.[1-2,22-24] Failure of thrombolytic therapy or a worsening clinical status warrants operation.[1] If therapy is successful, we still favor laparotomy since the extent and degree of intestinal ischemia cannot be accurately predicted by physical examination, laboratory studies, or diagnostic tests. Only eight patients with AMAI were treated with endovascular techniques at the Mayo Clinic through 1999.[2] Six had transcatheter vasodilator therapy for nonocclusive mesenteric ischemia. Of the two who had balloon angioplasty or catheter-directed thrombolysis, one required laparotomy. Whether percutaneous techniques will lower the mortality and morbidity is yet to be determined.[1-2]

Operative treatment of AMAI is dictated by the appearance of the intestine and the status of blood flow within the SMA. The goals of therapy include restoration of SMA blood flow and resection of nonviable bowel.[1] Importantly, the severity of ischemia to the bowel may be masked by its appearance. The bowel may be dull gray, lack peristalsis, or have patchy areas of cyanosis.[1] No SMA pulse is palpable at the base of the mesentery in patients with SMA thrombosis. A patient with an embolus may have a water-hammer pulse in the proximal artery but an absent pulse distally. Foul-smelling fluid or perforation is seen in advanced cases of ischemia. Extensive microemboli produce multiple patchy areas of ischemia throughout the entire small and large intestine and infarcts of the solid organs.[1]

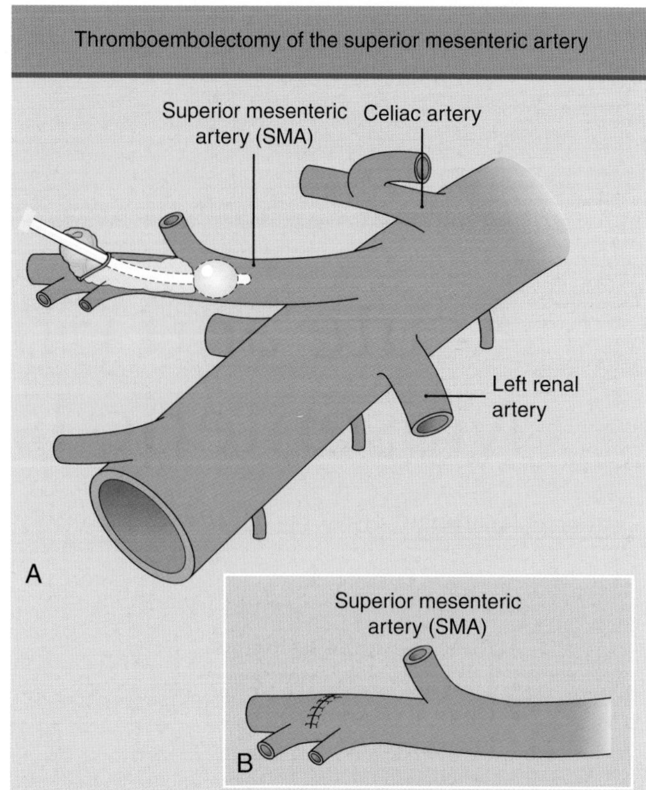

Figure 19-1. A, Thromboembolectomy of the superior mesenteric artery performed through a transverse incision. **B,** The incision is closed primarily.

Methods to restore blood flow to the SMA depend on the operative findings and the preoperative arteriogram or CTA, if one was obtained. The SMA is isolated at the base of the mesentery with the transverse colon retracted superiorly and the small intestine retracted toward the right side except for the distal duodenum or proximal jejunum.[1] If the artery is soft, it is opened transversely. Fogarty catheters (Nos. 3 and 4) are passed proximally and distally in the artery to extract the embolic material and thrombus (Figures 19-1 and 19-2). Passage of the Fogarty catheter into the main divisions of the artery must be done with care to avoid perforation of these segments. The artery should be opened longitudinally if clinical findings or the arteriogram suggests in situ thrombosis or if atherosclerotic disease is palpable in the SMA.[1] A longitudinal arteriotomy can be closed with a patch of saphenous vein, bovine pericardium, or prosthetic if excellent inflow is achieved. A transverse arteriotomy is closed primarily. A bypass to the artery is required if inflow is poor. The bypass may be performed retrograde from the infrarenal aorta or iliac artery or antegrade from the supraceliac aorta.[1-2] The group from Portland, Oregon, has championed the use of a retrograde graft from the distal infrarenal aorta or proximal common iliac artery, which is then looped in a C fashion so that the distal anastomosis of the graft is in an antegrade position vis-à-vis the SMA.[1,25] This graft orientation may minimize the chance of kinking or buckling, which is a problem with retrograde grafts performed by other methods.[1,25] A prosthetic bifurcated graft from the supraceliac aorta is used to reconstruct both the celiac artery and the SMA in stable patients

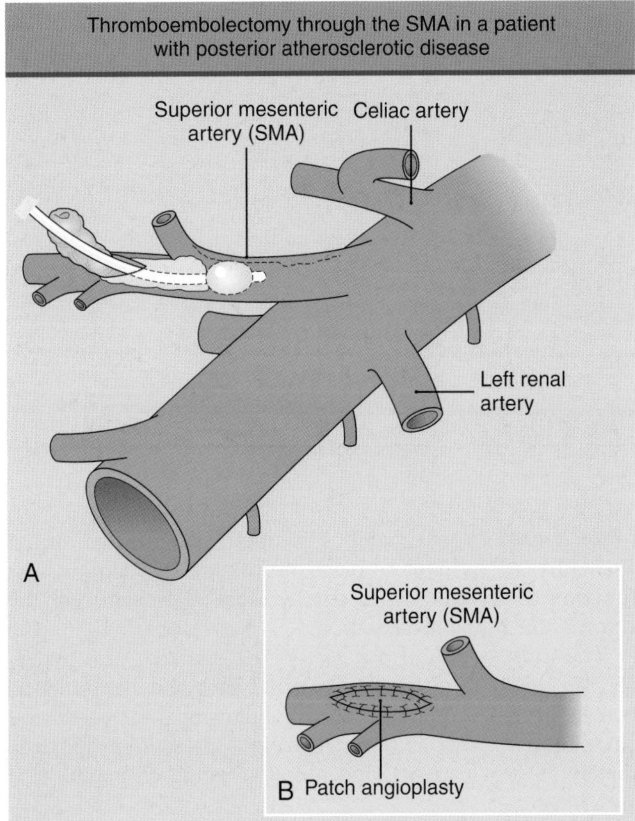

Figure 19-2. Thromboembolectomy through the superior mesenteric artery in a patient with posterior atherosclerotic disease. The artery is opened longitudinally **(A)** and closed with either an autogenous or a prosthetic patch **(B)**.

with severe occlusive disease of both arteries and no peritoneal contamination.[2] Celiac reconstruction should follow that of the SMA in this circumstance. However, saphenous vein graft can be based from the iliac artery in patients with gross contamination of the peritoneal cavity. This reconstruction is quicker than the creation of a pantaloon saphenous vein graft taken from the supraceliac aorta. Thromboendarterectomy of the celiac artery and of the SMA is rarely performed in the acute setting because the exposure is time consuming and the technique is demanding.[26] Wyers and associates recently reported the use of retrograde mesenteric stenting during laparotomy as an alternative to surgical bypass.[27] The infracolic SMA is exposed as noted earlier. The SMA origin is accessed in a retrograde fashion using a 6-French (Fr) sheath and a 0.035-inch system. The SMA lesion is predilated (using a 3-mm balloon) and then treated with a balloon-expandable stent.

Once blood flow is restored, an assessment of bowel viability is necessary. Clinical examination is helpful but less reliable than other techniques. The presence of pulse in the distal mesenteric arcades, return of peristalsis and normal color to the bowel, and audible Doppler flow on the mesenteric and antimesenteric borders of the intestine are encouraging signs.[1,28] Intravenous fluorescein with ultraviolet imaging is useful. Uniform perfusion under an ultraviolet lamp indicates a viable bowel, whereas patchy or no perfusion indicates an ischemic, nonviable bowel.[1-2,28-29] We have a low threshold to leave the abdomen open when bowel edema is significant to avoid an abdominal compartment syndrome.[1-2] Our preference has been to perform a second-look procedure within 24 hours in all but the rarest of cases, as we have had patients who remain hemodynamically stable despite progressive bowel ischemia. The decision to perform a second-look procedure is made at the first operation.

A few patients with advanced intestinal ischemia are hemodynamically unstable en route to the operating room even with aggressive fluid resuscitation. Abdominal exploration often reveals large segments of severely ischemic or gangrenous bowel. If a decision is made to attempt revascularization, these patients benefit from clamping (bowel clamps) of the venous outflow of the gangrenous bowel before isolation and reconstruction of the SMA. This reduces the washout of toxins into the portal circulation, which helps sterilize hemodynamics as restoration of blood flow to the SMA proceeds.

At the Mayo Clinic, 43 of 58 patients with AMAI had revascularization of the SMA.[2] The others could not be revascularized because of the extent of gangrenous bowel. Bypass grafting was performed in 22 patients, thromboembolectomy in 19, endarterectomy in 5, and reimplantation in 2. Eleven had patch angioplasty of the SMA. Of 22 patients with SMA bypass, 17 had polyester grafts, of which 10 were bifurcated. The other 5 patients had vein grafts. Inflow was from the supraceliac aorta in 15 patients and from the infrarenal aorta in 7. Only 23 patients (40%) had second-look procedures, but almost half of the patients had additional bowel resected.[2]

Summary

The mortality rate from AMAI is high (24% to 96%) and has changed little over the years (Table 19-1).[1-13] In the Mayo Clinic report, the 30-day mortality rate was highest for patients with nonocclusive AMAI (80%) but was 31% and 32% for patients with SMA embolism and thrombosis, respectively.[2] Major complications can be expected in one half to three fourths of patients, with respiratory failure and multiorgan system failure being most common.[2] Factors associated with increased mortality rate include multisystem organ failure (67%), recurrent mesenteric thrombosis during the same hospitalization (50%), and age over 70 years (40%). Long-term survival was only 59% at 1 year and 32% at 2 years. More than one third of patients died from recurrent mesenteric ischemia during late follow-up.[2]

CHRONIC MESENTERIC ISCHEMIA

A report from the Peter Bent Brigham Hospital by Dunphy in 1936 correlated fatal intestinal infarction and obstruction of the intestinal arteries to clinical histories of chronic recurrent abdominal pain. Of 12 patients who died of intestinal infarction, 7 (58%) had a history of recurrent abdominal pain, which preceded the fatal event by weeks, months, or years.[30]

Atherosclerotic disease of the mesenteric arteries usually affects their origins. The prevalence of disease ranges from 6% to 10% in random autopsy studies to 14% to 24% of patients undergoing aortography.[3,31-32] It is generally felt that at least two of the three intestinal arteries must be either occluded or tightly stenotic to cause symptoms because of the rich collateral network among the celiac artery, SMA, IMA, and hypogastrics.[31] We have treated several patients, however, with SMA disease alone who had relief of symptoms after single-vessel

Table 19-1
Clinical Results of Contemporary Series (1999 to 2007) of Acute Mesenteric Ischemia

Author (Year)	n	% Embolism	% Thrombosis	% Other	Mortality n (%)
Mamode et al. (1999)[4]	57	—	—	—	46 (81)
Foley et al. (2000)[25]	21	48	52	—	5 (24)
Endean et al. (2001)[14]	43	38	36	26	26 (60)
Park et al., Mayo Clinic (2002)[2]	53	28	64	8	17 (32)
Edwards et al. (2003)[15]	76	42	58	—	46 (62)
Char et al. (2003)[16]	22	—	—	—	8 (36)
Acosta-Merida et al. (2006)[17]	132	50	25	25	86 (65)
Kougias et al. (2007)[18]	72	33	67	—	19 (26)
Total	476				253 (53)

reconstruction. Importantly, these patients had poorly developed collaterals between their mesenteric arteries.

Data are limited regarding the natural history of asymptomatic patients found to have high-grade stenoses or occlusions of one or more visceral arteries. Data published by Thomas et al. from the University of Kansas provide some insight.[32] They reviewed 980 aortograms between 1989 and 1995 and found 60 patients (6%) who had significant visceral artery disease. Of these, 15 patients had involvement of all three visceral vessels. In addition, 4 of the 15 patients (27%) developed symptoms over a mean follow-up of 2.6 years and 1 died from intestinal infarction.[32] More recently, Wilson and associates reported the results of a prospective cohort study of 553 elderly patients who were screened for mesenteric arterial disease using duplex ultrasound. The prevalence of critical (more than 70%) stenosis or occlusion of the SMA, celiac axis, or both was 18%.[33] None of the 90 patients with mesenteric arterial disease developed symptoms at follow-up of 7 years. We have followed asymptomatic patients with significant three-vessel involvement closely and have a low threshold to treat them if they develop abdominal pain.[31] Intestinal ischemia or infarction has occurred after aortic reconstructions in patients who had no visceral ischemic symptoms preoperatively but in whom visceral artery stenosis or occlusion was documented.[31] Reconstruction of the SMA, reimplantation of the IMA, or hypogastric artery revascularization is necessary in such cases.[31]

Clinical Presentation

The typical patient with CMAI is between the ages of 40 and 70 years and is usually female. The classical symptoms include abdominal pain, weight loss, and food fear.[31,34] Pain is often postprandial and often begins within 10 to 30 minutes of meals. It is usually midabdominal in location, is crampy, and has a duration from minutes to hours.[34-36] We recently reviewed 229 consecutive patients treated for CMAI with open or endovascular revascularization.[37] Abdominal pain was documented in 96% of the patients (postprandial in 74%) and weight loss in 84%. Mean duration of symptoms before treatment was 15 months but ranged from 1 month to 5 years. At times, the clinical presentation is less specific, and patients may have vague midabdominal pain, nausea, vomiting, or a change in bowel habits without a classical postprandial component to the pain.[34] Approximately 10% of our patients had diffuse small ulcerations in the stomach or proximal duodenum, liver function abnormalities, or patchy areas of ischemia in the colon as the initial presentation.

The most common risk factors are smoking and hypertension.[31,33-34] Two thirds of patients have had symptomatic disease in the coronary, cerebrovascular, renal, or peripheral circulation.[31,34] An abdominal bruit is present in approximately 50% of patients, and muscle wasting or inanition is seen in severe cases.[31]

Diagnosis

Diagnosis of CMAI is suggested by the clinical history and physical examination, and confirmed by one or more studies such as duplex ultrasonography, magnetic resonance angiography, CTA, or biplane aortography.[3] Tests of intestinal absorptive and excretory function have not been useful.[3,38]

Duplex ultrasonography has been used to screen patients with abdominal pain or an epigastric bruit. The group at the Oregon Health Science University uses peak systolic velocities in the SMA of more than 275 cm/sec and velocities in the celiac artery exceeding 200 cm/sec to indicate stenoses of 70% or more.[3,39] While these velocities were initially derived from a retrospective comparative analysis of duplex scan and aortography, they were later confirmed in a blinded prospective study of 100 patients. This peak systolic velocity, as an indicator of more than 70% SMA stenosis, had a sensitivity of 92%, specificity of 96%, positive predictive value of 80%, and negative predictive value of 99%. A velocity of 200 cm/sec in the celiac artery as a predictor of a 70% stenosis had somewhat lower values.[3,39] End diastolic flow velocities of 45 cm/sec or higher in the SMA and reversal of blood flow in the hepatic and splenic arteries also indicate significant lesions in these vessels.[40-41] Preprandial versus postprandial blood flow velocities are not specific enough to distinguish physiologically appropriate from inappropriate blood flow responses.[3]

Magnetic resonance angiography and CTA are used most often to study patients with visceral lesions. Biplane aortography is used in select patients with long-segment stenosis or occlusion or in those suspected of having vasculitis. Biplane views of the aorta define the location, severity, and extent of visceral artery involvement; identify the presence of concomitant lesions in the renal or iliac arteries; and indicate

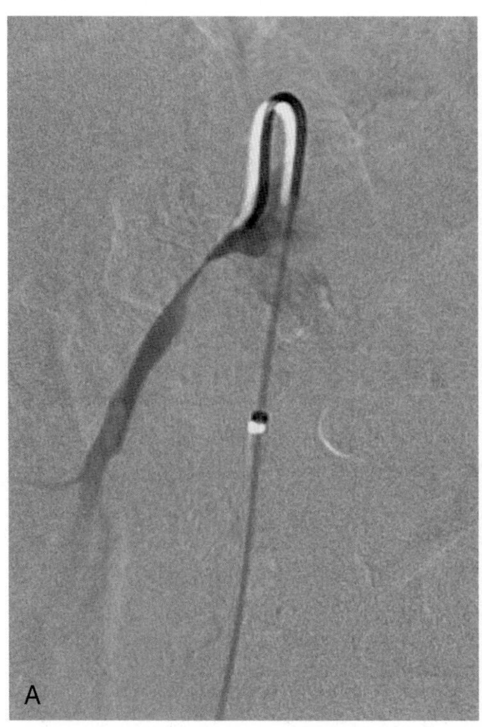

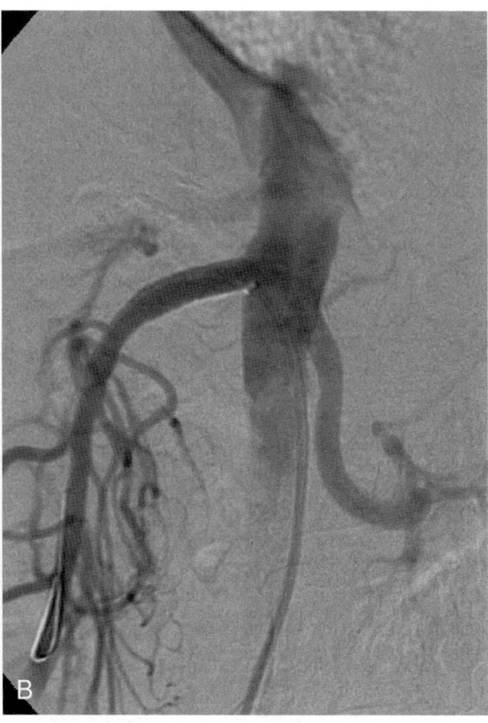

Figure 19-3. **A,** Abdominal aortogram reveals a high-grade, short-segment (less than 2 cm) stenosis of the superior mesenteric artery. **B,** Repeat angiography after placement of a balloon-expandable stent reveals no evidence of residual stenosis.

the suitability of the supraceliac or infrarenal aorta as inflow sites.[26,31] While extensive intestinal collaterals may be evident on arteriography or CTA, the presence or the absence of a collateral network cannot be used as the only means of determining hemodynamic significance of visceral artery lesions.[3] Arteriography in 98 patients operated upon at the Mayo Clinic for CMAI over the last 10 years showed occlusion or critical stenosis (70% to 99%) of the SMA in 92%, of the celiac artery in 83%, and of both arteries in 78%.[34]

More common conditions such as pancreatic cancer may have similar clinical presentations. Therefore, preoperative tests such as CT, upper and lower gastrointestinal endoscopy, or ultrasonography are necessary.[3,31,34]

Endovascular Treatment

Treatment of visceral artery stenoses and short-segment occlusion by balloon angioplasty or stent placement is attractive since many patients with CMAI are older and malnourished.[23] The main advantages are shorter length of hospital stay and potentially less morbidity and mortality. Recurrent stenosis has been the bane of this technique because the atherosclerotic lesions are an extension of intraaortic plaque.[42-45] Although no comparative data exist of angioplasty versus stenting for mesenteric artery stenosis, most interventionalists use primary stenting for mesenteric ostial lesions based on improved patency rates obtained with such an approach for renal artery stenosis. We currently recommend percutaneous treatment in older, higher-risk patients with significant cardiac, pulmonary, and renal comorbidities. This modality is also attractive as a bridge to surgical bypass in patients with significant malnutrition. Mesenteric stenting is also an option in good-risk patients with favorable anatomy. The ideal lesion is a short-segment (less than 2 cm) SMA stenosis without eccentric calcification or thrombus (Figure 19-3). Percutaneous treatment of more complex lesions, such as a long stenosis, tandem lesions, or occlusion, may be needed in some high-risk patients.

Technique

The goal of percutaneous treatment is primary stenting of the SMA. The risk of dissection, embolization, stent fractures, and residual stenosis is higher with treatment of celiac axis lesions because that trunk may be short and thick and is surrounded by fibromuscular tissue. Celiac axis intervention is only considered in high-risk patients if SMA recanalization is not possible or yields a suboptimal result (flow-limiting stenosis or dissection). In our experience, angioplasty of the IMA is associated with excessive risk of rupture, dissection, or embolization.

Preprocedure planning with CTA is paramount. Key factors include the angle of origin of the mesenteric vessels in relation to the aortic axis, the amount of calcium and thrombus load, and the presence of important collaterals in proximity to the target lesion. A brachial artery approach is preferred for patients with a very angulated SMA or in those with occlusion or long-segment lesions (Figure 19-4).

Aortography and mesenteric angiography are preferred using a 5-Fr sheath, 0.035-inch system. A 5-Fr diagnostic flush catheter is used for anteroposterior and lateral aortography, and a 5-Fr SOS catheter (femoral approach) or multipurpose angiographic (MPA) catheter (brachial approach) is used for selective mesenteric catheterization. The optimal projection to display the proximal celiac artery and SMA is a lateral view, and for the origin of the IMA it is a 15-degree right lateral–oblique view. Systemic heparinization (80 mg/kg) is used before intervention. An activated clotting time of greater than 250 seconds is maintained during the case. From the brachial approach, the 5-Fr sheath is exchanged to a 7-Fr, 90-cm Raabe sheath, which is positioned at the origin of the SMA. A 7-Fr MPA guide catheter combined with a 5-Fr MPA catheter

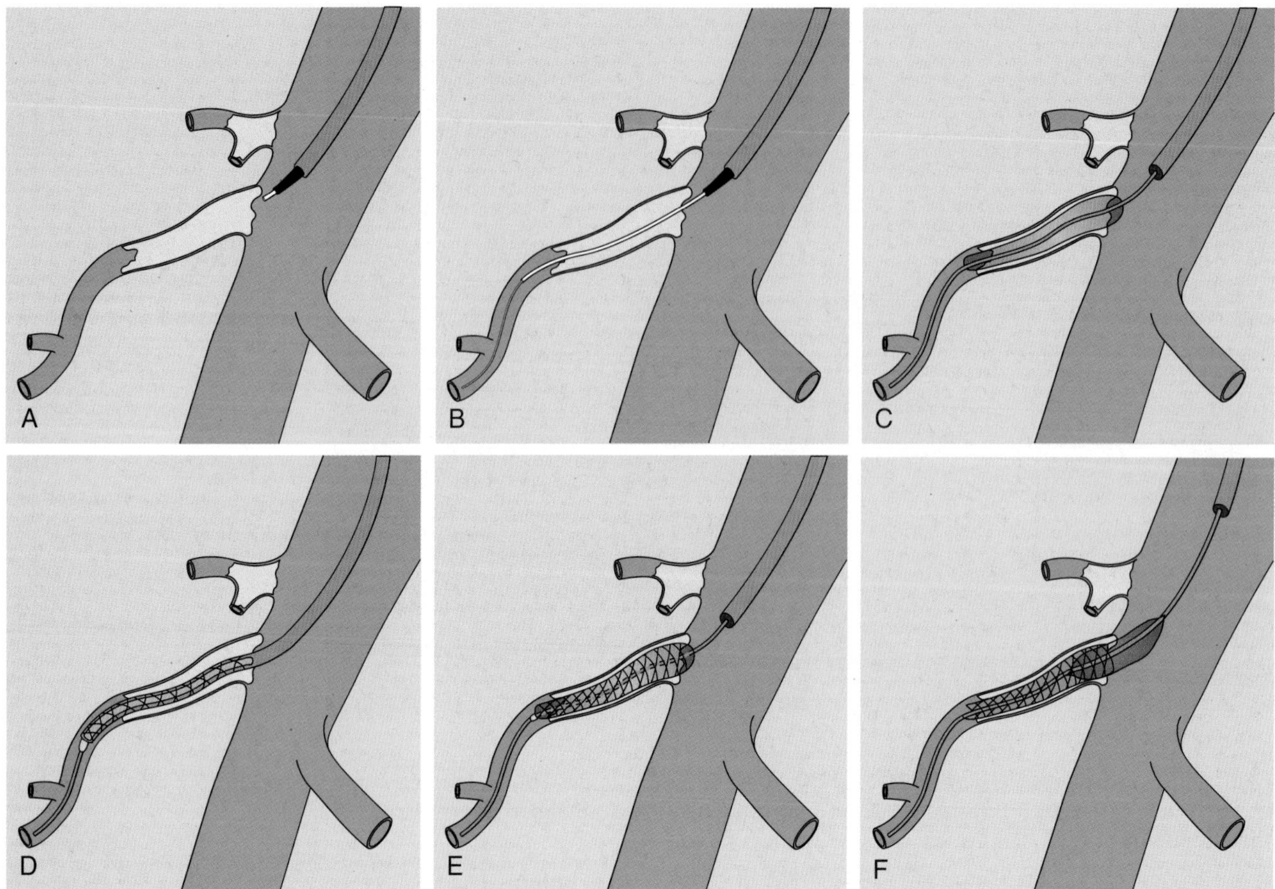

Figure 19-4. Illustration of technique of recanalization of superior mesenteric artery using brachial approach. **A,** A 7-Fr, 90-cm Raabe sheath combined with a 7-Fr multipurpose angiographic (MPA) guide catheter and a 5-Fr MPA catheter are advanced from the left brachial approach to provide support for selective catheterization. **B,** Following passage of the wire, the catheter is advanced across the lesion to confirm true lumen access. **C,** Predilatation is performed using a 3- to 4-mm angioplasty balloon. A balloon-expandable stent is advanced under protection of the sheath **(D)**, and the stent is deployed with minimal (1 to 2 mm) protrusion into the aortic lumen **(E)**. **F,** The proximal aspect of the stent may be flared using a larger balloon to facilitate reintubation in the event of restenosis.

allows sufficient support to cross a tight stenoses or occlusion, although most SMA stenosis can be crossed with a 5-Fr MPA catheter alone (Figure 19-4). The lesion is crossed with a 0.014- to 0.018-inch stiff wire (BMW or PT-II wire). The tip of the wire should be positioned within the main trunk of the SMA or within a large jejunal branch to avoid perforation and dissection. Predilatation using a 2- or 3-mm balloon is advised for tight stenosis or occlusion. A balloon-expandable stent (5 to 7 mm diameter) is deployed, covering the entire length of the lesion, with minimal (1 mm) protrusion into the aortic lumen. Ideally, the proximal aspect of the stent should be flared to minimize residual stenosis at the ostium and to facilitate recatheterization if the patients develops symptomatic restenosis. The use of a small-profile 0.014- to 0.018-inch system allows rapid exchange and more flexibility and trackability than a 0.035-inch system, while the 0.035-inch system has the advantages of more support, more hoop strength, better visualization, and less cost.

Clopidrogel is started the day of the intervention and continued for 8 weeks, after which patients are kept on aspirin. A duplex ultrasound scan is obtained before dismissal to serve as a baseline for future comparison. Patients are followed with clinical examination and duplex ultrasound every 6 months during the first year and annually thereafter.

Surgical Treatment

Open surgical repair for patients with symptomatic CMAI is offered to good-risk patients, especially those 70 years or younger.[31-37,46-51] Several operative techniques can be used to perform either single- or multiple-vessel reconstructions in an antegrade or a retrograde fashion. Each technique has advantages and disadvantages. Controversy surrounds the number of visceral vessels reconstructed, which artery is the most important to revascularize, and the configuration of the graft.[26,31,34]

Bypass Grafting

Reconstruction of the celiac artery and the SMA with a bifurcated prosthetic graft originating from the supraceliac aorta is performed in more than 80% of our patients.[24] The others have had either single-vessel reconstruction to the SMA or, rarely, had all three mesenteric arteries reconstructed by transaortic endarterectomy.[33,34]

The operation is done through an upper midline or bilateral subcostal incision, depending on the patient's body habitus and costal cartilage flare. The lesser omentum is opened, and the left lobe of the liver is retracted after division of the left triangular ligament. The esophagus is retracted toward the patient's left side with a nasogastric tube in place, and the stomach is gently retracted caudally. The diaphragmatic crura are divided, and the supraceliac aorta is dissected free to allow performance of the proximal graft anastomosis. Usually, only the celiac trunk and proximal hepatic and splenic arteries need isolation, but with more extensive disease, the common hepatic artery may require dissection toward the origin of the gastroduodenal artery. The left gastric artery is often small and may be divided without sequelae. This generally facilitates celiac anastomosis and makes tunneling of the SMA graft behind the pancreas easier.[26]

The SMA may be exposed above or below the pancreas depending on the extent of disease and the patient's anatomy. As much as 3 to 4 cm of the SMA may be dissected free by mobilization of the superior border of the pancreas. Otherwise, the artery is isolated at the base of the mesentery beyond the ligament of Treitz as discussed for patients with AMAI.[26]

Patients are given heparin and Mannitol before aortic cross-clamp. The use of two cross-clamps affords better exposure for the proximal aortic-graft anastomosis than a partial occlusion clamp. A straight or angled aortic clamp (Cherry supraceliac clamp) and a Wylie hypogastric clamp work well. Placed appropriately, occlusion of the lumbar vessels is achieved as well. A vertical or slightly oblique aortotomy is made. A 12 × 7 mm knitted polyester graft is sewn end to side to the aorta with permanent suture. Aortic cross-clamp time rarely exceeds 20 minutes and most often ranges from 12 to 15 minutes. The risks of renal ischemia or distal microembolization is low when patients are properly selected and have a relatively disease-free supraceliac aorta.[26]

The celiac artery anastomosis is performed end to end, most often with a tongue of graft extending onto one of the two major branch arteries, usually the hepatic. The anastomosis to the SMA is done end to end when performed above the pancreas but end to side when the anastomosis is performed at the base of the mesentery (Figure 19-5).[26] It is important to relax retraction when cutting the graft limbs to length to avoid angulation or kinking, whether antegrade or retrograde bypass is done.

Supraceliac-origin grafts are a poor choice in patients with compromised cardiac or pulmonary function or those with extensive atherosclerosis or circumferential calcification of the supraceliac aorta. In these cases, infrarenal sources of inflow are preferred.[26,31]

The infrarenal aorta, a prior infrarenal aortic graft, or the iliac artery are excellent inflow sources and have been preferred by the group from the Oregon Health Sciences University.[25,31] The infrarenal aorta may be replaced, if diseased, with retrograde reconstruction of the SMA based from the aortic graft.[26,31] In general, we reconstruct only one artery (the SMA) if a retrograde graft is used. The proximal anastomosis is performed (Pilling-Weck, Fort Washington, Pennsylvania) to the anterolateral wall of the aorta and can be done with either two cross-clamps or a partial occlusion clamp, depending on the aortic size and the presence of atherosclerosis or calcification within that segment.[26] A 6-mm coronary punch can be used to remove a portion or portions of the aortic wall. The Oregon group prefers the proximal anastomosis at the distal infrarenal aorta or the infrarenal aorta–right common iliac artery junction.[25,31] The key to avoiding elongation, angulation, or kinking of the graft is to cut it to length with the SMA in a nearly

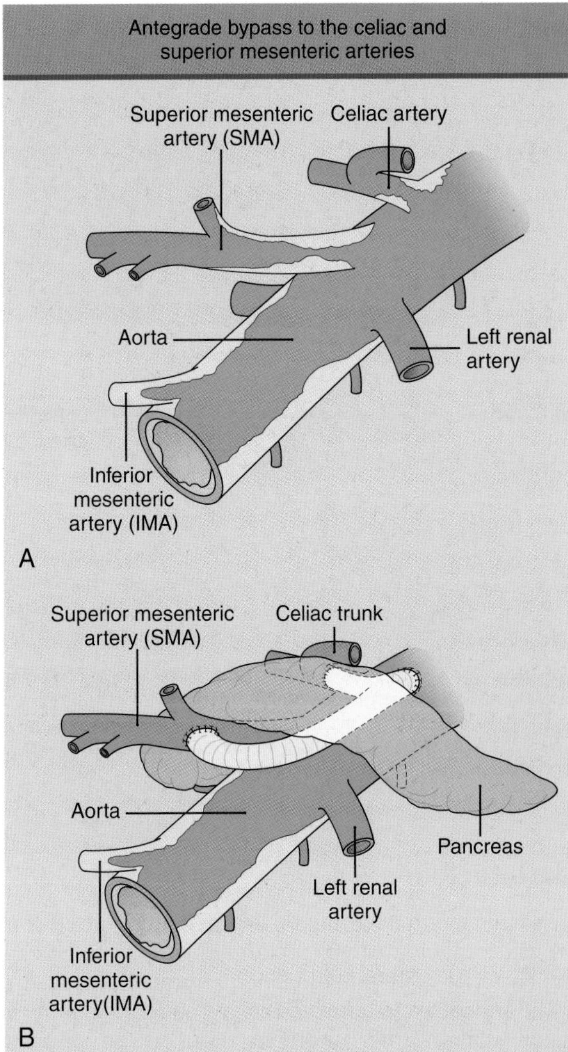

Figure 19-5. **A,** Patient with chronic mesenteric ischemia and high-grade stenoses of the celiac and superior mesenteric arteries. The patient was reconstructed with a bifurcated synthetic graft taken from the supraceliac aorta. **B,** The celiac anastomosis is done end to end, and the superior mesenteric artery anastomosis is done end to side. The latter graft limb is tunneled behind the pancreas.

anatomical position. If a short retrograde graft is performed, the distal anastomosis is done first, followed by the aortic graft anastomosis (Figure 19-6). The Portland group has favored a C-shaped graft configuration (as mentioned earlier)[25,31] and has had excellent results and few graft failures with this technique. In our most recent analysis, retrograde grafts worked as well as antegrade grafts, although the patients with the former were older and had reduced life spans.[26,34] Some patients have extensive circumferential aortic calcification but soft common or external iliac arteries, which can serve as good donor vessels. Either the right or the left common iliac artery can be chosen for inflow depending on the orientation of that artery to the normal anatomical position of the SMA.[26] Two-vessel reconstructions can be performed with retrograde grafts by doing a side-to-side anastomosis to the SMA and an end-to-side anastomosis to the common hepatic artery. These grafts may be passed on top of or beneath the pancreas and curved in a C shape toward the hepatic artery.

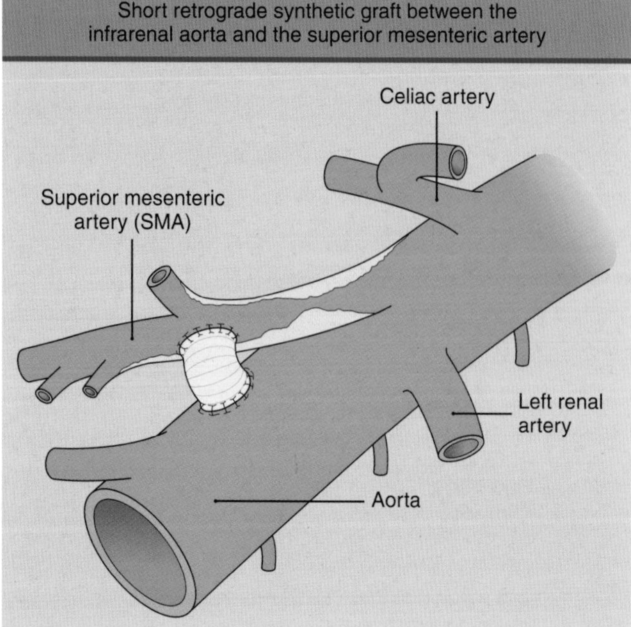

Figure 19-6. Short retrograde synthetic graft placed between the infrarenal aorta and the superior mesenteric artery (SMA). The graft length is usually 1 to 1.5 cm. The distal anastomosis to the SMA is done first, followed by the aortic anastomosis, to allow return of the SMA to its normal anatomical position.

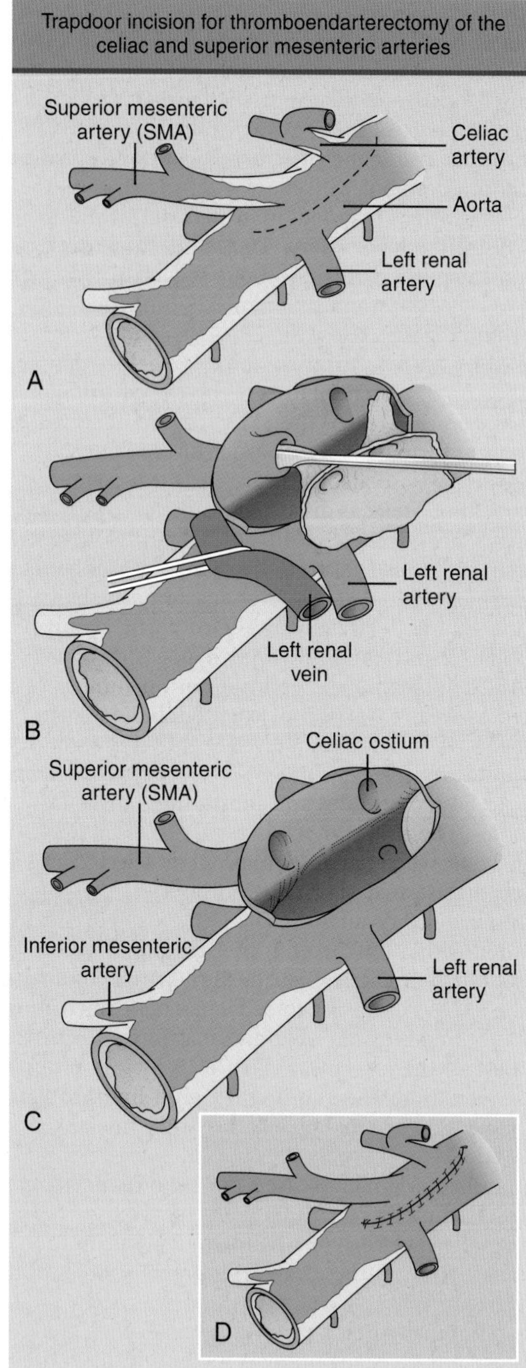

Figure 19-7. Thromboendarterectomy of the celiac and superior mesenteric arteries done after medial visceral rotation. **A,** The aortotomy can be made longitudinally or in a trapdoor fashion. **B,** The endarterectomy is done using an eversion technique. **C,** Distal tacking sutures are placed. **D,** The aortotomy is closed primarily.

Endarterectomy

Transaortic endarterectomy of the mesenteric arteries may be considered over other techniques of revascularization when bacterial contamination or perforated bowel, previous abdominal irradiation, extensive abdominal wall hernias, or other hostile conditions occur.[26] Our preference is to approach the paravisceral aorta through a full-length, midline abdominal or subcostal incision. These incisions carry lower pulmonary morbidity than a thoracoabdominal approach in these nutritionally depleted patients. Nonetheless, a thoracoabdominal incision may be useful for patients who have narrow costal flares, have rib cages that lay close to the iliac crest, or are truly obese.[26,47,52] Exposure with an abdominal incision alone in the latter patients is suboptimal because access to the origins of the visceral arteries is restricted, orientation from which to perform the endarterectomy is poor, and adequately retracting the costal margins is difficult.[26]

A medial visceral rotation is performed, but the left kidney is left in its bed, and the left renal vein is retracted caudally.[26,52] The SMA is dissected free over several centimeters. A longitudinal or trapdoor aortotomy is performed after the patient has been given heparin and diuretics and the supraceliac and infrarenal aortic clamps have been placed. An endarterectomy of the paravisceral aorta, the celiac artery, and the SMA is affected. The endarterectomy ends at the renal artery orifices. In rare patients with symptomatic renal artery stenoses, the aortotomy can be extended into the infrarenal aorta and the specimen can include the renal arteries. The distal endpoint may require tacking sutures to avoid aortic dissection. The aortotomy is closed longitudinally and rarely requires a patch (Figure 19-7). Endarterectomy of the celiac artery usually has an endpoint at its bifurcation, whereas SMA disease may extend beyond the limits that ostial endarterectomy allows. In this case, the aortotomy is closed, flow is restored through the distal aorta and celiac artery, and a completion endarterectomy of the SMA is effected.[26] The SMA may be opened transversely or longitudinally depending on the extent of residual distal disease, with the latter arteriotomy closed by prosthetic or autogenous patch.[26]

The use of intraoperative duplex scan to assess the technical outcomes of the reconstruction has reduced the number of our early postoperative graft failures.

Postoperative Management

Patients are monitored in an intensive care unit for 1 to 3 days. Patients with severe ischemia preoperatively, or a long operation, undergo major fluid shifts and have high volume requirements over the first 48 hours because of the loss of autoregulation of the mesenteric arterioles and the systemic inflammatory response. However, persistent hypotension, tachycardia, leukocytosis, reduction in urine output with elevated bladder pressures, or increase in abdominal pain may indicate graft occlusion, ischemic intestine, or abdominal compartment syndrome.[31,52] CT, abdominal reexploration, or both is needed to exclude these problems.

Return of oral intake varies by individual but may be prolonged. Thus, total parenteral nutrition may be required. The "food fear" many patients have preoperatively does not resolve quickly after operation, as it is often a "learned behavior."[31] Furthermore, the absorptive capacity of the gut changes and patients often experience diarrhea over the first few postoperative weeks. Medications that slow bowel motility or help thicken stool are often necessary.

Outcomes

Comparison of outcomes between patients treated with open and endovascular repair should include mortality, morbidity, freedom from restenosis, symptom recurrence, and reintervention (Tables 19-2 and 19-3). The interpretation of published reports is difficult because open repair traditionally has been used in healthier patients whereas endovascular therapy has been reserved for sicker patients and many reports lump outcomes for both AMAI and CMAI.

The mortality rate for patients undergoing open reconstruction for CMAI has improved over the years. In a report from the Mayo Clinic, in 2002, three patients died within 30 days of operation for a mortality rate of 3.1%; the overall in-hospital mortality rate was 5.1%. In a more recent review from our center, the outcomes of 229 patients with CMAI treated with open and endovascular reconstructions were analyzed and compared.[37] Patients were divided into a low- or high-risk category based on the presence of severe (Society for Vascular Surgery score greater than 2) cardiac, pulmonary, and/or renal disease. The mortality rate for open reconstruction was 0.9% for low-risk patients and 6.7% for high-risk patients. In the endovascular group, no deaths occurred among low-risk patients but a mortality rate of 4.2% was seen in high-risk patients.[37] All patients who died were older than 70 years, and cardiac ischemia accounted for 60% of those deaths.[34] The improvement in mortality is likely due to our patient selection, choice of reconstruction, improved anesthesia techniques and critical care, and focus on reconstruction of the mesenteric disease, along with avoidance of extensive nonessential aortic reconstructions.[26,31,34] In contrast to our early experience, where extensive concomitant aortic or renal revascularization was associated with a 19% mortality,[33] our current results suggest that aortic replacement does not increase morbidity and mortality provided that it is confined to the infrarenal aorta and used as a source of inflow.[34]

Successful long-term outcome is based on graft patency, relief of symptoms, and long-term survival. Assurance of graft patency begins in the operating room. Intraoperative duplex scan is an excellent method to identify technical defects either at the graft-arterial anastomoses or within the graft itself.[26,34] Early graft failure is rare if the intraoperative scan shows a widely patent reconstruction. We currently reimage the mesenteric grafts between 6 and 12 months postoperatively and then annually unless symptoms warrant.

The report by Park and the Mayo Clinic group identified restenosis of the celiac artery or SMA graft limb in 11 of 93 survivors.[35] Three had restenosis or occlusion of both graft limbs, and all underwent revision. Five patients had stenosis of the celiac limb. All of these had bifurcated grafts, and none needed reintervention. Three other patients developed stenosis of the SMA graft. One of these patients had a single graft to the SMA with moderate stenosis but was asymptomatic. The other two had bifurcated grafts, and one patient underwent revision for symptoms.

Reintervention was reserved for symptoms that occurred in six patients during follow-up.[34] All had abdominal pain, and two developed weight loss. Four of these patients had stenosis

Table 19-2
Clinical Results of Contemporary Series (1999 to 2007) of Open Surgical Revascularization for Chronic Mesenteric Ischemia*

				Percentage			
Author (Year)	n/vessels	Technical Success	Mortality	Morbidity	Recurrence	Restenosis	Primary Patency
Kihara (1999)[36]	42/52	100	10	35	10	24	65
Mateo (1999)[50]	85/n/r	100	8	33	20	23	71
Foley (2000)[25]	28/28	100	3	n/r	10	10	79
Leke (2002)[41]	17/25	100	6	41	0	0	100
Cho (2002)[51]	25/41	100	0	n/r	21	n/r	57
Park et al (2002)[35]	98/179	100	5	21	8	11	n/r
Modrall (2003)[45]	15/n/r	100	0	n/r	0	0	100
Illuminati (2004)[46]	11/12	100	0	27	10	10	90
Brown (2005)[61]	33/51	100	9	30	9	0	92
Sivamurthy (2006)[62]	41/68	100	15	41	32	17	83
Biebl (2007)[65]	26/48	100	8	29	11	n/r	n/r
Total	410/504	100	6	32	12	11	82

*IMA, inferior mesenteric artery; SMA, superior mesenteric artery.

Table 19-3
Clinical Results of Contemporary Series (1999 to 2007) of Endovascular Revascularization for Chronic Mesenteric Ischemia*

		%					
Author (Year)	n/Vessels	Technical Success	Mortality	Morbidity	Recurrence	Restenosis	Primary Patency
Sheeran et al. (1999)[54]	12/13	92	10	N/R	N/R	N/R	78
Kasirajan et al. (2001)[42]	28/32	100	11	18	39	27	73
Matsumoto et al. (2002)[43]	33/47	88	0	13	15	15	N/R
Cognet et al. (2002)[55]	16/17	90	0	15	13	13	N/R
Sharaefuddin et al. (2003)[56]	25/26	96	8	12	17	15	65
AbuRahma et al. (2003)[57]	22/24	96	0	0	39	70	30
Chahid et al. (2004)[58]	14/17	100	0	15	23	50	N/R
van Wanroij et al. (2004)[59]	27/33	93	0	11	33	19	81
Landis et al. (2005)[60]	29/34	97	6	10	45	45	70
Brown et al. (2005)[61]	14/18	93	0	0	57	57	N/R
Sivamurthy et al. (2006)[62]	19/21	95	21	19	71	39	68
Schaefer et al. (2006)[63]	19/23	96	11	N/R	53	40	60
Silva et al. (2006)[64]	59/79	97	2	N/R	17	37	71
Biebl et al. (2004)[65]	23/40	N/R	0	4	17	22	N/R
Total	340/424	95	5	12	34	35	66

*N/R, not reported.

or occlusion of a SMA graft, and the other two had patent grafts and normal findings on endoscopic and radiological evaluation of the gastrointestinal tract. The latter two were treated expectantly, and one patient later developed Crohn's disease. Two patients with graft stenosis underwent percutaneous angioplasty with symptom relief. The two with occluded SMA graft limbs were reoperated. One had thrombectomy and patch angioplasty of the graft, and the other underwent a redo two-vessel reconstruction after an initial attempt at angioplasty failed. Both patients had relief of symptoms.

Late pain relief was documented in 74 of 80 patients queried (93%), and weight gain was noted in 61 of 71 patients (86%) who had documented reference to weight change in the analysis. Symptom recurrent-free survival in the Mayo Clinic study was 98% at 90 days, 95% at 1 year, and 92% at 5 years.[34]

The most common cause of late death was cardiac. Two patients died of bowel infarction. Survival was 83% at 1 year, 62% at 5 years, and 55% at 8 years, all significantly worse than an age-matched, sex-matched control population. Survival was unaffected by the number of vessels bypassed or by graft orientation, even though patients with retrograde grafts were older (mean age 75 years) than those with antegrade grafts (mean age 65 years).[34]

Mesenteric angioplasty and stenting has clear short-term advantages. In our recent series, patients treated with endovascular procedures spent fewer days in the intensive care unit (0.7 ± 3.5 versus 4.6 ± 4.8 days; $p < 0.0001$) and in the hospital (3.3 ± 4.8 versus 12 ± 8 days; $p < 0.0001$), and had fewer complications (18% versus 36%; $p < 0.003$) as compared to patients treated with open reconstruction. The benefit of endovascular procedures is mostly due to a significant reduction in the incidence of cardiac (2% versus 10%; $p < 0.04$) and pulmonary problems (1% versus 15%; $p < 0.04$). The incidences of renal, gastrointestinal, or surgical complications were similar in both groups.

Results of collective retrospective series of 340 patients treated with mesenteric angioplasty or stenting since 1999 are summarized in Table 19-3.[21,43,54-65] The average 30-day mortality was 5% (0% to 21%), the 30-day morbidity rate was 12% (0% to 26%), late recurrence was 34% (13% to 71%), and the restenosis was rate 35% (13% to 70%).

The role of angioplasty or stenting as a "diagnostic" maneuver for patients with vague symptoms and moderate visceral artery stenoses of only one or two arteries has yet to be defined.

Summary

Our management of patients with CMAI has evolved over the years. Open revascularization should focus on mesenteric artery revascularization as the primary goal and should avoid extensive aortic or renal artery reconstruction in all but the rarest of cases. This approach has clearly lowered our mortality rate. However, infrarenal aortic replacement, if needed for inflow, can be safely done. Certainly patient selection, preoperative cardiac evaluation and treatment, and improvement in anesthesia and intensive care monitoring have contributed the lower mortality. Older, poor-risk patients may be best served by interventional techniques. SMA stenting is being used more as first-line therapy in good-risk patients with suitable artery and does not seem to preclude operation if it is needed later. Higher restenosis and reintervention rates should be anticipated compared to open revascularization. If operative repair is necessary in this group, single-vessel reconstruction to the SMA may be preferable.

We believe it is no longer necessary to revascularize all three mesenteric arteries.[34] However, we continue to favor antegrade two-vessel reconstruction to the SMA and the celiac artery in select patients because of the excellent durability and symptom-free survival achieved in this group. Since mesenteric disease involves multiple arteries, there may be some margin of safety in a two-vessel reconstruction should one limb occlude or become stenotic during follow-up.[24] Reconstruction of the SMA alone is certainly preferable for patients who present with AMAI-on-CMAI and for older, high-risk patients.[31] Retrograde versus antegrade reconstruction is not as important as careful patient selection and attention to detail during the operation to avoid technical pitfalls.

Since CMAI is rare, controlled clinical trials are unlikely to be able to determine the importance of any single variable in treatment.[26] Choice of intervention or operation should be dictated by patient age, comorbid conditions, and detailed assessment of the aortic and visceral artery anatomy.

References

1. Taylor LM, Moneta GL, Porter JM. Treatment of acute intestinal ischemia caused by arterial occlusions. In: Rutherford, ed. *Vascular surgery.* 5th ed. Philadelphia: WB Saunders; 2000:1512-1518.
2. Park WM, Gloviczki P, Cherry KJ, et al. Contemporary management of acute mesenteric ischemia: factors associated with survival. *J Vasc Surg* 2002;35:445-452.
3. Moneta GL. Diagnosis of intestinal ischemia. In: Rutherford, ed. Vascular surgery. 5th ed. Philadelphia: WB Saunders; 2000:1501-1510.
4. Mamode N, Pickford I, Leiberman P. Failure to improve outcome in acute mesenteric ischemia: seven year review. *Eur J Surg* 1999;165:203-208.
5. Ottinger LW. The surgical management of acute occlusion of the superior mesenteric artery. *Ann Surg* 1978;188:721-731.
6. Wilson C, Gupta R, Gilmour DG, et al. Acute superior mesenteric ischemia. *Br J Surg* 1987;74:279-281.
7. Boley SJ, Feinstein FR, Sammartano R, et al. New concepts in the management of emboli of the superior mesenteric artery. *Surg Gynecol Obstet* 1981;153:561-569.
8. Hertzer NR, Beven EG, Humphries AW. Acute intestinal ischemia. *Am Surg* 1978;44:744-749.
9. Batellier J, Kieny R. Superior mesenteric artery embolism: eighty-two cases. *Ann Vasc Surg* 1990;4:112-116.
10. Lazaro T, Sierra L, Gesto R, et al. Embolization of the mesenteric arteries: surgical treatment in twenty-three consecutive cases. *Ann Vasc Surg* 1986;1:311-315.
11. Smith S, Patterson LT. Acute mesenteric infarction. *Am J Surg* 1976;42:562-567.
12. Stoney RJ, Cunningham CG. Acute mesenteric ischemia. *Surgery* 1993;114:489-490.
13. Konturek A, Cichon S, Gucwa J, et al. Acute intestinal ischemia in material of the III Clinic of General Surgery Collegium Medicum at the Jagellonian University. *Przegl Lek* 1996;53:719-721.
14. Endean ED, Barnes SL, Kwolek CJ, et al. Surgical management of thrombotic acute intestinal ischemia. *Ann Surg* 2001;233(6):801-808.
15. Edwards MS, Cherr GS, Craven TE, et al. Acute occlusive mesenteric ischemia: surgical management and outcomes. *Ann Vasc Surg* 2003;17(1):72-79.
16. Char DJ, Cuadra SA, Hines GL, et al. Surgical intervention for acute intestinal ischemia: experience in a community teaching hospital. *Vasc Endovascular Surg* 2003; 37(4):245-252.
17. Acosta-Merida MA, Marchena-Gomez J, Hemmersbach-Miller M, et al. Identification of risk factors for perioperative mortality in acute mesenteric ischemia. *World J Surg* 2006; 30(8):1579-1585.
18. Kougias P, El Sayed HF, Zhou W, Lin PH. Management of chronic mesenteric ischemia: the role of endovascular therapy. *J Endovasc Ther* 2007;14(3):395-405.
19. Czerny M, Trubel W, Claeys L, et al. Acute mesenteric ischemia. *Zentralbl Chir* 1997;122:538-544.
20. Fock CM, Kullnig P, Ranner G, et al. Mesenteric arterial embolism: the value of emergency CT in diagnostic procedure. *Eur J Radiol* 1994;18:12-14.
21. Clark RA, Gallant TE. Acute mesenteric ischemia: angiographic spectrum. *Am J Roengenol* 1984;142:555-562.
22. Gallego AM, Ramirez P, Rodriquez JM, et al. Role of urokinase in the superior mesenteric artery embolism. *Surgery* 1996;120:111-113.
23. van Deinse WH, Zawacju JK, Phillips D. Treatment of acute mesenteric ischemia by percutaneous transluminal angioplasty. *Gastroenterology* 1986;91:475-478.
24. McBride KD, Gaines PA. Thrombolysis of a partially occluded superior mesenteric artery thromboembolus by streptokinase. *Cardiovasc Intervent Radiol* 1994;17:164-166.
25. Foley MI, Moneta GL, Abou-Zamzam AM, et al. Revascularization of the superior mesenteric artery alone for treatment of intestinal ischemia. *J Vasc Surg* 2000;32:37-47.
26. Cherry KJ Jr. Visceral revascularization for chronic visceral ischemia: transabdominal approach. In: Geroulakos G, Cherry KJ Jr, eds. *Disease of the visceral circulation.* New York: Arnold Publishing; 2002:94-100.
27. Wyers MC, Powell RJ, Nolan BW, Cronenwett JL. Retrograde mesenteric stenting during laparotomy for acute occlusive mesenteric ischemia. *J Vasc Surg* 2007;45:269-275.
28. Ballard JL, Stone WM, Hallett JW, et al. A critical analysis of adjuvant techniques used to assess bowel viability in acute mesenteric ischemia. *Am Surg* 1993;59:309-311.
29. Bergman RT, Gloviczki P, Welch TJ, et al. The role of intravenous fluorescein in the detection of colon ischemia during aortic reconstruction. *Ann Vasc Surg* 1992;6:74-79.
30. Dunphy JE. Abdominal pain of vascular origin. *Am J Med Sci* 1936;192:109.
31. Taylor LM, Moenta GL, Porter JM. Treatment of chronic visceral ischemia. In: Rutherford, ed. Vascular surgery. 5th ed. Philadelphia: WB Saunders; 2000:1532-1541.
32. Thomas JH, Blake K, Pierce GE, et al. The clinical course of asymptomatic mesenteric arterial stenosis. *J Vasc Surg* 1998;27:840-844.
33. Wilson DB, Mostafavi K, Craven TE, et al. Clinical course of mesenteric artery stenosis in elderly Americans. *Arch Intern Med* 2006;166(19):2095-2100.
34. McAfee MK, Cherry KJ, Naessens JM, et al. Influence of complete revascularization on chronic mesenteric ischemia. *Am J Surg* 1992;164:220-224.
35. Park WM, Cherry KJ, Chua HK, et al. Current results of open revascularization for chronic mesenteric ischemia: a standard for comparison. *J Vasc Surg* 2002;35:853-859.
36. Kihara TK, Blebea J, Anderson KM, et al. Risk factors for revascularization for chronic mesenteric ischemia. *Ann Vasc Surg* 1999 13(1):37-44.
37. Oderich GS, Sullivan TM, Bower TC, et al. Open versus endovascular revascularization for chronic mesenteric ischemia: risk-stratified outcomes. Presented at the 2006 Vascular Annual Meeting, June 1-4, 2006. Philadelphia, Pennsylvania. Abstract book, page 158.
38. Marston A. Chronic intestinal ischemia. In: *Vascular disease of the gastrointestinal tract: pathophysiology, recognition and management.* Baltimore: Williams & Wilkins; 1986:116.
39. Moneta GL, Lee RW, Yeager RA, et al. Mesenteric duplex scanning: a blinded prospective study. *J Vasc Surg* 1993;17:79.
40. Bowersox JC, Zwalak RM, Walsh DB, et al. Duplex ultrasonography in the diagnosis of celiac and mesenteric artery occlusive disease. *J Vasc Surg* 1991;14:780.
41. Leke MA, Hood DB, Rowe VL, et al. Technical consideration in the management of chronic mesenteric ischemia. *Am Surg* 2002;68(12):1088-1092.
42. Kasirajan K, O'Hara PJ, Gray BH, et al. Chronic mesenteric ischemia: open surgery versus percutaneous angioplasty and stenting. *J Vasc Surg* 2001;33:63-67.

43. Matsumoto AH, Tegtmeyer CJ, Fitzcharles EK, et al. Percutaneous transluminal angioplasty of visceral arterial stenoses: results and long-term clinical follow-up. *J Vasc Interv Radiol* 1995;6:165-174.
44. Allen RC, Martin GH, Rees RC, et al. Mesenteric angioplasty in the treatment of chronic mesenteric ischemia. *J Vasc Surg* 1996;24:415-423.
45. Modrall JG, Sadjadi J, Joiner DR, et al. Comparison of superficial femoral vein and saphenous vein as conduits for mesenteric arterial bypass. *J Vasc Surg* 2003;37(2):362-366.
46. lluminati G, Calio FG, D'Urso A, et al. The surgical treatment of chronic mesenteric ischemia: results of a recent series. *Acta Chir Belg* 2004;104(2):175-183.
47. Cunningham CG, Reilly LM, Rapp JH, et al. Chronic visceral ischemia. *Ann Surg* 1991;214:276-288.
48. Rapp JH, Reilly LM, Qvarfordt PG, et al. Durability of endarterectomy and antegrade grafts in the treatment of chronic visceral ischemia. *J Vasc Surg* 1986:799-806.
49. Moawad J, McKinsey JF, Wyble CW, et al. Current results of surgical therapy for chronic mesenteric ischemia. *Arch Surg* 1997;132:613-619.
50. Mateo RB, O'Hara PJ, Hertzer NR, et al. Elective surgical treatment of symptomatic chronic mesenteric occlusive disease: early results and late outcomes. *J Vasc Surg* 1999;29:821-832.
51. Cho JS, Carr JA, Jacobsen G, et al. Long-term outcome following mesenteric artery reconstruction: a 37-year experience. *J Vasc Surg* 2002;35:453-460.
52. Reilly LM, Ramos TK, Murray SP, et al. Optimal exposure of the proximal abdominal aorta: a critical appraisal of transabdominal medial visceral rotation. *J Vasc Surg* 1994;19:375-390.
53. Gewertz BL, Zarins CK. Postoperative vasospasm after antegrade mesenteric revascularization: a report of three cases. *J Vasc Surg* 1991;14:382.
54. Sheeran SR, Murphy TP, Khwaja A, et al. Stent placement for treatment of mesenteric artery stenoses or occlusions. *J Vasc Interv Radiol* 1999;10(7):861-867.
55. Cognet F, Ben Salem D, Dranssart M, et al. Chronic mesenteric ischemia: imaging and percutaneous treatment. *Radiographics* 2002;22(4):863-879. discussion, 879-880.
56. Sharafuddin MJ, Olson CH, Sun S, et al. Endovascular treatment of celiac and mesenteric artery stenoses: applications and results. *J Vasc Surg* 2003;38:692-698.
57. AbuRahma AF, Stone PA, Bates MC, Welch CA. Angioplasty/stenting of the superior mesenteric artery and celiac trunk: early and late outcomes. *J Endovasc Ther* 2003;10:1046-1053.
58. Chahid T, Alfidja AT, Biard M, et al. Endovascular treatment of chronic mesenteric ischemia: results in 14 patients. *Cardiovasc Intervent Radiol* 2004;27(6):637-642.
59. van Wanroij JL, van Petersen AS, Huisman AB, et al. Endovascular treatment of chronic splanchnic syndrome. *Eur J Vasc Endovasc Surg* 2004;28(2):193-200.
60. Landis MS, Rajan DK, Simons ME, et al. Percutaneous management of chronic mesenteric ischemia: outcomes after intervention. *J Vasc Interv Radiol* 2005;16(10):1319-1325.
61. Brown DJ, Schermerhorn ML, Powell RJ, et al. Mesenteric stenting for chronic mesenteric ischemia. *J Vasc Surg* 2005;42(2):268-274.
62. Sivamurthy N, Rhodes JM, Lee D, et al. Endovascular versus open mesenteric revascularization: immediate benefits do not equate with short-term functional outcomes. *J Am Coll Surg* 2006;202(6):859-867.
63. Schaefer PJ, Schaefer FK, Hinrichsen H, et al. Stent placement with the monorail technique for treatment of mesenteric artery stenosis. *J Vasc Interv Radiol* 2006;17(4):637-643.
64. Silva JA, White CJ, Collins TJ, et al. Endovascular therapy for chronic mesenteric ischemia. *J Am Coll Cardiol* 2006;47(5):944-950.
65. Biebl M, Oldenburg WA, Paz-Fumagalli R, et al. Endovascular treatment as a bridge to successful surgical revascularization for chronic mesenteric ischemia. *Am Surg* 2004;70(11):994-998.

chapter

20

Mesenteric Venous Thrombosis

Donald T. Baril, MD • Robert Y. Rhee, MD

Key Points

- Mesenteric venous thrombosis (MVT) is an uncommon but potentially lethal form of mesenteric ischemia secondary to thrombosis of the portomesenteric venous system.
- Signs and symptoms of MVT are typically nonspecific.
- A high index of suspicion is necessary, particularly in those patients with a prior history of a hypercoagulable state.
- The diagnostic test of choice is computed tomography scanning.
- Confirmation of MVT warrants immediate anticoagulation therapy.
- Peritonitis on presentation mandates immediate surgical exploration to rule out ischemic bowel.
- Second-look laparotomy should be performed liberally.
- If there are no contraindications, anticoagulation therapy should be continued indefinitely after the acute episode.
- Catheter-directed thrombolytic therapy offers an alternative therapeutic approach for patients with extensive MVT.

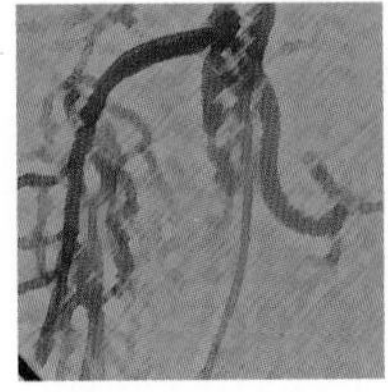

Mesenteric venous thrombosis (MVT) is an uncommon form of mesenteric ischemia, occurring far less often than mesenteric ischemia resulting from arterial embolism or thrombosis. It was first described by Elliot[1] in 1895 as intestinal gangrene resulting from "thrombosis of the portomesenteric venous system." This disorder is potentially lethal, with associated mortality rates of 15% to 40%.[2-5] Warren and Eberhard's historic report[6] in 1935 characterized MVT as a distinct clinical entity and emphasized its lethality, reporting a mortality rate of 34% following intestinal resection for thrombosed veins in the mesentery of the bowel. MVT comprises only 2% to 15% of all acute mesenteric ischemic cases reported in the literature.[7,8] Autopsy analysis reported 0.2% to 2% of the population having MVT.[6,8] However, its true incidence is not known since MVT may not be suspected on presentation. Abdu et al.[2] reported 372 total cases in the literature, identified from 1911 to 1984. The Mayo Clinic series[9] identified 72 cases from 1972 to 1993, comprising 6.2% of 1167 patients treated for mesenteric ischemic disorders during that period. In a study by Ottinger and Austen,[8] MVT consisted of only 0.006% of hospital admissions and less than 2% of autopsy cases. Intestinal infarction associated with MVT is estimated to be less than 1 in 1000 laparotomies for the acute abdomen.[10] Morasch et al.[11] reported only 31 cases of MVT over a 14-year period from a large tertiary academic medical center. In a population-based study by Acosta et al.,[12] the estimated incidence of MVT with transmural intestinal infarction was 1.8 per 100,000 person years.

ANATOMY AND PATHOLOGY

The portomesenteric venous system comprises the portal, superior mesenteric, inferior mesenteric, and splenic veins (Figure 20-1). The junction or confluence of the superior mesenteric and splenic veins forms the portal vein, posterior to the neck of the pancreas. The portal vein ascends superiorly and posterior to the first part of the duodenum at the level of the second lumbar vertebra. The portal vein is a relatively large vein, ranging from 1 to 3 cm in diameter and from 5 to 8 cm in length. It terminates into the left and right branches at the level of the porta hepatis. The portal vein typically passes behind the hepatic artery and the bile duct in the hepatoduodenal ligament. The inferior mesenteric vein arises from the splenic vein posterior to the midbody of the pancreas, before the junction of the superior mesenteric and splenic vein.

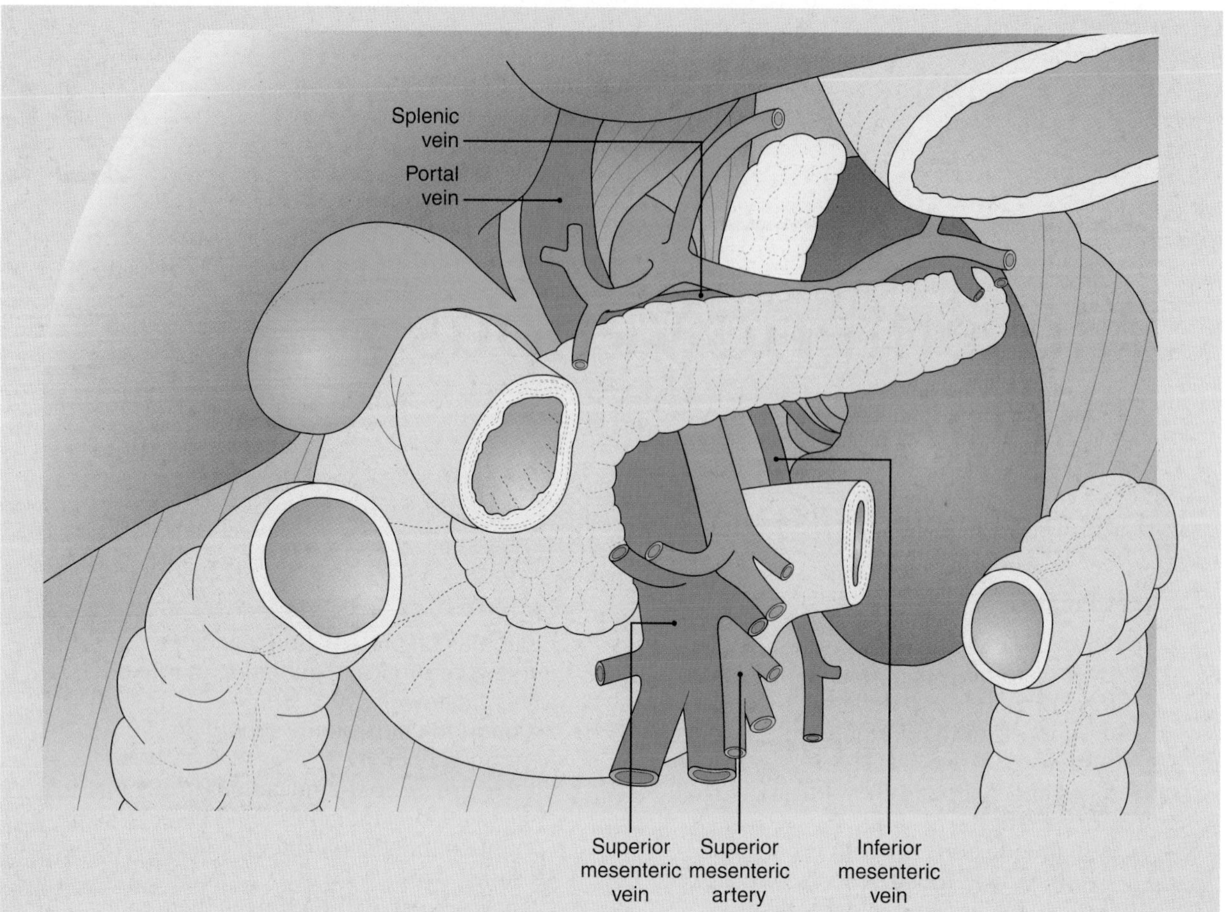

Figure 20-1. Locoregional anatomy of the portomesenteric venous system.

ETIOLOGY AND PATHOPHYSIOLOGY

MVT can be classified into primary and secondary. Primary MVT is defined as idiopathic, spontaneous thrombosis of the mesenteric veins not associated with any disease processes.[13] The incidence of primary MVT has decreased substantially over the past decade because of improvement in diagnosis and recognition of previously unknown thrombophilic conditions. An autopsy series reported by Johnson and Baggenstoss[14] identified 99 cases of MVT, of which only 8 patients (12.4%) did not have identifiable etiological factors associated with MVT.

Secondary MVT, representing most reported cases in the literature, is associated with known conditions that predispose the mesenteric venous system to a thrombotic process (Table 20-1). Abdu et al.[2] found that 81% of cases of MVT were secondary or related to an underlying condition. Multiple hypercoagulable conditions have been associated with MVT, the most common being polycythemia vera. Other causes of secondary MVT include neoplastic diseases, heparin-induced thrombocytopenia,[11] and oral contraceptive use[15-18] Thrombophilic disorders associated with MVT include protein C and S deficiency, antithrombin III deficiency, dysfibrinogenemia, abnormal plasminogen, thrombocytosis, sickle cell disease, the 20210A allele of the prothrombin gene, the factor V Leiden mutation, the JAK2 V617F mutation, and hyperhomocysteinemia.[13,19-25] In addition to these hypercoagulable states, inflammatory bowel disease has also been associated with MVT, both spontaneously and postoperatively.[26-27] MVT has also been described following almost every major intraabdominal operation, including appendectomy, gastric bypass, splenectomy, colectomy, and Nissen fundoplication.[28-31] In the Mayo series,[9] 42% had a documented hypercoagulable disorder, with polycythemia vera being the most common. Morasch et al.[11] reported that 56% of patients with MVT had an identifiable coagulopathy. The true incidence of hypercoagulability associated with MVT is likely to be higher than that currently reported in the literature because, before the last decade, many of these patients may not have been appropriately screened for any hypercoagulable conditions.[3,11]

In addition to the classification of primary and secondary MVT, Kumar and Kamath[32] have divided patients with MVT into two separate groups: those with splenic or portal vein involvement and those without. In their review, patients with isolated MVT (i.e., not involving the splenic or portal vein) were more difficult to diagnose and more likely to have hypercoagulable disorders.

Table 20-1
Conditions Associated with Mesenteric Venous Thrombosis (MVT)

Hypercoagulable states
Antithrombin III deficiency
Protein C and S deficiency
20210A allele of the prothrombin gene
Factor V Leiden gene mutation
Heparin-induced thrombocytopenia
Lupus anticoagulant
Polycythemia vera
Hyperhomocysteinemia
Oral contraceptive use
Neoplasms
Inflammatory bowel disease
Previous abdominal surgery
Intraabdominal inflammation
Previous MVT or deep venous thrombosis
Smoking
Alcohol abuse
Portal hypertension or cirrhosis

CLINICAL PRESENTATION

Acute MVT

Although patients with acute MVT present with clinical findings similar to those of patients with acute mesenteric arterial ischemia, the symptoms and signs are more subtle and can be misleading. Like acute mesenteric arterial ischemia, the delay in diagnosis is still common and is a significant contributory factor to the mortality rate of 13% to 50% reported in the literature.[2-5,32-34] Typically, patients with acute MVT may present with pain out of proportion to physical findings, nausea and vomiting, or diarrhea. The pain may be diffuse or intermittent, lasting for several days or even weeks. Mathews and White[35] found that about 50% of patients had experienced pain from 5 days to as much as 30 days before seeking evaluation, and as many as 27% reported having had pain for more than 1 month. In the Mayo series,[9] abdominal distention was the most common sign of acute MVT, albeit present in only 43% of patients. Only 4 of 53 patients presented with symptoms of less than 24 hours' duration. Of the patients, 75% had had symptoms present for more than 48 hours at the time of diagnosis, signifying the frequency in delay of diagnosis. Peritonitis was present in a little more than 33% of patients and fever in 25%. In more recent reports, Morasch et al.[11] found that only 16% of their patients had severe peritonitis, while Kumar and Kamath[32] reported abdominal tenderness in 83% of their patients with isolated MVT and peritoneal signs in 43%. Abdu et al.[2] found that the only true constant finding of MVT was pain out of proportion to the physical findings, with slow progression, often with steady low-grade symptoms, for more than 48 hours. Prior medical history or familial-related history of hypercoagulable syndromes associated with presenting complaints of abdominal pain may help suggest the diagnosis.[19-24,32] Furthermore, a diagnosis of MVT should be entertained in patients presenting with atypical complaints of abdominal pain who are taking oral contraceptives, have a history of inflammatory bowel disease, or have recently undergone a major intraabdominal operation. Morasch et al.[11] and the Mayo group[9] both found that 42% of patients in their series had some form of factor deficiency associated with hypercoagulability.[9]

Chronic MVT

Presentations with the chronic form vary widely, from subtle abdominal findings to asymptomatic. This is particularly true with patients who have incidental findings on abdominal computed tomography (CT) scanning performed for pathological processes unrelated to chronic MVT. Patients may present with dramatic symptoms related to extension of the MVT to the portal or splenic vein leading to esophageal or gastric variceal hemorrhage.

DIAGNOSTIC TECHNIQUES

Laboratory Tests

As in other mesenteric ischemic disorders, laboratory tests are not helpful in making the diagnosis of acute MVT—they can neither confirm nor exclude it—and should be used for screening purposes only. Boley et al.[5] reported that a white blood cell count greater than 12 (10×10^9/L) and bandemia were present in only two thirds of their patients. The Mayo series[9] reported elevated white blood cell counts in 49% of patients. Other biochemical variables such as serum lactate and amylase are not elevated in most patients. Although not useful as screening tests, measurement of coagulation factors and laboratory values associated with hypercoagulable states are of value once the diagnosis of MVT has been confirmed on imaging.

Radiographic Diagnosis

Before the advent of CT, the diagnosis of MVT had been difficult to establish objectively. Plain abdominal radiographs are abnormal in 50% to 75% of patients with MVT but demonstrate evidence of ischemic bowel in less than 5% of patients.[36] In general, abdominal x-rays are nonspecific and of little use in the diagnostic process except to rule out other causes of abdominal pain. Venous-phase mesenteric angiography was once the preferred nonoperative method for diagnosing MVT.[10,37] Most reports during this era diagnosed MVT at laparotomy or autopsy. Since then, because of improved image resolution of CT scanning and magnetic resonance imaging (MRI) with gadolinium, the disease process is diagnosed more readily. Venography may still play a role in patients suspected of having small-vessel MVT, although this should be performed only after CT scanning.

CT is currently the diagnostic test of choice in acute MVT.[38] Harward et al.[3] reported a 90% sensitivity in the 10 patients they studied. The most common positive finding is the demonstration of thrombus in the superior mesenteric vein, as shown in Figure 20-2. Associated findings that may suggest MVT include bowel wall thickening, pneumatosis, "streaky" mesentery, collateralization with splenomegaly, and ascites. Portal or mesenteric venous gas strongly suggests the presence of bowel infarction. Combining bowel ischemia and the presence of venous thrombosis, the sensitivity of CT in showing an abnormality was 100% in the Mayo series.[9] In the study by Morasch et al.,[11] CT was considered diagnostic in 18 of 20 patients (90%) who underwent the test, including 15 of 15 (100%) who presented with abdominal pain or diarrhea.

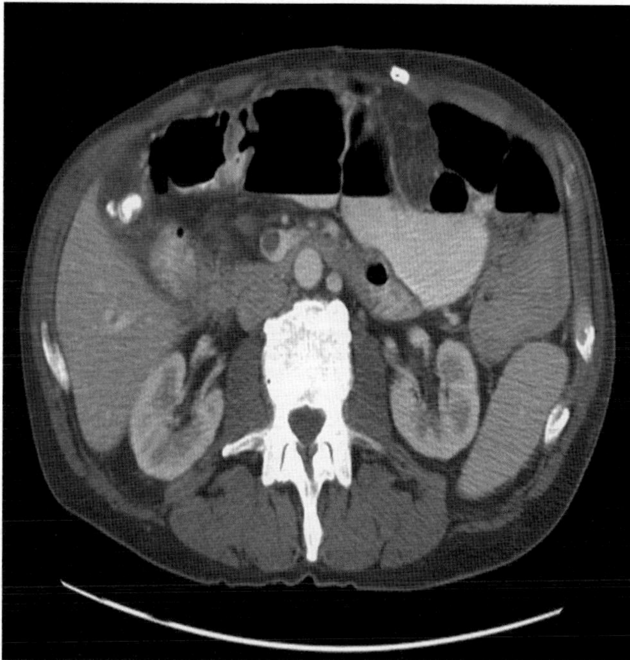

Figure 20-2. Computed tomography scan of a patient with acute superior mesenteric venous thrombosis.

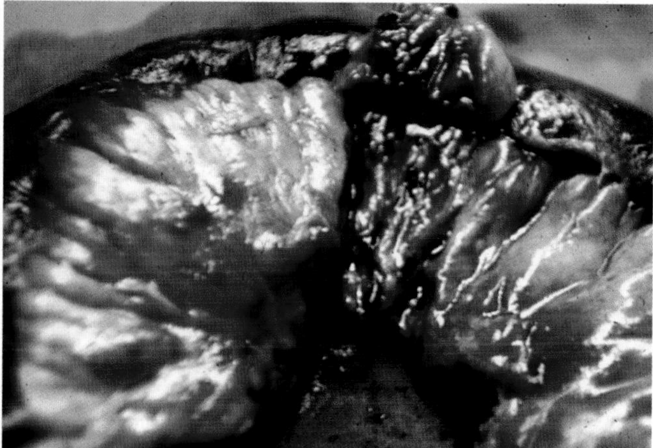

Figure 20-3. Gross pathology of a resected segment of small intestine in a patient with mesenteric venous thrombosis demonstrating thrombus formation in the smaller, distal mesenteric veins.

Similarly, Vogelzang et al.[39] diagnosed MVT using CT in all 14 patients studied and Grisham et al.[40] found MVT in 21 of 22 patients who underwent CT scanning.

Duplex ultrasonography and MRI are promising modalities. Duplex ultrasonography can be diagnostic only if obtained early.[41] The Mayo study[9] pointed to an 80% overall sensitivity demonstrating either a thrombus or an absence of flow in the mesenteric veins. In the acute setting, ultrasound is often limited by the large amount of overlying bowel gas from the associated ileus. In addition, in chronic presentations, the sensitivities are not as high because of the extensive collateralizations.

MRI, although expensive, is also sensitive. Gehl et al.[42] reported 100% sensitivity in diagnosing MVT with the use of MRI in 115 patients. Improved image resolution of high-speed CT scanning and use of gadolinium as a contrast agent in MRI for more accurate visceral evaluation improve the diagnostic capabilities in detecting MVT.

MANAGEMENT: ACUTE MVT

Various therapies exist for MVT, including surgical resection of bowel, thrombolytic therapy, and medical management. All patients require resuscitation and broad-spectrum antibiotic coverage. Anticoagulation with intravenous heparin and subsequently warfarin should be instituted to limit thrombosis, as well as to prevent recurrence. The sole objective of surgical therapy is to prevent or limit bowel gangrene. Patients who present with peritonitis should undergo immediate surgical exploration. Select patients may be candidates for laparoscopy rather than formal lapartomy.[43] Without findings of peritonitis, radiographic assessment may be warranted to delineate further abdominal pathology. In the Mayo series,[9] 64% (34/53) of patients with acute MVT eventually required abdominal exploration. Morasch et al.[11] reported that a total of 10 patients (32%) ultimately required exploration, while Grisham et al.[40] reported 4 of 23 (17%) requiring surgical intervention. Features of MVT include edema of the mesentery and cyanotic discoloration of the involved bowel. Infarction from MVT commonly involves the middle segment of the small intestine: the colon is usually not affected. Duodenal involvement suggests that bowel infarction is not venous in origin. The sites of thrombosis in most patients are located in the smaller, distal mesenteric veins (Figure 20-3). Once the diagnosis is made, either intraoperatively or preoperatively with radiographic assessments, immediate anticoagulation should be started. The risk of bleeding complications may be increased in the perioperative period. However, the benefit decreases the risk of rethrombosis and ultimately improves survival.[9]

At operation, minimal bowel resection and liberal use of second-look laparotomy after 24 hours is the primary goal. Up to 90% of patients present with transmural necrosis, with bowel perforation present in 20% of cases. The length of bowel resection can be fairly extensive. If initial ischemia is extensive, resection should be limited to bowel that is definitely infarcted. Recurrent infarction from repeated venous thrombosis involves the area adjacent to the bowel anastomosis in 60% of patients.[10] If any doubt remains about bowel viability, a second look is certainly warranted.[44] In most situations, a diverting ileostomy or colostomy may be preferred, although primary repair is possible in stable patients with local confined intestinal infarction. Intraoperative assessment of intestinal viability with Wood's light illumination, Doppler, or both may be difficult in this situation.[10]

Thrombectomy of the superior mesenteric vein has been previously described.[9,11,45] The vein is typically to the right of the artery. Access is standard and is obtained by lifting the transverse colon superiorly, displacing the small intestines to the right, and dividing the ligament of Treitz. Inahara[45] describes a linear venotomy, proximal thrombectomy, and removal of small clots of the distal venous mesentery by "milking" the veins of the bowel and mesentery. Fogarty catheters are also used to retrieve thrombi. Because of the high failure rate of mesenteric venous thrombectomy, we do not advocate this treatment in any situation. Most patients have such diffuse MVT with distal extent that a venous thrombectomy of the superior mesenteric vein does little in relieving the venous congestion in the mesentery. An alternative approach described for the treatment of chronic MVT is the use of an inferior mesenteric vein to renal vein bypass to allow decompression of the mesenteric outflow tracts,[46] a procedure that should be reserved only for patients who fail medical therapy.

The use of thrombolytic therapy in this setting remains controversial. Reports of thrombolysis[11,47-50] have described limited success, although the hemorrhagic complications make the option less appealing. Train et al.[49] described successful treatment of MVT by intraarterial lytic therapy. Intramesenteric venous lytic therapy using urokinase for MVT has also been reported.[50] Recently, multiple reports have demonstrated the use of percutaneous thrombectomy with pharmacological thrombolysis for the treatment of MVT approached most commonly via a transhepatic route (Figure 20-4).[51-55] Hollingshead et al.[54] reported 85% of patients had resolution of symptoms following transcatheter thrombolytic therapy but also reported that 60% of patients developed a major complication, primarily related to bleeding. Kim et al.[55] reported clinical success in 90% of their patients with no recurrent thrombosis at a mean follow-up of 42 months. Although these series are limited and the long-term follow-up data are scarce, with improvements in technology and the ability to limit the amount of systemic thrombolytics, this modality may increase in its applicability for select patients with MVT. In particular, patients who are hemodynamically stable, have no evidence of intestinal compromise on CT scan, and have minimal bleeding risk may be considered for such therapy.

Medical Therapy

Nonoperative medical management with anticoagulation and observation constitutes treatment of those patients who have not developed peritonitis, those with no evidence of ongoing bowel necrosis, and those with incidental findings of venous thrombosis on radiographic studies. Boley and colleagues[5] suggest that anticoagulation should be started at the time of diagnosis and maintained lifelong to decrease the incidence of recurrence unless significant risks exist of bleeding complications due to portal venous hypertension. A complete hypercoagulable workup should be undertaken at the time of diagnosis not only to treat the patient but also to identify relatives at risk for thrombotic complications.

Anticoagulation Therapy

The proper duration of anticoagulation is not known. Current recommendations suggest that anticoagulation should be continued indefinitely unless contraindications prevent use. Primary mesenteric ischemia should be treated with indefinite anticoagulation since the source may be an undefined or as-yet-undetected anticoagulation factor. Patients with secondary mesenteric ischemic disorders usually receive indefinite anticoagulation therapy, although a search for an occult underlying thrombophilia should be considered.

PROGNOSIS: ACUTE MVT

The natural history of MVT is not known. The 30-day mortality remains high (13% to 15%) and can be as high as 50%. Morasch et al.[11] reported a 30-day mortality of 23%, with only two patients dying of massive bowel infarction. Figure 20-4 depicts the survival curves of acute MVT for the Mayo series.[9] In that series, prolonged hospitalization was observed in patients who presented with peritonitis and required bowel resection. Mean stay for acute MVT was beyond 22 days, ranging from 1 to 98 days. Of the patients presenting with acute MVT, 38% (20/53) ultimately died due to disease progression. Anticoagulation was found to be the factor that altered early survival in that series. Late survival of acutely presenting patients with MVT was consistently poor. Patients treated surgically and with anticoagulation had improved survival.

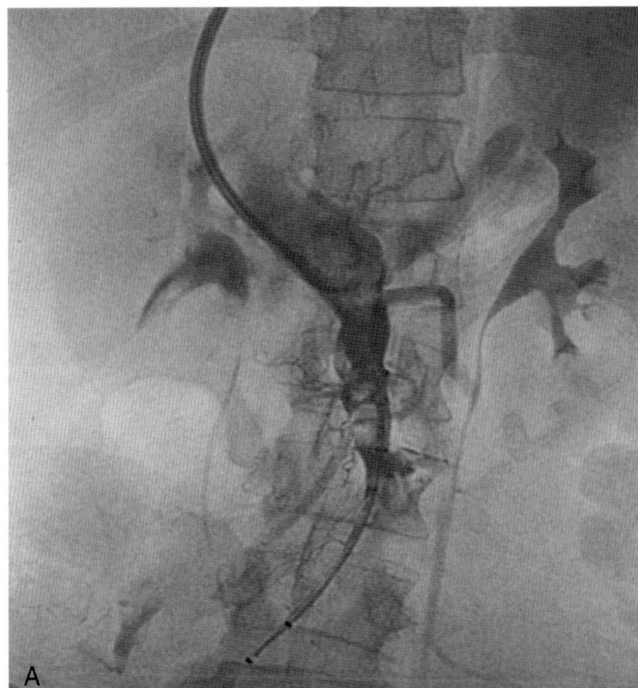

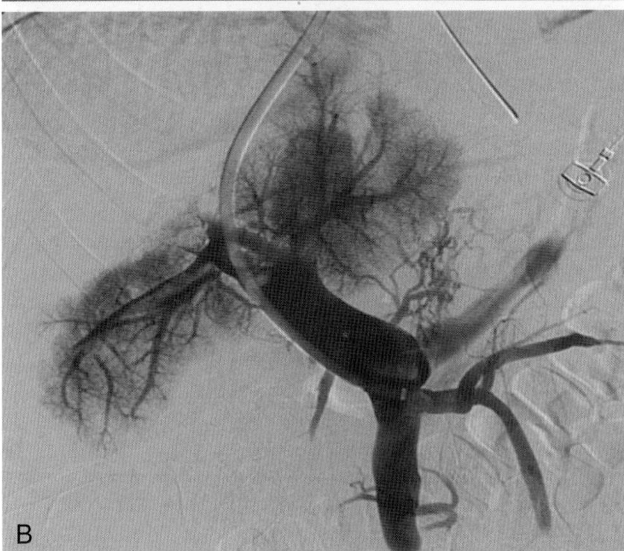

Figure 20-4. A, Venogram demonstrating extensive thrombus within the portal vein, occlusion of the superior mesenteric vein, and a patent inferior mesenteric vein in a young female patient with Crohn's disease after an ileocolic resection. **B,** Venogram following percutaneous mechanical thrombectomy and thrombolysis demonstrating patent superior mesenteric, inferior mesenteric, and portal veins. (Courtesy Alfio Carroccio, MD.)

In a review of the international literature by Abdu et al.,[2] similar benefits were seen for those without surgery, although not as good as for those with surgery with anticoagulation. The recurrence rate of acute MVT is generally high, and up to 14% who undergo bowel resection have recurrent MVT within 6 weeks.[2,9,11] The use of anticoagulation alone is associated with a higher recurrence rate than surgery with anticoagulation.[9] The cause of the MVT does not appear to affect survival. Furthermore, involvement of the splenic or portal veins does not appear to affect either 30-day mortality or long-term outcome.[32]

CHRONIC MVT

Patients presenting with MTV may be asymptomatic or may have symptoms ranging from vague abdominal pain to dramatic abdominal distention. Mild leukocytosis may be the only significant laboratory finding in these patients, but it was present in less than half of patients in the Mayo series.[9] The incidental finding of a thrombosed mesenteric venous system is not uncommon, in particular during evaluation of other abdominal pathology. In most cases of chronic MVT, collateral venous circulation is usually sufficient to maintain adequate drainage of the affected bowel.[9] Prognosis, however, is determined by the underlying abdominal disease, and late survival appears to be better than in those patients who present with acute MVT. A review by Orr et al. of 60 patients with chronic MVT reported overall 1-year and 5-year survival rates of 81.6% and 78.3%, respectively, and 1-year and 5-year survival rates of 85.7% and 82.1%, respectively, when excluding patients who died from malignancy-related causes.[56]

SUMMARY

MVT is an uncommon yet important cause of visceral ischemia. Suspicion should be high, particularly in those patients with prior histories of hypercoagulable disorders, including inflammatory bowel disease or recent intraabdominal surgery. Operative therapy is necessary to assure that the intestinal ischemia from venous thrombosis has not progressed to transmural infarction. If not, observation and anticoagulation therapy is appropriate. Lifelong anticoagulation therapy is necessary to decrease the frequency of recurrences.

The overall outcome for those patients who present acutely still remains fairly poor. The 30-day mortality rate is high and is comparable to that for its arterial counterpart causing visceral ischemia. Despite adequate anticoagulation and disease awareness, the recurrence rate is also high. Long-term prognosis for acute MVT, too, is poor. Overall outcome is better for the chronic form of MVT and appears to be determined by the underlying disease process. Unfortunately, despite advances in diagnostic modalities over the past quarter century, only a slight improvement has been seen in overall survival in those patients who suffer from MVT.

References

1. Elliot JW. The operative relief of gangrene of intestine due to occlusion of the mesenteric vessels. *Ann Surg* 1895;21:9-23.
2. Abdu R, Zakhour BJ, Dallis DJ. Mesenteric venous thrombosis: 1911 to 1984. *Surgery* 1987;101:383-388.
3. Harward TRS, Green D, Bergan JJ, et al. Mesenteric venous thrombosis. *J Vasc Surg* 1989;9:328-333.
4. Sack J, Aldrete JS. Primary mesenteric venous thrombosis. *Surg Gynecol Obstet* 1982;154:205-208.
5. Boley SJ, Kaleya RN, Brandt LJ. Mesenteric venous thrombosis. *Surg Clin North Am* 1992;72:183-201.
6. Warren S, Eberhard TP. Mesenteric venous thrombosis. *Surg Gynecol Obstet* 1935;61:102.
7. Kairaluoma MI, Karkola P, Heikkinen E, et al. Mesenteric infarction. *Am J Surg* 1977;133:188-193.
8. Ottinger LW, Austen WG. A study of 136 patients with mesenteric infarction. *Surg Gynecol Obstet* 1967;124:251-261.
9. Rhee RY, Gloviczki P, Mendonca CT, et al. Mesenteric venous thrombosis: still a lethal disease in the 1990s. *J Vasc Surg* 1994;20:688-697.
10. Kazmers A. Intestinal ischemia caused by venous thrombosis. In: Rutherford RB, ed. Vascular surgery. 5th ed. Philadelphia: WB Saunders; 2000: 1524-1531.
11. Morasch MD, Ebaugh JL, Chiou AC, et al. Mesenteric venous thrombosis: a changing clinical entity. *J Vasc Surg* 2001;34:680-684.
12. Acosta S, Ogren M, Sternby NH, et al. Mesenteric venous thrombosis with transmural intestinal infarction: a population-based study. *J Vasc Surg* 2005;41(1):59-63.
13. Kitchens CS. Evolution of our understanding of the pathophysiology of primary mesenteric venous thrombosis. *Am J Surg* 1992;163:346-348.
14. Johnson CC, Baggenstoss AH. Mesenteric vascular occlusion. I. Study of 99 cases of occlusion of the veins. *Proc Staff Meet Mayo Clinic* 1949;24:628.
15. Hassan HA. Oral contraceptive-induced mesenteric venous thrombosis with resultant intestinal ischemia. *J Clin Gastroenterol* 1999;29:90-95.
16. Nesbit RR Jr, Deweese JA. Mesenteric venous thrombosis and oral contraceptives. *South Med J* 1977;70:360-362.
17. Oliviero B, Di Micco P, Guarino G, et al. A case of thrombosis of the superior mesenteric vein occurring in a young woman taking oral contraceptives: full and fast resolution with low molecular weight heparin. *Clin Lab* 2007;53(3-4):167-171.
18. Bailey KA, Bass J, Nizalik E, et al. Unusual case of mesenteric venous thrombosis associated with oral contraceptive use in an adolescent girl. *Pediatr Dev Pathol* 2005;8(1):128-131.
19. Bontempo FA, Hassett AC, Faruki H, et al. The Factor V Leiden mutation: spectrum of thrombotic events and laboratory evaluation. *J Vasc Surg* 1997;25:271-275.
20. Inagaki H, Sakakibara O, Miyaika H, et al. Mesenteric venous thrombosis in familial free protein S deficiency. *Am J Gastroenterol* 1993;88: 134-138.
21. Ostermiller W Jr, Carter R. Mesenteric venous thrombosis secondary to polycythemia vera. *Am Surg* 1969;35:407.
22. Tollefson DFJ, Friedman KD, Marlar RA, et al. Protein C deficiency: a cause of unusual or unexplained thrombosis. *Arch Surg* 1988;123: 881-884.
23. Wilson C, Walker ID, Davidson JF, et al. Mesenteric venous thrombosis and antithombin III deficiency. *J Clin Pathol* 1987;40:906-908.
24. Colaizzo D, Amitrano L, Tiscia GL, et al. The JAK2 V617F mutation frequently occurs in patients with portal and mesenteric venous thrombosis. *J Thromb Haemost* 2007;5(1):55-61.
25. Tan KJ, Chow PK, Tan YM, et al. Portal vein thrombosis secondary to hyperhomocysteinemia: a case report. *Dig Dis Sci* 2006;51(7):1218-1220.
26. Fichera A, Cicchiello LA, Mendelson DS, et al. Superior mesenteric vein thrombosis after colectomy for inflammatory bowel disease: a not uncommon cause of postoperative acute abdominal pain. *Dis Colon Rectum* 2003;46(5):643-648.
27. Hatoum OA, Spinelli KS, Abu-Hajir M, et al. Mesenteric venous thrombosis in inflammatory bowel disease. *J Clin Gastroenterol* 2005;39(1): 27-31.
28. Noh KW, Wolfsen HC, Bridges MD, et al. Mesenteric venous thrombosis following laparoscopic antireflux surgery. *Dig Dis Sci* 2007;52(1): 273-275.
29. Swartz DE, Felix EL. Acute mesenteric venous thrombosis following laparoscopic Roux-en-Y gastric bypass. *JSLS* 2004;8(2):165-169.
30. Lam L, Acosta J. Abdominal pain after uncomplicated laparoscopic appendectomy. *J Am Coll Surg* 2007;204(1):177-178.
31. Stamou KM, Toutouzas KG, Kekis PB, et al. Prospective study of the incidence and risk factors of postsplenectomy thrombosis of the portal, mesenteric, and splenic veins. *Arch Surg* 2006;141(7):663-669.
32. Kumar S, Kamath PS. Acute superior mesenteric venous thrombosis: one disease or two? *Am J Gastroenterol* 2003;98(6):1299-1304.
33. Carr N, Jamison MH. Superior mesenteric venous thrombosis. *Br J Surg* 1981;68:343-344.

34. Clavien PA, Harder F. Mesenteric venous thrombosis. *Helv Chir Acta* 1988;55:29-34.
35. Mathews JE, White RR. Primary mesenteric venous occlusive disease. *Am J Surg* 1971;122:579-583.
36. Grendell JH, Ockner RK. Mesenteric venous thrombosis. *Gastroenterology* 1982;82:358-372.
37. Clemett AR, Chang J. The radiologic diagnosis of spontaneous mesenteric venous thrombosis. *Am J Gastroenterol* 1975;63(3):209-215.
38. Rahmouni A, Mathieu D, Golli M, et al. Value of CT and sonography in the conservative management of acute splenoportal and superior mesenteric venous thrombosis. *Gastrointest Radiol* 1992;17:135-140.
39. Vogelzang RL, Gore RM, Anschuetz SL, Blei AT. Thrombosis of the splanchnic veins: CT diagnosis. *Am J Roentgenol* 1988;150:93-96.
40. Grisham A, Lohr J, Guenther JM, et al. Deciphering mesenteric venous thrombosis: imaging and treatment. *Vasc Endovascular Surg* 2005;39(6):473-479.
41. Kidambi H, Herbert R, Kidambi AV. Ultrasonic demonstration of superior mesenteric and splenoportal venous thrombosis. *J Clin Ultrasound* 1986;14:199-201.
42. Gehl HB, Bohndorf K, Klose KC, et al. Two-dimensional MR angiography in the evaluation of abdominal veins with gradient refocused sequences. *J Comput Assist Tomogr* 1990;14:619-624.
43. Chong AK, So JB, Ti TK. Use of laparoscopy in the management of mesenteric venous thrombosis. *Surg Endosc* 2001;15(9):1042.
44. Levy PJ, Krausz MM, Manny J. The role of second-look procedure in improving survival time for patients with mesenteric venous thrombosis. *Surg Gynecol Obstet* 1990;170:287-291.
45. Inahara T. Acute superior mesenteric venous thrombosis treatment by thrombectomy. *Ann Surg* 1971;174:956-961.
46. Akingba AG, Mangalmurti CS, Mukherjee D. Surgical management of chronic mesenteric venous thrombosis: a case report. *Vasc Endovascular Surg* 2006;40(2):157-160.
47. Bilbao JI, Rodriguez-Cabello J, Longo J, et al. Portal thrombosis: percutaneous transhepatic treatment with urokinase—a case treated with thrombectomy. *Surgery* 1974;76:286.
48. Robin P, Gurel Y, Lang M, et al. Complete thrombolysis of mesenteric vein occlusion with recombinant tissue-type plasminogen activator. *Lancet* 1988;1:1391.
49. Train JS, Ross H, Weiss JD, et al. Mesenteric venous thrombosis: successful treatment by intraarterial lytic therapy. *J Vasc Interv Radiol* 1998;9:461-464.
50. Poplausky MR, Kaufman JA, Geller SC, et al. Mesenteric venous thrombosis treated with urokinase via the superior mesenteric artery. *Gastroenterology* 1996;110:1633-1635.
51. Ferro C, Rossi UG, Bovio G, et al. Transjugular intrahepatic portosystemic shunt, mechanical aspiration thrombectomy, and direct thrombolysis in the treatment of acute portal and superior mesenteric vein thrombosis. *Cardiovasc Intervent Radiol* 2007;30(5):1070-1074.
52. Zhou W, Choi L, Lin PH, et al. Percutaneous transhepatic thrombectomy and pharmacologic thrombolysis of mesenteric venous thrombosis. *Vascular* 2007;15(1):41-45.
53. Latzman GS, Kornbluth A, Murphy SJ, et al. Use of an intravascular thrombectomy device to treat life-threatening venous thrombosis in a patient with Crohn's disease and G20210A prothrombin gene mutation. *Inflamm Bowel Dis* 2007;13(4):505-508.
54. Hollingshead M, Burke CT, Mauro MA, et al. Transcatheter thrombolytic therapy for acute mesenteric and portal vein thrombosis. *J Vasc Interv Radiol* 2005;16(5):651-661.
55. Kim HS, Patra A, Khan J, et al. Transhepatic catheter-directed thrombectomy and thrombolysis of acute superior mesenteric venous thrombosis. *J Vasc Interv Radiol* 2005;16(12):1685-1691.
56. Orr DW, Harrison PM, Devlin J, et al. Chronic mesenteric venous thrombosis: evaluation and determinants of survival during long-term follow-up. *Clin Gastroenterol Hepatol* 2007;5(1):80-86.

chapter

21

Splanchnic Artery Aneurysms

John E. Rectenwald, MD • James C. Stanley, MD • Gilbert R. Upchurch Jr, MD

Key Points

- True aneurysms of the splanchnic arteries are a rare, but important disease.
- Morbidity and mortality associated with rupture of splanchnic artery aneurysms is high.
- Little is known about the natural history of these aneurysms.
- Splenic artery aneurysms remain the most common and compose 60% of all splanchic artery aneurysms.
- Splenic artery aneurysms are associated with female sex, multiparity, portal hypertension, splenomegally and chronic pancreatitis.
- Hepatic artery aneurysms account for 20% of all splanchnic artery aneurysms.
- Hepatic artery aneurysm may rupure into the bile duct causing hematobilia.
- Aneurysms of the celiac trunk, superior mesenteric, and gastroepiploic arteries are rare entities.
- Management of splanchnic artery aneurysms has traditionally been by open surgery, although endovascular treatment is being increasingly applied.

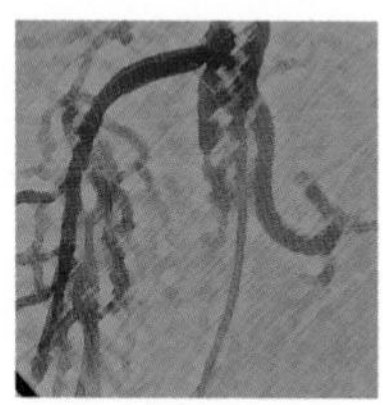

True aneurysms of splanchnic arteries are less common than visceral artery pseudoaneurysms, but they remain an important vascular disease.[1] Nearly 22% of these present as clinical emergencies, including 8.5% that result in death.[2] The pathogenesis and natural history of these aneurysms have been reassessed, and in most instances redefined, within the past three decades as advances in imaging technology and endovascular treatments have begun to influence diagnostic and management strategies. Recognition of splanchnic artery aneurysms has increased because of the greater availability and widespread use of advanced imaging capabilities such as high-resolution computed tomography (CT) scanning, magnetic resonance angiography (MRA), sophisticated ultrasonography, and angiography. Selective arteriography remains the most valuable examination in planning therapy,[3] but noninvasive imaging techniques for diagnosis and operative planning are becoming increasingly important.[4]

Although surgery remains the mainstay of therapy for most splanchnic aneurysms, especially in the setting of rupture,[5] many aneurysms (particularly those involving solid organs) are now treated with catheter-based interventions. Endovascular approaches are commonly used to control the bleeding that accompanies aneurysm rupture, and prophylactic treatment of incidentally discovered intact aneurysms has become common[6,7] (particularly those well-collateralized aneurysms that are imbedded within the pancreatic or hepatic parenchyma). Embolization has become the preferred treatment in patients at high surgical risk or for aneurysms in locations that are difficult to approach surgically.[8]

Inconsistencies appear in outcome following endovascular interventions. Early success with coil placement is reported to be as high as 92%, with 4% mortality at 1 month and only a single recurrence at 4 years. In another report, the early success rate was only 57%, and open operative therapy was needed in slightly more than 20% (with one patient dying before operation could be undertaken).[9,10] It is clear that a cautious approach to catheter-based management of splanchnic artery aneurysms should be employed,[11] but reports of failed procedures and a lack of long-term follow-up after have not tempered enthusiasm for endovascular treatment.[12-14]

More than 3000 splanchnic artery aneurysms have been documented in the literature, and the increasing discovery of these lesions supports the contention that they are more

Table 21-1
Relative Incidence of Aneurysms of the Splanchnic Arterial Circulation

Arterial Location	Incidence of Aneurysms
Splenic	60.0%
Hepatic	20.0%
Superior mesenteric	5.5%
Celiac	4.0%
Gastric or gastroepiploic	4.0%
Jejunal, ileal, or colic	3.0%
Pancreaticoduodenal or pancreatic	2.0%
Gastroduodenal	1.5%
Inferior mesenteric	Rare

common than previously claimed.[15] The distribution of aneurysms among splanchnic arteries has varied little during the past three decades (Table 21-1).[3,16-21] Anomalous arteries in the splanchnic circulation, such as a common celiacomesenteric trunk or replaced hepatic artery, may become aneurysmal, but there does not appear to be a predilection for this to occur.[22,23] Nearly a third of splanchnic artery aneurysms are associated with other nonvisceral aneurysms, involving, in decreasing frequency, the thoracic aorta, abdominal aorta, renal arteries, iliac arteries, lower extremity arteries, and intracranial arteries.[16] Cumulative experience with some aneurysms is so meager that discussion of them would be anecdotal. In other instances, evidence is sufficient to develop a rational basis for treatment.[24] Specific biological differences among individual aneurysms make it imperative to comment on them separately rather than collectively, although generally the repair of any splanchnic artery aneurysm greater than 2 cm in diameter should be considered.[10]

SPLENIC ARTERY ANEURYSMS

The most common abdominal visceral vessel affected by aneurysmal disease is the splenic artery. Aneurysms of the splenic artery make up 60% of all true splanchnic artery aneurysms. More than 1800 patients with splenic artery aneurysms have been described in previous publications, yet few clinical series of more than 20 patients from a single institution exist in the English literature.[25-29] The incidence of these lesions remains ill defined,[29a] ranging from 0.098% among nearly 195,000 autopsies[30] to 10.4% in a careful autopsy study of the splenic vessels in elderly patients.[31] Incidental demonstration of splenic aneurysms in 0.78% of nearly 3600 abdominal arteriographic studies at our institution may be a relatively accurate approximation of the actual frequency of these lesions in the population.[28] Macroaneurysms of the splenic artery usually are saccular. These lesions occur most often at bifurcations and are multiple in approximately 20% of patients.

In contrast to aneurysms of the abdominal aorta and lower extremity arteries, splenic artery aneurysms exhibit an unusual sex predilection, with a female-to-male ratio of 4:1. The propensity for aneurysm development in the splenic artery rather than in other splanchnic arteries has been attributed to acquired derangements of the vessel wall, including elastic fiber fragmentation, loss of smooth muscle, and internal elastic lamina disruption.

Three distinct phenomena may contribute to these changes. The first contributing factor to splenic artery aneurysms is the presence of systemic arterial fibrodysplasia. The recognized disruption of arterial wall architecture by medial dysplastic processes[32] is a logical forerunner of aneurysms, and patients with medial fibrodysplasia of the renal artery exhibit splenic artery aneurysms with a frequency six times greater than that seen in the normal population.[28]

The second contributing factor to the development of these splenic artery aneurysms is portal hypertension with splenomegaly.[33-38] Splenic artery aneurysms have been encountered in 10% to 30% of patients with portal hypertension and splenomegaly.[2,17,39] In these instances, aneurysms may have been sequelae of the apparent hyperkinetic process that causes increased splenic artery diameters in portal hypertension.[37,40,41] Whatever process underlies dilation of the artery, a similar process at vessel bifurcations would increase the likelihood of aneurysm formation. In this regard, aneurysm size in patients with portal hypertension has been directly correlated with splenic artery diameter.[39] Most of these aneurysms are multiple.[42] These particular splenic artery aneurysms are recognized most often in patients who have undergone orthotopic liver transplantation.[43] Screening for splenic artery aneurysms in all patients before undergoing liver transplantation has been recommended.[44]

The third contributing factor relevant to the evolution of splenic artery aneurysms is the vascular effects of repeated pregnancy.[17,28,29] In a large series from our institution, 40% of female patients with no obvious cause of their aneurysms had completed six or more pregnancies.[28] The importance of pregnancy in the genesis of these lesions receives further support because 45% of female patients with splenic artery aneurysms reported in the English-language literature from 1960 to 1970 (in whom parity was stated) were grand multiparous.[21] Gestational alterations in the vessel wall that are due to hormonal and local hemodynamic events may have a causal relation to medial defects and aneurysmal formation. Such effects may be similar to those underlying the vascular complications of pregnancy associated with Marfan's syndrome. The predilection for aneurysms to occur in the splenic artery instead of in other similar-sized muscular vessels may reflect increased splenic arteriovenous shunting during pregnancy with excessive blood flow, or it may represent preexisting structural abnormalities inherent to the splenic artery.

Certain splenic artery aneurysms appear to have evolved with arteriosclerotic weakening of the vessel wall.[45] However, frequent localization of calcific arteriosclerotic changes to aneurysms, without involvement of the adjacent artery, supports the contention that arteriosclerosis often occurs as a secondary process rather than a primary etiological event. The observation that calcific arteriosclerotic changes occur in some aneurysms arising from diseased splenic arteries lends further credence to this hypothesis.

Inflammatory processes adjacent to the splenic artery, particularly chronic pancreatitis with associated pseudocysts, are also known to cause aneurysms. Peripancreatic pseudoaneurysms occur in more than 10% of patients with chronic pancreatitis, and many of these involve the splenic artery.[46] Similarly, penetrating and blunt trauma may precipitate aneurysmal development. Infected (mycotic) lesions, often associated with subacute bacterial endocarditis in intravenous drug users, are being encountered more often in contemporary times. Microaneurysms of intrasplenic vessels are usually a manifestation of a connective tissue disease, such as periarteritis nodosa, and are of less surgical importance than macroaneurysms due to other causes.

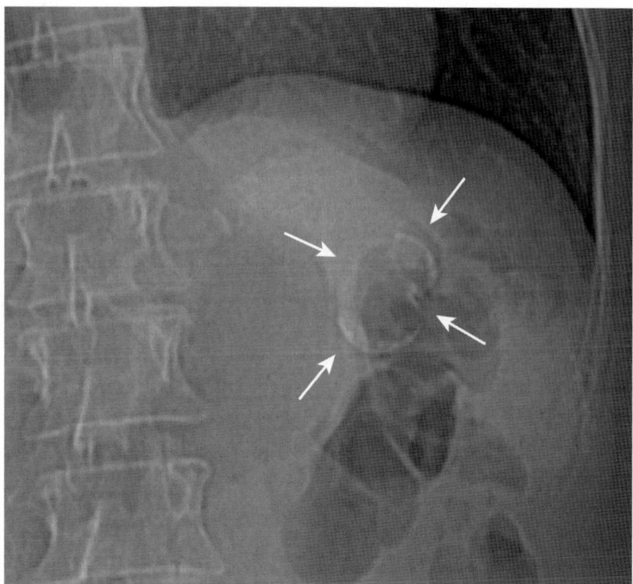

Figure 21-1. Splenic artery aneurysm on plain radiographic film. Curvilinear, signet ring–like calcifications in the upper-left quadrant are characteristic of splenic artery aneurysms. Calcified splenic artery aneurysm is between arrows.

The presence of a splenic artery aneurysm may be suspected with radiographic demonstration of curvilinear, signet ring–like calcifications in the upper-left quadrant on plain film x-rays (Figure 21-1) or CT scan (Figure 21-2). Plain x-ray findings have been reported in as many as 70% of cases.[47] However, diagnoses of these aneurysms are most often the result of conventional arteriography (Figure 21-3), ultrasonography, CT, (Figure 21-4A), or magnetic resonance imaging (MRI, Figure 21-4B)[42,48] in patients having imaging for other reasons.[28,49]

Splenic artery aneurysms usually are asymptomatic, although 17% and 20%, respectively, of patients in two large series allegedly had suggestive symptoms referable to these lesions.[47,50] Others have reported even higher rates of symptomatic aneurysms. A common complaint among symptomatic patients is vague upper-left quadrant or epigastric discomfort with occasional radiation to the left subscapular area. Acute expansion of splenic artery aneurysms intensifies these symptoms. Abdominal tenderness is an unlikely accompaniment of an intact aneurysm. A bruit ascribed to these lesions is more likely to arise from turbulent blood flow through the aorta and its branches than from splenic aneurysmal disease. Most splenic artery aneurysms are smaller than 2 cm in diameter; accordingly, pulsatile abdominal masses associated with these lesions are palpated rarely. A recent report raises possibility that circulating matrix metalloproteinase-9 levels in patients with these aneurysms may be a marker to monitor disease progression.[51]

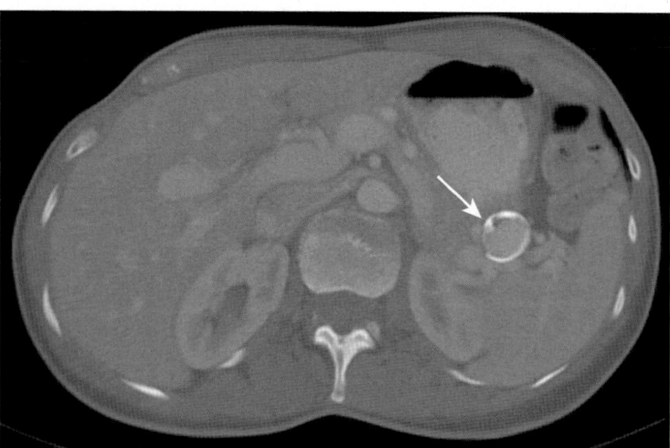

Figure 21-2. Typical appearance of a splenic artery aneurysm on a noncontrasted computed tomography scan. Again, note the curvilinear, signet ring calcifications in the upper-left quadrant *(white arrow)*.

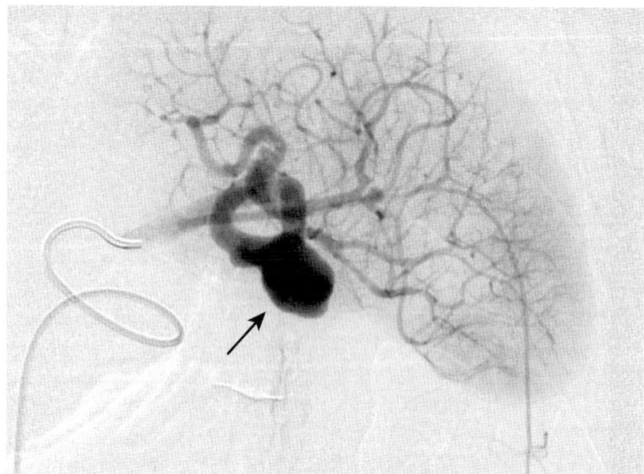

Figure 21-3. Selective splenic artery angiogram depicting a large splenic artery aneurysm *(black arrow)* of the main splenic artery.

Aneurysmal rupture with intraperitoneal hemorrhage accounts for the most dramatic clinical presentation of a splenic artery aneurysm and is associated with a mortality rate of approximately 40%. In nonpregnant patients, rupture often presents as an acute intraabdominal catastrophe with associated cardiovascular collapse. In most cases, bleeding initially occurs into the retrogastric area. Symptoms distant from the upper-left quadrant and epigastrium may follow as blood escapes through the foramen of Winslow. Hemorrhage invariably proceeds to severe intraperitoneal bleeding as lesser sac containment is lost. Such a "double rupture phenomenon" occurs in nearly 25% of cases and often provides an opportunity for treatment before the onset of fatal hemorrhage. In pregnant patients, aneurysmal rupture often mimics common obstetric emergencies, such as placental abruption, amniotic fluid embolization, or uterine rupture.[52-56]

Occasionally, intermittent gastrointestinal bleeding may reflect a communication between a splenic artery aneurysm and the intestinal tract or pancreatic ductal system.[57] These latter lesions are usually products of an inflammatory process, and the communication most often occurs directly, as with penetrating gastric ulcers. In cases associated with pancreatitis, bleeding may occur through the pancreatic ducts.[58] Splenic arteriovenous fistulae are an even more uncommon complication of aneurysmal rupture, but when they do occur, they are often associated with secondary portal hypertension.[59]

Life-threatening rupture appears to affect fewer than 2% of bland splenic artery aneurysms.[28] Factors contributing to rupture of previously asymptomatic splenic artery aneurysms remain poorly defined. No basis exists for the contention that rupture is less likely to occur in patients with calcified aneurysms, in normotensive as opposed to hypertensive patients, or in patients older than 60 years. It has been suggested that the use of beta-blockers may be associated with a lesser risk of rupture.[60] Aneurysms in patients who have received orthotopic liver transplants may be at greater risk of rupture than other

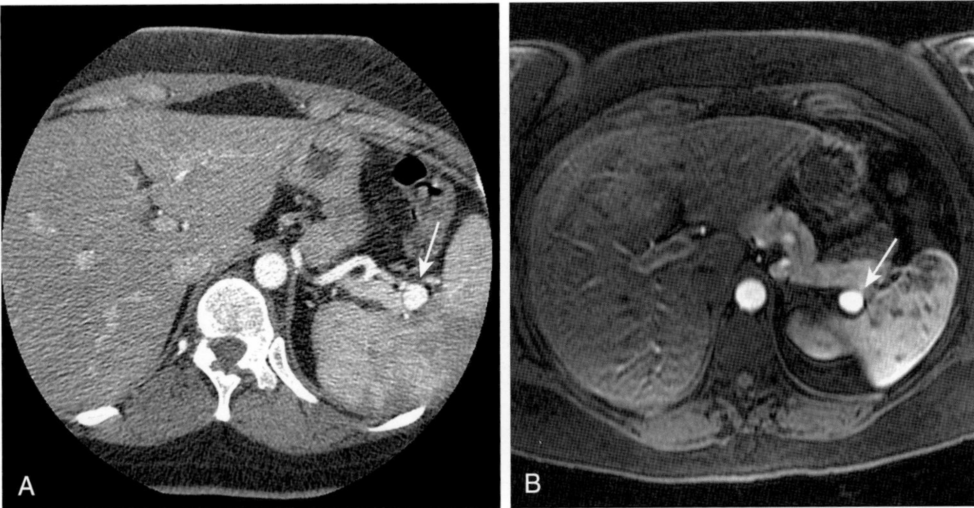

Figure 21-4. Typical appearance of splenic artery aneurysm on contrasted computed tomography **(A)** and magnetic resonance imaging **(B).** White arrow denoted splenic artery aneurysm on the image.

bland aneurysms.[35,43,61] The highest incidence of aneurysmal rupture occurs in young women during pregnancy. More than 95% of aneurysms discovered during pregnancy have ruptured.[28,52,55,62] Despite this observation, it is logical to believe that many splenic artery aneurysms develop during pregnancy and that most of these do not rupture during the pregnancy.

Indications for surgical therapy of splenic aneurysms have become better defined in recent years.[28,29,63] Symptomatic aneurysms warrant early surgical therapy. Operative intervention appears to be justified for splenic artery aneurysms encountered in pregnant patients or in females of childbearing age who subsequently may conceive. Splenic artery rupture during pregnancy is a catastrophic event associated with a maternal mortality of approximately 70% and fetal mortality exceeding 75%.[28,52-54,56] Survival of both mother and child following rupture of a splenic artery aneurysm, as of 1993, had been reported only 12 times.[52,54,64,65] In nonpregnant patients, operative mortality following surgical treatment for aneurysmal rupture is less than 25%.[21] The mortality following splenic artery aneurysm rupture in liver transplant patients is greater than 50%.[66]

Although rupture has been reported to occur in 3% to 9.6% of all patients with splenic artery aneurysms,[28,29,67] it is important to recall that disruption of bland lesions probably occurs in no more than 2% of cases. Thus, elective operation for bland splenic artery aneurysms is appropriate only when the predicted surgical mortality rate is no greater than 0.5%. This latter figure represents the product of the reported 2% incidence of rupture and the 25% mortality rate accompanying operative treatment of patients with ruptured aneurysms. In most instances, elective operation is recommended for good-risk patients with splenic artery aneurysms greater than 2 cm in diameter. In certain patients in whom operative therapy entails a prohibitively high risk, transcatheter embolization of the aneurysm may be the preferred treatment.[68,69] Several authors suggest that this may be the procedure of choice for splenic and indeed all splanchnic aneurysms. Temporizing enthusiasm for this approach is its 10% to 15% failure rate, the recognized complication of embolization, and continued enlargement of the aneurysm with potential for subsequent rupture.

Although there appears to be a slowly increasing role for endovascular techniques in the management of splenic artery aneurysms, open surgical techniques for treating splenic artery aneurysms have become standardized. Aneurysms of the proximal vessel may be treated by aneurysmectomy or simple ligation-exclusion without arterial reconstruction. Restoration of splenic artery continuity when treating aneurysms of this vessel is rarely indicated. Proximal splenic artery aneurysms are easily exposed through the lesser sac after the gastrohepatic ligament has been incised. Entering and exiting vessels are ligated, and these lesions usually are excised if they are not embedded within pancreatic tissue. Certain midsplenic artery aneurysms, especially those occurring as a result of pancreatic inflammatory disease, may not be removed so easily. Such false aneurysms, which often occur as a consequence of pancreatic pseudocyst erosion into the splenic artery, may be treated by arterial ligation from within the aneurysmal sac. Monofilament suture, such as polypropylene, is used to ligate vessels in this situation to lessen the risk of chronic infection that might occur in the presence of bacterial contamination of pseudocyst contents. Proximal splenic artery ligation or clamping, if easily accomplished, is recommended to lessen bleeding encountered upon opening the false aneurysm. Internal or external drainage of associated pseudocysts is often necessary following arterial ligation; later, extirpation of the diseased pancreas is often required. Distal pancreatectomy, including the affected artery, is preferred when treating inflammatory aneurysms involving the distal body and tail regions of the pancreas.

In the past, surgical therapy of aneurysms within the hilus of the spleen usually entailed a conventional splenectomy. Given the importance of splenic preservation in maintaining host resistance, simple suture obliteration, aneurysmorrhaphy, or excision of distal aneurysms may become favored over traditional splenectomy. Mortality following surgical therapy for pancreatitis-related bleeding arterial aneurysms, most commonly affecting the splenic artery, approaches 30%.[67] On the other hand, operative mortality following elective surgical treatment of bland noninflammatory splenic artery aneurysms, without concomitant vascular or gastrointestinal tract operations, has not been described among cases reported in the recent literature.[21,28,29] Laparoscopic treatment of these aneurysms, often guided by intraoperative ultrasound, is likely to decrease the expected blood loss and morbidity, as well as shorten the length of hospital stay accompanying conventional open procedures.[70,71]

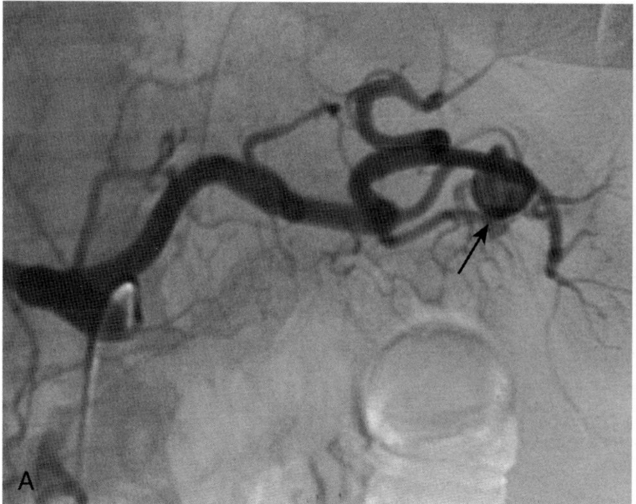

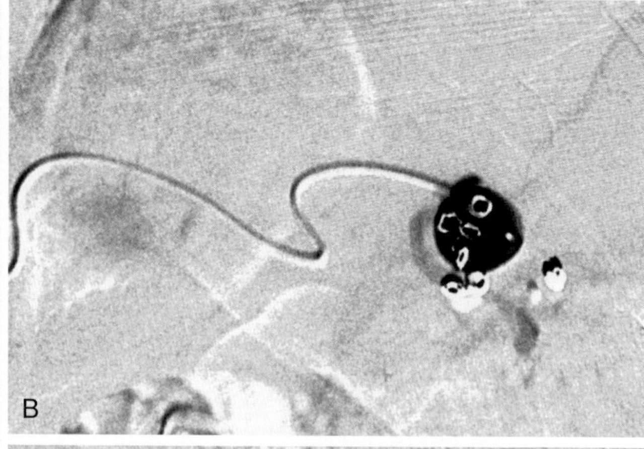

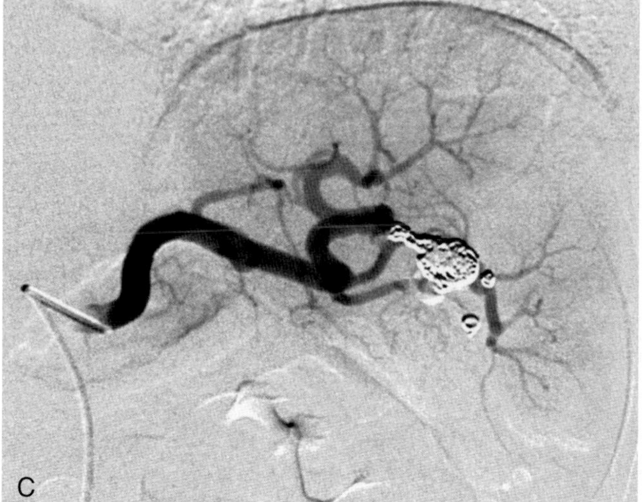

Figure 21-5. Splenic artery aneurysm. Arteriographic documentation of splenic artery aneurysm **(A;** *black arrow*) treated by coil embolization of the outflow branches of the splenic artery aneurysm, **(B)** followed by coil embolization of the aneurysm itself and the inflow artery to the aneurysm **(C)**.

Endovascular occlusion using coil embolization is becoming increasingly applied to splenic artery aneurysms and provides an alternative to operative intervention,[13,14,72-74] but splenic infarction (Figure 21-5), the possibility of splenic abscess formation, and the inability to ensure durable obliteration of the aneurysm mandate careful follow-up of patients treated in this fashion. Patients with multiple distal splenic artery aneurysms near the hilum of the spleen appear to particularly be at risk for major complications.[14] Migration of coils into the stomach following transcatheter coil embolization of a bleeding splenic artery aneurysm has been described.[75] The use of a stent graft to preserve splenic artery flow may be justified in rare clinical settings.[74,76-78] One such situation was reported in a patient in whom continued splenic artery flow was required in anticipation of creating a mesocaval shunt as a means of treating portal hypertension with bleeding jejunal varices.[76] Placement of a stent graft into such a tortuous artery is fraught with difficulty and, in the authors' experience, often results in thrombosis and occlusion of the splenic artery. This is due to dissection of the artery either from the placement of the larger diameter delivery catheter into the splenic artery or from the arterial wall occluding the lumen of the relatively stiff stent graft in an area of tortuosity—the so-called T-bar phenomenon. This problem may be overcome eventually with development of more flexible delivery catheters and stent grafts.

HEPATIC ARTERY ANEURYSMS

Aneurysmal disease of the hepatic artery accounts for 20% of aneurysms affecting splanchnic vessels.[79] Mycotic aneurysms, previously considered the most common type of hepatic artery aneurysm,[80] accounted for 16% of lesions described in the literature from 1960 to 1970.[21] At present, they represent only 10% of known hepatic artery aneurysms, occurring most often as a complication of intravenous drug use. Atheromatous changes have been encountered in approximately 32% of hepatic artery aneurysms. In most instances, however, atherosclerosis is considered not an etiological process but, rather, a secondary phenomenon.

Medial degeneration, including alterations similar to those encountered in many splenic artery aneurysms, has been documented in approximately 24% of these lesions. Medial defects appear to be acquired and are seemingly unrelated to congenital abnormalities. Specific events leading to the development of aneurysms in this latter setting are unknown. True aneurysms or pseudoaneurysms developing as a consequence of trauma represent an additional 22% of reported hepatic artery aneurysms, and the frequency of such lesions is increasing. Central hepatic rupture and deep parenchymal fractures subsequent to blunt abdominal injury or gunshot wounds are responsible for most traumatic aneurysms. Polyarteritis nodosa, cystic medial necrosis, and other more unusual arteriopathies have been associated with a few these aneurysms. A possible association between excessive oral amphetamine use and multiple visceral aneurysms has been reported. Both patients had hepatic and superior mesenteric artery aneurysms, and one also had a splenic artery aneurysm.[81] Lastly, periarterial inflammation, such as occurs with cholecystitis or pancreatitis, is a recognized but uncommon cause of hepatic artery aneurysms.

Hepatic artery aneurysms reported in surgical series have averaged greater than 3.5 cm in diameter.[82] Those larger than 2 cm usually are saccular in character. Smaller nontraumatic aneurysms tend to be fusiform. Of these lesions, 80% involve the extrahepatic vessels. The remaining 20% occur within the substance of the liver, with traumatic aneurysms dominating this latter group. A review of 163 aneurysms in which the specific site of the lesion could be ascertained revealed the following locations: common hepatic, 63%; right hepatic, 28%; left hepatic, 5%; and both right and left hepatic arteries, 4%.[21] Excluding multiple microaneurysms associated with inflammatory arteriopathies, such as polyarteritis nodosa,[83] most hepatic artery aneurysms are solitary. More than a third of aneurysms affecting the hepatic artery are associated with other visceral artery aneurysms, most commonly splenic aneurysms.[82]

Men with hepatic artery aneurysms outnumber women 2:1. Most of these lesions, excluding traumatic aneurysms, occur in patients who have entered their sixth decade of life. Most aneurysms remain asymptomatic. Among symptomatic patients with intact aneurysms, the most common complaint is upper-right quadrant or epigastric pain. Discomfort, although often vague, usually is persistent and is often attributed to cholecystitis. In most instances, this pain is not meal-related. Symptoms are most likely to evolve in patients with nonarteriosclerotic and multiple aneurysms. Expanding hepatic artery aneurysms usually cause severe upper abdominal discomfort, often with radiation to the back, similar to that accompanying pancreatitis. Exceedingly large aneurysms may compress the biliary tree and result in clinical manifestations similar to other forms of extrinsic extrahepatic bile duct obstruction. Pulsatile masses and abdominal bruits are uncommon findings in the presence of an intact aneurysm.

Rupture of hepatic artery aneurysms occurs into the hepatobiliary tract and the peritoneal cavity with equal frequency. Rupture into bile ducts often is responsible for the characteristic findings of hematobilia.[84-86] In such a setting, patients may complain of intermittent abdominal pain similar to that of biliary colic. Most exhibit massive gastrointestinal bleeding with periodic hematemesis.[47] More than half of these patients become jaundiced when blood clots obstruct their biliary ducts.

Most patients with hematobilia are febrile at some time during their illness. Symptoms of chronic anemia associated with insidious bleeding and melena are less common manifestations of aneurysmal communication with the biliary tree. Hematobilia occurs most often in the presence of traumatic intrahepatic pseudoaneurysms. Erosion of nontraumatic hepatic artery aneurysms into the stomach, duodenum, common bile duct, pancreatic duct, or portal vein is a recognized, but relatively rare, complication of these lesions. Intraperitoneal bleeding and exsanguinating hemorrhage, producing clinical signs of abdominal catastrophe, often accompany extrahepatic aneurysmal rupture.[47] In this regard, aneurysms associated with polyarteritis nodosa that rupture into the intraperitoneal cavity are most likely to arise from the hepatic artery.[87] Unfortunately, many patients destined to develop such complications do not exhibit prior symptoms and may present in extremis.

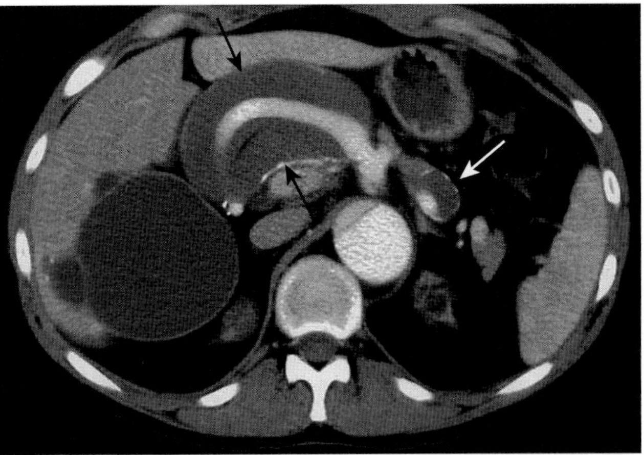

Figure 21-6. Hepatic artery aneurysm. Computed topographic image of a large common hepatic artery aneurysm in a patient with Marfan's syndrome (between *black arrows*). Additional findings on this image include a splenic artery aneurysm *(white arrow)*, an aortic dissection, and a large hepatic cyst (not marked).

In the past, the diagnosis of hepatic artery aneurysms was made most often at autopsy or at times of surgical exploration for major complications of these lesions. Historically, vascular calcifications in the upper abdomen and displacement of contiguous structures evident on barium studies or cholecystography suggested the presence of these aneurysms. More recently, arteriographic studies in patients with unknown causes of gastrointestinal hemorrhage and in those with major abdominal trauma have led to an increased recognition of hepatic artery aneurysms. Ultrasonography and CT may be valuable in screening patients for suspected hepatic artery aneurysms and in maintaining noninvasive follow-up[88] (Figure 21-6).

Excision or obliteration of all hepatic artery aneurysms appears justified unless unusual risks preclude operation. Although not every aneurysm eventually ruptures, rupture occurred in 44% of the lesions described in the literature from 1960 to 1970.[21] In some isolated experiences, high incidences of rupture have been reported,[89] but the overall rupture rate is probably less than 20%. Mortality associated with rupture continues to be exceedingly high and certainly is not less than the 35% previously reported.[62] An aggressive approach to managing these aneurysms seems appropriate.

Preoperative arteriographic delineation of the foregut and midgut arterial circulation is essential in planning optimal surgical therapy of these aneurysms.[90] Common hepatic artery aneurysms may often be treated by aneurysmectomy or aneurysmal exclusion without arterial reconstruction (depending on the status of the gastroduodenal artery). Extensive foregut collateral circulation to the liver through the gastroduodenal and right gastric arteries often provides adequate hepatic blood flow despite common hepatic artery interruption. However, if blood flow to the liver appears compromised following a 5-minute trial of intraoperative hepatic artery occlusion, then aneurysmorrhaphy or formal hepatic revascularization should be pursued (Figure 21-7). Failure to assess the adequacy of existing, collateral vessels may lead to hepatic necrosis.[91] Similarly, coexisting liver parenchymal disease makes ligation of the proximal hepatic artery less advisable and arterial reconstruction preferable.

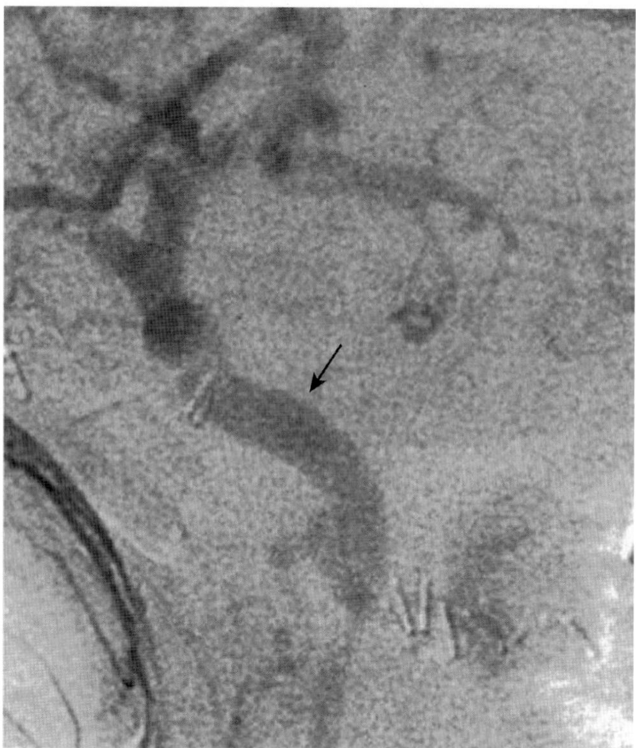

Figure 21-7. Vein graft repair of a common hepatic artery aneurysm. Selective superior mesenteric arteriogram showing a gastroduodenal to proper hepatic artery reverse saphenous vein graft *(black arrow)* to preserve arterial blood flow to the liver after aneurysmectomy and ligation of the common hepatic artery.

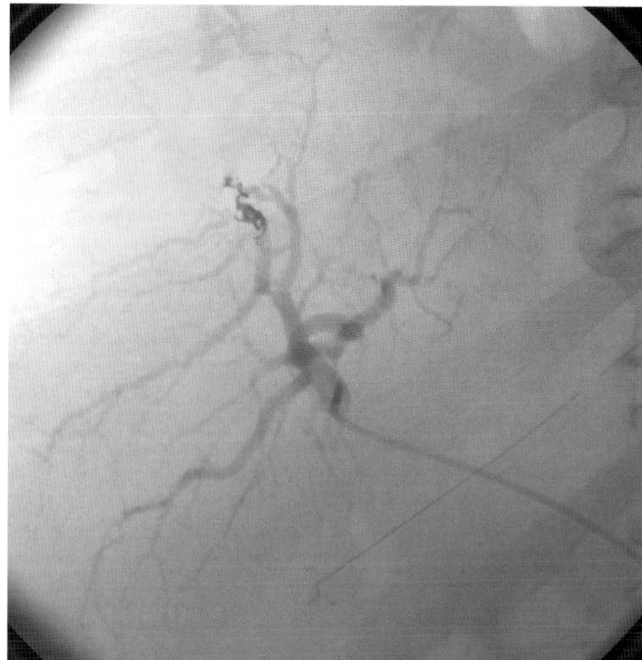

Figure 21-8. Intrahepatic artery aneurysm after coil embolization. Postembolization selective proper hepatic arteriogram shows the typical appearance of coils and occlusion of flow within the treated hepatic arterial segment.

Restoration of normal hepatic blood flow is important in the management of aneurysms involving the proper hepatic artery and its extrahepatic branches. Aneurysms of the hepatic artery are usually approached through an extended right subcostal or a vertical midline incision. Intact common hepatic artery aneurysms are easily isolated. However, proximal proper hepatic artery aneurysms should be cautiously dissected, especially near the gastroduodenal artery and its pancreaticoduodenal artery branch, which often cross over the common bile duct inferiorly. Similarly, distal proper hepatic or hepatic artery branch aneurysms must be carefully dissected to avoid bile duct injuries. Expeditious vascular control of entering and exiting vessels from within an aneurysm may be safer than dissecting the adjacent arteries when treating large or inflammatory aneurysms.

Several therapeutic alternatives exist in repairing aneurysmal hepatic arteries.[79] Aneurysmorrhaphy, with or without a vein patch closure, may be appropriate in managing select traumatic aneurysms. Fusiform and large saccular aneurysms that involve greater arterial circumferences are best treated by resection and arterial reconstruction (Figure 21-7). The use of an autogenous saphenous vein, despite occasional failures,[92] is preferred over synthetic prostheses in most circumstances. Anastomoses are best undertaken by spatulation of both the hepatic artery and the vein graft to provide an ovoid anastomosis less likely to become narrowed with healing. Interposition grafts within the hepatic arterial circulation are often possible; when not, an aortohepatic bypass may be undertaken. An extended Kocher's maneuver with medial visceral rotation allows exposure of the vena cava and aorta. A vein graft from the anterolateral aspect of the infrarenal aorta may then be carried behind the duodenum to the porta hepatis. After the aneurysmectomy has been performed, the spatulated vein is anastomosed end to end to either the common or the proper hepatic artery.

Resection of liver parenchyma for intrahepatic aneurysms that are not amenable to reconstruction is occasionally necessary. Control of bleeding intrahepatic aneurysms by simple ligation of the proximal vessel, despite the possibility of subsequent liver necrosis, may be preferable to undertaking a major liver resection in a critically ill patient. Similarly, percutaneous transcatheter balloon embolization with occlusion of hepatic artery aneurysms in high-risk cases may be an acceptable alternative to operative therapy[63,74,93-95] (Figure 21-8). This may be the preferred treatment for small intrahepatic pseudoaneurysms, especially in those patients with malignancies.[74] Noteworthy is a reported 42% recanalization rate following hepatic artery embolocclusion, mandating careful follow-up. Stent graft repair of a hepatic artery aneurysm has been described in the literature.[74,96] In our limited experience, stent grafts placed in the hepatic artery for treatment of aneurysm cause slowly progressive stenosis of the hepatic artery. The artery eventually occludes. In a few cases, sufficient hepatic collaterals to the liver develop by the time of occlusion and the liver parenchyma remains viable. The potential for migration of embolic material or stent graft occlusion with central lobular necrosis and abscess formation is also a recognized complication of transcatheter treatment of these aneurysms. Percutaneous thrombin injection of a hepatic artery pseudoaneurysm has been reported in a liver transplant patient following repair of a perforated duodenum in the setting of bile peritonitis.[97]

SUPERIOR MESENTERIC ARTERY ANEURYSMS

The third most common splanchnic artery aneurysm, accounting for 5.5% of splanchnic artery aneurysms, involves the main trunk of the superior mesenteric artery. These lesions, affecting the proximal 5 cm of this vessel, have been reported to be the most often infectious in etiology.[21,98,99] In this regard, the superior mesenteric artery harbors more infectious aneurysms than any other muscular arteries. Nonhemolytic *Streptococcus,* related to left-sided bacterial endocarditis, has been the organism reported most often in these lesions. Various other pathogens, especially staphylococcal organisms, have been described in aneurysms associated with noncardiac septicemia. A recent report suggested that an infectious etiology accounted for less than 5% of these aneurysms.[100] Syphilitic aneurysms, often described in early reports, have not been observed in contemporary times. Dissecting aneurysms associated with medial defects are rare[101] but affect this vessel more than any other splanchnic artery.[102] Arteriosclerosis, most likely representing a secondary event, is evident in approximately 20% of reported superior mesenteric artery aneurysms. Trauma is a rare cause.

Intermittent upper abdominal discomfort that progresses to persistent and severe epigastric pain often accompanies symptomatic mycotic superior mesenteric artery aneurysms. In certain cases, it may be difficult to distinguish symptomatology due to mesenteric ischemia from that due to aneurysmal expansion. It is noteworthy that a tender pulsatile abdominal mass that is not rigidly fixed has been discovered in nearly half of these patients.

Female patients were predominant in earlier series of superior mesenteric artery aneurysms. More recent experience has not confirmed such a sex predilection, and men and women are affected equally. Most mycotic aneurysms occur in patients under 50 years of age. Nonmycotic aneurysms of the superior mesenteric artery most often affect patients after the sixth decade of life. This older subgroup of patients often experiences prodromata of intestinal angina before aneurysm rupture. Superior mesenteric artery aneurysm rupture, although not common in earlier times, was reported in nearly 40% of patients from one recent series.[100]

Aneurysmal expansion with dissection, or propagation of intraluminal thrombus, beyond the vessel's inferior pancreaticoduodenal and middle colic branches, effectively isolates the superior mesenteric artery from the collaterals of the celiac and inferior mesenteric artery circulations. In such circumstances, any compromise of blood flow through the superior mesenteric artery may cause intestinal angina. Because of the critical location of most superior mesenteric artery aneurysms, the existence of asymptomatic lesions is not as common as with many other splanchnic aneurysms. Antemortem diagnosis of uncomplicated superior mesenteric artery aneurysms is therefore uncommon. In fact, recognition of asymptomatic solitary dissecting superior mesenteric artery aneurysms has not been reported.[101] Radiographic evidence of calcified mycotic aneurysms and abdominal angiograms made during studies for unrelated disease have been responsible for most antemortem diagnoses.

Surgical treatment of most superior mesenteric artery aneurysms appears justified in light of the seemingly common occurrence of rupture or arterial occlusion. Nearly a third of reported superior mesenteric artery aneurysms have been successfully treated by operation.[103] This includes fewer than 20 mycotic aneurysms of this vessel.[99] Operative exposure for more distal lesions may be obtained by a transmesenteric route or for proximal lesions by a retroperitoneal approach after the lateral parietes are incised, allowing the colon, pancreas, and spleen to be reflected medially. Since the first successful surgical treatment of a superior mesenteric artery aneurysm was reported nearly five decades ago,[98,104] the most common procedures attempted have been aneurysmorrhaphy and simple ligation, the latter having been undertaken in more than a third of cases. Ligation of the vessels entering and exiting these aneurysms without arterial reconstruction has proved to be an acceptable, simple means of treatment.[21,100,105] The existence of preformed collaterals involving the inferior pancreaticoduodenal and middle colic arteries allows this approach to be successful in most instances. Temporary occlusion of the superior mesenteric artery, with intraoperative assessment of bowel viability, offers a means of identifying cases in which mesenteric revascularization is necessary.

Superior mesenteric artery aneurysmectomy may prove hazardous because of the proximity of neighboring structures, such as the superior mesenteric vein and the pancreas. Endoaneurysmorrhaphy in selected patients with saccular aneurysms may be possible. Arterial reconstruction, with an interposition graft or aortomesenteric bypass after exclusion or excision of the aneurysm, has been rarely accomplished.[103,106,107] Use of synthetic prostheses, originating from the anterior aorta or intact proximal superior mesenteric artery and carried to the normal vessel beyond the aneurysm, is acceptable in the absence of a mycotic aneurysm or infarcted bowel. In the presence of infection, an autogenous saphenous vein is a more appropriate conduit for reconstruction. In such cases, long-term antibiotic therapy is also recommended. Contemporary surgical intervention for all types of superior mesenteric artery aneurysms carries a mortality of less than 15%.

Transcatheter occlusion of saccular aneurysms with discrete necks arising from the side of the superior mesenteric artery may occasionally be justified[63,73] and has been advocated by some in the patient with severe abdominal adhesions from prior laparotomies or at high risk for surgery.[108] In theory, endovascular coil occlusion of a superior mesenteric artery aneurysm may be an appropriate alternative to surgical ligation or repair, especially in the setting of a hostile abdomen such as that of acute pancreatitis.[109,110] Percutaneous stent graft treatment of a proximal superior mesenteric artery pseudoaneurysm[74] and traumatic pseudoaneurysm[111] has been described. This approach may shorten the length of hospital stay and avoid the excessive mortality associated with open surgical repair in the multitrauma patient. A recent report describes two superior mesenteric artery aneurysms successfully treated with stent grafts.[14] Stent graft treatment of a superior mesenteric artery pseudoaneurysm in the setting of infection, while described,[112] is not favored, and the long-term outcome of such treatment is unknown.

CELIAC ARTERY ANEURYSMS

Aneurysms of the celiac artery are unusual lesions that account for 4% of all splanchnic aneurysms. In 1985, only 108 celiac artery aneurysms had been described in the literature.[113] Arteriosclerosis and medial degeneration were the most common histological changes observed in these aneurysms. The former, noted in 27% of patients, probably represents a secondary rather than a primary causative process. A preexisting paucity of elastic tissue and smooth muscle at major branchings appears to be a contributing factor in an additional 17% of patients in whom developmental aneurysms were suspected.

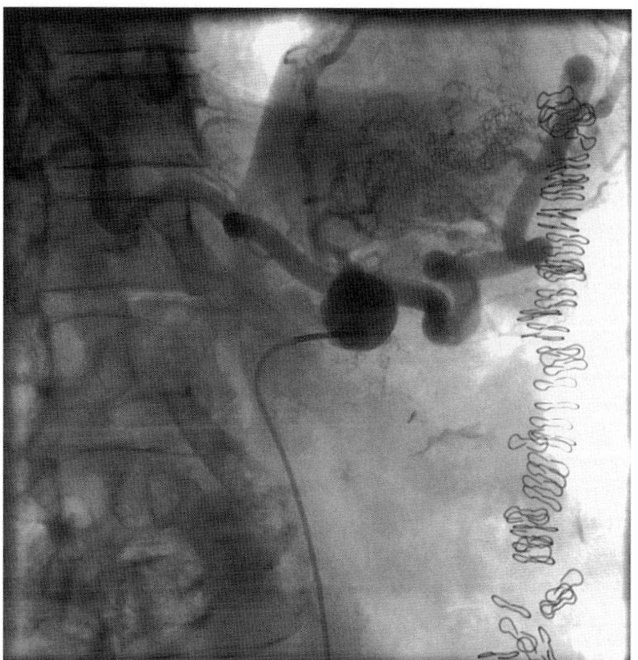

Figure 21-9. Celiac artery aneurysm. A selective celiac artery angiogram illustrating the appearance of a true aneurysm of the celiac artery. The main branches of the celiac, splenic, common hepatic, and left gastric arteries are clearly seen in this oblique projection.

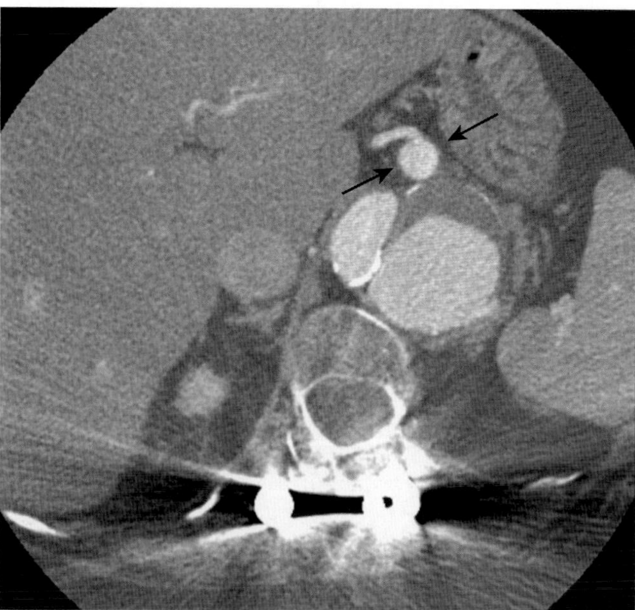

Figure 21-10. Computed topographic appearance of a celiac artery aneurysm. Contrasted computed topography scan of the abdomen showing a discrete celiac artery aneurysm (between *black arrows*) in a Marfan's patient with an aneurysmal dilation of a thoracoabdominal aortic artery dissection.

Traumatic aneurysms caused by penetrating injuries are uncommon. Poststenotic dilatation occasionally progresses to frank aneurysmal change but is an uncommon cause of these lesions. Mycotic celiac artery aneurysms are rare,[114] and in recent times syphilitic and tuberculous lesions have not been encountered. Associated aortic aneurysms were noted in 18% of patients with celiac artery aneurysms, and other splanchnic artery aneurysms affected 38% of these patients.[113]

Most celiac artery aneurysms are asymptomatic. Although males outnumber females among all reported cases, no sex predilection occurred in patients reported since the 1960s. The average age of patients reported before 1950 was 40 years, in contrast to an average age of 52 years reported since then.[109]

Abdominal discomfort localized to the epigastrium accompanies more than 60% of symptomatic celiac artery aneurysms. Intense discomfort, often with radiation to the back, as well as nausea and vomiting, has been attributed to aneurysmal expansion and may be confused with pancreatitis. Abdominal bruits are often heard in patients with celiac artery aneurysms, although these bruits are rarely due to the aneurysm. Celiac artery aneurysms are apparent as pulsatile abdominal masses in nearly 30% of cases.[109] Symptomatology suggestive of intestinal angina is a rare accompaniment of celiac artery aneurysms and, when present, is usually due to significant coexisting arteriosclerotic occlusive disease affecting the superior mesenteric and inferior mesenteric arteries.

The most serious clinical complication of celiac artery aneurysmal disease is rupture. Although nearly 80% of all previously reported lesions had ruptured, clinical experience over the past 25 years has documented a risk of rupture of 13%.[109] The contemporary incidence of rupture may be even lower.[115] Aneurysmal disruption is most often associated with intraperitoneal hemorrhage, although communication with the gastrointestinal tract can occur.

Recognition of most celiac artery aneurysms encountered before 1950 occurred at the time of autopsy. Currently, unexpected discovery of aneurysms during angiography accounts for nearly 65% of cases (Figure 21-9).[21,116,117] Calcification of the aneurysm, which affects 20% of these lesions, and displacement of contiguous structures are occasional radiographic findings that suggest the diagnosis. Ultrasonography and CT may be of diagnostic use in assessing certain lesions[117-120] and should be useful in longitudinal follow-up of nonoperative cases (Figure 21-10). Surgical treatment of celiac artery aneurysms is warranted except when operative risks contraindicate an abdominal operation.[115,117] Success in more than 90% of cases reported since the first successful surgical treatment 40 years ago supports operative management.[115,121]

Most patients, especially those with small, bland aneurysms, can be treated by the abdominal route alone. This approach is particularly applicable if a broad costal margin exists. In these instances, a medial visceral rotation of the left colon, spleen, and pancreas allow exposure of the aorta at the diaphragmatic hiatus. Transection of the crus and median arcuate ligament provides access to the origin of the celiac artery and adjacent aorta. Exposure of celiac artery aneurysms for symptomatic or large lesions is more difficult and may require a thoracoabdominal approach, with the incision extending from the midaxillary line on the left, usually in the seventh intercostal space, across the costal margin into the abdomen.

Aneurysmorrhaphy has been advocated in select cases. It is favored only for discrete saccular aneurysms in which the integrity of the remaining arterial wall appears normal. Aneurysmectomy with arterial reconstruction accounts for 50% of reported operations.[116] Aneurysmectomy and primary reanastomosis of the celiac artery trunk are sometimes possible but should only be undertaken in the presence of a relatively normal and lengthy proximal celiac artery. When reanastomosis is not feasible, an aortoceliac bypass with a synthetic prosthesis[115] or autogenous vein graft should be performed.

Celiac axis ligation with interruption of antegrade blood flow through the common hepatic, left gastric, and splenic vessels has been undertaken in 35% of reported operations.[116] Ligation is clearly preferred in certain settings, such as with Ehlers-Danlos syndrome, where vessel wall fragility precludes safe arterial reconstructions.[122] Although celiac artery ligation rarely results in hepatic necrosis, it should be undertaken only when no liver disease preexists and intraoperative findings suggest that hepatic blood flow will not be severely compromised.[123] Mortality for open operative treatment of patients with ruptured celiac artery aneurysms is 40%, compared with only 5% for those with nonruptured aneurysms.[116]

Glue embolic occlusion of the celiac trunk has been described[124] as a technique for endovascular management of celiac artery aneurysms.[74125,126] One report describes celiac artery occlusion in various aneurysms, including thoracoabdominal aortic aneurysm and dissections, as well as celiac artery aneurysms. The authors report treatment of three true aneurysms of the celiac artery, with coil embolization of the celiac branch vessels in two cases and of the celiac artery alone in one. No treatment-related complications occurred in any case, but care was taken to ensure that collateralization to the proper hepatic artery remained intact after celiac artery or branch embolization. Normal liver function was considered a prerequisite for embolic treatment of these aneurysms.[125] Successful treatment of a large (10 cm) saccular celiac artery pseudoaneurysm in a high-risk surgical patient by exclusion of the celiac artery with an aortic stent graft has also been described.[126] An example of stent graft placement for treatment of a celiac artery aneurysm from our institution is presented as an example of the results that can be obtained using this technique (Figure 21-11).

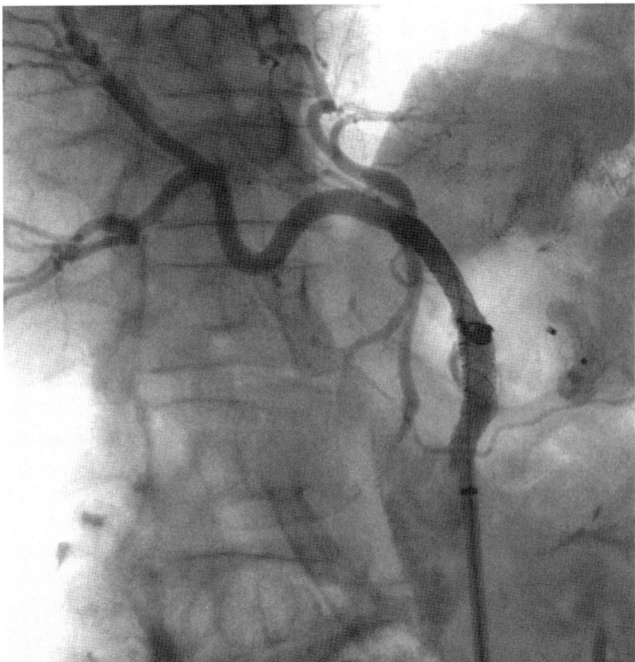

Figure 21-11. Stent graft repair of the celiac artery aneurysm presented in Figure 21-9. After coil embolization of the proximal left gastric and splenic arteries, a stent graft (Wallgraft) was placed from the origin of the celiac artery into the proper hepatic artery.

GASTRIC AND GASTROEPIPLOIC ARTERY ANEURYSMS

Aneurysms of gastric and gastroepiploic arteries account for approximately 4% of splanchnic aneurysms. These lesions appear to be acquired, although their exact cause remains undefined.[127] Histological evidence of arteriosclerosis in many aneurysms led to an earlier belief that this was an important etiological factor,[128] but it now seems likely that medial degeneration of undetermined origin or degeneration resulting from periarterial inflammation precedes the arteriosclerotic changes (making atherosclerosis a secondary event). Most clinically important aneurysms involving vessels to the stomach are solitary. Aneurysms of gastric arteries are nearly 10 times more common than those of gastroepiploic arteries. They are considered together because their natural history and management are similar.

Asymptomatic aneurysms of the gastric and gastroepiploic arteries are rare. Most aneurysms described in the literature have presented as vascular emergencies, with rupture at the time of diagnosis occurring in more than 90% of cases. Nearly 70% were associated with serious gastrointestinal bleeding. A few patients describe antecedent dyspeptic epigastric discomfort, but most have no abdominal pain before aneurysmal rupture. Intestinal bleeding in these cases is usually manifest by acute massive hematemesis,[129] although a few patients experience chronic occult gastrointestinal bleeding. Rupture of gastric and gastroepiploic artery aneurysms causes life-threatening intraperitoneal bleeding in approximately 30% of cases.[130,131] As is the case with intestinal bleeding, most patients are asymptomatic before the occurrence of acute intraperitoneal aneurysmal disruption. Most cases affect individuals in their sixth and seventh decades of life, and men outnumber women approximately 3:1.

Antemortem diagnosis of gastric and gastroepiploic artery aneurysms most often occurs during urgent operation for gastrointestinal or intraperitoneal bleeding. Intraoperative search for gastric and gastroepiploic aneurysms requires careful palpation and transillumination of the entire stomach. Arteriographic studies for unexplained gastrointestinal bleeding result in occasional preoperative recognition of these lesions. Mucosal alterations associated with these aneurysms are often minimal, and endoscopic recognition is difficult. Larger lesions may be mistaken for gastric ulcers or malignancies.

Treatment of gastric and gastroepiploic aneurysms is directed at controlling life-threatening hemorrhage. Approximately 70% of patients reported to have these lesions succumb following aneurysm rupture.[21] Early diagnosis and urgent operative intervention are necessary to improve survival. Ligation of aneurysmal vessels, with or without excision of the aneurysm, is appropriate treatment for extraintestinal lesions and for those aneurysms associated with inflammatory processes adjacent to the stomach. Intramural aneurysms and those associated with bleeding into the gastrointestinal tract should be excised with portions of the involved gastric tissue. Successful transcatheter coil embolization of a left gastric artery pseudoaneurysm after blunt abdominal trauma has been described.[132]

SUMMARY

Splanchnic artery aneurysms are rare; when they occur, they are usually complicated by rupture and are often fatal when rupture occurs. The presenting symptoms of splanchnic artery aneurysms are often vague and, given the low frequency of these aneurysms in the population, little is known about their natural history. Limited data on treatment of these aneurysms make management difficult. Open surgical repair of splanchnic artery aneurysms has been the standard of care, although endovascular techniques can be used when applicable. Close clinical follow-up of patients with endovascularly treated splanchnic artery aneurysms is mandatory given the relatively high rate of required secondary catheter-based procedures to permanently occlude these aneurysms.

ACKNOWLEDGMENTS

This chapter has been updated and modified from Upchurch GR Jr, Zelenock GB, and Stanley JC. Splanchnic artery aneurysms, Chapter 107, In: Cronenwett JL, Gloviczki P, Johnston KW, et al., eds. *Vascular surgery*. 6th ed. Philadelphia: Elsevier Saunders; 2005.

References

1. Upchurch GR, Zelenock GB, Stanley JC. Splanchnic artery aneurysms. In: Rutherford RB, ed. *Vascular surgery*. 6th ed. Philadelphia: Elsevier; Saunders, 2005:1565-1580.
2. Stanley JC. Abdominal visceral aneurysm. In. Haimovici H, ed. *Vascular emergencies*. New York: Appleton-Century-Crofts; 1981:387.
3. Hong Z, Chen F, Yang J, et al. Diagnosis and treatment of splanchnic artery aneurysms: a report of 57 cases. *Chin Med J* 1999;112(1):29-33.
4. Pilleul F, Beuf O. Diagnosis of splanchnic artery aneurysms and pseudoaneurysms, with special reference to contrast enhanced 3D magnetic resonance angiography: a review. *Acta Radiol* 2004;45(7):702-708.
5. Wagner WH, Allins AD, Treiman RL, et al. Ruptured visceral artery aneurysms. *Ann Vasc Surg* 1997;11(4):342-347.
6. Yamakado K, Nakatsuka A, Tanaka N, et al. Transcatheter arterial embolization of ruptured pseudoaneurysms with coils and n-butyl cyanoacrylate. *J Vasc Interv Radiol* 2000;11(1):66-72.
7. Salam TA, Lumsden AB, Martin LG, Smith RB, 3rd. Nonoperative management of visceral aneurysms and pseudoaneurysms. *Am J Surg* 1992;164(3):215-219.
8. Pasha SF, Gloviczki P, Stanson AW, Kamath PS. Splanchnic artery aneurysms. *Mayo Clin Proc* 2007;82(4):472-479.
9. Pilleul F, Dugougeat F. Transcatheter embolization of splanchnic aneurysms/pseudoaneurysms: early imaging allows detection of incomplete procedure. *J Comput Assist Tomogr* 2002;26(1):107-112.
10. Gabelmann A, Gorich J, Merkle EM. Endovascular treatment of visceral artery aneurysms. *J Endovasc Ther* 2002;9(1):38-47.
11. Raad E, Demaria R, Rouviere P, et al. Visceral artery aneurysms: multiple aneurysmal localization—a case report and literature review. *J Mal Vasc* 2007;32(4-5):216-220.
12. Ruiz-Tovar J, Martinez-Molina E, Morales V, et al. Evolution of the therapeutic approach of visceral artery aneurysms. *Scand J Surg* 2007;96(4):308-313.
13. Huang YK, Hsieh HC, Tsai FC, et al. Visceral artery aneurysm: risk factor analysis and therapeutic opinion. *Eur J Vasc Endovasc Surg* 2007;33(3):293-301.
14. Saltzberg SS, Maldonado TS, Lamparello PJ, et al. Is endovascular therapy the preferred treatment for all visceral artery aneurysms? *Ann Vasc Surg* 2005;19(4):507-515.
15. Miani S, Arpesani A, Giorgetti PL, et al. Splanchnic artery aneurysms. *J Cardiovasc Surg (Torino)* 1993;34(3):221-228.
16. Carr SC, Mahvi DM, Hoch JR, et al. Visceral artery aneurysm rupture. *J Vasc Surg* 2001;33(4):806-811.
17. Deterling RA Jr. Aneurysm of the visceral arteries. *J Cardiovasc Surg (Torino)* 1971;12(4):309-322.
18. Grego FG, Lepidi S, Ragazzi R, et al. Visceral artery aneurysms: a single center experience. *Cardiovasc Surg* 2003;11(1):19-25.
19. Jorgensen BA. Visceral artery aneurysms: a review. *Dan Med Bull* 1985;32(4):237-242.
20. Kanazawa S, Inada H, Murakami T, et al. The diagnosis and management of splanchnic artery aneurysms: report of 8 cases. *J Cardiovasc Surg (Torino)* 1997;38(5):479-485.
21. Stanley JC, Thompson NW, Fry WJ. Splanchnic artery aneurysms. *Arch Surg* 1970;101(6):689-697.
22. Bailey RW, Riles TS, Rosen RJ, Sullivan LP. Celiomesenteric anomaly and aneurysm: clinical and etiologic features. *J Vasc Surg* 1991;14(2):229-234.
23. Settembrini PG, Jausseran JM, Roveri S, et al. Aneurysms of anomalous splenomesenteric trunk: clinical features and surgical management in two cases. *J Vasc Surg* 1996;24(4):687-692.
24. Carr SC, Pearce WH, Vogelzang RL, et al. Current management of visceral artery aneurysms. *Surgery* 1996;120(4):627-633; discussion, 33-34.
25. Fukunaga Y, Usui N, Hirohashi K, et al. Clinical courses and treatment of splenic artery aneurysms: report of 3 cases and review of literatures in Japan. *Osaka City Med J* 1990;36(2):161-173.
26. Mattar SG, Lumsden AB. The management of splenic artery aneurysms: experience with 23 cases. *Am J Surg* 1995;169(6):580-584.
27. Moore SW, Lewis RJ. Splenic artery aneurysm. *Ann Surg* 1961;153: 1033-1046.
28. Stanley JC, Fry WJ. Pathogenesis and clinical significance of splenic artery aneurysms. *Surgery* 1974;76(6):898-909.
29. Trastek VF, Pairolero PC, Joyce JW, et al. Splenic artery aneurysms. *Surgery* 1982;91(6):694-699.

29a. Kreel L. The recognition and incidence of splenic artery aneurysms: a historical review. *Australas radiolo* 1972;16:126.

30. Moore SW, Guida PM, Schumacher HW. Splenic artery aneurysm. *Bull Soc Int Chir* 1970;29(4):210-218.
31. Bedford PD, Lodge B. Aneurysm of the splenic artery. *Gut* 1960;1: 312-320.
32. Stanley JC, Gewertz BL, Bove EL, et al. Arterial fibrodysplasia. Histopathologic character and current etiologic concepts. *Arch Surg* 1975;110(5):561-566.
33. Boijsen E, Efsing HO. Aneurysm of the splenic artery. *Acta Radiol Diagn (Stockh)* 1969;8(1):29-41.
34. Feist JH, Gajaraj A. Extra- and intrasplenic artery aneurysms in portal hypertension. *Radiology* 1977;125(2):331-334.
35. Gaglio PJ, Regenstein F, Slakey D, et al. α-1 Antitrypsin deficiency and splenic artery aneurysm rupture: an association? *Am J Gastroenterol* 2000;95(6):1531-1534.
36. Kobori L, van der Kolk MJ, de Jong KP, et al. Splenic artery aneurysms in liver transplant patients: liver transplant group. *J Hepatol* 1997;27(5):890-893.
37. Manenti F, Williams R. Injection studies of the splenic vasculature in portal hypertension. *Gut* 1966;7(2):175-180.
38. Scheinin TM, Vanttinen E. Aneurysms of the splenic artery in portal hypertension. *Ann Clin Res* 1969;1(3):165-168.
39. Puttini M, Aseni P, Brambilla G, Belli L. Splenic artery aneurysms in portal hypertension. *J Cardiovasc Surg (Torino)* 1982;23(6):490-493.
40. Nishida O, Moriyasu F, Nakamura T, et al. Hemodynamics of splenic artery aneurysm. *Gastroenterology* 1986;90(4):1042-1046.
41. Ohta M, Hashizume M, Ueno K, et al. Hemodynamic study of splenic artery aneurysm in portal hypertension. *Hepatogastroenterology* 1994;41(2):181-184.
42. Keehan MF, Kistner RL, Banis Jr J. Angiography as an aid in extraenteric gastrointestinal bleeding due to visceral artery aneurysm. *Ann Surg* 1978;187(4):357-361.
43. Ayalon A, Wiesner RH, Perkins JD, et al. Splenic artery aneurysms in liver transplant patients. *Transplantation* 1988;45(2):386-389.
44. Lee PC, Rhee RY, Gordon RY, et al. Management of splenic artery aneurysms: the significance of portal and essential hypertension. *J Am Coll Surg* 1999;189(5):483-490.
45. Owens JC, Coffey RJ. Aneurysm of the splenic artery including a report of 6 additional cases. *Int Abstr Surg* 1953;97(4):313-335.
46. Hofer BO, Ryan JA Jr, Freeny PC. Surgical significance of vascular changes in chronic pancreatitis. *Surg Gynecol Obstet* 1987;164(6):499-505.
47. Reber PU, Baer HU, Patel AG, et al. Life-threatening upper gastrointestinal tract bleeding caused by ruptured extrahepatic pseudoaneurysm after pancreatoduodenectomy. *Surgery* 1998;124(1):114-115.
48. Martin KW, Morian Jr JP, Lee JK, Scharp DW. Demonstration of a splenic artery pseudoaneurysm by MR imaging. *J Comput Assist Tomogr* 1985;9(1):190-192.

49. Shanley CJ, Shah NL, Messina LM. Common splanchnic artery aneurysms: splenic, hepatic, and celiac. *Ann Vasc Surg* 1996;10(3):315-322.
50. Pitkaranta P, Haapiainen R, Kivisaari L, Schroder T. Diagnostic evaluation and aggressive surgical approach in bleeding pseudoaneurysms associated with pancreatic pseudocysts. *Scand J Gastroenterol* 1991;26(1):58-64.
51. Ebaugh JL, Chiou AC, Morasch MD, et al. Staged embolization and operative treatment of multiple visceral aneurysms in a patient with fibromuscular dysplasia: a case report. *Vasc Surg* 2001;35(2):145-148.
52. Angelakis EJ, Bair WE, Barone JE, Lincer RM. Splenic artery aneurysm rupture during pregnancy. *Obstet Gynecol Surv* 1993;48(3):145-148.
53. Barrett JM, Caldwell BH. Association of portal hypertension and ruptured splenic artery aneurysm in pregnancy. *Obstet Gynecol* 1981;57(2):255-257.
54. Caillouette JC, Merchant EB. Ruptured splenic artery aneurysm in pregnancy: twelfth reported case with maternal and fetal survival. *Am J Obstet Gynecol* 1993;168(6 Pt 1):1810-1811: discussion, 1-3.
55. Macfarlane JR, Thorbjarnarson B. Rupture of splenic artery aneurysm during pregnancy. *Am J Obstet Gynecol* 1966;95(7):1025-1037.
56. O'Grady JP, Day EJ, Toole AL, Paust JC. Splenic artery aneurysm rupture in pregnancy: a review and case report. *Obstet Gynecol* 1977;50(5):627-630.
57. Wagner WH, Cossman DV, Treiman RL, et al. Hemosuccus pancreaticus from intraductal rupture of a primary splenic artery aneurysm. *J Vasc Surg* 1994;19(1):158-164.
58. Harper PC, Gamelli RL, Kaye MD. Recurrent hemorrhage into the pancreatic duct from a splenic artery aneurysm. *Gastroenterology* 1984;87(2):417-420.
59. Brothers TE, Stanley JC, Zelenock GB. Splenic arteriovenous fistula. *Int Surg* 1995;80(2):189-194.
60. Abbas MA, Stone WM, Fowl RJ, et al. Splenic artery aneurysms: two decades experience at Mayo Clinic. *Ann Vasc Surg* 2002;16(4):442-449.
61. Bronsther O, Merhav H, Van Thiel D, Starzl TE. Splenic artery aneurysms occurring in liver transplant recipients. *Transplantation* 1991;52(4):723-724.
62. Busuttil RW, Brin BJ. The diagnosis and management of visceral artery aneurysms. *Surgery* 1980;88(5):619-624.
63. Baker KS, Tisnado J, Cho SR, Beachley MC. Splanchnic artery aneurysms and pseudoaneurysms: transcatheter embolization. *Radiology* 1987;163(1):135-139.
64. Lowry SM, O'Dea TP, Gallagher DI, Mozenter R. Splenic artery aneurysm rupture: the seventh instance of maternal and fetal survival. *Obstet Gynecol* 1986;67(2):291-292.
65. Salo JA, Salmenkivi K, Tenhunen A, Kivilaakso EO. Rupture of splanchnic artery aneurysms. *World J Surg* 1986;10(1):123-127.
66. Gangahar DM, Carveth SW, Reese HE, et al. True aneurysm of the pancreaticoduodenal artery: a case report and review of the literature. *J Vasc Surg* 1985;2(5):741-742.
67. Spittell JA, Fairbairn JF, Kincaid CW, ReMine WH. Aneurysm of the splenic artery. *JAMA* 1961;174.
68. Mandel SR, Jaques PF, Sanofsky S, Mauro MA. Nonoperative management of peripancreatic arterial aneurysms: a 10-year experience. *Ann Surg* 1987;205(2):126-128.
69. Probst P, Castaneda-Zuniga WR, Gomes AS, et al. Nonsurgical treatment of splenic-artery aneurysms. *Radiology* 1978;128(3):619-623.
70. Arca MJ, Gagner M, Heniford BT, et al. Splenic artery aneurysms: methods of laparoscopic repair. *J Vasc Surg* 1999;30(1):184-188.
71. Hashizume M, Ohta M, Ueno K, et al. Laparoscopic ligation of splenic artery aneurysm. *Surgery* 1993;113(3):352-354.
72. McDermott VG, Shlansky-Goldberg R, Cope C. Endovascular management of splenic artery aneurysms and pseudoaneurysms. *Cardiovasc Intervent Radiol* 1994;17(4):179-184.
73. Ikeda O, Tamura Y, Nakasone Y, et al. Nonoperative management of unruptured visceral artery aneurysms: treatment by transcatheter coil embolization. *J Vasc Surg* 2008.
74. Sachdev U, Baril DT, Ellozy SH, et al. Management of aneurysms involving branches of the celiac and superior mesenteric arteries: a comparison of surgical and endovascular therapy. *J Vasc Surg* 2006;44(4):718-724.
75. Takahashi T, Shimada K, Kobayashi N, Kakita A. Migration of steel-wire coils into the stomach after transcatheter arterial embolization for a bleeding splenic artery pseudoaneurysm: report of a case. *Surg Today* 2001;31(5):458-462.
76. Arepally A, Dagli M, Hofmann LV, et al. Treatment of splenic artery aneurysm with use of a stent-graft. *J Vasc Interv Radiol* 2002;13(6):631-633.
77. Brountzos EN, Vagenas K, Apostolopoulou SC, et al. Pancreatitis-associated splenic artery pseudoaneurysm: endovascular treatment with self-expandable stent-grafts. *Cardiovasc Intervent Radiol* 2003;26(1):88-91.
78. Yoon HK, Lindh M, Uher P, et al. Stent-graft repair of a splenic artery aneurysm. *Cardiovasc Intervent Radiol* 2001;24(3):200-203.
79. Lumsden AB, Mattar SG, Allen RC, Bacha EA. Hepatic artery aneurysms: the management of 22 patients. *J Surg Res* 1996;60(2):345-350.
80. Guida PM, Moore SW. Aneurysm of the hepatic artery: report of five cases with a brief review of the previously reported cases. *Surgery* 1966;60(2):299-310.
81. Welling TH, Williams DM, Stanley JC. Excessive oral amphetamine use as a possible cause of renal and splanchnic arterial aneurysms: a report of two cases. *J Vasc Surg* 1998;28(4):727-731.
82. Abbas MA, Fowl RJ, Stone WM, et al. Hepatic artery aneurysm: factors that predict complications. *J Vasc Surg* 2003;38(1):41-45.
83. Parangi S, Oz MC, Blume RS, et al. Hepatobiliary complications of polyarteritis nodosa. *Arch Surg* 1991;126(7):909-912.
84. Erskine JM. Hepatic artery aneurysm. *Vasc Surg* 1973;7(2):106-125.
85. Harlaftis NN, Akin JT. Hemobilia from ruptured hepatic artery aneurysm: report of a case and review of the literature. *Am J Surg* 1977;133(2):229-232.
86. Jeans PL. Hepatic artery aneurysms and biliary surgery: two cases and a literature review. *Aust NZ J Surg* 1988;58(11):889-894.
87. Naito A, Toyota N, Ito K. Embolization of a ruptured middle colic artery aneurysm. *Cardiovasc Intervent Radiol* 1995;18(1):56-58.
88. Athey PA, Sax SL, Lamki N, Cadavid G. Sonography in the diagnosis of hepatic artery aneurysms. *AJR Am J Roentgenol* 1986;147(4):725-727.
89. Salo JA, Aarnio PT, Jarvinen AA, Kivilaakso EO. Aneurysms of the hepatic arteries. *Am Surg* 1989;55(12):705-709.
90. Weaver DH, Fleming RJ, Barnes WA. Aneurysm of the hepatic artery: the value of arteriography in surgical management. *Surgery* 1968;64(5):891-896.
91. Røkke O, Søndenaa K, Amundsen SR, et al. Successful management of eleven splanchnic artery aneurysms. *Eur J Surg* 1997;163(6):411-417.
92. Rutten AP, Sikkenk PJ. Aneurysm of the hepatic artery: reconstruction with saphenous vein-graft. *Br J Surg* 1971;58(4):262-266.
93. Goldblatt M, Goldin AR, Shaff MI. Percutaneous embolization for the management of hepatic artery aneurysms. *Gastroenterology* 1977;73(5):1142-1146.
94. Jonsson K, Bjernstad A, Eriksson B. Treatment of a hepatic artery aneurysm by coil occlusion of the hepatic artery. *AJR Am J Roentgenol* 1980;134(6):1245-1247.
95. Okazaki M, Higashihara H, Ono H, et al. Percutaneous embolization of ruptured splanchnic artery pseudoaneurysms. *Acta Radiol* 1991;32(5):349-354.
96. Larson RA, Solomon J, Carpenter JP. Stent graft repair of visceral artery aneurysms. *J Vasc Surg* 2002;36(6):1260-1263.
97. Patel JV, Weston MJ, Kessel DO, et al. Hepatic artery pseudoaneurysm after liver transplantation: treatment with percutaneous thrombin injection. *Transplantation* 2003;75(10):1755-1757.
98. De Bakey ME, Cooley DA. Successful resection of mycotic aneurysm of superior mesenteric artery: case report and review of literature. *Am Surg* 1953;19(2):202-212.
99. Friedman SG, Pogo GJ, Moccio CG. Mycotic aneurysm of the superior mesenteric artery. *J Vasc Surg* 1987;6(1):87-90.
100. Stone WM, Abbas M, Cherry KJ, et al. Superior mesenteric artery aneurysms: is presence an indication for intervention? *J Vasc Surg* 2002;36(2):234-237; discussion, 7.
101. Cormier F, Ferry J, Artru B, et al. Dissecting aneurysms of the main trunk of the superior mesenteric artery. *J Vasc Surg* 1992;15(2):424-430.
102. Guthrie W, Maclean H. Dissecting aneurysms of arteries other than the aorta. *J Path* 1972;108(3):219-235.
103. McNamara MF, Bakshi KR. Mesenteric artery aneurysms. In: Bergan JJ, Yao JS, eds. Aneurysms: diagnosis and treatment. New York: Grune & Stratton; 1981:285.
104. Kopatsis A, D'Anna JA, Sithian N, Sabido F. Superior mesenteric artery aneurysm: 45 years later. *Am Surg* 1998;64(3):263-266.
105. Geelkerken RH, van Bockel JH, de Roos WK, Hermans J. Surgical treatment of intestinal artery aneurysms. *Eur J Vasc Surg* 1990;4(6):563-567.
106. Violago FC, Downs AR. Ruptured atherosclerotic aneurysm of the superior mesenteric artery with celiac axis occlusion. *Ann Surg* 1971;174(2):207-210.
107. Wright CB, Schoepfle WJ, Kurtock SB, et al. Gastrointestinal bleeding and mycotic superior mesenteric aneurysm. *Surgery* 1982;92(1):40-44.

108. Jimenez JC, Lawrence PF, Reil TD. Endovascular exclusion of superior mesenteric artery pseudoaneurysms: an alternative to open laparotomy in high-risk patients. *Vasc Endovascular Surg* 2008;42(2):184-186.
109. Eckhauser FE, Stanley JC, Zelenock GB, et al. Gastroduodenal and pancreaticoduodenal artery aneurysms: a complication of pancreatitis causing spontaneous gastrointestinal hemorrhage. *Surgery* 1980;88(3):335-344.
110. Hama Y, Iwasaki Y, Kaji T, et al. Coil compaction after embolization of the superior mesenteric artery pseudoaneurysm. *Eur Radiol* 2002;12(Suppl 3):S189-S191.
111. Appel N, Duncan JR, Schuerer DJ. Percutaneous stent-graft treatment of superior mesenteric and internal iliac artery pseudoaneurysms. *J Vasc Interv Radiol* 2003;14(7):917-922.
112. Cowan S, Kahn MB, Bonn J, et al. Superior mesenteric artery pseudoaneurysm successfully treated with polytetrafluoroethylene covered stent. *J Vasc Surg* 2002;35(4):805-807.
113. Graham JM, McCollum CH, DeBakey ME. Aneurysms of the splanchnic arteries. *Am J Surg* 1980;140(6):797.
114. Werner K, Tarasoutchi F, Lunardi W, et al. Mycotic aneurysm of the celiac trunk and superior mesenteric artery in a case of infective endocarditis. *J Cardiovasc Surg (Torino)* 1991;32(3):380-383.
115. Stone WM, Abbas MA, Gloviczki P, et al. Celiac arterial aneurysms: a critical reappraisal of a rare entity. *Arch Surg* 2002;137(6):670-674.
116. Graham LM, Stanley JC, Whitehouse WM Jr., et al. Celiac artery aneurysms: historic (1745-1949) versus contemporary (1950-1984) differences in etiology and clinical importance. *J Vasc Surg* 1985;2(5): 757-764.
117. Haimovici H, Sprayregen S, Eckstein P, Veith FJ. Celiac artery aneurysmectomy: case report with review of the literature. *Surgery* 1976;79(5):592-596.
118. Herzler GM, Silver TM, Graham LM, Stanley JC. Celiac artery aneurysm: ultrasonic diagnosis. *J Clin Ultrasound* 1981;9(3):141-143.
119. Serafino G, Vroegindeweij D, Boks S, van der Harst E. Mycotic aneurysm of the celiac trunk: from early CT sign to rupture. *Cardiovasc Intervent Radiol* 2005;28(5):677-680.
120. Connell JM, Han DC. Celiac artery aneurysms: a case report and review of the literature. *Am Surg* 2006;72(8):746-749.
121. Shumacker HB Jr., Siderys H. Excisional treatment of aneurysm of celiac artery. *Ann Surg* 1958;148(6):885-889.
122. Parfitt J, Chalmers RT, Wolfe JH. Visceral aneurysms in Ehlers-Danlos syndrome: case report and review of the literature. *J Vasc Surg* 2000;31(6):1248-1251.
123. Michels NA. Collateral arterial pathways to the liver after ligation of the hepatic artery and removal of the celiac axis. *Cancer* 1953;6(4):708-724.
124. Schoder M, Cejna M, Langle F, et al. Glue embolization of a ruptured celiac trunk pseudoaneurysm via the gastroduodenal artery. *Eur Radiol* 2000;10(8):1335-1337.
125. Waldenberger P, Bendix N, Petersen J, et al. Clinical outcome of endovascular therapeutic occlusion of the celiac artery. *J Vasc Surg* 2007;46(4):655-661.
126. Atkins BZ, Ryan JM, Gray JL. Treatment of a celiac artery aneurysm with endovascular stent grafting: a case report. *Vasc Endovascular Surg* 2003;37(5):367-373.
127. Varekamp AP, Minder WH, Van Noort G, Wassenaar HA. Rupture of a submucosal gastric aneurysm: a rare cause of gastric hemorrhage. *Neth J Surg* 1983;35(3):100-103.
128. Millard M. Fatal rupture of gastric aneurysm: case report with review of the literature. *JAMA* 1955;59(3):363-371.
129. Mandelbaum I, Kaiser GC, Lempke RE. Gastric intramural aneurysm as a cause for massive gastro-intestinal hemorrhage. *Ann Surg* 1962;155: 199-203.
130. Jacobs PP, Croiset van Ughelen FA, Bruyninckx CM, Hoefsloot F. Haemoperitoneum caused by a dissecting aneurysm of the gastroepiploic artery. *Eur J Vasc Surg* 1994;8(2):236-237.
131. Thomford NR, Yurko JE, Smith EJ. Aneurysm of gastric arteries as a cause of intraperitoneal hemorrhage: review of literature. *Ann Surg* 1968;168(2):294-297.
132. Varela JE, Salzman SL, Owens C, et al. Angiographic embolization of a left gastric artery pseudoaneurysm after blunt abdominal trauma. *J Trauma* 2006;60(6):1350-1352.

VI

Renovascular Disease

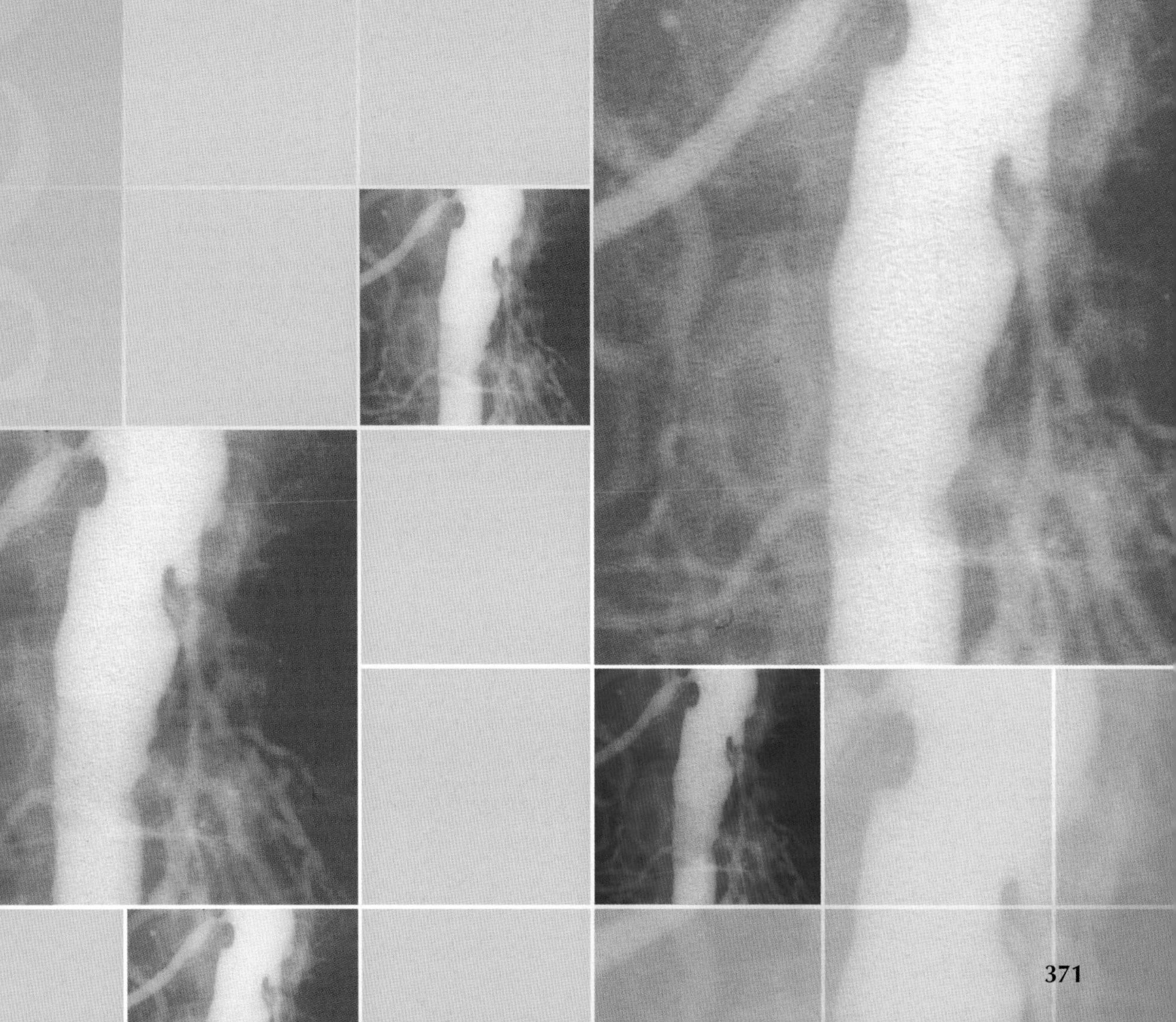

chapter

22

Pathophysiology and Evaluation of Renovascular Hypertension

Stephen C. Textor, MD

Key Points

- Renovascular hypertension refers to de novo development or acceleration of hypertension produced by high-grade vascular renal artery stenosis.
- Activation of the renin–angiotensin system occurs when renal artery perfusion falls.
- Mechanisms of sustained hypertension differ between one-kidney and two-kidney forms of renovascular hypertension, depending on the ability of the contralateral kidney to excrete sodium.
- Sustained rises in arterial pressure and vascular resistance develop despite a fall in renin activity, corresponding to recruitment of alternative pressor systems.
- Medical treatment of systemic hypertension may reduce poststenotic renal perfusion pressures to levels prone to induce ischemic nephropathy.
- Ischemic nephropathy refers to intrarenal tissue injury resulting from reduced renal perfusion.
- Renal injury beyond arterial stenosis results from oxidative stress, proinflammatory cytokine release, and disturbances of fibrotic mechanisms.
- The severity of renal injury appears to be modified by interactions with other factors, including age, dyslipidemias, and atheroembolic disease.
- Evaluation includes functional evaluation, including severity of vascular occlusion, and imaging procedures to define location, severity, and accessibility.
- Doppler imaging is inexpensive but operator dependent.
- Magnetic resonance angiography provides excellent imaging, but risks of gadolinium exposure limit use in subjects, with a glomerular filtration rate of less than 30 ml/min/1.73m^2.
- Computed tomography angiography provides excellent detail but has contrast and radiation exposure.
- Intensity of evaluation is determined by the clinical demands for renal revascularization, largely influenced by stability of blood pressure control and renal function.

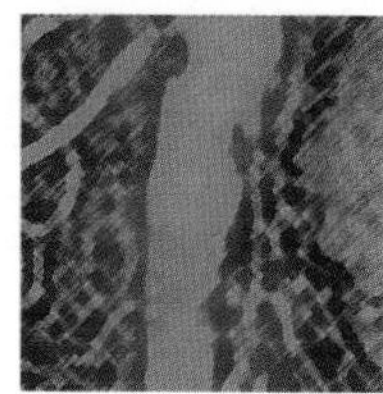

Renovascular hypertension refers to the rise in arterial pressure caused by reduced kidney perfusion. It can be produced by many vascular lesions, including segmental infarction or large-vessel lesions from fibromuscular dysplasia or atherosclerotic occlusive disease. It remains among the most common secondary forms of hypertension, particularly among the elderly with atherosclerotic disease elsewhere. When severe and prolonged, reduced kidney perfusion also can lead to loss of kidney size and function, often designated as ischemic nephropathy. Because these conditions can progress and can benefit from vascular intervention, it behooves clinicians caring for vascular disease to be familiar with their development and clinical manifestations.

Renovascular disease and ischemic nephropathy reflect complex pathogenic pathways. Some of these remain poorly understood. Advances in medical therapy and imaging procedures during the past decade have recalibrated the urgency for the diagnosis and for intervention in these disorders. Because effective antihypertensive therapy is available, protection of renal function from occlusive disease often becomes a dominant clinical issue. The precise role and timing for renal revascularization in the current era remain controversial. They are now the subject of several prospective trials. It should be emphasized from the outset that the intensity of evaluating renovascular disease often hinges on the clinical commitment to act on the results of diagnostic studies. This chapter summarizes current views regarding the pathophysiology and clinical evaluation of these syndromes.

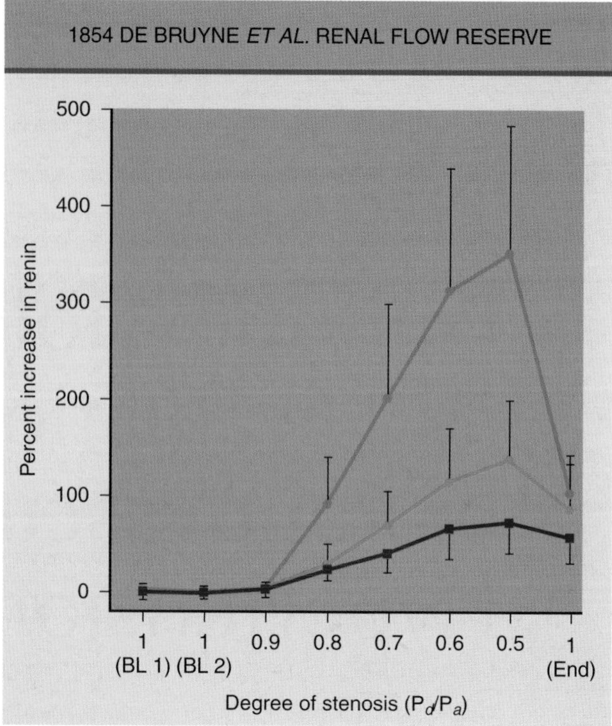

Figure 22-1. Relative increase in measured renin on renal vein renin obtained from the stenotic kidney *(closed circles)* during production of pressure gradient in human subjects. A balloon catheter was inflated until pressure fell by 10% (ratio of distal pressure / aortic pressure = 0.9) before any change could be detected. These observations argue that lesions that fail to produce a gradient are unlikely to activate pressor mechanisms causing renovascular hypertension. (From De Bruyne B, Manoharan G, Pijls NHJ, et al. *J Am Coll Cardiol* 2006;48:1851-1855.)

PRESSOR ROLE OF THE KIDNEYS

Seminal studies by Goldblatt and Loesch more than 70 years ago established the connection between kidneys and regulation of systemic blood pressure by producing sustained hypertension in dogs after placement of arterial occlusive clamps.[1] The basis for a rise in arterial pressure is complex and multifactorial, and it requires activation of the renin–angiotensin system. Recent studies in genetically modified mice indicate that an intact angiotensin receptor-1 is required to produce experimental hypertension, confirming previous studies using pharmacological blockade of the system. Careful studies using experimental kidney transplants between angiotensin receptor-1–deficient mice and wild-type mice indicate that both kidneys and systemic receptors participate in nearly equal degrees to the development of hypertension.[2] Human studies during partial occlusion of the renal artery using an inflatable balloon indicate that renin release from the poststenotic kidney relates closely to the severity of the gradient across the stenosis (Figure 22-1).[3] It should be emphasized that vascular lesions require substantial cross-sectional occlusion to impair blood flow or to produce a pressure gradient. In experimental situations, the degree of occlusion appears to require between 60% and 80% cross-sectional occlusion as determined by latex vascular casts.[4] Clinical revascularization for less advanced disease predictably fails to lower arterial pressure.

A simplified summary of components of the renin–angiotensin system is depicted in Figure 22-2. Reduced renal perfusion produces release of renin into the general circulation, where it enzymatically cleaves angiotensin I from its substrate. Angiotensin I is then cleaved further by angiotensin-converting enzyme (ACE) located in many vascular beds but most prominently in the lung to generate angiotensin II. The latter is a peptide with broad effects, including regulation of renal sodium balance, aldosterone production, and vascular resistance. Several decades of study have broadened our view of this system to indicate widespread actions in vascular smooth muscle remodeling and hypertrophy, interactions with the sympathetic nervous system and other pressor systems, and numerous regulatory functions for cardiac metabolism, hypertrophy, and fibrosis.[5] Remarkably, measurable activation of the renin–angiotensin system is often temporary. Over time, circulating levels of plasma renin activity fall, partly related to changes in sodium homeostasis and recruitment of alternate pressor systems, including oxidative stress pathways.[6]

RENIN-RELEASE, HYPERTENSION, AND KIDNEY ISCHEMIA

Reduced renal perfusion pressure initiates several compensatory mechanisms that sustain blood flow. Initial responses include a rise in systemic arterial pressure that restores poststenotic pressure and flow in the kidneys. When present, the contralateral kidney without vascular occlusion responds to elevated arterial pressure with suppression of renin release and exaggerated sodium excretion (termed pressure natriuresis) that tends to counteract the rise in pressure. It should be

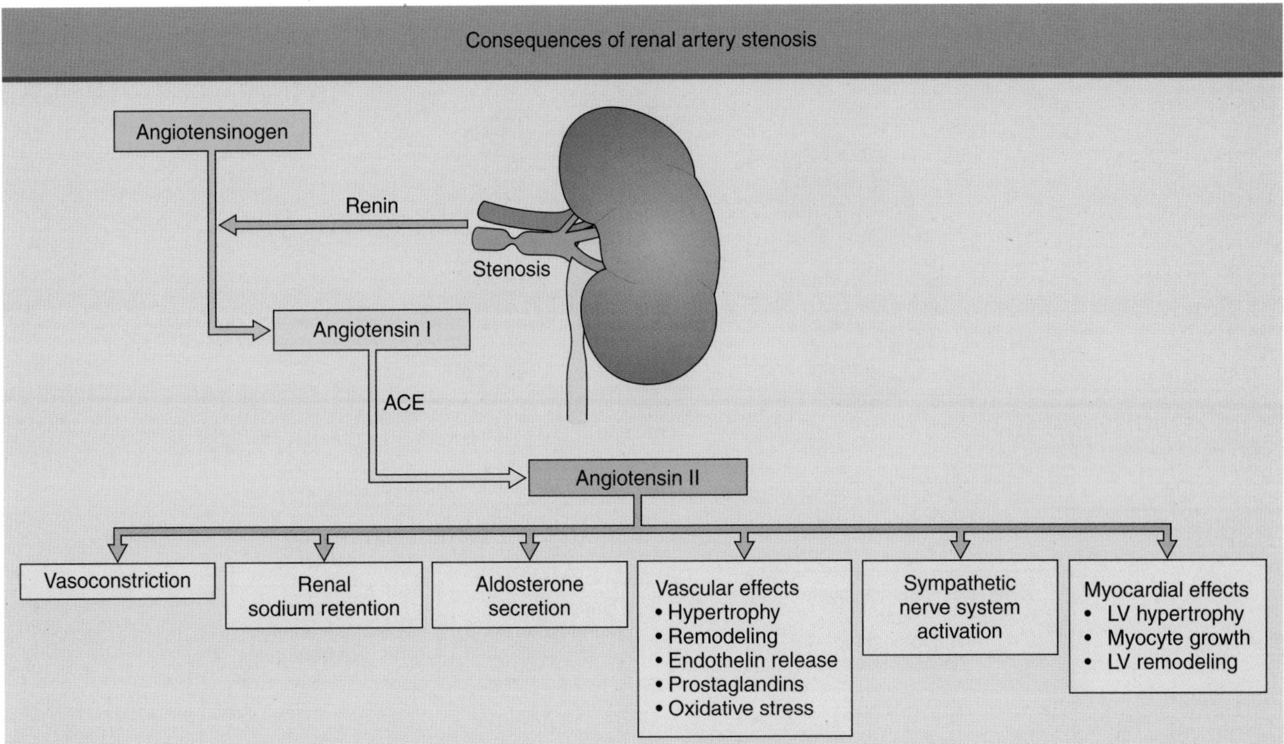

Figure 22-2. Consequences of renal artery stenosis. Reduction of perfusion pressure to the kidney leads to release of renin from juxtaglomerular cells in the afferent arteriole. This leads to a cascade eventually amplifying the signal to produce both local and systemic angiotensin II, whose actions are complex. Angiotensin II raises arterial pressure by direct vascular effects and by changing renal sodium homeostasis, in addition to having wide effects on other pressor systems, fibrosis, and remodeling. ACE, angiotensin-converting enzyme; LV, left ventricular.

emphasized that this phase may have normal renal blood flow to both kidneys, enhanced renin release from the poststenotic kidney, and elevated systemic pressure. Renal vein renin levels are elevated only on the side of the stenotic kidney, while measured levels of venous oxygen do not differ, indicating adequate blood flow to both kidneys.[7] An abundant literature during the era of surgical revascularization indicates that subjects with lateralization of renal vein renin values were most likely to lower arterial pressures after removing the stenotic lesion.

DIFFERENCES BETWEEN ONE-KIDNEY AND TWO-KIDNEY RENOVASCULAR HYPERTENSION

Experimental studies of renovascular hypertension identify important differences between one-kidney and two-kidney models (Figure 22-3). These studies indicate that two-kidney, one-clip hypertensive models present a paradigm of renovascular hypertension, with activation of restorative pressor mechanisms in the "affected" kidney that tend to be counterbalanced by a normal "contralateral" kidney. The release of renin from the affected side produces elevated arterial pressures, sodium retention in the underperfused kidney, and under some circumstances, reduced renal blood flow and glomerular filtration in the affected kidney. The contralateral kidney is exposed to elevated arterial pressures. As a result, release of renin is suppressed in the contralateral kidney, which undergoes "pressure natriuresis" and enhanced urinary excretion of sodium. The contralateral kidney, then, tends to work continually against the sodium-retaining actions of the poststenotic kidney. The resulting profile then can be established by comparing the function and hormonal status of one kidney with that of the other. The hallmarks of such an arrangement are persistently elevated levels of renin and angiotensin II, dependence of systemic hypertension on the pressor action of angiotensin II, and side-to-side differences during comparative studies of renal blood flow, sodium excretion, and glomerular filtration. Side-to-side differences have been employed in various preinterventional functional studies to predict the likelihood of blood pressure benefit or "cure" of renovascular hypertension.[8]

By contrast, one-kidney, one-clip hypertension represents a model reflecting the situation of the entire renal mass (both kidneys or a solitary functioning kidney, Figure 22-3B) being affected by vascular occlusive disease. Although reduced pressure to the kidney activates the renin–angiotensin system as with two-kidney models, the one-kidney model does not have a "normal" contralateral kidney. Sodium-retaining mechanisms are activated and expand circulatory volume, finally returning renal perfusion pressures to nearly normal. As a result, plasma renin activity falls and arterial pressure does not depend on the pressor effects of angiotensin II. Volume expansion is critical, as the dependence of hypertension on angiotensin can be demonstrated only after sodium depletion. Side-to-side comparisons cannot be made in this form of renovascular hypertension.

Many human clinical disease situations appear more closely to approximate the one-kidney, one-clip model of

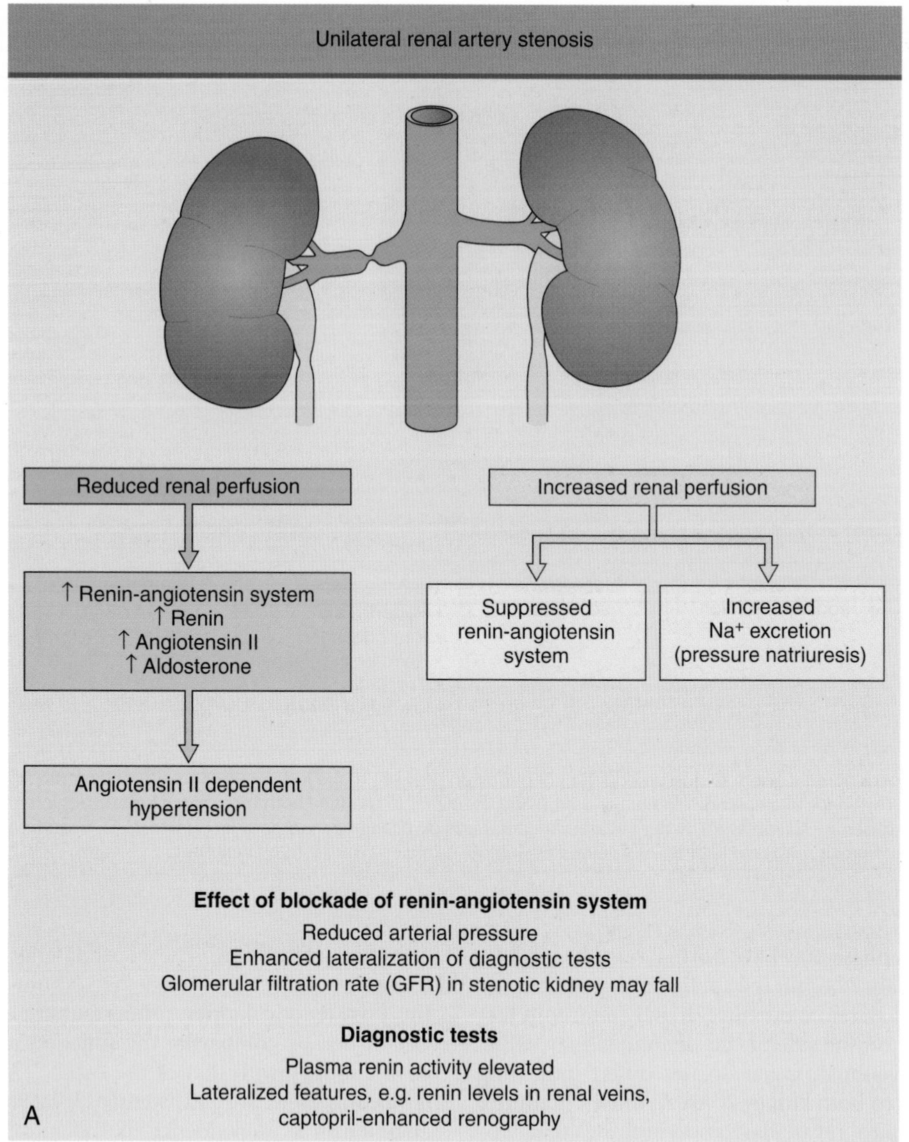

Figure 22-3. Differences between unilateral (one-clip, two-kidney; **A**) and bilateral (one-kidney, one-clip; **B**) renovascular hypertension. These figures illustrate the differences observed in models whereby a normal contralateral kidney is present or not. When two kidneys are present, differences in sodium excretion and renin activation favor angiotensin-dependent hypertension and lateralization of diagnostic tests (e.g., renal vein renin determinations). When both kidneys (or the entire renal mass, such as a solitary functioning kidney) are affected by vascular stenosis, sodium retention and volume expansion eventually suppress renin release, obscuring the role of the renin–angiotensin system (see text).

renovascular hypertension than the two-kidney model. This may be the case even when main renal artery stenosis (RAS) affects only one kidney. It may be argued that small-vessel changes in an otherwise normal contralateral kidney lead to volume retention and mask the angiotensin II–dependent status of two-kidney, one-clip forms of human hypertension in some instances.

ADDITIONAL MECHANISMS OF INJURY

Remarkably, renal arterial lesions produce widespread recruitment of additional mechanisms raising arterial pressure. Unlike other organs such as the heart or brain, the kidneys are oversupplied with oxygenated blood, since their major function is filtration. Basal renal metabolic requirements are met with less than 10% of blood flow. A moderate reduction in flow activates oxidative stress pathways that impair vasodilatory prostanoid and nitric oxide production in favor of vasoconstrictor isoprostanes.[9] Both fibromuscular and atherosclerotic lesions increase sympathetic adrenergic nerve traffic, leading to increased heart rate, blood pressure lability, and loss of circadian blood pressure patterns. These effects sometimes can be reversed after successful restoration of kidney perfusion.[10] Experimental studies indicate that the contralateral kidney also shifts to preferential production of vasoconstrictor eicosanoids. When stenotic lesions progress to higher levels of occlusion, blood flow to the kidney may fall sufficiently to activate fibrogenic pathways, leading to collagen deposition and parenchymal damage. Pathological samples demonstrate loss of glomerular volume, activation of

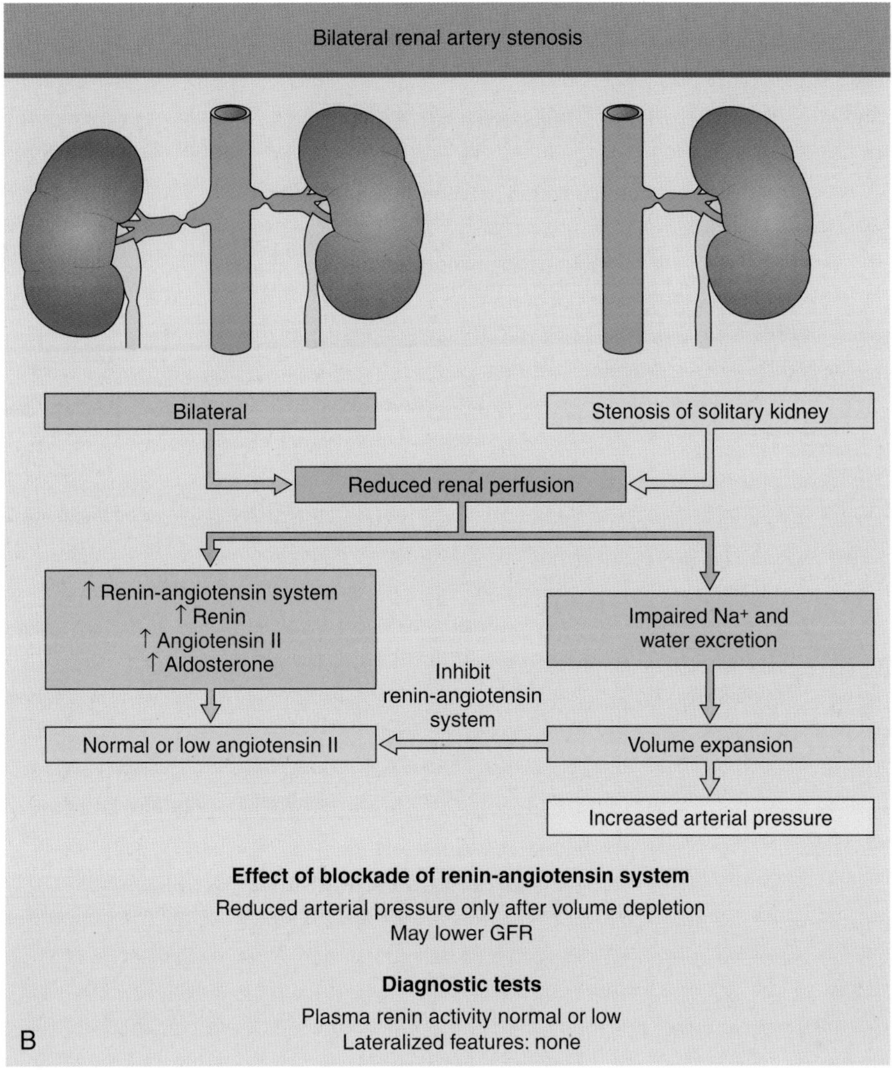

Figure 22-3—cont'd, Differences between unilateral (one-clip, two-kidney; **A**) and bilateral (one-kidney, one-clip; **B**) renovascular hypertension.

cytokines, inflammatory pathways, and interstitial fibrosis. One schematic representation of the pathways leading to long-term kidney injury is illustrated in Figure 22-4. While this has been termed ischemic nephropathy, it has not yet been established that actual oxygen deficits are required. The mechanisms by which reduction in renal perfusion activates tissue injury remain an active area of research and partly explain the difficulty in predicting recovery of the glomerular filtration rate (GFR) after renal revascularization. The degree to which each of these mechanisms participates in developing renovascular hypertension varies over time. Studies of experimental renovascular hypertension indicate that effects of stenotic lesions produce a series of transitional states, starting from an early phase with elevated angiotensin II levels and prompt reversal of hypertension after removal of the lesion.[11] Later, renal artery clip hypertension is associated with lower angiotensin II levels, despite sustained hypertension. This phase remains amenable to reversal of hypertension after removal of the stenotic lesion (Figure 22-5). Eventually, however, a late phase develops with sustained hypertension, normal levels of renin and angiotensin II, and no response to removal of the clip lesion. This observation suggests that mechanisms producing arterial hypertension sometimes undergo a transition to an irreversible stage. Whether such a set of transitions applies in human renovascular hypertension is not well understood. This paradigm has been invoked to explain treatment failures, although the date of onset for renovascular hypertension only rarely can be established with certainty. The best predictor of a favorable blood pressure response to renal revascularization is a "short duration" of hypertension (when known); clinicians are aware of patients with sustained, long-term hypertension that can be reversed with successful restoration of blood flow.[12]

The most common cause of renal artery occlusive disease is atherosclerosis. This tends to occur in older individuals with previous histories of essential hypertension, often with diabetes. In this instance, renal artery occlusion develops in the context of preexisting vascular injury. Recent studies suggest that the "atherosclerotic environment" (e.g., produced by cholesterol feeding in experimental animals) fundamentally accelerates tissue injury and alters the reactivity of kidney microvessels to vasodilatory and vasoconstrictor stimuli.[13] These features partly may explain why the results of renal revascularization may differ between patients with atherosclerotic disease and

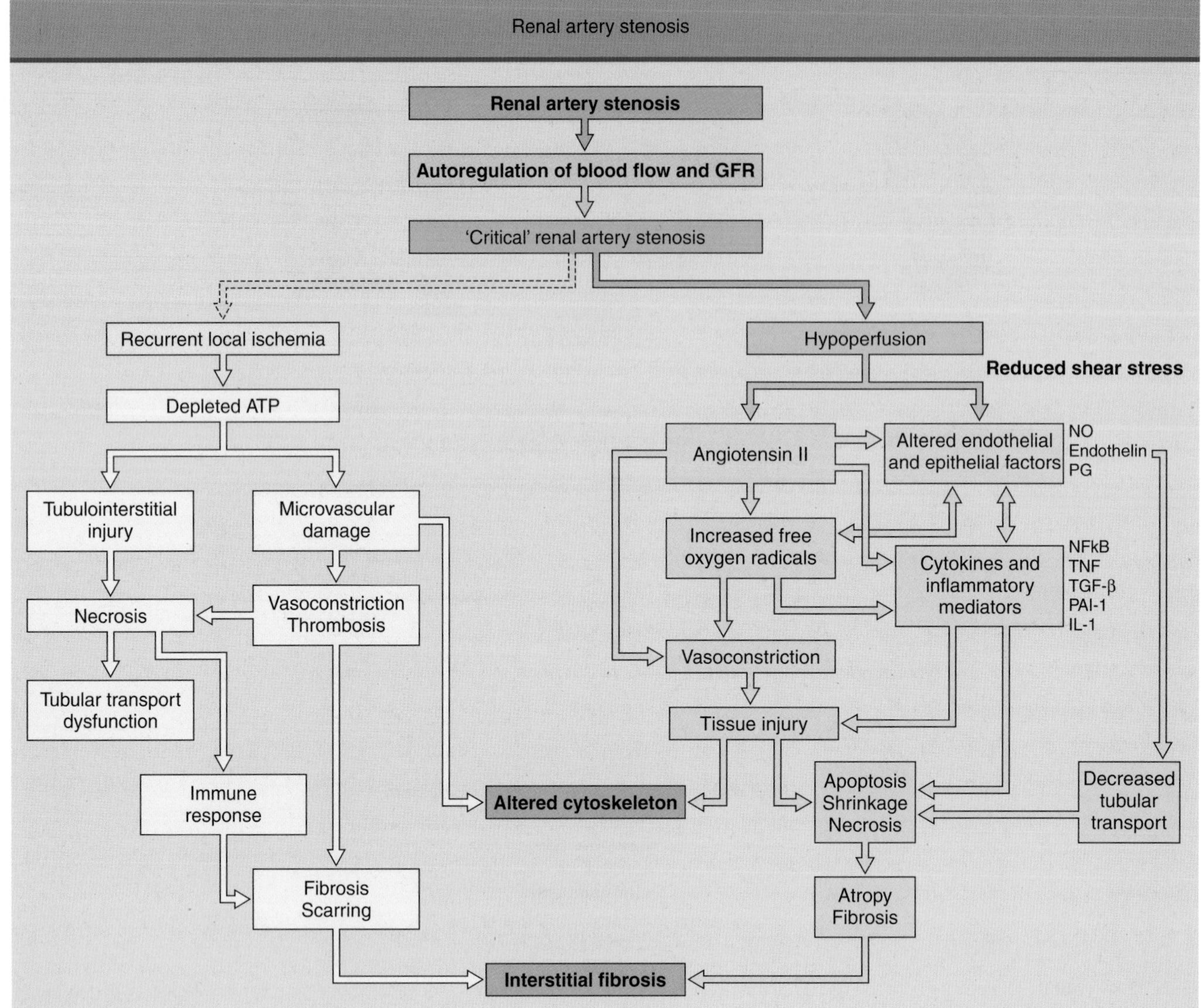

Figure 22-4. Renal artery stenosis (RAS). Summary of mechanisms by which "critical" RAS can produce both local hypoperfusion and activation of mechanisms inducing tissue injury. Alterations of endothelial function, oxidative stress, and cytokine production have been demonstrated and favor interstitial fibrosis, despite oversupply of oxygenated blood to the kidney as a whole. GFR, glomerular filtration rate; IL-1, interleukin-1; NO, nitric oxide; PAI-1, plasminogen activator inhibitor-1; PG, prostaglandin; TGF-β, transforming growth factor-β; TNF, tumor necrosis factor. (From Lerman L, Textor SC. *Urol Clin North Am* 2001;28:793-803.)

those with other causes, such as fibromuscular disease or traumatic renal artery occlusion.

ROLE OF THE RENIN–ANGIOTENSIN SYSTEM REGARDING GLOMERULAR FILTRATION

ACE inhibitors (and angiotensin II receptor blockers) now are administered widely for many reasons beyond treatment of high blood pressure. They produce survival benefits for patients with congestive cardiac failure and recurrent myocardial infarction. They also offer important advantages for proteinuric renal diseases, including diabetic nephropathy. It is likely that a new antihypertensive drug class, renin inhibitors such as aliskiren, will have similar effects. One result of these trends is that many individuals with unsuspected renal artery disease are being treated with agents capable of blocking the pathophysiological pathways associated with renovascular hypertension. It is important to recognize the effects this may have on both development and presentation of renal arterial disease (Figure 22-6).

One prominent effect of angiotensin II in the kidneys is the preferential constriction of the efferent arteriole at the glomerulus. Normally, vasodilation within the afferent arterioles is capable of sufficient autoregulation to preserve glomerular capillary blood flows and pressure over a range of conditions. As a result, the transcapillary pressures that determine the amount of filtrate formed as plasma traverses the glomerular vessels are high enough to generate adequate urine formation. Filtration does not depend much on efferent arteriolar resistance in this situation. However, when afferent pressures are reduced from preglomerular vascular disease, the transcapillary pressure gradient becomes dependent on increased

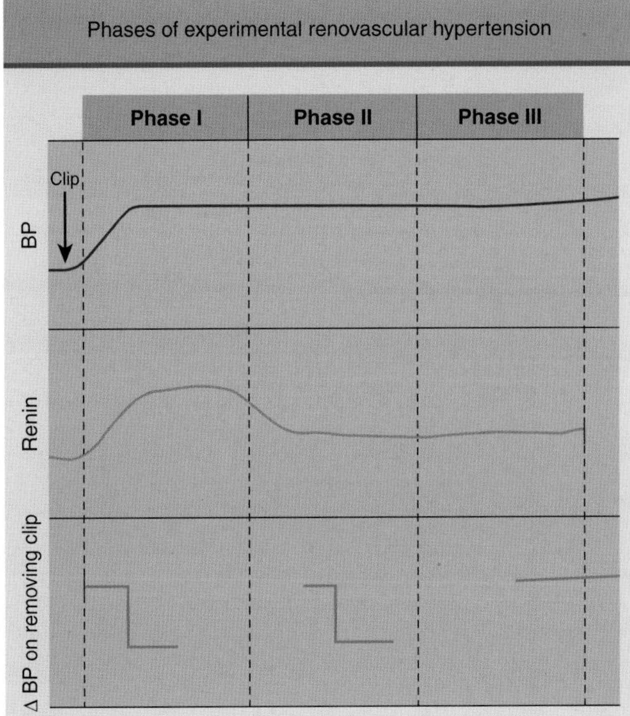

Figure 22-5. Phases of experimental renovascular hypertension. Transition occurs from an early "renin-dependent" but reversible phase to a final stage that is neither renin dependent nor reversible. These phases are difficult to define in clinical practice, but they highlight the recruitment of non-angiotensin-dependent mechanisms sustaining long-term renovascular hypertension.

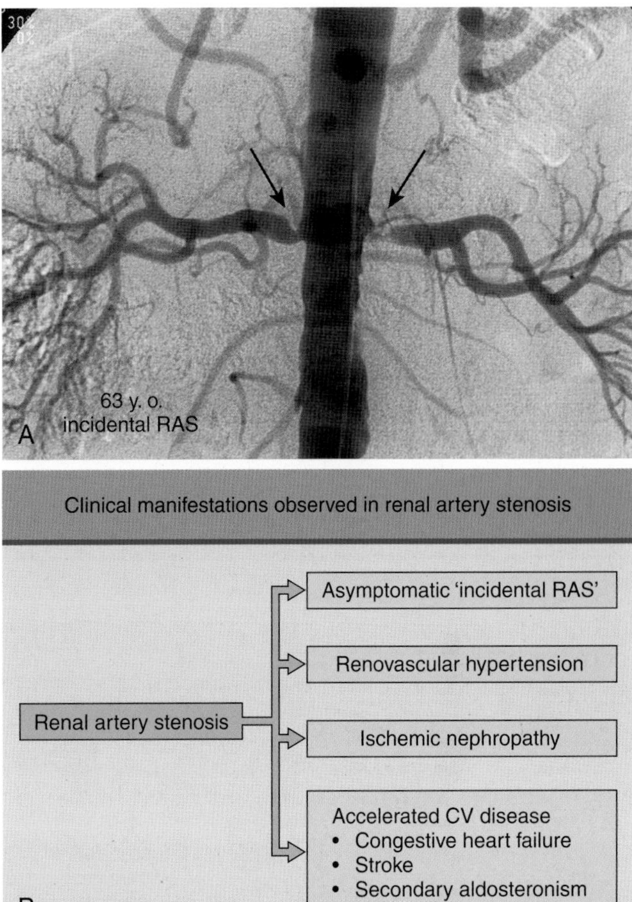

Figure 22-6. Renal artery lesions. **A,** Aortogram from a patient with moderate hypertension and normal renal function, demonstrating the potential for "incidental" renal artery stenosis (RAS) to be detected during angiography performed for other reasons. **B,** Spectrum of clinical manifestations observed with varying degrees of RAS. These range from "incidental" lesions with minimal hemodynamic effects to advanced renal failure and accelerated cardiovascular risk from congestive heart failure and stroke. Clinicians face the challenge of identifying the role of such lesions in individual patients.

efferent resistance. Filtration then depends on the presence of angiotensin II under these conditions, particularly when sodium intake is low. Blockade of the renin–angiotensin system under these conditions, either with ACE inhibitors or with angiotensin receptor blockers, has the potential to reduce transcapillary filtration pressures further. This leads to abrupt loss of glomerular filtration, so-called functional acute renal insufficiency (Figure 22-7).

This postglomerular hemodynamic effect is the basis for identification of major changes in the isotope renogram after administration of captopril and for reduction of proteinuria in patients with renal failure. Reduction of transcapillary pressures is fundamental to the reversal of glomerular "hyperfiltration" responsible for slowing the hydraulic injury attributed to elevated glomerular pressures.[14] It is also the basis for early decrements in glomerular filtration after starting these agents, particularly when high-grade RAS affects the entire renal mass.

Clinicians should be attuned to the possibility of this loss of GFR and understand its significance. A major fall in GFR should alert the physician to the possibility of bilateral disease or a solitary functioning kidney and highlight the need to define the circulation precisely. In some cases, the preglomerular vascular injury is not in major blood vessels but appears to be a residual parenchymal "small vessel" injury.[15] Glomerular filtration can recover if the efferent angiotensin effect (achieved by removal of ACE inhibition or angiotensin receptor blockade), adequate preglomerular pressures, or both are restored (by increasing kidney perfusion pressure). A minor decrement in GFR in one kidney may be difficult to detect, particularly since the contralateral kidney can increase filtration.[16]

PREVALENCE AND CLINICAL MANIFESTATIONS

As with other vascular occlusive lesions, clinicians recognize that simply finding RAS does not establish its functional significance. Vascular imaging studies obtained during coronary and peripheral angiography indicate that at least moderate RAS (more than 50%) can be identified in 20% to 30% of patients with atherosclerosis elsewhere. Earlier autopsy studies conducted in hypertensive individuals indicated that hypertensive individuals had some degree of RAS in nearly 60% of cases. Because mortality rates from stroke and cardiovascular disease continue to fall in Western countries, the prevalence of high-grade atherosclerotic renal artery lesions developing in older individuals appears to be increasing.

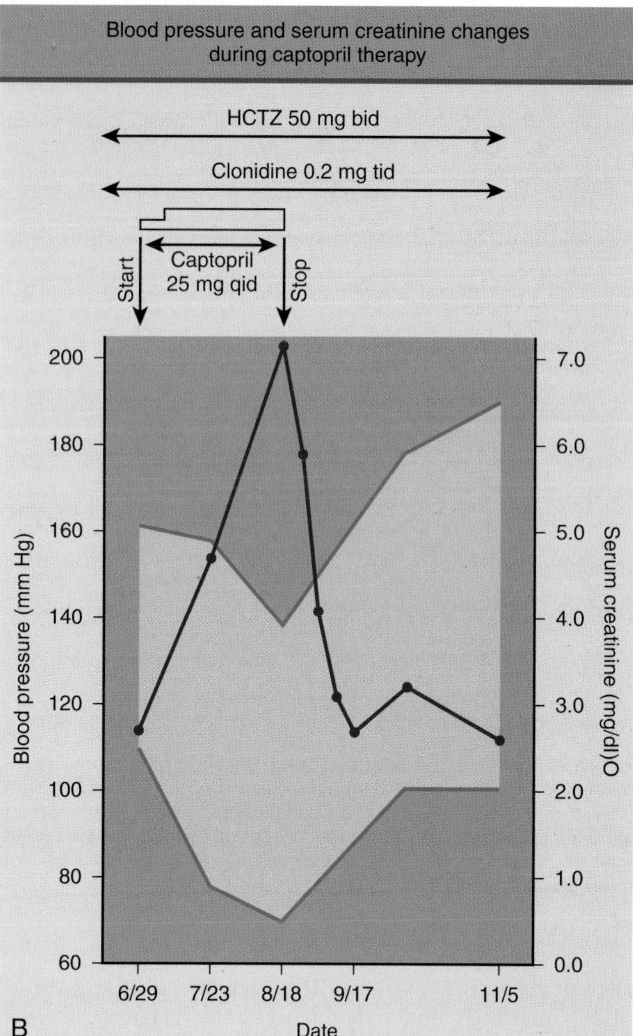

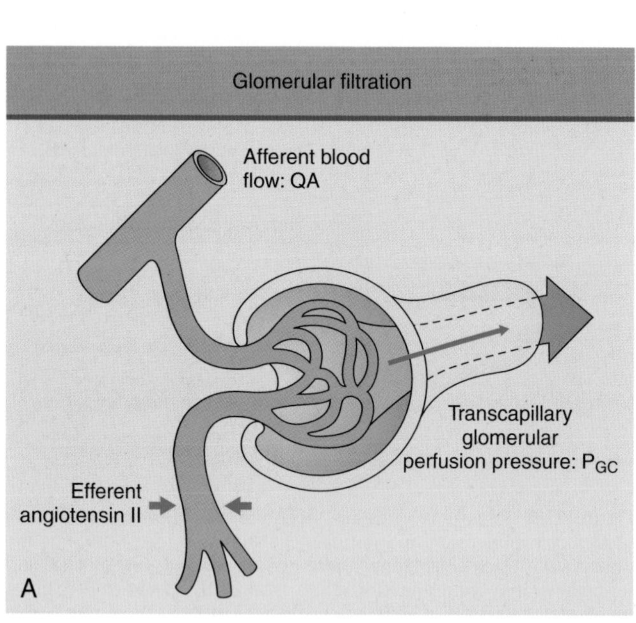

Figure 22-7. Blockade of the renin–angiotensin system in the kidney. **A,** Schematic of the glomerulus, illustrating the role of angiotensin II in maintaining efferent vascular tone and transcapillary filtration pressure. Removal of efferent vascular tone by blockade of the renin–angiotensin system may reduce filtration pressure and lower the glomerular filtration rate. When the entire renal mass is affected by renal artery stenosis (RAS), this effect can produce a "functional acute renal insufficiency." This is usually reversible upon withholding blockade of angiotensin. **B,** Example of acute renal insufficiency induced by blockade of angiotensin in a patient with RAS and renovascular hypertension. The rise in serum creatinine can be associated with preserved blood flow and thereby reflects primarily reduced filtration pressure. Such examples provide evidence that filtration can depend on angiotensin II under certain conditions and provide an impetus for restoring the renal blood supply by renal revascularization.

As a result, most cases of renovascular hypertension develop gradually and are superimposed on essential hypertension. Some authors suggest that up to 14% of patients reaching end-stage renal disease have renovascular disease as a primary etiological factor, although recent estimates suggest that this may be less than 5%.[17] Remarkably, fibromuscular diseases that activate pressor mechanisms and produce renovascular hypertension in younger individuals rarely produce renal parenchymal injury unless total occlusion develops. This observation has led some to suggest that other factors related to age and other diseases, such as nephrosclerosis or diabetes, may be required for irreversible tissue injury to occur (Figure 22-4). The physiological effects of renal artery lesions can vary widely, as illustrated in Figure 22-6. Many are "incidental" lesions with only minor hemodynamic effects.

Studies of vascular occlusion in which cross-sectional lumen was measured with latex cast indicate that detectable changes in either blood flow or blood pressure can be identified only after more than 70% to 80% lumen obstruction occurs (Figure 22-6A). When enough obstruction is present to reduce distal pressures, it is considered "critical" RAS. Hence, identification of a renal artery lesion alone is rarely enough to determine its role in a given patient. Once a gradient is established with reduced renal perfusion, a sequence of events (described later) ensues to restore renal perfusion pressure at the expense of elevated systemic arterial pressures (Figure 22-6B).

An important corollary of this observation is that renal perfusion is generally normal in untreated, early renovascular hypertension. Hence, the pressor effects of the poststenotic kidney restore blood flow and renal functional capacity, albeit at the expense of systemic hypertension. Progressive vascular obstruction, however, triggers further reduction to the kidney and further pressure elevation, which if unchecked can produce malignant-phase hypertension.

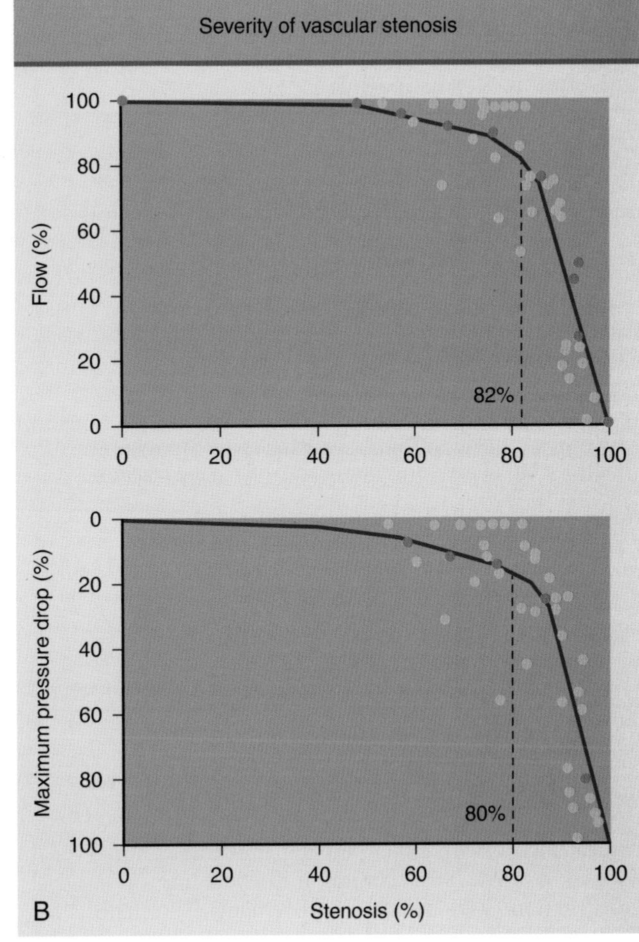

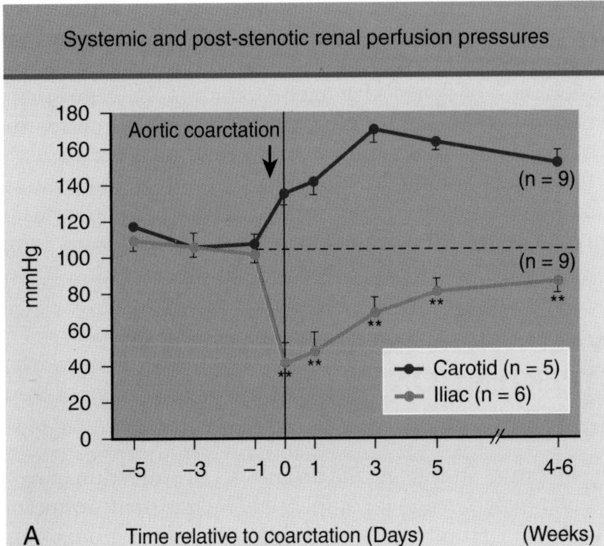

Figure 22-8. Hemodynamic effects of stenosis. **A,** Severity of vascular stenosis (as determined by latex casts of blood vessel lumen) and measured blood flow and pressure drop in the artery. These observations indicate that hemodynamic effects are sufficient to compromise flow only when lumen obstruction exceeds 70% to 80%. Many less severe lesions produce no clinical effects (see text). **B,** Systemic and poststenotic renal perfusion pressures measured after placement of an aortic clip between the renal arteries. The rise in systemic arterial pressure allows preservation of renal perfusion pressure to near normal levels. (From Textor SC, Smith-Powell L. *J Hypertens* 1988;6:311-319.)

A second corollary is that medical therapy of systemic hypertension with critical renovascular disease reduces perfusion to the poststenotic kidney. This can lead to activation of counterregulatory mechanisms, making antihypertensive therapy less effective, and in some situations to critical loss of blood flow in the affected kidney, leading to irreversible renal injury identified as ischemic nephropathy.[18]

Fibromuscular Dysplasia

Among younger individuals, various forms of fibromuscular disease of the renal arteries, traumatic disruption of renal vessels, or both are most common. The prevalence of occlusive vascular lesions affecting the kidneys varies widely with age. Cases of congenital aortic narrowing and varied fibromuscular dysplasias remain associated with younger age groups and appear most commonly as individual case reports. A prospective series of 96 mainly younger patients (mean age 54 years) addressed the value of structured search for secondary hypertension from a Hypertension Specialty Clinic in the United Kingdom. These individuals had only moderate blood pressure elevations, with an average level of 157/97 mm Hg determined by ambulatory blood pressure monitoring. The authors argue that a secondary cause surfaced in 18.1%, most commonly (75%) attributable to renovascular hypertension.[19] These cases appear commonly as rapidly progressive or severe hypertension, sometimes during pregnancy. In such cases, individuals benefit substantially from identification and restoration of blood flow, usually at low risk from the procedures. Most cases of fibromuscular disease and renovascular hypertension remain in women, with recent result of percutaneous transluminal renal angioplasty achieving primary patency in more than 90% and ongoing combined patency rates nearly 87% over up to 6 years of follow-up.[20] As expected, the mean age (44 years) of patients was young in this series. The authors acknowledge that a long duration of hypertension and the presence of branch vessel disease were unfavorable predictors for antihypertensive response after angioplasty.

In some countries, other conditions affecting large arteries produce renovascular hypertension, including Takayasu's arteritis. Reports from these countries indicate that either percutaneous or surgical restoration of blood flow in young individuals can be achieved with comparable results regarding blood pressure control and kidney salvage, although complex lesions require surgical revision.[21] A series of 85 patients (59 with Takayasu's and 26 with fibromuscular disease) indicates

Table 22-1
Goals of Diagnostic and Therapeutic Intervention in Renovascular Hypertension and Ischemic Nephropathy

Goals of Diagnostic Evaluation
Establish presence of renal artery stenosis: location and type of lesion
Establish whether unilateral or bilateral stenosis (or stenosis to a solitary kidney) is present
Establish presence and function of stenotic and nonstenotic kidneys
Establish hemodynamic severity of renal arterial disease
Plan vascular intervention, including degree and location of atherosclerotic disease
Goals of Therapy
Improve blood pressure control
Prevent morbidity and mortality of high blood pressure
Improve blood pressure control and reduce medication requirement
Preserve renal function
Reduce risk of renal adverse perfusion from use of antihypertensive agents
Reduce episodes of circulatory congestion ("flash" pulmonary edema)
Reduce risk of progressive vascular occlusion causing loss of renal function
Salvage renal function and recover glomerular filtration rate

From Brenner BM, ed. *Brenner and Rector's: the kidney*. 8th ed. Philadelphia: Saunders; 2008:1545, Table 43-5.

technical success with either percutaneous transluminal renal angioplasty (95%; 85% clinical improvement) or surgical reconstruction (94% clinical improvement).[21] Restenosis for lesions of Takayasu's reached 24%, whereas for fibromuscular disease restenosis developed in 10%.

Atherosclerotic renal artery stenosis (ARAS) is by far the most common lesion producing hypertension and most commonly treated with endovascular revascularization.[22] Recent epidemiological studies reconfirm the close association between renovascular disease and cardiovascular morbidity. A population-based cohort of 870 subjects older than age 65 was screened for ARAS using Doppler ultrasound and followed for 14 months. The prevalence of stenosis greater than 60% was 6.8% at baseline in this population. During a follow-up just over 1 year later, 68 (9.7%) experienced a coronary event (defined as hospitalization for angina, myocardial infarction, coronary revascularization, or a combination of these). The presence of ARAS conferred a 1.96 relative risk after adjusting for other risk factors, including blood pressure.[23] Kalra and colleagues reviewed Medicare claims data for 1,085,250 individuals without preexisting renovascular disease sampled between 1999 and 2001. The incidence of newly detected ARAS in this population during follow-up was 3.7 per 1000 patient years. Most importantly, subsequent claims for the next 2 years indicate that cardiovascular events in incident ARAS patients greatly exceed the general population (e.g., 304 versus 73 per 1000 patient years for atherosclerotic heart disease, $p < 0.01$).[24] Cardiovascular events far exceed claims related to renal dysfunction (304 versus 28 per 1000 patient years, $p < 0.001$). An additional cardiac angiography cohort study of 837 subjects identified by preset criteria (e.g., severe hypertension, unexplained renal dysfunction, congestive heart failure with hypertension, and severe atherosclerosis) were subjected to "drive-by" renal angiography. Renal artery atherosclerosis with more than 50% lumen obstruction was identified in 14.3%, with more severe lesions greater than 70%) in 7.3%. Multivariate analysis indicated that RAS was predicted by female gender, systolic hypertension, reduced creatinine clearance, and atherosclerotic disease in the carotid or peripheral beds.[25]

These observations underscore that renovascular disease carries substantial associated cardiovascular risk. It can produce an array of clinical symptoms. It most commonly presents as accelerating hypertension, often with disturbances of sympathetic adrenergic nerve stimulation and elevations in circulating catecholamines and augmented renal nerve traffic. Measurements of baroceptor sensitivity indicate reduced sensitivity that can improve after revascularization. Ambulatory blood pressure monitoring indicates more sustained hypertension and reduced day–night variation in renovascular hypertensive subjects as compared to essential hypertension. Left ventricular mass and cardiac arrhythmias are increased in this group, potentially contributing to increased cardiovascular mortality risk. Afferent nerve traffic is partly responsible for activation of the renin–angiotensin system and development of hypertension in the presence of RAS.[26]

EVALUATION OF RENOVASCULAR HYPERTENSION

Goals of Evaluation

The literature addressing the diagnosis and evaluation of renovascular hypertension is complex and inconsistent. Some confusion likely reflects the widely different patient groups being considered for evaluation and divergent goals for intervention. It behooves the clinician to carefully identify the objectives before initiating sometimes ambiguous and expensive studies. As with all tests, the reliability and value of diagnostic studies depend heavily on the pretest probability of disease. Furthermore, it is essential to consider from the outset exactly what is to be achieved. Is the major goal to exclude high-grade renal artery disease? Is it to exclude bilateral (as opposed to unilateral) disease? Is it to identify stenosis and estimate the potential for clinical benefit from renal revascularization? Is it to evaluate the role of renovascular disease in explaining deteriorating renal function? The specific approach to diagnosis differs depending on which of these is the predominant clinical objective (Table 22-1).

Noninvasive diagnostic tests for renovascular hypertension and ischemic nephropathy remain imperfect. For the purposes of this discussion, diagnostic tests fall into these general categories: (1) physiological and functional studies to evaluate the role of stenotic lesions, particularly related to activation of the renin–angiotensin system; (2) perfusion and imaging studies to identify the presence and degree of vascular stenosis; and (3) studies to predict the likelihood of benefit from invasive maneuvers, including renal revascularization.

Physiological and Functional Studies of the Renin–Angiotensin System

For more than 30 years, efforts have been made to establish the level of activation of the renin–angiotensin system as a marker of underlying renovascular hypertension. Peripheral plasma renin activity conducted under standardized conditions of sodium intake (renin-sodium profiling) and the response of renin to administration of an ACE inhibitor such as captopril have been proposed. While these studies are promising, when studied in patients with known renovascular hypertension, they have lower performance as diagnostic tests when applied to wider populations. In a series of 31 patients studied before percutaneous transluminal renal angioplasty, combined mathematical models to predict the clinical results indicate a sensitivity of 36% and accuracy of 43%, which are too low to be used as major determinants in decision making.[27] Plasma renin activity is sensitive to changes of sodium intake, volume status, renal function, and many medications. The sensitivity and specificity of such maneuvers depend heavily on the a priori probability of renovascular hypertension. In practice, the major utility of these studies depends on their negative predictive value, specifically the certainty with which the clinician can exclude significant renovascular disease if the test is negative. Since negative predictive value rarely exceeds 60% to 70%, these tests offer limited value in clinical decision making.

Measurement of renal vein renin levels has been widely applied in planning surgical revascularization for hypertension. These measurements are obtained by sampling renal vein and inferior vena cava blood individually. The level of the vena cava is taken as comparable to the arterial levels into each kidney and allows estimation of the contribution of each kidney to total circulating levels of plasma renin activity. Lateralization is defined usually as a ratio exceeding 1.5 between the renin activity of the stenotic kidney and that of the nonstenotic kidney. Some authors propose detailed examination not only of the relative ratio between kidneys but also of the degree of suppression of renin release from the nonstenotic or contralateral kidney.[28]

In general, the greater the degree of lateralization, the more probable that clinical blood pressure benefit will accrue from surgical or other revascularization. Results from many early studies support the observation that large differences between kidneys identify high-grade renal artery stenoses. These observations have been reinforced by recent studies of renal vein measurements before considering nephrectomy for refractory hypertension and advanced renovascular occlusive disease.[29]

As with many tests of hormonal activation, study conditions are crucial. Several measures to enhance renin release and magnify differences between kidneys have been proposed, including sodium depletion with diuretic administration, hydralazine, tilt-table stimulation, or captopril. A review of more than 50 studies of renal vein renin measurements indicated that when lateralization could be demonstrated clinical benefit regarding blood pressure control could be expected in more than 90% of cases. Failure to demonstrate lateralization, however, still was associated with significant benefit in more than 50% of cases.[4] More recent series reached similar conclusions, indicating that overall sensitivity of renal vein renin measurements was no better than 65% and that positive predictive value was 18.5%.[30]

For many reasons, renal vein assays are performed less commonly than in the past. An additional factor is that the goals of renal revascularization have shifted toward "preservation of renal function," rather than blood pressure control *per se*. In cases for which it is important to establish the degree of pressor effect of a specific kidney or site, such as before considering nephrectomy of a pressor kidney, measurement of renal vein renins can provide strong supportive evidence.

Studies of Individual Renal Function

Serum creatinine, iothalamate clearance, and other estimates of GFR are measures of total renal excretory function and do not address changes within each kidney. They may be influenced by numerous factors, including body mass, protein intake, and age. A large body of literature addresses the potential for individual "split" renal function studies to establish the functional importance of each kidney in renovascular disease.

Classical split renal function studies use separate ureteral catheters to allow individual urine collection for measurement of separate GFR, renal blood flow, sodium excretion, concentrating ability, and response to blockade of angiotensin II. These studies demonstrate that hemodynamic effects of renal artery lesions translate directly into functional changes, such as avid sodium retention, before major changes in blood flow occur. They emphasize that autoregulation of blood flow and GFR can occur over a range of pressures in man and may be affected in both stenotic and contralateral kidneys by the effects of angiotensin II. These studies require urinary tract instrumentation and provide only indirect information regarding the probability of benefit from revascularization. They are now rarely performed.

Separate renal functional measurements now can be obtained less invasively with radionuclide techniques. These methods use various radioisotopes (e.g., technetium-99-mercaptoacetyltriglycine or technetium-99-pentetic acid [diethylenetriaminepentaacetic acid]) to estimate fractional blood flow and filtration to each kidney. Administration of captopril beforehand magnifies differences between kidneys, primarily by delaying excretion of the filtered isotope due to removal of the efferent arteriolar effects of ACE inhibition. Some authors rely on such measurements to follow progressive renal artery disease and its effect on unilateral kidney function as a guide to consider revascularization.[8,31] Recent studies indicate that single-kidney GFR measurements by this method accurately reflect changes in three-dimensional volume parameters measured by magnetic resonance imaging.[32] These authors argue that demonstrating preserved "parenchymal volume" with disproportionate reduction in single-kidney GFR supports the concept of "hibernating" kidney parenchyma and might provide a predictive parameter for recovery of kidney function after revascularization.[32]

Imaging of the Renal Vasculature

Advances in Doppler ultrasound, radionuclide imaging, magnetic resonance angiography (MRA), and computed tomography angiography (CTA) continue to introduce major changes in the field of renovascular imaging. The details of these methods are beyond the scope of this discussion. They are addressed more fully elsewhere. What follows is a discussion of some specific merits and limitations of each modality as they apply to application in renovascular hypertension and ischemic nephropathy.[33]

Current practice in the United States favors reserving invasive arteriography to the occasion of endovascular intervention, e.g., stenting, angioplasty, or both. While angiography

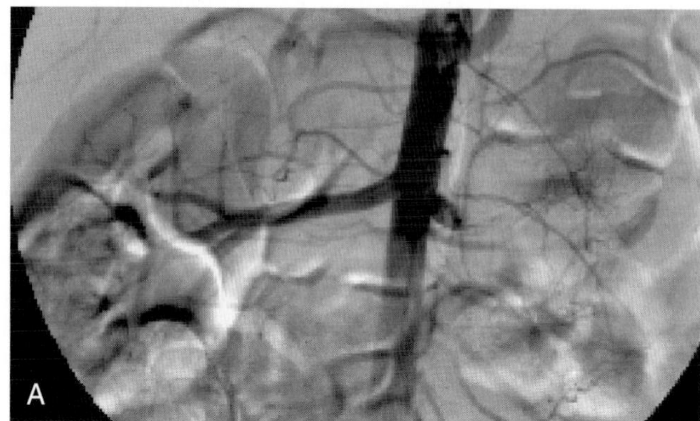

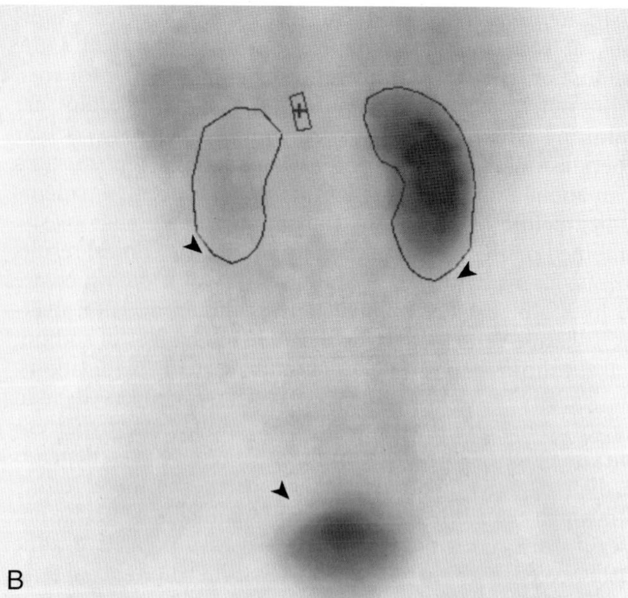

Figure 22-9. Radionuclide scan illustrating loss of filtration and perfusion to the left kidney in a 19-year-old with severe hypertension developing after a motor vehicle accident. Angiogram *(left)* demonstrates dissection and occlusion of the left renal artery. While renal scans do not provide direct viewing of the vasculature, they demonstrate changes in blood flow and filtration.

remains for many the gold standard for evaluation the renal vasculature, its invasive nature, potential hazards, and cost make it most suitable for those in whom intervention is planned, often during the same procedure. As a result, most clinicians favor preliminary noninvasive studies.

Noninvasive Imaging

Captopril Renography

Imaging the kidneys before and after administration of an ACE inhibitor (e.g., captopril) provides a functional assessment of the change in blood flow and GFR to the kidneys related to both changes in arterial pressure and removal of the efferent arteriolar effects of angiotensin II. The most commonly used radiopharmaceuticals are technetium-99-diethylenetriamine-pentaacetic acid and technetium-99-mercaptoacetyltriglycine. The latter agent has clearance characteristics similar to hippuran and is often taken as reflecting renal plasma flow. Both can be used, although specific interpretive criteria differ.[31] Both provide information regarding size and filtration of both kidneys (Figure 22-9), and the change in these characteristics after inhibition of ACE allows inferences regarding the dependence of glomerular filtration on angiotensin II. Several series of patients studied in patient groups with prevalence rates between 35% and 64% of subjects suggest that sensitivity and specificity range between 65% and 96% and 62% and 100%, respectively.[31]

These studies are less sensitive and specific for renovascular disease in the presence of renal insufficiency (usually defined as creatinine greater than 2.0 mg/dl).[34] These performance characteristics deteriorate for patients who cannot be prepared carefully, i.e., withdrawal of diuretics and ACE inhibitors for 4 to 14 days before the study.[31] It should be emphasized that renography provides functional information but no direct anatomical information, i.e., the location of renal arterial disease, the number of renal arteries, or associated aortic disease, ostial disease, or both. Some authors argue that renographic screening of patients using this technique is among the most cost-effective methods of identifying candidates for further diagnostic studies and is superior to functional studies of the renin–angiotensin system.[35] The prospective studies of renovascular disease from the Netherlands did observe changes in the renogram during follow-up but did not find captopril renography predictive of angiographic findings or outcomes.[36] A prospective study of 74 patients undergoing both renography and Doppler ultrasound evaluation before renal revascularization could identify only limited predictive value of scintigraphy (sensitivity 58% and specificity of 57%) regarding blood pressure outcomes.[37]

Doppler Ultrasound of the Renal Arteries

Duplex interrogation of the renal arteries provides measurements of localized velocities of blood flow. In many institutions, this provides an inexpensive means for measuring vascular occlusive disease at sequential time points to establish both the diagnosis of RAS and its progression.[38] After renal revascularization, Doppler studies are commonly used to monitor restenosis and target vessel patency[39,40] (Figure 22-10). Its main drawbacks relate to the difficulties of obtaining adequate studies in obese patients. The utility and reliability of Doppler ultrasound depend partly on the specific operator and the time allotted for optimal studies. These factors vary considerably among institutions.

The primary criteria for renal artery studies are a peak systolic velocity above 180 cm/sec and/or a relative velocity above 3.5 as compared to the adjacent aortic flow.[41] Using these criteria, sensitivity and specificity with angiographic estimates of lesions exceeding 60% can surpass 90% and 96%, respectively,[42,43] although not universally.[44] When main-vessel velocities cannot be determined reliably, segmental waveforms within the arcuate vessels in the renal hilum can provide additional information. Damping of these waveforms, labeled as "parvus" and "tardus" (Figure 22-10B), has been proposed

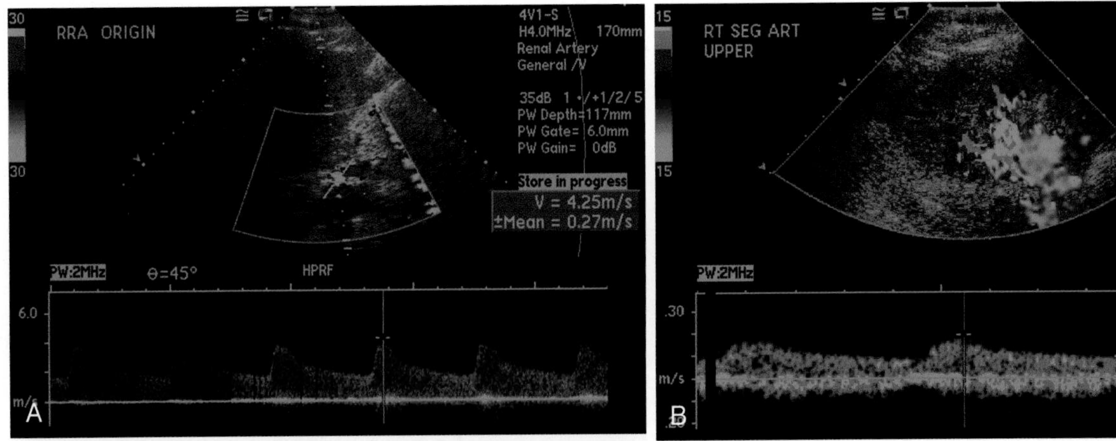

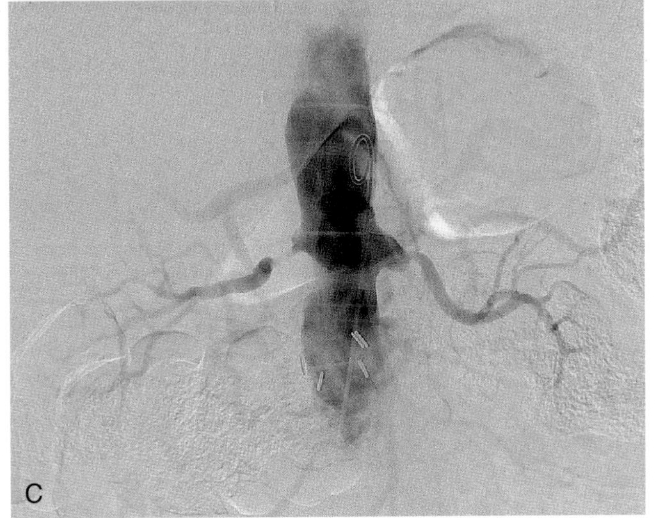

Figure 22-10. Doppler ultrasound. **A,** Doppler ultrasound examination of the proximal section of the right renal artery in a 71-year-old male with high-grade atherosclerotic occlusive disease. Flow velocity was 4.25 m/sec recorded at a Doppler angle of 45 degrees. Segmental interrogation of the distal vessels indicated a parvus tardus waveform **(B)** and a relatively low resistive index (RI = 0.51). **C,** Renal arteriogram from the same subject confirming the presence of a tight proximal stenosis. Serum creatinine fell from 4.5 mg/dl to 1.8 mg/dl within a week after renal revascularization in this patient.

as indirect signs of upstream vascular occlusive phenomena.[45] Some authors challenge the use of angiographic estimates of stenosis as a gold standard altogether.[46] These authors argue that Doppler velocities correlate highly (R = 0.97) with a truer estimate of vascular occlusion, specifically stenosis determined by intravascular ultrasound.

In our experience, Doppler study of the renal arteries is highly reliable when adequate imaging of the renal arteries can be obtained. Positive Doppler velocities in an artery clearly identified as the renal artery are rarely proven to be negative later. False-negative studies are more common. In subjects with accessible vessels, Doppler ultrasound provides the most practical means of following vessel characteristics sequentially over time. Drawbacks of renal artery Doppler include failure to identify accessory vessels.

Recent studies emphasize the potential for Doppler ultrasound to characterize the small-vessel flow characteristics within the kidneys. The resistive index provides an estimate of the relative flow velocities in diastole and systole. In a study of 138 patients with RAS, a resistive index above 80 provided a reliable tool for identification of parenchymal renal disease that did not improve after renal revascularization.[47] A sizable portion of this group eventually progressed to renal failure. A resistive index of less than 80 was associated with more than 90% favorable blood pressure response and stable or improved renal function. The authors emphasize that accurate predictive power depended on using the highest resistive index observed, even when present in the nonstenotic kidney. A subsequent report of 215 subjects with mean preintervention serum creatinine levels of 1.51 mg/dl failed to confirm the predictive value of resistive index measurements. Of 99 subjects with "improved" renal function after 1 year, 18% had resistive index above 0.8 before intervention, whereas 15% of 92 subjects with no improvement had index above 0.8 (NS). In this series, preintervention level of serum creatinine itself was the strongest predictor of improved renal function.[48]

Magnetic Resonance Angiography

Gadolinium-enhanced images of the abdominal and renal vasculature had become a mainstay of evaluating renovascular disease in many institutions until recently.[49] No radiation is used. Comparative studies indicate that sensitivity ranges from 83% to 100% and specificity from 92% to 97% in RAS.[50,51] Metaanalyses of published literature including 998 subjects support more than 97% sensitivity using gadolinium-enhanced imaging.[52] The nephrogram obtained from gadolinium filtration provides an estimate of relative function and filtration, as well as parenchymal volume.[53] Quantitative measurement of parenchymal volume determined by magnetic resonance imaging appears to correlate closely with isotopically determined single-kidney GFR in some institutions.[32]

Recent concerns regarding the potential role of gadolinium in the development of nephrogenic systemic fibrosis have severely reduced to the use of MRA as a diagnostic tool

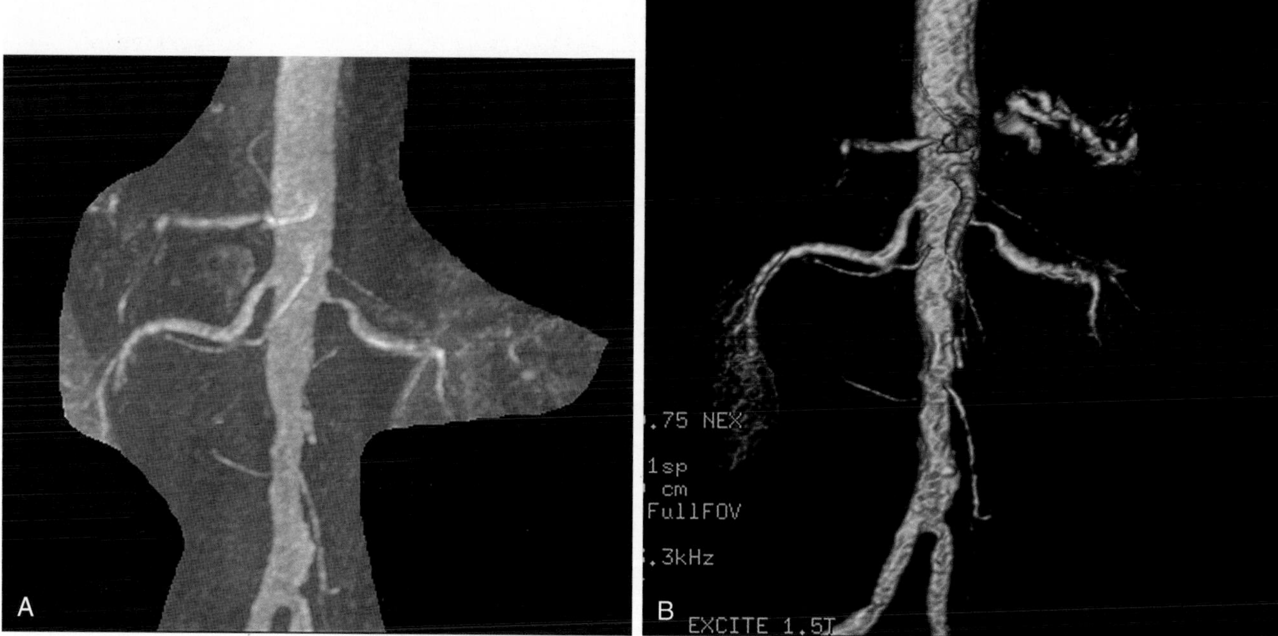

Figure 22-11. Magnetic resonance angiogram. Gadolinium-enhanced magnetic resonance angiogram **(A)** and volume reconstruction **(B)** illustrating high-grade renal artery stenosis in a 79-year-old male with renovascular hypertension. While gadolinium is relatively free of nephrotoxicity, concerns raised in 2006 regarding its potential role in producing nephrogenic systemic fibrosis led the U.S. Food and Drug Administration to issue a "black box" warning cautioning against its use in patients with reduced kidney function (estimated glomerular filtration rate less than 30 ml/min/1.73 m^2). As a result, use of gadolinium magnetic resonance angiography has declined considerably.

for patients with renal insufficiency. The precise incidence is not known, but this serious skin and muscle condition can be debilitating and sometimes fatal. As a result, the U.S. Food and Drug Administration has issued a "black box" warning effectively eliminating its use for patients with estimated GFR below 30 ml/min/1.73 m^2.[54]

Examples of MRA are shown in Figure 22-11. Additional drawbacks include expense and tendency to overestimate the severity of lesions, which appear as a signal void. The limits of resolution with current instrumentation make detection of small accessory vessels limited. Identifying fibromuscular lesions has been difficult. Both of these are improving with newer generations of scanners. High spatial resolution, three-dimensional, contrast-enhanced magnetic resonance scanners provide up to 97% sensitivity and 92% specificity for renal artery stenotic lesions.[55] Signal degradation in the presence of metallic stents renders MRA unsuitable for follow-up studies after endovascular procedures in which stents are used.

Recent efforts focus on using magnetic resonance to evaluate renovascular disease in other ways. Blood oxygen level–dependent magnetic resonance offers the potential to determine real-time changes in tissue oxygenation during maneuvers that change oxygen consumption.[56] These techniques are being investigated as potential tools to determine both tissue viability and salvageability of the kidneys beyond vascular occlusive disease without the requirement for gadolinium.

Computed Tomography Angiography

CTA using "helical" and/or multiple head scanners and intravenous contrast can provide excellent images of both the kidneys and the vascular tree. Resolution and reconstruction techniques render this modality capable of identifying smaller vessels, vascular lesions, and parenchymal characteristics, including stones[57] (Figure 22-12). When used for detection of RAS, CTA agrees well with conventional arteriography (correlation, 95%); sensitivity may reach 98% and specificity 94%.[57,58] While this technique offers a noninvasive examination of the vascular tree suitable for kidney donors and for individuals with vascular lesions including aneurysms, for example, it has the drawback of requiring iodinated contrast. As a result, it is less ideally suited for evaluation of renovascular hypertension or ischemic nephropathy for patients with impaired renal function.

One prospective study comparing both CTA and MRA with intraarterial studies in 402 subjects indicated substantially worse performance for detection of lesions with more than 50% stenosis than for those reported in other series.[59] In this study, CTA had sensitivity of 64% and specificity of 92%, whereas MRA had sensitivity of 62% and specificity of 84%. This was an unusual population, with only 20% of the screened population having stenotic lesions, nearly half of which were fibromuscular disease. The results of such studies reinforce the importance of careful patient selection for study and establishing the exact questions for which imaging is being undertaken in advance.[60]

Invasive Imaging

Intraarterial angiography remains the gold standard for definition of vascular anatomy and stenotic lesions in the kidneys. It is often completed at the time of a planned intervention, such as endovascular angioplasty, stenting, or both. What is the current role of including angiography of the renal arteries during imaging of other vascular beds, such as "drive-by" angiography during coronary artery imaging? Several studies confirm a high prevalence of renal artery lesions exceeding

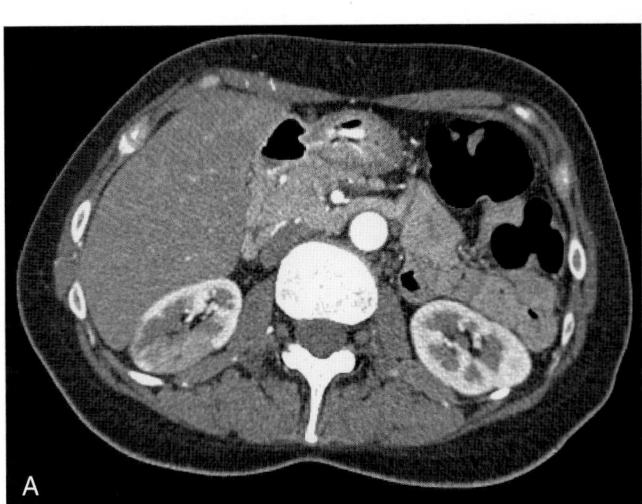

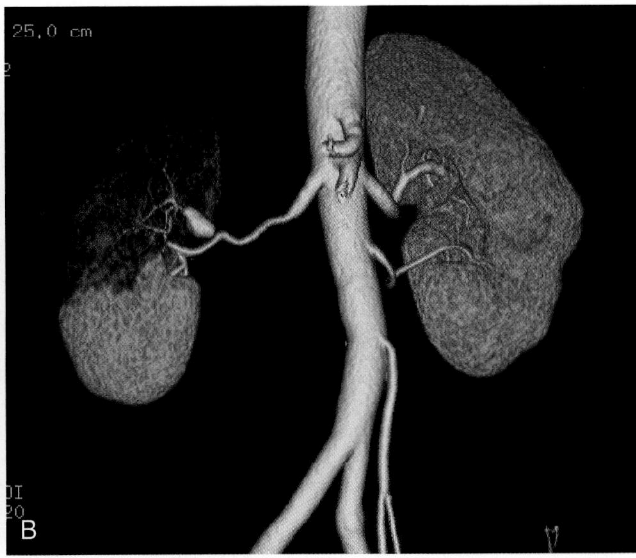

Figure 22-12. Computed tomography (CT) angiogram. **A,** CT angiogram demonstrating a cross-sectional view of both kidneys and illustrating areas of nonperfusion in the posterior segments of the right kidney. **B,** Reconstructed angiogram demonstrating a renal artery aneurysm producing thrombosis of the upper pole vessel to the right kidney, thus producing renovascular hypertension.

50% lumen occlusion in patients with hypertension and coronary artery disease, usually between 18% and 24%.[61] Some of these individuals (7% to 10%) have high-grade stenoses above 70%, and some are bilateral. Accepting that intraarterial puncture and catheterization of the aorta and coronary vessels produces some risk, the *added* risk of including aortography of the renal vessels appears to be almost negligible. Follow-up studies of individuals with identified "incidental" renal artery lesions suggest that the presence of these lesions does provide additive predictive risk for mortality.[62] No data to this point suggest that combining screening angiography with renal revascularization changes that risk. Hence, endovascular procedures for such lesions should be confined to individuals with strong indications for renal revascularization, as even ardent advocates of catheter-based intervention have suggested.[61]

Contrast toxicity remains an issue with conventional iodinated agents.[63] In many centers, gadolinium has been employed to reduce toxicity while still providing satisfactory imaging to complete endovascular procedures, particularly if the location and severity of the lesions have been preestablished. Concerns about development of nephrogenic systemic fibrosis in subjects with reduced kidney function (estimated GFR below 30 ml/min for every 1.73 m^2) limit this application. Intravascular ultrasound procedures have been undertaken using papaverine to evaluate "flow reserve" beyond stenotic lesions.[64] These studies confirm both reduction in absolute flow and impaired response to arterial vasodilators that reverse after successful revascularization in stenotic kidneys.

INTEGRATED EVALUATION AND MANAGEMENT OF RENAL ARTERY STENOSIS AND ISCHEMIC NEPHROPATHY

Considering the array of potential interventions that bear upon renovascular disease and the complexity of these patients, clinicians need to formulate a clear set of therapeutic goals. Because each mode of treatment—ranging from medical therapy alone to surgical revascularization—carries both benefits and risks, the clinician's task is to weigh the role of each of these within the context of the individual's comorbid disease risk.

It is rarely obvious how best to proceed. In most cases, long-term management of the patient with renovascular disease represents a balance between the pharmacological management of blood pressure and cardiovascular risk and the optimal timing of renal revascularization. It should be emphasized that consideration of renal artery disease takes place in the broad context of managing other cardiovascular risk factors, including withdrawal of tobacco use, reduction of cholesterol levels, and treatment of diabetes and obesity.

SUMMARY

Major reductions in mortality rates from coronary and cerebrovascular disease over the last three decades have given rise to longer life spans and an aging U.S. population. One result of these changes is a larger number of individuals reaching the seventh, eighth, and ninth decades of life and delayed onset of vascular disease. The mean age of interventional and surgical patient series is increasing. It is essential for clinicians to recognize that the syndromes of renovascular hypertension and ischemic nephropathy can develop at any age. They are more common now among older subjects than ever before. Advances in our understanding of these disorders and the antihypertensive agents available provide a wider set of options regarding effective blood pressure control. As a result, physicians must recognize the factors predisposing a patient to disease progression and the limitations of medical management for each patient.

With improved imaging and older patients, significant renal artery disease is detected more often than ever before. It is incumbent upon the clinician to evaluate both the role of renal artery disease in the individual patient and the potential risk–benefit ratio for renal revascularization. An algorithm to guide treatment and reevaluation of patients with ARAS is presented in Figure 22-13. This process relies heavily on

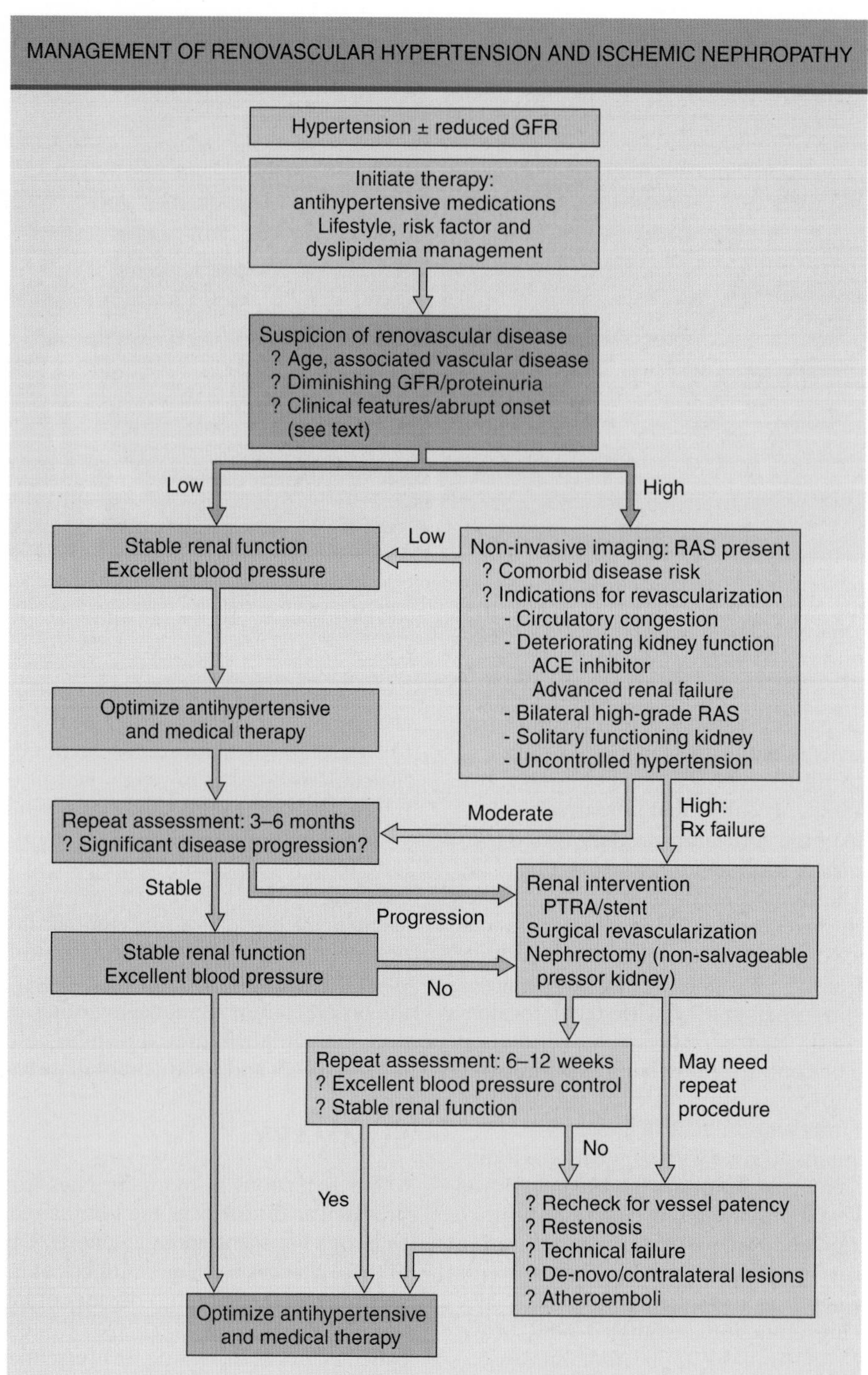

Figure 22-13. Algorithm for considering evaluation and intervention in subjects at risk for renovascular hypertension, ischemic nephropathy, or both. This approach emphasizes the primary goals of achieving satisfactory blood pressure control and stable renal function. These usually require effective antihypertensive therapy, including blockade of the renin–angiotensin system. Diagnostic studies to establish whether renovascular disease is present should be directed toward managing specific problems, e.g., refractory hypertension, circulatory congestion, or declining kidney function. Imaging studies can be selected to examine specific questions, e.g., whether the disease is unilateral or bilateral, whether it is progressing over time, and whether it is in a position suitable for endovascular or surgical intervention. (From Brenner BM, ed. *Brenner and Rector's: the kidney*. 8th ed. Philadelphia: Saunders; 2008:1528-1566.)

considering comorbid risks and the evolution of both blood pressure control and kidney function over a period. Management of cardiovascular risk and hypertension is the primary objective of medical therapy. For most patients, the realistic goals of renal revascularization are to reduce medication requirements and to stabilize renal function over time. Patients with bilateral disease or stenosis to a solitary functioning kidney may achieve lower risk of circulatory congestion ("flash" pulmonary edema or its equivalent) and lower risk for advancing renal failure. It is essential to appreciate the risks inherent in either surgical or endovascular manipulation of the diseased aorta. These include a hazard of atheroembolic complications and potential deterioration of renal function related to the procedure itself (estimated at 20%). Hence, the decision to undertake these procedures should include consideration of whether the potential gain warrants such risks. In many cases, improved blood pressure and recovery of renal function are justified. Follow-up of both blood pressure and renal function is important, particularly because of the potential for restenosis, recurrent disease, or both. Selection of the balance and timing of medical management and revascularization depends largely on the comorbid disease risks for each patient.

References

1. Goldblatt H, Lynch J, Hanzal RE, Summerville WW. Studies on experimental hypertension. I. the production of persistent elevation of systolic blood pressure by means of renal ischemia. *J Exp Med* 1934;59:347-379.
2. Crowley SD, Gurley SB, Oliverio MI, et al. Distinct roles for the kidney and systemic tissues in blood pressure regulation by the renin–angiotensin system. *J Clin Invest* 2005;115:1092-1099.
3. De Bruyne B, Manoharan G, Pijls NHJ, et al. Assessment of renal artery stenosis severity by pressure gradient measurements. *J Am Coll Cardiol* 2006;48:1851-1855.
4. Textor SC. Renovascular hypertension and ischemic nephropathy. In: Brenner BM, ed. Brenner and Rector's: the kidney. 8th ed. Philadelphia: Saunders; 2008:1528-1566.
5. Long DA, Price KL, Herrera-Acosta J, Johnson RJ. How does angiotensin II cause renal injury? *Hypertension* 2004;43:722-723.
6. Lerman LO, Nath KA, Rodriguez-Porcel M, et al. Increased oxidative stress in experimental renovascular hypertension. *Hypertension* 2001;37:541-546.
7. Wiecek A, Kokot F, Kuczera M, et al. Plasma erythropoietin concentration in renal venous blood of patients with unilateral renovascular hypertension. *Nephrol Dial Transplant* 1992;7:221-224.
8. Safian RD, Textor SC. Medical progress: renal artery stenosis. *N Engl J Med* 2001;344:431-442.
9. Lerman L, Textor SC. Pathophysiology of ischemic nephropathy. *Urol Clin North Am* 2001;28:793-803.
10. Miyajima E, Yamada Y, Yoshida Y, et al. Muscle sympathetic nerve activity in renovascular hypertension and primary aldosteronism. *Hypertension* 1991;17:1057-1062.
11. Brown JJ, Davies DL, Morton JJ, et al. Mechanism of renal hypertension. *Lancet* 1976;1:1219-1221.
12. Hughes JS, Dove HG, Gifford RW, et al. Duration of blood pressure elevation in accurately predicting cure of renovascular hypertension. *Am Heart J* 1981;101:408-413.
13. Chade AR, Rodriguez-Porcel M, Grande JP, et al. Mechanisms of renal structural alterations in combined hypercholesterolemia and renal artery stenosis. *Aterioscler Thromb Vascu Biol* 2003;23:1295-1301.
14. Mackenzie HS, Brenner BM. Prevention of progressive renal failure. In: Brady H, Wilcox C, eds. Therapy in nephrology and hypertension. 1st ed. Philadelphia: WB Saunders; 1999:463-473.
15. Toto RD, Mitchell HC, Lee HC, et al. Reversible renal insufficiency due to angiotensin converting enzyme inhibitors in hypertensive nephrosclerosis. *Ann Int Med* 1991;115:513-519.
16. Miyamori I, Yasuhara S, Takeda Y, et al. Effects of converting enzyme inhibition on split renal function in renovascular hypertension. *Hypertension* 1986;8:415-421.
17. Levin A, Linas SL, Luft FC, et al. Controversies in renal artery stenosis: a review by the American Society of Nephrology Advisory Group on Hypertension. *Am J Nephrol* 2007;27:212-220.
18. Textor SC. Ischemic nephropathy: where are we now? *J Am Soc Nephrol* 2004;15:1974-1982.
19. Little MA, O'Brien E, Owens P, et al. A longitudinal study of the yield and clinical utility of a specifically designed secondary hypertension investigation protocol. *Ren Fail* 2003;25:709-717.
20. Alhadad A, Mattiasson I, Ivancev K, et al. Revasularisation of renal artery stenosis caused by fibromuscular dysplasia: effects on blood pressure during 7-year follow-up are influenced by duration of hypertension and branch artery stenosis. *J Hum Hypertens* 2005;19:761-767.
21. Kumar A, Dubey D, Bansal P, et al. Surgical and radiological management of renovascular hypertension in a developing country. *J Urol* 2003;170:727-730.
22. Garovic V, Textor SC. Renovascular hypertension: current concepts. *Semin Nephrol* 2005;25:261-271.
23. Edwards MS, Craven TE, Burke GL, et al. Renovascular disease and the risk of adverse coronary events in the elderly: a prospective, population-based study. *Arch Int Med* 2005;165:207-213.
24. Kalra PA, Guo H, Kausz AT, et al. Atherosclerotic renovascular disease in United States patients aged 67 years or older: risk factors, revascularization and prognosis. *Kidney Int* 2005;68:293-301.
25. Buller CE, Nogareda JG, Ramanathan K, et al. The profile of cardiac patients with renal artery stenosis. *J Am Coll Cardiol* 2004;43:1606-1613.
26. Grisk O, Rettig R. Interactions between the sympathetic nervous system and the kidneys in arterial hypertension. *Cardiovasc Res* 2004;61:238-246.
27. Postma CT, van Oijen AH, Barentsz JO, et al. The value of tests predicting renovascular hypertension in patients with renal artery stenosis treated by angioplasty. *Arch Int Med* 1991;151:1531-1535.
28. Vaughan ED. Renovascular hypertension. *Kidney Int* 1985;27:811-827.
29. Kane GC, Textor SC, Schirger A, Garovic VD. Revisiting the role of nephrectomy for advanced renovascular disease. *Am J Med* 2003;114:729-735.
30. Roubidoux MA, Dunnick NR, Klotman PE, et al. Renal vein renins: inability to predict response to revascularisation in patients with hypertension. *Radiology* 1991;178:819-822.
31. Taylor A. Functional testing: ACEI renography. *Semin Nephrol* 2000;20:437-444.
32. Cheung CM, Shurrab AE, Buckley DL, et al. MR-derived renal morphology and renal function in patients with atherosclerotic renovascular disease. *Kidney Int* 2006;69:715-722.
33. Boudewijn G, Vasbinder C, Nelemans PJ, et al. Diagnostic tests for renal artery stenosis in patients suspected of having renovascular hypertension: a meta-analysis. *Ann Int Med* 2001;135:401-411.
34. Fernandez P, Morel R, Jeandot R, et al. Value of captopril renal scintigraphy in hypertensive patients with renal failure. *J Nucl Med* 1999;40:412-417.
35. Elliot WJ, Martin WB, Murphy MB. Comparison of two non-invasive screening tests for renovascular hypertension. *Arch Intern Med* 1993;153:755-764.
36. van Jaarsveld BC, Krijnen P, Pieterman H, et al. for the Dutch Renal Artery Stenosis Intervention Cooperative Study Group. The effect of balloon angioplasty on hypertension in atherosclerotic renal-artery stenosis. *N Engl J Med* 2000;342:1007-1014.
37. Soulez G, Therasse E, Qanadli SD, et al. Prediction of clinical response after renal angioplasty: respective value of renal Doppler sonography and scintigraphy. *AJR Am J Roentgenol* 2004;181:1029-1035.
38. Caps MT, Perissinotto C, Zierler RE, et al. Prospective study of atherosclerotic disease progression in the renal artery. *Circulation* 1998;98:2866-2872.
39. Bakker J, Beutler JJ, Elgersma OE, et al. Duplex ultrasonography in assessing restenosis of renal artery stents. *Cardiovasc Intervent Radiol* 1999;22:468-474.
40. Henry M, Amor M, Henry I, et al. Stents in the treatment of renal artery stenosis: long-term follow-up. *J Endovasc Surg* 1999;6:42-51.
41. Edwards JM, Zaccardi JM, Strandness DE. A preliminary study of the role of duplex scanning in defining the adequacy of treatment of patients with renal artery fibromuscular dysplasia. *J Vasc Surg* 1992;15:604-609.
42. Olin JW, Piedmonte MR, Young JR, et al. The utility of duplex ultrasound scanning of the renal arteries for diagnosing significant renal artery stenosis. *Ann Intern Med* 1995;122:833-838.
43. Spies KP, Fobbe F, El-Bedewi M, et al. Color-coded duplex sonography for noninvasive diagnosis and grading of renal artery stenosis. *Am J Hypertens* 1995;8:1222-1231.
44. Postma CT, van Aalen J, de Boo T, et al. Doppler ultrasound scanning in the detection of renal artery stenosis in hypertensive patients. *Brit J Radiol* 1992;65:857-860.
45. Stavros AT, Parker SH, Yakes WF, et al. Segmental stenosis of the renal artery: pattern recognition of tardus and parvus abnormalities with duplex sonography. *Radiology* 1992;184:487-492.
46. Radermacher J, Weinkove R, Haller H. Techniques for predicting favourable response to renal angioplasty in patients with renovascular disease. *Curr Opin Nephrol Hyper* 2002;10:799-805.
47. Radermacher J, Chavan A, Bleck J, et al. Use of Doppler ultrasonography to predict the outcome of therapy for renal-artery stenosis. *N Engl J Med* 2001;344:410-417.
48. Zeller T, Muller C, Frank U, et al. Stent angioplasty of severe atherosclerotic ostial renal artery stenosis in patients with diabetes mellitus and nephrosclerosis. *Catheter Cardiovasc Interv* 2003;58:510-515.

49. Spinosa DJ, Hagspiel KD, Angle JF, et al. Gadolinium-based contrast agents in angiography and interventional radiology: uses and techniques. *J Vasc Intervent Radiol* 2000;11:985-990.
50. Grist TM. Magnetic resonance angiography of renal artery stenosis. *Am J Kidney Dis* 1994;24:700-712.
51. Postma CT, Joosten FB, Rosenbusch G, Thien T. Magnetic resonance angiography has a high reliability in the detection of renal artery stenosis. *Am J Hypertens* 1997;10:957-963.
52. Tan KT, van Beek EJ, Brown PW, et al. Magnetic resonance angiography for the diagnosis of renal artery stenosis: a meta-analysis. *Clin Radiol* 2002;57:617-624.
53. Ros PR, Gauger J, Stoupis C, et al. Diagnosis of renal artery stenosis: feasibility of combining MR angiography, MR renography and gadopentetate-based measurements of glomerular filtration rate. *Am J Radiol* 1995;165:1447-1451.
54. Marckmann P, Skov L, Rossen K, et al. Nephrogenic systemic fibrosis: suspected causative role of gadodiamide used for contrast-enhanced magnetic resonance imaging. *J Am Soc Nephrol* 2006;17:2359-2362.
55. Fain SB, King BF, Breen JF, et al. High resolution contrast-enhanced MR angiography of the renal arteries: a prospective comparison to x-ray angiography. *Radiology* 2001;218:481-490.
56. Textor SC, Glockner JF, Lerman LO, et al. The use of magnetic resonance to evaluate tissue oxygenation in renal artery stenosis. *J Am Soc Nephrol* 2008;19:780-788.
57. Olbricht CJ, Paul K, Prokop M, et al. Minimally invasive diagnosis of renal artery stenosis by spiral computed tomography angiography. *Kidney Int* 1995;48:1332-1337.
58. Elkohen M, Beregi JP, Deklunder G, et al. Evaluation of the spiral computed tomography alone and combined with color Doppler ultrasonography in the detection of renal artery stenosis: a prospective study of 114 renal arteries. *Arch Mal Coeur Vaiss* 1995;88:1159-1164.
59. asbinder GBC, Nelemans PJ, Kessels AGH, et al. Accuracy of computed tomographic angiography and magnetic resonance angiography for diagnosing renal artery stenosis. *Ann Int Med* 2004;141:674-682.
60. Textor SC. Pitfalls in imaging for renal artery stenosis. *Ann Int Med* 2004;141:730-731.
61. White CJ. Catheter-based therapy for atherosclerotic renal artery stenosis. *Circulation* 2006;113:1464-1473.
62. Conlon PJ, Athirakul K, Kovalik E, et al. Survival in renal vascular disease. *J Am Soc Nephrol* 1998;9:252-256.
63. Gami AS, Garovic VD. Contrast nephropathy after coronary angiography. *Mayo Clin Proc* 2004;79:211-219.
64. Mounier-Vehier C, Cocheteux B, Haulon S, et al. Changes in renal blood flow reserve after angioplasty of renal artery stenosis in hypertensive patients. *Kidney Int* 2004;65:245-250.

chapter 23

Treatment of Renovascular Disease: Medical Therapy

Paul N. Harden, MB, ChB, FRCP

Key Points

- Atherosclerotic renal artery disease is common in arteriopaths.
- Vascular comorbidity and mortality are high.
- At 38%, the 2-year mortality rate is greater than that of many cancers.
- Tight lipid and blood pressure control should be standard therapy.
- Cardioprotective medical therapy should be used when possible.
- Angiotensin-converting enzyme inhibitors and angiotensin II receptor–blocking agents are the antihypertensive therapy of choice and can be used safely to control blood pressure in most cases.
- Nonpharmacological measures should be applied to reduce cardiovascular risk, e.g., smoking cessation and weight reduction.
- No direct evidence shows benefit of medical therapy on clinical outcomes in renovascular disease, although most patients have systemic arterial disease meriting medical modulation of cardiovascular risk factors.
- Early trial data suggest limited benefit of renal artery stenting over continued aggressive medical therapy in most cases.

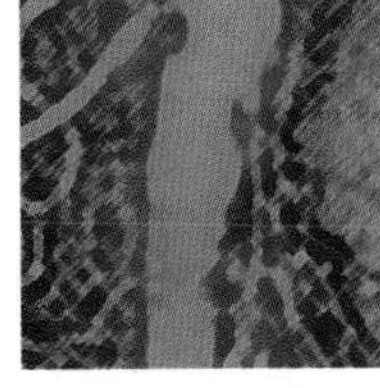

Atherosclerotic renal artery stenosis (ARAS) can cause hypertension and is increasingly recognized as a cause of progressive renal insufficiency.[1] The proximal part (first 10 mm) of the renal artery and the adjacent aorta (Figure 23-1) are involved in 85% of cases[2]; thus, the disease should be more correctly termed aortorenal atherosclerotic disease. The aorta is always diffusely involved with atherosclerotic disease, except in the extremely rare case of fibromuscular dysplasia causing more distal renal artery stenosis, which is often multiple (Figure 23-2). Progressive renal damage may also result from cholesterol embolization (from the aorta or proximal renal artery)[3] or disease of the intermediate and small renal vessels.

Atherosclerotic renovascular disease (ARVD) is associated with systemic vascular disease[4] and commonly coexists with significant coronary, carotid, or peripheral arterial disease.[5] The heavy burden of generalized atherosclerosis results in a high mortality rate—ranging from 29.7% at 3 years[4] to 38% at 2 years[5]—predominantly due to fatal cardiac events. The absolute risk of concomitant cardiovascular disease is heavily influenced by risk factors including age, gender, blood pressure (BP), and serum lipids.[6]

Medical treatment aims to prevent or retard the progression of atherosclerosis and to minimize the risks of progressive renal ischemia and death. Aggressive medical therapy has been shown to cause regression of atherosclerosis in other vascular beds.[7] In one nonrandomized study of 66 patients with ARVD and serum creatinine below 2 mg/dl, no significant difference appeared in renal function at 21 months of follow-up in patients treated with aggressive medical therapy (antihypertensives, statin and antiplatelet agent) versus patients receiving medical therapy and intervention.[8] This observation is supported by preliminary results of randomized, controlled trials of radiological intervention versus medical therapy alone in ARVD with chronic renal failure. Consequently, cardiovascular risk factor modification (including effective BP control and lipid lowering) is the cornerstone of current therapeutic strategy (Table 23-1). This chapter outlines therapeutic approaches that should be applied to all patients with ARVD, including those upon whom revascularization is performed.

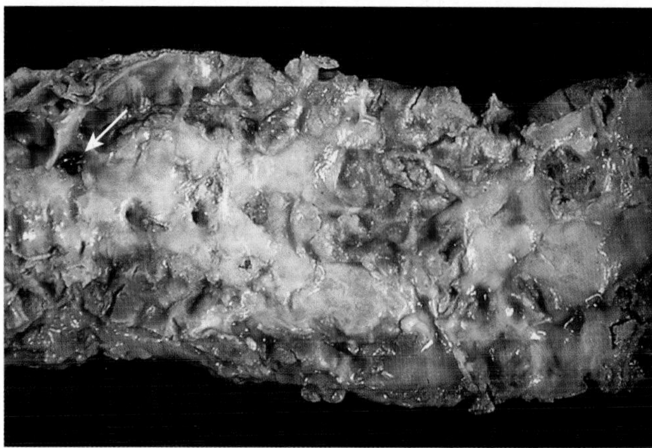

Figure 23-1. Generalized aortic atheroma associated with circumferential stenosis of the right renal artery, with patent Palmaz stent.

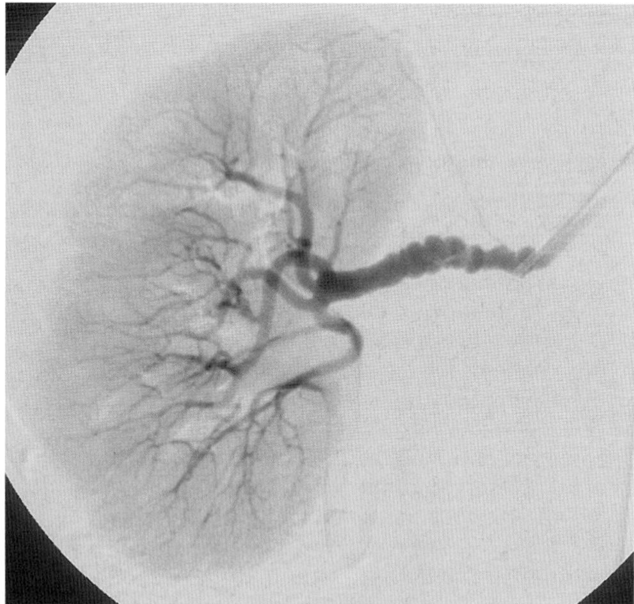

Figure 23-2. Multiple distal arterial stenoses due to fibromuscular dysplasia shown on selective renal angiography.

MEDICAL THERAPEUTIC OPTIONS

Medical therapy is targeted at modification of atherogenic risk factors (Table 23-1).

Hypertension

Persistent uncontrolled hypertension is an important cause of increased cardiovascular morbidity and mortality.[9,10] A kidney supplied by a normal renal artery in unilateral ARVD is at risk of progressive end-organ damage due to hypertension. Hypertensive renal damage may result whenever glomeruli are subjected to elevated perfusion pressures, which can occur even in the presence of a functionally insignificant proximal ARAS. Once the ARAS exceeds 70%, perfusion of the distal glomeruli is reduced, resulting in the production of renin by the juxtaglomerular apparatus and activation of the renin–angiotensin system (Figure 23-3). Angiotensin II causes efferent arteriolar constriction (to preserve glomerular perfusion and filtration) and systemic vasoconstriction. The result is renovascular hypertension. Angiotensin-converting enzyme (ACE) inhibitors and angiotensin II receptor–blocking agents (ARBs) are effective and safe antihypertensive agents in renovascular disease (Figure 23-3), as long as total glomerular filtration is not critically dependent on renal perfusion maintained by the activated renin–angiotensin system.[4,11,12] Other beneficial effects of ACE inhibitors are found in ARAS, as these agents reduce proteinuria[13] and prevent glomerular scarring in various renal diseases.[14,15] Introduction of these agents has greatly improved target BP control in renovascular hypertension: 35.3% achieved a target BP of less than 140/90 mm Hg, and 57.4% had BP of less than 160/95 mm Hg, exceeding the national average of 24% of patients with treated essential hypertension in the United States who achieve a target BP.[16] Caution and close clinical supervision are required in patients with renal failure (baseline serum creatinine of more than 130 mmol/L; glomerular filtration rate of less than 70 ml/min). Serial serum creatinine and potassium levels should be monitored before initiation of ACE inhibitors or ARBs, 5 days and again at 10 days after starting therapy, and thereafter every 4 to 6 months at clinical review. An initial rise in the serum creatinine of more than 15% is suspicious of functional renal artery disease, and the ACE inhibitor or ARB should be discontinued.[17] Acute deterioration in renal function can also occur in individuals with stable subcritical renal artery disease taking ACE inhibitors who develop dehydration with intravascular volume depletion due to gastrointestinal fluid losses or excessive use of diuretic therapy.[17] Patients with atherosclerotic renal artery disease taking ACE inhibitors or ARBs should be advised to withhold these drugs at times of gastrointestinal disturbances and to seek medical advice early. The acute deterioration in renal function is usually reversible with adequate fluid repletion and temporary suspension of the ACE inhibitor or ARB. Once renal function has recovered following the acute episode, the ACE inhibitor or ARB can usually be reintroduced with close monitoring of serum creatinine and potassium. Recurrent acute renal insufficiency suggests the development of critical renal artery stenosis, requiring further investigation and contraindicating ACE inhibitor or ARB use.

Table 23-1
Medical Therapeutic Approaches to Atherosclerotic Renal Artery Disease

- Blood pressure control
- Lipid-lowering therapy
- Antiplatelet agent
- Cessation of tobacco smoking and lifestyle modification

Often, more than one agent is required to achieve target BP control. A loop diuretic is an effective adjuvant to ACE inhibitor or ARB therapy through promotion of increased sodium excretion in the nephron. Loop diuretics have a good dose response curve in progressive renal failure, while thiazide diuretics are less effective in moderate-to-severe chronic renal failure. The various antihypertensives that can be employed, with details of mode of action, are shown in Table 23-2. β-Adrenoreceptor blockers can be used in the absence of critical peripheral vascular disease and have a beneficial effect on cardiac function in the presence of concurrent myocardial

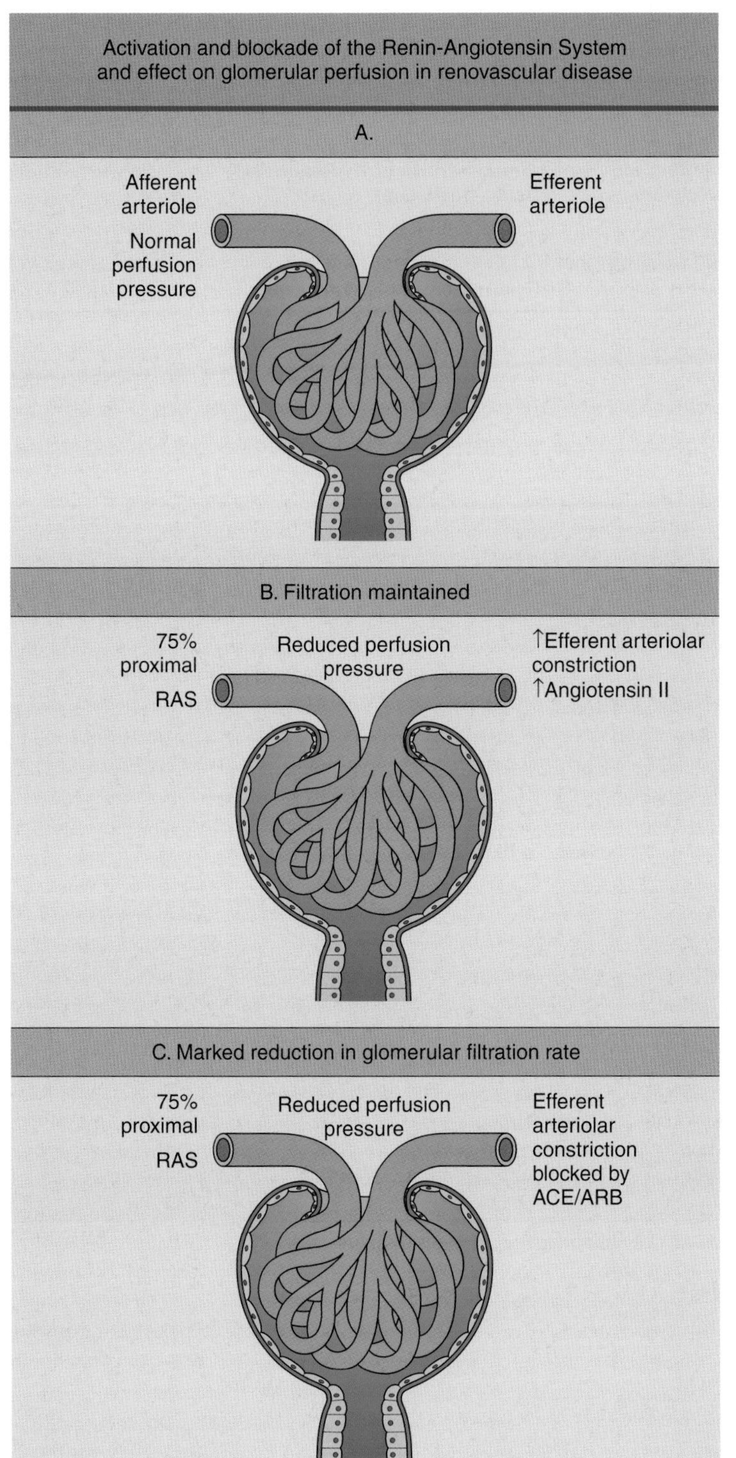

Figure 23-3. Activation and blockade of the renin–angiotensin system and effect on glomerular perfusion in renovascular disease. **A,** Normal renal perfusion. **B,** Maintenance of glomerular perfusion by angiotensin II–mediated efferent arteriolar constriction when renal artery perfusion is reduced in significant renal artery disease. **C,** Adverse effect of angiotensin-converting enzyme or angiotensin II receptor–blocking agent on renal perfusion in significant proximal renovascular disease.

damage. Doses should be reduced in elderly patients or those with renal failure due to impaired excretion.

Nonpharmacological measures of BP reduction should be actively employed but are rarely sufficient for achieving target BP control.[18] Targeted weight reduction to a body mass index corrected for age should be encouraged, coupled with reduction of salt intake, moderation of alcohol consumption, and increased regular exercise. It is essential to involve a dedicated dietician in the multidisciplinary team.

Target Blood Pressure

Many studies have demonstrated a reduction in cardiovascular morbidity and mortality achieved by good BP control.[19] Consensus groups in Europe and North America have developed target BP levels for the treatment of hypertension.[20,21] These targets (Table 23-3) are derived from the treatment of essential hypertension but are likely to benefit renovascular hypertension. Generalized atherosclerotic disease is associated

Table 23-2
Range of Antihypertensives, with Details of Mode of Action

Drug Class: Example	Mode of Action	Key Side Effects	Dose in CRF
Beta-blocker—atenolol, metoprolol	Selective beta$_1$-blockade	Lethargy, bronchospasm	50% decrease
Alpha-blocker—doxazosin	Postsynaptic alpha-blockade	Edema, orthostatic hypotension	Nil
Calcium channel antagonist—nifedipine, amlodipine	Blockade of T-type channel	Edema, headaches	Nil
ACE inhibitor—enalapril, lisinopril	Inhibit ACE	Raised K^+, cough	Caution, watch K^+
ARB—losartan	Block angiotensin II receptors	Raised K^+	Caution, watch K^+
Diuretic—furosemide	Natriuresis	Hyperuricemia, hyperglycemia	Increased doses

ACE, angiotensin-converting enzyme; ARB, angiotensin II receptor–blocking agent; CRF, chronic renal failure; K^+, potassium.

Table 23-3
Guidelines for the Treatment of Hypertension*

Joint British Recommendations

Lifestyle targets for all patients:
- Stop smoking
- Increase aerobic exercise: brisk walking for more than 30 minutes more than 3 times per week
- Limit alcohol intake to less than 3 units per day for men and less than 2 units per day for women
- Maintain a BMI between 20 and 25 kg/m^2
- Reduce intake of total and saturated fat
- Consume at least five portions of fresh fruit and vegetables per day
- Reduce salt intake to less than 100 mmol/day

Target blood pressure:
- Less than 140 mm Hg systolic and less than 85 mm Hg diastolic
- (diabetic: less than 130 mm Hg systolic and less than 80 mm Hg diastolic)

Target lipids:
- Total cholesterol of less than 3.5 mmol/L
- LDL cholesterol of less than 2 mmol/L

Cardioprotective drug treatment:
- Aspirin, 75 mg daily for all patients
- Beta-blockers after MI for more than 3 years
- Statin to achieve total serum cholesterol level of less than 3.5 mmol/L
- ACE inhibitors in heart failure after MI or ejection fraction of less than 40%

Anticoagulants:
- Large anterior infarcts
- Severe heart failure

U.S. Guidelines: Joint National Committee VII

Blood pressure (systolic/diastolic) (mm Hg)	130-139/85-89	140-159/90-99	>160/100
Risk group A†	Modify lifestyle	Modify lifestyle	Drug therapy
Risk group B‡	Modify lifestyle	Modify lifestyle up to 6 months	Drug therapy
Risk group C§	Drug therapy	Drug therapy	Drug therapy

*ACE, angiotensin-converting enzyme; BMI, body mass index; LDL, low-density lipoprotein; MI, myocardial infarction.
†Risk group A: No risk factors, target organ damage, or complications.
‡Risk group B: At least one risk factor; no target damage or complications.
§Risk group C: Target organ damage or complications with or without diabetes.

with stiffening of the major arterial tree, with reduced compliance, and with an increased incidence of systolic hypertension. First-line therapy should include an ACE inhibitor or ARB, with a loop diuretic if required. This regimen is well tolerated in most patients with subcritical ARAS and may adequately control BP. Many patients with ARAS are elderly and therefore more susceptible to postural hypotension, which can limit the use of vasodilating agents. Often, these arteriopaths have concurrent coronary artery disease, which may require therapy withselective beta-blockade, nitrates, or calcium channel blockade. All of these agents have antihypertensive effects that contribute to target BP control. Individuals who continue to have poor BP control despite the use of three or four antihypertensive agents may have poor drug compliance or, rarely, require the addition of centrally acting antihypertensives. Refractory hypertension is seldom controlled by revascularization procedures[22] unless a critical level of stenosis has developed causing ipsilateral impairment of glomerular filtration and resultant intolerance of ACE inhibitors and ARBs. In this specific circumstance, successful revascularization can afford the safe reintroduction of ACE inhibitors or ARBs with effective BP control.[12]

Lipid-Lowering Therapy

Patients with atherosclerotic renal artery disease have a high incidence of coexisting ischemic heart disease, cerebrovascular disease, and peripheral vascular disease.

Evidence from large multicenter trials shows a significant reduction in secondary cardiovascular events and mortality with lipid-lowering therapy.[23,24] Although no direct evidence supports an effect of lipid control on the progression of renal artery disease, tight control of total and low-density lipoprotein (LDL) cholesterol is justified to reduce cardiovascular morbidity and mortality. Hemorrhage into unstable atheromatous plaques may result in rupture, surface thrombosis, and reduction of functional vessel diameter. A pool of lipid in atheromatous plaques is amenable to removal with lipid-lowering therapy.[25] Target cholesterol levels have been set in Europe[26] and North America (Table 23-3). Most patients with renal artery disease have elevated total and LDL cholesterol, with a detrimentally low high-density lipoprotein fraction.[27] Individuals with coexisting diabetes mellitus often have hypertriglyceridemia. Dietary modification is rarely successful, as rigorous dietary compliance can only reduce cholesterol levels by 10%. Most patients require specific drug therapy to achieve target cholesterol levels.

3-Hydroxy-3-methylglutaryl–coenzyme A reductase inhibitors effectively reduce total and LDL cholesterol, with some increase in high-density lipoprotein cholesterol, and have a lesser effect on the reduction of triglycerides. 3-Hydroxy-3-methylglutaryl–coenzyme A reductase inhibitors (statins) promote stabilization of atherosclerotic plaques by multiple effects, including inhibition of cholesterol synthesis in hepatocytes, inhibition of proliferation of vascular smooth muscle cells and fibroblasts, and suppression of inflammation.[28] Statins are well tolerated, although they rarely are hepatotoxic and can cause myositis. Serum liver enzyme levels should be checked at baseline and 2 weeks after initiation of therapy; statins should be discontinued if a rise occurs in liver enzymes. The dose should be titrated upward at monthly intervals until the target total and LDL cholesterol levels are achieved or the maximum daily dose is reached. Statins are potent, with an average cholesterol-lowering potential of 20% to 30% over baseline levels. Rarely, a fibrate is required when hypertriglyceridemia is the predominant lipid abnormality; these agents can also provoke myositis and should be used with caution in patients with chronic renal failure.

Antiplatelet Therapy

Platelet activation is implicated in the pathogenesis of atherosclerosis and is associated with elevated serum levels of thromboglobulin and P-selectin.[29] Atheromatous plaques in renal artery disease, fibrinogen, and damaged endothelial cells may trigger or promote the formation of platelet thrombi, which in turn promote the local release of inflammatory cytokines and chemoattractants. Elevated fibrinogen levels correlate with the severity of peripheral vascular disease and angina.[30] Antiplatelet therapy has been shown to reduce the risk of secondary events in patients with ischemic heart disease[31] and carotid disease. No trials directly support a beneficial effect of antiplatelet therapy on progression of renal arterial disease. However, the close association of significant coronary and peripheral vascular disease merits the administration of antiplatelet therapy in most cases.

Smoking Cessation

Smoking cessation should be encouraged in all patients with renovascular disease as an important means of reducing cardiovascular risk and reducing progression of generalized atherosclerosis.

Other Cardiovascular Risk Factors

Elevated levels of serum homocysteine are associated with increased cardiovascular risk and may occur in renovascular patients. Homocysteine levels can be reduced using oral folic acid,[32] although the effect of this reduction on renal artery disease is unknown. Increasingly, generalized atherosclerosis is considered a systemic inflammatory disease associated with inflammatory markers like C-reactive protein.[33] A reduction in the levels of acute-phase proteins occurs in patients treated with statins and is associated with improved cardiovascular outcomes,[34] although there is no evidence to date for the use of other antiinflammatory agents. Recently, intraarterial recombinant basic fibroblast growth factor-2 has been shown to significantly increase peak walking time at 90 days in patients with moderate-to-severe peripheral vascular disease.[35] It is not clear whether targeted angiogenesis could likewise improve renal ischemia in atherosclerotic renal artery disease.

THERAPEUTIC OPTIONS

All patients with atherosclerotic renal artery disease should have (1) a thorough clinical assessment of total burden of atherosclerotic disease and (2) appropriate cardiovascular risk factor modification. Often, a multidisciplinary team approach is used, with active contributions from clinicians managing cardiac, renal, neurological, and peripheral vascular disease. It is important to have close coordination among these services to optimize holistic care, preferably with a lead clinician in a specialized vascular risk clinic.

Macrovascular renovascular disease has been shown to progress in studies using sequential angiography or Doppler ultrasound; 10% of renal artery stenoses greater than 60% went on to occlusion over 2 years on sequential Doppler studies,[36] and 14% of renal artery stenoses greater than 75% occluded over 2 years at repeat angiography.[37] Risk of progression has encouraged many centers to undertake surgical or radiological intervention to preserve vessel patency,[38,39] although only limited trial evidence supports intervention for the control of renovascular hypertension.[23] The natural history of ARVD is poorly understood, with a variable decline in glomerular filtration demonstrated in a group of patients with renal artery stenosis greater than 50% bilaterally or in a solitary functioning kidney.[4] Recent results of an international randomized, controlled trial (Angioplasty and Stent for Renal Artery Lesions Trial) of radiological intervention versus continued medical therapy in patients with chronic renal failure and radiologically proven renal artery stenosis of more than 50% reveals no difference in renal function in the two arms at 12 months follow-up.[40] Three further trials in progress are designed to assess the benefit of revascularization over medical therapy in ARVD.[41-43]

It remains uncertain whether radiological intervention improves morbidity or mortality in most cases of ARVD, but overwhelming evidence shows that good BP and lipid control can improve clinical outcomes in patients with various forms of cardiovascular disease, including ARVD.

References

1. Mailloux LU, Napolitano B, Bellucci AG, et al. Renal vascular disease causing end-stage renal disease: incidence, clinical correlates and outcomes—a 20-year clinical experience. *Am J Kidney Dis* 1994;24:622-629.
2. Greco BA, Breyer JA. Atherosclerotic ischemic renal disease. *Am J Kidney Dis* 1997;29:176-187.
3. Meyrier A, Buchet P, Simon P, et al. Atheromatous renal disease. *Am J Med* 1988;85:139-146.
4. Chabova V, Schirger A, Stanson AW, et al. Outcomes of atherosclerotic renal artery stenosis managed without revascularization. *Mayo Clin Proc* 2000;75:437-444.
5. Baboolal K, Evans C, Moore RH. Incidence of end-stage renal disease in medically treated patients with severe bilateral atherosclerotic renovascular disease. *Am J Kidney Dis* 1998;31:971-977.
6. Anderson KV, Odell PM, Wilson PWF, Kannel WB. Cardiovascular disease risk profiles. *Am Heart J* 1991;121:293-298.
7. Loscalzo J. Regression of coronary atherosclerosis. *N Engl J Med* 1990;323:337-339.
8. Haazel G, Balon H, Wong O, et al. Prospective evaluation of aggressive medical therapy for atherosclerotic renal artery stenosis with renal stenting reserved for previously injured heart, brain or kidney. *Am J Cardiol* 2005;96:1322-1327.
9. MacMahon S, Peto R, Cutler J, et al. Blood pressure, stroke, and coronary heart disease. I. Prolonged differences in blood pressure: prospective observational studies corrected for the regression dilution bias. *Lancet* 1990;335:754-774.
10. Systolic Hypertension in the Elderly Program Cooperative Research Group. Prevention of stroke by antihypertensive drug treatment in older persons with isolated systolic hypertension. Final results of the Systolic Hypertension in the Elderly Program (SHEP). *JAMA* 1991;265:3255-3264.
11. Textor SC. ACE inhibitors in renovascular hypertension. *Cardiovasc Drugs Ther* 1990;4:229-235.
12. Goldsmith DJA, Reidy J, Scoble J. Renal arterial intervention and angiotensin blockade in atherosclerotic nephropathy. *Am J Kidney Dis* 2000;36:837-843.
13. Lewis EJ, Hunsicker LG, Bain RP, Rohde RD. The effect of angiotensin-converting enzyme inhibition on diabetic nephropathy. *N Engl J Med* 1993;329:1456-1462.
14. Maschio G, Alberti D, Janin G, et al. Effect of the angiotensin-converting enzyme inhibitor benazepril on the progression of chronic renal insufficiency. *N Engl J Med* 1996;334:939-944.
15. Reggenenti P, Perna A, Gherardi G, et al. Renoprotective properties of ACE-inhibition in non-diabetic nephropathies with non-nephrotic proteinuria. *Lancet* 1999;354:359-364.
16. Joint National Committee on Prevention. *The sixth report of the Joint National Committee on Prevention. NIH publication 98-4080.* Bethesda, MD: National Institutes of Health; 1997.
17. Kalra PA, Kumwenda M, MacDowall P, Roland MO. ACE-inhibitor usage and monitoring in general practice: the need for guidelines to prevent renal failure. *BMJ* 1999;318:234-237.
18. Alderman MH. Non-pharmacological treatment of hypertension. *Lancet* 1994;344:307-311.
19. Hansson L, Zanchetti A, Carruthers SG, et al. Effects of intensive blood pressure lowering and low-dose aspirin in patients with hypertension: principal results of the Hypertension Optimal Treatment (HOT) randomised trial. *Lancet* 1998;351:1755-1762.
20. Williams B, Poulter NR, Brown MJ, et al. Working party guidelines for management of hypertension: report of the fourth working party of the British Society of Hypertension 2004—BHS IV. *J Hum Hypertens* 2004;18:139-185.
21. Chobanian AV, Bakris GI, Black HR, et al. The seventh report of the Joint National Committee on prevention, detection, evaluation and treatment of high blood pressure: the JNC 7 report. *JAMA* 2003;289:2560-2567.
22. van Jaarsveld BC, Krijnen P, Pieterman H, et al. The effect of balloon angioplasty on hypertension in atherosclerotic renal artery stenosis. *N Engl J Med* 2000;342:1007-1014.
23. LaRosa JC, He J, Vupputuri S. Effect of statins on risk of coronary disease: meta-analysis of randomized controlled trials. *JAMA* 1999;282:2340-2346.
24. West of Scotland Coronary Prevention Group. West of Scotland Coronary Prevention Study: identification of high-risk groups and comparison with other cardiovascular intervention trials. *Lancet* 1996;348:1339-1342.
25. Brown BG, Zhou XQ, Sacco DE, Albers JJ. Lipid lowering and plaque regression: new insights into plaque disruption and clinical events in coronary artery disease. *Circulation* 1993;87:1781-1791.
26. Joint British recommendations on prevention of coronary heart disease in clinical practice: summary. British Cardiac Society, British Hyperlipidaemia Association, British Hypertension Society, British Diabetic Association. *BMJ* 2000;320:705-708.
27. Scoble JE, deTakats D, Ostermann ME, et al. Lipid profiles in patients with atherosclerotic renal artery stenosis. *Nephron* 1999;83:117-121.
28. Rosenson RS, Tangney CC. Anti-atherothrombotic properties of statins: implications for cardiovascular event reduction. *JAMA* 1998;279:1643-1650.
29. Wu KK. Platelet activation mechanisms and markers in arterial thrombosis. *J Intern Med* 1996;239:17-34.
30. Fowkes FGR, Lowe GDO, Housley E, et al. Cross-linked fibrin degradation products, progression of peripheral vascular arterial disease, and risk of coronary heart disease. *Lancet* 1993;342:84-86.
31. Antiplatelet Trialists' Collaboration. Secondary prevention of vascular disease by prolonged anti-platelet treatment. *BMJ (Clin Res Ed)* 1988;296:320-331.
32. Hankey GJ, Eikelboom JW. Homocysteine and vascular disease. *Lancet* 1999;354:407-413.
33. Stenvinkel P, Heimburger O, Paultre F, et al. Strong association between malnutrition, inflammation, and atherosclerosis in chronic kidney failure. *Kidney Int* 1999;(55):1899-1911.
34. Ridker PM, Rifai N, Pfeffer MA, et al. Long-term effects of pravastatin on plasma concentration of C-reactive protein: the Cholesterol and Recurrent Events (CARE) investigators. *Circulation* 1999;100:230-235.
35. Lederman RJ, Mendelsohn FO, Anderson RD, et al. Therapeutic angiogenesis with recombinant fibroblast growth factor-2 for intermittent claudication (the Traffic study): a randomised trial. *Lancet* 2002;359:2053-2058.
36. Zierler RE, Bergelin RO, Davidson RC, et al. A prospective study of disease progression in patients with atherosclerotic renal artery stenosis. *Am J Hypertens* 1996;9:1055-1061.
37. Schreiber MJ, Pohl MA, Novick AC. The natural history of atherosclerotic and fibrous renal artery disease. *Urol Clin North Am* 1984;11:383-392.
38. Harden PN, MacLeod MJ, Rodger RSC, et al. Effect of renal artery stenting on progression of renovascular renal failure. *Lancet* 1997;349:1133-1136.
39. Plouin PF, Chantellier G, Darne B, et al. Blood pressure outcome of angioplasty in atheromatous renal artery stenosis: a randomised trial: Essai Multicentrique Medicaments vs Angioplastie (EMMA) Study Group. *Hypertension* 1998;31:823-829.
40. Mistry S, Ives N, Harding J, et al. ASTRAL rationale, methods and results so far. *J Hum Hypertens* 2007;7:511-515.
41. Scarpioni R, Michieletti E, Cristinelli L, et al. Atherosclerotic renovascular disease: medical therapy versus medical therapy plus renal artery stenting in preventing renal failure progression. The rationale and study design of a prospective multicenter randomized controlled trial (NITER). *J Nephrol* 2005;18:423-428.
42. Bax L, Mali WP, Buskens E, et al. The benefit of stent placement and blood pressure and lipid lowering for the prevention of progression of renal dysfunction caused by atherosclerotic ostial stenosis of the renal artery: the STAR-study rationale and study design. *J Nephrol* 2003;16:807-812.
43. Cooper CJ, Murphy TP, Matsumoto A, et al. Stent revascularization for the prevention of cardiovascular and renal events among patients with renal artery disease and systolic hypertension: rationale and design of the CORAL trial. *Am Heart J* 2006;152:59-66.

chapter 24

Endovascular Therapy of Renovascular Disease

Jonathan G. Moss, MBChB, FRCS, FRCR

Key Points

- Renal artery stenosis is divided into atheromatous and nonatheromatous etiologies.
- Atheromatous lesions are 10 times more prevalent than nonatheromatous lesions.
- Percutaneous transluminal angioplasty (PTA) is the procedure of choice for nonatheromatous lesions.
- The improvement of blood pressure control in nonatheromatous lesions is good to excellent following PTA.
- Most atheromatous lesions are ostial.
- Stents have a higher technical success rate compared with PTA in atheromatous ostial lesions (AHA: A).
- Stents have a higher patency rate compared with PTA in atheromatous ostial lesions (AHA: A).
- Improvement of blood pressure control in atheromatous lesions following PTA is marginal but may reduce the drug burden for the patient (AHA: B).
- Results in atheromatous patients with renal insufficiency following PTA or stenting are variable, with no consensus.
- Three randomized, controlled trials are currently comparing stenting with best medical treatment measuring renal and cardiovascular outcomes.

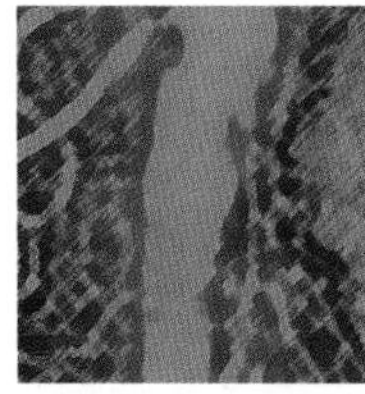

Renal artery stenosis (RAS) is an anatomical description of a lesion that may lead to various pathophysiological disease processes or simply exist as a silent lesion throughout life. To add more confusion, the disease entities hypertension, renal insufficiency, and pulmonary edema are common and have myriad etiologies, only one of which is RAS. It is often difficult to determine how much contribution the RAS is making to the symptomatology, if any.

RAS is caused by either atheromatous disease (of the aorta) or various disparate entities, which include fibromuscular disease, neurofibromatosis, and Takayasu's arteritis. Fibromuscular disease usually affects young females and children, and the presenting feature is hypertension. It is rare for renal function to be impaired. The lesions almost never involve the renal artery ostium but predominate in the middle to distal main vessel and can extend out to the first- and second-order side branches. Although rare, the arteritides are rewarding to treat, usually responding well to percutaneous transluminal angioplasty (PTA), with 10-year cumulative patency of 87% and cure rates for hypertension approaching 50%.[1,2]

Atherosclerotic renal artery stenosis (ARAS) is a common disorder, prevalent in the population of patients encountered with coronary, carotid, and peripheral vascular disease. Although much of the original research focused on renovascular hypertension, a renewed interest has focused on renal impairment. ARAS is now the commonest cause of end-stage renal failure (ESRF) in patients older than 60 years on renal replacement therapy, accounting for at least 25% of this group.[3] ARAS is known to be a progressive disorder, with a cumulative incidence of progression to occlusion of 5% per annum in stenoses equal to or greater than 60%.[4] Renal revascularization by either an endovascular or an open surgical method has the potential to alter this process and prevent progression to ESRF. Three randomized, controlled trials (RCTs)—Angioplasty and Stent for Renal Artery Lesions (ASTRAL) Trial (United Kingdom),[5] STAR (Holland), and Cardiovascular Outcomes with Renal Atherosclerotic Lesions (CORAL) Study (United

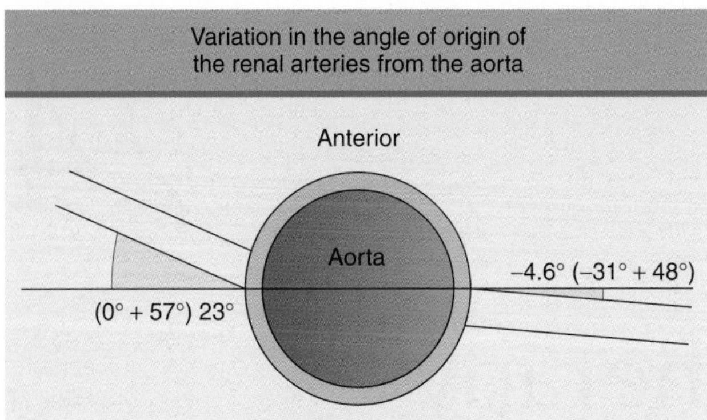

Figure 24-1. Variation in the angle of origin of the renal arteries from the aorta. The right arises anterior to the midcoronal plane (0 to 57 degrees). The left is more variable and can arise to either side of the midcoronal plane (−31 to +48 degrees).

States)[6]—are comparing renal stenting with best medical treatment to test this hypothesis. ASTRAL will report early results in March 2008.

PREOPERATIVE PREPARATION

It is essential patients are appropriately worked up and prepared for renal revascularization. The following should be addressed:

- Noninvasive imaging
- Adequate hydration
- Renoprotective drugs

Noninvasive Imaging

It is no longer acceptable to attempt renal revascularization without adequate noninvasive imaging. This should include images in the coronal, oblique, and transverse planes. Until the emergence of nephrogenic fibrosing dermopathy in 2006[7] (described later), magnetic resonance angiography was the preferred imaging modality, with computed tomography angiography (CTA) as the second choice. Noninvasive imaging allows advanced planning of the revascularization procedure, and the transverse images are invaluable in setting the C-arm to the appropriate angle so that the renal artery ostium is seen in tangential profile ensuring accurate stent placement (Figure 24-1).[8,9,16] In addition, renal size can be measured, multiple vessels can be detected, and a decision can be made regarding the feasibility of using a protection device. Occasionally, other pathologies are detected.[9,10]

Nephrogenic Fibrosing Dermopathy

A pivotal report in January 2006 linked gadolinium exposure during magnetic resonance examinations to the development of nephrogenic fibrosing dermopathy.[7] This is a rare but occasionally fatal condition that causes woody induration of legs, thighs, hands, and forearms with severe loss of motion and flexion contractures in multiple joints. It only occurs where renal function is impaired and the gadolinium cannot be excreted rapidly from the body. Current guidelines suggest gadolinium should not be given to those with an estimated glomerular filtration rate of less than 60 ml/min. The next fall-back imaging procedure is CTA. This carries the more benign risk of contrast-induced nephropathy, which is almost always self-limiting.

Adequate Hydration

It is essential that patients with impaired renal function are not dehydrated before revascularization, as this increases the susceptibility to iodinated contrast nephropathy. A randomized trial has shown that intravenous infusion of 0.45% saline (100 to 150 ml/hr) for 12 hours before and 12 hours after intervention reduces the incidence of contrast nephropathy.[11] Acetylcysteine may have a renoprotective benefit if given prophylactically (1200 mg before and after iodinated contrast administration). Acetylcysteine appears to work by improving renal hemodynamics and having antioxidant properties. Although the first RCT showed a beneficial effect,[12] subsequent trials have given conflicting opinions. Finally, it should be remembered the ideal way to avoid iodinated contrast nephropathy is to avoid such contrast altogether. It is now feasible to carry out renal revascularization using carbon dioxide exclusively or with at most 5 to 10 cm^3 of iodinated contrast.[13] Gadolinium is another alternative contrast agent but is "off label" when used intraarterially. With the recognition of nephrogenic fibrosing dermopathy, it is now seldom indicated.[14]

Technique

Traditionally, renal angioplasty or stenting has been performed using so-called standard-platform technology. This uses 0.035-inch guide wires with 5-French (Fr) angioplasty balloons. Increasingly over the last 5 years, a inexorable swing has occurred toward "small platform" technology, which uses 0.014- to 0.018-inch wires and 2.5- to 4-Fr balloons. This technology has been plagiarized from the coronary field and carries several potential advantages. The puncture site sheath diameter can be reduced to 5 Fr (previously 7 to 8 Fr), and the finer guide wires, balloons, and stents are likely to be less traumatic when crossing the stenosis, reducing the risk of distal embolization and dissection. Not all operators are familiar with or wish to use this new technology; hence, both platforms are described here.

Standard-Platform Renal Angioplasty

Usually, a femoral approach is used for standard-platform renal angioplasty. However, if the noninvasive imaging shows a severely caudally angulated renal artery or severely diseased aortoiliac segments, then an arm approach should be chosen. When using an arm approach, either the left brachial or the left radial is the first choice. Longer guide wires, catheters, and balloons are also required to reach the renal artery from the arm.

Having placed a 6-Fr sheath, intravenous heparin is administered and the renal artery is catheterized with an appropriately shaped 4- to 5-Fr catheter. From a femoral approach, the most useful configuration is the "reverse curve" or "shepherd's crook," such as the SOS Omni (Angiodynamics, Queensbury, NY) (Figure 24-2). Occasionally, the femorovisceral or "cobra shape" catheter is a useful alternative (Figure 24-2B). Once the wire is across the lesion, the reverse curve catheter is gently withdrawn, which advances it across the stenosis. The guide wire should only be advanced a couple of centimeters beyond the lesion, as distal guide wire placement can invoke spasm or

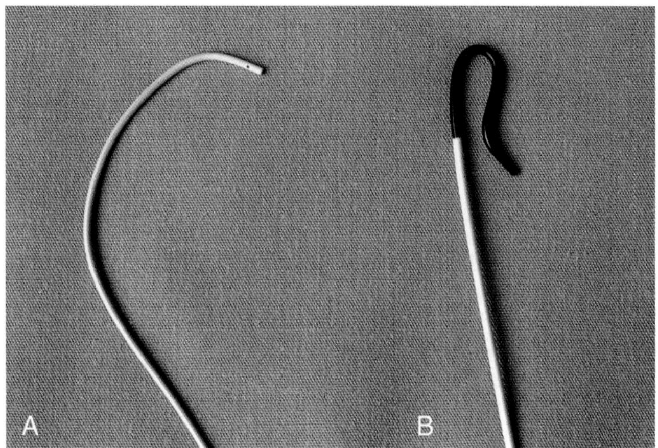

Figure 24-2. Catheters. **A,** Cobra catheter; **B,** Sos Omni catheter.

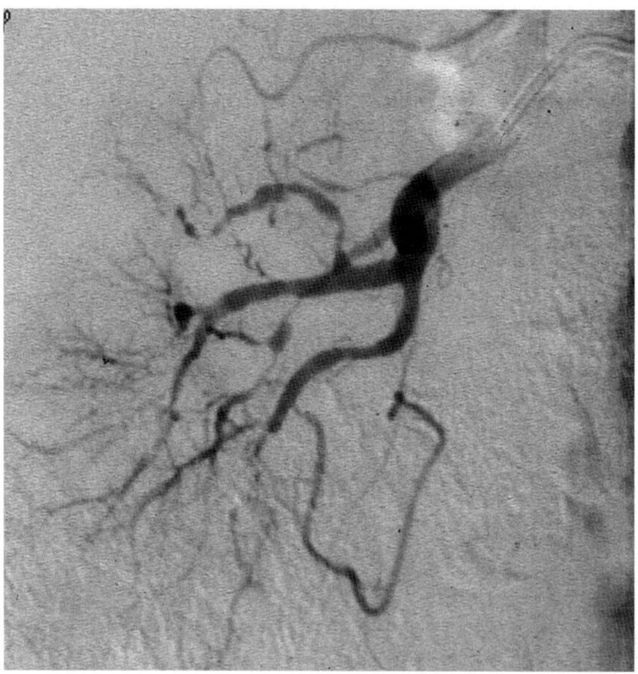

Figure 24-3. Angiogram showing severe intrarenal small-vessel disease not suitable for revascularization.

even perforate the kidney. At this stage, a proprietary vasodilator (e.g., glycerol trinitrate, 150 to 500 mg) is given through the catheter into the renal circulation to minimize the risk of spasm. A selective renal angiogram is then performed. If this shows severe intrarenal disease, then the procedure should probably be abandoned, as revascularization is unlikely to bring about any therapeutic benefit (Figure 24-3). At present, noninvasive imaging is rarely able to accurately image the intrarenal circulation.

The stenosis should be dilated with a short-tipped (2 cm) balloon, the diameter matching that of the normal renal artery. A completion angiogram should be done using a 4-Fr pigtail alongside the guide wire in the sheath, maintaining access across the lesion should the decision be made to place a stent.

Small-Platform Renal Angioplasty

Many common themes are associated with the standard-platform procedure regarding choice of access and imaging. There are two types of small-platform device, the coaxial system and the "rapid exchange" system. The coaxial system is identical to the standard platform except a 2.5- to 4-Fr balloon is used over a 0.014- or 0.018-inch guide wire. Rapid exchange systems require a guiding sheath or catheter preshaped to suit the renal artery angle (usually renal double curve). Through this, the 0.014- or 0.018-inch wire and balloon are passed across the stenosis. The guiding catheter does not cross the lesion. The rapid exchange systems have some advantages in that catheter exchanges are faster and shorter wires are used. The necessary guiding catheter also helps stabilize the gear, improving torquability, and permits contrast injections, ensuring accurate placement.

Renal Stenting Technique

Two renal stenting methods are in use: the first uses conventional 0.035-inch guide wire technology (standard platform, Figure 24-4), whereas the more recent small-platform systems use 0.014- to 0.018-inch guide wires. Both are described; they are similar to PTA, as described earlier.

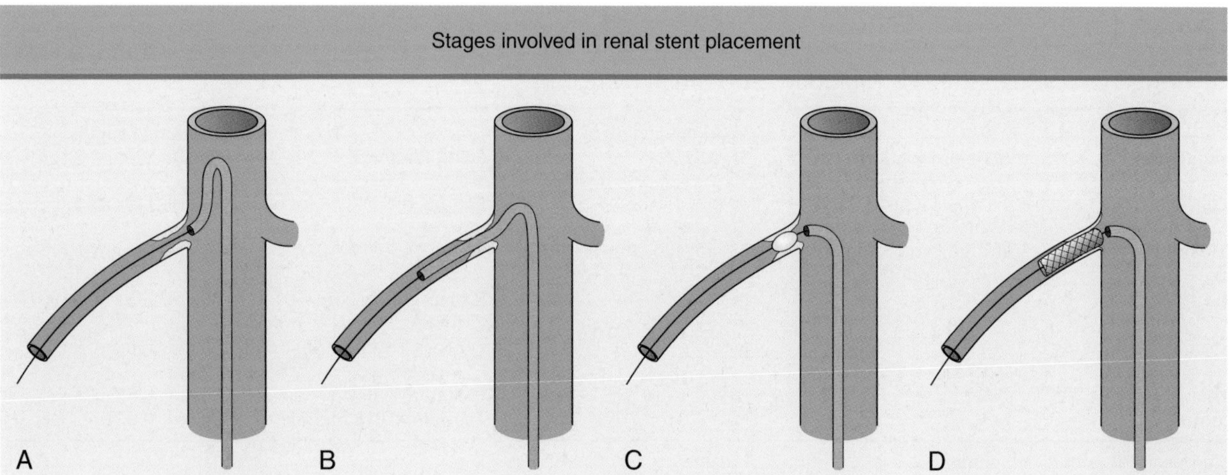

Figure 24-4. Stages involved in renal stent placement. **A,** Crossing the stenosis with a wire. **B,** Advancing the catheter across the lesion. **C,** Balloon dilatation. **D,** Stent deployment.

Table 24-1
Pros and Cons of a Femoral versus Arm Approach for Renal Angioplasty and Stenting

Route	Angulation	Distance to vessel	Diameter of access vessel	Aortic plaque	Access vessel damage
Femoral	+	++	+++	+	++
Arm	+++	+	++	++	+

Standard Platform

As with PTA, femoral access is the commonest access site. Recently, a radial artery approach has been described.[15] Each has its advocates, and the advantages and disadvantages are shown in Table 24-1. The C-arm should be rotated to profile the renal artery ostium as dictated on the noninvasive imaging.

Having crossed the lesion as described earlier, the stenosis is predilated using a 3-mm balloon. Predilatation is thought to produce less atheroembolization than full or no dilation. A renal stent (Table 24-2) is then placed using either a 7- to 8-Fr renal double curve (RDC) guiding catheter or a 45-cm-long 6-Fr sheath. Both provide support and allow small volumes (5 ml) of contrast to be injected alongside the stent to ensure accurate placement. It is not necessary—and is undesirable—to access the other groin to inject large volumes of contrast through a pigtail catheter. The clinician should ensure that the renal ostium is fully covered, which necessitates leaving approximately 1 to 3 mm of stent protruding into the aorta. Figure 24-5 shows a restenosis caused by inadequate covering of the ostium due to incorrect C-arm angulation. Stent diameter should match that of the normal vessel, and the length should be just enough to cover the stenosis (usually 15 to 18 mm). Balloon-expandable stents should always be used as they permit a more accurate placement than self-expanding stents. Recently, carbon-covered and drug-eluting stents have become available; their role in the renal artery remains unclear.

If using a brachial approach, the following equipment should be available:

- 90-cm sheath or 90-cm multipurpose shape guiding catheter
- Exchange length wires (260 cm)
- 120-cm shaft balloons

Small Platform

Like small-platform PTA, small-platform stents are gaining popularity and likely to become the norm. Potential advantages of small-platform systems include the following:

- Less traumatic 0.014- to 0.018-inch guide wires
- Less traumatic 2.5- to 4-Fr shaft balloons
- Superior trackability
- Smaller puncture site (5-Fr sheath or 7-Fr introducer catheter)
- Rapid exchange systems, avoiding need for long wires

It is assumed that these smaller systems cause less risk of atheroembolism and reduce local groin complications. They may be particularly advantageous when using a brachial or radial approach. Most evidence is anecdotal and comes from the carotid territory, where it is relatively easy to measure atheroembolic events using transcranial Doppler.

The technique is basically the same as for standard-platform stenting. The correct choice of guide wire is important with these systems, and some recommended choices are shown in Table 24-3. Available stents are shown in Table 24-2. A 7-Fr introducer guide is the preference for delivery of the stent; again, this should not cross the lesion.

Troubleshooting

Although most renal arteries are relatively straightforward to stent, some can be exceedingly difficult and, on occasion, impossible.

If the wire will not cross the stenosis, consider the following:

1. Try a curved hydrophilic wire. These should be used with great care as they can easily dissect the vessel without the operator being aware.
2. Try a different access approach (usually the left brachial).
3. Change the catheter shape.
4. Try a 0.014- to 0.018-inch guide wire.

If nothing will follow the wire, take the following steps:

1. Try a 4-Fr hydrophilic cobra catheter (Terumo, Surrey, United Kingdom).
2. Try a 4-Fr Van Andel tapered catheter (Cook, Limerick, Ireland).

Table 24-2
Renal Stents Available in the EEC (Standard and Small Platform)*

Manufacturer	Standard Platform	Working Lengths, Sheath Size	Small Platform	Working Lengths, Sheath Size
Cordis	Palmaz Genesis 0.035 inches	80 cm, 135 cm, 6-7 Fr‡	Palmaz Blue 0.014 inches†	80 cm, 142 cm, 5-6 Fr‡
Medtronic	Bridge Extra Support 0.035 inches	75 cm, 120 cm, 7 Fr	Racer RX 0.014 + 0.018 inches†	75 cm, 120 cm, 6 Fr
Abbott	NA	NA	RX Herculink Elite 0.014 inches†	80 cm, 135 cm, 5 or 6 Fr‡
Boston	NA	NA	Express Vascular SD 0.018 inches	90 cm, 150 cm, 5 Fr
Cook	NA	NA	Formula 414	80 cm, 135 cm, 5 Fr
Terumo	NA	NA	Tsunami 0.018 inches	90 cm, 150 cm, 5-6 Fr

EEC, European Economic Community.
*NA, not available.
†Cobalt chromium stents.
‡Where two sheath sizes are quoted, the largest only applies to the 6.5- to 7-mm-diameter stents.

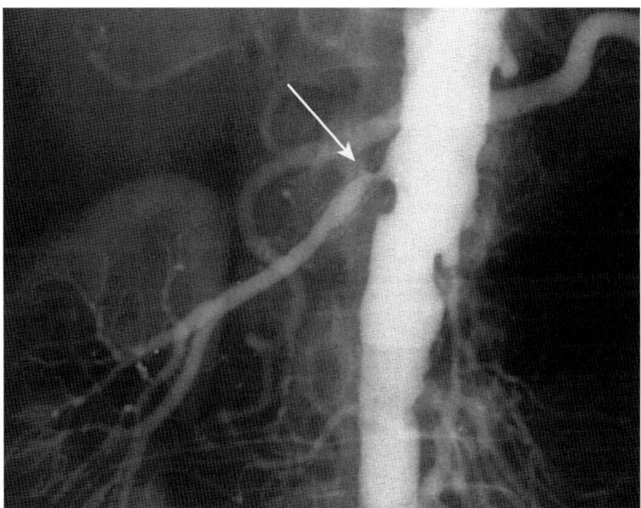

Figure 24-5. Six-month angiogram showing restenosis of the original lesion due to the stent not adequately covering the renal ostium *(arrow)*. This was treated by placing a second stent.

3. If you are not already using a guiding catheter, use one for extra support.
4. Use a small-platform system.

Postprocedure

A 6-Fr sheath and an 8-Fr guiding catheter both make the same size hole in the access vessel, i.e., 8 Fr. To prevent groin complications, a closure device should be strongly considered, particularly if the patient is hypertensive, has renal impairment (which increases the bleeding time), or both. It may not be necessary to use a closure device with the small-platform systems.

Intravenous hydration should be continued for 12 hours, and blood pressure and renal function should be carefully monitored for 24 to 48 hours. The real risk of labile blood pressure swings and temporary renal deterioration make day case renal stenting an unrealistic option in most circumstances.

Antiplatelet therapy (aspirin, 75 to 325 mg daily) should be routinely given lifelong. If the patient is intolerant to aspirin, then clopidogrel (75 mg daily) can be used.

Nonatheromatous Lesions

Nonatheromatous lesions invariably respond to simple PTA, and stenting is rarely required.

Nonbranch Lesions

Nonbranch lesions are usually relatively simple to treat, and either a standard- or a small-platform system can be used.

Table 24-3
Small-Platform Guide Wires for Renal Angioplasty and Stenting

Manufacturer	Guide Wire
Boston Scientific	Platinum Plus 0.018 inches
Cordis	SV-5 0.018 inches
Guidant	Spartacore 0.014 inches 130, 190, 300 cm

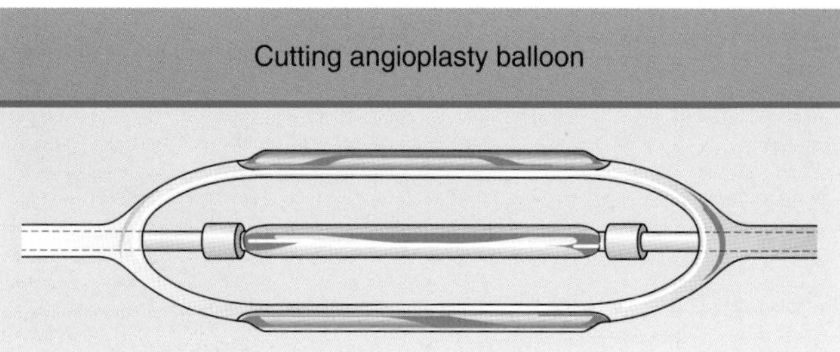

Figure 24-6. Cutting angioplasty balloon with three blades attached at 120-degree intervals.

If the lesion is difficult to cross (which can occur in the classical "string of beads" appearance), then changing to one of the hydrophilic wires is usually successful. The stenosis should be dilated with a short (2 cm) balloon, the diameter matching that of the normal renal artery. Some arteritides can be resistant to PTA, and it may be necessary to use high-pressure balloons. Another alternative is a cutting balloon, which has recently become available and licensed for renal use (Boston Scientific, St. Albans, United Kingdom). This consists of three blades attached to the balloon surface at 120-degree intervals (Figure 24-6). The blades are protected by the wrap of the balloon material, permitting atraumatic passage across the stenosis. As the balloon is inflated, the exposed blades relieve the "hoop stress" by making three small, controlled incisions into the vessel wall. The expanded balloon then flattens or dilates the cut area with the minimal amount of trauma (Figure 24-7). These cutting balloons are available in diameters up to 8 mm.

Finally, when dilating the beaded type of fibromuscular lesion, the angiographic appearance may not change much following PTA, but, usually, measurement of the pressure gradient demonstrates a marked improvement (Figure 24-8).

Branch Lesions

Branch lesions are more complex and technically demanding. The small-platform systems should be used. A twin-port Tuohy-Borst adaptor is also needed if twin balloons are to be used. If possible, the guiding catheter is placed in the proximal renal artery, then the appropriate balloon and wire are placed and the lesion is crossed. The second balloon and wire are then placed in a "kissing" manner. Before inflating the balloons, the clinician must check the measurements and ensure that the main vessel proximal to the branch is not smaller in diameter than the sum of both balloon diameters (Figure 24-9). If this is the situation, then the balloons must only be inflated individually. Contrast can be injected through the guiding catheter at any stage to check position and post-PTA appearances. Again, if required, cutting balloons can be used but should not be placed in a "kissing" fashion as they can burst the adjacent balloon.

Atheromatous Lesions

Atheromatous lesions differ from nonatherosclerotic lesions in that most are ostial, which is defined as lying within 10 mm of the opacified aortic wall on an arteriogram.[29] Even when such lesions appear to be nonostial on angiography, studies using

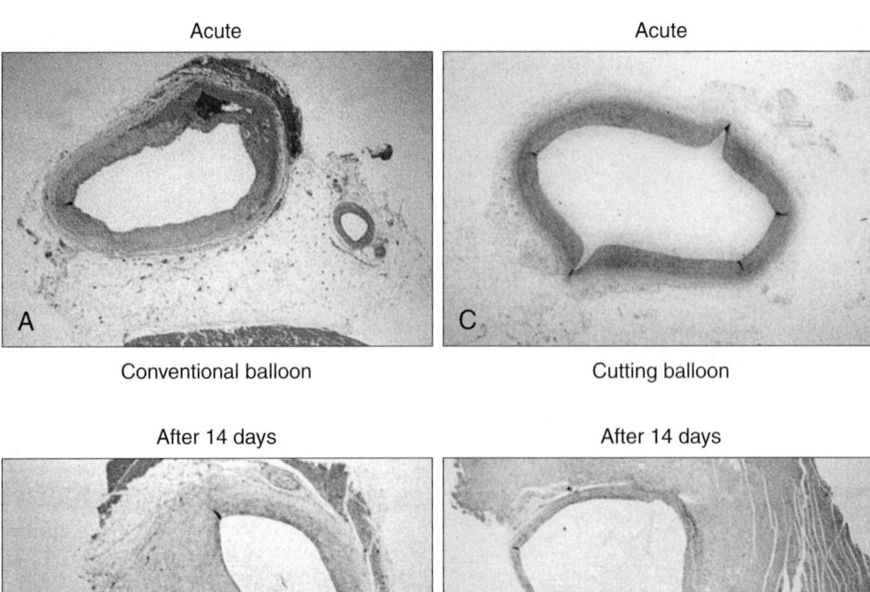

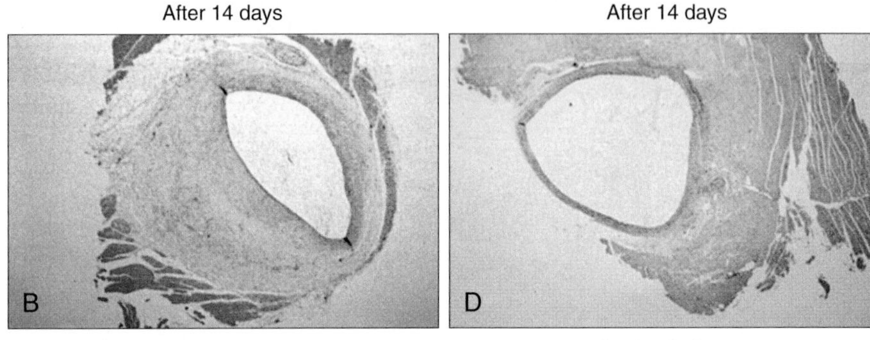

Figure 24-7. Percutaneous transluminal angioplasty (PTA). Photomicrographs of an artery having undergone PTA with a standard balloon **(A, B)** and a cutting balloon **(C, D).**

CTA have shown that they are in fact ostial.[29] A randomized trial[17] (see the next section) has demonstrated a clear technical advantage of stenting over PTA for these lesions. Few operators would now use PTA alone for atheromatous lesions.

Restenosis

Restenosis following renal stenting is less common than after PTA and occurs in 15% of stents at 6 months, as determined by angiography. Its treatment is more difficult, however, and no consensus exists regarding the optimal approach. The pathological process is due to neointimal hyperplasia. In general, simple PTA of this tissue leads to suboptimal results, due to almost immediate recoil and a later neointimal tissue response. Recently, cutting balloons have been advocated as an alternative, but data are insufficient to make any firm recommendation on their use at present.[15-18]

Much enthusiasm exists for drug-eluting stents in the coronary circulation, where dramatic reductions in binary restenosis rates have been reported. The GREAT Trial[19] compared sirolimus-eluting renal stents with bare-metal renal stents in a small ($n = 106$), nonrandomized trial. Results showed a trend favoring sirolimus-eluting renal stents, but none of the measures reached statistical significance, possibly due to underpowering.

Renal Protection Devices

There is little doubt that cholesterol embolization occurs during all stages of a renal stenting procedure[20] and indeed occurs commonly as a spontaneous event in atherosclerotic patients. These embolic particles invoke an inflammatory response and damage renal tissue, resulting in nephron loss that is usually permanent. It seems likely that cholesterol embolization at

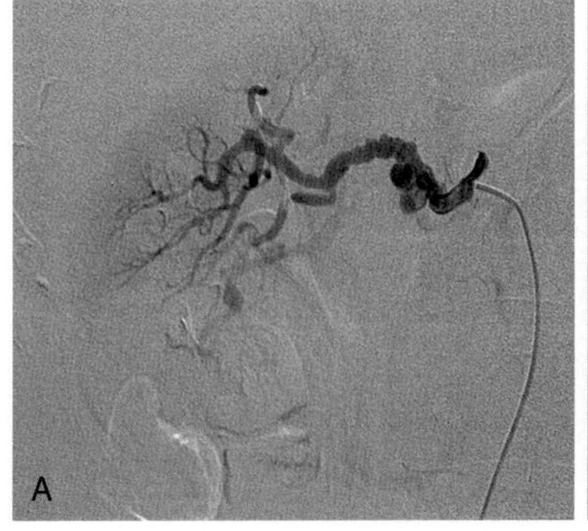

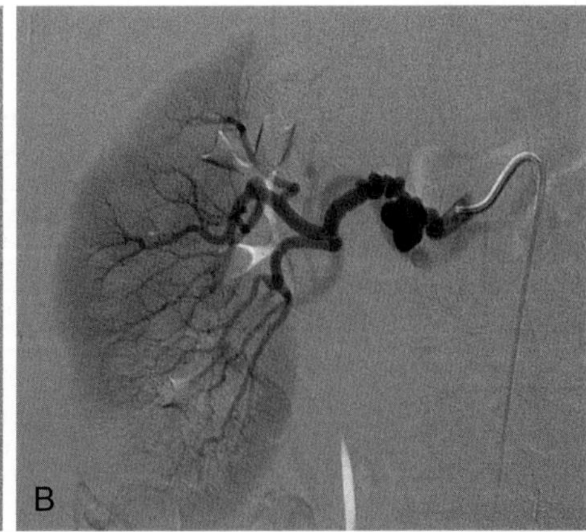

Figure 24-8. Beaded type of fibromuscular lesion. **A,** Angiogram showing a classical "string of beads" appearance. **B,** Following percutaneous transluminal angioplasty, no angiographic improvement occurred but the pressure gradient dropped from 44 mm Hg to 5 mm Hg.

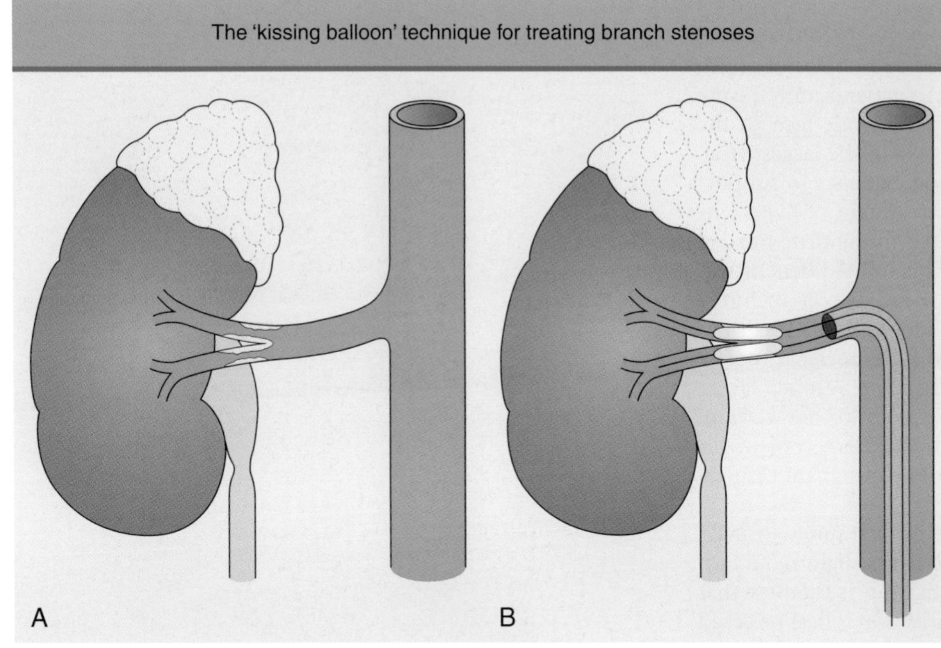

Figure 24-9. The "kissing balloon" technique for treating branch stenoses. Two small-platform balloons are simultaneously placed through a guiding catheter and inflated.

least partly explains the significant minority of patients (up to 30%) in whom the renal function deteriorates after renal stenting. It seems reasonable therefore to propose that an embolic protection device may help prevent or minimize this risk. There are no renal protection devices currently approved for renal use, and early experience reflects off-label use of the carotid devices (both filters and balloon occlusion devices). It is not possible to use these in all situations, and cases with early branching or poststenotic dilatation of more than 7 mm compromise the protection afforded. In addition, protection devices undoubtedly add significant complexity and cost to the procedure. The limited literature of 242 patients from four centers[21-27] suggests high technical success rates (60% to 100%) and rates of renal deterioration as low as zero. Further work is needed to confirm this early encouraging work. The RESIST Trial is a randomized trial comparing protection devices with glycoprotein 11a/111b inhibitors in renal arteries; it awaits publication.[28]

SELECTION OF THERAPY

Arteritides

Arteritide patients are often young females with hypertension and normal renal function. Although an abdominal bruit may be present, most renal artery lesions are detected on conventional catheter angiography. Selective views may be necessary to detect subtle branch lesions. The decision to offer the patient PTA should be a team judgment, involving the blood pressure physician, vascular radiologist, and vascular surgeon. Although the pharmacological control of hypertension has improved over the last 20 years, the potential of PTA to cure hypertension makes a strong case for intervention. However, occasionally, the distribution and number of lesions may make PTA hazardous, and the risk of causing permanent renal damage must be balanced against the potential benefits. In these circumstances, the decision should be made on an individual and depends on factors that include the center's experience and results. The results of PTA are good, with 10-year cumulative patency rates of 87%; up to 50% of patients are cured of their hypertension, with the remainder having a reduced drug burden and improved blood pressure control.[1,2] If, however, the patient is asymptomatic, a more expectant policy can be adopted. Although fibromuscular disease has been reported to progress in up to a third of patients, occlusion and loss of renal function is rare. There may be an argument for routine follow-up and possibly imaging, but prophylactic PTA is difficult to justify.

Takayasu's arteritis is a nonspecific inflammatory disease that mainly affects large arteries such as the aorta and its main branches, including the renal artery. It is the most common cause of renovascular hypertension in India and China, in contrast to Western countries. Most patients can be managed medically with corticosteroids, monitoring disease activity using the erythrocyte sedimentation rate. When in the chronic inactive stage, renovascular hypertension can be successfully managed by PTA, with good clinical results.[16]

Atheromatous Disease

The selection of patients for treatment by revascularization in the atheromatous group is difficult and still contentious. Widely differing views are held, ranging from those who rarely advocate stenting to those who treat all lesions. Several small, recent RCTs have helped the decision making a little, although many questions still remain, particularly regarding renal insufficiency.

The goals of therapy are to improve or cure hypertension, to improve or prevent deterioration in renal function, or both. It is easiest to look at these two objectives separately.

Hypertension

Three RCTs have compared revascularization (essentially PTA) with best medical treatment.[30-32] The trials were small: the largest recruited 106 patients. Many patients were excluded before randomization, and slow recruitment restricted patient numbers. Blood pressure is notoriously difficult to measure and reproduce, and the three trials used different measurement criteria. All reported only short-term results (3 to 54 months). Of the total 210 patients, only 2 were treated with stents. Patient crossover from one arm to the other was common and occurred in 44% in the largest trial. None of these trials produced any good evidence to support the routine use of angioplasty in the treatment of hypertension, although some reduction occurred in the drug burden in the PTA arm in all three studies. This limited benefit was countered by the complications of PTA, which included one nephrectomy. However, the confidence limits in all trials were wide; consequently, they had little power to detect moderate but potentially worthwhile benefits. A much larger trial would be required to answer this question for certain. These impressions have been supported by a recent meta-analysis conducted by the University of Birmingham Clinical Trials Unit.[33]

Consensus is growing that hypertension is rarely, if ever, cured by PTA or stenting in ARAS and that a slight reduction in either blood pressure or drug medication is the best that can be hoped for. Therefore, revascularization is best reserved for patients with poorly controlled hypertension despite maximum drug treatment or for those who cannot take the appropriate medications due to side effects.

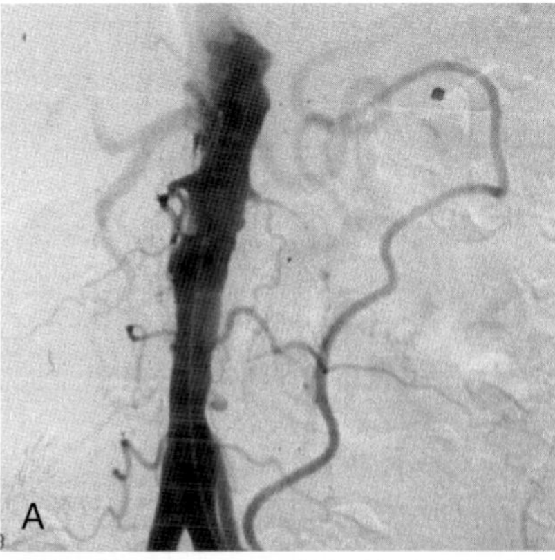

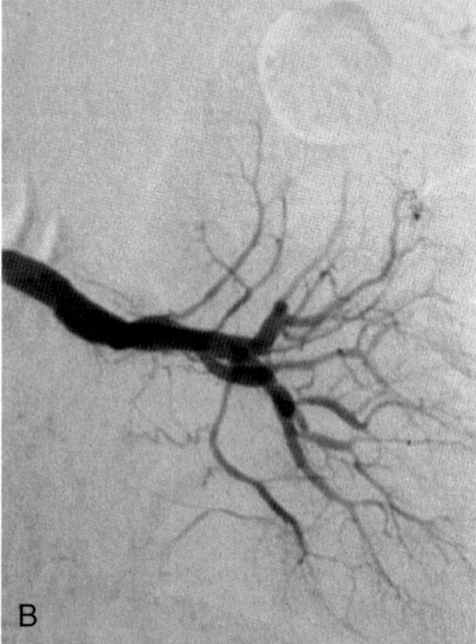

Figure 24-10. Renal insufficiency. **A,** Bilateral renal artery occlusion presenting with acute renal failure. **B,** The left renal artery was stented and renal function was recovered, allowing the patient to discontinue dialysis.

Renal Insufficiency

The aim of treatment in the renal insufficiency group is to improve or stabilize renal function. Even slowing the rate of deterioration is of benefit, as it may delay or prevent the need for renal replacement therapy.[34]

Once patients have reached ESRF, recoverable renal function following revascularization is uncommon. A rare exception to this is the patient who presents in acute renal failure with bilateral renal artery occlusions but at least one reasonable-sized kidney (Figure 24-10). Provided that the occlusion can be crossed and stented, there is at least a 50% chance of regaining sufficient function to obviate the need for dialysis. If the lesion cannot be stented, then a surgical bypass should be considered if the patient is fit.[35] Although hugely rewarding for both doctor and patient, these are rare situations. Renal arteries usually progress to occlusion in an insidious, asymptomatic way, with permanent loss of renal mass and function.[36] It is not clear at what stage in the progressive stenotic process the doctor should intervene. Two recent publications have failed to demonstrate any relationship between severity of stenosis and renal function.[24,25] Zierler et al. were the first to accurately measure this process and showed that renal arteries with 60% stenosis have a cumulative risk of occlusion of 5% per year.[4] This is much less than was originally postulated from retrospective cohort studies. It is possible that the widespread use of statins and other lipid-lowering agents in atherosclerotic disease has modulated the disease process in recent years.[39]

The strongest indications for renal stenting comprise are as follows:

- Difficult-to-control hypertension despite full medical treatment, or intolerance to the drugs
- Angiotensin-converting enzyme inhibitor–induced renal insufficiency, with a good clinical indication to remain on the inhibitors
- Rapidly deteriorating renal function
- Acute renal failure with renal artery occlusion and a good-sized kidney
- Flash pulmonary edema

Uncertain indications for renal stenting include the following:

- Stable but impaired renal function
- Moderately severe hypertension
- Stenosis in a single kidney (other kidney not functioning)
- Bilateral high-grade stenoses
- Patients with high-grade stenoses undergoing coronary surgery

The evidence for renal insufficiency is less clear-cut than for hypertension. Although all three blood pressure RCTs measured renal function in various ways, none was powered to detect an improvement in renal function.[30-32] Two of the trials excluded patients with moderate to severe renal impairment. None of the trials showed any clear benefit for PTA in terms of serum creatinine or creatinine clearance. Because of the weak power of the studies, however, a modest but important benefit from PTA may not have been detected. Stents were only used in 1% of the revascularized patients. A much larger study is needed, and the ASTRAL, STAR, and CORAL trials are

Table 24-4
Complications of Renal Arteris Angioplasty and Stenting[*]

	PTRA (n = 512 procedures)		Stents (n = 512 patients)	
Complication	***n* (%)**	**Mortality**	***n* (%)**	**Mortality**
Major				
Permanent renal insufficiency	2 (0.3)		10 (1.9)	
Renal artery occlusion	1 (0.15)		5 (1)	
Renal artery damage	10 (1.5)		4 (0.8)	2[†]
Segmental infarct embolization	2 (0.3)		7 (1.4)	
Retroperitoneal hematoma	5 (0.75)		7 (1.4)	
Groin complications	8 (1.2)		10 (2)	1[†]
MI/stroke	6 (0.8)	1[†]		
Other	3 (0.4)		2 (0.4)	
Total	47 (7)		45 (8.8)	
Minor				
Temporary renal insufficiency	25 (3.7)		16 (3.1)	
Segmental infarct	6 (0.9)			
Retroperitoneal hematoma	1 (0.15)		1 (0.2)	
Groin complications	8 (1.2)		14 (2.7)	
Other	4 (0.46)		8 (1.6)	
Total	44 (6.5)		39 (7.6)	
Radiological	1 (0.15)		33 (6.4)	

[*]PTRA, percutaneous transluminal renal angioplasty; MI, myocardial infarction.
[†]deaths.
[*]Compilation of published results from 10 percutaneous transluminal renal angioplasty (PTRA) and 14 stent series.

Table 24-5
Management and Prevention of Endovascular Complications[*]

Complication	Prevention	Treatment
Groin related	Small-platform systems Closure devices	Supportive Thrombin injection
Contrast nephropathy	Minimize contrast load Use carbon dioxide Acetylcysteine	Supportive
Cholesterol embolization	Minimize manipulations Small-platform systems Protection devices	Supportive
Renal artery perforation	Correct balloon size	Balloon tamponade Covered stent (Jomed, United Kingdom)
Retroperitoneal bleed (perirenal)	Avoid stiff-tipped guide wire Avoid distal guide wire placement	Supportive

currently under way. The ASTRAL trial randomized more than 800 patients and will report in March 2008.[5]

The decision to treat should be made by a multidisciplinary team involving the nephrologist or blood pressure physician, vascular radiologist, and surgeon. The risks of damaging the kidney should be balanced against the perceived benefits, which should be realistic. Until the trials report, patients should understand that the evidence for revascularization remains weak.

Endovascular or Surgical Revascularization?

Only one RCT (AHA: A) has compared PTA with surgical (mainly endarterectomy) revascularization.[40] This small study (n = 58) found that the technical success rate was higher in the surgical group (97% versus 83%) and that the primary 2-year patency was superior (96% versus 75%). However, the secondary patency rates were similar, and the authors suggested that PTA should be the first-choice treatment, provided adequate surveillance and reintervention was available. This trial, from 1993, predated the stent era.

Angioplasty or Stents?

A single RCT (AHA: A) compared PTA with stenting in 85 patients with ostial lesions.[17] The technical success rate of stents was superior to that of PTA (88% versus 55%) and primary 6-month patency was likewise superior (75% versus 29%). The trial was stopped following an interim analysis of the data.

The clinical outcomes in the two groups were similar, although the study was not powered to detect differences in blood pressure or renal function. The results of this trial came as no surprise to many radiologists, who recognized the poor technical results that PTA gave when dealing with ostial disease, which is due to recoil of the aortic plaque.[41]

Stents or Surgery?

No trials answer the question of stents or surgery, and it seems doubtful there ever will be such a trial, as the two treatments are so different in nature that patient recruitment would be difficult. Although it is unlikely that the patency rates of any endovascular technique will match those of surgical reconstruction, the increased morbidity and mortality of surgery will restrict its use to the young and fit with a long life expectancy. These patients are uncommon in the atherosclerotic renovascular field. A rare indication for surgery is a stent technical failure, which most commonly occurs when attempting to treat complete occlusions. Some complications such as cholesterol embolization may be less common with a surgical revascularization, as usually no instrumentation of the lesion occurs.

COMPLICATIONS

The endovascular approach offers some obvious advantages over a conventional surgical reconstruction. These include the avoidance of a general anesthetic and the morbidity associated with an abdominal incision in what is often a high-risk population with other comorbid vascular disease. However, it would be naïve to assume that that an endovascular procedure is risk free.

The literature quotes complication rates ranging from 0% to 66% for renal PTA or stenting. Most of the series are retrospective, and there are no agreed reporting standards or

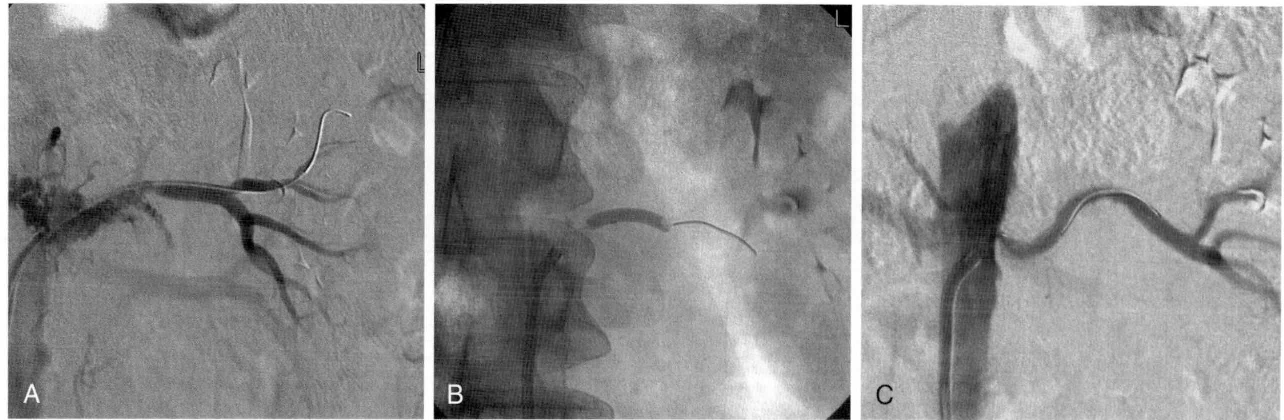

Figure 24-11. Perforation of a renal artery following percutaneous transluminal angioplasty **(A).** Balloon tamponade for 5 minutes **(B)** achieved vascular stasis **(C).**

definitions. It has been suggested to classify complications as follows:

- Major—serious complications requiring active management
- Minor—complications that usually require expectant observation only
- Radiological—technical complications occurring during the procedure that produce no adverse clinical symptoms.[42]

It is difficult to compare the complication rates with surgical series as these usually report events up to 30 days whereas radiological papers often report complications within a shorter time window. In the single RCT (AHA: A) comparing surgery with PTA,[36] the major complication rate following PTA was 17%, versus 31% after surgery, with minor complications in 48% of the PTA group versus 7% of the surgical group. These differences were not statistically significant. The Dutch RCT (AHA: A) comparing PTA with stenting reported a 39% complication rate following PTA compared with 43% following stenting.[17] Although most of these complications were minor and groin related, more serious complications such as vessel rupture and cholesterol embolization can have grave consequences for the patient.

Table 24-4 shows complications compiled from 10 published PTA and 14 published stent studies. No difference occurs between the complications rates of PTA and those of stenting. Many complications can be avoided by good technique and can be treated by endovascular methods (Table 24-5). Surgical salvage should be rarely required and often is too late to save a kidney, due to the relatively short warm ischemic time of this organ (approximately 90 minutes).

Perforation of the renal artery is a dreaded complication but can usually be treated either by simple balloon tamponade or by placing a stent graft (Figure 24-11).

Deterioration in renal function (usually temporary) is one of the commonest complications. It is usually due to the effects of iodinated contrast and appears in the first 24 to 48 hours (Figure 24-12). Efforts to minimize this have been discussed previously, but once it does occur, supportive treatment usually suffices. Only about 1% of cases require dialysis, although the outcome is poor. More worrying is cholesterol atheroembolism, which occurs due to simple catheter manipulation in the aorta, crossing the stenosis, balloon inflation, stent placement or more likely all of these. The onset is more insidious (over 1 to 3 weeks; Figure 24-13) and may be

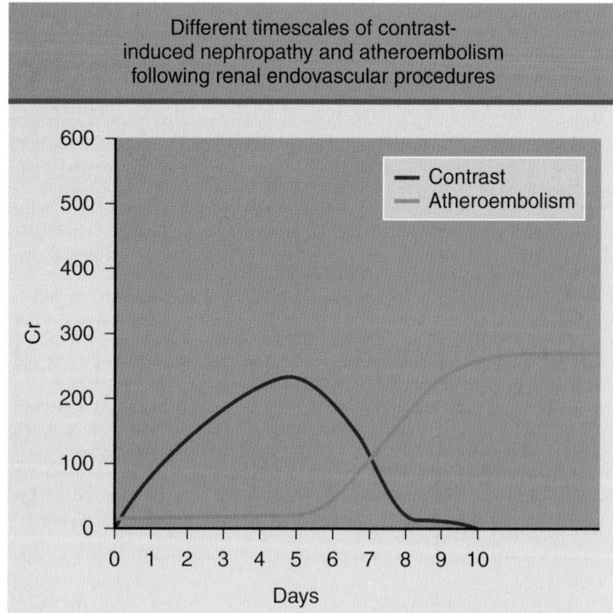

Figure 24-12. Different timescales of contrast-induced nephropathy and atheroembolism following renal endovascular procedures.

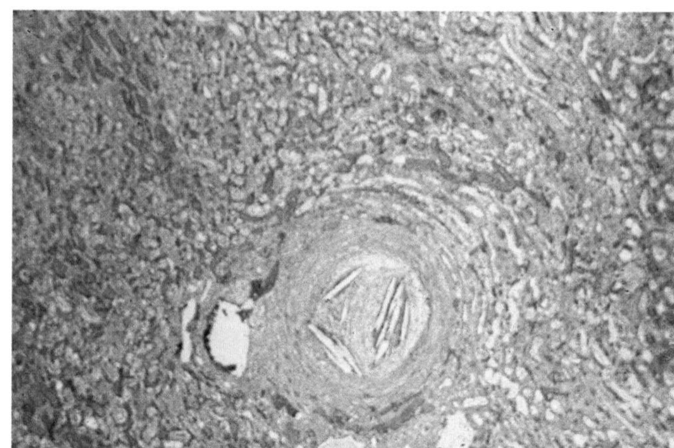

Figure 24-13. Photomicrograph of a renal biopsy, showing cholesterol crystals in a medium-sized arteriole.

associated with an elevated erythrocyte sedimentation rate, eosinophilia, and typical livedo reticularis skin rash. Atheroembolism is probably more common than previously thought and often goes undetected in patients with a normal contralateral kidney, normal renal function, or both. It should be remembered that 50% of renal functional mass has to be lost before the serum creatinine begins to rise above normal levels. However, once renal function does deteriorate following cholesterol embolization, the prognosis is guarded and little can be done beyond general supportive measures. Some patients progress to ESRF as a result. As discussed earlier, it remains to be seen whether protection devices will prevent this complication, but the early results appear promising.[21-27]

SUMMARY

Atherosclerotic renovascular disease is a complex multifactorial entity. It is naïve to think of it as being simply due to a flow-limiting stenosis, which can be treated by revascularization. Atheroembolism, small-vessel atheroma, and hypertensive nephropathy often coexist. The three randomized hypertension trials comparing PTA with medical treatment have demonstrated little useful gain from PTA other than a possible drug-sparing effect. Research has now turned toward renal function and whether revascularization can improve or stabilize renal function. It is hoped the ASTRAL, CORAL, and STAR trials will answer this question. ASTRAL reports in 2008.

The preferred method of revascularization—endovascular versus surgical—remains contentious, and enthusiasm for an RCT to answer this question seems unlikely. The perceived advantages of an endovascular approach seem obvious to many, particularly in the aging high-risk vasculopath. The Dutch RCT has demonstrated the technical superiority of stents over PTA in ostial lesions, and stenting has become the standard endovascular technique in those undergoing renal revascularization for atherosclerotic disease.

Although not evidence based, a strong intellectual basis is increasing for using a protection device during renal stenting in atheromatous patients.

References

1. Tegtmeyer CJ, Selby JB, Hartwell GD, et al. Results and complications of angioplasty in fibromuscular disease. *Circulation* 1991;83(2 Suppl): I155-I161.
2. Tegtmeyer CJ, Matsumoto AH, Angle JF. Percutaneous transluminal angioplasty in fibrous dysplasia and children. In: Novick A, Scoble J, Hamilton G, eds. *Renal vascular disease.* 1st ed. London: WB Saunders; 1996:363-383.
3. Mailloux LU, Napolitano B, Bellucci AG, et al. Renal vascular disease causing end-stage renal disease, incidence, clinical correlates and outcomes: a 20 year clinical experience. *Am J Kidney Dis* 1994;24:622-629.
4. Zierler RE, Bergelin RO, Isaacson JA, Strandness DE Jr. Natural history of atherosclerotic renal artery stenosis: a prospective study with duplex ultrasonography. *J Vasc Surg* 1994;19:250-258.
5. Mistry S, Ives N, Harding J, et al. Angioplasty and Stent for Renal Artery Lesions (ASTRAL Trial): rationale, methods and results so far. *J Hum Hypertens* 2007;21:511-515.
6. Murphy TP, Cooper CJ, Dworkin LD, et al. The Cardiovascular Outcomes with Renal Atherosclerotic Lesions (CORAL) Study: rationale and methods. *J Vasc Interv Radiol* 2005;16:1295-1300.
7. Grobner T, Prischl FC. Gadolinium and nephrogenic systemic fibrosis. *Kidney Int* 2007;72(3):260-264.
8. Verschuyl E-J, Kaatee R, Beek FJA, et al. Renal artery origins: best angiographic projection angles. *Radiology* 1997;205:115-120.
9. Weigner M, Pruessmann KP, Kassner A, et al. Contrast-enhanced 3D MRA using SENSE. *J Magn Reson Imaging* 2000;12:671-677.
10. Roditi G. Contrast-enhanced magnetic resonance angiography. *Br J Surg* 2002;89:817-820.
11. Solomon R, Werner C, Mann D, et al. Effects of saline, mannitol and furosemide on acute decreases in renal function induced by radiocontrast agents. *N Engl J Med* 1994;331:1416-1420.
12. Tepel M, van der Giet M, Schwarzfeld C, et al. Prevention of radiographic contrast agent induced reductions in renal function by acetylcysteine. *N Engl J Med* 2000;343:180-184.
13. Spinosa DJ, Matsumoto AH, Angle JF, et al. Safety of CO_2^- and gadodiamide-enhanced angiography for the evaluation and percutaneous treatment of renal artery stenosis in patients with chronic renal insufficiency. *AJR Am J Roentgenol* 2001;176:1305-1311.
14. Reyes R, Carreira JM, Pardo MD, et al. Utility of gadolinium as a contrast medium in endovascular therapeutic procedures. *Radiologia* 2001;43: 435-438.
15. Kessel DO, Robertson I, Patel JV. Transradial renal artery intervention. *Cardiovasc Intervent Radiol* 2003;26:146-149.
16. Kaatee R, Beek FJA, Verschuyl EJ, et al. Atherosclerotic renal artery stenosis: ostial or truncal? *Radiology* 1996;199:637-640.
17. Van de ven PJG, Kaatee R, Beutler JJ, et al. Arterial stenting and balloon angioplasty in ostial atherosclerotic renovascular disease: a randomised trial. *Lancet* 1999;353:282-286.
18. Munneke GJ, Engelke C, Morgan RA, Belli A-M. Cutting balloon angioplasty for resistant renal artery in-stent restenosis. *J Vasc Interv Radiol* 2002;13:327-331.
19. Zahringer M, Sapoval M, Pattynama PM, et al. Sirolimus-eluting versus bare-metal low-profile stent for renal artery treatment (GREAT Trial): angiographic follow-up after 6 months and clinical outcome up to 2 years. *J Endovasc Ther* 2007;14:460-468.
20. Hiramoto J, Hansen KJ, Pan XM, et al. Atheroemboli during renal artery angioplasty: an ex vivo study. *J Vasc Surg* 2005;41:1026-1030.
21. Henry M, Klonaris C, Henry I, et al. Protected renal stenting with the PercuSurge GuardWire device: a pilot study. *J Endovasc Ther* 2001;8: 227-237.
22. Henry M, Henry I, Klonaris C, et al. Renal angioplasty and stenting under protection: the way for the future? *Catheter Cardiovasc Interv* 2003;60:299-312.
23. Holden A, Hill A. Renal angioplasty and stenting with distal protection of the main renal artery in ischemic nephropathy: early experience. *J Vasc Surg* 2003;38:962-968.
24. Hagspiel KD, Stone JR, Leung DA. Renal angioplasty and stent placement with distal protection: preliminary experience with the FilterWire EX. *J Vasc Interv Radiol* 2005;16:125-131.
25. Edwards MS, Craven BL, Stafford J, et al. Distal embolic protection during renal artery angioplasty and stenting. *J Vasc Surg* 2006;44:128-135.
26. Holden A, Hill A, Jaff MR, Pilmore H. Renal artery stent revascularization with embolic protection in patients with ischemic nephropathy. *Kidney Int* 2006;70:948-955.
27. Edwards MS, Corriere MA, Craven TE, et al. Atheroembolism during percutaneous renal artery revascularisation. *J Vasc Surg* 2007;46:55-61.
28. Cooper CJ, Haller ST, Coyler W, et al. *RESIST:* embolic protection and platelet inhibition during renal artery stenting. Presented at the American College of Cardiology Meeting. New Orleans: Louisiana May 15, 2007.
29. Tyagi S, Singh B, Kaul UA, et al. Balloon angioplasty for renovascular hypertension in Takasayu's arteritis. *Am Heart J* 1993;125:1386-1393.
30. Plouin P-F, Chatellier G, Darne B, et al. Blood pressure outcome of angioplasty in atherosclerotic renal artery stenosis. *Hypertension* 1998;31:823-829.
31. Webster J, Marshall F, Abdalla M, et al. Randomised comparison of percutaneous angioplasty vs continued medical therapy for hypertensive patients with atheromatous renal artery stenosis. *J Hum Hypertens* 1998;12:329-335.
32. Van Jaarsveld BC, Krijnen P, Pieterman H, et al. The effects of balloon angioplasty on hypertension in atherosclerotic renal artery stenosis. *N Engl J Med* 2000;342:1007-1014.
33. Ives N, Wheatley K, Stowe RL, et al. Continuing uncertainty about the value of percutaneous revascularisation in atherosclerotic renovascular disease: a meta-analysis of randomised trials. *Nephrol Dial Transplant* 2003;18:298-304.
34. Harden PN, Macleod MJ, Rodger RSC, et al. Effect of renal artery stenting on progression of renovascular renal failure. *Lancet* 1997;349:1133.
35. Schefft P, Novick AC, Stewart BH, et al. Renal revascularisation in patients with total occlusion of the renal artery. *J Urol* 1980;124:184-186.
36. Guzman RP, Zierler RE, Isaacson JA, et al. Renal atrophy and arterial stenosis: a prospective study with duplex ultrasound. *Hypertension* 1994;23:346-350.

37. Deleted in proof.
38. Deleted in proof.
39. Bianchi S, Bigazzi R, Caiazza A, Campese VM. A controlled, prospective study of the effects of atorvaststin on proteinuria and progression of kidney disease. *Am J Kidney Dis* 2003;41:565-570.
40 Weibull H, Bergqvist D, Bergentz S-E, et al. Percutaneous transluminal renal angioplasty versus surgical reconstruction of atherosclerotic renal artery stenosis: a prospective randomised study. *J Vasc Surg* 1993;18: 841-852.
41. Cicuto KP, McLean GK, Oleaga JA, et al. Renal artery stenosis: anatomical classification for percutaneous transluminal angioplasty. *AJR Am J Roentgenol* 1981;137:599-601.
42. Beek FJA, Kaatee R, Beutler JJ, et al. Complications during renal artery stent placement for atherosclerotic ostial stenosis. *Cardiovasc Intervent Radiol* 1997;20:184-190.

chapter

25

Surgical Management of Atherosclerotic Renal Artery Disease

Matthew S. Edwards, MD • Matthew A. Corriere, MD • Kimberley J. Hansen, MD

Key Points

- Atherosclerotic renovascular disease may be clinically silent or may contribute to severe, secondary hypertension and renal insufficiency (i.e., ischemic nephropathy).
- Renovascular disease progression occurs in about one third of patients but is more accelerated when systolic blood pressure is more than 160 mm Hg and diabetes mellitus is present.
- No justification can be made for prophylactic renal artery intervention in patients with controlled hypertension and normal renal function.
- Greater than 95% of hemodynamically significant atherosclerotic renal artery lesions are ostial (i.e., aortic in origin).
- A beneficial blood pressure can be expected in approximately 85% of selected patients with surgical renal artery repair.
- With surgical revascularization, approximately 60% of patients with ischemic nephropathy stabilize or improve.
- Surgeons performing renal artery surgery should be familiar with and trained in the diverse options of open surgical revascularization.

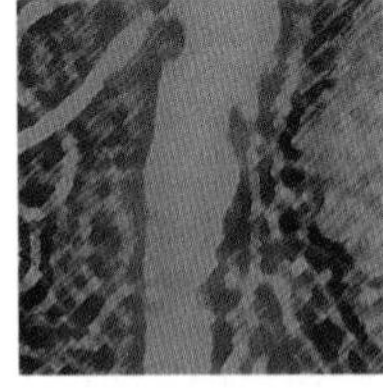

The introduction of more potent antihypertensive agents and percutaneous endovascular techniques has influenced surgical intervention for atherosclerotic renovascular disease.[1-3] Many physicians currently limit surgical intervention to the following:

- Patients with severe hypertension despite maximal medical therapy
- Failures or disease patterns not amenable to percutaneous transluminal renal angioplasty (PTRA)
- Renovascular disease associated with excretory renal insufficiency (i.e., ischemic nephropathy)

As a result, the patient population selected for operative management is characterized by ostial renal artery atherosclerosis (85%) superimposed on diffuse extrarenal atherosclerotic disease (95%) in combination with renal insufficiency.[1,4-6]

Although several operative methods can correct atherosclerotic renal artery disease, no single technique predominates. Optimal methods of renal reconstruction vary with the patient, the pattern of renal artery disease, and the clinical significance of associated aortic lesions.

PREVALENCE, EVALUATION, AND DIAGNOSIS

Prevalence and Natural History

Until recently, no prospective, population-based data have defined the prevalence and natural history of atherosclerotic renovascular disease. Past assumptions regarding atherosclerotic renal artery lesions were extrapolated from case series angiographic and ultrasound examinations, from retrospective reviews, or from prospective studies of select hypertensive patients.

Retrospective angiographic clinical studies are summarized in Table 25-1.[7-12] The early studies by Wollenweber et al.,[12] Meaney et al.,[9] and Schreiber et al.[10] demonstrated dramatic progression of renovascular disease. However, the applicability of these early observations to the population at large is

Table 25-1
Natural History of Atherosclerotic Renal Artery Stenosis: Retrospective Angiographic Studies*

	Year	Patients (*n*)	Renal Arteries (*n*)	Mean Follow-up (Months)	Anatomical Progression (% of Patients)	Progression to Occlusion (% of Arteries)	Blood Pressure Change	Decrease in Renal Length (% of Patients)	SCr Increase (% of Patients)†	GFR Decline (% of Patients)
Wollenweber et al.[12]	1968	109	252	42	59					
Meaney et al.[9]	1968	39	78	34	36	4				
Schreiber et al.[10]	1984	85	126	52	44	11	NS	46†	38	
Tollefson and Ernst[11]	1991	48		54	53‡	9‡				
Crowley et al.[8]	1998	1178		30	11	0.3			§	
Chabova et al.[7]	2000	68		39			NS		15	

*GFR, glomerular filtration rate; NS, nonsignificant; SCr, serum creatinine.
†There is a 1.5-cm discrepancy in renal length.
‡Percentage of renal arteries with baseline stenosis or stenosis in follow-up.
§SCr increased among patients with anatomical progression to more than 75% stenosis.
From Pearce JD, Craven BL, Craven TE, et al. *J Vasc Surg* 2006;44 (5):955-962.

probably flawed. These studies reported on selected groups of patients with significant clinical disease that demonstrated clinical progression prompting serial invasive imaging. Renovascular hypertension was suspected in nearly all of these subjects, and worsening hypertension was the most common indication for repeat study. It is doubtful whether the same rate of progression would apply to all individuals with renovascular disease.

Prospective angiographic clinical studies are summarized in Table 25-2, which shows results from randomized trials that have compared renal artery intervention to medical management.[13-17] These data reflect the analysis of medical treatment arms from these studies to provide an indication of disease progression. For those patients, three studies demonstrated that hypertension was stable or improved during trial participation.[15-17] One of the studies provided angiographic follow-up at 12 months. Of the 25 patients in the Dutch Renal Artery Stenosis Intervention Cooperative Trial with serial angiographic imaging, 5 had a more than 20% increase in stenosis, 16 had no change, and 4 had a 20% reduction in stenosis.[16]

Prospective duplex ultrasound studies are summarized in Table 25-3.[18-22] Renal duplex sonography (RDS) is both accurate and reproducible. Serial imaging involves minimal risk and less expense than angiography, magnetic resonance angiography, or computed tomographic angiography. Consecutive papers from investigators at the University of Washington have described a prospective investigation of progression of atherosclerotic renovascular disease in four separate reports.[18,19,21,22] Of these, a report by Caps et al. in 1998 is perhaps the most informative.[18] At 5-year follow-up on 170 patients (295 kidneys) were provided. Disease progression was defined by a increase of more than 100 cm/sec in renal artery peak systolic velocity compared with baseline values. Disease progression was detected in 91 (31%) of the renal arteries in this study. For renal arteries without ipsilateral or contralateral stenosis, in a nondiabetic patient with systolic blood pressure of less than 160 mm Hg, the calculated risk of progression was 7%. Conversely, in a diabetic patient with a systolic blood pressure of more than 160 mm Hg, the risk was estimated at 65%. In a separate report on this cohort, Caps and colleagues observed a decrease of more than 1 cm in renal length in 16% of kidneys followed over 33 months.[19]

When considered collectively, the retrospective and prospective angiographic studies and prospective duplex studies reviewed previously are commonly interpreted to support inevitable progression of an atherosclerotic renal artery lesion,

Table 25-2
Natural History of Atherosclerotic Renal Artery Stenosis: Prospective Angiographic Studies*

	Year	Patients (*n*)	Renal Arteries (*n*)	Mean Follow-up (Months)	Anatomical Progression (% of Patients)	Progression to Occlusion (% of Arteries)	Blood Pressure Change	Decrease in Renal Length (% of Patients)	SCr Increase (% of Patients)†	GFR Decline (% of Patients)‡
Dean et al.[13]	1981	41		44	17	12		37	46	3†
Plouin et al.[15]	1998	26		6			−24/+12		NS	NS
Webster et al.[17]	1998	30			13‡	0§	−28/−16†		NS	
van Jaarsveld et al.[16]	2000	50	100	12	20	5	−17/−7		NS	NS
Pillay et al.[14]	2002	85	159	30			NS	NS	¶	

*GFR, glomerular filtration rate; NS, nonsignificant; SCr, serum creatinine.
†More than 50% increase, data for 30 patients.
‡Of eight patients with serial angiography.
§From referral to last follow-up.
¶Unilateral group had significant increase; bilateral group did not.
From Pearce JD, Craven BL, Craven TE, et al. *J Vasc Surg* 2006;44(5):955-962.

Table 25-3
Natural History of Atherosclerotic Renal Artery Stenosis: Prospective Duplex Sonography Studies*

	Year	Patients *(n)*	Renal Arteries *(n)*	Mean Follow-up (Months)	Anatomical Progression (% of Patients)	Progression to Occlusion (% of Arteries)	Blood Pressure Change	Decrease in Renal Length (% of Patients)	SCr Increase (% of Patients)†	GFR Decline (% of Patients)
Zierler et al.[21]	1994	80	134	13	8	3		8		
Zierler et al.[22]	1996	76	132	32	20	7				
Caps et al.[18]	1998	170	295	33	31	3				
Caps et al.[19]	1998	122	204	33		2		16	†	
Pearce et al.[20]	2006	119	235	96	4	0	+9/−8	‡	§	

*GFR, glomerular filtration rate; SCr, serum creatinine.
†Seven subjects with bilateral atrophy increased 0.33 mg/dl the remainder were nonsignificant.
‡Mean decrease of 0.37 cm reported for entire group.
§Mean increase of 0.29 mg/dl reported for entire group.
Adapted from Pearce JD, Craven BL, Craven TE, et al. *J Vasc Surg* 2006;44(5):955-962.

with inevitable decline in kidney size and kidney function. This view is used to support intervention for atherosclerotic renovascular disease whenever it is discovered, particularly during performance of unrelated catheter-based procedures.

In contrast to this pessimistic view, recent prospective, population-based data in the elderly suggest that the rate of anatomical progression of renovascular disease in patients without renovascular hypertension is low.[20] From 1995 to 1996, 834 participants in the Cardiovascular Health Study (CHS) underwent RDS to define the presence or absence of significant renal artery disease. The CHS is a multicenter, longitudinal cohort study of cardiovascular risk factors, morbidity, and mortality among men and women older than 65 years. Between 2002 and 2005, a second RDS study was performed in 119 participants, providing 235 renal arteries for analysis. The mean interval between the first and the second duplex studies was 8.0 ± 0.8 years. Prevalent disease was defined as significant renovascular disease at the first RDS, and incident disease was defined as new, significant renovascular disease at the second RDS. Significant change in renovascular disease was defined as a change in renal artery peak systolic velocity of greater than two times the standard deviation of expected change over time (i.e., 45 cm/sec), regardless of hemodynamic significance or progression to renal artery occlusion.

By the preceding criteria, no prevalent renovascular disease progressed to occlusion after 8 years of follow-up. However, nine kidneys demonstrated incident disease (eight new stenoses; one new occlusion). Controlling for within-subject correlation, the overall estimated annual change in renovascular disease to hemodynamically significant renal artery stenosis was only 4%, providing an annualized rate of 0.5% per year. Considered in terms of a significant change in peak systolic velocity, a significant change in renovascular disease was observed in 12% of kidneys on follow-up at 8 years, for an annualized rate of 1.5% per year. These prospective data in the elderly would argue against prophylactic renal artery intervention in the absence of renovascular hypertension.

The term prophylactic repair describes renal revascularization that is performed before any pathological or clinical sequelae related to the lesion. By definition, therefore, the patient considered for prophylactic renal artery repair has neither hypertension nor reduced renal function. Correction of the renal artery lesion in this setting assumes that a significant percentage of these asymptomatic patients will survive to the point that the renal lesion will cause hypertension or renal dysfunction. Furthermore, prophylactic intervention assumes that preemptive correction is necessary to prevent a clinically adverse event either for which the patient cannot be treated or for which reoperative treatment would be unduly hazardous.

In the absence of hypertension, the clinician has to assume that a renal artery lesion must progress anatomically to become functionally significant (i.e., produce hypertension). Considering the rate of progression in patients with established or presumed renovascular hypertension,[10] progression of a renal artery lesion to produce renovascular hypertension could be expected in approximately 44% of normotensive patients. If we assume that the subsequent development of renovascular hypertension is managed medically, then the next consideration is the frequency of decline in renal function. Among 41 patients with renovascular hypertension (i.e., renal artery lesions with severe hypertension and lateralizing functional studies) randomized to medical management, significant loss of renal function, manifest by at least a 25% decrease in estimated glomerular filtration rate (EGFR) or loss of renal length, occurred in 41% of patients during a follow-up period of 15 to 24 months.[13] These patients were considered failures of medical management and submitted to operative renal artery repair. However, 13% of those patients who were subsequently submitted to operation continued to exhibit progressive deterioration in renal function. Therefore, of the patients with renovascular hypertension randomized to medical management, only 36% had potentially preventable loss of renal function by means of an earlier operation. Novick et al. have reported that, among patients who demonstrate a decline in kidney function during medical management, 67% of properly selected patients have renal function restored by renal artery repair.[23]

The relevance of these issues to prophylactic renal revascularization can be demonstrated by considering 100 hypothetical patients without hypertension who have an unsuspected renal artery lesion detected by angiography before either an open operative aortic repair or a catheter-based intervention. Table 25-4 demonstrates the unique benefits and adverse outcomes associated with prophylactic renal artery revascularization (open aortorenal reconstruction, as well as percutaneous intervention). If the renal artery lesion is not repaired prophylactically, 44 patients may eventually develop renovascular hypertension. Of these 44 patients, 16 (36%) may experience

Table 25-4
Comparison of Benefit to Risk of Renal Revascularization in 100 Hypothetical Normotensive Patients

Benefit or Risk	Patients (n)
Benefit (prior estimates)	
Progression to renovascular hypertension (44%)	44
Patients with renovascular hypertension who lose renal function (36%)	16
Renal function restored by later intervention (67%)	11
Renal function not restored by later intervention (33%)	5
Unique benefit	5
Risk (open aortorenal bypass combined with aortic reconstruction)	
Operative mortality (5.5%)	5
Early technical failure (0.5%)	1
Late failure of revascularization (4%)	4
Adverse outcome	10
Risk (percutaneous renal artery angioplasty with endoluminal stent)	
Mortality (0.3%)	0
Early technical failure (1%)	1
Late (12 month) failure (17%)	17
Adverse outcome	18

a preventable reduction in renal function during follow-up. However, delayed operation would restore function in 11 (67%) of these 16 patients. In theory, therefore, only 5 of these 100 hypothetical patients would receive unique benefit from prophylactic intervention.

This unique benefit must be considered in context of the associated morbidity and mortality associated with both open combined surgical repair and endovascular intervention. The operative mortality associated with the surgical treatment of isolated renal artery disease at our institution is 1.6%; however, combined aortorenal reconstruction is associated with a 5% to 7% perioperative mortality.[24,25] If direct aortorenal methods of reconstruction are employed, in conjunction with intraoperative completion duplex sonography, the early technical failure rate is approximately 0.8%, with 3.6% late failure on follow-up.[26] In all, early and late failures of reconstruction can be expected in 4% to 5% of renal artery repairs.[6] While percutaneous renal revascularization offers lower procedure-associated mortality, the potential value of prophylactic repair is diminished by the higher rate of late technical failure with this technique.[27] As demonstrated in Table 25-4, the risk of adverse outcome for both combined aortorenal reconstruction and combined percutaneous intervention far outpaces the unique benefit. *On the basis of available data, we can cite no justification for prophylactic renal artery intervention, either as an open operative procedure performed with aortic repair or as an independent catheter-based procedure.* These conclusions are supported by the findings of Williamson et al.[28]

In contrast to prophylactic renal revascularization, empirical renal artery repair is appropriate under select circumstances.

Evaluation and Diagnosis

Cross-sectional study of the CHS participants has demonstrated a 6.8% prevalence of hemodynamically significant renal artery stenosis or occlusion in elderly Americans.[29] If the prevalence of anatomical disease is similarly low in the population of all hypertensives, the dilemma becomes the identification of a renal lesion contributing to hypertension. In this latter regard, the key clinical characteristic defining a subpopulation with significant prevalence of important renal artery disease is defined by severe hypertension. Although its prevalence in patients with mild hypertension (diastolic blood pressure below 95 mm Hg) is low, renovascular disease is a common finding in patients with severe hypertension. Among patients older than 60 years with diastolic blood pressure greater than 110 mm Hg, approximately 50% have significant renal artery stenosis or occlusion. When associated with an elevated serum creatinine of more than 2 mg/dl, the prevalence increases to 70%, with half of these latter patients demonstrating bilateral renal artery disease.

These data suggest the probability of finding clinically significant renal artery disease correlates with the patient's age, the severity of hypertension, and the presence and severity of renal insufficiency. With this in mind, the researcher should search for renovascular disease in everyone with severe hypertension, especially when this is found in combination with excretory renal insufficiency.

A noninvasive screening test that accurately identifies renal artery disease in all individuals does not yet exist.[30] Currently available tests can be characterized broadly as functional or anatomical. With the exception of captopril renography, studies that rely on activation of the renin–angiotensin axis have been associated with an unacceptable rate of false-negative results. Current isotope renography uses various radiopharmaceuticals before and after exercise or angiotensin-converting enzyme inhibition.[31] However, the methods employed and the criteria for interpretation have been continuously modified in an effort to improve their sensitivity and specificity.[30,32-35] Consequently, direct screening methods are preferable.[36] RDS is the preliminary study of choice for both renovascular hypertension and ischemic nephropathy. Through continued improvements in software and probe design, renal duplex has proven to be an accurate method to identify hemodynamically significant renal artery occlusive disease, with a 91% sensitivity, 96% specificity, and 92% overall accuracy.[37,38] The examination poses no risk to residual excretory renal function, and overall accuracy is not affected by concomitant aortoiliac disease. In addition, preparation is minimal (an overnight fast), and antihypertensive medications do not need to be altered.

Previous results suggest that a negative renal duplex effectively excludes ischemic nephropathy since the primary consideration is global renal ischemia based on main renal artery disease to both kidneys. However, when renal duplex is used to screen for renovascular hypertension, multiple or polar renal arteries and their associated disease pose a potential limitation. Despite enhanced recognition of multiple arteries provided by Doppler color flow, only 49% of these accessory renal vessels are currently identified by renal duplex examination.[37] Consequently, our group proceeds with conventional angiography when hypertension is severe or poorly controlled, despite a negative duplex result.

When a unilateral renal artery lesion is confirmed by angiography, its functional significance should be defined. Both renal vein renin assays and split renal function studies have proven valuable in assessing the functional significance of renovascular disease. Renal vein renin assays should demonstrate a ratio of renin activity exceeding 1.5:1.0 between involved and uninvolved sides before a diagnosis of renovascular hypertension is established. Unfortunately, neither functional study has great value when severe bilateral disease or disease to a solitary kidney is present. Therefore, the decision for empirical intervention is based on the severity of the renal artery lesions, the severity of hypertension, and the degree of associated renal insufficiency. In this latter instance, issues determining recovery of excretory renal function in patients with ischemic nephropathy remain ill defined. Our center's experience with more than 210 patients who have severe hypertension and preoperative serum creatinine of 1.8 mg/dl has demonstrated a significant association between an improved renal function response after operative intervention and the site of renal artery disease, the extent of renovascular repair, and the rate of decline in preoperative renal function.[1,39-42] Global renal disease submitted to complete renal artery repair after rapid decline in excretory renal function is associated with the best opportunity for recovery of renal function.[1,39,41,42] Moreover, improved renal function after operation is the primary determinant of dialysis-free survival.[1,4,43]

Management of renal artery disease discovered incidentally during evaluation of aneurysmal or occlusive disease of the abdominal aorta is controversial.[44] In this setting, the surgeon must address the need for additional diagnostic study and decide whether to perform combined aortic and renal artery reconstruction.

In contrast to prophylactic renal revascularization, empirical renal artery repair with surgical intervention for aortic disease is appropriate under select circumstances. The term empirical repair implies that hypertension, renal dysfunction, or both are present, although a causal relationship between the renal artery lesion and these clinical sequelae has not been established by functional studies.

Repair of unilateral renal artery disease may be appropriate as a combined aortorenal procedure in the absence of functional studies (i.e., renal vein renin assays) in the following situations:

- Hypertension is severe
- The patient is without significant risk factors for operation
- The probability of technical success is greater than 95%

In these circumstances, correction of a renal artery lesion may be justified to eliminate all possible causes of hypertension and renal dysfunction. However, because the probability of blood pressure benefit is lower in such a patient, morbidity from the procedure must also be predictably low.

When a patient has bilateral renal artery stenoses and hypertension, the decision to combine renal artery repair with correction of the aortic disease is based on severity of the hypertension and the renovascular lesions. If the renal artery lesions consist of severe disease on one side and only mild or moderate disease on the contralateral side, then the patient is treated as if only a unilateral lesion exists. If both lesions are only moderately severe (65% to 80% diameter-reducing stenosis), then renal revascularization is undertaken only if the hypertension is severe. In contrast, if both renal artery lesions are severe (more than 80% stenosis) and the patient has drug-dependent hypertension, bilateral simultaneous renal revascularization is performed. Hypertension secondary to severe bilateral renal artery stenoses is often particularly severe and difficult to control. Furthermore, at least mild excretory renal insufficiency is often present. Since renal insufficiency usually parallels the severity of hypertension, a patient who presents with severe renal insufficiency but only mild hypertension usually has renal parenchymal disease. Characteristically, renovascular hypertension associated with severe renal insufficiency or dialysis dependence is also associated with severe bilateral stenoses or total renal artery occlusions. When considering combined repair of incidentally defined renal artery disease with correction of aortic disease, the clinician should evaluate the clinical status with respect to this characteristic presentation. In such situations, combined renal artery repair at the time of aortic surgery is indicated to improve excretory renal function, with beneficial blood pressure response a secondary goal. Such indications appear justified in light of the observed increase in dialysis-free survival associated with improved renal function despite the increased morbidity and mortality of a combined aortorenal procedure in this patient population.

MANAGEMENT OPTIONS

Optimal management of renal artery disease has become increasingly controversial. In the absence of prospective randomized trials, advocates of medical management, renal angioplasty and stenting, and operative management cite selective clinical data that support their views. Most of the medical community evaluates patients for renovascular disease only when medications are not tolerated or hypertension remains severe and uncontrolled. The study by Hunt and Strong[45] remains the most informative study available to assess the comparative value of medical therapy and operation. In their nonrandomized study, the results of operative treatment in 100 patients were compared with the results of drug therapy in 114 similar patients. After 7 to 14 years of follow-up, 84% of the operated group were alive, as compared with 66% in the drug therapy group. Of the 84 patients alive in the operated group, 93% were cured or significantly improved, compared with 16 (21%) of the patients alive in the drug therapy group. Death during follow-up was twice as common in the medically treated group as in the surgically managed group. Antihypertensive agents in current use provide improved blood pressure control compared with those in this earlier era. However, additional data regarding medical therapy for renovascular hypertension suggest that decreases in kidney size and renal function occur despite satisfactory blood pressure control.[13]

In patients with functionally significant renal artery lesions and severe hypertension, the detrimental changes that occur during medical therapy alone, combined with the excellent results of operative management, argue for an aggressive attitude toward renal artery intervention.[1,5,43] Our indications for operation include all patients with severe, difficult-to-control hypertension. This includes patients with complicating factors such as branch lesions and extrarenal vascular disease and patients with associated cardiovascular disease that would be improved by blood pressure reduction. Age, type of lesion, medical comorbidity, and aortic disease must be considered in selecting patients for open surgical or endovascular management. While primary angioplasty and stenting of atherosclerotic renal artery disease has been applied with increasing frequency, this management strategy is associated with greater frequency of both restenosis and periprocedural decline in renal function versus open revascularization.[27] Consequently, for most patients with ostial atherosclerosis and renal insufficiency, we believe that operative repair remains the best treatment. Nevertheless, the decision for interventional therapy for atherosclerotic renovascular disease must be individualized. In this regard, predictors of accelerated death on follow-up (e.g., clinical congestive heart failure, longstanding diabetes mellitus, and uncorrectable azotemia) are considered before any intervention is made.

Operative Management

General Issues

The presence of hypertension is considered a prerequisite for renal artery intervention. In general, functional studies are used to guide the management of unilateral lesions. Empirical renal artery repair is performed without functional studies when hypertension is severe, renal artery disease is bilateral, or the patient has ischemic nephropathy.[1,5,6] As described earlier, prophylactic renal artery repair in the absence of hypertension, whether as an isolated procedure or combined with aortic reconstruction, is not recommended. During surgical reconstruction, all hemodynamically significant renal artery disease is corrected in a single operation, with the exception of disease requiring bilateral ex vivo reconstructions, which are staged. Having observed beneficial blood pressure and renal function responses regardless of kidney size or histological pattern on renal biopsy, nephrectomy is reserved for unreconstructable renal artery disease to a nonfunctioning kidney (i.e., 10% function by renography).[6,39,41,42] Direct aortorenal reconstructions are preferred over indirect methods since concomitant disease of the celiac axis is present in 40% to 50% of patients and bilateral repair is required in half.[5,42] Failed renal artery repair is associated with a significantly increased risk of dialysis dependence.[6] To minimize these failures, intraoperative duplex is used to evaluate the technical results of surgical repair.[26]

Preoperative Preparation

Antihypertensive medications are reduced during the preoperative period to the minimum necessary for blood pressure control. Patients requiring large doses of multiple medications often have reduced requirements while hospitalized and resting in bed. If continued therapy is required, selective β-adrenergic blocking agents and vasodilators are the agents of choice. If the diastolic blood pressure exceeds 120 mm Hg, operative treatment is postponed until the pressure is brought under control. In this instance, the combination of intravenous nitroprusside and esmolol is administered in an intensive care setting.

Operative Techniques

Various operative techniques have been used to correct renal artery atherosclerosis. From a practical standpoint, three basic operations have been used most often:

- Aortorenal bypass
- Renal artery thromboendarterectomy
- Renal artery reimplantation

Although each method may have its proponents, no single approach provides optimal repair for all types of renal artery disease. Aortorenal bypass, preferably with saphenous vein, is probably the most versatile technique; however, thromboendarterectomy is especially useful for ostial atherosclerosis involving multiple renal arteries. When the artery is sufficiently redundant, reimplantation is probably the simplest technique and one particularly appropriate for combined repairs of aortic and renal pathology.

Certain measures are used in almost all renal artery operations. Mannitol is administered intravenously in 12.5-g doses early, and repeated before and after periods of renal ischemia, up to a total dose of 1 g per kilogram body weight. Just before renal artery occlusion, 100 units of heparin per kilogram body weight are given intravenously, and systemic anticoagulation is verified by activated clotting time. Unless required for hemostasis, protamine is not routinely administered for reversal of heparin at the completion of the operation.

Mobilization and Dissection

A xiphoid-to-pubis midline abdominal incision is made for operative repair of atherosclerotic renal artery disease. The last 1 to 2 cm of the proximal incision coursing to one side of the xiphoid are important in obtaining full exposure of the upper abdominal aorta and renal branches. Some form of fixed mechanical retraction is also advantageous, particularly when combined aortorenal procedures are required. Otherwise, extended flank and subcostal incisions are reserved for ex vivo reconstructions or splanchnorenal bypass.

When the supraceliac aorta is used as an inflow source for aortorenal bypass, an extended flank incision is useful. With the flank elevated, the incision extends from the semilunar line into the flank, bisecting the abdominal wall between the costal margin and the iliac crest. A visceral mobilization allows access to the renal vasculature and the aortic crus. If necessary, the crus can be divided and an extrapleural dissection of the descending thoracic aorta can provide access to the T9 to T10 thoracic aorta for proximal control and anastomosis.

When the midline xiphoid-to-pubis incision is used, the posterior peritoneum overlying the aorta is incised longitudinally and the duodenum is mobilized at the ligament of Treitz (Figure 25-1). During this maneuver, it is important to identify visceral collaterals that course at this level. Finally, the duodenum is reflected to the patient's right, to expose the left renal artery. By extending the posterior peritoneal incision to the left along the inferior border of the pancreas, an avascular plane posterior to the pancreas can be entered (Figure 25-1) to expose the entire renal hilum on the left.

This exposure is of special significance when distal renal artery lesions need to be managed (Figure 25-2A). The left renal artery lies behind the left renal vein. In some cases, the vein can be retracted cephalad to expose the artery; in other cases, caudal retraction of the vein provides better access. Usually, the gonadal and adrenal veins, which enter the left renal vein, must be ligated and divided to facilitate exposure of the distal artery. Often, a lumbar vein enters the posterior wall of the left renal vein and can be easily avulsed unless special care is taken while mobilizing the renal vein (Figure 25-2B). The proximal portion of the right renal artery can be exposed through the base of the mesentery by ligating two or more pairs of lumbar veins and retracting the left renal vein cephalad and the vena cava to the patient's right (Figure 25-2C). However, the distal portion of the right renal artery is best exposed by mobilizing the duodenum and right colon medially. Then, the right renal vein is mobilized and usually retracted cephalad to expose the artery (Figure 25-3).

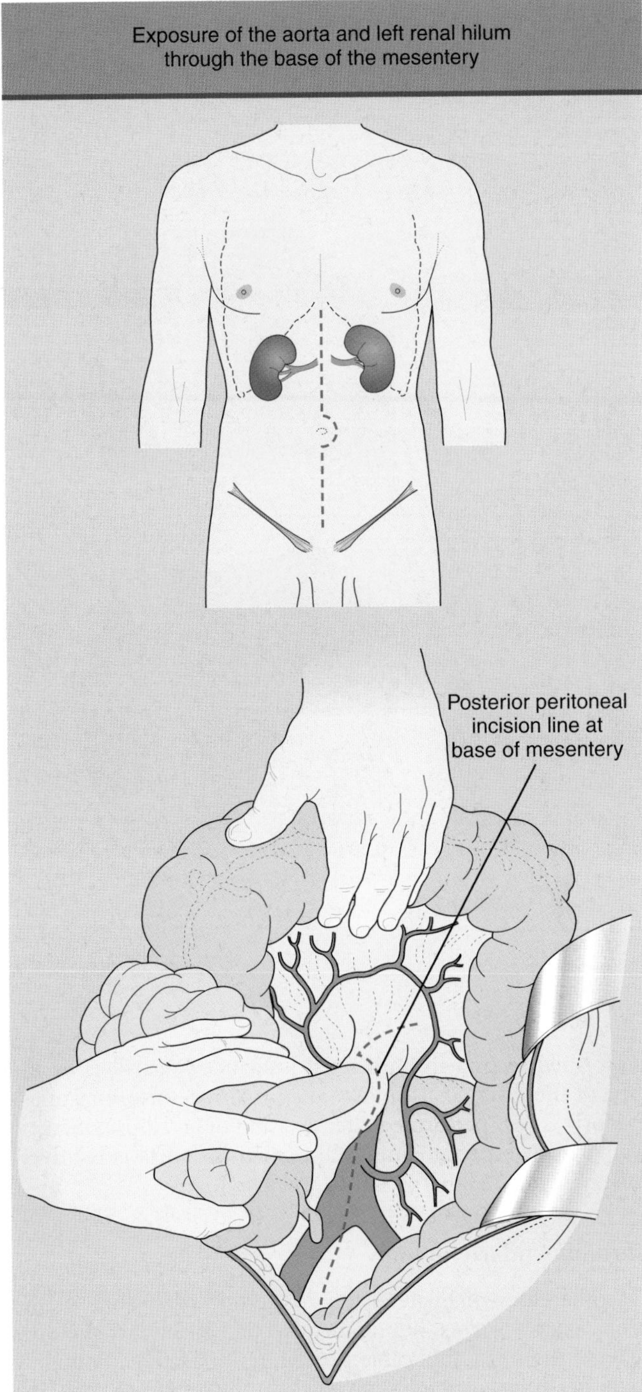

Figure 25-1. Exposure of the aorta and left renal hilum through the base of the mesentery. Extension of the posterior peritoneal incision to the left, along the inferior border of the pancreas, provides entry to an avascular plane behind the pancreas. This allows excellent exposure of the entire left renal hilum, as well as the proximal right renal artery.

Exposure of the distal right renal artery is achieved by hepatic and duodenal mobilization. First, the hepatic flexure is mobilized at the peritoneal reflection. With the right colon retracted medially and inferiorly, a Kocher maneuver mobilizes the duodenum and pancreatic head to expose the inferior vena cava and right renal vein. Typically, the right renal artery is located just inferior to the accompanying vein, which can be retracted superiorly to provide the best exposure. Although accessory vessels may arise from the aorta or iliac vessels at any level, all arterial branches coursing anterior to the vena cava should be considered accessory renal branches and carefully preserved (Figure 25-3).

When bilateral renal artery lesions are to be corrected in combination with aortic reconstruction, these exposure techniques can be modified. Extended exposure may be provided by mobilizing the base of the small bowel mesentery to allow complete evisceration of the entire small bowel and ascending and transverse colon. For this extended exposure, the posterior peritoneal incision begins with division of the ligament of Treitz, proceeds along the base of the mesentery to the cecum, and then moves up the lateral gutter to the foramen of Winslow (Figure 25-4). The inferior border of the pancreas is fully mobilized to enter a retropancreatic plane, thereby exposing the aorta to a point above the superior mesenteric artery. Through this modified exposure, simultaneous bilateral renal endarterectomize, aortorenal grafting, or renal artery attachment to the aortic graft can be performed with wide visualization of the entire area.

Aortorenal Bypass

Three types of materials are available for aortorenal bypass:

- Autologous saphenous vein
- Autologous hypogastric artery
- Synthetic prosthetic

The decision as to which graft should be used depends on several factors. We use the saphenous vein preferentially. However, if the vein is small (less than 4 mm in diameter) or sclerotic, the hypogastric artery or a synthetic prosthesis may be preferable. A 6-mm, thin-walled polytetrafluoroethylene or Dacron polyester graft is satisfactory when the distal renal artery is of large caliber (4 mm).

When an end-to-side renal artery bypass is used, the anastomosis between the renal artery and the graft is performed first (Figure 25-5A). Silastic slings can be used to occlude the renal artery distally. This method of vessel occlusion is especially applicable to this procedure. In contrast to vascular clamps, these slings are essentially atraumatic to the delicate renal artery and avoid the presence of clamps in the operative field. Furthermore, when tension is applied to the slings, they lift the vessel out of the retroperitoneal soft tissue for better visualization. The length of the arteriotomy should be at least three times the diameter of the smaller conduit to guard against late suture line stenosis (Figure 25-5B). A 6-0 or 7-0 polypropylene suture is employed with loupe magnification. After the renal artery anastomosis is completed, the occluding clamps and slings are removed from the artery and a small bulldog clamp is placed across the vein graft adjacent to the anastomosis. The aortic anastomosis is then performed (Figure 25-5C) after removing an ellipse of the anterolateral aortic wall. If the graft is too long, kinking of the vein and subsequent thrombosis may result. In this instance, the aortic anastomosis should be taken down and revised after appropriate orientation of the graft. In most instances, and end-to-end anastomosis between the graft and the renal artery provides a better reconstruction (Figure 25-5D). We routinely employ end-to-end renal artery anastomosis when combining aortic replacement with renal revascularization. In this circumstance, the proximal anastomosis is performed first and the distal renal anastomosis is

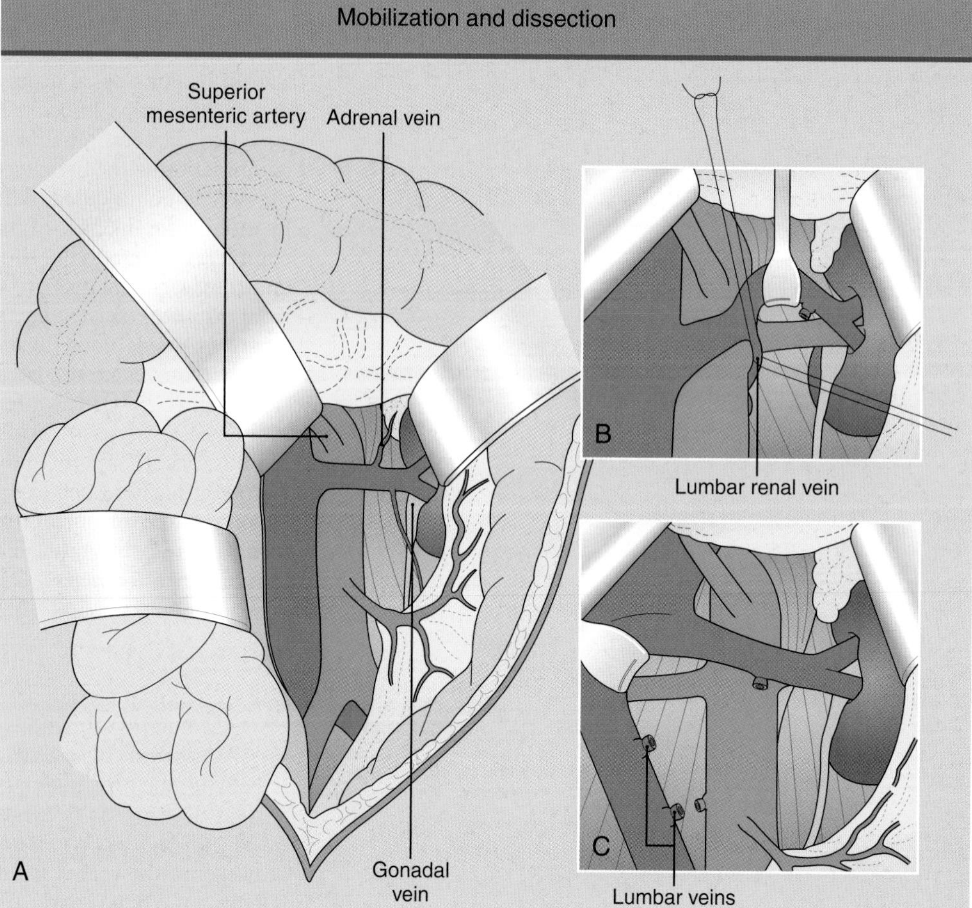

Figure 25-2. Mobilization and dissection. **A,** Exposure of the proximal right renal artery through the base of the mesentery. **B,** Mobilization of the left renal vein by ligation and division of the adrenal, gonadal, and lumbar–renal veins allows exposure of the entire left renal artery to the hilum. **C,** Two pairs of lumbar vessels have been ligated and divided to allow retraction of the vena cava to the right, revealing adequate exposure of the proximal renal artery.

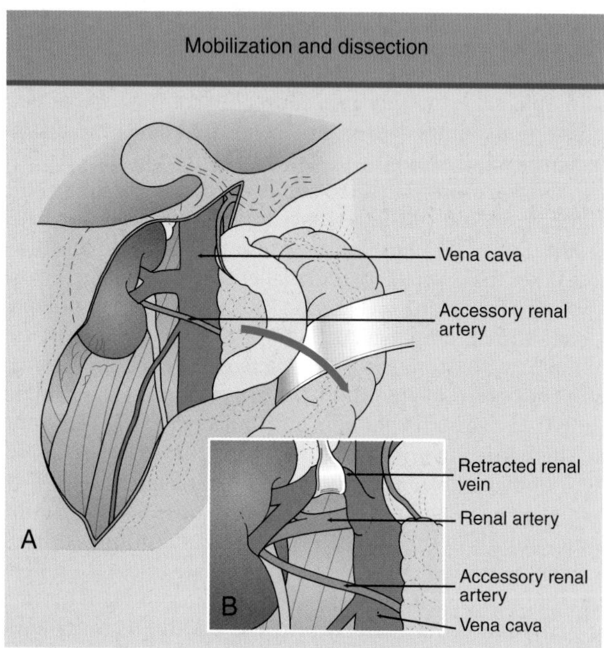

Figure 25-3. Mobilization and dissection. **A,** Not uncommonly, an accessory right renal artery arises from the anterior aorta and crosses anterior to the vena cava. **B,** The right renal vein is typically mobilized superiorly for exposure of the distal renal artery.

performed second to limit renal ischemia. Regardless of the type of the distal anastomosis, the proximal aortorenal anastomosis is best performed after excision of an ellipse of aortic wall. This is especially important when the aorta is relatively inflexible due to atherosclerotic involvement.

Thromboendarterectomy

In some cases of bilateral atherosclerotic occlusions of the renal artery origins, simultaneous bilateral endarterectomy may be the most applicable procedure. Endarterectomy may be either transaortic or transrenal. In the latter instance, the aortotomy is made transversely and is carried across the aorta and into the renal artery to a point beyond the visible disease (Figure 25-6A). With this method, the distal endarterectomy can be assessed and tacked down with mattress sutures under direct vision if necessary. Following completion of the endarterectomy, the arteriotomy is closed. In most patients, this closure is performed with a Dacron patch to ensure the proximal renal artery is widely patent (Figure 25-6B and 25-6C). In most instances, the transaortic endarterectomy technique is used. The transaortic method is particularly applicable in patients with multiple renal arteries that demonstrate orificial disease. Transaortic endarterectomy is performed through a longitudinal aortotomy with sleeve endarterectomy of the aorta and renal arteries (Figure 25-7). When combined aortic

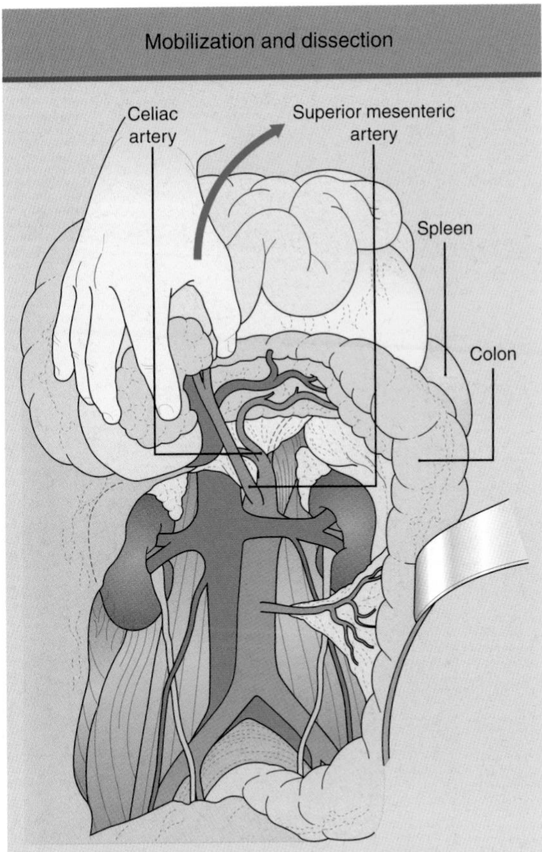

Figure 25-4. Mobilization and dissection. For complex bilateral renal artery reconstruction, wide exposure can be obtained with mobilization of the cecum and ascending colon. The entire small bowel and right colon are then mobilized to the right upper quadrant and placed onto the chest wall. Division of the diaphragmatic crura exposes the origin of the mesenteric vessels.

replacement is planned, the transaortic endarterectomy is performed through the transacted aorta (Figure 25-8). When using the transaortic technique, it is important to mobilize the renal arteries extensively to allow eversion of the vessel into the aorta. This allows the distal endpoint to be completed under direct vision.

Renal Artery Reimplantation

After the renal artery has been dissected from the surrounding retroperitoneal tissue, the vessel may be somewhat redundant. When the renal artery stenosis is orificial and vessel length is sufficient, the renal artery can be transected and reimplanted into the aorta at a slightly lower level. The renal artery must be spatulated and a portion of the aortic wall removed as in renal artery bypass.

Splanchnorenal Bypasses

Splanchnorenal bypass and other indirect procedures have been used as alternative methods for renal revascularization.[46,47] In general, we do not believe that these procedures are comparable with direct reconstructions, but they are useful in a selected subgroup of high-risk patients.

Hepatorenal Bypass

A right subcostal incision is used to perform the hepatorenal bypass.[46] The lesser omentum is incised to expose the hepatic artery both proximal and distal to the gastroduodenal artery (Figure 25-9). Next, the descending duodenum is mobilized by Kocher's maneuver, the inferior vena cava and right renal vein are identified, and the right renal artery is encircled where it is found, either immediately cephalad or caudad to the renal vein.

A greater saphenous vein graft is used to construct the bypass. The hepatic artery anastomosis of the vein graft can be placed at the site of the amputated stump of the gastroduodenal artery; however, this vessel may serve as important collateral for intestinal perfusion. Therefore, the proximal anastomosis is usually made from the common hepatic artery. After completion of the anastomosis, the renal artery is transacted and brought anterior to the inferior vena cava for end-to-end anastomosis to the graft (Figure 25-10).

Splenorenal Bypass

Splenorenal bypass can be performed through a midline or a left subcostal incision. The posterior pancreas is mobilized by reflecting the inferior border cephalad. A retropancreatic plane is developed, and the splenic artery is mobilized from the left gastroepiploic artery to the level of its branches. The left renal artery is exposed cephalad to the left renal vein after division of the adrenal vein. After the splenic artery has been mobilized, it is divided distally, spatulated, and anastomosed end to end to the transected renal artery (Figure 25-11).

Ex Vivo Reconstruction

Operative strategy for renal artery branch vessel repair is partly determined by the required exposure and anticipated period of renal ischemia. When reconstruction can be accomplished with less than 30 minutes of ischemia, an in situ repair is undertaken without special measures for renal preservation. When longer periods of ischemia are anticipated, one of two techniques for hypothermic preservation of the kidney is considered:

- Renal mobilization without renal vein transaction
- Ex vivo repair and anatomical replacement in the renal fossa

For atherosclerotic renovascular disease, these techniques are most commonly required after failure or complications of PTRA.

Ex vivo management is necessary when extensive exposure is required for extensive periods. This includes the following cases:

- Patients with fibromuscular dysplasia and aneurysms or stenosis involving the renal artery branches
- Patients with fibromuscular dysplasia and renal artery dissection and branch occlusion
- Patients with congenital arteriovenous fistulae of renal artery branches requiring partial dissection
- Patients with degeneration of previously placed grafts to the distal renal artery

Several methods of ex vivo hypothermic perfusion and reconstruction are also available.[48] A midline xiphoid-to-pubis incision is used for most renovascular procedures and is

Technique for end-to-side and end-to-end aortorenal bypass grafting

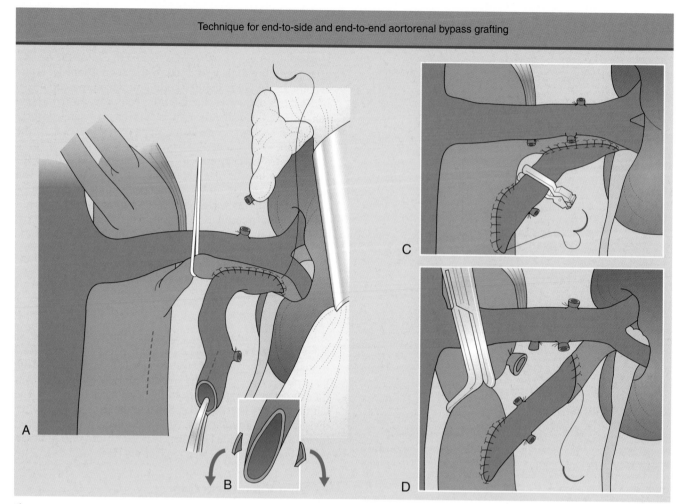

Figure 25-5. Technique for end-to-side **(A-C)** and end-to-end **(D)** aortorenal bypass grafting. The length of the arteriotomy is at least three times the diameter of the artery to prevent recurrent anastomotic stenosis. For the anastomosis, 6-0 or 7-0 monofilament polypropylene sutures are used continuously under loupe magnification. If the apex sutures are placed too deeply or with excess advancement, stenosis can be created, posing a risk of late graft thrombosis.

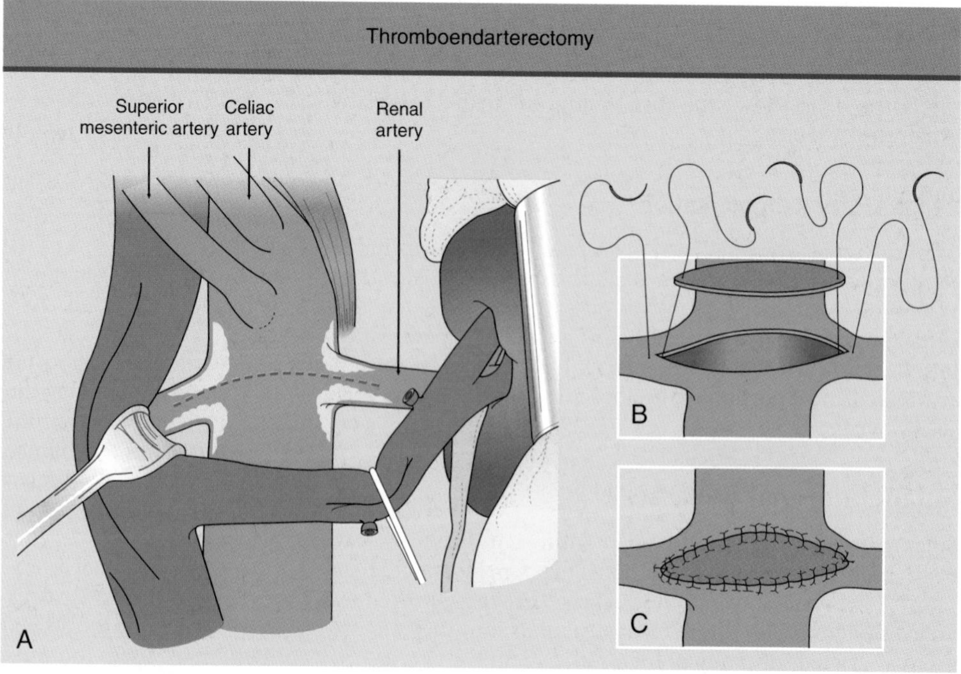

Figure 25-6. Thromboendarterectomy. **A,** Exposure of the juxtarenal aorta and renal arteries in preparation for transrenal endarterectomy. **B,** Transverse aortotomy is used in some instances, being certain to carry the incision out onto the renal artery to a point beyond the stenosis. **C,** Following completion of the endarterectomy, the arteriotomy is usually closed with a Dacron patch angioplasty to ensure that the newly repaired renal artery is left widely patent.

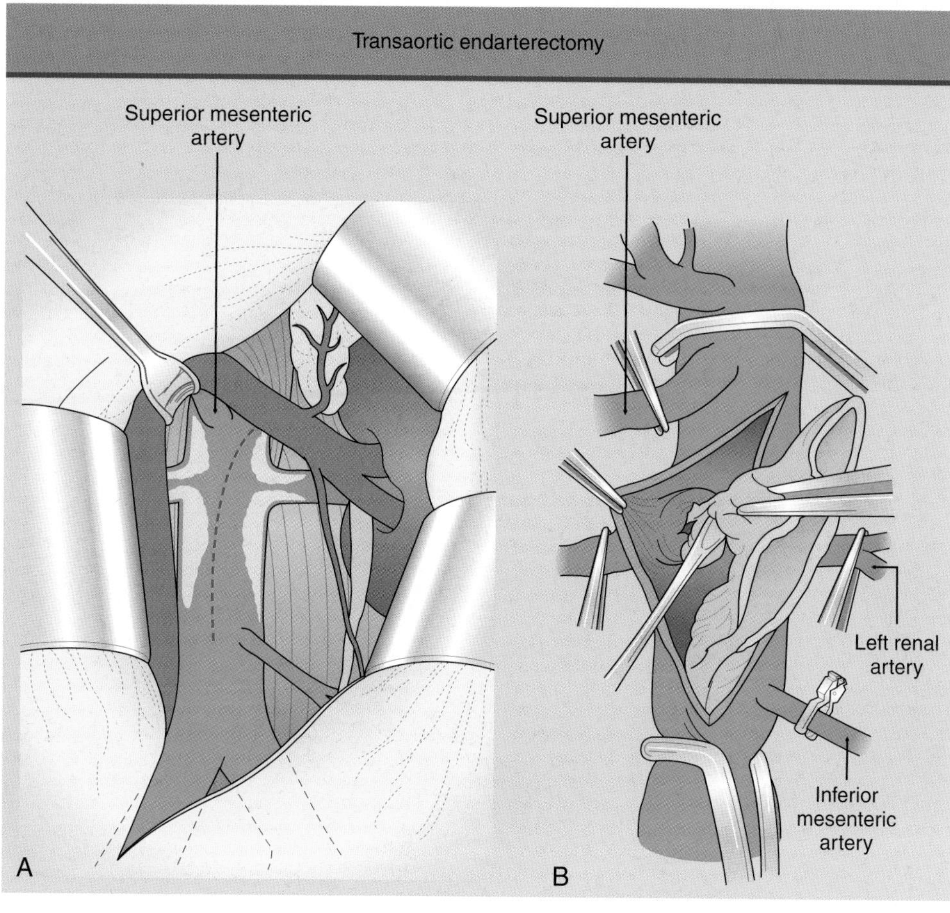

Figure 25-7. Transaortic endarterectomy. Exposure for a longitudinal transaortic endarterectomy is through the standard transperitoneal approach. The duodenum is mobilized from the aorta laterally in standard fashion, or for more complete exposure, the ascending colon and small bowel are mobilized. **A,** The dotted line shows the location of the aortotomy. **B,** The plaque is transected proximally and distally, and with eversion of the renal arteries, the atherosclerotic plaque is removed from each renal ostium. The aortotomy is typically closed with a running 4-0 or 5-0 polypropylene suture.

preferred when autotransplantation of the reconstructed kidney or combined aortic reconstructions are to be performed. For isolated branch renal artery repairs, an extended flank incision is made parallel to the lower rib margin and carried to the posterior axillary line. This is our preferred approach for ex vivo reconstructions. The ureter is mobilized to the pelvic brim but left intact, and an elastic sling or noncrushing clamp is placed around the ureter to prevent collateral perfusion and subsequent renal rewarming.

Gerota's fascia is opened with a cruciate incision, the kidney is mobilized, and the renal vessels are divided (Figure 25-12A). The kidney is placed on the abdominal wall and perfused with a chilled renal preservation solution. Continuous perfusion during the period of total renal ischemia is possible with perfusion pump systems and may be superior for prolonged renal preservation. However, simple intermittent flushing with a chilled preservation solution provides equal protection during the shorter periods (2 to 3 hours) required for ex vivo dissection and branch renal artery reconstructions. For this technique, we refrigerate the preservative overnight, add the additional components immediately before use to make up a liter of solution, and hang the chilled (5° C to 10° C) solution at a height of at least 2 m. Immediately after its removal from the renal fossa, 300 to 500 ml of solution are flushed through the kidney until the venous effluent is clear. As each anastomosis is completed, the kidney is perfused with an additional 150 to 200 ml of solution. Besides maintaining satisfactory hypothermia, periodic perfusion demonstrates suture-line leaks, which are repaired before reimplantation.

In addition to perfusion, surface hypothermia is used during ex vivo renal artery reconstruction. Our method of surface hypothermia consists of the following steps. We place liter bottles of normal saline solution in ice slush overnight. When we elevate the kidney, we place it in a watertight plastic sheet, which serves as a barrier from which excess saline solution can be suctioned. Laparotomy pads are placed over the kidney, keeping it cool and moist by a constant drip of chilled saline solution. With this technique, we can maintain renal core temperatures of 10° C to 15° C throughout the period of reconstruction.

Autotransplantation to the iliac fossa is unnecessary for most ex vivo reconstructions. Reduction in the magnitude of operative exposure, manual palpation of the transplanted kidney, and ease of removal when treatment of rejection fails are all practical reasons for placing the transplanted kidney into the recipient's iliac fossa, but none of these advantages apply to the patient requiring ex vivo reconstruction. In this latter patient group, the most important factors relate to those favoring the long-term patency after renal artery repair. Because many ex vivo procedures are performed in relatively young patients, the durability of operation must be measured in terms of decades. For this reason, attachment of the kidney to the iliac arterial system within or below sites that are susceptible to atherosclerotic occlusive disease subjects the repaired vessels to atherosclerotic disease that may threaten their long-term patency. Moreover, subsequent management of peripheral vascular disease may be complicated by the presence of the autotransplanted kidney. Finally, if the kidney is replaced in

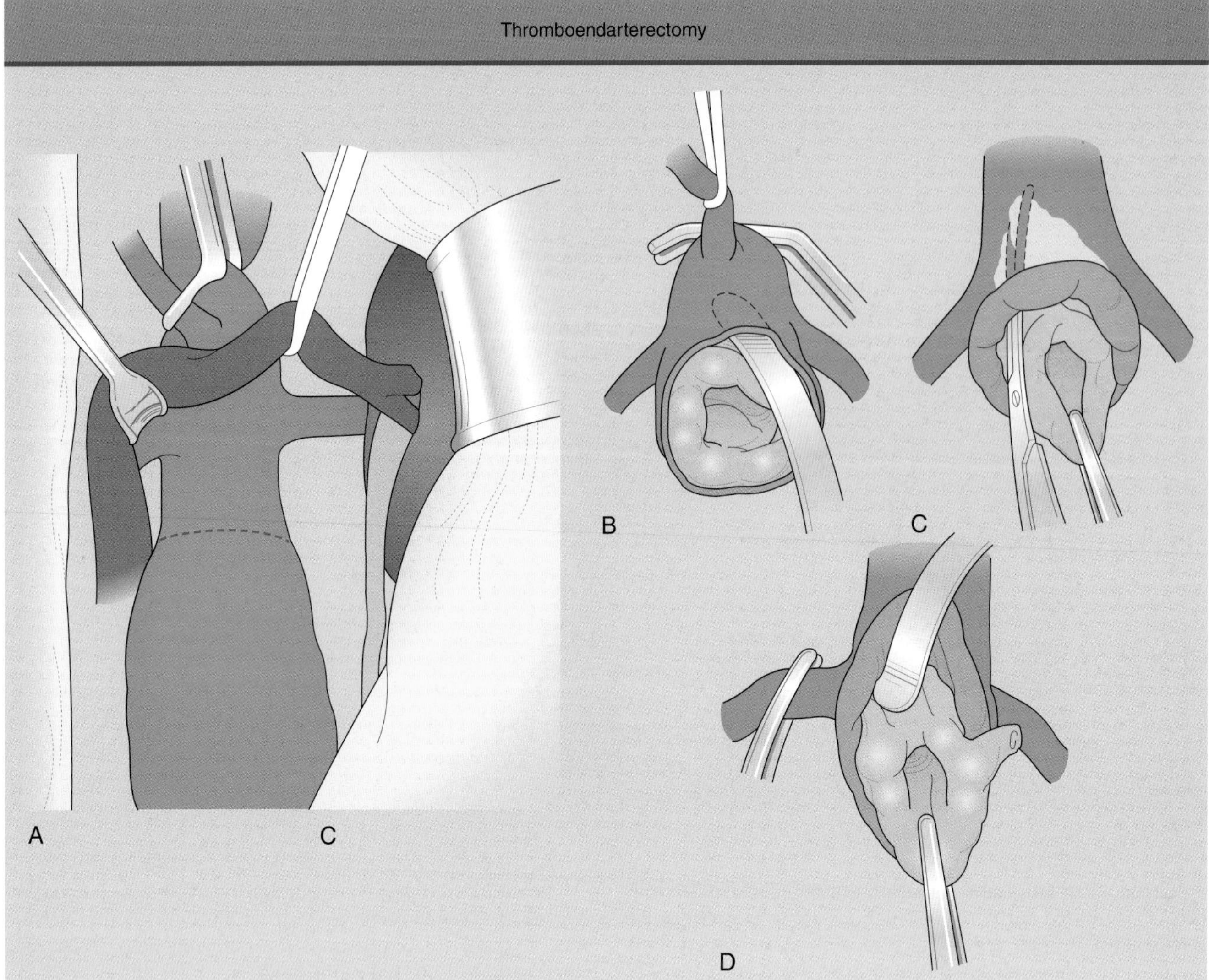

Figure 25-8. Thromboendarterectomy. For aortic repair and bilateral ostial stenosis of the renal arteries, thromboendarterectomy is most commonly performed through the divided aorta.

the renal fossa and the renal artery graft is properly attached to the aorta at a proximal infrarenal site, the result should mimic that of the standard aortorenal bypass and thus carry a high probability of technical success and long-term durability.

For replacement of the kidney in its original site, a large vascular clamp is placed to partially occlude the vena cava, where it is entered by the renal vein. An ellipse of vena cava containing the entrance site of the renal vein is then excised, and the kidney is removed for ex vivo perfusion and reconstruction (Figure 25-12A). When the renal artery–graft anastomoses are completed and the kidney is replaced in its bed, the ellipse of vena cava is reattached (Figure 25-12B). This technique protects against stenosis of the renal vein anastomosis. The renal artery-to-aorta anastomosis is made in the standard manner (Figure 25-12C).

Intraoperative Duplex Sonography

Provided that the best method of reconstruction is chosen for renal artery repair, the short course and high blood flow rates characteristic of renal reconstructions favor their patency. Consequently, flawless technical repair plays a dominant role in determining postoperative success. The negative impact of technical errors unrecognized and uncorrected at operation is implied because we have observed no late thromboses of renovascular reconstruction free of disease after 1 year.

Intraoperative assessment of most arterial reconstructions has been made by intraoperative angiography. This method has serious limitations, however, when applied to upper aortic and branch aortic reconstruction. At these locations, intraoperative angiography requires additional suprarenal or supraceliac aortic occlusion. The study obtained provides static images in the absence of pulsatile blood flow and provides anatomical evaluation in only one projection.[49] In addition, arteriolar vasospasm in response to cross-clamp ischemia and contrast injection may falsely suggest distal vascular occlusion. Finally, coexisting renal insufficiency is often present, increasing the risk of postoperative contrast nephropathy.

These risks and the inherent limitations of completion angiography are not demonstrated by intraoperative duplex sonography. Because the ultrasound probe can be placed immediately adjacent to the vascular repair, high carrying

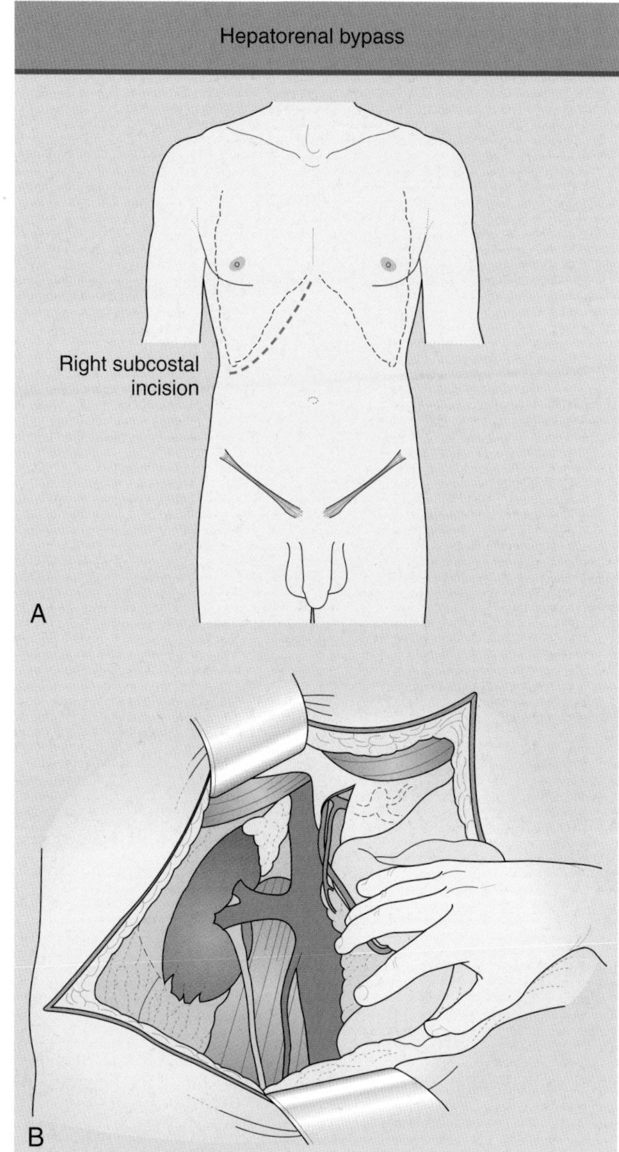

Figure 25-9. Hepatorenal bypass. In preparation for extraanatomical reconstruction of the right renal artery, the common hepatic artery and proximal gastroduodenal artery are exposed within the hepatoduodenal ligament. Exposure would typically be through a right subcostal skin incision.

frequencies may be used that provide excellent B-scan detail sensitive to anatomical defects of less than 1 mm. Once imaged, defects can be viewed in a multitude of projections during conditions of uninterrupted, pulsatile blood flow. Intimal flaps not apparent during static conditions are easily imaged while avoiding the adverse effects of additional renal ischemia. In addition to excellent anatomical detail, important hemodynamic information is obtained from the spectral analysis of the Doppler-shifted signal proximal and distal to the imaged defect.[26] The freedom from static projections, the absence of potentially nephrotoxic contrast material or additional ischemia, and the hemodynamic data provided by Doppler spectral analysis make duplex sonography a useful intraoperative method to assess renovascular repairs.

To realize the advantages of intraoperative duplex, close cooperation between the vascular surgeon and the vascular technologist is required for accurate intraoperative assessment. Although the surgeon is responsible for manipulating the probe head to acquire optimal B-scan images of the vascular repair at likely sites of technical error, proper power and time gain adjustments are best made by an experienced technologist. Close cooperation is likewise required to obtain complete pulse-Doppler and color flow sampling associated with abnormalities on the B-scan. While the surgeon images the area of interest at an optimal insonation angle, the technologist sets the Doppler sample depth and volume and estimates the blood flow velocities from the Doppler spectrum analysis. Finally, the participation of the vascular technologist during the intraoperative assessment enhances the technologist's ability to obtain satisfactory surveillance duplex studies during follow-up. Our technique of intraoperative assessment with the routine participation of a vascular technologist has yielded a scan time of 7 to 10 minutes and a 98% study completion rate.[26]

Currently, we use a 15.0/7.0-MHz compact linear array probe with Doppler color flow designed specifically for intraoperative assessment. The probe is placed within a sterile sheath with a latex tip containing sterile gel. After the operative field is flooded with warm saline, B-scan images are first obtained in longitudinal projection. Care is taken to image the entire upper abdominal aorta and renal artery origins along the length of the repair. All defects seen in longitudinal projection are imaged in transverse projection to confirm their anatomical presence and to estimate the associated luminal narrowing. Doppler samples are then obtained just proximal and distal to imaged lesions in longitudinal projection, determining their potential contribution to flow disturbance. Our criteria for major B-scan defects associated with 60% diameter-reducing stenosis have been validated in a canine model of graded renal artery stenosis (Table 25-5).

We studied 249 renal artery repairs with anatomical follow-up evaluation.[40] Intraoperative assessment was normal in 157, while 84 (35%) repairs demonstrated one or more B-scan defects. Of these defects, 25 (10%) had focal increases in estimated peak systolic velocity of 2.0 m/sec with turbulent distal waveform and were defined as major. Each major B-scan defect prompted immediate operative revision, and in each case a significant defect was discovered. B-scan defects defined as minor were not repaired. At 12-month follow-up, renal artery patency free from critical stenosis was demonstrated in 97% of normal studies, 100% of minor B-scan defects, and 88% of revised major B-scan defects, providing an overall patency of 97%. Among the five failures with normal B-scan studies, three occurred after ex vivo branch renal artery repair.

RESULTS OF OPERATIVE REPAIR

Demographics and Perioperative Management

From January 1987 through December 1999, 626 patients had operative renal artery repair at our center.[1] Of these, 500 patients underwent repair for atherosclerotic renovascular disease, while 126 patients were treated for nonatherosclerotic renovascular disease, including congenital lesions, renal artery aneurysms, and fibromuscular dysplasia.

The atherosclerotic patients consisted of 254 women and 246 men, with a mean age of 65 ± 9 years. Their mean blood pressure was 200 ± 35/104 ± 21 mm Hg, with a mean duration of hypertension of 10 years. Preoperative mean and

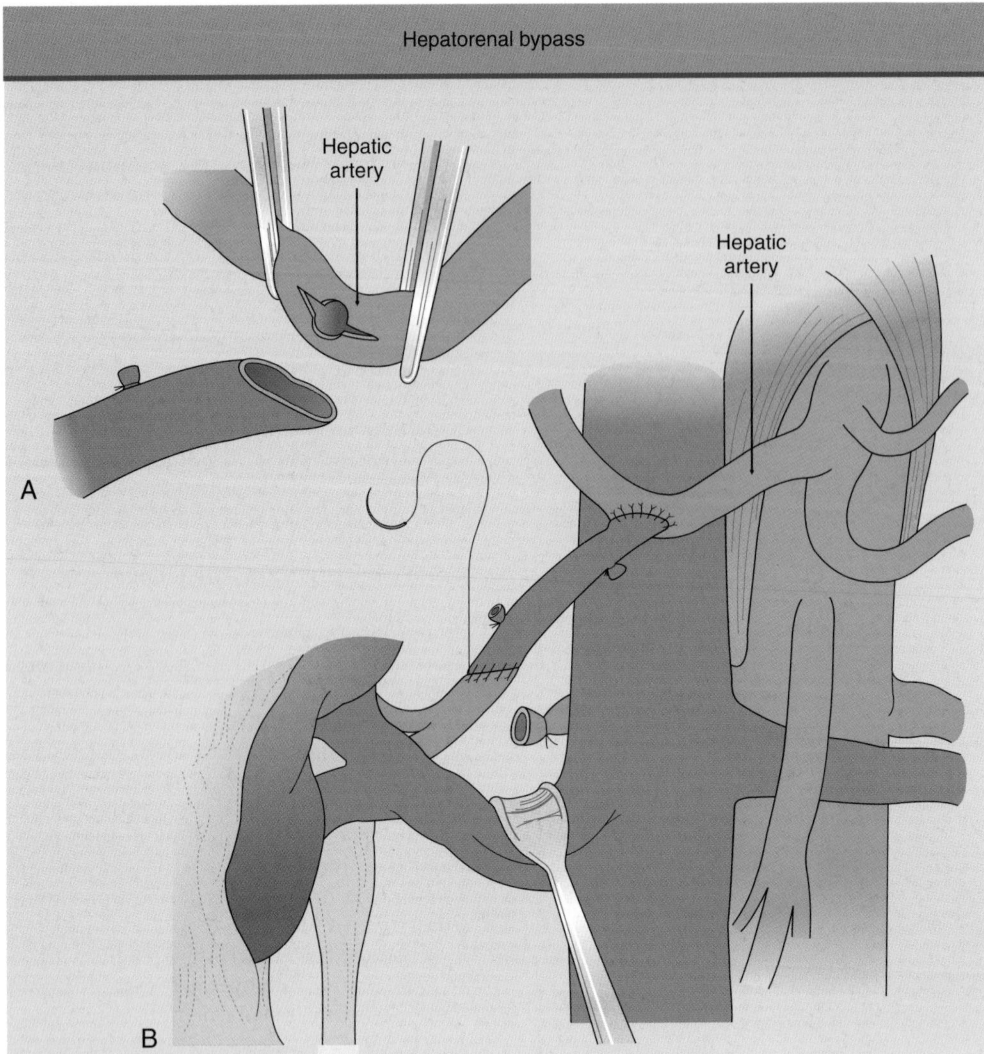

Figure 25-10. Hepatorenal bypass. The reconstruction is completed using a saphenous vein interposition graft between the side of the hepatic artery **(A)** and the distal end of the transected right renal artery **(B).**

median serum creatinine were 2.6 mg/dl and 1.7 mg/dl, respectively, with a mean EGFR of 40.5 ± 23.2 ml/min/m^2. As a group, patients with atherosclerosis had widespread disease, with 70% demonstrating at least one manifestation of cardiac disease, including angina, prior myocardial infarction, left ventricular hypertrophy, or a prior coronary intervention. In addition, 32% demonstrated prior history significant for transient ischemic attack, cerebrovascular infarct, or carotid endarterectomy. Overall, 90% of patients exhibited some clinical manifestation of extrarenal atherosclerosis. Finally, as evidenced by a serum creatinine of 1.8 mg/dl or greater, 49% were considered to have ischemic nephropathy, including 40 patients who were dialysis dependent.

Angiography demonstrated significant (80% ostial stenosis or occlusion) unilateral renal artery disease in 41% of patients and bilateral disease in 59% of patients with atherosclerotic renovascular disease. Most stenotic lesions (more than 95%) were ostial, and renal artery occlusions were noted in 31% of patients. Of the patients, 26% had abdominal aortic aneurysms and 51% demonstrated severe aortoiliac occlusive disease.

Among 720 renal artery reconstructions, aortorenal bypass was performed in 384 instances, with 204 vein grafts, 159 polytetrafluoroethylene, and 21 Dacron prosthetic grafts (Table 25-6). Splanchnorenal bypass was performed in 13 instances. Renal artery reimplantation was performed in 56 instances, while renal artery thromboendarterectomy was performed in 267 instances. Revascularization was combined with aortic or mesenteric reconstruction in 41% of patients. A total of 56 nephrectomies were performed for a total of 776 kidneys that underwent operation.

Operative Morbidity and Mortality

Perioperative morbidity occurred in 81 patients (16%). These morbid events included myocardial infarction (15 patients), stroke (5 patients), significant arrhythmia (22 patients), and pneumonia (36 patients). In addition, 5 patients had worsening renal function after operation that resulted in permanent hemodialysis dependence within 1 month of surgery. The mean preoperative serum creatinine and EGFR for these 5 patients were 3.4 mg/dl and 20.2 ml/min/m^2, respectively. Finally, 9 patients on dialysis before renal revascularization continued to require renal replacement therapy after operation.

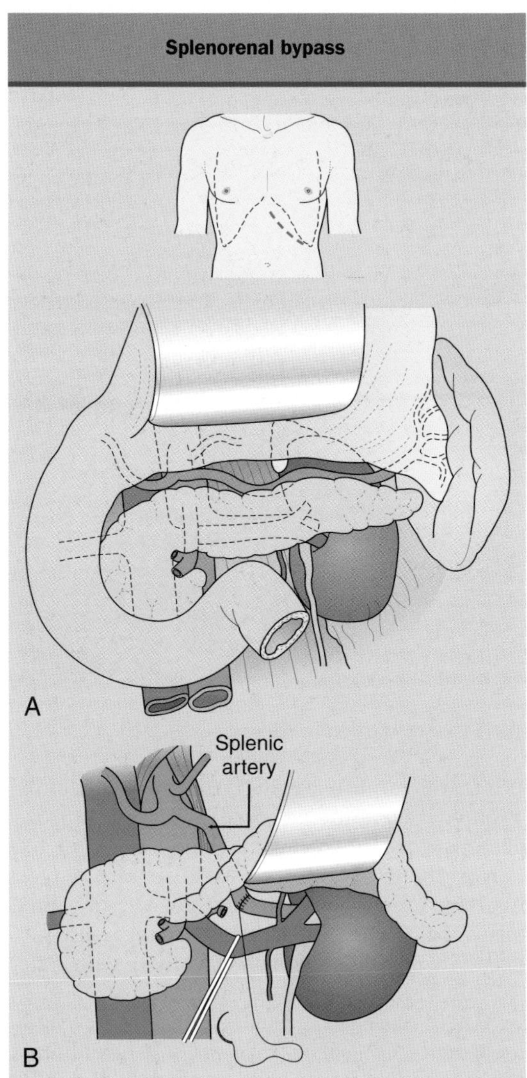

Figure 25-11. Splenorenal bypass. **A,** Exposure of the left renal hilum in preparation for splenorenal bypass. **B,** The pancreas has been mobilized along its inferior margin and retracted superiorly to reveal the posterior surface. The transected splenic artery is tunneled behind the pancreas and anastomosed end to end to the transected left renal artery. A splenectomy is not routinely performed.

Perioperative mortality, defined as in-hospital death or death within 30 days of surgery, occurred in 23 patients (4.6%). All but one death occurred following bilateral renal artery reconstruction or renal reconstruction and simultaneous aortic or mesenteric artery repair. Mortality following isolated renal artery repair (0.8%) differed significantly from mortality following combined or bilateral repair (6.9%). Perioperative mortality demonstrated significant associations with advanced age and clinical congestive heart failure.

Blood Pressure Response

Using previously published criteria,[39] blood pressure measurements and medication requirements at least 1 month after operative intervention were used to define blood pressure response. Among all surgical survivors, 85% were cured or improved, while 15% were considered failed (Table 25-7). When compared with blood pressure improved or failed, blood pressure cured was significantly associated with an improved dialysis-free survival. Although improved blood pressure was associated with significant postoperative decreases in blood pressure and medication requirements (205/107 versus 147/81 mm Hg and 2.8 versus 1.7 medications respectively), these differences were not associated with increased dialysis-free survival. Product limit estimates of dialysis-free survival according to postoperative blood pressure response are depicted in Figure 25-13.

Renal Function Response

Considering all surgical survivors, renal function improved significantly after operation (preoperative versus postoperative mean EGFR, 41.1 ± 23.9 versus 48.2 ± 25.5 ml/min/m^2, $p < 0.0001$). For individual patients, a significant change in excretory renal function was defined as a change in EGFR of 20% obtained at least 3 weeks after repair. Patients were classified as improved if they were removed from dialysis or if their EGFR increased by 20%. Patients were considered worsened if their EGFR decreased by 20%. All others were considered unchanged. Of patients with ischemic nephropathy (preoperative serum creatinine of 1.8 mg/dl), 58% were improved, including 28 patients who were removed from dialysis. Another 35% remained unchanged, while 7% had worsened renal function.[1,42] The proportion of patients improved increased with increasing severity of preoperative renal dysfunction, with 70% of dialysis-dependent patients removed from dialysis (Table 25-8). This association between increased preoperative serum creatinine and improved postoperative renal function was significant ($p < 0.0001$).

Significance of Blood Pressure and Renal Function Benefit

Progression to death or dialysis demonstrated significant associations with both preoperative parameters and postoperative blood pressure and renal function response. Preoperative factors significantly associated with death or dialysis included diabetes mellitus, severe aortic occlusive disease, poor renal function, and high systolic blood pressure. Significant associations were noted for blood pressure cured compared with blood pressure improved or worsened. Moreover, improved postoperative renal function demonstrated significant associations with increased dialysis-free survival compared with renal function unchanged. The relationship between each category of renal function response and dialysis-free survival demonstrated significant interactions with preoperative renal function. For patients with renal function unchanged, an increased risk for death or dialysis was observed for patients with poor preoperative renal function. For patients worsened, an increased risk of death or dialysis was significant for those with preoperative renal function at median values of EGFR or greater. These significant interactions are shown for predicted dialysis-free survival according to postoperative renal function response in Figure 25-14.

COMBINED AORTIC AND RENAL RECONSTRUCTION

To assess the management philosophy of combined repair described earlier, we reviewed the subset of 133 patients who had combined aortic and renovascular procedures at

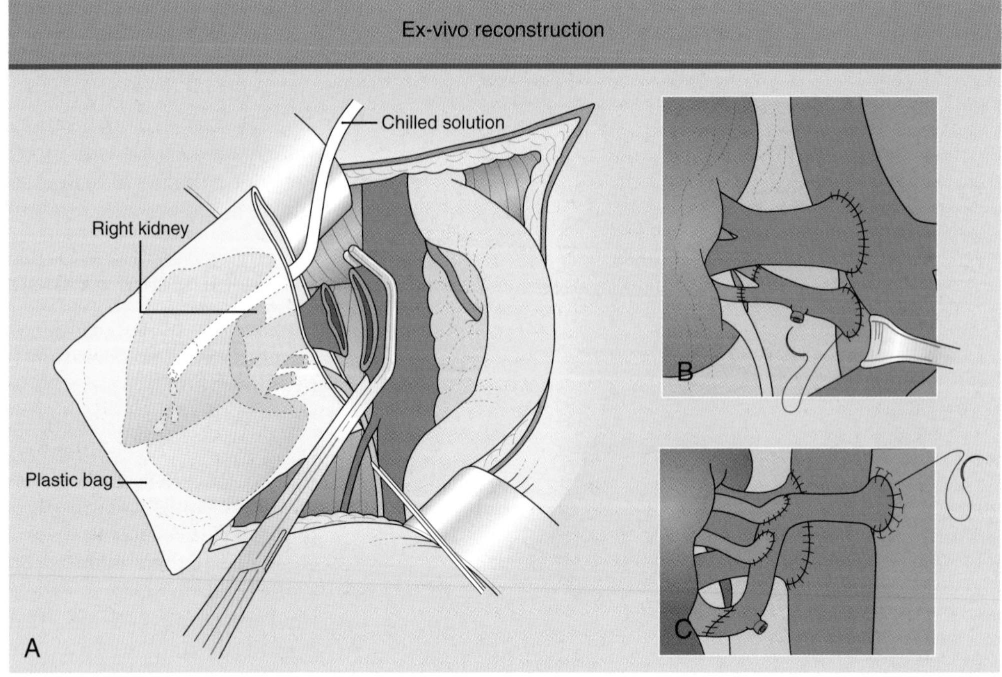

Figure 25-12. Ex vivo reconstruction. **A,** An ellipse of the vena cava containing the renal vein origin is excised by placement of a large partially occluding clamp. After ex vivo branch repair, the renal vein can be reattached without risk of anastomotic stricture. **B,** The kidney is repositioned in its native bed after ex vivo repair. Gerota's fascia is reattached to provide stability to the replaced kidney. Arterial reconstruction can be accomplished via end-to-end anastomosis—as in panel B—or with a combination of end-to-end and end-to-side anastomoses **(C).**

our center.[24] Patients requiring extraanatomical or ex vivo renal artery reconstruction or repair combined with supraceliac, thoracic, thoracoabdominal, or extraanatomical aortic repair were excluded, as were patients with ruptured aneurysms. Aortic replacements (29% tube grafts, 71% bifurcated grafts) were combined with unilateral renal artery repair in 63 patients (47%); 70 (53%) had bilateral repair. These combined aortorenal procedures were compared with results from 182 consecutive patients who had isolated in situ repair for atherosclerotic renovascular disease and 562 patients who underwent isolated elective aortic reconstruction during the same period.

Perioperative mortality after combined repair was 5.3%, which differed significantly from that observed for the "renal surgery alone" group (1.6%) and the "aortic surgery alone" group (0.7%).

Regarding blood pressure response (defined using blood pressure measurements and medication requirements at least 8 weeks after operation), 2% of surgical survivors in the combined group were considered cured, 63% were improved, and 35% demonstrated no beneficial blood pressure response. Based on a change of at least 20% in serum creatinine, excretory renal function was improved in 33% of patients with combined repair, while 53% had no change and 14% were worsened. These results compare favorably with other large series of combined aortorenal repair (Table 25-9).[24,25,50-61] Compared with renal artery repair alone, however, both blood pressure benefit (63% versus 95%, $p < 0.001$) and renal function response (33% versus 58% improved, $p = 0.01$) were significantly decreased. These differences suggest that simultaneous aortic and renal artery repair should only be performed empirically for strong clinical indications. As stated previously, prophylactic repair of clinically silent disease is not supported by these results or available natural history data.[44]

Table 25-5
Intraoperative Doppler Velocity Criteria for Renal Artery Repair*

B-Scan Defect	Doppler Criteria
Minor (<60% diameter-reducing stenosis)	PSV from entire artery <2.0 m/sec
Major (≥60% diameter-reducing stenosis)	Focal PSV ≥2.0 m/sec and distal turbulent waveform
Occlusion	No Doppler-shifted signal from renal artery B-scan image
Inadequate study	Failure to obtain Doppler samples from entire arterial repair

*PSV, peak systolic velocity.
From Hansen KJ, O'Neil EA, Reavis SW, et al. *J Vasc Surg* 1991;14(3):364-374.

Table 25-6
Summary of Operative Management for Atherosclerotic Renovascular Disease*†

Procedure	Number of Kidneys
Aortorenal bypass	384
Vein	204
PTFE	159
Dacron	21
Splanchnorenal bypass	13
Reimplantation	56
Endarterectomy	267
Nephrectomy	56
Primary	13
Contralateral	43
Total kidneys operated	776

*PTFE, polytetrafluoroethylene.
†$N = 500$ patients.
From Cherr GS, Hansen KJ, Craven TE, et al. *J Vasc Surg* 2002;35(2):236-245.

Table 25-7
Blood Pressure Response to Operation*

Response	Number of Patients (%)	Preoperative Blood Pressure (mm Hg)	Postoperative Blood Pressure (mm Hg)	Preoperative Number of Medications	Postoperative Number of Medications
Cured	57 (12)	195 ± 35/103 ± 22	137 ± 16/78 ± 9†	2.0 ± 1.1	0 ± 0†
Improved	345 (73)	205 ± 35/107 ± 21	147 ± 21/81 ± 11†	2.8 ± 1.1	1.7 ± 0.8†
Failed	70 (15)	182 ± 30/87 ± 13	158 ± 28/82 ± 12‡	2.0 ± 0.9	2.0 ± 0.9
All	472 (100)	201 ± 35/104 ± 22	148 ± 22/81 ± 11†	2.6 ± 1.1	1.6 ± 0.9†

*$N = 472$ patients. Blood pressure and medication data displayed represent mean ± standard deviation.
†$p < 0.0001$ compared with preoperative value.
‡$p = 0.001$ compared with preoperative value.
From Cherr GS, Hansen KJ, Craven TE, et al. *J Vasc Surg* 2002;35(2):236-245.

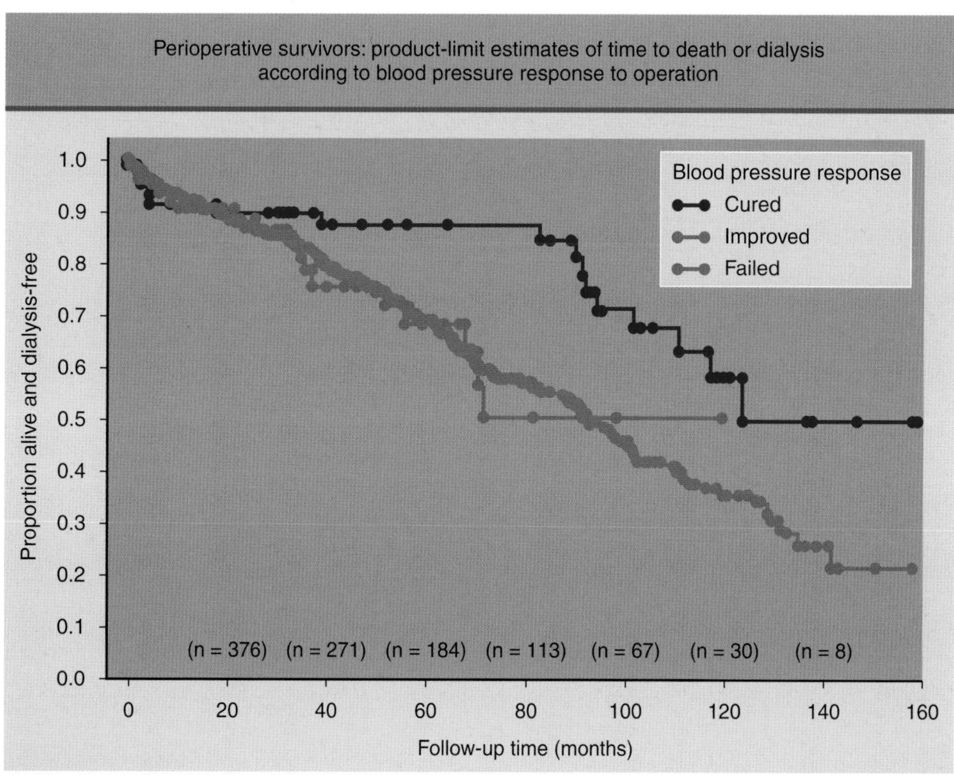

Figure 25-13. Perioperative survival: product-limit estimates of time to death or dialysis ($n = 472$) according to blood pressure response to operation. (From Cherr GS, Hansen KJ, Craven TE, et al. *J Vasc Surg* 2002;35(2):236-245.)

BRANCH RENAL ARTERY REPAIR

To determine the influence of more complex renal artery repairs, we examined a group of 77 consecutive patients undergoing branch renal artery repair with cold perfusion (including both ex vivo and in situ methods) at our center.[48] Six of these branch repairs were performed on patients who had previous failed PTRA (F-PTRA). Perioperative death and complication rates were 1.3% and 5.1%, respectively. Among patients with anatomical follow-up, 12-month primary patency was 85%, with a 12-month assisted primary patency rate of 93%. A 5.2% perioperative complication rate and one perioperative death (1.3%) were reported. Blood pressure response to branch repair was cured in 15% of patients, improved in 65%, and failed in 20%. Based on a 20% change in EGFR, postoperative renal function was improved in 35%, unchanged in 48%, and worsened in 17%. Based on these results, we feel that branch renal artery repair performed at experienced centers confers blood pressure and renal function benefits similar to those associated with less complex repairs without significant increases in perioperative morbidity or mortality.

OPERATIVE FAILURES AND CONSEQUENCES OF SECONDARY REPAIR

A renal artery repair eventually fails in approximately 5% of patients. Blood pressure response after secondary operative intervention is often equivalent to that observed among patients with primary intervention only. However, patients requiring secondary renal artery intervention have a significantly greater risk of worsened renal function (40% versus 13%), including eventual dialysis dependence (35% versus 4%). Furthermore, patients requiring secondary intervention demonstrate decreased dialysis-free survival. Use of PTRA following failed primary renal intervention potentially avoids technical challenges related to secondary operative

Table 25-8
Renal Function Response Based on Preoperative Serum Creatinine (SCr)*

Renal Function Response	Preoperative SCr (mg/dl) <1.8	1.8-3.0	≥3.0	Dialysis Dependent	Total
Improved (column %)	71 (29)	75 (54)	29 (58)	28 (76)	203 (43)
No change (column %)	142 (58)	52 (38)	17 (34)	9 (24)	220 (47)
Worse (column %)	31 (13)	11 (8)	4 (8)	0 (0)	46 (10)

*N = 469 patients.
From Cherr GS, Hansen KJ, Craven TE, et al. *J Vasc Surg* 2002;35(2):236-245.

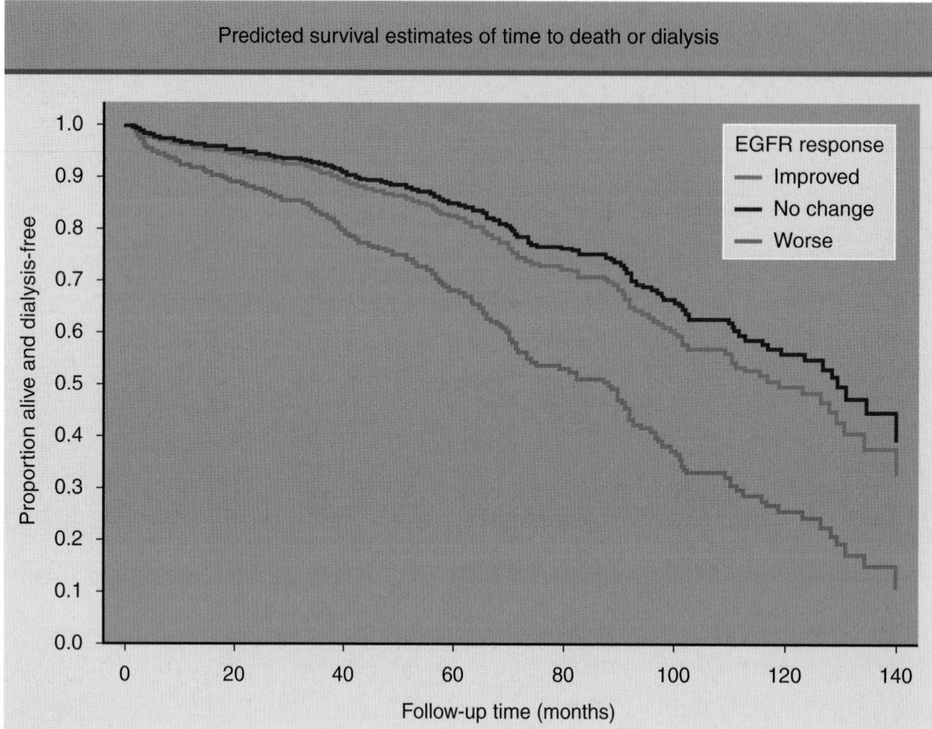

Figure 25-14. Predicted survival estimates to time of death or dialysis. The interaction between preoperative estimated glomerular filtration rate (EGFR) and renal function response for dialysis-free survival was significant. Preoperative EGFR was 38 ml/min/m^2 (median). (From Cherr GS, Hansen KJ, Craven TE, et al. *J Vasc Surg* 2002;35(2):236-245.)

Table 25-9
Combined Aortic and Renal Artery Repair: Results from Selected Series*

	Year	Patients	Bilateral Repair (%)	Hypertension Response (%)	Renal Function Response (%)	Perioperative Mortality (%)
Chaikof et al.[53]	1994	50	42	50	42	2
Cambria et al.[25]	1995	170	15	86		6.5
Clair et al.[55]	1995	43	70	83	14	4.7
Dougherty et al.[56]	1995	52	42	70		0
Benjamin et al.[24]	1996	133	53	63	33	5.3
Ballard et al.[51]	1996	50		43		10
Chaikof et al.[54]	1996	32	34	18		3.1
Kulbaski et al.[58]	1998	43	47	50		4.7
Taylor et al.[60]	2000	31	32	100		6.5
Hassen-Khodja et al.[57]	2000	39	31	61	57	2.6
Tsoukas et al.[61]	2001	73	21	63	18	5.5

*Hypertension and renal function responses displayed are percentages of patients with respective follow-up data available.

intervention, but evidence is inadequate to determine whether this advantage translates into improved outcomes, decreased procedure-associated morbidity, or both.

Our experience with failed renal artery repairs reinforces two important issues. First, significant hypertension is considered a prerequisite for renovascular intervention.[1,24,42] The irretrievable loss of excretory renal function observed after failed renal artery repair supports the view that renal revascularization should be performed for clear clinical indications, not as a "prophylactic" procedure in the absence of either hypertension or renal insufficiency. Second, the direct aortorenal reconstructions in these patients are characterized by their short length and high blood flow, favoring prolonged patency. Early failures of repair reflect errors in surgical technique or operative judgment.

SURGERY AFTER FAILED PTRA

We examined the influence of previous F-PTRA on methods of secondary surgical management, as well as both blood pressure and excretory renal function response to operation. Among 32 patients with atherosclerosis and history of F-PTRA, 25 had unilateral and 7 had bilateral PTRA (including two solitary kidneys). Before PTRA, 31 patients had significant hypertension (mean blood pressure 188 ± 32/102 ± 15 mm Hg) and 19 patients had ischemic nephropathy (mean serum creatinine 2.0 ± 1.3 mg/dl, range 1.3 to 6.6 mg/dl). Twenty patients had ischemic nephropathy after F-PTRA (mean serum creatinine 2.0 ± 0.8 mg/dl, range 1.3 to 4.1 mg/dl, excluding two dialysis-dependent patients). Excluding the three emergency operative procedures, the interval between F-PTRA and surgical repair ranged from 3 weeks to 12 years (mean 24.8 ± 32.6 months, median 9 months).

Secondary operative repair was considered complicated by F-PTRA in 19 patients (59%). In all, four nephrectomies were required. Bilateral procedures were performed in 20 patients. Aortorenal bypass was performed most commonly. Renal artery reimplantation, renal artery thromboendarterectomy, and combined aortic reconstruction were other successful options.

Blood Pressure Response

Among the 28 operative survivors with atherosclerotic renovascular disease and hypertension repaired after F-PTRA, 7% were considered cured, 50% were improved, and 43% were considered failed. Compared with patients treated by operative repair only, F-PTRA was associated with significantly decreased blood pressure benefit (57% versus 89% benefited, $p < 0.001$).

Renal Function Response

Among operative survivors with preoperative renal insufficiency, 41% were considered improved and 59% were unchanged. Compared with patients treated with operative repair only, the proportion of patients with improved renal function after surgery was similar ($p = 0.804$).

CONCLUSIONS

With proper patient selection and preparation, operative repair of atherosclerotic renovascular disease results in both blood pressure and renal function benefit. Improvement in renal function is associated with a significant increase in dialysis-free survival independent of other comorbidities. The application of intraoperative duplex ultrasound to assess renal artery reconstruction has resulted in long-term primary patency exceeding 96%. However, when failure of operative repair does occur, eventual renal function is worsened, culminating in an increased risk of dialysis dependence and death. In addition, the requirements of operative reconstruction after failed angioplasty are significant; our experience demonstrates increased complexity of repair, as well as inferior blood pressure benefit. Therefore, we recommend operative repair of ostial atherosclerosis and renal artery occlusion associated with severe hypertension and renal insufficiency.

References

1. Cherr GS, Hansen KJ, Craven TE, et al. Surgical management of atherosclerotic renovascular disease. *J Vasc Surg* 2002;35(2):236-245.
2. Knipp BS, Dimick JB, Eliason JL, et al. Diffusion of new technology for the treatment of renovascular hypertension in the United States: surgical revascularization versus catheter-based therapy, 1988-2001. *J Vasc Surg* 2004;40(4):717-723.
3. Murphy TP, Soares G, Kim M. Increase in utilization of percutaneous renal artery interventions by Medicare beneficiaries, 1996-2000. *AJR Am J Roentgenol* 2004;183(3):561-568.
4. Cambria RP, Brewster DC, L'Italien GJ, et al. Renal artery reconstruction for the preservation of renal function. *J Vasc Surg* 1996;24(3):371-380.
5. Hansen KJ, Starr SM, Sands RE, et al. Contemporary surgical management of renovascular disease. *J Vasc Surg* 1992;16(3):319-330.
6. Hansen KJ, Deitch JS, Oskin TC, et al. Renal artery repair: consequence of operative failures. *Ann Surg* 1998;227(5):678-689.
7. Chabova V, Schirger A, Stanson AW, et al. Outcomes of atherosclerotic renal artery stenosis managed without revascularization. *Mayo Clin Proc* 2000;75(5):437-444.
8. Crowley JJ, Santos RM, Peter RH, et al. Progression of renal artery stenosis in patients undergoing cardiac catheterization. *Am Heart J* 1998;136(5):913-918.
9. Meaney TF, Dustan HP, McCormack LJ. Natural history of renal arterial disease. *Radiology* 1968;91(5):881-887.
10. Schreiber MJ, Pohl MA, Novick AC. The natural history of atherosclerotic and fibrous renal artery disease. *Urol Clin North Am* 1984;11(3):383-392.
11. Tollefson DF, Ernst CB. Natural history of atherosclerotic renal artery stenosis associated with aortic disease. *J Vasc Surg* 1991;14(3):327-331.
12. Wollenweber J, Sheps SG, Davis GD. Clinical course of atherosclerotic renovascular disease. *Am J Cardiol* 1968;21(1):60-71.
13. Dean RH, Kieffer RW, Smith BM, et al. Renovascular hypertension: anatomic and renal function changes during drug therapy. *Arch Surg* 1981;116(11):1408-1415.
14. Pillay WR, Kan YM, Crinnion JN, Wolfe JHN. Prospective multicentre study of the natural history of atherosclerotic renal artery stenosis in patients with peripheral vascular disease. *Br J Surg* 2002;89(6):737-740.
15. Plouin PF, Chatellier G, Darne B, Raynaud A. Blood pressure outcome of angioplasty in atherosclerotic renal artery stenosis: a randomized trial. *Hypertension* 1998;31(3):823-829.
16. van Jaarsveld BC, Krijnen P, Pieterman H, et al. The effect of balloon angioplasty on hypertension in atherosclerotic renal-artery stenosis. *New Engl J Med* 2000;342(14):1007-1014.
17. Webster J, Marshall F, Abdalla M, et al. Randomised comparison of percutaneous angioplasty vs continued medical therapy for hypertensive patients with atheromatous renal artery stenosis. *J Hum Hypertens* 1998;12(5):329-335.
18. Caps MT, Perissinotto C, Zierler RE, et al. Prospective study of atherosclerotic disease progression in the renal artery. *Circulation* 1998;98(25):2866-2872.
19. Caps MT, Zierler RE, Polissar NL, et al. Risk of atrophy in kidneys with atherosclerotic renal artery stenosis. *Kidney Inter* 1998;53(3):735-742.
20. Pearce JD, Craven BL, Craven TE, et al. Progression of atherosclerotic renovascular disease: a prospective population-based study. *J Vasc Surg* 2006;44(5):955-962.
21. Zierler RE, Bergelin RO, Isaacson JA, Strandness Jr DE. Natural history of atherosclerotic renal artery stenosis: a prospective study with duplex ultrasonography. *J Vasc Surg* 1994;19(2):250-257.

22. Zierler RE, Bergelin RO, Davidson RC, et al. A prospective study of disease progression in patients with atherosclerotic renal artery stenosis. *Am J Hypertens* 1996;9(11):1055-1061.
23. Novick AC, Pohl MA, Schreiber M, et al. Revascularization for preservation of renal function in patients with atherosclerotic renovascular disease. *J Urol* 1983;129(5):907-912.
24. Benjamin ME, Hansen KJ, Craven TE, et al. Combined aortic and renal artery surgery: a contemporary experience. *Ann Surg* 1996;223(5):555-565.
25. Cambria RP, Brewster DC, L'Italien G, et al. Simultaneous aortic and renal artery reconstruction: evolution of an eighteen-year experience. *J Vasc Surg* 1995;21(6):916-924.
26. Hansen KJ, O'Neil EA, Reavis SW, et al. Intraoperative duplex sonography during renal artery reconstruction. *J Vasc Surg* 1991;14(3):364-374.
27. Leertouwer TC, Gussenhoven EJ, Bosch JL, et al. Stent placement for renal arterial stenosis: where do we stand? A meta-analysis. *Radiology* 2000;216(1):78-85.
28. Williamson WK, bou-Zamzam AM Jr, Moneta GL, et al. Prophylactic repair of renal artery stenosis is not justified in patients who require infrarenal aortic reconstruction. *J Vasc Surg* 1998;28(1):14-20.
29. Hansen KJ, Edwards MS, Craven TE, et al. Prevalence of renovascular disease in the elderly: a population-based study. *J Vasc Surg* 2002;36(3):443-451.
30. Svetkey LP, Himmelstein SI, Dunnick NR, et al. Prospective analysis of strategies for diagnosing renovascular hypertension. *Hypertension* 1989;14(3):247-257.
31. Nally JV, Barton DP. Contemporary approach to diagnosis and evaluation of renovascular hypertension. *Urol Clin North Am* 2001;28(4):781-791.
32. Clorius JH, Allenberg J, Hupp T, et al. Predictive value of exercise renography for presurgical evaluation of nephrogenic hypertension. *Hypertension* 1987;10(3):280-286.
33. Huot SJ, Hansson JH, Dey H, Concato J. Utility of captopril renal scans for detecting renal artery stenosis. *Arch Intern Med* 2002;162(17): 1981-1984.
34. Hupp T, Clorius JH, Allenberg JR. Renovascular hypertension: predicting surgical cure with exercise renography. *J Vasc Surg* 1991;14(2):200-207.
35. Mudun A, Falay O, Eryilmaz A, et al. Can exercise renography be an alternative to ACE inhibitor renography in hypertensive patients who are suspicious for renal artery stenosis? *Clin Nucl Med* 2004;29(1):27-34.
36. Hansen KJ. Renovascular disease: an overview. In: Rutherford RB, ed. *Vascular surgery*. 6 ed. Philadelphia: Elsevier Saunders; 2006: 1763-1772.
37. Hansen KJ, Tribble RW, Reavis SW, et al. Renal duplex sonography: evaluation of clinical utility. *J Vasc Surg* 1990;12(3):227-236.
38. Motew SJ, Cherr GS, Craven TE, et al. Renal duplex sonography: main renal artery versus hilar analysis. *J Vasc Surg* 2000;32(3):462-469.
39. Dean RH, Tribble RW, Hansen KJ, et al. Evolution of renal insufficiency in ischemic nephropathy. *Ann Surg* 1991;213(5):446-455.
40. Hansen KJ, Ditesheim JA, Metropol SH, et al. Management of renovascular hypertension in the elderly population. *J Vasc Surg* 1989;10(3):266-273.
41. Hansen KJ, Thomason RB, Craven TE, et al. Surgical management of dialysis-dependent ischemic nephropathy. *J Vasc Surg* 1995;21(2): 197-209.
42. Hansen KJ, Cherr GS, Craven TE, et al. Management of ischemic nephropathy: dialysis-free survival after surgical repair. *J Vasc Surg* 2000;32(3):472-481.
43. Hansen KJ, Cherr GS, Dean RH. Dialysis-free survival after surgical repair of ischemic nephropathy. *Cardiovasc Surg* 2002;10(4):400-404.
44. Corriere MA, Edwards MS, Hansen KJ. Abdominal aortic aneurysm and renal artery stenosis. *Vasc Dis Manag* 2008;5(1):16-21.
45. Hunt JC, Strong CG. Renovascular hypertension: mechanisms, natural history and treatment. *Am J Cardiol* 1973;32(4):562-574.
46. Moncure AC, Brewster DC, Darling RC, et al. Use of the splenic and hepatic arteries for renal revascularization. *J Vasc Surg* 1986;3(2):196-203.
47. Gill IS, Novick AC, Hodge EE. Extraanatomic renal revascularization in patients with renal-artery stenosis and abdominal aortic occlusion. *Urology* 1993;42(6):630-634.
48. Crutchley TA, Pearce JD, Craven TE, et al. Branch renal artery repair with cold perfusion protection. *J Vasc Surg* 2007;46(3):405-412.
49. Okuhn SP, Reilly LM, Bennett JB, et al. Intraoperative assessment of renal and visceral artery reconstruction: the role of duplex scanning and spectral analysis. *J Vasc Surg* 1987;5(1):137-147.
50. Allen BT, Rubin BG, Anderson CB, et al. Simultaneous surgical management of aortic and renovascular disease. *Am J Surg* 1993;166(6):726-732.
51. Ballard JL, Hieb RA, Smith DC, et al. Combined renal artery stenosis and aortic aneurysm: treatment options. *Ann Vasc Surg* 1996;10(4):361-364.
52. Branchereau A, Espinoza H, Magnan PE, et al. Simultaneous reconstruction of infrarenal abdominal aorta and renal arteries. *Ann Vasc Surg* 1992;6(3):232-238.
53. Chaikof EL, Smith RB III, Salam AA, et al. Ischemic nephropathy and concomitant aortic disease: a ten-year experience. *J Vasc Surg* 1994;19(1): 135-146.
54. Chaikof EL, Smith RB III, Salam AA, et al. Empirical reconstruction of the renal artery: long-term outcome. *J Vasc Surg* 1996;24(3):406-414.
55. Clair DG, Belkin M, Whittemore AD, et al. Safety and efficacy of transaortic renal endarterectomy as an adjunct to aortic surgery. *J Vasc Surg* 1995;21(6):926-933.
56. Dougherty MJ, Hallett JW Jr, Naessens J, et al. Renal endarterectomy vs. bypass for combined aortic and renal reconstruction: is there a difference in clinical outcome? *Ann Vasc Surg* 1995;9(1):87-94.
57. Hassen-Khodja R, Sala F, Declemy S, et al. Renal artery revascularization in combination with infrarenal aortic reconstruction. *Ann Vasc Surg* 2000;14(6):577-582.
58. Kulbaski MJ, Kosinski AS, Smith RB III, et al. Concomitant aortic and renal artery reconstruction in patients on an intensive antihypertensive medical regimen: long-term outcome. *Ann Vasc Surg* 1998;12(3): 270-277.
59. McNeil JW, String ST, Pfeiffer Jr RB. Concomitant renal endarterectomy and aortic reconstruction. *J Vasc Surg* 1994;20(3):331-336.
60. Taylor SM, Langan EM III, Snyder BA, et al. Concomitant renal revascularization with aortic surgery: are the risks of combined procedures justified? *Am Surg* 2000;66(8):768-772.
61. Tsoukas AI, Hertzer NR, Mascha EJ, et al. Simultaneous aortic replacement and renal artery revascularization: the influence of preoperative renal function on early risk and late outcome. *J Vasc Surg* 2001;34(6): 1041-1049.

chapter 26

Hemodialysis Access: Placement and Management of Complications

Brendon Quinn, MD • David L. Cull, MD • Christopher G. Carsten, MD

Key Points

- The National Kidney Foundation/Dialysis Outcome Quality Initiative (DOQI) has published evidence-based clinical practice guidelines for vascular access and established specific clinical goals to assess and improve the quality of vascular access.
- A long-term strategy that anticipates and plans for multiple access procedures should be developed for each patient.
- Duplex ultrasonography can assess arterial inflow, determine the diameter and quality of superficial extremity veins, and confirm patency of central veins. Duplex ultrasonography is also helpful in the selection of the most appropriate site for arteriovenous (AV) access placement.
- Autogenous AV accesses require fewer interventions to maintain long-term patency compared to nonautogenous AV accesses.
- Surgeons who provide vascular access should be familiar and facile with various autogenous and nonautogenous AV access procedures and should understand their relative advantages and disadvantages.
- Although DOQI guidelines recommend a routine monitoring or surveillance program for evaluating AV access dysfunction and prophylactic intervention for hemodynamically significant stenoses, the benefits and cost effectiveness of such an approach are as yet unproven.

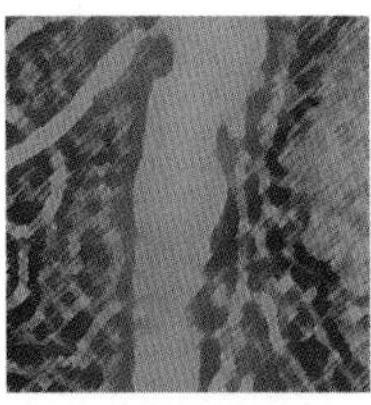

Chronic hemodialysis became a feasible treatment for end-stage renal disease in 1960 after Quinton and Scribner devised an external shunt that provided repetitive access to the circulation. The subsequent development of vascular access techniques and devices now permits patients to be maintained on dialysis for decades. The ideal vascular access system would provide the following:

- Reliable, repetitive access to the circulation
- Flow rates sufficient to deliver efficient dialysis
- Prolonged patency
- A low complication rate

However, the significant morbidity and cost associated with the establishment and maintenance of vascular access in the hemodialysis patient population is an indication of how far we are from achieving the "ideal" vascular access system. It is ironic that the breakthroughs that allowed access to the circulation that were so crucial to the development of chronic dialysis nearly 50 years ago are responsible for much of the cost and morbidity associated with dialysis today. Hemodialysis access failure is the most common cause of hospitalization and is responsible for the greatest number of hospitalized days for the patient on hemodialysis.[1] Vascular access establishment and maintenance account for nearly 17% of total Medicare spending for hemodialysis patients in the United States.[2] The societal impact of vascular access failure has been magnified by the dramatic growth in the number of patients with end-stage renal disease over the past decade. Between 1991 and 2001, the number of patients in the Medicare

Table 26-1
Dialysis Access Method: Advantages and Disadvantages*

Method	Advantages	Disadvantages
Dialysis catheter	• Easily inserted and removed • Immediately available for use • Hemodynamic effects of AV shunt (heart failure, steal) do not occur • Placement possible in nearly all patients	• Highest risk for infection • Incites central venous thrombosis or stenosis that may preclude use of extremities for AV access • Inconsistently provides blood flow rates adequate for optimum dialysis
Autogenous AV access	• Fewer secondary procedures required to maintain equivalent patency • Resistant to infection	• More difficult to cannulate • Early failure rate higher compared to bridge grafts • Requires prolonged maturation period • Hemodynamic effects (heart failure, steal) may occur • Anatomy may preclude procedure in some patients
Nonautogenous (prosthetic) AV access	• Available for use in 2-3 weeks • Easy to cannulate • Superior early technical success in patients with small or diseased vasculature • Placement possible in most patients	• Infection often requires removal • Hemodynamic effects (heart failure, steal) may occur • Multiple secondary procedures usually required to maintain patency

*AV, arteriovenous.

End-Stage Renal Disease Program doubled from 207,000 to more than 400,000, and this population is expected to continue to expand well into the twenty-first century.[3]

A technological breakthrough that would significantly reduce the morbidity and cost associated with vascular access does not appear to be on the horizon. The methods and devices available today for vascular access are fundamentally the same as those available 20 years ago. With this realization in mind, recent efforts have focused on developing algorithms to better define patient selection criteria for each access method and surveillance techniques to identify the failing vascular access.

METHODS OF VASCULAR ACCESS FOR CHRONIC HEMODIALYSIS

Vascular access for hemodialysis is obtained by one of the following methods: (1) placement of a temporary or permanent double lumen central venous catheter, (2) creation of an autogenous arteriovenous (AV) access (native or natural fistula), or (3) placement of a nonautogenous AV access (bridge AV graft). Although the most appropriate access option for a particular patient depends on several factors, such as patient age, comorbid diseases, vascular anatomy, previous access procedures, and timing of hemodialysis, several generalizations regarding each access method can be made (Table 26-1).

SITE SELECTION

The surgeon must consider numerous factors when planning dialysis access placement. Patients with end-stage renal disease often have comorbidities such as coronary artery disease, peripheral vascular disease, and diabetes mellitus that may increase the risk of surgery and adversely affect the long-term function of the access. The patient's medical condition should be optimized before surgery. For patients in tenuous medical condition, it is often prudent to perform dialysis via a catheter until they can be stabilized and the operation more safely performed.

A major determinant of AV access success is the diameter and quality of the arterial inflow and venous outflow. The arterial inflow should be evaluated by obtaining a history to elicit symptoms of arterial insufficiency. The axillary, brachial, radial, and ulnar pulses should be carefully palpated and the upper extremity blood pressures should be compared. Competence of the palmar arch is assessed with the Allen's test. If a lower extremity access is planned, the femoral, popliteal, and pedal pulses are palpated. If doubt exists as to the adequacy of the donor artery inflow or runoff, arterial duplex ultrasonography may clarify the anatomy. The radial artery should be evaluated with Duplex ultrasonography before selecting it as a donor artery for AV access, because AV accesses created with radial arteries that are highly calcified or less than 1.6 mm in diameter are unlikely to mature.[4] In selected patients, an arteriogram that shows the entire arterial anatomy of the limb may be necessary.

Venous outflow is assessed by history and physical examination. A history of thrombophlebitis, central venous catheterization, or placement of pacemaker wires via the subclavian vein or physical examination findings of arm edema or a prominent venous pattern of the shoulder and chest wall should alert the surgeon to the possibility of central venous stenosis or occlusion. Such findings should prompt preoperative venography. The size and quality of the superficial veins are determined by carefully palpating them with and without a tourniquet on the upper arm. If the vein cannot be visualized because of overlying subcutaneous fat, the superficial veins should be assessed with duplex ultrasonography. The technique for upper extremity duplex ultrasound vein

Table 26-2
Order of Preference For AV Access Placement*

	New Nomenclature	Traditional Nomenclature
First choice	Autogenous radial–cephalic direct wrist access	Brescia-Cimino fistula
	Autogenous posterior radial branch–cephalic direct access	Snuff box fistula
Second choice	Autogenous brachial–cephalic direct access	Brachiocephalic fistula
	Autogenous radial–basilic forearm transposition	Superficial forearm vein transposition
	Autogenous ulnar–basilic forearm transposition	Superficial forearm vein transposition
	Autogenous radial–cephalic forearm transposition	Superficial forearm vein transposition
	Autogenous ulnar–cephalic forearm transposition	Superficial forearm vein transposition
	Autogenous brachial–basilic upper arm transposition	Basilic vein transposition
Third choice	Prosthetic radial–antecubital forearm access	Forearm straight bridge AV graft
	Prosthetic brachial–antecubital forearm loop access	Forearm loop bridge AV graft
Fourth choice	Prosthetic brachial–axillary upper arm access	Upper arm straight bridge AV graft
	Prosthetic axillary–axillary upper arm access	Upper arm loop bridge AV graft
Fifth choice	Prosthetic popliteal–greater saphenous straight access	Thigh straight bridge AV graft
	Prosthetic femoral–greater saphenous looped access	Thigh looped bridge AV graft
	Autogenous popliteal–superficial femoral transposition	Superficial femoral vein transposition
Sixth choice	Prosthetic brachial–axillary chest access	Brachioaxillary straight bridge AV graft
	Prosthetic brachial–internal jugular access	Brachiojugular straight bridge AV graft
	Prosthetic axillary–axillary chest loop access	Axilloaxillary loop bridge AV graft
	Prosthetic axillary–internal jugular chest loop access	Axillojugular loop bridge AV graft
	Prosthetic axillary–axillary straight chest loop access	Axilloaxillary straight bridge AV graft
Seventh choice	Prosthetic axillary–femoral access	Axillofemoral bridge AV graft

*AV, arteriovenous.

mapping and criteria for selection of superficial veins for autogenous AV access creation have been reported by Silva et al.[5] A tourniquet is placed on the arm and the superficial veins are insonated with a 5- or 7-MHz scanning probe. Veins are assessed for compressibility and diameter. Patency of the axillary and subclavian veins are also confirmed with the study. A superficial vein diameter exceeding 2.5 mm without segmental sclerosis, stenosis, or occlusion is considered suitable for autogenous AV access creation.

An important factor to be considered when determining the optimal site for access placement is the influence of that site selection on subsequent access procedures. Each access procedure invariably fails, and some patients may outlive their available access sites. The ill-timed use of an access site may compromise future use of alternative sites in that extremity when the access fails. The surgeon should therefore develop a long-term management strategy for each patient that anticipates and plans for the possibility of multiple access procedures.

Although access procedures of the proximal extremity tend to have longer patency than those placed distally, the access should generally be placed as distally in the extremity as practical. This approach preserves more sites in the limb for subsequent access procedures. In addition, the more distally placed access procedures are associated with fewer hemodynamic complications such as arterial steal and congestive heart failure. Should surgical intervention for ischemic steal syndrome (ISS) or infection become necessary, accesses located in the distal extremity are easier to treat than those located proximally. The order of preference for AV access placement using the new and traditional nomenclature is shown in Table 26-2.[6,7]

A movement in the United States to enhance autogenous AV access utilization has resulted in the publication of several strategies or algorithms.[6,8-10] These algorithms have emphasized the following principles:

- Preoperative upper extremity vein assessment with duplex ultrasonography
- Use of the cuffed dialysis catheter as a bridge to autogenous AV access maturation
- Use of "secondary" AV access procedures such as the brachial–cephalic or venous transposition procedures
- Timely revision of failing autogenous AV accesses and thorough reevaluation of the patient for autogenous AV access creation should uncorrectable access failure occur

EVIDENCE-BASED DATA RELATED TO VASCULAR ACCESS

Although the published literature on the patency and complication rates of vascular access procedures is extensive, the outcome and conclusions of these studies are often conflicting. Hodges et al. identified several factors responsible for these conflicts.[11] First, no large, prospective, randomized studies compare the outcomes of vascular access procedures. Second, the access literature, until recently, lacked a standard reporting method that would allow comparison of access outcomes. For example, some reports exclude early autogenous AV access failures or those that do not mature from patency analysis. These less-strict definitions of success tend to tilt reported results heavily in favor of the autogenous AV access procedures. Furthermore, vascular access procedure outcome reports often use different statistical methods to report patency and fail to differentiate between primary and secondary patency. Finally, the comparison of studies is also complicated by inconsistent use of terms to describe vascular access procedures and by differences among studies in graft materials and configurations, quality of the arterial inflow or venous outflow, and patient risk factors. The Committee on Reporting Standards of the Society of Vascular Surgery (SVS) has published reporting standards

Table 26-3
Nomenclature for AV Access*

Naming AV access based on the following:
Conduit
Autogenous AV access—An access created by a connection between an artery and a vein whereby the vein serves as an accessible conduit. This type of access was previously referred to as a native or natural fistula.
Nonautogenous AV access—An access created by connecting an artery to a vein with a graft. This access can be divided into prosthetic (e.g., polytetrafluoroethylene or Dacron) and biograft (e.g., bovine heterograft or human umbilical vein).
Location—The arterial site of the AV access is reported first, followed by a hyphen and then the venous outflow site. When the arterial location may be ambiguous (e.g., brachial artery), a broader anatomical reference is included, such as forearm or upper arm (e.g., prosthetic brachial–antecubital forearm loop access).
Configuration
Transposition—Used when the peripheral portion of the vein is moved from its original position (usually to a more superficial tunnel) and connected to the artery. The more central portion of the vein remains intact in its native location (e.g., autogenous brachial–basilic transposition).
Translocation—A vein that has been disconnected both proximally and distally and is placed in a position remote from its origin (e.g., autogenous brachial–cephalic saphenous vein looped translocation).
Looped and straight—The course of the conduit.
Terms used for reporting results of AV access:
Patency
Primary patency—The interval from the time of access placement until any intervention designed to maintain or reestablish patency or functionality.
Assisted primary patency—The interval from the time of access placement until access thrombosis, including intervening manipulations, such as balloon angioplasty, designed to maintain the functionality of a patent access.
Secondary patency—The interval from the time of access placement until access abandonment, including intervening manipulations, such as thrombectomy, designed to reestablish functionality in thrombosed access.

*AV, arteriovenous.
From the Committee of Reporting Standards of the Society of Vascular Surgery and the American Association for Vascular Surgery.

for vascular access placement and revision.[7] This document provides preferred nomenclature for vascular access procedures and standardized methods for reporting patency and complications. The adoption of these standards should permit meaningful comparison of studies reporting the outcome of vascular access procedures.

In an effort to standardize reported or expected outcomes in this chapter, we have chosen to use the nomenclature recommended by the SVS/American Association for Vascular Surgery (AAVS) Reporting Standards for Vascular Accesses[7] (Table 26-3). We have therefore deliberately chosen to cite only those articles that report patency using the criteria established by these reporting standards. Patency results for each of the autogenous and nonautogenous AV access procedures are shown in Tables 26-4,[12-16] 26-5,[17-21] 26-6,[21-26] and 26-7.[22,24,27-36]

Outcome of Autogenous Versus Nonautogenous AV Access Procedures

Despite the limitations of the vascular access literature, compelling evidence exists that autogenous AV accesses have better long-term patency rates and require fewer interventions to maintain patency than nonautogenous AV accesses. Autogenous AV accesses also are less likely to become infected than nonautogenous AV accesses. However, for vascular access surgeons to select the most appropriate vascular access procedure for their patients, they must consider the magnitude of the relative benefit of the autogenous AV access. For example, if the benefits of autogenous AV accesses over nonautogenous AV accesses are great, an approach that emphasizes autogenous AV access creation in nearly every case is warranted. On the other hand, if the benefits of an autogenous AV access over a nonautogenous access are more modest, it might be prudent to place a nonautogenous access when an autogenous access is not likely to mature. For the reasons outlined earlier, determining the magnitude of the benefit of autogenous accesses over nonautogenous accesses is difficult given the range of outcomes reported for each of the vascular access procedures. One study that provides some clarity to this issue is a recently published metaanalysis comparing the outcome of upper extremity autogenous and nonautogenous AV accesses. This review identified only 34 studies in the literature that reported patency results using the criteria established by the SVS/AAVS Reporting Standards for AV Accesses. A metaanalysis of those studies demonstrated an 18-month primary patency rates for autogenous and prosthetic upper extremity AV accesses of approximately 51% and 33%, respectively; corresponding secondary patency rates were approximately 77% and 55% (Figure 26-1).[37] This same study was unable to accurately determine complication rates for upper extremity AV accesses from the available literature because either complications were not described or reporting methods were inconsistent among the studies.

These findings suggest that indeed an access survival advantage exists for autogenous compared to nonautogenous accesses. However, this advantage is not dramatic and would be nullified if the early failure or nonmaturation rates of the autogenous accesses were excessive. Careful patient selection for access type and site is thus crucial if the benefits of an autogenous access over a nonautogenous access are to be realized. Table 26-8 shows factors that have been implicated in early failure or nonmaturation of autogenous accesses.

DIALYSIS OUTCOME QUALITY INITIATIVE CLINICAL PRACTICE GUIDELINES FOR VASCULAR ACCESS

In an effort to control the cost and reduce the morbidity associated with vascular access, several initiatives are being implemented by government agencies and private organizations

Table 26-4
Summary of Results of Wrist Direct AV Access*

Study	Study Design	*n*	Cumulative Patency (%) 1 Year	2 Years	3 Years	Infection (%)
Wolowczyk et al.[12]	Retrospective SBDA	210	65	58	55	0
Golledge et al.[13]	Retrospective RCDA	107	70	63	—	—
Burger et al.[14]	Prospective RCDA	208	79	68	59	—
Leapman et al.[15]	Retrospective RCDA	150	56	50	45	—
Palder et al.[16]	Retrospective RCDA	99	65	50	—	1

*AV, arteriovenous; RCDA, radial–cephalic direct AV access; SBDA, snuffbox radial–cephalic direct AV access.

Table 26-5
Summary of Results of Brachial–Cephalic Direct AV Access*

Study	Study Design	*n*	Cumulative Patency (%) 1 Year	2 Years	3 Years	Infection (%)
Dunlop et al.[17]	Retrospective	81	70	57	—	2
Sparks et al.[18]	Retrospective	111	—	80	—	—
Livingston et al.[19]	Retrospective	39	70	—	—	2
Bender et al.[20†]	Retrospective	73	84	78	78	1
Ascher et al.[21]	Retrospective	109	72	—	—	0

*AV, arteriovenous.
†Patency not defined.

Table 26-6
Summary of Results of Brachial–Basilic Transposition*

		Patients (*n*)		Cumulative Patency (%) 1 Year		2 Years		Infection (%)	
Study	Study Design	BBT	PTFE	BBT vs.	PTFE	BBT vs.	PTFE	BBT vs.	PTFE
Coburn and Carney[22]	Retrospective BBT vs. PTFE	59	47	90	87	86	64†	3	16†
Rivers et al.[23]	Retrospective BBT	65	—	—	—	49	—	2	—
Matsuura et al.[24]	Retrospective BBT vs. PTFE	30	68	88	78	70	51†	0	10
Oliver et al.[25]	Retrospective BBT vs. PTFE	59	82	65	63	—	—	2	13†
Murphy et al.[26]	Retrospective BBT	61	—	55	—	35	—	4	—
Ascher et al.[21]	Retrospective BBT	63	—	70	—	—	—	0	—

*BBT, brachial–basilic transposition; PTFE, polytetrafluoroethylene arteriovenous access.
†Differences are statistically significant.

Table 26-7
Results of Prosthetic Arteriovenous Access Using Polytetrafluoroethylene*

Author	Location	Study Design	*n*	Primary Patency (%) 1 Year	2 Years	Secondary Patency (%) 1 Year	2 Years	Infection (%)	Steal (%)
Lenz et al.[27]	FA-L	Prospective	56	49	38	92	59	2	?
Rizzuti et al.[28]	FA-L	Retrospective	111	—	—	80	70	10	
Rizzuti et al.[28]	FA-S	Retrospective	68	—	—	70	47	—	
Bosman et al.[29]	FA	Retrospective	67	40	—	63	—	13	
Steed et al.[30]	UA	Retrospective	20	84	67	—	—	10	
Staramos et al.[31]	UA	Retrospective	64	—	—	80	64	—	
Coburn and Carney[22]	UA	Retrospective	47	70	49	87	64	16	8
Matsuura et al.[24]	UA	Retrospective	68	68	46	78	51	10	
Cull et al.[32]	T	Retrospective	116	34	19	68	54	41	
Khadra et al.[33]	T	Retrospective	74	—	—	74	63	16	3
Bhandari et al.[34]	T	Retrospective	49	—	—	85	82	35	
Vega et al.[35]	BJ	Retrospective	51	57	43	74	63	2	
McCann[36]	AA, AJ	Retrospective	40	63	43	85	68	3	

*AA, axillary–axillary; AJ, axillary–internal jugular; BJ, brachial–jugular; FA-L, forearm loop; FA-S, forearm straight; T, thigh; UA, upper arm.

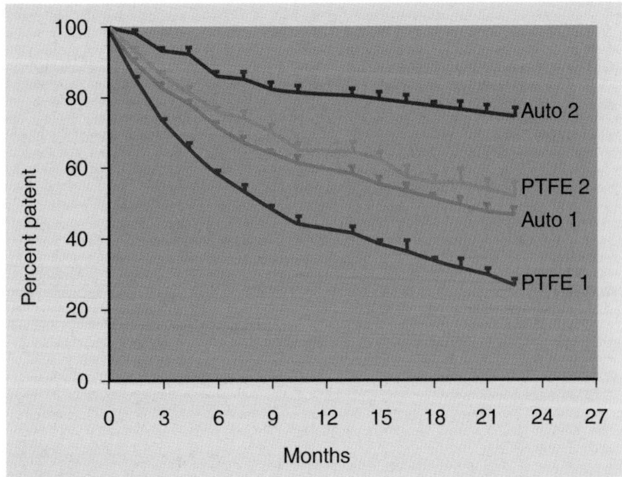

Figure 26-1. Metaanalysis of the patency rates for upper extremity autogenous and nonautogenous AV accesses.

to standardize the approach to vascular access management. The principle focus of these efforts is an attempt to change the practice pattern among surgeons in the United States from primary placement of prosthetic AV accesses to creation of autogenous AV accesses. The most influential of these efforts is the National Kidney Foundation (NKF)/ Dialysis Outcome Quality Initiative (DOQI) guidelines, which were first published in 1997 and most recently updated in 2006.[6,38] The DOQI Clinical Practice Guidelines for Vascular Access were developed by a multidisciplinary team of surgeons, nephrologists, and dialysis nurses who evaluated the credibility of the vascular access–related literature. They used the best available literature to develop evidence-based clinical practice guidelines for vascular access. In addition, for situations in which solid evidence was not available, several clinical practice recommendations were adopted based on group consensus. In addition to provision of guidelines and recommendations for standardizing the approach to vascular access management, the DOQI guidelines have established several specific clinical outcome goals to assess and improve quality. A summary of the Clinical Outcome Goals for Vascular Access established by the NKF/DOQI Guidelines Update 2006 is shown in Table 26-9.

Implications and Limitations of the DOQI Guidelines

The DOQI guidelines have significantly influenced vascular access practice patterns in the United States. In 1997, the DOQI guidelines recommended that "primary" AV fistulae be constructed in at least 50% of all new patients with end-stage renal disease who elect to receive hemodialysis and that AV fistulae be used in 40% of patients on hemodialysis.[38] In the decade since these benchmarks were established, the AV fistula creation and utilization rates have increased substantially, thereby confirming the influence of this document in changing surgeon practice patterns in the United States. Unfortunately, many have interpreted the DOQI guidelines to mean that the significant advantages of an AV fistula over an AV graft almost always justify attempts at AV fistula creation. Furthermore, many consider the attainment of the DOQI guideline benchmark of 50% AV fistula creation rate to be an ad hoc measure of vascular access quality. Such a stance may be responsible for negative and unintended consequences. At least one study has suggested that the AV fistula nonmaturation rate has increased since the publication of the DOQI guidelines.[39] Furthermore, a dramatic increase occurred in the use of cuffed dialysis catheters, presumably a result of the use of the catheter as a bridge to fistula maturation.[40] We must be cautious in using the DOQI fistula creation benchmark as an important quality-of-care measure. Surgeons can create AV fistulae in nearly 100% of patients; however, many of these fistulae will never mature. Selecting a patient for the most appropriate access is one of the most challenging aspects of vascular access surgery because the dialysis population is not uniform and many factors influence AV fistula maturation. Since early thrombosis or failure of an AV fistula to mature can have significant adverse effects, including the need for prolonged use of a cuffed dialysis catheter and loss of potential AV access sites, the fistula maturation rate must also be considered an important quality-of-care measure. To date, the DOQI guidelines have neither made recommendations regarding patient selection for specific AV access procedures nor suggested a benchmark for primary failure rates of AV fistulae because to do so "might discourage AV fistula creation."[6]

The DOQI Guidelines Update 2006 also includes a section titled the "Clinical Outcome Goals for Vascular Access," which provides additional benchmarks not supported by evidence-based data but, rather, reached by the opinion of the Vascular Access Work Group (Table 26-9). Undoubtedly, at least a few of these benchmarks will be considered by the Centers for Medicare Services and managed care providers as performance-quality measures for vascular access. Further work is needed to improve and implement the practice guidelines, as well as to decrease the morbidity and improve the quality of life of the growing population of patients with end-stage renal disease.

Table 26-8
Possible Factors Adversely Influencing Autogenous Arteriovenous Access Maturation

Vein size <2.5-3.0 mm	African American race
Artery size <1.6 mm	Peripheral vascular disease
Diabetes mellitus	Obesity
Elderly	Female
Surgeon inexperience	Previous failed access

AUTOGENOUS AV ACCESS

Autogenous Radial–Cephalic Direct Wrist Access (Radiocephalic Fistula, Brescia–Cimino Fistula, Snuffbox Fistula)

General Considerations

The radial–cephalic direct wrist access is often referred to as the "gold standard" for hemodialysis access because its creation is associated with a low complication rate and excellent long-term patency for those patients who develop a mature access. Its major limitation is a relatively high early failure rate that has been reported in up to 50% of cases. Early failure is more common in patients with diabetes mellitus and in elderly, female, and obese patients. Patients with cephalic

Table 26-9
Clinical Outcome Goals for Vascular Access: NKF/DOQI Guidelines 2006 Update*

1. Each center should establish a database and process to track the types of accesses created and complication rates of these accesses. The goals for permanent hemodialysis access placement should include the following:
   a. Prevalent functional AVF placement rate of greater than 65% of patients
   b. Cuffed catheter for permanent dialysis access (not a bridge to chronic access) in less than 10% of patients; long-term catheter access is defined as the use of a dialysis catheter of more than 3 months in the absence of a maturing permanent access graft or fistula
2. The primary access failure rates of hemodialysis accesses in the following locations and configurations should not be more than the following:
   a. Forearm straight grafts—15%
   b. Forearm loop grafts—10%
   c. Upper-arm grafts—5%
   d. Tunneled catheters with blood flow less than 300 ml/min—5%
3. Access complications and performance should be as follows:
   a. Fistula complications or performance should be as follows:
      1. Fistula thrombosis—fewer than 0.25 episodes per patient-year at risk
      2. Fistula infection—less than 1% during the use-life of the access
      3. Fistula patency greater than 3.0 years (by life-table analysis)
   b. Graft complications or performance should be as follows:
      1. Graft thrombosis—fewer than 0.5 thrombotic episodes per patient-year at risk
      2. Graft infection—less than 10% during the use-life of the access
      3. Graft patency greater than 2 years (by life-table analysis)
      4. Graft patency after PTA—longer than 4 months
   c. Catheter complications or performance should be as follows:
      1. Tunneled catheter-related infection less than 10% at 3 months and less than 50% at 1 year
      2. The cumulative incidence of insertion complications (e.g., pneumothorax, air embolism, and hemothorax) should not exceed 1% of all catheter placements
4. Efficacy of corrective intervention—the rate of certain milestones after correction of thrombosis or stenosis should be as follows:
   a. AVF patency after PTA—greater than 50% unassisted patency at 6 months
      AVF patency following surgery—greater than 50% unassisted patency at 1 year
   b. AVG patency after PTA—a primary patency of 50% at 6 months
      AVG patency after surgery—a primary patency of 50% at 6 months

*AVF, arteriovenous fistula; AVG, arteriovenous graft; NFK/DOQI, National Kidney Foundation/Dialysis Outcome Quality Initiative; PTA, percutaneous transluminal angioplasty.

veins measuring less than 2.5 mm by preoperative vein mapping with duplex ultrasonography are also less likely to develop a mature access. As the demographics of the hemodialysis population shift to older and sicker patients, fewer are considered candidates for this access. The benefits of the radial–cephalic direct wrist access probably warrant consideration of its creation in most patients who are referred for vascular access months in advance of the anticipated need for dialysis. Failure of the access in this situation does not "burn any bridges" for subsequent access procedures and may result in dilatation of the more proximal vein, thereby increasing success of subsequent procedures should the radial–cephalic direct wrist access fail.[41]

Patients who are referred late for vascular access warrant a more selective approach. The likelihood of successful access maturation based on patient factors and vein size and the risk of prolonged dialysis catheter use while awaiting maturation must be considered. Patency for the autogenous radial–cephalic direct wrist access ranges between 56% and 79% at 1 year (Table 26-4).[12-16]

Technique

The radial–cephalic direct wrist access procedure involves creation of an anastomosis between the radial artery and the cephalic vein at the wrist. Several anastomotic configurations have been described; however, anastomosis from the end of the vein to the side of the artery is most commonly used because it provides superior blood flow rates compared to end-to-end anastomosis and minimizes the risk of venous hypertension associated with side-to-side anastomosis.

In most instances, the operation is performed with local anesthesia. A transverse incision is made over the radial artery and cephalic vein at the level of the head of the radius. The cephalic vein is mobilized for 3 to 4 cm. To achieve adequate mobilization, it may be necessary to ligate and divide several venous tributaries. To prevent inadvertent twisting, the anterior surface of the vein is carefully marked with ink before its transection. A superficial sensory branch of the radial nerve lies laterally to the brachioradialis muscle. Injury to this nerve during dissection should be avoided. The radial artery is exposed by longitudinally incising the deep forearm fascia over the arterial pulse. A 2 cm length of artery is mobilized. The cephalic vein is ligated as far distally as possible and divided, and the proximal vein is gently flushed with heparinized saline. If the vein does not flush easily, it is probed with a 2.5-mm coronary artery dilator. The inability to advance the dilator should prompt an intraoperative venogram before performing the vascular anastomosis. A stenosis of the cephalic vein, if identified, should be corrected. If the location or length of a venous stenosis precludes revision, an alternative site for vascular access should be considered. After administration of systemic heparin, fine vascular clamps are applied to the artery. The pneumatic tourniquet can be used to avoid clamp injury to the vessel.[42] The vein is spatulated for approximately 5 mm. If the venous anatomy permits, a side tributary of the vein can be used to create a patchlike end of the vein (Figure 26-2). A 5-mm arteriotomy is made, and

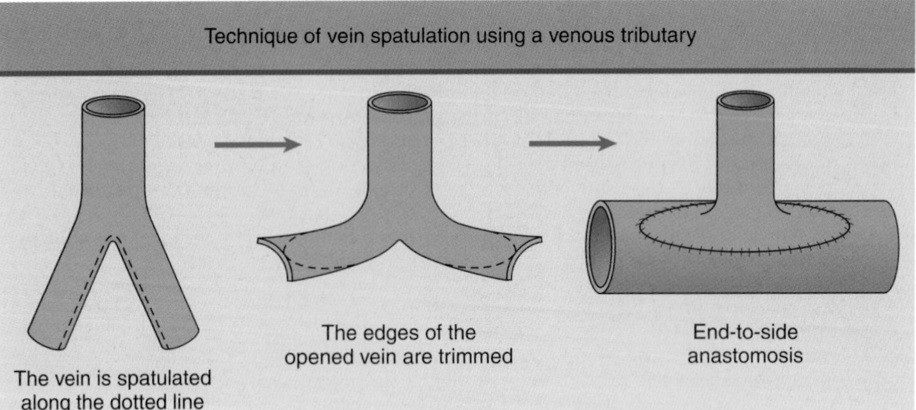

Figure 26-2. Technique of vein spatulation using a venous tributary.

the anastomosis is performed in the standard fashion using a continuous running 6-0 polypropylene suture. Following release of the vascular clamps, an easily palpable thrill over the cephalic vein is expected. A weak or absent thrill is indicative of either anastomotic stenosis or arterial spasm. Proximal obstruction of the vein should be suspected if the fistula is strongly pulsatile. If an abnormality is suspected, an intraoperative fistulogram should be obtained.

An alternative exposure of the radial artery and cephalic vein for fistula creation is in the anatomical snuffbox. A longitudinal incision is made between the tendons of the extensor pollicis longus and brevis. At this location, the cephalic vein and the radial artery are in close proximity. The cephalic vein is mobilized. The radial artery lies beneath a fascial layer that must be incised. The same anastomotic technique described for standard radial–cephalic direct wrist access creation is used (Figure 26-3).

Autogenous Brachial–Cephalic Direct Access (Brachiocephalic Fistula)

General Considerations

The brachial–cephalic direct access is often referred to as a "secondary" vascular access procedure. This label is meant to emphasize the status of the radial–cephalic direct wrist access as the gold standard for access procedures. Unfortunately, this label tends to minimize significant advantages of the brachial–cephalic direct access over other access procedures. First, owing to the larger artery and vein at the antecubital fossa, the early failure rate is lower and the blood flow rate is greater with this access compared to the rates for the autogenous wrist accesses. Second, the effects of age, female gender, and diabetes mellitus do not appear to negatively affect the maturation of upper arm autogenous accesses. Consequently, the percentage of dialysis patients who are candidates for autogenous AV access creation can be significantly increased if the upper arm autogenous AV access procedures are considered.

Like the direct wrist AV access, the brachial–cephalic direct access is resistant to infection. The patency for the brachial–cephalic direct AV access ranges between 70% and 84% at 1 year (Table 26-5).[17-21] The disadvantages of the brachial–cephalic direct access include a slightly greater incidence of ISS compared to the wrist accesses. Also, the access may not be accessible in obese patients with significant subcutaneous fat overlying the cephalic vein in the upper arm. We have salvaged many brachial–cephalic direct accesses that lie too deep with an operation called the fistula elevation procedure. Using local anesthesia, the access is mobilized from the antecubital fossa to the proximal upper arm. The subcutaneous fat is closed beneath the access with interrupted 3-0 polyglycolic suture. The skin is closed with a running subcuticular closure with 4-0 polyglycolic suture. After healing, the fistula is accessed directly through the cicatrix that overlies the AV access (Figure 26-4).[43]

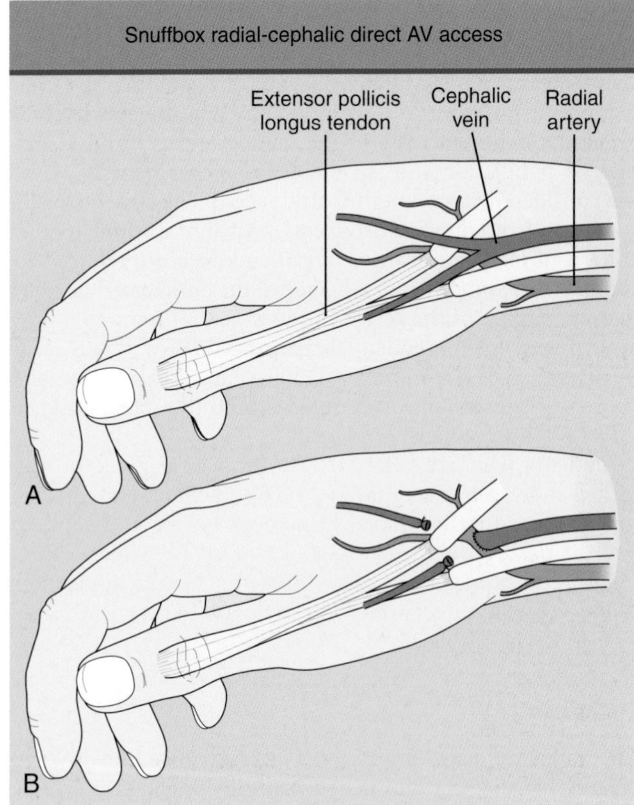

Figure 26-3. Snuffbox radial–cephalic direct AV access. Before access construction **(A)** and after access construction **(B)**, showing the cephalic vein and the radial artery between the dissected extensor pollicis tendons.

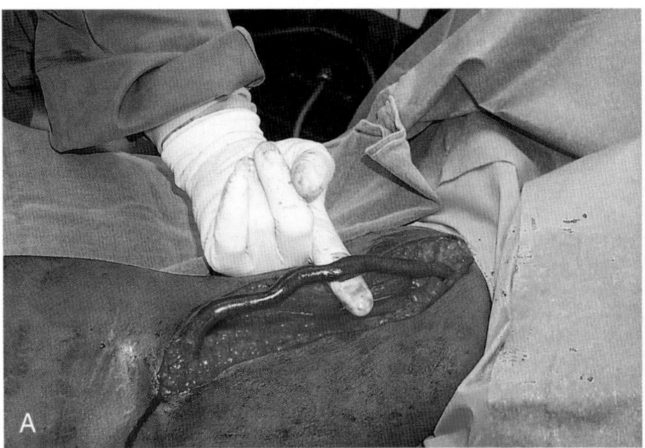

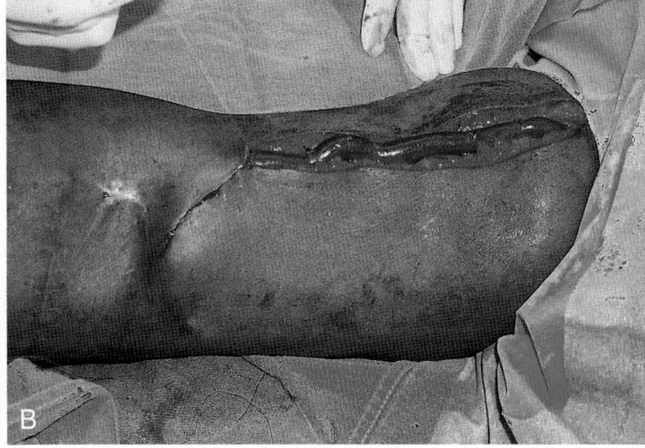

Figure 26-4. Fistula elevation procedure. **A,** The brachial–cephalic direct AV access is mobilized. **B,** The subcutaneous tissue is approximated beneath the AV access. A subcuticular closure is used to approximate the skin over the access.

Technique

The brachial–cephalic direct access operation is performed using local anesthesia. A 6-cm transverse incision is made approximately one fingerbreadth distal to the antecubital crease. The superficial veins in the antecubital fossa are exposed. The superficial venous anatomy of the antecubital fossa is variable (Figure 26-5). Often, several vein sites can be used for the venous anastomosis. The most appropriate site is determined by the vein size, quality, and position relative to the artery. If the anatomy permits, a venous tributary can be spatulated such that a vein patch is created and incorporated into the arterial anastomosis (Figure 26-2).

The brachial artery lies beneath the bicipital aponeurosis. This fascia is incised transversely. The brachial artery is dissected for a distance of approximately 3 cm. Care is taken to avoid injury to the median nerve, located medially and posteriorly to the artery. After systemic heparin is administered, the vessels are clamped. The vein is marked with ink to prevent rotation, transected, and gently flushed with heparinized saline. If the surgeon perceives any resistance to flow while flushing the vein, the patency and quality of the proximal vein must be investigated as described previously. The AV anastomosis is limited to approximately 5 mm in length and is completed with a 6-0 polypropylene continuous running suture.

Occasionally, preoperative vein mapping or physical examination identifies a large, patent cephalic vein in the upper arm immediately above thrombosed or sclerotic veins in the antecubital fossa. This finding often occurs after thrombosis of a forearm prosthetic AV access. The technique for creating a brachial–cephalic direct access in this situation is modified. Longitudinal incisions over the cephalic vein and the brachial artery proximal to the antecubital crease are made. The cephalic vein and brachial artery are mobilized. The cephalic vein is ligated distally and transected. The vein is tunneled subcutaneously to the brachial artery. An end-to-side anastomosis is constructed as described previously (Figure 26-6).

Autogenous Transposition AV Accesses

Autogenous transposition AV accesses comprise the following:

- Forearm vein transposition
- Brachial–basilic transposition (basilic vein transposition)
- Popliteal–superficial femoral transposition

General Considerations

Transposition procedures are considered secondary, or as in the case of the popliteal–superficial femoral transposition, tertiary vascular access procedures. This is because the operations are more extensive and require more time to perform than other autogenous AV access procedures and most prosthetic AV access procedures. Each of the procedures requires long incisions to expose and mobilize the vein. The vein is transposed to a more superficial position through a subcutaneous tunnel. An end-to-side anastomosis is created between the vein and an inflow artery. Although we use local anesthesia in most cases for the forearm and brachial–basilic transpositions, many prefer axillary block for anesthesia. Epidural or general anesthesia is required for the popliteal–superficial femoral transposition.

The brachial–basilic transposition was first described by Dahger more than 25 years ago.[20a] The basilic vein is usually of greater diameter than the cephalic vein and is rarely damaged by previous venopuncture because of its deep location in the upper arm. Several studies have shown superior patency and resistance to infection of the brachial–basilic transposition compared to prosthetic AV accesses (Table 26-6).[21-26] The major criticism of the brachial–basilic transposition is that it uses a proximal upper extremity vein, which may preclude use of veins more distally in the arm for forearm prosthetic AV access placement if the brachial–basilic transposition fails. However, we suggest that a failed brachial–basilic transposition does not preclude subsequent forearm or upper arm prosthetic AV access placement. The cephalic, brachial, and axillary veins usually remain patent and can be used for venous outflow of other AV access procedures in the extremity. Another disadvantage of the basilic vein transposition procedure is an increased incidence of arterial steal syndrome compared to the other upper extremity AV access procedures, likely due to increased vein caliber.

We believe that the inherent advantages of enhanced patency and resistance to infection warrant the use of the brachial–basilic transposition in preference to forearm prosthetic AV access placement if the following criteria are met. The first criterion is that preoperative vein mapping indicates the basilic vein is of adequate size and quality for use. The size of the vein at the level of the antecubital fossa is important because extensive branching of the vein can occur, rendering

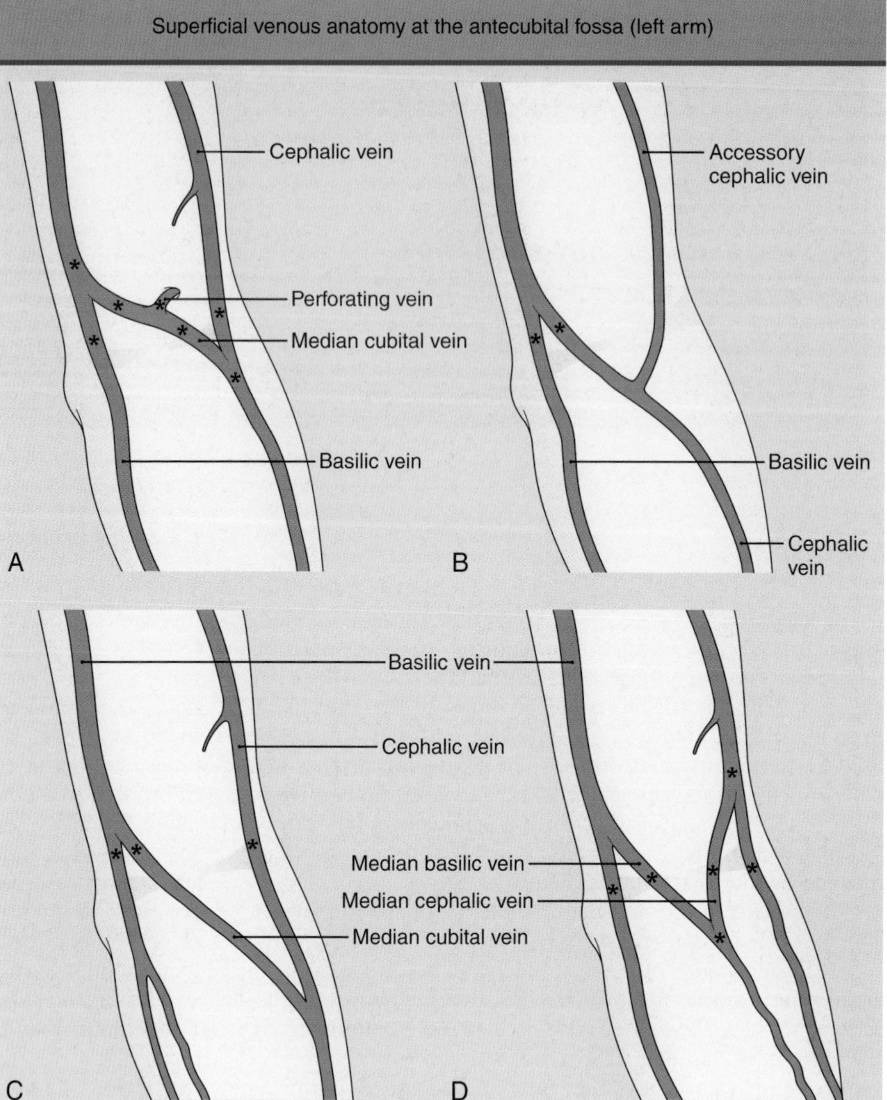

Figure 26-5. Superficial venous anatomy at the antecubital fossa (left arm). **A,** Standard superficial venous anatomy. **B-D,** Variations in the superficial venous anatomy. * denotes possible venous sites for autogenous direct AV access creation.

it too small for use. The vein diameter should exceed 2.5 mm by duplex ultrasound vein mapping. Also, in approximately 5% of cases, the basilic vein empties into the brachial vein at the middle of the upper arm rather than at the axilla. This anatomical variation may be identified by preoperative duplex ultrasonography and usually precludes the procedure because the length of vein is inadequate to transpose. The second criterion is that the patient's medical condition must permit the more extensive procedure required to perform the operation.

Silva et al. reported results of a technique for transposing veins in the forearm for autogenous AV access creation that is similar to the brachial–basilic transposition.[44] The procedure is used when preoperative vein mapping indicates that a forearm vein is of adequate caliber (more than 2.5 mm) and quality for fistula creation; however, the vein lies too deep to facilitate easy needle cannulation. The technique of forearm vein transposition is shown in Figure 26-7. In Silva and colleagues' series of 89 patients who underwent the procedure, the primary cumulative patency rate was 84% at 1 year and 69% at 2 years.[44] In another report, the primary patency of forearm vein transposition was 62% at 1 year.[45]

Two published reports have described the technique of autogenous AV access construction with transposed superficial femoral vein.[46,47] The extensive nature of the procedure tends to limit its indications. The authors have used the procedure in young patients in whom all upper extremity sites for AV access have been exhausted. To have an adequate length of vein for needle cannulation after vein transposition, the vein must be mobilized from the popliteal fossa to its origin at the common femoral vein and the patient must be thin. Symptoms of significant lower extremity venous hypertension are rare; however, it is important that the profunda vein be preserved. The cumulative patency in a limited series of 25 patients reported by Gradman et al. was 73% at 1 year.[46] The procedure is associated with major wound complications in nearly one third of patients and is also associated with a high incidence of arterial steal. The length of the arterial anastomosis must be limited to minimize the risk of steal.

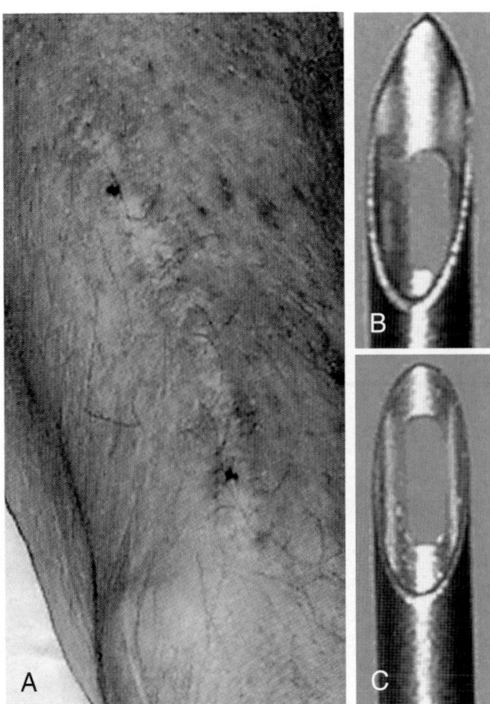

Figure 26-14. Buttonhole technique of autogenous AV access cannulation. **A,** Repetitive cannulation at same site and angle results in the development of a scar tract. **B,** Traditional sharp-tipped needle used for access cannulation. **C,** Blunt-tipped needle used for cannulating the access once the scar tracts are developed.

Patients are instructed to notify the surgeon immediately if they develop hand numbness or pain. Failure to promptly recognize and correct significant arterial steal can result in permanent neurological injury. The patient is also instructed to regularly palpate the access for presence of a thrill. Loss of the thrill usually indicates the access has thrombosed. Early thrombectomy and revision may salvage the access.

HEMODIALYSIS CATHETERS

The complication rate for hemodialysis catheters is higher than other chronic vascular access options. Therefore, except in extraordinary cases, hemodialysis catheters are used as a temporary means of access until an autogenous or nonautogenous access can be established. To prevent prolonged dialysis catheter use, adequate planning on the part of the primary care physician, the nephrologist, and the surgeon is required. Patients at risk for development of end-stage renal disease should be identified and referred to a nephrologist to maximize medical management and to a surgeon for evaluation and placement of permanent access. Every effort should be made to provide a functioning autogenous or nonautogenous AV access before the initiation of hemodialysis. This ideal, however, is often not realized, and a significant number of patients with end-stage renal disease require hemodialysis via a dialysis catheter.

Dialysis catheters can be used immediately after their placement for hemodialysis. The uncuffed dialysis catheter is generally reserved for situations in which the anticipated need for hemodialysis is less than 3 weeks. Cuffed dialysis catheters can be used from several months to years if necessary. Patients who require dialysis via a dialysis catheter usually fall into one of several categories. Those with access malfunction or infection may need a short-term method of dialysis, which can be provided with an uncuffed catheter, until the access is revised or the infection cleared. Patients with acute renal failure in whom recovery of renal function is uncertain are best dialyzed with a cuffed dialysis catheter. If permanent dialysis becomes necessary, an autogenous or nonautogenous AV access can be placed and the dialysis catheter used until the AV access is ready for cannulation. Cuffed dialysis catheters are also used in patients with chronic renal insufficiency who present with an acute exacerbation of their renal failure and require urgent hemodialysis. The cuffed catheter is used as a bridge for dialysis until permanent access is available. Finally, patients who have exhausted all peripheral sites for AV access or with poor cardiac output or hypercoagulable disorders in whom AV access cannot be maintained can be dialyzed long term with a cuffed dialysis catheter.

The veins commonly used for dialysis catheter insertion are the internal jugular vein, external jugular vein, subclavian vein, femoral vein, and inferior vena cava. The right internal jugular vein is the most ideal vein for dialysis catheter insertion for the following reasons:

- It has the straightest course to the superior vena cava and right atrium, which is the target for the tip of the catheter
- The anatomical landmarks identifying its location are easily identified
- Tunneling of the cuffed catheter to an infraclavicular position allows for maximum patient mobility and comfort[1,74,75]

The left internal jugular vein is the second choice for dialysis catheter insertion. It is associated with lower catheter flow rates and higher rates of catheter malfunction compared to the right internal jugular vein.[1,74,75] The left internal jugular venous catheter also places the left upper extremity at risk for venous outflow obstruction, since the catheter crosses the innominate vein and can precipitate its stenosis or occlusion. The use of the subclavian vein for dialysis catheter placement should be avoided because of the significant rate of central venous stenosis associated with its use. Studies have shown that up to 50% of patients who have had central venous access via the subclavian vein develop a significant stenosis, potentially rendering the ipsilateral upper extremity unusable for AV access placement.[76-79] The femoral vein is easily accessible and often used for temporary catheter placement; however, it is associated with a significantly higher rate of infection than internal jugular or subclavian venous catheters. Dialysis catheters placed via the femoral vein must be at least 19 cm long to prevent recirculation.[80] If the internal jugular and subclavian veins have been exhausted, however, the femoral vein can be used for cuffed dialysis catheter placement.[81,82] The translumbar approach to the inferior vena cava is used for dialysis catheter placement when all other peripheral and central sites for catheter insertion have been exhausted. Catheters placed via this approach have a higher incidence of catheter dislodgement and infection than other sites and are technically more difficult to place.[83,84]

Cuffed dialysis catheters are inserted percutaneously or by surgical cutdown. If surgical cutdown technique is used, hemostasis should be obtained by placing a purse-string suture

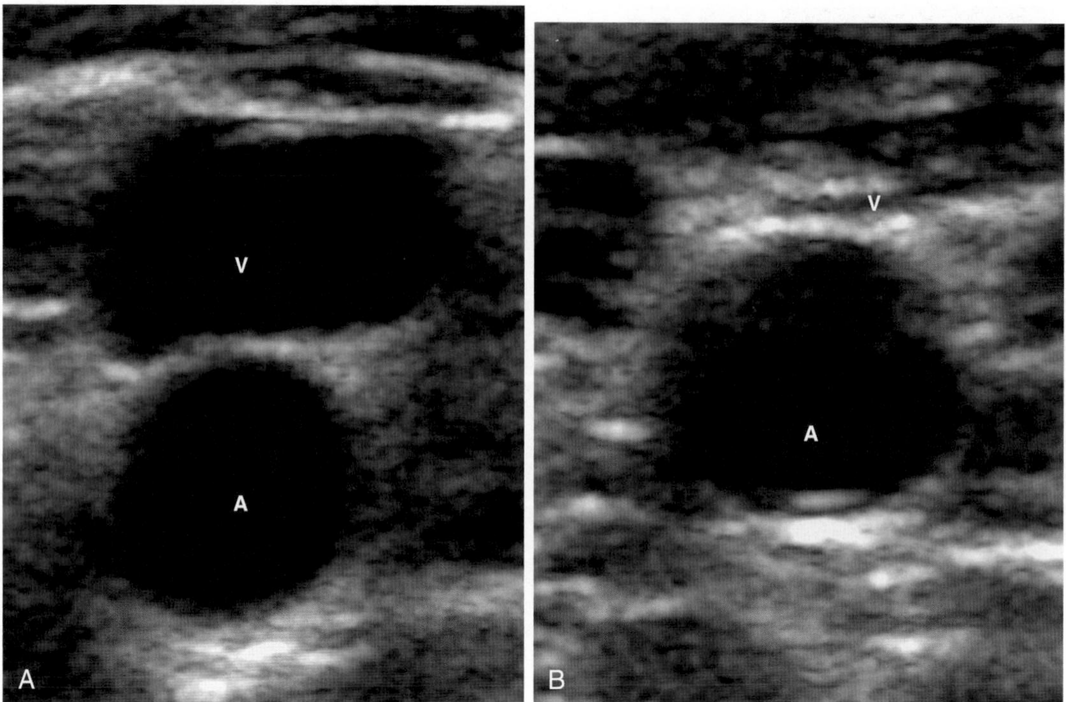

Figure 26-15. Use of the ultrasound to facilitate dialysis catheter placement. **A,** Ultrasound image of the internal jugular vein and carotid artery. **B,** The vessels are differentiated by using the ultrasound probe to compress the neck. The vein flattens with compression.

in the vessel around the catheter rather than placing proximal and distal ligatures, which precludes the future use of the vessel for dialysis access when the catheter is removed. The percutaneous placement of dialysis catheters may be performed blindly using only anatomical landmarks. Although this is the traditional method taught to most surgeons, ultrasound guidance offers significant advantages to blind placement. Patients with end-stage renal disease have often had multiple catheters placed previously, and one or more of the access veins may be thrombosed.[85,86] Thrombosis of the internal jugular, external jugular, and femoral veins are easily identified with ultrasonography. Ultrasonography can also identify variations of the venous anatomy that can occur in 26% to 35% of patients.[87,88] One study showed that ultrasound guidance decreases the number of punctures required, decreases the time required, and improves the success rate of dialysis catheter placement.[89]

The uncuffed dialysis catheters are stiffer than cuffed dialysis catheters. When placed from the jugular or subclavian approach, the tip of the uncuffed catheter should be positioned in the superior vena cava rather than the right atrium to minimize the risk of cardiac perforation. Uncuffed catheters placed in the femoral vein should be left in for no more than 5 days, and the patients should be kept at bed rest.

Insertion of the cuffed dialysis catheters is more technically challenging than that of the uncuffed catheters. To place a cuffed dialysis catheter via the internal jugular vein, the patient's neck and chest are prepped and draped. Intravenous antibiotics are administered preoperatively. Sterile insonation gel is placed on the neck. The ultrasound probe is covered with a sterile sheath and used to visualize the internal jugular vein (Figure 26-15). Local anesthesia is infiltrated over the vein. The ultrasound image is used to guide a large-gauge needle into the vein. A flexible guide wire is inserted through the needle using the Seldinger technique. A 1- to 2-cm incision is placed at the guide wire insertion site in the neck. Another 1-cm incision is placed on the chest in the lateral infraclavicular region. The dialysis catheter is passed through a subcutaneous tunnel from the chest incision to the neck. The tract into the jugular vein is serially dilated over the guide wire, followed by placement of the dilator–introducer complex. The wire and dilator are removed. The catheter is inserted through the introducer sheath, and the sheath is peeled away. Air embolism during the procedure is prevented by maintaining the patient in a "head down" position. The procedure is performed with fluoroscopic guidance to confirm accurate positioning of the catheter tip. Optimal flow rates are obtained with the catheter tip positioned in the right atrium.[74] The course of the catheter must be inspected with fluoroscopy to insure the catheter is not kinked (Figure 26-16). If the catheter is the "stepped tip" design, care must be taken to orient the longer venous limb along the outer curve of the catheter (Table 26-11). Early catheter failure is most often due to technical problems such as kinks in the course of the catheter or catheter tip malposition.[85-90]

Complications of dialysis catheters can be categorized as early or late (Table 26-12). Aside from mechanical failure, the early complications include pneumothorax, arterial puncture or laceration, hematoma, and air embolism. These early complications may be decreased if the catheter is placed using ultrasound guidance.[89]

Infection is one of the most serious late complications and is a primary reason for catheter loss. In a large prospective study, dialysis catheter–related bacteremia occurred once

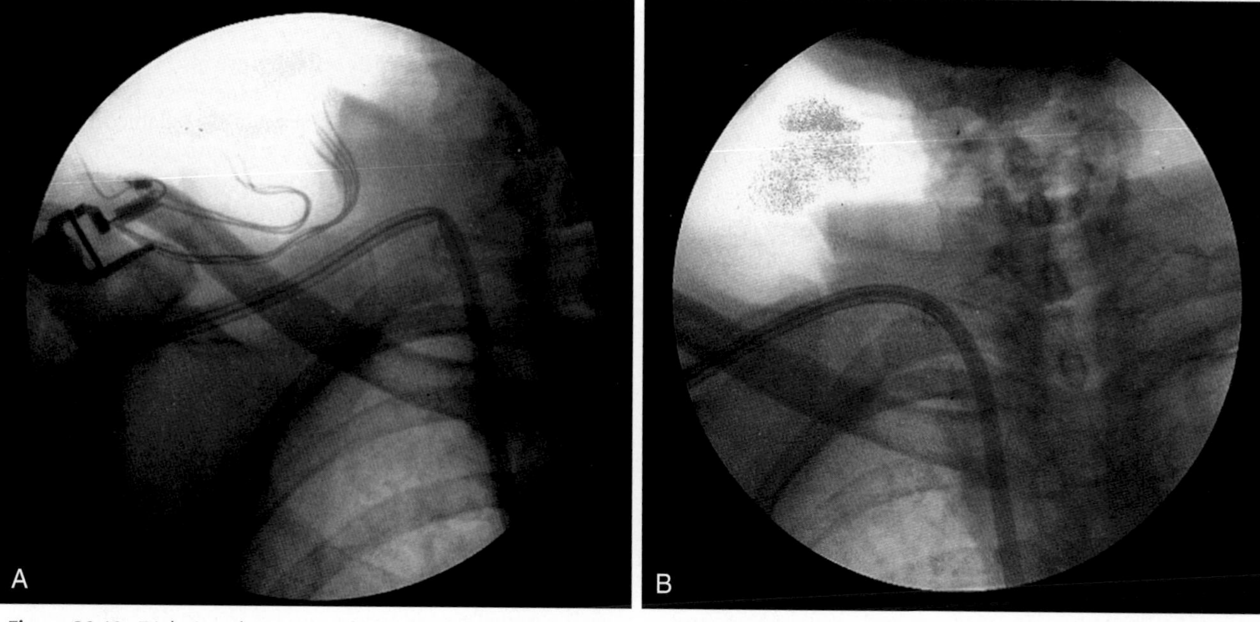

Figure 26-16. Dialysis catheter. **A,** Radiograph of a kinked, tunneled dialysis catheter. **B,** Radiograph of a dialysis catheter tunneled correctly.

every 256 catheter days.[91] Retrospective studies have reported catheter-associated bacteremia rates ranging from 0.72 to 5.5 episodes per 1000 catheter days.[92,93] Catheter infection may present in one of four fashions:

- Exit site infection
- Tunnel infection
- Bacteremia
- Systemic sepsis

The management of each of these is somewhat different.

Exit site infections represent infections between the Dacron cuff and the skin and present with redness, crusting, and an exudate. Blood cultures are negative. Local wound care with topical antibiotics is often sufficient to clear the infection. If the infection fails to respond to local measures, then parenteral antibiotic therapy may be necessary.

Tunnel tract infection and catheter-related bacteremia are more difficult to treat. Intravenous antibiotic therapy alone is associated with a low rate of catheter salvage and a significant incidence of metastatic infection.[94,95] This is probably related to poor antibiotic penetration of the fibrin sheath that forms on the catheter. The definitive treatment for tunnel tract infection and catheter-related bacteremia is catheter removal and intravenous antibiotics. The catheter access site can be salvaged with guide wire exchange of the catheter in patients who rapidly respond to intravenous antibiotics by becoming afebrile and who do not develop other signs of systemic sepsis. All patients treated with catheter exchange require at least 3 weeks of culture directed antibiotic therapy and should be monitored for evidence of recurrent infection.[96] In one report, 83% of these catheter infections were successfully treated with antibiotics and guide wire exchange of the catheter; this is similar to results achieved with catheter removal and subsequent replacement using a new site.[96,97] Catheters with associated erythema and tenderness along the tunnel tract in patients without bacteremia can also undergo guide wire exchange; however, a new tunnel and exit site must be created. The steps of this procedure are as follows:

1. Cut down on the catheter at its insertion in the jugular vein in the neck.
2. Divide the catheter.

Table 26-11
Tips for Tunneled Dialysis Catheter Placement via the Internal Jugular or Subclavian Vein

Venous access is obtained using ultrasound guidance.
The patient is positioned "head down" to prevent air embolism.
The catheter position is confirmed with fluoroscopy at the time of insertion.
The catheter tip is positioned in the right atrium.
The "stepped tip" catheter is oriented with the longer limb (venous limb) along the outer curve.

Table 26-12
Complications of Central Venous Catheterization

Early Complications	Late Complications
Mechanical obstruction of the catheter	Infection
Pneumothorax	Catheter thrombosis
Arterial puncture or laceration	Central venous stenosis or occlusion
Hematoma	Endocarditis or metastatic infection
Hemothorax or hemomediastinum	Catheter fracture or embolization
Thoracic duct injury	Catheter dislodgement
Nerve injury	
Cardiac arrhythmia	
Cardiac perforation	
Air embolism	

3. Remove the subcutaneous catheter and cuff.
4. Cover the old exit site with an occlusive dressing.
5. Tunnel a new catheter through an uninfected field.
6. Insert a guide wire through the central portion of the catheter.
7. Remove the remainder of the old catheter, leaving the guide wire in place.
8. Place the new catheter through the introducer sheath as previously described.

Catheters with tunnel tract involvement and bacteremia should be removed immediately, and intravenous antibiotics should be administered for 3 weeks. A cuffed catheter can be inserted at a new site after the patient has been afebrile for 48 to 72 hours and when blood cultures are negative.[6] Although most catheter infections are caused by gram-positive organisms, gram-negative and mixed flora infections are not uncommon.[93]

Catheter malfunction is a problem associated with dialysis catheters. The catheter patency rate varies widely in the literature and may be affected by the type of catheter placed and its tip configuration.[92,98-100] Retrospective data suggest that catheters with both side and end holes have improved patency rates.[92] Although a randomized, prospective study found improved catheter survival with a "split-tip" compared to a "step-tip" design, others found no difference in survival among three catheter types.[101,102] Evidence is insufficient to support the use of one catheter over another.

Late catheter occlusion is most often caused by thrombus formation within the tip of the catheter or formation of a sleeve of fibrin that envelops the catheter. Thrombus formation may be related to inadequate heparinization of the catheter following use.

A chest radiograph is obtained in patients with catheter occlusion to exclude the possibility of kinking of the catheter or catheter tip malposition. Once excluded, thrombolytic agents have proven beneficial in restoring the patency of occluded catheters. Both urokinase and tissue plasminogen activator (tPA) have been used to restore catheter patency; however, in a blinded, randomized, prospective trial, tPA was superior to urokinase.[103] Several protocols have been used. The usual dose of tPA is 2 mg, which is allowed to dwell in the catheter for 2 hours.[104]

If thrombolysis fails to reestablish catheter patency, radiological stripping of the catheter to remove the pericatheter fibrin sheath may be successful. A nitinol gooseneck snare is introduced through the femoral vein to snare the catheter and strip the sheath. Symptomatic embolization related to catheter stripping is rare. The initial success of this procedure is reported to be 94% to 100%.[85,105] Failure of this method mandates catheter replacement, which often can be accomplished with a guide wire exchange.

Although dialysis catheters provide an invaluable method of access in a difficult group of patients, they are at best a secondary form of access. Efforts should be made to limit the duration of dialysis catheter use by promptly providing patients with a functioning autogenous or nonautogenous AV access.

PEDIATRIC DIALYSIS ACCESS

Every year, 13 children per million of the U.S. population develop chronic renal failure.[106] Although this translates into a relatively small number of children each year who require dialysis access, considerable time and resources are consumed in planning and providing their access. The limited number of pediatric patients with renal failure also means that single institutions rarely have significant experience providing access for children. Thus, few large series are available in the literature that report results of pediatric dialysis access. Those series that are published tend to be single institutional retrospective reviews acquired over many years. Consequently, little level I data is available to guide planning of dialysis access in children.

Children have been successfully dialyzed since the mid-1950s. Initially, children were dialyzed using separate arterial and venous catheters or a single catheter positioned in the inferior vena cava via the saphenous vein. With time, the management of children with chronic renal failure began to more closely parallel that of adults.

The ultimate therapy for a child with chronic renal failure is kidney transplantation. Children who undergo transplantation have fewer hospitalizations, improved quality of life, and improved growth characteristics compared to children who undergo dialysis. Unfortunately, the 5-year transplant graft survival rate is as low as 38% in certain pediatric populations.[106] Thus, many children with transplants ultimately present with failed grafts needing dialysis access.

Peritoneal dialysis is the most common method of dialysis in the pediatric population. It is used in 95% of infants requiring dialysis.[107] Peritoneal dialysis is preferred in the pediatric population for the following reasons:

- A functional peritoneal dialysis access is easier to establish than a hemodialysis access.
- Peritoneal dialysis is more convenient for families who live a long distance from the dialysis center.
- Growth of the child may be superior compared to with hemodialysis.
- School attendance is not interrupted by dialysis center schedules.
- Frequent needle sticks are avoided.
- Fewer fluid and dietary limitations are necessary.[106,108]

Despite these advantages, no data support the physiological superiority of peritoneal dialysis over hemodialysis in the pediatric population.

Peritoneal dialysis is performed using cuffed or noncuffed catheters that are placed surgically or percutaneously within the peritoneal cavity. Noncuffed catheters can be placed percutaneously at the bedside and used immediately. Since they are associated with an increased incidence of infectious and thrombotic complications, the noncuffed catheters are considered only a temporary means for dialysis access. The cuffed dialysis catheters require surgical placement. They have single or double cuffs that are positioned in the subcutaneous tissue of the abdominal wall. The double cuff peritoneal dialysis catheter may have a lower infection rate compared to the single cuff catheter.[109] Several techniques for peritoneal dialysis catheter placement have been described that may affect catheter survival and influence infection rates.[94,110]

Hemodialysis is performed via a central venous dialysis catheter, an autogenous direct AV access, or a nonautogenous AV access. The method of hemodialysis access used is often dictated by the clinical situation and institutional preference. Dialysis catheters are used for hemodialysis access in 60% to 75% of the pediatric patient population.[94,110] These cuffed silastic catheters are placed in the internal jugular, subclavian, or femoral vein percutaneously or by surgical cutdown. If the cutdown method is used, hemostatic control of the vessel is obtained by placing a purse-string suture around the catheter rather than placing ligatures proximal and distal to the vessel puncture site. Avoiding the use of ligatures may maintain vessel patency after catheter removal, potentially preserving a site for future dialysis access. Several series have demonstrated the superiority of the right internal jugular vein for dialysis catheter placement in adults; however, such data are lacking in the pediatric literature.[94] The North American Pediatric Renal Transplant Cooperative Study showed that the subclavian vein was chosen for 77% of percutaneously placed catheters, whereas only 15% of catheters were placed in the jugular vein.[110] Despite the lack of data in the pediatric population regarding catheter site complications, the high incidence of central venous stenosis associated with subclavian venous catheters in adults is a cause for concern and should be considered when planning catheter-based hemodialysis access in children. Infection and thrombosis are the major complications associated with hemodialysis catheters in children.[111] Nearly half of the dialysis catheters placed in the pediatric population become nonfunctional or infected within 1 year. Catheters that provide poor flow rates or occlude may be salvaged with catheter exchange over a guide wire. Infection, manifesting as either exit-site drainage or bacteremia, may be treated initially with antibiotics in stable patients. If the tunnel or exit site is not involved, catheter salvage has been reported with guide wire exchange and intravenous antibiotics.[112]

The autogenous AV access is considered the optimal access for hemodialysis in the pediatric patient population. Originally described for use in adults by Brescia in 1966, the radial–cephalic direct AV access was soon used in the pediatric population.[112a] Although its early use was limited to larger children, modern microsurgical techniques have allowed for the successful creation and use of the access in children who weigh less than 10 kg.[95] Ulnar–basilic direct AV access and radial–basilic transposed AV access procedures have been used in the pediatric population.[113,114] Davis reported 2-year patency rates of 83% for the brachial–basilic transposition AV access in pediatric patients.[115] The same considerations and diagnostic modalities used to select the appropriate hemodialysis access in the adult are employed in the child. The techniques used for AV access placement in the child are the same as those in the adult with two important exceptions: First, AV access creation is facilitated in the pediatric patient through microsurgical techniques using microsurgical instruments and adequate magnification. The AV anastomosis is performed with 8-0 to 10-0 polypropylene suture. Second, to minimize vessel dissection and vasospasm, vascular control is obtained with use of a sterile tourniquet.[116]

The reported patency rates for AV accesses in the pediatric population vary widely and are mostly retrospective reviews of limited series.[108,110,111,113-115] Secondary patency rates as high as 85% at 12 months are reported for autogenous AV accesses.[114] Lerner et al. reported a median survival for autogenous AV accesses of 805 days.[110] The patency rates of autogenous AV accesses in children weighing more than 15 kg was 70% at 48 months in a series reported by Bagolan et al.[116] The patency of autogenous AV accesses in children in Lumsden and colleagues' series, however, was only 6 months, compared to 11 months for prosthetic AV accesses placed in the upper arm.[111]

In conclusion, the pediatric patient presents significant challenges for the surgeon tasked to provide dialysis access. The ultimate goal in all of these patients is renal transplantation. For small children in whom vascular access is more difficult, peritoneal dialysis is advisable. Peritoneal dialysis also affords older children a more normal lifestyle, allowing them to participate more readily in school and other activities. Hemodialysis can be provided with percutaneously or surgically placed catheters; however, infectious and thrombotic complications are common. Ideally, pediatric patients needing hemodialysis should be considered for an autogenous AV access placed as distally as possible in the extremity. If the superficial vasculature is unsuitable for an autogenous AV access, a prosthetic AV access can be placed with acceptable results.

COMPLICATIONS OF AV ACCESS

Thrombosis

Pathophysiology

Thrombosis is the most common complication associated with AV access and is the most common cause for access abandonment. Multiple etiologies exist for access thrombosis, including systemic hypotension, poor arterial inflow, hypercoagulability, access infection, central venous stenosis or occlusion, and external compression of the access. The most common etiology of access thrombosis for both autogenous and prosthetic AV accesses is the development of a venous stenosis. A venous stenosis has been identified after thrombectomy of prosthetic AV accesses in more than 90% of cases.[117] Most venous stenoses that develop in prosthetic AV accesses occur within 1 cm of the venous anastomosis (Figure 26-17).[118] The stenosis is often found more centrally in autogenous AV accesses near areas of vein bifurcation, pressure points, and venous valves.[1] Histopathological examination of the wall of stenotic veins removed from failing dialysis accesses has revealed progressive intimal smooth muscle cell proliferation and extracellular matrix secretion.[119] The etiology for the development of the venous stenosis after access placement is probably related to venous trauma from one or all of the following:

- Compliance mismatch between the prosthetic graft and the vein
- The effect of increased blood pressure in the venous system
- Injury related to the AV anastomosis creation
- Turbulent blood flow within the vein[120]

If fistulography fails to detect a stenosis, another etiology for access thrombosis must be considered. Dialysis personnel and records should be queried to determine whether the thrombotic episode could have been caused by hypotension or excessive postdialysis needle site compression. Recurrent episodes of access thrombosis may also result from an underlying hypercoagulable disorder, including protein C or S deficiency, antithrombin III deficiency, factor V Leiden mutation, and the presence of anticardiolipin antibodies. Patients with these disorders or in whom a cause for access failure cannot be determined are treated with chronic oral anticoagulation.

Treatment AV Access Thrombosis

Historically, treatment of access thrombosis involved abandonment of the access, with placement of a new access in a different anatomical location. This approach, however, quickly exhausts venous sites for hemodialysis. Over time,

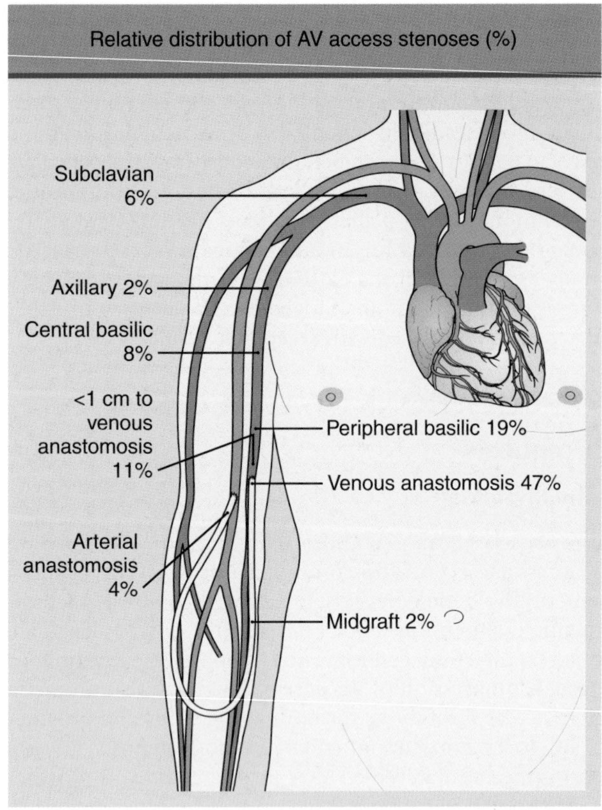

Figure 26-17. Relative distribution of AV access stenoses (%).

both surgical and percutaneous methods have been developed to salvage thrombosed AV accesses. Critical steps in the treatment of a thrombosed AV access include the following:

- Removal of the thrombus from the access
- Fistulography to identify the cause for access failure
- Correction of the underlying access or venous outflow stenosis

Surgical Techniques

Surgical thrombectomy of an AV access is accomplished by exposing a segment of the access and by mechanically removing the thrombus with a Fogarty embolectomy catheter. The technical success of surgical thrombectomy ranges from 82% to 94%.[121-124]

Several elements of the surgical technique are key for prosthetic AV access thrombectomy. First, the incision over the graft should be carefully planned. Since most prosthetic AV access thromboses are caused by the development of a stenosis near the venous anastomosis, the graftotomy should be preferentially made over the venous limb. This position facilitates passage of a wire through a tight venous stenosis if the surgeon elects to treat the stenosis with angioplasty. It also enables the surgeon to easily perform a segmental bypass of a venous stenosis with PTFE. The graftotomy should be made no closer than 2 cm from the venous anastomosis because doing so can prevent clear visualization of a venous anastomotic stenosis on fistulogram. Incisions should never be made over the regions where the access is regularly cannulated because the numerous puncture sites can thwart attempts to close the graftotomy and obtain hemostasis after thrombectomy.

Second, the clot should be carefully inspected for the presence of the arterial plug after thrombectomy of the arterial limb. If the plug is not identified in the clot, it probably has not been completely dislodged and is still in the graft. Every attempt should be made to remove this plug from the graft.

Finally, a complete fistulogram should be obtained in every case, regardless of the quality of the arterial inflow or the venous back bleeding. The fistulogram should clearly visualize the arterial anastomosis, the entire graft, the venous anastomosis, the venous outflow, and central veins. Not only is complete visualization important to adequately treat the immediate cause of access failure, but the information gained is also important in planning future access placement in the extremity.

It may be quite difficult to completely remove clot from an autogenous access that is tortuous or aneurysmal. Consequently, surgical thrombectomy of autogenous AV accesses is thought by many to be a fruitless endeavor. The percutaneous or surgical treatment of these accesses is usually unsuccessful because of an inability to pass either a guide wire or an embolectomy catheter through the access. We recently reported a technique of surgical thrombectomy for autogenous AV accesses that has proven to be successful even for tortuous or aneurysmal accesses. The surgical technique involves the following steps: (1) The fistula is exposed close to the arterial anastomosis. A generous transverse fistulotomy is made within 2 or 3 cm of the arterial anastomosis. This permits the surgeon to remove the arterial plug with forceps under direct vision if it cannot be dislodged with a Fogarty catheter. (2) After arterial inflow is established, a vascular clamp is placed across the access near the anastomosis. (3) The thrombus in the distal access is removed by manually "milking" the thrombus in a retrograde fashion through the fistulotomy. This maneuver requires vigorous manipulation and pressure over the fistula and may require further sedation of the patient during this part of the operation. (4) The embolectomy catheter now usually passes easily up the fistula and can be used to remove any residual thrombus. Fistulography should then be performed to identify and treat the cause for access failure.[125]

Percutaneous Techniques

Several percutaneous techniques have been developed to restore AV access patency. Continuous infusion of thrombolytic agents into the access was used initially; however, the technical success of this method was inferior to surgical thrombectomy, required prolonged infusion times, and was associated with bleeding complications.[126] To shorten infusion times, several methods have been developed to mechanically disrupt the thrombus, thus exposing a greater surface area of thrombus to the thrombolytic agent. These include pharmacomechanical methods of "lacing" the thrombus with a high dose of thrombolytic agent or forcefully injecting it into the thrombus (the "pulse-spray" technique). Others have reported the use of external massage, balloon maceration, and balloon clot displacement to disrupt the thrombus before infusion of the thrombolytic agent. The addition of pharmacomechanical and mechanical methods of thrombus disruption has resulted in much lower infusion times and technical success rates that are equivalent to surgical thrombectomy.[127,128]

More recently, percutaneous techniques have been developed to mechanically remove thrombus from AV accesses without thrombolytic agents. These techniques involve the use of thrombectomy devices that strip or pulverize the thrombus, which can then be aspirated out of the access or flushed into the venous system. Advocates for these devices claim their use avoids the cost and risk associated with thrombolytic agents. The technical success rates reported with these devices are similar to those achieved with surgical thrombectomy and pharmacomechanical thrombolysis.[123,124,129-131]

The basic steps of the percutaneous treatment of AV access thrombosis are as follows:

1. A crossing wire technique is used. A 4-French (Fr) introducer sheath is percutaneously placed into the arterial limb of the prosthetic AV access approximately 3 to 4 cm from the arterial anastomosis. A second 4-Fr introducer sheath is inserted into the venous limb of the prosthetic AV access approximately 3 to 4 cm from the venous anastomosis. Systemic heparin should be administered (Figure 26-18A).
2. Thrombus within the graft is macerated and removed from the graft using one of several mechanical or pharmacomechanical techniques (Figure 26-18B).
3. A fistulogram of the venous anastomosis, venous outflow, and central veins is obtained by injecting contrast through the introducer sheath. Hemodynamically significant stenoses identified by fistulogram should be crossed with a 0.035-inch wire and dilated with a high-pressure, noncompliant angioplasty balloon. If the stenosis is resistant to dilation, alternative percutaneous (use of a cutting balloon or stent) or surgical intervention should be used to treat the stenosis (Figure 26-18C).
4. The thrombus plug at the arterial anastomosis is dislodged using a 4-Fr embolectomy catheter to establish arterial inflow into the graft (Figure 26-18D).
5. A completion fistulogram is obtained. Residual thrombus within the graft is macerated and removed with the embolectomy catheter.

Results of Surgical versus Percutaneous Treatment of AV Access Thrombosis

Since 90% of all access thromboses are associated with a hemodynamically significant stenosis, clot removal alone is inadequate therapy; fistulography and repair of any identified stenosis are mandatory[132] to avoid high early failure rates. Stenoses identified by fistulography can be treated with either surgical revision or balloon angioplasty.

Most studies that report results of balloon angioplasty for AV access stenosis do not stratify patients based on lesion characteristics; however, short-segment and anastomotic stenoses appear to respond better to balloon angioplasty than long-segment stenoses or occlusions.[133]

Intravascular stents have been used to treat access-related stenosis. Several reports have examined the utility of stents for salvage of a failed angioplasty, particularly for lesions with significant elastic recoil. These reports have shown patency rates similar to balloon angioplasty.[134,135] Reports comparing balloon angioplasty alone and balloon angioplasty with stenting as primary treatment of venous stenoses have shown no improvement in patency and increased cost with stenting.[136,137] At present, stenting of access-related stenoses should not routinely be used. Stenting may be helpful if balloon angioplasty has failed and the position of the access is unfavorable for surgical revision, such as an access located in the proximal upper arm.

Comparative outcomes for the surgical and percutaneous treatment of thrombosed prosthetic AV accesses have been evaluated by several studies (Table 26-13).[121,124,129,131,133,138-140] A recent metaanalysis of prospective trials comparing patency rates of surgical thrombectomy and percutaneous treatment of AV access thrombosis demonstrated the superiority of surgery at all time periods.[141] However, based on the conflicting results obtained from these studies, the 2006 updated DOQI guidelines concluded that a clear difference between the two treatments has not been established and both the surgical and the percutaneous techniques are effective for the treatment of thrombosed AV accesses.[6] Therefore, a major consideration regarding treatment selection should be based on which intervention can be performed the most expeditiously, since a delay can result in unnecessary hospitalization and a need for temporary dialysis catheter placement.

Proponents of the percutaneous methods for the management of AV access thrombosis emphasize that these techniques are less invasive than surgical thrombectomy and revision. The procedures are performed on an outpatient basis in the radiology suite, which is often more accessible than the operating room. Since the percutaneous methods treat the stenosis with dilatation rather than bypass, vein is preserved for future access revision or new AV access placement. A potential risk of percutaneous intervention, particularly for the mechanical thrombectomy techniques, is the embolism of disrupted thrombus into the pulmonary circulation. Lung perfusion scans after percutaneous thrombectomy have shown that a high percentage of these patients have detectable emboli.[142] Although fatal pulmonary emboli have been reported, most are not clinically significant and their relevance is unclear.[142,143] It has been out practice to surgically revise those accesses that fail balloon angioplasty early or those that have long-segment venous stenoses or occlusions that do not respond well to balloon angioplasty.

Infection

Background

Access infection accounts for 20% of all hemodialysis-related complications and is a major cause of morbidity and mortality in the dialysis patient population. It results in up to 10% of all deaths in these patients, ranking second only to cardiovascular disease as the most common cause of death.[144]

Multiple systemic and local factors are responsible for this high incidence of infection. The adverse effects of uremia and chronic renal failure on the immune system are well documented. Studies have demonstrated decreased phagocytosis and cellular killing by polymorphonuclear cells and inhibited lymphocyte transformation in patients with chronic renal failure.[145,146]

Access infections in the immediate postoperative period are most often caused by a break-in sterile technique that leads to bacterial seeding of the graft. An infection remote from the surgical site can also lead to early graft seeding. Meticulous intraoperative technique and use of prophylactic antibiotics have reduced the incidence of early graft infection to less than 4%.[147]

Wounds heal poorly in patients on chronic hemodialysis. In the setting of a recent access placement, poor healing can lead to wound breakdown and graft exposure. Excessive edema can also lead to breakdown of incisions, as well as blistering and cellulitis. Seroma or hematoma increase the potential for postoperative wound and graft infection.

Infections that develop after initial wound healing and graft incorporation are usually related to local graft manipulation, in particular to recurrent needle cannulation. Puncture of the skin during access cannulation is a potential source of bacterial introduction. Poor hemostasis following needle removal can lead to hematoma or pseudoaneurysm formation and subsequent infection. Access thrombectomy or revision also presents an opportunity for graft contamination and infection.

Most vascular access infections are caused by bacteria that comprise normal skin flora. *Staphylococcus aureus* is the most common pathogen cultured from infected AV access wounds. The high rate of *S. aureus* infections may be partly due to skin colonization, which has been reported in 60% of the patients on chronic hemodialysis, as well as in 30% of the dialysis staff. These figures compare to a colonization rate of 10% to 14% in the general population.[148]

The AV access method and location play a significant role in the incidence of access infection. The incidence of infection ranges between 0% and 5% for autogenous AV accesses and between 6% and 35% for nonautogenous AV accesses.[21-26,33,34] Accesses located in the thigh are associated with a higher rate of infection than those located in the upper extremity or chest wall.[32-34]

An infected dialysis access can present with various signs and symptoms. Local signs of infection include erythema, warmth, and tenderness over the access. Autogenous AV accesses tend to manifest infection only as cellulitis, whereas nonautogenous AV accesses usually present with perigraft fluid, fluctuance over the graft, or a draining sinus. *Staphylococcus epidermidis* may cause a chronic, indolent graft infection. Patients with *S. epidermidis* graft infections present with perigraft fluid or anastomotic pseudoaneurysms and may otherwise exhibit no manifestations of infection. Access infection may also be complicated by the development of distant sites of infection or systemic sepsis syndrome. Endocarditis, osteomyelitis, septic arthritis, and septic pulmonary emboli have all been reported in conjunction with AV access infection.[149]

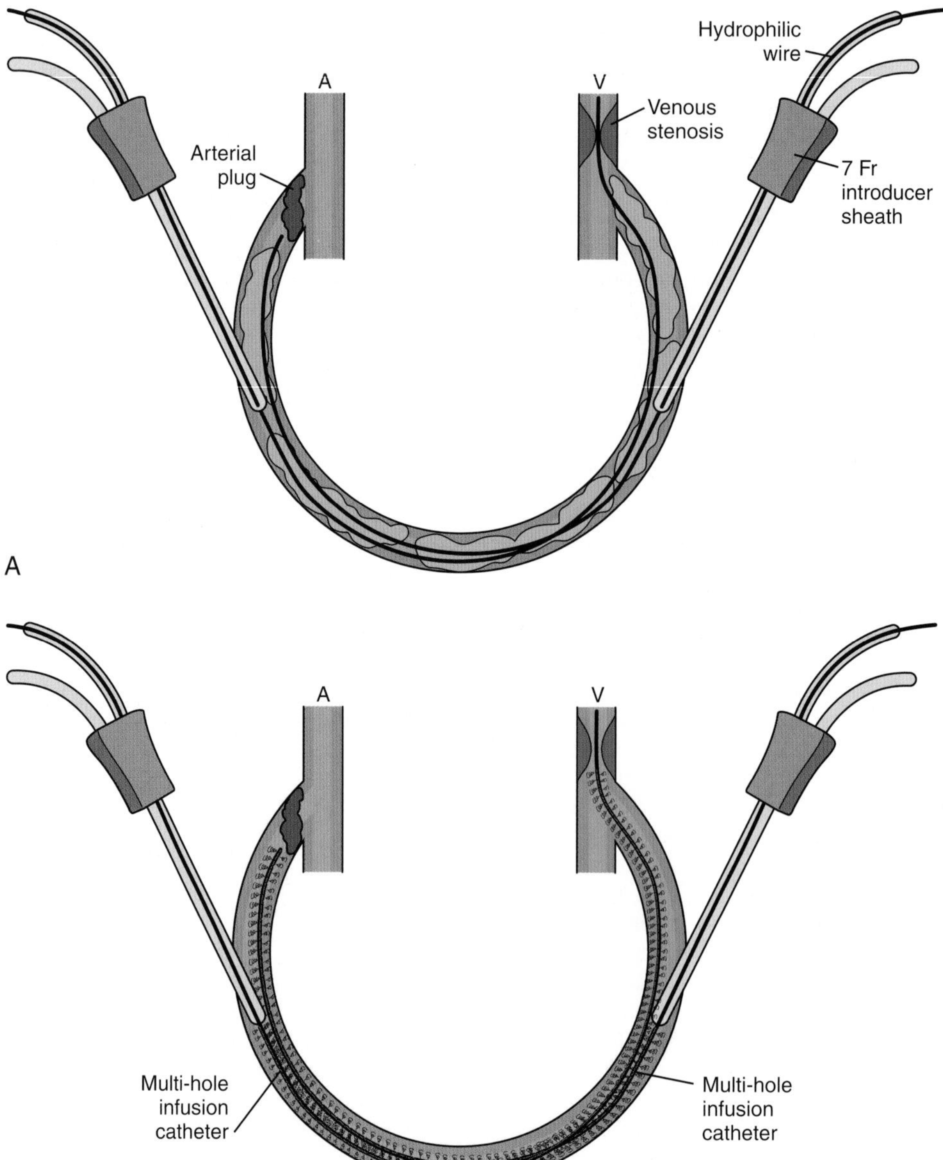

Figure 26-18. Percutaneous treatment of AV access thrombosis. Crossing wire technique. **A,** The 4-Fr introducer sheaths are inserted into the arterial and venous limbs of the prosthetic AV access. **B,** Pharmacomechanical lysis of the thrombus is performed by forcefully injecting a high-dose thrombolytic agent into the graft through a multihole infusion catheter (pulse-spray technique; shown) or macerating the thrombus with an embolectomy balloon catheter.

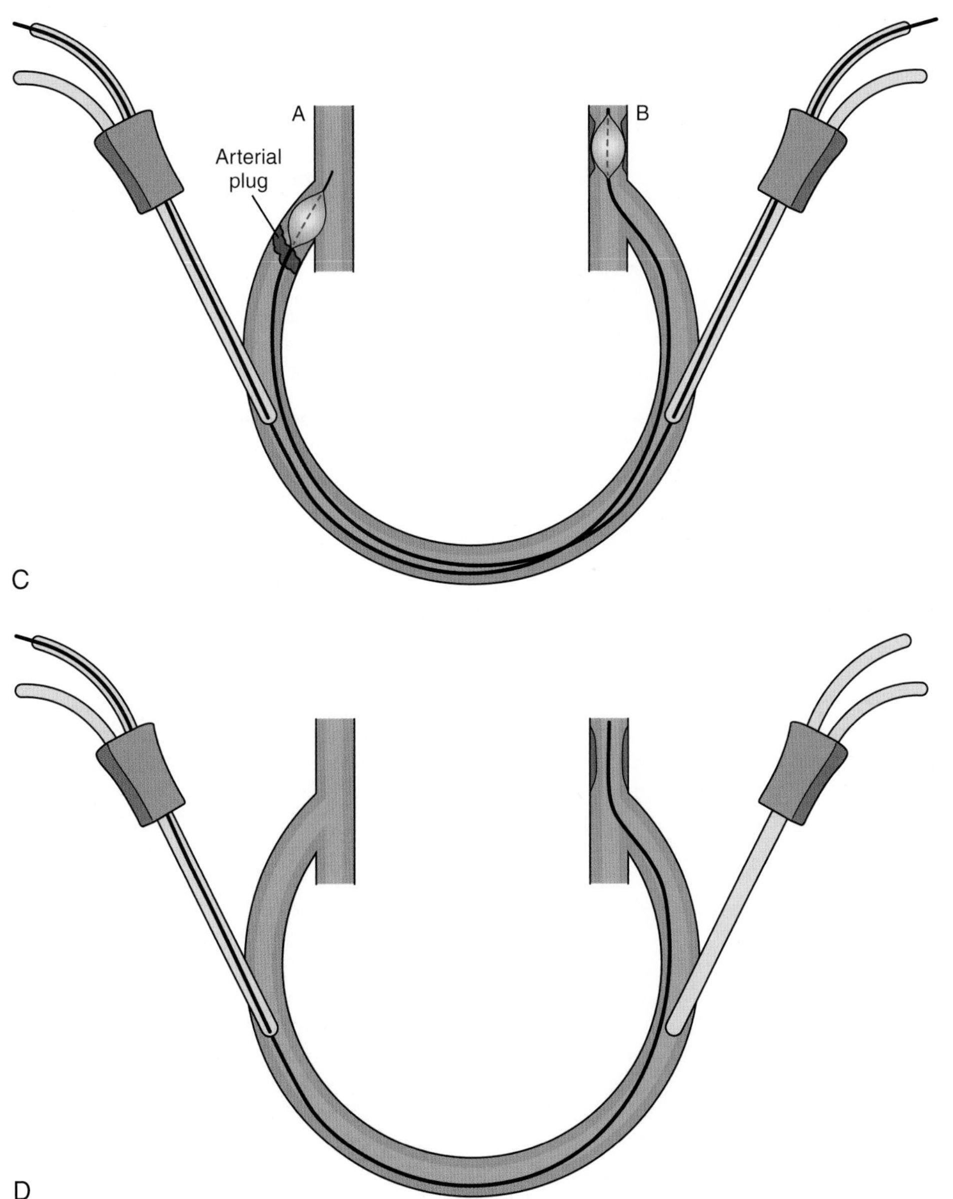

Figure 26-18—cont'd, C, A fistulogram is obtained. Stenoses that are identified by fistulography are angioplastied using a high-pressure, noncompliant angioplasty balloon. **D,** The thrombus plug at the arterial anastomosis is dislodged using a 4-Fr embolectomy catheter. A completion fistulogram is obtained.

The diagnosis of access-related infections relies heavily on clinical judgment. Blood cultures or local fluid cultures are obtained to determine responsible pathogens and to confirm the success of treatment. Cultures are often negative, particularly if antibiotics are started before blood cultures are obtained. Once a treatment course has been completed, blood cultures should be repeated because a continued positive culture is highly predictive of infection recurrence.[144] Duplex ultrasonography of the access can identify findings suggestive of access infection, such as perigraft fluid or pseudoaneurysm.

Treatment

Treatment of access-related infection begins with antibiotics. Due to the high percentage of cultures that are positive for methicillin-resistant *S. aureus,* most authors recommend empirical vancomycin therapy.[144,148] An antibiotic effective against gram-negative organisms is also added initially. Once cultures return, antibiotic therapy is tailored appropriately. If no gram-positive organisms are present or if methicillin-sensitive organisms are found, the vancomycin should be stopped to minimize development of resistant organisms. The optimal duration of antibiotic therapy is not well defined by the literature, and recommendations vary depending on the extent of infection.

Autogenous AV access infections usually present with cellulitis that can be effectively treated with antibiotics alone. Infected pseudoaneurysms or abscesses that directly involve the vein require ligation or segmental bypass of the access.

Nonautogenous AV access infection may be localized to a segment of the graft or may involve the entire graft. Graft removal offers the best chance for complete eradication of the infection; however, since sites for vascular access are limited, the decision to remove an infected access requires careful consideration. Early graft infection that develops before tissue ingrowth has occurred usually involves the entire graft, and treatment mandates complete graft excision.

Table 26-13
Results of Treatment for Failing and Failed AV Access

Study	Study Design	Indication	Access Type	Method	N	Tech Success (%)	Primary Patency (%) 1 Month	6 Months	12 Months
Schwartz et al.[121]	Retrospective	Thrombosis	Prosthetic	Surg T/Rev	24	87	60	30	13
Dougherty et al.[138]	Prospective/rand	Thrombosis	Prosthetic	Surg T/Rev	41	—	—	—	26
				PMT/BA	39	—	—	—	14
Marston et al.[124]	Prospective/rand	Thrombosis	Prosthetic	Surg T/Rev	56	82	61	34	24
				PMT/BA	59	71	44	11	9
Trerotola et al.[129]	Retrospective	Thrombosis	Prosthetic	MT/BA	34	94	56	20	0
Overbosch et al.[131]	Retrospective	Thrombosis	Prosthetic/autogenous	MT/BA	65	89	71	36	—
Brooks et al.[139]	Prospective/rand	Malfunction	Prosthetic	Surg Rev	19	—	—	68	62
				PTA	24	—	—	34	24
Lumsden et al.[140]	Retrospective	Malfunction	Prosthetic	PTA	40	—	76	27	10
Beathard[133]	Retrospective	Malfunction	Prosthetic/autogenous	PTA	285	—	91	61	38

MT/BA, percutaneous mechanical thrombectomy/balloon angioplasty; PMT/BA, pharmacomechanical thrombectomy/balloon angioplasty; PTA, percutaneous transluminal angioplasty; rand, randomized; Surg Rev, surgical revision; Surg T/Rev, surgical thrombectomy/revision.

Successful graft salvage of localized infections with incision and drainage, long-term antibiotics, and wound packing has been reported.[150] This treatment modality may result in wound contraction and fixation of the graft at or above skin level that precludes any chance for wound epithelialization and long-term cure. Coverage of exposed AV graft segments has been achieved with skin or muscle flaps.[151,152] These techniques are reported as isolated cases, with no large series.

Another treatment for localized graft infection is segmental bypass and partial graft excision. The procedure is performed by making a cutdown on the graft proximal and distal to the infected graft segment at sites that appear remote from the infection. The graft at each of these sites is assessed for infection. If the graft is unincorporated or if perigraft fluid is present at either of these sites, the graft is excised. If the graft is well incorporated and does not appear infected, it is divided and the ends of the infected graft segment and tunnel are oversewn. Graft continuity is restored with an interposition graft that is tunneled through clean tissue planes around the infected graft segment. The interposition graft is sewn end to end to the old graft. The incisions are closed and covered with an occlusive dressing. The infected graft segment is excised, and the open wound is packed. If an adequate length of the initial graft remains to allow cannulation away from the new graft segment, the graft can be used immediately (Figure 26-19). Schwab et al. reviewed 17 patients treated with this technique and reported a 94% late graft salvage rate, with no perioperative deaths and no major morbidity.[153]

Aneurysm and Pseudoaneurysm

Long-term AV access use can be complicated by formation of pseudoaneurysms. Less commonly, true aneurysmal dilation of the access can occur. Pseudoaneurysm formation is most often due to poor access cannulation technique, either from repeated needle sticks in a limited area of the access or from poor hemostasis after needle removal. Although little scientific evidence supports it, prosthetic AV accesses are generally not cannulated for 2 weeks after placement to minimize the risk for pseudoaneurysm formation due to lack of graft incorporation into the surrounding soft tissue.

Infection may either be a primary cause for development of an AV access pseudoaneurysm or occur later as a secondary event. Distinguishing between a sterile and an infected pseudoaneurysm can be difficult as the local effects of a pseudoaneurysm on skin temperature and color can mimic changes secondary to infection. Other complications of aneurysms include thrombosis and rupture.

Most small, asymptomatic aneurysms do not require treatment. Treatment becomes mandatory for large aneurysms that appear at risk for rupture and for aneurysms complicated by thrombosis or infection. If the skin overlying an aneurysm becomes ulcerated or ischemic, surgical revision or ligation of the access is indicated. Sterile pseudoaneurysms of a prosthetic AV access can be locally excised, and the graft can be repaired. Multiple, close pseudoaneurysms may require partial graft excision and interposition bypass. Infected pseudoaneurysms can be treated with segmental bypass and partial excision, as described previously, with good result.[153] There have been case reports and small series of percutaneously placed stent grafts across sterile pseudoaneurysms.[154-157] Reported results of this approach have been mixed. At present, open repair remains the primary treatment.

High-Output Congestive Heart Failure

An AV access can have marked effects on the cardiovascular system. The establishment of a high-flow connection between the arterial and the venous systems causes an immediate and significant drop in peripheral arterial resistance. To maintain blood pressure, cardiac output rises due to increased heart rate and stroke volume. Although this response is well tolerated in most patients, congestive heart failure may occur in patients who have poor cardiac reserve. Today's dialysis machines require flow rates up to 600 ml/min. Flow rates in this range rarely cause cardiac failure except in the patient with minimal

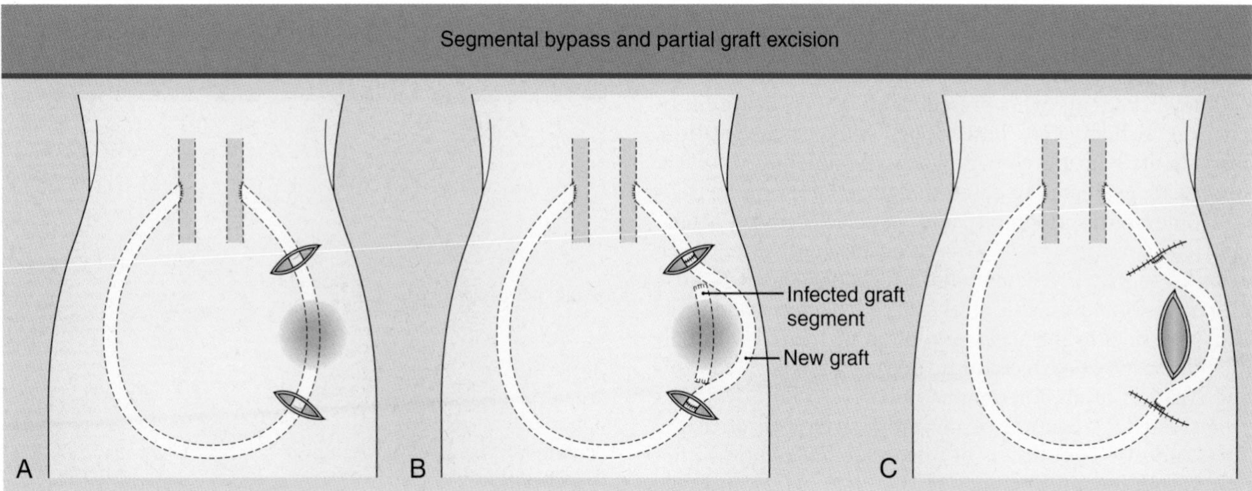

Figure 26-19. Technique of segmental bypass and partial graft excision for localized prosthetic AV access infection. **A,** The graft is exposed proximal and distal to the infected graft segment at sites remote from the infection. **B,** The ends of the infected graft segment and tunnel are oversewn. A graft is tunneled through clean tissue planes around the infected graft segment and sewn end to end to the old graft. **C,** The incisions are closed and dressed. The infected graft segment is excised, and the open wound is packed.

cardiac reserve. AV access flow rates in excess of 1000 ml/min are generally required for cardiac failure to ensue. Such high flow rates are more commonly encountered when the larger vessels of the upper arm or proximal thigh are used for AV access, rather than the smaller vessels of the forearm.

Since congestive heart failure related to volume overload, anemia, severe hypertension, and cardiac dysfunction occurs often in the dialysis patient population, the role of the AV access is often overlooked as a potential cause of congestive heart failure. By recognizing those patients at risk for development of access-related congestive heart failure and using appropriate diagnostic maneuvers and testing, the clinician can identify those patients who may benefit from correction or removal of the access.

Decreased cardiac reserve must be present to develop symptoms. Patients at risk include those with coronary artery disease, severe hypertension, and hypertrophic cardiomyopathy.[158] Systemic hypertension may increase flow through the low-resistance access and exacerbate the stress on the heart.

Diagnosis requires documentation of a drop in cardiac output with fistula compression. In patients with congestive heart failure secondary to an AV access, the precompression volume of flow through the access is usually greater than the subsequent drop in cardiac output with compression of the access.[158]

Although ligation of the access is the most definitive treatment, there are reports of successful treatment of access-related congestive heart failure with banding or narrowing of the access, which reduces AV shunting.[159] Flow through the access can be assessed as it is narrowed. The goal is to decrease the flow rate to less than 1000 ml/min, as measured by intraoperative or postoperative duplex examination.

Ischemic Steal Syndrome

Symptomatic extremity ischemia after creation of an AV access is uncommon. This complication more often occurs with accesses that are located in the proximal extremity, such as the upper arm or thigh. It is also more commonly seen with prosthetic than autogenous AV accesses. Patients with diabetes mellitus who have atherosclerotic occlusive disease are especially susceptible to access-related ischemia.

Steal syndrome is caused by a drop in distal extremity perfusion pressure resulting from creation of a proximal low-resistance AV shunt. The difference in resistance between the shunt and the runoff bed can cause reversal of flow in the native artery distal to the access that shunts blood away from the distal extremity. In patients who have adequate flow through collaterals, this flow reversal does not result in the development of symptomatic steal. Physiological steal (reduced digital blood flow) can be detected by vascular laboratory studies in approximately 80% of patients following construction of an AV access. Most patients remain asymptomatic due to compensatory flow via collaterals and distal vasodilation. In patients with vascular occlusive disease or in those patients in whom the access flow rate is high, collateral flow can be inadequate to compensate and signs and symptoms of limb ischemia may ensue. Reversal of blood flow does not necessarily result in symptoms, as studies have shown that clinically silent retrograde flow occurs in up to 67% of autogenous radial–cephalic AV accesses and in 86% of prosthetic upper arm AV accesses.[160] Ischemia can occur without flow reversal as well, especially in cases of severe peripheral occlusive disease and from embolic events. Flow reversal by itself is therefore neither necessary nor sufficient to cause access-induced ischemia. Patients with ISS may present with various symptoms, ranging from hand coolness or paresthesias that occur only during dialysis to severe ischemia with tissue necrosis. Patients may complain of pain, stiffness, or swelling of the fingers or hand weakness. On examination, the fingers may be cool, with delayed capillary refill and decreased sensation. The radial pulse is usually absent. Compression of the access may result in relief of symptoms and return of a radial pulse and is diagnostic of access-induced ISS. Objective documentation of the presence and severity of steal can be obtained in the vascular laboratory by demonstrating flat or low pulsatility digital waveforms and reduced digital artery pressures that augment significantly with access compression.

Treatment of ISS is based on the anatomy and symptom severity. Mild symptoms that occur early after access placement are observed and treated conservatively. Most resolve with time.[161] Patients who present with severe, acute limb-threatening ischemia are best treated with access ligation. Those patients who develop progressive moderate to severe symptoms are evaluated to determine the etiology of the ischemia. Duplex ultrasonography and, in selected cases, arteriography can identify inflow arterial occlusive disease, which contributes to distal ischemia after access placement in 20% to 30% of cases.[162] Ischemic steal caused by an arterial inflow stenosis proximal to the access can often be treated with balloon angioplasty, endarterectomy, or arterial bypass. ISS following creation of an autogenous radial–cephalic AV access may be treated by ligation of the radial artery distal to the AV anastomosis. The success of this treatment requires normal arterial inflow and patency of the ulnar artery and palmar arch; it should not be used in patients who rely solely on the radial artery for hand perfusion. Various techniques have been developed for the prevention or treatment of ISS by attempting to increase flow resistance in the AV access to increase distal arterial perfusion. Access banding, plication, and tapered interposition grafts have all been used to increase the flow resistance through the access.[161,163,164] This treatment approach has met with limited success. It is difficult to objectively determine intraoperatively the degree of graft narrowing necessary to relieve symptoms of hand ischemia while simultaneously maintaining sufficient flow to ensure continued access patency.[165] An alternative method for treating access-related vascular steal is the distal revascularization with interval ligation procedure first described by Schanzer et al.[166] The procedure increases collateral circulation to the ischemic limb by the creation of a large-caliber, low-resistance bypass from the artery proximal to the AV access to the artery distal to the access. To prevent retrograde arterial flow, the native artery is ligated between the access and the distal anastomosis of the bypass (Figure 26-20). This procedure has been effective in relieving symptoms of limb ischemia in more than 90% of patients with access-related ISS.[161,167,168] Recently, several alternative bypass procedures conceptually similar to the distal revascularization with interval ligation procedure have been described. Although the reported early outcomes look promising, experience with these procedures is limited.[169,170]

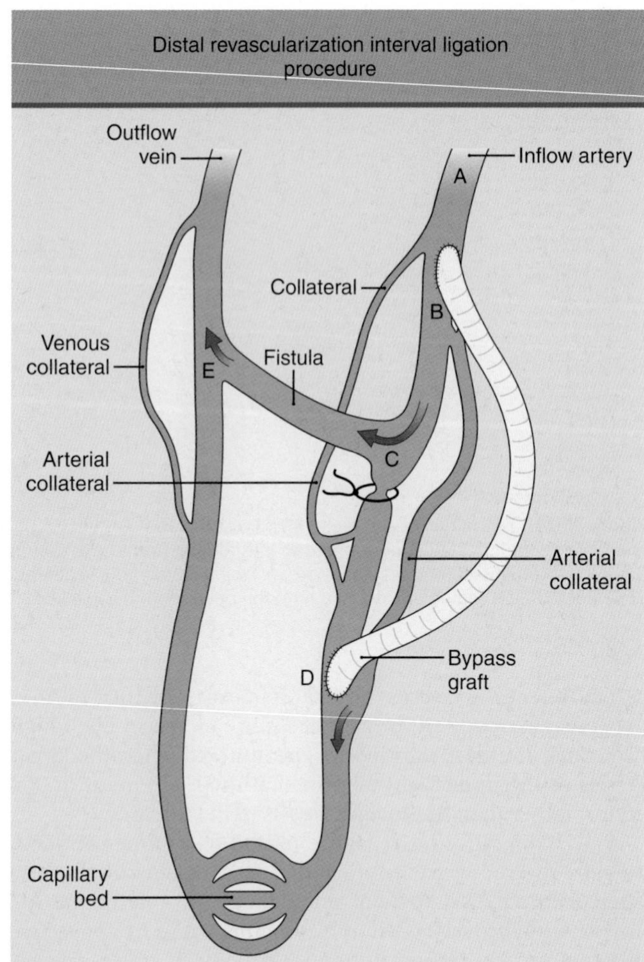

Figure 26-20. Technique of distal revascularization interval ligation. A critical component of technical success is the location of the bypass origin in relation to the origin of the access. This distance should be at least 3 cm. A ligature is placed around the artery just distal to the access to prevent retrograde flow.

Peripheral Neuropathy

Placement of a vascular access can lead to peripheral neuropathy. The etiology for this complication is multifactorial and includes ischemia, venous hypertension, and local compression. As with ischemic complications, the presenting symptoms can vary widely. The diagnosis and treatment depend on the severity of symptoms and the underlying causative factors.

Ischemic Monomelic Neuropathy

Ischemic monomelic neuropathy (IMN) is characterized by pain, weakness, and paralysis of the muscles of the forearm and hand that develops minutes to hours after placement of an antecubital AV access. Sensory loss may also be present. In contrast to access-related ISS, which results in global ischemia of the distal extremity, IMN results in isolated neural ischemia and develops in the immediate postoperative period. It is probably caused by nerve ischemia in the vascular "watershed area" for the radial, ulnar, and median nerves at the antecubital fossa.

IMN is a rare complication of AV access creation, although the actual incidence is probably underreported in the literature.[171] Patients at risk are older and almost exclusively have diabetes mellitus. Patients who have preexisting peripheral neuropathy and peripheral vascular disease are prone to this complication. It only occurs with accesses placed at the antecubital position.

The classic presentation of IMN is the development of weakness of all or most muscles of the forearm and hand, paresthesias, and numbness along the distribution of the radial, ulnar, and median nerves. Usually, minimal findings of distal limb ischemia occur. Generally, the hand is warm and a radial pulse is present. Objective examination of distal perfusion generally reveals a digital pressure greater than 50 mm Hg and a digital–brachial index greater than 0.3. Nerve conduction studies show axonal loss and reduced motor and sensory nerve conduction velocities of the radial, ulnar, and median nerves.[172]

Table 26-14
Methods of Access Surveillance: Advantages and Disadvantages

Methods	Advantages	Disadvantages
Flow rate measurement	• Most predictive of access failure • Serial measurements obtainable	• Not available at all institutions • Duplex methods not performed in dialysis unit and requires experienced technologist
Venous pressure measurement	• Performed in the dialysis unit • Inexpensive • Serial measurements easily obtained	• Unable to detect inflow and in-graft stenosis • Significant overlap between venous pressures obtained in failing and normal grafts
Urea recirculation measurement	• Serial measurements easily obtained • Performed in the dialysis unit	• Relatively late predictor access dysfunction • Threshold value for intervention is not well defined
Duplex ultrasonography	• Accurate in identifying more than 50% stenosis • Serial measurements easily obtained	• Duplex methods not performed in a lysis unit and requires experienced technologist • Not shown to reliably predict access failure

Treatment requires immediate access ligation, with restoration of distal perfusion. Even with prompt action, neurological deficits may not be reversible.[172,173] Due to the low incidence of IMN, and because many of the symptoms are confused with routine postoperative complaints, the diagnosis of IMN is often delayed. The routine performance of a thorough neurological examination in the perioperative period may distinguish those patients with localized pain or single nerve dysfunction due to edema or compression from those patients with IMN.

Local Compression and Carpal Tunnel Syndrome

A postoperative fluid collection, such as a seroma, hematoma, or abscess, can cause nerve compression and result in neuropathy. Motor and sensory deficits in the distribution of a single nerve combined with the presence of a local fluid collection adjacent to the nerve make it straightforward to distinguish this entity from IMN or vascular steal. The treatment is decompression of the space-occupying fluid collection. If the diagnosis is established and the nerve is decompressed promptly, full recovery of neurological function is likely.

A pathological entity that has been described but is not fully understood is access-related carpal tunnel syndrome. Multiple causes for the syndrome have been proposed, including elevated venous pressure, steal leading to ischemia of the median nerve, and thickening of the flexor synovium. The diagnosis can be confirmed by demonstrating decreased median nerve conduction velocities across the carpal ligament. Successful treatment of the syndrome has been reported with release of the carpal ligament.[173]

SURVEILLANCE OF AV ACCESS

The DOQI Clinical Practice Guidelines for Vascular Access recommend that an organized monitoring and surveillance program for AV accesses be established to detect AV access dysfunction and that the program include an evaluation of each AV access at least monthly.[6] The rationale for this recommendation is based on the following facts and underlying assumptions:

- Most access thromboses are associated with the development of a venous stenosis.
- AV access thrombosis is associated with significant morbidity and cost.
- If the underlying cause for AV access dysfunction can be identified and corrected before thrombosis, the AV access thrombosis rate, patient morbidity, and cost will be reduced and AV access longevity will be increased.

Although this concept intuitively makes sense, the success of a surveillance program in increasing AV access longevity and reducing the morbidity and cost of AV access failure has not verified by the literature.

Physical findings such as extremity edema, prolonged bleeding at the needle puncture site, and changes in the characteristics of the access thrill can be helpful in predicting access dysfunction and should prompt a fistulogram to detect a significant AV access stenosis. However, the DOQI guidelines also recommend the use of more objective screening methods to identify hemodynamically significant stenosis. The advantages and disadvantages of the available methods of surveillance are shown in Table 26-14.

Although low-access blood flow rates or a downward trend in flow rates appears to be the preferred method for access surveillance, a metaanalysis of 12 studies that evaluated blood flow nor the rate as a predictor of prosthetic AV access thrombosis showed that neither the blood flow rate or a change in blood flow rate provided adequate sensitivity and specificity to be useful as a screening test.[174] In another study that evaluated the performance of blood flow monitoring and both static and dynamic venous pressure monitoring in 71 dialysis patients with PTFE AV accesses, pressure measurements were not predictive of graft failure and receiver operating curve analysis showed poor performance of graft flows in predicting graft failure. The authors concluded, "the lack of sensitivity and specificity makes clinical decision making based on results of graft blood flows alone difficult."[175]

Color flow duplex ultrasonography has been used as a screening tool to identify hemodynamically significant access stenosis. Studies that have correlated color flow duplex ultrasonography with angiography have demonstrated it to be accurate in identifying hemodynamically significant AV access stenoses.[140,176] It has not been conclusively shown, however, that prophylactic intervention on prosthetic AV accesses with a stenosis identified with duplex ultrasonography extend access function. Lumsden et al. found no difference in long-term patency rates between treatment and observation groups of patients shown to have greater than 50% stenosis in functioning PTFE grafts[140]; however, none of the grafts in this study had any prior evidence of dysfunction. Therefore, the significance of a stenosis identified with duplex ultrasonography or angiography without associated evidence of access dysfunction, such as decreasing graft flow rates, elevated venous pressures, or prolonged needle-puncture bleeding, remains unclear.

Although the latest DOQI guidelines recommend that a surveillance program for AV accesses be established and that hemodynamically significant stenoses identified by fistulography be treated, the literature suggests that the available methods of access monitoring lack the sensitivity and specificity necessary to both identify accesses at risk for thrombosis and minimize unnecessary interventions. Although there is no debate that access thrombosis is associated with significant morbidity and expense, the cost effectiveness of routine access surveillance with the existing monitoring techniques has not been established.

SUMMARY

The substantial cost and morbidity associated with the maintenance of hemodialysis access will continue to stimulate the efforts of industry, managed care providers, and researchers to solve the vexing problem of AV access failure. Population-based studies show reduced morbidity associated with autogenous AV accesses and significant regional variations in autogenous access utilization are likely. Such studies prompt government and managed care providers to exert pressure to increase their placement. The DOQI guideline goal stating that 65% of patients starting dialysis have an autogenous access placed will likely be used by the centers for Medicare services and by managed care providers as a quality benchmark for vascular access.

Further work is needed to define the role of AV access surveillance. Methods that directly measure AV access blood flow seem to hold the greatest promise. However, the cost effectiveness of implementing a surveillance program for the entire dialysis population has yet to be established. Although surveillance can detect AV access stenosis and can significantly improve access patency, this improved patency is obtained at the cost of many additional procedures. Perhaps the cost effectiveness of surveillance will be achieved by developing methods of identifying and surveying only those patients at greatest risk for AV access failure.

Industry continues to modify the structure and configuration of PTFE and to develop new biomaterials for AV access use in an attempt to create the ideal conduit. The limitations of available prosthetic conduits are as follows:

- A susceptibility to infection
- An inability to cannulate the access immediately after implantation
- A propensity for development of stenosis at or near the venous anastomosis

The development of new biomaterials that have improved perigraft tissue ingrowth, perhaps with concomitant advances in gene therapy, and the use of vascular endothelial growth factors may result in methods to increase graft endothelialization, thereby reducing access infection and stenosis.

Recent innovations that reduce stent restenosis following coronary angioplasty are being investigated to determine whether they are effective in blocking the venous hyperplastic response responsible for 80% to 90% of AV access thromboses. Rapamycin, a macrolide antibiotic, and paclitaxel, a new class of anticancer agent, have been shown to inhibit vascular smooth muscle cell proliferation and migration. These drugs can be bonded to vascular stents. These drug-eluting stents have been somewhat effective in preventing the restenosis associated with standard coronary angioplasty and stenting. Trials are under way to determine whether the drug-eluting stents will prevent the venous stenosis associated with AV access. Although the results that have been achieved thus far in the coronary circulation with this modality are a cause for optimism, the pathophysiology associated with myointimal hyperplasia in the coronary arteries following angioplasty is quite different from that associated with AV accesses. The stimulus to smooth muscle cell proliferation is presumably over after the initial injury with coronary balloon angioplasty, whereas the stimulus to smooth muscle cell proliferation in AV accesses is ongoing. It remains to be seen whether these innovative technologies that have shown promise in the coronary circulation will result in enhanced survival of AV accesses.

References

1. National Kidney Foundation. NKF/DOQI clinical practice guidelines for vascular access, 2000. *Am J Kidney Dis* 2001;37(Suppl 1):S137-S181.
2. U.S. Renal Data System USRDS 1997 annual data report. X. The economic cost of ESRD vascular access procedures and Medicare spending for alternative modalities of treatment. *Am J Kidney Dis* 1997;30:S160-S177.
3. U.S. Renal Data System. USRDS 2002 annual data report: atlas of chronic kidney disease and end-stage renal disease in the United States. Bethesda, Maryland: National Institutes of Health, National Institute of Diabetes and Digestive and Kidney Diseases; 2002.
4. Malovrh M. Native arteriovenous fistula: preoperative evaluation. *Am J Kidney Dis* 2002;39:1218-1225.
5. Silva Jr MB, Hobson II RW, Pappas PJ, et al. A strategy for increasing use of hemodialysis access procedures: impact of preoperative noninvasive evaluation. *J Vasc Surg* 1998;27:302-308.
6. Vascular Access Work Group. Clinical practice guidelines for vascular access. *Am J Kidney Dis* 2006;48:S248-S278.
7. Sidawy AN, Gray R, Besarab A, et al. Recommended standards for reports dealing with arteriovenous hemodialysis accesses. *J Vasc Surg* 2002;35:603-610.
8. Ascher E, Gade P, Hingorami A, et al. Changes in the practice of angioaccess surgery: impact of dialysis outcome and quality initiative recommendations. *J Vasc Surg* 2000;31:84-92.
9. Beathard GA. Strategy for maximizing the use of arteriovenous fistulae. *Semin Dial* 2000;13:291-299.
10. Miller A, Holzenbein TJ, Gottlieb MN, et al. Strategies to increase the use of autogenous arteriovenous fistula in end-stage renal disease. *Ann Vasc Surg* 1997;11:397-405.
11. Hodges TC, Fillinger MF, Zwolak RM, et al. Longitudinal comparison of dialysis access methods: risk factors for failure. *J Vasc Surg* 1997;26:1009-1019.
12. Wolowczyk L, Williams AJ, Donovan KL, et al. The snuffbox arteriovenous fistula for vascular access. *Eur J Vasc Endovasc Surg* 2000;19:70-76.
13. Golledge J, Smith CJ, Emery J, et al. Outcome of primary radiocephalic fistula for haemodialysis. *Br J Surg* 1999;86:211-216.

14. Burger H, Kluchert BA, Kootstra G, et al. Survival of arteriovenous fistulas and shunts for haemodialysis. *Eur J Surg* 1995;161:327-334.
15. Leapman SB, Boyle M, Pescovitz MD, et al. The arteriovenous fistula for hemodialysis access: gold standard or archaic relic? *Am Surg* 1996;62:652-657.
16. Palder SB, Kirkman RL, Whittemore AD. Vascular access for hemodialysis: patency rates and results of revision. *Ann Surg* 1985;202:235-239.
17. Dunlop MG, Mackinlay JY, Jenkins AM. Vascular access: experience with the brachiocephalic fistula. *Ann R Coll Surg Engl* 1986;68: 203-206.
18. Sparks SR, VanderLinden JL, Gnanadev DA, et al. Superior patency of perforating antecubital vein arteriovenous fistulae for hemodialysis. *Ann Vasc Surg* 1997;11:165-167.
19. Livingston CK, Potts JR. Upper arm arteriovenous fistulas as a reliable access alternative for patients requiring chronic hemodialysis. *Am Surg* 1999;65:1038-1342.
20. Bender MHM, Bruyninckx CMA, Gerlag PGG. The Gracz arteriovenous fistula evaluated: results of the brachiocephalic elbow fistula in haemodialysis angio-access. *Eur J Vasc Endovasc Surg* 1995;10:294-297.
20a. Dagher F, Gelber R, Ramos E, Sadler J. The use of basilic vein and brachial artery as an A-V fistula for long term hemodialysis. *J Surg Res* 1976;20:373-376.
21. Ascher E, Hingorani A, Gunduz Y, et al. The value and limitations of the arm cephalic and basilic vein for arteriovenous access. *Ann Vasc Surg* 2001;15:89-97.
22. Coburn MC, Carney Jr WI . Comparison of basilic vein and polytetrafluoroethylene for brachial arteriovenous fistula. *J Vasc Surg* 1994;20: 896-902.
23. Rivers SP, Scher LA, Sheehan E, et al. Basilic vein transposition: an underused autologous alternative to prosthetic dialysis angioaccess. *J Vasc Surg* 1993;18:391-397.
24. Matsuura JH, Rosenthal D, Clark M, et al. Transposed basilic vein versus polytetrafluoroethylene for brachial-axillary arteriovenous fistulas. *Am J Surg* 1998;176:219-221.
25. Oliver MJ, McCann RL, Indridason OS, et al. Comparison of transposed brachiobasilic fistulas to upper arm grafts and brachiocephalic fistulas. *Kidney Int* 2001;60:1532-1539.
26. Murphy GJ, White SA, Knight AJ, et al. Long-term results of arteriovenous fistulas using transposed autologous basilic vein. *Br J Surg* 2000;87:819-823.
27. Lenz BJ, Veldenz HC, Dennis JW, et al. A three-year follow-up on standard versus thin wall ePTFE grafts for hemodialysis. *J Vasc Surg* 1998;28:464-470.
28. Rizzuti RP, Hale JC, Burkart TE. Extended patency of expanded polytetrafluoroethylene grafts for vascular access using optimal configuration and revisions. *Surg Gynecol Obstet* 1988;166:23-27.
29. Bosman PJ, Blankestign PJ, van der Graaf Y, et al. A comparison between PTFE and denatured homologous vein grafts for hemodialysis access: a prospective randomized multicentre trial. *Eur J Vasc Endovasc Surg* 1998;16:126-132.
30. Steed DL, McAuley CE, Rault R, et al. Upper arm graft fistula for hemodialysis. *J Vasc Surg* 1984;1:660-663.
31. Staramos DN, Lazarides MK, Tzilalis VD, et al. Patency of autologous and prosthetic arteriovenous fistulas in elderly patients. *Eur J Surg* 2000;166:777-781.
32. Cull JD, Cull DL, Taylor SM, et al. Prosthetic thigh arteriovenous access: outcome with SVS/AAVS reporting standards. *J Vasc Surg* 2004;39:381-386.
33. Khadra MH, Dwyer AJ, Thompson JF. Advantages of polytetrafluoroethylene arteriovenous loops in the thigh for hemodialysis access. *Am J Surg* 1997;73:280-283.
34. Bhandari S, Wilkinson A, Sellors L. Saphenous vein forearm grafts and Gore-Tex thigh grafts as alternative forms of vascular access. *Clin Nephrol* 1995;44:325-328.
35. Vega D, Polo JR, Polo J, et al. Brachial–jugular expanded PTFE grafts for dialysis. *Ann Vasc Surg* 2001;15:553-556.
36. McCann RL. Axillo-axillary (necklace) grafts for hemodialysis access. In Henry ML, ed. *Vascular access for hemodialysis VI*. Chicago: WL Gore & Associates, Precept Press; 1999:197-202.
37. Huber TS, Carter JW, Carter RL, Seeger JM. Patency of autogenous and polytetrafluoroethylene upper extremity arteriovenous hemodialysis accesses: a systematic review. *J Vasc Surg* 2003;38:1005-1011.
38. National Kidney Foundation/Dialysis Outcome Quality Initiative. NKF/DOQI clinical practice guidelines for vascular access. *Am J Kidney Dis* 1997;30:S150-S191.
39. Patel ST, Hughes J, Mills JL Sr. Failure of arteriovenous fistula maturation: an unintended consequence of exceeding Dialysis Outcome Quality Initiative guidelines for hemodialysis access. *J Vasc Surg* 2003;38:439-445.
40. U.S. Renal Data System. USRDS 2007 annual data report: atlas of chronic kidney disease and end-stage renal disease in the United States. Bethesda, Maryland: National Institutes of Health, National Institute of Diabetes and Digestive and Kidney Diseases; 2007.
41. Keoghane SR, Kar Leow C, Gray DWR. Routine use of arteriovenous fistula construction to dilate the venous outflow prior to insertion of an expanded polytetrafluoroethylene (PTFE) loop graft for dialysis. *Nephrol Dial Transplant* 1993;8:154-156.
42. Dickson CS, Gregory RT, Parent FN, et al. A new technique for hemodialysis access surgery: use of the pneumatic tourniquet. *Ann Vasc Surg* 1996;10:373-377.
43. Bronder CM, Cull DL, Kuper SG, et al. The fistula elevation procedure: experience with 295 consecutive cases over a seven year period. *JACS* in press.
44. Silva MB, Hobson RW, Pappas PJ, et al. Vein transposition in the forearm for autogenous hemodialysis access. *J Vasc Surg* 1997;26:981-988.
45. Gefen JY, Fox D, Giangola G, et al. The transposed forearm loop arteriovenous fistula: a valuable option for primary hemodialysis access in diabetic patients. *Ann Vasc Surg* 2002;16:89-94.
46. Gradman WS, Cohen W, Hagi-Aghaii M. Arteriovenous fistula construction in the thigh with transposed superficial femoral vein: our initial experience. *J Vasc Surg* 2001;33:968-975.
47. Jackson MR. The superficial femoral–popliteal vein transposition fistula: description of a new vascular access procedure. *J Am Coll Surg* 2000;191:581-584.
48. Ethier JH, Lindsay RM, Barre PE, et al. Clinical practice guidelines for vascular access: Canadian Society of Nephrology. *J Am Soc Nephrol* 1999;10(Suppl 1):S297-S305.
49. Lazarides MK, Iatrou CE, Karanikas IO, et al. Factors affecting the lifespan of autologous and synthetic arteriovenous access routes for hemodialysis. *Eur J Surg* 1996;162:297-301.
50. Hylander B, Fernstrom A, Swedenborg J. Interposition graft fistulas for hemodialysis. *Acta Chir Scand* 1988;154:107-110.
51. Hurt AV, Batello-Cruz M, Skipper BJ, et al. Bovine carotid artery heterographs versus polytetrafluoroethylene grafts. *Am J Surg* 1983;146:844-847.
52. Lilly L, Ngheim D, Mendez-Picon G, et al. Comparison between bovine heterografts and expanded PTFE grafts for dialysis access. *Am Surg* 1980;46:694-696.
53. Butler HG, Baker LD, Johnson JM. Vascular access for chronic hemodialysis: polytetrafluoroethylene (PTFE) versus bovine heterografts. *Am J Surg* 1977;134:791-793.
54. Reese JC, Esterl R, Lindsey L, et al. A prospective randomized comparison of bovine heterografts versus Impra grafts for chronic hemodialysis. In Henry ML, Fergusen RM, eds. *Vascular access for hemodialysis III*. Chicago: WL Gore & Associates, Precept Press; 1993:57-163.
55. May J, Harris J, Fletcher J. Long-term results of saphenous vein graft arteriovenous fistulas. *Am J Surg* 1980;140:387-390.
56. Jenkins AM, Buist TAS, Glover SD. Medium-term follow-up of forty autogenous vein and forty polytetrafluoroethylene (Gore-Tex) grafts for vascular access. *Surgery* 1980;88:667-672.
57. Matsuura JH, Johansen KH, Rosenthal D, et al. Cryopreserved femoral vein grafts for difficult hemodialysis access. *Ann Vasc Surg* 2000;14: 50-55.
58. Bolton W, Cull DL, Taylor SM, et al. The use of cryopreserved femoral vein grafts for hemodialysis access in patients at high risk for infection: a word of caution. *J Vasc Surg* 2002;36:464-468.
59. Dardik H, Ibrahim IM, Dardik I. Arteriovenous fistulas constructed with modified human umbilical cord vein graft. *Arch Surg* 1976;111: 60-62.
60. Karkow WS, Cranley JJ, Cranley RD, et al. Extended study of aneurysm formation in umbilical vein grafts. *J Vasc Surg* 1986;4:486-492.
61. Jamil Z, O'Donnell JA, Merk EA, Hobson RW. A comparison of knitted Dacron velour and bovine heterograft for hemodialysis access. *J Surg Res* 1979;26:423-429.
62. Burdick JF, Scott W, Cosimi AB. Experience with Dacron graft arteriovenous fistulas for dialysis access. *Ann Surg* 1978;187:262-266.
63. Levowitz BS, Flores L, Dunn I, et al. Prosthetic arteriovenous fistula for vascular access in hemodialysis. *Am J Surg* 1976;132:368-372.
64. Farmer DL, Goldstone J, Lim RC, et al. Failure of glow-discharge polymerization onto woven Dacron to improve performance of hemodialysis grafts. *J Vasc Surg* 1993;18:570-576.

65. Hiranaka T. Tapered and straight grafts for hemodialysis access: a prospective, randomized, comparison study. In: Henry ML, ed. *Vascular access for hemodialysis VII*. Chicago: WL Gore & Associates, Precept Press; 2001:219-224.
66. Shaffer D. A prospective randomized trial of 6-mm versus 4-7-mm PTFE grafts for hemodialysis access in diabetic patients. In: Henry ML, Ferguson RM, eds. *Vascular access for hemodiaysis V*. Chicago: WL Gore & Associates, Precept Press; 1997: 91-94.
67. Huber TS, Buhler AG, Seegar JM. Evidence based data for the hemodialysis access surgeon. *Semin Dial* 2004;17:217-223.
68. Kakkos SK, Haddad R, Haddad GK, et al. Results of aggressive graft surveillance and endovascular treatment on secondary patency rates of Vectra vascular access grafts. *J Vasc Surg* 2007;45:974-980.
69. Kiyama H, Imazeki T, Kurihara S, Yoneshima H. Long-term follow-up of polyurethane vascular grafts for hemoaccess bridge fistulas. *Ann Vasc Surg* 2003;17:516-521.
70. Allen RD, Yuill E, Nankivell BJ, Francis DM. Australian multicentre evaluation of a new polyurethane vascular access graft. *Aust NZ J Surg* 1996;66:738-742.
71. Jaffers G, Angstadt JD, Bowman JS III. Early cannulation of plasma TFE and Gore-Tex grafts for hemodialysis: a prospective randomized study. *Am J Nephrol* 1991;11:369-373.
72. Haag BW, Paramesh V, Roberts T. Early use of polytetrafluoroethylene grafts for hemodialysis access. In: Sommer BG, Henry ML, eds. *Vascular access for hemodialysis II*. Chicago: WL Gore & Associates, Precept Press; 1990:173-178.
73. Hakaim AG, Scott TE. Durability of early prosthetic dialysis graft cannulation: results of a prospective nonrandomized clinical trial. *J Vasc Surg* 1997;25:1002-1006.
74. McLaughlin K, Jones B, Mactier R, et al. Long-term vascular access for hemodialysis using silicon dual-lumen catheters with guidewire replacement of catheters for technique salvage. *Am J Kidney Dis* 1997;29: 553-559.
75. Oliver MJ, Edwards LJ, Treleaven DJ, et al. Randomized study of temporary hemodialysis catheters. *Int J Artif Organs* 2002;25:40-44.
76. Schillinger F, Schillinger D, Montagnac R, et al. Post-catheterization vein stenosis in haemodialysis: comparative angiographic study of 50 subclavian and 50 internal jugular accesses. *Nephrol Dial Transplant* 1991;6:722-724.
77. Surratt RS, Picus D, Hicks ME, et al. The importance of preoperative evaluation of the subclavian vein in dialysis access planning. *AJR Am J Roentgenol* 1991;156:623-625.
78. Hernandez D, Diaz F, Rufino M, et al. Subclavian vascular access stenosis in dialysis patients: natural history and risk factors. *J Am Soc Nephrol* 1998;9:1507-1510.
79. Barrett N, Spencer S, McIvor J, et al. Subclavian stenosis: a major complication of subclavian dialysis catheters. *Nephrol Dial Transplant* 1988;3:423-425.
80. Kelber J, Delmez JA, Windus DW. Factors affecting delivery of high-efficiency dialysis using temporary vascular access. *Am J Kidney Dis* 1993;22:24-29.
81. Montagnac R, Bernard C, Guillaumie J, et al. Indwelling silicone femoral catheters: experience of three haemodialysis centres. *Nephrol Dial Transplant* 1997;12:772-775.
82. Weitzel WF, Boyer CJ, El-Khatib MT, et al. Successful use of indwelling cuffed femoral vein catheters in ambulatory hemodialysis patients. *Am J Kidney Dis* 1993;22:426-429.
83. Biswal R, Nosher JL, Siegel RL, et al. Translumbar placement of paired hemodialysis catheters (Tesio catheters) and follow-up in 10 patients. *Cardiovasc Intervent Radiol* 2000;23:75-78.
84. Lund GB, Trerotola SO, Scheel Jr PJ. Percutaneous translumbar inferior vena cava cannulation for hemodialysis. *Am J Kidney Dis* 1995;25:732-737.
85. Suhocki PV, Conlon Jr PJ, Knelson MH, et al. Silastic cuffed catheters for hemodialysis vascular access: thrombolytic and mechanical correction of malfunction. *Am J Kidney Dis* 1996;28:379-386.
86. Lund GB, Trerotola SO, Scheel PF, et al. Outcome of tunneled hemodialysis catheters placed by radiologists. *Radiology* 1996;198:467-472.
87. Lin BS, Kong CW, Tarng DC, et al. Anatomical variation of the internal jugular vein and its impact on temporary haemodialysis vascular access: an ultrasonographic survey in uraemic patients. *Nephrol Dial Transplant* 1998;13:134-138.
88. Forauer AR, Glockner JF. Importance of U.S. findings in access planning during jugular vein hemodialysis catheter placements. *J Vasc Interv Radiol* 2000;11:233-237.
89. Lin BS, Huang TP, Tang GJ, et al. Ultrasound-guided cannulation of the internal jugular vein for dialysis vascular access in uremic patients. *Nephron* 1998;78:423-428.
90. Obialo CI, Conner AC, Lebon LF. Tunneled hemodialysis catheter survival: comparison of radiologic and surgical implantation. *ASAIO J* 2000;46:771-774.
91. Marr KA, Sexton DJ, Conlon PJ, et al. Catheter-related bacteremia and outcome of attempted catheter salvage in patients undergoing hemodialysis. *Ann Intern Med* 1997;127:275-280.
92. Meester JD, Vanholder R, De Roose J, et al. Factors and complications affecting catheter and technique survival with permanent single-lumen dialysis catheters. *Nephrol Dial Transplant* 1994;9:678-683.
93. Saad TF. Bacteremia associated with tunneled, cuffed hemodialysis catheters. *Am J Kidney Dis* 1999;34:1114-1124.
94. Warady BA, Bunchman TE. An update on peritoneal dialysis and hemodialysis in the pediatric population. *Curr Opin Pediatr* 1996;8: 135-140.
95. Bourquelot P, Wolfeler L, Lamy L. Microsurgery for haemodialysis distal arteriovenous fistulae in children weighing less than 10 kg. *Proc Eur Dial Transplant Assoc* 1981;18:537-541.
96. Robinson D, Suhocki P, Schwab SJ. Treatment of infected tunneled venous access hemodialysis catheters with guidewire exchange. *Kidney Int* 1998;53:1792-1794.
97. Tanriover P, Carlton D, Saddekni S, et al. Bacteremia associated with tunneled dialysis catheters: comparison of two treatment strategies. *Kidney Int* 2000;57:2151-2155.
98. Moss AH, Vasilakis C, Holley JL, et al. Use of silicone dual-lumen catheter with a Dacron cuff as a long-term vascular access for hemodialysis patients. *Am J Kidney Dis* 1990;16:211-215.
99. Tesio F, De Baz H, Panarello G, et al. Double catheterization of the internal jugular vein for hemodialysis: indications, techniques, and clinical results. *Artif Organs* 1994;18:301-304.
100. Trerotola SO, Shah H, Johnson M, et al. Randomized comparison of high-flow versus conventional hemodialysis catheters. *J Vasc Interv Radiol* 1999;10:1032-1038.
101. Trerotola SO, Kraus M, Shah H, et al. Randomized comparison of split tip versus step tip high-flow hemodialysis catheters. *Kidney Int* 2002;62:282-289.
102. Richard HT III, Hastings GS, Boyd-Kranis RL, et al. A randomized, prospective evaluation of the Tesio, Ash Split, and Opti-flow hemodialysis catheters. *J Vasc Interv Radiol* 2001;12:431-435.
103. Haire WD, Arkinson JB, Stephens LC, et al. Urokinase versus recombinant tissue plasminogen activator in thrombosed central venous catheters: a double-blinded, randomized trial. *Thromb Haemost* 1994;72:543-547.
104. Daeihagh P, Jordan J, Chen GJ, et al. Efficacy of tissue plasminogen activator administration on patency of hemodialysis access catheters. *Am J Kidney Dis* 2000;36:75-79.
105. Crain MR, Mewissen MW, Ostrowski GJ, et al. Fibrin sleeve stripping for salvage of failing hemodialysis catheters: technique and initial results. *Radiology* 1996;198:41-44.
106. U.S. Renal Data System. USRDS 1999 annual data report. Bethesda, Maryland: National Institutes of Health, National Institute of Diabetes and Digestive and Kidney Diseases; 1999.
107. Beanes SR, Kling KM, Fonkalsrud EW, et al. Surgical aspects of dialysis in newborns and infants weighing less than 10 kilograms. *J Pediatr Surg* 2000;35:1543-1548.
108. Bunchman TE. Pediatric hemodialysis: lessons from the past, ideas for the future. *Kidney Int* 1996;49:S64-S67.
109. Stone MM, Fonkalsrud EW, Salusky IB, et al. Surgical management of peritoneal dialysis catheters in children: five-year experience with 1,800 patient-month follow-up. *J Pediatr Surg* 1986;21:1177-1181.
110. Lerner GR, Warady BA, Sullivan EK, et al. Chronic dialysis in children and adolescents. *Pediatr Nephrol* 1999;13:404-407.
111. Lumsden AB, MacDonald MJ, Allen RC, et al. Hemodialysis access in the pediatric patient population. *Am J Surg* 1994;168:197-201.
112. Sharma A, Zilleruelo G, Abitbol C, et al. Survival and complications of cuffed catheters in children on chronic hemodialysis. *Pediatr Nephrol* 1999;13:245-248.
112a. Brescia MJ, Cimino JE, Appel K, Hurwich BJ. Chronic hemodialysis using venipuncture and a surgically created arteriovenous fistula. *N Engl J Med* 1966;275:1089-1092.
113. Sanabia J, Polo JR, Morales MD, et al. Microsurgery in gaining-paediatric vascular access for haemodialysis. *Microsurgery* 1993;14: 276-279.

114. Brittinger WD, Walker G, Twittenhoff WD, et al. Vascular access for hemodialysis in children. *Pediatr Nephrol* 1997;11:87-95.
115. Davis JB, Howell CG, HumphriesJr AL. Hemodialysis access: elevated basilic vein arteriovenous fistula. *J Pediatr Surg* 1986;21:1182-1183.
116. Bagolan P, Spagnoli A, Ciprandi G, et al. A ten-year experience of Brescia-Cimino arteriovenous fistula in children: technical evolution and refinements. *J Vasc Surg* 1998;27:640-644.
117. Beathard GA. Mechanical versus pharmacomechanical thrombolysis for the treatment of thrombosed dialysis access grafts. *Kidney Int* 1994;45:1401-1406.
118. Kanterman RY, Vesely TM, Pilgrim TK, et al. Dialysis access grafts: anatomic location of venous stenosis and results of angioplasty. *Radiology* 1995;195:135-139.
119. Swedberg SH, Brown BG, Sigley R. Intimal fibromuscular hyperplasia at the venous anastomosis of PTFE grafts in hemodialysis patients: clinical, immunocytochemical, light, and electron microscopic assessment. *Circulation* 1989;80:1726-1736.
120. Krysl J, Kumpe DA. Failing and failed hemodialysis access sites: management and percutaneous catheter methods. *Semin Vasc Surg* 1997;10: 175-183.
121. Schwartz CJ, McBrayer CV, Sloan JH, et al. Thrombosed dialysis grafts: comparison of treatment with transluminal angioplasty and surgical revision. *Radiology* 1995;194:337-341.
122. Schuman E, Quinn S, Standage B, et al. Thrombolysis versus thrombectomy for occluded hemodialysis grafts. *Am J Surg* 1994;167:473-476.
123. Uflacker R, Rajagopalan PR, Vujic I, et al. Treatment of thrombosed dialysis access grafts: randomized trial of surgical thrombectomy versus mechanical thrombectomy with the Amplatz device. *J Vasc Interv Radiol* 1996;7:185-192.
124. Marston WA, Criado E, Jaques PF, et al. Prospective randomized comparison of surgical versus endovascular management of thrombosed dialysis access grafts. *J Vasc Surg* 1997;26:373-380.
125. Palmer RM, Cull DL, Kalbaugh C, et al. Is surgical thrombectomy to salvage failed autogenous arteriovenous fistulae worthwhile? *Am Surg* 2006;72:1231-1233.
126. Gray RJ. Percutaneous intervention for permanent hemodialysis access: a review. *J Vasc Interv Radiol* 1997;8:313-327.
127. Berger MF, Aruny JE, Skibo LK. Recurrent thrombosis of polytetrafluoroethylene dialysis fistulas after recent surgical thrombectomy and salvage by means of thrombolysis and angioplasty. *J Vasc Interv Radiol* 1994;5:725-730.
128. Valji K, Bookstein JJ, Roberts AC, et al. Pulse-spray pharmacomechanical thrombolysis of thrombosed hemodialysis access grafts: long-term experience and comparison of original and current techniques. *AJR Am J Roentgenol* 1995;164:1495-1500.
129. Trerotola SO, Lund GB, Scheel Jr PJ, et al. Thrombosed dialysis access grafts: percutaneous mechanical declotting without urokinase. *Radiology* 1994;191:721-726.
130. Sofocleous CT, Cooper SG, Schur I, et al. Retrospective comparison of the Amplatz thrombectomy device with modified pulse-spray pharmacomechanical thrombolysis in the treatment of thrombosed hemodialysis access grafts. *Radiology* 1999;213:561-567.
131. Overbosch EH, Pattynama PM, Aarts HJ, et al. Occluded hemodialysis shunts: Dutch multicenter experience with the hydrolyser catheter. *Radiology* 1996;201:485-488.
132. Beathard GA, Welch BR, Maidment HJ. Mechanical thrombolysis for the treatment of thrombosed hemodialysis access grafts. *Radiology* 1996;200:711-716.
133. Beathard GA. Percutaneous transvenous angioplasty in the treatment of vascular access stenosis. *Kidney Int* 1992;42:1390-1397.
134. Patel RI, Peck SH, Cooper SG, et al. Patency of Wallstents placed across the venous anastamosis of hemodialysis grafts after percutaneous recanalization. *Radiology* 1998;209:365-370.
135. Hood DB, Yellin AE, Richman MF, et al. Hemodialysis graft salvage with endoluminal stents. *Am Surg* 1994;60:733-737.
136. Hoffer EK, Sultan S, Herskowitz MM, et al. Prospective randomized trial of a metallic intravascular stent in hemodialysis graft maintenance. *J Vasc Interv Radiol* 1997;8:965-973.
137. Quinn SF, Schuman ES, Demlow TA, et al. Percutaneous transluminal angioplasty versus endovascular stent placement in the treatment of venous stenoses in patients undergoing hemodialysis: intermediate results. *J Vasc Interv Radiol* 1995;6:851-855.
138. Dougherty MJ, Calligaru KD, Schindler N, et al. Endovascular versus surgical treatment for thrombosed hemodialysis grafts: a prospective randomized trial. *J Vasc Surg* 1999;30:1016-1023.
139. Brooks JL, Sigley RD, May KJ, et al. Transluminal angioplasty versus surgical repair for stenosis of hemodialysis grafts. *Am J Surg* 1987;153: 530-531.
140. Lumsden AB, MacDonald MJ, Kikeri D, et al. Prophylactic balloon angioplasty fails to prolong patency of expanded polytetrafluoroethylene arteriovenous grafts: results of a prospective randomized study. *J Vasc Surg* 1997;26:382-392.
141. Green LD, Lee DS, Kucey DS. A metaanalysis comparing surgical thrombectomy, mechanical thrombectomy, and pharmacomechanical thrombolysis for thrombosed dialysis grafts. *J Vasc Surg* 2002;36:939-945.
142. Swan TL, Smyth SH, Ruffenach SJ, et al. Pulmonary embolism following hemodialysis access thrombolysis/thrombectomy. *J Vasc Interv Radiol* 1995;6:683-686.
143. Smits HF, Van Rijk PP, Van Isselt JW, et al. Pulmonary embolism after thrombolysis of hemodialysis grafts. *J Am Soc Nephrol* 1997;8: 1451-1461.
144. Sexton DJ. Vascular access infections in patients undergoing dialysis with special emphasis on the role and treatment of. *Staphylococcus aureus. Infect Dis Clin North Am* 2001;15:731-742.
145. Alexiewicz JM, Smogorzewski M, Fadda GZ, et al. Impaired phagocytosis in dialysis patients; studies on mechanisms. *Am J Nephol* 1991;11: 102-111.
146. Pederson JO, Knudsen F, Nielsen AH, Grunnet N. The ability of uremic serum to induce neutrophil chemotaxis in relation to hemodialysis. *Blood Purif* 1987;5:24-28.
147. Albers FJ. Clinical considerations in hemodialysis access infection. *Adv Ren Replace Ther* 1996;3:208-217.
148. Kudva A, Hye RJ. Management of infectious and cutaneous complications in vascular access. *Semin Vasc Surg* 1997;10:184-190.
149. Butterly DW, Schwab SJ. Dialysis access infections. *Curr Opin Nephrol Hypertens* 2000;9:631-635.
150. Bhat DJ, Tellis VA, Kohlberg WI, et al. Management of sepsis involving polytetrafluoroethylene grafts for hemodialysis access. *Surgery* 1980;87:445-450.
151. Tellis VA, Weiss P, Matas AJ. Skin-flap coverage of polytetrafluoroethylene vascular access graft exposed by previous infection. *Surgery* 1988;103:118-121.
152. McKenna PJ, Leadbetter MG. Salvage of chronically exposed Gore-Tex vascular access grafts in the hemodialysis patient. *Plast Reconstr Surg* 1988;82:1046-1049.
153. Schwab DP, Taylor SM, Cull DL, et al. Isolated arteriovenous dialysis access graft segment infection: the results of segmental bypass and partial graft excision. *Ann Vasc Surg* 2000;14:63-66.
154. Hausegger KA, Tiessenhausen K, Klimpfinger M, et al. Aneurysms of hemodialysis access grafts: treatment with covered stents: a report of three cases. *Cardiovasc Intervent Radiol* 1998;21:334-337.
155. Sapoval MR, Turmel-Rodrigues LA, Raynaud AC, et al. Cragg covered stents in hemodialysis access: initial and midterm results. *J Vasc Interv Radiol* 1996;7:335-342.
156. Najibi S, Bush RL, Terramani TT, et al. Covered stent exclusion of dialysis access pseudoaneurysms. *J Surg Res* 2002;106:15-19.
157. Rhodes ES, Silas AM. Dialysis needle puncture of wallgrafts placed in polytetrafluoroethylene hemodialysis grafts. *J Vasc Interv Radiol* 2005;16:1129-1134.
158. Engelberts I, Tordoir JH, Boon ES, et al. High-output cardiac failure due to excessive shunting in a hemodialysis access fistula: an easily overlooked diagnosis. *Am J Nephrol* 1995;15:323-326.
159. Tzanakis I, Hatziathanassiou A, Kagia S, et al. Banding of an overfunctioning fistula with a prosthetic graft segment. *Nephron* 1999;81: 351-352.
160. Miles AM. Vascular steal syndrome and ischaemic monomelic neuropathy: two variants of upper limb ischemia after hemodialysis vascular access surgery. *Nephrol Dial Transplant* 1999;14:297-300.
161. Rivers SP, Scher LA, Veith FJ. Correction of steal syndrome secondary to hemodialysis access fistulas: a simplified quantitative technique. *Surgery* 1992;112:593-597.
162. Wixon CL, Mills JL, Berman SS. Distal revascularization-interval ligation for maintenance of dialysis access and restoration of distal perfusion in ischemic steal syndrome. *Semin Vasc Surg* 2000;13:77-82.
163. West JC, Bertsch DJ, Peterson SL, et al. Arterial insufficiency in hemodialysis access procedures: correction by banding technique. *Transplant Proc* 1991;23:1838-1840.
164. Rosental JJ, Bell DD, Gaspar MR, et al. Prevention of high flow problems of arteriovenous grafts: development of a new tapered graft. *Am J Surg* 1980;140:231-233.

165. Valentine RJ, Bouch CW, Scott DJ, et al. Do preoperative finger pressures predict early arterial steal in hemodialysis access patients? A prospective analysis. *J Vasc Surg* 2002;36:351-356.
166. Schanzer H, Skladany M, Haimov M. Treatment of angioaccess-induced ischemia by revascularization. *J Vasc Surg* 1992;16:861-866.
167. Berman SS, Gentile AT, Glickman MH, et al. Distal revascularization-interval ligation for limb salvage and maintenance of dialysis access in ischemic steal syndrome. *J Vasc Surg* 1997;26:393-404.
168. Knox RC, Berman SS, Hughes JD, et al. Distal revascularization-interval ligation: a durable and effective treatment for ischemic steal syndrome after hemodialysis access. *J Vasc Surg* 2002;36:250-255.
169. Minion DJ, Moore E, Endean E. Revision using distal inflow: a novel approach to dialysis-associated steal syndrome. *Ann Vasc Surg* 2005;19:625-628.
170. Zanow J, Kruger U, Scholz H. Proximalization of the arterial inflow: a new technique to treat access-related ischemia. *J Vasc Surg* 2006;43:1216-1221.
171. Hye RJ, Wolf YG. Ischemic monomelic neuropathy: an under-recognized complication of hemodialysis access. *Ann Vasc Surg* 1994;8:578-582.
172. Miles AM. Upper limb ischemia and vascular access surgery: differential diagnosis and management. *Semin Dial* 2000;13:312-315.
173. Redfern AB, Zimmerman NB. Neurologic and ischemic complications of upper extremity vascular access for dialysis. *J Hand Surg* 1995;20:199-204.
174. Paulson WD, Ram SJ, Birk CG, et al. Does blood flow accurately predict thrombosis or failure of hemodialysis synthetic grafts? A meta-analysis. *Am J Kidney Dis* 1999;34:478-485.
175. McDougal G, Agarwall R. Clinical performance characteristics of hemodialysis graft monitoring. *Kidney Int* 2001;60:762-766.
176. Middleton WD, Picus DD, Marx MV, et al. Color Doppler sonography of hemodialysis vascular access: comparison with angiography. *Am J Radiol* 1989;152:633-639.

Section

VII

Aneurysmal Disease

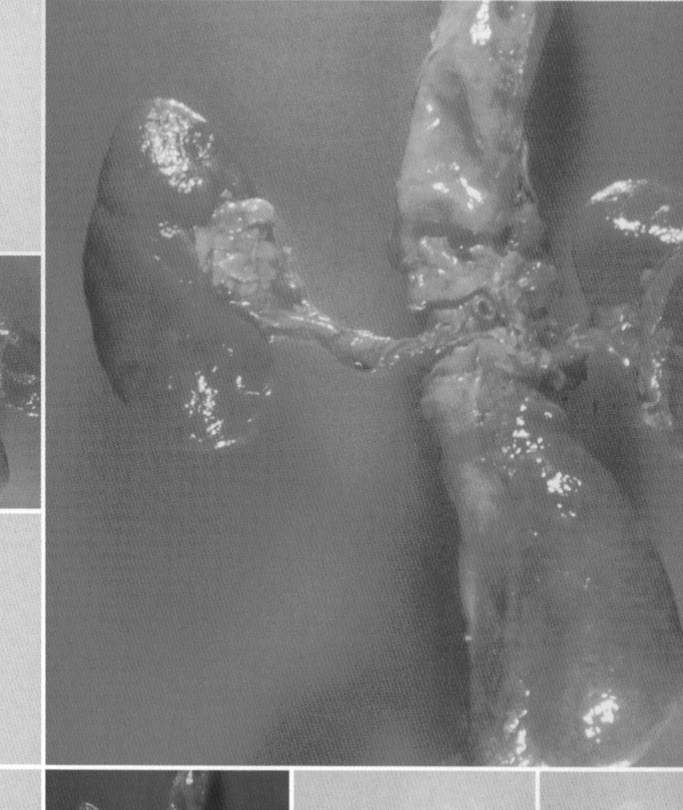

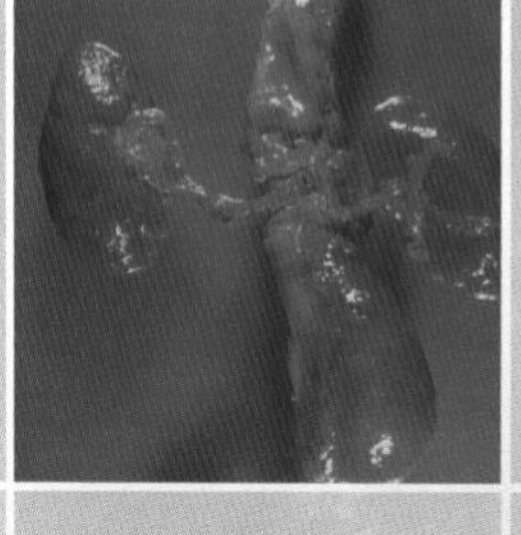

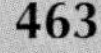

chapter 27

Pathogenesis of Aortic Aneurysms

B. Timothy Baxter, MD • Jason MacTaggart, MD

Key Points

- Arterial aneurysms are generally described as an increase greater than 50% in the normal diameter of the particular artery.
- Etiologies are diverse, but the final common pathway is degeneration of the structural integrity of the artery.
- Smoking has a much stronger relationship to the development of an abdominal aortic aneurysm (AAA) than any other risk factor.
- AAA development is a multifactorial disorder without a single inheritance mode.
- Inflammation is present in AAAs and plays an important role in cause and outcome.
- Enzymatic degradation of the aortic wall by matrix metalloproteinases is well documented.
- Wall stress leading to rupture is more complex than the law of Laplace.
- Better understanding of the pathogenesis of aneurysms should lead eventually to effective pharmacological approaches for clinical practice.

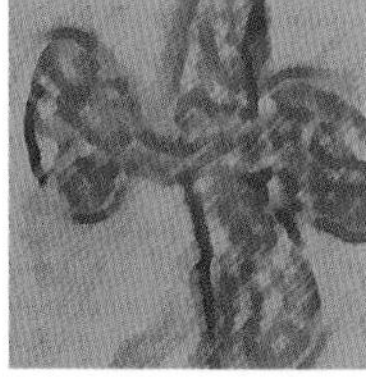

An aneurysm is a permanent, localized dilation encompassing all three layers of a blood vessel wall and defined by an increase greater than 50% in the diameter compared with the expected normal diameter.[1] Aneurysms are usually classified based on their etiology and anatomical location. Intracranial aneurysms, while common, are etiologically distinct from extracranial aneurysms with the exception of those associated with systemic connective disorders. Vessel wall degeneration is the common etiology; its cause is usually idiopathic but less commonly can be ascribed infection, poststenotic dilation, trauma, arteritis, and various connective tissue defects (Ehlers-Danlos type IV and Marfan's syndrome). Aneurysms occur throughout the arterial tree, but the predominant extracranial location for aneurysms is the infrarenal aorta. Aneurysms may cause arterial occlusion or distal embolization of thrombus, but tissue failure, rupture, and exsanguination are the most deadly outcome, accounting for at least 15,000 deaths a year in the United States.[2] Thoracic aortic aneurysms are diverse in etiology, although evidence is accumulating that there may be a common pathway in the later stages of the process. Most work on the etiology of extracranial aneurysms is related to abdominal aortic aneurysms (AAAs), and this work is the focus of this chapter.

CLINICAL FACTORS ASSOCIATED WITH AAA

AAA has been ascribed to atherosclerosis in the past because of shared risk factors, predisposition for atherosclerosis in the abdominal aorta, and concurrent atherosclerosis (coronary artery disease and cardiovascular disease). Several analyses in recent years have called the association into question. Smoking has been found to have a much stronger relationship with AAA than atherosclerosis.[3] Diabetes mellitus, known a risk factor associated with accelerated and diffuse atherosclerosis, is inversely related to the presence of AAA.[4] The relationship between cholesterol level and AAA is less clear, although some evidence shows that statin therapy might affect aneurysm expansion rate.[5-7] This epidemiological information lends evidence to the school of thought that AAA is a process distinct from atherosclerosis. The clinical impact of AAA has also been recognized by the Centers for Medicare and Medicaid Services through their authorization of ultrasound screening for AAA in men who have smoked. In its review, the U.S. Preventive Services Task Force concluded that this screening could reduce AAA mortality by 43% in men age 65 to 75 years.[8]

INTERPRETING ANEURYSM RESEARCH

While studies cited in this chapter have allowed us to better understand the causes of AAA, they should be interpreted in the context their inherent limitations. Human AAA tissue for study is typically obtained at operation for aneurysms more than 5 cm in diameter. At this point, most samples exhibit features of advanced, late-stage disease. The earlier juncture in the transition from a normal aorta, the stage that would best help identify key pathogenic events, is essentially unknown. Small animal models can fill in this gap and thus complement human tissue studies by allowing sequential study at the early stage of the process. Currently, three well-characterize mouse models exist of AAA.[9-11] Each results in aneurysm formation in a relatively acute time frame, and none can completely reproduce the entire spectrum of pathology found in human AAA. Aneurysm formation is triggered in these models through artificial means (elastase infusion, calcium chloride, angiotensin infusion) that converge toward similar end-stage processes. Thus, AAA research should be evaluated within the context of these limitations. Based on the increasing number of publications related to AAA pathogenesis from human studies (systemic markers and aneurysm tissue) and animal models, new information is available almost daily.

HERITABILITY OF AAA

The study of the genetics of AAA serves two purposes. The first objective is that by locating and characterizing genes suspected in AAA pathogenesis investigators may uncover additional pathways for more detailed study. These pathways may also provide potential new targets for pharmacological intervention. The second, and perhaps most important, objective is development of a test to identify patients at risk for AAA early in the course of the disease.

The initial studies describing the familial tendency of AAA were small cohort studies identifying the increased prevalence of AAA in a first-degree relative of a patient.[12,13] These studies did not use genetic models to determine the specific inheritance pattern of AAA. Two studies have used segregation analyses of large pedigrees, and both have concluded that the genetic transmission of AAA is best explained by a single gene rather than by multiple factors. However, these studies do not agree on whether the gene inheritance is recessive[14] or dominant.[15] In contrast, Kuivaniemi et al. published their pedigree analysis of 233 families with at least two affected members. They concluded that AAA is a multifactorial disorder without a single inheritance model.[16]

New tools in molecular biology make it possible to simultaneously evaluate expression of thousands of genes. Interpreting such a vast data set requires advanced computer technology and techniques for analysis. Two studies using complementary DNA microarrays have analyzed the gene expression profiles of human AAA tissue compared to normal and atherosclerotic aortas. AAA tissue demonstrated a pattern showing chronic inflammation, smooth muscle cell depletion, atherosclerosis, and extracellular matrix degradation that was significantly different from the normal aorta.[17,18] The significance of these observations is lessened to a degree in that most key findings reflect changes in cell populations within AAA tissue (increased numbers of macrophages, loss of smooth muscle cells) compared to normal aorta. DNA studies using whole genome scanning and linkage analysis of 36 AAA families found possible susceptibility loci on chromosomes 4 and 19. Further study of candidate genes from among numerous genes in these loci is required to validate such findings.[19]

In searching for a gene that might explain AAA, considerable work has focused on the genes regulating matrix protein

Table 27-1
Polymorphisms Associated with Abdominal Aortic Aneurysm (AAA)*

Gene	Polymorphism	Reference
Angiotensin II type 1 receptor	AGTR1 1166C	Jones et al.[22]
IL-6 polymorphism	L-6-572 G > C	Smallwood et al.[23]
IL-10 polymorphism	1082 "A"	Brown et al.[24]
MMP-3	5A/5A	Deguara et al.[25]
MMP-2	– 1306 C > T	Powell[26]
MMP-3	– 1171 5A > 6A	
MMP-9	– 1562 C > T	
MMP-12	– 82 A > G	
TIMP-1	– 372 C > T	
PAI-1	– 675 4G > 5G, –847 A > G	
HLA	DQA1*0102 allele	Ogata et al.[27]
MMP-2	None with AAA	Hinterseher et al.[28]
MMP-9	C-1562T	Jones et al.[29]

*IL, interleukin; MMP, matrix metalloproteinase; PAI, plasminogen activator inhibitor; TIMP, tissue inhibitor of metalloproteinase.

metabolism, inflammation, and immune function. With the exception of uncommon cases of type III collagen mutations,[20] no known mutations in matrix proteins can account for AAAs.[21] Polymorphisms, or variants in the promoter regions of potential AAA-associated genes, have been implicated in AAA. Specific polymorphisms alter gene expression. Polymorphisms in protease, cytokine, and other immunoregulatory genes thought to be associated with AAA are shown in Table 27-1. Most of these studies are small and lack the statistical power to provide definitive information, so the contribution of each to AAA pathogenesis remains to be clarified.

INFLAMMATION AND AAA

Histological examination of human AAA tissue demonstrates an inflammatory cell infiltrate consisting of T cells, B cells, dendritic cells, plasma cells, and macrophages.[30-32] These cells are typically located throughout the intima, media, and adventitia and in extreme cases produce what is termed an "inflammatory" AAA. In contrast to the panmural inflammation of AAA, the microscopic appearance of an atherosclerotic aorta shows an infiltrate of T cells and macrophages located within the intima and media.[32] In comparing larger versus smaller AAAs, Freestone et al. found that as aneurysm size increased so did the intensity of the inflammatory cell infiltrate.[33] Figure 27-1 illustrates the role of inflammation and potential targets for therapy.

Animal models of AAA confirm the importance of inflammation in the aorta during aneurysm formation. In the elastase infusion model of AAA, pressurized infusion of the infrarenal aorta with pancreatic elastase immediately renders the aorta larger through mechanical disruption of the elastic lamellae. The subsequent 300% increase in diameter parallels the inflammatory cell infiltration.[34] Cyclosporine or methylprednisolone treatments block this inflammation and subsequent dilatation.[35] White cell depletion or anti-inflammatory medications attenuate aneurysm formation.[36] A second, commonly used mouse model employing the periaortic application of calcium chloride to the outer aortic surface shows a similar inflammatory cell (macrophage and lymphocyte) infiltrate preceding aortic enlargement.[9] Thus, the prominent

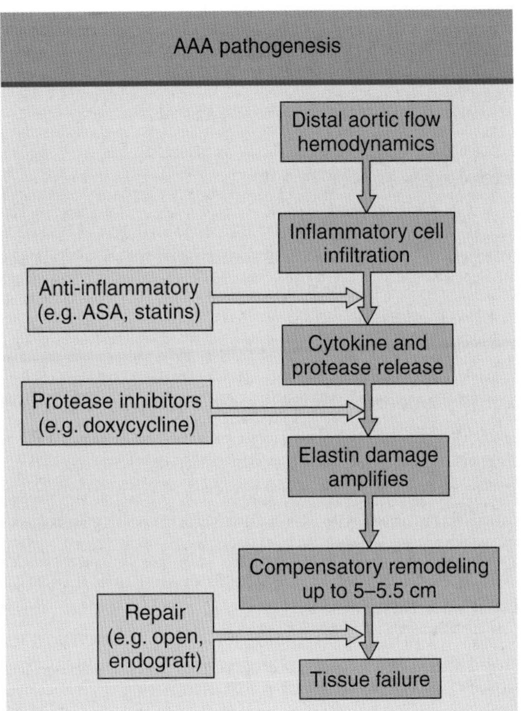

Figure 27-1. The role of inflammation and potential targets for therapy.

inflammation observed in human AAA tissues has been shown, through the use of animal models, to play an important causal role in AAA.

Recruitment of the Inflammatory Cell Infiltrate

The stimulus for the recruitment of the inflammatory cells into the aorta and initiation of matrix degradation is unknown and is an area of ongoing research. Once this begins, specific epitopes that had been shielded from the immune system may be exposed. The vigorous immune response potentiates inflammatory cell invasion. Supporting experimental evidence comes from Hance et al. who studied soluble elastin degradation fragments from human AAA tissue. These peptides attract mononuclear phagocytes in vitro through a specific interaction with a 67-kDa elastin-binding protein receptor on the phagocytes.[37] Elastin degradation products have also been found to induce angiogenesis in the adventitia of rat aortas.[38] What remains to be explained is the inciting event leading to initial elastin breakdown. Clearly, once elastin degradation is initiated, the elastin-derived peptides amplify the immune response in AAAs.

Studies of human AAA tissue reveal characteristics consistent with an autoimmune process, namely, large amounts of immunoglobulin G[39] and the presence of plasma cells.[30] In addition, a proposed autoantigen, a 40-kDa protein similar to an extracellular matrix component that specifically binds to antibodies isolated from human AAA has been identified and characterized.[40] However, two more recent studies have cast doubt on this autoimmune hypothesis by demonstrating that AAA lymphocytes are responding to an array of antigens.[41,42]

Infection with *Chlamydia pneumoniae* has been suggested as a possible contributor in the formation of AAA. In one early study, investigators found that chlamydial antigens were present in most human AAA tissue samples compared with healthy control aortas.[43] Subsequent studies have confirmed that chlamydia, or chlamydial antigens, are often present in AAA tissue.[44,45] In another study by Tambiah and Powell using a rabbit model of AAA, topical treatment of the aorta with chlamydial antigens enhanced aneurysm formation through a process that could be attenuated by treatment with azithromycin.[46] In this instance, the mere presence of the chlamydial antigens was sufficient to enhance aneurysm development without active infection, leading the investigators to suggest that azithromycin most likely worked through an anti-inflammatory mechanism. Furthermore, positive chlamydia titers do not affect AAA expansion rates.[47] Roxithromycin inhibits AAA expansion, but this is unrelated to the presence or absence of chlamydial antigens.[48] Taken together and considering the high prevalence of chlamydial infection in the general population,[49] strong evidence of specificity for AAA initiation or progression is lacking.

Another possible recruitment mechanism involves the action of chemokines, a related family of low-molecular-weight cytokines that control leukocyte trafficking. Compared to controls, human AAA tissue contains greater amounts of the chemokines interleukin-8 (IL-8) and monocyte chemotactic protein-1 (MCP-1).[50] In mice, work using the elastase infusion model has demonstrated an increased production of the chemokines MCP-1 and RANTES in aneurysmal tissue. Notably, the expression of these chemokines by the aortic smooth muscle cells preceded the influx of inflammatory cells during the experimental AAA development.[51] As with elastin degradation peptides, however, the events that initially upregulate these chemokines have not been identified but they are clearly involved in the subsequent propagation of the prominent immune response.

Cytokines and AAA

Once inflammatory cells transmigrate into tissues, their subsequent course of action can be variable. The direction of the ongoing immune response is regulated by cytokines, which can be produced both by invading inflammatory cells and by resident mesenchymal cells. A dichotomous murine immune response, directed by cytokine secretion from a subset of lymphocytes (CD4), results in a proinflammatory response (Th1) or an anti-inflammatory response (Th2). Human AAA tissue has been evaluated to determine whether a polarization occurs toward a Th1 or a Th2 response. Studies of homogenized AAA tissue and culture of AAA tissue explants have demonstrated overexpression of proinflammatory cytokines, such as tumor necrosis factor-α, IL-6, and IL-1β.[52,53] The Th1 cytokine interferon-γ (IFN-γ) has also been implicated in human AAA,[52] and elevated circulating levels of IFN-γ appear to correlate with more rapid aneurysm expansion.[54] Furthermore, transgenic mice deficient in IFN-γ are resistant to aneurysm formation. Aneurysms were regenerated by transplantation of normal splenocytes capable of producing IFN-γ.[55]

These findings contrast with recent work implicating the Th2 cytokine response. Schonbeck et al. examined the cytokine profile of human AAA tissue and found no evidence for Th1 or IFN-γ pathway activation but did find an abundance of IL-4, IL-5, and IL-10, all Th2 cytokines.[56] Extending these observations into an animal model, researchers transplanted wild-type mouse aortas into mice deficient in IFN-γ receptors. Despite the absence of IFN-γ receptors in all cells save for the transplanted aorta, these chimeric mice were able to form large aneurysms. Upon treatment with anti-IL-4 antibody, however, these transplanted mice were unable to form aneurysms, a finding confirmed in IL-4 knockout mice.[57] These findings suggest that invading inflammatory cells depend on Th2 signaling pathways for aneurysm development. It is difficult to explain these contradictory results. One possible explanation is a transition from a Th1-dominated response early in AAA to a Th2 response in the later stages of the disease. Few human diseases fit conveniently into this Th1–Th2 scheme, with most showing some mix of cytokines from each pathway, a response known as a Th0 response.

Smooth Muscle Cell Depletion

The presence of inflammatory cells and the cytokine environments they produce are thought to be responsible for another unique feature found in AAA—decreased medial smooth muscle cell density. Histological examination of AAA specimens reveals a paucity of medial smooth muscle cells when compared to normal and atherosclerotic aortas.[58,59] In addition, many of the smooth muscle cells present show features consistent with apoptosis.[58] The significance of these findings cannot be underestimated. The smooth muscle cell is critical to the vasomotor function of the arterioles. In the large capacitance vessels such as the aorta, matrix content and structure impart the critical strength and expansile function to the aorta. The important role of the smooth muscle cells was illustrated using an aortic xenograft model in which seeding of the graft with vascular smooth muscle cells resulted in protection of the graft from inflammation, proteolysis, and aneurysm formation.[60]

Role of Prostaglandins

Several studies have examined the role of prostaglandin E_2 (PGE_2) in aneurysm formation. In these studies, researchers have found an increased expression of cyclooxygenase-2 (Cox-2) localizing primarily to infiltrating macrophages. Cox-2 is thought to be responsible for the increased PGE_2 levels found in both human aneurysm tissue and conditioned media from aortic tissue culture.[61,62] PGE_2 could influence aneurysm pathogenesis by altering matrix metalloproteinase (MMP) activity, cytokine expression, and smooth muscle cell viability. Indomethacin, a nonspecific Cox inhibitor, decreases PGE_2 and attenuates aneurysm expansion in experimental aneurysms.[63]

Oxidative Stress

Inflammatory cells can also be a significant source of reactive oxygen species. These toxic substances, which may also be produced by mesenchymal cells and endothelial cells, are capable of inducing apoptosis of smooth muscle cells and activating proteases.[64,65] Miller et al. have shown that reactive oxygen species and evidence of oxidative damage are increased in human AAA tissue.[66] Investigators have shown in the elastase infusion model that genes associated with oxidative stress, such as those encoding inducible nitric oxide synthase and heme oxygenase, are upregulated during aneurysm development.[67] Inhibition of inducible nitric oxide synthase, one of many enzymes capable of producing nitric oxide, attenuated aneurysm development.[68] However, this same study also found that mice lacking the gene for inducible nitric oxide synthase were able to form aneurysms in a similar manner to controls, casting doubt on the importance of this enzyme in AAA pathogenesis.[69]

PROTEASES AND AAA

The two principle functions of the aorta, blood transport and transmission of pulsatile energy, demand both tensile strength and elasticity in its structure. These properties are provided mainly by collagen and elastin, two connective tissue proteins synthesized and maintained primarily by resident mesenchymal cells in the aortic wall. Because the normal structure and function of the aorta are so dependent upon these two proteins, the study of elastin, collagen, and their metabolism has provided valuable insight into the pathogenesis of AAA.

Because disruption of collagen and elastin is necessary for, and well documented in, AAA pathogenesis, investigators have focused intensely on studying the enzymes capable of degrading them. In the early 1980s, researchers began studying the proteolytic activity within human AAA tissue.[70-72] Since then, numerous studies have demonstrated the importance of the enzymatic degradation of the aortic wall in the development of AAA. Although many enzymes are capable of degrading these proteins in vivo, particular emphasis has been placed on the study of MMPs.

Matrix Metalloproteinases

MMPs are a family of structurally related enzymes that are capable of digesting the various components of the extracellular matrix. They are produced by most cell types native to the aorta, such as endothelial cells, smooth muscle cells, and adventitial fibroblasts, and are produced by invading inflammatory cells, such as macrophages. The normal physiological function of these enzymes is thought to be primarily extracellular matrix remodeling, although participation in other functions, such as cell motility and cell signaling, are also known.[73] Most MMPs are secreted from cells in a proenzyme form and require some type of processing to become fully activated. Other MMPs are anchored to cell surfaces to help concentrate their activities close to the cell. Regulation of MMP synthesis and activity occurs through several mechanisms. MMP synthesis is primarily regulated at the level of transcription. Activity level may be regulated by the processing of the proenzyme form to its active form. Endogenous inhibitors (tissue inhibitors of metalloproteinases) and interaction with specific extracellular matrix components can also affect activity.[74] Dysregulation of MMP activity has been linked not only with vascular disease but also with malignancy, rheumatoid arthritis, and a host of other pathological conditions.

Matrix Metalloproteinase-9

MMP-9, also known as gelatinase B, is one of the most extensively studied MMPs within AAA research. It has the capacity to degrade both elastin and partially hydrolyzed collagen. Using zymography and immunohistochemistry, studies of human AAA tissue have demonstrated increased amounts of MMP-9 compared to control tissue.[75] Furthermore, this MMP-9 localizes to areas surrounding infiltrating macrophages in the aortic wall. Using the elastase infusion model in mice, Pyo et al.[10] showed that mice lacking the gene for MMP-9 were resistant to

AAA formation. In addition, they were able to show that the key source of MMP-9 was the infiltrating macrophage, as infusion of bone marrow cells from mice with the MMP-9 gene into the MMP-9 knockout mice permitted aneurysm formation.

Matrix Metalloproteinase-2

MMP-2, or gelatinase A, is another MMP found to be important in AAA pathogenesis. It too has the capacity to degrade elastin, but unlike MMP-9, it can degrade intact fibrillar collagen.[76] MMP-2 also differs from MMP-9 in that processing of MMP-2 to its activated form requires the presence of other membrane-bound MMPs.[73] Like MMP-9, MMP-2 levels and activity have been found to be greater in human AAA tissue compared to controls.[68,77] However, whereas MMP-9 is typically not present in disease free aortas,[75] MMP-2 is constitutively produced by resident mesenchymal cells even in histologically normal aortas.[68] Confirmation of MMP-2's importance to AAA development has come from the calcium chloride mouse model of AAA. In this study, Longo et al. were able to show that the targeted deletion of the MMP-2 gene inhibited AAA formation and that the key source of MMP-2 production was not invading inflammatory cells but resident mesenchymal cells.[9] The stimulus for the increased production and activation of MMP-2 in aneurysmal aortas remains unknown.

Other Matrix Metalloproteinases

MMP-12, sometimes referred to as macrophage elastase, is also elevated in human AAA tissue compared to controls. Importantly, immunohistochemical analysis has localized the enzyme to areas of elastin destruction.[78] In contrast to MMP-9 and MMP-2, however, MMP-12 has not been shown to be required for aneurysm generation in knockout mice.[10] Levels of other MMPs are altered in AAA as well, but current studies have not documented a definitive role for these enzymes in AAA development.

Other Proteases

Other proteases and their endogenous inhibitors besides MMPs have been suggested as potential contributors to AAA pathogenesis. Cystatin C, an endogenous inhibitor of cysteine proteases, appears to be reduced in human AAA tissue.[79] Serine proteases, particularly neutrophil elastase, have been hypothesized to play a role in AAA formation due to their potent elastase activities. However, no supporting experimental evidence currently exists. Other serine proteases, such as those from the plasminogen activator family, have been shown to play a role in AAA formation. The main pathogenic mechanism involving these enzymes, however, appears to be activation of MMPs.[80]

BIOMECHANICAL WALL STRESS

The infrarenal aorta is subjected to unique hemodynamic flow patterns and possesses specific structural characteristics that are thought to predispose it toward aneurysm formation. Reflected pressure waves from the aortic bifurcation and the presence of large renal and splanchnic artery takeoffs result in disturbed flow patterns.[81] The elastin-to-collagen ratio decreases distally, translating into increased stiffness in this section of the aorta.[82] In addition, the absence of vasa vasorum in the normal abdominal aortic media[83] and the presence of a thick intraluminal thrombus are thought to impair oxygen and nutrient delivery to the aneurysmal aorta.[84] All of these observations are plausible reasons for the development and progression of disease in the infrarenal aorta.

Aortic Wall Stress

Stress on the aortic wall is one of the key factors involved in the rupture of AAAs. The law of Laplace is often used to explain the propensity for larger aneurysms to rupture, as it predicts wall tension to be directly proportional to the product of the radius of a tubular, thin-walled structure (AAA diameter) and its intraluminal pressure (patient blood pressure). This may be an oversimplification, however, as AAAs are often asymmetrical, are thick walled, and become more spherical as their size increases.[85] Because of this, researchers are developing improved methods to help determine the patterns of stress on the aneurysmal aortic wall, as well as the effect of stress on the pathogenesis of AAA.

Raghavan et al. recently used a method termed finite element analysis to noninvasively determine AAA wall stress distribution and AAA rupture risk.[86] Application of this method comparing calculated stress values obtained from patients

Table 27-2
Potential medical therapies for AAA

Intervention	References	Effect on AAA Growth	Level of Evidence	Proposed Mechanism
Propanolol	Lindholt et al.,[88] Propanolol Aneurysm Trial Investigators[89]	No inhibition	Level I	Hemodynamic
Macrolides	Vammen et al.[48]	Inhibition	Level II	Antiinfectious Anti-inflammatory
Tetracyclines	Mosorin et al.[90]	Inhibition†	Level II	Antiinfection Anti-inflammatory Protease inhibitor
Statins	Sukhija et al.,[6] Schouten et al.[7]	Inhibition	Level II	Anti-inflammatory Protease inhibitor
ACE inhibitors	Sukhija et al.,[6] Schouten et al.,[7] Habashi et al.[91]	No inhibition	Level II	Hemodynamic Protease inhibitor
AR receptor blocker	Daugherty et al.,[11] Rizzoni et al.[92]	Inhibition	Animal	Hemodynamic Protease inhibitor

*AAA, abdominal aortic aneurysm; ACE, angiotensin-converting enzyme; AR, angiotensin receptor.
†Inhibition at 6 and 12 months after 3 months of treatment.

near the time of rupture of their AAA, to size-matched, electively repaired AAA patients, showed significantly elevated stress values in the ruptured AAA group.[87] Although still investigational, these methods could have an important impact on determining the indications for operative repair of AAAs.

POTENTIAL THERAPEUTIC TARGETS FOR AAA

The work outlined earlier has led to evaluation of several potential therapeutic targets for inhibiting aneurysm growth. Three important features of AAA lend themselves to medical treatment: (1) inexpensive and accurate methods for detection, (2) long period of surveillance before intervention, and (3) life expectancy of the affected population.

Increased public awareness and availability of screening will lead to increased aneurysm detection in the next decade. Of aneurysms detected at screening, 90% are below the threshold for immediate repair, and aneurysm expansion is gradual. A reduction of the expansion rate of a 4.0-cm AAA by 50% potentially increases the time before surgical intervention to 10 years, which exceeds the life expectancy of many aneurysm patients. The current standard of care for these small AAAs is "watchful waiting." The provision of a relatively benign and efficacious medical therapy to these patients may reverse the diminished quality of life associated with detection of a potentially life-threatening condition for which no immediate treatment is offered. Based on the studies outlined earlier, several therapies might influence the growth of aortic aneurysm. Table 27-2 outlines these therapies and what is known of their effectiveness.

CONCLUSION

Significant progress has been made over the past 20 years in delineating the pathogenesis of AAA. Both clinicians and basic scientists will continue to play important roles in understanding this complex process. With continued progress, the coming decade should offer improved diagnostics and a medical therapy to impede the growth of small AAA.

References

1. Johnston KW, Rutherford RB, Tilson MD, et al. Suggested standards for reporting on arterial aneurysms: Subcommittee on Reporting Standards for Arterial Aneurysms, Ad Hoc Committee on Reporting Standards, Society for Vascular Surgery and North American Chapter, International Society for Cardiovascular Surgery. *J Vasc Surg* 1991;13(3):452-458.
2. The Center for Disease Control Deaths, percent of total deaths, and death rates for the 15 leading causes of death. Available at: www.cdc.gov/nchs/data/statab/lcwk9.pdf. Accessed March 30, 2008.
3. Lederle FA, Nelson DB, Joseph AM. Smokers' relative risk for aortic aneurysm compared with other smoking-related diseases: a systematic review. *J Vasc Surg* 2003;38(2):329-334.
4. Lederle FA, Johnson GR, Wilson SE, et al. Prevalence and associations of abdominal aortic aneurysm detected through screening: Aneurysm Detection and Management (ADAM) Veterans Affairs Cooperative Study Group. *Ann Intern Med* 1997;126(6):441-449.
5. Evans J, Powell JT, Schwalbe E, et al. Simvastatin attenuates the activity of matrix metalloprotease-9 in aneurysmal aortic tissue. *Eur J Vasc Endovasc Surg* 2007;34(3):302-303.
6. Sukhija R, Aronow WS, Sandhu R, et al. Mortality and size of abdominal aortic aneurysm at long-term follow-up of patients not treated surgically and treated with and without statins. *Am J Cardiol* 2006;97(2):279-280.
7. Schouten O, van Laanen JH, Boersma E, et al. Statins are associated with a reduced infrarenal abdominal aortic aneurysm growth. *Eur J Vasc Endovasc Surg* 2006;32(1):21-26.
8. Fleming C, Whitlock EP, Beil TL, et al. Screening for abdominal aortic aneurysm: a best-evidence systematic review for the U.S. Preventive Services Task Force. *Ann Intern Med* 2005;142(3):203-211.
9. Longo GM, Xiong W, Greiner TC, et al. Matrix metalloproteinases 2 and 9 work in concert to produce aortic aneurysms. *J Clin Invest* 2002;110(5):625-632.
10. Pyo R, Lee JK, Shipley JM, et al. Targeted gene disruption of matrix metalloproteinase-9 (gelatinase B) suppresses development of experimental abdominal aortic aneurysms. *J Clin Invest* 2000;105(11):1641-1649.
11. Daugherty A, Manning MW, Cassis LA. Angiotensin II promotes atherosclerotic lesions and aneurysms in apolipoprotein E–deficient mice. *J Clin Invest* 2000;105(11):1605-1612.
12. Tilson MD, Seashore MR. Fifty families with abdominal aortic aneurysms in two or more first-order relatives. *Am J Surg* 1984;147(4):551-553.
13. Clifton MA. Familial abdominal aortic aneurysms. *Br J Surg* 1977;64(11):765-766.
14. Majumder PP, St. Jean PL, Ferrell RE, et al. On the inheritance of abdominal aortic aneurysm. *Am J Hum Genet* 1991;48(1):164-170.
15. Verloes A, Sakalihasan N, Koulischer L, et al. Aneurysms of the abdominal aorta: familial and genetic aspects in three hundred thirteen pedigrees. *J Vasc Surg* 1995;21(4):646-655.
16. Kuivaniemi H, Shibamura H, Arthur C, et al. Familial abdominal aortic aneurysms: collection of 233 multiplex families. *J Vasc Surg* 2003;37(2):340-345.
17. Armstrong PJ, Johanning JM, Calton WC Jr, et al. Differential gene expression in human abdominal aorta: aneurysmal versus occlusive disease. *J Vasc Surg* 2002;35(2):346-355.
18. Tung WS, Lee JK, Thompson RW. Simultaneous analysis of 1176 gene products in normal human aorta and abdominal aortic aneurysms using a membrane-based complementary DNA expression array. *J Vasc Surg* 2001;34(1):143-150.
19. Shibamura H, Olson JM, van Vlijmen-Van Keulen C, et al. Genome scan for familial abdominal aortic aneurysm using sex and family history as covariates suggests genetic heterogeneity and identifies linkage to chromosome 19q13. *Circulation* 2004;109(17):2103-2108.
20. Kontusaari S, Tromp G, Kuivaniemi H, et al. A mutation in the gene for type III procollagen (COL3A1) in a family with aortic aneurysms. *J Clin Invest* 1990;86(5):1465-1473.
21. Tromp G, Wu Y, Prockop DJ, et al. Sequencing of cDNA from 50 unrelated patients reveals that mutations in the triple-helical domain of type III procollagen are an infrequent cause of aortic aneurysms. *J Clin Invest* 1993;91(6):2539-2545.
22. Jones GT, Thompson AR, van Bockxmeer FM, et al. Angiotensin II type 1 receptor 1166C polymorphism is associated with abdominal aortic aneurysm in three independent cohorts. *Arterioscler Thromb Vasc Biol* 2008;28(4):764-770.
23. Smallwood L, Allcock R, van Bockxmeer F, et al. Polymorphisms of the interleukin-6 gene promoter and abdominal aortic aneurysm. *Eur J Vasc Endovasc Surg* 2008;35(1):31-36.
24. Bown MJ, Lloyd GM, Sandford RM, et al. The interleukin-10-1082 "A" allele and abdominal aortic aneurysms. *J Vasc Surg* 2007;46(4):687-693.
25. Deguara J, Burnand KG, Berg J, et al. An increased frequency of the 5A allele in the promoter region of the MMP3 gene is associated with abdominal aortic aneurysms. *Hum Mol Genet* 2007;16(24):3002-3007.
26. Powell JT. Genes predisposing to rapid aneurysm growth. *Ann NY Acad Sci* 2006;1085:236-241.
27. Ogata T, Gregoire L, Goddard KA, et al. Evidence for association between the HLA-DQA locus and abdominal aortic aneurysms in the Belgian population: a case control study. *BMC Med Genet* 2006;7:67.
28. Hinterseher I, Krex D, Kuhlisch E, et al. Tissue inhibitor of metalloproteinase-1 (TIMP-1) polymorphisms in a Caucasian population with abdominal aortic aneurysm. *World J Surg* 2007;31(11):2248-2254.
29. Jones GT, Phillips VL, Harris EL, et al. Functional matrix metalloproteinase-9 polymorphism (C-1562T) associated with abdominal aortic aneurysm. *J Vasc Surg* 2003;38(6):1363-1367.
30. Beckman EN. Plasma cell infiltrates in atherosclerotic abdominal aortic aneurysms. *Am J Clin Pathol* 1986;85(1):21-24.
31. Bobryshev YV, Lord RS, Parsson H. Immunophenotypic analysis of the aortic aneurysm wall suggests that vascular dendritic cells are involved in immune responses. *Cardiovasc Surg* 1998;6(3):240-249.

32. Koch AE, Haines GK, Rizzo RJ, et al. Human abdominal aortic aneurysms. Immunophenotypic analysis suggesting an immune-mediated response. *Am J Pathol* 1990;137(5):1199-1213.
33. Freestone T, Turner RJ, Coady A, et al. Inflammation and matrix metalloproteinases in the enlarging abdominal aortic aneurysm. *Arterioscler Thromb Vasc Biol* 1995;15(8):1145-1151.
34. Anidjar S, Dobrin PB, Eichorst M, et al. Correlation of inflammatory infiltrate with the enlargement of experimental aortic aneurysms. *J Vasc Surg* 1992;16(2):139-147.
35. Dobrin PB, Baumgartner N, Anidjar S, et al. Inflammatory aspects of experimental aneurysms: effect of methylprednisolone and cyclosporine. *Ann NY Acad Sci* 1996;800:74-88.
36. Ricci MA, Strindberg G, Slaiby JM, et al. Anti-CD 18 monoclonal antibody slows experimental aortic aneurysm expansion. *J Vasc Surg* 1996;23(2):301-307.
37. Hance KA, Tataria M, Ziporin SJ, et al. Monocyte chemotactic activity in human abdominal aortic aneurysms: role of elastin degradation peptides and the 67-kD cell surface elastin receptor. *J Vasc Surg* 2002;35(2):254-261.
38. Nackman GB, Karkowski FJ, Halpern VJ, et al. Elastin degradation products induce adventitial angiogenesis in the Anidjar/Dobrin rat aneurysm model. *Surgery* 1997;122(1):39-44.
39. Brophy CM, Reilly JM, Smith GJ, et al. The role of inflammation in nonspecific abdominal aortic aneurysm disease. *Ann Vasc Surg* 1991;5(3):229-233.
40. Gregory AK, Yin NX, Capella J, et al. Features of autoimmunity in the abdominal aortic aneurysm. *Arch Surg* 1996;131(1):85-88.
41. Yen HC, Lee FY, Chau LY. Analysis of the T cell receptor V β-repertoire in human aortic aneurysms. *Atherosclerosis* 1997;135(1):29-36.
42. Walton LJ, Powell JT, Parums DV. Unrestricted usage of immunoglobulin heavy chain genes in B cells infiltrating the wall of atherosclerotic abdominal aortic aneurysms. *Atherosclerosis* 1997;135(1):65-71.
43. Juvonen J, Juvonen T, Laurila A, et al. Demonstration of *Chlamydia pneumoniae* in the walls of abdominal aortic aneurysms. *J Vasc Surg* 1997;25(3):499-505.
44. Halme S, Juvonen T, Laurila A, et al. *Chlamydia pneumoniae* reactive T lymphocytes in the walls of abdominal aortic aneurysms. *Eur J Clin Invest* 1999;29(6):546-552.
45. Meijer A, van Der Vliet JA, Roholl PJ, et al. *Chlamydia pneumoniae* in abdominal aortic aneurysms: abundance of membrane components in the absence of heat shock protein 60 and DNA. *Arterioscler Thromb Vasc Biol* 1999;19(11):2680-2686.
46. Tambiah J, Powell JT. *Chlamydia pneumoniae* antigens facilitate experimental aortic dilatation: prevention with azithromycin. *J Vasc Surg* 2002;36(5):1011-1017.
47. Lindholt JS, Ashton HA, Scott RA. Indicators of infection with *Chlamydia pneumoniae* are associated with expansion of abdominal aortic aneurysms. *J Vasc Surg* 2001;34(2):212-215.
48. Vammen S, Lindholt JS, Ostergaard L, et al. Randomized double-blind controlled trial of roxithromycin for prevention of abdominal aortic aneurysm expansion. *Br J Surg* 2001;88(8):1066-1072.
49. Kalayoglu MV, Libby P, Byrne GI. *Chlamydia pneumoniae* as an emerging risk factor in cardiovascular disease. *JAMA* 2002;288(21):2724-2731.
50. Koch AE, Kunkel SL, Pearce WH, et al. Enhanced production of the chemotactic cytokines interleukin-8 and monocyte chemoattractant protein-1 in human abdominal aortic aneurysms. *Am J Pathol* 1993;142(5):1423-1431.
51. Colonnello JS, Hance KA, Shames ML, et al. Transient exposure to elastase induces mouse aortic wall smooth muscle cell production of MCP-1 and RANTES during development of experimental aortic aneurysm. *J Vasc Surg* 2003;38(1):138-146.
52. Szekanecz Z, Shah MR, Pearce WH, et al. Human atherosclerotic abdominal aortic aneurysms produce interleukin (IL)–6 and interferon-γ but not IL-2 and IL-4: the possible role for IL-6 and interferon-γ in vascular inflammation. *Agents Actions* 1994;42(3-4):159-162.
53. Newman KM, Jean-Claude J, Li H, et al. Cytokines that activate proteolysis are increased in abdominal aortic aneurysms. *Circulation* 1994;90 (5 Pt 2):II224-II227.
54. Juvonen J, Surcel HM, Satta J, et al. Elevated circulating levels of inflammatory cytokines in patients with abdominal aortic aneurysm. *Arterioscler Thromb Vasc Biol* 1997;17(11):2843-2847.
55. Xiong W, Zhao Y, Prall A, et al. Key roles of CD4+ T cells and IFN-γ in the development of abdominal aortic aneurysms in a murine model. *J Immunol* 2004;172(4):2607-2612.
56. Schonbeck U, Sukhova GK, Gerdes N, et al. T(H)2 predominant immune responses prevail in human abdominal aortic aneurysm. *Am J Pathol* 2002;161(2):499-506.
57. Shimizu K, Shichiri M, Libby P, et al. Th2-predominant inflammation and blockade of IFN-γ signaling induce aneurysms in allografted aortas. *J Clin Invest* 2004;114(2):300-308.
58. Henderson EL, Geng YJ, Sukhova GK, et al. Death of smooth muscle cells and expression of mediators of apoptosis by T lymphocytes in human abdominal aortic aneurysms. *Circulation* 1999;99(1):96-104, 5-12.
59. Lopez-Candales A, Holmes DR, Liao S, et al. Decreased vascular smooth muscle cell density in medial degeneration of human abdominal aortic aneurysms. *Am J Pathol* 1997;150(3):993-1007.
60. Allaire E, Muscatelli-Groux B, Mandet C, et al. Paracrine effect of vascular smooth muscle cells in the prevention of aortic aneurysm formation. *J Vasc Surg* 2002;36(5):1018-1026.
61. Holmes DR, Wester W, Thompson RW, et al. Prostaglandin E_2 synthesis and cyclooxygenase expression in abdominal aortic aneurysms. *J Vasc Surg* 1997;25(5):810-815.
62. Walton LJ, Franklin IJ, Bayston T, et al. Inhibition of prostaglandin E_2 synthesis in abdominal aortic aneurysms: implications for smooth muscle cell viability, inflammatory processes, and the expansion of abdominal aortic aneurysms. *Circulation* 1999;100(1):48-54.
63. Miralles M, Wester W, Sicard GA, et al. Indomethacin inhibits expansion of experimental aortic aneurysms via inhibition of the cox2 isoform of cyclooxygenase. *J Vasc Surg* 1999;29(5):884-892; discussion, 892-883.
64. Li PF, Dietz R, von Harsdorf R. Reactive oxygen species induce apoptosis of vascular smooth muscle cell. *FEBS Lett* 1997;404(2-3):249-252.
65. Rajagopalan S, Meng XP, Ramasamy S, et al. Reactive oxygen species produced by macrophage-derived foam cells regulate the activity of vascular matrix metalloproteinases in vitro. Implications for atherosclerotic plaque stability. *J Clin Invest* 1996;98(11):2572-2579.
66. Miller FJ Jr., Sharp WJ, Fang X, et al. Oxidative stress in human abdominal aortic aneurysms: a potential mediator of aneurysmal remodeling. *Arterioscler Thromb Vasc Biol* 2002;22(4):560-565.
67. Yajima N, Masuda M, Miyazaki M, et al. Oxidative stress is involved in the development of experimental abdominal aortic aneurysm: a study of the transcription profile with complementary DNA microarray. *J Vasc Surg* 2002;36(2):379-385.
68. McMillan WD, Patterson BK, Keen RR, et al. In situ localization and quantification of seventy-two-kilodalton type IV collagenase in aneurysmal, occlusive, and normal aorta. *J Vasc Surg* 1995;22(3):295-305.
69. Lee JK, Borhani M, Ennis TL, et al. Experimental abdominal aortic aneurysms in mice lacking expression of inducible nitric oxide synthase. *Arterioscler Thromb Vasc Biol* 2001;21(9):1393-1401.
70. Busuttil RW, Abou-Zamzam AM, Machleder HI. Collagenase activity of the human aorta: a comparison of patients with and without abdominal aortic aneurysms. *Arch Surg* 1980;115(11):1373-1378.
71. Busuttil RW, Rinderbriecht H, Flesher A, et al. Elastase activity: the role of elastase in aortic aneurysm formation. *J Surg Res* 1982;32(3): 214-217.
72. Cannon DJ, Read RC. Blood elastolytic activity in patients with aortic aneurysm. *Ann Thorac Surg* 1982;34(1):10-15.
73. Visse R, Nagase H. Matrix metalloproteinases and tissue inhibitors of metalloproteinases: structure, function, and biochemistry. *Circ Res* 2003;92(8):827-839.
74. Nagase H, Woessner JF Jr.. Matrix metalloproteinases. *J Biol Chem* 1999;274(31):21491-21494.
75. Thompson RW, Holmes DR, Mertens RA, et al. Production and localization of 92-kilodalton gelatinase in abdominal aortic aneurysms: an elastolytic metalloproteinase expressed by aneurysm-infiltrating macrophages. *J Clin Invest* 1995;96(1):318-326.
76. Aimes RT, Quigley JP. Matrix metalloproteinase-2 is an interstitial collagenase: inhibitor-free enzyme catalyzes the cleavage of collagen fibrils and soluble native type I collagen generating the specific ¾- and ¼-length fragments. *J Biol Chem* 1995;270(11):5872-5876.
77. Davis V, Persidskaia R, Baca-Regen L, et al. Matrix metalloproteinase-2 production and its binding to the matrix are increased in abdominal aortic aneurysms. *Arterioscler Thromb Vasc Biol* 1998;18(10): 1625-1633.
78. Curci JA, Liao S, Huffman MD, et al. Expression and localization of macrophage elastase (matrix metalloproteinase-12) in abdominal aortic aneurysms. *J Clin Invest* 1998;102(11):1900-1910.
79. Shi GP, Sukhova GK, Grubb A, et al. Cystatin C deficiency in human atherosclerosis and aortic aneurysms. *J Clin Invest* 1999;104(9):1191-1197.
80. Carmeliet P, Moons L, Lijnen R, et al. Urokinase-generated plasmin activates matrix metalloproteinases during aneurysm formation. *Nat Genet* 1997;17(4):439-444.

81. Moore JE Jr, Ku DN, Zarins CK, et al. Pulsatile flow visualization in the abdominal aorta under differing physiologic conditions: implications for increased susceptibility to atherosclerosis. *J Biomech Eng* 1992;114(3):391-397.
82. Peterson L, Jensen RE, Parnell J. Mechanical properties of arteries in vivo. *Circ Res* 1960;8:622-633.
83. Wolinsky H, Glagov S. Comparison of abdominal and thoracic aortic medial structure in mammals: deviation of man from the usual pattern. *Circ Res* 1969;25(6):677-686.
84. Vorp DA, Lee PC, Wang DH, et al. Association of intraluminal thrombus in abdominal aortic aneurysm with local hypoxia and wall weakening. *J Vasc Surg* 2001;34(2):291-299.
85. Vorp DA, Raghavan ML, Webster MW. Mechanical wall stress in abdominal aortic aneurysm: influence of diameter and asymmetry. *J Vasc Surg* 1998;27(4):632-639.
86. Raghavan ML, Vorp DA, Federle MP, et al. Wall stress distribution on three-dimensionally reconstructed models of human abdominal aortic aneurysm. *J Vasc Surg* 2000;31(4):760-769.
87. Fillinger MF, Raghavan ML, Marra SP, et al. In vivo analysis of mechanical wall stress and abdominal aortic aneurysm rupture risk. *J Vasc Surg* 2002;36(3):589-597.
88. Lindholt JS, Henneberg EW, Juul S, et al. Impaired results of a randomised double-blinded clinical trial of propranolol versus placebo on the expansion rate of small abdominal aortic aneurysms. *Int Angiol* 1999;18(1): 52-57.
89. Propanolol Aneurysm Trial Investigators. Propranolol for small abdominal aortic aneurysms: results of a randomized trial. *J Vasc Surg* 2002;35(1):72-79.
90. Mosorin M, Juvonen J, Biancari F, et al. Use of doxycycline to decrease the growth rate of abdominal aortic aneurysms: a randomized, double-blind, placebo-controlled pilot study. *J Vasc Surg* 2001;34(4):606-610.
91. Habashi JP, Judge DP, Holm TM, et al. Losartan, an AT1 antagonist, prevents aortic aneurysm in a mouse model of Marfan syndrome. *Science* 2006;312(5770):117-121.
92. Rizzoni D, Rodella L, Porteri E, et al. Effects of losartan and enalapril at different doses on cardiac and renal interstitial matrix in spontaneously hypertensive rats. *Clin Exp Hypertens* 2003;25(7):427-441.

chapter 28

Abdominal Aortic Aneurysm Screening and Evaluation

Frank A. Lederle, MD

Key Points

- Abdominal aortic aneurysms (AAAs) that rupture are often unknown to the patient until the day of the rupture.
- Consequently, earlier AAA detection by screening is reasonable in patients at risk for aneurysms.
- Four risk factors increase the likelihood of an AAA: age (more than 65 years old), male gender, history of smoking, and family history of AAA.
- Four randomized trials of AAA screening have reported results that collectively show a substantial reduction in AAA-related mortality.
- The U.S. Preventive Services Task Force has recommended one-time AAA screening with ultrasound for men 65 to 75 years old.
- The U.S. Congress added a Medicare benefit for AAA screening that went into effect on January 1, 2007.
- The sensitivity of abdominal palpation to detect an AAA large enough to be considered for repair is high, especially if the abdominal girth is less than 40 inches.
- Abdominal ultrasound is the initial diagnostic test of choice to confirm a clinical suspicion of AAA.
- Two recent randomized clinical trials found no survival advantage of repair of AAAs smaller than 5.5 cm. Periodic ultrasound surveillance with repair reserved for AAAs that are 5.5 cm is less costly than repairing all AAAs equal to 4.0 cm.

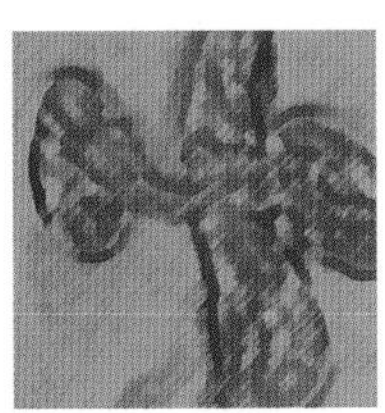

BACKGROUND AND RATIONALE

Screening for abdominal aortic aneurysms (AAAs) was first reported in 1966 by Schilling and colleagues.[1] Using physical examination and lateral abdominal radiography, they detected 26 AAAs of 3.6 cm in 873 men 55 to 64 years old, a prevalence of 3.1%.[1,2] The study received little attention, but in 1983, Cabellon and colleagues reported using ultrasound and abdominal palpation to find AAAs in 7 of 73 asymptomatic patients with vascular disease.[3] This study was followed by numerous similar studies and later by reports of larger, community-based programs. Since that time, screening for AAAs with ultrasound has been advocated by various authors and groups and debated extensively in the literature. Four randomized trials have reported results, and screening for AAA has become accepted practice in the United States.[4]

Early detection of disease through screening is an inherently appealing idea. However, screening must be undertaken with caution because the risks and costs apply to many whereas the benefits affect few and in some instances may even be negligible compared with usual care. Cochrane and Holland[5] argued that when the practitioner initiates screening procedures, an ethical requirement exists for greater certainty regarding benefit than for routine health care in which the patient asks the practitioner for help. In 1975, Frame and Carlson[6] proposed the following criteria for an acceptable screening program:

1. The disease must have a significant effect on the quality or quantity of life.
2. Acceptable methods of treatment must be available.
3. The disease must have an asymptomatic period during which detection and treatment significantly reduce morbidity, mortality, or both.
4. Treatment in the asymptomatic phase must yield a therapeutic result superior to that obtained by delaying treatment until symptoms appear.

Table 28-1
Prevalence of Abdominal Aortic Aneurysms (AAAs) by Diameter in Male Veterans 50 to 79 Years Old*

AAA Diameter	AAAs (*n*)	%
≥3.0 cm	5283	4.2
≥4.0 cm	1644	1.3
≥5.0 cm	571	0.45
≥5.5 cm†	342	0.27
≥6.0 cm	212	0.17
≥7.0 cm	76	0.06
≥8.0 cm	32	0.03

*n = 126,196.
†Adapted from Lederle FA, Johnson GR, Wilson SE, et al., and the ADAM VA Cooperative Study Investigators. *Arch Intern Med* 2000;160:1425-1430.

5. Tests must be available at reasonable cost to detect the condition in the asymptomatic period.
6. The incidence of the condition must be sufficient to justify the cost of screening.

Screening for AAA appears to meet these criteria. AAAs are common in older men, with AAAs of 3.0 cm occurring in 4% to 8%.[7,8] The prevalence of AAA, and hence the yield from screening, depends both on the population considered and on how AAA is defined. No widely accepted method exists of defining the cutoff point between AAA and normal. Most authors have used unadjusted aortic diameter (e.g., 3.0 cm), which is known to be associated with the risk of rupture.[9] While such a one-size-fits-all method could exaggerate the prevalence of AAA in larger people, we have found that age, gender, race, and body size have little influence on normal aortic diameter, suggesting that their use in defining AAA may not offer sufficient advantage to be warranted.[10]

Small AAAs are more common than large AAAs. Data from a large screening study conducted in older veterans show that with each 1 cm decrease in AAA diameter, the number of AAAs of that diameter or larger more than doubles (Table 28-1). Aortic aneurysm is the 15th leading cause of death in the United States,[11] and most of these deaths are due to rupture of AAAs.[12] Small AAAs enlarge at an average rate of 1 cm every 3 years,[13,14] so usually at least 5 years lapse from the time that the abdominal aorta reaches 3 cm in diameter (the most common definition of AAA) until symptoms of rupture develop, usually after the AAA is 6 cm. During this period, AAAs are nearly always asymptomatic and elective repair can be carried out with relatively low operative mortality (2% to 5%) by experienced surgeons, whereas once rupture occurs, only a fifth of patients survive.[15] The screening tests that have been proposed (ultrasound or abdominal palpation with confirmatory ultrasound) are safe, inexpensive, and acceptable to patients.[16]

The great difficulty in justifying screening programs is in demonstrating that early detection improves outcome compared with usual care without screening. Because of the many possibilities for bias, randomized trials are usually necessary to make this determination. Several randomized trials confirm the benefit of AAA screening in terms of both patient survival and cost of care.[17]

SCREENING MODALITIES

The diagnosis of asymptomatic AAA in the absence of screening must be incidental as the result of a physical examination or imaging test done for reasons other than to detect AAA.

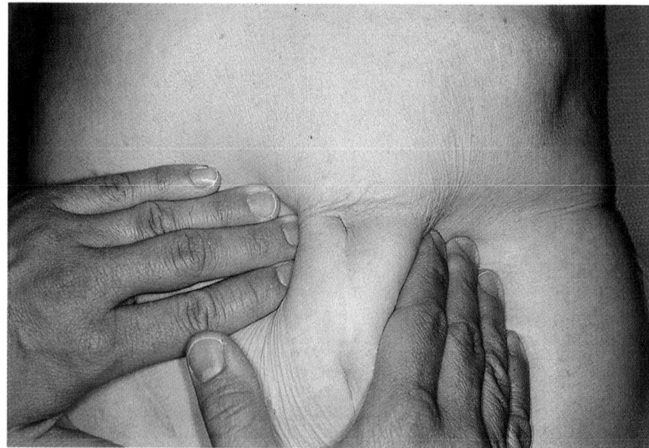

Figure 28-1. Abdominal palpation.

The frequency of incidental diagnoses of AAA led to attempts to systematically apply tests to high-risk populations for the purpose of detecting asymptomatic AAA. Abdominal palpation is the oldest method of AAA detection. Few aneurysms are found by "routine" palpation of the abdomen,[18] but deliberate and careful evaluation of the aorta detects most clinically important AAAs.[19] During the examination, the patient should be supine with the abdomen relaxed and the knees flexed to relax the anterior abdominal muscles. The examiner places both hands palms down on the abdomen between the xiphoid process and the umbilicus and palpates deeply to detect the aorta pulsation between the two index fingers. Ample skin should be included between the two index fingers, and it is often helpful initially to probe for one side of the aorta at a time (Figure 28-1).

The width, and not the intensity, of the aortic pulsation determines the diagnosis; a normal aorta is often readily palpable in thin patients or those with loose abdominal muscles. The aorta is normally less than 1 inch (2.5 cm) in diameter, and aortas larger than this (after allowing for skin thickness) warrant further investigation, usually with ultrasound. Findings of abdominal or femoral bruits or absent femoral pulses do not contribute to the diagnosis of asymptomatic AAA.[18] As Osler observed: "No pulsation, however forcible, no thrill, however intense, no bruit, however loud—singly or together—justify the diagnosis of an aneurysm of the abdominal aorta, only the presence of a palpable expansile tumour."[20]

The sensitivity of abdominal palpation for detecting AAA depends on the diameter of both aneurysm and patient. Three quarters of AAAs that are 5.0 cm in diameter are detectable by abdominal palpation, whereas less than one quarter of AAAs 3.0 to 3.9 cm are palpable.[19] The sensitivity of palpation is also much lower in patients with an abdominal girth of more than 100 cm (a 40-inch waist) compared with thinner patients.[18,21] The sensitivity of palpation to detect AAAs large enough to be considered for repair (5 cm) is quite high (100% in one small series of 12 cases[21]). Agreement among different examiners has been shown to be "fair to good" (κ of 0.53).[21] Only about one third of elderly men suspected of having an enlarged aorta on abdominal palpation are found to actually have AAA. This number (the positive predictive value) is much lower in women and young men[19] but is not of great concern because ultrasound provides a safe and inexpensive confirmatory test. Thus, while abdominal palpation is not an ideal diagnostic

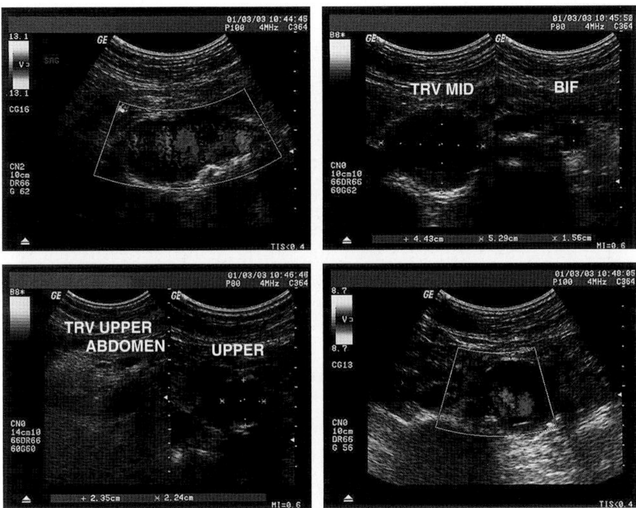

Figure 28-2. Ultrasound of abdominal aortic aneurysm.

test, many physicians consider it among the most worthwhile components of the physical examination, especially if ultrasound screening for AAA is not available.

Various abdominal imaging procedures accurately diagnose AAA, but virtually all screening programs undertaken or considered to date have involved the use of ultrasound. Ultrasound is particularly useful because of its accuracy (Figure 28-2), low cost, patient acceptance, lack of radiation exposure, and general availability. Various studies have shown the sensitivity and specificity of ultrasound for AAA to be nearly 100%.[18,22] Small portable ultrasonography equipment has increased the feasibility of mobile or temporary screening centers.

Plain radiography is a common means of incidental diagnosis of AAA and often provides early diagnostic clues to rupture, e.g., calcification, soft tissue mass, or loss of psoas or renal outlines.[23] However, plain radiography should not be used to confirm or exclude the diagnosis because many AAAs are missed due to insufficient calcification, resulting in sensitivities as low as 25%.[24] Computed tomography, angiography, magnetic resonance imaging, and their variants are all useful for detailed preoperative evaluation of AAA but offer no advantage over ultrasound for initial diagnosis and are more expensive.

PATIENT SELECTION

For screening to be efficient, it must target the population most likely to benefit. Published screening studies provide detailed information on factors associated with having an AAA detected at screening (Figure 28-3). The factors that have been most important are gender and age. AAA is primarily a disease of men. Numerous studies have found that men are about four times as likely as women to have AAA.[7] Even after adjustment for other risk factors, men are still more than twice as likely to have AAA.[25] As a result, most published population screening programs and randomized trials of screening have not included women.[4] Age is an equally important consideration. Like most diseases, AAAs are more common in older people. Prevalence increases throughout life, but incidence may peak at age 65.[26] Few people younger than 50 years of

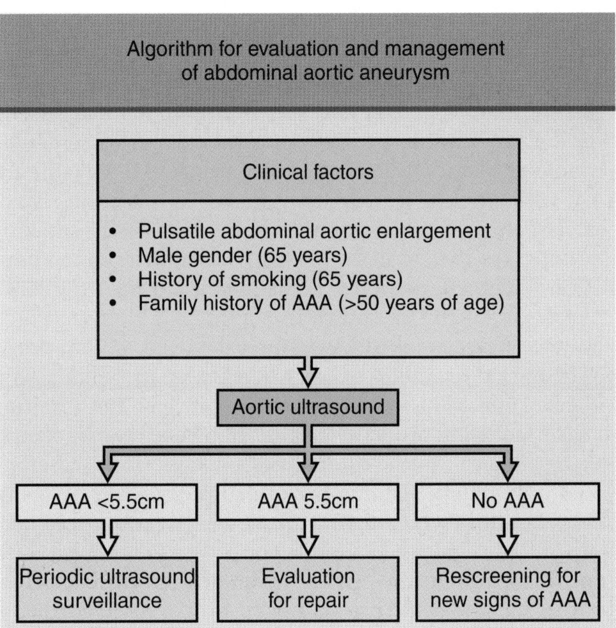

Figure 28-3. Algorithm for evaluation and management of abdominal aortic aneurysm.

age have AAA, but the prevalence increases sharply afterward (Figure 28-4). Targeting young people results in low yield, but targeting the very old is also of little value because many of those found to have AAA are not candidates for repair or do not live long enough after repair to realize any benefit. AAA incidence and prevalence, death rates, and screening compliance rates from several population-based screening studies in

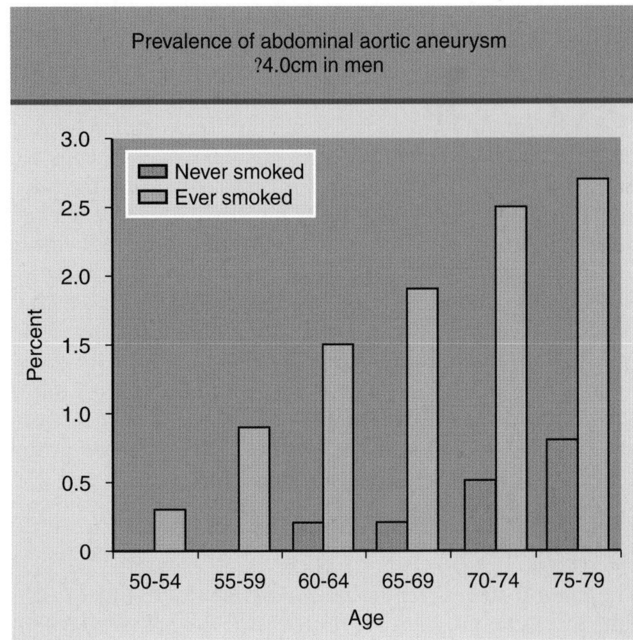

Figure 28-4. Prevalence of abdominal aortic aneurysms of 4.0 cm in men by age and smoking history. (Adapted from Lederle FA, Johnson GR, Wilson SE, et al., for the Aneurysm Detection and Management (ADAM) Veterans Affairs Cooperative Study Group. Prevalence and associations of abdominal aortic aneurysm detected through screening. *Ann Intern Med* 1997;126:441-449. Redrawn with permission from Chesler E, ed. *Clinical cardiology in the elderly*. 2nd ed. Armonk, New York: Futura; 1999.)

England have led their directors to conclude that the preferred age for AAA screening is 65,[27,28] and none of the study groups have proposed screening those more than 80 years old.

In addition to gender and age, another potentially useful criterion for defining a target population for AAA screening is smoking history. Smoking is the strongest risk factor for AAA, with smokers having more than five times the risk of nonsmokers.[25] The excess prevalence associated with smoking accounted for 75% of all the AAAs of 4.0 cm in a veteran population.[25] The effects of age and smoking on the prevalence of AAAs of 4.0 cm are shown in Figure 28-4 Note that men who have never smoked have a prevalence of 4.0-cm AAAs well below 1% regardless of age, whereas men in their 70s who had ever smoked had a prevalence greater than 2%. Limiting an AAA screening program to those who have ever smoked is therefore logical, but excluding nonsmokers from screening would only reduce the number of people screened by about 30%.[29] Limiting screening to current smokers cannot be recommended, as most AAAs in the population would be missed using this requirement.[29] Other moderately strong risk factors for AAA include white race; family history of AAA; coronary, cerebral, or peripheral artery disease; and absence of diabetes.[25] However, efforts to further select a target population beyond that of men aged 65 to 80 years have not been found to be worthwhile.[29,30]

EVIDENCE THAT SCREENING IS BENEFICIAL

Assessment of the benefit of screening is difficult because of the large numbers of patients required and the difficulty of ascertaining AAA-related deaths, particularly in the unscreened group.[31] Nevertheless, four randomized trials of AAA screening have published results.[4] The four trials randomly assigned patients from a population list: half were invited to an ultrasound screening, and the other half served as controls. Analysis was by intention to treat, and all four trials defined AAA as having a maximum diameter of 3.0 cm or larger. Of the invited groups, 60% to 80% attended the screening. Of the men attending, 4% to 8% had an AAA, and elective AAA repair was increased several fold in the invited groups compared with in the control groups. In a metaanalysis of these four trials for the U.S. Preventive Services Task Force (USPSTF),[4] invitation to screening was associated with a significant reduction in AAA-related mortality in men (odds ratio 0.57, confidence interval 0.45 to 0.74). The first trial, from Chichester, United Kingdom, included 9342 women. No benefit was seen from screening in women, with 10 ruptures in the screened group versus 9 in controls at 10 years of follow-up.[32]

RESCREENING

The randomized screening trials describe the results of one-time screening programs. A related issue is whether rescreening at specified intervals would be worthwhile. Although no randomized trials have addressed this question, some information on the yield of rescreening is available. In one study, 2622 veterans who had aortic diameters less than 3.0 cm by ultrasound at age 50 to 79 underwent repeat ultrasound after 4 years.[33] At that time, 58 (2.2%) had aortic diameters of 3.0 cm (meeting the usual definition of AAA), of which 3 were equal to 4.0 cm. Rescreening at 4 years was not considered worthwhile because of the low yield and small diameters of the AAAs detected. Crow et al.[28] described 223 men who had aortic diameters less than 2.6 cm by ultrasound at age 65 and were then rescreened after 5 and 12 years. Six men had aortic diameters of 3.0 to 3.6 cm (meeting the usual definition of AAA) at rescreening, but because of their age, none of these patients were considered likely to ever require elective repair. Based on these studies, it appears that screening, if implemented, need only occur once. As noted previously, the ideal time for one-time screening appears to be at age 65.

COST EFFECTIVENESS

Unlike many other screening programs, most of the cost of an ultrasound program of AAA screening results from treatment of detected AAA, with only about 15% coming from diagnosis.[34] Thus, the benefit of screening would appear to be closely linked to the benefit of treatment—that is, if repairing an AAA is worthwhile, then spending 15% more to detect it is probably also worthwhile.

Five of six older cost-effectiveness models of ultrasound screening for AAA published for men over age 60[34,35] found screening to be beneficial at costs ranging from about $2000 to $41,550 per year of life saved. A review of published studies on costs of screening conducted by the Oregon Evidence-based Practice Center (in conjunction with its evidence synthesis for the USPSTF) estimated the cost effectiveness of AAA screening to be $14,000 to $20,000 per quality-adjusted life year.[36] Two recent analyses using Markov models have concluded that AAA screening of older men is cost effective in Sweden[37] and in the United States,[38] where the cost was less than $20,000 per quality-adjusted life year.

In the 7-year follow-up of the largest screening trial, the Multicentre Aneurysm Screening Study, the cost effectiveness of ultrasound screening prevented AAA-related deaths at a cost that was estimated to be about $19,500 per year of life saved based on AAA-related deaths or $7600 per year of life saved based on all-cause mortality.[39] In addition, a randomized trial of ultrasound screening from Viborg, Denmark, reported that ultrasound screening prevented AAA-related deaths at a cost of 9057 Euros per year of life saved at 5 years,[40] and 2301 Euros per death (year of life saved was not calculated) at 10 years.[41] Cost-effectiveness ratios up to $40,000 per year of life saved are consistent with currently funded programs, and those under $20,000 are considered to be "very attractive."[34] Screening with abdominal palpation and confirmatory ultrasound has been calculated to be more cost effective than screening with ultrasound.[42]

MISCELLANEOUS CONCERNS REGARDING SCREENING

Screening identifies many small AAAs that are unlikely to rupture in the patient's lifetime. Adverse consequences for these patients include needless worry and risk from unnecessary procedures. Limited data are available on the possible adverse psychological effects of screening in general, but false-positive results have been associated with depression[43] and with increased anxiety that persists even after further testing rules out the disease.[44] Regarding AAA screening, a report

Table 28-2
Results of Recent AAA Screening Programs In the U.S.

Program	Screened (*n*)	Prosportion of Women (%)	Prevalence of AAA ≥ 3.0 cm (%)	
			Men	Women
AVA[48]	7,841	60	4.5	0.85
DARE to CARE[49]	12,055	59	3.2	0.5
Life Line[50]	17,540	57	3.9	0.7

n = AVA; CARE; DARE.

of no difference in anxiety and depression scores between screened and unscreened subjects is encouraging[45] but may not be reliable because the groups were small and dissimilar (the unscreened group had fewer married men). Another study reported that anxiety levels dropped after screening, regardless of whether AAA was detected.[46] Unfortunately, anxiety levels from before the screening invitation were not available for comparison.

More concerning for those with small AAAs detected at screening is the risk from unnecessary procedures. Despite publication of the two trials demonstrating that survival is not improved by elective repair of AAAs smaller than 5.5 cm even in good operative candidates,[13,14] the inclination to repair smaller AAAs remains strong, at least in the United States. About 4500 deaths are attributed to AAA rupture in the United States each year,[12] indicating that postoperative deaths constitute nearly a quarter of all AAA mortality. In the Multicentre Aneurysm Screening Study,[39] the largest and most influential screening trial, AAA repair was not undertaken unless the AAA was 5.5 cm or larger, a possible key to the success of that trial. If screening in the United States leads to a large increase in elective repair in patients whose AAA would never have ruptured, the expected benefit of screening on AAA-related mortality may never be realized.

CURRENT RECOMMENDATIONS

Following publication of four randomized trials that collectively showed that ultrasound screening was associated with a significant reduction in AAA-related mortality, the USPSTF recommended one-time AAA screening with ultrasound for men 65 to 75 years old who have ever smoked.[17] The task force made no recommendation for men who had never smoked and recommended against routine screening for AAA in women.

CURRENT PRACTICE

After the USPSTF report, the U.S. Congress added a Medicare benefit for AAA screening that went into effect on January 1, 2007. It provides a free, one-time, ultrasound test for men who have smoked and for men and women with a family history of AAA. The ultrasound test must be ordered within the first 6 months of Medicare eligibility (i.e., age 65 to 65 ½).

A consensus statement published by three American vascular societies proposed criteria for screening eligibility considerably broader than those recommended by the USPSTF or used in the randomized trials of screening.[47] The vascular societies' criteria include men aged 60 to 85, women aged 60 to 85 with cardiovascular risk factors, and anyone over age 50 with a family history of AAA, unless the subject is unfit for any intervention. Descriptions of several recent free ultrasound screening programs conducted in the United States have been published and are shown in Table 28-2.

The Life Line program[50] used criteria similar to those proposed by the vascular societies, whereas the AVA[48] and DARE to CARE[49] programs had only a minimum age criterion. As shown in Table 28-2, most subjects screened in all three programs were women, despite a fivefold lower prevalence of AAA. The USPSTF had recommended against screening women because the only randomized trial to include women showed not only low prevalence but also no favorable trend in AAA-related mortality.[32] Furthermore, in the DARE to CARE program, 439 screenees were younger than 40 years, another 433 were 40 to 49, and 788 were 80 to 95. These reports suggest that the many screening programs operating in the United States outside of Medicare are likely to be considerably less cost effective than those done in the randomized trials in Europe.

Acceptance rates for AAA screening invitations have been reported for several investigational programs. Community screening programs using letters sent by the patients' general practitioner have reported acceptance rates of about 75%.[8,51] Acceptance rates are higher at age 65 than in more elderly patients.[51] A lower acceptance rate of 30% was observed when letters were sent to veterans from physicians whom they did not know.[52] More recently, letters sent to randomly selected Medicare beneficiaries from the referral region of three university-affiliated hospitals resulted in an attendance rate of only 7%.[53]

EVALUATION AND FOLLOW-UP

The success of a screening program depends largely on how patients are managed after the screening test. For those who test negative, being actively informed of the negative results is more reassuring than telling the patient that "no news is good news."[43] For patients who screen positive for an AAA by ultrasound, the first consideration is whether to recommend elective repair. As noted earlier, two randomized trials have demonstrated that survival is not improved by elective repair of AAAs below 5.5 cm, even in good operative candidates. Therefore, asymptomatic AAAs should be considered for repair when they are 5.5 cm in good surgical candidates, and repair should be further deferred in patients with high operative risk until the risk of rupture outweighs that risk in the opinion of the attending vascular surgeon. For most patients with an AAA detected at screening, the management plan is periodic imaging surveillance of the AAA until the AAA diameter crosses the threshold for elective repair in that patient. The patient and family must be educated that periodic follow-up is essential to the patient's safety. Patients with unrepaired AAAs who are potential operative candidates should have AAA measurement, usually with ultrasound, at intervals of 6 months for AAA 4.0 to 5.4 cm.[14] Intervals of 2 to 3 years have been proposed for smaller AAA.[54,55] Variations in AAA measurement of 0.5 cm or more are not uncommon, and this should be taken into account in management decisions.[56]

The natural history of AAA is usually one of progressive slow growth, with the risk of rupture increasing with the size of the aneurysm. AAAs of 4.0 to 5.5 cm enlarge at a mean rate of 0.3 cm per year, with less than 25% enlarging faster than 0.5 cm per year.[13,14] Less than one third of AAAs eventually rupture, and most patients with AAAs die of other causes, especially coronary artery disease.[57] Continued smoking is associated with increased AAA growth rate[58] and possibly with an increased likelihood of rupture.[59]

CONCLUSIONS

Many large AAA remain undetected until rupture, and many small AAA that will never rupture are detected incidentally and repaired, with some resulting morbidity and mortality. Both scenarios contribute to aortic aneurysms remaining a leading cause of death. Recent randomized trials have demonstrated a substantial reduction in AAA-related mortality from ultrasound screening (and resulting elective AAA repair). Now that the USPSTF has recommended AAA screening and Medicare has led the way in providing coverage, the era of AAA screening has begun. If screening is accompanied by prudent criteria for elective repair, the mortality associated with AAA may at last be reduced.

References

1. Schilling FJ, Hempel HF, Becker WH, Christakis G. Asymptomatic aortic aneurysms detected on the abdominal roentgenogram. *Circulation* 1966;33(Suppl 3):209.
2. Schilling FJ, Christakis G, Hempel HH, Orbach A. The natural history of abdominal aortic and iliac atherosclerosis as detected by lateral abdominal roentgenograms in 2663 males. *J Chronic Dis* 1974;27:37-45.
3. Cabellon S, Moncrief CL, Pierre DR, Cavanaugh DG. Incidence of abdominal aortic aneurysms in patients with atheromatous arterial disease. *Am J Surg* 1983;146:575-576.
4. Fleming C, Whitlock E, Beil T, Lederle FA. Screening for abdominal aortic aneurysm: a systematic review and meta-analysis for the U.S. Preventive Services Task Force. *Ann Intern Med* 2005;142:203-211.
5. Cochrane AL, Holland WW. Validation of screening procedures. *Br Med Bull* 1971;27:3-8.
6. Frame PS, Carlson SJ. A critical review of periodic health screening using specific screening criteria. I. Selected diseases of respiratory, cardiovascular, and central nervous systems. *J Fam Pract* 1975;2:29-36.
7. Lederle FA, Johnson GR, Wilson SE, for the Aneurysm Detection and Management Veterans Affairs Cooperative Study. Abdominal aortic aneurysm in women. *J Vasc Surg* 2001;34:122-126.
8. Boll AP, Verbeek AL, van de Lisdonk EH, van der Vliet JA. High prevalence of abdominal aortic aneurysm in a primary care screening programme. *Br J Surg* 1998;85:1090-1094.
9. Nevitt MP, Ballard DJ, Hallett JW. Prognosis of abdominal aortic aneurysms: a population-based study. *N Engl J Med* 1989;321:1009-1014.
10. Lederle FA, Johnson GR, Wilson SE, et al., and the ADAM VA Cooperative Study Investigators. Relationship of age, gender, race, and body size to infrarenal aortic diameter. *J Vasc Surg* 1997;26:595-601.
11. Hoyert DL, Arias E, Smith BL, Murphy SL, Kochanek KD. Deaths: final data for 1999. *Natl Vital Stat Rep* 2001;49:1-113.
12. Centers for Disease Control and Prevention, National Center for Health Statistics. CDC WONDER On-line Database, compiled from Compressed Mortality File 1999-2004 Series 20 No. 2J, 2007. Available at: http://wonder.cdc.gov. Accessed November 2007.
13. U.K. Small Aneurysm Trial Participants. Mortality results for randomised controlled trial of early elective surgery or ultrasonographic surveillance for small abdominal aortic aneurysms. *Lancet* 1998;352:1649-1655.
14. Lederle FA, Wilson SE, Johnson GR, et al., for the Aneurysm Detection and Management (ADAM) Veterans Affairs Cooperative Study Investigators. Immediate repair compared with surveillance of small abdominal aortic aneurysms. *N Engl J Med* 2002;346:1437-1444.
15. Adam DJ, Mohan IV, Stuart WP, et al. Community and hospital outcome from ruptured abdominal aortic aneurysm within the catchment area of a regional vascular surgical service. *J Vasc Surg* 1999;30:922-928.
16. Lindholt JS, Juul S, Henneberg EW, Fasting H. Is screening for abdominal aortic aneurysm acceptable to the population? Selection and recruitment to hospital-based mass screening for abdominal aortic aneurysm. *J Public Health Med* 1998;20:211-217.
17. U.S. Preventive Services Task Force. Screening for abdominal aortic aneurysm: recommendation statement. *Ann Intern Med* 2005;142: 198-202.
18. Lederle FA, Walker JM, Reinke DB. Selective screening for abdominal aortic aneurysms with physical examination and ultrasound. *Arch Intern Med* 1988;148:1753-1756.
19. Lederle FA, Simel DL. The rational clinical examination: does this patient have abdominal aortic aneurysm? *JAMA* 1999;281:77-82.
20. Osler W. Aneurysm of the abdominal aorta. *Lancet* 1905;2:1089-1096.
21. Fink HA, Lederle FA, Roth CS, et al. The accuracy of physical examination to detect abdominal aortic aneurysm. *Arch Intern Med* 2000;160: 833-836.
22. Nusbaum JW, Freimanis AK, Thomford NR. Echography in the diagnosis of abdominal aortic aneurysm. *Arch Surg* 1971;102:385-388.
23. Loughran CF. A review of the plain abdominal radiograph in acute rupture of abdominal aortic aneurysms. *Clin Radiol* 1986;37:383-387.
24. Roberts A, Johnson N, Royle J, et al. The diagnosis of abdominal aortic aneurysms. *Aust NZ J Surg* 1974;44:360-362.
25. Lederle FA, Johnson GR, Wilson SE, et al., the ADAM VA Cooperative Study Investigators. The Aneurysm Detection and Management Study screening program: validation cohort and final results. *Arch Intern Med* 2000;160:1425-1430.
26. Vardulaki KA, Prevost TC, Walker NM, et al. Incidence among men of asymptomatic abdominal aortic aneurysms: estimates from 500 screen detected cases. *J Med Screen* 1999;6:50-54.
27. Scott RA, Vardulaki KA, Walker NM, et al. The long-term benefits of a single scan for abdominal aortic aneurysm (AAA) at age 65. *Eur J Vasc Endovasc Surg* 2001;21:535-540.
28. Crow P, Shaw E, Earnshaw JJ, et al. A single normal ultrasonographic scan at age 65 years rules out significant aneurysm disease for life in men. *Br J Surg* 2001;88:941-944.
29. Spencer CA, Jamrozik K, Norman PE, Lawrence-Brown MM. The potential for a selective screening strategy for abdominal aortic aneurysm. *J Med Screen* 2000;7:209-211.
30. Lindholt JS, Henneberg EW, Fasting H, Juul S. Mass or high-risk screening for abdominal aortic aneurysm. *Br J Surg* 1997;84:40-42.
31. Lederle FA. Screening for snipers: the burden of proof. *J Clin Epidemiol* 1990;43:101-104.
32. Scott RA, Bridgewater SG, Ashton HA. Randomized clinical trial of screening for abdominal aortic aneurysm in women. *Br J Surg* 2002;89(3): 283-285.
33. Lederle FA, Johnson GR, Wilson SE, et al., the ADAM VA Cooperative Study Investigators. Yield of repeated screening for abdominal aortic aneurysm after a four-year interval. *Arch Intern Med* 2000;160:1117-1121.
34. Lederle FA. Looking for asymptomatic abdominal aortic aneurysms. *J Gen Intern Med* 1996;11:774-775.
35. Pentikainen TJ, Sipila T, Rissanen P, et al. Cost-effectiveness of targeted screening for abdominal aortic aneurysm: Monte Carlo–based estimates. *Int J Technol Assess Health Care* 2000;16:22-34.
36. Meenan RT, Fleming C, Whitlock EP, et al. Cost-effectiveness analyses of population-based screening for abdominal aortic aneurysm: evidence synthesis. AHRQ Publication No. 05-0569-C, February 2005. Agency for Healthcare Research and Quality, Rockville, Maryland. Available at: http://www.ahrq.gov/clinic/uspstf05/aaascr/aaacost.htm. Accessed April 13, 2009.
37. Henriksson M, Lundgren F. Decision–analytical model with lifetime estimation of costs and health outcomes for one-time screening for abdominal aortic aneurysm in 65-year-old men. *Br J Surg* 2005;92:976-983.
38. Silverstein MD, Pitts SR, Chaikof EL, Ballard DJ. Abdominal aortic aneurysm (AAA): cost-effectiveness of screening, surveillance of intermediate-sized AAA, and management of symptomatic AAA. *Proc (Bayl Univ Med Cent)* 2005;18:345-367.
39. Kim LG, Scott RAP, Ashton HA, Thompson SG. for the Multicentre Aneurysm Screening Study Group. A sustained mortality benefit from screening for abdominal aortic aneurysm. *Ann Intern Med* 2007;146(10):699-706.
40. Lindholt JS, Juul S, Fasting H, Henneberg EW. Cost-effectiveness analysis of screening for abdominal aortic aneurysms based on five year results from a randomised hospital based mass screening trial. *Eur J Vasc Endovasc Surg* 2006;32:9-15.
41. Lindholt JS, Juul S, Fasting H, Henneberg EW. Preliminary ten year results from a randomised single centre mass screening trial for abdominal aortic aneurysm. *Eur J Vasc Endovasc Surg* 2006;32:608-614.
42. Frame PS, Fryback DG, Patterson C. Screening for abdominal aortic aneurysm in men ages 60 to 80 years: a cost-effectiveness analysis. *Ann Intern Med* 1993;119:411-416.

43. Marteau TM. Psychological costs of screening. *BMJ* 1989;299:527.
44. Stewart-Brown S, Farmer A. Screening could seriously damage your health. *BMJ* 1997;314:533-534.
45. Khaira HS, Herbert LM, Crowson MC. Screening for abdominal aortic aneurysms does not increase psychological morbidity. *Ann R Coll Surg Engl* 1998;80:341-342.
46. Lucarotti ME, Heather BP, Shaw E, Poskitt KR. Psychological morbidity associated with abdominal aortic aneurysm screening. *Eur J Vasc Endovasc Surg* 1997;14:499-501.
47. Kent KC, Zwolak RM, Jaff MR, et al. Society for Vascular Surgery, American Association of Vascular Surgery, Society for Vascular Medicine and Biology. Screening for abdominal aortic aneurysm: a consensus statement. *J Vasc Surg* 2004;39:267-269.
48. Flinn WR, Silva MB, Pearce WH, Hobson RW. Ultrasound screening for abdominal aortic aneurysms in women. Available at: http://mvss.vascularweb.org/MVSS_Contribution_Pages/Annual_Meeting/Abstracts_Program/Abstracts/2005/Ultrasound_Screening_for_Abdominal_Aortic_Aneurysms_in_Women.html. Accessed April 13, 2009.
49. Hupp JA, Martin JD, Hansen LO. Results of a single center vascular screening and education program. *J Vasc Surg* 2007;46:182-187.
50. Derubertis BG, Trocciola SM, Ryer EJ, et al. Abdominal aortic aneurysm in women: prevalence, risk factors, and implications for screening. *J Vasc Surg* 2007;46:630-635.
51. Khoo DE, Ashton H, Scott RA. Is screening once at age 65 an effective method for detection of abdominal aortic aneurysms? *J Med Screen* 1994;1:223-225.
52. Lederle FA, Johnson GR, Wilson SE, et al., for the Aneurysm Detection and Management (ADAM) Veterans Affairs Cooperative Study Group. Prevalence and associations of abdominal aortic aneurysm detected through screening. *Ann Intern Med* 1997;126:441-449.
53. Schermerhorn M, Zwolak R, Velazquez O, et al. Ultrasound screening for abdominal aortic aneurysm in Medicare beneficiaries. *Ann Vasc Surg* 2007;22(1):16-24.
54. Santilli SM, Littooy FN, Cambria RA, et al. Expansion rates and outcomes for the 3.0-cm to the 3.9-cm infrarenal abdominal aortic aneurysm. *J Vasc Surg* 2002;35:666-671.
55. Grimshaw GM, Thompson JM, Hamer JD. A statistical analysis of the growth of small abdominal aortic aneurysms. *Eur J Vasc Surg* 1994;8:741-746.
56. Lederle FA, Wilson SE, Johnson GR, et al., for the Abdominal Aortic Aneurysm Detection and Management Veterans Administration Cooperative Study Group. Variability in measurement of abdominal aortic aneurysms. *J Vasc Surg* 1995;21:945-952.
57. Darling RC, Messina CR, Brewster DC, Ottinger LW. Autopsy study of unoperated abdominal aortic aneurysms: the case for early resection. *Circulation* 1977;56(Suppl 2):161-164.
58. MacSweeney ST, Ellis M, Worrell PC, et al. Smoking and growth rate of small abdominal aortic aneurysms. *Lancet* 1994;344:651-652.
59. Brown LC, Powell JT. Risk factors for aneurysm rupture in patients kept under ultrasound surveillance: UK Small Aneurysm Trial Participants. *Ann Surg* 1999;230:289-296.

chapter

29

Abdominal Aneurysms: Endovascular Aneurysm Repair

Marc R.H.M. van Sambeek, MD, PhD • Philippe Cuypers, MD, PhD • Johanna M. Hendriks, MD, PhD • Jaap Buth, MD, PhD

Key Points

- Endovascular aneurysm repair (EVAR) for abdominal aortic aneurysms offers an important new alternative to open surgical procedure.
- Compared with conventional open surgery, EVAR reduces operating time, blood transfusions, intensive care requirements, and length of hospital stay.
- Perioperative mortality rates after EVAR in asymptomatic abdominal aortic aneurysms in the randomized trials is between 1.2% and 1.7%.
- The perioperative survival advantage with endovascular repair as compared with open repair is not sustained after the first year.
- Long-term reports are not available, but midterm follow-up of EVAR reveals a higher incidence of reinterventions compared to open surgical repair.
- The perplexing problems of endoleaks and graft failure continue to be challenges that technological innovations must address.
- Until solutions for endoleaks, endotension, and stent failure are found, EVAR remains an imperfect long-term treatment and requires regular, lifelong graft surveillance.
- Based on the available evidence, EVAR is an appropriate treatment for selected patients.

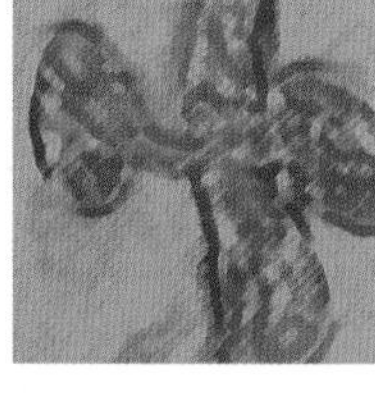

In the last 10 to 15 years, the interest in minimally invasive surgery has grown. The same trend can be observed in vascular surgery and interventional radiology, leading to what is commonly referred as endovascular surgery. Although the 1990s represent a decade of technological revolution, it is a mistake to consider endovascular treatment as a recent development. In 1947, João Cid Dos Santos described thromboendarterectomy[1]; this technique was modified by Jorg Vollmar in 1964 to a semiclosed endarterectomy using ringstrippers.[2] In the same year, other pioneers, including Charles Dotter and Melvin Judkins, published preliminary results on what they called "angioplasty" of the femoropopliteal artery using coaxial catheters.[3] This technique was modified by Grüntzig and Hophoff in 1974, who replaced the coaxial catheters with dilatation balloons.[4] In the early 1990s, Volodos et al. and Parodi et al. introduced endovascular treatment of abdominal aortic aneurysm (AAA) with a device composed of a Dacron graft and a balloon-expandable stent.[5,6]

Since the first use of a stent graft for the endovascular exclusion of an AAA, the use of endovascular treatment of AAA has greatly expanded and has become a mainstay in the repair of AAA. Randomized trials have shown a perioperative survival benefit of endovascular repair over open surgical repair, with fewer complications and shorter recovery. Nevertheless, concerns still surround the long-term durability of the endovascular repair, the increasing risk of late rupture with endovascular repair, and the necessity of more common reinterventions, including conversion to open surgical repair.

The transabdominal approach and replacement of the aneurysmal aorta by a prosthesis are inevitable in open surgical repair. Because the procedure may cause stress to both physical and mental health, quality of life decreases for up to 3 months after the operation.

With endovascular treatment of AAA, a laparotomy is not required. The endovascular graft can be implanted from a remote access site in the groin with less anesthetic requirement. The endovascular graft is advanced over guide wires up the femoral and iliac arteries. Once in position, the graft is deployed immediately distal from the renal arteries. The aorta is not clamped, and the blood loss is less than with open surgery.

Many terms are used to describe the prostheses that are implanted during an endovascular procedure; these include endovascular graft, stent graft, grafted stent, endoprosthesis, transluminally placed endovascular graft, and endograft. The graft material creates a barrier that excludes the AAA, and the stent or metallic ultrastructure positions the graft precisely, without the need for a surgical anastomosis. At the same time, the stent provides a certain level of support.

PATIENT SELECTION AND PREOPERATIVE IMAGING FOR REGULAR ENDOVASCULAR AAA REPAIR

Not all patients with an AAA are suitable for endovascular repair. Preprocedural assessment must reject unsuitable patients, identify potential difficulties, and allow selection of an appropriate stent graft. The main criteria for patient selection apply to anatomical details of the vascular tree between the renal arteries and the external iliac artery. Endovascular aneurysm repair (EVAR) brings many new challenges for preoperative imaging. Unlike with conventional surgery, with endovascular repair the anatomical configuration of the infrarenal aorta must be known to a high degree of accuracy. Regardless of which kind of stent graft is to be used, a similar series of measurements must be obtained for each patient. Every company, every study, and every registry has its own worksheet that can be filled out to record the most relevant details. One of the most commonly used is the worksheet from the European Collaborators on Stent-Graft Techniques for Abdominal Aortic Aneurysm Repair (EUROSTAR) Registry (Figure 29-1).[7]

The most common reasons to reject a patient based on anatomical configurations are listed here.

Visceral and Renal Supply

Patency of the celiac axis and superior mesenteric artery should be assessed before a patent inferior mesenteric artery (IMA) can be overstented. Renal arteries and accessory renal arteries should be identified.

Diameter of Proximal Neck

Depending on the device used, an infrarenal neck with a diameter of more than 30 mm is considered unsuitable. Newer-generation stent grafts are capable of accommodating even lager infrarenal diameters. All stent grafts need to achieve a seal between the device and the aortic wall. Usually, the stent graft is oversized by 10% to 20% compared with the diameter of the proximal neck.

Length of Proximal Neck

To achieve a good seal between the stent graft and the aortic wall, a snug apposition over a lengthof 10 to 15 mm is required. Some limitations of the large diameter and short length of the infrarenal neck are overcome with the introduction of fenestrated and branched stent grafts.

Angulation of the Proximal Neck

Angulation of the proximal neck is possible and is more often seen with larger aneurysms (more than 60 mm). Aortic neck angulation appears to be an important determinant of outcome after EVAR. Mild angulation (less than 40 degrees) is associated with favorable outcome, whereas those with moderate (40 degrees to 59 degrees) and severe (more than 60 degrees) angulation have a higher risk of adverse events, especially type I endoleaks.[8]

Conical Nature of the Proximal Neck

A contour change of the proximal neck of more than 10% is associated with a higher proximal endoleak rate and therefore considered unfavorable (Figure 29-2).[9]

Calcification and Mural Thrombus in Proximal Neck

Calcification and mural thrombus in the proximal neck are expressed in degrees of circumference. Mural thrombus in the neck of more than 90 degrees is considered a risk factor for endoleak, whereas extended calcification increases the probability of stent graft migration.

Diameter of Iliac Artery

In general, the stent graft ends in the common iliac artery. Therefore, a size limitation arises from the diameter of the common iliac artery, depending on the device used. If the diameter of the common iliac artery is too large, the stent graft can be extended to the external iliac artery. In such a case, it is advisable to coil-embolize the hypogastric artery, since retrograde flow from the hypogastric artery can cause an endoleak. Currently, newer-generation stent grafts have the option of a hypogastric side branch. In this situation, the stent graft is extended to the external iliac artery. The patency of the hypogastric artery can be preserved with covered side branch.

Length of Distal Sealing Zone

In a similar way to the proximal sealing zone, a snug apposition over a length of 10 to 15 mm is required.

Tortuosity of Iliac Arteries

The introducer systems are large (16 to 28 French [Fr] in diameter) and relatively inflexible. If the iliac arteries are small, calcified, and tortuous, it is difficult for the delivery system to pass without causing damage to the iliac tract. No strict criteria are available in this matter, and a decision should be made based on the diameter and flexibility of the delivery system and the surgeon's experience.

Almost all imaging modalities have been used in the diagnostic workup of a patient. Ultrasound is most commonly used to establish the diagnosis of an AAA.

Spiral Computed Tomography Angiography

High-quality contrast-enhanced computed tomography angiography (CTA) is essential and is currently the imaging technique of choice for EVAR. It provides detailed information on vascular anatomy and thus helps in selecting suitable patients and the right stent graft. The patient should not have oral

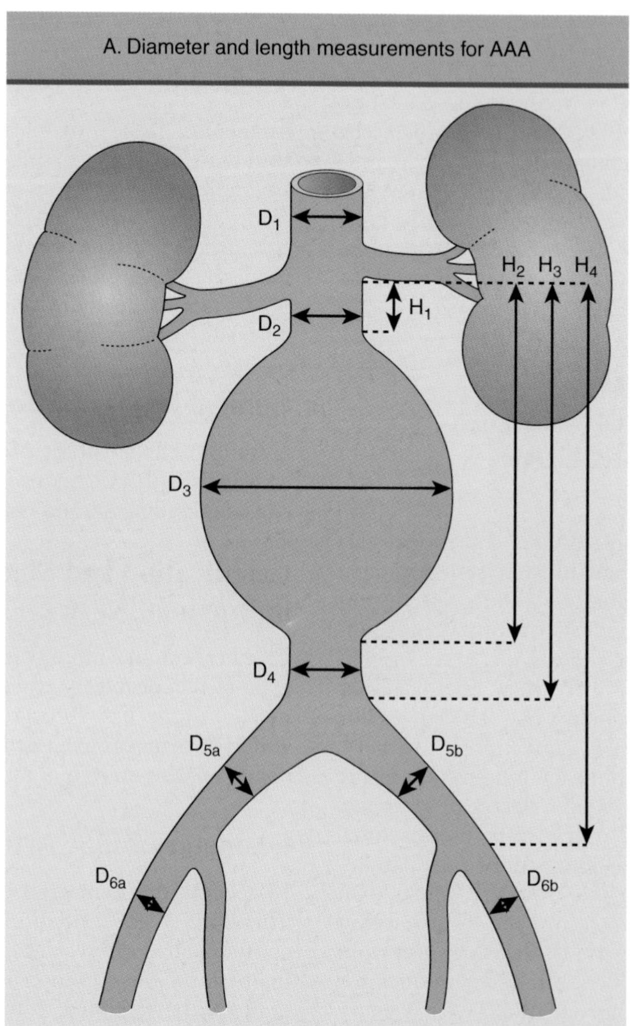

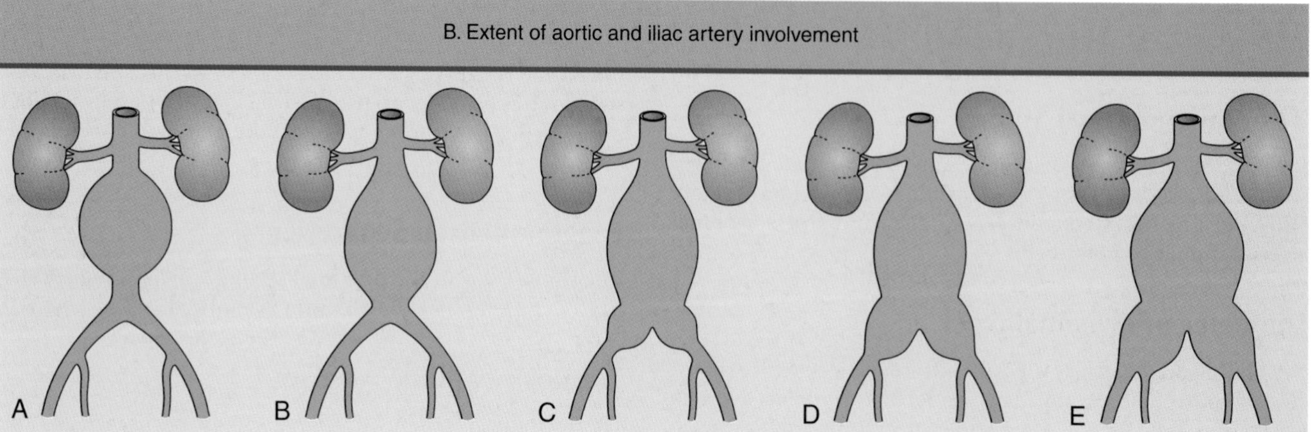

Figure 29-1. Endovascular repair of the aorta. **A,** Worksheet for documentation of diameters and length measurements for abdominal aortic aneurysms. **B,** Worksheet for documentation of iliac artery involvement.

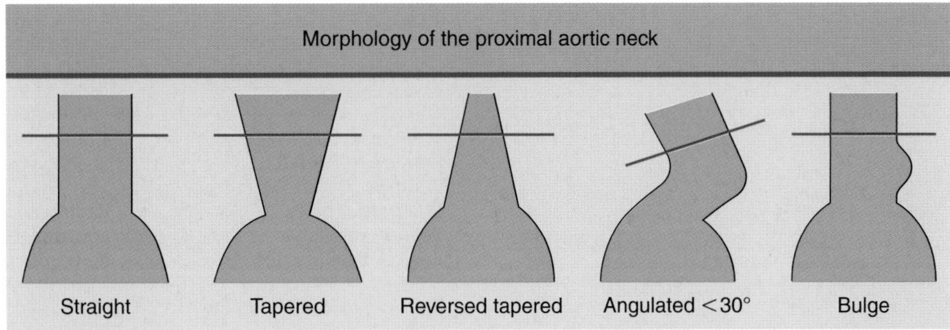

Figure 29-2. Worksheet for documentation of the morphology of the proximal aortic neck.

contrast as this may interfere with three-dimensional reconstructions. The scan must image from the celiac axis to the common femoral artery. CTA protocols vary considerably, but most require a large volume of iodinated contrast agent (100 to 150 ml), narrow collimation (3 to 5 mm), and reformatting of overlapping axial slices at short (2 to 4 mm) intervals.

A potential pitfall can occur when assessing axial scans. As the aorta expands, it can also lengthen. This can cause the aneurysm neck to deviate anteriorly and laterally. Axial scanning does not take this into account, and the neck or aneurysm may appear oval rather than round in cross section. This can result in a tendency to overestimate the neck diameter and underestimate the neck length (Figure 29-3). Mistakes in assessment can be overcome with image processing on a workstation. Curved linear reformats can be used for accurate assessment of the diameters and length of the potential attachment zones in the aorta and iliac arteries. Unlike axial computed tomography images, curved linear reformats allow visualization of the aortic and iliac lumen in a plane perpendicular to the central arterial axis. By avoiding oblique projection, the images represent the true cross-sectional shape of the aorta. Curved linear reformats perpendicular to the vessel axis can be acquired using central lumen lines, which can be created by positioning markers in the center of the aorta and iliac arteries at several levels (Figure 29-4).[10]

Dedicated computer programs are available to facilitate multiplanar reconstructions from CTA data set.

Arterial Angiography

Arterial angiography can provide additional information. It is superior to CTA in the assessment of the grade of stenosis of major branches of the aorta. By itself, it is insufficient for patient selection because thrombus in the aneurysm and arteriosclerotic disease of the arterial wall are not displayed.

For many years, arterial angiography was mandatory in the preoperative workup for endovascular procedures, especially to perform accurate length measurements. With the dedicated computer programs currently available, the arterial angiography has become redundant.

If the arteries are tortuous and not too calcified during the angiography, the surgeon can try to straighten the iliac artery by passing a superstiff guide wire through the pigtail catheter.

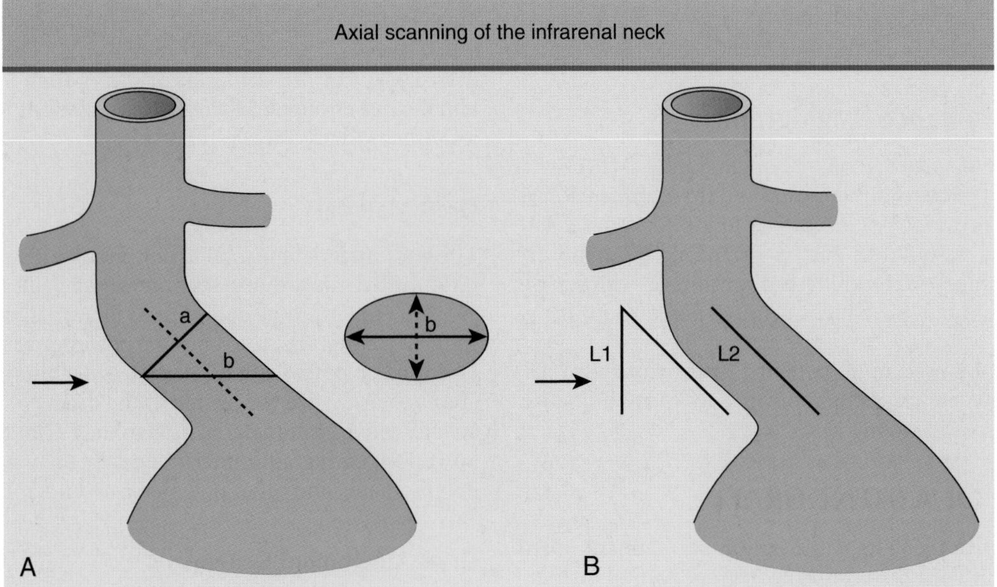

Figure 29-3. Axial scanning of the infrarenal neck. **A,** With axial scanning of an angulated infrarenal neck, the neck may appear elliptical. Assessment of the largest diameter includes overestimation of the "real" diameter. **B,** With axial scanning, the length of the infrarenal neck (L1) includes an underestimation of the "real" length (L2).

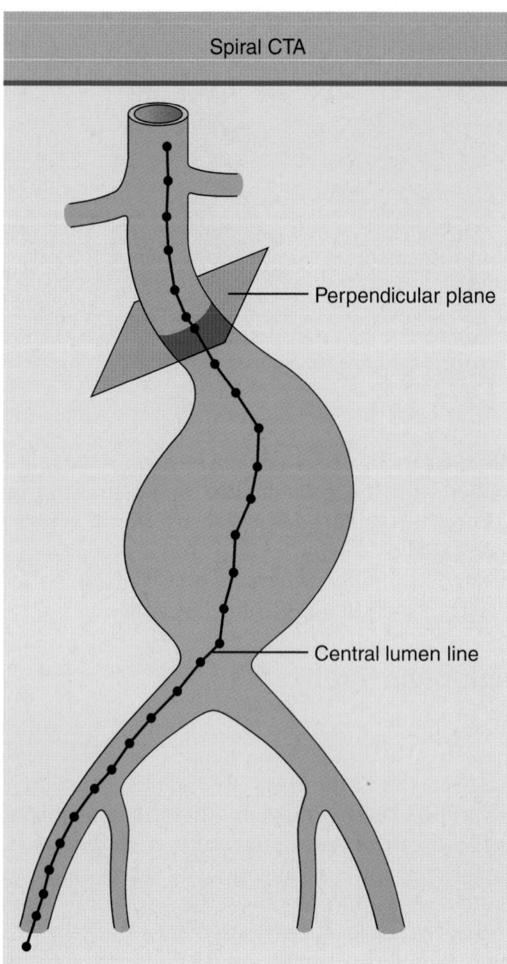

Figure 29-4. Spiral computed tomography angiography. Curved linear reformats (created by imaging processing on a workstation) allow visualization in a plane perpendicular to the central lumen line. Oblique projections are avoided.

If the wire does not pass or the artery does not straighten, a stent graft delivery is unlikely to succeed.

Magnetic Resonance Angiography

Like spiral CTA, magnetic resonance angiography (MRA) can produce multiplanar two-dimensional and three-dimensional images. Although MRA is currently inferior to spiral CTA regarding spatial resolution, and is technically demanding and time consuming, it certainly has advantages worthy of mention. For example, the patient is not exposed to ionizing radiation.

MRA cannot be used in all patients. Approximately 10% to 15% of patients are claustrophobic or have metal implants that make it impossible to use MRA.

SELECTION OF A STENT GRAFT

The minimally invasive therapeutic option of treatment of an AAA is of great interest to various medical specialties, including cardiovascular surgery, interventional radiology, and interventional cardiology. Each year, approximately 50,000 patients undergo open repair for AAA in the United States

Table 29-1
Characteristics of the Ideal Stent Graft

Low Overall Cost	User Friendliness
Stent graft size range	Column strength
Durability (metallic ultrastructure + graft material)	Sealing capacity
Biocompatibility	Radioopacity
Sealing capacity	Low thrombogenicity
Lowest delivery device size	Lowest delivery device profile
Delivery device flexibility	Delivery device reliability
Radial force stability	Excellent apposition of graft
Customization	

alone. With such a large potential market, most important companies that manufacture endovascular products now produce and distribute stent grafts.

Various materials have been tested, and all major producers now use the two materials most often used in surgery: polyester weaves and polytetrafluoroethylene (PTFE). Ideally, if stent grafts are to provide the advantages they potentially offer over conventional surgery, they must have certain characteristics (Table 29-1).[11] Each device must have as many of these characteristics as possible to warrant a safe implantation, high rates of immediate technical success, and excellent long-term clinical success.

Following the early use of improvised, noncommercial endovascular grafts for AAA, several commercially produced endovascular grafts have become available (Table 29-2).

Components of Endovascular Devices

Delivery Systems

Stent grafts are delivered in the vascular tree using introducer sheaths, trocars, deployment capsules, and retractable covers. The profile of the introducer sheaths must be small enough to pass through the iliac tract without causing vascular damage. However, the introducer sheaths must be wide enough for easy passage of the stent graft, rigid enough to resist kinking, and flexible enough to follow the angulations in the iliac arteries. A hemostatic valve is mandatory.

Graft Material

The graft material must be strong enough to resist late deterioration and damage due to friction with metallic parts of the stent yet thin enough to be compressed in a small delivery catheter. In most stent grafts, conventional polyester has been preferred. Over time, companies have started using thinner polyester variations to downsize the profile of the delivery systems. PTFE is an alternative graft material used in the Excluder endograft and Powerlink endograft. Other materials, such as polycarbonate, polyurethane, and other polymers, are under investigation.

Graft Attachment Systems

Vascular stents can be constructed from stainless steel, Elgiloy, tantalum, or nitinol. Friction with the vessel wall is the main mechanism of attachment, but hooks, anchors, and

Table 29-2
Available Endovascular Grafts*

Name (Company)	Graft Material	Stent Material	Introducer Size (OD)	Device Composition	Expansion	Fixation
AneuRx (Medtronic AVE)	Polyester	Nitinol	22 Fr	Modular	Self-expanding	Friction
Talent (Medtronic AVE)	Polyester	Nitinol	18-22 Fr	Modular	Self-expanding	Friction + juxtarenal bare stent
Excluder (WL Gore)	PTFE	Nitinol	18 Fr	Modular	Self-expanding	Friction + hooks
Zenith (Cook)	Polyester	Stainless steel	22 Fr	Modular	Self-expanding	Hooks + juxtarenal bare stent
Powerlink (Endologix)	PTFE	Stainless steel	18-20 Fr	Unibody	Self-expandable	Friction
Anaconda (Vascutek)	Polyester	Nitinol	18-23 Fr	Modular	Self-expandable	Friction

*FR, French; OD, outside diameter; PTFE, polytetrafluoroethylene.

barbs are used in addition to secure a better fixation and seal inside the artery.

Deployment Accessories

Regular tools of interventional radiology are essential accessories for a successful stent graft placement. Among these are floppy to superstiff guide wires, angiographic and guiding catheters, dilatation balloons, snares, and power injectors.

Various structural differences among the different devices are potentially associated with both beneficial and deleterious effects. While most of these structural differences are considered to be important, until now no evidence has shown whether they are beneficial or not. Polyester weaves are claimed to be stronger materials than PTFE, especially in contact with the metallic skeleton. However, PTFE has a lower thrombogenicity, is thinner, and has a better graft apposition.[12] Another issue is the use of a metallic exo- or endoskeleton (stent frame at the outside or inside of the graft). Whereas an exoskeleton might be associated with better embedding into the vessel wall and with better fixation of the graft, an endoskeleton might have the advantage of better graft apposition to the wall and less potential turbulence. In addition, an ongoing discussion concerns the unibody and modular design of stent grafts. A unibody design may give rise to better overall stent graft stability, with no risk of dislodgement of any components, and may bear a closer resemblance to surgical grafts. Modular designs have the advantage of increased size combinations and the possibility of “tailoring” the stent graft during the procedure. Suprarenal fixation creates a better fixation of the stent graft and therefore decreases the risk of stent graft migration. This technique could be particularly useful when the aortic neck is short or has unfavorable features such as irregular shape, mural thrombus, or extensive calcification. Opponents of suprarenal fixation fear a more complicated procedure in case of a conversion.[13] To date, no evidence indicates that suprarenal fixation is associated with a higher incidence of renal infarction.[14]

TECHNIQUE OF ENDOVASCULAR REPAIR

Endovascular repair of an AAA can be performed in the operating theater, radiological angiosuite, or catheterization laboratory under general, regional, and even local anesthesia. The choice of one of these locations is subjective and is influenced by the preference of the interventionist. If the procedure is not performed in an operating theater, it should meet the standards of hygiene and sterility associated with the latter.

Radiological Requirements

Minimum radiological requirements for fluoroscopy are a mobile C-arm image intensifier with possibilities for cine loop angiography, digital subtraction, roadmap, and frame-by-frame replay. Ceiling- or floor-mounted fluoroscopy equipment has several advantages over the portable image intensifier. Most important are a better field size–spatial resolution ratio and a suitable radiolucent table that can be adjusted to the fluoroscopic field.

The typical aorta at the infrarenal level has a slight anterior angulation (10 to 15 degrees) due to lordosis of the lumbar vertebrae. This angulation is more pronounced in most patients with AAA (the angle can vary from 10 to 60 degrees), because the aneurysm raises the aorta from the vertebral column. Fluoroscopy with the C-arm in the anteroposterior position produces projection errors, and this may lead to less optimal or inaccurate placement of the stent graft in the infrarenal aortic neck (Figure 29-5).[15,16] In addition to an angulation of the C-arm, sometimes a rotation of the C-arm is required for optimal projection of the orifice of the renal arteries. It is essential to have aortic angulation and rotation data available preoperatively. Only lateral angiograms or CTA reconstructions can give an indication of neck angulation.

Operating Team

The patient should be positioned on a radiolucent operating table and draped for emergent open repair in the event of failed endovascular repair or occurrence of complications needing conversion.

The locations of the operating team and fluoroscopy equipment are illustrated in Figure 29-6. An endovascular procedure should be performed by at least two interventionists and one scrub nurse–radiology technician. There should be two monitors so that both interventionists have an unobstructed view of a monitor. Since the delivery devices are long (usually longer than 100 cm), long guide wires (180 to 300 cm) are required. Therefore, it is advisable to extend the operating table with an extension table to enable safe manipulation of the devices.

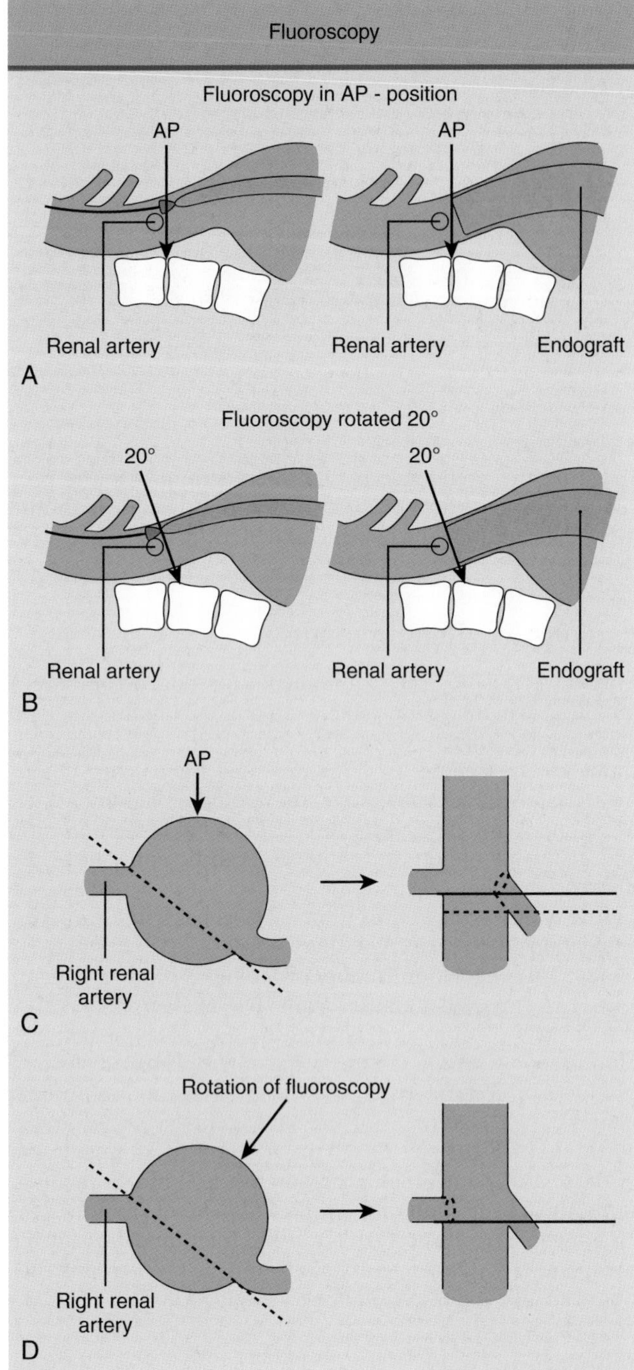

Figure 29-5. Fluoroscopy. Fluoroscopy in the anteroposterior position produces projection errors that could lead to less accurate placement of the stent graft in the infrarenal aortic neck **(A** and **C)**. Angulation and rotation of the C-arm may be required for optimal projection **(B** and **D)** of the infrarenal neck and renal artery orifice.

Graft Insertion

The common femoral artery in the ipsilateral groin is exposed through a surgical cut-down, and intravenous heparin is given to the patient. In some institutions, there is extensive experience in percutaneous access. In general, a closure device is "preloaded" before the introducer sheath is inserted.[17] A 6- to 8-Fr introducer sheath is inserted, and a flexible guide wire is positioned in the suprarenal aorta. With the use of a (straight) diagnostic catheter, the flexible guide wire is exchanged for a superstiff guide wire, which is positioned in the descending aorta. At the same time, another introducer sheath (6 to 8 Fr) is inserted into the contralateral common femoral artery, either percutaneously or through a groin cut-down. With the use of a flexible guide wire, a pigtail catheter is positioned at the level of the renal arteries. The introducer sheath in the ipsilateral common femoral artery is removed, and a transverse arteriotomy is performed in such a way that the superstiff guide wire is situated within the arteriotomy. A large introducer sheath (depending on the device used) or the delivery device and stent graft within it are introduced under fluoroscopic control until the superior end of the prosthesis is at the assumed level of the renal arteries. If necessary, the image intensifier is angulated, rotated, and moved into place the superior end of the stent graft in the center of the field to eliminate errors caused by parallax. Magnification can be advantageous in identifying the superior end of the stent graft in relation to the orifice of the renal arteries. At this time, the first aortogram is performed with the use of a power injector by injecting 20 ml of contrast at 10 ml/sec, imaging at two frames per second. Rotation of the stent graft and repositioning can be performed. It is usually necessary to perform several aortograms to properly position the stent graft.

Once it has been ascertained that the stent graft is in the optimal position, immediately distal from the renal arteries, the pigtail catheter is pulled distally (Figure 29-7). The trunk and ipsilateral limb of the stent graft can be deployed under fluoroscopic control. If balloon dilatation of the proximal and distal attachment side is required, this is performed at this time. After dilatation, a guide wire from the contralateral femoral artery is directed into the short contralateral stump of the stent graft. This can usually be achieved with a "freestyle" catheterization using an angled guiding catheter. If difficulty is experienced, a guide wire can be passed from the ipsilateral side, through the ipsilateral limb of the stent graft, and with the aid of a "crossover" guiding catheter, over the bifurcation in the contralateral short limb into the aneurysm sac. With a snare catheter from the contralateral femoral artery, the guide wire can be retrieved. An approach from the brachial artery can also be used if the freestyle catheterization of the short contralateral stump fails. The brachial approach can be used in the case of extreme tortuosity in the iliac tract. After retrieval of the brachial wire with the snare catheter, tension can be applied at the brachial and femoral ends. This technique of "body-flossing" results in considerable straightening of the iliac arteries.

After cannulation of the contralateral short stump, the guide wire is exchanged for a superstiff guide wire. The 6- to 8-Fr introducer sheath is exchanged for a larger sheath, and the contralateral limb is directed under fluoroscopic control to a position within, and overlapping, the contralateral stump. The position of the hypogastric artery can be assessed by regular angiography or retrograde angiography through the introducer sheath. The contralateral limb is deployed under fluoroscopic control. The overlapping attachment site and distal attachment site can be dilated.

A pigtail catheter is reintroduced, and a postintervention digital subtraction aortogram is performed several times for the detection of the presence of extravasation of contrast,

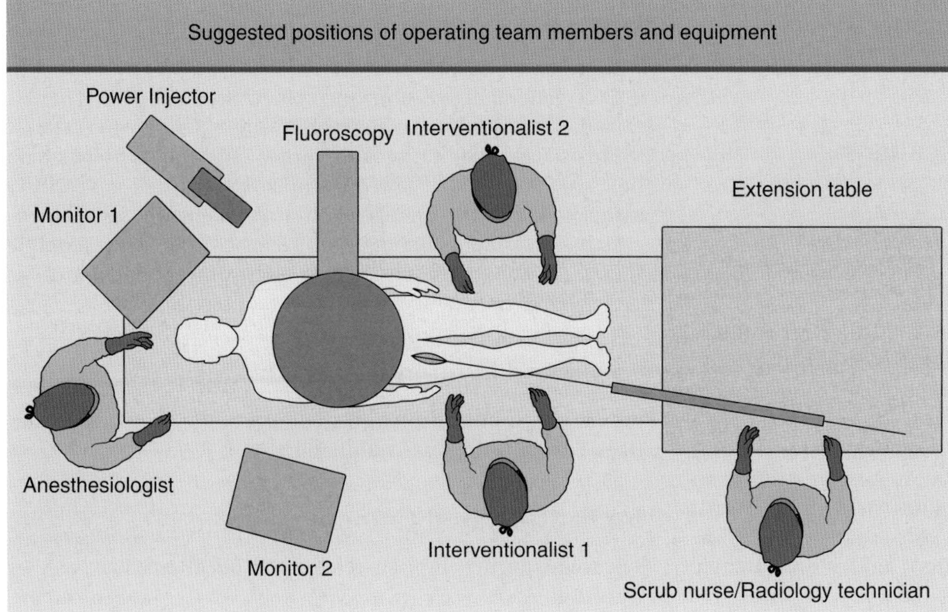

Figure 29-6. Suggested positions of operating team members and equipment.

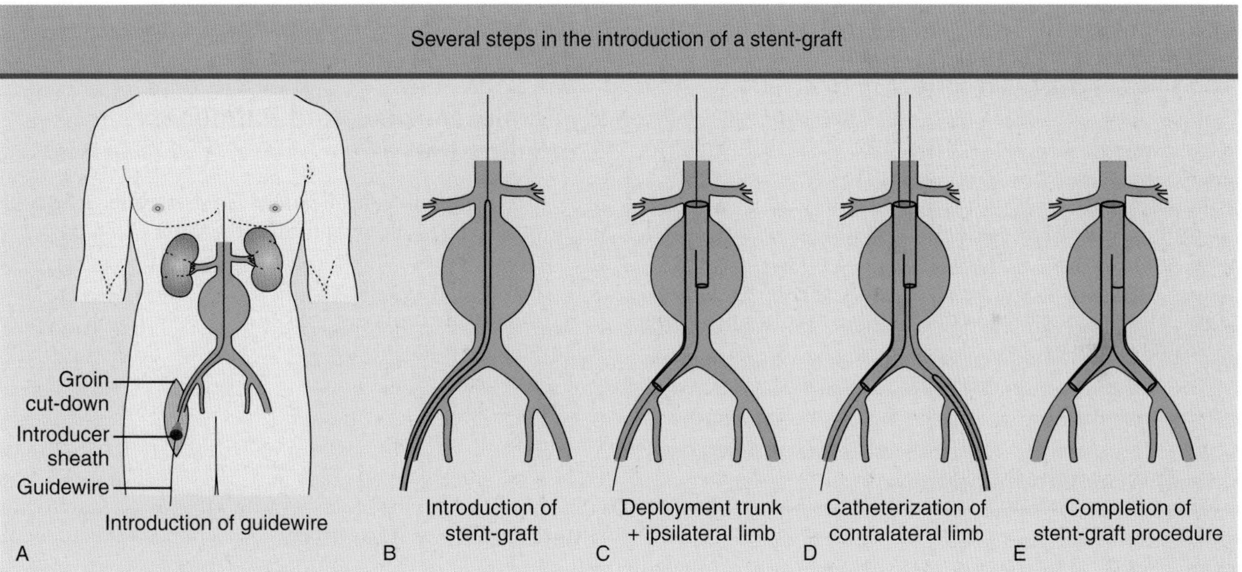

Figure 29-7. Several steps in the introduction of a stent graft. **A,** After a cut-down in the groin, a guide wire is introduced through an introducer sheath. **B,** The delivery system is positioned under fluoroscopic control. **C,** The trunk and ipsilateral limb are deployed. **D,** The contralateral stump is catheterized, and the contralateral limb is introduced. **E,** The contralateral limb is deployed, and the stent graft is completed.

which can indicate an endoleak. Stent graft limbs and iliac arteries are examined for kinking or twisting.

The technique for introduction and deployment differs for every individual stent graft; discussion of these differences is beyond the scope of this chapter. For individual techniques of introduction and deployment, refer to the relevant specialized manuals.

PERIOPERATIVE COMPLICATIONS

Standardized reporting of deaths and complications is necessary to establish stent graft exclusion as safe and effective therapy for AAA. Complications may be deployment related, groin and wound related, implant related, or systemic (cardiac and pulmonary).

According to the current reporting standards, deployment-related complications can be classified into the following sections[18]:

Failed deployment with or without conversion
Operative bleeding
Aortic dissection
Arterial perforation or rupture
Access artery injury
Peripheral microembolization
Access site hematoma or false aneurysm
Access site lymphocele or lymphedema

Access site infection
Postimplant fever eci
Some of these sections are described here in more detail.

Deployment-Related Complications

Access Artery Injury

Damage to the access vessels can easily occur due to the passage of large-bore catheters, containing stent grafts. This may result in rupture, particularly in tortuous and diseased iliac arteries. The surgeon should be aware that the large catheter can have a tamponading effect and the bleeding may only become apparent after removal of the catheter. Newer stent grafts can be introduced through iliac arteries with a high degree of tortuosity and in the presence of extensive circumferential calcification. Visceral organs can be damaged by an uncontrolled introduction of (stiff) guide wires into the renal and suprarenal arteries. Therefore, it is mandatory that guide wires and catheters are only introduced under fluoroscopic control.

Peripheral Microembolization

Manipulation of endovascular devices within the aneurysm sac can result in microembolization and death from renal failure.[19] Every effort should be made to reduce catheter and balloon manipulations at the renal and suprarenal level, especially when mural thrombus is present at the renal and suprarenal level.

Distal embolization resulting in ischemia is also a recognized complication. Dislodgement of emboli from the mural thrombus in the aneurysm sac can be prevented by the use of stiff guide wires. Using the latter, the delivery device follows the guide wires more easily, with a reduced risk of impinging on the mural thrombus.

Table 29-3
Groin and Wound Complications

(Post)operative bleeding
Access site hematoma
Access site false aneurysm
Access site lymphocele, lymphorrhea, or lymphedema
Wound infection

Postimplant Fever Eci

Postimplant syndrome is characterized by febris eci (up to 40° C), general depression, and sometimes back pain. There is no leukocytosis or other signs of infection. Symptoms can last up to 10 days. The cause is unknown, and the incidence may be as high as 50%.[20] The postimplant syndrome is probably associated with thrombosis within the aneurysm sac. In general, it is considered benign: some consider it to be a favorable sign, signifying thrombosis of the aneurysm sac and complete exclusion of the aneurysm.

Groin and Wound Complications

Numerous groin and wound complications can occur, and these complications are outlined in Table 29-3.

Implant-Related Complications

The following are implant-related complications:
Ruptured AAA
Stent graft migration
Device erosion through vessel wall
Intraoperative stent graft limb obstruction
Postoperative stent graft obstruction
Buttock–leg claudication–ischemia

Systemic, Cardiac, and Pulmonary Complications

The final types of complications are systemic, cardiac, and pulmonary. The following fit into the latter category:
Renal insufficiency
Cerebrovascular complications
Deep venous thrombosis
Pulmonary embolism
Coagulopathy
Bowel ischemia
Spinal cord ischemia
Erectile dysfunction

Postoperative Mortality

The option of having a less invasive treatment choice has been accepted favorably by the medical community and has been gaining consensus since its introduction. EVAR can be

Table 29-4
Comparative Results after EVAR and Conventional Open Repair*

Author	Journal (Year)	EVAR Mortality (%)	Open Repair Mortality (%)	p
Brewster et al.[24]	*J Vasc Surg* (1998)	0	0	NS
Goldstone et al.[21]	*Proceedings* (1998)	1.1	3.8	NS
May et al.[23]	*J Vasc Surg* (1998)	5.6	5.6	NS
Zarins et al.[22]	*J Vasc Surg* (1999)	2.6	0	NS
De Virgilio et al.[25]	*Arch Surg* (1999)	3.6	4.7	NS
Beebe et al.[26]	*J Vasc Surg* (2001)	1.5	3.1	NS
May et al.[27]	*J Vasc Surg* (2001)	2.7	5.9	NS
Zarins et al.[28]	*Proceedings* (2001)	0.5	3.5	<0.05
Prinssen et al.[29]	*N Engl J Med* (2004)	1.2	4.6	NS
Greenhalgh et al.[30]	*Lancet* (2004)	1.7	4.7	0.009

*EVAR, endovascular aneurysm repair; NS, not significant.

undertaken under local anesthesia; it can reduce operative risk and shorten recovery time. Mortality and morbidity increase in patients with significant comorbidities and in the elderly population.

Comparative studies on mortality with EVAR and conventional open surgery have been carried out in single centers in the form of case control studies, and concurrent single or multicentric prospective nonrandomized comparisons. The most published series report similar intraoperative mortality rates after EVAR and open repair (Table 29-4).[21-30]

ENDOLEAKS AND LATE COMPLICATIONS

Endoleaks

An endoleak is a condition associated with endovascular stent grafts, defined by persistent blood flow outside the lumen of the stent graft but within the aneurysm sac or adjacent vascular segment being treated by the stent graft.[31,32] An endoleak is evidence of incomplete exclusion of the aneurysm from the circulation. Evidence indicates that an endoleak may resolve spontaneously, but a proportion of those that do persist are associated with late aneurysm rupture.[33-35] Although intrasac pressure may approach systemic arterial pressure in the presence of an endoleak, some type II endoleaks have been associated with a decrease in aneurysm volume and intrasac pressures that are substantially less than systemic pressures.[36]

An endoleak can be classified according to the time of occurrence.[31] An endoleak first observed during the perioperative (less than 30 days) period is defined as a "primary endoleak," and detection thereafter is termed a "secondary endoleak." Further categorization requires precise information regarding the course of the blood flow into the aneurysm sac (Figure 29-8).[18]

A type I endoleak is indicative of a persistent perigraft channel of blood flow caused by inadequate seal at either the proximal (Ia) or the distal (Ib) stent graft end or attachment zones. In the case of an aortomonoiliac prosthesis, a type I endoleak may also refer to blood flow around an iliac occluder plug (Ic).

A type II endoleak is attributed to retrograde flow from the IMA (IIa), lumbar arteries (IIb), or other collateral vessels. Origin and outflow sources of a type II endoleak should be specified, such as lumbar and lumbar, lumbar and IMA, accessory renal and lumbar or IMA, hypogastric and lumbar or IMA, or undefined. It should be emphasized that any connection with a proximal or distal attachment zone classifies the endoleak as a type I endoleak.

A type III endoleak is caused by component disconnection (IIIa) or fabric tear, fabric disruption, or graft disintegration (IIIb). A type IIIb endoleak can be further stratified as minor (less than 2 mm) or major (more than 2 mm).

A type IV endoleak is caused by blood flow through an intact but otherwise porous fabric, observed during the first 30 days after stent graft implantation. This definition is not applicable to fabric-related endoleaks observed after the first 30-day period.

If an endoleak is visualized in imaging studies but the precise source cannot be determined, the endoleak is categorized as an endoleak of undefined origin.

It is recognized that an AAA can continue to enlarge after endovascular repair, even in the absence of a detectable endoleak, and that this enlargement may lead to aneurysm rupture. This phenomenon is currently defined as "endotension."[37,38] Explanations for persistent or recurrent pressurization of an aneurysm sac include blood flow that is below the sensitivity limits of detection with current imaging modalities or pressure transmission through thrombus or stent graft material.[39-41]

The incidence of endoleak has been reported as between 10% and 44%.[42-44] If left untreated, an endoleak may seal spontaneously by thrombosis. This occurred in almost 50% of the cases reported by Moore et al., resulting in a permanent endoleak rate of approximately 20%.[42] Spontaneous sealing of an endoleak results in a decrease in the size of the aneurysm sac. Conversely, the size of an AAA can increase when a secondary endoleak develops in a previously excluded AAA after endovascular repair. Type II endoleaks are more likely to seal than types I or III endoleaks. It has also been suggested that an AAA with a type II endoleak is less likely to rupture. This assumption is dangerous, since late ruptures of an AAA treated with a stent graft and with a type II endoleak have been reported. However, persistent type I and III endoleaks are more prone to causing a rupture following an endograft.[33]

Endoleaks may be managed by observation, a further endovascular procedure, endoscopic treatment, and conversion.

As some endoleaks seal spontaneously, most interventionists are prepared to disregard endoleaks despite the

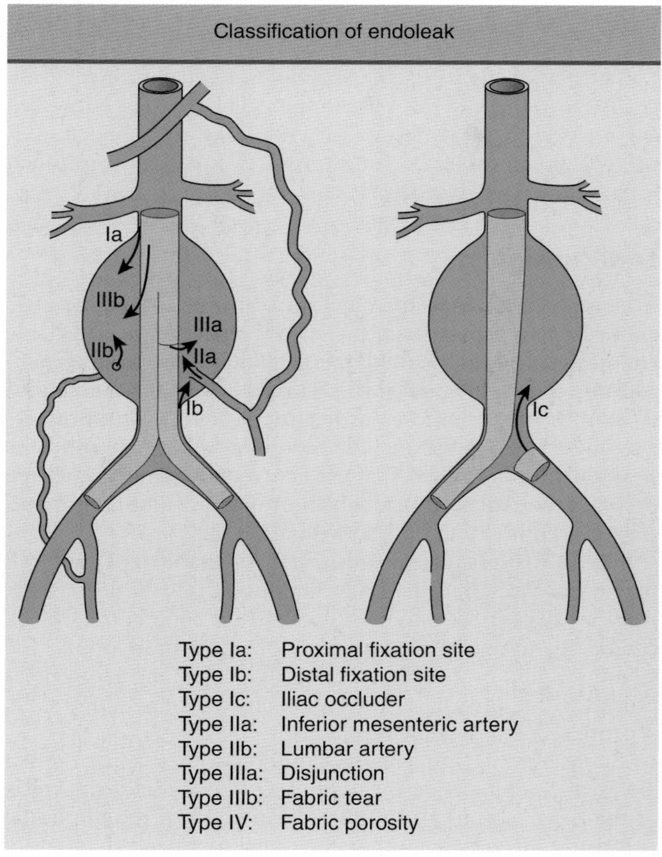

Figure 29-8. Classification of endoleaks.

knowledge that aneurysm rupture may occur. Although no proof shows that spontaneous sealing of an endoleak by thrombosis decreases pressure within the aneurysm sac, some evidence indicates that this is the case, as a reduction in the diameter of treated aneurysms has been observed. The duration of the observation period varies according to the size of the aneurysm and the interventionist's personal experience and preference.

Type I endoleaks can be treated by secondary endoluminal interventions. A balloon dilatation, to compress the device against the vessel wall, is the most appropriate first step. If this fails, application of a "giant" Palmaz stent is likely to be successful in resolving a proximal endoleak if the stent graft has been positioned correctly. If migration of the proximal or distal attachment occurs, or when these fixations are in a less-than-optimal position, a secondary intervention to extend the stent graft with an extension cuff is indicated. The same procedure can be performed in the case of type III endoleaks. Surgical-band ligature has been used; it involves open exposure and placement of an external ligature around the proximal attachment site.[45] Although this technique necessitates a laparotomy or endoscopic approach, it is less disturbing hemodynamically than conversion in high-risk patients with a type I endoleak.

Type II endoleaks arising from the lumbar arteries or IMA may be treated by coil embolization with superselective catheterization of the superior gluteal artery or superior mesenteric artery. The aneurysm can also be punctured by the translumbar or transperitoneal route. In this way, thrombogenic material can be injected directly into the aneurysm.

Retroperitoneal endoscopic ligation of the IMA and all lumbar arteries remains a popular alternative for the treatment of persistent type II endoleaks if the less invasive possibilities are not applicable or have failed.[46]

The perplexing problems of endoleaks will continue to be a challenge to the success of EVAR and will have to be addressed aggressively. Until solutions for endoleaks are found, EVAR will remain an imperfect long-term treatment and continued follow-up will be mandatory.[47]

Endotension

It is appreciated that an AAA can continue to enlarge after endovascular repair even in the absence of a detectable endoleak and that this enlargement may lead to aneurysm rupture. This phenomenon is currently indicated as endotension.[48,49] Explanations for persistent or recurrent pressurization of an AAA sac include blood flow that is beyond the sensitivity limits of detection with current imaging modalities, pressure transmission through thrombus or stent graft material, or accumulation of fluid within the sac.

Fluid and pressure transmission through the stent graft wall may occur with graft materials that are porous or permeable. Another reason for endotension without apparent endoleak can be due to in situ accumulation of excess fluid around the stent graft and eventual formation of a hygroma. Hyperfibrinolysis within the sac, and consequently a hyperosmotic state, is proposed as a possible mechanism.

Endotension is not a benign condition. Enlargement of the AAA can eventually result in rupture. Continued expansion of the AAA sac can also result in dilatation of the infrarenal neck, iliac arteries, or both, which may threaten the integrity of proximal and distal anastomotic seals.

Graft Limb Thrombosis

First-generation stent grafts with unsupported fabric were prone to thrombosis of the limbs of the graft due to kinking and twisting within the native arteries. This problem required primary stenting during the initial procedure or a secondary procedure to reopen or expand a limb in the iliac artery.[50] The problem can also occur in stent grafts with full support of the limbs. Successful EVAR results in a reduction in the size of the AAA, both in length and in transverse diameter. The morphological changes in the AAA may lead to kinking of the previously straight limbs, with possible progression to thrombosis. X-ray studies in anteroposterior and lateral planes are required at regular intervals to identify the problem of kinking in supported limbs and to prevent graft limb thrombosis. With unsupported limbs, a color flow duplex ultrasonography may be required to identify the problem.

Stent Graft Infection

Stent graft infection is a rare phenomenon, and the incidence is reported in less than 1%. There has been one report of the development of an aortoenteric fistula after EVAR.[51] Over the last 10 years, stent grafts have been used on a larger scale. The apparent low incidence of infection at this stage may suggest that the devices are more resistant to infection than conventional grafts placed by open surgery.

Device Failure

One of the negative aspects of EVAR is the unknown long-term outcome. The durability of prostheses in the long term is, as yet, unknown. Despite extensive premarketing fatigue testing of stent grafts, reports of structural failure throughout a range of device types continue to be noted with some frequency, including fractures of nitinol frames and Elgiloy hooks and disruption of stent graft fabrics within 4 years of implantation. Many patients who underwent EVAR with one of the first-generation devices are currently encountering serious complications requiring surgical explantation.[52] Some first-generation devices have been taken off the market, and some encountered problems have been solved by using another choice of materials or a complete redesign of the stent graft or delivery systems.

Dilatation of the Proximal Neck

Morphological characteristics of the proximal neck influence the effectiveness of aneurysm exclusion and the durability of the stent graft attachment. Gradual dilatation of the aorta at the level of the attachment systems may cause an endoleak and stent graft migration. Studies in healthy people have shown that the infrarenal aortic diameter increases approximately 25% between 25 and 70 years of age.[53] After conventional AAA repair, higher rates of increase have been described.[54-56]

Some studies have shown dilatation of the proximal neck following endovascular repair.[57-61] Two possible explanations can be given for the continued growth of the infrarenal neck after endovascular repair: it can be a continuation of the aneurysmal process or an effect of the outward force generated by the endovascular stent onto the aortic wall. If the outward force is the predominant cause of postoperative neck dilatation, the diameter will probably not stretch beyond the nominal stent size.

Late Rupture

The most significant outcome measure of EVAR is the absence of AAA rupture. Prevention of rupture is the reason for which EVAR is undertaken. A recently published large series of patients treated with EVAR reported late rupture rates up to 1.5% per year.[62-65] Multivariate analysis of risk factors for rupture has identified only three that are statistically significant: the last diameter measurement of the aneurysm (relative risk 1.057), midgraft endoleak (relative risk 7.5), and stent graft migration (relative risk 5.3).[63] A type I endoleak was a significant risk factor for late rupture on univariate analysis but dropped out on multivariate analysis, indicating that late type I endoleaks are usually secondary to migration.

Several reported late ruptures in all mentioned studies occurred in compassionate cases treated with first-generation devices. On the basis of a decreasing trend, we can hypothesize that, with new-generation devices and meticulous follow-up with state-of-art imaging, concerns of rupture may lessen.

QUALITY OF LIFE

Utilities for a given health state represent the preference that individuals have for a certain health state. Utilities can be conceptualized as a single summary measure of health-related quality of life on a scale with anchors of one corresponding to perfect health and zero corresponding to death. Utilities are usually used to estimate quality-adjusted life years, providing a generic health-related outcome measure for comparison of different treatments for different patient groups.

In chronic disease states, where the quality of life of patients is impaired for a prolonged period, incorporating utilities into economic evaluation can significantly influence the cost effectiveness of the intervention.

In most studies, utilities were calculated with the help of EuroQuol EQ-D. Comparison between the two larger randomized trials is not that easy, because the Dutch Randomized Endovascular Aneurysm Management (DREAM) Trial reported differences in mean scores at baseline and after intervention.[66,67] But both studies demonstrated an initial dip in utilities due to the invasive nature of the intervention. They showed different levels of improvement after that. With open surgical repair, the dip in utilities is more than that with endovascular repair at 4 to 6 weeks after the intervention. After 12 months, the utilities returned to baseline for both endovascular and open repair with the exception of the DREAM Trial, where utility scores for open surgical repair were slightly better than for endovascular repair.[68]

ECONOMICS

EVAR is a less invasive method for the treatment of AAAs compared to conventional open surgery. The potential benefits of EVAR include increased patient acceptance, less resource utilization, and hopefully, cost saving. The cost analysis of this technology is critically dependent on the potential to reduce morbidity and mortality rates, relative to conventional open surgery. EVAR is expensive due to the high cost of the devices and the need for close postintervention surveillance and secondary interventions. The main possibility for cost savings are reduced requirements for blood transfusion, a shorter intensive care unit and hospital stay, a lower 30-day mortality, and a lower systemic–remote complication rate.

Several studies have been carried out to evaluate the cost effectiveness of EVAR compared to conventional open surgery (Table 29-5).[66,67,69-78] In most of these studies, only the hospital cost was included. Both randomized trials (EVAR Trial 1 and DREAM) have showed that the cost for endovascular repair is higher than for open surgical repair. During follow-up, the cost for the endovascular group is increased mainly due to the more stringent imaging requirements and more common reinterventions.

FOLLOW-UP

As the long-term outcome of endovascular repair is, as yet, unknown, careful and indefinite follow-up is required. Physical examination and CTA are recommended within 1 month of the procedure; at 6, 12, and 18 months after the intervention; and annually thereafter. CTA may fail to identify an endoleak if delayed images are not obtained after infusion of contrast.[79] Although conflicting studies exist, most investigations suggest that the sensitivity of CTA is superior to that of other noninvasive imaging techniques, such as duplex ultrasonography, for endoleak detection.[80,81] Color duplex ultrasonography is operator dependent but does have the advantages of showing blood flow within the aneurysm sac, not requiring contrast, and being less costly.

Besides the search for endoleaks, changes in the dimension of the aneurysm sac may assist in defining the success or failure of aneurysm exclusion. Aneurysm growth after endovascular repair is an indicator of incomplete aneurysm exclusion and therefore a continued risk for late aneurysm rupture.[82] Aneurysm size should be expressed as either maximum diameter or volume. The maximum diameter should be measured perpendicular to the central lumen line of the vessel with three-dimensional reconstructed CTA images. Because the aneurysm cross section often appears elliptical on axial images, the minor axis of the ellipse (smallest diameter) is generally a closer assessment of the maximum aneurysm diameter.[83] Intraobserver and interobserver variability of diameter measurements obtained from CTA range between 2 and 5 mm.[84] Therefore, only a diameter change of 5 mm or more is considered significant.

Total aneurysm volume comprises luminal aneurysm volume and nonluminal aneurysm volume. An aneurysm can be considered excluded if the nonluminal aneurysm volume is less than 10% of the original nonluminal aneurysm volume noted after endograft implantation. The intraobserver and interobserver variability of volume measurements have ranged between 3% and 5%. Therefore, a volume change of 5% or more is considered significant.[85]

A plain abdominal x-ray in four planes should be obtained at regular intervals to assess kinking and migration of the stent graft and to assess the integrity of the support system. Structural failures have been reported in most devices within 4 years from implantation. These structural failures include hook fractures, disintegration of the metal frame, wireform fractures, and lateral bar and proximal spring fractures.

CONVERSION

Conversions should be differentiated as primary conversions (at the original operation or within 30 days) or secondary conversions (at a later operation).

The current indications for primary conversion include vascular damage to the access vessels, iliac or aortic rupture, stent graft migration with obstruction of renal or iliac arteries, and device-related problems (deployment failures, entrapment of the delivery catheter).

Secondary conversion might be indicated in persistent endoleak, growing aneurysm, graft thrombosis, graft infection, renal artery obstruction, and migration of the stent graft.

The conversion rate in most series is 2% to 15%. Several studies have evaluated the secondary conversion rate. In the EUROSTAR Registry, the secondary conversion rate of aneurysms treated with first-generation stent grafts was 7.1%.[86] Kaplan-Meier analysis from the Lifeline Registry of EVAR revealed freedom from surgical conversion in 95% of the patients at year 6.[87] Nearly 80% of the conversions were performed in the first postoperative month (primary conversion). Primary conversion was mostly due to access problems and device migration. Secondary conversions were performed for rupture and for a persistent endoleak, with or without aneurysmal growth. Patients who required primary conversion had an 18% mortality rate. Secondary conversion was associated with a perioperative mortality of 27% and, when performed for rupture, a mortality of 50%.

At conversion, the aorta can be cross-clamped at a suprarenal or subdiaphragmal level. If it is impossible to cross-clamp the aorta, control can be obtained with an occluding balloon at the level of the visceral arteries. The aneurysm sac can be opened and the stent graft removed by traction. After removal of the stent graft, the clamp can be applied infrarenally and reconstruction can be continued. If the graft is incorporated in the aortic wall (e.g., suprarenal fixation), the stent graft can be cut through the metal frame. The proximal part of the stent graft remains in situ, and a surgical anastomosis can be performed on the remaining stent graft.

Due to extensive variations in stent graft configurations, and the complications pending conversion, conversion needs a flexible intraoperative attitude toward clamping techniques and stent graft extraction.

EVIDENCE

The EVAR Trial 1 included 1082 patients with AAA who were healthy enough to be suitable candidates for surgery.[66] The 30-day mortality in this randomized, controlled trial was 1.7% in the endovascular group and 4.7% in the open surgical group ($p < 0.001$). At 4 years, the aneurysm-related mortality rate in the endovascular group was 4% compared to 7% in the open surgical group ($p < 0.04$). No significant difference was found in causes of mortality (26% for EVAR versus 29% for open surgical repair, $p = 0.46$). The proportion of patients with postoperative complications within 4 years of randomization was 41% in the endovascular group and 9% in the open surgical group. Reinterventions were 20% for endovascular repair versus 6% for open surgical repair.

The DREAM Trial had a design similar of the EVAR Trial 1 but was much smaller (351 patients).[67] Two years after randomization, the cumulative survival rates were 89.6% for open repair, and 89.7% for endovascular repair ($p = 0.86$). The cumulative rates for aneurysm-related death 2 years after randomization were 5.7% in the open-repair group and 2.1% in the endovascular repair group ($p = 0.005$). Two years after randomization, the rates of survival free of severe events were 80.6% for open repair and 83.1% for endovascular repair ($p = 0.39$). Kaplan-Meier estimates of the likelihood of freedom from reinterventions were 95% for open repair and 87% for endovascular repair.

Similar results were found in a large systematic review and metaanalysis including 28,862 patients[88] and a propensity-score matched Medicare analysis including 22,830 patients.[89]

From the metaanalysis, it became clear that the annual rates of operative mortality, rupture, and endoleak have fallen between 1992 and 2002.

Table 29-5
Is Endovascular Aneurysm Repair Cost Effective?

Author	Journal (Year)	
Holzenbein et al.[69]	*Eur J Vasc Endovasc Surg* (1997)	Yes
Ceelen et al.[70]	*Acta Chir Belg* (1999)	Equal
Patel et al.[71]	*J Vasc Surg* (1999)	Yes
Seiwert et al.[72]	*Am J Surg* (1999)	Equal
Quinones-Baldrich[73]	*J Vasc Surg* (1999)	No
Sternbergh et al.[74]	*J Vasc Surg* (2000)	No
Clair et al.[75]	*J Vasc Surg* (2000)	No
Birch et al.[76]	*Aus NZ J Surg* (2000)	No
Turnipseed et al.[77]	*J Vasc Surg* (2001)	No
Bosch et al.[78]	*Radiology* (2001)	No
Greenhalgh et al.[66]	*Lancet* (2005)	No
Prinssen et al.[92]	*J Vasc Surg* (2007)	No

FUTURE DEVELOPMENTS

Commercially available stent grafts have limitations with respect to unfavorable anatomy, which most often include a short (less than 15 mm) and angulated (more than 60 mm) proximal neck and a reversed, cone-shaped neck. Fenestrated and branched devices have been proposed as means to address the proximal neck limitations.[90]

Internal iliac artery inflow obstruction can cause hip claudication and may predispose patients to higher incidence of colon, spinal cord, or pelvic ischemia. Endovascular internal iliac artery branch grafts were designed to prevent these complications.[91]

The experience with fenestrated and branched stent grafts is limited, and only highly specialized centers are using these techniques. Technical issues lead to the complexity of these procedures. Nevertheless, promising results have been reported. As these procedures mature, long-term results and randomized clinical trials will ultimately be required to determine the safety and efficacy of these procedures.

References

1. Dos Santos JC. Sur la desobstruction des thrombose arterielle anciennes. *Med Acad Chir* 1947:409-411.
2. Vollmar J. Rekonstruktive chirurgie der arterien. *Stuttgart* 1967;24-27:264-270.
3. Dotter CT, Judkins MP. Transluminal treatment of arteriosclerotic obstruction: description of a new technique and a preliminary report of its application. *Circulation* 1964;30:654-670.

4. Grüntzig A, Hophoff H. Perkutane rekanlisation chronischer arterieller verschlüsse mit einem neuen dilatationskatheter: modification der dotter-technik. *Dtsch Med Wochenschr* 1974;99:2502-2505.
5. Volodos N, Karpovich I, Trojan V, et al. Clinical experience in the use of self-fixing synthetic prosthesis for remote endoprosthetics of the thoracic and abdominal aorta and iliac arteries through the femoral artery and as intraoperative endoprosthesis for aorta reconstruction. *Vasa* 1991;33:93-95.
6. Parodi JC, Palmaz J, Barone H. Transfemoral intraluminal graft implantation for abdominal aortic aneurysms. *Ann Vasc Surg* 1991;5:491-499.
7. Harris PL, Buth J, Miahle C, et al. The need for clinical trials of endovascular abdominal aortic repair: the EUROSTAR Project—European Collaborators on Stent-Graft Techniques for Abdominal Aortic Aneurysm Repair. *J Endovasc Surg* 1997;1:72-77. discussion, 78-79.
8. Sternbergh WC III, Carter G, York JW, et al. Aortic neck angulation predicts adverse outcome with endovascular abdominal aortic aneurysm repair. *J Vasc Surg* 2002;35:482-486.
9. Stanley BM, Semmens JB, Mai Q, et al. Evaluation of patient selection guidelines for endoluminal AAA repair with the Zenith stent-graft: the Australian experience. *J Endovasc Ther* 2001;8:457-464.
10. Broeders IAMJ, Balm R, Blankensteijn JD, et al. Preoperative sizing of grafts for transfemoral endovascular aneurysm management; a prospective comparative study of spiral CT angiography, arterial angiography and conventional CT imaging. *J Endovasc Surg* 1997;4:252-261.
11. Capasso P. Abdominal and thoracic aortic stent-grafts. *Semin Interv Radiol* 2001;18:299-319.
12. Palmaz JC. Biopolymers for endovascular use. *Semin Interv Radiol* 1998;15:13-19.
13. Malina M, Lindh M, Ivancev K, et al. The effect of endovascular aortic stents placed across the renal arteries. *Eur J Vasc Endovasc Surg* 1997;13:207-213.
14. Kramer SC, Seifarth H, Pamler R, et al. Renal infarction following endovascular aortic aneurysm repair: incidence and clinical consequences. *J Endovasc Ther* 2002;9:98-102.
15. Beebe HG. Imaging modalities for aortic endografting. *J Endovasc Surg* 1997;4:111-123.
16. Broeders IAMJ, Blankensteijn JD. A simple technique to improve the accuracy of proximal AAA endograft deployment. *J Endovasc Ther* 2000;7:389-393.
17. Torsello GB, Kasprzak B, Klenk E, et al. Endovascular suture versus cutdown for endovascular aneurysm repair: a prospective randomized pilot study. *J Vasc Surg* 2003;38:78-82.
18. Chaikof EL, Blankensteijn JD, Harris PL, et al. Reporting standards for endovascular aneurysm repair. *J Vasc Surg* 2002;35:1048-1060.
19. Parodi JC. Endovascular repair of abdominal aortic aneurysms and other arterial lesions. *J Vasc Surg* 1995;21:549-555.
20. May J, White GH. Endovascular treatment of aortic aneurysms. In: Rutherford R, ed. *Vascular surgery*. 5th ed. Philadelphia: WB Saunders; 1999:1281-1295.
21. Goldstone J, Brewster DC, Chaikoff EL, et al. Endoluminal repair versus standard open repair of abdominal aortic aneurysms: early results of a prospective clinical comparison trial. Proceedings of the 46th Scientific Meeting of the NA Chapter of the International Society for Cardiovascular Surgery. San Diego: California, 1998.
22. Zarins CK, White RA, Schwarten D, et al. Investigators of the Medtronic AneuRx Multicenter Clinical Trial: AneuRx stent graft versus open surgical repair of abdominal aortic aneurysms—multicenter prospective clinical trial. *J Vasc Surg* 1999;29:292-308.
23. May J, White GH, Yu W, et al. Concurrent comparison of endoluminal versus open repair in the treatment of abdominal aortic aneurysms: analysis of 303 patients by life table method. *J Vasc Surg* 1998;27:213-221.
24. Brewster DC, Geller CS, Kaufmann JA, et al. Initial experience with endovascular aneurysm repair: comparison of early results with outcome of conventional open repair. *J Vasc Surg* 1998;27:992-1003.
25. De Virgilio C, Bui H, Donayre C, et al. Endovascular vs open abdominal aortic aneurysm repair. *Arch Surg* 1999;134:947-951.
26. Beebe HG, Cronewett JL, Katzen BT, et al. Results of an aortic endograft trial: impact of device failure beyond 12 months. *J Vasc Surg* 2001;33:S55-S63.
27. May J, White GH, Waugh R, et al. Improved survival after endoluminal repair with second generation prostheses compared with open repair in the treatment of abdominal aortic aneurysms: a 5-year concurrent comparison using life table method. *J Vasc Surg* 2001;33:S21-S26.
28. Zarins CK, Arko FR, Lee WA, et al. Effectiveness of endovascular versus open repair in prevention of aneurysm related death. Proceedings of the 49th Scientific Meeting of the American Association for Vascular Surgery. Baltimore: Maryland, 2001.
29. Prinssen M, Verhoeven ELG, Buth J, et al. A randomized trial comparing conventional and endovascular repair of abdominal aortic aneurysms. *N Engl J Med* 2004;351:1607-1618.
30. Endovascular Aneurysm Repair Trial Participants. Comparison of endovascular repair with open repair in patients with abdominal aortic aneurysm (EVAR Trial 1), 30-day operative mortality results: randomised controlled trial. *Lancet* 2004;364:843-848.
31. White GH, Yu W, May J, et al. Endoleaks as a complication of endoluminal grafting of abdominal aortic aneurysms: classification, incidence, diagnosis and management. *J Endovasc Surg* 1997;4:152-168.
32. White GH, May J, Waugh R, et al. Type I and type II endoleak: a more useful classification for reporting results of endoluminal repair of AAA (Letter). *J Endovasc Surg* 1998;5:189-191.
33. Lumsden AB, Allen RC, Chaikof EL, et al. Delayed rupture of aortic aneurysms following endovascular stent grafting. *Am J Surg* 1995;170:174-178.
34. White GH, Yu W, May J, et al. Three-year experience with the White-Yu endovascular GAD graft for transluminal repair of aortic and iliac aneurysms. *J Endovasc Surg* 1997;4:124-136.
35. Torsello GB, Klenk E, Kasprzak B, et al. Rupture of abdominal aortic aneurysm previously treated by endovascular stentgraft. *J Vasc Surg* 1998;28:184-187.
36. Malina M, Ivancev K, Chuter TAM, et al. Changing aneurysmal morphology after endovascular grafting: relation to leakage or persistent perfusion. *J Endovasc Surg* 1997;4:23-30.
37. Gilling-Smith G, Brennan G, Harris PL, et al. Endotension after endovascular repair: definition, classification and implications for surveillance and intervention. *J Endovasc Surg* 1999;6:305-307.
38. White GH, May J, Petrasek P, et al. Endotension: an explanation for continued AAA growth after successful endoluminal repair. *J Endovasc Surg* 1999;6:308-315.
39. Schurink GW, Aarts N, Wilde J, et al. Endoleakage after stent-graft treatment of abdominal aneurysms: implications on pressure and imaging: an in vitro study. *J Vasc Surg* 1998;28:234-241.
40. Faries PL, Sanchez LA, Marin ML, et al. An experimental model for the acute and chronic evaluation of intra-aneurysmal pressure. *J Endovasc Surg* 1997;4:290-297.
41. Schurink GW, van Baalen JM, Visser MJ, et al. Thrombus within an aortic aneurysm does not reduce pressure on the aneurysmal wall. *J Vasc Surg* 2000;31:501-506.
42. Moore WS, Rutherford RB, for the EVT Investigators. Transfemoral endovascular repair of abdominal aortic aneurysm: results of the North American EVT phase 1 trial. *J Vasc Surg* 1996;23:543-553.
43. Blum U, Voshage G, Lammer J, et al. Endoluminal stent-grafts for infrarenal abdominal aortic aneurysms. *N Engl J Med* 1997;336:13-20.
44. May J, White GH, Yu W, et al. Repair of abdominal aortic aneurysms by endoluminal method: outcome in the first 100 patients. *Med J Aust* 1996;165:549-551.
45. Yusuf SW, Whitaker SC, Chuter TA, et al. Early results of endovascular aortic aneurysm surgery with aortouniiliac graft, contralateral occlusion and femoro-femoral bypass. *J Vasc Surg* 1997;25:165-172.
46. Wisselink W, Cuesta MA, Berends PJ, et al. Retroperitoneal endoscopic ligation of lumbar and inferior mesenteric artery as a treatment of persistent endoleak after endovascular aortic aneurysm repair. *J Vasc Surg* 2000;31:1240-1244.
47. Veith FJ, Baum RA, Ohki T, et al. Nature and significance of endoleaks and endotension: summary of opinions expressed at an international conference. *J Vasc Surg* 2002;35:1029-1035.
48. Deleted in proof.
49. Deleted in proof.
50. Cuypers PW, Laheij RJ, Buth J. Which factors increase the risk of conversion to open surgery following endovascular abdominal aortic aneurysm repair? The EUROSTAR collaborators. *Eur J Vasc Endovasc Surg* 2000;20:183-189.
51. Norgren L, Jernby B, Engellau L. Aortoenteric fistula caused by a ruptured stent-graft: a case report. *J Endovasc Surg* 1998;5:269-272.
52. Schlensak C, Doenst T, Moreno JB, et al. Serious complications requiring surgical interventions after endoluminal stent graft placement for the treatment of infrarenal aortic aneurysms. *J Vasc Surg* 2001;34:198-203.
53. Sonesson B, Lanne T, Hansen F, et al. Infrarenal aortic diameter in the healthy person. *Eur J Vasc Surg* 1994;8:89-95.
54. Lipski DA, Ernst CB. Natural history of the residual infrarenal aorta after infrarenal abdominal aortic aneurysm repair. *J Vasc Surg* 1998;27:805-811.
55. Sonesson B, Resch T, Lanne T, et al. The fate of the infrarenal aorta after open aneurysm surgery. *J Vasc Surg* 1998;28:889-894.

56. llig KA, Green RM, Ouriel K, et al. Fate of the proximal aortic cuff: implications for endovascular aneurysm repair. *J Vasc Surg* 1997;26:492-499.
57. Sonesson B, Malina M, Ivancev K, et al. Dilatation of the infrarenal aneurysm neck after endovascular exclusion of abdominal aortic aneurysm. *J Endovasc Surg* 1998;5:195-200.
58. Matsumura JS, Chaikof EL. Continued expansion of aortic necks after endovascular repair of abdominal aortic aneurysms: EVT Investigators. *J Vasc Surg* 1998;28:422-430.
59. May J, White GH, Yu W, et al. A prospective study of anatomico-pathological changes in abdominal aortic aneurysms following endoluminal repair: is the aneurysmal process reversed. *Eur J Vasc Endovasc Surg* 1996;12:11-17.
60. Wever JJ, de Nie AJ, Blankensteijn JD, et al. Dilatation of the proximal neck of infrarenal aortic aneurysms after endovascular AAA repair. *Eur J Vasc Endovasc Surg* 2000;19:197-201.
61. Prinssen M, Wever JJ, Mali WP, et al. Concerns for the durability of proximal AAA endograft fixation from a 2-year and 3-year longitudinal CT angiography study. *J Vasc Surg* 2001;33:S64-S69.
62. Zarins CK, White RA, Moll FL, et al. Aneurysm rupture after endovascular repair using the AneuRx stent graft. *J Vasc Surg* 2000;31:960-970.
63. Harris PL, Vallabhaneni SR, Desgranges P, et al. Incidence and risk factors of late rupture, conversion, and death after endovascular repair of infrarenal aortic aneurysms: the EUROSTAR experience. *J Vasc Surg* 2000;32:739-749.
64. Zarins CK, White RA, Moll Fl, et al. The AneuRx stent graft: four-year results and worldwide experience 2000. *J Vasc Surg* 2001;33:S135-S145.
65. Makaroun MS. The Ancure endografting system: an update. *J Vasc Surg* 2001;33:S129-S134.
66. Endovascular Aneurysm Repair Trial Participants. Endovascular repair versus open repair in patients with abdominal aortic aneurysm (EVAR Trial 1): randomised controlled trial. *Lancet* 2005;365:2179-2186.
67. Blankensteijn JD, de Jong SECA, Prinssen M, et al. Two-year outcomes after conventional or endovascular repair of abdominal aortic aneurysms. *N Engl J Med* 2005;352:2398-2405.
68. Muszbek N, Thompson MM, Soong CV, et al. Systematic review of utilities in abdominal aortic aneurysm. *Eur J Vasc Endovasc Surg* 2008;36(3): 283-289.
69. Holzenbein J, Kretschmer G, Glanzl R, et al. Endovascular AAA treatment: expensive prestige or economic alternative?. *Eur J Vasc Endovasc Surg* 1997;14:265-272.
70. Ceelen W, Sonneville T, Randon C, et al. Cost-benefit analysis of endovascular versus open abdominal aortic aneurysm treatment. *Acta Chir Belg* 1999;99:64-67.
71. Patel ST, Haser PB, Bush Jr HL, et al. The cost-effectiveness of endovascular repair versus open surgical repair of abdominal aortic aneurysms: a decision analysis model. *J Vasc Surg* 1999;29:958-972.
72. Seiwert AJ, Wolfe J, Whalen RC, et al. Cost comparison of aortic aneurysm endograft exclusion versus open surgical repair. *Am J Surg* 1999;178: 117-120.
73. Quinones-Baldrich WJ. Achieving cost-effective endoluminal aneurysm repair. *Semin Vasc Surg* 1999;12:220-225.
74. Sternbergh WC III, Money SR. Hospital cost of endovascular versus open repair of abdominal aortic aneurysms: a multicenter study. *J Vasc Surg* 2000;31:237-244.
75. Clair DG, Gray B, O'Hara PJ, et al. An evaluation of the cost to health care institutions of endovascular aortic aneurysm repair. *J Vasc Surg* 2000;32:148-152.
76. Birch SE, Stary DR, Scott AR. Cost of endovascular versus open surgical repair of abdominal aortic aneurysms. *Aust NZ J Surg* 2000;70: 660-666.
77. Turnipseed WD, Carr SC, Tefera G, et al. Minimal incision aortic surgery. *J Vasc Surg* 2001;34:47-53.
78. Bosch JL, Lester JS, McMahon PM, et al. Hospital costs for elective endovascular and surgical repairs of infrarenal abdominal aortic aneurysms. *Radiology* 2001;220:492-497.
79. Deleted in proof.
80. McWilliams RG, Martin J, White D, et al. Detection of endoleaks with enhanced ultrasound imaging: comparison with biphasic computed tomography. *J Endovasc Ther* 2002;9:170-179.
81. Sato DT, Goff CD, Gregory RT, et al. Endoleak after aortic stent graft repair: diagnosis by color duplex ultrasound versus computed tomography. *J Vasc Surg* 1998;28:657-663.
82. Matsumura JS, Moore WS. Clinical consequences of periprosthetic leak after endovascular repair of abdominal aortic aneurysm. *J Vasc Surg* 1998;27:606-613.
83. Ouriel K, Green RM, Donayre C, et al. An evaluation of new methods of expressing aortic aneurysm size: relationship to rupture. *J Vasc Surg* 1992;15:12-20.
84. Aarts NJ, Schurink GW, Schultze Kool LJ, et al. Abdominal aortic aneurysm for endovascular repair: intra- and interobserver variability of CT measurements. *Eur J Vasc Endovasc Surg* 1999;18:475-480.
85. Singh-Ranger R, McArthur T, Corte MD, et al. The abdominal aortic aneurysm sac after endoluminal exclusion: a medium term morphologic follow-up based on volumetric technology. *J Vasc Surg* 2000;31: 490-500.
86. Leurs LJ, Buth J, Laheij RJF. Long-term results of endovascular abdominal aortic aneurysm treatment with the first generation of commercially available stent grafts. *Arch Surg* 2007;142:33-41.
87. Lifeline Registry of Endovascular Aneurysm Repair Publications Committee. Lifeline registry of endovascular aneurysm repair: long-term primary outcome measures. *J Vasc Surg* 2005;42:1-10.
88. Franks SC, Sutton AJ, Bown MJ, et al. Systematic review and meta-analysis of 12 years of endovascular abdominal aortic aneurysm repair. *Eur J Vasc Endovasc Surg* 2007;33:154-171.
89. Shermerhorn ML, O'Malley AJ, Jhaveri A, et al. Endovascular vs open repair of abdominal aortic aneurysm in the Medicare population. *N Engl J Med* 2008;385:464-474.
90. Muhs BE, Verhoeven ELG, Zeebregts CJ, et al. Mid-term results of endovascular aneurysm repair with branched and fenestrated endografts. *J Vasc Surg* 2006;44:9-15.
91. Haulon S, Greenberg RK, Pfaff K, et al. Branched grafting for aortoiliac aneurysms. *Eur J Vasc Endovasc Surg* 2007;33:567-574.
92. Prinssen M, Buskens E, de Jond SE, et al. Costeffectiveness of conventional and endovasular repair of abdominal aortic aneurysms: Results of a randomized trial. *J Vasc Surg* 2007;46:883-890.

chapter

30

Infrarenal Abdominal Aortic Aneurysm: Open Repair

Patrick J. O'Hara, MD, FACS • Norman R. Hertzer, MD, FACS

Key Points

- Open repair is the direct surgical replacement of an infrarenal abdominal aortic aneurysm using a transperitoneal or retroperitoneal incision.
- Key features include nearly universal applicability, low mortality and morbidity rates, and exceptional durability.
- Clinical considerations include the proximal and distal extent of the aneurysm, patient selection, and associated comorbidities.
- A preoperative strategy is used to treat all relevant aneurysmal or occlusive disease.
- The incision should be tailored to suit the anatomy.
- A straightforward bifurcated graft is preferred to a difficult tube graft.
- The proximal end-to-end anastomosis is constructed near the renal arteries.
- Preserve at least one hypogastric artery or implant the inferior mesenteric artery.
- Avoid embolization.
- Assure that distal perfusion is adequate before leaving the operating room.

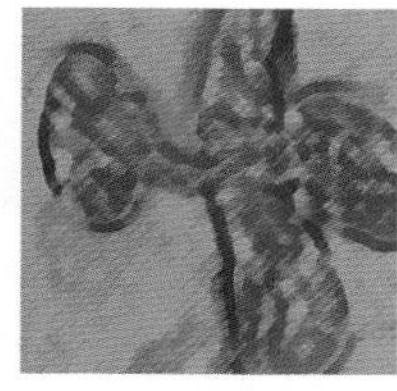

Most arterial aneurysms for which surgical intervention is necessary are located in the infrarenal aorta (Figure 30-1). As an example, Figure 30-2 illustrates the distribution of all 2326 true aneurysms that were treated either with open operations or with endovascular intervention by members of the Department of Vascular Surgery at the Cleveland Clinic from January 2002 through December 2007 (unpublished data). Approximately 60% of these aneurysms involved the infrarenal aorta, the iliac arteries, or both. Suprarenal and thoracoabdominal aortic aneurysms together consisted of only 19% of the aneurysms, while femoral (6.4%), popliteal (2.2%), and other miscellaneous aneurysms (15%) were even less common. The prevalence of each lesion may vary slightly from one center to the next, but the Cleveland Clinic experience probably is representative.

Dubost et al.[1] reported the first surgical repair of an infrarenal abdominal aortic aneurysm (AAA) using an arterial homograft more than 55 years ago. Since that time, countless advances in preoperative assessment, surgical technique, anesthetic management, and postoperative care have led to a dramatic reduction in the early risk of this procedure. In addition, the development of modern synthetic materials has been associated with excellent long-term patency rates and a low incidence of late graft-related complications.[2-4] For nearly four decades, definitive AAA repair could not be done without direct exposure of the abdominal aorta. Parodi et al.[5] then introduced another therapeutic alternative in 1991 with their landmark description of endovascular aneurysm repair (EVAR) using a transfemoral catheter-based approach and homemade stent grafts in five high-risk cases. Several commercial over-the-wire devices have since been refined to the point that EVAR now can be performed in increasingly larger numbers of patients worldwide with operative mortality and complication rates that are generally lower—although not always significantly so—than those for open repair of either asymptomatic or ruptured AAAs.[6-8]

Despite such encouraging results, EVAR also has been found to have a unique set of late complications that require lifelong surveillance with follow-up imaging studies. These include stent fractures, device migration, and most often,

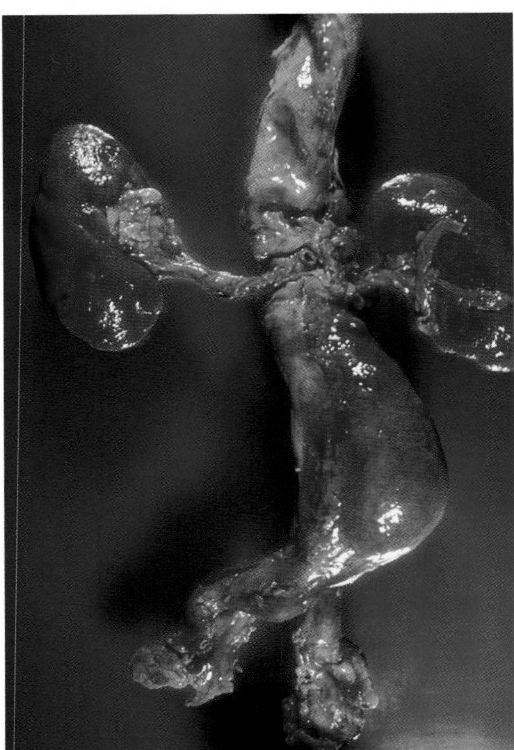

Figure 30-1. Infrarenal aortic aneurysm. As in this pathological specimen, most abdominal aortic aneurysms are located below the renal arteries.

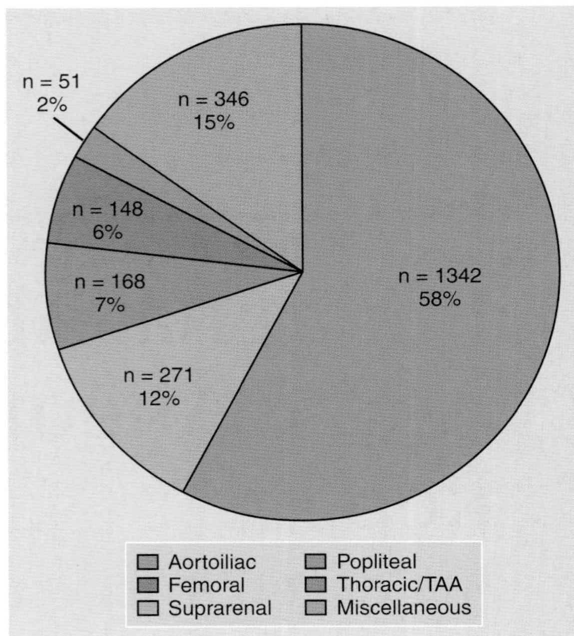

Figure 30-2. Distribution of arterial aneurysms. Anatomical location of 2326 true aneurysms treated either with open operations or with endovascular intervention at the Cleveland Clinic from January 2002 through December 2007. TAAs, thoracoabdominal aortic aneurysms.

endoleaks at graft fixation sites or from collateral branch vessels that continue to maintain pressure within the excluded aneurysm sac. The most serious endoleaks (types I and III) occur at fixation sites and may contribute to the annual rupture rate of 1% occurring after EVAR unless steps are taken to correct them by further endovascular intervention or occasionally even by complete explantation of the endoprosthesis. In comparison, the risk of rupture caused by collateral blood flow into the aneurysm sac (type II endoleaks) appears to be quite low.[9] Nevertheless, given the collective uncertainties about its durability, there seems to be a consensus that EVAR still should be reserved primarily for high-risk patients and that conventional open repair is not obsolete.[10]

INDICATIONS

The principal risk of an AAA is progressive expansion with eventual rupture, exsanguination, and death. Much less commonly, an AAA can undergo complete thrombosis or cause distal emboli, either of which can provoke critical limb ischemia. Consequently, the therapeutic objectives of open repair are the prevention of death by rupture and, secondarily, the preservation of adequate arterial perfusion to the pelvis and lower extremities. Urgent surgical treatment ordinarily can be justified for any ruptured or clearly symptomatic AAA, irrespective of its size, provided that the patient does not have a preexisting medical condition, such as widespread metastatic cancer, that already is considered terminal. In comparison, symptomatic AAAs should be repaired whenever their risk to rupture predictably exceeds the risk of an elective operation itself. Therefore, the decision to operate on an asymptomatic AAA must be tailored to its diameter and its documented expansion rate, as well as to the age of the patient and the presence of associated comorbidities.

Until recently, the traditional threshold for open repair had been a maximum diameter of 5 cm or more based on estimated rupture and survival rates, a few of which are presented in Table 30-1. These historical data suggest that rupture eventually occurs in approximately 20% of AAAs that are more than 5 cm in diameter, 40% of those that measure at least 6 cm, and as many as 50% of those that exceed 7 cm. Taylor and Porter[15] concluded from their collective review in 1986 that the annual rupture rates for AAAs in these relative size ranges were about 4%, 7%, and 20%. In comparison, the long-term rupture rate for AAAs with a baseline diameter of less than 4 cm appears to be quite low, perhaps because older patients often do not survive long enough for such truly small AAAs to enlarge to a size that rupture would become more likely. In 2001, Hallin et al.[17] performed another literature search and reported expansion rates of 0.2 to 0.4 cm per year for AAAs smaller than 4 cm, 0.2 to 0.5 cm per year for those 4 to 5 cm in diameter, and 0.3 to 0.7 cm per year for those larger than 5 cm. The risk for AAA rupture at 4 years was 2%, 10%, and 22%, respectively.

Randomized Clinical Trials

Beginning in the mid-1990s, the U.K. Small Aneurysm Trial (UKSAT) and the Veterans Administration Aneurysm Detection and Management (ADAM) Trial were conducted to compare early elective surgery versus ultrasound surveillance for AAAs measuring 4.0 to 5.4 cm in diameter. Per protocol, surgical treatment was not offered to patients who were assigned to surveillance in these two randomized trials unless their AAAs became symptomatic or enlarged to at least 5.5 cm

Table 30-1
Estimated Rupture and Survival Rates According to Abdominal Aortic Aneurysm Diameter*

	Year	Aneurysm Diameter	Follow-Up Interval	Rupture (%)	Survival (%)
Case Series					
Szilagyi et al.[11]	1966	6 cm or less (n = 82)	34 months (mean)	19	45
		More than 6 cm (n = 141)	17 months (mean)	43	10
Hertzer et al.[12]	1987	Less than 6 cm (n = 24)	5 years	20	38
		6 cm or more (n = 18)	5 years	69	(overall)
Nevitt et al.[13]	1989	Less than 5 cm (n = 130)	5 years	0	NA
		5 cm or more (n = 46)	5 years	25	NA
Conway et al.[14]	2001	5.5-5.9 cm (n = 23)	25 months (mean)	22	39
		6-7 cm (n = 62)	25 months (mean)	34	32
		More than 7 cm (n = 21)	16 months (mean)	52	5.0
Collective Reviews					
Taylor and Porter[15]	1986	5 cm	NA	4.1 annually	NA
		5.7 cm	NA	6.6 annually	NA
		7 cm	NA	19 annually	NA
Hollier et al.[16]	1992	Less than 5 cm (n = 349)	5 years	4.6	NA
		More than 5 cm (n = 90)	5 years	30	NA
Hallin et al.[17]	2001	Less than 4 cm (n = 43)	4 years	2.0	NA
		4-5 cm (n = 30)	4 years	10	NA
		More than 5 cm (n = 23)	4 years	22	NA

*NA, not available.

in diameter on serial imaging studies.[18-21] Selected data from both investigations are summarized in Table 30-2, using information reported from the UKSAT at three follow-up intervals (mean 4.6, 8.0, and 12 years) and from the ADAM trial at a mean of 4.9 years. The principal demographic difference between the two study populations was that women made up less than 1% of the ADAM Trial, whereas they represented a more typical 17% of the patients in the UKSAT. All but two patients who received early surgery in either trial underwent open repair rather than EVAR, with 30-day operative mortality rates of 5.5% in the UKSAT and 2.1% in the ADAM Trial.

At a mean follow-up of 4.9 years, early repair provided no significant benefit with respect to the incidence of either AAA-related deaths or deaths from all causes in the ADAM Trial.[21] These same conclusions initially were reached at a mean follow-up of 4.6 years in the UKSAT.[18] The annual rupture rate was only 0.6% for surveillance in the ADAM Trial and ranged from 1.6% to 3.2% in the UKSAT. Rupture was more likely to occur among women under surveillance in the UKSAT (odds ratio 4.0, 95% confidence interval [CI] 2.0 to 7.9, $p < 0.001$), accounting for 14% of their deaths compared to 4.6% of all deaths in men ($p < 0.001$). Early surgery had a lower overall mortality rate than surveillance at a mean follow-up of 8 years in the UKSAT ($p = 0.03$), but this was attributed largely to a higher rate of smoking cessation.[19] Baseline AAA size failed to influence the risk for rupture in the UKSAT or the long-term mortality rate in either trial. Adjusted hazard ratios tended to favor early surgery for younger patients, for men and for larger AAAs in the UKSAT, but these trends were not found to be statistically significant on interaction testing.[20] More than 60% of all patients who were under surveillance in the ADAM Trial underwent repair for AAA enlargement within 4 years of randomization, including 81% of those whose AAAs were 5.0 to 5.4 cm in diameter at the time they entered the trial. The final repair rate was 76% at 12 years of follow-up for all patients who had been randomized to surveillance in the UKSAT; 26 (6.5%) of these 401 procedures were done using EVAR.

Both randomized trials concluded that AAAs measuring 4.0 to 5.4 cm in diameter should be kept under surveillance. Nevertheless, more than 80% of the AAAs that were at least 5 cm in diameter were repaired in 4 years or less in the ADAM Trial, which could be viewed as confirmation that the traditional threshold of 5 cm still may be appropriate for intervention in younger, good-risk patients. Furthermore, the finding that rupture was four times more likely to occur in the women under surveillance in the UKSAT adds perspective to a lingering controversy concerning whether, because of the smaller diameter of their normal aorta, the size criteria for early repair should be slightly more liberal in women than in men. Brewster et al.[10] addressed both of these issues in a comprehensive guidelines document in 2005, adding that several other factors—e.g., severe chronic obstructive pulmonary disease (COPD), multiple familial aneurysms, poorly controlled hypertension, saccular AAAs, and rapid enlargement while under observation—also are associated with higher-than-average rupture rates and, like patient age and gender, may need to be balanced against the risk of elective repair for some AAAs that are smaller than 5.5 cm.

TECHNIQUE

The ideal goal of open AAA repair is to treat all aneurysms and incidental aortoiliac occlusive disease that are identified on preoperative imaging studies, but judgment is necessary to modify the optimal plan according to the particular circumstances. Depending on such clinical considerations as the urgency of operation and the presence of medical comorbidities, objectives must be prioritized and accomplished as time and circumstances permit. Important precautions include close monitoring of arterial blood pressure and intravascular volume, both of which are facilitated by routine placement of radial artery lines and pulmonary artery catheters. The use of epidural anesthesia with a general anesthetic greatly enhances postoperative pain management and seems especially

Table 30-2
Intention-to-Treat Outcome of Early Elective Surgery versus Ultrasound Surveillance for Asymptomatic Abdominal Aortic Aneurysms Measuring 4.0 to 5.5 cm in Diameter in the U.K. Small Aneurysm Trial (UKSAT)[18-20] and the Veterans Administration Aneurysm Detection and Management (ADAM) Trial[21]*

		UKSAT		ADAM
Randomized patients	1090			1136
Early surgery	563			569
Open	561			567
Endovascular	2			2
Surveillance	527			567
Men	902			1127
Women	188			9
Mean age	69 ± 4 years			68 ± 6 years
Operative mortality rate for early surgery	5.5% (30 days)			2.1% (30 days) 2.7% (in-hospital)
Follow-up period	Range 3-7 years Mean 4.6 years	Range 6-10 years Mean 8 years	12 years	Range 3-8 years Mean 4.9 years
Survival Rate				
Early surgery	64%	57%	36%	75%
Surveillance	64%	52% ($p = 0.03$)	33%	78%
Rupture rate while under surveillance	1.6% annually	3.2% annually	4.4% crude	0.6% annually
Men	NA	OR 1.0 (reference set)	NA	NA
Women	NA	OR 4.0 95% CI 2.0-7.9 ($p < 0.001$)	NA	NA
Eventual Repair				
Early surgery cohort	520 (92%)	520 (92%)	528 (94%)	527 (93%)
Surveillance cohort	321 (61%)	327 (62%)	401 (76%)	349 (62%)
Surveillance Outcome According to Diameter				
Survival rate	NA	4.0-4.4 cm: 57% 4.5-4.8 cm: 54% 4.9-5.5 cm: 43%	4.0-4.4 cm: 38% 4.5-4.8 cm: 35% 4.9-5.5 cm: 26%	4.0-4.4 cm: 79% 4.5-4.9 cm: 78% 5.0-5.4 cm: 68%
Eventual repair rate	NA	NA	NA	4.0-4.4 cm: 27% 4.5-4.9 cm: 53% 5.0-5.4 cm: 81%

*CI, confidence interval; NA, not available; OR, odds ratio.

important in the care of patients who have advanced COPD. The cost effectiveness of intraoperative blood salvage and autotransfusion remains uncertain, but a recent metaanalysis of four randomized trials found that autotransfusion was associated with a significant reduction (37%, $p = 0.03$) in the homologous blood requirement at the time of elective open AAA repair.[22] The combination of autotransfusion and readministration of one or two units of autologous blood already donated by the same patient is another efficient way to reduce the need for banked blood.[23]

Choice of Incision

A midline transperitoneal incision from the xiphoid process to just above the pubis (Figure 30-3A) allows the opportunity for exploration of the intraabdominal viscera and has the advantage of giving ample exposure of the distal right common iliac artery and its bifurcation vessels when they are involved by aneurysms or incidental occlusive disease. An alternative retroperitoneal incision extending toward the tip of the 11th rib in the left flank (Figure 30-3B) may be better suited to obese patients and for other specific situations, such as juxtarenal AAAs, horseshoe kidneys, and "hostile" abdomens resulting from previous operations or infections. Two single-center randomized trials have produced conflicting results concerning whether a retroperitoneal flank incision might be superior to a transperitoneal approach for infrarenal aortic reconstruction in all cases. Sicard et al.[24] randomized 145 patients and reported that the flank incision was associated with a lower incidence of prolonged gastrointestinal ileus ($p = 0.013$) and small bowel obstruction ($p = 0.05$), as well as with a shorter stay in the intensive care unit ($p = 0.006$) and lower hospital costs ($p = 0.017$). There was no significant difference in the number of pulmonary complications or the total length of hospital stay. In a similar randomized trial that had been done only 5 years earlier, however, Cambria et al.[25] found no differences in blood, fluid, or narcotic requirements; pulmonary complications; gastrointestinal function; or length of stay in a total of 113 patients. On balance, neither of these trials may have been large enough to reach a convincing conclusion.

A low thoracoretroperitoneal incision through the 10th intercostal space (Figure 30-3B) rarely is necessary for infrarenal aortic aneurysm repair, but there is an exception for which this approach may be indispensable—i.e., an unusually short and sometimes angulated visceral aortic segment located so near the left hemidiaphragm that it can be exceedingly difficult to isolate the neck of the aneurysm through any other incision. This potential problem could influence the course of the entire operation, so it should be identified whenever possible

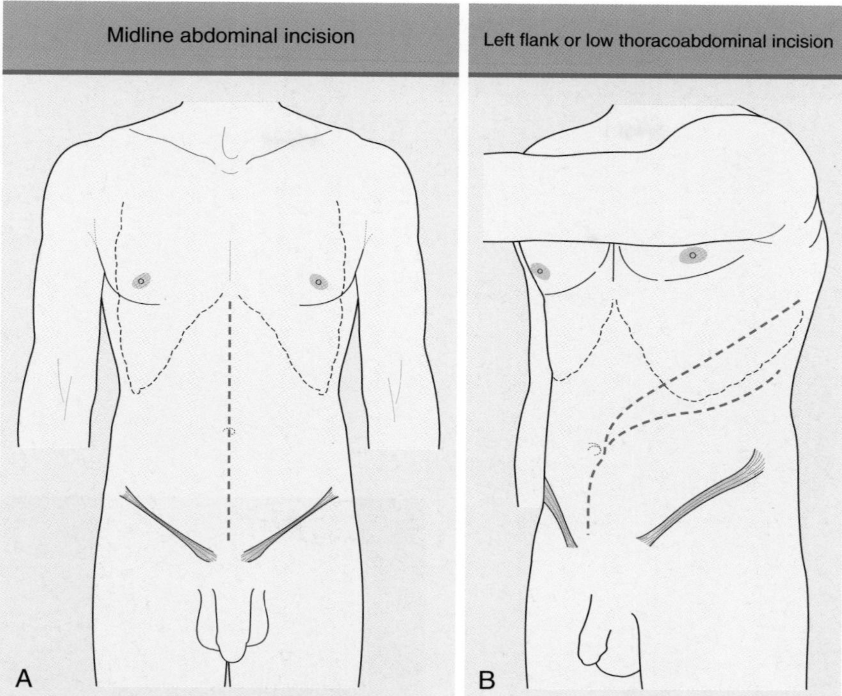

Figure 30-3. Incisions for open aneurysm repair. **A,** Midline transabdominal. **B,** Left flank and low thoracoretroperitoneal, the latter for juxtarenal or visceral aortic exposure.

on the preoperative imaging studies. The left kidney can be mobilized anteriorly through either a low thoracoretroperitoneal incision or a flank incision if more proximal exposure of the visceral aortic segment is required, for instance, for suprarenal or supraceliac clamp control of a juxtarenal AAA.

Intact Aneurysms

Deep exposure is obtained with as little direct manipulation of the AAA as possible in an attempt to minimize the risk for distal embolization of mural thrombus or other debris, a precaution that is especially important if the patient already has had prior embolic events. For the same reason, once heparin has been administered, it usually is preferable to apply the outflow clamps before placing the proximal aortic clamp. The aneurysm sac then is incised along its right anterolateral aspect, avoiding the autonomic nerve plexus that weaves anteriorly and along the left side of the aorta, encircles the origin of the inferior mesenteric artery (IMA) and crosses the left common iliac artery (Figure 30-4). Preservation of this plexus is important in men who still are sexually active, since its injury may lead to retrograde ejaculation.[26] Once the bulk of mural thrombus has been removed without allowing any fragments to dislodge into the iliac arteries where they could become a hidden source of emboli, patent lumbar arteries are stripped of calcium and oversewn with nonabsorbable suture material. Provided the IMA is backbleeding vigorously, it also may be oversewn from within the aneurysm. If any doubt exists about the adequacy of retrograde bleeding, however, the IMA should be controlled with an elastic vessel loop or a small vascular clamp and preserved until the appearance of the sigmoid colon can be reassessed after flow has been restored to the pelvis through the new aortic graft.

The synthetic replacement graft may be fabricated from woven or knitted Dacron, usually with hemostatic collagen coating, or from polytetrafluoroethylene, perhaps the most important feature being that its size should appropriately match the diameter of the aneurysm neck and the outflow vessels. The proximal anastomosis can be done formally end to end after dividing a long infrarenal neck (Figure 30-5A), but more often it is performed from inside the open aneurysm sac without transection of the posterior aortic wall (Figure 30-5B). Using either technique, the proximal anastomosis should be constructed close to the level of the renal arteries to reduce the chance for a future aneurysm in the infrarenal aortic cuff remaining above the graft. In the case of juxtarenal AAAs, the suture line actually may incorporate the lower rim of the renal artery ostia. Continuous monofilament sutures ordinarily are used for this anastomosis, but they may warrant additional reinforcement with a strip of Teflon felt when the aorta is either flimsy or heavily calcified (Figure 30-5C).[27] If the quality of the aorta is particularly poor or the residual aortic cuff is ectatic, the proximal anastomosis instead can be done using interrupted, evenly spaced horizontal mattress sutures buttressed with Teflon felt pledgets (Figure 30-5D).

Provided that the AAA terminates at an adequate distance above the aortic bifurcation and the iliac arteries are free of aneurysms or occlusive disease, an aortic interposition (or "tube") graft may be adequate (Figure 30-6A). The distal anastomosis then can be done using the techniques that are shown in Figure 30-5. The distal aorta often is prohibitively calcified, however, particularly in its posterior wall. Under these circumstances, it usually is better to perform a straightforward aortoiliac bifurcation graft rather than to attempt a

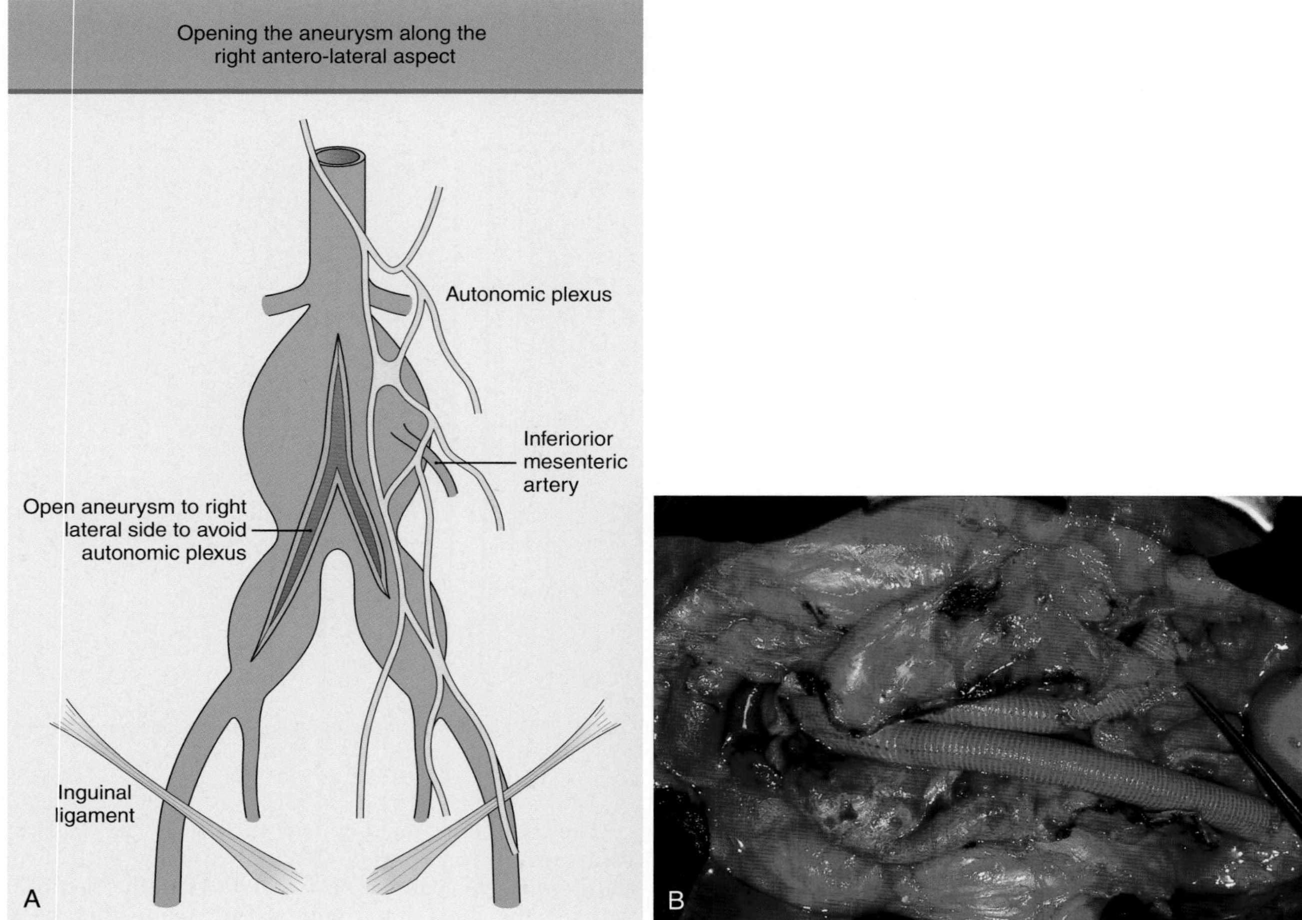

Figure 30-4. Preservation of autonomic nerves. **A,** The aneurysm is opened along its right anterolateral aspect in an attempt to avoid injury to the autonomic plexus, which is swept lateral to the left common iliac artery. **B,** Operative photograph of the plexus, indicated by the forceps.

difficult tube graft. The aortic stem of the bifurcation graft should be cut short enough to discourage the iliac limbs from kinking. An end-to-end configuration is preferred for the outflow anastomoses, which should be performed near the origins of the external iliac and hypogastric arteries (Figure 30-6B) whenever the common iliac arteries contain aneurysms or severe occlusive disease. While aortofemoral bypass occasionally expedites the management of ruptured AAAs in the presence of large retroperitoneal hematomas obscuring regional anatomy, extensive occlusive disease is sufficiently unusual in most patients with aneurysms that aortofemoral grafts rarely are necessary for nonruptured AAAs.

Every possible effort should be made to restore perfusion to at least one and ideally to both of the hypogastric arteries to reduce the incidence of postoperative colon ischemia, buttock claudication, or sexual dysfunction.[26] This may require sequential branch grafting in the pelvis (Figure 30-6C). Reimplantation of the IMA into the aortic graft or, if necessary, into the left limb of a bifurcation graft offers further protection from colon ischemia in certain cases where neither hypogastric artery is patent, backbleeding from the IMA seems inadequate, or the sigmoid colon still appears dusky after all clamps have been removed and antegrade flow has been returned to the pelvis. The Carrel patch technique is useful for this purpose (Figure 30-6D), keeping the button of native aorta that contains the IMA small enough to avoid a subsequent patch aneurysm.

Circulating heparin is neutralized with protamine sulfate only after perfusion to the colon and both lower extremities has been shown to be adequate and after reclamping of the graft is no longer necessary. The color of the sigmoid colon and the filling of its arterial arcades should be carefully assessed, and either the surgeon or an experienced assistant should inspect both feet from beneath the drapes to confirm that pedal pulses (or Doppler signals) are consistent with those that were present preoperatively. Once complete hemostasis has been obtained, the aneurysm sac is closed over the graft and the retroperitoneum is reconstructed so that it is watertight to insure separation of the synthetic graft from the duodenum and the other abdominal viscera, thus minimizing the potential for graft-enteric erosion (Figure 30-7A). If the aneurysm sac and the retroperitoneum are inadequate to cover the graft reliably, a pedicle of omentum should be mobilized, together with its nutrient artery; drawn through an opening at the base of the transverse mesocolon within the lesser peritoneal sac; and secured over the new graft (Figure 30-7B). The incision then is closed in a standard fashion and the patient is transferred

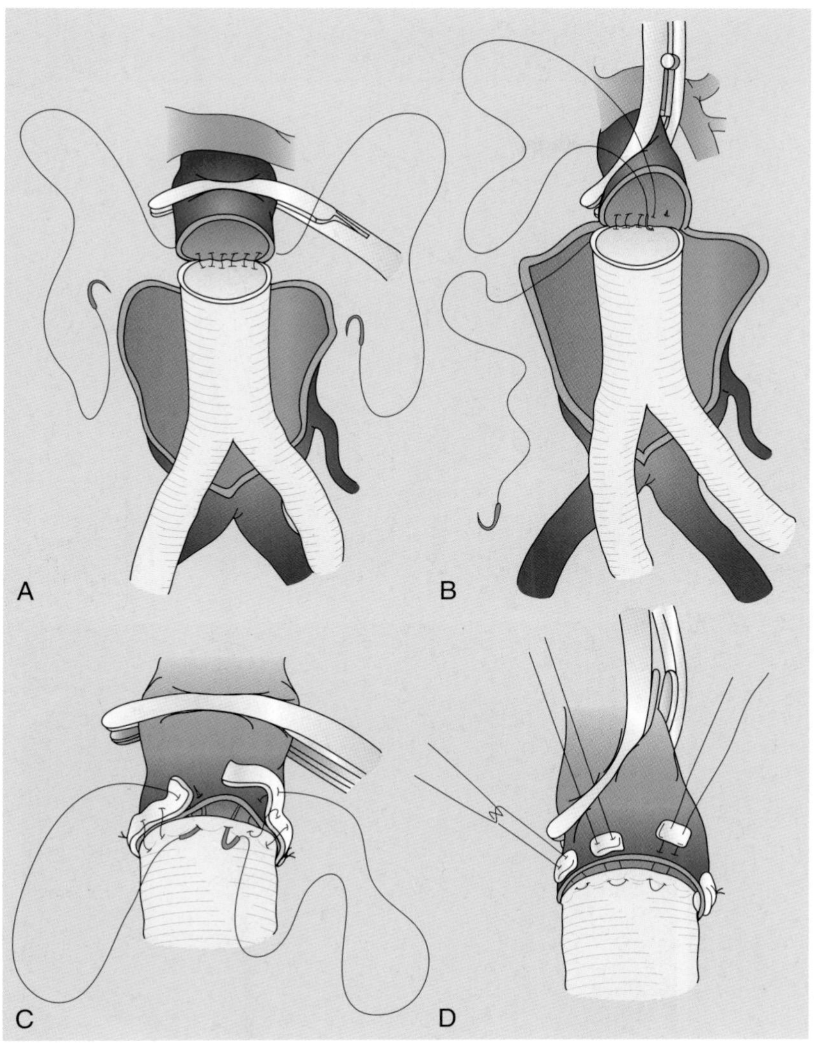

Figure 30-5. Anastomotic techniques. **A,** Formal end-to-end proximal anastomosis after dividing the neck of the aneurysm. **B,** Functional end-to-end proximal anastomosis without transection of the posterior wall of the aneurysm sac. **C,** Reinforcement of a continuous suture line with Teflon® strips tends to reduce needle-hole bleeding from flimsy or heavily calcified aortic walls. **D,** An anastomosis using interrupted mattress sutures may be appropriate for an ectatic aortic neck and can be reinforced with Teflon® pledgets. (From the Cleveland Clinic, Cleveland, Ohio.)

to the recovery room or the intensive care unit for monitoring and support.

Ruptured Aneurysms

A ruptured AAA is an abdominal catastrophe. If the rupture is directed anteriorly into the free peritoneal cavity, it usually is not possible to salvage the patient from rapid exsanguination unless prompt control of the aorta proximal to the rupture site is achieved in the operating room—literally within minutes. Bleeding temporarily may be contained if the rupture occurs posteriorly into the retroperitoneal space, but an urgent operation remains necessary because the expanding hematoma still can perforate into the peritoneal cavity. No time can be wasted in this situation. The patient should be prepared and draped while other members of the surgical team establish adequate volume replacement lines. The incision usually must be made immediately after the induction of anesthesia, since abrupt hemodynamic decompensation often occurs once reflex muscular tamponade of the hematoma is lost when paralytic agents are given for endotracheal intubation.

Rapid proximal control often is facilitated by manual compression of the supraceliac aorta or by applying a vertical aortic clamp at the level of the diaphragmatic crura. This clamp then can be moved to below the renal arteries (Figure 30-8) after carefully exposing the neck of the aneurysm without injury to any of its surrounding veins. Proximal control also can be obtained above the renal arteries by using an intraaortic balloon catheter inserted either through the aneurysm or via a transfemoral or left brachial approach. Judgment is necessary to choose an appropriate method for proximal control that requires the least amount of time. For instance, in some patients much of the dissection around the neck of the aneurysm already has been done by the hematoma itself. In such cases, it often is possible to identify the aneurysm neck using fingertip exploration within the hematoma while an assistant positioned to the left of the surgeon manually compresses the supraceliac aorta against the spine. A single infrarenal clamp then can be applied.

As shown in Figure 30-8, distal control is much easier to obtain using balloon embolectomy catheters or conventional instruments. The remainder of the repair is identical to that already described for intact AAAs, but Rasmussen et al.[28] have reported that delayed abdominal closure using synthetic mesh appears to have reduced the incidence of abdominal compartment syndromes and multisystem organ failure after repair of ruptured AAAs at the Mayo Clinic.

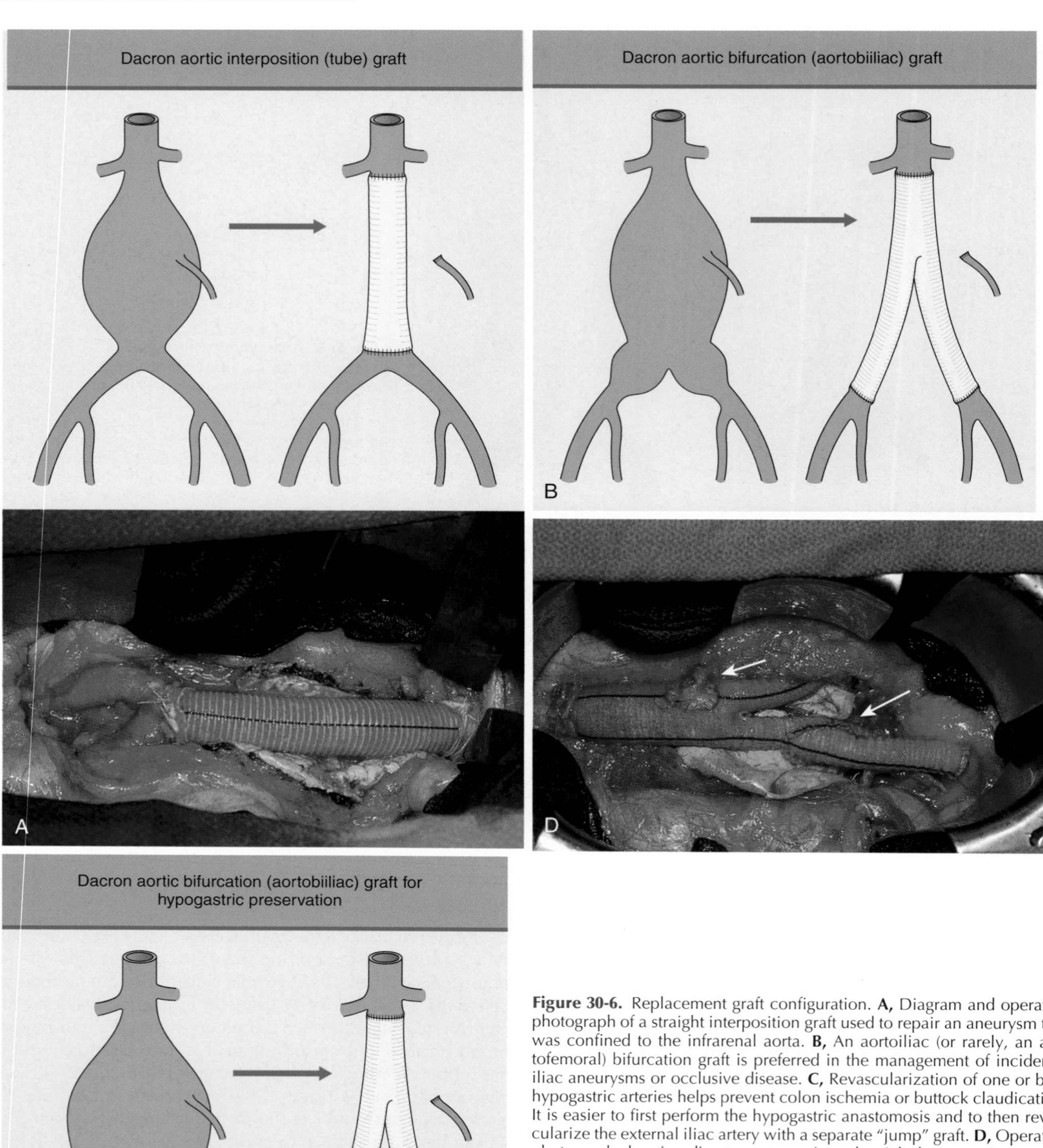

Figure 30-6. Replacement graft configuration. **A,** Diagram and operative photograph of a straight interposition graft used to repair an aneurysm that was confined to the infrarenal aorta. **B,** An aortoiliac (or rarely, an aortofemoral) bifurcation graft is preferred in the management of incidental iliac aneurysms or occlusive disease. **C,** Revascularization of one or both hypogastric arteries helps prevent colon ischemia or buttock claudication. It is easier to first perform the hypogastric anastomosis and to then revascularize the external iliac artery with a separate "jump" graft. **D,** Operative photograph showing direct anastomosis to the right hypogastric artery, a jump graft to the ipsilateral external iliac artery, and reimplantation of the inferior mesenteric artery into the aortic stem of the bifurcation graft.

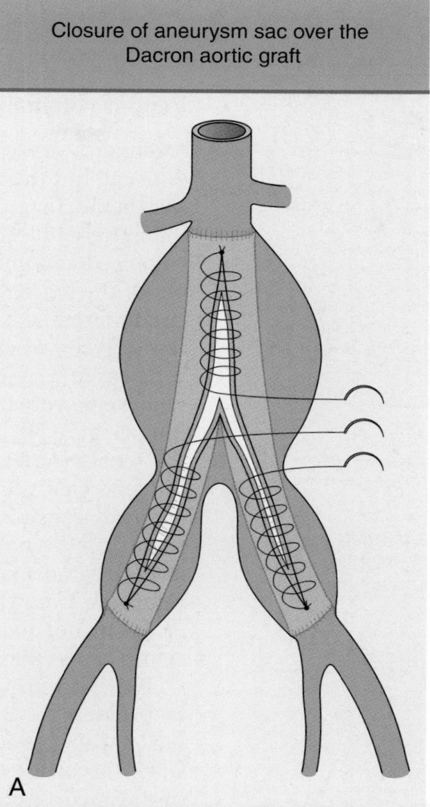

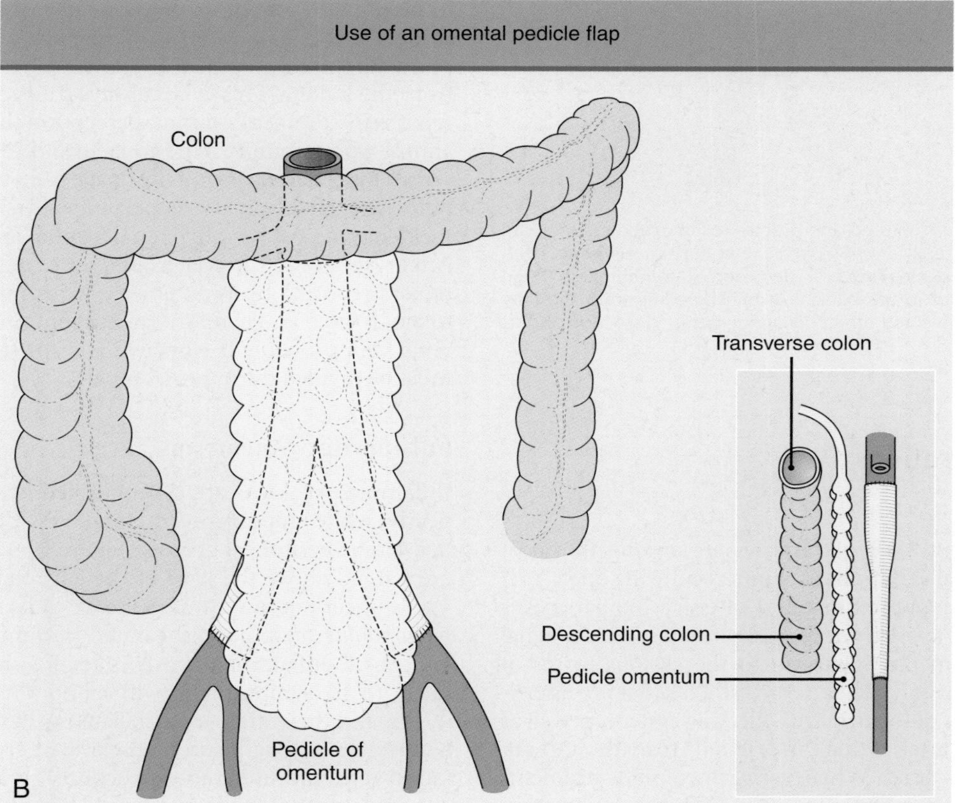

Figure 30-7. Retroperitoneal graft coverage. **A,** Closure of the aneurysm sac and the posterior parietes ordinarily is sufficient to isolate the aortic replacement graft from the intestine. **B,** It sometimes is necessary to mobilize a pedicle of greater omentum with an adequate arterial supply and pass it through an avascular rent at the base of the transverse mesocolon to obtain satisfactory graft coverage in thin patients or during aortic reoperations.

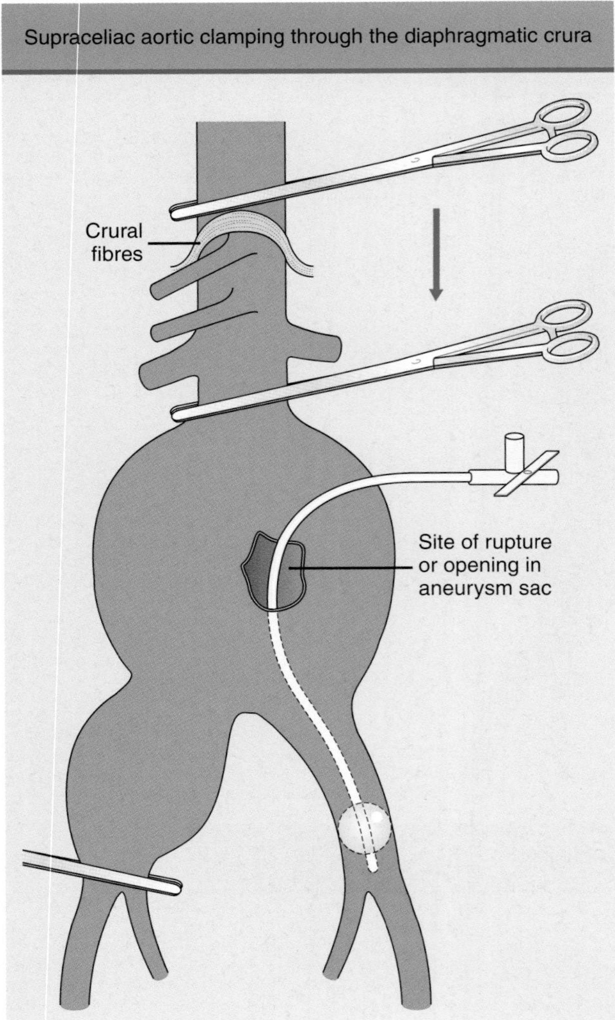

Figure 30-8. Control of ruptured aneurysms. A supraceliac clamp can be moved below the renal arteries once the aneurysm neck has been fully defined, thus restoring visceral perfusion. Intraluminal balloon catheters may be useful in the control of backbleeding from the iliac arteries without extensive and time-consuming pelvic dissection and its attendant blood loss.

Other Considerations

Renal Anomalies

Anomalies involving the renal arteries are among the most common anatomical variations encountered during open AAA repair; they occur in approximately 1 of every 200 patients.[29] They range in complexity from the presence of accessory renal arteries arising from the aneurysm to the various forms of renal ectopia and fusion, the latter of which often are associated with anomalies of the urinary collecting system, as well as with aberrant renal arteries that can originate from the aorta or the common iliac arteries. Whenever such complex problems are detected on computed tomography (CT) scans or by other preoperative imaging studies, they usually are best managed using a retroperitoneal or thoracoretroperitoneal incision.[30-32] This approach allows the renal mass and the collecting system to be displaced anteriorly, and it facilitates the reimplantation of anomalous renal arteries into the replacement graft from inside the open aneurysm sac (Figure 30-9).

Venous Anomalies

Anomalies of the major intraabdominal veins are relatively unusual, but their injury during AAA repair can lead to massive hemorrhage that typically is more difficult to control than arterial bleeding. Aljabri et al.[33] reviewed 1788 contrast-enhanced abdominal and pelvic CT scans and found anomalies of the left renal vein to be most common. Retroaortic or circumferential left renal veins were present in 3.2% or 1.6%, respectively, whereas left-sided (Figure 30-10) or duplicated vena cavae were identified in less than 1%. A retroaortic left renal vein ordinarily can be detected by preoperative CT scanning (Figure 30-11A) but also should be suspected whenever the renal arteries come into view without first encountering the left renal vein while exposing the aneurysm through an anterior transperitoneal incision (Figure 30-11B). Most retroaortic left renal veins enter the vena cava at a more caudad level than normal, coursing obliquely down and toward the right side from the left renal hilus. Considerable care should be taken not to damage this vein while placing a proximal clamp across the neck of the aneurysm.

Either a retroaortic or a circumferential left renal vein can be problematic if the left kidney is mobilized anteriorly during retroperitoneal or thoracoretroperitoneal AAA repair, since this tends to rotate the vein directly around the neck of the aneurysm. If a circumferential left renal vein is known to be present, one of its divisions probably can be sacrificed to obtain adequate exposure under the assumption that the remaining division still will allow adequate venous outflow from the kidney. This is not always true with an unpaired left renal vein despite a common perception that it can be divided almost with impunity if the gonadal and adrenal veins are preserved for collateral venous drainage from the kidney. Division of the left renal vein was associated with a significantly higher incidence of postoperative renal insufficiency in the Canadian Aneurysm Study[34] as well as in a series of 247 pararenal AAA repairs reported by West et al.[35] (odds ratio 3.0, 95% CI 1.1 to 8.6, $p = 0.04$). Therefore, an attempt to reconstruct the left renal vein probably is worthwhile if for some good reason it must be divided during AAA repair.

Inflammatory Aneurysms

Inflammatory AAAs are distinguished by their characteristic pearly white appearance, a markedly thickened wall, and dense retroperitoneal fibrosis (Figure 30-12A and B) that may not extend above the level of the left renal vein. Their etiology is uncertain, but some evidence links them to *Chlamydia pneumoniae* or to an exaggerated immune response to viral antigens.[36] Inflammatory AAAs tend to be larger and more likely to be symptomatic with abdominal pain than other AAAs, and they often are associated with familial aneurysms, a current smoking history, an elevated erythrocyte sedimentation rate, and ureteral obstruction.[36,37] It the latter is present, urological consultation should be obtained and the use of retrograde stents should be considered for ureteral protection during open AAA repair. Like the ureters, the duodenum often is involved by the inflammatory fibrosis and can be so adherent to the aorta that it seems to be incorporated within the wall of

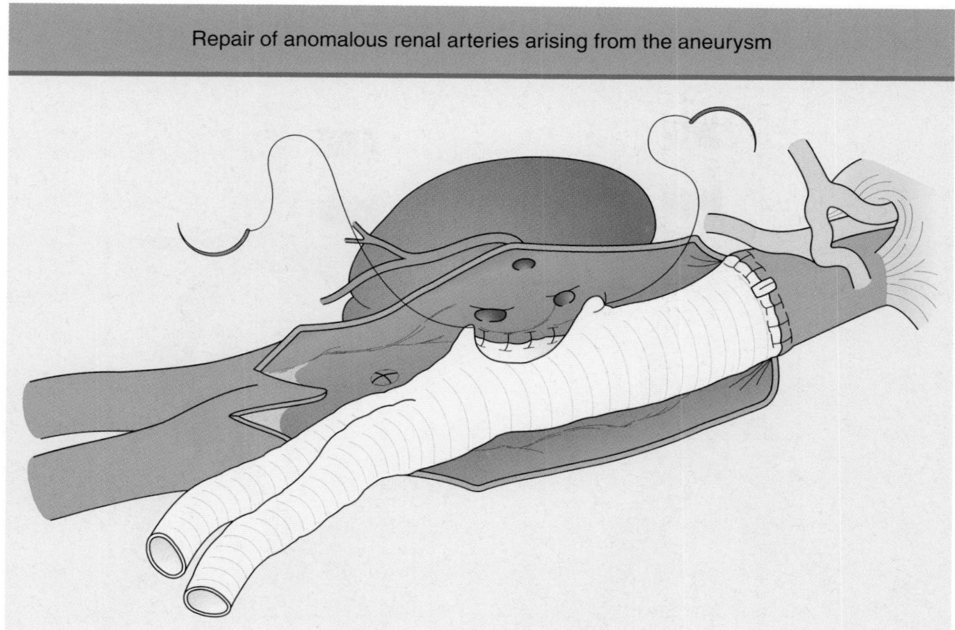

Figure 30-9. Anomalous renal arteries. Anomalous renal arteries arising from the aneurysm sac or supplying a horseshoe kidney may be reimplanted into the replacement graft most easily by using a retroperitoneal incision in the left flank. (From the Cleveland Clinic, Cleveland, Ohio.)

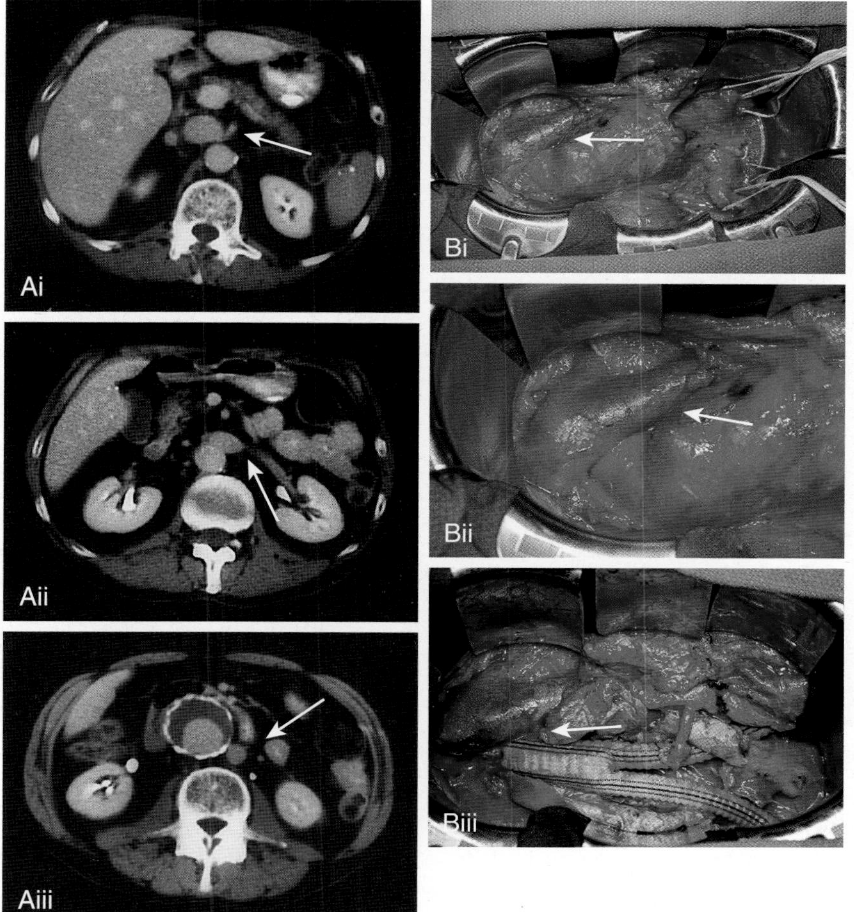

Figure 30-10. Left-sided vena cava. Computed tomography scans **(A)** and intraoperative photographs **(B)** showing a left-sided vena cava *(arrows)*. In this particular patient, the inferior mesenteric artery was reimplanted into the left limb of the bifurcated replacement graft **(Biii).**

Continued

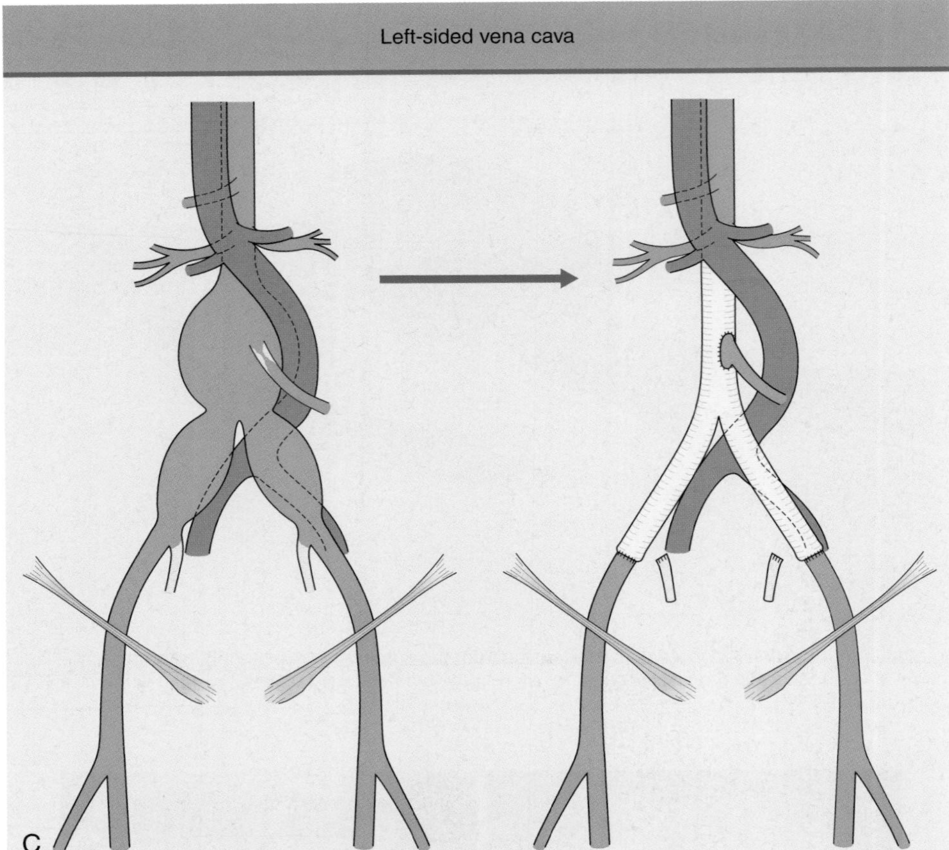

Figure 30-10—cont'd, C, Schematic depiction of a left-sided vena cava.

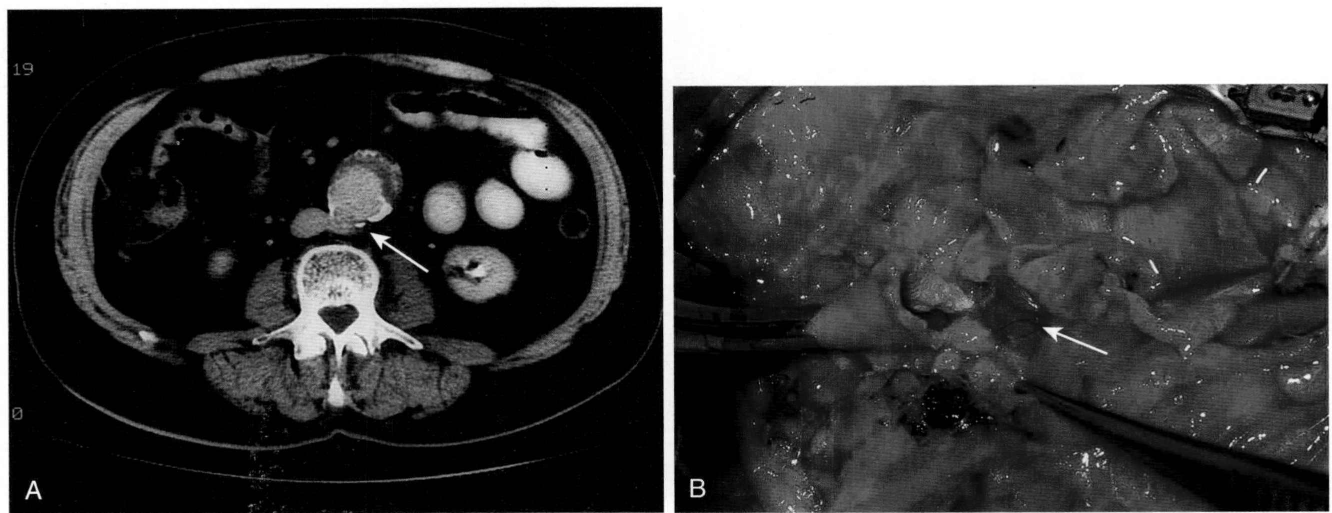

Figure 30-11. Retroaortic left renal vein. **A,** Computed tomography scan demonstrating a retroaortic left renal vein *(arrow)*. **B,** Operative photograph showing the same finding *(arrow)*. Note the absence of a renal vein in its usual position anterior to the aorta.

the aneurysm (Figure 30-12C). Exposure of the neck of the aneurysm can be difficult and time consuming for this reason, especially from an anterior approach. Attempts to dissect the duodenum away from the AAA should be avoided, however, because they can lead to duodenal injury and contamination of the surgical field. Once proximal control has been attained either below or, in some cases, above the renal arteries and the AAA has been opened, the aneurysm sac and the adherent duodenum can be retracted laterally before constructing a conventional replacement graft. The decision then must be

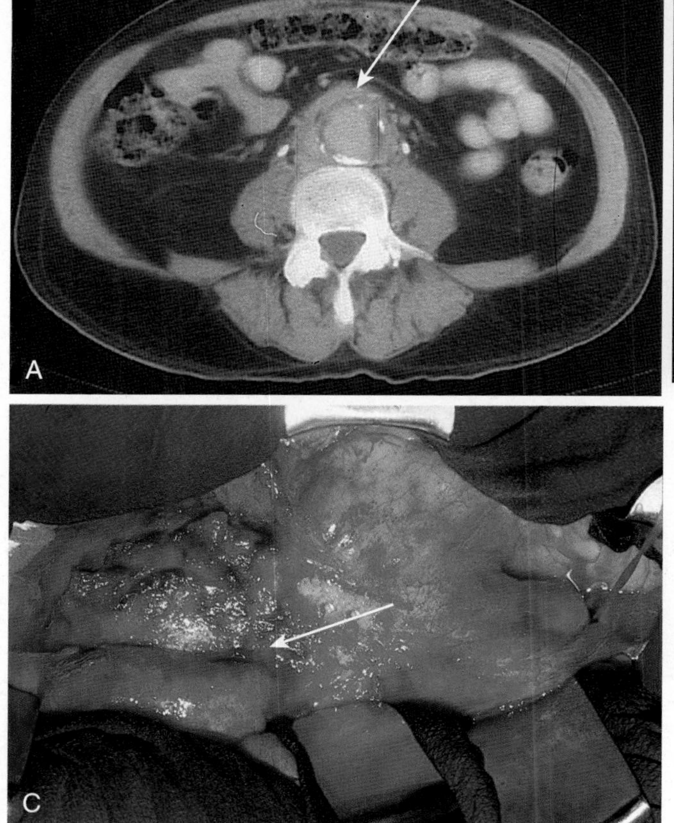

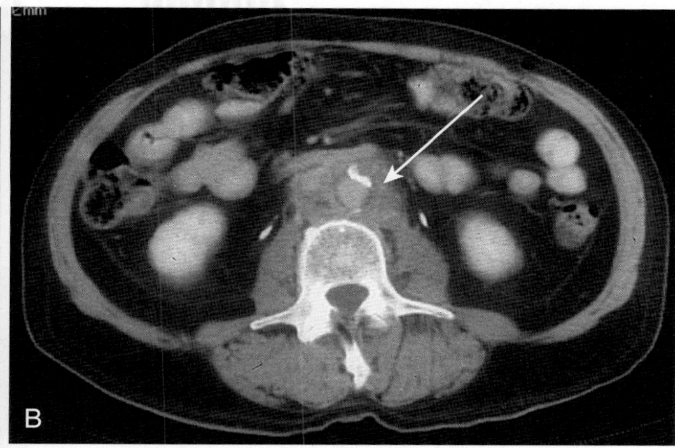

Figure 30-12. Inflammatory aortic aneurysm. **A,** Computed tomography scan showing thick fibrosis *(arrow)* anterior to an inflammatory infrarenal aortic aneurysm. **B,** The fibrotic process *(arrow)* extends as far distally as the origins of the common iliac arteries. **C,** Operative photograph after limited exposure of the proximal neck of an inflammatory aneurysm. Note the closely adherent duodenum *(arrow)* that should not be mobilized.

made with a urologist regarding whether simultaneous ureterolysis also should be done in patients who have ureteral obstruction, since some element of periureteral fibrosis persist in about half of these patients even after their inflammatory AAAs have been repaired.[37]

Complementary Renal Revascularization

Despite the proximity of the renal arteries to the neck of an AAA, a substantial amount of additional dissection is necessary to perform complementary renal revascularization using a bypass graft. On the left side, exposure of the renal artery often requires division of the adrenal vein, the gonadal vein, or both to mobilize the renal vein. On the right side, only a short segment of the renal artery is accessible near the aorta before it passes posterior to the vena cava on its way to the renal hilum. Consequently, the ascending colon often must be mobilized medially to isolate an adequate length of the right renal artery for bypass purposes. It has not been shown whether patency rates are better with synthetic grafts or vein grafts in the unique setting of combined operations, but a synthetic graft is convenient and does tend to resist kinking when used in a retrograde configuration deep in the abdomen (Figure 30-13).

The operative mortality rate for simultaneous aortic reconstruction and renal revascularization exceeds the additive risks of each operation performed alone and is even higher in patients who require bilateral renal artery bypass grafts or when the baseline serum creatinine is 2.0 mg/dl or more.[38-40] Cambria et al.[40] have reported that bilateral renal revascularization can be done with a lower mortality rate using transaortic endarterectomy but concede that it requires more extensive dissection of the visceral aortic segment. Indications for complementary renal revascularization are relatively clear when renal artery disease already is associated with refractory hypertension or deteriorating renal function, but the management of incidental asymptomatic lesions has long been controversial. Williamson et al.[41] and many others have discouraged simultaneous renal revascularization for asymptomatic renal artery stenosis during aortic reconstruction, citing no greater long-term risk for renal insufficiency, dialysis, or death if asymptomatic lesions are left untreated. It seems worth noting that the initial interest in combined operations was generated during an era when, if not done at the time of aortic reconstruction, renal revascularization would require a difficult reoperation if it ever did become necessary. This is not always the case now that percutaneous renal artery stenting is widely available, so aortic surgeons may be willing to adopt a more conservative attitude toward asymptomatic renal artery lesions in the future.

Nonvascular Procedures

Coexistent intraabdominal pathology, such as gallstones or colon cancer, occasionally is discovered preoperatively or even unexpectedly during AAA repair if a transperitoneal approach is employed. According to some estimates, up to 7% of patients with AAAs also have cholelithiasis[42] and 0.5% have colorectal malignancies.[43] The avoidance of a catastrophic

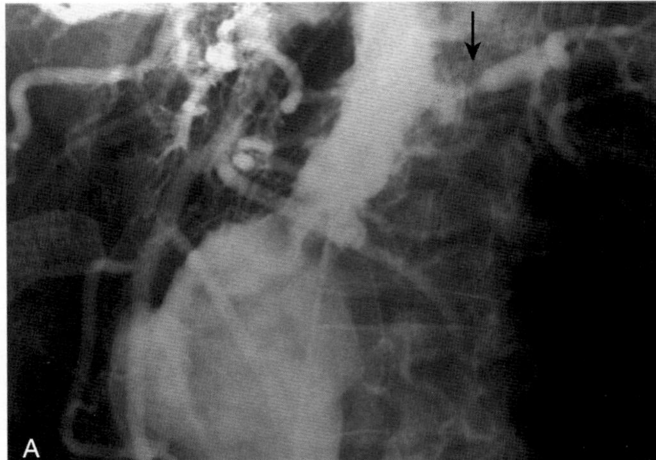

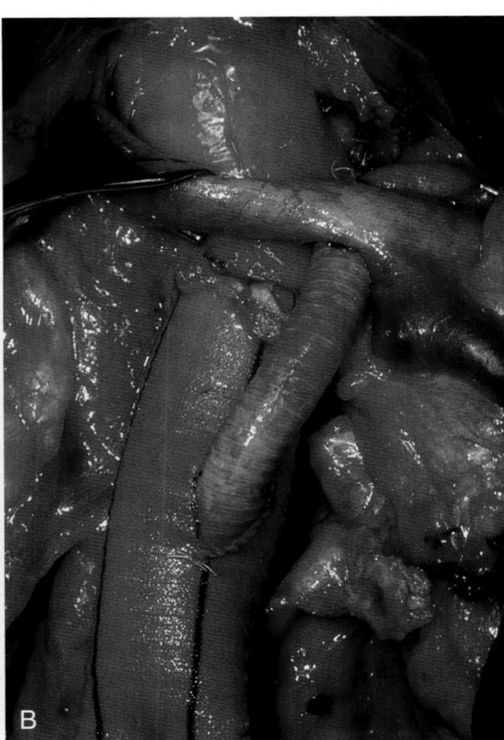

Figure 30-13. Simultaneous renal revascularization. **A,** Preoperative arteriogram showing severe stenosis of the left renal artery *(arrow)* to a solitary kidney in addition to an infrarenal aortic aneurysm. **B,** Operative photograph after aneurysm repair and a synthetic bypass graft to the renal artery.

aortic graft infection is a critical consideration with respect to the management of incidental nonvascular lesions, however, and it seems unwise to perform additional procedures that could pose a risk for such an infection at the same time as AAA repair without a compelling reason. For example, it has been reported that bile is colonized with bacteria in as many as 46% of patients with gallstones.[44] Spillage of contaminated bile at the time of cholecystectomy thus has the potential to inoculate a synthetic graft with bacteria. Although concomitant colon cancer occurs much less often than gallstones, its implications are even more ominous regarding graft contamination, as well as long-term survival. Furthermore, the scant data that are available on this topic suggest that AAA rupture is a leading cause of death in patients who first undergo resection of their colon cancer.[43,45] The conundrum of an AAA and synchronous colon cancer is difficult to resolve with complete confidence,[45] but it seems reasonable (1) to treat each lesion at a separate procedure to minimize the risk of graft infection and (2) to correct the more threatening problem first. Therefore, in the absence of bleeding or obstruction from the colon cancer, AAA repair usually should precede colectomy, especially if the aneurysm is large and certainly if it is symptomatic.

Hostile Abdomen

Patients who have had multiple prior abdominal operations or have a history of previous abdominal adhesions from sepsis or radiotherapy predictably are at greater risk for bowel or ureteral injury if they undergo subsequent AAA repair using a transperitoneal approach. In this setting, the ureters may need to be protected by temporary stents placed cystoscopically in the operating room before the abdominal incision. Alternatively, either retroperitoneal incision shown in Figure 30-3B avoids the hostile intraperitoneal environment yet allows direct AAA repair with its demonstrated durability. Within the universe of open operations, this solution is much preferable to ligation of the aneurysm neck in conjunction with extraanatomical bypass grafting, an option that has been associated with late AAA rupture caused by continued pressurization of the AAA by patent collateral vessels.[46] This is identical to the mechanism for rupture after other "exclusionary" open procedures,[47] as well as for further expansion related to some persistent type II endoleaks following EVAR. Nevertheless, the hostile abdomen unquestionably represents one of the most valuable applications of EVAR in patients who are anatomically suitable for it.

Coronary Artery Disease

Advanced age, coronary artery disease (CAD), and renal insufficiency always have been associated with lower survival rates after open AAA repair,[34,48-50] but unlike old age and poor renal function, CAD is a risk factor that often can be altered. In an attempt to improve survival, preoperative coronary arteriography was performed in 1000 nonrandomized patients who were scheduled for elective peripheral vascular operations at the Cleveland Clinic from 1978 until 1982.[51] Paul et al.[52] later reviewed the data set for this study and determined that 119 (14%) of the 878 patients whose coronary arteriograms had been obtained within 6 months of their vascular surgery had at least 70% stenosis involving the left main coronary artery or all three coronary arteries, either of which still would have satisfied the criteria for coronary artery bypass grafting (CABG)

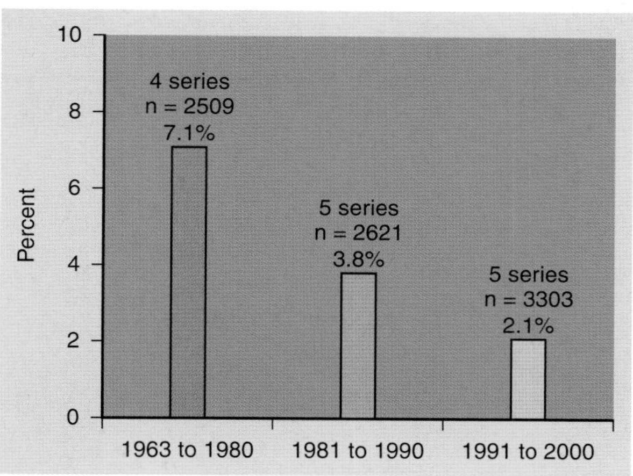

Figure 30-14. Trends in operative mortality. The declining operative mortality rate for open repair of nonruptured infrarenal abdominal aortic aneurysms at certain tertiary referral centers is illustrated by these selected data from three consecutive study periods concluding in 1963 to 1980,[11,48,57,58] 1981 to 1990,[51,59-62] and 1991 to 2000.[24,63-66] (From Hertzer NR. *Ann NY Acad Sci* 2006;1085:175.)

or percutaneous transluminal coronary angioplasty (PTCA) in 1996.

On the basis of their arteriographic findings, preliminary CABG was performed for 28% of the 246 patients who had AAAs in the Cleveland Clinic series. The operative mortality rate was 1.8% for subsequent AAA repair in these patients, and their 5-year survival rate was 75%. In comparison, the 5-year survival rate was only 29% in a small group of 16 patients with severe uncorrected or inoperable CAD.[12] Nuclear myocardial scanning and stress echocardiography eventually replaced arteriography as screening tools for CAD and, because of their value in predicting postoperative cardiac complications or death in patients with myocardial ischemia, have been widely used to evaluate cardiac risk before open AAA procedures. The therapeutic yield of routine noninvasive testing has been relatively low, however, since it generally has led to some kind of prophylactic coronary intervention in fewer than 10% of patients.[53]

The Coronary Artery Revascularization Prophylaxis (CARP) Trial was a randomized Veterans Administration study that was intended to determine whether preliminary CABG or PTCA is associated with improved survival rates after contemporary peripheral vascular operations.[54] It consisted of a total of 510 patients (98% men) who were scheduled for open AAA repair (n = 169, 33%) or lower extremity revascularization and underwent preoperative coronary arteriography because a consultant cardiologist felt they were at risk for a postoperative cardiac complication. This decision was based on clinical factors in many cases, but nuclear stress tests also were done in 316 patients (62%). Of these scans, 20 (6.3%) were interpreted as normal, but 253 (80%) revealed reperfusion ischemia and 43 (14%) demonstrated fixed defects.[53] Patients who had at least 70% stenosis in one or more coronary arteries then were randomized to receive coronary intervention (CABG, n = 99; PTCA, n = 141) plus medical management or medical management alone. Perioperative beta-blockade was administered to 85% of all patients, aspirin to 72%, statin drugs to 53%, and intravenous nitroglycerine to 32%. Coronary intervention had a low mortality rate (CABG 2.0%, PTCA 1.4%), but no significant differences appeared in operative mortality rates for vascular procedures (3.1% versus 3.4%) or in overall late survival rates at a median follow-up interval of 2.7 years (78% versus 77%) between patients who were assigned to intervention and those who were not. The CARP trialists concluded that coronary artery revascularization could not be recommended for patients with stable cardiac symptoms.

The results of the CARP Trial appear to represent yet another example of the benefit of modern medical management with beta-blockade and statin therapy in patients who have peripheral vascular disease.[55] Its conclusions apply specifically to those having stable cardiac symptoms, however, so surgeons still may want to obtain preoperative cardiac imaging, cardiology consultation, or both before open AAA repair in other patients with a recent history of angina pectoris, myocardial infarction, or congestive heart failure.

RESULTS

Operative Mortality

The results of open AAA repair have been collected and analyzed for more than half a century from various sources. These include single-center case series, cooperative multicentered registries, regional (often statewide) audits, the Veterans Administration and large administrative data sets from the Medicare system, the National Hospital Discharge Survey, and the Nationwide Inpatient Sample. Judging by selected case series, the operative mortality rate for open repair of nonruptured AAAs has declined steadily to the point that it has been performed with an early risk of approximately 2% at certain tertiary referral centers during the last 10 to 15 years.[56] This is illustrated in Figure 30-14, using data from De Bakey et al.,[57] Szilagyi et al.,[11] Thompson et al.,[58] and Crawford et al.[49] for study periods before 1980 and subsequently from 10 other experienced centers like the Mayo Clinic,[59] Brigham and Women's Hospital,[60,66] Albany Medical College,[63] and the Cleveland Clinic.[51,61,65] In comparison, Hallin et al.[17] and Drury et al.[7] have reported aggregate operative mortality rates ranging from 3.9% to 5.5% in their collective reviews of the literature. Unfortunately, operative mortality rates probably are unknown at many hospitals and, even when documented, are not likely to be submitted for publication if they are poor. Therefore, information gathered through impartial audits of population-based data sets may reflect the risk of nonruptured AAA repair most accurately.

Several representative examples of this kind of information are given in Table 30-3. Although Cronenwett et al.[76] recently reported an operative mortality rate of 2.9% among participants in the Vascular Study Group of Northern New England, the weighted mean mortality rate was 6.4% for a total of 98,516 open AAA procedures in nine previous statewide audits[67-75] and was 6.3% for 390,908 procedures in the National Hospital Discharge Survey.[80,81] Additional weighted mean mortality rates were 4.6% in Veterans Administration data (n=8021),[77-79] 4.0% in the Nationwide Inpatient Sample (n = 30,337),[82,83] and 4.2% in international studies (n = 8686).[62,84-87] Some results from statewide audits and the National Hospital Discharge Survey are disappointing yet remain vastly superior to the average mortality rate for repair of ruptured AAAs, which,

Table 30-3
Population-Based Mortality Rates for Open Repair of Nonruptured Abdominal Aortic Aneurysms

	Year	Data Source (Study Period)	*n*	Operative Mortality (%)
Regional Audits				
Hannan et al.[67]	1992	New York State (1982-1987)	6042	7.6
Katz et al.[68]	1994	Michigan (1980-1990)	8185	7.5
Manheim et al.[69]	1998	California (1982-1994)	35,130	7.6
Dardik et al.[70]	1999	Maryland (1990-1995)	2335	3.5
Pearce et al.[71]	1999	Florida (1992-1996)	13,415	5.7
Sollano et al.[72]	1999	New York State (1990-1995)	9847	5.5
Anderson et al.[73]	2004	New York State (2000-2002)	3064	4.0
Leon et al.[74]	2005	Illinois (1995-2003)	10,720	6.0
Rigberg et al.[75]	2006	California (1995-1999)	9778	4.0
Cronenwett et al.[76]	2007	Vascular Study Group of Northern New England (2003-2006)	667	2.9
National Datasets				
Kazmers et al.[77]	2001	Veterans Administration (1991-1995)	5833	4.5
Axelrod et al.[78]	2001	Veterans Administration (1997-1998)	1001	3.7
Bush et al.[79]	2006	Veterans Administration (2001-2003)	1187	5.6
Lawrence et al.[80]	1999	National Hospital Discharge Survey (1994)	32,389	8.4
Heller et al.[81]	2000	National Hospital Discharge Survey (1979-1997)	358,521	5.6
Huber et al.[82]	2001	Nationwide Inpatient Sample (1994-1996)	16,450	4.2
Dimick et al.[83]	2002	Nationwide Inpatient Sample (1996-1997)	13,887	3.8
International Studies				
Johnston and Scobie[84]	1988	Canadian Aneurysm Group (1986)	Elective ($n = 541$)	3.9
			Symptomatic ($n = 125$)	7.2
			Total ($n = 666$)	4.5
Wen et al.[85]	1996	Ontario Aneurysm Study (1988-1992)	5492	3.8
Kantonen et al.[86]	1997	Finland Vascular Registry (1992-1996)	929	5.1
Koskas and Kieffer[62]	1997	French Association for Academic Research in Vascular Surgery (1989)	1107	4.8
Bradbury et al.[87]	1998	Edinburgh Vascular Registry (1976-1996)	492	6.1

despite having improved by about 3.5% per decade since the mid-1950s, still was 48% (95% CI 46% to 50%) in 2002.[88]

Volume–Outcome Relationships

Ever since the initial work of Luft et al.[89] nearly 30 years ago, considerable interest has focused on whether the observation that high-volume hospitals or surgeons often have lower mortality rates for certain operations is related to "practice makes perfect" (Do busy providers get good?) or to selective referral patterns (Do good providers get busy?). Whatever the answer to this question—and it may be a little of both—a few examples of the volume–outcome relationships for open AAA repair are given in Table 30-4. Several of these studies found highly significant correlations between high volume and low mortality rates for open repair of nonruptured AAAs, some of which were as important as those that correlated with medical comorbidities.[68,90] The high risk of ruptured AAAs often is determined by hypovolemic shock and multisystem organ failure, but it also was influenced ($p = 0.0026$) by low hospital volume in Michigan[68] and marginally ($p = 0.05$) by low surgeon volume in Maryland.[93] Pearce et al.[71] have calculated that a doubling of surgeon volume was associated with an 11% reduction in the incidence of unfavorable outcomes after AAA repair in Florida, and Young et al.[95] have estimated from their metaanalysis of surgeon caseloads that an annual volume of 13 open AAA cases is necessary to attain a low mortality rate with nonruptured AAAs. Khuri et al.[96] caution against using arbitrary volume thresholds as a surrogate for quality of care, however. They encountered no risk-adjusted volume–outcome relationships for elective open AAA repair or for seven other common operations in the Veterans Administration National Surgical Quality Improvement Program and instead believe that adherence to process measures and prospective outcome assessment is as important for good results as case volume.

Gender and Age

Women have not had higher operative mortality rates than men for open AAA repair at the Cleveland Clinic,[53,61,65] but this is not always the case in large population-based studies. Katz et al.[68] documented mortality rates of 11% in women and 6.8% in men ($p < 0.001$) after all open operations for nonruptured or ruptured AAAs in Michigan throughout the 1980s, and both Huber et al.[82] and Dimick et al.[83] have reported significantly higher mortality rates for women on the basis of Nationwide Inpatient Sample data from the mid-1990s. Working with a 5% Medicare inpatient sample during the decade from 1994 through 2003, Dillavou et al.[97] discovered that the number of surgical procedures for ruptured AAAs declined by 29% in men but only by 12% in women ($p < 0.001$). Furthermore, the mortality rate for all elective interventions (open or EVAR) fell from 5.6% to 3.2% in men but only from 7.5% to 5.5% in women ($p < 0.001$).

Table 30-4
Volume–Outcome Relationships Associated with the Operative Mortality Rate for Open Repair of Abdominal Aortic Aneurysms*

	Year	Data Source (Study Period)	*n*	Operative Mortality (%)		
				Overall	Hospital Volume	Surgeon Volume
Nonruptured Aneurysms						
Hertzer et al.[90]	1984	Northeastern Ohio (1978-1981)	840	6.5	NA	Low: 4.7 Medium: 16 High: 2.9 ($p < 0.001$)
Hannan et al.[67]	1992	New York State (1982-1987)	6042	7.6	Low: 12 Medium: 6.8 High: 5.6 ($p < 0.05$)	Low: 11 Medium: 7.3 High: 5.6 ($p < 0.05$)
Katz et al.[68]	1994	Michigan (1980-1990)	8185	7.5	Low: 8.9 High: 6.2 ($p < 0.001$)	NA
Kazmers et al.[91]	1996	Veterans Administration (1991-1993)	3419	4.9	Low: 6.7 High: 4.2 ($p < 0.05$)	NA
Dardik et al.[70]	1999	Maryland (1990-1995)	2335	3.5	Low: 4.3 Medium: 4.2 High: 2.5 ($p = 0.08$)	Very low: 9.9 Low: 4.9 Medium: 2.8 High: 2.9 Very high: 3.8 ($p = 0.01$)
Birkmeyer et al.[92]	2003	Center for Medicare and Medicaid Services (1998-1999)	NA	NA	Low: 5.4 High: 4.3	Low: 6.2 Medium: 4.6 High: 3.9 ($p < 0.001$)
Dimick et al.[93]	2003	Nationwide Inpatient Sample (1997)	3912	4.2	Low: 5.5 High: 3.0 ($p < 0.001$)	Low: 5.6 High: 2.5 ($p < 0.001$)
Ruptured Aneurysms						
Hertzer et al.[90]	1984	Northeastern Ohio (1978-1981)	213	33	NA	Low: 32 Medium: 39 High: 27 (p = NS)
Katz et al.[68]	1994	Michigan (1980-1990)	1829	50	Low: 54 High: 46 ($p = 0.0026$)	NA
Dardik et al.[94]	1998	Maryland (1990-1995)	527	47	Low: 46 Medium: 49 High: 47 (p = NS)	Low: 51 Medium: 47 High: 36 ($p = 0.05$)

*NA, not available; NS, not significant.

The results from selected case series suggest that the operative mortality rate for open AAA repair is less than 2% in patients who are 65 years of age or younger,[56,64] and Dimick et al.[83] have proved this to be a realistic expectation even in a larger data set of 13,887 patients in the Nationwide Inpatient Sample. They found that the overall mortality rate for open repair of nonruptured AAAs was only 1.8% in patients of this age from 1996 to 1997 and was even lower (1.0%) at high-volume hospitals where 30 or more operations were done annually. Conversely, advanced age and the comorbidities that often accompany it are associated with higher operative mortality rates after open repair in virtually every published series. However, age alone rarely becomes a prohibitive factor, even in octogenarians. A total of 114 octogenarians had open repair of asymptomatic AAAs (mean 6.7 cm) at the Cleveland Clinic from 1984 through 1993.[98] The overall mortality rate was 9.6% in this series, but only two deaths (3.8%) occurred among the 53 asymptomatic patients who had their operations during the second 5 years of the study period. During the same 5 years, the comparable mortality rate was 31% in a small group of 13 patients who had ruptured and/or symptomatic AAAs. Ballotta et al.[99] subsequently reported a series of 111 octogenarians who underwent open AAA repair from 1992 through 2005 with an operative mortality rate of just 1.8% and remarkable survival rates of 67% at 5 years and 59% at 10 years. The 5-year survival rate was only 48% for a total of 97 operative survivors in the Cleveland Clinic series, but it was significantly better (80% versus 38%, $p = 0.0077$) for the 27 patients who had a history of previous myocardial revascularization than for the other 70 patients who did not (Figure 30-15).

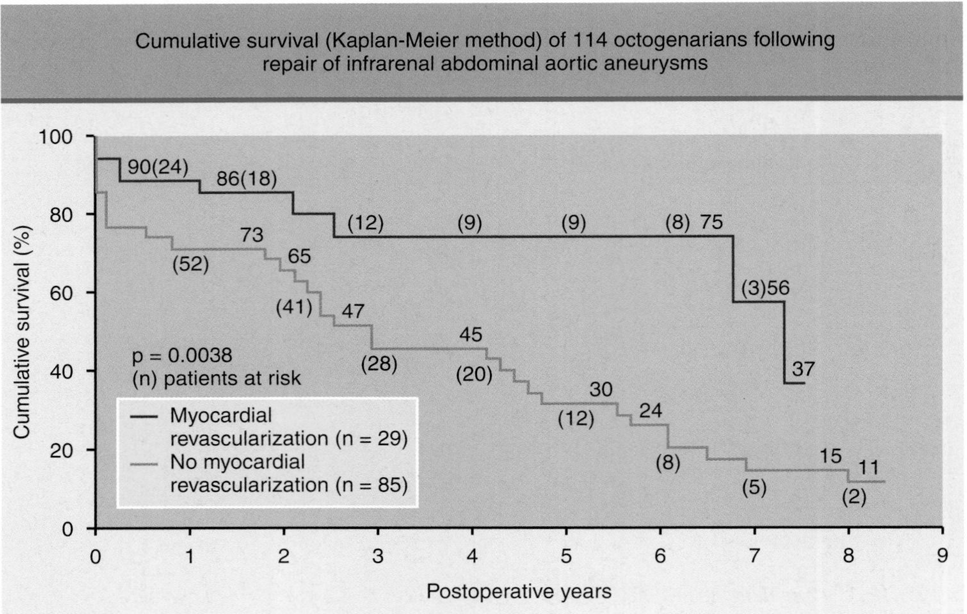

Figure 30-15. Survival in octogenarians. Kaplan-Meier estimates of survival following open infrarenal aortic aneurysm repair in 114 consecutive octogenarians. Late survival rates were significantly better ($p = 0.0038$) for patients who had previous myocardial revascularization. (From O'Hara PJ, Hertzer NR, Krajewski LP, et al. *J Vasc Surg* 1995;21:830.)

Late Survival

De Bakey et al.[57] were among the first to express late survival using life-table methods during a pioneering experience with open AAA repair more than 40 years ago. Their cumulative 5-year and 10-year survival rates of 67% and 43%, respectively, have been improved only slightly in the modern era. The representative 5-year and 10-year survival rates reported from the Cleveland Clinic[65] in 2002 (75% and 49%) and from the Massachusetts General Hospital[4] in 2007 (71% and 44%) are not too dissimilar from those described by De Bakey and his associates in 1964. Fifteen-year survival ranges from 16% to 18% in the few series for which this length of follow-up is available.[3,49,53] The survival rate for patients who had ruptured AAAs (22%) was substantially worse than the survival rate for patients with nonruptured AAAs (60%) 6 years after open repair in the Canadian Aneurysm Study,[50,100] and Kazmers et al.[77] found that patients who were discharged alive from a Veterans Administration hospital and lived 30 days or more after open repair of ruptured AAAs still had a higher 2-year mortality rate (odds ratio 1.74, 95% CI 1.3 to 2.3, $p < 0.001$) than patients who were discharged alive and lived 30 days or more after open repair of nonruptured AAAs. Observations such as these conceivably could be explained by the presence of serious medical comorbidities that either contributed directly to AAA rupture (e.g., hypertension or COPD) or discouraged elective repair long enough for rupture finally to occur.

Older age ($p < 0.001$), impaired renal function ($p < 0.001$), COPD ($p = 0.012$), and large aneurysm diameter ($p = 0.036$) were the only patient-related risk factors that significantly influenced the late survival rate in the experience of one of the authors (Hertzer) with open AAA repair in 855 consecutive asymptomatic patients during nearly 30 years at the Cleveland Clinic.[53] This may be related to a history of previous coronary intervention in 335 (39%) of these patients, including 100 (15%) who received preliminary CABG ($n = 78$) or PTCA ($n = 22$) in preparation for their AAA procedures. The risk for any postoperative or late death was lower in patients who had preliminary CABG or PTCA (hazard ratio 0.76, 95% CI 0.59 to 0.98, $p = 0.035$) even when a separate multivariable model was fit to accommodate nine other patients who also had preliminary CABG or PTCA but developed symptomatic AAAs before open repair could be done (hazard ratio 0.78, 95% CI 0.61 to 0.99, $p = 0.044$). Overall, late survival rates were 70% at 5 years, 36% at 10 years, and 16% at 15 years. As illustrated in Figure 30-16, late survival rates for patients who were 65 years of age or younger at the time of their operations (77% at 5 years, 52% at 10 years, and 29% at 15 years) were significantly better than for those in older age groups ($p < 0.001$).

Late Complications

Graft Complications

Perhaps the greatest advantage of open AAA repair is its durability. The risk for graft-related complications or secondary graft intervention after open AAA repair is sufficiently low that it attracted little attention in the literature before the introduction of EVAR. In a report often cited elsewhere, Hallett et al.[2] retrospectively reviewed 307 patients who underwent open repair from 1957 to 1990 at the Mayo Clinic or in the surrounding community of Olmsted County. Of these patients, 140 underwent follow-up imaging of their aortic grafts with ultrasound or CT scans. Late graft complications eventually were recognized in 21 (6.8%) of the 307 patients at a mean of 5.8 years, with a cumulative 10-year incidence of 3% for graft thrombosis, 4% for anastomotic pseudoaneurysm, and 5% for graft-enteric erosion, graft infection, or both.

Biancari et al.[3] encountered a slightly higher incidence of graft complications (15%) at a median follow-up 8 years after

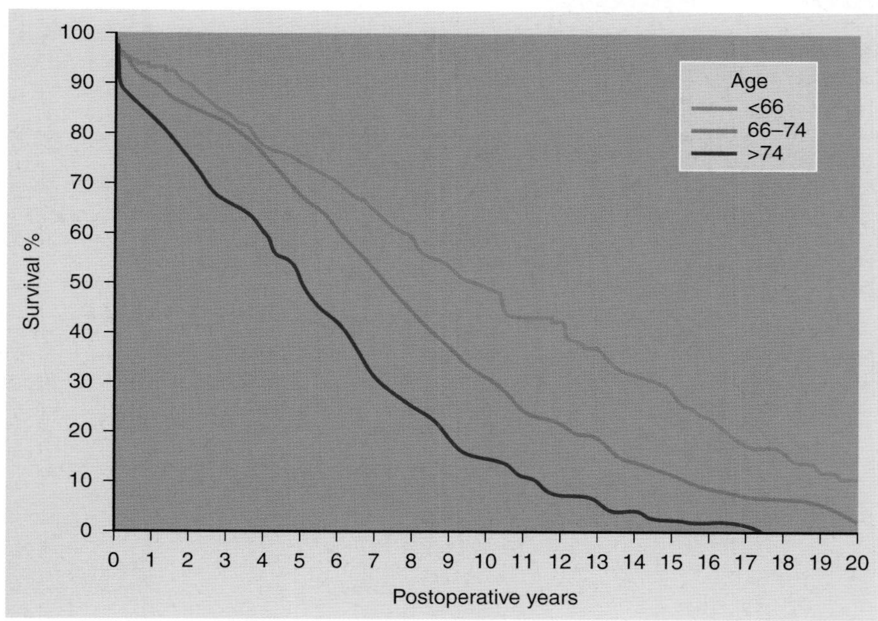

Figure 30-16. Age-related survival rates. Kaplan-Meier estimates of survival following elective open repair of asymptomatic infrarenal aortic aneurysms according to patient age (65 years or younger, $n = 272$; 66 to 74 years, $n = 375$; 75 years or older, $n = 208$). Differences were statistically significant at $p < 0.001$. (From Hertzer NR, Mascha EJ. *J Vasc Surg* 2005;42:898.)

open AAA repair in 208 patients, including graft limb occlusions in 5.3%, proximal anastomotic pseudoaneurysms in 2.9%, and distal anastomotic pseudoaneurysms in 8.7%. However, aortofemoral grafts were used for an unusually large number of the treated limbs in this series (203 of 414, or 49%) and accounted for 17 of the 18 late distal pseudoaneurysms. Conrad et al.[4] employed aortofemoral grafts in only 12% of their series of 540 open AAA repairs at the Massachusetts General Hospital, 152 of which were kept under postoperative surveillance by CT scanning. Only 13 graft complications occurred in 11 patients (2.0%) at a mean follow-up period of 87 months, comprising four graft limb occlusions, seven pseudoaneurysms (four proximal, three distal), and two graft infections. New arterial aneurysms were discovered in 68 (45%) of the 152 patients who received surveillance imaging, most of which involved the iliac arteries and required no treatment because they were less than 2.5 cm in diameter. Of the 152 patients, 15 (10%) had new aneurysms exceeding 5.5 cm in diameter in either the visceral aortic segment ($n = 6$) or the thoracic aorta ($n = 9$), and 7 of these eventually were repaired.

Experience at the Cleveland Clinic has been similar. Aortofemoral grafts have been used during AAA repair in fewer than 10% of cases, and the incidence of recognized graft complications has remained low despite relatively routine postoperative surveillance with CT scans at 1 year and every 3 to 5 years thereafter during the past decade.[53,65] According to unpublished data from the personal series of one of the authors,[53] only 12 (1.4%) of the 855 patients who had open repair of asymptomatic AAAs are known to have had late graft complications, represented by anastomotic pseudoaneurysms in 6 and graft limb occlusions, aortoenteric fistulas, or infection each in 2 patients. Proximal aortic aneurysms have been discovered in 51 patients (6.0%). In addition, 5 patients developed iliac aneurysms measuring at least 3.0 cm in diameter, and 6 others sustained aortic dissections unrelated to aneurysms. Reoperations for graft complications ($n = 10$), proximal aortic aneurysms ($n = 18$), or dissections ($n = 2$) have been performed in a total of 30 patients (3.5%).

Other Complications

Graft-related complications are not the only unfavorable late events that can occur after open AAA repair, especially when performed using a transperitoneal approach. Like any intraabdominal operation, open repair also is associated with a low but measurable risk for incisional hernias and adhesive intestinal obstruction. In a propensity analysis of 45,660 Medicare beneficiaries who underwent either open repair or EVAR from 2001 through 2004, Schermerhorn et al.[101] found that the incidence of laparotomy-related complications requiring intervention within 4 years was significantly higher after open repair (9.7% versus 4.1%, $p < 0.001$). This included the repair of abdominal wall hernias (5.8% versus 1.1%, $p < 0.001$), lysis of adhesions (1.5% versus 0.5%, $p < 0.001$), and to a lesser extent, small- or large-bowel resection (3.4% versus 3.0%, $p = 0.02$). The hospitalization rate also was higher after open repair (14.0% versus 8.1%, $p < 0.001$) for laparotomy-related complications that did not need lysis or bowel resection and presumably were related to conservative management of partial intestinal obstruction.

Comparative Trials

Endovascular AAA repair is the topic of the previous chapter, but the results of two randomized clinical trials also are presented here because they reflect the results of open AAA repair as much as those of EVAR. These are EVAR Trial 1, a study in which a total of 1082 patients who had asymptomatic AAAs and were deemed fit for either form of treatment were randomized to open repair or EVAR at 34 centers in the United Kingdom,[102,103] and the smaller Dutch Randomized Endovascular Aneurysm Management (DREAM) Trial, in which 351 similar patients were randomized to open repair or EVAR at 28 centers in the Netherlands and Belgium.[104,105] Table 30-5 summarizes a few of the disclosures that presently are available from these investigations concerning operative mortality and patient survival during 2 to 4 years of

Table 30-5
Survival Outcomes in Endovascular Aneurysm Repair (EVAR) Trial 1[102,103] and the Dutch Randomized Endovascular Aneurysm Management (DREAM) Trial[104,105] Comparing Open Repair versus EVAR for Nonruptured Abdominal Aortic Aneurysms

	EVAR Trial 1		DREAM Trial	
	Open	**EVAR**	**Open**	**EVAR**
Randomized patients	539	543	178	173
Men	489	494	161	161
Women	50	49	17	12
Mean age (years ± SD)*	74.0 ± 6.1	74.2 ± 6.0	69.6 ± 6.8	70.7 ± 6.6
Mean aneurysm diameter (cm ± SD)*	6.5 ± 1.0	6.5 ± 0.9	6.0 ± 0.8	6.1 ± 0.9
Operative Mortality Rates Based on Treatment Actually Received				
30-day	4.7% (24/516)	1.7% (9/531) $p = 0.009$	4.6%† (8/174)	1.2%† (2/171) $p = 0.10$
In-hospital	6.2% (32/516)	2.1% (11/531) $p = 0.001$		
Follow-up interval	2.9 years (median)	2.9 years (median)	21 months (mean)	22 months (mean)
All-Cause Mortality Rates				
Crude	20% (109/539)	18% (100/543) $p = 0.46$	10% (18/178)	12%‡ (20/173)
Cumulative (Kaplan-Meier)	29% (4 years)	26% (4 years) $p > 0.20$	11% (2 years)	11% (2 years) $p = 0.86$
Aneurysm-Related Mortality Rates				
Crude	6.3% (34/539)	3.5% (19/543) $p = 0.04$	4.5% (8/178)	1.2%‡ (2/173)
Cumulative (Kaplan-Meier)	7% (4 years)	4% (4 years) $p > 0.20$	5.7% (2 years)	2.1% (2 years) $p = 0.05$

*SD, standard deviation.
†Deaths within 30 days or during the same hospital admission, whichever was longer.
‡Level of statistical significance not available in the original report.

follow-up.[56] Although EVAR had a lower operative mortality rate than open repair in each study, this difference was statistically significant only in the larger EVAR Trial 1 and has not been associated with improvement in intermediate-term survival in either trial. All-cause mortality rates are similar for EVAR and for open repair in both trials, and a marginal difference in aneurysm-related mortality at 2 years in the DREAM Trial has been interpreted by the trialists simply to reflect the lower operative mortality rate of EVAR.

Open repair was associated with significantly longer operative time, greater blood loss, and more transfusions compared to EVAR ($p < 0.001$),[104] but it also was significantly less likely to require reintervention during the original hospital admission (5.8% versus 9.8%, $p = 0.02$).[102] The cumulative incidence of graft-related complications (9% versus 41%, $p < 0.0001$) and secondary interventions (6% versus 20%, $p < 0.0001$) was significantly lower for open repair than for EVAR at 4 years of follow-up in EVAR Trial 1. Although the immediate quality of life was worse after open repair, this disadvantage lasted only for 3 months.[103] Finally, the principal investigators for both the EVAR Trial 1 and the DREAM Trial have calculated that open AAA repair costs significantly less than EVAR and provides as many if not more quality-adjusted life years.[106,107]

SUMMARY

Open repair is an exceptionally versatile and durable approach that can be tailored to a variety of circumstances in the management of infrarenal AAAs. Even in an era of rapidly evolving technology for catheter-based intervention, open repair still appears to be the treatment of choice for patients who are 65 years of age or younger because of their low operative risk and their comparatively long life expectancy. More than a half century since it first was described, open AAA repair remains a signature procedure in the field of vascular surgery.

References

1. Dubost C, Allary M, Oeconomos N. Resection of an aneurysm of the abdominal aorta: reestablishment of the continuity by a preserved human arterial graft, with result after five months. *Arch Surg* 1952;64:405.
2. Hallett Jr JW, Marshall DM, Petterson TM, et al. Graft-related complications after abdominal aortic aneurysm repair: reassurance from a 36-year population-based experience. *J Vasc Surg* 1997;25:277.
3. Biancari F, Ylönen K, Anttila V, et al. Durability of open repair of infrarenal abdominal aortic aneurysm: a 15-year follow-up study. *J Vasc Surg* 2002;35:87.
4. Conrad MF, Crawford RS, Pedraza JD, et al. Long-term durability of open abdominal aortic aneurysm repair. *J Vasc Surg* 2007;46:669.
5. Parodi JC, Palmaz JC, Barone HD. Transfemoral intraluminal graft implantation for abdominal aortic aneurysms. *Ann Vasc Surg* 1991;5:491.

6. Katzen BT, Dake MD, MacLean AA, et al. Endovascular repair of abdominal and thoracic aortic aneurysms. *Circulation* 2005;112:1663.
7. Drury D, Michaels JA, Ayiku L. Systematic review of recent evidence for the safety and efficacy of elective endovascular repair in the management of infrarenal abdominal aortic aneurysms. *Br J Surg* 2005;92:937.
8. Mastracci TM, Garrido-Olivares L, Cinà CS, et al. Endovascular repair of ruptured abdominal aortic aneurysms: a systematic review and meta-analysis. *J Vasc Surg* 2008;47:214.
9. Heikkinen MA, Arko FR, Zarins CK. What is the significance of endoleaks and endotension. *Surg Clin North Am* 2004;84:1337.
10. Brewster DC, Cronenwett JL, Hallett Jr JW, et al. Guidelines for the treatment of abdominal aortic aneurysms: report of a subcommittee of the Joint Council of the American Association for Vascular Surgery and Society for Vascular Surgery. *J Vasc Surg* 2003;37:1106.
11. Szilagyi DE, Smith RF, DeRusso FJ, et al. Contribution of abdominal aortic aneurysmectomy to prolongation of life. *Ann Surg* 1966;164:678.
12. Hertzer NR, Young JR, Beven EG, et al. Late results of coronary bypass in patients with infrarenal aortic aneurysms: the Cleveland Clinic Study. *Ann Surg* 1987;205:360.
13. Nevitt MP, Ballard DJ, Hallett Jr JW. Prognosis of abdominal aortic aneurysms: a population-based study. *N Engl J Med* 1989;321:1009.
14. Conway KP, Byrne J, Townsend M, et al. Prognosis of patients turned down for conventional abdominal aortic aneurysm repair in the endovascular and sonographic era: Szilagyi revisited? *J Vasc Surg* 2001;33:752.
15. Taylor Jr LM, Porter JM. Basic data related to clinical decision making in abdominal aortic aneurysms. *Ann Vasc Surg* 1987;1:502.
16. Hollier LH, Taylor LM, Ochsner J. Recommended indications for operative treatment of abdominal aortic aneurysms: report of a subcommittee of the Joint Council of the Society for Vascular Surgery and the North American Chapter of the International Society for Cardiovascular Surgery. *J Vasc Surg* 1992;15:1046.
17. Hallin A, Bergqvist D, Holmberg L. Literature review of surgical management of abdominal aortic aneurysm. *Eur J Vasc Endovasc Surg* 2001;22:197.
18. U.K. Small Aneurysm Trial Participants. Mortality results for randomised controlled trial of early elective surgery or ultrasonographic surveillance for small abdominal aortic aneurysms. *Lancet* 1998;352:1649.
19. U.K. Small Aneurysm Trial Participants. Long-term outcomes of immediate repair compared with surveillance of small abdominal aortic aneurysms. *N Engl J Med* 2002;346:1445.
20. U.K. Small Aneurysm Trial Participants. Final 12-year follow-up of surgery versus surveillance in the U.K. Small Aneurysm Trial. *Br J Surg* 2007;94:702.
21. Lederle FA, Wilson SE, Johnson GR, et al. Immediate repair compared with surveillance of small abdominal aortic aneurysms. *N Engl J Med* 2002;346:1437.
22. Takagi H, Sekino S, Kato T, et al. Intraoperative autotransfusion in abdominal aortic aneurysm surgery: meta-analysis of randomized controlled trials. *Arch Surg* 2007;142:1098.
23. O'Hara PJ, Hertzer NR, Krajewski LP, et al. Reduction in the homologous blood requirement for abdominal aortic aneurysm repair by the use of preadmission autologous blood donation. *Surgery* 1994;115:69.
24. Sicard GA, Reilly JM, Rubin BG, et al. Transabdominal versus retroperitoneal incision for abdominal aortic surgery: report of a prospective randomized trial. *J Vasc Surg* 1995;21:174.
25. Cambria RP, Brewster DC, Abbott WM, et al. Transperitoneal versus retroperitoneal approach for aortic reconstruction: a randomized prospective study. *J Vasc Surg* 1990;11:314.
26. O'Hara PJ. Aortoiliac revascularization. In: Montague DK, ed. *Disorders of male sexual function*. Chicago: Year Book Medical Publishers; 1987.
27. Hertzer NR. Teflon reinforcement of an uninterrupted aortic anastomosis. *Surg Gynecol Obstet* 1983;157:480.
28. Rasmussen TR, Hallett Jr JW, Noel AA, et al. Early abdominal closure with mesh reduces multiple organ failure after ruptured abdominal aortic aneurysm repair: guidelines from a 10-year case-control study. *J Vasc Surg* 2002;35:246.
29. Hallett Jr JW. Management of aneurysms. In: Strandness JE, van Breda A, eds. Vascular diseases. New York: Churchill Livingstone; 1994.
30. Crawford ES, Coselli JS, Safi HJ, et al. The impact of renal fusion and ectopia on aortic surgery. *J Vasc Surg* 1988;8:375-383.
31. Hollis Jr HW, Rutherford RB, Crawford GJ, et al. Abdominal aortic aneurysm repair in patients with pelvic kidney: technical considerations and literature review. *J Vasc Surg* 1989;9:404.
32. O'Hara PJ, Hakaim AG, Hertzer NR, et al. Surgical management of aortic aneurysm and coexistent horseshoe kidney: review of a 31-year experience. *J Vasc Surg* 1993;17:940.
33. Aljabri B, MacDonald PS, Satin R, et al. Incidence of major venous and renal anomalies relevant to aortoiliac surgery as demonstrated by computed tomography. *Ann Vasc Surg* 2001;15:615.
34. Johnston KW. Multicenter prospective study of nonruptured abdominal aortic aneurysm. II. Variables predicting morbidity and mortality. *J Vasc Surg* 1989;9:437.
35. West CA, Noel AA, Bower TC, et al. Factors affecting outcomes of open surgical repair of pararenal aortic aneurysms: a 10-year experience. *J Vasc Surg* 2006;43:921.
36. Tang T, Boyle JR, Dixon AK, et al. Inflammatory abdominal aortic aneurysms. *Eur J Vasc Endovasc Surg* 2005;29:353.
37. Nitecki SS, Hallett Jr JW, Stanson AW, et al. Inflammatory abdominal aortic aneurysms: a case-control study. *J Vasc Surg* 1996;23:860.
38. Tarazi RY, Hertzer NR, Beven EG, et al. Simultaneous aortic reconstruction and renal revascularization: risk factors and late results in eighty-nine patients. *J Vasc Surg* 1987;5:707.
39. Tsoukas AI, Hertzer NR, Mascha EJ, et al. Simultaneous aortic replacement and renal artery revascularization: the influence of preoperative renal function on early risk and late outcome. *J Vasc Surg* 2001;34:1041.
40. Cambria RP, Brewster DC, L'Italien GL, et al. Simultaneous aortic and renal artery reconstruction: evolution of an eighteen-year experience. *J Vasc Surg* 1995;21:916.
41. Williamson WK, Abou-Zamzam Jr AM, Moneta GL, et al. Prophylactic repair of renal artery stenosis is not justified in patients who require infrarenal aortic reconstruction. *J Vasc Surg* 1998;28:14.
42. Thomas JH. Abdominal aortic aneurysmorrhaphy combined with biliary or gastrointestinal surgery. *Surg Clin North Am* 1989;69:807.
43. Nora JD, Pairolero PC, Nivatvongs S, et al. Concomitant abdominal aortic aneurysm and colorectal carcinoma: priority of resection. *J Vasc Surg* 1989;9:630.
44. Csendes A, Burdiles P, Maluenda F, et al. Simultaneous bacteriologic assessment of bile from gallbladder and common bile duct in control subjects and patients with gallstones and common duct stones. *Arch Surg* 1996;131:389.
45. Morris HL, da Silva AF. Co-existing abdominal aortic aneurysm and intra-abdominal malignancy: reflections on the order of treatment. *Br J Surg* 1998;85:1185.
46. Pevec WC, Holcroft JW, Blaisdell FW. Ligation and extraanatomic arterial reconstruction for the treatment of aneurysms of the abdominal aorta. *J Vasc Surg* 1994;20:629.
47. Darling III RC Ozsvath K, Chang BB, et al. The incidence, natural history, and outcome of secondary intervention for persistent collateral flow in the excluded abdominal aortic aneurysm. *J Vasc Surg* 1999;30:968.
48. Hertzer NR. Fatal myocardial infarction following abdominal aortic aneurysm resection: three hundred forty-three patients followed 6-11 years postoperatively. *Ann Surg* 1980;192:667.
49. Crawford ES, Saleh SA, Babb III JW, et al. Infrarenal abdominal aortic aneurysm: factors influencing survival after operation performed over a 25-year period. *Ann Surg* 1981;193:699.
50. Johnston KW. Nonruptured abdominal aortic aneurysm: six-year follow-up results from the multicenter prospective Canadian Aneurysm Study. *J Vasc Surg* 1994;20:163.
51. Hertzer NR, Beven EG, Young JR, et al. Coronary artery disease in peripheral vascular patients: a classification of 1000 coronary angiograms and results of surgical management. *Ann Surg* 1984;199:223.
52. Paul SD, Eagle KA, Kuntz KM, et al. Concordance of preoperative clinical risk with angiographic severity of coronary artery disease in patients undergoing vascular surgery. *Circulation* 1996;94:1561.
53. Hertzer NR, Mascha EJ. A personal experience with factors influencing survival after elective open repair of infrarenal aortic aneurysms. *J Vasc Surg* 2005;42:898.
54. McFalls EO, Ward HB, Moritz TE, et al. Coronary-artery revascularization before elective major vascular surgery. *N Engl J Med* 2004;351:2795.
55. Hirsch AT, Haskal ZJ, Hertzer NR, et al. ACC/AHA guidelines for the management of patients with peripheral arterial disease (lower extremity, renal, mesenteric, and abdominal aortic): a collaborative report from the American Association for Vascular Surgery/Society for Vascular Surgery, Society for Cardiovascular Angiography and Interventions, Society for Vascular Medicine and Biology, Society of Interventional Radiology, and the ACC/AHA Task Force on Practice Guidelines. *Circulation* 2006;113:1474 and *J Am Coll Cardiol* 2006;47:1239. (Joint publication.)
56. Hertzer NR. Current status of endovascular repair of infrarenal abdominal aortic aneurysms in the context of 50 years of conventional repair. *Ann NY Acad Sci* 2006;1085:175.
57. De Bakey ME, Crawford ES, Cooley DA, et al. Aneurysm of abdominal aorta: analysis of results of graft replacement therapy one to eleven years after operation. *Ann Surg* 1964;160:622.

58. Thompson JE, Hollier LH, Patman RD, et al. Surgical management of abdominal aortic aneurysms: factors influencing mortality and morbidity: a 20-year experience. *Ann Surg* 1975;181:654.
59. Riegel MM, Hollier LH, Kazmier FJ, et al. Late survival in abdominal aortic aneurysm patients: the role of selective myocardial revascularization on the basis of clinical symptoms. *J Vasc Surg* 1987;5:222.
60. Golden MA, Whittemore AD, Donaldson MC, et al. Selective evaluation and management of coronary artery disease in patients undergoing repair of abdominal aortic aneurysms: a 16-year experience. *Ann Surg* 1990;212:415.
61. Starr JE, Hertzer NR, Mascha EJ, et al. Influence of gender on cardiac risk and survival in patients with infrarenal aortic aneurysms. *J Vasc Surg* 1996;23:870.
62. Koskas F, Kieffer E. Long-term survival after elective repair of infrarenal abdominal aortic aneurysm: results of a prospective multicenter study, Association for Academic Research in Vascular Surgery (AURC). *Ann Vasc Surg* 1997;11:473.
63. Lloyd WE, Paty PS, Darling III RC, et al. Results of 1000 consecutive elective abdominal aortic aneurysm repairs. *Cardiovasc Surg* 1996;4:724.
64. Aune S. Risk factors and operative results of patients aged less than 66 years operated on for asymptomatic abdominal aortic aneurysm. *Eur J Vasc Endovasc Surg* 2001;22:240.
65. Hertzer NR, Mascha EJ, Karafa MT, et al. Open infrarenal abdominal aortic aneurysm repair: the Cleveland Clinic experience from 1989 to 1998. *J Vasc Surg* 2002;35:1145.
66. Menard MT, Chew DKW, Chan RK, et al. Outcome in patients at high risk after open surgical repair of abdominal aortic aneurysm. *J Vasc Surg* 2003;37:285.
67. Hannan EL, Kilburn Jr H, O'Donnell JF, et al. A longitudinal analysis of the relationship between in-hospital mortality in New York State and the volume of abdominal aortic aneurysm surgeries performed. *Health Serv Res* 1992;27:517.
68. Katz DJ, Stanley JC, Zelenock GB. Operative mortality rates for intact and ruptured abdominal aortic aneurysms in Michigan: an eleven-year statewide experience. *J Vasc Surg* 1994;19:804.
69. Manheim LM, Sohn MW, Feinglass J, et al. Hospital vascular surgery volume and procedure mortality rates in California, 1982-1994. *J Vasc Surg* 1998;28:45.
70. Dardik A, Lin JW, Gordon TA, et al. Results of elective abdominal aortic aneurysm repair in the 1990s: a population-based analysis of 2335 cases. *J Vasc Surg* 1999;30:985.
71. Pearce WH, Parker MA, Feinglass J, et al. The importance of surgeon volume and training in outcomes for vascular surgical procedures. *J Vasc Surg* 1999;29:768.
72. Sollano JA, Gelijns AC, Moskowitz AJ, et al. Volume–outcome relationships in cardiovascular operations: New York State, 1990-1995. *J Thorac Cardiovasc Surg* 1999;117:419.
73. Anderson PL, Arons RR, Moskowitz AJ, et al. A statewide experience with endovascular abdominal aortic aneurysm repair: rapid diffusion with excellent early results. *J Vasc Surg* 2004;39:10.
74. Leon Jr LR, Labropoulos N, Laredo J, et al. To what extent has endovascular aneurysm repair influenced abdominal aortic aneurysm management in the state of Illinois? *J Vasc Surg* 2005;41:568.
75. Rigberg DA, Zingmond DS, McGory ML, et al. Age stratified, perioperative, and one-year mortality after abdominal aortic aneurysm repair: a statewide experience. *J Vasc Surg* 2006;43:224.
76. Cronenwett JL, Likosky DS, Russell MT, et al. A regional registry for quality assurance and improvement: the Vascular Study Group of Northern New England (VSGNNE). *J Vasc Surg* 2007;46:1093.
77. Kazmers A, Perkins AJ, Jacobs LA. Aneurysm rupture is independently associated with increased late mortality in those surviving abdominal aortic aneurysm repair. *J Surg Res* 2001;95:50.
78. Axelrod DA, Henke PK, Wakefield TW, et al. Impact of chronic obstructive pulmonary disease on elective and emergency abdominal aortic aneurysm repair. *J Vasc Surg* 2001;33:72.
79. Bush RL, Johnson ML, Collins TC, et al. Open versus endovascular abdominal aortic aneurysm repair in VA hospitals. *J Am Coll Surg* 2006;202:577.
80. Lawrence PF, Gazak C, Bhirangi L, et al. The epidemiology of surgically repaired aneurysms in the United States. *J Vasc Surg* 1999;30:632.
81. Heller JA, Weinberg A, Arons R, et al. Two decades of abdominal aortic aneurysm repair: have we made any progress? *J Vasc Surg* 2000;32:1091.
82. Huber TS, Wang JG, Derrow AE, et al. Experience in the United States with intact abdominal aortic aneurysm repair. *J Vasc Surg* 2001;33:304.
83. Dimick JB, Stanley JC, Axelrod DA, et al. Variation in death rate after abdominal aortic aneurysmectomy in the United States: impact of hospital volume, gender, and age. *Ann Surg* 2002;235:579.
84. Johnston KW, Scobie TK. Multicenter prospective study of nonruptured abdominal aortic aneurysms. I. Population and operative management. *J Vasc Surg* 1988;7:69.
85. Wen SW, Simunovic M, Williams JI, et al. Hospital volume, calendar age, and short term outcomes in patients undergoing repair of abdominal aortic aneurysms: the Ontario experience, 1988-92. *J Epidemiol Community Health* 1996;50:207.
86. Kantonen I, Lepantalo M, Salenius JP, et al. Mortality in abdominal aortic aneurysm surgery: the effect of hospital volume, patient mix and surgeon's case load. *Eur J Vasc Endovasc Surg* 1997;14:375.
87. Bradbury AW, Adam DJ, Makhdoomi KR, et al. A 21-year experience of abdominal aortic aneurysm operations in Edinburgh. *Br J Surg* 1998;85:645.
88. Bown MJ, Sutton AJ, Bell PRF, et al. A meta-analysis of 50 years of ruptured abdominal aortic aneurysm repair. *Br J Surg* 2002;89:714.
89. Luft HS, Bunker JP, Enthoven AC. Should operations be regionalized? The empirical relation between surgical volume and mortality. *N Engl J Med* 1979;301:1364.
90. Hertzer NR, Avellone JC, Farrell CJ, et al. The risk of vascular surgery in a metropolitan community: with observations on surgeon experience and hospital size. *J Vasc Surg* 1984;1:13.
91. Kazmers A, Jacobs L, Perkins A, et al. Abdominal aortic aneurysm repair in Veterans Affairs medical centers. *J Vasc Surg* 1996;23:191.
92. Birkmeyer JD, Stukel TA, Siewers AE, et al. Surgeon volume and operative mortality in the United States. *N Engl J Med* 2003;349:2117.
93. Dimick JB, Cowan Jr JA, Stanley JC, et al. Surgeon specialty and provider volumes are related to outcome of intact abdominal aortic aneurysm repair in the United States. *J Vasc Surg* 2003;38:739.
94. Dardik A, Burleyson GP, Bowman H, et al. Surgical repair of ruptured abdominal aortic aneurysms in the state of Maryland factors influencing outcome among 527 recent cases. *J Vasc Surg* 1998;28(3):413-420.
95. Young EL, Holt PJE, Poloniecki JD, et al. Meta-analysis and systematic review of the relationship between surgeon annual caseload and mortality for elective open abdominal aortic aneurysm repairs. *J Vasc Surg* 2007;46:1287.
96. Khuri SF, Daley J, Henderson W, et al. Relation of surgical volume to outcome in eight common operations: results from the VA National Surgical Quality Improvement Program. *Ann Surg* 1999;230:414.
97. Dillavou ED, Muluk SC, Makaroun MS. A decade of change in abdominal aortic aneurysm repair in the United States: have we improved outcomes equally between men and women? *J Vasc Surg* 2006;43:230.
98. O'Hara PJ, Hertzer NR, Krajewski LP, et al. Ten-year experience with abdominal aortic aneurysm repair in octogenarians: early results and late outcome. *J Vasc Surg* 1995;21:830.
99. Ballotta E, Da Giau G, Bridda A, et al. Open abdominal aortic aneurysm repair in octogenarians before and after the adoption of endovascular grafting procedures. *J Vasc Surg* 2008;47:23.
100. Johnston KW. Ruptured abdominal aortic aneurysm: six-year follow-up results of a multicenter prospective study. *J Vasc Surg* 1994;19:888.
101. Schermerhorn ML, O'Malley AJ, Jhaveri A, et al. Endovascular vs. open repair of abdominal aortic aneurysms in the Medicare population. *N Engl J Med* 2008;358:464.
102. Endovascular Aneurysm Repair Trail Participants. Comparison of endovascular aneurysm repair with open repair in patients with abdominal aortic aneurysm (EVAR Trial 1): 30-day operative mortality results—randomised controlled trial. *Lancet* 2004;364:843.
103. Endovascular Aneurysm Repair Trial Participants. Endovascular aneurysm repair versus open repair in patients with abdominal aortic aneurysm (EVAR Trial 1): randomised controlled trial. *Lancet* 2005;365:1179.
104. Prinssen M, Verhoeven ELG, Buth J, et al. A randomized trial comparing conventional and endovascular repair of abdominal aortic aneurysms. *N Engl J Med* 2004;351:1607.
105. Blankensteijn JD, de Jong SECA, Prinssen M, et al. Two-year outcomes after conventional or endovascular repair of abdominal aortic aneurysms. *N Engl J Med* 2005;352:2398.
106. Epstein EM, Sculpher MJ, Manca A, et al. Modelling the long-term cost-effectiveness of endovascular or open repair for abdominal aortic aneurysm. *Br J Surg* Sep 2008;95:183.
107. Prinssen M, Buskens E, De Jong SE, et al. Cost-effectiveness of conventional and endovascular repair of abdominal aortic aneurysms: results of a randomized trial. *J Vasc Surg* 2007;46:883.

chapter 31

Aortic Dissection

Kenneth J. Cherry Jr, MD • Michael D. Dake, MD

Key Points

- General considerations
- Classification
- Natural history
- Clinical presentation
- Diagnosis
- Anatomical pattern of the dissection lumen
- Related conditions
- Traditional management
- Initial therapy for type B dissection
- Complication-specific therapy
- Surgery for complicated acute type B dissections
- Results of surgery for acute type B dissections
- Endovascular options
- Surgery for chronic type B dissection
- Surgical technique tips
- Hybrid surgical and endovascular procedures
- Current approach to chronic type B aortic dissection
- Endovascular management of subacute dissections
- Endovascular era
- Timing of intervention
- Recent endovascular experience
- Current perspective on endovascular therapy

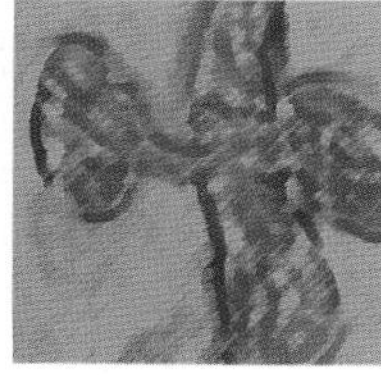

GENERAL CONSIDERATIONS

Aortic dissection results from a tear in the aortic intima allowing arterial blood to flow between the layers of the intima and the media, creating a second false lumen. At least two lumens are formed by this process (Figure 31-1). In some complex dissections, more than two lumens may form. A cleavage plane develops between these layers, allowing the dissection to propagate antegrade or retrograde or in both directions, although most extend antegrade or distally.

A septum, or dissection flap, is created and is composed of intima and a thin layer of media. Acutely, the dissection flap is friable and may appear wavy on computed tomography angiography (CTA). Chronically, it thickens and becomes leathery. On CTA it is a straight or curvilinear structure (Figure 31-2).

Dissections have been thought to occur at sites in the aorta where some form of medial degeneration exists. The most common causes for this degeneration are hypertension, connective tissue disorders (e.g., Marfan syndrome and Ehlers-Danlos syndrome), and traumatic transections. A great deal of current research looks into the etiology of dissections and medial degenerative conditions. Matrix metalloproteases, structural degradation of collagen and elastin, mutant fibrillin, and growth factors are being studied to identify molecular and genetic bases for dissections. Pregnancy associated with preeclampsia, power weight lifting, and the use of cocaine are also associated with aortic dissection.[1] Some dissections remain idiopathic.

CLASSIFICATION

Classically, dissections of the aorta are classified by the site of origin of the primary tear. Two major classification systems are used.

The *DeBakey system* recognizes three types (Figure 31-3): type I dissections begin in the proximal ascending aorta and involve both the ascending and the descending thoracic aorta, type II De Bakey dissection is confined to the ascending aorta, and type III involves the descending thoracic aorta and distal sites only. Type IIIa involves the descending thoracic aorta only. Type IIIb involves the descending thoracic and abdominal aortas, the latter for variable distances, even extending down to the iliac and femoral artery levels.

The *Stanford classification* has two types (Figure 31-3): type A dissection involves the ascending aorta, and type B dissection involves the descending thoracic aorta. The Stanford system is currently the most widely employed system, although it has its limitations. As an example, if the primary tear is in the descending thoracic aorta but extends retrograde into the transverse arch or the ascending thoracic aorta, the classification system fails to describe adequately the risks and possible complications.

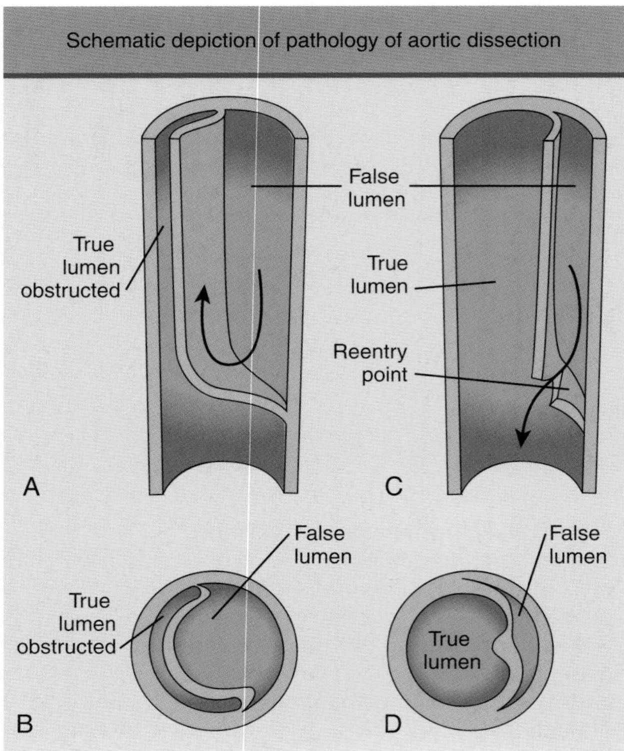

Figure 31-1. Schematic depiction of the pathology of aortic dissection. If the false lumen is not decompressed distally back into the true lumen, the false lumen may expand dynamically to narrow or obliterate the true lumen. Reentry of the false lumen distally or surgical or interventional fenestration usually allows flow to continue to varying degrees through the true lumen.

NATURAL HISTORY

Aortic dissection is a more common problem than is ruptured abdominal aortic aneurysm. Two population-based studies indicated incidences of 2.9 and 3.5 acute aortic dissections per 100,000 person years.[2,3] It is seen more often in men, with a ratio of 5:1. Type B patients are typically 10 years older than type A patients, with a peak incidence between 60 and 70 years for type B and 50 to 60 years for type A.[4]

Hypertension is present in approximately 75% of type B patients. Pain is the most common presenting symptom, occurring in approximately 95% of patients, and is usually described as sudden in onset.[2]

Acute aortic dissection is highly lethal if not recognized and treated aggressively. Approximately 20% of patients with acute aortic dissection die before reaching the hospital. Mortality for an untreated dissection is about 25% at 6 hours and 50% by 24 hours. Within 1 week, two thirds of patients die if untreated.[5] Of these deaths, 75% occur in the first 2 weeks. Consequently, the arbitrary distinction of acute dissection is less than 14 days, and chronic dissections are those surviving more than 2 weeks. The rule of thumb has been a mortality of 1% per hour in the acute stage. The two independent risk factors most often identified with type B dissections are hypertension and age.[6,7]

Despite improvements in surgical, anesthetic, interventional, and medical techniques, even the mortality and morbidity of treated patients remain high. According to the International Registry of Aortic Dissection (IRAD), a worldwide registry of 21 centers with consecutively enrolled patients, the in-hospital mortality for all dissections is 27%. Mortality and morbidity differ significantly for type A and B dissections and depends

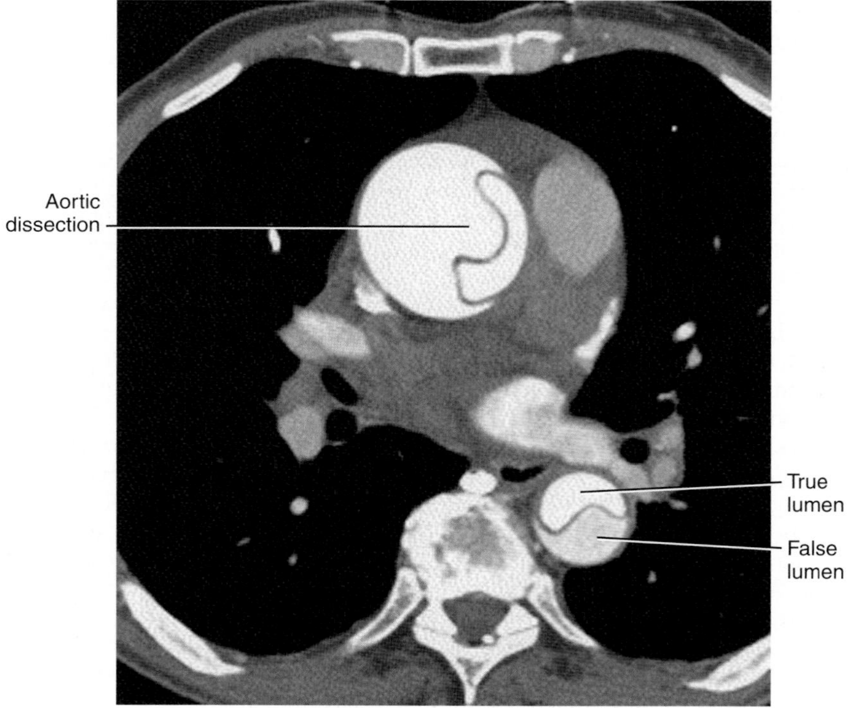

Figure 31-2. Computed tomography of an aortic dissection.

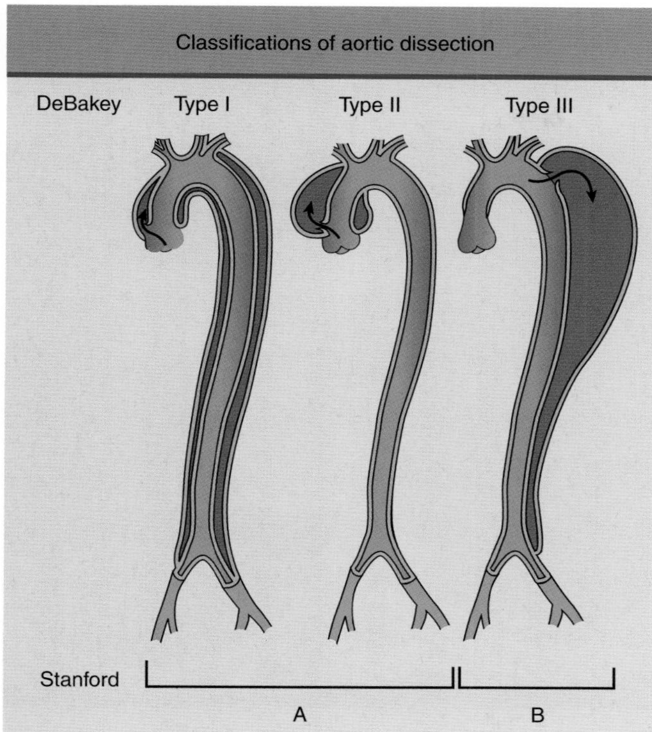

Figure 31-3. DeBakey and Stanford classifications of aortic dissection.

on the type of therapy and the medical comorbidities of the patients.

Patients with type A treated medically have a mortality of 58%, whereas mortality for surgical treatment of type A dissections is 26%. Type A is a more immediately life-threatening problem than is type B. These patients die of pericardial tamponade, rupture, aortic valve dysfunction, or malperfusion of the coronary arteries. Patients who present with syncope are more likely to have a type A dissection than a type B; syncope is associated with cardiac tamponade, stroke, and death.[8]

In contrast, the mortality for type B dissections is initially about 10% to 12% for patients who can be treated medically. Surgical or endovascular therapy is indicated for complications including progressive pain and dissection extension, rupture, and compromise of limb or organ perfusion. Patients with such complications necessitating intervention have a higher mortality of at least 30%.[4]

PRIMARY FOCUS OF THIS CHAPTER

This chapter deals primarily with De Bakey type III or Stanford type B dissections that involve the descending thoracic aorta where newer endovascular therapies are playing an innovative role in management. The Stanford nomenclature is used.

CLINICAL PRESENTATION

The classical clinical presentation is one of acute, severe tearing chest or back pain unlike any experienced previously by the patient. Severe hypertension is often present, and other signs of peripheral organ malperfusion may be present. Examples of the obstructive effects of the dissection may include stroke, acute limb ischemia, or mesenteric or renal perfusion insufficiency. Careful measurement of blood pressures in both arms, abdominal palpation for tenderness, assessment of urinary output, and evaluation of lower-limb pulses and neurological examination are essential components of the initial evaluation of any patient suspected of an aortic dissection.

DIAGNOSIS

Computed tomography with contrast (CTA) is the most commonly employed diagnostic test according to IRAD.[4] Axial images with and without contrast are obtained. When dissection is suspected, the study should include the chest, abdomen, and pelvis to determine the extent of the dissections. Invasive conventional arteriography for diagnosis, which has been considered the gold standard in the past, is used much less often now.

The pressures associated with injection into the true lumen are important. High injection pressures may falsely inflate the true lumen and consequently underdiagnose dynamic malperfusion syndromes. False-negative studies are also seen with thrombosis of the false lumen.[9]

The early criticisms of CTA for diagnosing dissection were (1) lack of definition in the area of the ascending aorta and (2) lack of clarity in the area of the ligamentum arteriosum. However, both radiologists and surgeons have become more proficient at interpretation, and the resolution of computed tomography (CT) scanners continues to improve dramatically. Thus, problems in diagnosis and interpretation of the dissection extent are less common today.

Significant advances in CTA are attributable to improvements in scanner technology, particularly the advent of multidetector scanners with 64 or greater channels. This technology allows for rapid acquisition of large-coverage volumetric data sets with isotropic voxels, cube volume elements with submillimeter dimensions, producing high-resolution images in *all planes* that were previously only obtainable in the *axial plane.*

Transesophageal echocardiography (TEE) is employed often, especially in patients suspected of having a type A dissection. In the IRAD studies, it was the second most commonly used test.[4] TEE is complementary to CTA, especially in the ascending aorta. CTA has a sensitivity in the ascending aorta of less than 80% in contrast to its greater than 95% sensitivity elsewhere.

Most primary tears, or entry sites, are transverse rather than linear. Approximately two thirds of primary tears occur in the ascending aorta, and most of these are located within the first 2 cm of the ascending aorta (Figure 31-3).[4] The second most common site is at the isthmus of the descending thoracic aorta beyond the subclavian artery at the ligamentum arteriosum. Dissection may also be seen in the descending thoracic aorta at other sites, in the aortic arch, and in the abdominal aorta. About 20% to 35% of dissections are in the descending thoracic aorta.[10] Ten percent occur in the aortic arch or the abdominal aorta.

Secondary tears, or reentry sites, are often seen with aortic dissection. These generally occur at the ostia of branch vessels and allow equalization of flow. With the exposure of the medial and adventitial layers, thrombosis is more likely in the false channel. The exposed medial and adventitial layers are less resistant to thrombosis than the intima. The false channel may become thrombosed either completely or partially.

Compression of the true lumen by the newly pressurized false lumen is often apparent and may be the cause of either acute or chronic complications. Tsai et al. have reported that partial thrombosis of the false lumen may be a more dangerous event than either continuous patency or full thrombosis, with a late mortality in their type B patients of 33%.[11] These investigators performed ex vivo experiments indicating that the presence of an entry tear was associated with significantly decreased systolic pressure in the false lumen, whereas the absence of a distal reentry tear resulted in a significant increase in false lumen diastolic pressure. They surmised that the false lumen, less distensible and elastin poor, bears the load during the longer diastolic phase of the cardiac cycle. Consequently, impaired outflow from the false lumen, as seen with partial thrombosis, may be a cause for false lumen expansion.[12] Most authors have felt that continued patency of the false lumen is a predictor of later aneurysmal degeneration,[13,14] but not all agree. Juvonen et al. reported that continued false lumen patency was not associated with an increased rate of rupture in medically treated patients.[15]

ANATOMICAL PATTERN OF THE DISSECTION LUMEN

The course of the Stanford type B dissection is extremely, but not perfectly, predictable in the thoracic aorta. The false channel courses along the lateral outer aspect of the descending aorta. The late E. Stanley Crawford emphasized that this lateral position of the false lumen was a relatively constant feature at operation. While performing a left lateral thoracotomy or thoracoabdominal incision, the surgeon encounters the false lumen first when opening the aorta.[16]

We agree with this prescient observation. At the University of Virginia, we have seen only two patients whose thoracic aortic false lumens were medial along the inner surface. Because of this lateral tracking of the false lumen in the thoracic aorta, the celiac artery, the superior mesenteric artery, and the right renal artery often arise from the true lumen and the left renal artery from the false lumen. Commonly, the dissection may end in the ostia of the celiac, superior mesenteric, or both types of arteries, extending into those vessels for variable distances. These lateral aortic tracking patterns of the false lumen do have some variance. The actual dissection patterns may be complex. For example, the dissection may spiral as it continues distally rather than extending in a single axial plane. Consequently, the relative medial and lateral positioning of the two lumens is not as predictable in the abdominal aorta as in the thoracic aorta.

RELATED CONDITIONS

Intramural hematoma and penetrating atheromatous ulcer are closely related syndromes and may represent dissection at different, perhaps earlier stages (Figure 31-4).[14] A penetrating aortic ulcer protrudes through the surface of an atherosclerotic plaque into the media without frank dissection. Penetrating atheromatous ulcers are often seen in multiple locations that may enlarge and even coalesce. In contrast, an intramural hematoma occurs in the aortic wall without a clear aortic tear or entry site as seen with a classical aortic dissection. Approximately 70% to 80% of penetrating ulcers progress to

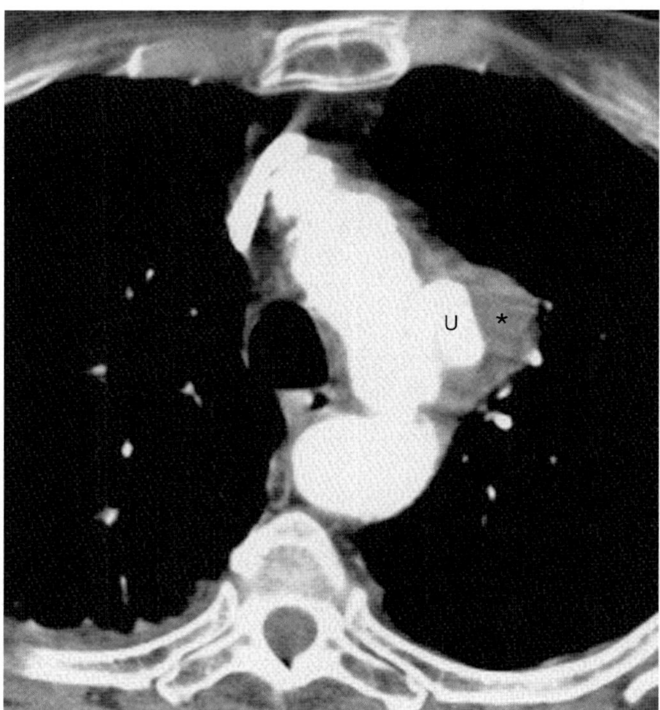

Figure 31-4. Penetrating ulcer of the aorta.

an intramural hematoma. These two entities are seen in about 5% of patients initially suspected of aortic dissection. They occur generally in patients who are about 10 years older than the usual patient with a type B dissection.

Both of these entities occur more commonly in the descending thoracic aorta compared to the ascending thoracic aorta. In particular, 90% affect the descending thoracic aorta. Both are associated with atherosclerosis, especially penetrating ulcers. Another interesting clinical association is that 40% of patients with a penetrating aortic ulcer have been treated previously for an abdominal aortic aneurysm. These two entities may coexist. Both are more worrisome when seen in an already-dilated aorta, particularly greater than 4 cm.

Both entities may progress to frank dissection, aneurysm, or rupture, or they may regress. Progress to forme fruste dissection occurs in 16% to 36% of patients with intramural hematoma. These patients are treated as type B patients. With complications, they undergo intervention. The other indication in this particular subset of patients is increase in the size of the hematoma.

TRADITIONAL MANAGEMENT

Modern surgical management began in 1955 with the report of DeBakey et al. describing the first three patients operated successfully for aortic dissection.[17] Surgical repair remains the primary therapy for ascending Stanford type A dissections. However, Wheat and colleagues in 1965 shifted the management of Stanford type B descending thoracic aortic dissections toward a medical regimen that emphasizes beta-blockade to decrease blood pressure and slow heart rate.[18]

Beta-blockers change pressure over time (dP/dT) or, as it is currently termed, force impact. Reductions in both blood pressure and force impact are the mainstays of the initial

management of nonruptured type B dissections. Antihypertensive therapy stabilizes the dissection, reduces movement of the septum, relieves dynamic obstruction (discussed later), and alleviates the pain of dissection.

Beta-blockade is the most important element in the long-term medical management of all patients with dissection, whether treated medically or interventionally. Although many types of antihypertensives are available, beta-blockers are usually an integral part of any medical regimen for dissection. Genoni et al. reported that freedom from later aortic events was 80% for patients at 4.2 years when treated with beta-blockers versus 47% for patients treated with different antihypertensive regimens.[5]

INITIAL THERAPY FOR TYPE B DISSECTION

Type B dissection is initially treated medically with beta-blockage and analgesics. If the patient responds favorably and no complicating features intervene, medical management is continued. The current debate is whether endovascular treatment of uncomplicated type B dissections would yield a more favorable long-term outcome than medical management alone. We address this important controversy later in this chapter.

We also want to add a word of caution about so-called failed medical management for type B dissections. Our observation is that some of these "failures" have not been treated adequately before surgical or endovascular intervention. A "normal" blood pressure of 140/80 is not adequate treatment for these patients. Estrera et al. at the University of Texas describe the primary goal as a systolic pressure of less than 140 mm Hg, and a secondary goal of less than 120 mm Hg for those with continued pain. With these parameters, they reported an early intervention rate of 16.2%.[19] Tefera et al. from the University of Wisconsin describe the effective medical therapy as a systolic pressure of less than 120 mm Hg and a heart rate of less than 70 beats/minute. Only 23% of their patients required emergency operation, but none were for back pain.[20]

In our experience, the following guidelines should be emphasized. Patients with acute type B dissection should be in an intensive care unit. Their blood pressure should be reduced to systolic ranges of 90 to 110 depending on the patient's cognition and renal function, i.e., without signs of malperfusion to the patient's central nervous system, abdominal viscera, or lower extremities. This aggressive pressure management usually alleviates their severe pain in a short period. Januzzi et al. report that pain is the softest of the indications for operation with type B dissection. They report that only 4% of patients have a complicated course. In the absence of clinical or radiographic deterioration, intense antihypertensive therapy is sufficient for initial management in most patients with type B dissections.[21]

There is one cautionary note: beta-blockade should be started before administering nitroprusside to prevent a reflex sympathetic reaction to the pharmacologically induced vasodilation with a consequent unwanted increase in force impact.[9]

The usual indications for operation or intervention in acute type B or descending thoracic aortic dissections were mentioned on page 519 but need reemphasis. They include (1) persistent or recurrent intractable pain, (2) rapidly enlarging aortic diameter (aneurysmal degeneration), (3) progression of the dissection, (4) aortic rupture, and (5) end-organ ischemia.

End-organ ischemia, affecting the abdominal viscera, the spinal cord, or the lower extremities, represents branch vessel compromise and is currently termed malperfusion syndrome. Such malperfusion may be dynamic or static. Malperfusion occurs in anywhere from 30% to 40% of patients. It may result from compression of the true lumen, compromise of the branch arteries, or thrombosis. Patients may present with end-organ ischemia of their spinal cord. This complication is seen more commonly with type B dissection but fortunately only occurs in 2% to 3% of patients. The most lethal and feared of the malperfusion syndromes is mesenteric ischemia. Acute lower-extremity arterial ischemia is an indication of a more extensive dissection involving the iliac arteries. Malperfusion may result from compression or partial collapse of the true aortic lumen.

Malperfusion is often dynamic, changing over time and with fluctuations in blood pressure, heart rate, and force impact. Arterial branch compromise may be a result of this dynamic aortic obstruction in which the compressed true aortic lumen cannot supply nonischemic levels of blood flow to the aortic branches, even though these vessels are not themselves dissected. Dynamic obstruction accounts for 80% of such cases of malperfusion. In essence, or in simplistic terms, dynamic obstruction may be thought of as aortic false lumen obstruction with compression of the aortic true lumen by the pressurized false lumen. This mechanism is "dynamic" because changes in blood pressure, heart rate, and peripheral resistance may change the symptom complex and can be altered favorably by medical management. Estrera et al. observed that this dynamism allowed spontaneous resolution with medical management of paraplegia in 62% of their patients and of limb ischemia in 57%.[19] The amount of aortic circumference involved in the dissection also contributes to the dynamic nature of these obstructions.

Static obstruction, occurring in about 20% of cases, is the result of obstruction by the blind end of the dissection or false lumen. The blind end may be either thrombosed or not and may extend into the ostium of a branch vessel and restrict flow. This obstructive phenomenon may represent prolapse of the aortic septum into the ostium or extension of the dissection from the aorta into the branch artery lumen. This anatomical problem is fixed or static and does not respond as well to medical therapy. Intervention is usually necessary.

False lumen thrombosis occurs spontaneously in 2% to 3% of those patients treated medically and in about 15% to 30% of those treated surgically. Continued false lumen patency may be a risk factor for aneurysmal degeneration over time and for dissection extension. Aneurysmal enlargement requiring intervention is seen in approximately a third of patients 4 years following initial management.

COMPLICATION-SPECIFIC THERAPY

Elefteriades et al. described the concept of "complication-specific therapy" in 1992.[22] Rather than performing central aortic repair initially in all patients, including type A, they addressed severe end-organ ischemia first, especially mesenteric ischemia. They delayed reconstruction of the proximal aorta dissection until the patient was stable from repair of the complicating problem.

This concept appears to have improved surgical results. At Baylor-Houston, the mortality for operation in complicated acute type B patients is 22%.[23] At the University of Texas-Houston, the initial mortality for aortic dissection with organ or limb ischemia is 17%.[19] These two groups of experienced surgeons using this approach of complication-specific therapy encourage us all to study the details of their innovative approach.

Additional support for complication-specific therapy, especially for type B dissections, comes from the Massachusetts General Hospital. Between 1965 and 1986, the rupture rate at this hospital was 18% and the mortality 37%. In the interim between 1990 and 1999, the rupture rate had dropped to 6% and the mortality to 18%.[9] They attributed this improvement to earlier diagnosis, aggressive medical care, and adherence to the tenets of complication-specific care.

SURGERY FOR COMPLICATED ACUTE TYPE B DISSECTIONS

Surgery for acute type B dissection is performed for patients with complications mentioned previously: (1) pain not responsive to adequate reduction in blood pressure and impulse force, (2) retrograde dissection in the ascending aorta, (3) continuing dissection, (4) aneurysmal dilation, (5) malperfusion of an organ or limb, or (6) rupture. Malperfusion is the most common indication for intervention. Frank rupture for type B dissections has declined and currently occurs in only 5% of patients. Continuing pain is the least common indication for intervention.[4]

Surgical mortality is higher for acute type B dissections than is medical mortality (30% versus 10%). This significant risk of operation must be understood by everyone involved with the patient, especially the patient and family. Several surgical concepts help reduce the mortality and morbidity. For example, the shortest segment of aorta should be replaced for aneurysmal degeneration. Extensive replacement of the thoracic aorta should be avoided if possible because of the risk of spinal cord ischemia. Aortic dissection extending the full length of the descending thoracic and abdominal aortas, in combination with aneurysmal degeneration, has a significant risk of paraplegia in the range of 30% to 40%.[9,14]

In other words, the goal of operation is treatment of the aneurysm, not resection of all dissected aorta. Excluding the primary entry site from pulsatile blood flow reduces blood volume in the false lumen and allows reexpansion of the true lumen. Distal reconstructions may still need to be performed, depending on the resultant true lumen flow, the extent of dissection, the presence of thrombosis, and the reentry sites. Most importantly, the presence of dynamic versus static dissection flaps as the cause of distal malperfusion must be treated effectively.

RESULTS OF SURGERY FOR ACUTE TYPE B DISSECTIONS

Results of surgery for acute type B dissection continue to improve. Nonetheless, 25% to 50% of patients who are treated acutely with central aorta replacement can still be expected to have chronic persistent false lumen flow.[14] Consequently, they must be monitored with long-term CT surveillance for aneurysmal degeneration. Two recent technical details may help seal the false lumen: (1) felt pledgets to reinforce suture lines and (2) biological glues to seal suture lines and obliterate false lumens. Several major cardiovascular centers have reported mortality for surgical management of acute complicated type B aortic dissections in the 16% to 18% range.[9,19,23]

ENDOVASCULAR OPTIONS

Currently, the most controversial question facing the surgeon taking care of patients with complicated acute type B aortic dissection is open reconstruction versus endovascular reconstruction. When possible, we employ endograft techniques if the patient's anatomy and clinical status are appropriate. Usually, dynamic obstruction responds to aortic endografting. Static obstruction usually requires additional branch artery stent grafting or aortic fenestration. Cognizant of the lack of long-term data, we believe the short-term reduction in both early mortality justifies this endovascular approach.

Two possible exceptions to our preference for endovascular therapy must be emphasized. The first is frank rupture. Fortunately, the incidence of rupture with acute type B dissections is declining. The other exception may be acute mesenteric malperfusion, which presents unique challenges and is not as well treated by endovascular techniques.

Mesenteric malperfusion is highly lethal, with a mortality of 80% to 90%, even greater than the mortality of rupture.[9] If patients have a clinical picture consistent with acute bowel ischemia, they are often best treated with open laparotomy and open reconstruction, most usually with fenestration of the paravisceral aorta. If mesenteric malperfusion is treated by endovascular techniques, a timely subsequent laparotomy is recommended to ascertain the persistence and extent of bowel ischemia, to locate perforations if present, and to allow any needed bowel resection. This approach is analogous to a second-look operation that follows an initial open reconstruction.

Many surgeons feel open fenestration for mesenteric malperfusion is preferable because of its definitive nature, and that has been the opinion of the surgeon-author until recently. The surgeon can also inspect the bowel and deal with any dead gut before perforation leads to sepsis. Consequently, many patients with acute mesenteric malperfusion are still treated via open operation, even in this endovascular era. The celiac and superior mesenteric arteries may be approached by retroperitoneal exposure, thoracoabdominal exposure, thoracoretroperitoneal exposure, or medial visceral rotation.

The choice is based on the surgeon's experience and on the patient's body habitus and vascular anatomy. The septum is resected widely, leaving only a rim on the outer aortic wall between the supraceliac and the distal clamps. Fenestration is carried into the mesenteric, renal, or both types of arteries as necessary. Such fenestration is fortunately rarely necessary. Of 857 patients studied at the Mayo Clinic, 81 had malperfusion and only 14 patients of that 857 underwent paravisceral aortic fenestration.[24]

Aortic fenestration for mesenteric or renal malperfusion provides good results. At the Massachusetts General Hospital, mortality in patients with mesenteric ischemia was reduced from 87% to 37% with adherence to complication-specific

treatment, i.e., dealing with mesenteric ischemia as the first priority in this open manner.[9] The open approach is durable. Elefteriades and colleagues found no aneurysmal degeneration in their series of fenestrations, nor did the surgeons from the Mayo Clinic.[24,25] At the Mayo Clinic, the mortality for fenestration in the acute setting was 43%, contrasted with the historical 87% mortality. Having said this, we have recently treated two young patients with complicated type B dissections, one with a contained thoracic rupture, gut malperfusion, and limb malperfusion and the other with gut malperfusion. Both had dynamic obstructions, both were treated by thoracic stent grafting and immediate laparotomy, and both survived. Our view, therefore, on the treatment of type B dissections with malperfusion syndromes may be considered to be in a state of evolution with more reliance on endovascular techniques than in the past.

SURGERY FOR CHRONIC TYPE B DISSECTION

Over long-term follow-up, aneurysms develop in 30% to 40% of patients with type B dissection who are treated initially with only antihypertensive therapy. These aneurysms may occur in the thoracic or abdominal areas of the dissection. The basic methods of dealing with all these aneurysms are dealt with elsewhere in the book. The size indications for operations on aortic aneurysms due to chronic aortic dissections may be less stringent than they are for degenerative aneurysms. Most aortic centers offer operation for aneurysms secondary to dissections at lesser aortic diameters than the usual 6 cm for degenerative thoracic aortic aneurysms and 5.5 cm for abdominal aortic aneurysms. These aneurysms associate with dissections, with their *unintact* layers, may be more prone to rupture. For example, Crawford reported that 23% of ruptured thoracic aortic aneurysms due to chronic type B dissections were less than 6 cm in size.[26] At Mount Sinai, the last median measurement of these aneurysms before rupture was 5.4 cm.[27] Consequently, once aneurysms associated with dissection reach 5 cm, most experienced surgeons offer open operation or endovascular intervention.

SURGICAL TECHNIQUE TIPS

Our surgical experience highlights some comments concerning how the true and false lumens should be handled to achieve optimal results (Figure 31-5). If the aneurysm arises just at the origin of the dissection, the proximal anastomosis is performed to nondissected normal caliber aorta. If the aneurysm arises below a relatively normal sized but dissected aorta, a surgical fenestration is performed at the time of anastomosis. The septum is resected to the side wall, leaving only a rim, and back to the proximal clamp.

Grafting is performed to the aortic circumference encompassing both lumens. It is the surgeon-author's preference to use a continuous circumferential felt pledget and horizontal mattress sutures of polypropylene in these situations. Distally, one aortic lumen can be created again by tacking the dissected septum to the appropriate overlying medial and adventitial layers. However, the decision is multifactorial.

If the false channel is providing excellent blood flow to the distal organs, if there are not distal aneurysmal changes, and if no reentry points are visible, compromising the false lumen blood flow by closing the false channel is problematic. Contrariwise, if blood flow would be improved to the distal organs by eradicating the false lumen, then an anastomosis to the recreated single lumen would be preferable and should be performed. If the dissection is left intact, a distal fenestration to the level of the distal clamp is performed. The multiplicity of reentry points often makes closure of the distal false lumen futile. The false lumen persists in 25% to 50% of patients. All of these patients, no matter the particular operation chosen, need to be followed for future aneurysmal degeneration.

HYBRID SURGICAL AND ENDOVASCULAR PROCEDURES

Surgery for chronic type B dissections now includes left subclavian artery reconstruction before thoracic aortic endografting. In general, we favor subclavian reconstruction before endografting of the descending aorta rather than stent graft coverage without reconstruction. This approach may not be possible in acute situations. In chronic patients undergoing descending thoracic aortic endografting, a dominant left vertebral artery mandates reconstruction. Furthermore, if most or all of the descending thoracic aorta will be covered by the endografts with a consequent loss of the intercostal artery radicular blood supply to the spinal cord, preservation of the vertebral artery and its thyrocervical contributions to the anterior and posterior spinal arteries is important.

CURRENT APPROACH TO CHRONIC TYPE B AORTIC DISSECTION

Endovascular methods are rapidly replacing open operations for managing the complications of all dissections of the descending and thoracoabdominal aorta. The stage or age of the dissections is important in determining whether open or endovascular therapy would be best for any given patient.

ENDOVASCULAR MANAGEMENT OF SUBACUTE DISSECTIONS

Aortic dissection is usually classified as acute (less than 14 days) or chronic (more than 2 weeks). A subacute heading (great than 14 days to several months) had been largely abandoned until the present endovascular era. Recently, Kasirajan et al. have proposed resurrection of a subacute phase terminology. They suggest "acute" for the first 3 months, "subacute" for 3 to 12 months, and "chronic" for greater than 1 year. This classification is based their observation of behavior of the septum as dynamic (acute), compliant (subacute), and noncompliant (chronic), respectively.[28] Consequently, subacute terminology is coming back into usage and may be relevant to whether newer endovascular treatments may benefit the patient.

ENDOVASCULAR ERA

The most exciting element of treatment for aortic dissection is endovascular therapy. The current endovascular era began just 9 years ago with two reports appearing in the same issue of the *New England Journal of Medicine* on the use of aortic stent grafting to treat complicated aortic dissection.[29,30] Those reports stimulated great enthusiasm and widespread application of endovascular techniques to both acute and chronic aortic dissections and to noncomplicated type B patients. Interest has been renewed in the pathophysiology and the anatomy of dissection, its natural and treated histories, outcomes research, and the causes and the genetics of dissection.

In 1999, those two concurrently published studies by Dake et al. and Nienaber et al. proposed endovascular stent grafting as an effective alternative to traditional therapies for acute type B aortic dissection.[29,30] These reports supported a new treatment modality that is less invasive than open thoracotomy and holds the potential for a more durable approach than medical therapy alone. However, evidence-based data from randomized clinical studies for acute type B aortic dissection are slow to accumulate. In addition, attempts to stratify patient groups based upon differential outcomes are effectively lacking.

As recently as 2005, the consensus remained that uncomplicated type B dissections are best managed medically. Endovascular interventions, even with the promise of a sustained effectiveness similar to long-term open surgical results, appear to offer no validated survival benefits over medical regimens in stable patients.[31] In 2005, Tsai et al. discussed the potential for endovascular treatment of uncomplicated type B dissections. However, they emphasized that "patients with uncomplicated aortic dissections confined to the descending aorta are presently best treated with medical therapy."[32]

Nonetheless, other interventionalists and surgeons, including ourselves, continue to explore endovascular opportunities to improve clinical results in various subgroups of patients with dissection. Indeed, better noninvasive imaging modalities and newer endovascular therapeutic alternatives for acute, complicated type B lesions have increased interest in using more endovascular techniques for early phases of aortic dissection. Moreover, the prospect of aortic remodeling in the chronic phase of disease has reinvigorated this debate. After endograft placement for dissection, the risk of aneurysmal degeneration may be lessened (Figure 31-6).

Much of the early attention directed at therapeutic advances has focused on improving the results of patients with complicated, acute type B dissection. This subgroup is associated with levels of clinically relevant morbidities and mortality related to open surgical repair that are important targets for better

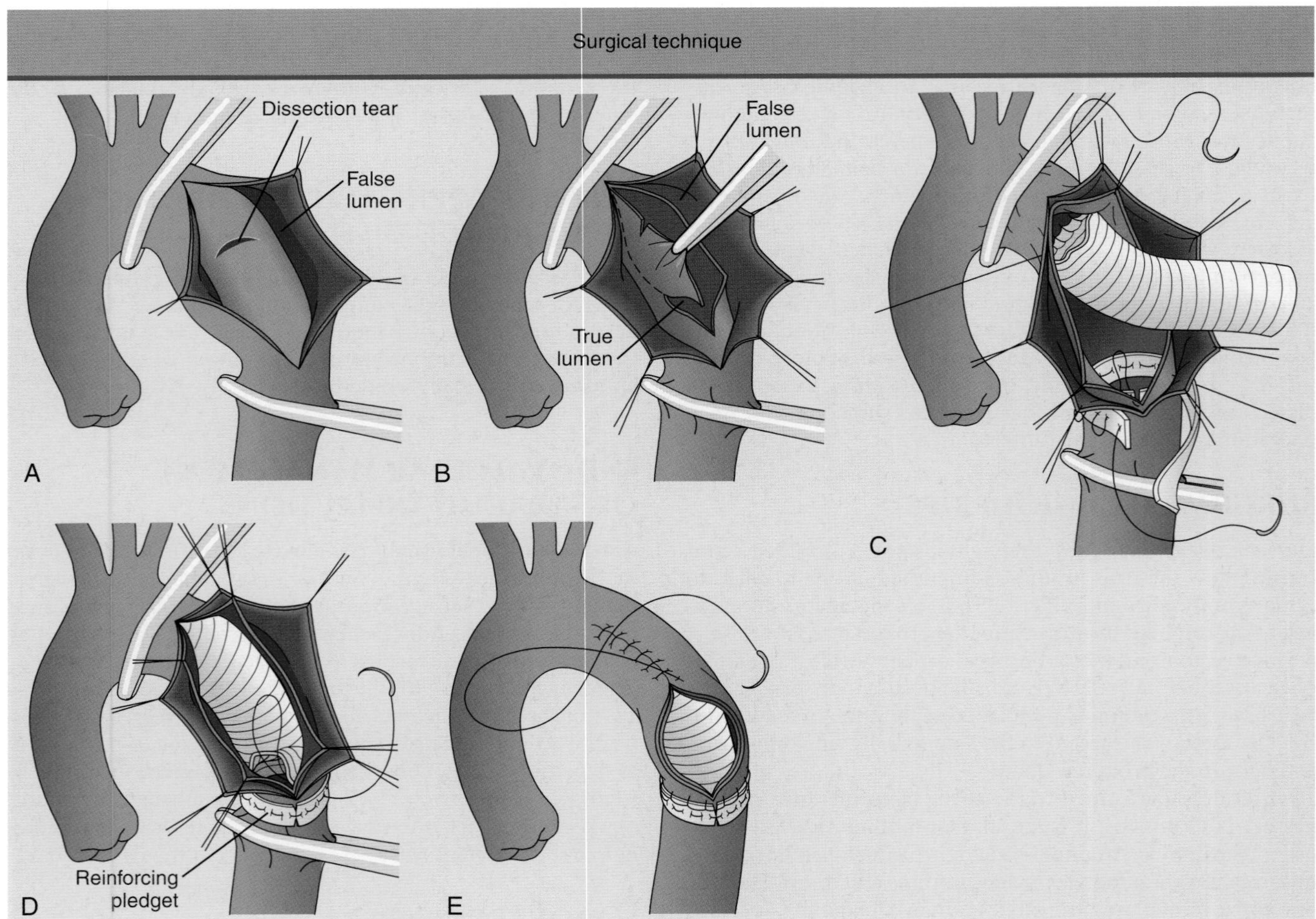

Figure 31-5. Surgical technique. **A,** The first lumen entered when the lateral aortic wall is incised is almost always the false lumen when the original dissection tear may or may not be seen. **B,** The edges of the false lumen are excised. **C,** The proximal anastomosis is constructed to normal aorta. **D,** Reinforcing felt pledgets to obliterate the distal false lumen are used to reinforce the distal anastomosis and to restore flow into the true lumen. **E,** The aortic wall is closed around the graft if possible.

patient outcomes. Indeed, some longstanding aortic centers have integrated endograft therapy prominently in managing acute dissection cases complicated by symptomatic aortic branch vessel involvement (Figure 31-7). This therapy is now widely accepted for this indication. However, the role of stent graft placement in the setting of uncomplicated, acute type B dissection remains contentious.

Indeed, the early application of endovascular therapy for acute, uncomplicated type B dissections must be weighed against the relative effectiveness of optimal medical therapy alone. The two most attractive reasons for early endotherapy are (1) a more durable prevention of aneurysm or recurrence and (2) prevention of the occasional aortic dissection that ruptures within 2 weeks after apparently effective medical management. However, these goals have not yet been proved by clinical trials and are advocated mainly by anecdotal reports.

For early endovascular therapy to succeed, stent grafts therapy must cover and seal the entry site (Figure 31-8).[33] Experimental models indicate that proper placement of the stent graft results in false lumen thrombosis, an event known to be associated with an improved prognosis. In contrast, patency of the false lumen is associated with late mortality.[34-37] A properly positioned stent graft with occlusion of the proximal tear results in decompression of the false lumen and reexpansion of the true lumen. Thrombosis of the false lumen typically occurs within 3 months.[29] Aortic remodeling occurs quickly after stent graft placement[29,34] and has the potential to reverse branch vessel ischemia and inhibit recanalization of the thrombosed false lumen.[34]

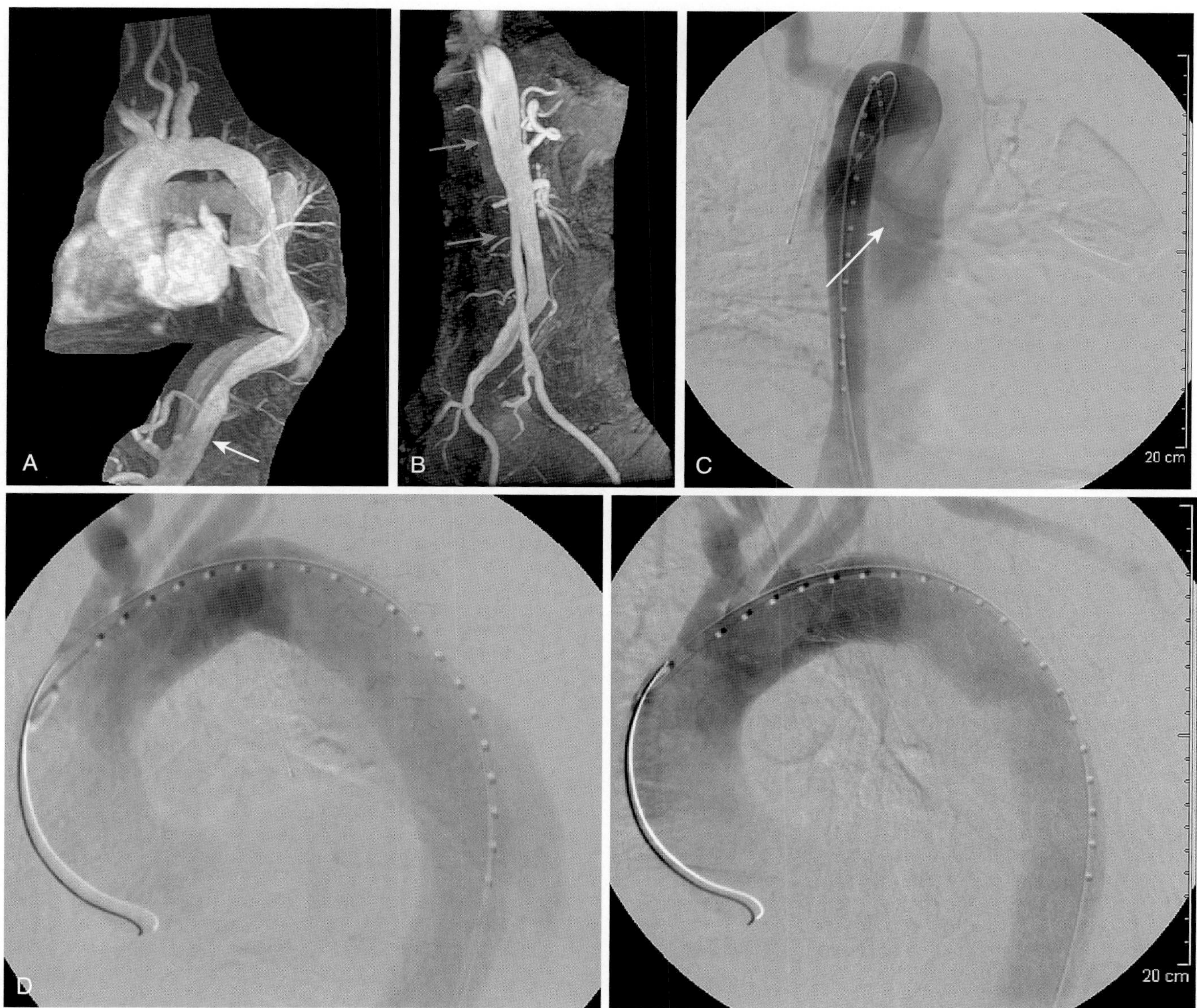

Figure 31-6. 63-year-old man with type B aortic dissection and enlarging false lumen managed by stent graft placement. **A,** Axial computed tomography (CT) image at the level of the aortic arch delineates type B dissection with intimal flap in a patient with acute back pain and hypertension. **B,** Follow-up study performed 30 days after the initial CT details marked increase in false lumen with associated pleural fluid. **C,** Aortogram with evidence of entry tear jet of contrast media between true lumen and false lumen in the proximal descending thoracic aorta. **D,** A comparison of pre– and post–stent graft placement aortograms documents the lack of persistent false lumen flow following device deployment.

Continued

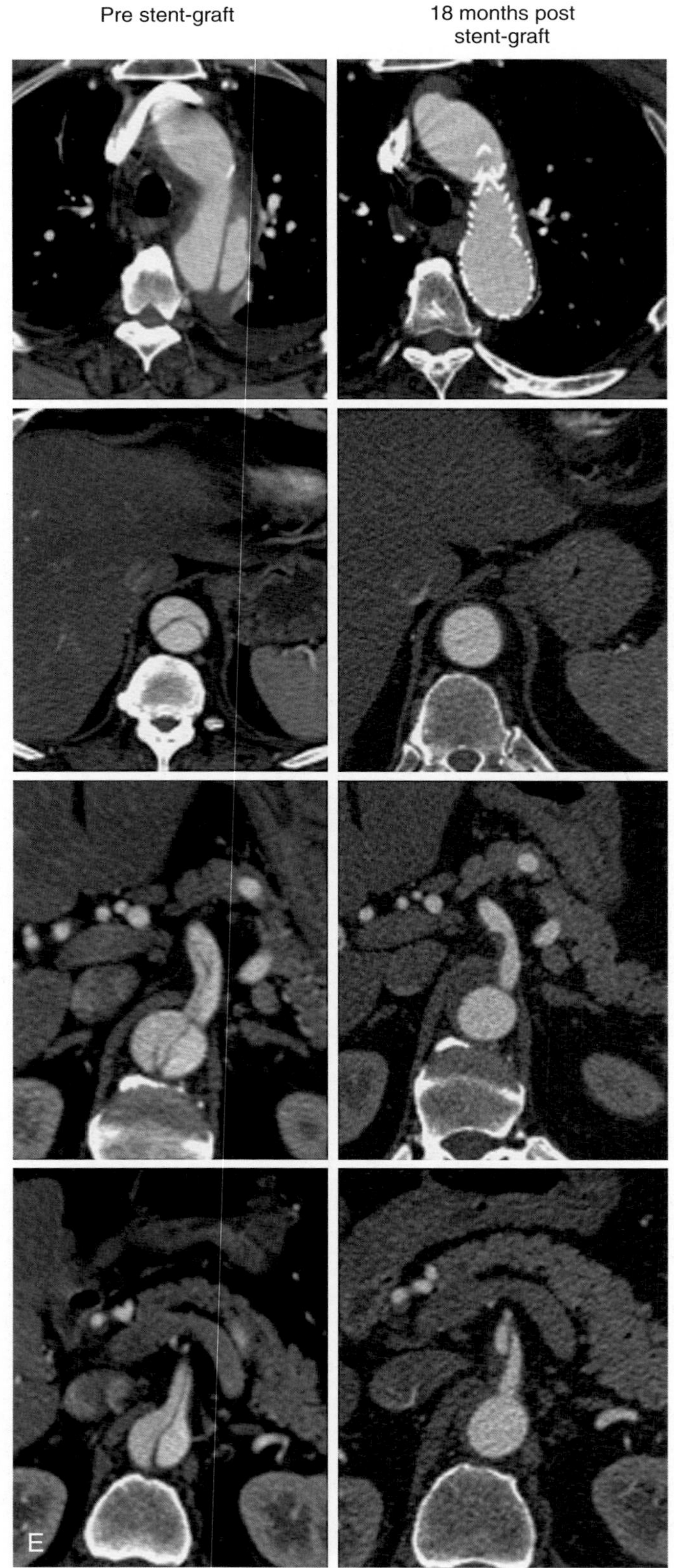

Figure 31-6—cont'd E, Comparison of CT images at similar anatomical levels (arch, distal descending, celiac, superior mesenteric artery) over an 18-month interval after the onset of the dissection shows the evolution in the appearance of the aorta and its branches with thrombosis of the aortic false lumen, "healing" of the flap within the celiac trunk, and persistent flap within the superior mesenteric artery. The patient remains asymptomatic.

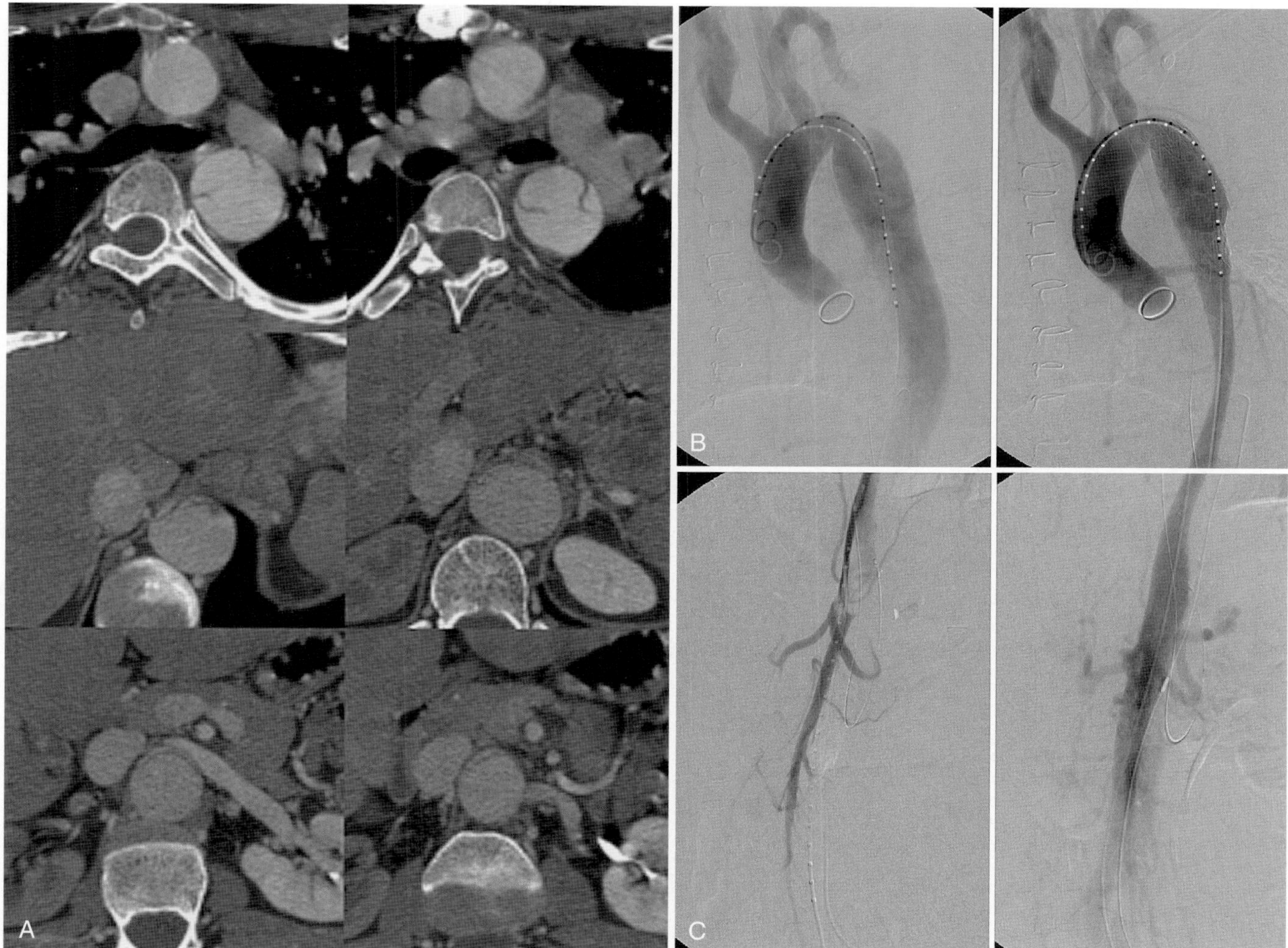

Figure 31-7. Stent graft treatment of a 27-year-old man with Marfan syndrome and newly diagnosed type B aortic dissection. He had his ascending aorta replaced in the remote past and recently experienced back pain for 5 days and acute abdominal pain for 12 hours before coming to the emergency room. **A,** Selected images from a computed tomography scan document a type B dissection with a large proximal entry tear and true lumen collapse distally. The true lumen is obliterated at the level of the abdominal aortic branch vessels. Only the left kidney is supplied by flow from the false lumen and appears well perfused. **B,** Aortograms performed before and after implantation of a stent graft within the thoracic aortic true lumen over the entry tear demonstrate good coverage of the communication and a lack of contrast media opacification of the false lumen following endograft deployment. **C,** Abdominal aortograms before and following stent graft placement over the primary tear show interval enlargement of the true lumen and good flow to the previously poorly perfused branches. The patient recovered without further intervention and left the hospital on day 3 following the procedure.

TIMING OF INTERVENTION

The optimal time for endovascular intervention of all type B dissections remains debatable. A retrospective study performed by Bortone et al. in 2002 strongly defends immediate intervention, as defined as procedures performed within 2 weeks of the initial diagnosis.[38] Stent graft placement was successful in all patients referred for intervention within the first 2 weeks. Conversely, 62% patients referred after 2 weeks failed to undergo stent graft placement. The causes of failure include a tortuous course of the dissection and multiple sites of communication between the true and the false lumens. Moreover, a thick and fibrotic dissection flap may impede adequate stent graft expansion.[34] Despite these impediments, multiple groups have reported successful stent graft management in chronic dissections treated after 2 weeks.[33,34,39-41]

As described previously, rapid intervention in the acute phase is also associated with its own complications. The adventitia and dissection flap are weak and vulnerable to injury induced by placement of a stent graft. Various groups have argued for greater than 1 week to 1 month elapsed time before intervention.[42,43] Interestingly, the inclusion criteria of the immediate versus delayed endovascular treatment for posttraumatic aortic pseudoaneurysm and type B dissections (Investigation of Stent Grafts in Patients with Type B Aortic Dissection, or INSTEAD) trial require intervention between 2 and 52 weeks. This range of time may enlighten us on the optimal timing for endovascular therapy. While the optimal time for endovascular intervention may lie in the acute or subacute phases, the exact timing must take into account the patient's underlying medical comorbidities and the specific dissection anatomy.

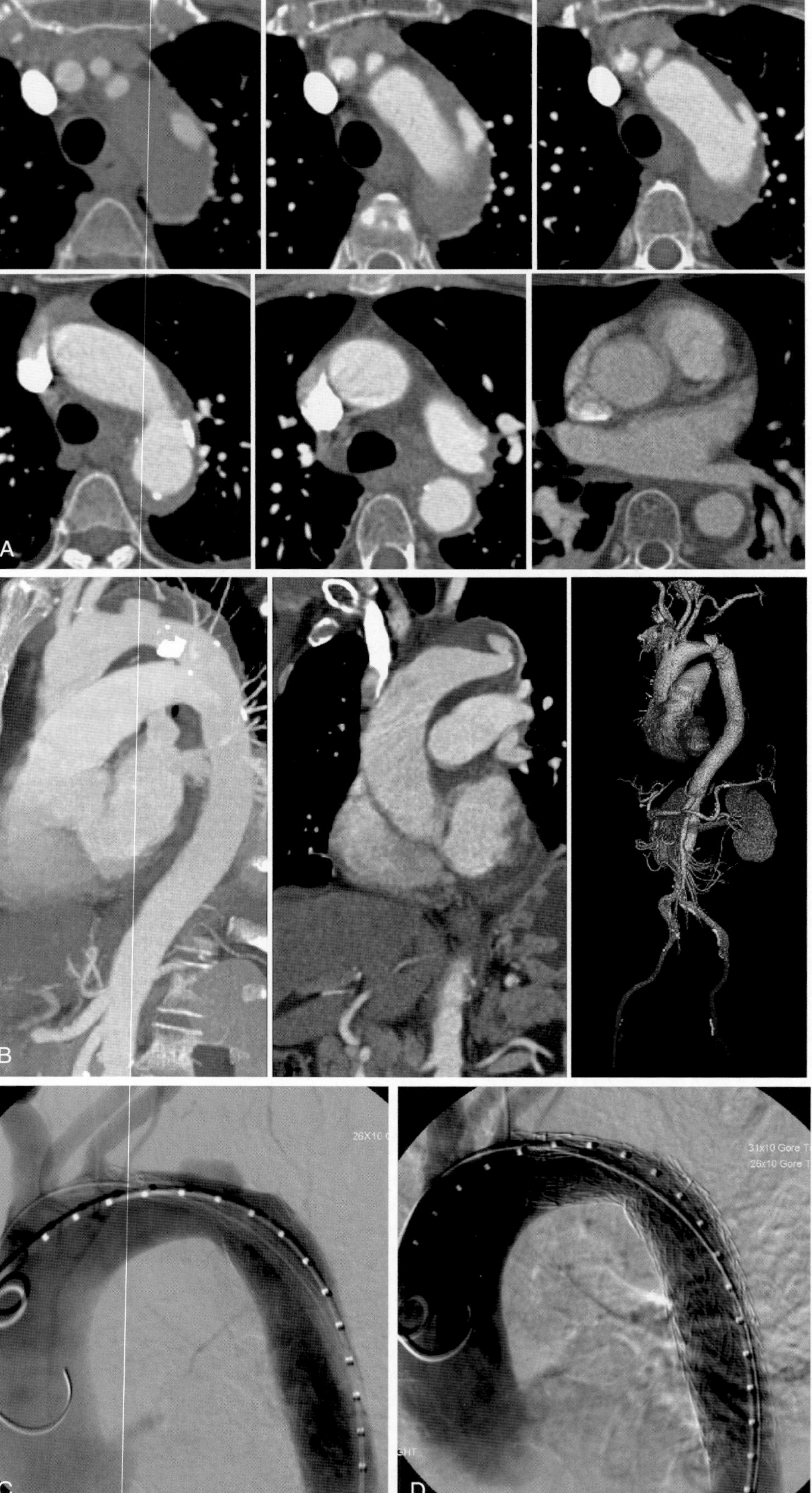

Figure 31-8. A 65-year-old woman with acute aortic syndrome and dissection variant; manifestations include back pain and hypertension associated with an ulcer-like projection in the aortic arch and intramural hematoma. **A,** Axial computer tomography (CT) images demonstrate a breach in the intimal integrity along the greater curvature of the arch with associated thick circumferential hematoma within the wall of the aorta. **B,** Three-dimensional reconstructions of the CT data display the lesion in a typical location for a primary entry tear in type B dissection. **C,** Aortogram in the left anterior oblique projection delineates the abnormality before placement of the proximal stent graft. **D,** Completion study shows a good result following stent graft deployment over the defect.

RECENT ENDOVASCULAR EXPERIENCE

To date, randomized clinical trials comparing early endovascular therapy versus medical therapy for uncomplicated type B aortic dissections are lacking. However, multiple clinical cohort reports include patients treated initially with endovascular therapy. These reports are providing insight into what we may expect from early endotherapy.

In 2001, Hausegger reported five patients with type B aortic dissection who were treated successfully with endovascular stent grafting.[44] However, only two of five patients had uncomplicated cases. No immediate or late complications developed in these patients. Furthermore, no aneurysms developed in the uncomplicated patients. In contrast, an aneurysm was reported in one of the complicated patients who initially had intractable pain. Although limited by a small sample size and use of a single device (Talent, Medtronic, Santa Rosa, California), this study introduced the prophylactic use of endovascular stent grafts in uncomplicated type B dissections.

Between 1996 and 2001, Palma et al. studied 70 patients who were treated for aortic dissection.[45] They found that 58 had type B dissections but only 3 of the 58 patients were performed electively for uncomplicated cases (large flow volume in the false lumen). Although this study did not independently assess uncomplicated cases, it did demonstrate the efficacy of stent graft placement for type B dissection and a low complication rate.

Technical success for endovascular therapy as defined by exclusion of the false lumen was 93%. Complications included conversion to open surgery (2), procedural-related deaths (2), delayed left subclavian artery compromise (1), stroke (2), access site vessel injury (2), deep venous thrombosis (1), mild transient renal failure (15), wound or dialysis catheter infection (3), and fever (15). No paraplegia occurred despite the use of multiple stent grafts in many patients. The authors concluded that endovascular stent grafting is an ideal option for both complicated and uncomplicated type B dissections, with considerably less risk than conventional open surgery.

In another study, Kato et al. reported the outcomes of 38 patients between 1997 and 2002.[42] There were 28 type B dissections, 8 with acute uncomplicated, 6 with acute complicated, and 14 were chronic type B dissections. Of the total, 24 patients underwent treatment within 1 month of diagnosis, while 14 underwent treatment between 1 month and 30 years after the initial diagnosis.

While the primary purpose of this study was to investigate the long-term outcomes of stent graft therapy for both acute and chronic dissection, several important observations regarding uncomplicated dissections deserve emphasis. The immediate outcome mortality (less than 30 days), intraoperative complications (stroke, intimal injury), and postoperative complications (aorta and nonaorta related) were significantly higher in patients with complicated dissection compared to those with uncomplicated dissection. The early and late complication rates were significantly lower in chronic cases as compared to acute cases (complicated or uncomplicated). In addition, late complications (aorta and nonaorta related) were comparable between complicated and uncomplicated patients. We contend that uncomplicated cases are best treated after 1 month when the adventitia and aortic flap are not so fragile as in the acute phase.

In a study conducted at a single institution in Italy, Totaro et al. reported 32 patients with either descending thoracic aneurysm or type B dissection who underwent endovascular stent graft repair.[43] The researchers enrolled 25 patients with type B dissection. Five underwent repair in the acute phase (defined as less than 2 weeks) and 20 underwent repair during the subacute phase (defined as more than 2 weeks and less than 2 months).

Although limited by use of a single stent graft (Excluder, WL Gore, Flagstaff, Arizona), the study yielded a 100% technical success rate and a low complication rate. Complications included 1 intraoperative retrograde dissection, 10 cases of primary endoleak (7 successfully treated, 3 with subsequent spontaneous thrombosis), and 8 cases of access site infection. As demonstrated in numerous other studies, there were no cases of paraplegia. To reduce complications, the authors argue strongly for a week of antihypertensive therapy before intervention in the setting of acute, uncomplicated type B aortic dissection. Unlike most, this group uses endovascular therapy as a first-line approach for all uncomplicated type B dissections.[46]

Between 1997 and 2000, Shimono et al. of Japan reported another 37 patients with acute and chronic aortic dissection treated with endotherapy.[39] The primary goals for treating acute dissections were to lower the complication risk of an emergent operation and to prevent subsequent aortic aneurysmal dilatation. Of the 37 patients, 24 were acute and 13 were chronic. Within the acute subset, 8 were without complication. Acute uncomplicated cases were treated if the aortic size was more than 40 mm, which increases the risk of continued aneurysmal dilation in the chronic phase. Chronic dissections were treated if they contained ulcer-like projections or maintained a maximal diameter greater than 50 mm. Complicated cases received intervention on the day of admission, but uncomplicated cases were treated electively following extensive evaluation with noninvasive imaging.

Follow-up evaluation with CT was performed at 4 weeks, 3 and 6 months, and yearly, with a mean follow-up of 24.5 months. There was a single death, likely related to preoperative morbidities. No early complications were observed in the uncomplicated acute onset group, in contrast to 18.8% in the complicated acute group and 7.7% in the chronic group. Endoleaks were more common in the acute onset cases than in the chronic cases. Complications related to the stent graft were more common in the complicated acute group (20%) relative to the uncomplicated acute group (12.5%) and the chronic group (0%). In addition, final CT imaging (mean follow-up 21.5 months) revealed complete or partial thrombosis of the false lumen in 94% overall, with a reduction (more than 5 mm) in aortic diameter observed in 88% of uncomplicated acute patients in contrast to 93% of acute complicated patients and 85% of chronic dissections.

All of these studies validated the efficacy of stent grafting not only in the chronic dissections but also in acute uncomplicated dissections. One additional study encouraged the final decision to proceed with the INSTEAD Trial. In 2002, Bortone et al. described the outcomes of acute and chronic type B aortic dissections treated electively.[38] While not explicitly stated, the elective nature of these procedures suggests that these were not complicated dissections. A single mortality was reported on a patient with substantial comorbidities that received delayed stent graft intervention. Technical success rate was achieved in

100% of patients who underwent endovascular repair within 2 weeks of the initial diagnosis. The complication rate was low, with no immediate life-threatening complications. No paraplegia occurred. Closure of the false lumen was attained in all patients at 3 months. The high technical success and relatively low complication rate in this study provided the foundation for the later INSTEAD Trial.

The European INSTEAD Trial is a seven-center, prospective, randomized trial investigating the use of stent grafts with adjunctive medical therapy versus medical therapy alone in patients with uncomplicated type B aortic dissections.[33] Although limited by the exclusive use of the Medtronic Talent stent graft, this trial is the most comprehensive study to date evaluating the use of stent grafts in this population. For the trial, 136 patients will be enrolled and followed at 3-, 12-, and 24-month intervals. Patients must have an uncomplicated type B dissection with a patent false lumen older than 2 weeks and less than 52 weeks. Dissections less than 14 days of age often thrombose spontaneously, thus conferring a better prognosis. In addition, those greater than 52 weeks of age are less amenable to intervention secondary to a thickened, fibrotic dissection flap.[33,34]

Early results are encouraging. Christoph Nienaber reported a near-100% initial success of tear-entry closure with no procedural mortality.[40] True lumen enlargement occurred in 92% and reduction of the false lumen in 63% of patients. Although 16% of patients in the stent graft arm experienced overall aortic expansion of greater than 5 mm, none required surgical or endovascular revision before discharge. At 3 months, five deaths were reported in the stent graft arm but only two were attributable to dissection or other aortic complications. No deaths occurred in the medical therapy group. At 3 months, 52% of patients had total thrombosis of the false lumen, while 27% had partial thrombosis. At the primary endpoint assessment of all-cause mortality at 1 year, no statistically significant difference appeared between the two groups. However, a definite trend favored medical management. The death rate at 1 year in the medical control group was 3% (2 out of 66) compared 10% (7 out of 70) in the endograft group. The 30-day postimplant mortality rate was 5.7% (4 out of 70).

Many variables affect the interpretation of these results. The mean time between diagnosis of dissection and randomization for the stent graft cohort was 57.3 days. This means that many patients enrolled did not have stent graft placement until 2 months from initial diagnosis. In addition, more than 80% of the enrolled patients were asymptomatic. Thus, this does not allow a comparison of treatments for the patients who are arguably at increased risk of deterioration despite their initial uncomplicated course, i.e., those with persistent symptoms and those within the first 2 weeks after the onset of symptoms. If you envision a subgroup of uncomplicated, acute type B patients who might benefit from an interventional approach beyond medical therapy, it would most likely consist of symptomatic individuals within the first 2 weeks of diagnosis who have imaging evidence of aortic enlargement over this initial period of observation.

In addition, over the first 12 months of follow-up, seven patients (10% to 12%) crossed over from medical therapy to have stent graft placement. The reasons for crossover to the interventional arm were visceral malperfusion, aortic expansion, and aortic rupture. No patient who crossed over to the stent graft therapy from the medical arm died in the first year of follow-up. In the stent graft group, 95% of the patients had thrombosis of the thoracic aortic false lumen (partial or complete) observed on imaging studies at 1 year.

The preliminary conclusions of the INSTEAD investigators for this heterogeneous group of chronic, uncomplicated type B dissections are (1) initial antihypertensive medical treatment, (2) serial imaging to identify developing complications of aneurysm and malperfusion, and (3) deferred stent graft implantation as an option for patients failing to respond to medical therapy. This study is one step in defining the legitimate roles of medical, interventional, and open surgical therapies in clearly delineated subgroups of aortic dissection.

CURRENT PERSPECTIVE ON ENDOVASCULAR THERAPY

The studies reviewed in this chapter demonstrate that endovascular stent grafting is a promising approach to uncomplicated type B dissections. The advantages may be reducing short-term mortality and avoiding late complications, including redissection, rupture, and late surgical repair.[41]

Despite the endovascular trends in managing type B aortic dissections, medical therapy as a first-line treatment in uncomplicated type B dissections remains relatively unchallenged. This approach reflects the adequacy of this medical tactic for short-term results. However, approximately 20% to 30% of patients with uncomplicated dissections are ultimately complicated by aneurysmal dilatation, which underscores the need for a long-term focus.[5,15,47]

Essential to successful stent grafting is proper patient selection, appropriate technique, and optimal timing. Preliminary work suggests that patients with uncomplicated dissections should be stratified based on their likelihood of long-term complications. Risk stratification for late aneurysmal development and rupture based on aortic diameter supports this practice.[39,41] Moreover, appropriate case selection based on the dissection anatomy (tortuosity and involvement of branch vessels), adequate peripheral access, and patient comorbidities is essential for achieving good results.

Endovascular technique is critical for success. Appropriate technique mandates proximal occlusion of the entry tear for decompression of the false lumen. Moreover, minimization of the angle between the inferior portion of the stent graft and the native aortic wall minimizes iatrogenic stress, thus lowering subsequent aneurysmal dilatation. Undoubtedly, innovations in stent graft technology with greater customization and flexibility will improve technical outcomes. The future role of endovascular therapy in managing type B aortic dissections is assured with advances in technology and technique.

References

1. Wong DR, Lermaire SA, Coselli JS. Managing dissections of the thoracic aorta. *Am Surg* 2008;74(5):364-380.
2. Clouse WD, Hallett JW, Schaff H, et al. Acute aortic dissections: the most common aortic catastrophe? *Mayo Clin Proc* 2003;79:176-180.
3. Meszaros I, Morocz J, Szlavi J, et al. Epidemiology and clinicopathology of aortic dissection. *Chest* 2000;117:1271-1278.
4. Hagan PG, Nienaber CA, Isselbacher EM, et al. The International Registry of Acute Aortic Dissection (IRAD): new insights into an old disease. *JAMA* 2000;283:897-903.
5. Genoni M, Paul M, Jenn R, et al. Chronic beta-blocker therapy improves outcome and reduces treatment costs in chronic type B dissection. *Eur J Cardiothorac Surg* 2001;19:606-610.

6. Mehta RH, Manfredini R, Hassan F, et al. Chronobiological patterns of acute aortic dissection. *Circulation* 2002;106:1110-1115.
7. Reed D, Reed C, Stemmerman G, et al. Are aortic aneurysms caused by atherosclerosis? *Circulation* 1992;85:205-211.
8. Nallamothu BK, Kofias TJ, Eagle KA. Of nicks and time. *N Engl J Med* 2001;345:359-363.
9. Atkins MD, Black JH, Cambria RP. Aortic dissection: perspective in the era of stent-graft repair. *J Vasc Surg* 2006;43(Suppl 2):A30-A43.
10. Tsai TT, Fattori R, Trimarchii S, et al. for the International Registry of Acute Aortic Dissection (IRAD). Long-term survival in patients presenting with type A acute aortic dissection. *Circulation* 2006;114(21):2226-2231.
11. Tsai TT, Evangelista A, Nienaber CA, et al. for the International Registry of Acute Aortic Dissection Partial thrombosis of the false lumen in patients with acute type B dissection. *N Engl J Med* 2007;357:349-359.
12. Tsai TT, Schlicht MS, Khanafer K, et al. Tear size and location impacts false lumen pressure in an ex vivo model of chronic type B aortic dissection. *J Vasc Surg* 2008;47(4):844-851.
13. Greenberg R. Treatment of aortic dissections with endovascular stent grafts. *Semin Vasc Surg* 2002;15:122-127.
14. Svensson LG, Kouchoukos NT, Miller DC, et al., for the Society of Thoracic Surgeons Endovascular Surgery Task Force. Expert consensus document on the treatment of descending thoracic aortic disease using endovascular stent-grafts. *Ann Thorac Surg* 2008;85(Suppl 1):S1-S41.
15. Juvonen T, Ergin MA, Galla JD, et al. Risk factors for rupture of chronic type B dissections. *J Thorac Cardiovasc Surg* 1999;117(4):776-786.
16. Personal communication to Kenneth Cherry, 1983.
17. De Bakey ME, Cooley DA, Creech O Jr. Surgical considerations of dissecting aneurysm of the aorta. *Ann Surg* 1955;142:586-610.
18. Wheat MW Jr, Palmer RF, Bartley TD, Seelman RC. Treatment of dissecting aneurysms of the aorta without surgery. *J Thorac Cardiovasc Surg* 1965;50:364-373.
19. Estrera AL, Miller CC, Goodrick J, et al. Update on outcomes of acute type B aortic dissection. *Ann Thorac Surg* 2007;83(2):5842-5845, discussion, 5846-5850.
20. Tefera G, Acher CW, Hoch JR, et al. Effectiveness of intensive medical therapy in type B aortic dissection: a single-center experience. *J Vasc Surg* 2007;45(6):1114-1119.
21. Januzzi H, Movsowitz HD, Choi J, et al. Significance of recurrent pain in acute type B aortic dissection. *Am J Cardiol* 2001;87:930-933.
22. Elefteriades JA, Hartleroad J, Gusberg RJ, et al. Long-term experience with descending aortic dissection: the complication-specific approach. *Ann Thorac Surg* 1992;53(1):11-21.
23. Bozinovski J, Coselli JS. Outcomes and survival in surgical treatment of descending thoracic aorta with acute dissection. *Ann Thorac Surg* 2008;85(3):965-970. discussion, 970-971.
24. Panneton JM, Teh SH, Cherry KJ, et al. Aortic fenestration for acute or chronic aortic dissection: an uncommon but effective procedure. *J Vasc Surg* 2000;32(4):711-721.
25. Elefteriades JA, Hammond GL, Gusberg RJ, et al. Fenestration revisited: a safe and effective procedure for descending aortic dissection. *Arch Surg* 1990;125:786-790.
26. Crawford ES. The diagnosis and management of aortic dissections. *JAMA* 1990;264:2537-2541.
27. Lansman SL, Hagl C, Fink D, et al. Acute type B aortic dissection: surgical therapy. *Ann Thorac Surg* 1833-1835;2002(Suppl):74, discussion, 1857-1863.
28. Kasirajan K, Milner R, Veeraswamy R, Chaikof E. *Thoracic endografts for chronic type B dissection. Presented at the Society for Vascular Surgery Annual Meeting*. San Diego: California; June 2008.
29. Dake MD, Kato N, Mitchell RS, et al. Endovascular stent-graft placement for the treatment of acute aortic dissection. *N Engl J Med* 1999;340:1546-1552.
30. Nienaber CA, Fattori R, Lung G, et al. Nonsurgical reconstruction of thoracic aortic dissection by stent-graft placement. *N Engl J Med* 1999;340:1539-1545.
31. Mukherjee D, Eagle KA. Aortic dissection: an update. *Curr Probl Cardiol* 2005;30:287-325.
32. Tsai TT, Nienaber CA, Eagle KA. Acute aortic syndromes. *Circulation* 2005;112:3802-3813.
33. Nienaber CA, Zannetti S, Barbieri B, et al. Investigation of stent grafts in patients with type B aortic dissection: design of the INSTEAD trial—a prospective, multicenter European randomized trial. *Am Heart J* 2005;149(4):592-599.
34. Wang DS, Dake MD. *Abrams' angiography interventional radiology.* 2nd ed. Baum S, Pentecost MJ, eds. Philadelphia: Lippincott Williams & Wilkins; 2006:415-455.
35. Erbel R, Oelert H, Meyer J, et al. Effect of medical and surgical therapy on aortic dissection evaluated by transesophageal echocardiography: implications for prognosis and therapy—the European Cooperative Study Group on Echocardiography. *Circulation* 1993;87:1604-1615.
36. Ergin MA, Phillips RA, Galla JD, et al. Significance of distal false lumen after type A dissection repair. *Ann Thorac Surg* 1994;57:820-824, discussion, 825.
37. Williams DM, Andrews JC, Marx MV, et al. Creation of reentry tears in aortic dissection by means of percutaneous balloon fenestration: gross anatomic and histologic considerations. *J Vasc Interv Radiol* 1993;4:75-83.
38. Bortone AS, Schena S, D'Agostino D, et al. Immediate versus delayed endovascular treatment of post-traumatic aortic pseudoaneurysms and type B dissections: retrospective analysis and premises to the upcoming European trial. *Circulation* 2002;106:234-240.
39. Shimono T, Kato N, Yasuda F, et al. Transluminal stent graft placements for the treatments of acute onset and chronic aortic dissection. *Circulation* 2002;106(Suppl 1):I241-I247.
40. Nienaber CA, Ince H, Petzsch M, et al. Endovascular treatment of acute aortic syndrome. *Endovasc Today* 2003;(Suppl):12-15.
41. Kato N, Hirano T, Shimono T, et al. Treatment of chronic type B aortic dissection with endovascular stent graft placement. *Cardiovasc Intervent Radiol* 2000;23:60-62.
42. Kato N, Shimono T, Hirano T, et al. Midterm results of stent graft repair of acute and chronic aortic dissection with descending tear: the complication-specific approach. *J Thorac Cardiovasc Surg* 2002;124:306-312.
43. Totaro M, Mazzesi G, Marullo AG, et al. Endoluminal stent grafting of the descending thoracic aorta. *Ital Heart J* 2002;3(6):366-369.
44. Hausegger KA, Tisenhausen K, Schedlbauer P, et al. Treatment of acute aortic type B dissection with stent grafts. *Cardiovasc Intervent Radiol* 2001;24:306-312.
45. Palma JH, Marcondes de Souza JA, Rodrigues Alves CM, et al. Self-expandable aortic stent grafts for treatment of descending aortic dissections. *Ann Thorac Surg* 2002;73:1138-1142.
46. Totaro M, Miraldi F, Fanelli F, Mazzesi G. Emergency surgery for retrograde extension of type B dissection after endovascular stent graft repair: case report. *Eur J Cardiothorac Surg* 2001;20:1057-1058.
47. Grabenwoger M, Fleck T, Czerny M, et al. Endovascular stent graft placement in patients with acute thoracic aortic syndromes. *Eur J Cardiothorac Surg* 2003;23:788-793.

chapter

32

Laparoscopic Abdominal Aortic Surgery

Olivier Goëau-Brissonnière, MD, PhD • Marc Coggia, MD

Key Points

- Videoscopic training
- Videoscopic approaches of the abdominal aorta
- Transperitoneal videoscopic approaches
- Transperitoneal retrocolic approach
- Transperitoneal retrorenal approach
- Transperitoneal direct approach
- Retroperitoneoscopic approach
- Choice of videoscopic approach
- Videoscopic aortic repair
- Videoscopic repair for abdominal aortic aneurysms through a transperitoneal retrorenal approach
- Tube graft implantation
- Juxtarenal abdominal aortic aneurysms
- Technical variations
- Aortic repair through transperitoneal retrocolic and transperitoneal direct approaches
- Aortic repair through a retroperitoneoscopic approach
- Conversion to open direct repair
- Conclusion

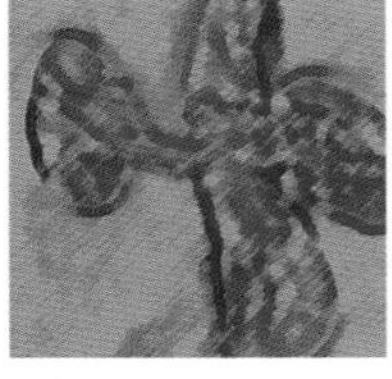

Open direct repair (ODR) is still considered the most reliable and durable technique to treat severe aortoiliac occlusive disease (AIOD) and abdominal aortic aneurysms (AAAs).[1,2] Postoperative mortality is less than 5%, and long-term results are excellent. However, the systemic morbidity of ODR remains substantial.[2] Complications are related to the surgical approach in about 30% of cases. The underlying premise of minimally invasive techniques, either endovascular or videoscopic, is to decrease operative trauma related to ODR and to reduce perioperative morbidity. Endovascular techniques have been increasingly used since 1990.[3] Their benefits in terms of postoperative morbidity and mortality have been demonstrated. They are now considered by their advocates to be the treatment of choice for most AIOD patients. For AAA, uncertainties remain concerning the mid- and long-term benefits of endovascular repair in patients suitable for ODR.[4-10]

Videoscopy recently entered the field of vascular surgery. As in other specialties, its basic concept is to decrease operative trauma by avoidance of large abdominal or lumbar incisions. Potential benefits of videoscopy are faster recovery, reduced pain, and decreased incidence of abdominal, intestinal, and pulmonary complications. In the field of minimally invasive aortic surgery, videoscopy has a major advantage over endovascular techniques, which is the performance of a proven and durable surgical technique. In addition, we can expect excellent long-term results similar to those of ODR. However, except for some pioneers,[11-24] few vascular teams have entered this new field of aortic surgery, especially for AAA repair. Specific difficulties of aortic surgery have discouraged vascular surgeons because most of them lack of advanced videoscopic skills. Nevertheless, videoscopic aortic surgery is feasible, with excellent results once training has been undertaken and the learning curve has been overcome.

VIDEOSCOPIC TRAINING

Gaining videoscopic skills is of particular importance for vascular surgeons because they generally lack training and experience in videoscopic surgery. It is important to remember that performance of anastomoses under videoscopy is probably the most difficult step during general, urological, or vascular surgery. Additional challenges in vascular surgery relate to the time required for videoscopic anastomosis, with attendant increases in aortic clamping time, resultant lower limb ischemia, and cardiac afterload. Moreover, aortoprosthetic anastomosis requires strict adherence to technical principles to avoid immediate leakage and to ensure strength, patency, and durability. This technical challenge has discouraged most vascular surgeons, while others are awaiting the development of anastomotic devices with either clips or staples. Use of such devices is still under evaluation and is limited by properties of the diseased aortic wall, especially if brittle or calcified. Moreover, anastomotic devices are only useful for the performance of videoscopic anastomoses. It is important to remember that a videoscopic aortic procedure cannot be confined to the aortoprosthetic anastomoses. Other important videoscopic skills are necessary, especially exposure of the aorta and preparation of anastomotic sites.

Videoscopic suturing requires thorough training to gain all requisite videoscopic skills. The equipment needs are simple:

- Videoscope, camera, monitor, and light, but a compact system is manufactured by Storz (Medipack), and a homemade video system is usable with a simple camcorder
- Needle holder, grasping forceps, and scissors
- Pelvitrainer with the same ergonomics as human aortic procedures
- Prostheses and stitches

Training consists of practicing the performance of end-to-end, end-to-side, or both types of anastomoses similar to those of human procedures and with the same preparation of stitches. Such training is possible in the office, in the operating room, or at home. We recommend daily training for a minimum of 3 months before performing the first human procedure. Once baseline expertise is gained, it is possible to proceed with discontinuous training periods, but this depends on the surgeon's skill set. Long-term, ongoing training is essential because vascular surgeons lack the simple weekly laparoscopic procedures such as cholecystectomy that serve to maintain their level of expertise.

Training on animals or cadavers is also important to gain expertise in all steps of videoscopic aortic procedures. Such training is usually organized during courses and workshops. We encourage vascular surgeons to attend such courses.

VIDEOSCOPIC APPROACHES OF THE ABDOMINAL AORTA

Videoscopic approaches to the abdominal aorta use the same anatomical landmarks and surgical dissection planes as open surgery. These approaches are well known by vascular surgeons, either transperitoneal or retroperitoneal. Four approaches have been described (Figure 32-1): transperitoneal retrocolic (TPRC), transperitoneal retrorenal (TPRR), transperitoneal direct (TPD), and retroperitoneoscopic (RP). The main differences among pioneers who reported these videoscopic approaches were the technical tools used to achieve and maintain a stable aortic exposure. Dion and Gracia reported on the peritoneal apron technique in 1997.[11] In this technique, the patient is slightly tilted to the right and the operator stands

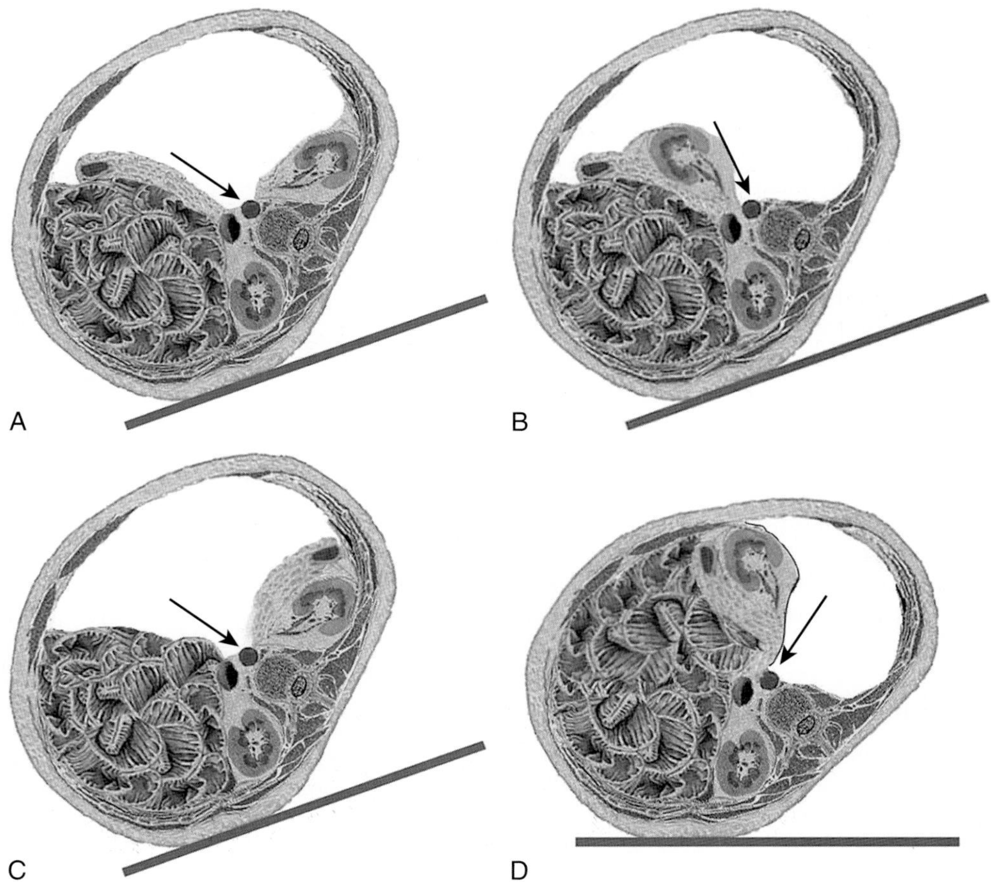

Figure 32-1. Transverse sections showing the videoscopic approaches to the abdominal aorta. **A,** Transperitoneal left retrocolic. **B,** Transperitoneal left retrorenal. **C,** Transperitoneal direct. **D,** Retroperitoneoscopic.

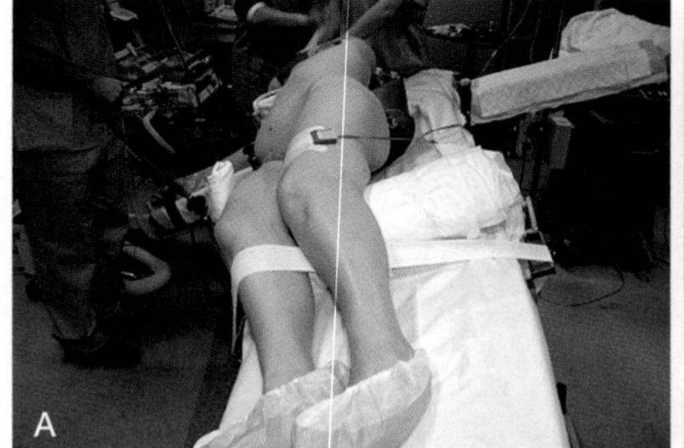

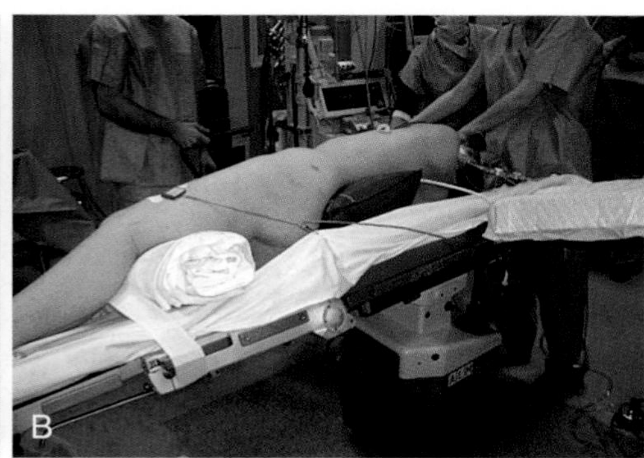

Figure 32-2. Operative views showing the positioning of the patient in the right lateral decubitus position with the use of an inflatable pillow.

on the left side of the patient. A peritoneal apron is made with the left parietal peritoneum sutured to the right abdominal wall. After creation of the peritoneal apron, the aorta is approached through a left retroperitoneal route. The kidney is only freed on its inferior and lateral surface, and its lower pole is mobilized cephalad. In 2003, Dion and colleagues modified the approach using the apron technique with a TPRC.[25] More recently, Stadler et al.[26] described the use of the apron technique for TPD. They made the peritoneal apron with the peritoneum lying on the left mesocolon.

Alimi et al.,[27] Barbera et al.,[28] and Cau et al.[29] described various intestinal retractors to allow a TPD. In the technique described by Barbera et al., the patient is tilted in Trendelenburg position and the small bowel is retracted upward. Alimi et al. and Cau et al. used intestinal retractors to maintain the small bowel in the right part of the abdomen, with the patient slightly tilted to the right and the operator standing on the left, just as in open surgery. In 1999, Said et al.,[30] in a cadaver study, used a TPRC with retractors to maintain the left mesocolon. In this technique, the patient was slightly tilted to the right and operator stood on the left of the patient. In 2002, we and our colleagues described a new and simple tool to maintain the viscera out of the operative field, which was positioning the patient in 80-degree right lateral decubitus (RLD).[21] With this installation, viscera drop into the right part of the abdomen and the operative field remains free from intrusion of intraabdominal organs. Additional tools are unnecessary to maintain exposure. With the patient in RLD, the surgeon stands on the right side of the patient and is not bothered by the orientation of surgical instruments. Initially, we described RLD for TPRC.[21] In 2004 and 2005, we reported RLD for TPRR[31] and TPD,[32] respectively.

The final videoscopic approach to the aorta is RP, first reported by Edoga.[32a] During the RP approach, no special tools are required. Edoga first used this approach for videoscopically assisted AAA repair. We reported RP for total AAA and AIOD repair in 2005.[33]

Transperitoneal Videoscopic Approaches

For transperitoneal approaches, we always use the RLD. The patient is placed in dorsal decubitus position with an inflatable pillow (Pelvic-Tilt, OR Comfort, Glen Ridge, New Jersey) placed behind the left flank. Insufflation of the pillow gives a 50- to 60-degree rotation of the abdomen. A maximal right rotation of the operating table affords an abdominal slope of 80 degrees (Figure 32-2). The operator faces the patient's abdomen and is unencumbered by orientation of surgical instruments. The assistant camera stands in front of the operator. The second assistant stands to the right of the operating surgeon (Figure 32-3).

We usually use a blind technique to create the pneumoperitoneum. A Veress needle is introduced 3 cm below the costal margin in the left midclavicular line, and the pneumoperitoneum is insufflated up to 14 mm Hg. In cases of previous abdominal scars, the first port is positioned using an open technique in the left anterior axillary line just below the costal margin. This port is used both to create the pneumoperitoneum and to introduce the endoscope (Storz-France, Paris, France). The major drawback of the open technique is that port site moves downward and medially during insufflation of the pneumoperitoneum.

Transperitoneal Retrocolic Approach

Positioning of ports depends on the aortic lesion type.[21] We use only 10-mm ports because of the need for large instruments. For AIOD, port 1 is positioned 3 cm below the costal margin in the anterior axillary line. Ports 2 and 3, about 8 cm

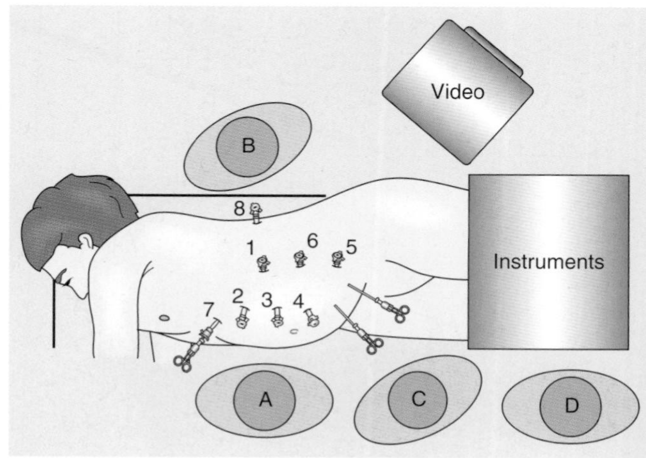

Figure 32-3. Basic operating room setup. **A,** Operating surgeon. **B,** Assistant for the laparoscope. **C,** Assistant for the instrumentation. **D,** Nurse. **1,** A 10-mm port for the laparoscope. **2** and **3,** The 10-mm ports for operator instruments. **4** and **5,** The 10-mm ports for assistant instrumentation. **6,** A 10-mm port for large aneurysms used for assistant instrumentation, laparoscope, or operator instruments. **7,** A 10-mm port for the endoretractor or proximal laparoscopic clamp. **8,** A 10-mm port for the proximal laparoscopic clamp.

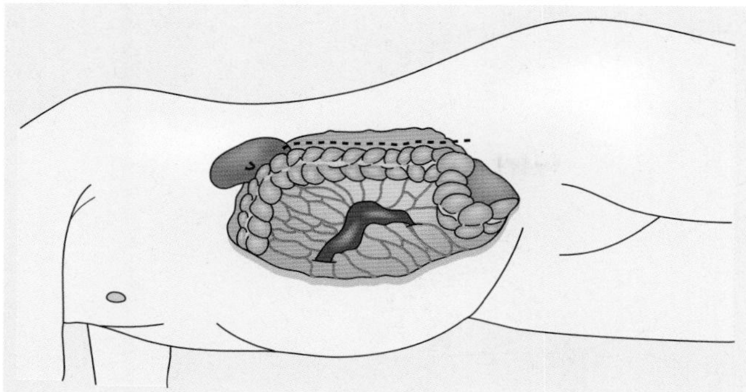

Figure 32-4. Incision of the parietal pneumoperitoneum in the left paracolic gutter during transperitoneal retrorenal and transperitoneal retrocolic procedures.

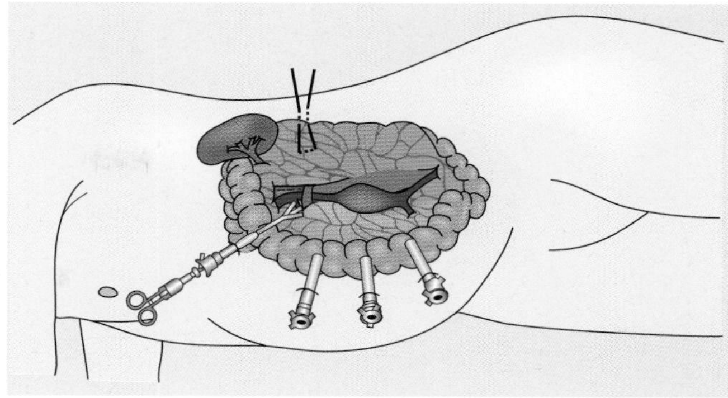

Figure 32-6. Exposure of the abdominal aortic aneurysm via the transperitoneal retrocolic approach.

apart, are placed at the supraumbilical and left paramedian level to insert operator instruments. Port 4 is positioned below the navel to introduce assistant instruments and the distal aortic clamp. Port 5 is placed in the left lower abdomen to insert assistant instruments. Finally, port 6 is placed in the subxiphoid area. It has two functions. At the beginning of the procedure, an endoretractor (Endoretract II, USSC, Autosuture, Elancourt, France) is introduced through this port to maintain the left mesocolon. During aortic repair, this port is used to introduce the proximal aortic clamp.

For AAA repair, port 1 is placed just below the costal margin, especially if the aortic neck is short or angulated. Just before the introduction of this port, abdominal pressure is elevated to 20 mm Hg to increase parietal strength and to avoid aortic injury. Once the first port is placed, pneumoperitoneal pressure is decreased to 14 mm Hg. An additional port (port 7) is introduced between ports 1 and 5 to insert instruments, an endoscope, or both, especially if distal aortic or common iliac anastomoses are needed.

A peritoneal incision is made in the left paracolic gutter up to the splenic flexure (Figure 32-4). By elevating and displacing the left colon, the avascular plane of the Toldt fascia is entered and developed medially to reach the internal edge of the kidney. The left gonadal vein provides a useful landmark because it leads to the left renal vein. Once the left renal vein is visualized, we always perform two steps to maintain the exposure. First, an endoretractor (Endoretract II) is positioned through port 7, which allows the surgeon to contain the left mesocolon. Then we place a stitch in Gerota's fascia and pull it out through the left abdominal wall. Traction on this stitch allows retraction of the kidney and opens the operative field in front of preaortic ganglia (Figure 32-5). Due to the RLD, the small bowel and left mesocolon drop to the right side of the abdomen. Dissection of the aorta is then conducted cranially to the left renal artery and caudally to the left iliac artery.

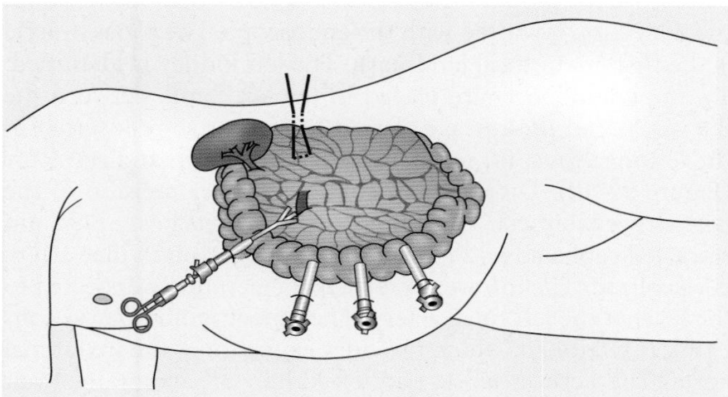

Figure 32-5. Two steps of the transperitoneal retrocolic approach: (1) an endoretractor is positioned through port 7 to contain the left mesocolon and (2) a stitch is placed in Gerota's fascia and pulled out through the left abdominal wall.

The inferior mesenteric artery is dissected and directed toward the mesocolon. The final step is exposure of the right common iliac artery, either to prepare the graft limb tunnel or to perform an anastomosis. For this step, we always perform the same maneuvers. The assistant introduces the endoretractor through port 4 and the suction device in port 5. The assistant points these two instruments toward the common iliac artery and retracts the left mesocolon. The operator conducts the dissection as far distally as possible, until the right ureter is crossed. Once this dissection is complete, exposure of the aorta is maintained by traction on additional stitches placed in the paraaortic fat (Figure 32-6).

After achieving exposure, the patient is returned to the dorsal decubitus position. The pillow is deflated and the operating table is rotated to the left, which allows a conventional approach to iliac or femoral arteries if needed.

Transperitoneal Retrorenal Approach

Positioning of ports for TPRR is quite similar to the positioning for TPRC.[31] Port 1 is positioned 2 cm medially from the line of the anterosuperior iliac spine. Other ports are positioned in the same way as for TPRC but slightly translated laterally. We do not place port 6 at the beginning of the procedure because we wait for positioning of the spleen after completion of the mediovisceral rotation. A peritoneal incision is made in the left paracolic gutter up to the level of the diaphragm. We enter the retroperitoneal plane in the iliac fossa and visualize the left ureter and iliac artery. Left retrorenal dissection is conducted cranially and medially from the psoas muscle after incision of the retrorenal fascia. We perform a complete rather than a partial right medial visceral rotation to avoid a capsular tear of the spleen during visceral retraction. Moreover, this maneuver increases working space. Due to the RLD, the small bowel, the left mesocolon, the left kidney, and the spleen drop

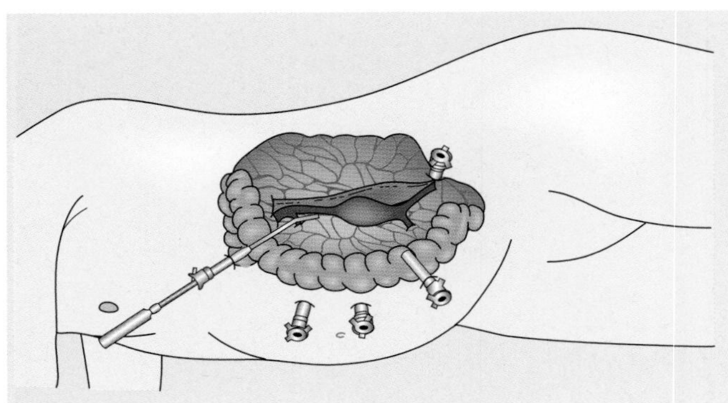

Figure 32-7. Exposure of the abdominal aortic aneurysm via the transperitoneal retrorenal approach. An endoretractor is placed through port 7 to contain the viscera.

into the right part of the abdomen (Figure 32-7). We place a stitch in the left perirenal fat and pull it out through the right abdominal wall. It allows the viscera to be contained. Dissection of the aorta is conducted cranially from the left iliac to the left renal artery. We section the left lumbar splanchnic nerve, which overlies the left side of the aorta. Just below the left renal artery, the renoazygolumbar venous trunk often crosses the left side of the aorta; its transection provides (1) complete retraction of the kidney without risk of bleeding and (2) dissection of the juxtarenal aorta. If needed, we develop the dissection cranially proximal to the left renal artery until the left crus of the diaphragm is reached. Division of the left crus provides exposure of the aortic visceral segment. Exposure of the right iliac artery is conducted as during a TPRC.

After achieving the dissection, subcostal port 6 is placed, taking care to avoid an iatrogenic injury to the spleen. We introduce an endoretractor (Endoretract II) through this port to contain the left kidney. The tip of the retractor is placed just below the left renal artery, which provides stable exposure of the juxtarenal aorta.

Transperitoneal Direct Approach

Positioning of ports for TPD is similar to the positioning for TPRC.[32] After abdominal exploration, the transverse mesocolon is elevated with a stitch pulled out through the left subcostal abdominal wall. A longitudinal incision of the retroperitoneum overlying the anterior aortic wall is made just

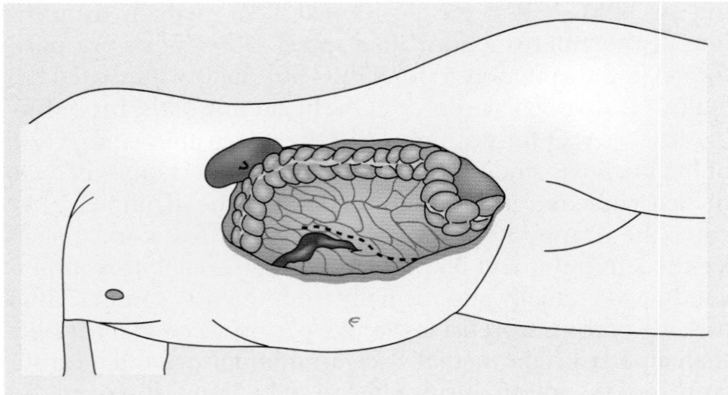

Figure 32-8. Incision of the posterior pneumoperitoneum during a transperitoneal direct procedure.

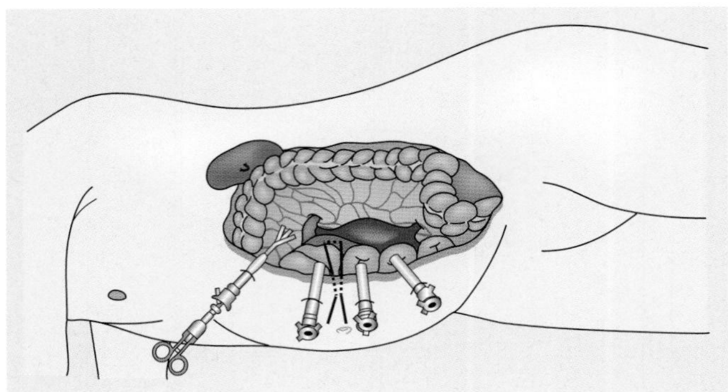

Figure 32-9. Exposure of the abdominal aortic aneurysm via a transperitoneal direct approach.

to the left of the mesentery (Figure 32-8). This incision is carried down to the iliac arteries. Another stitch is placed on the posterior peritoneum, near the duodenum, and pulled out through the right abdominal wall. If needed, an additional port is used to allow retraction of the small bowel (Endoretract II), introduced in the left flank or in the pelvis, in the right paramedian line. Intestinal retractors such as those described by Alimi et al.[27] or Cau et al.[29] can also be used to contain the small bowel. The aortic periadventitial plane is freed, and circumferential aortic dissection is performed from iliac arteries up to the left renal vein (Figure 32-9). After achieving aortoiliac dissection, the pillow is deflated and the operating table is rotated to the left, which enables conventional approaches to the femoral arteries. The patient is then returned to an RLD position for aortoiliac videoscopic reconstruction.

Retroperitoneoscopic Approach

With the RP approach, the patient is under general anesthesia and placed in a dorsal decubitus position with an inflatable pillow (Pelvic-Tilt) behind the left flank, which gives a 30-degree rotation of the abdomen.[33] The surgeon stands on the patient's left side, and the video monitor is viewed distally from the right side. The port is used to introduce the 45-degree endoscope (Storz-France), which is positioned using an open technique halfway between the costal margin and the anterosuperior iliac spine. A retroperitoneal blunt dissection is first performed to prepare the working space. After insufflation, the dissection is started with the endoscope. The psoas muscle is the first anatomical landmark. The left kidney is identified. Two operator ports are placed in the left flank, between the iliac crest and the ribcage. Two 10-mm ports are inserted in the left iliac fossa for assistant instrumentation and retractor (Figure 32-10). Dissection is conducted after incision of the left retrorenal fascia. The kidney is freed on its lower pole and retracted cephalad and medially. The left common iliac artery is visualized. The infrarenal aorta is then cranially dissected to the level of the left renal artery. The renoazygolumbar venous trunk is sectioned, which provides exposure of the juxtarenal aorta. The peritoneal sac and left kidney are maintained out of harm's way with a retractor (Endoretract II). The anterior surface of the right common iliac artery is dissected over a length of 3 to 5 cm if needed. As in conventional surgery, ligation of an occluded inferior mesenteric artery can expand the

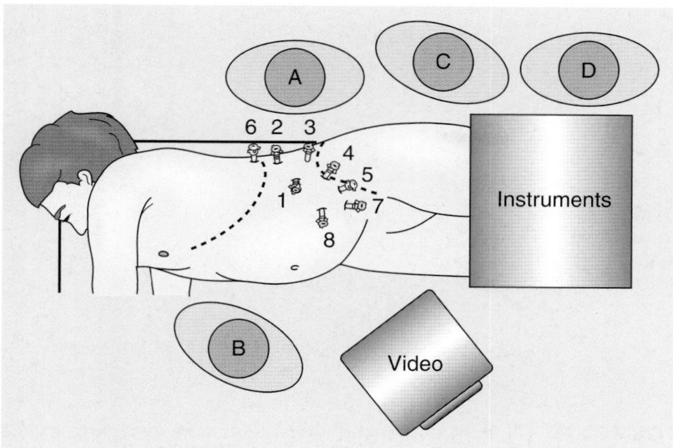

Figure 32-10. Basic operating room setup for the retroperitoneoscopic approach of the abdominal aorta. **A,** Operating surgeon. **B,** Assistant for the laparoscope. **C,** Assistant for the instrumentation. **D,** Nurse. **1,** A 10-mm port for the laparoscope. **2** and **3,** The 10-mm ports for operator instruments. **4** and **5,** The 10-mm ports for the assistant instrumentation. **6** to **8,** The 10-mm ports for proximal and iliac laparoscopic aortic clamps.

exposure of the right common iliac artery. After achieving the dissection, the pillow is deflated, which allows a conventional approach to femoral arteries if needed.

Choice of Videoscopic Approach

The approach is selected based on anatomical and patient considerations. TPRR is now our first choice. It provides broad exposure, especially when control of the juxtarenal aorta is needed. Dissection of the suprarenal or celiac aorta is conducted in line with the left side of the aorta after section of the left crus of the diaphragm. Unlike TPRC or TPD, neither the kidney nor the mesocolon blinds exposure of the left side of the aorta. This is of particular importance for control of lumbar arteries during AAA repair. At the end of the procedure, the viscera are permitted to fall back into place, providing optimal covering of the prosthesis.

TPRR is contraindicated in cases of perisplenic adhesions, the presence of a retroaortic left renal vein, or both. In such cases, we use the TPRC. TPRC is also indicated for concomitant left renal or superior mesenteric videoscopic bypass.[34]

In cases of hostile abdomen, we use the RP.[33] However, working space with RP is reduced, either externally for placement of ports or internally behind the peritoneal sac. For AAA repair, this approach is feasible but exceptionally difficult, and in such cases, conversion to open repair is often necessary. For these reasons, RP is rarely indicated, and even in cases of previous abdominal scars, we often try to enter the peritoneal cavity to perform a transperitoneal approach.

Finally, in a few selected cases we use the TPD.[18] This approach is theoretically the simplest approach, using common landmarks for vascular surgeons. However, this approach needs careful dissection close to intestine. Upward retraction of the transverse mesocolon is not always simple and needs two or more stitches. Exposure of the juxtarenal aorta is then difficult, especially for AAA with short or angulated necks. Use of different tools is essential to avoid the frequent prolapse of bowel loops into the operative field. The primary drawback of TPD is achieving coverage of the prosthesis, especially when the patient is thin. For these reasons, we only use TPD in cases of previous left nephrectomy when retrorenal and retrocolic dissection planes are blocked.

VIDEOSCOPIC AORTIC REPAIR

Videoscopic aortic repair is the second step of the procedure after completing the aortic arch. The two main challenges during this step are minimizing aortic cross-clamp time and reducing blood loss. We consider AAA repair through a TPRR to be the gold standard technique. We discuss specific technical tips and tricks using other videoscopic approaches.

Before aortic repair, we prepare specific stitches for anastomoses. We prepare two types of stitches using 3-0 or 4-0 polypropylene (Prolene Ethicon, Johnson-Johnson, Brussels, Belgium). Stitches for running sutures are between 18 and 22 cm in length and knotted on 10 × 10-mm Teflon or prosthetic pledgets. Stitches for single sutures are between 8 and 12 cm and knotted on small pledgets.

Videoscopic Repair for Abdominal Aortic Aneurysms through a Transperitoneal Retrorenal Approach

We describe as a gold standard a videoscopic aneurysmorrhaphy with tube graft implantation and then technical variations for other types of AAA.

Tube Graft Implantation

Once the aortic exposure is stable, three steps are prepared before clamping:

1. A stitch is placed through the right abdominal wall, and its needle is left free in the iliac fossa. It is later used for retraction of the aneurysmal sac.
2. Iliac clamps are introduced percutaneously in the left iliac fossa.
3. A conventional Dacron graft (Gelweave or Gelsoft Plus, Vascutek-Terumo, Inchinnan, Scotland) is prepared for an end-to-end anastomosis, and the body of the graft is secured to the distal extremity with a stitch.

Once these steps are achieved, proximal videoscopic clamp (Storz-France) is positioned either through subcostal port 6 or through an additional port placed via the left flank (Figures 32-11 and 32-12). After proximal clamping, we proceed methodically for all subsequent steps. We place a stitch into the aneurysmal sac and pull it out through the right abdominal wall (Figure 32-13). Traction on this stitch allows retraction of the aneurysmal sac to the right, facilitating complete dissection of the left and posterior aspects of the aorta. We control lumbar and medial sacral arteries with hemoclips (Ligaclip ERCA, Ethicon Endosurgery, Johnson-Johnson, Brussels, Belgium) before opening the aneurysmal sac (Figures 32-14 and 32-15). A clip or a bulldog clamp is used to occlude the inferior mesenteric artery. Iliac clamping is performed with the videoscopic clamps previously placed in the left iliac fossa. Videoscopic detachable clamps (Storz-France) can also be used, but they do not allow simple clamping and unclamping, especially during retrograde flushes. Moreover, unlike detachable clamps, straight clamps

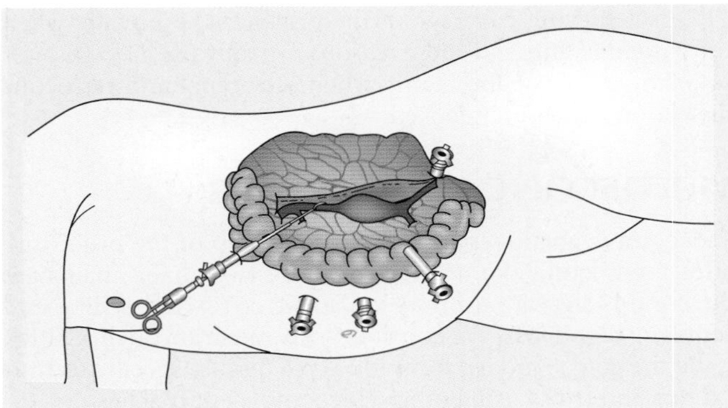

Figure 32-11. Part of the first step of abdominal aortic aneurysm repair via a transperitoneal retrorenal (TPRR) approach: Positioning of proximal laparoscopic clamp through subcostal port (port 7) via TPRR.

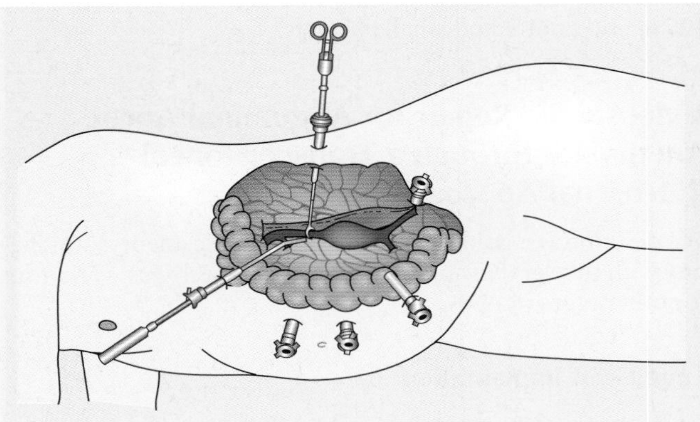

Figure 32-12. Part of the first step of abdominal aortic aneurysm repair via a transperitoneal retrorenal (TPRR) approach: Positioning of proximal laparoscopic clamp through flank port (port 8) via TPRR. An endoretractor is placed through port 7 to contain the viscera.

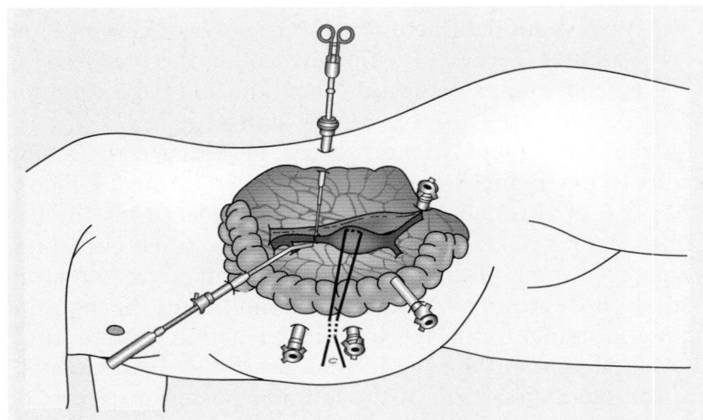

Figure 32-13. The second step of abdominal aortic aneurysm repair via a transperitoneal retrorenal approach: Placement of a stitch in the aneurysmal sac.

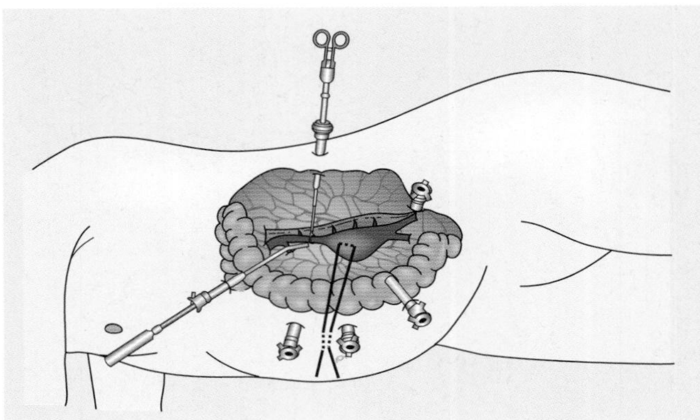

Figure 32-14. The third step of abdominal aortic aneurysm repair via a transperitoneal retrorenal approach: traction on the stitch to expose the left side of the aorta and externally control the lumbar arteries.

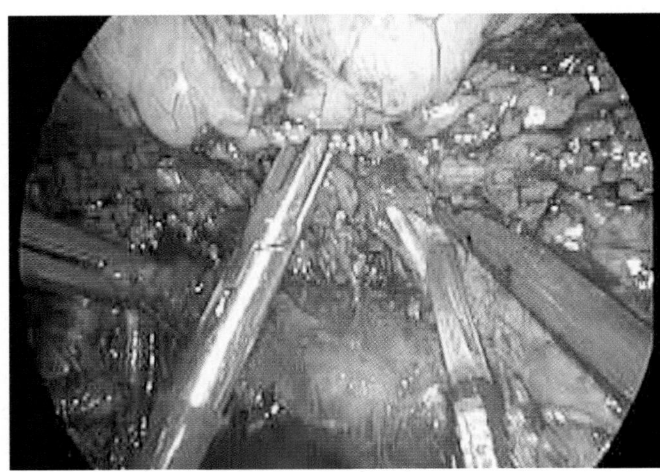

Figure 32-15. Operative view showing external control of lumbar arteries.

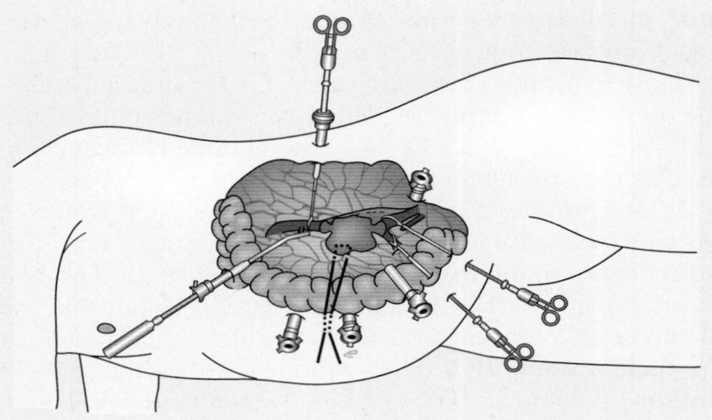

Figure 32-16. The aneurysmorrhaphy. Traction on the stitch allows opening the aneurysmal sac after the aortotomy.

stabilize the left mesocolon into position and allow a stable exposure during the performance of endoaneurysmorrhaphy and creation of anastomoses.

A longitudinal aortotomy is performed on the left side on the aorta. Traction on the stitch, which was previously placed in the aortic wall, allows opening of the aneurysmal sac (Figure 32-16). Mural thrombus is removed and placed temporarily in the left hypochondrium. It is removed at the end of the procedure and placed into a container. In cases of residual bleeding from the aneurysmal sac, lumbar arteries

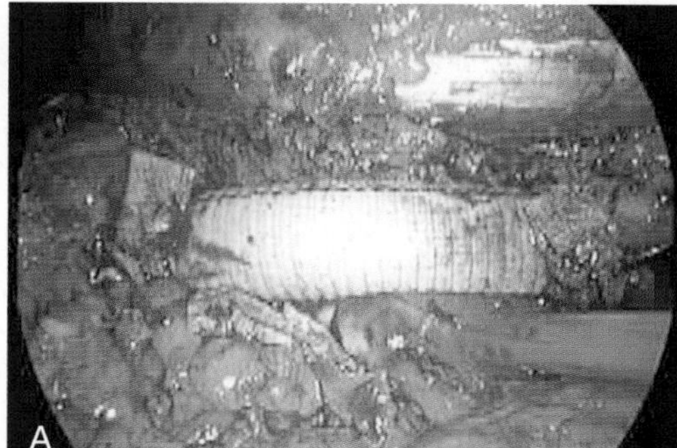

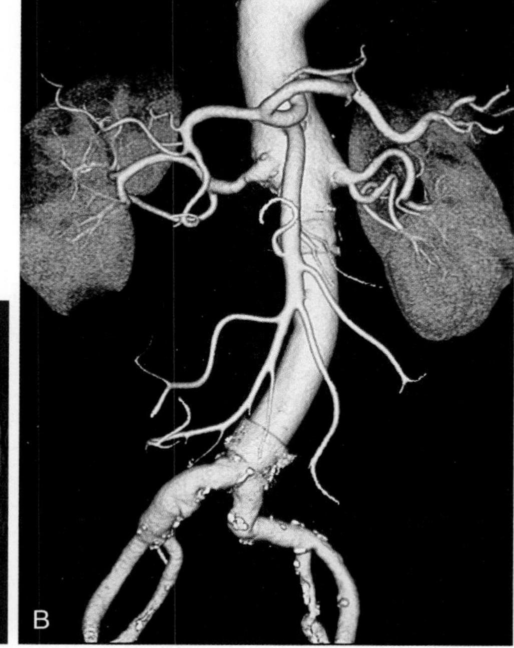

Figure 32-17. Operative **(A)** and computed tomography scan **(B)** views showing a tube graft after laparoscopic abdominal aortic aneurysm repair.

are controlled either externally with clips or internally with staples (EMS, Ethicon Endosurgery, Johnson-Johnson, Brussels, Belgium) or polypropylene stitches. As in Creech's original open technique,[1] the proximal aortic neck is usually completely transected. Whenever possible, the distal aorta is also transected for tube graft implantation. In the case of dense adhesions between the distal aorta and the inferior vena cava, we keep the right aortic wall in place to avoid inferior vena cava injury during its dissection. The prosthesis is introduced into the abdomen through one of the ports. Proximal and distal anastomoses are performed with hemicircumferential running sutures previously knotted on pledgets. At the end of each anastomosis, both ends of the thread are tied together intracorporally (Figure 32-17). Retrograde flushing from both common iliac arteries is checked before closing the suture line.

At the end of the procedure, we perform a videoscopic inspection of the left colon to assess its viability. Backbleeding from the inferior mesenteric artery and intraoperative Doppler ultrasound (Ultrasonic Doppler Flow Detector, model 811b, Parks Medical Electronics, Aloha, Oregon) are used to assess the adequacy of collateral blood flow to the left mesocolon. Should reimplantation of the inferior mesenteric artery be necessary, it can be performed laparoscopically[35] or via a minilaparotomy. Hemostasis is checked, especially within the aneurysmal sac to detect backbleeding from lumbar arteries after unclamping of iliac arteries. On closure, a suction drain is positioned near the prosthesis. Reattaching viscera is unnecessary because they fall back into place once the patient is returned to a dorsal decubitus position. The aneurysmal wall covers the graft when the kidney falls into place. Ports are removed under videoscopic control to confirm the lack of parietal bleeding. The abdominal fascia of port holes is closed with absorbable sutures.

Bifurcated Graft Implantation

When a bifurcated graft is indicated, specific steps are performed. After achieving laparoscopic exposure, the patient is rotated back into the dorsal decubitus position. The pillow is deflated and the operating table is rotated to the left, which allows a conventional approach to iliac–femoral arteries. A knot is placed as a landmark on the left prosthetic limb. We always proceed methodically for the steps that follow.

The right tunnel is first initiated from the groin–iliac incision. At the abdominal level, the assistant exposes the right common iliac artery with an endoretractor in the left hand (port 4) and a suction device in the right hand (port 5). The primary operating surgeon introduces an aortic clamp from the groin with its tip anterior to the right common iliac artery under abdominal videoscopic control. Once the clamp is positioned, the vascular prosthesis is introduced into the abdomen through one of the ports and the right limb is easily brought to the groin incision. The left prosthetic limb is similarly brought down with the aid of an aortic clamp introduced through the left groin. Unlike the right side, the left tunnel is short and widely open due to the displacement of the intraabdominal organs toward the right. Care must be taken to avoid an excessively large tunnel because of risk of gas leakage.

The technical steps differ somewhat for bifurcated grafts. If distal anastomoses to the common iliac arteries are feasible, the entire procedure is performed through the abdominal route. In cases of external iliac anastomoses, we prefer to perform a separate RP approach in the iliac fossa, especially on the right side. Blood flow to the internal iliac arteries is ensured, either by retrograde perfusion or reimplantation. In such cases, we use videoscopy for the left side but an open approach for the right side. The main technical point for bifurcated grafts is a strategy used to decrease clamping time. Whenever possible, once graft limbs are tunneled, distal iliac, femoral, or both

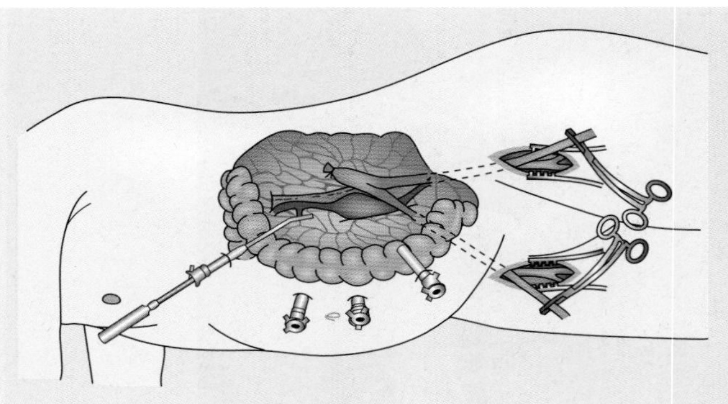

Figure 32-18. The positioning of the bifurcated graft before performing distal anastomosis, which is performed first.

anastomoses are performed first (Figure 32-18). Using such an approach, total aortic clamping time is only required for aneurysmorrhaphy and proximal anastomosis.

Juxtarenal Abdominal Aortic Aneurysms

Laparoscopic juxtarenal AAA aneurysmorrhaphy uses steps similar to those employed for infrarenal AAA repair.[36] In summary, the proximal laparoscopic clamp (Storz-Endoscopie France, Guyancourt, France) is placed through the flank port (Figure 32-19). We place a stitch into the left part of the aneurysmal sac. It is used (1) to retract the aorta to the right during external control of lumbar and sacral medial arteries and (2) to open the aneurysmal sac after the aortotomy. The right and left iliac arteries are occluded with laparoscopic clamps introduced percutaneously in the left iliac fossa. We use sequential steps for suprarenal clamping to decrease renal ischemic time. Once the juxtarenal aorta is freed of thrombus, we first perform infrarenal clamping. After aneurysmorrhaphy, we place a second clamp above the renal arteries and remove the first clamp. This maneuver allows a target zone for creation of the proximal anastomosis close to the renal arteries. The renal ischemic time is then only the time needed for completion of the proximal anastomosis. Whenever the juxtarenal aorta is unsuitable for clamping before aneurysmorrhaphy, we first perform suprarenal clamping. If preparation

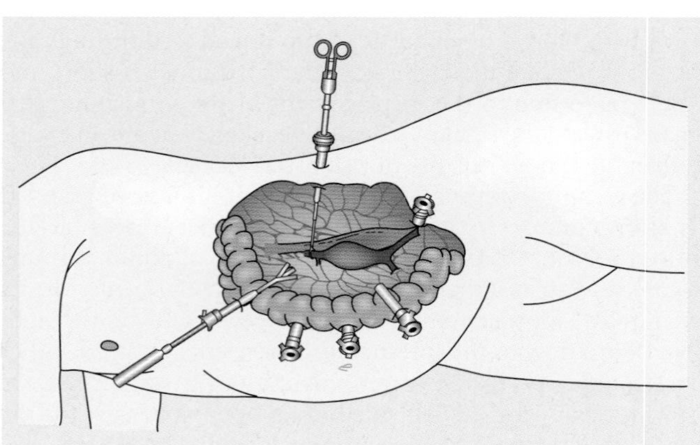

Figure 32-19. Proximal laparoscopic clamping for laparoscopic juxtarenal abdominal aortic aneurysm repair.

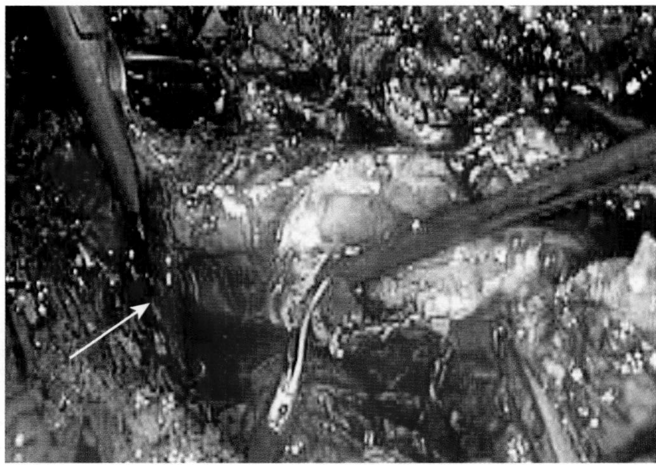

Figure 32-20. The laparoscopic abdominal aortic aneurysm repair via a transperitoneal retrocolic approach: aortic and iliac laparoscopic clamps stabilize the left mesocolon and maintain stable exposure.

of the target zone of the proximal anastomosis is of sufficient length below the renal arteries, we place a second infrarenal clamp and remove the suprarenal clamp. The renal ischemic time is the time needed to perform the proximal anastomosis. If preparation of the infrarenal aorta does not allow enough length to move the clamp after aneurysmorrhaphy (Figure 32-20), we then also perform the proximal anastomosis with suprarenal clamping.

Technical Variations

Aortic Repair through Transperitoneal Retrocolic and Transperitoneal Direct Approaches

Aortic repair through TPRC and TPD uses the same steps as TPRR. The main differences are clamp positioning and graft limb tunneling. Positioning of the proximal aortic clamp uses the subxiphoid port (port 6) after removal of the endoretractor. This clamp stabilizes the left mesocolon (Figure 32-21). Tunneling of graft limbs for aortobifemoral bypass grafts is the same as for TPRC than TPRR. For the right side, there are

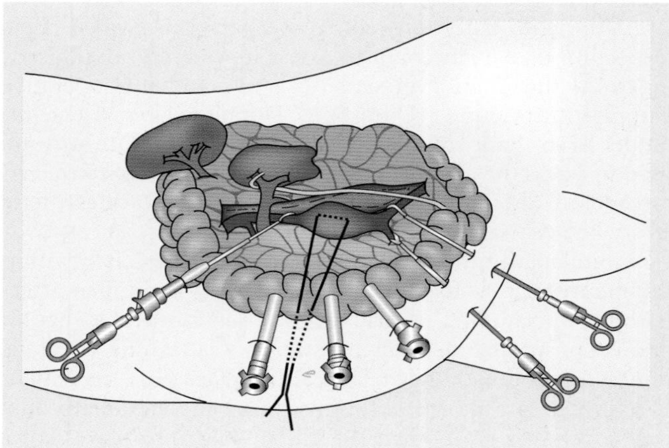

Figure 32-21. The abdominal incision for conversion to open repair between ports 1 and 5. Patient is left in the right lateral decubitus position.

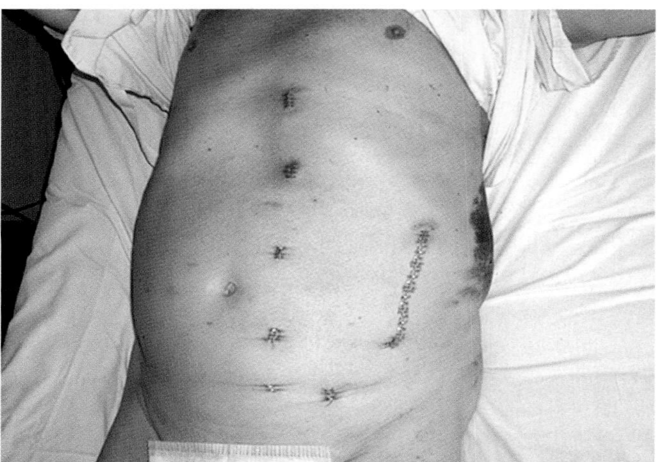

Figure 32-22. Postoperative view showing a patient after conversion to open repair.

no differences. For the left side through TPRC, the operator moves the clamps from the groin toward the aorta under videoscopic control. The operating surgeon advances the clamp tip beneath the ureter, which overlies the iliac artery.

Through TPD, creating the left graft limb tunnel is more demanding. Videoscopic dissection along the anterior aspect of the left iliac artery is blinded by the left mesocolon and does not allow enough exposure to be sure that tunnel is strictly behind the ureter. We recommend a short peritoneal incision in the left iliac fossa with retroperitoneal dissection and exposure of the distal common iliac artery. With such an exposure, tunneling is simple and the operator moves the clamp beneath the ureter under strict videoscopic control.

Aortic Repair through a Retroperitoneoscopic Approach

The proximal clamp is introduced through a sixth port placed above the left twelfth rib. The distal clamp is positioned through a seventh port placed in the left iliac fossa. For AAA repair, right iliac clamping can be performed with a detachable clamp or with an additional clamp introduced 3 cm below the navel, which stabilizes the peritoneal sac into position. Aortoprosthetic anastomoses use same principles but are in a reverse shape compared to transperitoneal exposures.

Conversion to Open Direct Repair

Conversion to ODR through a short incision should not be viewed as a failure; it is a safe and reasonable strategy when difficulties arise during total videoscopic procedures. Making such a decision is sometimes difficult for surgeons, especially at the beginning of their experience. Dialogue and joint decision making with the anesthesiologists is essential to decide when to convert. Usual indications for conversion are (1) difficult reconstruction with prolonged aortic cross-clamp time; (2) extensive calcification with an unclampable aorta; (3) difficult or unstable exposure of the abdominal aorta, especially during the RP approach, small abdominal cavities, unexpected adhesions, and extensive dilatation of the small bowel; (4) iatrogenic injuries to structures adjacent to the aorta such as small bowel, inferior vena cava or iliac veins. Relative indications are (1) the need for inferior mesenteric artery reimplantation, (2) difficult control of the endarterectomy endpoint in the iliac or visceral arteries and (3) lack of sufficient precision and visibility for bleeding control.

The technique for conversion is relatively simple. The patient is still in RLD, and we conduct a short vertical laparotomy between the laparoscope and the assistant's ports (ports 1 and 5; Figure 32-22). If needed, this laparotomy is extended. Exposure through the initial direct, retrocolic, or retrorenal route is maintained with autostatic retractors or valves. Completion of the procedure uses the same principles as conventional ODR. Sometimes it is useful to use laparoscopic clamps, which are less cumbersome than conventional aortic clamps. Another useful tool is the percutaneous introduction of clamps, either conventional or laparoscopic.

CONCLUSION

Total laparoscopic AAA repair is feasible but requires advanced expertise in laparoscopic suturing. Surgeons who want to set up a laparoscopic program for AAA repair must perform intensive training and complete basic training courses to gain this expertise. The learning curve is long and difficult. We encourage surgeons to gain laparoscopic vascular skills with aortobifemoral bypass procedures before attempting to perform AAA repair. The assistance of experienced proctors is also essential at the beginning.

References

1. Creech O Jr. Endo-aneurysmorrhaphy and treatment of aortic aneurysm. *Ann Surg* 1966;164:935-946.
2. Brewster DC, Cronenwett JL, Hallett JW Jr, et al. Guidelines for the treatment of abdominal aortic aneurysms: report of a subcommittee of the Joint Council of the American Association for Vascular Surgery and Society for Vascular Surgery. *J Vasc Surg* 2003;37:1106-1117.
3. Parodi JC, Palmaz JC, Barone HD. Transfemoral intraluminal graft implantation for abdominal aortic aneurysms. *Ann Vasc Surg* 1991;5:491-499.
4. Terramani TT, Chaikof EL, Rayan SS, et al. Secondary conversion due to failed endovascular abdominal aortic aneurysm repair. *J Vasc Surg* 2003;38:473-477.
5. Ricco JB, Goëau-Brissonnière O, Rodde-Dunet MH, et al. Use of abdominal aortic endovascular prostheses in France from 1999 to 2001. *J Vasc Surg* 2003;38:1273-1281.
6. Prinssen M, Verhoeven EL, Buth J, et al. A randomized trial comparing conventional and endovascular repair of abdominal aortic aneurysms. *N Engl J Med* 2004;351:1607-1618.
7. Greenhalgh RM, Brown LC, Kwong GP, et al. Comparison of endovascular aneurysm repair with open repair in patients with abdominal aortic aneurysm (EVAR Trial 1), 30-day operative mortality results: randomised controlled trial. *Lancet* 2004;364:843-848.
8. Blankensteijn JD, de Jong SE, Prinssen M, et al. Two-year outcomes after conventional or endovascular repair of abdominal aortic aneurysms. *N Engl J Med* 2005;352:2398-2405.
9. Endovascular Repair Trial Participants. Endovascular aneurysm repair versus open repair in patients with abdominal aortic aneurysm (EVAR Trial 1): randomised controlled trial. *Lancet* 2005;365:2179-2186.
10. Endovascular Repair Trial Participants. Endovascular aneurysm repair and outcomes in patients unfit for open repair of abdominal aortic aneurysm (EVAR Trial 2): randomised controlled trial. *Lancet* 2005;365:2187-2192.
11. Dion YM, Gracia CR. A new technique for laparoscopic aortobifemoral grafting in occlusive aortoiliac disease. *J Vasc Surg* 1997;26:685-692.
12. Kline RG, D'Angelo AJ, Chen MH, et al. Laparoscopically assisted abdominal aortic aneurysm repair: first 20 cases. *J Vasc Surg* 1998;27:81-87.

13. Jobe BA, Duncan W, Swanstrom LL. Totally laparoscopic abdominal aortic aneurysm repair. *Surg Endosc* 1999;13:77-79.
14. Cerveira JJ, Cohen JR. Laparoscopically assisted abdominal aortic aneurysm repair. *Surg Clin North Am* 1999;79:541-550.
15. Nott DM, Crinnion J, Benson J, et al. Laparoscopically assisted abdominal aortic aneurysm repair. *Lancet* 1999;22:1765-1766.
16. Castronuovo JJ Jr, James KV, Resnikoff M, et al. Laparoscopic-assisted abdominal aortic aneurysmectomy. *J Vasc Surg* 2000;32:224-233.
17. Kolvenbach R, Cheshire N, Pinter L, et al. Laparoscopy-assisted aneurysm resection as a minimal invasive alternative in patients unsuitable for endovascular surgery. *J Vasc Surg* 2001;34:216-221.
18. Dion YM, Gracia CR, Ben El Kadi H. Totally laparoscopic abdominal aortic aneurysm repair. *J Vasc Surg* 2001;33:181-185.
19. Alimi YS, Di Molfetta L, Hartung O, et al. Laparoscopy-assisted abdominal aortic aneurysm endoaneurysmorrhaphy: early and mid-term results. *J Vasc Surg* 2003;37:744-749.
20. Matsumoto Y, Nishimori H, Yamada H, et al. Laparoscopy-assisted abdominal aortic aneurysm repair: first case reports from Japan. *Circ J* 2003;67:99-101.
21. Coggia M, Bourriez A, Javerliat I, Goëau-Brissonnière O. Totally laparoscopic aortobifemoral bypass: a new and simplified approach. *Eur J Vasc Endovasc Surg* 2002;24:274-275.
22. Coggia M, Javerliat I, Di Centa I, et al. Total laparoscopic bypass for aortoiliac occlusive lesions: a 93-case experience. *J Vasc Surg* 2004;40:899-906.
23. Coggia M, Javerliat I, Di Centa I, et al. Total laparoscopic infrarenal aortic aneurysm repair: preliminary results. *J Vasc Surg* 2004;40:448-454.
24. Coggia M, Di Centa I, Javerliat I, et al. Total laparoscopic abdominal aortic aneurysm repair. *J Cardiovasc Surg* 2005;46:407-414.
25. Dion YM, Thaveau F, Fearn SJ. Current modifications to totally laparoscopic apron technique. *J Vasc Surg* 2003;38:403-406.
26. Stadler P, Sebesta P, Vitasek P, et al. A modified technique of transperitoneal direct approach for totally laparoscopic aortoiliac surgery. *Eur J Vasc Endovasc Surg* 2006;32:266-269.
27. Alimi YS, Hartung O, Cavalero C, et al. Intestinal retractor for transperitoneal laparoscopic aortoiliac reconstruction: experimental study on human cadavers and initial clinical experience. *Surg Endosc* 2000;14:915-919.
28. Barbera L, Ludemann R, Grossefeld M, et al. Newly designed retraction devices for intestine control during laparoscopic aortic surgery: a comparative study in an animal model. *Surg Endosc* 2000;14:63-66.
29. Cau J, Ricco JB, Deelchand A, et al. Totally laparoscopic aortic repair: a new device for direct transperitoneal approach. *J Vasc Surg* 2005;41:902-906.
30. Said S, Mall J, Peter F, Muller JM. Laparoscopic aorto-femoral bypass grafting: human cadaveric and initial clinical experiences. *J Vasc Surg* 1999;29:639-648.
31. Coggia M, Di Centa I, Javerliat I, et al. Total laparoscopic aortic surgery: transperitoneal left retrorenal approach. *Eur J Vasc Endovasc Surg* 2004;28:619-622.
32. Di Centa I, Coggia M, Javerliat I, et al. Total laparoscopic aortic surgery: transperitoneal direct approach. *Eur J Vasc Endovasc Surg* 2005;30:494-496.
32a. Edoga JK, Asgarian K, Singh D et al. Laparoscopic surgery for abdominal aortic aneurysms. Technical elements of the procedure and a preliminary report of the first 22 patients. *Surg Endosc* 1998;12:1064-1072.
33. Javerliat I, Coggia M, Di Centa I, et al. Total videoscopic aortic surgery: left retroperitoneoscopic approach. *Eur J Vasc Endovasc Surg* 2005;29:244-246.
34. Javerliat I, Coggia M, Bourriez A, et al. Total laparoscopic aortomesenteric bypass. *Vascular* 2004;12:126-129.
35. Javerliat I, Coggia M, Di Centa I, et al. Total laparoscopic abdominal aortic aneurysm repair with reimplantation of the inferior mesenteric artery. *J Vasc Surg* 2004;39:1115-1117.
36. Coggia M, Cerceau P, Di Centa I, et al. Total laparoscopic juxtarenal abdominal aortic aneurysm repair. *J Vasc Surg* 2008;48:37-42.

chapter

33

Complex Aortic Aneurysm: Pararenal, Suprarenal, and Thoracoabdominal

W. Darrin Clouse, MD, FACS • Richard P. Cambria, MD, FACS

Key Points

- Complex aortic aneurysms represent a continuum of disease involving multiple aortic segments.
- Patient-specific variables that may enhance rupture risk include chronic obstructive pulmonary disease, renal insufficiency, smoking, hypertension, prior stroke, Marfan syndrome, pain or symptoms attributable to the aneurysm, and female gender.
- Aneurysm-specific variables that enhance rupture risk include aneurysm size, dissection, extent of disease, and expansion rate.
- The decision to undertake operative reconstruction in patients with complex aortic aneurysms is made by weighing the preceding characteristics with the patient's overall medical condition.
- Refinements in computed tomography and helical reconstruction have made this the imaging modality of choice and often the only study required for evaluating complex aneurysmal disease.
- Results of open reconstruction have improved due to the multiplicity of operative strategies and adjuncts applied attempting to minimize the principal complications.
- Debranching procedures facilitating endovascular repair are described but will likely be supplanted by fenestrated and branched endograft constructs with less morbidity and mortality.
- Endovascular repair of complex aortic aneurysm, including arch branch and the visceral aortic segment, via several technical methods are feasible and have become part of management strategies.
- Endovascular repair of thoracic aortic aneurysms has quickly become commonplace, and the acceptable maturing results obtained in clinical trials have provided momentum for changes in treatment paradigms, as well as therapy for those who would previously been denied repair.

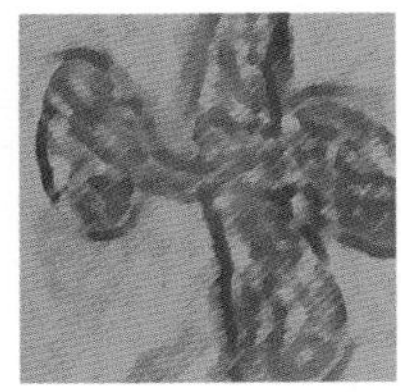

While most degenerative aortic aneurysms are isolated infrarenal lesions, some 7% to 15% involve segments at or above the renal arteries. These lesions represent varying points on an anatomical continuum of aneurysmal disease, and multiple aortic segments are commonly affected. For example, most studies examining natural history data for thoracic aortic aneurysms indicate that between 20% and 30% of these patients will also be found to have aneurysms of the abdominal aorta (AAAs).[1-3] Our experience indicates that roughly 20% of patients undergoing thoracoabdominal aortic aneurysm (TAA) repair proceed to have expansion of remaining aortic segments.[4] In a large Mayo Clinic series encompassing nearly 6000 aortic resections for aneurysmal disease, 2% of patients undergoing AAA repair and 18% of patients with TAA underwent multiple aneurysm repairs.[5] Crawford and Cohen noted in a series of 1500 patients treated for AAA that some 12.5% harbored aneurysms in other aortic segments.[6]

Aside from the obvious, more proximal extent of aorta involved, TAA can be distinguished from the more routine AAA because of differing etiologies and shifts in patient demographic profiles. While most are degenerative in nature and occur in association with hypertension, smoking, and often evidence of vascular disease in other territories, up to 20% of TAAs in most series result from chronic aortic dissection.[7-11] Furthermore, the male-to-female sex ratio of TAA is 1:1, whereas AAA patients have a 5:1 male-to-female ratio. Others have noted the tendency for aneurysmal disease in females to involve proximal aortic segments more often, and women appear to be at increased risk of rupture.[12-14]

Successful operation on an abdominal aneurysm involving the visceral aortic segment was first reported by Etheredge et al. in 1955.[15] Thereafter, DeBakey and colleagues reported Dacron graft aortic replacement with multiple sidearms for visceral vessel reconstruction.[16] The modern era of successful surgical management of TAA began with the pioneering work of E. Stanley Crawford and his technical modifications. Crawford described a simplified operative approach using the inclusion technique wherein visceral and intercostal vessels were reconstructed from within the aneurysm directly anastomosing openings in the main Dacron graft to the aortic origin of these vessels.[17,18] Despite various surgical and adjunctive strategies applied in different centers to minimize overall operative morbidity, the state of the art in contemporary management still entails a 5% to 10% risk of perioperative mortality, morbidity, or both in the form of renal, respiratory, and spinal cord ischemic complications. Given this fact, and while acknowledging conventional surgical repair remains the only treatment option in many environments, endovascular repair using techniques providing for preserved side-branch flow is altering the treatment of pararenal aneurysms and TAA.[19,20] While a number of endovascular concepts focused on treating complex aortic aneurysmal disease have developed, we concentrate this chapter on aneurysm definitions, natural history, operative selection, techniques, and results of open repair, incorporating a detailed review of these endovascular techniques.

Aneurysm Extent

While a degree of confusion exists regarding the terms juxtarenal and pararenal aneurysm, the Ad Hoc Committee on Reporting Standards of the Society for Vascular Surgery and the American Association for Vascular Surgery have identified *pararenal* as synonymous with *juxtarenal* (Figure 33-1).[21] Juxtarenal and pararenal aneurysms are those that extend cephalad sufficiently close to the renal arteries (less than a 1-cm neck) to require suprarenal, or higher, aortic cross-clamping to create an infrarenal anastomosis. The term suprarenal aneurysm implies that at least one renal artery arises from the aneurysm, yet it does not extend proximally to involve the superior mesenteric artery (SMA). Further extension cephalad to involve the visceral vessels is considered a total abdominal aneurysm or, synonymously, a type IV TAA, as described later. Thus, lesions simultaneously involving the thoracic and abdominal aorta, as well as those that include the visceral aortic segment, are termed thoracoabdominal aortic aneurysms.

TAAs are classified according to the scheme originally devised by Crawford, which, in the most basic terms, considers whether the lesion is primarily a caudal extension of a descending thoracic aneurysm, or a cephalad extension of a total abdominal aneurysm (Figure 33-1).[18] This classification is clinically useful since it has direct implications for both the technical conduct of operation and the incidence of operative complications, in particular, spinal cord ischemia (SCI). There is considerable variation in the spectrum and overall scope of operation required to deal with aneurysms within the classification of TAA. For example, in contemporary practice, management of the type IV aneurysm should be accomplished with an overall morbidity and mortality not significantly different from the management of routine AAA.[22] Delineating between a suprarenal aneurysm and a type IV TAA amounts to no more than a few centimeters of the visceral aortic segment. We define type IV repair as one in which it is necessary to extend the graft proximal to the celiac axis.

Type I and type II lesions are more extensive and require resection of the entire descending thoracic aorta. Repair of these aneurysms typically requires a clamp placed at or even proximal to the left subclavian artery. We reserve the designation type II aneurysm for those patients in whom the entire descending thoracic and abdominal aorta is involved. Type III aneurysms involve variable lengths of the descending aorta and abdominal aorta. Furthermore, the aneurysm should be classified according to the extent of aorta resected during a single procedure. For example, it is commonplace to resect a type I aneurysm into a prior infrarenal aneurysm repair. Such lesions should be classified as type I rather than type II aneurysms.

Considerable variation is reported in the literature with respect to the distribution of TAA. While this reflects, to a degree, referral biases, the issue of precision in aneurysm classification, as discussed earlier, likely also accounts for some variability. Displayed in Table 33-1 are data from representative contemporary series regarding the relative distribution of TAA extent. Virtually all major clinical series of TAA reconstruction emphasize a significant incidence of prior aortic resections, and in our experience this is seen in nearly one third of patients presenting for TAA resection.[27] The most common pattern is the patient who has undergone a prior infrarenal AAA repair (60% of total prior resections). However, virtually every pattern can be seen, including prior proximal thoracic aortic grafts and prior TAA resections in which part of the visceral aortic segment was encompassed in the original operation.[28,29]

The classification scheme outlined in Figure 33-1 does not consider the patient with concomitant discontinuous aneurysm of parts or all of the ascending aorta and aortic arch. While synchronous proximal aneurysm is noted in 6% to 13% of TAA patients, contiguous arch aneurysm is rare, typically occurring only in patients with a prior DeBakey type I aortic dissection, especially those with Marfan syndrome.[30] Patients with incontinuity arch–TAA usually require complex, staged procedures.[31,32] Since patients with degenerative TAA or prior distal dissections most often have an aneurysm "neck" in the region of the aortic isthmus, TAA resection is usually, and more safely, performed staged after surgical correction of ascending–arch aneurysms when both require resection.

Etiology

Most pararenal aneurysms, suprarenal aneurysms, and TAAs are degenerative in nature, and most authorities agree that the terms atherosclerotic and degenerative may be used interchangeably. With the exception of the rare primary abdominal aortic dissection or infected aneurysm, abdominal aneurysm etiology is limited to degenerative disease and

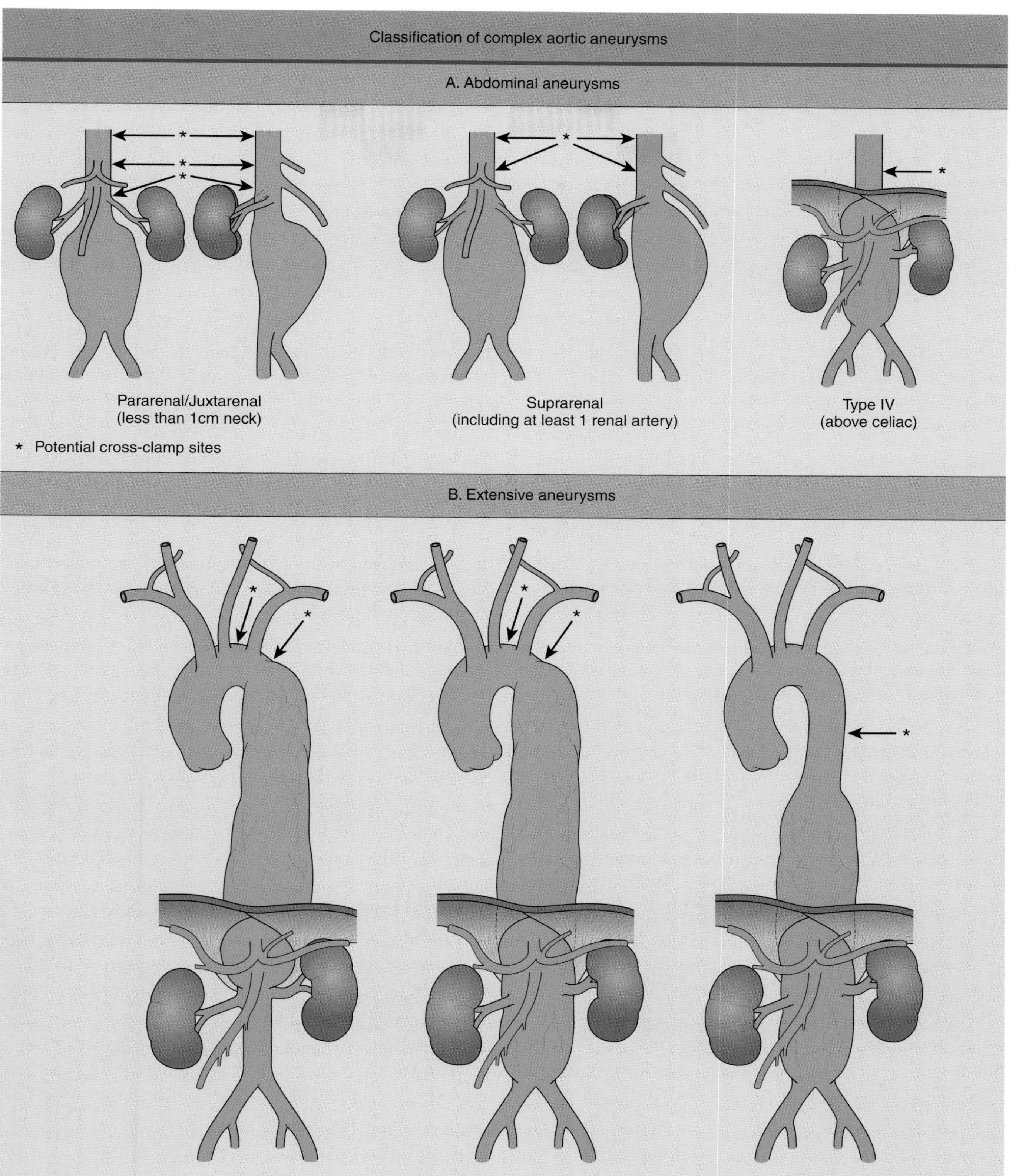

Figure 33-1. Classification of complex aortic aneurysms. **A,** Abdominal aneurysms: pararenal with infrarenal neck of less than 1 cm, suprarenal with at least one renal artery involved in aneurysm, and total abdominal or type IV thoracoabdominal aortic aneurysm (TAA) when it is necessary to carry graft above celiac axis. **B,** Extensive TAA: types I to III. Notice potential aortic cross-clamp sites for each extent.

Table 33-1
Aneurysm Extent (Crawford Classification) Among Major Series of Patients Undergoing Thoracoabdominal Aneurysm Repair

Reference	Year	Repairs (*n*)	Type I *n* (%)	Type II *n* (%)	Type III *n* (%)	Type IV *n* (%)
Svensson et al.[8]	1993	1509	378 (25)	442 (29)	343 (23)	346 (23)
Grabitz et al.[23]	1996	260	68 (26.2)	81 (31.2)	87 (33.5)	24 (9.2)
Acher et al.[7]	1998	176	35 (19.9)	66 (37.5)	29 (16.5)	46 (26.1)
Hamilton et al.[24]	1998	265	40 (15.1)	74 (27.9)	78 (29.4)	73 (27.5)
Safi et al.[25]	2003	696	213 (31)	205 (29)	133 (19)	145 (21)
Schepens et al.[26]	2007	500	110 (22)	234 (46.8)	103 (20.6)	53 (10.6)
Coselli et al.[9]	2007	2286	706 (31)	762 (33)	391 (17)	427 (19)
Conrad et al.[11]	2007	455	121 (27)	69 (15)	164 (36)	101 (22)
Total		6147	1671 (27)	1933 (31)	1328 (22)	1215 (20)

paraanastomotic pseudoaneurysm. In contrast, some 20% of TAAs are the sequelae of chronic aortic dissection.[7-11] Of patients experiencing acute aortic dissection, 25% to 40% progress to have aneurysmal dilation of the dissected aorta.[33-37] DeBakey et al.[38] found this phenomenon occurred in 30% of more than 500 aortic dissection patients treated surgically. Recently, Marui et al.[39] reported that 43% of patients initially treated medically during the acute phase of type III dissection progressed to have aortic enlargement. Moreover, dilation to 6 cm or greater occurred in nearly 30%. Factors that appear to have a significant impact on chronic aneurysm development after dissection include poorly controlled hypertension, maximal aortic diameter of at least 4 cm in the acute phase, and continued patency of the false lumen.[39-42] Furthermore, some 10% to 20% of those with dissection subsequently experience rupture.[33,37] Confounding this issue is that some patients with degenerative lesions go on to develop dissection within the preexisting aneurysm, an inherently unstable condition.[14,43]

Aneurysms that are the sequelae of chronic dissection tend to be more extensive and occur in younger patients compared with degenerative aneurysms. Patients with true cystic medial necrosis, such as those with Marfan syndrome, have an increased risk of aneurysm and dissection formation. Marfan syndrome is an autosomal, dominant, inherited mutation of the fibrillin-1 gene leading to disarrayed microfibrillar connective tissue formation and subsequent aortic degeneration. In addition to disorders of other connective tissue, cystic medial degeneration of the aorta, perhaps caused by smooth muscle cell apoptosis mediated by angiotensin II receptors, leads to a spectrum of aortic pathology, including root and sinotubular aneurysm, annuloaortic ectasia, and acute and chronic dissection.[44] While aortic disease has traditionally led to early death in patients with Marfan syndrome, the surgical and diagnostic advances in aortic disease during the last three decades have allowed their life expectancy to approach that of the population at large.[45,46] These patients often have either total aortic ectasia or multiple aneurysms. Ascending aortic and aortic valve disease is the most common lesion addressed, with 90% of initial operations occurring in this segment. However, up to 40% proceed to a second aortic procedure, which typically involves the thoracoabdominal aorta.[47,48] Aggressive beta-blockade has been shown to retard the growth of the aortic root and may have a similar effect on the thoracoabdominal aorta.[49]

Aortitis leading to aneurysm development is rare. Lesions secondary to the sequelae of giant cell arteritis are typically seen in women. Aneurysms can result from either Takayasu's disease or giant cell aortitis. Evans et al.[50] found that patients with giant cell arteritis were 17.3 and 2.4 times more likely to develop thoracic and abdominal aneurysms, respectively, when compared with the general population. There may be no known prior diagnosis of aortitis or other associated collagen vascular disease. Such aneurysms can be either focal or diffuse along the thoracoabdominal aorta and are often associated with other known sequelae of inflammatory aortitis, namely, visceral and renal artery occlusive disease. TAAs secondary to infectious processes present challenging management issues because the dual goals of eradication of sepsis and arterial reconstruction typically demand an in situ type of reconstruction (i.e., placement of a prosthetic graft in a contaminated field). The term mycotic aneurysm continues to be applied to these lesions, although, as originally described by Osler,[51] this term more precisely relates to aneurysms secondary to embolization from an infected cardiac vegetation. A more proper term is infected aneurysm. In contemporary practice, the pathogenesis of these lesions is usually hematogenous seeding of atherosclerotic plaque, the development of focal aortitis with dissolution of the aortic wall, and the formation of a false aneurysm. All such aneurysms are contained ruptures of false aneurysms.

In summary, the distribution of TAA etiology is approximately 80% degenerative, 15 to 20% secondary to chronic dissection (including those with familial connective tissue diseases), 2% infectious, and 1 to 2% resulting from aortitis.[27,28]

Natural History

Natural history data aid balancing aneurysm rupture risk with surgical morbidity. The expected natural history of pararenal aneurysms and TAA is progressive enlargement and eventual rupture regardless of etiology. Since these aneurysms are uncommon compared with AAA, fewer natural history studies are available. Furthermore, studies of degenerative TAA are confused by inclusion of patients with acute aortic dissection, many of whom succumb in the acute phase of the disease.[1,12] Size criteria for operation in TAA are not as clearly defined compared with AAA. Since rupture risk and factors associated with rupture of pararenal aneurysms are similar to those for AAA described elsewhere in this text, herein we concentrate on natural history studies of TAA.

Population-based studies, since they are exempt from the inherent bias of referral center series, offer the best insight. Two studies performed 20 years ago form the foundation of thoracic aneurysm epidemiology. Bickerstaff and colleagues from the Mayo Clinic reported an incidence of 5.9 thoracic aortic aneurysms per 100,000 person years over a 30-year period (1951 to 1980) in Rochester, Minnesota.[1] They found that rupture occurred in 74% of their patients and was nearly always fatal. Actuarial 5-year survival was a mere 13%. If patients with aortic dissection were eliminated, the prognosis of degenerative thoracic aortic aneurysm in the first 3 years after diagnosis was considerably worse when compared with a prior Mayo Clinic study of unoperated AAAs.[52] Similar data with respect to the incidence of concomitant AAAs (25%), the higher risk of rupture with aortic dissection, and a substantial rupture risk for thoracic aneurysm were reported by McNamara and Pressler.[2] The latter study is valuable since no patients were operated on and the 3-year survival of patients with degenerative thoracic aortic aneurysm was only 35%. Almost half of the deaths were related to aneurysm rupture.

Clouse and associates reevaluated the prognosis of degenerative thoracic aortic aneurysms found in Olmsted County, Minnesota, between 1980 and 1994[14] and compared this experience to Bickerstaff's prior communication.[1] The descending aorta was the principal segment affected in 60% of patients. The incidence of degenerative aneurysm had nearly tripled and the 5-year survival had improved to 56% in the 15 years of study. This was attributed to the development of computed tomography (CT) and echocardiography, with earlier diagnosis, and potentially improved surgical techniques. Notably, the overall 5-year rupture risk was 20%. Nearly 80% of ruptures occurred in women, and female gender was independently associated with rupture risk (relative risk 6.8, 95% confidence interval [CI] 2.3 to 19.9, $p = 0.01$). Aneurysm-specific variables also strongly correlated with rupture and included symptoms attributable to the aneurysm and dissection developing within the degenerative aneurysm, further establishing their importance in surgical decision making.[45,53] Increasing aneurysm size led to higher rupture risk (Figure 33-2). Rupture accounted for 30% of all deaths and occurred with an incidence of 3.5 per 100,000 patient years.[54] The 30-day mortality for elective repair was 8%, versus 54% for emergent cases. The authors suggested 6 cm as the size criterion for intervention in appropriate-risk, asymptomatic patients. Johansson et al.[12] also reported the incidence of ruptured thoracic aortic aneurysm in two separate time intervals (1989 and 1980). The incidence of presentation for treatment of ruptured thoracic aortic aneurysm was 5 per 100,000 patient years. The incidence was stable over the decade examined, and rupture was usually fatal. Interestingly, these investigators found an equal sex distribution among patients with ruptured thoracic aortic aneurysm.

Although natural history data from referral center populations are biased, such studies remain valuable since issues surrounding the selection of patients for operative therapy are considered. Crawford and DeNatale reported on nearly 100 patients referred for, but subsequently denied, surgical treatment for TAA, usually related to advanced age or associated comorbid conditions.[53] Survival at 2 years was only 24%, and half of all deaths were related to aneurysm rupture. Interestingly, chronic obstructive pulmonary disease (COPD) was noted in 80% of patients denied reconstruction. Not surprisingly, the 2-year survival in these authors' comparative series of surgically treated patients (70%) was far superior to the observed survival in the nonoperated cohort.[53] Size criteria for recommending operation were initially inferred from another report from Crawford's group.[55] In a series of 117 patients

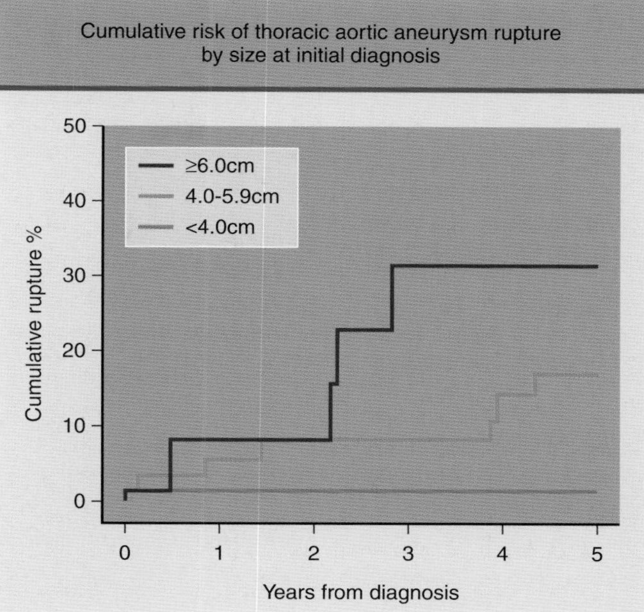

Figure 33-2. Cumulative risk of thoracic aortic aneurysm rupture by size at initial diagnosis. Five-year rupture risk for aneurysms 6.0 cm or larger, 31%; for 4 to 5.9 cm, 16%; and for those less than 4 cm, 0%. (Adapted from Clouse WD, Hallett JW, Schaff HV, et al. *JAMA* 1998;280: 1926-1929.)

treated for ruptured thoracic aortic aneurysm or TAA, they found 80% of all ruptures occurred in aneurysms less than 10 cm, dispelling the previously held myth that only exceedingly large thoracic aneurysms rupture. Rupture occurred in smaller aneurysms when acute dissection was the pathology. Rupture occurred with equal frequency in the chest and abdominal cavities, and 60% of all TAA ruptures occurred in cases where the abdominal component was less than 8 cm in diameter. Since rupture was observed in some 10% of patients with aneurysms less than 6 cm in diameter, the authors recommended elective operation for TAA when a 5-cm-diameter threshold was exceeded.[55]

Recent referral center reports give further insight into the expected natural history and rupture risk in patients considered for TAA resection. These valuable data have delineated both patient-specific and aneurysm-specific factors that are important elements in aneurysm prognosis (Table 33-2). TAAs appear to expand at more rapid rates as they become larger, and several investigators have correlated increased expansion rates with rupture.[58,60,64,66,67] Furthermore, these studies indicate that TAA rupture risk is negligible in aneurysms less than 5 cm, is equivalent to the risk of surgical morbidity in the 5 to 6 cm range, and increases substantially at aneurysm diameters above 6 cm and growth rates of 10 mm/year.

SELECTION FOR OPERATION

These natural history observations have led us to use 6 cm as a generally appropriate size threshold to recommend intervention for extent I to III TAA. In view of recent Society for Vascular Surgery guidelines for AAA treatment, 5.5 cm is used for abdominal lesions.[68] Increasing expansion rate is used as an indicator of heightened rupture risk, and consideration

Table 33-2
Referral Center Reports Describing Thoracic–Thoracoabdominal Aortic Aneurysm Prognosis*

Reference	Prognostic Factors (Endpoint)	
	Aneurysm Specific	Patient Specific
Cambria et al.[56]	Size ≥5 cm (rupture)	COPD (expansion, rupture trend) Chronic renal failure (rupture trend)
Dapunt et al.[57]	Size ≥5 cm (expansion, survival)	Smoking (expansion)
Perko et al.[13]	Dissection (rupture) Size ≥6 cm (rupture, survival)	Hypertension (survival) Respiratory insufficiency (survival) Renal failure (rupture, survival)
Masuda et al.[58]	Size (expansion) Abdominal aneurysmal disease (expansion)	Diastolic hypertension (expansion) Renal failure (expansion)
Griepp et al.[59]	Dissection (rupture, survival) Smaller maximum size (dissection, rupture) Increasing extent (rupture)	Age (rupture) Hypertension (dissection, rupture) COPD (rupture) Pain—even atypical (rupture)
Coady et al.[60,61]	Size ≥6 cm (rupture or dissection)	
Bonser et al.[62]	Intraluminal thrombus (expansion) Mid descending aorta (expansion)	Smoking (expansion) Prior stroke (expansion) Peripheral vascular disease (expansion)
Juvonen et al.[40,63]	Size ≥5 cm (smaller maximum for dissection, rupture)	Age (rupture) COPD (rupture) Pain—even atypical (rupture) Hypertension (dissection, rupture)
Lobato et al.[64]	Size ≥5 cm (rupture) Expansion (rupture)	
Davies et al.[65]	Size ≥5 cm (rupture) Size ≥6 cm (rupture or acute dissection) Descending aorta (survival) Elective repair (survival) Expansion (rupture trend)	Female gender (rupture or acute dissection) Prior stroke (rupture or acute dissection) Marfan syndrome (rupture or acute dissection)

*COPD, chronic obstructive pulmonary disease.

is given to earlier operation, while in chronic dissection and patients with Marfan syndrome, a 5-cm size threshold is maintained due to rupture tendency at smaller sizes.[40,59,60,63,66]

Asymptomatic presentation with radiographic detection is common, yet symptoms due to aneurysm expansion, rupture, and local compression are seen and should be quickly evaluated in view of enhanced rupture potential. Juvonen et al.[63] noted even the presence of atypical symptoms was an independent rupture correlate. The usual dismissal of such complaints, if they are chronic, is inappropriate in patients with known TAA. Typical symptoms reported include back pain localized to the left lower hemithorax or, when the aortic hiatus is significantly involved, a typical midback pain, epigastric pain, or both. When the aneurysm erodes into the thoracolumbar spine or chest wall, complaints of chest and back pain can be both prominent and present for weeks to months, as they nearly always represent contained rupture. Depending on the topography of the aneurysm, other symptoms may be referable to various compression phenomena, erosion phenomena, or both. New onset of hoarseness related to left recurrent laryngeal nerve palsy; compression or erosion of the tracheobronchial tree or pulmonary parenchyma producing cough, hemoptysis, or dyspnea; and dysphagia are all possible but uncommon symptomatic manifestations of TAA.[69] Similar to AAA, distal embolization of atheromatous debris can be observed but has constituted a rare indication for operation in our experience. Perhaps due to reluctance recommending elective operation secondary to threat of surgical morbidity, between 40% and 70% of TAA patients present with symptoms.[8,9,11,27,70,71] This explains the higher proportion of patients treated for rupture when compared with AAA. Up to 25% of patients are treated in urgent or emergent circumstances, with half presenting with frank rupture.[7-11,27,70,71]

Comorbid conditions associated with diffuse atherosclerosis and global vascular disease are commonplace in patients with TAA. A familial aneurysm history is present in about 10% of patients. Prior aortic grafting for aneurysmal disease is seen in nearly one third of patients with TAA. The most common scenario is a previous infrarenal aneurysm repair. Coselli et al. detailed experience in 123 patients undergoing TAA resection after prior infrarenal AAA repair. These patients presented for TAA repair a mean of 8 years after the initial AAA operation.[28] While many of these represent de novo development of a second aneurysm, it is also clear that an inadequate initial infrarenal operation creates the necessity for a second, more definitive procedure. Our experience with TAA has corroborated that remaining segments of aneurysmal aorta predict need for further intervention.[4] The presence of a previous infrarenal or more proximal thoracic aortic graft does not unduly complicate the subsequent TAA repair. Coselli and colleagues have indicated that TAA operation after a prior aortic graft produces results similar to those seen with de novo TAA resection, although a prior proximal graft appears to increase the risk of SCI.[29] Patients treated for degenerative aneurysm generally have advanced diffuse atherosclerosis, with an average age of 70 years. Hypertension is nearly universal. Cerebrovascular disease, prior stroke, and lower extremity arterial occlusive disease occur in 20% to 25% of patients. Associated renovisceral occlusive disease occurs in 30% to 40% of patients, with nearly 35% requiring endarterectomy or bypass of these vessels.[27] About 15% of patients have significant renal insufficiency (serum creatinine of more than 1.8 mg/dl).[11,25,27,72,73] Renal dysfunction accompanied by renal artery occlusive disease has important implications for both accurate assessment of perioperative risk and long-term preservation of renal function. Some of these patients have the potential for retrieval or salvage of renal function with renal artery reconstruction. The presence of an abnormal preoperative serum creatinine correlates with perioperative mortality and renal failure, potentially SCI, and poorer long-term survival.[11,25,73] As a result, investigating renal function and associated renovascular disease becomes an important component of preoperative patient evaluation and surgical decision making. Preoperative azotemia (serum creatinine of more than 2.5 mg/dl) constitutes a relative contraindication to elective, open operation unless preoperative studies indicate renal artery reconstruction may possibly salvage or recover renal function.

An accurate assessment of cardiopulmonary function and associated comorbid conditions is mandatory to guide appropriate decision making with respect to recommending operation. Cigarette smoking, significant COPD, or both are often encountered. Pulmonary function tests are recommended in all such patients. Approximately one third of patients have moderately compromised pulmonary function, with 15% having severe COPD manifested by a forced expiratory volume in the first second of less than 50% predicted. In patients with clinically evident heart disease, some type of noninvasive cardiac testing is often appropriate given the usual risk factors and activity tolerance in these patients. Preoperative beta-blockade should be instituted. In addition, patients with a history or symptoms suggestive of heart failure should have an assessment of left ventricular function. Advanced age must be considered if it is accompanied by overall fragility and impaired functional status. Accordingly, advanced age is not an absolute reason to deny operation.[74,75]

Preoperative hydration is critical, especially in patients with impaired renal function. In the past, preoperative dopamine infusion was used in patients with renal insufficiency; however, preliminary results with intravenous infusion of the D_1-selective dopamine agonist, fenoldopam, suggest a salutary effect on postrepair renal function, and some now use this adjunct when any degree of renal impairment is present. Patients may undergo mechanical and antibiotic bowel preparation, based on evidence indicating that bacterial translocation during supraceliac clamping may contribute to disorders of blood coagulation.[76,77]

Nonoperative therapy may be selected initially in frail patients, those with modest-size aneurysms, and those for whom associated comorbid conditions make the short-term risk of open surgery prohibitive, life expectancy is limited to a degree that surgical treatment is not rational, or both. Should anatomy and expertise for the given aneurysm complexity be available, endovascular means of repair may be considered. Patients selected for nonoperative therapy should be treated aggressively with beta-blockade, hypertension control, and cessation of cigarette smoking.[78,79]

Imaging

Accurate and complete radiographic evaluation is mandatory. Based on review of preoperative studies, there should be no equivocation in the surgeon's mind as to the proximal and distal extent of resection. In contemporary practice, a dynamic, fine-cut, contrast-enhanced CT scan with or without helical reconstruction provides the surgeon with the following:

- The location of proximal aortic cross-clamping and anastomosis
- A qualitative assessment of the aorta in the region of the proximal cross-clamp
- The assessment of patency and orificial stenosis of the visceral vessels
- The topography of the renal artery origins in relation to aneurysm contour, in addition to kidney size and adequacy of perfusion
- The distal extent of the resection, including major aneurysmal disease of the iliac vessels

Traditionally, complete contrast arteriography has also been used to evaluate patients treated in elective settings to assist in examination of the aortic arch and renovisceral vessels. Furthermore, surgeons who use retrograde transfemoral aortic perfusion have routinely used pelvic arteriography to exclude significant iliac occlusive disease. However, in conjunction with its ability to provide the best topographic information, refinements in helical CT reconstruction have made renovisceral and iliac evaluation by this means more than adequate (Figure 33-3). Magnetic resonance angiography may also be used for renovisceral evaluation. Contrast arteriography remains beneficial in selected situations. Chronic dissection generally requires complete arteriography. It is critical to understand preoperatively exactly how each renovisceral and iliac orifice is related to the true and false lumens. When distal aortic reconstruction is required in patients with previous colon resection, arteriography may also provide useful information about the remaining collateral colonic blood supply. Patients with rare anatomical variants such as horseshoe kidneys and anomalous arterial anatomy generally require arteriography. Furthermore, arteriography may be useful in providing some assessment of the number and location of patent intercostal vessels. While decisions about intercostal vessels are ultimately made intraoperatively, knowledge of multiple patent arteries in the critical aortic segment (T8 to L1) can prepare the surgeon for their reconstruction and potentially save operative and clamp time and lessen neurological morbidity. Kieffer et al.[80] have commented on spinal cord arteriography safety and efficacy in 480 patients. They reported complications in 6 (1.2%) patients, with only 2 (0.4%) being spinal cord related. Adamkiewicz's artery was identified in 86% of cases, and the anterior spinal artery was able to be completely or partially visualized in 89%. Magnetic resonance angiography and computed tomography angiography technologies are other noninvasive imaging options now evolving to identify intercostal and spinal vessels with similar success.[81,82] Contrast studies should be minimized in patients with any degree of renal insufficiency, as should catheter manipulation in patients with excessive atherosclerotic debris in the visceral aortic segment. All elective iodinated contrast diagnostic studies should be performed well in advance of surgery. Serum creatinine should be rechecked after contrast-related imaging, and operative repair should be delayed until renal function is stable.

OPERATIVE MANAGEMENT

Standard central venous access, including selective pulmonary artery catheter or mixed venous monitor use, and arterial lines appropriate for the site of anticipated cross-clamping are

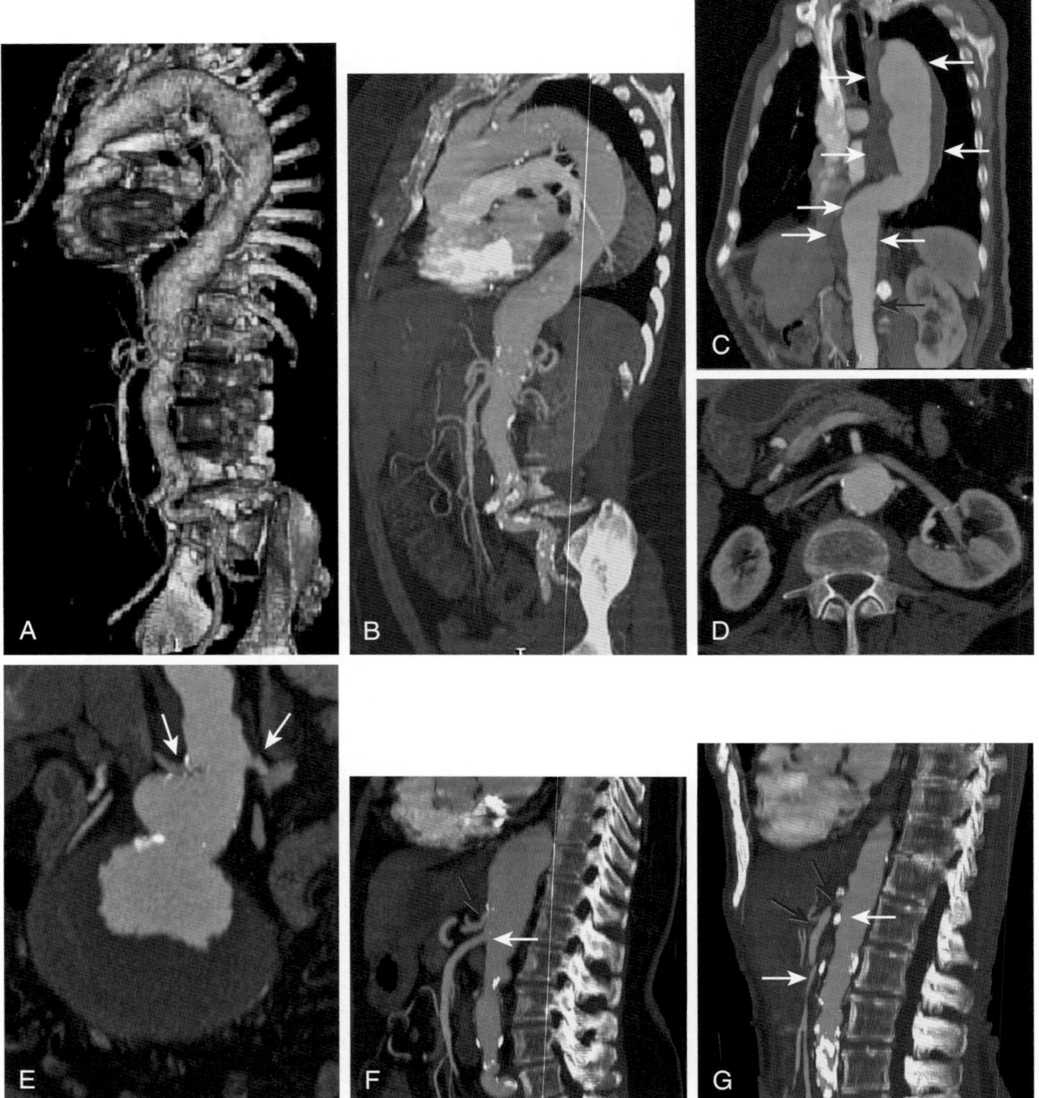

Figure 33-3. Computed tomography (CT) reformat. **A** and **B,** CT reformat and three-dimensional reconstruction of type I thoracoabdominal aortic aneurysm (TAA) showing aneurysm extent. Note clear visualization of aortic bifurcation and iliac arteries without significant disease. **C,** CT reformat revealing type I TAA aneurysm extent *(white arrows)* and where the aorta returns to normal caliber at the visceral aortic segment *(red arrow)*. **D** and **E,** Axial cut and CT reformat of pararenal aortic aneurysm, allowing evaluation of the proximal neck. Note less than 1 cm of neck appears below the renal arteries *(white arrows)*. **F,** CT reformat of the celiac *(red arrow)* and superior mesenteric artery (SMA) *(white arrow)* in a type I TAA, delineating no significant occlusive disease. **G,** Severe celiac stenosis *(red arrows)* and occlusion of the SMA at its calcific origin with distal reconstitution *(white arrows)*.

essential. Fluid warming and passive external warming devices should be standard to avoid systemic hypothermia. An epidural catheter is recommended for intraoperative anesthesia and postoperative analgesia. When epidural cooling or spinal drainage is used, a lower thoracic epidural catheter is necessary, and a cerebrospinal fluid (CSF) drainage catheter should be placed in the lower lumbar area and connected to a pressure transducer.

Packed red blood cells and fresh frozen plasma are started early as the primary fluid replacement; platelets are administered when the visceral or distal aortic anastomoses are completed. Autotransfusion is routinely used to retrieve shed blood and generally accounts for half the red blood cell volume returned to the patient. In preparation for aortic cross-clamping, 12.5 to 25 g of mannitol, furosemide, or both is administered to promote diuresis. Patients with renal insufficiency are maintained on dopamine or fenoldopam infusions. When CSF drainage, epidural cooling, or both are in place, 20 ml of CSF are removed before clamping. Operative cases involving a difficult proximal aortic reconstruction or significant renal dysfunction preoperatively may benefit from partial left heart bypass and distal aortic perfusion.

Aortic cross-clamping proceeds slowly, and the epidural anesthetic is often reinforced to aid in lowering the blood pressure before aortic clamping. Sequential clamping of the left iliac and visceral vessels before proximal aortic clamping facilitates a more controlled blood pressure manipulation with vasodilator agents. With more proximal TAA, lower blood pressures are required during the cross-clamp time. While some controversy exists regarding the spinal cord blood flow effects of vasodilators, particularly sodium nitroprusside, for control of proximal hypertension during aortic cross-clamping, we continue to use nitroprusside as the principal afterload reducing agent.[83-85] It provides rapid and easily reversible manipulation of arterial pressure. CSF is removed to maintain preclamp baseline CSF pressures. Aortic unclamping is associated with significant hemodynamic alterations during two stages—visceral reperfusion and distal reperfusion. Sodium bicarbonate is given before visceral vessel unclamping unless an inline mesenteric shunt (Figure 33-4) has been used, and may be needed with distal unclamping. The temporary use of vasopressors may also be required during these times. Repeat administration of mannitol is given, and renal-dose dopamine or fenoldopam is continued. Further dosing through the epidural catheter may be discontinued so that a lower extremity neurological examination can be done at the procedure's end. Emergence from anesthesia usually requires therapy for hypertension. In the intensive care unit, the blood pressure should be maintained in the upper levels of normal and hypotension should be aggressively treated. When used, CSF catheters must be transduced and pressures maintained at less than 10 to 12 mm Hg for 24 to 48 hours after operation.

Abdominal Aneurysms (Pararenal, Suprarenal, and Type IV TAA)

Operative decision making includes the aortic clamp site in relation to the renal and visceral vessels, necessary renovisceral reconstructions, and proper proximal and distal graft configurations. Complete resection of the aneurysm is the objective. Too often, resection is confined to the infrarenal aorta, placing suture lines in diseased, aneurysmal aorta and creating the milieu for eventual graft failure and reintervention. Adequate operative exposure is the sine qua non of a complete and safe reconstruction. Adjuncts for spinal cord and visceral protection are not routinely used in repair of these lesions. Proximal clamp times for reestablishing visceral flow can be 20 to 30 minutes with type IV TAA. In addition, most pararenal lesions allow positioning the proximal aortic clamp to provide flow in at least one mesenteric artery and occasionally one renal artery. Similar to more extensive aneurysmal disease, a cross-clamp time more than 30 minutes has been associated with postoperative renal dysfunction.[86-88] Mannitol and, if necessary, furosemide should be used to maintain diuresis intraoperatively. Dopamine and fenoldopam infusion may benefit those with renal insufficiency. Furthermore, cold renal perfusion is recommended when access to the renal ostia is safe. Several options exist for exposure of abdominal aneurysms. They can be divided into anterior and lateral approaches.

Anterior Approaches

Transperitoneal Approach with Supraceliac Clamping

The traditional midline transperitoneal approach supplemented by supraceliac aortic clamping is adequate for some juxtarenal aneurysms (Figure 33-5). Adequate exposure starts by extending the midline incision onto the xiphoid process. Inferior traction on the stomach with division of the lesser omentum and mobilization with rightward retraction of the left lateral liver segment provide access to the aorta at the hiatus. Nasogastric intubation assists in esophageal identification. A clamp may be placed with the tips against the vertebral column posteriorly, or circumferential control with a tape may facilitate improved aortic clamping. The clear disadvantage of this approach is discontinuous exposure of the visceral segment with repositioning of the retractors and transverse colon. Thus, it is only useful for juxtarenal aneurysms where exposure and treatment of visceral occlusive disease are not necessary. The left renal vein may hinder adequate aneurysm exposure. However, mobilization and retraction of this vein is possible in most cases (Figure 33-6). We eschew division of the vein.

Transperitoneal Approach with Medial Visceral Rotation

Medial visceral rotation from the left, introduced by Sauer and Stoney, provides exposure of the entire abdominal aorta without the theoretic morbidity of a combined thoracoabdominal approach.[89] A full-length laparotomy is made. The small bowel is wrapped and retracted superiorly and to the right, as with all transperitoneal approaches. The left colon is mobilized along the line of Toldt. Cephalad, the phrenocolic and splenorenal ligaments are divided. A plane may be developed anterior to the kidney, ureter, and adrenal gland while rotating the stomach, colon, spleen, and pancreas medially (Figure 33-7). Control and mobilization of the left renal vein may be enhanced with this exposure specifically by ligating the adrenal, gonadal, and renal–lumbar branches (Figure 33-6). Alternatively, the plane may be developed posterior to the left kidney, thus rotating venous structures to the midline and allowing unimpeded access to the suprarenal aorta (Figure 33-7). Splenic, pancreatic, or both types of injury are a potential complication of this technique.[90] During medial visceral rotation from the right, the small bowel mesentery is mobilized from its retroperitoneal attachments. This is extended to include right colon medialization in continuity with the duodenum and pancreatic head. Dissection along the posterior pancreatic border with superior displacement of the viscera reveals the SMA origin 90 degrees to the anterior surface of the aorta (Figure 33-8). Division of the autonomic tissue surrounding the SMA and division of the left diaphragmatic crus allow clamping above the renal arteries or above the SMA. The right-sided rotation provides excellent visualization for pararenal aneurysm repair, with particular advantages when full right renal artery or right iliac artery visualization is essential. When continuous exposure of the visceral aortic segment is required, however, we opt for the lateral approaches.

Lateral Approaches

Retroperitoneal–Thoracoabdominal Approach

We reserve the term retroperitoneal for those incisions no higher than the eleventh rib where the peritoneum is not entered and consider incisions higher than the tenth interspace thoracoabdominal irrespective of peritoneal entry (Figure 33-9). In our view, it is now obsolete to debate the merits of lateral versus anterior approaches. Both randomized and uncontrolled studies delineate the merits of both.[91-93] Certain technical and anatomical circumstances dictate the

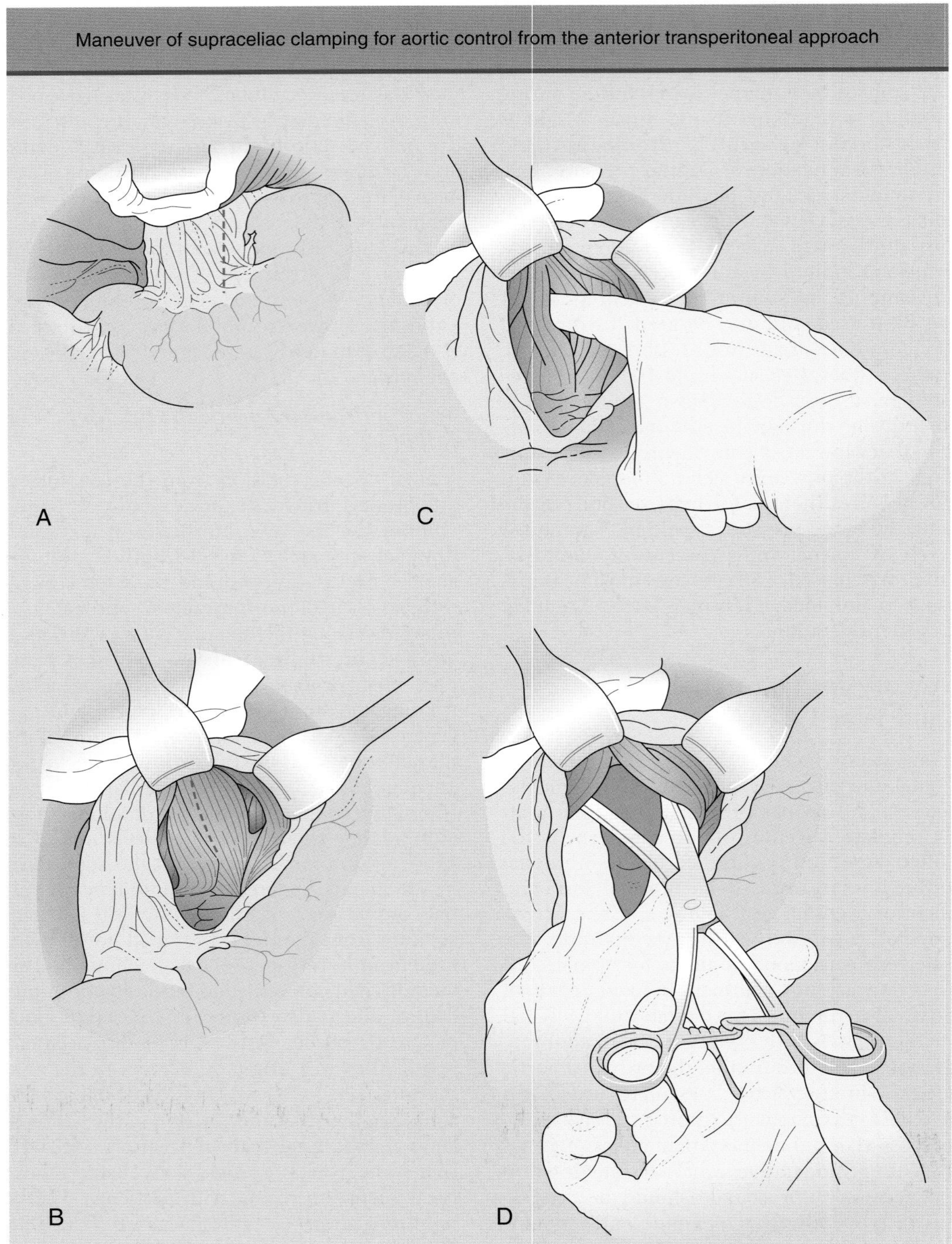

Figure 33-4. Maneuver of supraceliac clamping for aortic control from the anterior transperitoneal approach. The lesser omentum is opened and the crus divided. The periaortic tissue is cleared with a finger and the aortic clamp placed with tips against the vertebral bodies.

use of lateral approaches. For patients with significant visceral segment disease and true type IV lesions where distal thoracic control is required, it is the method of choice. It is clearly advantageous in obese patients or those with multiple prior abdominal procedures and adhesive obliteration of the peritoneal space. The main disadvantage is poor access to right-sided aortic branches.

The main considerations when using this type of exposure is the level of the flank incision necessary and whether the left kidney and ureter are to remain in anatomical position or swept medially with the peritoneum and its contents. For pararenal aneurysms, the incision is somewhat higher than for infrarenal repairs. If full supraceliac exposure is required, then extension into the ninth or even eighth interspace is used. The left pleural space is usually entered on these approaches, and the diaphragm may need to be partially divided. For type IV TAA, extension into the eighth interspace with costal margin division and a phrenic-sparing incision provides excellent

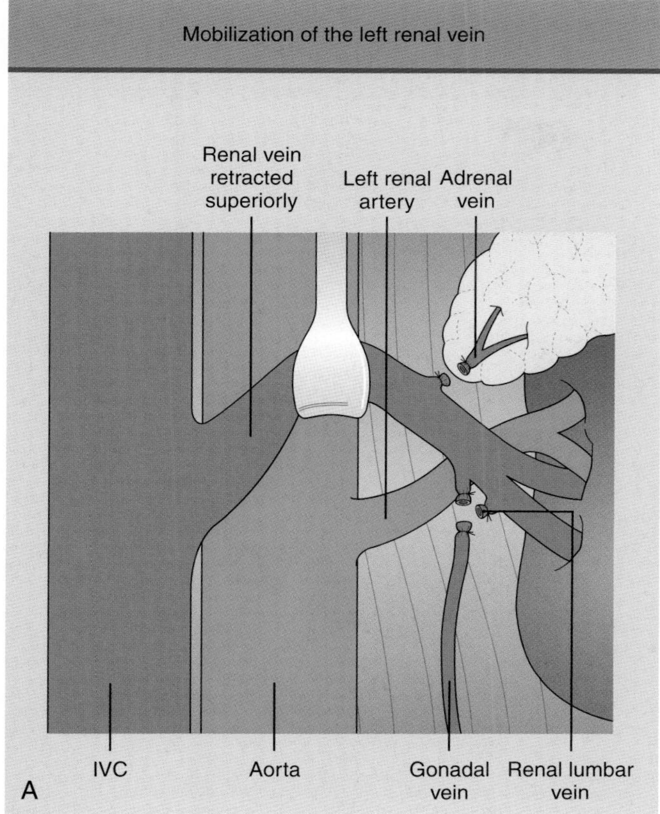

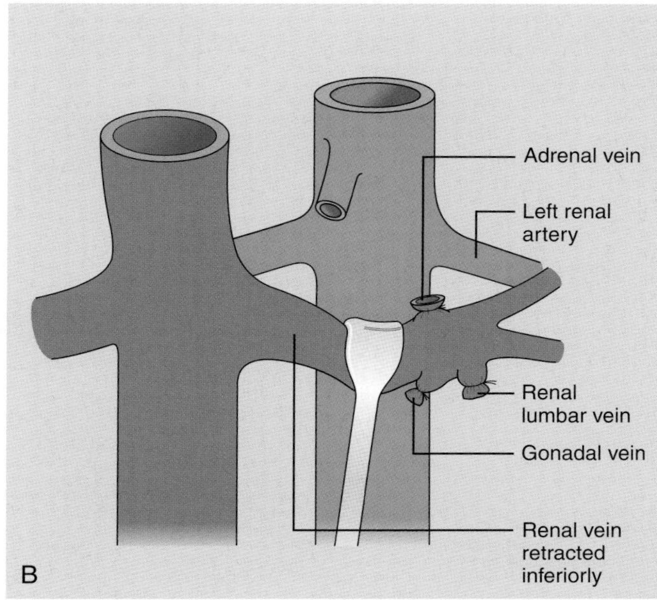

Figure 33-5. Mobilization of the left renal vein. **A,** Ligation of the adrenal, gonadal, and renal-lumbar veins. **B,** The left renal artery usually courses behind the vein.

visualization. The patient is placed on an air-vacuum Styrofoam beanbag in a right lateral decubitus position with the torso at a 65- to 70-degree rotation, with the hips and lower extremities rotated back as close as possible to horizontal. The table is jackknifed to open the left flank. The incision is carried through the abdominal wall musculature and transversalis fascia until the preperitoneal space is entered laterally. The peritoneal sac is swept anteromedially, defining the retroperitoneal space (Figure 33-9). This is continued until the peritoneal envelope is dissected over the aneurysmal segments. Ligation of the inferior mesenteric artery facilitates full inferior exposure. As with left medial visceral rotation, a plane anterior or posterior to the kidney may be developed. For most aneurysm surgery, a retrorenal plane is preferred, with the exception of a retroaortic left renal vein. The left diaphragmatic crus is divided, completing exposure of the entire suprarenal aorta (Figure 33-9). The retroperitoneal approach with renal elevation is preferable for pararenal aneurysm repair as it facilitates dissection, aortic control, and reconstruction. For type IV lesions or those where any significant visceral segment work must be accomplished, thoracoabdominal exposure with peritoneal entry for visceral inspection and distal vessel palpation is ideal.

Aortic Clamping

Clamping above the renal arteries and below the SMA is possible in many pararenal aneurysms. However, this may not be ideal in some patients due to associated side-branch occlusive disease, aortic calcification and thrombus, and differences in anatomical spacing of the branch vessels. When clamping between the renal artery and the SMA is feasible, construction of the proximal anastomosis can be accomplished with less involved proximal dissection and potentially less cardiac strain and hemodynamic compromise, as visceral flow remains open. It may also decrease coagulation disturbances, as supraceliac clamping with hepatic and bowel ischemia with bacterial translocation have been implicated in this process.[76,77,94,95] The advantages of clamping below the celiac have been challenged by Green and co-workers. They found less renal dysfunction with supraceliac clamping in their aneurysm experience.[96,96a] In contradistinction, Sarac and colleagues have scrutinized their operative technique for juxtarenal aneurysm. Using a supravisceral clamp was an independent predictor of operative mortality and renal dysfunction.[97] Renal dysfunction may be related to atheromatous embolization during clamping or surgical dissection of diseased aortic segments, as the supraceliac aorta is usually less involved by atherosclerotic disease. Also, mechanical or hemodynamic factors related to clamping near the renal orifices are potential factors. These considerations must be weighed when evaluating preoperative imaging studies. Helical CT with and without contrast allows for critical evaluation of aortic calcification and mural thrombus, aiding in choosing the most appropriate clamp location. However, clamp site location may occasionally require intraoperative decision-making and aortic exposure, or the site may change during the conduct of operation. The vascular surgeon dealing with complex abdominal aneurysms should be familiar with all exposures and clamping maneuvers. The Henry Ford Hospital pararenal aneurysm experience revealed 7% of clamps

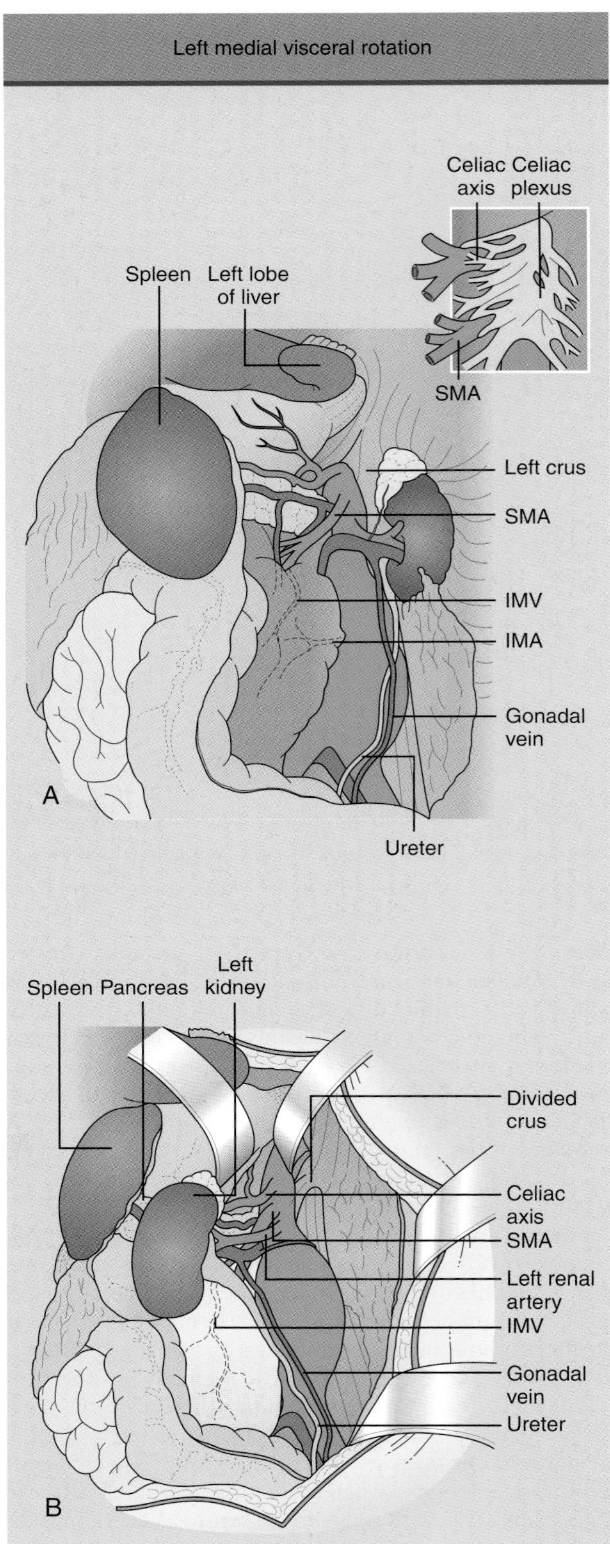

Figure 33-6. Left medial visceral rotation. **A,** Approach with left kidney remaining in retroperitoneum. **B,** Approach with kidney mobilized and rotated anteriorly with other viscera. Note renal-lumbar vein courses across the aorta near the left renal artery.

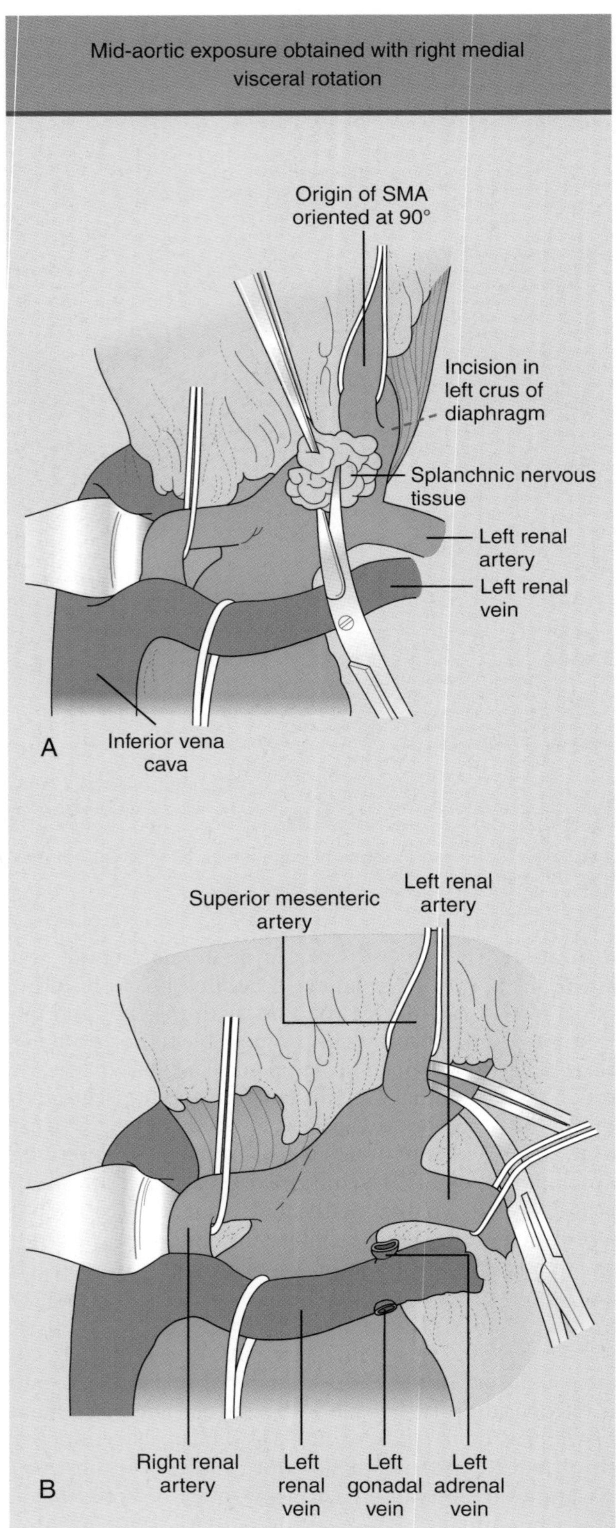

Figure 33-7. Mid-aortic exposure obtained with right medial visceral rotation. **A,** Note superior mesenteric artery elevated to 90° angle with aorta. **B,** After left renal vein mobilization, excellent access to the pararenal aorta is obtained.

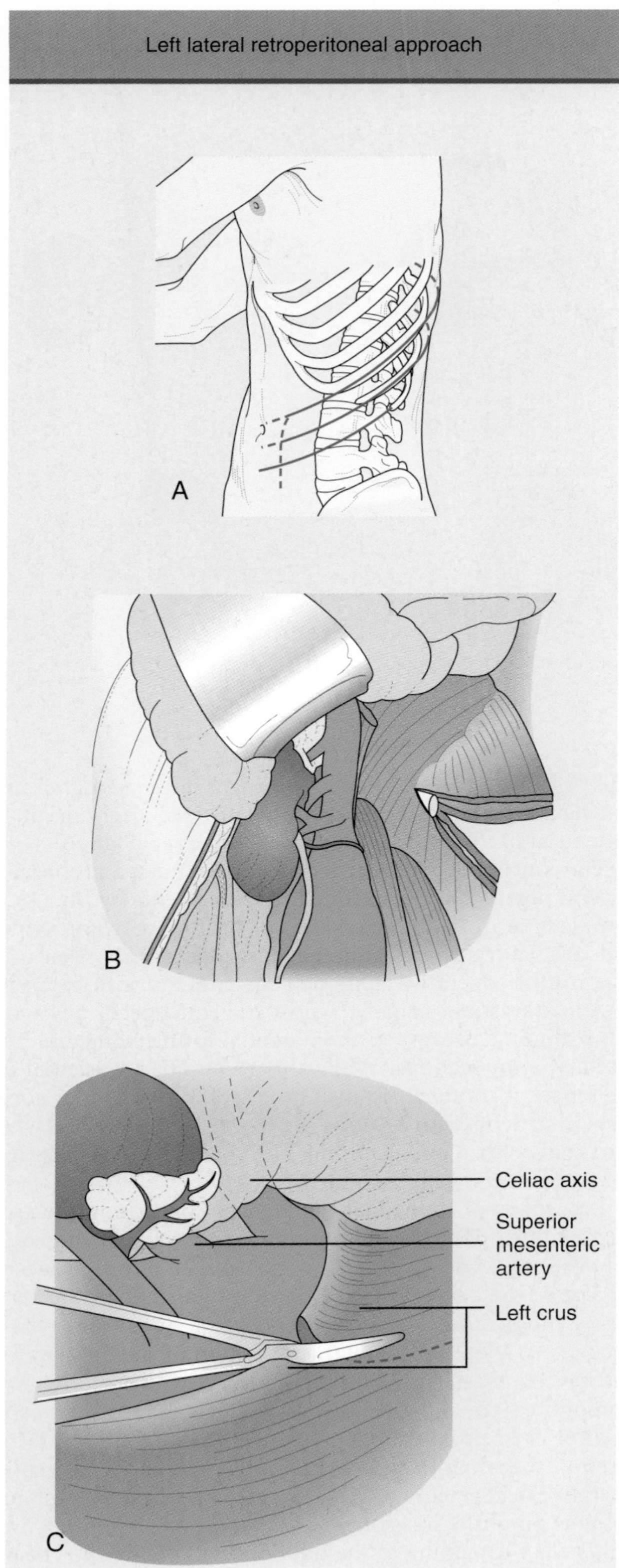

Figure 33-8. Left lateral retroperitoneal approach. **A,** Various levels of incision depend upon extent of aneurysmal disease. The abdominal portion is not carried to midline so as to keep the viscera intraperitoneal, to decrease evaporative and heat losses. **B,** Excellent contiguous exposure to the visceral aortic segment is obtained. Again note the renal-lumbar vein at the level of the left renal artery. **C,** Division of the left crus at the aortic hiatus facilitates supraceliac aortic exposure.

between the celiac artery and the SMA, 17% between the two renal arteries, 36% between the renal arteries and the SMA, and 40% at the supraceliac level.[98] Constructs for configuration of the proximal anastomosis vary according to the extent of proximal aneurysmal disease (Figures 33-10 and 33-11).

Extensive TAA (Type I to III)

Consensus indicates that the inclusion technique, refined by Crawford, is the preferred operative method for replacement of extensive TAA (Figure 33-4).[17,18] Crawford also emphasized operative expediency and simplicity without the use of external shunts or bypasses, minimal cross-clamp times, minimal dissection on the anterior aspects of the aorta, and avoidance of systemic anticoagulation because of its potential contribution to intraoperative bleeding complications.[99]

These general principles of operation are recommended with certain modifications. The two general approaches involve a clamp-and-sew technique versus the use of distal aortic perfusion combined with a sequential clamping technique (Figure 33-4). The rationale for distal aortic perfusion is the reduction of ischemic times to the spinal cord and viscera since their vascular beds are perfused during creation of the proximal anastomosis. Some surgeons use an initial right axillary–to–femoral bypass graft to provide passive distal aortic perfusion.[100] However, most authors who prefer distal aortic perfusion use active distal perfusion with atrial–femoral bypass using the Bio-Medicus pump. This centripetal, motorized pump is used with heparin-impregnated tubing and can be placed without systemic heparin.[101] But most surgeons prefer systemic heparin if using atrial–femoral bypass. Partial left heart bypass using a femoral vein to femoral artery technique becomes more complicated because of the necessity to add an inline oxygenator and higher doses of heparin. Although reports continue to suggest potential benefit,[9,10,25,75,102,103] the atrial–femoral bypass technique with sequential clamping only saves the cross-clamp time required to complete the proximal aortic anastomosis, which is a minimum of the overall clamp time. After constructing the proximal aortic anastomosis, reconstruction of critical intercostal vessels and visceral aortic segment must then proceed, with distal perfusion providing only retrograde pelvic perfusion and some additional spinal cord circulation via the lateral sacral branches of the hypogastric vessels. However, selective visceral perfusion by various catheter arrangements may be used (Figure 33-4). These have the disadvantage of interfering with surgical exposure. The pressure–flow relationships of multiple small catheters may be problematic. At least two studies have demonstrated a paradoxical detrimental effect on renal function using multiple selective visceral perfusion catheters.[70,104]

While some have been aggressive about the application of distal perfusion methods for all TAA,[10,25,75] others advocate their use only in the more extensive type I and type II aneurysms. Still others use atrial–femoral bypass and distal aortic perfusion selectively in accordance with individual patient anatomy.[102,105] Currently, we favor the selective use of atrial–femoral bypass. Since its principal advantage is visceral–spinal cord protection during the performance of the proximal aortic reconstruction, distal aortic perfusion is most beneficial when the proximal reconstruction is likely to be complex, for example, in patients with chronic dissection. Clearly, comparable results have been achieved in contemporary

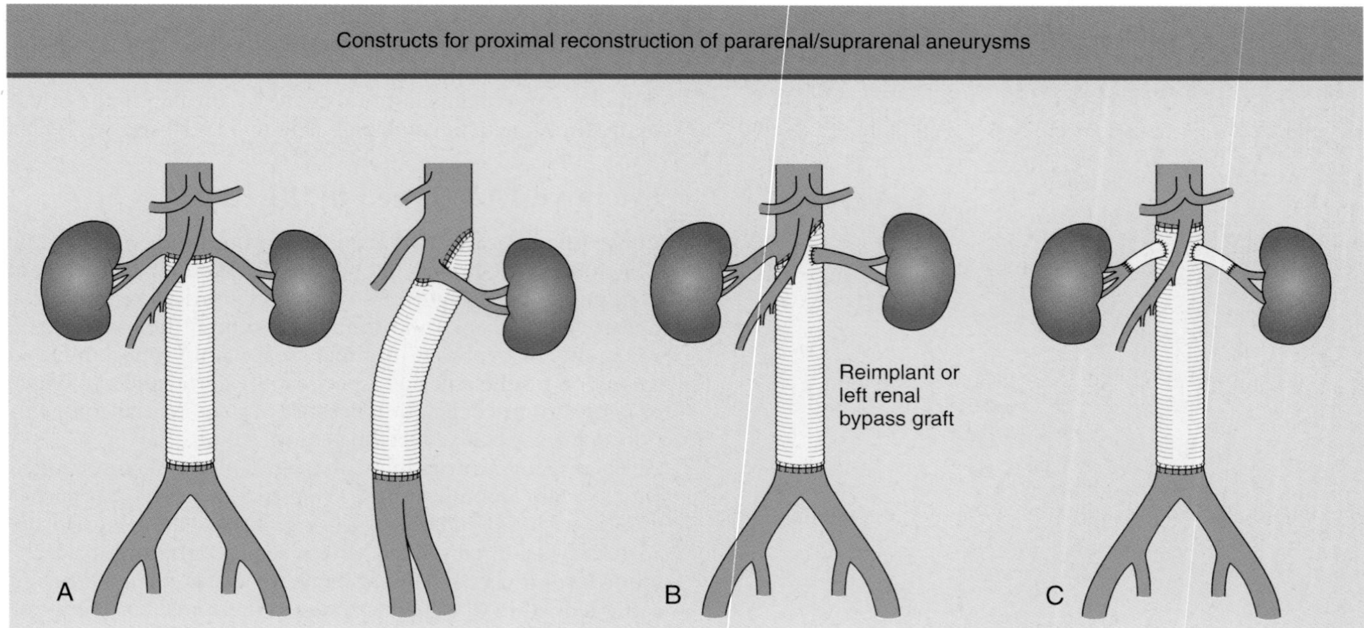

Figure 33-9. Constructs for proximal reconstruction of pararenal/suprarenal aneurysms. **A,** Posterior bevel. **B,** Left lateral bevel with left renal reconstruction. **C,** Suprarenal flush graft with bilateral renal artery reconstruction.

practice using both clamp–sew and distal perfusion techniques.[9-11,66,75,106,107] In addition, atrial–femoral bypass provides easily titratable mechanical unloading of the left ventricle, which may be desirable in patients with significant valvular or left ventricular dysfunction.

Our general approach to the technical conduct of operation involves a clamp–sew technique with specific adjuncts for spinal cord, visceral, and renal protection (Figure 33-4). We have developed a technique to provide for regional hypothermic protection to that segment of the spinal cord typically at risk for ischemic injury during TAA repair.[108-111] As schematized in Figure 33-4, this epidural cooling system uses an iced saline epidural infusion that provides moderate (25° C to 27° C) hypothermia to the spinal cord during the critical period when the aorta is cross-clamped. Direct installation of renal preservation fluid (4° C lactated Ringer's solution with 25 g/L of mannitol and 1 g/L of methylprednisolone) into the renal artery ostia is performed after the aorta is opened. Initially, 250 cc of this solution is instilled into each renal artery ostium, and a continuous drip of the same is begun through perfusion balloon-tipped catheters. Experience has shown that such an infusion results in a rapid decline of renal parenchymal temperature to 15° C after the bolus infusion and it remains at roughly 25° C during the continuous infusion.

The final adjunct in our overall approach involves inline mesenteric shunting. As displayed in Figure 33-4, a 10-mm Dacron sidearm graft is sewn to the main aortic graft so as to be located just beyond the region of the proximal anastomosis. A 20- to 24-French (Fr) arterial perfusion cannula is attached to the sidearm graft, and immediately after completion of the proximal anastomosis, prograde pulsatile perfusion can be established into either the celiac axis or SMA to minimize visceral ischemic time. In our experience, pulsatile arterial perfusion can thus be reestablished to the mesenteric circulation within 25 minutes of initial aortic cross-clamp placement.[112]

This system can be modified by using a bifurcated graft and placing a separate cannula into the left renal artery origin in patients at particular risk for perioperative renal failure.

The concept of hypothermic protection for spinal cord and visceral organs can be extended to the extreme by the use of complete cardiopulmonary bypass, profound hypothermia, and circulatory arrest. Although this method has been used as a routine operative approach for patients with extensive TAA in at least one center,[113] most surgeons specifically avoid this technique because of the potential for bleeding and pulmonary complications. While this technique is essential for the repair of complex lesions of the ascending aorta or aortic arch, in patients with TAA, its use is only recommended when proximal control and clamping of the aorta is either hazardous or not technically possible.[114]

Regardless of individual preferences concerning the conduct of operation, broad continuous exposure of the entire left posterolateral aspect of the aorta is key to technical success (Figure 33-12). The posterior portion of a standard posterolateral thoracotomy is only necessary for type I and type II aneurysms. We keep the thoracic portion of the incision low and have found the fifth or sixth interspace with posterior division of the sixth and seventh ribs provides adequate exposure in most even proximal aneurysms. A self-retaining retractor system is essential to have continuous exposure of the entire operative field (Figure 33-12). We prefer to keep the abdominal portion of the incision well lateral on the abdominal wall rather than extending to the midline. This allows the visceral contents to lie within the abdominal cavity and decreases evaporative fluid and heat losses. The abdominal portion of the incision is transperitoneal to allow direct inspection and assessment of the visceral circulation at the conclusion of operation. Exposure of the abdominal aorta is obtained by entering the plane posterior to the spleen, left kidney, and left colon. Located topographically close to the renal–lumbar vein as it

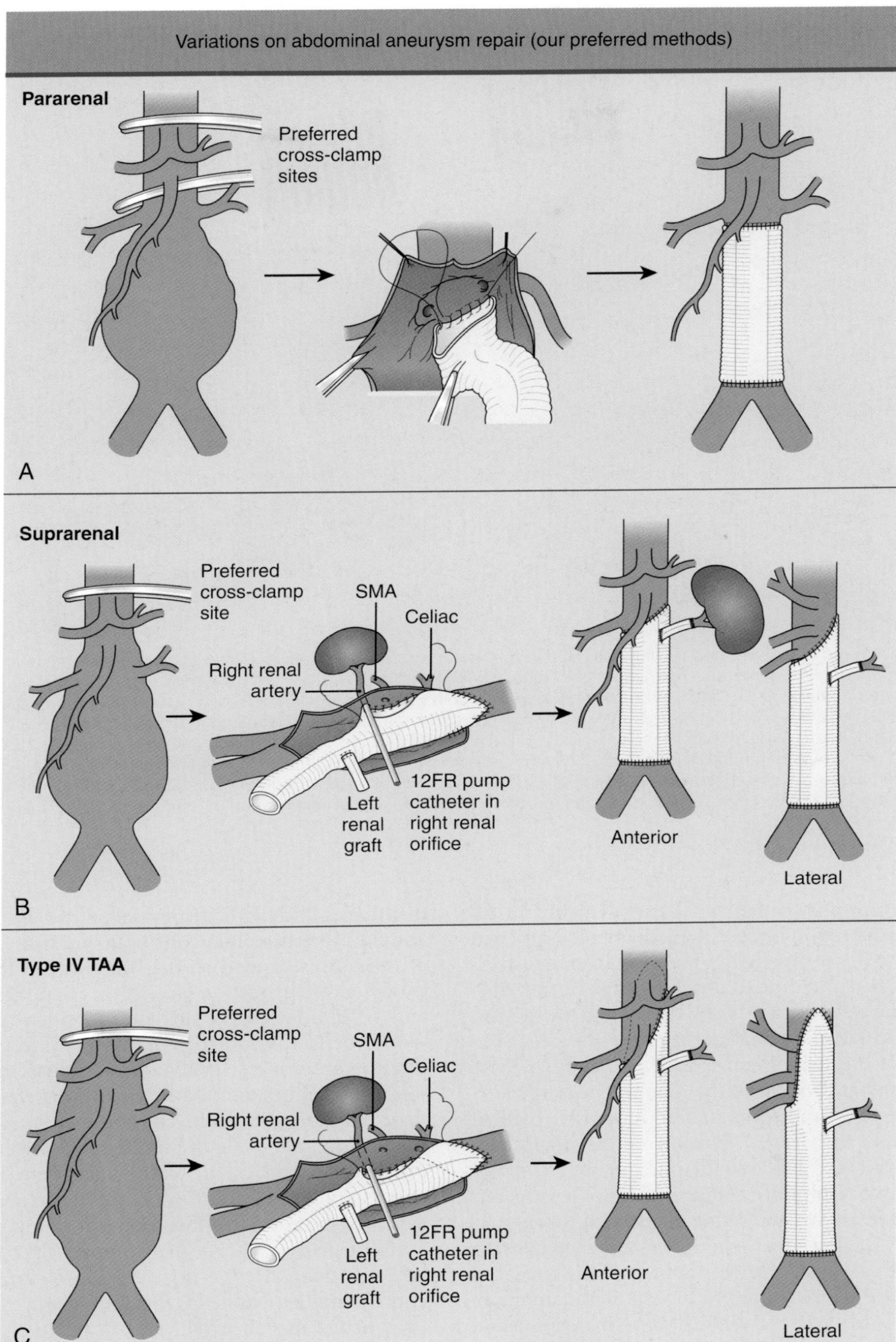

Figure 33-10. Variations on abdominal aneurysm repair (our preferred methods). **A,** Pararenal aneurysm. Cross-clamp: supraceliac or suprarenal inframesenteric depending upon aortic disease and renovisceral artery spacing. *Inset*: sewing proximally to the cuff of aorta at the renal artery orifices. **B,** Suprarenal aneurysm. Cross-clamp: supraceliac. *Inset:* beveled proximal anastomosis with 12F perfusion catheter as stent-of-sorts in the right renal artery to inhibit orificial compromise. Left renal artery reconstruction with 6mm polytetrafluoroethylene (PTFE) pre-attached to aortic prosthesis. **C,** Type IV. Cross-clamp: thoracic aorta. *Inset*: beveled proximal anastomosis encompassing the entire visceral segment and pre-attached left renal artery PTFE graft. When sewing to the visceral aortic segment, care must be taken to place the suture line as close to the visceral vessels as possible, to exclude diseased aorta.

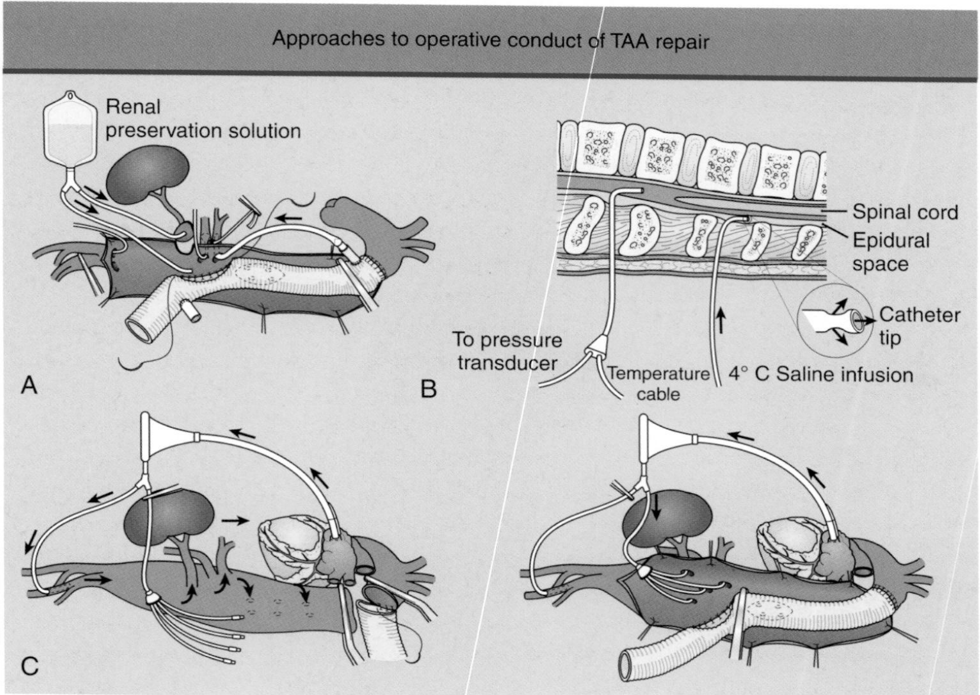

Figure 33-11. Approaches to operative conduct of thoracoabdominal aneurysm repair. **A,** Our modified clamp-and-sew technique with in-line mesenteric shunting after proximal anastomosis completion, providing pulsatile arterial flow that can be inserted into either the celiac axis (as depicted) or the superior mesenteric artery (SMA), and cold renal perfusion into both kidneys. Critical intercostal reconstruction and single inclusion button anastomosis of the celiac axis, SMA, and right renal artery with 6mm polytetrafluoroethylene sidearm graft for the left renal reconstruction. **B,** Epidural cooling for regional spinal cord hypothermia is accomplished with 4°C saline infusion via an epidural catheter, achieving 25°C prior to clamping. CSF temperature and pressure are monitored simultaneously with a separate intrathecal catheter. **C,** Repair with atriofemoral bypass and sequential aortic clamping. Two clamps are placed proximally to initially allow proximal anastomosis completion with retrograde, transfemoral aortovisceral perfusion. Subsequently, the distal clamp is moved caudad to allow critical intercostal reconstruction while renovisceral perfusion is provided by 'octopus' catheters.

courses across the aorta is the left renal artery (Figure 33-6). A key point in the dissection is identifying the renal artery and dissecting it back to its aortic origin. This is a convenient starting point for cephalad and caudad division of the retroperitoneal tissues over the aorta inferiorly and division of the median arcuate ligament and diaphragmatic crura superiorly.

The incision in the diaphragm can be by one of several methods. Direct radial division of the diaphragm to the aortic hiatus is the quickest and simplest, and it affords excellent exposure. However, such radial division of the diaphragm irrevocably paralyzes the left hemidiaphragm and contributes to postoperative respiratory compromise. Some surgeons prefer a circumferential division of the diaphragm through its muscular portion, leaving a few centimeters attached laterally to the chest wall. Engle et al.[115] have emphasized the benefit of preserving the phrenic innervation to the left hemidiaphragm by dividing only a portion lateral to the phrenic nerve insertion and then taking down the muscular fibers of the aortic hiatus. A large Penrose drain can be passed around the diaphragm pedicle for retracting superiorly and inferiorly during different stages of the subsequent reconstruction (Figure 33-13). We have applied this method liberally, particularly in patients with evidence of preoperative pulmonary compromise.

Following deflation of the left lung, the thoracic component of the dissection is usually straightforward. The mediastinal pleura over the aneurysm and proximal aorta are divided. Additional mobility on the vagus nerve can be obtained by dividing it distal to the origin of the left recurrent nerve. Should more proximal control be necessary, the ligamentum arteriosum is divided on the aorta, and in this region, care is taken to keep dissection directly on the underside of the aortic arch to avoid injury to the left pulmonary artery. In patients with degenerative aneurysm, dissection in this area is generally straightforward. When chronic dissection is the pathology, the prior inflammation from the dissecting process makes dissection more difficult. The aorta is surrounded with a vessel tape on either side of the left subclavian artery depending on the proximal extent of the aneurysm. Sufficient normal aorta should be cleared with blunt dissection on the posterior aspect of the aorta to allow room for clamp placement and an accurate proximal aortic anastomosis. External control of the left subclavian artery is not necessary as intraluminal balloon control can be obtained if the cross-clamp needs to be placed proximal to the left subclavian artery.

The aneurysm is opened initially in the abdomen, atherothrombotic debris is evacuated, and backbleeding from the right iliac or distal aorta is controlled with balloon catheters. In cases in which the entire descending thoracic aorta is resected, proximal intercostal vessel orifices between T4 and T8 are typically vigorously backbleeding and are rapidly oversewn. Intercostal arteries in the critical T8 to L1 aortic segment are evaluated for potential reimplantation into the graft, and these vessels are balloon occluded to prevent both backbleeding and the negative "sump" effect on net spinal cord perfusion that

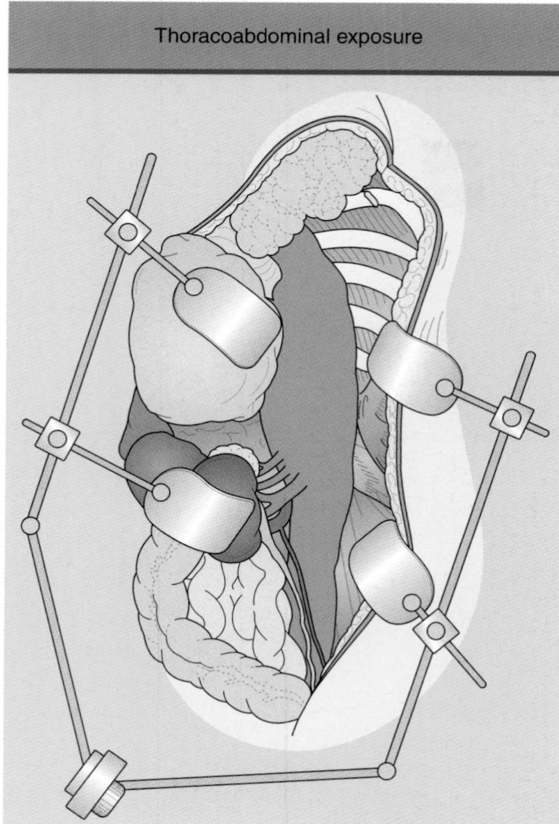

Figure 33-12. Thoracoabdominal exposure is achieved similarly to the retroperitoneal abdominal approach, with extension of a posterolateral thoracotomy into the sixth or even seventh interspace for extensive aneurysms. The Omnitract self-retaining retractor is placed opposite the patient's back to allow unimpeded access to the field. Again, the abdominal portion is not extended to midline so as to keep the peritoneal contents intraabdominal; however, the peritoneum is opened to provide an avenue to assess visceral perfusion and arterial flow.

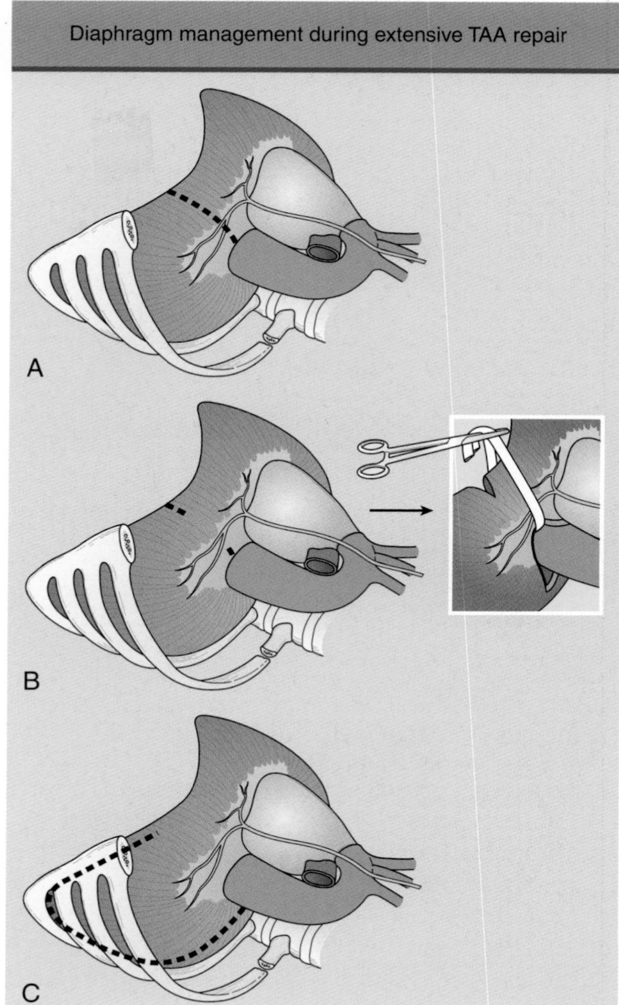

Figure 33-13. Diaphragm management during extensive thoracoabdominal repair. **A,** Radial division provides rapid, direct, and uncompromised aortic exposure but causes left hemidiaphragm paralysis. **B,** Partial division under the costal margin and dissection of the aortic hiatus preserves the phrenic nerve, and the diaphragmatic pedicle can be mobilized with a large Penrose drain. **C,** Circumferential division of the muscular diaphragm is time consuming and less hemostatic but spares the phrenic nerve.

can result from these orifices being exposed to atmospheric pressure.[116] The proximal aortic neck is prepared for reconstruction, and circumferential division of the aorta is mandatory if chronic dissection is present at the site of proximal anastomosis. If the anastomosis is carried out in the distal arch, division of the aneurysm neck is helpful in preventing late suture line–esophageal erosion.

Reconstruction of intercostal vessels in the T8 to L1 segment is usually the next step in the operation. The most common technique used is an inclusion button anastomosis. Intercostal vessels in the region of a proximal or distal aortic anastomosis can be reconstructed by use of a long beveled suture line (Figure 33-14). Depending on the topography of intercostal vessel origins, it may be possible to defer intercostal vessel reconstruction until after completion of the visceral vessel anastomosis by using partial occluding clamps on the main aortic graft. Since we have the protective effect of regional spinal cord hypothermia until all aspects of the reconstruction have been completed, there is no urgency to reestablish intercostal blood flow. The important intercostal vessels are those in the T8 to L1 segment; therefore, it is common for the intercostal inclusion button to nearly overlap (on the opposite side of the aorta) the visceral segment inclusion button.

Visceral and renal artery reconstruction is subsequently carried out. Significant occlusive lesions of the right renal and mesenteric arteries should be treated with orificial or visceral segment endarterectomy (Figure 33-15A). This method involves incising the diseased intima and media and entering the correct endarterectomy plane typically evidenced by the pinkish color of the inner adventitia. Sufficient length of the SMA and celiac artery should be dissected out to facilitate countertraction from the external side of the vessel, although this is not possible with the right renal artery. Should the calcified end of the obstructing lesion not break off easily, sharp division under direct vision is the preferred method. The most common method of visceral–renal artery reconstruction, which has been applied in the overwhelming majority of our cases, is a single inclusion button to encompass the origins of the celiac artery, SMA, and right renal artery (Figure 33-15B). If the aneurysm is excessively large in the visceral

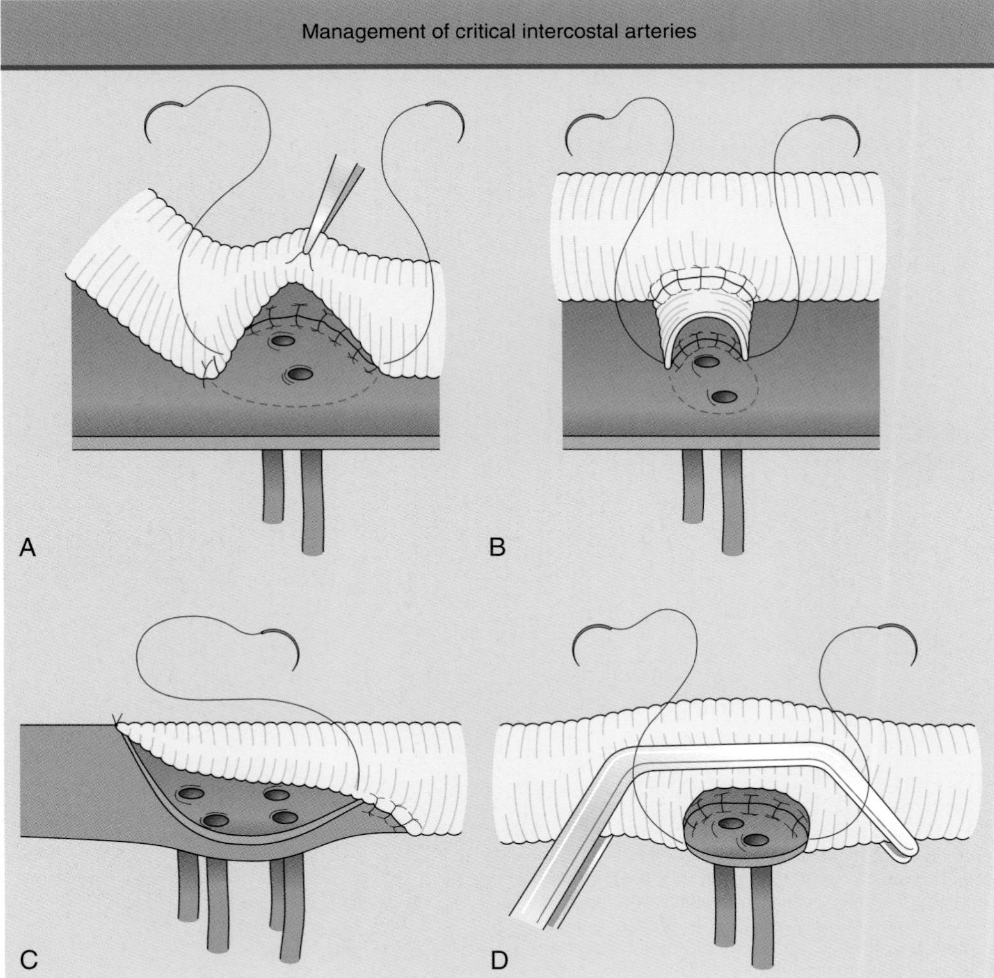

Figure 33-14. Methods of management of critical intercostal arteries. **A,** Inclusion button anastomosis. **B,** Separate sidearm graft. **C,** Beveled anastomosis preservation when possible. **D,** Carrell patch mobilization and direct reimplantation into the graft.

aortic segment, wide separation of the visceral–renal ostia may necessitate individual inclusion button anastomoses or grafts. Suture bites should be close to the visceral vessel origins to avoid leaving too much aneurysmal aortic wall. As the posterior aspect of this suture line continues around the inferior border of the right renal artery, we exchange the 6-Fr perfusion catheter for a 12-Fr perfusion catheter to serve as a stent of sorts in the right renal artery origin. This catheter is gently agitated up and down as the suture line moves around the renal artery to ensure that the latter is not compromised by the suture bites. The topography and course of the right renal artery should be interrogated with this indwelling catheter because, in circumstances when the right renal artery drapes over a large infrarenal component of the aneurysm, occlusion of the right renal artery is a definite technical complication of operation (Figure 33-15B). Just before completion of this suture line, backbleeding and patency of the celiac artery, SMA, and right renal artery are verified and the inline mesenteric shunt is clamped and removed.

Reconstruction of the left renal artery is now accomplished with a separate sidearm graft of 6-mm polytetrafluoroethylene (PTFE). This allows a direct, deliberate end-to-end anastomosis and permits flexibility in dealing with the spectrum of occlusive lesions, multiple renal arteries, and so forth that may be encountered. As noted in Figure 33-15, care must be taken to place this sidearm graft in an orientation where it will not kink when returned to its anatomical position. Some surgeons prefer to use a single inclusion button to encompass both renal arteries along with the visceral vessels, but in our experience, this includes too great an area of aneurysmal aorta unless the aneurysm is exceedingly small in the visceral aortic segment. Allowing too much diseased aorta remain in the visceral patch risks aneurysmal change over time.[4,117,118] When a single, pristine left renal artery and orifice are encountered, direct reimplantation may be entertained. The clamp is then moved again to a position inferior to the origin of the left renal artery graft, and the distal aortic anastomosis is carried out. We make every effort to perform tube reconstructions to the aortic bifurcation unless there is gross aneurysmal disease of the proximal common iliac arteries. After reestablishment of flow to the lower extremities and verification of adequate perfusion by intraoperative pulse volume recordings, Doppler signals in the left renal, celiac, and superior mesenteric vessels are checked, in addition to palpation of the SMA pulse in the root of the mesentery. Hemostasis usually is adequate at this point, but infusions of platelets and fresh frozen plasma are typically increased, when a final check for hemostasis is made. Careful inspection of the inferior aspect of the aneurysm sac in both the chest and the abdomen is necessary to detect backbleeding of lumbar vessels, intercostal vessels, or both, which can be an important source of postoperative hemorrhage. The redundant aneurysm sac is then sutured securely over the aortic prosthesis in the abdomen and the chest. Occasionally, in patients with modest-size aneurysms, chronic dissections, or prior proximal thoracic aortic grafts, the aneurysm wall is insufficient to cover the proximal suture line and aortic graft. In selected cases, we have used a PTFE patch to exclude the aortic prosthesis from the left lung. The left kidney is returned to its bed, and perinephric fat usually suffices to provide adequate coverage of the aortic graft in the region of the visceral aortic segment. During closure, renal artery reconstructions are interrogated one final time. As displayed in Table 33-3, clamp times, blood turnover, and blood component replacement vary as a function of aneurysm extent, but overall operative time can be kept in the 5- to 6-hour range for most patients.

ENDOVASCULAR RECONSTRUCTION

Initial success with endoluminal treatment for isolated infrarenal aortic aneurysms (endovascular aneurysm repair, or EVAR) was described by Parodi et al. in Argentina.[119] The feasibility of isolated thoracic aortic stent grafting (thoracic endovascular aneurysm repair, or TEVAR) was introduced 3 years later, in 1994, by Dake et al.[120] Endografting in these positions has steadily continued the refining process and is now commonplace. Reduced operative morbidity and mortality compared to surgical repair is recognized. Transrenal fixation for proximal seating of endovascular aortic grafts is also now performed regularly.[121] Although longer-term effects of suprarenal fixation are largely unknown, currently undergoing study, and remain controversial, this method appears to assists proximal graft fixation.[122]

The visceral segment has been a formidable technical barrier to contiguous endovascular repair of the descending thoracic and abdominal aorta, and thus complex aneurysms. Fenestrated, scalloped, and branched endografts continue to mature and are undergoing trials. Hybrid procedures such as combining open infrarenal repair, retrograde visceral reconstruction, and TEVAR are well known (Figure 33-16). Both open surgical arch and abdominal debranching maneuvers have been described to augment seal zones and to allow complete endovascular repair while maintaining aortic branch perfusion without aortic clamping. Arch repair with dedicated endograft constructs, as well as double-barrel and fenestration techniques, is being developed and reported. A trial is ongoing to decipher what role endovascular repair plays in aortic

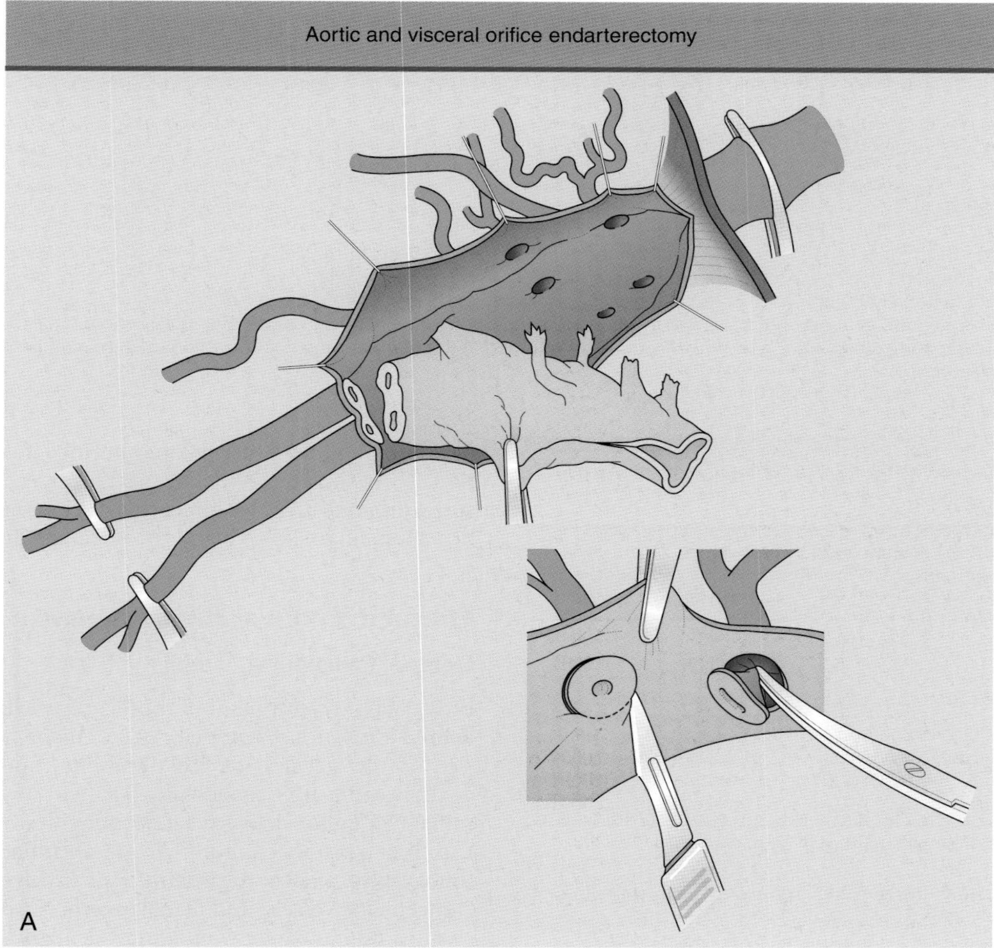

Figure 33-15. Renovisceral occlusive disease. **A,** This may be dealt with by transaortic visceral segment endarterectomy or, when limited in nature, by orificial endarterectomy.

Continued

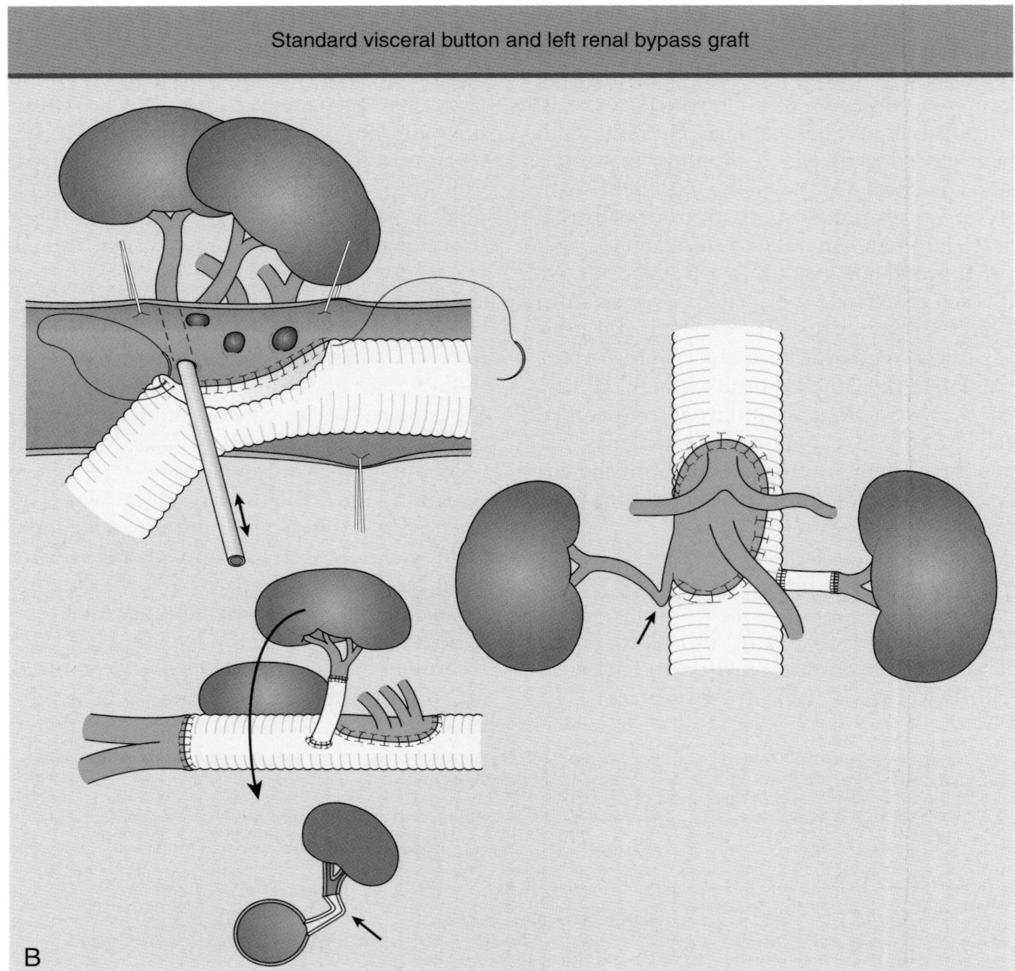

Figure 33-15—cont'd B, Creation of a standard visceral button inclusion anastomosis of the celiac axis, SMA, and right renal artery and a 6-mm polytetrafluoroethylene sidearm bypass for left renal artery reconstruction. When performing this, we use a 12-Fr perfusion catheter as a stent of sorts in the right renal artery to prevent compromise of its orifice as the anastomosis is carried around these arterial origins. Care must be taken with both renal reconstructions. If the infrarenal portion of the aneurysm is large and the right renal artery drapes over this portion, once reconstructed the right renal may kink against the aortic graft. Also, when the left kidney is returned to the retroperitoneum, unless the sidearm graft has been trimmed to the precise length, it may kink.

Table 33-3
Operative Characteristics in 337 Thoracoabdominal Aneurysm Repairs*

	Type I and II	Type III and IV	
Intraoperative Data	(n = 151)	(n = 186)	p
OR time (minutes)	329 ± 95	298 ± 93	0.0025
Visceral XC time (minutes)	52.5 ± 16.8	42.7 ± 11.4	<0.0001
Total XC time (minutes)	72.7 ± 28.8	76.1 ± 23.7	0.22
Total transfusion (cm^3)	3341 ± 2035	2301 ± 1755	<0.0001
FFP (units)	6.4 ± 4.2	4.4 ± 3.8	<0.0001
Platelets (units)	10.1 ± 5.9	5.6 ± 5.5	<0.0001

From Cambria RP, Clouse WD, Dorer DJ, et al. *Ann Surg* 2002;216:471-479.
*FFP, fresh frozen plasma; OR, operating room; XC, cross-clamping.

dissection and the potential for altering late aneurysm formation.[123] As Chapter 29 delineates current progress and issues surrounding EVAR, we direct this discussion on complex aortic aneurysm to TEVAR and the visceral segment.

Thoracic Endovascular Aneurysm Repair

General Procedural Aspects

Proprietary development of thoracic aortic devices has lagged behind those for infrarenal AAA. This is largely due to the size of the devices, device durability, and several notable anatomical factors challenging TEVAR. These concerns culminate in either delivery access difficulty or poor endograft seal and treatment failure. Aortic and iliac tortuosity, arch topography, aneurysm proximity or involvement of the brachiocephalic vessels, and iliac size or occlusive disease all may create a milieu whereby endograft delivery and proper seal is compromised. Proximal and distal attachment zones should be at least 2 cm in length to ensure adequate fixation and seal.

Depending on the population studied, some 5% to 30% of patients with TAA may not allow these criteria for adequate seal zones.[66,124] Currently developed devices require delivery platforms of at least 20 to 26 Fr; thus, a minimal iliac diameter of 7.6 to 9.1 mm is required. In the presence of significant calcification and narrowing, operative conduits are often required. Further confounding iliac access for endografting in the thoracic position is the larger relative proportion of female patients afflicted with thoracic aortic disease as they usually have smaller iliac systems.[14] To wit, 9% to 30% of patients require conduit access to allow successful endograft platform delivery.[125-130]

Perhaps more so than in the abdominal aorta, oversizing of thoracic endografts has unmasked serious troubles with graft infolding, graft collapse, aortic thrombosis, and failure.[124,131] Thoracic endografts should, therefore, only be oversized by roughly 10% of the aortic diameter. The arch configuration is critical to proper endograft placement. The posterior aortic arch genu creates an angulation along the inner aortic curvature such that the proximal edge of the endograft may not conform to the aortic wall at this position and project into the lumen. This can lead to graft collapse, migration, endoleak, thrombosis, stroke, and graft failure in this extremely high flow, shear force location. When graft protrusion takes place in conjunction with infolding secondary to graft oversizing, it portends poor durability and outcomes. As humans age, the arch enlarges and elongates leading to a more acute posterior angle. This has clearly been identified in experiences with endovascular treatment of degenerative aortic disease. When angulation causes difficulties in accomplishing thoracic endografting, brachial access, either right or left depending on morphology and desired proximal placement, can help in a couple of areas. First, it can assist in visualization and landmarking without hindering deployment. Also, when a long, stiff guide wire is snared and traverses from the brachial to the iliofemoral access, it straightens the angulation somewhat and may aid in device tracking and pushability.

To circumvent these collective adversities of the proximal aorta, more proximal seal length has been gained along a less angulated zone by intentionally placing the endograft across the left subclavian origin with or without adjunctive revascularization.[132,133] In our experience, this has been necessary in 20% of those undergoing TEVAR for aneurysmal disease.[130,133]

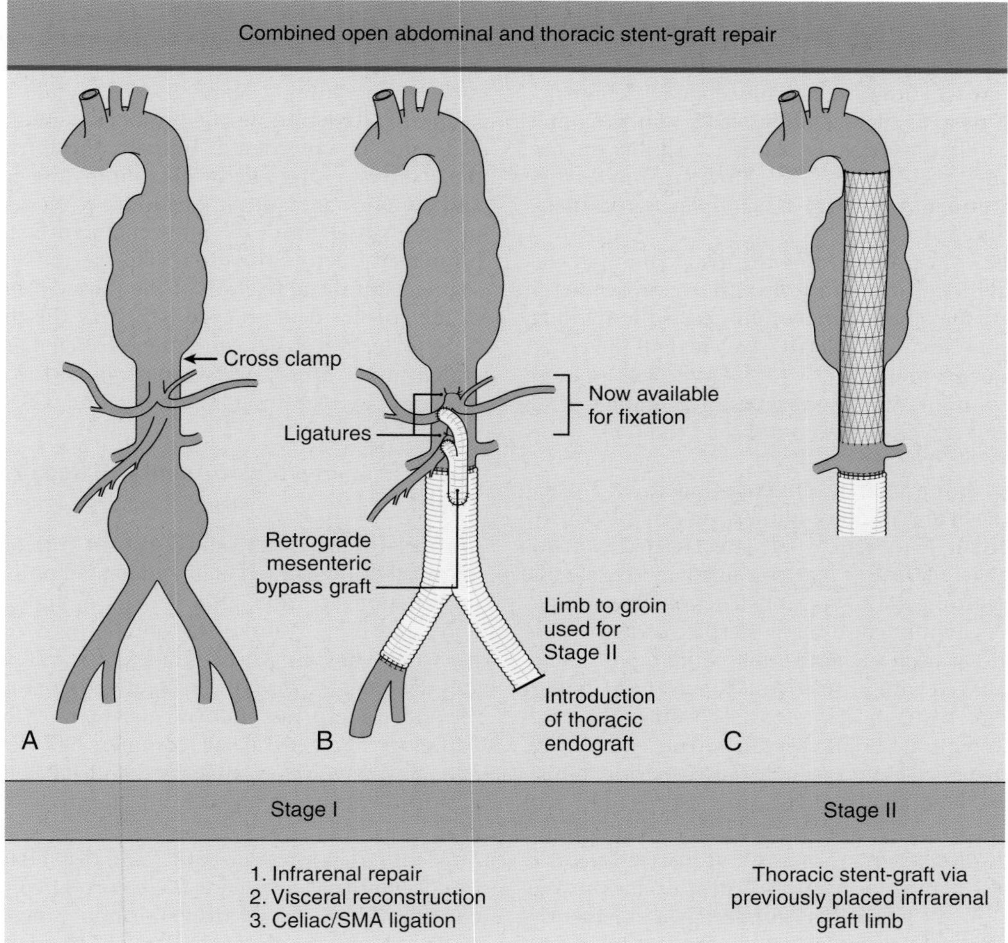

Figure 33-16. Combined open abdominal and thoracic stent graft repair. **A,** Thoracoabdominal aortic aneurysm with sparing of the visceral segment, or the so-called dumbbell aneurysm. **B,** Initial standard open repair of the infrarenal abdominal portion is performed using a bifurcated prosthesis accompanied by retrograde mesenteric reconstruction using a bifurcated graft to the celiac and superior mesenteric artery, followed by ligation of these vessels. Then the visceral aortic segment may be used as the distal fixation site for the thoracic endograft. **C,** This is performed in stages, allowing spinal cord perfusion to accommodate, using one limb of the prior placed infrarenal graft for adequate access.

Most TEVAR trial protocols require left subclavian reconstruction in these instances, yet we have performed this in only 57% of our cases with little consequence. It is rare for a patient to have significant left arm ischemia with this approach, and it has been widely accepted and viewed as benign. A cautionary note, however: recent data by the European Collaborators on Stent Graft Techniques for Aortic Aneurysm Repair investigators showed intentional coverage of the left subclavian artery without revascularization during endovascular repair of thoracic aortic pathologies as a significant independent predictor of SCI (odds ratio 3.9, $p = 0.027$).[134] Consequently, we have changed our approach and now revascularize the left subclavian before TEVAR should the operative plan include coverage of this artery for proper proximal steal.

Stroke also appears more prevalent when proximal extension requiring left subclavian coverage and revascularization is undertaken.[127,134,135] This likely represents more involved manipulation of the aortic arch and carotid systems in these situations. Rarer neurological sequelae are hemodynamic vertebrobasilar insufficiency or acute posterior fossa stroke, but preoperative attention to the status of the vertebral arteries is important to avoid these complications. The risk of stroke is roughly 5% with surgical ligation of the vertebral artery, and this must be considered and speaks to the need for proper cerebrovascular arteriography before these cases.[136,137] Collectively, it is apparent that cavalier coverage of the left subclavian artery during TEVAR is no longer acceptable. Furthermore, open extraanatomical brachiocephalic debranching, with varying degrees of ascending, arch, and proximal descending endograft coverage, is gaining visibility in the treatment of degenerative diseases.[138-142] How these endeavors will fit into the treatment paradigm for complex aortic aneurysms is being defined.

Should there be concern regarding the distal landing zone and the location of the celiac origin, a visceral selective catheter can be inserted into the celiac from femoral access for marking purposes. Some now advocate selective coverage of the celiac with little consequence during TEVAR.[143] We have not yet adopted such an outlook. Varying degrees of debranching of the visceral segment can also be accomplished to increase the distal seal zone.[139,140,144-149]

Specific factors implicated in contributing to SCI after TEVAR include the extent of descending aorta excluded, previous or concomitant AAA repair, left subclavian coverage, hypogastric coverage, the use of iliac conduits, and renal failure.[66,134,150,151] Regarding the AAA reconstruction, it is unclear whether infrarenal clamping or lumbar sacrifice contribute to ischemic injury. It has been suggested that patients with these risk factors be managed with protective adjuncts. As SCI after TEVAR is more related to critical intercostal coverage and cord under perfusion, epidural cooling serves no role, while CSF drainage is likely beneficial in these high-risk scenarios. While the benefit of such an adjunct remains statistically unproven, it has been our practice to preoperatively place spinal drains in those with acute dissections, prior aortic grafts, stable aortic ruptures, and grafts planned for long-segment exclusion. We place them post-TEVAR when this is undertaken emergently and patients are relatively unstable.

Although an early concern with first-generation devices, the "windsock" effect of ventricular ejection, leading to inaccurate proximal deployment (particularly when performed near the arch), has now been overcome by superior design attributes. Early in thoracic endografting, many found this to be a significant problem in achieving successful treatment. Poor graft expansion and movement were seen with disastrous consequences. Before deployment, the blood pressure should be lowered to a mean arterial pressure of 50 to 70 mm Hg. This allows for deployment without a billowing effect on the expanding graft and more accurate placement. Means to accomplish this include mechanical and pharmacological manipulations. Pharmacological methods use rapid onset antihypertensive medications and adenosine administration. Adenosine is attractive as it allows for short-term asystole and no fluctuations in pressure during deployment. This induced cardiac arrest seems relatively harmless from both a systemic and a neurological standpoint.[152] Placement of a transvenous pacemaker with tachycardic, hypotensive manipulation is also being used to achieve reduced mean arterial pressure mechanically, but this must be used sensibly in those with significant coronary artery disease or heart failure.[153,154] Another described method of mechanically induced hypotension for accurate thoracic endograft placement is temporary caval occlusion.[155] Regardless of the method chosen, it appears thus far that induction of hypotension to aid in deployment is safe and useful. We have found nothing more than pressure control and reduction to be necessary in most situations.

Moreover, we have had success with our hybrid repair experience of combining open abdominal repair with thoracic endografting (Figure 33-16). While combined repair is an attractive option in "dumbbell" aneurysms, the risk of SCI must be considered. Initially, the infrarenal portion of the aneurysm is repaired with a bifurcated graft. Before celiac and superior mesenteric ligation, retrograde reconstruction of these vessels from the infrarenal graft is performed with a bifurcated Dacron prosthesis. This permits use of the visceral segment for distal fixation of the thoracic endograft. Because of the current data on cord ischemia, the thoracic endograft is performed in stages, with one infrarenal graft limb used for endoluminal access and reanastomosed at the appropriate level once endografting is complete.

Thoracic Endovascular Aneurysm Repair Device Trials

European collaborators and registries preceded administrative approval in the United States and aided production of needed information. In 2005, after 7 years of clinical trials, the U.S. Food and Drug Administration approved commercial use of the Gore Thoracic Aortic Graft (TAG; WL Gore and Associates, Flagstaff, Arizona). This first approval ushered in the era of more widespread endovascular therapy for thoracic aortic pathology. In general, all commercially developed thoracic endografts involve prosthetic (expanded PTFE, fluorinated ethylene propylene, or polyester) attached to self-expanding nickel titanium (nitinol) or stainless steel stents with seal dependent on stent radial force, proximal and distal barbs, or both. The multicenter trials involving these current commercial thoracic endografts have provided an enormous amount of data.

The WL Gore phase II (PIVOTAL) trial is a prospective, nonrandomized, multicenter trial comparing TEVAR using the TAG endoprosthesis to open repair of thoracic aortic aneurysms. The studies endpoint purposes were to assess the safety and efficacy of the TAG device in both short-term and long-term evaluation.[127,135] Thus, 140 patients were assigned TEVAR and 94 open surgical repair. Perioperative (30-day) mortality occurred significantly less often in the TEVAR group (2.1% versus 11.7%, $p = 0.007$), as did respiratory failure (4% versus 20%, $p < 0.001$), renal failure (1% versus 13%, $p = 0.01$), and SCI (3% versus 14%, $p = 0.003$). Peripheral vascular complications were more prominent in the TAG group (14% versus 4%, $p = 0.015$). Lengths of hospital and intensive care unit stay were significantly less in the TEVAR cohort. Of the TAG group, 98% had successful implantation of the endograft, as 3 patients were delivery failures due to iliac access. In addition, 21 patients (15%) required operative conduit for device delivery. At 3 years, freedom from aneurysm-related mortality was 97% in those undergoing TEVAR and 90% in the open surgical controls ($p = 0.024$). All-cause mortality was no different between groups.[156,157]

Recently, the 5-year data from this trial have been released.[158] The noted benefits of TEVAR appear to be maintained in the long term. While all-cause mortality remains similar between groups, aneurysm-related death continues to be significantly less in those repaired endoluminally (2.8% versus 11.7%, $p = 0.008$). All aneurysm-related deaths occurred in the first year after treatment. Within the TAG group, significantly fewer major adverse events were seen at 5 years ($p = 0.004$). Endoleak has been identified at some point in 10.6% of the cohort. However, only five patients (3.6%) have required aneurysm-related reintervention and one open conversion. Indeed, overall aneurysm-related secondary procedures were performed less often in the TAG group compared to the open surgical controls over the 5 years ($p = 0.01$). Only one case of endograft migration of 10 mm or more was noted (0.7%).

Other devices currently in U.S. trials have been available elsewhere for some time. The Talent thoracic endovascular graft (Medtronic AVE, Santa Rosa, California) has now evolved into a third generation, the Medtronic Valiant thoracic endograft. In 2005, the Vascular Talent Thoracic Stent Graft System for the Treatment of Thoracic Aortic Aneurysms (VALOR) trial using the Talent system completed enrollment.[125,159,160] It includes three arms: PIVOTAL data group, phase II; high-risk patients; and a registry group. Historical literature was used for comparison to open repair. In the high-risk group (Society for Vascular Surgery comorbidity of 3 or deemed nonsurgical candidates), most were treated for degenerative pathology (82% TAA, 9% aneurysmal change in chronic dissection). Operative mortality was 8.4%, stroke was 8%, and an SCI rate of 5.5% was found. Endoleak was present in 10%, and some 2.6% required secondary intervention by 6 months. These results are reasonable and compare favorably to contemporary open repair outcomes. Recently, 1-year data from the PIVOTAL cohort was released. In these good-surgical-risk degenerative aneurysm patients, 159 of the 195 enrolled had completed protocol. Successful deployment was achieved in 99.5%. The 30-day mortality was 2.1%, with SCI and stroke occurring in 1.5% and 3.6%, respectively. All-cause mortality was 16.1%, and aneurysm-related mortality was 3.1%. Successful aneurysm treatment without growth or endoleak was present in 89.2%. Currently, VALOR II is recruiting to further evaluate the Valiant thoracic endograft, which is the third-generation Medtronic thoracic endograft.

The Study of Thoracic Aortic Aneurysm Repair with the Zenith TX2 TAA Endovascular Graft (STARZ) trial using the Cook Zenith TX2 thoracic endovascular graft (William Cook Europe, ApS, Bjaeverskov, Denmark) has recently published data from the first year of the trial.[161,162] It involves 160 patients undergoing TEVAR compared to 70 patients anatomically unfit for TEVAR. The 30-day mortality (1.9% versus 5.7%) was lower with TEVAR, and major perioperative adverse events were less common (9.4%% versus 33%, $p < 0.01$). Specifically, cardiovascular, pulmonary, and vascular complications were significantly less in the TEVAR cohort. Stroke, paraplegia, and paraparesis tended to occur less often in the TEVAR group (2.5% versus 8.6%, $p = 0.07$; 1.3% versus 5.7%, $p = 0.07$; and 4.4% versus 0%, $p = 0.10$, respectively). Endoleaks were present 13% at discharge, and this decreased to 2.6% at 6 months and 3.9% at 1 year. Over the year after repair, secondary intervention was similarly necessary in the TEVAR and open groups (4.4% TEVAR versus 5.7% open, $p = 0.74$). No statistical difference was seen in all-cause mortality and aneurysm-related mortality between the groups. Ventilator use, intensive care unit stay, time to ambulation, bowel function, and hospital discharge were all significantly less in those undergoing TEVAR. Endograft migration has been found in three (2.8% of those with follow-up) patients.

In concert with multicenter trials, ongoing reports from registries and institutional experiences have also helped solidify TEVAR results.[128,129,134,163-165] Our experience at the Massachusetts General Hospital comparing TEVAR with open repair for thoracic aortic pathology during the period encompassing January 1, 1996, to November 30, 2005, has recently been delineated.[130] Despite nearly 28% of the TEVAR group being deemed unfit for open repair, the perioperative mortality was 7.6% compared to 15.1% in the open cohort ($p = 0.09$). Conduit access was necessary in 24%. SCI developed in 6.7% of the TEVAR group and was not statistically different from the open repair group (8.6%, $p = 0.44$). Reintervention was required in some 10% of both groups, and actuarial freedom from reintervention was 80% at 2 years. No difference was found in the risk of perioperative stroke, operative time, late survival, or aneurysm-related mortality. These outcomes are seen throughout the experience of those performing both open and endovascular repair.[166]

Methods of Visceral Aortic Segment Management

Debranching

Anatomical constraints currently challenging endovascular repair of complex aortic aneurysms, particularly short fixation zones, as well as the significant risks of open repair, have provided an impetus to develop extension of endovascular technology. To wit, hybrid procedures providing extraanatomical aortic arch and visceral segment revascularization with aortic branch ligation have been described to lengthen and stabilize fixation zones. Reported success with such aortic "debranching" and staged endovascular reconstruction has led to interest in these maneuvers.

Proximal, or arch, debranching may involve anatomical ascending aorta–based brachiocephalic reconstruction or any combination of extraanatomical, extrathoracic reconstructions.[138-141] Visceral segment debranching may involve direct distal aortovisceral bypass or retrograde unilateral or bilateral iliovisceral bypass. Potential inflow from a celiac–based reconstruction (hepatic and splenic) may be considered depending on aneurysm morphology and areas of needed endograft fixation.[139,149] To date, this technique remains descriptive without comparative studies. While these procedures seem shrewd and logical in patients deemed high risk for standard operative repair, these open debranching operations are not benign. They are challenging, involved open revascularizations. Case series of debranching procedures with follow-on aortic endografting indicate broad ranges of morbidity and mortality. However, perioperative mortalities of up to 30% are seen, and perioperative complications occur in up to 33%.[140,144-148] These indeed seem comparable to the contemporary experience with open repair.

The procedure requires many technical steps. The early primary patency of the visceral bypasses appears quite satisfactory, with rates of more than 95% at 8 to 12 months reported.[146,147] Longer-term durability information is lacking. In addition, the durability of these endovascular repairs and any potential migratory or thrombotic effects on visceral branches remains undefined. However, minimal paraplegia is noted. This is likely this procedure's major benefit and a product of visceral flow maintenance, as the accompanying physiological insults of visceral ischemia and aortic clamping during open repair are attenuated. Thus far, the preliminary collective experience suggests the use of debranching techniques is feasible but at significant remaining risk and speaks to the need for refinements in total endovascular reconstruction of the visceral segment.

Endovascular Repair Incorporating the Visceral Segment

To date, two methods for incorporation of the renovisceral vessels in endograft repair have been developed: graft fenestration and side-branch extension grafts. The construct, feasibility, and implantation technique of fenestrated visceral segment endografts was introduced in 1996 and further developed by Anderson et al.[19] Based on preoperative 1-mm interval CT scanning with reconstruction, each endograft is custom made with fenestrations placed at specific, measured locations for the renovisceral ostia (Figure 33-17). These fenestrations are radiopaquely marked. The device itself is based on the Zenith system. It is modular (unilimbed and a contralimb extension) with an uncovered Gianturco Z-stent (William Cook Europe, Bjaeverskov, Denmark) for proximal fixation. No stent wiring crosses the fenestrations, and radiopaque markers are placed on the posterior and anterior graft surface for proper axial placement. Apposition of the renal fenestrations to the ostia in these early cases was provided by modified Palmaz P204 stents (Cordis Endovascular, Warren, New Jersey). These stents are placed with a small portion in the endograft lumen. The modification consists of laser cutting to facilitate flaring to 90 degrees in one end of the stent. This provides for graft-wall approximation and the ability to endoluminally access the renal arteries. The graft is loaded with the prongs of the proximal stent separately capped and deployable to allow manipulation and positioning of the graft in the neck. In a series of 13 patients, Anderson's group initially communicated feasibility and technical success in 100% of 19 renal arteries, five accessory renal arteries, and nine SMAs targeted for fenestration. Two type II endoleaks occurred.[19]

Since these early phases of fenestration technology, much work has been accomplished, including further communication from groups in Australia and Europe.[167-172] The fenestrated endograft based on the Cook Zenith system continues to undergo minor modifications. It has become more commercially custom made, and various balloon-expandable stents, both covered and uncovered, have been used for ostial fixation with flaring on the luminal side of the endograft by progressive dilation with increasing sizes. Fenestration has now been applied specifically to pararenal aneurysms and those that are more extensive. In the United States, this treatment is available in a few, select centers, and a phase I trial is forthcoming. Greenberg and colleagues have led the introduction of fenestration in the United States, and their experience at the Cleveland Clinic continues.[173-175] They recently presented 119 patients encompassing varying degrees of renovisceral vessel coverage.[174] They found that 302 vessels were below the proximal level of the endograft, with the most common construct being bilateral renal artery and SMA incorporation. Graft placement was successful in all patients, and no renovisceral vessel was lost intraprocedurally. One perioperative death occurred. Type I and III endoleaks occurred in 11 patients (9%). These were treated aggressively with reintervention. At 30 days, endoleak was present in 10% of patients and all were type II in nature. During follow-up, 10 renal artery occlusions, 12 renal artery stenoses, and an SMA stenosis were noted. Five patients required hemodialysis, and 25% of those treated sustained at least transient renal dysfunction. At 19 months mean follow-up, there were no aneurysm-related deaths and no conversions to open repair.

A second method to permit even more proximal endograft placement using multiple side-branch grafts has been described by Chuter et al.[20] Using this system, they initially grafted a type III TAA; however, the patient suffered delayed paraplegia, again reinforcing the continued potential of ischemic cord injury with endovascular technology.[176] Recent depiction of Chuter's evolving experience with this complex procedure using the next-generation customized branched graft (Cook Australia, Brisbane, Australia) has been published.[177] The device construct is modular and consists of a proximal attachment portion; a narrowed visceral graft segment incorporating stumps, or cuffs, for renovisceral vessel extensions; and a distal attachment segment. Stumps for the celiac and SMA are 18 mm long and 6 to 8 mm in diameter and are marked with radiopaque material. Fluency PTFE covered nitinol stents (C.R. Bard, Tempe, Arizona) 60 mm in length are used as bridging renovisceral grafts from a left brachial approach. Each of these is then reinforced with Wallstents (Boston Scientific, Natick, Massachussets) oversized compared to the fluency to prevent kinking. Chuter has deployed this graft in 22 patient with extension grafts into 81 visceral vessels. All underwent CSF drainage. Procedural success was achieved in 100%. Perioperative death occurred in 2 (9.1%) patients. One was due to paraplegia and renal failure. Significant complications occurred in 9 (41%). Three surviving patients experienced transient SCI (15%). No paraplegia, stroke, or myocardial infarction occurred in survivors. One branch vessel occlusion occurred at 1 month; hence, a 99% branch patency at 1 month was achieved. Two (9.1%) of patients required reintervention during surveillance thus far.

Although progress in fenestration and branch graft technology has rendered endovascular complex aneurysm repair possible, such work has, to date, been preliminary and continues at the province of a few acknowledged innovators in stent

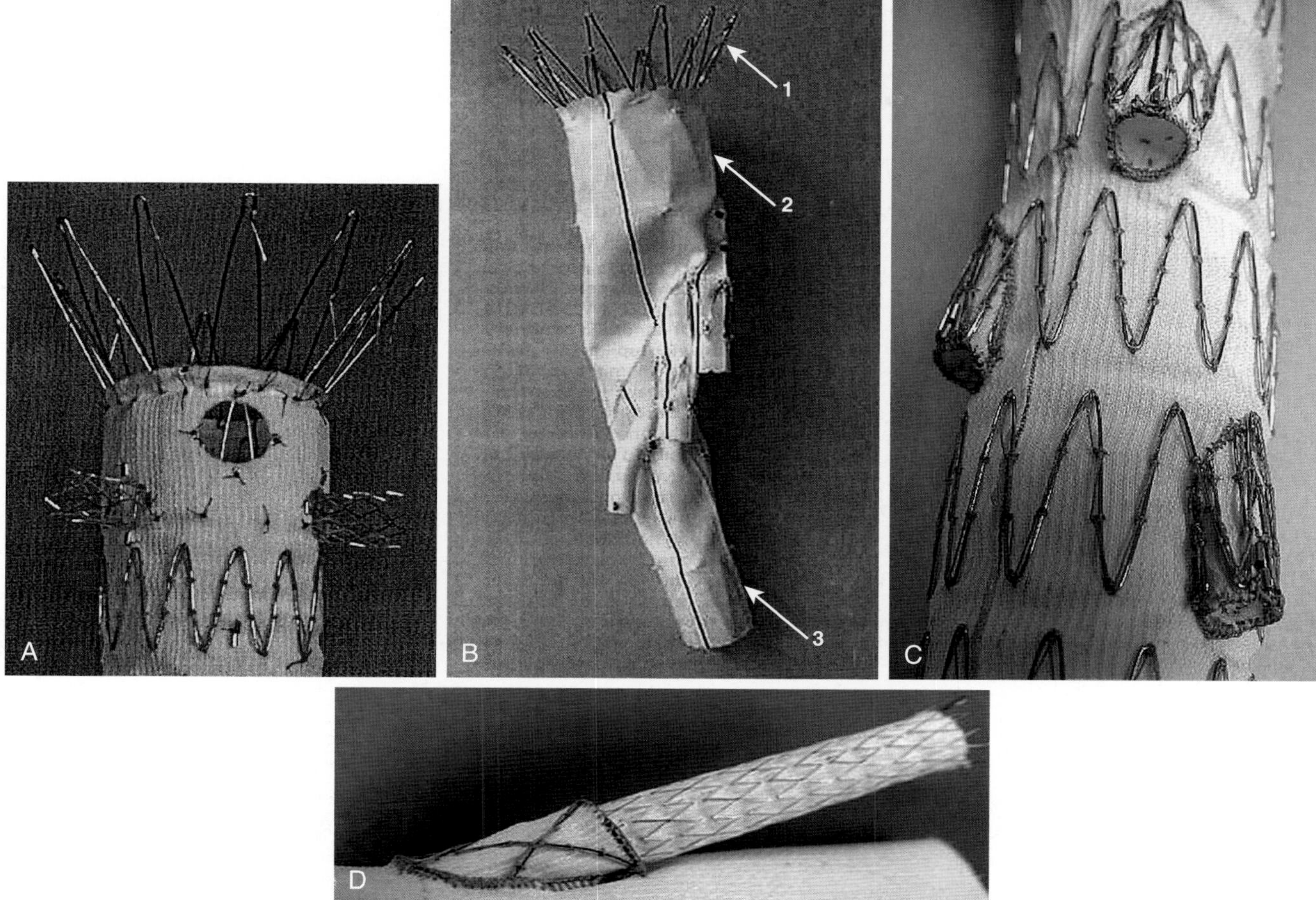

Figure 33-17. Endovascular constructs used for repair of aneurysms involving the visceral aortic segment. **A,** Custom fenestrated device used by Anderson et al. in their initial experience. Based upon preoperative imaging, the fenestrations are made and surrounded by radiopaque markers. The renal fenestrations are supported by modified Palmaz-204 stents that flare and approximate the graft to the renal orifices. **B,** Side-branch extension type graft developed by Chuter et al. Note the active, proximal fixation stent (1) and the distal segment (3) in which a standard AAA endovascular graft is placed for completion of distal reconstruction. **C,** Newer custom-made, proprietary branched device with premade renovisceral access cuffs (Cook Australia, Inc., Brisbane, Australia). **D,** Renovisceral cuffs are selected from brachial access and Fluency covered stents (C.R. Bard, Inc; Tempe, AZ) docked into the renovisceral arteries, then supported by Wallstents (Boston Scientific Corp., Natick, MA). (**A,** Anderson JL, Berce M, Hartley DE. Endoluminal aortic grafting with renal and superior mesenteric artery incorporation by graft fenestration. *J Endovasc Ther* 2001;8:3-8. **B,** Chuter TAM, Gordon RL, Reilly LM, et al. An endovascular system for thoracoabdominal aortic aneurysm repair. *J Endovasc Ther* 2001;8:25-33. **C,** Chuter TAM, Rapp JH, Hiramoto JS, et al. Endovascular treatment of thoracoabdominal aortic aneurysms. *J Vasc Surg* 2008;48:6-16.

graft technology. Tempered by promising early to midterm results, the ongoing outcomes obtained, however, suggest an expanded role for endovascular reconstruction of the visceral aortic segment in complex aortic aneurysms. Concerns remain regarding overall graft durability, branch vessel outcomes, and renal events.[172,178] As these technologies improve and allow a more generalized expertise. it is likely they will replace hybrid debranching in high-risk patients.

OPEN SURGICAL RESULTS AND COMPLICATIONS

Operative Mortality

Pararenal aneurysmorraphy operative mortality approaches 5%, while in large clinical series of TAA repair it averages roughly 10% (Table 33-4). However, other reports detail considerably higher perioperative mortality in TAA.[187-189] Several preoperative patient characteristics may influence the patient's ultimate outcome regardless of operative conduct. The circumstances of clinical presentation are a dominant factor associated with operative mortality in pararenal–suprarenal aneurysms and TAA. In the recent update of our experience, operative mortality was 6.8% for elective TAA operations, while it increased to 12.9% in nonelective situations (p = 0.06).[11] Similar data have been reported by others, regardless of aneurysm extent.[7,8,25,75,105,182,186,190]

Although not universal, some contemporary series have demonstrated an increased operative mortality in elderly patients undergoing either complex abdominal or extensive TAA repair.[7,8,70,75,150,190] The presence of increasing numbers of comorbid conditions can naturally be expected to increase overall operative risk. Individual series variously demonstrate increased operative risks with patients with coronary artery disease, COPD, and renal insufficiency. Dysfunction in these respective organ systems increases the risks of organ-specific

Table 33-4
Operative Series of Complex Aortic Aneurysm: Morbidity and Mortality*

Reference	Patients (n)	Aneurysm Extent	Early Mortality n (%)	Paraplegia or Paraparesis n (%)	Renal Failure n (%)
Qvarfordt et al.[179]	77	Pararenal	1 (1.3)	0	2 (2.5)†
Crawford et al.[180]	101	Pararenal	8 (7)	‡	7 (7)
Poulias et al.[86]	38	Pararenal	2 (5.2)	0	5 (13)†
Nypaver et al.[98]	53	Pararenal	2 (3.5)	0	3 (5.6)†
Faggioli et al.[182]	50	Pararenal	6 (12)	0	1 (2)
Allen et al.[181]	65	Pararenal or suprarenal	1 (1.5)	1 (1.5)	2 (3)†
Jean-Claude et al.[183]	257	Pararenal or suprarenal	15 (5.8)	1 (0.4)	18 (7)†
Sarac et al.[97]	138	Pararenal	7 (5.1)	‡	8 (5.8)†
Shortell et al.[184]	112	Pararenal	7 (6)	0	4 (3)†
West et al.[185]	247	Pararenal	6 (2.5)	0	9 (4)†
Knott et al.[88]	126	Pararenal	1 (0.8)	0	6 (5)†
Chiesa et al.[87]	85	Pararenal	4 (4.7)	0	5 (5.8)†
Chiesa et al.[87]	34	Suprarenal	1 (2.9)	0	2 (5.8)†
Martin et al.[186]	57	Suprarenal	1 (1.8)	0	1 (2, elective only)†
Svensson et al.[8]	1509	TAA	155 (10)	234 (16)	269 (18)
Coselli et al.[9]	2286	TAA	150 (6.6)	87 (3.8)	129 (5.6)†
Schepens et al.[75]	402	TAA	44 (10.9)	45 (11.3)	24 (6.1)†
Hamilton et al.[24]	265	TAA	21 (7.9)	12 (4.5)	‡(§9)
Grabitz et al.[23]	260	TAA	37 (14.2)	39 (15)	27 (10.4)†
Acher et al.[7]	217§	TAA	21 (9.7)	17 (7.8)	4 (3.8)†
Safi et al.[10,25]	1106§	TAA	162 (14.6)	36 (3.3)	73 (¶7.9)
Conrad et al.[11]	455	TAA	39 (8.2)	60 (13.2)	21 (4.6)†

*TAA, thoracoabdominal aneurysm.
†Only those requiring hemodialysis.
‡Not reported.
§Includes descending thoracic aneurysms.
¶Strict criteria; based upon glomerular filtration rate <29 ml/min/1.73 m² or on dialysis.

complications after operation. Patients who sustain major neurological deficits, postoperative renal failure, and cardiopulmonary complications have a significantly increased risk of operative mortality.[7,8,25,27] Previously, we reported the risk of operative mortality with TAA repair was increased more than sixfold in patients with postoperative renal failure and increased by a factor of 16 in those with paraplegia.[27,72] These continue in our ongoing experience with renal failure (odds ratio 7.8; 95% CI, 3.4 to 17.9; $p < 0.0001$) and SCI (odds ratio 3.1, 95% CI 1.2 to 7.8, $p = 0.02$) portending operative mortality. Visceral ischemic time during repair has been shown to enhance plasma concentrations of proinflammatory mediators and thus predispose to multiple system organ failure.[191] Thirty to fifty percent of in-hospital deaths after TAA repair are associated with multiple system organ failure.[27,75] These data emphasize the importance of minimizing such complications.

Perioperative Hemorrhage

Intraoperative bleeding complications can occur from technical mishaps and from dilutional coagulopathy caused by excessive blood turnover, and they previously were an important source of early mortality. Blood turnover in extensive aneurysm cases is, of necessity, significant, since large type II aneurysms, for example, can contain up to several liters of blood in the aneurysm sac alone. This is routinely returned to the patient in the form of autotransfused blood. Approximately half the blood turnover during TAA resection is returned to the patient by autotransfusion methods. Total blood transfusion for resection of the more extensive type I and type II aneurysms averages more than 3 L, and this figure varies with the extent of aortic replacement (Table 33-3). An expected correlation exists among blood turnover, aneurysm extent, and perioperative mortality. In our experience, operative transfusion requirement is an independent correlate of perioperative mortality (odds ratio 1.4, 95% CI 1.1 to 1.7, $p = 0.0015$).[11,27]

Before restoration of visceral and lower extremity perfusion, blood component replacement with fresh frozen plasma and platelet transfusions alleviates coagulopathic bleeding. Minimizing systemic heparin and careful hemostasis throughout the course of operation also reduce coagulopathic bleeding. Hepatic and mesenteric ischemia contributes to intraoperative coagulopathic bleeding.[76,77,102,192-195] Significant depletion of coagulation factors occurs during supraceliac aortic clamping. These changes are quantitatively more severe when compared with an infrarenal aortic cross-clamp.[94,196] Regardless of whether the mechanism of coagulopathic bleeding is hepatic ischemia or bacterial translocation in ischemic gut, experimental data and clinical observations suggest that minimizing mesenteric ischemia is critical in avoiding coagulopathic bleeding.[194,196] Minimizing the supraceliac cross-clamp duration, along with the use of adjuncts to achieve mesenteric blood flow during repair (see the Operative Management section), is also an important component of operative success (Figure 33-4).[112,197]

Reexploration for bleeding complications has a highly significant impact on overall operative mortality.[8] Currently, bleeding complications occur in roughly 2% to 5% of TAA patients and should be less with pararenal aneurysmorrhaphy.[9,10,27,87,97,186] Postoperative splenic bleeding and undetected backbleeding from intercostal or lumbar vessels have been the principal sources of postoperative hemorrhage.

A careful search of the entire aneurysm sac, after all suture lines have been completed, and an aggressive posture toward splenectomy for even apparently trivial splenic tears should prevent these complications.

Respiratory Insufficiency

Despite emphasis on spinal cord ischemic complications and renal failure in most clinical series, postoperative respiratory failure is the most common complication after TAA resection, occurring in 25% to 45% of patients.[8,11,27,70,75,189] While the incidence may be somewhat less after pararenal and suprarenal aneurysm repair, it remains one of the most often encountered postoperative problems.[87,88,97,183-185] A slow wean from ventilatory support, often planned to proceed over several days, is appropriate management in patients with baseline pulmonary insufficiency. Most patients can be extubated within 48 hours of operation.

Variables predictive of postoperative pulmonary insufficiency include active cigarette smoking, baseline COPD, and cardiac, renal, or bleeding complications and aneurysm rupture.[27,115,198-201] Before elective operation, the patient should discontinue tobacco use for a minimum of a month. Preoperative consultation with a pulmonologist for optimization of bronchodilator therapy and pulmonary toilet is an important component in the management of patients with significant COPD. It is intuitive that paralysis of the left diaphragm by its radial division to the aortic hiatus significantly contributes to postoperative respiratory failure. Accordingly, a diaphragm-sparing technique should be applied and has been reported to ameliorate pulmonary compromise after repair (Figure 33-13).[115]

Perioperative Renal Insufficiency

Various criteria have been used to define postoperative renal failure. Doubling of the baseline serum creatinine level or an absolute postoperative creatinine level of more than 3.0 mg/dl is a definition applied in many clinical series. Factors important in the development of postoperative renal failure include the duration of renal ischemia, baseline renal dysfunction, cholesterol embolization from surgical manipulation in the region of the renal artery orifices, and renal artery reconstruction failure. Transient and modest decreases in overall excretory function are the inevitable consequence of some obligatory period of renal ischemia. In many patients, postoperative renal insufficiency is both nonoliguric and reversible with maintenance of intravascular volume (Table 33-5). Preoperative renal insufficiency is the most powerful predictor of postoperative renal failure. Abnormal preoperative serum creatinine, estimated glomerular filtration rate, and prolonged aortic cross-clamp time increase the risk of postoperative renal failure substantially.[7,8,70,73,104,202]

The risk of postoperative renal insufficiency is higher for reconstructions involving pararenal aneurysms compared with infrarenal lesions.[86,88,98,179,183-185] As aortic aneurysmal extent increases, so does the risk of renal complications (Table 33-4).[27,107] In Crawford's experience, significant postoperative renal failure occurred in about 20% of patients, with dialysis being required in half. The risk of operative mortality increased fivefold in patients sustaining postoperative renal failure.[8] We previously reviewed more than 180 TAA operations and found that in the 8% of patients who sustained significant postoperative renal failure the risk of mortality was increased almost tenfold (odds ratio 9.1, 95% CI 2.5 to 33, $p < 0.005$).[201] About one third of patients who develop significant postoperative renal dysfunction die perioperatively.[11,27]

Table 33-5
Stratification, by Postoperative Renal Function, of 334 Patients Undergoing Thoracoabdominal Aneurysm Repair

	n (%)
0-50% elevation in baseline creatinine	195 (58.4)
50-100% elevation in baseline creatinine	77 (23)
>100% elevation in baseline creatinine	19 (5.7)
Doubling and creatinine rising to >3.0 mg/dl	27 (8)
Dialysis	16 (4.8)

From Schepens MAAM, Kelder JC, Morshuis WJ, et al. *Ann Thorac Surg* 2007;83:S851-S855.

The most important maneuver to minimize the risk of postoperative renal failure is minimizing renal ischemic time. Some authors prefer the use of distal aortic perfusion and a sequential clamping technique so that the renal arteries can be perfused during construction of the proximal aortic anastomosis. The addition of individual visceral–renal perfusion catheters from the atrial femoral bypass circuit, at least in theory, provides for continuous renal artery perfusion during all phases of the operation (Figure 33-4). However, the size of such catheters may not permit adequate perfusion pressure or flow to the renal vessels, and an apparent paradoxical detrimental effect on overall renal function with this technique has been suggested.[70,104] We prefer cold crystalloid-based renal perfusion, and other authorities have found this superior to warm blood.[203] The other often-applied intraoperative adjunct, and the one preferred on our service, is selective hypothermic renal artery perfusion (Figure 33-4). While such regional renal hypothermia is likely unnecessary in patients with normal renal function and with renal ischemic times less than 1 hour, it can provide a margin of safety in circumstances of either technical difficulty or prolongation of renal ischemia. An additional intraoperative adjunct employed to minimize the risk of postoperative renal failure is correction of renal artery occlusive lesions.[70,204] Perioperative continuous infusions of dopamine or fenoldopam may benefit patients with renal insufficiency.[205-207] Management of perioperative renal failure is usually conservative if the patient remains nonoliguric. Patients taking diuretic medications preoperatively generally require some in the postoperative period, and renal-dose dopamine or fenoldopam infusions are appropriate to aid diuresis. We prefer to avoid the use of hemodialysis therapy unless clear-cut indications exist on either a metabolic or an intravascular volume basis. Conventional hemodialysis is accompanied by a substantial risk of hemodynamic instability after TAA resection, and we have observed such hypotension precipitating spinal cord ischemic events even weeks after surgery. Continuous venovenous hemodialysis may provide a smoother hemodynamic course than conventional hemodialysis. Currently, some 2% to 9% of patients require hemodialysis for renal failure postoperatively.[8,9,11,27,70,75,202]

Spinal Cord Ischemic Complications

Two morphological factors referable to human spinal cord circulation explain ischemic risk to the spinal cord during TAA.[111,208] The first is the anatomical vagaries of the anterior spinal artery, which is variable both in caliber and in continuity. Angiographic studies have shown that the anterior spinal artery may be discontinuous, with the typical pattern being extreme narrowing cephalad to its joining the greater radicular artery. The second factor is that the radiculomedullary arterial supply to the human spinal cord is inconsistent. Although radicular arteries are contributed at each segmental level, only a few actually go on to contribute medullary (i.e., actually reaching the cord) components. The cervical thoracic territory is richly supplied with radiculomedullary arteries, but the middle thoracic segment has but one or two such arteries. However, the anterior spinal artery in this region remains well developed. The thoracolumbar watershed region is at highest risk for ischemic injury because this region is typically supplied by a single radiculomedullary artery, the artery of Adamkiewicz, or the greater radicular artery. This artery enters the vertebral canal between the ninth and the twelfth thoracic vertebral segments in 75% to 80% of individuals and arises between T8 and L1 in 86%. Angiographic studies confirm that one or more intercostal arteries can contribute to it and, in some three quarters of patients, it arises from the left side.[80]

In the presence of an aneurysm, additional anatomical variability may be added by mural thrombus, obliterating many or all intercostal vessels. Such gradual obliteration of intercostal vessels in a chronic degenerative aneurysm establishes antecedent collateral circulation before surgical correction. Most authors agree that the risk of cord injury is considerably less in patients where intercostal vessels in the critical T8 to L1 zone have been obliterated by mural thrombus.[71,209] In aneurysms caused by chronic dissection, the typical pattern is aneurysmal dilatation of the false lumen and a narrow, compressed true lumen giving rise to multiple patent intercostals. Furthermore, obliteration of intercostals in a chronic degenerative aneurysm is virtually never accompanied by spontaneous cord injury, while sudden obliteration of multiple intercostal vessels, as might be seen in acute aortic dissection, can cause acute paraplegia.[210] This difference in intercostal patency between degenerative and dissecting aneurysms accounts for the increased risk of cord ischemia when dissection is the etiology.

Despite improvements in surgical and adjunctive techniques, SCI remains an unsolved problem and is the most feared and devastating nonfatal complication of TAA reconstruction. The pathogenesis of spinal cord injury after aortic replacement is likely multifactorial but ultimately results from ischemic insult caused by temporary or permanent interruption of spinal cord blood supply. Debate continues about the relative importance of the initial ischemic insult versus reperfusion injury. Spinal cord ischemic complications manifest along a clinical spectrum from complete flaccid paraplegia to varying degrees of temporary or permanent paraparesis. The clinical observation of delayed deficits has led some to speculate that swelling in the rigid bony spinal canal, accompanied by relative increases in CSF pressure, are the pathogenesis of such delayed deficits.[211-213] Others have speculated that the initial ischemic insult in the operating room creates the milieu for programmed neuronal cell death as an inevitable consequence.[214] We and others have noted the striking correlation between perioperative hypotension and delayed-onset neurological deficit, suggesting that the principal and collateral circulation to the cord may be in a delicate balance for some time after operation.[27,72,209] Indeed, delayed deficits occur nearly as often as those evident on emergence from anesthesia.[11,190,209,213] Careful attention to maintain adequate perfusion pressure in the days following TAA resection is important in limiting the occurrence of delayed deficit, but other mechanisms such as thrombosis of reconstructed vessels and microembolization may contribute to subsequent delayed deficits. Efforts to minimize SCI have been the principal driving force in the development and application of a variety of operative approaches. Svensson et al.,[8] in reviewing Crawford's experience, reported a 16% incidence of lower extremity neurological deficits. As detailed in Table 33-4, contemporary results from centers of excellence find a valuable decrease in the overall incidence of SCI comparatively. While good functional outcome after delayed deficit is commonly possible, some 30% to 60% of patients experiencing SCI suffer total paraplegia without any hope of meaningful recovery.[8,10,27,70,211,213]

The main difficulty in interpreting literature regarding spinal cord ischemic complications revolves around differing study populations based on operative urgency, aneurysm extent, and etiology, as well as individual operative approaches using multiple adjuncts. The general consensus is that the clinical variables of aortic cross-clamp duration, aneurysm extent, emergency operations, and dissection increase spinal cord injury risk, although the latter has recently been disputed.[10,25,27,70,213] In our series of 455 reconstructions,[11] as well as Coselli's interim series of 1220 repairs[70] and Safi's recent report in 1106 operations,[10,25] dissection did not augment the risk of SCI. Crawford initially demonstrated that with increasing TAA extent, risk of cord injury increased with longer aortic cross-clamp duration.[8] We have reported that a visceral cross-clamp time longer than 60 minutes was significantly associated with ischemic cord injury.[210] In our recent interim analysis, total aortic and visceral clamp times increased ischemic cord injury risk. Total clamp time was an independent predictor for SCI.[27]

Clinically significant SCI with pararenal–suprarenal aneurysm repair is rare. However, the incidence clearly increases in treatment for more extensive aneurysms. Svensson and colleagues noted a 24% incidence of cord injury in treatment of type I and type II TAA, as opposed to a 5.5% incidence for type III and type IV TAA.[8] While absolute rates were improved, Coselli most recent report described increasing aneurysm extent still correlated with cord ischemia, as 6.3% of type II patients and 1.4% of type IV patients suffered paraplegia or paraparesis.[9,70] Similar results have been conveyed by Safi's group.[10,25] We also have detected substantial ischemic risk in reconstructions for type I and type II TAA compared with those for less extensive aneurysms.[11,27]

The circumstances of clinical presentation have great bearing on cord injury risk. In Crawford's experience, cord injury rates doubled in treatment for ruptured versus intact aneurysms.[8] In our earlier data, operation for acute presentation (half for frank rupture, dissection, or both) was independently associated with postoperative lower extremity neurological deficit (odds ratio 7.7, 95% CI 1.7 to 37.7, $p = 0.009$).[8] Rupture itself has been proven an independent predictor of SCI.[27]

This has been maintained into our most recent analysis with urgent–emergent operation independently associated with SCI (odds ratio 2.1, 95% CI 1.1 to 4.0, $p = 0.02$) Also, most authors contend that sacrifice of critical intercostal arteries, the inability to reperfuse these arteries in a timely fashion, or both are important factors in the pathogenesis of ischemic cord injury. Griepp et al.[215] noted that cord ischemia increased dramatically when 10 or more intercostal pairs were sacrificed (i.e., resection of the entire descending thoracic aorta). It has been demonstrated that sacrifice of intercostal vessels in the critical T8 to L1 zone correlates with postoperative cord injury.[27,70,71,108,209] In our experience, sacrifice of patent intercostal arteries in the critical zone is an independent predictor of cord ischemia.[27]

Various clinical strategies and adjuncts have been applied in an effort to prevent ischemic spinal cord injury.[111,208] These methods can be divided into two general categories. The first of these are surgical or adjunctive methods designed to preserve relative spinal cord perfusion pressure. Localization techniques (preoperative imaging such as arteriography, magnetic resonance angiography, and computed tomography angiography and intraoperative evoked potentials or polargraphic) act as guides for the surgeon to preserve or reconstruct critical intercostal arteries. Preoperative spinal imaging can demonstrate the location and intercostal feeder vessels to the greater radicular artery in 65% to 85% of TAA patients studied.[80-82] However, except for predicting the risk of cord injury when the resection needs to encompass the critical aortic segment, clinical benefit of preoperative spinal arteriography has been debatable.[80,216] The hydrogen ion polargraphic technique, described by Svensson, has been elegantly documented with postoperative angiographic studies but has not been applied clinically by others.[217] Evoked potential monitoring evaluates the ability of the long tracks of the spinal cord to conduct an impulse during the cross-clamp period. Variations in the latency and amplitude of recorded potentials imply ischemia of the cord. Somatosensory evoked potentials was the original technique used, but this method has been plagued by lack of sensitivity and specificity, likely related to the peripheral nerve recording electrode being located distal to the cross-clamp.[218] Newer techniques used for evoked potential monitoring, such as epidural electrode spinal cord stimulation and motor evoked potentials have shown promise both in correlation between cord deficits and intraoperative evoked potential abnormalities and as a guide for application of intraoperative adjuncts when detected with initial cross-clamping.[75,219-221]

Intercostal vessel reanastomosis is the most commonly applied surgical maneuver used to preserve spinal cord perfusion. When excessive atheroma or acute dissection surrounds intercostal vessel origins, this may be technically challenging. Furthermore, the critical intercostal zone is in topographic proximity to the visceral aortic segment, and separate reconstruction to minimize intercostal clamp time may be impossible. Also, the surgeon typically faces the intraoperative dilemma of expending total aortic cross-clamp time to reattach intercostal vessels. Some authors have suggested expending aortic clamp time for this is a worthless maneuver and routinely oversew or occlude all intercostal vessels, often using other adjuncts directed against SCI.[7,215] As described, we rapidly oversew the backbleeding intercostals in the T4 to T8 region and balloon occlude those intercostals selected for reconstruction in the critical T8 to L1 zone. Svensson's and Safi's groups have previously detailed specifics of intercostal management during operation.[71,209]

It must be acknowledged, however, that intercostal reattachment is a "blind" maneuver unless some reliable method of preoperative or intraoperative critical vessel localization is applied.[221] Documentation detailing the merit of directed intercostal vessel reattachment was provided by Grabitz et al. using spinal cord somatosensory evoked potentials. These investigators reported more neurological deficits when rapid loss of spinal cord somatosensory evoked potentials occurred after aortic cross-clamping. Furthermore, neurological outcome for each group of somatosensory evoked potential responses correlated with achieving rapid evoked potential return by early intercostal reimplantation.[23] Jacobs and co-workers, using motor evoked potentials to guide intercostal reconstruction or sacrifice, demonstrated this modality can provide rapid detection of intraoperative SCI and its reversal by either hemodynamic manipulations or intercostal reconstruction.[220,221] These authors initially obtained an impressive 2.7% neurological deficit rate using this strategy in 184 patients with type I to III TAA.[220] Their subsequent report has delineated a 4.2% early SCI rate and a 2.9% delayed deficit occurrence.[221] Schepens, using a similar operative conduct, reduced neurological sequelae from 17% to 5.4%.[75] The supposition that motor evoked potentials may be more useful than somatosensory evoked potentials in guiding intraoperative preventive strategies has also been supported by van Dongen and associates.[219] It appears, however, restoring intercostal perfusion may be inadequate as a standalone adjunct simply because it cannot be performed rapidly enough.

The rationale for CSF pressure monitoring and drainage relates to the concept of spinal cord perfusion pressure as the difference between distal arterial pressure below the clamp and CSF pressure. Thoracic aortic clamping results in an abrupt increase in intracerebral blood flow, which is likely the principal mechanism leading to increases in CSF pressure that may accompany clamping. However, the absolute degree of this rise is typically modest,[23,22] and Kazama et al. found CSF drainage favorably influenced spinal cord blood flow only when CSF pressure was experimentally elevated to four times baseline values.[223] Thus, assumptions on which theoretic benefit of CSF drainage are based may not be valid. Several studies have failed to demonstrate benefit for CSF drainage.[224,225] However, elevated CSF pressure has correlated with delayed-onset deficit in particular, and many authors continue to use CSF drainage either alone or more typically with other strategies since it is simple and safe.[7,9,10-11,75] Furthermore, reversal of delayed deficits by CSF drainage has been reported, and chances of delayed deficit reversal appear greater than those of reversing immediate deficits.[213] Coselli's group recently reported a prospective, randomized trial of CSF drainage in type I and II repairs. Of those without drainage, 13% experienced clinically significant SCI while this occurred in significantly fewer (only 2.6%) drained patients.[226] Moreover, Cina and colleagues have provided a metaanalysis of the literature and further substantiated the positive impact CSF drainage has on SCI.[227]

The second preventive method, neuroprotective adjuncts, is intended to increase spinal cord tolerance to ischemia. Two general categories of such adjuncts exist: systemic or regional hypothermia and pharmacological agents. The latter can be classified according to intended mechanisms of actions:

- *Nonspecific neuroprotective agents* (e.g., steroids, prostaglandins, magnesium, and barbiturates)[228-233]
- *Excitatory neurotransmitter inhibitors* such as naloxone and[234,235] calcium channel blockers[236]
- *Oxygen free radical scavengers*[237]

Other agents continue to undergo study in laboratory models.[238] Furthermore, determining benefits of these agents in the clinical setting is difficult because they are typically used in combination with other strategies. The preeminent clinical experience involving this general strategy has been reported by Acher et al., applying endorphin receptor blockade with naloxone with CSF drainage and routine intercostal ligation. Using this technique in patients with thoracic aneurysms and TAA, these authors have reported overall spinal cord ischemic injury rates of 3.5%.[7]

Oxygen requirements of spinal cord tissue decrease 6% to 7% for each degree Celsius reduction in cord temperature. Hypothermia for cord protection during TAA surgery can be either regional (i.e., confined to the spinal cord itself) or systemic. The protective effect of hypothermia is presumed due to decreased tissue metabolism. However, the mechanism may be more complex, involving membrane stabilization and attenuation of excitatory neurotransmitter release.[239] Hypothermic spinal cord protection may ablate the hyperemic phase of cord reperfusion, resulting in less edema after circulation is restored.[240,241] The specifics of applying hypothermic protection range from modest systemic hypothermia, simply achieved by passively cooling the operating room and allowing evaporative and respiratory heat losses, to profound hypothermia (15° C to 18° C), with complete cardiopulmonary bypass and temporary circulatory arrest. Lesser degrees can be achieved actively by adding a heat exchanger to a partial cardiopulmonary bypass circuit. This technique provides for active systemic hypothermia, the degree of which is limited by cardiac arrhythmias. Regional hypothermia has the distinct advantage of avoiding systemic hypothermia, a concept we believe critical to the operative management of TAA patients. Systemic hypothermia has been independently associated with the development of complications after elective abdominal aortic surgery.[242] Regional hypothermia can be indirectly administered via the doubly clamped thoracic aorta[243] or directly onto the spinal cord.[110] Our experience with the rate and volume of cooled epidural perfusate necessary to achieve moderate regional cord hypothermia indicates that effective cooling through intercostal vessels alone is likely not feasible. Application of regional hypothermic techniques is based on convincing experimental data revealing near complete protection against cord injury.[244] Marsala and colleagues established a clinically applicable closed epidural infusion system that achieved moderate (26° C to 28° C) cord hypothermia and was 100% effective against SCI induced by double thoracic aortic clamping in a dog model.[245] Moreover, newer experimental evidence indicates moderate regional cord hypothermia is compatible with motor evoked potential monitoring and does not lessen its ability to detect cord ischemia in pigs.[246]

Stimulated by these data and the potential to fit regional hypothermia into our operative strategy, we developed a clinically applicable epidural cooling system and have used it since 1993. The mechanics of this clinically applicable system as

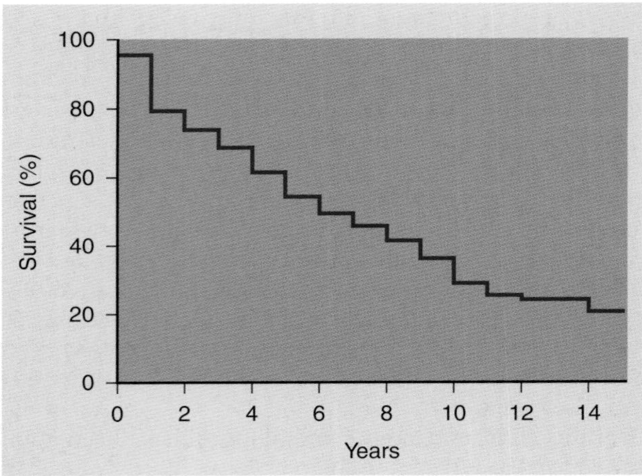

Figure 33-18. Recent evaluation of long-term survival in patients undergoing 455 TAA reconstructions. Actuarial estimates of 54% 5-year, 29% 10-year and 21% 15-year survival. (Conrad MF, Crawford RS, Davison JK, et al. Thoracoabdominal aneurysm repair: a 20-year perspective. *Ann Thorac Surg* 2007;83:S856-S861.)

displayed in Figure 33-4 are straightforward, with an epidural catheter used for infusion of 4° C saline and a separate intrathecal catheter used to measure CSF temperature and pressure. It is necessary to maintain a continuous infusion to achieve moderate (approximately 25° C) levels of cord hypothermia, and the infusion must be initiated some 45 minutes before the anticipated application of the cross-clamp. Technically, the principal limitation of the system is pressure increases during epidural infusion—averaging twice baseline in our patients—and is a significant concern relative to spinal cord perfusion above the cooling level. It therefore is necessary to maintain an arbitrary 30 to 40 mm Hg between mean arterial pressure and mean CSF pressure by either decreasing the epidural infusion rate or increasing systemic arterial pressure. Neurological outcomes in our first 70 patients using this method were significantly improved compared with institutional controls. Those without regional cord hypothermia experienced nearly a tenfold increase in ischemic cord injury.[72] In subsequent evaluation, devastating neurological deficits after 170 thoracic aneurysm or extensive TAA (types I, II, and III) resections were reduced to the 2% to 3% range with use of epidural cooling.[109] In recent examinations of our overall experience with TAA repair, use of epidural cooling produced a significant reduction in cord ischemia in types I to III aneurysms (odds ratio 0.42, 95% CI 0.2 to 0.87, $p = 0.02$).[11,27]

Late Survival

Late survival in patients after complex abdominal aortic repair has been reported to be 40% to 75% at 5 years.[80,180,182,186,247] Svensson et al. indicated survival projections in the 60% range at 5 years after TAA operation.[8] Displayed in Figure 33-18 is our initial late survival data from 2002 indicating a 5-year survival of 67.2% (95% CI 59% to 77%).[27] Recent actuarial life-table analysis in our ongoing series of 455 patients describes a 5-year, 10-year, and 15-year survival of 54%, 29%, and 21%, respectively. Long-term actuarial survival rates in various clinical series are displayed in Table 33-6. Results are comparable regardless of aneurysm extent. The contemporary

Table 33-6
Long-Term Survival in Series of Repaired Aortic Aneurysms of Various Extent*

Reference	Year	Aneurysm Extent	5-Year Survival (%)
Svensson et al.[8]	1993	TAA	61
Schwartz et al.[22]	1996	Type IV	50
Hallett et al.[248]	1997	AAA	67
Faggioli et al.[182]	1998	Pararenal	40
Martin et al.[186]	2000	Suprarenal or type III or IV	50
Coselli et al.[70]	2000	TAA	72
Cambria et al.[27]	2002	TAA	67.2
Biancari et al.[249]	2002	AAA	66.8
Back et al.[247]	2005	Pararenal or suprarenal type IV	70
Conrad et al.[250]	2007	TAA	54
Conrad et al.[250]	2007	AAA	70.7
Schepens et al.[26]	2007	TAA	63
Knott et al.[88]	2008	Pararenal	78.3

*AAA, abdominal aortic aneurysm; TAA, thoracoabdominal aneurysm.

5-year results achieved signify that the substantial resource investments required to support complex aneurysm patients through successful operation and recovery is an appropriate expenditure of such resources.

Many operative survivors return to their preoperative independent living status, but some do not.[189,201] Cardiac events are the most common source of late mortality.[8,26,186,201] Furthermore, the negative impact of postoperative lower extremity neurological deficit and dialysis dependence on perioperative survival remains significant as these patients also have distinctly inferior late survival.[8] In Schepens' et al recent evaluation of 500 patients after repair, long-term survival depended on ventricular function, age at repair, postoperative neurological and renal sequelae, and urgency of operation.[26] Some 10% of patients go on to have another aortic event, whether it be remote aneurysm or graft related, and rupture of another aneurysm has accounted for approximately 10% of late deaths.[4,26,201] In determining long-term aortic outcome in our patients, we have found 10.5% of patients went on to have a second aortic event at an average of just over 2 years after repair.[4] Interestingly, aortic disease–related events occurred in 7% of patients and accounted for 71% of late events, with most being repair of another aneurysm (n = 20, 87%). Graft-related complications occurred in only 3% of repairs and accounted for the remaining 29% of late aortic events. Clinically evident renovisceral occlusion was the most common graft-related event (n = 5, 56%). Inclusion anastomosis pseudoaneurysm, graft infection, and graft–esophageal fistula were rare, occurring in less than 1% of patients. One-year and 5-year freedom from another aortic event was 96% and 71%, respectively. Independent predictors of late aortic events were female gender, initial aneurysm rupture, partial aneurysmal disease resection, and expansion of remaining aortic segments on imaging surveillance. This evaluation suggests TAA repair is durable with few long-term sequelae related to grafting. However, these patients are at risk for further aortic problems, and aortic surveillance after successful TAA reconstruction is important, particularly in those with the preceding risk factors.

SUMMARY

Substantial progress has been made in the overall results of operative treatment of pararenal, suprarenal, and thoracoabdominal aortic aneurysms. Given the unfavorable natural history of these lesions, an aggressive posture toward graft replacement is clearly justified in environments with demonstrated surgical expertise. The multiplicity of surgical strategies and adjuncts applied in efforts to minimize the principal complications of operation for complex aortic aneurysms indicate that the evolution of surgical sophistication is, as of yet, incomplete. Similar to the maturation in surgical treatment of standard infrarenal AAA, an increase in the percentage of patients treated in elective circumstances improves overall results. Endovascular repair of complex aortic aneurysms via several technical methods is feasible and has become part of management strategies. Debranching of the arch and visceral segment, as well as improving fenestrated and branched endografts will enrich aneurysm treatment.

References

1. Bickerstaff LK, Pairolero PC, Hollier LH, et al. Thoracic aortic aneurysms: a population-based study. *Surgery* 1982;92:1103-1108.
2. McNamara JJ, Pressler VM. Natural history of arteriosclerotic thoracic aortic aneurysms. *Ann Thorac Surg* 1978;26:468-473.
3. Svensjö S, Bengtsson H, Bergqvist D. Thoracic and thoracoabdominal aortic aneurysm and dissection: an investigation based on autopsy. *Br J Surg* 1996;83:68-71.
4. Clouse WD, Marone LK, Davison JK, et al. Late aortic and graft-related events after thoracoabdominal aneurysm repair. *J Vasc Surg* 2003;37:254-261.
5. Gloviczki P, Pairolero P, Welch T, et al. Multiple aortic aneurysms: the results of surgical management. *J Vasc Surg* 1990;11:19-28.
6. Crawford ES, Cohen ES. Aortic aneurysm: a multifocal disease. *Arch Surg* 1982;117:1393-1400.
7. Acher CW, Wynn MM, Hoch JR, Kranner PW. Cardiac function is a risk factor for paralysis in thoracoabdominal aortic replacement. *J Vasc Surg* 1998;27:821-830.
8. Svensson LG, Crawford ES, Hess KR, et al. Experience with 1509 patients undergoing thoracoabdominal aortic operations. *J Vasc Surg* 1993;17:357-370.
9. Coselli JS, Bozinovski J, LeMaire SA. Open surgical repair of 2286 thoracoabdominal aortic aneurysms. *Ann Thorac Surg* 2007;83:S862-S864.
10. Safi HJ, Estrera AL, Miller CC, et al. Evolution of risk for neurologic deficit after descending and thoracoabdominal aortic repair. *Ann Thorac Surg* 2005;80:2173-2179.
11. Conrad MF, Crawford RS, Davison JK, et al. Thoracoabdominal aneurysm repair: a 20-year perspective. *Ann Thorac Surg* 2007;83:S856-S861.
12. Johansson G, Markstrom U, Swedenborg J. Ruptured thoracic aortic aneurysms: a study of incidence and mortality rates. *J Vasc Surg* 1995;21:985-988.
13. Perko MJ, Norgaard M, Herzog TM, et al. Unoperated aortic aneurysm: a survey of 170 patients. *Ann Thorac Surg* 1995;59:1204-1209.
14. Clouse WD, Hallett JW, Schaff HV, et al. Improved prognosis of thoracic aortic aneurysms. *JAMA* 1998;280:1926-1929.
15. Etheredge SN, Yee J, Smith JV, et al. Successful resection of large aneurysm of the upper abdominal aorta and replacement with homograft. *Surgery* 1955;38:1071-1081.
16. DeBakey ME, Creech O Jr, Morris CG. Aneurysms of the thoracoabdominal aorta involving the celiac, superior mesenteric, and renal arteries: report of four cases treated by resection and homograft replacement. *Ann Surg* 1956;44:549-573.
17. Crawford ES. Thoracoabdominal and abdominal aortic aneurysm involving renal, superior mesenteric and celiac arteries. *Ann Surg* 1974;179:763-772.
18. Crawford ES, Crawford JL, Safi H, et al. Thoracoabdominal aortic aneurysms: preoperative and intraoperative factors determining immediate and long term results of operation in 605 patients. *J Vasc Surg* 1986;3:389-404.

19. Anderson JL, Berce M, Hartley DE. Endoluminal aortic grafting with renal and superior mesenteric artery incorporation by graft fenestration. *J Endovasc Ther* 2001;8:3-8.
20. Chuter TAM, Gordon RL, Reilly LM, et al. An endovascular system for thoracoabdominal aortic aneurysm repair. *J Endovasc Ther* 2001;8: 25-33.
21. Johnston KW, Rutherford RB, Tilson MD, et al. Ad Hoc Committee on Reporting Standards, SVS/NAISCVS: suggested standards for reporting on arterial aneurysms. *J Vasc Surg* 1991;13:452-458.
22. Schwartz LB, Belkin M, Donaldson M, et al. Improvements in results of repair of type IV thoracoabdominal aortic aneurysms. *J Vasc Surg* 1996;24:74-81.
23. Grabitz K, Sandmann W, Stuhmeirer K, et al. The risk of ischemic spinal cord injury in patients undergoing graft replacement for thoracoabdominal aortic aneurysms. *J Vasc Surg* 1996;23:230-240.
24. Hamilton IN Jr, Hollier LH. Adjunctive therapy for spinal cord protection during thoracoabdominal aortic aneurysm repair. *Semin Thorac Cardiovasc Surg* 1998;10:35-39.
25. Safi HJ, Miller CC III, Huynh TT, et al. Distal aortic perfusion and cerebrospinal fluid drainage for thoracoabdominal and descending thoracic aortic repair. *Ann Surg* 2003;238:372-381.
26. Schepens MAAM, Kelder JC, Morshuis WJ, et al. Long-term follow-up after thoracoabdominal aortic aneurysm repair. *Ann Thorac Surg* 2007;83:S851-S855.
27. Cambria RP, Clouse WD, Dorer DJ, et al. Thoracoabdominal aortic aneurysm repair: results with 337 operations performed over a 15-year interval. *Ann Surg* 2002;216:471-479.
28. Coselli JS, LeMaire SC, Buket S, et al. Subsequent proximal aortic operations in 123 patients with previous infrarenal abdominal aortic aneurysm surgery. *J Vasc Surg* 1995;22:59-67.
29. Coselli JS, Poli de Figuerrado LF, LeMaire SA. Impact of previous thoracic aneurysm repair on thoracoabdominal aortic aneurysm management. *Ann Thorac Surg* 1997;64:639-650.
30. Panneton JM, Hollier LM. Basic data underlying clinical decision making. I. Non-dissecting thoracoabdominal aortic aneurysms. *Ann Vasc Surg* 1995;9:503-514.
31. Safi HJ, Miller CC III, Estrera AL, et al. Optimization of aortic arch replacement: two-stage approach. *Ann Thorac Surg* 2007;83:S815-S818.
32. Safi HJ, Miller CC III, Estrera A, et al. Staged repair of extensive aortic aneurysms: morbidity and mortality in the elephant trunk technique. *Circulation* 2001;104:2938-2942.
33. Neya K, Omoto R, Kyo S. Outcome of Stanford type B acute aortic dissection. *Circulation* 1992;86(Suppl 5):II1-II7.
34. Schor JS, Yerlioghu ME, Galla JD, et al. Selective management of acute type B aortic dissection: long-term follow-up. *Ann Thorac Surg* 1996;61:1339-1341.
35. Fattori R, Bacchi-Reggiani L, Bertaccini P, et al. Evolution of aortic dissection after repair. *Am J Cardiol* 2000;86:868-872.
36. Iguchi A, Tabayashi K. Outcome of medically treated Stanford type B aortic dissection. *Jpn Circ J* 1998;62:102-105.
37. Kato M, Bai H, Sato K, et al. Determining surgical indications for acute type B dissection based on enlargement of aortic diameter during the chronic phase. *Circulation* 1995;92(Suppl 2):II107-II112.
38. De Bakey ME, McCollum CH, Crawford ES, et al. Dissection and dissecting aneurysms of the aorta: twenty-year follow-up of five hundred twenty-seven patients treated surgically. *Surgery* 1982;92: 1118-1134.
39. Marui A, Mochizuki T, Mitsui N, et al. Toward the best treatment for uncomplicated patients with type B acute aortic dissection: a consideration for sound surgical indication. *Circulation* 1999;100(Suppl 2): 275-280.
40. Juvonen T, Ergin MA, Galla JD, et al. Risk factors for rupture of chronic type B dissections. *J Thorac Cardiovasc Surg* 1999;117:776-786.
41. Bernard Y, Zimmermann H, Chocron S, et al. False lumen patency as a predictor of late outcome in aortic dissection. *Am J Cardiol* 2001;87:1378-1382.
42. Kozai Y, Watanabe S, Yonezawa M, et al. Long-term prognosis of acute aortic dissection with medical treatment: a survey of 263 unoperated patients. *Jpn Circ J* 2001;65:359-363.
43. Cambria RP, Brewster DC, Moncure AC, et al. Spontaneous aortic dissection in the presence of coexistent or previously repaired atherosclerotic aortic aneurysm. *Ann Surg* 1988;208:619-624.
44. Nagashima H, Sakomura Y, Aoka Y, et al. Angiotensin II type 2 receptor mediates vascular smooth muscle cell apoptosis in cystic medial degeneration associated with Marfan's syndrome. *Circulation* 2001;104 (Suppl 1):I282-I287.
45. Murdoch JL, Walker BA, Halpern BL, et al. Life expectancy and causes of death in the Marfan syndrome. *N Engl J Med* 1972;286:804-808.
46. Silverman DI, Burton KJ, Gray J, et al. Life expectancy in the Marfan syndrome. *Am J Cardiol* 1995;75:157-160.
47. Finkbohner R, Johnston D, Crawford ES, et al. Marfan syndrome: long-term survival and complications after aortic aneurysm repair. *Circulation* 1995;91:728-733.
48. Carrel T, Beyeler L, Schnyder A, et al. Reoperations and late adverse outcome in Marfan patients following cardiovascular surgery. *Eur J Cardiothorac Surg* 2004;25:671-675.
49. Shores J, Berger KR, Murphy EA, et al. Progression of aortic dilatation and the benefit of long-term beta-adrenergic blockade in Marfan's syndrome. *N Engl J Med* 1994;330:1335-1341.
50. Evans JM, O'Fallon WM, Hunder GG. Increased incidence of aortic aneurysms and dissection in giant cell (temporal) arteritis. *Ann Intern Med* 1995;122:502-507.
51. Osler W. The Gulstonian lectures on malignant endocarditis. *BMJ* 1885;1:467.
52. Estes JE Jr. Abdominal aortic aneurysm: a study of one hundred and two cases. *Circulation* 1950;2:258-264.
53. Crawford ES, DeNatale RW. Thoracoabdominal aortic aneurysm: observations regarding the natural course of the disease. *J Vasc Surg* 1986;3:578-582.
54. Clouse WD, Hallett JW, Schaff HV, et al. Acute aortic dissection: population-based incidence compared with degenerative aortic aneurysm rupture. *Mayo Clin Proc* 2004;79:176-180.
55. Crawford ES, Hess KR, Cohen JS, et al. Ruptured aneurysm of the descending thoracic and thoracoabdominal aorta. *Ann Surg* 1991;213:417-426.
56. Cambria RA, Gloviczki P, Stanson A, et al. Outcome and expansion rate of 57 thoracoabdominal aortic aneurysms managed nonoperatively. *Am J Surg* 1995;170:213-217.
57. Dapunt OE, Galla JD, Sadeghi AM, et al. The natural history of thoracic aortic aneurysms. *J Thorac Cardiovasc Surg* 1994;107:1323-1333.
58. Masuda Y, Takanashi K, Takasu J, et al. Expansion rate of thoracic aortic aneurysms and influencing factors. *Chest* 1992;102:461-466.
59. Griepp RB, Ergin MA, Galla JD, et al. Natural history of descending thoracic and thoracoabdominal aneurysms. *Ann Thorac Surg* 1999;67: 1927-1930.
60. Coady MA, Rizzo JA, Hammond GL, et al. Surgical intervention criteria for thoracic aortic aneurysms: a study of growth rates and complications. *Ann Thorac Surg* 1999;67:1922-1926.
61. Coady MA, Rizzo JA, Hammond GL, et al. What is the appropriate size criterion for resection of thoracic aortic aneurysms? *J Thorac Cardiovasc Surg* 1997;113:476-491.
62. Bonser RS, Pagano D, Lewis ME, et al. Clinical and patho-anatomical factors affecting expansion of thoracic aortic aneurysms. *Heart* 2000;84:277-283.
63. Juvonen T, Ergin MA, Galla JD, et al. Prospective study of the natural history of thoracic aortic aneurysms. *Ann Thorac Surg* 1997;63: 1533-1545.
64. Lobato AC, Puech-Leao P. Predictive factors for rupture of thoracoabdominal aortic aneurysm. *J Vasc Surg* 1998;27:446-453.
65. Davies RR, Goldstein LJ, Coady MA, et al. Yearly rupture or dissection rates for thoracic aortic aneurysms: simple prediction based on size. *Ann Thorac Surg* 2002;73:17-28.
66. Svensson LG, Kouchoukos NT, Miller DC, et al. Expert consensus document on the treatment of descending thoracic aortic disease using endovascular stent grafts. *Ann Thorac Surg* 2008;85:S1-S41.
67. Galla JD, Ergin MA, Lansman SL, et al. Identification of risk factors in patients undergoing thoracoabdominal aneurysm repair. *J Cardiovasc Surg* 1997;12:292-299.
68. Brewster DC, Cronenwett JL, Hallett JW, et al. Guidelines for the treatment of abdominal aortic aneurysms. *J Vasc Surg* 2003;37:1106-1117.
69. Cooke J, Cambria RP. Simultaneous tracheobronchial and esophageal obstruction secondary to thoracoabdominal aneurysm. *J Vasc Surg* 1993;18:90-94.
70. Coselli JS, LeMaire SA, Miller CC III, et al. Mortality and paraplegia after thoracoabdominal aortic aneurysm repair: a risk factor analysis. *Ann Thorac Surg* 2000;69:409-414.
71. Safi HJ, Miller CC III, Carr C, et al. Importance of intercostal artery reattachment during thoracoabdominal aortic aneurysm repair. *J Vasc Surg* 1998;27:58-68.
72. Cambria RP, Davison JK, Zannetti S, et al. Thoracoabdominal aneurysm repair: perspectives over a decade with the clamp-and-sew technique. *Ann Surg* 1997;226:294-305.

73. Huynh TT, van Eps RGS, Miller CC III, et al. Glomerular filtration rate is superior to serum creatinine for prediction of mortality after thoracoabdominal aortic surgery. *J Vasc Surg* 2005;43:206-212.
74. Huynh TT, Miller CC, Estrera AL, et al. Thoracoabdominal and descending thoracic aortic aneurysm surgery in patients aged 79 years and older. *J Vasc Surg* 2002;36:469-475.
75. Schepens MA, Dossche K, Morshuis W, et al. Introduction of adjuncts and their influence on changing results in 402 consecutive thoracoabdominal aortic aneurysms repairs. *Eur J Cardiothorac Surg* 2004;25:701-707.
76. Cohen JR, Angus L, Asher A, et al. Disseminated intravascular coagulation as a result of supraceliac clamping: implications for thoracoabdominal aneurysm repair. *Ann Vasc Surg* 1987;1:552-557.
77. Cohen JR, Sardari F, Paul J, et al. Increased intestinal permeability: implications for thoracoabdominal aneurysm repair. *Ann Vasc Surg* 1991;6:433-437.
78. Gadowski GR, Pilcher DB, Ricci MA. Abdominal aortic aneurysm expansion rate: effects of size and beta-adrenergic blockade. *J Vasc Surg* 1994;19:727-731.
79. Genoni M, Paul M, Jenni R, et al. Chronic beta-blocker therapy improves outcomes and reduces treatment costs in chronic type B aortic dissection. *Eur J Cardiothorac Surg* 2001;19:606-610.
80. Kieffer E, Fukui S, Chiras J, et al. Spinal cord arteriography: a safe adjunct before descending thoracic or thoracoabdominal aortic aneurysmectomy. *J Vasc Surg* 2002;35:262-268.
81. Hyodoh H, Kawaharada N, Akiba H, et al. Usefulness of preoperative detection of artery of Adamkiewicz with dynamic contrast-enhanced MR angiography. *Radiology* 2005;236:1004-1009.
82. Nijenhuis RJ, Jacobs MJ, Jaspers K, et al. Comparison of magnetic resonance with computed tomography angiography for preoperative localization of the Adamkiewicz artery in thoracoabdominal aortic aneurysm patients. *J Vasc Surg* 2007;45:677-685.
83. Cernaianu A, Olah A, Cilley JJ, et al. Effect of sodium nitroprusside on paraplegia during cross-clamping of the thoracic aorta. *Ann Thorac Surg* 1993;56:1035-1038.
84. Shine T, Nugent M. Sodium nitroprusside decreases spinal cord perfusion pressure during descending thoracic aortic cross-clamping in the dog. *J Cardiothorac Anesth* 1990;4:185-193.
85. Simpson J, Eide T, Schiff G, et al. Isoflurane versus sodium nitroprusside for the control of proximal hypertension during thoracic aortic cross-clamping: effects on spinal cord ischemia. *J Cardiothorac Vasc Anesth* 1995;9:491-496.
86. Poulias GE, Doundalikis N, Skoutas B, et al. Juxtarenal abdominal aneurysmectomy. *J Cardiovasc Surg* 1992;127:520-524.
87. Chiesa R, Marone EM, Brioschi C, et al. Open repair of pararenal aortic aneurysms: operative management, early results, and risk factor analysis. *Ann Vasc Surg* 2006;20:739-746.
88. Knott AW, Kalra M, Duncan AA, et al. Open repair of juxtarenal aortic aneurysms remains a safe option in the era of fenestrated grafts. *J Vasc Surg* 2008;47(4):695-701.
89. Sauer L, Stoney RJ. Transabdominal exposure of the pararenal and suprarenal aorta by medial visceral rotation. *Semin Vasc Surg* 1989;2: 209-213.
90. Goldstone J. Aneurysms of the aorta and iliac arteries. In: Moore WS, ed. Vascular surgery: a comprehensive review. 7th ed. Philadelphia: WB Saunders; 2006:488-511.
91. Cambria RP, Brewster DC, Abbott WM, et al. Transperitoneal versus retroperitoneal approach for aortic reconstruction: a randomized prospective study. *J Vasc Surg* 1990;11:314-325.
92. Kirby LB, Rosenthal D, Atkins CP, et al. Comparison between the transabdominal and retroperitoneal approaches for aortic reconstruction in patients at high risk. *J Vasc Surg* 1999;30:400-406.
93. Sicard GA. Surgical techniques for repair of abdominal aortic aneurysms. In: Gewertz BL, Schwartz LB, eds. Surgery of the aorta and its branches. Philadelphia: WB Saunders; 2000:124-175.
94. Gertler JP, Cambria RP, Laposata M, et al. Coagulation changes during thoracoabdominal aneurysm repair. *J Vasc Surg* 1996;24:936-945.
95. llig KA, Green RM, Ouriel K, et al. Primary fibrinolysis during supraceliac aortic clamping. *J Vasc Surg* 1997;25:244-254.
96. Green RM. Supraceliac aortic clamping for infrarenal aortic surgery: value and technical precautions. In Veith FJ, ed. *Current critical problems in vascular surgery,* vol. 4. St. Louis: Quality Medical; 1992:211-216.
96a. Green RM, Ricotta JJ, Ouriel K, DeWeese JA. Results of supraceliac aortic clamping in the difficult elective resection of infrarenal aortic aneurysms. *J Vasc Surg* 1989;9:124-34.
97. Sarac TP, Clair DG, Hertzer NR, et al. Contemporary results of juxtarenal aneurysm repair. *J Vasc Surg* 2002;36:1104-1111.
98. Nypaver TJ, Shepard AD, Reddy DJ, et al. Repair of pararenal abdominal aortic aneurysms: an analysis of operative management. *Arch Surg* 1993;128:803-813.
99. Crawford ES, Mizrahi EM, Hess KR, et al. The impact of distal perfusion and somatosensory evoked potential monitoring on prevention of paraplegia after aortic aneurysm operation. *J Thorac Cardiovasc Surg* 1988;95:357-366.
100. Comerota AJ, White JV. Reducing morbidity of thoracoabdominal aneurysm repair by preliminary axillofemoral bypass. *Am J Surg* 1995;170:218-222.
101. Connolly J, Wakabayashi A, German J, et al. Clinical experience with pulsatile left heart bypass without anticoagulation for thoracic aneurysms. *J Thorac Cardiovasc Surg* 1971;62:568-576.
102. Coselli JS, LeMaire SA. Left heart bypass reduces paraplegia rates after thoracoabdominal aortic aneurysm repair. *Ann Thorac Surg* 1999;67:1931-1934.
103. Schepens MAA, Vermeulen FEE, Morshuis WJ. Impact of left heart bypass on the results of thoracoabdominal aortic aneurysm repair. *Ann Thorac Surg* 1999;67:1963-1967.
104. Safi HJ, Harlin SA, Miller CC III. Predictive factors for acute renal failure in thoracic and thoracoabdominal aortic aneurysm surgery. *J Vasc Surg* 1996;24:338-345.
105. Coselli JS, LeMaire SA, Poli de Figueiredo L, et al. Paraplegia after thoracoabdominal aortic aneurysm repair: is dissection a risk factor? *Ann Thorac Surg* 1997;63:28-36.
106. Mauney M, Tribble C, Cope J, et al. Is clamp and sew still viable for thoracic aortic resection? *Ann Surg* 1996;223:534-543.
107. LeMaire SA, Miller CC III, Conklin LD, et al. A new predictive model for adverse outcomes after elective thoracoabdominal aortic aneurysm repair. *Ann Thorac Surg* 2001;71:1233-1238.
108. Cambria RP, Davison JK, Zannetti S, et al. Clinical experience with epidural cooling for spinal cord protection during thoracic and thoracoabdominal aneurysm repair. *J Vasc Surg* 1997;25:234-243.
109. Cambria RP, Davison JK, Carter C, et al. Epidural cooling for spinal cord protection during thoracoabdominal aneurysm repair: a five-year experience. *J Vasc Surg* 2000;31:1093-1102.
110. Davison J, Cambria R, Vierra D, et al. Epidural cooling for regional spinal cord hypothermia during thoracoabdominal aneurysm repair. *J Vasc Surg* 1994;20:304-310.
111. Cambria RP, Giglia J. Prevention of spinal cord ischemic complications after thoracoabdominal aortic surgery. *Eur J Vasc Endovasc Surg* 1998;15:96-109.
112. Cambria RP, Davison JK, Giglia JS, et al. Mesenteric shunting decreases visceral ischemic time during thoracoabdominal aneurysm repair. *J Vasc Surg* 1998;27:745-749.
113. Kouchoukos NT, Masetti P, Murphy SF. Hypothermic cardiopulmonary bypass and circulatory arrest in the management of extensive thoracic and thoracoabdominal aortic aneurysms. *Semin Thorac Cardiovasc Surg* 2003;15:333-339.
114. Safi HJ, Muller CC, Subramanian MH, et al. Thoracic and thoracoabdominal aortic aneurysm repair using cardiopulmonary bypass, profound hypothermia and circulatory arrest via left side of the chest incision. *J Vasc Surg* 1998;28:591-598.
115. Engle J, Safi HJ, Miller CC III, et al. The impact of diaphragm management on prolonged ventilator support following thoracoabdominal aortic repair. *J Vasc Surg* 1999;29:150-156.
116. Wadouh F, Arndt C, Oppermann E, et al. The mechanism of spinal cord injury after simple and double aortic cross-clamping. *J Thorac Cardiovasc Surg* 1986;92:121-127.
117. Tshomba Y, Melissano G, Civilini E, et al. Fate of the visceral aortic patch after thoracoabdominal aortic repair. *Eur J Vasc Endovasc Surg* 2005;29:383-389.
118. Dardik A, Perler BA, Roseborough GS, et al. Aneurysmal expansion of the visceral patch after thoracoabdominal aortic replacement: an argument for limiting patch size? *J Vasc Surg* 2001;34:405-409.
119. Parodi JC, Palmaz JC, Barone HD. Transfemoral intraluminal graft implantation for abdominal aortic aneurysms. *Ann Vasc Surg* 1991;5:491-499.
120. Dake MD, Miller DC, Semba CP, et al. Transluminal placement of endovascular stent grafts for the treatment of descending thoracic aortic aneurysms. *N Engl J Med* 1994;331:1729-1734.
121. Greenberg RK, Chuter TA, Lawrence-Brown M, et al. Analysis of renal function after aneurysm repair with a device using suprarenal fixation (Zenith AAA endovascular graft) in contrast to open surgical repair. *J Vasc Surg* 2004;39:1219-1228.

122. Walsh SR, Boyle JR, Lynch AG, et al. Suprarenal endograft fixation and medium-term renal function: systematic review and meta-analysis. *J Vasc Surg* 2008;47(6):1364-1370.
123. Nienaber CA, Zannetti S, Barbieri B, et al. Investigation of stent grafts in patients with type B aortic dissection: design of the INSTEAD trial—a prospective, multicenter, European randomized trial. *Am Heart J* 2005;149:592-599.
124. Jackson BM, Carpenter JP, Fairman RM, et al. Anatomic exclusion from endovascular repair of thoracic aortic aneurysm. *J Vasc Surg* 2007;45:662-666.
125. Fattori R, Nienaber CA, Rousseau H, et al. Results of endovascular repair of the thoracic aorta with the Talent thoracic stent graft: the Talent thoracic retrospective registry. *J Thorac Cardiovasc Surg* 2006;132(2): 332-339.
126. Criado F. Technical strategies to expand stent graft applicability in the aortic arch and proximal descending thoracic aorta. *J Endovasc Ther* 2002;9(Suppl II):II32-II38.
127. Makaroun MS, Dillabou ED, Kee ST, et al. Endovascular treatment of thoracic aortic aneurysms: results of the phase II multicenter trial of the Gore TAG thoracic endoprosthesis. *J Vasc Surg* 2005;41:1-9.
128. Leurs LJ, Bell R, Degrieck Y, et al. Endovascular treatment of thoracic aortic diseases: combined experience from the EUROSTAR and United Kingdom Thoracic Endograft registries. *J Vasc Surg* 2004;40:670-680.
129. Demers P, Miller DC, Mitchell RS, et al. Midterm results of endovascular repair of descending thoracic aortic aneurysms with first-generation stent grafts. *J Throac Cardiovasc Surg* 2004;127:664-673.
130. Stone DH, Brewster DC, Kwolek CJ, et al. Stent graft versus open surgical repair of the thoracic aorta: mid-term results. *J Vasc Surg* 2006;44:1188-1197.
131. Muhs BE, Balm R, White GH, Verhagen HJM. Anatomic factors associated with acute endograft collapse after Gore TAG treatment of thoracic aortic dissection or traumatic rupture. *J Vasc Surg* 2007;45:655-661.
132. Rehders TC, Petzsch M, Ince H, et al. Intentional occlusion of the left subclavian artery during stent graft implantation in the thoracic aorta: risk and relevance. *J Endovasc Ther* 2004;11(6):659-666.
133. Conrad MF, Cambria RP. Contemporary management of descending thoracic and thoracoabdominal aortic aneurysms: endovascular versus open. Circulation 208;117:841–852.
134. Buth J, Harris PL, Hobo R, et al. Neurologic complications associated with endovascular repair of thoracic aortic pathology: incidence and risk factors—a study from the European Collaborators on Stent Graft Techniques for Aortic Aneurysm Repair (EUROSTAR) Registry. *J Vasc Surg* 2007;46:1103-1111.
135. Bavaria JE, Appoo JJ, Makaroun MS, et al. Endovascular stent grafting versus open surgical repair of descending thoracic aortic aneurysms in low-risk patients: a multicenter comparative trial. *J Thorac Cardiovasc Surg* 2007;133:369-377.
136. Steinberg GK, Drake CG, Peerless SJ. Deliberate basilar or vertebral artery occlusion in the treatment of intracranial aneurysms: immediate results and the long-term outcome in 201 patients. *J Neurosurg* 1993;79:161-173.
137. Woo EY, Bavaria JE, Pochettino A, et al. Techniques for preserving vertebral artery perfusion during thoracic aortic stent grafting requiring arch landing. *Vasc Endovasc Surg* 2006;40:367-373.
138. Criado F. Technical strategies to expand stent graft applicability in the aortic arch and proximal descending thoracic aorta. *J Endovasc Ther* 2002;9(Suppl II):II32-II38.
139. Eskandari MK. Aortic debranching procedures to facilitate endografting. *Perspect Vasc Endovasc Ther* 2006;18:287-292.
140. Zhou W, Reardon M, Peden EK, et al. Hybrid approach to complex thoracic aortic aneurysms in high-risk patients: surgical challenges and clinical outcomes. *J Vasc Surg* 2006;44:688-693.
141. Saleh H, Inglese L. Combined surgical and endovascular treatment of aortic arch aneurysms. *J Vasc Surg* 2006;44:460-466.
142. Sanchez LA. Managing proximal arch vessels. *J Vasc Surg* 2006;43:A78-A80.
143. Vaddineni SK, Taylor SM, Patterson MA, et al. Outcome after celiac artery coverage during endovascular thoracic aortic aneurysm repair: preliminary results. *J Vasc Surg* 2007;45:467-471.
144. Gawenda M, Aleksic M, Heckenkamp J, et al. Hybrid procedures for the treatment of thoracoabdominal aortic aneurysms and dissections. *Eur J Vasc Endovasc Surg* 2007;33:31-77.
145. Chiesa R, Tshomba Y, Melissano G, et al. Hybrid approach to thoracoabdominal aortic aneurysms in patients with prior aortic surgery. *J Vasc Surg* 2007;45:1128-1135.
146. Black SA, Wolfe JHN, Clark M, et al. Complex thoracoabdominal aortic aneurysms: endovascular exclusion with visceral revascularization. *J Vasc Surg* 2006;43:1081-1089.
147. Lee WA, Brown MP, Martin TD, et al. Early results after staged hybrid repair of thoracoabdominal aortic aneurysms. *J Am Coll Surg* 2007;205:420-431.
148. Resch TA, Greenberg RK, Lyden SP, et al. Combined staged procedures for the treatment of thoracoabdominal aneurysms. *J Endovasc Ther* 2006;13:481-489.
149. Farber MA. Visceral vessel relocation techniques. *J Vasc Surg* 2006;43:A81-A84.
150. Gravereaux EC, Faries PF, Burks JA, et al. Risk of spinal cord ischemia after endograft repair of thoracic aortic aneurysms. *J Vasc Surg* 2001;34:997-1003.
151. Khoynezhad A, Donayre CE, Bui H, et al. Risk factors of neurologic deficit after thoracic aortic endografting. *Ann Thorac Surg* 2007;83:S882-S889.
152. Plaschke K, Boeckler D, Schumacher H, et al. Adenosine-induced cardiac arrest and EEG changes in patients with thoracic aorta endovascular repair. *Br J Anaesth* 2006;96:310-316.
153. Pornratanarangsi S, Webster MW, Alison P, Nand P. Rapid ventricular pacing to lower blood pressure during endograft deployment in the thoracic aorta. *Ann Thorac Surg* 2006;81(5):e21-e23.
154. Nienaber CA, Kische S, Rehders TC, et al. Rapid pacing for better placing: comparison of techniques for precise deployment of endografts in the thoracic aorta. *J Endovasc Ther* 2007;14:506-512.
155. Ishiguchi T, Nishikimi N, Usui A, Ishigaki T. Endovascular stent-graft deployment: temporary vena caval occlusion with balloons to control aortic blood flow—experimental canine study and initial clinical experience. *Radiology* 2000;215:594-599.
156. Cho JS, Haider S, Makaroun MS. Endovascular therapy of thoracic aneurysms: Gore TAG trial results. *Semin Vasc Surg* 2006;19:18-24.
157. Cho JS, Haider S, Makaroun MS. U.S. multicenter trials of endoprostheses for endovascular treatment of descending thoracic aneurysms. *J Vasc Surg* 2006;43:12A-19A.
158. Makaroun MS, Dillavou ED, Wheatley GH, et al. Five-year results of endovascular treatment with the Gore TAG device compared with open repair of thoracic aortic aneurysms. *J Vasc Surg* 2008;47(5):912-918.
159. Kwolek CJ, Fairman R. Update on thoracic aortic endovascular grafting using the Medtronic Talent device. *Semin Vasc Surg* 2006;19:25-31.
160. Fairman RM, Farber M, Kwolek CJ, et al. Pivotal results of the Medtronic Vascular Talent Thoracic Stent Graft System for patients with thoracic aortic disease: the VALOR Trial. Vascular Annual Meeting. Baltimore: Maryland; June 7-10, 2007.
161. Hassoun HT, Matsumura JS. The Cook TX2 thoracic stent graft: preliminary experience and trial design. *Semin Vasc Surg* 2006;19:32-39.
162. Matsumura JS, Cambria RP, Dake MD, et al. International controlled clinical trial of thoracic endovascular aneurysm repair with the Zenith TX2 endovascular graft: 1-year results. *J Vasc Surg* 2008;47:247-257.
163. Greenberg RK, O'Neill S, Walker E, et al. Endovascular repair of thoracic aortic lesions with the Zenith TX1 and TX2 thoracic grafts: intermediate-term results. *J Vasc Surg* 2005;41:589-596.
164. Wheatley GH, Gurbuz AT, Rodriguez-Lopez JA, et al. Midterm outcome in 158 consecutive Gore TAG thoracic enodprostheses: single center experience. *Ann Thorac Surg* 2006;81(5):1570-1577.
165. Ellozy SH, Carroccio A, Minor M, et al. Challenges of endovascular tube graft repair of thoracic aortic aneurysm: midterm follow-up and lessons learned. *J Vasc Surg* 2003;38:676-683.
166. Walsh SR, Tang TY, Sadat U, et al. Endovascular stenting versus open surgery for thoracic aortic disease: systematic review and meta-analysis of perioperative results. *J Vasc Surg* 2008;47(5):1094-1098.
167. Verhoeven ELG, Prins TR, Tielliu IFJ, et al. Treatment of short-necked infrarenal aortic aneurysms with fenestrated stent-grafts: short-term results. *Eur J Vasc Endovasc Surg* 2004;27:477-483.
168. Anderson JL, Adam DJ, Berce M, et al. Repair of thoracoabdominal aortic aneurysms with fenestrated and branched endovascular stent grafts. *J Vasc Surg* 2005;42:600-607.
169. Muhs BE, Verhoeven ELG, Zeebregts CJ, et al. Mid-term results of endovascular aneurysm repair with branched and fenestrated endografts. *J Vasc Surg* 2006;44:9-15.
170. Semmens JB, Lawrence-Brown MD, Hartley DE, et al. Outcomes of fenestrated endografts in the treatment of abdominal aortic aneurysm in Western Australia. *J Endovasc Ther* 2007;13:320-329.
171. Ziegler P, Avgerinos ED, Umscheid T, et al. Fenestrated endografting for aortic aneurysm repair: a 7-year experience. *J Endovasc Ther* 2007;14:609-618.

172. Halak M, Goodman MA, Baker SR. The fate of target visceral vessel after fenestrated endovascular aortic repair: general considerations and mid-term results. *Eur J Vasc Endovasc Surg* 2006;32:124-128.
173. Greenberg RK, Haulon S, O'Neill S, et al. Primary endovascular repair of juxtarenal aneurysms with fenestrated endovascular grafting. *Eur J Vasc Endovasc Surg* 2004;27:484-491.
174. O'Neill S, Greenberg RK, Haddad F, et al. A prospective analysis of fenestrated endovascular grafting: intermediate-term outcomes. *Eur J Vasc Endovasc Surg* 2006;32:115-123.
175. Roselli EE, Greenberg RK, Pfaff K, et al. Endovascular treatment of thoracoabdominal aortic aneurysms. *J Thorac Cardiovasc Surg* 2007;133:1474-1482.
176. Chuter TAM, Gordon RL, Reilly LM, et al. Multi-branched stent-graft for type III thoracoabdominal aortic aneurysm. *J Vasc Interv Radiol* 2001;12:391-392.
177. Chuter TAM, Rapp JH, Hiramoto JS, et al. Endovascular treatment of thoracoabdominal aortic aneurysms. *J Vasc Surg* 2008;48:6-16.
178. Haddad F, Greenberg RK, Walker E, et al. Fenestrated endovascular grafting: the renal side of the story. *J Vasc Surg* 2005;41:181-190.
179. Qvarfordt PG, Stoney RJ, Reilly LM, et al. Management of pararenal aneurysms of the abdominal aorta. *J Vasc Surg* 1986;3:84-93.
180. Crawford ES, Beckett WC, Greer MS. Juxtarenal infrarenal aortic aneurysm: special diagnostic and therapeutic considerations. *Ann Surg* 1986;203:661-670.
181. Allen BT, Anderson CB, Rubin BG, et al. Preservation of renal function in juxtarenal and suprarenal abdominal aortic aneurysm repair. *J Vasc Surg* 1993;17:948-959.
182. Faggioli G, Stella A, Freyrie A, et al. Early and long-term results in the surgical treatment of juxtarenal and pararenal aortic aneurysms. *Eur J Vasc Endovasc Surg* 1998;15:205-211.
183. Jean-Claude JM, Reilly LM, Stoney RJ, et al. Pararenal aortic aneurysms: the future of open aortic aneurysm repair. *J Vasc Surg* 1999;29:902-912.
184. Shortell CK, Johansson M, Green RM, et al. Optimal operative strategies in repair of juxtarenal abdominal aortic aneurysms. *Ann Vasc Surg* 2003;17:60-65.
185. West CA, Noel AA, Bower TC, et al. Factors affecting outcomes of open surgical repair of pararenal aortic aneurysms: a 10-year experience. *J Vasc Surg* 2006;43:921-928.
186. Martin GH, O'Hara PJ, Hertzer NR, et al. Surgical repair of aneurysms involving the suprarenal, visceral, and lower thoracic aortic segments: early results and late outcome. *J Vasc Surg* 2000;31:851-862.
187. Cowan JA, Dimick JB, Henke P, et al. Surgical treatment of intact thoracoabdominal aortic aneurysms in the United States: hospital and surgeon volume related outcomes. *J Vasc Surg* 2003;37:116-174.
188. Rigberg DA, McGory ML, Zigmond DS, et al. Thirty-day mortality statistics underestimate the risk of repair of thoracoabdominal aortic aneurysms: a statewide experience. *J Vasc Surg* 2006;43:217-223.
189. Rectenwald JE, Huber TS, Martin TD, et al. Functional outcome after thoracoabdominal aortic aneurysm repair. *J Vasc Surg* 2002;35:640-671.
190. Estrera AL, Miller CC III, Huynh TTT. Neurologic outcome after thoracic and thoracoabdominal aortic aneurysm repair. *Ann Thorac Surg* 2001;72:1225-1231.
191. Welborn MB, Oldenburg SA, Hess PJ, et al. The relationship between visceral ischemia proinflammatory cytokines, and organ injury in patients undergoing thoracoabdominal aneurysm repair. *Crit Care Med* 2000;28:3191-3197.
192. Safi H, Hess KR, Randel M, et al. Cerebrospinal fluid drainage and distal aortic perfusion: reducing neurologic complications in repair of thoracoabdominal aortic aneurysms, type I and type II. *J Vasc Surg* 1996;23:223-228.
193. Cambria R, Brewster D, Moncure A, et al. Recent experience with thoracoabdominal aneurysm repair. *Arch Surg* 1989;124:620-624.
194. Cohen JR, Schroder W, Leal J, et al. Mesenteric shunting during thoracoabdominal aortic clamping to prevent disseminated intravascular coagulation in dogs. *Ann Vasc Surg* 1988;2:261-267.
195. Safi HJ, Miller CC III, Yawn DH, et al. Impact of distal aortic and visceral perfusion on liver function during thoracoabdominal and descending thoracic aortic repair. *J Vasc Surg* 1998;27:145-153.
197. Anagnostopoulos PV, Shepard AD, Pipinos II, et al. Hemostatic alterations associated with supraceliac aortic cross-clamping. *J Vasc Surg* 2002;35:100-108.
197a. Gertler JP, Cambria RP, Makary MA, et al. Correction of coagulation defect in thoracoabdominal aneurysm repair by mesenteric shunting. The 24th Meeting of the New England Society for Vascular Surgery, September 18-19, 1997, Bolton Landing, NY (abstract).
198. Money SR, Rice K, Crockett D, et al. Risk of respiratory failure after repair of thoracoabdominal aortic aneurysms. *Am J Surg* 1994;168: 152-155.
199. Svensson LG, Hess KR, Coselli JS, et al. A prospective study of respiratory failure after high-risk surgery on the thoracoabdominal aorta. *J Vasc Surg* 1991;14:271-282.
200. Etz CD, Di Luozzo G, Bello R, et al. Pulmonary complications after descending thoracic and thoracoabdominal aortic aneurysm repair: predictors, prevention, and treatment. *Ann Thorac Surg* 2007;83:S870-S876.
201. Schepens MA, Dekkar E, Hanerlijnck RP, et al. Survival and aortic events after graft replacement for thoracoabdominal aortic aneurysm. *Cardiovasc Surg* 1996;4:713-719.
202. Kashyap VS, Cambria RP, Davison JK, et al. Renal failure after thoracoabdominal aortic surgery. *J Vasc Surg* 1997;26:949-957.
203. Köksoy C, LeMaire SA, Curling PE, et al. Renal perfusion during thoracoabdominal aortic operations: cold crystalloid is superior to normothermic blood. *Ann Thorac Surg* 2002;73:730-738.
204. Svensson LG, Crawford ES, Hess KR, et al. Thoracoabdominal aortic aneurysms associated with celiac, superior mesenteric and renal artery occlusive disease: methods and analysis of results in 271 patients. *J Vasc Surg* 1992;16:378-390.
205. DeLasson L, Hanson HE, Juhl B, et al. A randomized, clinical study on the effect of low-dose dopamine on central and renal hemodynamics in infrarenal aortic surgery. *Eur J Vasc Endovasc Surg* 1995;10:82-90.
206. Oliver WC Jr, Nuttall GA, Cherry KJ, et al. A comparison of fenoldopam with dopamine and sodium nitroprusside in patients undergoing cross-clamping of the abdominal aorta. *Anesth Analg* 2006;103: 833-840.
207. Halpenny M, Rushe C, Breen P, et al. The effects of fenoldopam on renal function in patients undergoing elective aortic surgery. *Eur J Anaesthesiol* 2002;19:32-39.
208. Cambria RP, Davison JK. Spinal cord ischemic complications after thoracoabdominal aortic surgery. In: Gewertz BL, Schwartz LB, eds. Surgery of the aorta and its branches. Philadelphia: WB Saunders; 2000: 212-230.
209. Svensson LG, Hess KR, Coselli JS, et al. Influence of segmental arteries, extent and atriofemoral bypass on postoperative paraplegia after thoracoabdominal aortic operations. *J Vasc Surg* 1994;20:255-262.
210. Lauterbach SR, Cambria RP, Brewster DC, et al. Contemporary management of aortic branch compromise resulting from acute aortic dissection. *J Vasc Surg* 2001;33:1185-1192.
211. Azizzadeh A, Huynh TTT, Miller CC III, et al. Postoperative risk factors for delayed neurologic deficit after thoracic and thoracoabdominal aortic aneurysm repair: a case-control study. *J Vasc Surg* 2003;37: 750-754.
212. Estrera AL, Miller CC III, Huynh TT, et al. Preoperative and operative predictors of delayed neurologic deficit following repair of thoracoabdominal aortic aneurysm. *J Thorac Cardiovasc Surg* 2003;126: 1288-1294.
213. Wong DR, Coselli JS, Amerman K, et al. Delayed spinal cord deficits after thoracoabdominal aortic aneurysm repair. *Ann Thorac Surg* 2007;83:1345-1355.
214. Rokkas CK, Kouchoukos NT. Profound hypothermia for spinal cord protection in operations on the descending and thoracoabdominal aorta. *Semin Thorac Cardiovasc Surg* 1998;10:57-60.
215. Griepp RB, Ergen MA, Galla JD, et al. Looking for the artery of Adamkiewicz: a quest to minimize paraplegia after operations for aneurysm of the descending thoracic and thoracoabdominal aorta. *J Thorac Cardiovasc Surg* 1996;112:1202-1215.
216. Heinemann MK, Brassel F, Herzog T, et al. The role of spinal angiography in operations on the thoracic aorta: myth or reality? *Ann Thorac Surg* 1998;65:346-351.
217. Svensson LG. Intraoperative identification of spinal cord blood supply during repairs of descending aorta and thoracoabdominal aorta. *J Thorac Cardiovasc Surg* 1996;112:1455-1461.
218. Cunningham JJ, Laschinger JC, Spencer FC. Monitoring of somatosensory evoked potentials during surgical procedures on the thoracoabdominal aorta. IV. Clinical observations and results. *J Thorac Cardiovasc Surg* 1987;94:275-285.
219. van Dongen EP, Schepens MA, Morshuis WJ, et al. Thoracic and thoracoabdominal aortic aneurysm repair: use of evoked potential monitoring in 118 patients. *J Vasc Surg* 2001;34:1035-1040.
220. Jacobs MJ, de Mol BA, Elenbaas T, et al. Spinal cord blood supply in patients with thoracoabdominal aortic aneurysms. *J Vasc Surg* 2002;35:30-37.

221. Jacobs MJ, Mess W, Mochtar B, et al. The value of motor evoked potentials in reducing paraplegia during thoracoabdominal aneurysm repair. *J Vasc Surg* 2006;43:239-246.
222. Svensson LG, Grum DF, Bednarski M, et al. Appraisal of cerebrospinal fluid alterations during aortic surgery with intrathecal papaverine administration and cerebrospinal fluid drainage. *J Vasc Surg* 1990;11:423-429.
223. Kazama S, Masaki Y, Maruyama S, et al. Effect of altering cerebrospinal fluid pressure on spinal cord blood flow. *Ann Thorac Surg* 1994;58: 112-115.
224. Crawford ES, Svensson LG, Hess KR, et al. A prospective randomized study of cerebrospinal fluid drainage to prevent paraplegia after high risk surgery on the thoracoabdominal aorta. *J Vasc Surg* 1991;13:36-46.
225. Murray MJ, Bower TC, Oliver WCJ, et al. Effects of cerebrospinal fluid drainage in patients undergoing thoracic and thoracoabdominal aortic surgery. *J Cardiothorac Vasc Anesth* 1993;7:266-272.
226. Coselli JS, LeMaire SA, Köksoy C, et al. Cerebrospinal fluid drainage reduces paraplegia after thoracoabdominal aortic aneurysm repair: results of a randomized clinical trial. *J Vasc Surg* 2002;35:631-639.
227. Cina CS, Abouzahr L, Arena GO, et al. Cerebrospinal fluid drainage to prevent paraplegia during thoracic aortic aneurysm surgery: a systematic review and meta-analysis. *J Vasc Surg* 2004;40:36-44.
228. Hollier L, Money SR, Naslund TC, et al. Risk of spinal cord dysfunction in patients undergoing thoracoabdominal aortic replacement. *Am J Surg* 1992;164:210-213.
229. Fowl R, Patterson R, Gewirtz R, et al. Protection against postischemic spinal cord injury using a new 21-aminosteroid. *J Surg Res* 1990;48: 597-600.
230. Francel P, Long B, Malik J, et al. Limiting ischemic spinal cord injury using a free radical scavenger 21-aminosteroid and/or cerebrospinal fluid drainage. *J Neurosurg* 1993;79:742-751.
231. Laschinger J, Cunningham JJ, Cooper MM, et al. Prevention of ischemic spinal cord injury following aortic cross-clamping: use of corticosteroids. *Ann Thorac Surg* 1984;38:500-507.
232. Nylander W, Plunkett RJ, Hammon JW Jr, et al. Thiopental modification of ischemic spinal cord injury in the dog. *Ann Thorac Surg* 1982;33:64-68.
233. Simpson I, Eide T, Schiff G, et al. Intrathecal magnesium sulfate protects the spinal cord from ischemic injury during thoracic aortic crossclamping. *Anesthesiology* 1994;81:1493-1499.
234. Acher CW, Wynn MM, Hoch JR, et al. Combined use of cerebral spinal fluid drainage and naloxone reduces the risk of paraplegia in thoracoabdominal aneurysm repair. *J Vasc Surg* 1994;19:236-248.
235. Follis F, Miller K, Scremin O, et al. NMDA receptor blockade and spinal cord ischemia due to aortic crossclamping in the rat model. *Can J Neurol Sci* 1994;21:227-232.
236. Gelbfish J, Phillips T, Rose D, et al. Acute spinal cord ischemia: prevention of paraplegia with verapamil. *Circulation* 1986;74:I5-I10.
237. Agee JM, Flanagan T, Blackbourne LH, et al. Reducing postischemic paraplegia using conjugated superoxide dismutase. *Ann Thorac Surg* 1991;51:911-915.
238. Casey PJ, Black JH, Szabo C, et al. Poly(adenosine diphosphate ribose) polymerase inhibition modulates spinal cord dysfunction after thoracoabdominal aortic ischemia-reperfusion. *J Vasc Surg* 2005;41:88-107.
239. Rokkas C, Cronin C, Nitta T, et al. Profound systemic hypothermia inhibits the release of neurotransmitter amino acids in spinal cord ischemia. *J Thorac Cardiovasc Surg* 1995;110:27-35.
240. Allen BT, Davis C, Osborne D, et al. Spinal cord ischemia and reperfusion metabolism: the effect of hypothermia. *J Vasc Surg* 1994;19:332-340.
241. Rokkas C, Sundaresan S, Shuman TA, et al. Profound systemic hypothermia protects the spinal cord in a primate model of spinal cord ischemia. *J Thorac Cardiovasc Surg* 1993;106:1024-1035.
242. Bush HJ, Hydo LJ, Fischer E, et al. Hypothermia during elective abdominal aortic aneurysm repair: the high risk of avoidable morbidity. *J Vasc Surg* 1995;21:392-400.
243. Fehrenbacher J, McCready R, Hormuth D, et al. One-stage segmental resection of extensive thoracoabdominal aneurysms with left-sided heart bypass. *J Vasc Surg* 1993;18:366-371.
244. Wisselink W, Becker M, Nguyen J, et al. Protecting the ischemic spinal cord during aortic clamping: the influence of selective hypothermia and spinal cord perfusion pressure. *J Vasc Surg* 1994;19:788-796.
245. Marsala M, Vanicky I, Galik J, et al. Panmyelic epidural cooling protects against ischemic spinal cord damage. *J Surg Res* 1993;55:21-31.
246. Meylaerts SA, de Haan P, Kalkman CJ, et al. The influence of regional spinal cord hypothermia on transcranial myogenic motor-evoked potential monitoring and the efficacy of spinal cord ischemia detection. *J Thorac Cardiovasc Surg* 1999;118:1038-1045.
247. Back MR, Bandyk M, Bradner M, et al. Critical analysis of outcome determinants affecting repair of intact aneurysms involving the visceral aorta. *Ann Vasc Surg* 2005;19:648-656.
248. Hallett JW, Marshall DM, Petterson TM, et al. Graft-related complications after abdominal aortic aneurysm repair: reassurance from a 36-year population-based experience. *J Vasc Surg* 1997;25:277-286.
249. Biancari F, Ylönen K, Anttila V, et al. Durability of open repair of infrarenal abdominal aortic aneurysm: a 15-year follow-up study. *J Vasc Surg* 2002;35:87-93.
250. Conrad MF, Crawford MS, Pedraza JD, et al. Long-term durability of open abdominal aortic aneurysm repair. *J Vasc Surg* 2007;46:669-675.

chapter 34

Peripheral Aneurysms

Matthew T. Menard, MD • Michael Belkin, MD

Key Points

- An aneurysm is a permanent localized (i.e., focal) dilation of an artery, having at least a 50% increase in diameter compared with the expected normal diameter of the artery in question.
- Arteriomegaly is diffuse enlargement involving several arterial segments (i.e., nonfocal), with an increase in diameter of greater than 50% compared with the expected normal diameter.
- Ectasia is characterized by dilation, with an increase in diameter of less than 50% of the normal arterial diameter.
- Popliteal artery aneurysms are the most common of peripheral aneurysms, exhibit a strong male predominance, and are commonly associated with aneurysms at other sites.
- Diagnosis is made by physical examination or ultrasound, while angiography is useful for operative planning.
- Given the high rate of complications, early operative intervention with autologous saphenous vein is recommended whenever possible.
- Femoral artery aneurysms, like popliteal aneurysms, are usually atherosclerotic in origin.
- Upper extremity aneurysms are rarely encountered, with subclavian–axillary artery aneurysms arising from compression against a congenital bony abnormality being the most common.
- Evidence of emboli to the hand should trigger a search for a causative aneurysm more proximally.
- Careful monitoring of all patients with peripheral aneurysms is indicated given the high prevalence of additional aneurysms.

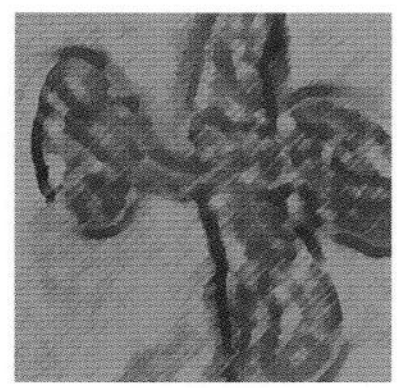

LOWER EXTREMITY ANEURYSMS

Popliteal Aneurysms

History

Since popliteal aneurysms were first described in early Greek manuscripts, a colorful literature has documented their evolving management over the centuries. Antyllus' initial report in 200 BC described ligation and open packing of the aneurysm sac. Philagrius' eighteenth century proposals for aneurysm excision led to Pott's recommendation of above-knee amputation in 1779. Amputation was later supplanted by compression therapy, notably illustrated by Parker's deployment in the nineteenth century of teams of medical students instructed to apply continuous pressure over several days.[1] Linton subsequently popularized sequential lumbar sympathectomy and extirpation of the aneurysm.

Since Edward's first recommendations in 1969, popliteal artery exclusion and surgical bypass with saphenous vein have remained the mainstays of operative repair. In recent years, endovascular exclusion with a covered stent graft has significantly grown in popularity as an alternative therapeutic option.[2,3] In general, the incidence of lower extremity aneurysms appears to be increasing, perhaps due to better surveillance of the aging population, as does the ratio of aneurysms in the periphery to those in the abdominal aorta.[4-6]

Although much less often encountered than aortic aneurysms, popliteal aneurysms are the most common peripheral aneurysm, representing nearly 80% of cases. Male predominance is strong, with an average male–female ratio of 30:1. Popliteal aneurysms typically occur in men in their fifth and sixth decades, while women with popliteal aneurysms are usually in their eighth decade. They are associated with aortic aneurysms 40% of the time and are bilateral in 50% to 70% of cases. Patients with bilateral aneurysms have a 70% chance of a concomitant abdominal aortic aneurysm, and the overall rate of second aneurysms in patients with popliteal aneurysms is nearly 80%.[6] Popliteal aneurysms are almost exclusively atherosclerotic in etiology. Trauma, cystic degeneration of the adventitia, entrapment, and infection are occasional causes.

A high rate of associated atherosclerotic disorders occurs in this population, with myocardial dysfunction present in up to 40%, hypertension in up to 66%, smoking in 50% to 75% and diabetes mellitus in 15% of patients.[7,8]

Signs and Symptoms

Peripheral aneurysms can be asymptomatic or can present with significant complications. The most common clinical presentation of popliteal aneurysms is one of thrombosis, embolism, or both with resultant acute limb ischemia. Early symptoms may be limited to petechial hemorrhage or localized digital gangrenous changes secondary to microemboli. Claudication as a first symptom has typically been found in 30% to 45% of patients in case series of popliteal aneurysms, although Bouhoutsos and Martin[9] reported 73% of 116 patients had initial claudication. As the aneurysm grows in the absence of developed collaterals, acute dissection of mural thrombus or propagation of clot can precipitate severe, often irreversible ischemia. Left untreated, the incidence of future thromboembolic events in initially asymptomatic aneurysms is high; in one series of popliteal aneurysms managed conservatively, only 32% of patients were without complication at 5 years.[5] Similarly, in a study of 26 asymptomatic aneurysms followed for an average of 3 years, 31% developed limb-threatening complications; 2 required amputation, and 2 developed rest pain.[7] Rarely, the initial symptoms are secondary to popliteal nerve compression from a growing aneurysm, leading to parasthesias, neuropraxia, and muscular dysfunction. Popliteal vein compression can lead to thrombosis, manifest by leg swelling, superficial varicosities, or phlebitis. In the unlikely event of popliteal aneurysm rupture, ischemia from arterial compression by the contained hematoma is more typical than exsanguination. Isolated case reports also describe arteriovenous fistula formation following aneurysm rupture into the popliteal vein.[10]

Diagnosis

Although smaller aneurysms or those protected by the suprageniculate or infrageniculate muscles may not readily be detectable on palpation, a careful physical examination leads to the diagnosis in most popliteal aneurysms. A prominent pulsatile mass typically is identified with the knee slightly flexed. Such masses are most often located at or just above the level of the knee joint. In the event of thrombosis, the mass may be firm and nonpulsatile. Widened pulses detected in the contralateral leg, or elsewhere on examination, are additional clues to the presence of a popliteal aneurysm. Cutaneous stigmata of distal embolism or the presence of severe lower extremity ischemia from an acute thromboembolic event in this setting should always raise the suspicion of a newly symptomatic popliteal aneurysm.

When the physical examination is not definitive, ultrasound can often confirm the presence or absence of a popliteal aneurysm. Scanning of the contralateral leg, as well as other sites of concomitant aneurysmal change, should always be performed given the high likelihood of detecting extrapopliteal or bilateral aneurysms. When the aneurysm wall is calcified, a plain x-ray of the knee may suggest the diagnosis. Computed tomography and magnetic resonance imaging (Figure 34-1) are both highly accurate in establishing the diagnosis of popliteal aneurysms. These modalities are particularly helpful in distinguishing aneurysms from other entities (e.g., Baker's cysts) in the differential diagnosis of a popliteal fossa mass. Angiography done during the workup for extremity ischemia can uncover a previously unsuspected aneurysm. But in the presence of occlusion or extensive laminated intramural thrombus, angiography can also be misleading in underestimating the size or even presence of a popliteal aneurysm. The principal role of angiography in the management of popliteal aneurysm is for planning the intervention. Specifically, it can usually delineate both the status of the inflow and outflow vasculature and the full axial extent of the aneurysm.

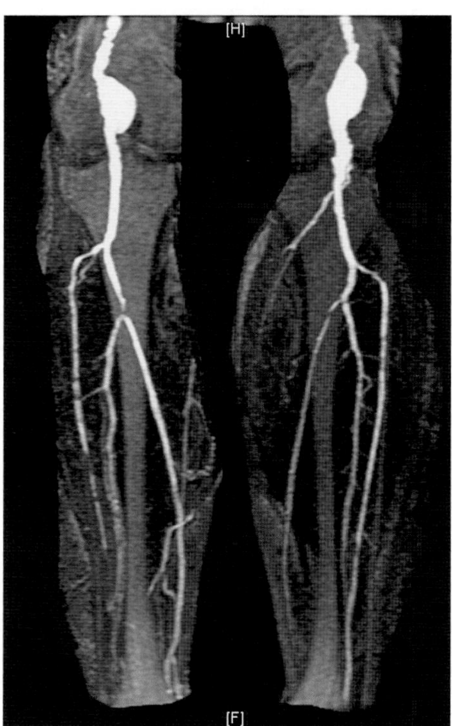

Figure 34-1. Magnetic resonance arteriography demonstrating bilateral popliteal aneurysms and disease of the tibial arteries.

Management

It is generally agreed that all symptomatic aneurysms should undergo operative repair, given the high rate of limb loss with conservative management. In patients with acute symptoms, the degree of leg ischemia determines the management. Patients with any sensory loss or motor weakness need urgent revascularization and in most cases cannot tolerate the additional time needed for angiography and thrombolysis. In contrast, if motor and sensory function is preserved, angiography is recommended to help clarify the inflow status and the extent of aneurysmal change and to identify a patent runoff vessel appropriate for a distal bypass (Figure 34-2).

The natural history of untreated asymptomatic popliteal aneurysms, on the other hand, is poorly defined. The indications for repair of a small, incidentally noted, asymptomatic popliteal aneurysm remain controversial. Lowell and colleagues[11] reported 94 asymptomatic aneurysms followed for nearly 7 years: 18% eventually developed symptoms (25% acute, 75% chronic) and 3 (4%) required amputation after attempted repair. Aneurysm size above 2 cm, the presence

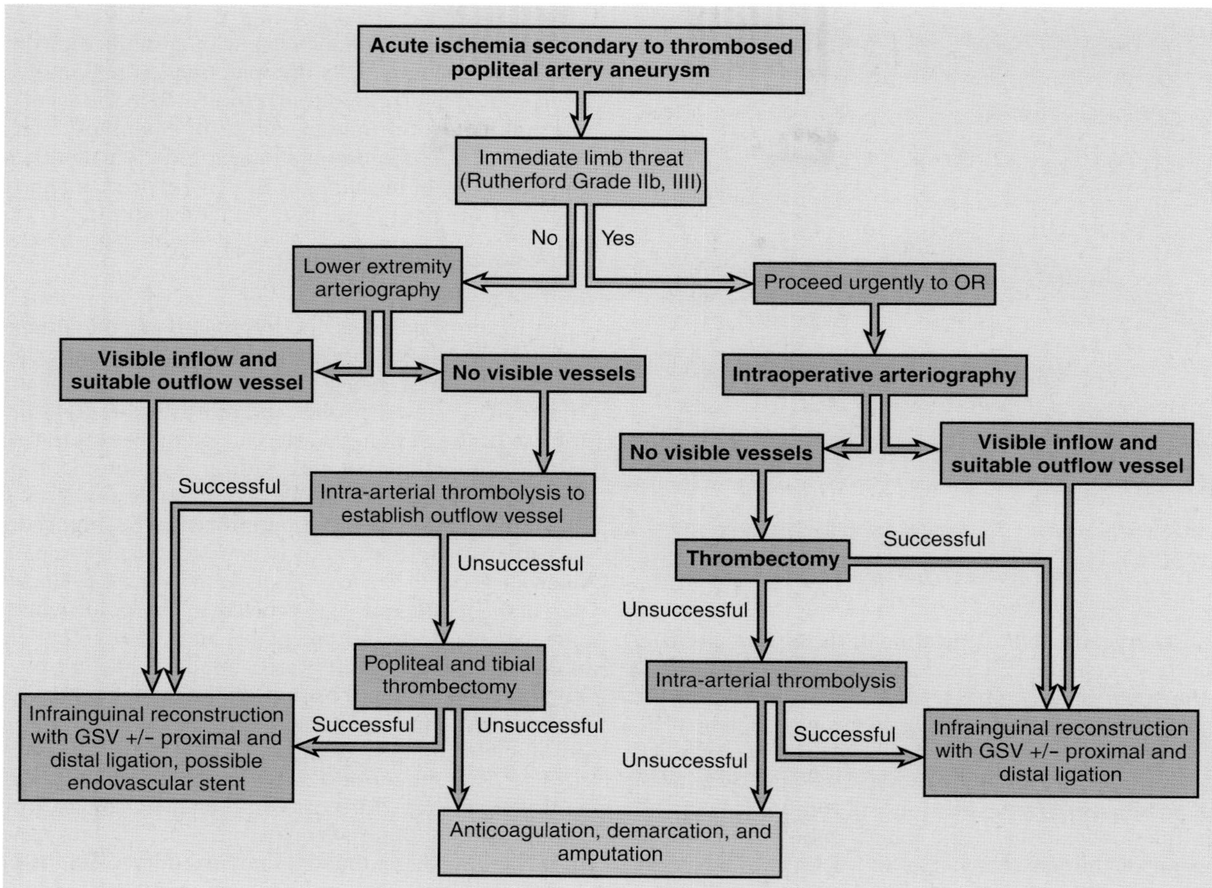

Figure 34-2. Proposed management algorithm for acute limb ischemia secondary to popliteal artery aneurysm.

of thrombus, and poor distal runoff were significant predictors of the development of symptoms in this study. In a review of the available literature between 1980 and 1994 involving 1673 patients with 2445 popliteal aneurysms, Dawson and coworkers[12] found that on average 35% of patients treated nonoperatively ultimately developed ischemic complications and, of those in whom surgical repair was later attempted, 25% went on to require amputation. In another single institution report of a cohort of popliteal aneurysm patients followed expectantly, 100% developed symptoms of ischemia over time and required surgery, half within 2 years of initial presentation.[13] When statistical modeling was applied to determine outcomes in operatively versus nonoperatively managed patients, intermediate-term results clearly favored surgical treatment.[14]

In view of these collective results, and the generally unfavorable long-term limb salvage rate following conservative treatment, most authors recommend surgical repair of asymptomatic popliteal aneurysms above 2 cm in diameter in all but high-risk patients. Some surgeons have modified these recommendations when autogenous vein is unavailable for use as a bypass conduit, given the poorer results with prosthetic reconstruction in the distal popliteal and tibial position, or in the rare cases when suitable runoff is lacking. Similarly, given the overall limited life expectancy of patients with multiple aneurysms (16% 10-year survival compared to 66% for those with a single aneurysm at initial presentation), other authors support conservative management in this subset of patients.[15]

Intervention for popliteal aneurysm is principally directed at excluding the aneurysm from the circulation, thereby eliminating the potential development of limb-threatening ischemia and providing adequate distal arterial flow. For typical aneurysms of small or modest size in which compression is not part of the presenting symptom profile, the aneurysm need not be opened or excised. It is often advantageous to avoid direct dissection of the aneurysm sac to avert injury to the adjacent nerves and veins that may be densely adherent from associated chronic inflammation. The aneurysm is usually ligated both proximally and distally, and a bypass graft is fashioned from autogenous great saphenous vein. While a prosthetic conduit can be used, 5-year patency rates with synthetic grafts have consistently failed to match the rates of 75% to 100% demonstrated when saphenous or arm vein is used.[12,16] When significant atherosclerotic or aneurysmal disease of the superficial femoral artery occurs, the proximal anastomosis should originate at the level of the common femoral artery. If the aneurysm is limited to the popliteal segment, the bypass graft may originate from the above-knee popliteal artery or, more typically, from the distal superficial femoral artery just proximal to the adductor canal. The site of the distal anastomosis is guided by the presence or degree of propagated thrombus in the below-knee popliteal segment; the tibial or peroneal arteries may be employed as dictated by the angiographic findings (Figure 34-3). The aneurysm usually thromboses to the level of the geniculate arteries, or the point of proximal ligation.

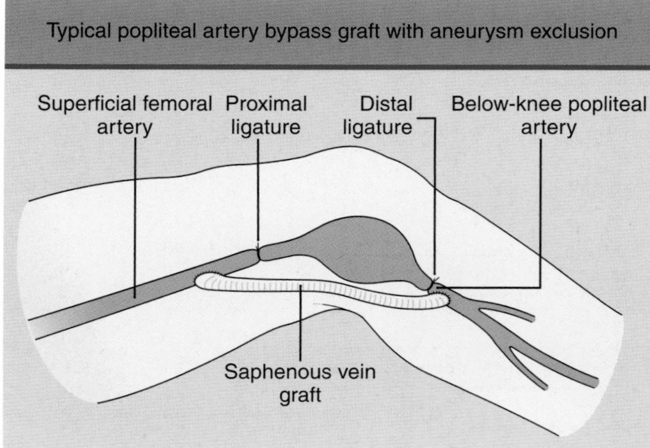

Figure 34-3. Typical popliteal artery aneurysm bypass graft, extending from the distal superficial femoral artery to the below-knee popliteal artery, with suture ligation proximal and distal to the aneurysm.

While most surgeons advocate ligation of the distal superficial femoral artery or suprageniculate popliteal artery just proximal to the aneurysmal segment, some defer this step in the hope of preserving collateral flow through superior geniculate branches. This maneuver is associated with a risk of continued perfusion and pressurization of the bypassed aneurysm, with the small possibility of late expansion and rupture.[17]

When the popliteal aneurysm is large enough to result in compression of the adjacent nerve and vein, it is advisable to expose and open the sac and to perform an endoaneurysmorrhaphy similar to that done for an abdominal aortic aneurysm. Thrombus is removed and all bleeding geniculate branches are ligated from within the sac, but excision of the sac is avoided. Although feasible through a medial approach, a posterior approach with the patient prone affords optimal exposure, particularly when the aneurysm is limited to the popliteal fossa. Harvesting of the small saphenous vein if it is of adequate size avoids the need for an additional incision when using this approach. The sequence of repair in patients with multiple aneurysms is dictated by the severity of symptoms. In the absence of limb-threatening complications from a popliteal aneurysm, the repair of a concomitant abdominal aortic aneurysm would generally take precedence.

Thrombolysis

Intraarterial thrombolytic therapy has become an important adjunct in the management of acute ischemia resulting from popliteal aneurysm.[18,19] Patients that present with thromboembolic complications may have obliteration of their popliteal artery outflow tract, with potential involvement of all three tibial vessels and the more distal microcirculation. Attempts at intraoperative thromboembolectomy may be insufficient to clear the clot burden and obtain vessel patency, severely limiting the surgical options. Intraoperative use of thrombolytic agents may restore a suitable runoff vessel and enhance distal outflow, thereby improving the success of subsequent bypass surgery.[20] Similarly, patients stable enough to undergo preoperative angiography in whom no visible runoff vessel is identifiable may be rendered appropriate for bypass surgery following a successful preoperative infusion of thrombolysis (Figure 34-2). Several reports have documented lower amputation and higher patency rates with combined thrombolysis and surgery, compared with open operation alone.[21,22] It has been argued that amputation is indicated in the event of failed thrombolysis for acute thrombosis of a popliteal aneurysm,[23] but this is not a common strategy. Elderly patients, those at increased risk of bleeding, or those who need urgent revascularization are poor candidates for lytic therapy.

Endovascular Treatment

Enthusiasm has been increasing in recent years for endovascular repair of popliteal aneurysm with an endolumenal stent graft.[24-26] While outcomes with early-generation percutaneous devices were poor, renewed interest has followed the introduction of newer, lower-profile, and more flexible grafts dedicated for use in the peripheral arterial system. Several recent series mostly comprising patients with an asymptomatic popliteal aneurysm have demonstrated comparable midterm patency and equivalent or reduced periprocedural complication rates in patients who had endovascular treatment compared with open surgery.[3,25,26] These results lend support to the view that percutaneous therapy has evolved to the point where it can now be regarded as an acceptable alternative in patients with nonurgent and uncomplicated popliteal aneurysms. Higher rates of periprocedural complications, stent fracture, and graft thrombosis reported in some series, however, underscore continued caution over this approach by some vascular surgeons.[27] Patients considered for popliteal stent grafting should not have excessive tortuosity in the aneurysmal segment and should have both an adequate proximal landing zone and a distal landing target that does not extend beyond the popliteal artery. Results of the accumulated experience to date do not yet support routine stent grafting for urgent or symptomatic aneurysms. Patients in whom a suitable autogenous vein is not available or those medically unfit for surgical intervention may warrant consideration. Until satisfactory long-term data are available, the overall role of endovascular treatment for popliteal aneurysms will remain undefined.

Outcome

The results of operative repair of popliteal aneurysms vary considerably, depending on the preoperative status of the patient and the type of conduit employed. For asymptomatic aneurysms with good outflow, long-term patency is excellent.[16,28-31] In one recent study, 5-year primary patency rates for saphenous vein grafts were 92%, compared with 66% for a matched cohort of patients who had bypass for occlusive disease.[32] Ten-year patency was approximately 80%, and limb salvage rates were higher still, surpassing 95% at 10 years.[13,28] The results of urgent surgical intervention have been variable. In the setting of a thrombosed aneurysm or an extremity with severely reduced outflow, 5- and 10-year patency rates of 60% and 48% and limb salvage rates of 60% and 80%, respectively, have been reported.[13,28] Highlighting the importance of the status of the tibial runoff vessels on patency rates, one series observed 5-year patency rates of 91% for asymptomatic compared with 54% for symptomatic popliteal aneurysms, with a direct correlation of outcome to the quality of the distal outflow.[29] In contrast to these results, another recent review demonstrated equivalent 5-year secondary patency rates approaching 97% in popliteal aneurysms treated emergently

Table 34-1
Patients Undergoing Preoperative Thrombolysis for Acute Ischemia Due to Popliteal Artery Aneurysm*

Author	Year	Patients (*n*)	Agent	Failure (%)	Hemorrhagic Complications (*n*)	Mortality (%)	Early Graft Patency (%)	Limb Salvage (%)
Debing et al.[33]	1997	2	UK	0	0	0	100	100 (5 years)
Taurino et al.[34]	1998	8		13	0			87
Greenberg et al.[35]	1998	6	rtPA	0	0	0	83	100 (2 years)
Marty et al.[23]	2002	13	UK	23		15	68	83 (30 days)
Dorigo et al.[18]	2002	14	UK	28	0	0	74	86 (30 days)
Ravn and Bjorck[19]	2007	41	UK, SK, tPA					90 (1 year)

*UK, urokinase; rtPA, recombinant tissue plasminogen activator; SK, streptokinase.

compared with those treated electively.[16] Table 34-1 lists the periprocedural and postoperative results of thrombolysis for patients with limb ischemia secondary to popliteal artery aneurysms in the most recent published series.

Long-term patency rates of saphenous vein grafts are nearly four times that of prosthetic alternatives. In one representative study, 7 of 31 popliteal repairs done using a prosthetic graft resulted in amputation, compared with only 1 of 42 done with saphenous vein.[11] Results from other reported series of prosthetic bypass for popliteal aneurysm are equally as poor, with 5-year primary patency rates ranging from 29% to 40%.[5,13,16,36] Of note, saphenous vein grafts done for popliteal aneurysm tend to dilate over time, in contrast to those performed for occlusive disease, whose diameter tends to remain static.[32]

Individual series have documented equivalent intermediate-term primary and secondary patency and survival rates in patients undergoing elective endovascular compared with open popliteal aneurysm repair.[3,25,26] A metaanalysis of published reports to date comparing endovascular with open repair of nonthrombosed popliteal aneurysms concluded that while medium-term results are similar, early graft thrombosis and reintervention rates are higher with endovascular treatment.[27] Notably, five of the eight initially identified series were excluded from the analysis due to insufficient data. The perioperative mortality associated with popliteal aneurysm repair is generally low; in a multicenter study conducted in the United Kingdom, a mortality rate of less than 2.0% was reported, with outcome influenced by the initial presentation.[37]

Femoral Aneurysms

History

Femoral artery aneurysms are the second most prevalent peripheral artery aneurysm after those in the popliteal artery. Their relative clinical rarity is highlighted by population studies that indicate a combined incidence of both femoral and popliteal aneurysms in the United States population of 7.39 per 100,000 hospitalized men and 1.00 per 100,000 hospitalized women.[38] True aneurysms are primarily atherosclerotic and are most often located in the common femoral artery. The femoral artery is also the most common site of pseudoaneurysms, including mycotic and anastomotic aneurysms and those secondary to trauma and percutaneous cannulation of the femoral artery. As with peripheral aneurysms elsewhere, femoral aneurysms are commonly associated with both abdominal aortic aneurysms and extremity aneurysms at other sites. In their review of patients with multiple aneurysms, Dent at al.[6] found that of those with a common femoral aneurysm, 95% had a second aneurysm, 92% had an aortoiliac aneurysm, and nearly 60% had bilateral femoral aneurysms. Conversely, the incidence of femoral and popliteal aneurysms in patients with an abdominal aortic aneurysm is low and ranges from 3.1% to 14%.[6,39] Notably, in the report by Diwan and colleagues,[39] patients with both an abdominal aortic aneurysm and a lower extremity aneurysm were all men, and only one had a family history of aneurysm disease. The presence of peripheral arterial occlusive disease in men with an isolated aortic aneurysm was the only factor that differentiated them from men with multiple aneurysms.[39] Other investigators have confirmed the predilection for men to develop lower extremity aneurysms compared to women. Graham et al.[40] reported a male–female ratio 15:1 for femoral artery aneurysms, a higher ratio than that typically seen with abdominal aortic aneurysms. Different biological and genetic processes for peripheral aneurysms are presumably responsible for this strong gender disparity. A murine strain with known X-chromosome mutations and abnormal elastin function has been shown to have a marked tendency to aneurysm development but as yet no particular predisposition for peripheral aneurysms over those of the aorta.[41]

The factors that lead to the development of a femoral artery aneurysm are not clearly delineated. One explanation is that constriction at the level of the inguinal ligament leads to relative turbulence in the poststenotic common femoral artery. Consistent with this, femoral artery aneurysms rarely extend proximally to involve the external iliac artery. Repetitive hip flexion with resulting shear stress and vessel distortion proximal to a major branch has also been suggested as a contributing factor. Others have investigated the role of inflammatory cells, or a more systemic defect in vessel architecture, to explain the multiplicity of peripheral aneurysms. The incidence is high of concomitant coronary artery disease and hypertension in patients with femoral aneurysms and a common history of cigarette smoking. Some authors have noted a particularly low incidence of lower extremity aneurysms in patients with diabetes mellitus,[42] perhaps due to the counterbalancing effect of vessel wall calcification seen with this disease.

Recognizing the more technically challenging nature of aneurysms involving the profunda femoris, femoral aneurysms have been classified as either type I, limited to the common femoral artery, or type II, extending to the profunda femoris artery. In their initial series describing 55 common femoral aneurysms, Cutler and Darling[42] found a distribution of 44% type I and 56% type II aneurysms. Isolated profunda artery aneurysms are uncommon, comprising only 2% of all femoral aneurysms. Similarly, aneurysms limited to the superficial femoral artery are unusual, with most being mycotic or traumatic in etiology. Aneurysms in the superficial femoral artery tend to present at a later age than other femoral and popliteal aneurysms and are more typically seen in patients with generalized degenerative enlargement of the entire superficial femoral artery, a situation known as arteriomegaly.[43]

Signs and Symptoms

Asymptomatic femoral artery aneurysms, representing 30% to 40% of cases in reported series, are often noted incidentally during routine physical examination. Palpation of a smooth, pulsatile, fusiform, and nontender groin mass is sufficiently diagnostic in most cases. Local pain, swelling, and tenderness are typical features when the femoral artery aneurysm becomes symptomatic. Pain as the sole symptom is present in 20% of cases[40] and is characterized by mild and focal groin or anterior thigh pain secondary to chronic compression of the femoral nerve. Compression of the femoral vein by a slowly expanding aneurysm can lead to lower extremity edema, phlebitis, and venous stasis changes.

Complications of femoral artery aneurysms include embolization, thrombosis, and rupture. In one series of 45 patients with 63 aneurysms, nearly half (47%) of the patients had suffered a major complication by the time of first presentation.[42] Of these, 32% had thrombosed while another 10% had ruptured. The rate of embolic complications from a femoral aneurysm is reported to be between 5% and 10%.[40,42,44] Acute thrombosis can result in critical ischemia with a sensorimotor deficit or frank gangrene, particularly if the profunda is also occluded. Patients with subacute or chronic thrombosis and who have had intervening collateral recruitment, on the other hand, typically present with claudication. Investigation has failed to correlate thrombosis of a femoral aneurysm with prolonged postural change, exercise, or any other identifiable cause.

Emboli from femoral artery aneurysms can either be clinically silent or cause symptoms such as foot or calf pain or distal cutaneous stigmata. The result of a few small emboli may be limited to petechial hemorrhage evident on the distal aspect of the toes or a transient skin pattern of livedo reticularis. More severe or recurrent episodes of embolism can result in greater degrees of ischemia, ranging from end-digit gangrene seen with blue toe syndrome to limb-threatening ischemia. As the fibrous femoral sheath serves to confine the femoral artery, rupture of a femoral aneurysm is a rare event, and exsanguination following rupture even more so. When rupture does occur, however, it is heralded by groin ecchymosis, local pain, and pressure effects due to the limited space in the femoral sheath. All told, 40% of patients with a femoral artery aneurysm have some manifestation of either acute or chronic ischemia. Of note, it can at times be difficult to determine to what degree concomitant arterial occlusive disease or an associated popliteal or aortic aneurysm is responsible for the presenting symptoms.

Diagnosis

When the diagnosis is not clear after physical examination, duplex ultrasonography is a reliable means of documenting both the presence and the size of femoral artery aneurysms and sac morphology. Ultrasound can also be used to screen for associated popliteal or aortoiliac aneurysms. Computed tomography or magnetic resonance imaging are additional highly accurate diagnostic modalities that can provide additional information concerning the status of the proximal and distal arteries. Once the diagnosis is secure, however, angiography can be used to delineate the extent of thromboembolic disease and optimize preoperative planning by detailing the patency of both the inflow and the lower extremity outflow. In an urgent situation, without time for formal preoperative arteriography, computed tomography angiography is available in most centers; alternatively, an intraoperative angiogram can provide the necessary anatomical information.

Management

There is little disagreement that patients with a symptomatic femoral artery aneurysm should undergo operative repair, particularly for rest pain or tissue loss. Claudication resulting from thromboembolic sequelae of a femoral aneurysm and not from associated occlusive disease also warrants intervention given the risk of recurrent embolism and progression of ischemia. Patients with aneurysms that cause pain from local expansion or evidence of venous compromise should be offered surgery if they are otherwise medically fit. Finally, surgical repair should be considered for aneurysms that enlarge on serial ultrasound monitoring.

In common with all peripheral aneurysms elsewhere, the indications for intervention for an asymptomatic femoral aneurysm remain an area of active controversy. Conservative authors argue that the risk of thromboembolic complications is much less than for popliteal aneurysms. Furthermore, little evidence correlates the size of a femoral artery aneurysm to the rate of ischemic complications. However, others cite the potential for adverse outcomes in patients that have been followed nonoperatively and the unacceptably high rate of limb loss following acute thromboembolism to support a more aggressive operative policy. The literature generally supports an active approach. In one study of 12 patients with a femoral aneurysm followed for 10 years, 5 (43%) thrombosed and all required amputation.[45] Similarly, in a series of 44 patients from the Mayo Clinic treated nonoperatively, a 16% rate of amputation was secondary to complications from the femoral aneurysm.[46] In practice, most surgeons consider repair appropriate for a femoral aneurysm reaching 2.5 to 3.0 cm in a fit patient. Additional factors that would encourage intervention are the presence of a popliteal aneurysm or distal occlusive disease.

The most common surgical treatment for a femoral aneurysm is replacement with a short interposition graft. Aneurysm resection is rarely indicated (except for mycotic femoral aneurysms), and the sac is usually opened and debrided of its thrombus but left in situ. Following reconstruction, the sac walls can then be closed over the interposition graft. The specific configuration of the replacement graft is determined by the anatomical extent of the aneurysm. The proximal anastomosis is typically at the level of the distal external iliac artery or proximal common femoral artery. Occasionally, it is necessary to obtain proximal control of the iliac artery via a retroperitoneal flank incision. Extension of the aneurysm into both the profunda and the superficial femoral arteries requires either reimplantation of the more distal, nonaneurysmal profunda

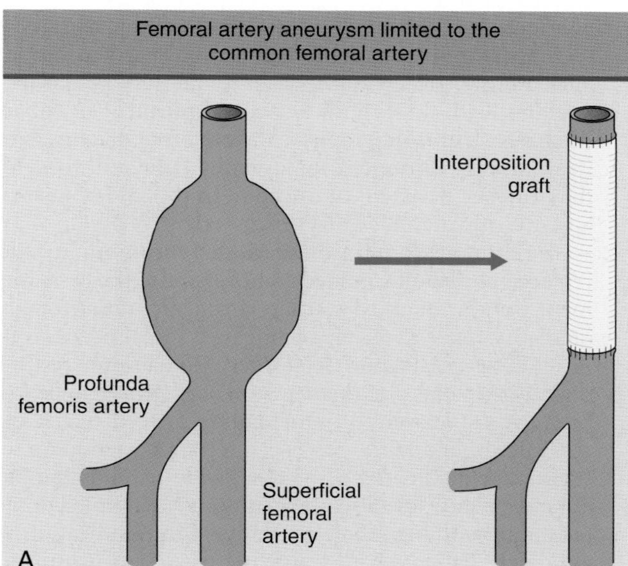

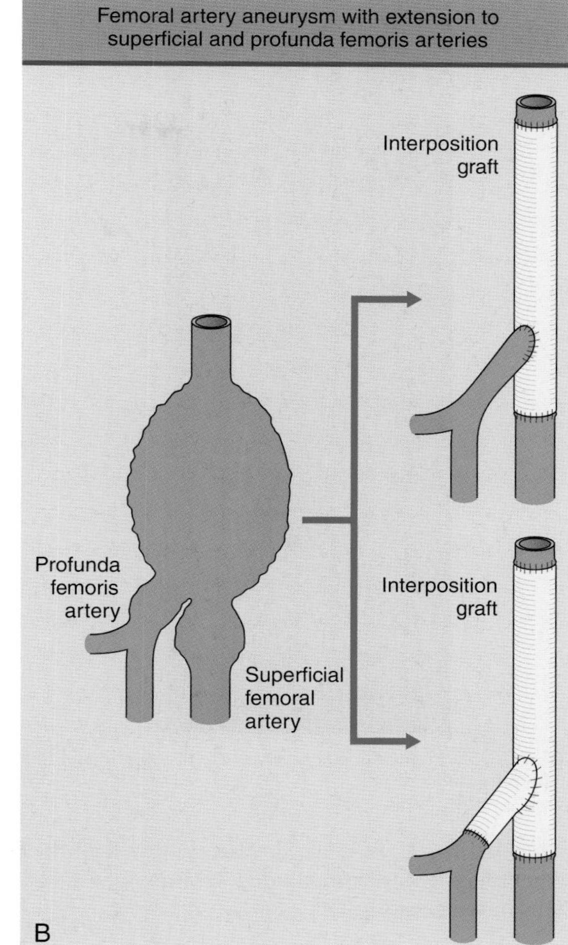

Figure 34-4. A, Femoral artery aneurysm limited to the common femoral artery. Typical operative reconstruction with end-to-end interposition graft. **B,** Femoral artery aneurysm with extension to superficial and profunda femoris arteries. Reconstructive options include interposition grafting to the superficial femoral artery with reimplantation of nonaneurysmal profunda or use of a sidearm graft to the profunda.

into a common-to-superficial femoral artery interposition graft or a second sidearm graft to the profunda (Figure 34-4). Alternatively, the interposition graft can be sutured directly into a reconstructed bifurcation fashioned by suturing a new common wall between the profunda and the superficial femoral arteries, a technique known as syndactilization.

If the entire superficial femoral artery is arteriomegalic or aneurysmal, or in the event of a concomitant popliteal artery aneurysm or significant superficial femoral artery occlusive disease, the distal anastomosis will be at the level of the popliteal or tibial arteries. In these cases, it is often advisable to fashion a separate common femoral artery interposition graft from which the proximal anastomosis of the planned distal graft can be based. The effect of graft thrombosis on the leg may not then be so catastrophic if the profunda element remains patent. The choice of conduit for femoral aneurysm reconstruction can be left to surgeon preference. For reconstructions limited to the common femoral artery, size considerations may confer a benefit to a synthetic graft. For more distal bypasses, however, both synthetic and saphenous vein grafts have been used with equivalent efficacy.

Outcome

In general, the results of operative repair of femoral artery aneurysm are excellent. Minimal perioperative mortality is found in published series, and the long-term patency rates in asymptomatic patients are in the 80% to 95% range.[40,42] When preoperative claudication, rest pain, or gangrene was present, however, the clinical outcome was satisfactory in only 70% of patients after mean follow-up of 2 years.[40]

Profunda Femoris Artery Aneurysms

As mentioned earlier, isolated profunda aneurysms are rare and usually arise secondary to penetrating trauma or iatrogenic groin cannulation. Based largely on isolated case reports, they have a reputation for relatively rapid enlargement and rupture compared to other femoral and popliteal aneurysms. It is unclear whether this reputation is deserved given the possibility that many profunda aneurysms may go undetected. Although 50% of isolated profunda femoral artery aneurysms in one review of 20 patients were treated with ligation and resection alone, the long-term outcome of these patients was

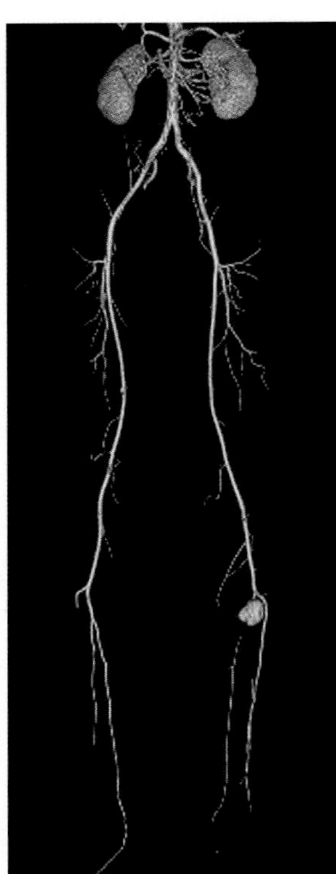

Figure 34-5. A 3.7-cm mycotic aneurysm of the tibioperoneal trunk in a patient with prior endocarditis.

poorly documented.[47] In general, resection or ligation with reconstruction is the recommended treatment strategy for aneurysms in this location.[48]

Infrapopliteal Aneurysms

Aneurysms of the tibial and pedal arteries are also uncommon. Although a small proportion are degenerative in etiology, most are pseudoaneurysms that arise following trauma or infection (Figure 34-5) or as a delayed complication of balloon catheter embolectomy.[49-51] Tibial artery aneurysm has also been reported in association with polyarteritis nodosa.[52] Tibial artery aneurysms are often asymptomatic and are discovered during routine arteriography undertaken for other reasons. Alternatively, they may present as a painful mass or with digital or calf ischemia secondary to thromboembolism. Small, asymptomatic aneurysms may safely be observed, while symptomatic lesions should be treated surgically. If the remaining tibial vessels are healthy, ligation of the aneurysm or percutaneous embolization are acceptable. In the presence of diabetes or concomitant atherosclerosis in the remaining infrageniculate vessels, however, ligation or excision with saphenous vein bypass is recommended.

Femoral Pseudoaneurysms

The femoral artery is the commonest site for pseudoaneurysm, and etiologies are numerous: iatrogenic, anastomotic, traumatic, and mycotic origins are the most often encountered. Their increasing incidence is mainly due to the expanding use of catheter-based interventions in the treatment of cardiovascular disease; pseudoaneurysms are reported to occur after 0.2% of all femoral arterial access procedures.[53] Longer procedures, larger-bore catheters, thrombolytic or anticoagulation therapy, and use of multiple catheters are risk factors for pseudoaneurysm development.[54] Intravenous drug misuse and greater use of arterial closure devices following needle cannulation are in turn responsible for an increasing incidence of infected femoral false aneurysms. Femoral suture-line pseudoaneurysms occur after 3% of all femoral anastomoses and 6% to 8% of aortofemoral anastomoses,[55] presenting an average of 6 years following graft placement. They have been found to be six times more likely to occur after insertion of a prosthetic graft compared with a vein graft.[56]

Usually detected as a pulsatile groin mass following percutaneous intervention, femoral pseudoaneurysms may be asymptomatic or associated with neuropathic pain secondary to femoral nerve compression from rapid expansion. Mycotic aneurysms typically appear as a tender, erythematous groin swelling, with or without associated purulent or sanguinous discharge. Ultrasonography is the preferred diagnostic modality, although computed tomography is helpful to determine the presence or extent of infection in the case of anastomotic and mycotic pseudoaneurysms.

In recent years, ultrasound-guided thrombin injection has replaced ultrasound-guided compression as the first-line treatment option for most routine iatrogenic, noninfected pseudoaneurysms.[57] Typically, a 22-gauge spinal needle is used to inject between 100 and 3000 international units of thrombin directly into the pseudoaneurysm sac. Repeat injections can be given in the event of initial failure or recurrence, and success rates of up to 98% have been reported in modern series.[57] Pseudoaneurysms fed by a short, wide-necked channel have a higher risk of distal embolization as a complication of the technique and represent a relative contraindication to this approach. Patients with traumatic pseudoaneurysms unsuitable for injection or compression, or in whom less invasive treatment fails, can still undergo surgery. Operative treatment of the technically more challenging mycotic and anastomotic pseudoaneurysms usually entails reconstruction with an interposition vein or prosthetic graft, respectively. Proximal and distal control may be simplified by using balloon catheters or suprainguinal clamping, but ensuring patency of the relevant outflow vessels is an important challenge.

UPPER EXTREMITY ANEURYSMS

History

Aneurysms of the arm are relatively uncommon. In their review of nearly 1500 patients documenting the incidence of multiple aneurysms, Dent et al.[6] observed a 3.5% incidence of peripheral aneurysms but only 2 cases of subclavian artery aneurysm and 1 with a brachial artery aneurysm. Reviewing the world literature, Hobson et al.[58] discovered only 195 cases of subclavian and axillary aneurysms, representing approximately 1% of all peripheral aneurysms. Eighty-eight percent of these were located in the subclavian artery. There are three main causes of subclavian artery aneurysm: atherosclerotic aneurysms of the proximal vessel, subclavian–axillary artery aneurysms typically associated with poststenotic enlargement from thoracic outlet syndrome, and those associated with aberrant anatomy. Mayo was the first to report a subclavian aneurysm in proximity to a first rib exostosis and resultant thoracic outlet syndrome in 1813, and Coote was the first to perform a cervical rib resection to decompress the subclavian artery in 1861. Based on a canine experimental model, Halsted in 1916 first postulated a connection between poststenotic dilatation and the formation of aneurysms.[59]

Proximal arm aneurysms have various clinical sequelae, ranging from exsanguinating rupture to compressive neuropathy or ischemia induced by thromboembolism. While clot propagation with distal ischemia is far more common, the risk of cerebral ischemia from retrograde propagation has been recognized since Symond's first description in 1927. Aneurysms located more distally in the arm are mainly complicated by thromboembolism. As with lower extremity aneurysms, intervention before the development of limb-threatening complications is generally recommended, given the potential long-term morbidity.

Proximal Subclavian Artery Aneurysms

Aneurysms of the proximal subclavian artery represent less than 25% of all subclavian aneurysms. While cystic medial necrosis, trauma, infection from syphilis or tuberculosis, and congenital factors are all well-documented causes, most aneurysms in this location are atherosclerotic in origin. They typically occur in patients older than 60 years and are slightly more common in men. Additional diagnostic and management features are included in the discussion that follows on subclavian–axillary aneurysms.

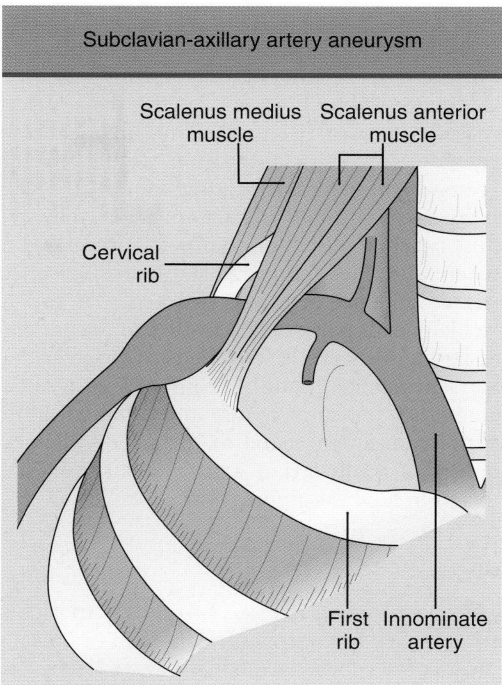

Figure 34-6. Compression of the subclavian artery from an abnormal cervical rib can lead to formation of a subclavian–axillary artery aneurysm.

Subclavian–Axillary Aneurysms

Aneurysms of the distal subclavian artery often extend into the axillary artery and are typically classified as subclavian–axillary artery aneurysms. They are the most common subset and represent 75% of all subclavian aneurysms. They usually occur in younger patients; in one series of 31 patients from the Mayo Clinic, patients' mean age was 47.[60] Other institutional reviews of aneurysms in this location consistently demonstrate a slight female predominance and a slight predilection for the right subclavian. This may be because cervical ribs are more often found in women, and right-handedness, being more common, is associated with bigger right-sided thoracic outlet muscle mass with subsequent impingement on the adjacent vessel. Between 33% and 45% of patients with subclavian–axillary aneurysms have a second aneurysm, usually in the abdominal aorta.[60,61]

Subclavian–axillary artery aneurysms are nearly always secondary to longstanding compression of the vessel against a congenital bony abnormality. Cervical ribs, present in 0.6% of the population and bilateral in up to 80%, are the predominant anatomical element responsible for compression (Figure 34-6). Abnormal first ribs, congenital bands, and malalignment following clavicular fracture are less common causes of arterial thoracic outlet syndrome. Vascular complications are rare and are estimated to occur in fewer than 5% of patients with thoracic outlet syndrome. Of note, in a large review by Halsted[59] of 716 patients with a cervical rib, only 4% had an associated subclavian–axillary artery aneurysm. Complete cervical ribs articulate with a tubercle on the superior aspect of the first rib behind the distal insertion point of the anterior scalene muscle. Longstanding compression where the artery crosses the first rib results in a localized stenosis, as well as angulation of the distal subclavian artery. Repeated mechanical trauma from shoulder movement leads to inflammation and fibrotic scarring of the vessel wall. Ultimately, turbulence develops as a consequence of both the angulation and the intrinsic luminal narrowing, and these alterations in vessel wall shear stress give rise to poststenotic dilation and aneurysm formation. Rarely, localized jet flow from a very tight lesion can produce a saccular aneurysm.

Signs and Symptoms

It is sometimes possible to diagnosis subclavian–axillary aneurysms before they cause symptoms by detection of a pulsatile palpable mass in the supraclavicular fossa or axilla. In the absence of complete thrombosis, an associated loud bruit and thrill are usually present. Isolated neurological symptoms stemming from compression of the brachial plexus by a cervical rib or other bony abnormality may also prompt a radiographic workup revealing an asymptomatic aneurysm. Most often, however, the presence of a subclavian–axillary aneurysm is heralded by the development of thromboembolic complications. Up to 90% of patients in reported series are symptomatic at the time of presentation.[58] Digital ischemia from embolization of laminated thrombus is the most common symptom and occurs in 70% of symptomatic cases.[58] It is typically manifest as small, punctate, cyanotic lesions focused in the fingers or the palm. The straighter course of the radial artery results in a preponderance of thumb and index finger involvement. Platelet aggregates at the site of an intimal disruption or at the point of impact of a poststenotic jet are believed to be another source of microemboli contributing to vasospasm mimicking Raynaud's syndrome. Episodic pallor and cyanosis, pain, and marked cold sensitivity are hallmarks of this common component of the disease; it is important not to forget these when seeing a patient with upper limb vasospasm. More severe ischemia may result from repeated embolism with progressive obliteration of the distal arterial bed. This may lead to loss of distal radial and ulnar pulses and the development of forearm claudication, digital ulceration, or limb-threatening tissue loss, the latter seen in 10% of cases.[58]

An enlarging subclavian–axillary aneurysm may stretch the fibers of the brachial plexus or adjoining soft tissues, producing persistent shoulder pain or distal neurological sequelae. The reported incidence of pain is between 20% and 40%,[58,60] while brachial plexus palsy is seen in 10% of the patients. If the recurrent laryngeal nerve is stretched by a right-sided aneurysm, hoarseness may result. Thrombosis of a subclavian–axillary aneurysm is relatively rare and often without serious symptomatic consequence due to the good collateral blood flow. Rupture of a subclavian–axillary aneurysm is also rare but can result in fatal exsanguination.

Diagnosis

Occasionally, a proximal subclavian aneurysm is diagnosed on plain x-ray, seen as an upper mediastinal or apical mass. If the diagnosis of a subclavian–axillary aneurysm is suspected from the history or physical examination, ultrasonography can confirm the presence of arterial compression and poststenotic dilatation, as well as detail the presence of mural thrombus, thrombosis, or collateral development. Computed tomography is also valuable to diagnose bony abnormalities and associated aneurysmal change in this region. For both diagnosis and preoperative planning, however, the imaging modality of choice for subclavian-level aneurysms remains arteriography. It is usually performed through a femoral approach and at times requires additional maneuvers such as dynamic imaging to fully demonstrate subtle degrees of stenosis or a thrombus-lined aneurysm in the presence of thoracic outlet syndrome. The administration of a vasodilator can be used to elucidate the full extent of collateral blood flow, as well as any digital artery embolic disease, especially in the presence of Raynaud's syndrome.

Management

In general, the presence of a subclavian aneurysm is sufficient indication to proceed to operative repair. In the setting of either acute or chronic ischemia of the arm stemming from thromboembolic sequelae, few disagree that surgery is warranted. Although several approaches have been described, including transaxillary and transclavicular, the supraclavicular approach is optimal in most patients. When thoracic outlet syndrome is present, this incision allows full decompression of the arterial channel through resection of the involved cervical rib, first rib, or both; anterior scalenectomy; and lysis of any constricting fibrous bands. Clavicular resection is unnecessary and leads to disabling shoulder instability. If the aneurysm is localized to the proximal subclavian artery, a median sternotomy for right-sided lesions or a left thoracotomy for left-sided lesions affords optimal exposure. Occasionally, additional access to the axillary artery is necessary through a separate transaxillary or deltopectoral incision.

After mobilization and resection of the subclavian–axillary aneurysm, a primary reconstruction of the artery is carried out if possible. An interposition graft is often necessary, and both autogenous saphenous vein and synthetic (Dacron or polytetrafluoroethylene) grafts have been used successfully. Generally, a prosthetic graft is preferred for subclavian artery reconstruction, while autogenous conduit is thought more appropriate for replacement of the smaller axillary artery.

An alternative approach to the treatment of aneurysms of this location favored by some surgeons is distal ligation with axilloaxillary bypass. This option is particularly well suited for high-risk patients or those with technically challenging proximal subclavian aneurysms. Alternatively, if the aneurysm is large or adherent, the sac may be opened and left in place and the aneurysm repaired via an inclusion technique. Proximal and distal ligation alone without reconstruction has also been described but resulted in forearm claudication in 25% of cases in one report.[60]

The optimal management of small, asymptomatic aneurysms with mild poststenotic dilatation but no clinical or radiographic evidence of mural thrombus remains a source of debate.[60,62] Blank and Connar[63] have suggested that thoracic outlet decompression alone may suffice and result in return of the artery to a normal caliber. Others favor operative repair of the artery given that the risk of subsequent aneurysmal dilatation or serious embolic complications is not insignificant and that few cases of actual regression have been documented.[62,64] It has been suggested that the artery should be explored surgically to rule out subtle intimal disease or mural thrombus, reserving the possibility of resection and reconstruction if appropriate.

If a subclavian–axillary aneurysm is complicated by occlusive embolic disease with significant ischemia, intraoperative thromboembolectomy should be the initial step. This usually entails separate access at the level of the brachial artery bifurcation or wrist. Preoperative thrombolysis, although less well supported in the literature, is another often effective way to optimize brachial and forearm outflow. If clearance of subacute or chronic thrombus proves impossible, an upper extremity bypass procedure is required at the same time as definitive treatment of the aneurysm. Autogenous vein, preferably distal saphenous, is the conduit of choice,[65] and in such cases the aneurysm can be simply resected or ligated. Given the documented risk of retrograde embolization, proximal, as well as distal, ligation should be performed. Analogous to the situation in the leg, when the proximal superficial outflow is compromised, revascularizing the deep brachial artery often suffices to perfuse the hand adequately, provided collateral flow through the elbow joint is intact. If bypass is necessary to the level of the forearm vessels, and the radial or ulnar arteries are unsuitable, the interosseous artery is often an acceptable outflow target. When restoration of adequate flow to the hand is not possible, especially in the setting of vasospasm or distal tissue loss, a cervicodorsal sympathectomy may provide symptom relief. In general, however, the once-preeminent role of sympathectomy has diminished as the efficacy of more definitive revascularization has become evident.

Outcome

Although few modern series are available, the published results of operative treatment of subclavian aneurysms are favorable, particularly in the absence of distal vessel occlusion. In one study of 18 patients undergoing aneurysm resection and reconstruction without distal bypass, graft or arterial patency was 100% after an average 9-year follow-up.[60] No operative mortality occurred and recurrent aneurysms were found among those repaired primarily. In a review of 33 bypass grafts for upper extremity ischemia, of which only 6 were for complications of thoracic outlet syndrome, patency of reconstructions in the entire cohort was 73% at 2 years and 67% at 3 years. Of limited value given the mixed nature of the study population, 2-year patency was 83% for grafts at or above the brachial artery and only 53% for grafts distal to the brachial bifurcation.[65] Upper limb loss is rare in the reported literature and usually follows multiple unsuccessful attempts to revascularize the arm in the face of an obliterated outflow tract. A single forearm amputation was required in the 31 patients reported by Pairolero et al.[60]

Aberrant Subclavian Artery Aneurysms

An aberrant subclavian artery arising from the proximal descending thoracic aorta is the most often encountered anomaly of the aortic arch and is present in 0.5% of normal adults. It is rarely associated with aneurysmal change at the vessel origin, a phenomenon referred to as Kommerell's diverticulum since the original description in 1936 (Figure 34-7). Although predominantly asymptomatic and detected on routine chest radiography as an incidental mediastinal mass, such aneurysms are a well-recognized cause of esophageal compression, a condition known as dysphasia lusoria. Other presenting symptoms include dyspnea or coughing from tracheal compression, chest pain from aneurysmal expansion, or right arm ischemia from thromboembolic complications. Given the risk of potentially fatal rupture or associated complications, surgical repair is recommended. Several techniques have been described, including resection of the aneurysm via either a right or a left thoracotomy or median sternotomy, and reconstruction of the subclavian artery either from the ascending aortic arch or via an end-to-side anastomosis with the right common carotid artery. A separate supraclavicular incision becomes necessary for this latter step when a left thoracotomy approach is used. Highlighting the technical challenge these cases represent, Kieffer et al.[66] reported a 30% operative mortality in the largest series to date of patients with Kommerell's diverticulum.

The considerable perioperative morbidity and mortality associated with traditional open repair have led to a growing enthusiasm for novel, less invasive endovascular treatment alternatives. Isolated case reports have documented successful percutaneous exclusion of subclavian aneurysms and pseudoaneurysms using covered stent grafts.[67,68] Hybrid therapeutic techniques have also been described for aberrant subclavian artery aneurysms, involving a combination of subclavian–carotid bypass grafting and endolumenal stent graft exclusion of the arch aneurysm. Such less-invasive treatment options are particularly suited for patients thought to be at high surgical risk.[69]

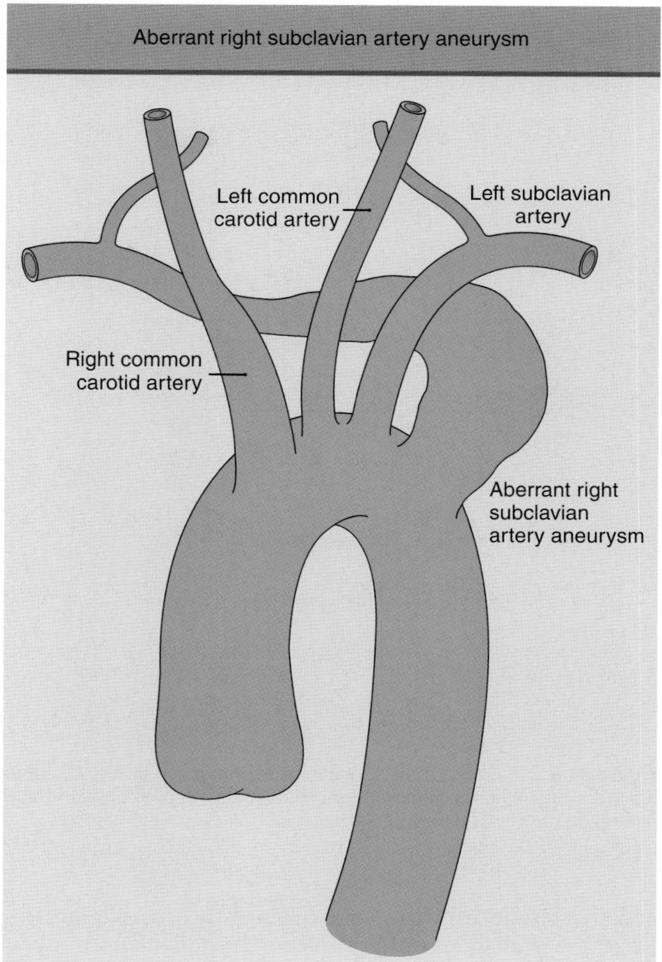

Figure 34-7. An aberrant right subclavian artery typically arises from the proximal descending thoracic aorta. When it is aneurysmal, it is known as Kommerell's diverticulum.

Distal Upper Extremity Aneurysms

Isolated axillary artery aneurysms are rare and predominantly of traumatic origin. Crutch-induced aneurysmal dilation of the axillary artery is well recognized and is typically heralded by acute ischemia from thrombosis or embolism to the brachial artery or more distal vessels. Pseudoaneurysms in this area usually follow penetrating trauma or are distant sequelae of humeral fracture or shoulder dislocation. Undetected aneurysm-related hemorrhage into the axillary sheath can lead to compression of the brachial plexus and significant neurological impairment. Surgical excision with vein interposition grafting has been the mainstay of treatment of these aneurysms, although more recently endolumenal stent grafts have also been employed successfully.[67]

The hypothenar hammer syndrome, or dilatation of the ulnar artery following repeated use of the hand in a pushing, pounding, or twisting motion, is another well-described syndrome. Typically occurring in male laborers, repetitive damage leads to medial degeneration and aneurysm formation. Subsequent thrombosis, embolism, or both produces varying degrees of digital ischemia. The pathophysiology results from the unique anatomical course of the distal ulnar artery; the aneurysmal changes invariably arise at a point beyond where the artery leaves the protection of the volar carpal ligament, known as Guyon's canal, and lies relatively unprotected just anterior to the hook of the hamate bone (Figure 34-8). It is an often-overlooked cause of secondary Raynaud's phenomenon, differing slightly in that the thumb is characteristically spared

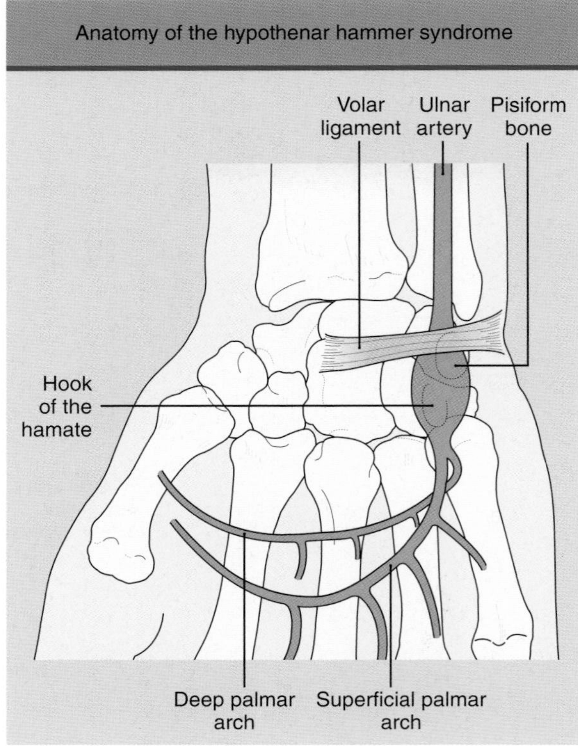

Figure 34-8. Anatomy of the hypothenar hammer syndrome. Distal to the volar ligament, the ulnar artery lies relatively unprotected and vulnerable to trauma in a position anterior to the hook of the hamate.

and the classic triphasic color changes are usually absent. Resection with microsurgical reconstruction offers the best chance for optimal digital perfusion and removes the painful source of ulnar nerve compression.[70] Cervicodorsal sympathectomy and thrombolytic therapy are adjunctive maneuvers that have been used in selected patients to further improve outcome.[71,72]

Isolated aneurysms of the brachial, radial, and more proximal ulnar artery, as well as aneurysms of the palmar arch, are rare and often the focus of individual case reports. Most stem from recreational or occupational trauma, although some are of mycotic origin. Unless small and asymptomatic, they are usually best treated with resection followed by revascularization with a vein bypass.[71,73]

References

1. Galland RB. History of the management of popliteal artery aneurysms. *Eur J Vasc Endovasc Surg* 2008;35:466-472.
2. Antonello M, Frigatti P, Battocchio P, et al. Open repair versus endovascular treatment for asymptomatic popliteal artery aneurysm: results of a prospective randomized study. *J Vasc Surg* 2005;42:185-193.
3. Curi MA, Geraghty PJ, Merino OA, et al. Mid-term outcomes of endovascular popliteal artery aneurysm repair. *J Vasc Surg* 2007;45:505-510.
4. Ravn H, Wanhainen A, Bjorck M. Risk of new aneurysms after surgery for popliteal aneurysm. *Br J Surg* 2008;95:571-575.
5. Szilagyi DE, Schwartz RL, Reddy DJ. Popliteal arterial aneurysms: their natural history and management. *Arch Surg* 1981;116:724-728.
6. Dent TL, Lindenauer MS, Ernst CB, et al. Multiple arteriosclerotic arterial aneurysms. *Arch Surg* 1972;105:338-344.
7. Vermilion BD, Kimmins SA, Pace WG, et al. A review of one hundred forty-seven popliteal aneurysms with long-term follow-up. *Surgery* 1981;90(6):1009-1014.
8. Reilly MK, Abbott WM, Darling RC. Aggressive surgical management of popliteal artery aneurysms. *Am J Surg* 1983;145:498-502.
9. Bouhoutsos J, Martin P. Popliteal aneurysm: a review of 116 cases. *Br J Surg* 1974;61(6):469-475.
10. Reed MK, Smith BM. Popliteal aneurysm with spontaneous arteriovenous fistula. *J Cardiovasc Surg* 1991;32:482-484.
11. Lowell RC, Gloviczki P, Hallett JW, et al. Popliteal artery aneurysms: the risk of nonoperative management. *Ann Vasc Surg* 1994;8:14-23.
12. Dawson I, Sie RB, Van Bockel JH. Atherosclerotic popliteal aneurysm. *Br J Surg* 1997;84:293-299.
13. Roggo A, Brunner U, Ottinger LW, et al. The continuing challenge of aneurysms of the popliteal artery. *Surg Gynecol Obstet* 1993;177:565-572.
14. Michaels JA, Galland RB. Management of asymptomatic popliteal aneurysms: the use of a Markov decision tree to determine the criteria for a conservative approach. *Eur J Vasc Surg* 1993;7:136-143.
15. Dawson I, Van Bockel JH, Brand R, et al. Popliteal artery aneurysms: long-term follow-up of aneurysmal disease and results of surgical treatment. *J Vasc Surg* 1991;13(3):398-407.
16. Aulivola B, Hamdan AD, Hile CN, et al. Popliteal artery aneurysms: a comparison of outcomes in elective versus emergent repair. *J Vasc Surg* 2004;39:1171-1177.
17. Ebaugh JL, Morasch MD, Matsumura JS, et al. Fate of excluded popliteal artery aneurysms. *J Vasc Surg* 2003;37:954-959.
18. Dorigo W, Pulli R, Turini F, et al. Acute leg ischaemia from thrombosed popliteal artery aneurysms: role of preoperative thrombolysis. *Eur J Vasc Endovasc Surg* 2002;23:251-254.
19. Ravn H, Bjorck M. Popliteal artery aneurysm with acute ischemia in 229 patients: outcome after thrombolytic and surgical therapy. *Eur J Vasc Endovasc Surg* 2007;33:690-695.
20. Wyffels PL, DeBord JR, Marshall JS, et al. Increased limb salvage with intraoperative and postoperative ankle level urokinase infusion in acute lower extremity ischemia. *J Vasc Surg* 1992;15:771-779.
21. Hoelting T, Paetz B, Richter GM, et al. The value of preoperative lytic therapy in limb-threatening acute ischemia from popliteal artery aneurysm. *Am J Surg* 1994;168:227-231.
22. Carpenter JP, Barker CF, Roberts B, et al. Popliteal artery aneurysms: current management and outcome. *J Vasc Surg* 1994;19:65-72. discussion, 72-73.
23. Marty B, Wicky S, Ris HB, et al. Success of thrombolysis as a predictor of outcome in acute thrombosis of popliteal aneurysms. *J Vasc Surg* 2002;35:487-493.
24. Henry M, Amor M, Henry I, et al. Percutaneous endoluminal treatment of peripheral aneurysms: a single center experience with a series of 35 aneurysms. *J Vasc Interv Radiol* 1998;9(2 Supp 1):183-184.
25. Tielliu IF, Verhoeven EL, Zeebregts CJ, et al. Endovascular treatment of popliteal artery aneurysms: results of a prospective cohort study. *J Vasc Surg* 2005;41:561-567.
26. Mohan IV, Bray PJ, Harris JP, et al. Endovascular popliteal aneurysm repair: are the results comparable to open surgery? *Eur J Vasc Endovasc Surg* 2006;32:149-154.
27. Lovegrove RE, Javid M, Magee TR, et al. Endovascular and open approaches to non-thrombosed popliteal aneurysm repair: a meta-analysis. *Eur J Vasc Endovasc Surg* 2008;36(1):96-100.
28. Anton GE, Hertzer NR, Beven EG, et al. Surgical management of popliteal aneurysms: trends in presentation, treatment, and results from 1952 to 1984. *J Vasc Surg* 1986;3(1):125-134.
29. Lilly MP, Flinn WR, McCarthy WJ, et al. The effect of distal arterial anatomy on the success of popliteal aneurysm repair. *J Vasc Surg* 1988;7:653-660.
30. Pulli R, Dorigo W, Troisi N, et al. Surgical management of popliteal artery aneurysms: which factors affect outcomes? *J Vasc Surg* 2006;43:481-487.
31. Huang Y, Gloviczki P, Noel AA, et al. Early complications and long-term outcome after open surgical treatment of popliteal artery aneurysms: is exclusion with saphenous vein bypass still the gold standard? *J Vasc Surg* 2007;45:706-713; discussion, 713-715.
32. Upchurch GR, Gerhard-Herman MD, Sebastian MW, et al. Improved graft patency and altered remodeling in infrainguinal vein graft reconstruction for aneurysmal versus occlusive disease. *J Vasc Surg* 1999;29(6):1022-1030.
33. Debing E, Van den Brande P, van Tussenbroek F, et al. Intra-arterial thrombolysis followed by elective surgery for thrombo-embolic popliteal aneurysms. *Acta Chir Belg* 1997;97:137-140.
34. Taurino M, Calisti A, Grossi R, et al. Outcome after early treatment of popliteal artery aneurysms. *Int Angiol* 1998;17:28-33.
35. Greenberg R, Wellander E, Nyman U, et al. Aggressive treatment of acute limb ischemia due to thrombosed popliteal aneurysms. *Eur J Radiol* 1998;28:211-218.

36. Hagino RT, Fujitani RM, Dawson DL, et al. Does infrapopliteal arterial runoff predict success for popliteal artery aneurysmorrhaphy? *Am J Surg* 1994;168(6):652-658.
37. Varga ZA, Locke-Edmunds JC, Baird RN. A multicenter study of popliteal aneurysms. *J Vasc Surg* 1994;20(2):171-177.
38. Lawrence PF, Lorenzo-Rivero S, Lyon JL. The incidence of iliac, femoral, and popliteal artery aneurysms in hospitalized patients. *J Vasc Surg* 1995;22(4):409-416.
39. Diwan A, Sarkar R, Stanley JC, et al. Incidence of femoral and popliteal artery aneurysms in patients with abdominal aortic aneurysms. *J Vasc Surg* 2000;31(5):863-869.
40. Graham LM, Zelenock GB, Whitehouse WM, et al. Clinical significance of arteriosclerotic femoral artery aneurysms. *Arch Surg* 1980;115:502-507.
41. Brophy CM, Tilson JE, Braverman IM, et al. Age of onset, pattern of distribution, and histology of aneurysm development in a genetically predisposed mouse model. *J Vasc Surg* 1988;8(1):45-48.
42. Cutler BS, Darling RC. Surgical management of arteriosclerotic femoral aneurysms. *Surgery* 1977;74(5):764-773.
43. Rigdon EE, Monajjem N. Aneurysms of the superficial femoral artery: a report of two cases and review of the literature. *J Vasc Surg* 1992;16(5):790-793.
44. Baird RJ, Gurry JF, Kellam J, et al. Arteriosclerotic femoral artery aneurysms. *Can Med Assoc J* 1977;117:1306-1307.
45. Tolstedt GE, Radhe HM, Bell JW. Late sequelae of arteriosclerotic femoral aneurysms. *Angiology* 1961;12:601-602.
46. Pappas G, Janes JM, Bernatz PE, et al. Femoral aneurysms. *JAMA* 1964;190(6):489-493.
47. Tait WF, Vohra RK, Carr HMH, et al. True profunda femoris aneurysms: are they more dangerous than other atherosclerotic aneurysms of the femoropopliteal segment? *Ann Vasc Surg* 1991;5:92-95.
48. Harbuzariu C, Duncan AA, Bower TC, et al. Profunda femoris artery aneurysms: association with aneurysmal disease and limb ischemia. *J Vasc Surg* 2008;47(1):31-35.
49. Cronenwett JL, Walsh DB, Garret HE. Tibial artery pseudoaneurysms: delayed complication of balloon catheter embolectomy. *J Vasc Surg* 1988;8:483-488.
50. Monig SP, Walter M, Sorgatz S, et al. True infrapopliteal artery aneurysms: report of two cases and literature review. *J Vasc Surg* 1996;24(2):276-278.
51. McKee TI, Fisher JB. Dorsalis pedis artery aneurysm: case report and literature review. *J Vasc Surg* 2000;31(3):589-591.
52. Borozan PG, Walker HSJ, Peterson GJ. True tibial artery aneurysms: case report and literature review. *J Vasc Surg* 1989;10(4):457-459.
53. Messina LM, Brothers TE, Wakefield TW, et al. Clinical characteristics and surgical management of vascular complications in patients undergoing cardiac catheterization: interventional versus diagnostic procedures. *J Vasc Surg* 1991;13(5):593-600.
54. Skillman JJ, Ducksoo K, Baim DS. Vascular complications of percutaneous femoral cardiac interventions: incidence and operative repair. *Arch Surg* 1988;123:1207-1212.
55. Biancari F, Ylonen K, Anttila V, et al. Durability of open repair of infrarenal abdominal aortic aneurysm: a 15-year follow-up study. *J Vasc Surg* 2002;35(1):87-93.
56. Szilagyi DE, Smith RF, Elliott JP, et al. Anastomotic aneurysms after vascular reconstruction: problems of incidence, etiology, and treatment. *Surgery* 1975;78(6):800-816.
57. Hirsch AT, Haskal ZJ, Hertzer NR, et al. ACC/AHA 2005 guidelines for the management of patients with peripheral arterial disease. *J Am Coll Cardiol* 2006;47(6):1239-1312.
58. Hobson RW Israel MR II, Lynch TG. Axillosubclavian arterial aneurysms. In Bergan JJ, Yao JST, eds: *Aneurysms: diagnosis and treatment.* New York. Grune and Stratton; 1982:435-447.
59. Halsted WS. An experimental study of circumscribed dilation of an artery immediately distal to a partially occluding band, and its bearing on the dilation of the subclavian artery observed in certain cases of cervical rib. *J Exp Med* 1916;24:271.
60. Pairolero PC, Walls JT, Payne S, et al. Subclavian–axillary artery aneurysms. *Surgery* 1981;90(4):757-763.
61. McCollum CH, Da Gama AD, Noon GP, et al. Aneurysm of the subclavian artery. *J Cardiovasc Surg* 1979;20(2):159-164.
62. Scher LA, Veith FJ, Samson RH, et al. Vascular complications of thoracic outlet syndrome. *J Vasc Surg* 1986;3(3):565-568.
63. Blank RH, Connar RG. Arterial complications associated with thoracic outlet syndrome. *Ann Thor Surg* 1974;17(4):315-324.
64. Banis JC, Rich N, Whelan TJ Jr. Ischemia of the upper extremity due to noncardiac emboli. *Am J Surg* 1977;134(1):131-139.
65. McCarthy WJ, Flinn WR, Yao JST, et al. Result of bypass grafting for upper limb ischemia. *J Vasc Surg* 1986;3(5):741-746.
66. Kieffer E, Bahnini A, Koskas F. Aberrant subclavian artery: surgical treatment in thirty-three adult patients. *J Vasc Surg* 1994;19(1):100-111.
67. Sullivan TM, Bacharach JM, Perl J, et al. Endovascular management of unusual aneurysms of the axillary and subclavian arteries. *J Endovasc Surg* 1996;3(4):389-395.
68. Bukhari HA, Saadia R, Hardy BW. Urgent endovascular stenting of subclavian artery pseudoaneurysm caused by seatbelt injury. *Can J Surg* 2007;50(4):303-304.
69. Shennib H, Diethrich EB. Novel approaches for the treatment of the aberrant right subclavian artery and its aneurysms. *J Vasc Surg* 2008;47:1066-1070.
70. Kalisman M, Laborde K, Wolff TW. Ulnar nerve compression secondary to ulnar artery false aneurysm at the Guyon's canal. *J Hand Surg* 1982;7(2):137-139.
71. Clark ET, Mass DP, Bassiouny HS, et al. True aneurysmal disease in the hand and upper extremity. *Ann Vasc Surg* 1991;5(3):276-281.
72. Lawhorne TW Jr, Sanders RA. Ulnar artery aneurysm complicated by distal embolization: management with regional thrombolysis and resection. *J Vasc Surg* 1986;3(4):663-665.
73. Nehler MR, Dalman RL, Harris EJ, et al. Upper extremity arterial bypass distal to the wrist. *J Vasc Surg* 1992;16(4):633-642.

Section

VIII

Cerebrovascular Disease

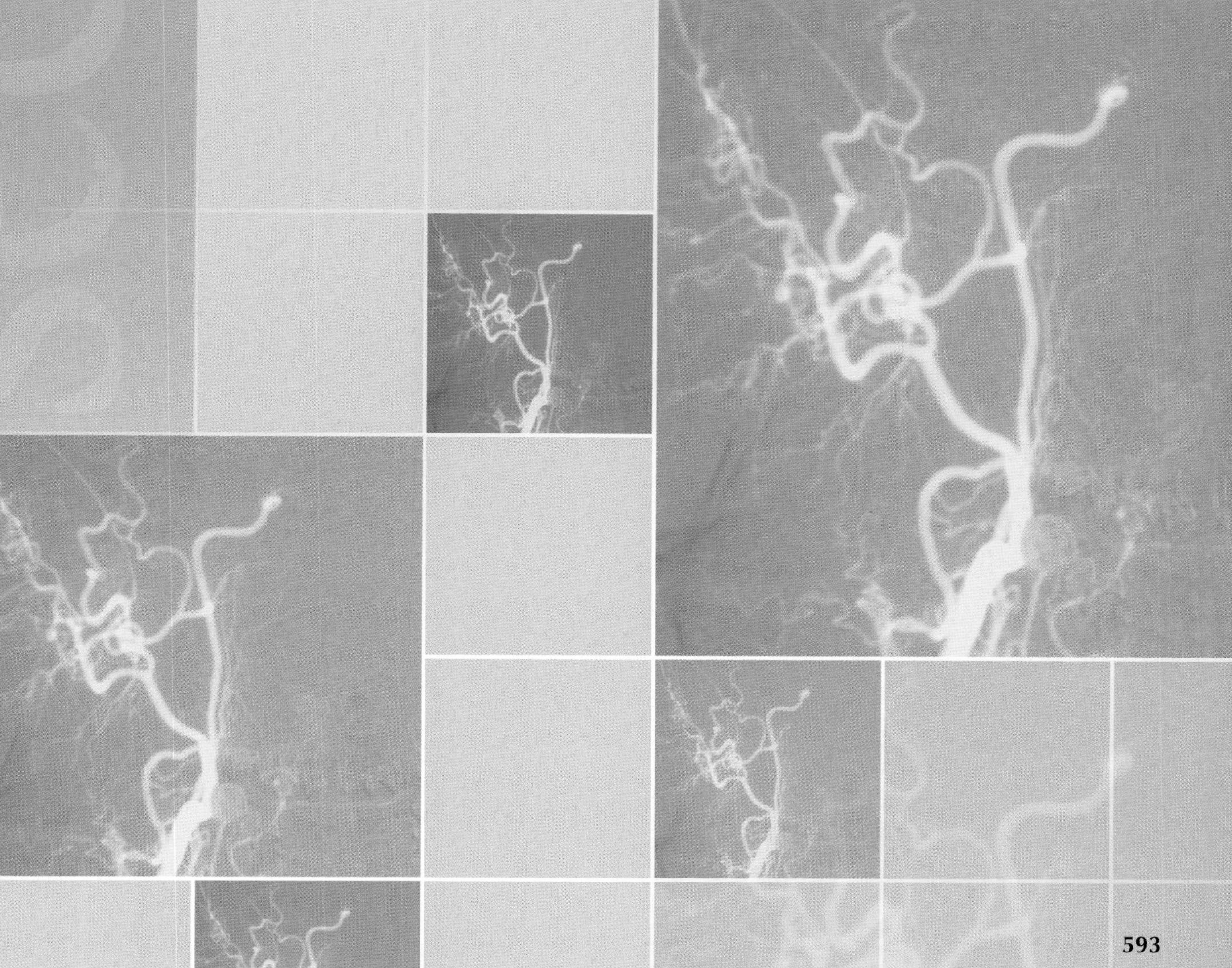

chapter 35

Carotid Artery Disease: Natural History and Diagnosis

William C. Mackey, MD, FACS • Desarom Teso, MD

Key Points

Natural History

- Carotid plaque progression and degeneration determine clinical natural history.
- The clinical natural history is well described for patients with transient ischemic attack or stroke related to carotid disease.
- The clinical natural history for asymptomatic patients is less well understood.
- Improved understanding of clinical natural history in asymptomatic patients awaits improved understanding of plaque evolution and degeneration.
- Treatment with aspirin or other antiplatelet agents and, in selected patients, carotid endarterectomy improves the clinical outcome in patients with carotid disease.

Diagnosis

- Duplex ultrasound is the best study currently available for the diagnosis of carotid disease.
- Magnetic resonance angiography, computed tomography angiography, and standard contrast angiography have a role in selected patients.
- Brain imaging is not routinely required as a part of the diagnostic evaluation but has an important role in selected patients.

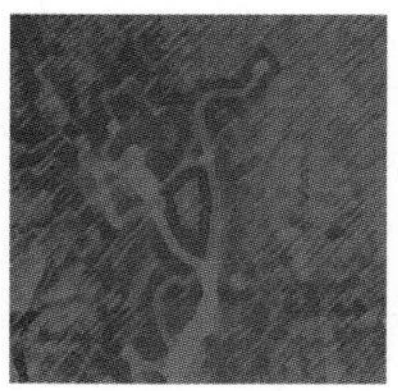

While substantial progress has been made in the understanding of the evolution of atherosclerotic plaques at the carotid bifurcation, the pathophysiological events that result in plaque instability, rupture, embolization, or arterial occlusion and that lead to transient cerebral ischemia or stroke remain somewhat obscure. Until knowledge improves about the events that trigger plaque instability, understanding the natural history of carotid disease will depend on information from clinical studies of patients with carotid disease subjected to various treatments. Over the past 12 years, many scientifically valid clinical studies have been carried out that have improved knowledge about the clinical course of both symptomatic and asymptomatic carotid lesions. Until the basic mechanisms underlying carotid plaque evolution and degeneration are better understood, however, this knowledge will be incomplete and the resulting management protocols imperfect.

Diagnostic imaging for carotid disease has changed significantly over the past decade. Once the gold standard in the diagnostic evaluation of patients with carotid disease, conventional contrast arteriography is now required in fewer than 10% of all patients being evaluated for carotid endarterectomy (CEA). Duplex ultrasonography provides a reliable noninvasive modality for the assessment of degree of stenosis in nearly all patients and for the assessment of plaque characteristics in many. Magnetic resonance angiography (MRA) provides a more comprehensive flow chart of the carotid circulation, including arch, proximal common carotid, and intracranial vessels. Coupled with magnetic resonance imaging (MRI) of the brain, MRA gives a detailed image of the cerebral circulation plus cerebral anatomy and pathology. Computed tomography (CT) techniques can provide cross-sectional and reconstructed three-dimensional data regarding plaque burden, plaque anatomy, and detailed anatomical assessment of nonatherosclerotic lesions of the carotid artery, as well as the brain. Conventional contrast arteriography, now with digitized images, allows detailed anatomical assessment of the entirety of the cerebral circulation. Because of its associated risks and costs, angiography is appropriate only in patients undergoing endovascular treatment of their carotid lesion or in the rare patient for whom the other techniques provide insufficient data for diagnosis, surgical planning, or both.

CLINICAL SYNDROMES ASSOCIATED WITH CAROTID ARTERY DISEASE

Many clinical syndromes are associated with symptomatic carotid disease. Events related to carotid artery lesions are usually classified as either a transient ischemic attack (TIA) or a stroke. TIA is defined as a focal neurological event that is sudden in onset without preceding aura, resolves completely within 24 hours to leave the patient at neurological baseline, and is referable to a definable vascular distribution of the central nervous system. TIA may be caused by hypoperfusion related to vascular stenoses or occlusions or, more commonly, to embolization. Stroke is the result of infarction of central nervous system tissue as a result of hypoperfusion, embolization, or intracranial hemorrhage. Reversible ischemic neurological deficit (RIND) is a term used to describe a focal neurological event lasting longer than 24 hours but resolving completely within 1 week. The duration of symptoms in patients with RIND suggests that a degree of structural damage to the brain must have occurred, although it may be limited and undetectable by clinical imaging.

TIA, RIND, and stroke are descriptions of clinical events. The correlation of these events with findings on brain imaging is imprecise. Approximately 24% of patients with clinical events consistent with TIA are found to have infarction in an anatomical distribution consistent with the transient neurological event.[1]

Occasionally, the differentiation between TIA and stroke can be less than clear. Patients presenting with frequent severe TIAs (crescendo TIAs) can be difficult to distinguish from patients presenting with acute or evolving stroke. Early in the course of these events, brain imaging studies may not be helpful since the anatomically detectable lesions evolve after the clinical events. MRI of the brain has improved the ability to detect early brain infarction and may allow a more precise differentiation of these clinical syndromes.

Carotid TIA may result in speech deficits (dysarthria, dysphasia, or aphasia). Motor manifestations range from mild clumsiness of a single limb to hemiplegia of the side contralateral to the carotid lesion. Sensory manifestations may include numbness or paresthesia, also on the contralateral side. Headache, mild confusion, and light-headedness may accompany the preceding symptoms, but these nonspecific and nonlocalizing symptoms occurring alone are not symptoms of carotid TIA.

Carotid territory TIA can involve the eye only (transient monocular blindness or transient monocular visual field defects). This is termed amaurosis fugax. More insidious chronic monocular visual deterioration can be associated with critical stenosis or occlusion of the ipsilateral internal carotid artery (ocular ischemic syndrome).

Stroke deficits related to carotid disease are similar to the temporary deficits seen with TIA. Permanent monocular blindness, aphasia, mono or hemiparesis, hemiplegia, and hemisensory deficits are the most common manifestations of carotid disease–related stroke.

Occasionally, patients with carotid disease can present with symptoms consistent with more global cerebral hypoperfusion. Patients with critical stenosis or occlusion of several extracranial vessels can present with decreased mental acuity, orthostatic presyncope, or even vertebrobasilar-like symptoms. In the context of severe hemodynamic compromise related to multiple vascular lesions, these global symptoms may be properly attributed to carotid disease.

Table 35-1
Signs and Symptoms Unlikely to be Related to Carotid Disease

Unconsciousness (including syncope)
Tonic or clonic activity
Sensory deficit
Vertigo alone
Dysphagia alone
Dysarthria alone
Bowel or bladder incontinence
Visual loss with alteration of consciousness
Focal symptoms with migraine
Scintillating scotoma
Confusion alone
Amnesia alone

From Toole JF, Dibert SW, Harpold GJ. In: Moore W, ed. *Surgery for cerebrovascular disease.* 2nd ed. Philadelphia, WB Saunders; 1996:73.

Of equal importance with the recognition of symptoms likely to be related to carotid disease is the recognition of symptoms unlikely to be carotid related. Common symptoms not likely to be related to carotid territory TIA or stroke are shown in Table 35-1.[2] Most of these symptoms are more likely to be manifestations of cardiac arrhythmias, seizures, migraine, or other nonvascular-related conditions.

NATURAL HISTORY OF ASYMPTOMATIC CAROTID DISEASE

The presence of carotid artery atherosclerosis predisposes patients to TIAs and strokes, and the risk of these events is roughly correlated with the severity of the carotid disease. Chambers and Norris followed 500 patients with neck bruits and varying severities of carotid stenosis confirmed and graded by Doppler ultrasound.[3] At 1 year, TIA or stroke had occurred in 5 of 239 (2.1%) of patients with 0 to 29% stenosis, in 9 of 157 (5.7%) of patients with 30% to 74% stenosis, and in 22 of 113 (19.5%) of patients with 75% to 100% stenosis. The authors further noted that the incidence of cardiac ischemic events correlated with the severity of carotid stenosis in this cohort.[3]

O'Holleran et al. also noted that TIA and stroke risk were related to the degree of carotid stenosis.[4] In their study, 60% of 121 patients with more than 75% stenosis by B-mode ultrasound had a stroke or TIA during a 5 year follow-up. Only 12.6% of patients with less than 75% stenosis suffered a neurological event during similar follow-up. These authors further correlated clinical outcome with the echogenicity of the carotid lesions. Calcified plaques were much less likely to be associated with symptoms than soft, primarily echolucent plaques (Table 35-2).[4]

From these data, it is apparent that both degree of stenosis and plaque density, as determined by ultrasound characteristics, correlated with clinical outcome.

Plaque progression was also noted to correlate with outcome. Roederer et al. found that in asymptomatic patients who initially had less than 80% stenosis progression to more than 80% was associated with a high incidence of stroke, TIA, or progression to carotid occlusion.[5] These authors noted a

Table 35-2
Neurological Event Risk and Carotid Plaque Characteristics

Ultrasound Characteristics	*N*	Transient Ischemic Attack (%)	Stroke (%)
Stenosis			
Calcified			
>75%	37	4 (11%)	1 (3%)
<75%	53	0	0
Dense			
>75%	42	23 (55%)	4 (10%)
<75%	76	7 (9%)	1 (1%)
Soft			
>75%	42	32 (76%)	9 (21%)
<75%	46	10 (21%)	4 (9%)

Modified from O'Holleran LW, Kennelly MM, McClurken M, Johnson JM. *Am J Surg* 1987;154:659-662.

35% risk of ischemic symptoms or carotid occlusion within 6 months of disease progression and a 46% incidence within 12 months. Conversely, only 1.5% of patients whose plaques remained stable developed symptoms over a 12-month follow-up.[5]

Further natural history data are available from the control, nonsurgical groups in the more recent randomized trials of asymptomatic carotid disease. These data reflect not the natural history of carotid disease but rather the outcome associated with best medical management. In the Veterans Administration Cooperative Trial, medical management of asymptomatic carotid lesions (at least 50% stenosis) resulted in a 20.6% incidence of ipsilateral TIA or stroke within 4 years.[6] Similarly, in the Asymptomatic Carotid Atherosclerosis Study (ACAS), medical management of at least 60% carotid stenosis was associated with a 19.2% estimated risk of TIA, stroke, or death over 5 years.[7]

Carotid plaques clearly place asymptomatic patients at risk for TIA and stroke. Degree of stenosis, plaque density, and plaque progression are correlates of the risk related to carotid artery atherosclerotic lesions. Patients at highest risk of TIA or stroke are those with more than 80% stenosis caused by a soft, echolucent plaque or those whose plaque progresses from less than 80% to more than 80% stenosis during follow-up. These clinical findings are consistent with the current understanding of plaque evolution and degeneration. Benign fatty streaks progress to fibrous plaques. Continued lipid infiltration into the arterial wall leads to macrophage infiltration and chronic inflammation with a slow increase in plaque mass. Macrophage lysis with release of proteolytic enzymes, coupled with further lipid infiltration, results in the complex plaque with areas of lipid accumulation, ongoing chronic inflammation, and calcification. Neovascularity within the arterial wall and overlying plaque results from this cycle of ongoing inflammation and healing. Intraplaque hemorrhage resulting from neovascularity in the unstable plaque is the critical event that causes sudden plaque expansion with thrombosis and arterial occlusion, or rupture of the fibrous cap overlying the lipid pool or area of intraplaque hemorrhage, with potential for embolization (Figure 35-1). Given the current understanding of the pathogenesis of cerebrovascular events based on this scenario, it is understandable that low-density plaques (more lipid pool or intraplaque hemorrhage), plaques causing greater stenosis,

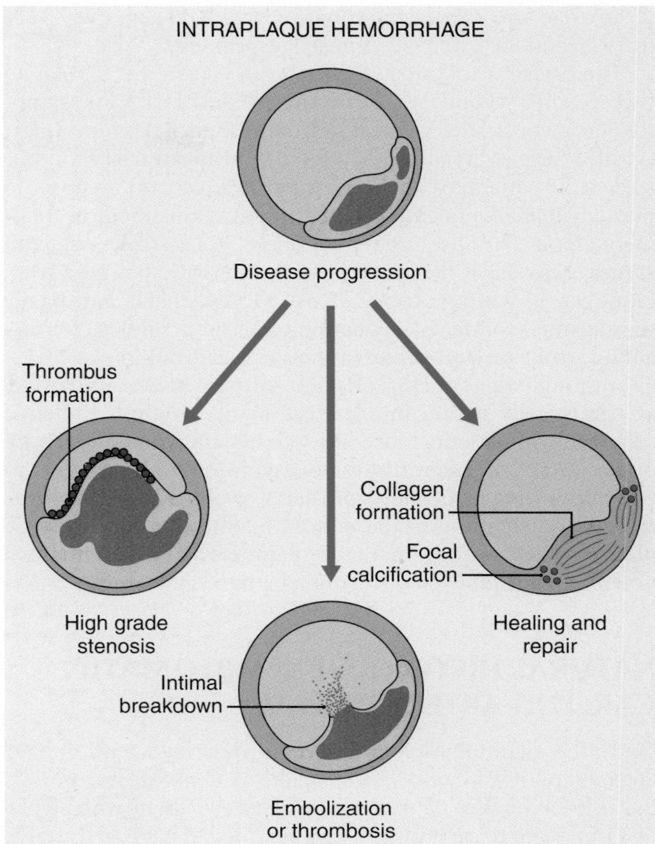

Figure 35-1. Intraplaque hemorrhage may result in sudden plaque expansion resulting in high grade stenosis or occlusion, in plaque rupture with distal embolization, or in arterial wall fibrosis and calcification. (Adapted from Bergan and Yao, eds. Cerebrovascular Insufficiency. New York: Grune & Stratton;1983:51.)

or plaques showing progression are associated with a greater risk of cerebrovascular events.

Medical therapy can favorably alter the natural history of asymptomatic carotid disease. Reductase inhibitors may slow the progression of carotid plaques and decrease the incidence of TIA and stroke even in individuals with normal cholesterol levels.[8] The role of aspirin or other antiplatelet agents in patients with asymptomatic carotid lesions has been established from several large-scale trials demonstrating a reduction in several cardiovascular endpoints (cardiac death, stroke death, stroke, and nonfatal myocardial infarction) both in patients with known atherosclerosis and in those at risk of atherosclerosis.

In addition, medical management of asymptomatic carotid disease has been compared with medical management plus CEA in several large-scale randomized trials. In ACAS, surgery was marginally, but statistically significantly, beneficial for patients with 60% or greater carotid stenosis.[7] The 5-year ipsilateral stroke risk in the surgically treated group was 5.1%, including perioperative stroke or death. In the medically treated cohort, the 5-year stroke risk was 11% (p = 0.004).[7] While this result suggested an advantage for surgery, it was meager: 100 carotid endarterectomies have to be performed in this group of patients to prevent 6 strokes over a 5-year interval. Subgroup analysis of the ACAS patients did not reveal greater benefit in patients with greater carotid stenosis. The relative stroke-risk reductions attributable to surgery were

45%, 67%, and 45% in the subgroups with 60% to 69%, 70% to 79%, and 80% to 89% stenosis, respectively.[7]

The 5-year stroke-risk reduction in ACAS was similar to that seen in a second large randomized trial of CEA for asymptomatic stenosis: the Medical Research Council Asymptomatic Carotid Surgery Trial (ACST).[9] This European trial randomized 3120 patients with more than 60% carotid stenosis to immediate CEA plus medical treatment versus medical treatment alone. The absolute reduction in 5-year stroke risk with surgery was 5.3% (95% confidence interval 3.0% to 7.8%). However, in contrast to ACAS, ACST reported a statistically significant absolute risk reduction of 2.5% ($p = 0.004$) for disabling stroke or fatal stroke in the surgical group.[9]

Although the benefits of CEA seen in ACAS and ACST are statistically significant, they are small. Attempts to define subgroups of patients more likely to benefit from surgery are under way.[10] The identification of asymptomatic patients who will derive greater benefit from CEA awaits a more sophisticated understanding of the natural history of atherosclerotic plaques. The key question that remains is what differentiates a potentially unstable plaque from a benign stable one.

NATURAL HISTORY OF SYMPTOMATIC CAROTID ARTERY DISEASE

Once the pathophysiological events described earlier have taken place, resulting in TIA or stroke, patients are at continuing risk for further neurological events. A patient with stroke or TIA related to carotid disease is assumed to have an unstable plaque that may remain unstable. Most studies of symptomatic carotid disease use stroke and death as endpoints. The natural history of symptomatic carotid disease cannot be discerned from recent studies for the simple reason that TIA and stroke are generally accepted to be compelling indications for intervention. A randomized study of the management of TIA or stroke that includes a medical control group is unlikely to be allowed by modern human investigation review committees. The basis for the certainty that TIA or stroke require treatment lies in several older studies. First, the Canadian Cooperative study showed that in 139 symptomatic patients placebo treatment was associated with a 22% risk of stroke or death over a mean follow-up of 26 months.[11] Similarly, in an American trial of aspirin for patients with symptomatic cerebrovascular disease, Fields et al. found a stroke or death risk of 21% at 2 years in the placebo group.[12] Finally in a French trial, placebo treatment of symptomatic patients was associated with a 3-year stroke or mortality risk of 19%.[13] In each of these trials, medical therapy with aspirin significantly reduced the risk of stroke. These studies clearly established that TIA and minor stroke are associated with a high risk of stroke, death, or both within a few years after the index event. These studies included no sophisticated brain or carotid imaging studies, so they may have included some strokes and TIAs unrelated to carotid disease.

Because the placebo-controlled trials clearly demonstrated the high risk of subsequent stroke and death associated with untreated TIA or minor stroke, and because aspirin and more recently clopidogrel have been shown to reduce this risk, all modern trials are conducted without placebo control. Current studies compare medically, with medically plus surgically treated carotid lesions. Future studies will compare outcomes of medical and surgical management with endovascular management.

Table 35-3
Risk Factors for Stroke in Medically Managed Symptomatic Patients*

Risk Factors	
Age >70	Ulcerated plaque
Systolic blood pressure >160	History of tobacco use
Diastolic blood pressure >90	Diabetes
Recent stroke	Claudication
Stenosis >80%	Hyperlipidemia
Stroke Risk at 2 Years	
Low risk (0-5 factors)	17%
Moderate risk (6 factors)	23%
High risk (>6 factors)	39%
Stroke Risk at 2 Years Based on Carotid Stenosis	
70-79%	12%
80-89%	18%
90-99%	26%

From North American Symptomatic Carotid Endarterectomy Trial Collaborators (NASCET). *New Engl J Med* 1991;325:445-453.
*For patients with symptomatic severe carotid disease managed medically, the risk of stroke is high and predictable based on well-established risk factors and on the severity of carotid stenosis. More recently, the NASCET collaborators have better defined the outcomes of moderate and mild carotid disease.[15] Medically managed patients with 50% to 69% and less than 50% stenosis had 5-year ipsilateral stroke risks of 22.2% and 18.7%, respectively.[15]

The North American Symptomatic Carotid Endarterectomy Trial (NASCET) revealed a remarkable amount about the stroke risk associated with symptomatic carotid atherosclerosis.[14] Stroke risk in NASCET-eligible patients randomized to medical therapy (aspirin plus risk factor management using lipid-lowering agents, antihypertensives, etc.) was correlated with the presence of risk factors identified at the time of study entry (Table 35-3).

Similar results were noted in the European Carotid Surgery Trial (ECST), which like NASCET compared outcomes in symptomatic carotid artery disease treated with medical management alone versus medical management plus surgery.[16] The results of NASCET and ECST are not directly comparable because the method of computing degree of stenosis in the two trials was quite different, such that 80% and 90% stenoses in the ECST were approximately equivalent to 61% and 80% stenoses, respectively, in NASCET. Even with this difference, the outcome in medically managed patients in ECST was similar to those in NASCET (Table 35-4). As in NASCET, stroke risk was high and correlated with degree of stenosis. In addition, stroke risk was greatest in the first year following presentation and declined over time. The finding that the risk of stroke after TIA or minor stroke is highest in the early aftermath of herald events is common to several studies, including the earliest studies of aspirin therapy. In the aspirin trial conducted by Fields et al., the placebo group had a 17.3% risk of cerebral or retinal infarction in the first year following randomization but only a 5% risk in the second year.[12] In NASCET, the ipsilateral stroke risk in the medically managed cohort was approximately 18% in the first year and 8% in the second.[14]

From all current randomized studies comparing medical management alone with CEA plus medical management for symptomatic severe carotid disease, it is clear that surgery favorably alters the natural history of medically treated disease. In NASCET, the 2-year ipsilateral stroke risk in all

Table 35-4
Three-Year Stroke Risk in Medically Managed Symptomatic Patients from the European Carotid Surgery Trial

	Annual Risk of Stroke (%)			
Stenosis (%)	Year 1	Year 2	Year 3	Cumulative 3-Year Risk (%)
70-79	6	6	5	17
80-89	11	6	3	20
90-99	18	14	3	35

From European Carotid Surgery Trialists' Collaborative Group. *Lancet* 1991;337:1235-1243.

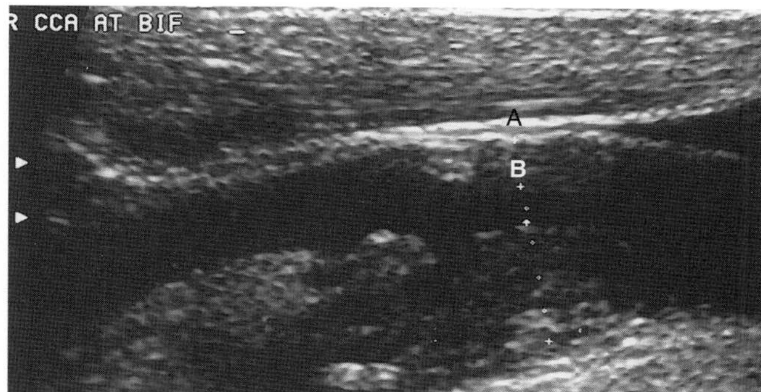

Figure 35-3. Duplex image of soft, smooth echolucent plaque at carotid bifurcation. Peak systolic velocity of 275 is indicative of 50% to 75% stenosis.

medically managed patients with 70% to 99% stenosis was 26%. CEA plus medical management was associated with a 2-year stroke risk of 9% (including perioperative risk of 5.5%) in these patients ($p < 0.001$).[14] In ECST, ipsilateral stroke was noted in 20.6% of medically managed patients and in 6.8% of patients undergoing surgery with 80% to 99% stenosis ($p < 0.0001$).[17] Less benefit was seen for NASCET patients with 50% to 69% stenosis with ipsilateral stroke risk at 5 years of 15.7% and 22.2% for surgically and medically treated patients, respectively ($p = 0.045$).[14] In NASCET patients with lesser degrees of stenosis, surgery had no beneficial effect on stroke risk.[15] In ECST, CEA had no beneficial effect on stroke risk in those with less than 70% stenosis and offered only marginal benefit for those with 70% to 80% stenosis.[17]

In summary, the risk of stroke in asymptomatic individuals is determined by the degree of carotid stenosis, plaque density, and plaque progression. The natural history of asymptomatic carotid lesions can be influenced favorably by medical therapy (reductase inhibitors and antiplatelet agents). Selected individuals with asymptomatic carotid disease can gain additional benefit from CEA, although at present the identification of exactly who will benefit from endarterectomy is imprecise. Accurate selection awaits a better understanding of those factors that create carotid plaque instability. In symptomatic patients, the natural history of carotid atherosclerosis is well defined. Both medical and surgical management offer significant benefit. In symptomatic carotid disease with 70% or greater (NASCET) or 80% or greater stenosis (ECST) criteria, CEA offers significant benefit over medical management alone. For 50% to 70% stenosis (NASCET) criteria, surgery provides modest benefit, but there is no advantage for patients with less than 50% stenosis. The potential benefit of surgery in reducing the stroke risk in both asymptomatic and symptomatic carotid disease is contingent on the safety of the surgical procedure itself. Excessive surgery-related stroke morbidity would offset any potential advantage.

DIAGNOSIS AND EVALUATION OF CAROTID DISEASE

The goals of the evaluation of patients with carotid atherosclerosis are to confirm the presence of the disease, to assess its severity, to determine whether or not the carotid lesion is responsible for the patient's symptoms, to assess the potential operability of the carotid lesion, and to seek any unusual features.[18] These goals must be achieved while subjecting the patient to minimal risk and to be cost effective. No single carotid evaluation protocol is appropriate for all patients. MRI or CT imaging of the brain is required in selected patients. Contrast angiography is now rarely indicated except when carotid angioplasty and stenting are being considered.

Because duplex ultrasound is noninvasive, risk free, relatively inexpensive, and accurate in determining the degree of stenosis and in assessing plaque density and progression, it is the appropriate initial imaging modality. It is also the best means of follow-up. The degree of stenosis is accurately assessed by Doppler-derived velocity data, while density and other morphological characteristics are assessed with high resolution ultrasound imaging (Figures 35-2 through 35-5).

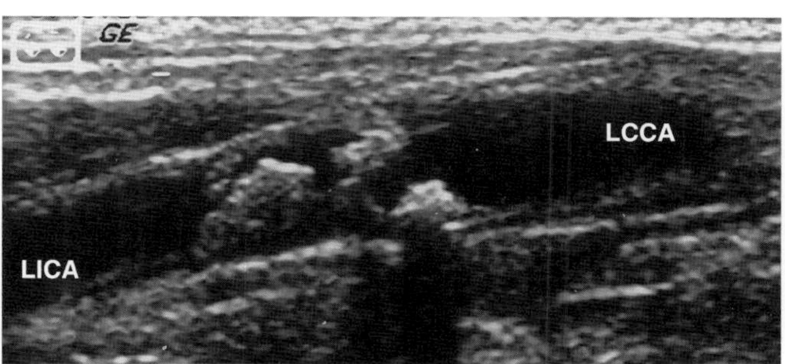

Figure 35-2. Duplex image of a highly irregular and ulcerated plaque in a patient with repeated episodes of transient monocular blindness. Peak systolic velocity of 204 cm/sec is consistent with 50% to 79% stenosis.

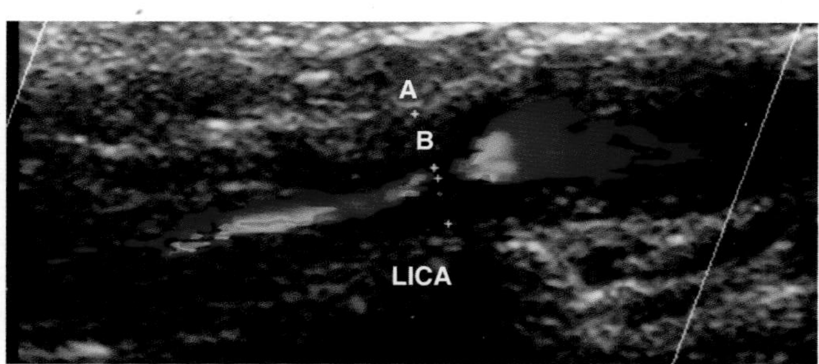

Figure 35-4. Color flow duplex image of apparent high-grade stenosis of left internal carotid origin in a patient with a minor hemispheric stroke. Peak systolic velocity of 500 cm/sec and end diastolic velocity of 153 cm/sec are indicative of 80% to 99% stenosis.

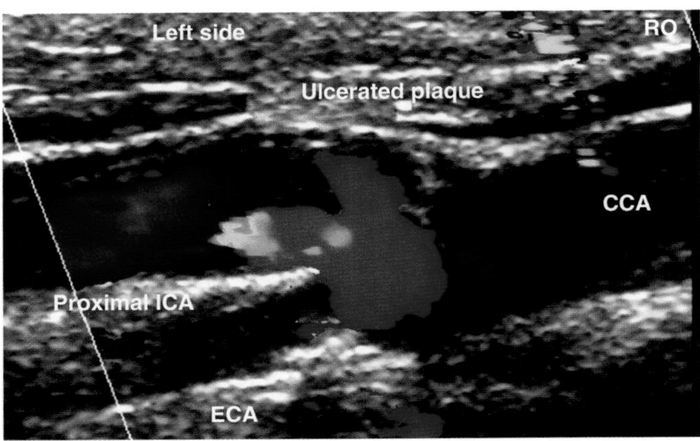

Figure 35-5. Color flow duplex image of an ulcerated plaque at the left internal carotid origin. Note flow into ulcer cavity. Peak systolic velocity of 589 cm/sec and end diastolic velocity of 173 cm/sec are indicative of 80% to 99% stenosis. The patient had multiple episodes of right arm weakness.

In color flow duplex, velocity data are color coded and superimposed over the ultrasound image to create a flow map.

Duplex ultrasound velocity data are reliable in the assessment of the degree of carotid stenosis. In Boston, we have found velocity criteria modified from the University of Washington studies provided the best correlation with angiographic or operative findings (Table 35-5).[5,19,20]

While these velocity criteria are accurate, they are not completely helpful in selecting patients for surgery based on the NASCET or ACAS criteria. Moneta et al. found that an internal carotid artery to common carotid artery peak systolic velocity ratio of 4.0 detected 70% or greater internal carotid stenosis by NASCET criteria with 91% sensitivity, 87% specificity, 76% positive predictive value, 96% negative predictive value, and 88% overall accuracy.[21] The velocity ratio of 4.0 provided the best overall accuracy in the detection of 70% or greater carotid stenosis by NASCET criteria.

Similarly, for asymptomatic patients, these same authors evaluated the 60% internal carotid artery stenosis threshold used to determine ACAS eligibility. They found that the combination of peak systolic velocity of at least 290 cm/sec and end diastolic velocity of at least 80 cm/sec predicted 60% or greater stenosis with sensitivity of 78%, specificity of 96%, positive predictive value of 95%, negative predictive value of 84%, and overall accuracy of 88%.[22] While this finding is of interest, most carotid surgeons still select only patients with more critical (at least 80% stenosis) for endarterectomy for asymptomatic disease.

Table 35-5
Duplex Velocity and Doppler Waveform Criteria for Carotid Stenosis*

Stenosis (%)	PSV (cm/sec)	EDV (cm/sec)	Turbulence
<30	<120	Any	Minimal
30-50	<120	Any	Present
50-79	>120	<140	Present
80-99	>120	>140	Present

*EDV, end diastolic velocity; PSV, peak systolic velocity.

Duplex ultrasound is also useful in evaluating plaque density and surface morphology. Plaque density and surface morphology data are not currently quantified for routine clinical use (Figures 35-2 and 35-3). El-Barghouty et al. attempted to use the gray-scale median as a means of quantifying plaque density.[23] While they have shown that less dense plaques (higher lipid content or higher incidence of intraplaque hemorrhage) with gray-scale medians of 32 or less are more often associated with stroke than are more dense plaques (calcified), their correlation is imprecise. At present, the clinical use of density and morphology data is limited to a qualitative appreciation of their relevance in determining clinical outcome. More precise assessment of their significance awaits a practical, precise, and clinically relevant means for quantifying these plaque attributes.

Duplex is also useful in detecting carotid artery occlusion and, therefore, in obviating the need for surgical intervention. Sensitivity and specificity of 97% for the detection of internal carotid occlusion were reported even in early experience with duplex.[19] Criteria for diagnosis of occlusion include absence of flow in the internal carotid artery, blunted diastolic flow (end diastolic velocity of 0) in the common carotid artery and accelerated flow in the external carotid artery. Transcranial Doppler (TCD) assessment of the ophthalmic artery for detection of reversal of flow provides additional evidence of internal carotid occlusion.

Duplex ultrasound has two major shortcomings. First, the quality of duplex data depends on the ultrasound technician's experience and diligence. Second, duplex cannot image the aortic arch, great vessel origins, distal internal carotid artery, or intracranial vasculature. Information regarding the intracranial circulation can be obtained noninvasively using TCD, although anatomical variability in the cranial acoustic windows and other technical limitations may result in less than a complete survey of the intracranial circulation. TCD can provide useful data confirming the hemodynamic significance of intracranial lesions detected by MRA or other modalities, but the TCD may be most useful as a means of detecting embolic events in the intracranial vessels.

Because of the shortcomings of duplex ultrasound and despite its proven accuracy in grading stenosis, some clinicians are hesitant to base decisions on ultrasound data alone. Through the 1980s, duplex was used primarily as a screening tool and was followed by contrast angiography in cases where surgical intervention was contemplated. Because of the risk and invasive nature of contrast angiography, a noninvasive study complementary to duplex was sought. MRA can image the arch, great vessel origins, distal internal carotid artery, and intracranial circulation. Like duplex, MRA gives a flow chart, rather than an image of the arterial wall, but the data can be rendered into images that closely mimic the anatomical data familiar from traditional contrast angiography. Furthermore, MRA data can be acquired along with MRI brain imaging data, allowing detailed assessment of the brain parenchyma and assessment of the cerebral circulation.

MRA depends on the detection of the differences in energy emitted from moving versus stationary protons after application of radiofrequency energy pulses within a magnetic field. This technique is called time-of-flight technology. In two-dimensional time-of-flight (2D TOF) MRA, images are acquired in thin 2- to 3-mm cross-sections and reassembled to give an image of the flowing blood. In three-dimensional

Table 35-6
Sensitivity and Specificity of Magnetic Resonance Angiography in Detection of Carotid Stenosis (70% to 99%) and Occlusion (Contrast Angiography as Standard for Comparison)*

Reference	Stenosis	Sensitivity (%)	Specificity (%)	Method
Young et al.[24]	70-99%	86	93	2D + 3D
Patel et al.[25]	70-99%	84	75	2D
Patel et al.[25]	70-99%	94	85	3D
Turnipseed et al.[26]	70-99%	100	93	2D
Mittl et al.[27]	70-99%	92	75	2D
Patel et al.[25]	Occlusion	100	100	2D + 3D
Young et al.[24]	Occlusion	80	99	2D + 3D

*2D, two dimensional; 3D, three dimensional.

time-of-flight (3D TOF) MRA, an entire vessel segment is subjected to the energy pulses at once and then partitioned for later reconstruction. The differences in these two data acquisition modes result in different image characteristics. The use of 2D and 3D modes in a complementary manner enhances the reliability of MRA, and most current MRA studies use both to insure optimal images. In general, 2D TOF MRA is better at imaging of longer arterial segments and therefore is preferred for imaging the proximal common carotid artery and distal internal carotid artery. Motion-related image degradation is less of a problem with 2D TOF because the images are acquired in thin slices and reconstructed later. Also, because each cross-sectional segment is energized individually, signal loss is minimized and sluggish flow can be differentiated from no flow. This makes the 2D mode more sensitive than 3D in differentiating occlusive from preocclusive lesions. In 3D mode, the reconstructed cross-sectional segments are thinner, yielding better spatial resolution and allowing a more accurate assessment of degree of stenosis. Furthermore, because in 3D mode the volume to be imaged is energized simultaneously and not in sequenced perpendicular slices, tortuous vessels and areas of turbulent flow are better imaged.

The sensitivity and specificity of MRA in the detection of carotid stenoses and occlusions are shown in Table 35-6.

In these studies, duplex was also assessed for sensitivity and specificity versus the standard of contrast angiography. In most studies, the sensitivity and specificity for duplex were similar to those of MRA.

In current practice, a normal or near-normal MRA virtually eliminates the possibility of a hemodynamically significant carotid stenosis (Figures 35-5 through 35-7). On the other hand, the specificity of MRA has been somewhat inconsistent. Turbulence related to moderate stenosis may result in more random motion of blood such that the axis of flow is inconsistent and no longer perpendicular to the imaging plane. Signal dropout may occur as a result of turbulence, resulting in a flow void (Figure 35-3). In 2D TOF mode, a flow void may represent anything from 30% to 99% stenosis. Riles et al. observed that using 2D TOF the sensitivity and the specificity for detecting 50% to 99% stenosis were 100% and 60%, respectively.[28] An MRA that revealed minimal disease was virtually certain to be accurate, but an MRA that predicted 50% to 99% stenosis was accurate only 60% of the time. This tendency to overread

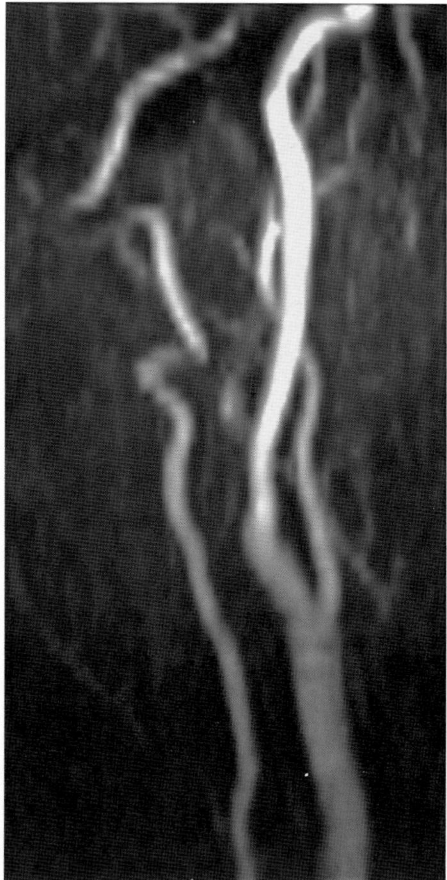

Figure 35-6. Two-dimensional time-of-flight magnetic resonance angiography of near-normal carotid and small tortuous vertebral artery.

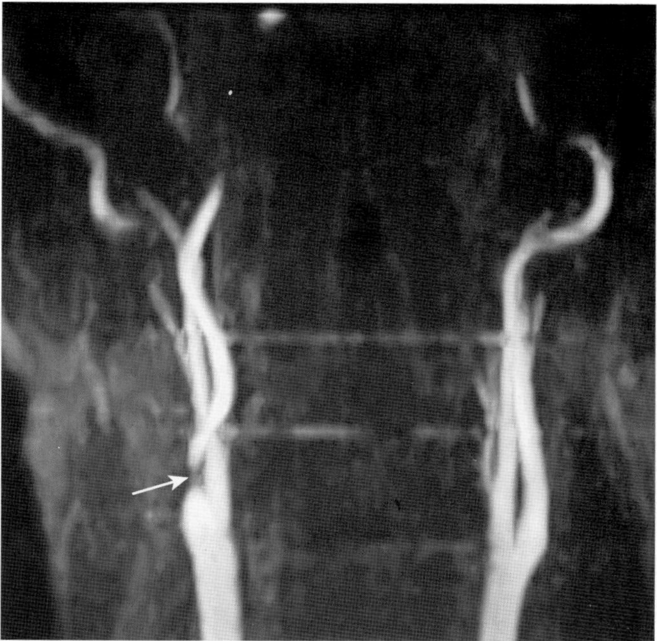

Figure 35-7. Magnetic resonance angiography showing both cervical carotid arteries. The left is normal, and the right has moderate to severe stenosis at the internal carotid origin.

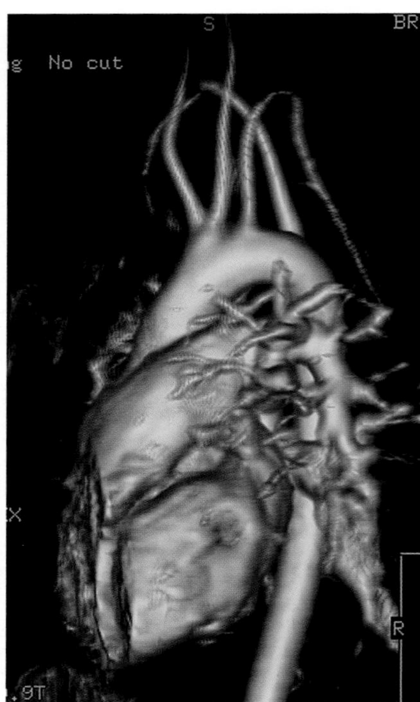

Figure 35-8. Magnetic resonance angiography (MRA) of heart and great vessels illustrating capability of MRA to visualize proximal portions of common carotid arteries. In this case the common carotids are normal, but an aberrant origin of the right subclavian artery explains this patient's dysphagia.

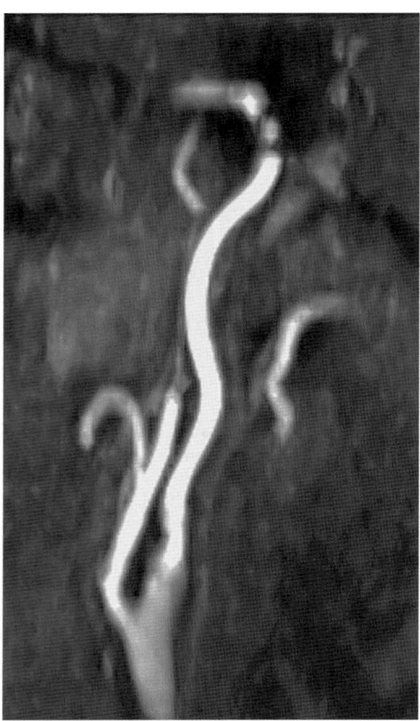

Figure 35-9. Magnetic resonance angiography (MRA) done to evaluate right hemispheric stroke in a patient with minimal disease at the carotid bifurcations by duplex. Study shows significant lesions in right carotid siphon region. MRA is useful in diagnosing intracranial vascular disease.

the degree of stenosis because of the flow void phenomenon limits the value of 2D TOF MRA in surgical decision-making because it does not allow accurate discrimination among minimal (30% to 49%), moderate (50% to 69%), and critical (70% to 99%) stenoses. Improved sensitivity has been achieved using 3D TOF, although specificity for diagnosis of 70% to 99% stenosis in some series employing 3D TOF is as low as 78% to 85%.[25,29]

The lack of specificity in the diagnosis of critical carotid stenosis remains a shortcoming for MRA and limits its value as a screening tool, where duplex remains preeminent. Most clinicians who employ MRA for clinical decision-making use it with duplex imaging (Figures 35-8 and 35-9). In their study, Patel et al. found that the diagnostic accuracy of MRA and duplex for determining a stenosis of 70% to 99% were 86% and 88%, respectively. However, when the two studies were concordant, the diagnostic accuracy increased to 94%.[25]

Rapid acquisition spiral CT allows image acquisition to be timed with contrast administration, and enhanced computer image reconstruction gives CT angiograms nearly the same anatomical detail and resolution as standard contrast angiography. Furthermore, the cross-sectional source images give added information on plaque morphology not available with standard arteriograms. The use of multidetector row computed tomography angiography (CTA) in the evaluation of carotid stenosis has been rapidly expanding in recent years. This is due to advances in the ability to perform multiplanar scanning at submillimeter slices and subsecond rotations, thus allowing for a quick and more anatomically accurate assessment of carotid stenosis than previous generations of scanners.[30] Recent prospective studies comparing the concordance rate of combined methods in noninvasive imaging revealed no statistical differences between duplex ultrasound plus MRA versus duplex plus CTA.[31] However, data supporting the routine use of CTA before carotid surgery are scant. Another drawback of CTA is the difficulty in interpreting stenosis in heavily calcified vessels. This is due to the inability to distinguish calcified vessel wall from luminal contrast in the postprocessing volume-rendering technique for 3D reconstruction (Figure 35-10). As more is learned about the influence of plaque morphology on natural history and as plaque morphology comes to play a greater role in patient selection, CT angiography may become a routine part of patient assessment.

For many, contrast angiography remains the standard against which all other diagnostic studies are measured. Newer digital imaging systems have enhanced image quality allowing multiplanar high-resolution images of the aortic arch, carotid, vertebral, and intracranial arteries (Figures 35-11 through 35-14). Arteriography, however, is subject to significant interobserver variability in interpretation. The discrepancy between the NASCET and the ECST methods for determining the severity of carotid stenosis highlights the potential for significant variability in image interpretation. In NASCET, the degree of stenosis was calculated as the ratio of the diameter at the narrowest point to the diameter at the point at which the internal carotid artery walls again become parallel, beyond the area of poststenotic dilatation. In ECST, the degree of stenosis was calculated as the ratio of the diameter at the narrowest point to the carotid bulb diameter, reconstructed as if there were no disease. This leads to significant differences in angiographic interpretation such that a 60% stenosis in ECST is only an 18% stenosis in NASCET, a 70% stenosis in ECST

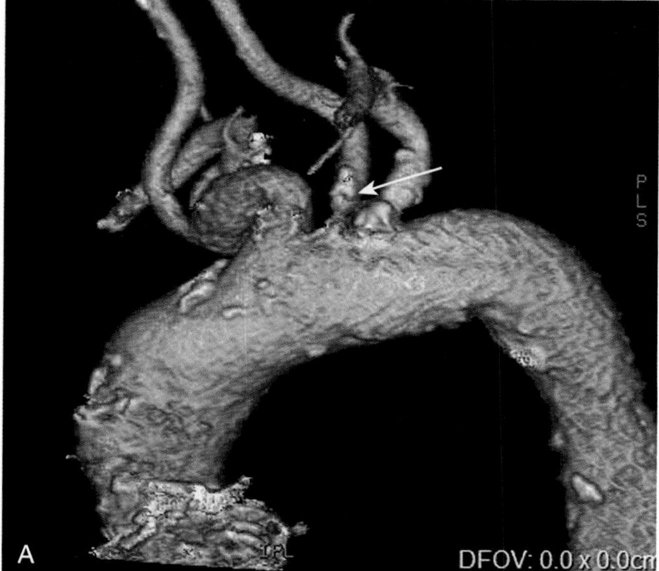

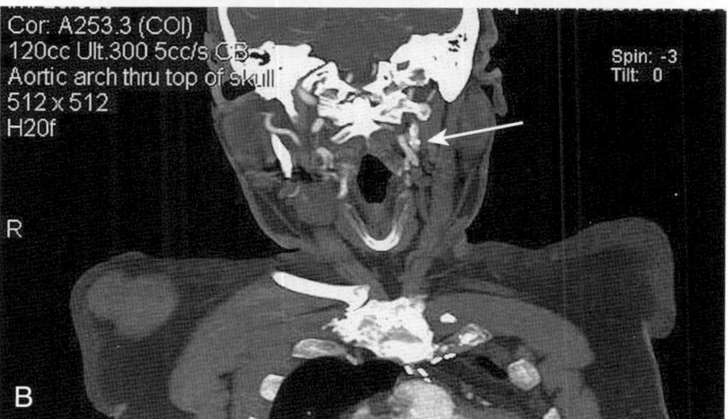

Figure 35-10. Computed tomography angiogram of proximal left common carotid lesion **(A)** and left carotid bifurcation lesion **(B),** each shown by an arrow. This patient underwent combined endovascular stenting of the common carotid and endarterectomy of the internal carotid artery.

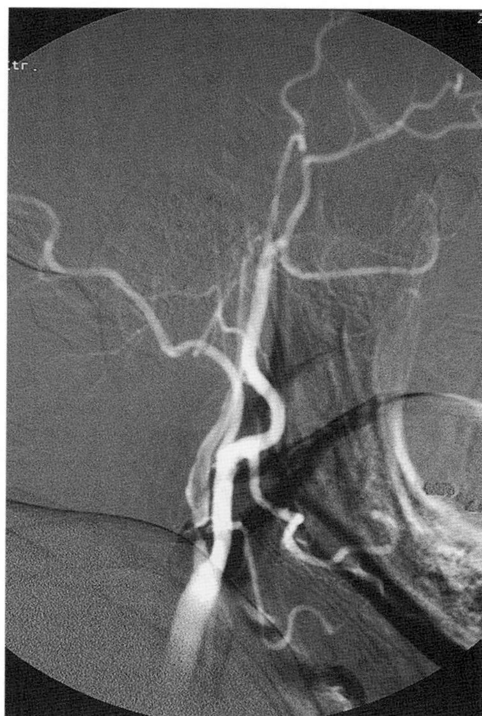

Figure 35-11. Critical internal carotid stenosis with tail of thrombus extending into more distal internal carotid artery. Patient had an evolving stroke. Duplex image suggested critical stenosis, but velocities were damped (peak systolic velocity = 55, end diastolic velocity = 17), and no patent distal vessel could be identified. Endarterectomy was carried out uneventfully with excellent neurological recovery.

is a 40% stenosis in NASCET, an 80% stenosis in ECST is a 61% stenosis in NASCET, and a 90% stenosis in ECST is an 80% stenosis in NASCET. Even if the method of calculation is agreed, the interobserver variability for contrast angiography can be significant and nearly as great as that for MRA.[24] While no one questions the ease with which contrast angiograms can be reviewed and their reliable depiction of carotid anatomy, contrast angiography should no longer be regarded uncritically as the standard assessment of carotid disease.

In addition to interobserver variability, potential morbidity and cost limit the applicability of contrast angiography. Contrast allergy and nephrotoxicity remain significant issues, despite newer contrast agents and improved protocols for prevention of anaphylaxis and renal failure. Arterial puncture can be a cause of significant morbidity from hemorrhage, pseudoaneurysm formation, and arterial thrombosis. Selective angiography by direct carotid artery puncture carries a small but significant risk of stroke which in ACAS was 1.2%.[7] Contrast angiography is also more expensive than ultrasound imaging and even MRA in most hospitals.

Neither CT nor MRI is indicated routinely in patients being evaluated for CEA. While evidence of previous stroke may be

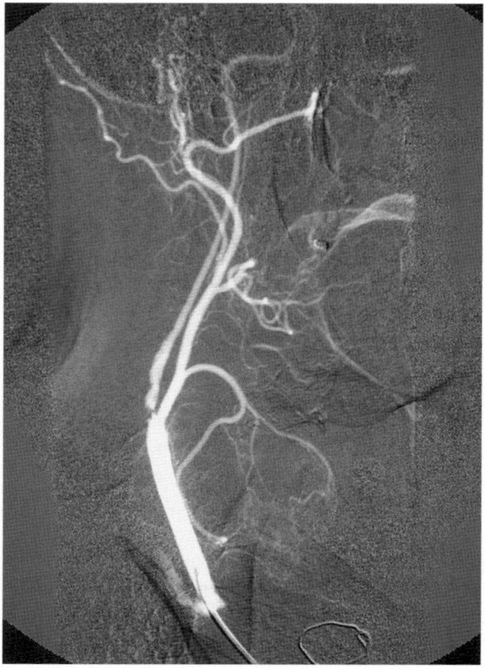

Figure 35-12. Carotid arteriogram showing critical carotid stenosis with small underperfused distal internal carotid artery (string sign). Duplex had been unable to rule out internal carotid artery occlusion.

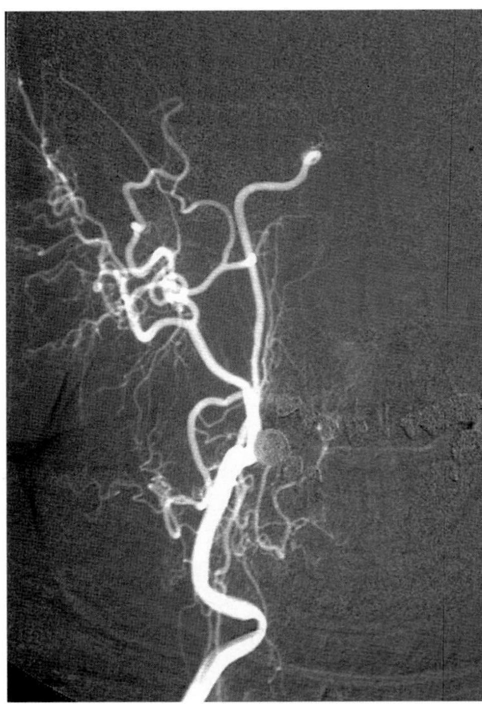

Figure 35-13. Carotid arteriogram revealing moderate bifurcation disease, a small internal carotid artery, and occlusion of the intracranial internal carotid artery (ICA) in a patient with a middle cerebral artery stroke. Duplex had shown moderate ICA stenosis by image but sluggish ICA velocities (peak systolic velocity = 25, end diastolic velocity = 6).

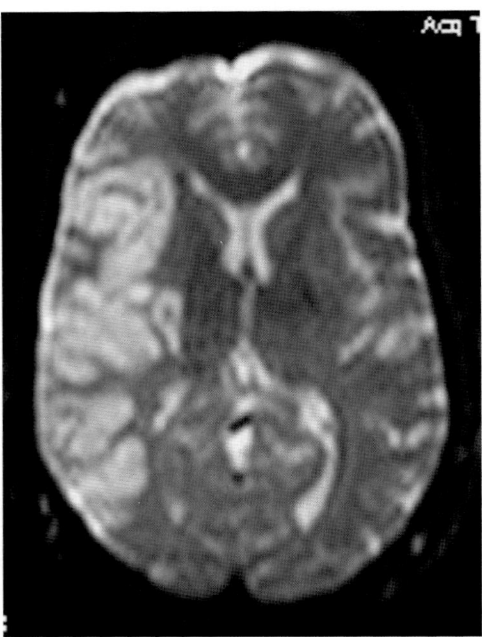

Figure 35-14. Brain imaging showing extensive acute infarct on diffusion-weighted magnetic resonance imaging. This patient is not a candidate for emergent operative intervention.

detected on brain imaging in up to 16% of asymptomatic and 35% of symptomatic patients, it appears this finding seldom alters surgical outcomes or influences surgical decisions.[32] Some authors have reported increased neurological morbidity associated with the presence of silent infarcts found on CT or MRI,[33,34] but others reported that incidentally discovered infarcts had no prognostic significance.[35,36] Martin et al. performed routine CT on 469 patients being considered for CEA.[35] Scans were abnormal in 62 patients with a history of previous stroke but in only 14% of patients with no history. No incidental tumors, arteriovenous malformations, intracranial aneurysms, or other significant brain lesions were identified. The CT did not alter clinical judgment with respect to patient selection in any case. The perioperative stroke rate for the 230 CEAs performed in this series was 1.3%.[33]

While not necessary routinely, preoperative brain imaging is important in selected conditions. Acute or evolving stroke, atypical neurological signs or symptoms, and history of significant head injury or intracranial lesions are all indications. A remote history of stroke may be an indication for preoperative imaging, especially in the presence of a residual neurological deficit. Of course, in patients undergoing MRA for evaluation of the cervical and intracranial arteries, MRI can be performed with no added morbidity or inconvenience and with little additional cost. In this case, it is hard to argue against brain imaging, although the anticipated influence of the MRI on surgical decisions is minimal.

Recently, the use of diffusion-weighted MRI has proved helpful in determining border zone infarct. Compared with regular MRI, diffusion-weighted brain imaging can be used to discriminate recent versus old infarct.[37] In addition, perfusion weighted imaging MRI can be used to identify individuals with acute cerebral ischemia within hours of its onset. Perfusion weighted imaging lesions are often larger than diffusion-weighted imaging abnormalities. Thus, identifying the areas of perfusion–diffusion-weighted imaging mismatch could potentially be used to distinguish between ischemic but viable brain and infarcted brain[38] (Figure 35-14).

Preoperative imaging should be tailored to the needs of each patient. Selected patients may undergo CEA based on duplex data alone, while others require more detailed evaluation, including contrast angiography and brain imaging.

References

1. Murros KE, Evans GW, Toole JF, et al. Cerebral infarction in patients with transient ischemic attacks. *J Neurol* 1989;236:182-186.
2. Toole JF, Dibert SW, Harpold GJ. Transient ischemic attacks and stroke in the distribution of the carotid artery: clinical manifestations. In: Moore W, ed. *Surgery for cerebrovascular disease*. 2nd ed. Philadelphia, WB Saunders; 1996:73.
3. Chambers BR, Norris JW. Outcome in patients with asymptomatic neck bruits. *New Engl J Med* 1986;315:860-865.
4. O'Holleran LW, Kennelly MM, McClurken M, Johnson JM. Natural history of asymptomatic carotid plaque. *Am J Surg* 1987;154:659-662.
5. Roederer GO, Langlois YE, Jager KA, et al. The natural history of carotid arterial disease in asymptomatic patients with cervical bruits. *Stroke* 1984;15:605-613.
6. Hobson RW, Weiss DG, Fields WS, et al. Efficacy of carotid endarterectomy for asymptomatic carotid stenosis. *New Engl J Med* 1993;328: 221-227.
7. Executive Committee for Asymptomatic Carotid Atherosclerosis Study. Endarterectomy for asymptomatic carotid artery stenosis. *JAMA* 1995;273:1421-1428.
8. Crouse JR, Byington RP, Hoen HM, Furberg CD. Reductase inhibitor monotherapy and stroke prevention. *Arch Int Med* 1997;157:1305-1310.
9. Nicolaides AN. Asymptomatic carotid stenosis and risk of stroke: identification of a high-risk group. *Int Angiol* 1995;14:21-28.

10. Medical Research Council Asymptomatic Carotid Surgery Trial Collaborative Group. Prevention of disabling and fatal strokes by successful carotid endarterectomy in patients without recent neurological symptoms: randomized controlled trial. *Lancet* 2004;363:1491-1502.
11. Canadian Cooperative Study Group. A randomized trial of aspirin and sulfinpyrazone in threatened stroke. *New Engl J Med* 1978;299:53-59.
12. Fields WS, Lemak NA, Frankowski RF, Hardy RJ. Controlled trial of aspirin in cerebral ischemia. *Stroke* 1977;8:301-315.
13. Bousser MG, Eschwege E, Haguenau M, et al. "AICLA" controlled trial of aspirin and dipyridamole in secondary prevention of athero-thrombotic cerebral ischemia. *Stroke* 1983;14:5-14.
14. North American Symptomatic Carotid Endarterectomy Trial Collaborators. Beneficial effect of carotid endarterectomy in symptomatic patients with high-grade carotid stenosis. *New Engl J Med* 1991;325:445-453.
15. Barnett HJM, Taylor DW, Eliaziw M, et al. Benefit of carotid endarterectomy in patients with symptomatic moderate or severe stenosis. *New Engl J Med* 1998;339:1415-1425.
16. European Carotid Surgery Trialists' Collaborative Group. MRC European Carotid Surgery Trial: interim results for patients with severe (70-99%) or mild (0-29%) carotid stenosis. *Lancet* 1991;337:1235-1243.
17. European Carotid Surgery Trialists' Collaborative Group. Randomised trial of endarterectomy for recently symptomatic carotid stenosis: final results of the MRC European Carotid Surgery Trial (ECST). *Lancet* 1998;351:1379-1387.
18. Wolf PA, Kannel WB, Sorlie P, McNamara P. Asymptomatic carotid bruit and risk of stroke: the Framingham study. *JAMA* 1981;245:1442-1445.
19. Roederer GO, Langlois YE, Chan ATW, et al. Ultrasonic duplex scanning of the extracranial carotid arteries: improved accuracy using new features of the common carotid artery. *J Cardiovasc Ultrasonography* 1982;1:373-380.
20. Moneta GL, Taylor DC, Nicholls SC, et al. Operative versus nonoperative management of asymptomatic high-grade internal carotid artery stenosis: improved results with endarterectomy. *Stroke* 1987;18:1005-1010.
21. Moneta GL, Edwards JM, Chitwood RW, et al. Correlation of North American Symptomatic Carotid Endarterectomy Trial (NASCET) angiographic definition of 70-99% internal carotid artery stenosis with duplex scanning. *J Vasc Surg* 1993;17:152-159.
22. Moneta GL, Edwards JM, Papanicolaou G, et al. Screening for asymptomatic internal carotid artery stenosis: duplex criteria for discriminating 60-99% stenosis. *J Vasc Surg* 1995;21:989-994.
23. El-Barghouty N, Geroulakos G, Nicolaides A, et al. Computer assisted carotid plaque characterization. *Eur J Vasc Endovasc Surg* 1995;9:389-393.
24. Young GR, Humphrey PRD, Nixon TE, et al. Variability in measurement of extracranial internal carotid artery stenosis as displayed by both digital subtraction and magnetic resonance angiography: an assessment of three caliper techniques and visual impression of stenosis. *Stroke* 1996;27:467-473.
25. Patel MR, Kuntz KM, Klufas RA, et al. Pre-operative assessment of the carotid bifurcation: can magnetic resonance angiography and duplex ultrasonography replace contrast angiography? *Stroke* 1995;26:1753-1758.
26. Turnipseed WD, Kennell TW, Turski PA, et al. Magnetic resonance angiography and duplex scanning: non-invasive tests for selecting symptomatic carotid endarterectomy candidates. *Surgery* 1993;114:643-648.
27. Mittl RL, Broderick M, Carpenter JP, et al. Blinded reader comparison of magnetic resonance angiography and duplex ultrasonography for carotid bifurcation stenosis. *Stroke* 1994;25:4-10.
28. Riles TS, Eidelman EM, Litt AW, et al. Comparison of magnetic resonance angiography, conventional angiography, and duplex scanning. *Stroke* 1992;23:341-346.
29. Anderson CM, Lee RE, Levin DL, et al. Measurement of internal carotid artery stenosis from source MR angiograms. *Radiology* 1994;193:219-226.
30. Takhtani D. CT neuroangiography: a glance at the common pitfalls and their prevention. *AJR Am J Roentgenol* 2005;185(3):772-783.
31. CARMEDAS Study Group. Concordance rate differences of 3 noninvasive imaging techniques to measure carotid stenosis in clinical routine practice: results of the CARMEDAS muticenter study. *Stroke* 2004;35(3):682-686.
32. Street D, O'Brien M, Ricotta J, et al. Observations on cerebral computed tomography in patients having carotid endarterectomy. *J Vasc Surg* 1988;7:798-801.
33. Graber J, Vollman R, Levine H, et al. Stroke following carotid endarterectomy: risk predicted by preoperative CT scan. *Am J Surg* 1984;147:492-497.
34. Vollman R, Eldrup-Jorgensen J, Hoffman M. The role of computed tomography in carotid surgery. *Surg Clinics North Am* 1986;66:255-268.
35. Martin J, Valentine R, Myers S, et al. Is routine CT scanning necessary in the preoperative evaluation of patients undergoing carotid endarterectomy? *J Vasc Surg* 1991;14:267-270.
36. Ricotta J, Ouriel K, Green R, DeWeese J. Use of computerized cerebral tomography in selection of patients for elective and urgent carotid endarterectomy. *Ann Surg* 1985;202:783-787.
37. Kang DW, Kwon SU, Yoo SH, et al. Early recurrent ischemic lesions on diffusion-weighted imaging in symptomatic intracranial atherosclerosis. *Arch Neurol* 2007;64(1):50-54.
38. Neumann-Haefelin T, Wittsack HJ, Fink GR, et al. Diffusion- and perfusion-weighted MRI: influence of severe carotid artery stenosis on the DWI/PWI mismatch in acute stroke. *Stroke* 2000;31(6):1311-1317.

chapter

36

Surgical Treatment of Carotid Disease

A. Ross Naylor, MBChB, MD, FRCS

Key Points

- Several major randomized clinical trials have informed vascular surgeons that carotid endarterectomy is an operation justified by a firm evidence base.
- Carotid endarterectomy has the potential to reduce the risk of stroke, particularly in selected high-risk patients with neurological symptoms and a tight internal carotid artery stenosis.
- Careful patient selection and obsessive attention to operative detail improve the results from surgery and enhance the benefit of carotid endarterectomy to the population.
- Areas of controversy remain, such as the exact role of carotid endarterectomy in asymptomatic patients and in patients undergoing coronary artery bypass.
- Carotid surgeons should be familiar with several rare syndromes and conditions that they may occasionally be called on to manage.

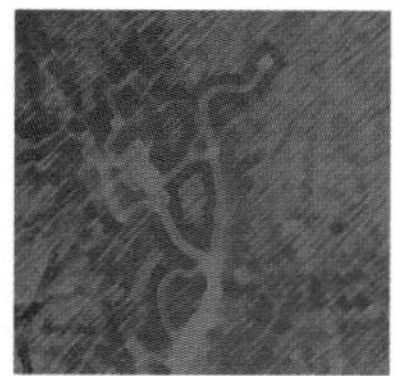

ATHEROSCLEROTIC CAROTID DISEASE

Atherosclerosis at the origin of the internal carotid artery (ICA) accounts for up to 50% of ischemic carotid territory strokes. This chapter summarizes the principles of treatment, with emphasis on the selection for, technique, and outcomes of carotid endarterectomy (CEA).

Guidelines for CEA have largely evolved from four studies.[1-4] For symptomatic patients, these are the European Carotid Surgery Trial (ECST) and the North American Symptomatic Carotid Endarterectomy Trial (NASCET), both of which were published in 1991. The 1995 Asymptomatic Carotid Atherosclerosis Study (ACAS) and the 2004 Asymptomatic Carotid Surgery Trial (ACST) were the most important trials to evaluate the role of CEA in asymptomatic patients. However, the rationale underlying individual management decisions inevitably reflects local, national, international, and cost-based factors. Where possible, discrepancies in practice are discussed.

International Trials

No operation has been subjected to more scientific scrutiny than CEA. The main trials have provided level I evidence to guide overall practice and have been the foundation for almost every guideline developed worldwide. However, surgeons have occasionally tended to generalize the results of these trials uncritically into clinical practice. It should be remembered that the results were attributable specifically to those clinicians, surgeons, and centers that randomized patients. It has, however, become customary to assume that all surgeons perform CEA with similar outcomes, that all patients receive optimal medical therapy, and that the trial cohorts still represent the current population of patients at risk. None of these assumptions is entirely valid. For example, provision of best medical therapy has improved greatly since 1991. Fewer than 0.5% of CEAs performed in North America between 1988 and 1989 were actually randomized within NASCET,[5] and 94% of CEAs in the United States are now performed in non-NASCET centers that report a significantly higher mortality rate than NASCET centers.[6] Community-based and other randomized trials in the United States and Europe also suggest that the operative risk is generally worse than was observed in ECST and NASCET.[6-8] Accordingly, interpretation of the data, grading of evidence, and recommendations for practice must take into account the additional effect of the individual surgeon's operative risk.

Symptomatic Trials

ECST and NASCET randomized 6462 patients with ipsilateral carotid territory symptoms in the preceding 6 months.[9] All underwent angiography, computed tomography (CT), and neurological assessment. Randomization was stratified for degree of stenosis, but the measurement method differed (Figure 36-1). Both trials measured the luminal diameter (the numerator). The ECST denominator was the estimated diameter of the carotid bulb. In NASCET, this was the diameter of disease-free ICA above the stenosis. In practice, a 50% NASCET stenosis approximates to a 75% ECST stenosis. It is crucial that the measurement method being used in noninvasive laboratories is known to doctors making management decisions. In a recent audit of U.K. practice, it became clear that considerable uncertainty surrounded whether the NASCET or the ECST measurement method was being used.[11]

The Carotid Endarterectomy Trialists Collaboration (CETC) has combined the ECST, NASCET, and The Veterans Affairs (VA) Trial data, having first remeasured all prerandomization angiograms using the NASCET measurement method.[12-14] This is now the most comprehensive database of outcomes, and these data should now be cited in preference to outcomes from the constituent studies. Table 36-1 presents the principle findings from the CETC database. In summary, no evidence shows that CEA should not be recommended to symptomatic patients with a NASCET stenosis of less than 50%. Patients with 50% to 69% stenoses do gain a small yet significant benefit from surgery, but endarterectomy confers its maximum benefit in patients with 70% to 99% stenoses.

To participate in the trials, each surgeon had to submit a track record and only those with a low complication rate were allowed to randomize patients. However, evidence suggests that the operative risk in current practice may be significantly higher[6-9] and could even nullify any long-term benefit. Not surprisingly, the higher the 30-day death or stroke rate, the lower the long-term benefit. Accordingly, surgeons cannot just implement the trial results without at least considering how their own operative risk affects the overall clinical effectiveness of the procedure.

Asymptomatic Trials

Table 36-2 summarizes the principle results from ACAS and ACST. CEA confers a small but significant reduction in the risk of late stroke, amounting to about 1% per annum. This benefit, however, is inextricably linked to the initial operative risk. If it exceeds 4%, no benefit accrues to the patient. However, real-world audits again suggest that outcomes may be worse than the 3% threshold recommended by the American Heart Association.[15] For example, in a recent 10-state review of practice in the United States in 2001, 7 states reported 30-day death or stroke rates in excess of 3% after CEA. More importantly, if patients with remote symptoms (more than 6 months prior) and those

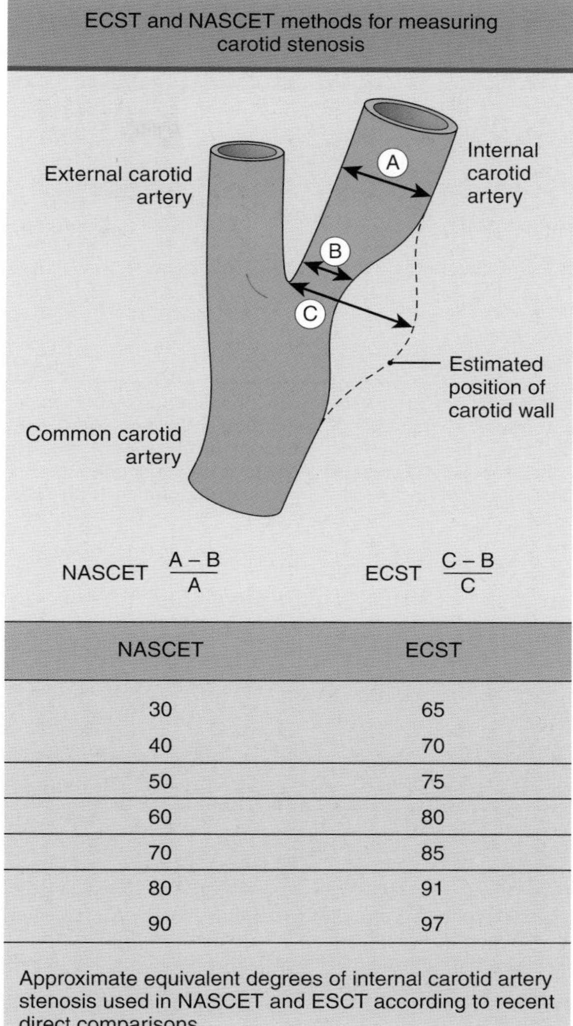

NASCET	ECST
30	65
40	70
50	75
60	80
70	85
80	91
90	97

Approximate equivalent degrees of internal carotid artery stenosis used in NASCET and ESCT according to recent direct comparisons

Figure 36-1. European Carotid Surgery Trial and North American Symptomatic Carotid Endarterectomy Trial methods for measuring carotid stenosis. The table indicates how the two measurement methods compare. (From Donnan GA, Davis SM, Chambers BR, Gates PC. *Lancet* 1998;351:1372-1373.)

with "nonhemispheric" or vertebrobasilar symptoms were excluded (i.e., they now fulfilled ACST entry criteria), the procedural risk rose to 5.9% in 2001, declining slightly to 5.4% when repeated in 2004.[16]

Extracranial–Intracranial Study

The extracranial–intracranial (EC-IC) bypass study[17] recruited 1377 patients with ICA occlusion who were randomized to best medical therapy or EC-IC bypass (revascularization of the ipsilateral middle cerebral artery with inflow from the superficial temporal artery). The rationale was that this might prevent stroke ipsilateral to the occluded carotid artery. This study found that surgery conferred no early or late benefit. The trial methodology did, however, arouse much debate and renewed calls for a better designed study. It has been suggested that if the new trial only included patients with ICA occlusion and exhausted hemodynamic reserve then surgery might have

Table 36-1
CETC: 5-Year Risk of Any Stroke (Including 30-Day Stroke or Death) from the Combined VA, ECST, and NASCET Trials*†

Trial	Stenosis	*n*	30-Day CEA Risk (%)	5-Year Risk: Surgery (%)	5-Year Risk: Medical (%)	ARR (%)	RRR (%)	NNT	Strokes Prevented per 1000 CEAs at 5 Years‡
CETC	<30%	1746	Unknown	18.36	15.71	−2.6	N/B	N/B	None
CETC	30-49%	1429	6.7	22.80	25.45	+2.6	10	38	26
CETC	50-69%	1549	8.4	20.00	27.77	+7.8	28	13	78
CETC	70-99%	1095	6.2	17.13	32.71	+15.6	48	6	156
CETC	String sign	262	5.4	22.40	22.30	−0.1	N/B	N/B	None

*Data derived from the CETC[12-14] with all prerandomization angiograms remeasured using NASCET method.
†ARR, absolute risk reduction; CEA, carotid endarterectomy; CETC, Carotid Endarterectomy Trialists Collaboration; ECST, European Carotid Surgery Trial; NASCET, North American Symptomatic Carotid Endarterectomy Trial; N/B, no benefit conferred by CEA; NNT, number of CEAs required to prevent one stroke at 5 years; RRR, relative risk reduction.
‡Number of strokes prevented at 5 years by performing 1000 CEAs.

Table 36-2
5-Year Risk of Stroke (Including 30-Day Stroke or Death) from the Asymptomatic Randomized Trials*†

Trial	Stenosis (%)	*n*	30-Day CEA Risk (%)	5-Year Risk: Surgery (%)	5-Year Risk: Medical (%)	ARR (%)	RRR (%)	NNT	Strokes Prevented per 1000 CEAs at 5 Years‡
ACAS	60-99	1662	2.3	5.1	11.0	+5.9	53	17	59
ACST	60-99	3120	2.8	6.4	11.8	+5.4	46	19	53

*In ACAS,[3] the 5-year stroke data refer to ipsilateral stroke. In ACST,[4] the 5-year data refer to any stroke.
†ACAS, Asymptomatic Carotid Atherosclerosis Study; ACST, Asymptomatic Carotid Surgery Trial; ARR, absolute risk reduction; CEA, carotid endarterectomy; NNT, number of CEAs required to prevent one stroke at a specified period; RRR, relative risk reduction.
‡Number of strokes prevented at 5 years by performing 1000 CEAs.

significant benefit. Until then, patients should not undergo EC-IC bypass routinely.

SELECTION OF PATIENTS FOR CAROTID SURGERY

Asymptomatic Patients

The management of asymptomatic disease continues to arouse much debate, largely because of a failure to address several inconvenient truths exposed by ACAS and ACST.[18] The general interpretation of the literature is that, provided a patient is anticipated to remain in good health and the surgeon has a low audited operative risk (less than 3%), it is appropriate to recommend CEA. Not surprisingly, this one-size-fits-all attitude has led to a huge increase in the number of procedures being performed worldwide.

However, it is also important to recognize that several practices still may be hard to justify following closer inspection of the evidence. For example, ACAS showed no apparent benefit for CEA in women, even if those suffering a procedural stroke or death were then excluded.[19] ACST did claim that they demonstrated significant benefit in women, but that was only if the 30-day risk of death or stroke was excluded. Second, neither ACAS nor ACST was able to demonstrate any relationship between stenosis severity and late stroke risk; similarly, in neither trial was there an association between severe bilateral carotid disease (including occlusion) and increased risk of late stroke. These latter two findings were opposite to what had been found in the earlier symptomatic trials. Third, the patient should be expected to survive 5 years to gain maximum benefit, yet in some states the largest single increase in the number of CEAs was in the elderly.[20] ACST found no evidence that CEA conferred any benefit in patients older than 75 years, even when the procedural risk was excluded.

Symptomatic Patients

What Is the Degree of Stenosis?

Using the NASCET measurement method, no evidence shows that symptomatic patients with a stenosis of less than 50% should be offered CEA. The only exception might be the rare patient with repeated transient ischemic attacks (TIAs) despite optimal medical therapy. In this situation (not least for medicolegal reasons), the surgeon should seek the input of a neurologist or stroke physician. Patients with a NASCET 50% to 69% stenosis gain a small yet significant benefit from CEA. However, this benefit is inextricably linked to the operative risk. Unequivocal evidence shows that patients with NASCET

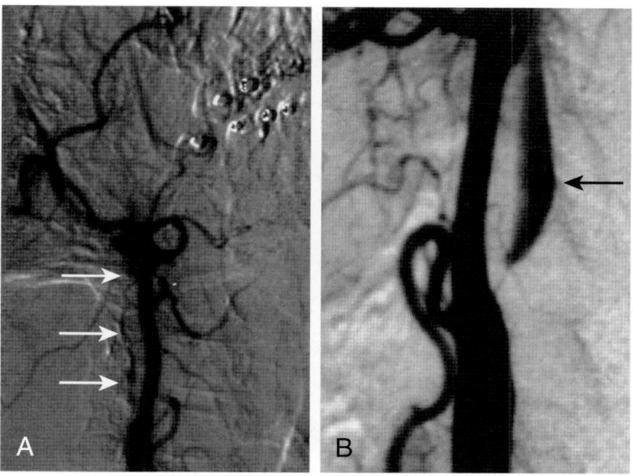

Figure 36-2. **A,** Near occlusion with a string sign is defined as a 95% to 99% stenosis with underfilling or nonvisualization or collapse of the distal internal carotid artery (ICA; *arrows*). **B,** Near occlusion with no string sign. Here, the distal ICA opens into a normal-caliber vessel *(arrow)*.

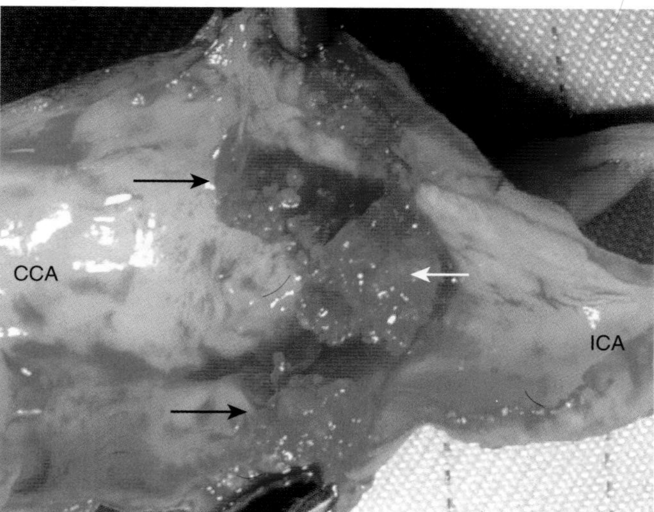

Figure 36-3. Opened carotid endarterectomy specimen in a patient presenting with crescendo transient ischemic attacks. The transected stenosis *(black arrows)* contains loose debris. Immediately distal to the stenosis is adherent fresh thrombus *(white arrow)*.

70% to 99% stenoses (an approximate ECST of 80% to 99%) benefit from CEA, although the magnitude of benefit varies according to certain patient and surgical factors (see later). Any patient with carotid territory symptoms and a severe ipsilateral stenosis should at least be considered for surgery. Exceptions include those with life-threatening comorbidity or senility, but even these patients benefit from optimization of risk factor management.

Concerns have arisen that patients older than 75 years may not benefit from CEA because it is perceived that their increased operative risk outweighs any long-term benefit. In fact, secondary analyses from NASCET[21] suggest that patients older than 75 years gain the most benefit, especially those with the severest grades of disease (absolute risk ratio 29% at 2 years, three CEAs to prevent one stroke). Accordingly, CEA should not be denied on the basis of chronological age; general fitness and biological age should always be the principal determinants.

Management of Patients with the "String Sign"

A string sign (otherwise known as near occlusion) is defined as a critical stenosis with underfilling or collapse of the distal ICA (Figure 36-2). Near occlusion with no string sign implies that the ICA opens into a normal-caliber vessel. Patients with the string sign have previously been considered to be at high risk for stroke, and any suspicion of this type of lesion on duplex imaging prompted urgent contrast angiography (with its attendant risks). Thereafter, these patients were heparinized and submitted to urgent exploration.

The CETC[12] undertook a separate analysis of outcomes in patients with an angiographic diagnosis of the string sign (Table 36-1). As can be seen, surgery did not confer any reduction in the 5-year risk of stroke in this situation. More importantly, no medically treated patient with a string sign in NASCET suffered a stroke within 30 days. These data therefore suggest that there is no need to consider emergency surgery in patients exhibiting the string sign; time is available for a more thorough evaluation. In Leicester, United Kingdom, these patients are now anticoagulated unless they are having ongoing cerebral events. This is because it is believed that the long-term embolic risk is very low. Moreover, because NASCET data suggested that two thirds of patients with a string sign have already recruited intracranial collateral pathways,[22] the risk of hemodynamic stroke must also be low.

Timing of CEA after the Most Recent Cerebral Event

Timing is one of the most topical subjects of the moment. ECST and NASCET recruited patients who reported ipsilateral symptoms within the preceding 6 months, and this has been used as the accepted threshold for treating symptomatic patients ever since. However, evidence increasingly shows that symptomatic patients need to be evaluated and treated more quickly. It is conventionally taught that the risk of stroke after presenting with a TIA or minor stroke is only about 1% to 2% at 7 days and 2% to 4% at 30 days. However, these data were derived from cohort studies that had several inherent biases. More recently, a review of 524 stroke patients who had reported a preceding TIA observed that 17% of TIAs occurred on the day of the stroke, 9% on the day before while 43% happened in the 7 days before the stroke.[23] Similarly, a metaanalysis of three population-based studies (which used face-to-face follow-up) observed that the risk of stroke following presentation with a stroke or TIA was 6.7% at 2 days and was 10.4% at 7 days.[24]

These risks are significantly higher than previously thought and suggest that a significant population of patients develop symptoms but then suffer their stroke before any of them can be offered surgery. The reason for the clustering of symptoms is because carotid stenoses are more likely to have overlying thrombus in the first week or so after onset of symptoms (Figure 36-3). More evidence supporting the need for expedited surgical intervention comes from the CETC, which performed subgroup analyses on the effect of delay to surgery on stroke prevention.[13,14] Figure 36-4 indicates the absolute risk reduction in the 5-year risk of ipsilateral stroke conferred

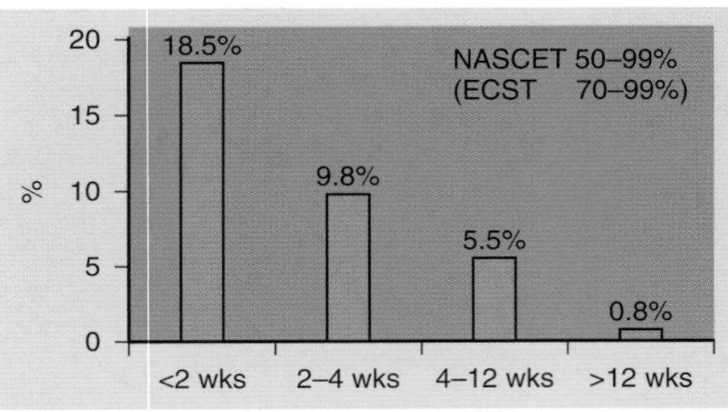

Figure 36-4. Absolute risk reduction (%) in ipsilateral stroke–conferred carotid endarterectomy (over best medical therapy) in symptomatic patients with 50% to 99% North American Symptomatic Carotid Endarterectomy Trial stenoses, stratified for delay from symptom onset to surgery in the international trials. (From Naylor AR. *Surgeon* 2007;5: 23-30. Data derived from the Carotid Endarterectomy Trialists Collaboration.[12-14])

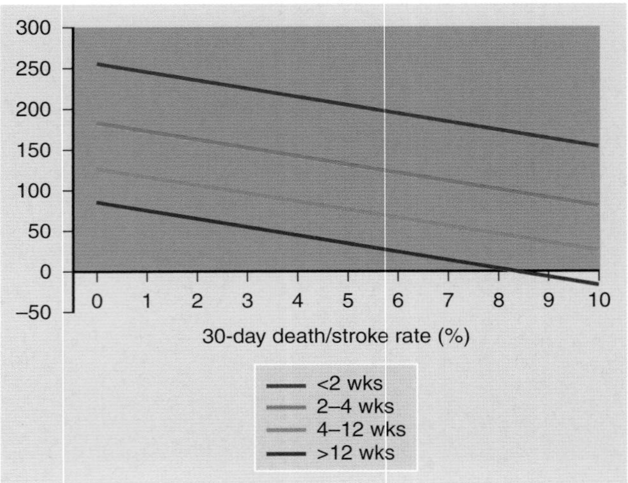

Figure 36-5. Number of ipsilateral strokes prevented at 5 years by performing 1000 carotid endarterectomies in symptomatic patients with North American Symptomatic Carotid Endarterectomy Trial 50% to 99% stenoses, stratified for delay to surgery and variations in the 30-day risk of death or stroke. (From Naylor AR. Time is brain! *Surgeon* 2007;5:23-30. Data derived from the Carotid Endarterectomy Trialists Collaboration.[12-14])

by CEA, stratified for the delay to surgery in patients with NASCET 50% to 99% stenoses. Note that the maximum benefit gained was when surgery was performed within 2 weeks of onset of symptoms. More worrying, however, is the lack of benefit conferred if surgery was delayed by more than 12 weeks.[13,25]

Of course, worries exist that expedited surgery will be associated with an increased procedural risk.[26] However, the available evidence suggests that even if this did happen, it would still be offset by the greater number of strokes prevented. Figure 36-5 models the number of ipsilateral strokes prevented at 5 years by performing 1000 CEAs with stratification for the delay to surgery and (most importantly) the procedural risk. Accordingly, were a surgeon to perform endarterectomy on patients within 2 weeks of onset of symptoms with a 10% procedural risk (which many consider excessive), the surgeon would still prevent more strokes in the long-term than by waiting 4 weeks and then operating with no risk.[25]

In the United Kingdom, the government has recommended that TIA or minor stroke should be treated as an emergency, with access to expedited CEA being available within 48 hours of onset of symptoms.[27] This threshold is going to be difficult to achieve because most health systems are currently incapable of meeting this kind of target. However, if a 7-day threshold for surgery became standard practice, this would result in a major improvement in long-term stroke prevention.

Timing of CEA after Stroke and Crescendo TIA

In the 1960s, there was a vogue for performing emergency CEA in patients with acute stroke secondary to carotid occlusion. This practice was associated with hemorrhagic transformation of the infarct in up to 60% of patients.[28] Since then, emergency CEA has largely been abandoned. The only exceptions (apart from in a trial) would be the immediate treatment of acute thrombotic stroke after CEA or carotid angioplasty.

In contrast to emergency CEA, urgent operation (within 24 hours) should be considered in patients with crescendo TIA or stroke in evolution. The former implies that the patient is suffering repeated TIAs, with full neurological recovery between attacks. Stroke in evolution suggests that partial recovery of the deficit is followed by repeated deterioration but never complete neurological recovery. It is assumed that both syndromes follow repeated embolization from an unstable plaque (Figure 36-3).

Following recognition that emergency CEA conferred no benefit after acute thrombotic stroke, it became customary to defer CEA for up to 8 weeks in all patients who had presented with a stroke (no matter how minor). This strategy has now been challenged, and a recent metaanalysis has shown that performing CEA on patients presenting with a minor stroke within 4 weeks was not associated with an increase in the procedural risk.[29] The key, of course, is careful patient selection. Expedited surgery should be reserved for patients who make a rapid early neurological recovery, achieve a neurological plateau, or both; who are Rankin score 0 to 2; and who do not have extensive middle cerebral artery territory infarctions on CT. Patients with extensive neurological deficits, carotid occlusion, intracranial hemorrhage, mental disorientation, and large areas of infarction on CT should not undergo early surgery.

Who Gains the Most Benefit from CEA?

An overview of the secondary analyses from NASCET and ECST has been helpful in identifying which patients gain the most (and least) benefit from CEA.[9] Table 36-3 details the absolute risk ratio conferred by CEA, together with the number of CEAs required to prevent one stroke in various situations. This table should be used to determine not who should be denied surgery but rather who needs fast tracking.

CEA conferred the maximum benefit in patients with a 95% carotid stenosis (but not near occlusion) plus plaque ulceration, or a 70% to 99% stenosis with contralateral occlusion (absolute risk ratio 47% to 54%). Only two operations were required to prevent one stroke at 2 years. Other clinical factors predictive of increased benefit from surgery include male sex, age greater than 75 years, cortical stroke presentation, and repeated symptoms for more than 6 months. Angiographic features associated with increased benefit from CEA include

Table 36-3
Relative Scale of Benefit for CEA over Best Medical Therapy in Symptomatic Patients from NASCET*

Stenosis	ARR	NNT	Stenosis	ARR	NNT
50-69% (all patients)	7% at 3 years	15	70-99% (all patients)	20% at 3 years	5
70-79% (all patients)	8% at 1 year	12	70-99% + contralateral 70-99% stenosis	20% at 2 years	5
50-99% + lacunar stroke	9% at 3 years	11	70-84% + intracranial disease	23% at 3 years	4
95-99% + no string	9% at 1 year	11	90-94% (all patients)	26% at 1 year	4
70-99% + patient <65 years	10% at 2 years	10	70-99% + patient >75 years	28% at 2 years	3
80-89% (all patients)	10% at 1 year	10	70-99% + >7 concurrent risk factors	30% at 2 years	3
70-99% + symptom onset <6 m	11% at 2 years	9	70-99% + recurrent events >6 months	30% at 2 years	3
75% + no plaque ulceration	11% at 2 years	9	85-99% + no intracranial collaterals	31% at 2 years	3
85% + no plaque ulceration	11% at 2 years	9	85% + plaque ulceration	32% at 2 years	3
95% + no plaque ulceration	11% at 2 years	9	85-99% + intracranial disease	37% at 3 years	3
50-99% + cortical stroke	15% at 3 years	7	70-99% + contralateral occlusion	47% at 2 years	2
70-99% + patient 65-74 years	15% at 3 years	7	95% + plaque ulceration	54% at 2 years	2

*ARR, actual risk reduction; CEA, carotid endarterectomy; NASCET, North American Symptomatic Carotid Endarterectomy Trial; NNT, number of CEAs required to prevent one stroke at a specified period.

plaque irregularity or ulceration and contralateral occlusion. Intracranial markers of increased stroke risk in medically treated patients include intracranial disease and a failure to recruit collaterals.

Should Staged or Synchronous CEA be Used in Patients with Severe Cardiac Disease?

With increasing awareness that aortic arch disease is probably the most important cause of stroke after coronary artery bypass grafting (CABG), debate has been renewed as to the value of staged or synchronous CEA. In a recent systematic review,[30] it was observed that 2% of patients suffered a stroke after CABG. Factors predictive of an increased risk of operative stroke included (1) carotid bruit (hazard ratio 3.6), (2) a history of stroke or TIA (hazard ratio 3.6), and (3) carotid stenosis of more than 50% or occlusion (hazard ratio 4.3). Interestingly, the first and third of these predictive features are also recognized to be highly predictive of aortic arch disease. This review also observed that about 85% of patients who suffered a stroke after CABG did not have significant carotid disease, while 60% had territorial infarctions on CT or autopsy that were incompatible with the underlying carotid disease. The review did indicate that the risk of stroke increased with the degree of carotid stenosis but was maximal (7% to 11%) in those with carotid occlusion. The stroke risk in patients who underwent a CABG (but no CEA) with asymptomatic bilateral 50% to 99% stenoses was only about 5%. Unfortunately, little quality data exist regarding the risk of stroke in patients with more severe grades of stenosis.

In practice, patients usually fall into one of two categories: patients undergoing CABG with asymptomatic carotid disease and symptomatic carotid patients with severe ischemic heart disease. In these situations, management strategies must be based on the available evidence and clinical reason for doing the operation. Most patients awaiting CEA do not need coronary revascularization. Symptomatic patients with severe cardiac disease are, however, at increased risk of perioperative myocardial events. The first-line strategy should always be optimization of medical management. For those in whom medical management is already considered optimal, the second-line approach is to see whether the coronary lesions are amenable to angioplasty, thereby enabling the surgeon to proceed with discrete CEA. This could also pose a logistical problem if the patient had to remain on clopidogrel after angioplasty. If angioplasty was not possible, the surgeon then has to decide between CEA under either local or regional anesthesia, staged CEA-CABG, or synchronous CEA-CABG. Synchronous procedures are currently preferred in Leicester, but no randomized trial evidence supports this strategy.

The main controversy, however, relates to the treatment of patients scheduled for CABG and who are found to have asymptomatic carotid disease. Metaanalyses suggest that staged (CEA-CABG), reverse staged (CABG-CEA), and synchronous CEA+CABG carry similar, quite considerable risks (Table 36-4) but that the magnitude of risk varies according to which procedure is performed first.[31] Reverse-staged (CABG-CEA) procedures incur a higher risk of stroke, whereas staged operations (CEA-CABG) have a higher incidence of cardiac events. Results for synchronous operations lie midway between. It should also be noted from Table 36-4 that synchronous and staged procedures incur considerable cumulative risk. In a large metaanalysis, the 30-day risk of death or stroke or myocardial infarction following synchronous CEA and CABG was 11.5%.[31] Staged procedures incurred a slightly lower cumulative risk, but this subgroup tended to have fewer patients with acute cardiological and neurological symptoms,

Table 36-4
Perioperative Outcomes for Synchronous and Staged CEA CABG*

	Operative Mortality	Ipsilateral Stroke	Any Stroke	Myocardial Infarction	Death +/− Ipsilat CVA	Death +/− Any CVA	Death +/− Any CVA +/− MI
Synchronous CEA+CABG							
Observed risk	359/7753	167/5643	333/7206	173/4800	413/5563	635/7260	513/4463
Risk (%)	4.6	3.0	4.6	3.6	7.4	8.7	11.5
95% CI	4.1-5.2	2.4-3.5	3.9-5.4	3.0-4.2	6.5-8.3	7.7-9.8	10.1-12.9
Heterogeneity *(p)*	0.0048	0.0002	<0.0001	0.0174	0.0001	<0.0001	<0.000
Staged CEA-CABG							
Observed risk	36/917	20/809	25/917	53/817	39/809	56/917	72/709
Risk (%)	3.9	2.5	2.7	6.5	4.8	6.1	10.2
95% CI	1.1-6.7	1.3-3.6	1.6-3.9	3.2-9.7	2.8-6.8	2.9-9.3	7.4-13.1
Heterogeneity *(p)*	<0.0001	<0.0001	<0.0001	0.9968	<0.0001	<0.0001	<0.0001
Staged CABG-CEA							
Observed risk	6/302	5/87	19/302	2/221	3/87	22/302	11/221
Risk (%)	2.0	5.8	6.3	0.9	3.4	7.3	5.0
95% CI	0.0-6.1	0.0-14.3	1.0-11.7	0.5-1.4	0.0-9.80	1.7-12.9	0.0-10.6
Heterogeneity *(p)*	<0.0001	0.2190	0.1784	<0.0001	0.0060	<0.0001	0.0102

From Naylor AR, Cuffe R, Rothwell PM, Bell PRF. *Eur J Vasc Endovasc Surg* 2003;25:380-389.
*CABG, coronary artery bypass grafting; CEA, carotid endarterectomy; CI, confidence interval; CVA, cerebral vascular accident; MI, myocardial infarction.

i.e., there is considerable potential for bias. The American Heart Association[15] currently sanctions CEA (staged or synchronous) in patients with asymptomatic carotid disease provided that the surgeon has an operative risk of less than 5% for discrete CEA in asymptomatic patients. Surgeons must therefore review their outcomes regularly, and management decisions must be made individually.

MANAGEMENT OF CAROTID DISEASE

Best Medical Management

All patients benefit from optimization of risk factors and introduction of antiplatelet- and lipid-lowering therapy. This role should not be delegated to the most junior member of the team as this aspect of patient care involves more than simply advising patients to stop smoking and take aspirin.

Ischemic heart disease was the main cause of death in ECST and NASCET. Accordingly, cardiac status should be evaluated and therapy for angina optimized. Controversy relates to whether routine preoperative cardiological assessment is necessary. This is more commonly practiced in North America. In the United Kingdom, cardiac referral is normally reserved for patients with cardiac failure and poor functional capacity, recent myocardial infarction (within 8 weeks), severe or unstable angina, severe valvular disease, symptomatic arrhythmias, or recurrence of symptoms after cardiac surgery or angioplasty.

Treatment of hypertension remains the cornerstone of stroke prevention. Treatment thresholds vary among countries and by age. In practice, patients less than 60 years old with a blood pressure (BP) higher than 140/90 mm Hg require treatment. As the patient ages, a slight relaxation in thresholds is permissible. Metaanalyses suggest that for every 5-mm Hg reduction in diastolic BP there is a 15% relative reduction in stroke.[31] Moreover, no patient should undergo CEA with a systolic BP of more than 180 mm Hg (unless clinically indicated) as this is an independent risk factor for operative stroke.[33]

Wherever possible, patients should be on antiplatelet therapy. Aspirin (cyclooxygenase pathway inhibitor) confers a 15% reduction in late stroke in patients presenting with TIA or stroke.[34] The optimal dose of aspirin is controversial. NASCET suggested that higher doses (600 to 1200 mg) were associated with a lower risk of operative events.[2] However, a large randomized trial has now clearly shown the converse to be true.[35] Although clopidogrel (adenosine diphosphate inhibitor) confers a small but significant reduction in any vascular event, no evidence shows that it specifically reduces the risk of stroke.[36] It does, however, significantly increase the bleeding time.[37] This should be borne in mind in patients scheduled for surgery. Metaanalyses suggest that the combination of aspirin plus dipyridamole reduces the risk of stroke by 23%. Unfortunately, up to 25% of patients have to stop treatment because of adverse side effects.[38] Thus, for all practical purposes, the evidence suggests that all patients should be on 75 to 300 mg of aspirin and that this should not be stopped before surgery. Clopidogrel is probably the second-line drug in those unable to take aspirin. Some surgeons stop clopidogrel treatment several days before CEA, particularly in patients taking the combination of clopidogrel and aspirin.

Careful control of blood glucose in diabetic patients is essential for the avoidance of diabetic complications. However, no evidence[39] shows that tight glycemic control actually reduces the risk of stroke. The U.K. Prospective Diabetes Study Group[40] has reported that type 2 diabetic patients require extremely tight control of BP (mean of less than 144/82 mm Hg). Evidence suggests that this reduces the risk of late stroke by up to 44%.

Treatment of hyperlipidemia is now much less controversial. The Medical Research Council/British Heart Foundation Heart Protection Study randomized more than 20,000 patients and showed that 40 mg of simvastatin daily conferred a 12% reduction in total mortality, a 17% reduction in vascular mortality, a 24% reduction in coronary events, and a 27% reduction in stroke.[41] This trial has changed practice throughout the world, especially as significant benefit was conferred

Table 36-5
Preoperative Surgical Checklist

- Is the reason for surgery clearly documented?
- Are there any atypical symptoms warranting further investigation?
- Is the degree of stenosis appropriate for surgery?
- Have the perioperative risks been documented in the notes?
- Is the patient on optimal medical therapy?
- Consider rescanning the carotid arteries before surgery.
- Is high carotid disease anticipated?
- Assess cranial nerve status in all patients with previous neck surgery.
- Mark the operation side with an indelible marker.

irrespective of age, gender, or cholesterol level. The latter observation suggests that some benefit conferred by statins is probably via a pleiotrophic effect. Accordingly, unless there is a contraindication, patients with symptomatic and asymptomatic carotid artery disease should be prescribed a statin or other type of lipid-lowering agent.

In the past, concerns existed that patients with multiple comorbidity gained less benefit from CEA, either because of an increased operative risk or because the patient was unlikely to live long enough to gain clinical advantage. NASCET has now shown that the presence of increasing comorbidity does not influence the long-term risk of stroke after CEA. By contrast, the presence of multiple risk factors significantly increased the risk of stroke in medically treated patients with severe carotid disease.[2] Little compelling evidence, however, exists that asymptomatic patients with significant medical comorbidity benefit from intervention.

PRINCIPLES OF SURGICAL MANAGEMENT

Preoperative Checklist

Before submitting a patient to surgery, it is important that the surgeon completes a checklist to minimize morbidity and mortality and potential exposure to medicolegal criticism (Table 36-5). In particular, the reasons for performing the operation should be documented clearly in the case notes, together with a review of the procedural risks (stroke, death, cranial nerve injury). The surgeon must also ensure that the patient is receiving optimal medical therapy.

The status of the cranial nerves should be reviewed. Any patient who has previously undergone thyroid surgery, radical neck surgery, or contralateral CEA should undergo indirect laryngoscopy and evaluation of hypoglossal and glossopharyngeal nerve function before undertaking CEA on the other side. Bilateral recurrent laryngeal or hypoglossal nerve injury is potentially fatal. If any evidence of injury appears, the surgeon should review the indication for surgery. It might, for example, be appropriate to abandon CEA in an asymptomatic patient with laryngoscopic evidence of contralateral vocal cord palsy or, alternatively, to consider angioplasty. If surgery is still deemed necessary, the patient must be warned of the potential for emergency (even permanent) tracheotomy.

In the United Kingdom and many parts of Europe, it is considered good practice to repeat the duplex examination immediately before operation. In North America, this is less commonly undertaken. Repeat duplex imaging enables the level of the bifurcation to be marked and ensures that the ICA has not occluded while awaiting surgery (thereby avoiding an unnecessary procedure). It also serves as a validation study against which the original magnetic resonance angiography, duplex imaging, angiogram, or resected plaque can be compared. In addition, it enables a regular review of duplex technologist practice (internal validation and quality control). Finally, it provides the surgeon with a last chance to exclude unexpected inflow and outflow disease or unrecognized distal disease extension. It is essential to anticipate high internal carotid disease.

TECHNIQUE OF CAROTID ENDARTERECTOMY

Position

The patient lies supine with the head extended and rotated away from the operation side. A sandbag beneath the shoulders and a head ring facilitate this. To reduce venous congestion, the head of the table is raised (Figure 36-6A). A urethral catheter minimizes discomfort from a full bladder, which can aggravate postoperative hypertension. The patient should receive perioperative intravenous antibiotic prophylaxis.

Choice of Anesthesia

Carotid surgery has traditionally been performed under general anesthesia, largely because the surgeon finds it less stressful, the operation does not need to be rushed (especially when supervising trainees), patient movement is avoided, and theoretical benefits exist regarding reduced cerebral metabolic requirements. More recently, there has been a vogue toward CEA under either local or regional anesthesia—hereafter to be described as locoregional anesthesia (LRA)—because it is the optimal method for neurological monitoring and selective shunting. Anesthesia is produced by varying combinations of local infiltration, deep and superficial cervical plexus blockade with 0.5% bupivacaine, or both. Light intravenous sedation may also be employed if a patient is agitated or anxious.

The evidence regarding LRA versus general anesthesia is conflicting. Few randomized trials have been performed, and none has shown that LRA reduces the overall stroke or cardiovascular risk.[42] However, an updated metaanalysis of nonrandomized studies suggested that LRA may be associated with a reduction in the rate of perioperative stroke, myocardial infarction, and pulmonary complications.[42] This debate will be helped immeasurably by the 2008 publication of the General Anaesthetic Local Anaesthetic (GALA) Trial. This trial is destined to become the largest randomized trial of CEA (more than 3000 patients) and should demonstrate whether choice of anesthesia influences outcome.

Is Distal Disease Extension a Possibility?

The possibility that the disease process might extend distally up the ICA must be anticipated in advance, not least because the operative risks increase (especially cranial nerve injury). It is not possible to perform temporomandibular subluxation once the procedure is under way.

Simple measures to facilitate distal ICA access include nasolaryngeal intubation (Figure 36-6B), which opens the angle

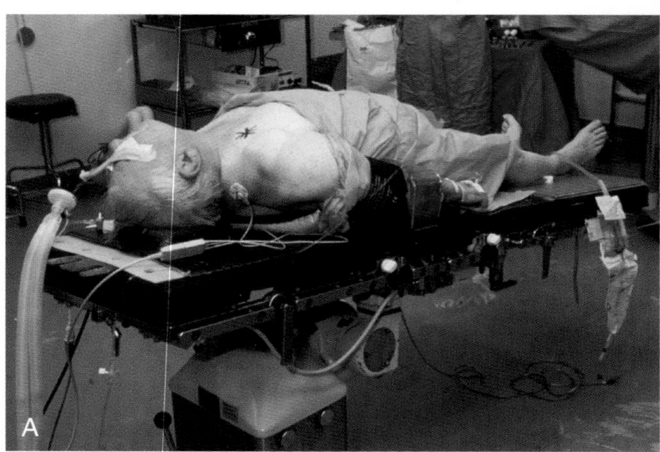

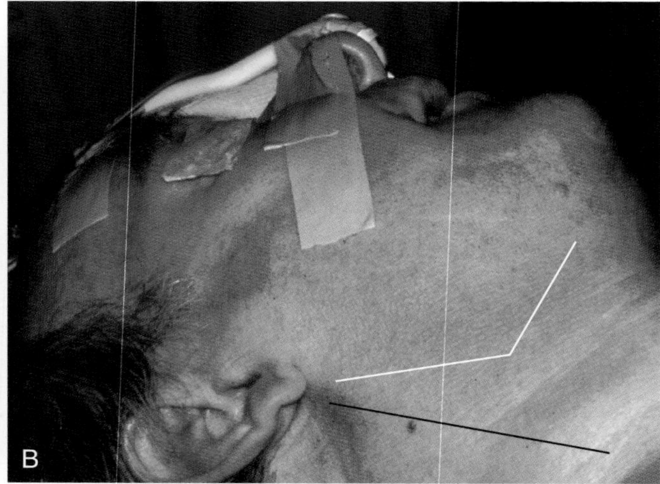

Figure 36-6. **A,** The side of the operation should be clearly marked. The patient is positioned head up to reduce venous congestion, and the table is slightly rotated away from the operative side. **B,** Patients with a "short neck" or suspected high disease extension benefit from nasolaryngeal intubation. This opens up the angle of access between the mastoid process or sternomastoid *(black line)* and the mandible *(white line)*.

between the mandible and the mastoid process. Temporomandibular dislocation has largely been replaced by subluxation. Here, the condyle is pulled anteriorly to rest under the articular eminence and stabilized by intraoral fixation wires, which are removed at the end of the procedure. Mandibular subluxation is associated with few complications and surprisingly little postoperative and long-term discomfort. An aid to accessing the upper reaches of the carotid artery once surgery is under way is discussed later in this chapter.

Exposure of the Carotid Bifurcation

The skin incision is made over the anterior border of sternomastoid, preserving the great auricular nerve superiorly. Alternatively, a transverse skin crease skin incision is used. No evidence shows that either is preferable. Skin edge bleeding is minimized by infiltrating the skin and subcutaneous tissues preoperatively with 0.5% bupivacaine with adrenaline. Dissection continues anterior to sternomastoid. The common facial vein traverses the operative field and overlies the carotid bifurcation. This is divided, and dissection continues in a plane immediately medial to the internal jugular vein. Some surgeons expose the ICA by dissecting laterally along the internal jugular vein. This obviates the need to divide the common facial vein and is said to allow easier exposure of the distal ICA. Comparative trials do not yet exist.

In individuals with a fat neck, a large pad of fat and lymph nodes often overlie the common facial vein and carotid bifurcation. The fat pad should be mobilized toward the operating surgeon. This minimizes troublesome bleeding and exposes a relatively avascular triangle bounded superiorly by digastric muscle. The bifurcation can also become slightly rotated, and branches may appear to emerge at unusual angles. Confusion can be avoided by remembering to mobilize all external carotid artery (ECA) branches toward the first assistant. (Remember: lymph nodes toward you, branches away.)

Access to the ICA just distal to the bifurcation is facilitated by (1) division of the digastric muscle (Figure 36-7A); (2) division of the sternomastoid branch of the ECA (plus vein), which tethers the hypoglossal nerve (Figure 36-7B); and (3) careful retraction of the hypoglossal nerve. This is aided by dividing the ansa cervicalis. A suture tie placed on the divided ansa acts as a useful retractor or elevator of the hypoglossal nerve and avoids the damage associated with a sling (Figure 36-7C). Finally, more distal branches of the ECA may have to be divided (Figure 36-7D) to mobilize the hypoglossal nerve and expose the diseased segment of the ICA completely.

Dissection continues until the ICA, common carotid artery (CCA), and ECA are mobilized above and below the disease (Figure 36-8). The bifurcation should not be skeletonized as this predisposes to functional elongation and kinking and increases the risk of embolization during the dissection phase. The patient is given 5000 units of heparin intravenously. Few centers measure coagulation profiles as no evidence shows that modifying the heparin dose alters outcome.

Minimizing Cranial Nerve Injury

The keys to minimizing cranial nerve injury are (1) knowledge of the anatomy, (2) care not to divide any neural tissue traversing the bifurcation (Figure 36-9) apart from the ansa (Figure 36-7B and 36-7C), (3) avoiding inclusion of the vagus nerve in the carotid clamps, (4) avoiding diathermy in the vicinity of the cranial nerves, and (5) careful division of the tissue between the hypoglossal and the glossopharyngeal nerves (Figure 36-10). This filmy, membranous tissue plane contains small motor branches from the vagus, and damage to them is probably the commonest reason for swallowing problems postoperatively.

Whether to Shunt

Insertion of a plastic shunt between the CCA and the ICA during endarterectomy can maintain cerebral flood flow. Surgeons tend to be routine, selective, or never shunters. An overview of the randomized trials by the Cochrane Collaboration[43] has failed to show that one strategy is better than another. However, the consensus is that routine or selective shunting is preferable to never shunting. Surgeons who shunt routinely

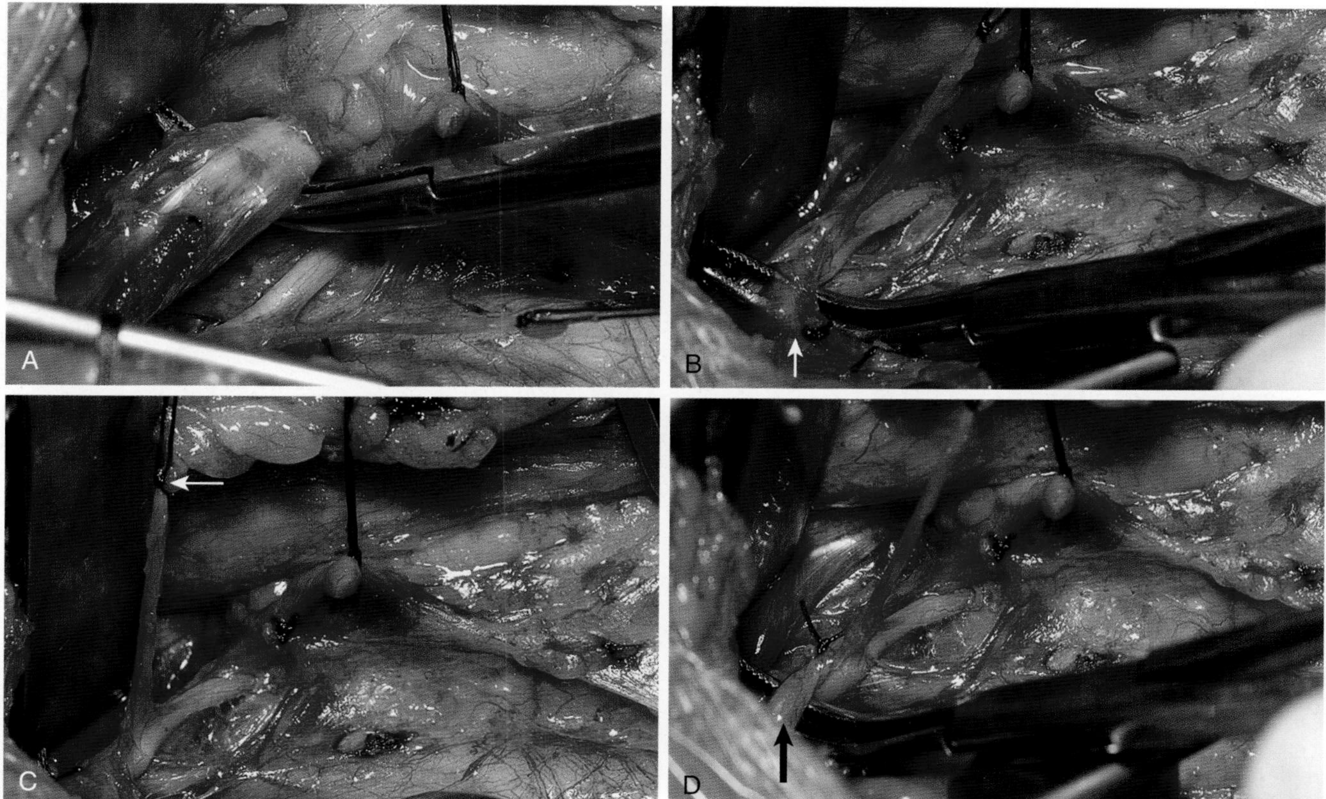

Figure 36-7. Distal internal carotid artery access is facilitated by several maneuvers. **A,** Division of digastric, here seen overlying the hypoglossal nerve. **B,** Division of sternomastoid artery or vein *(white arrow),* which tethers the hypoglossal nerve. The ansa cervicalis *(white arrow)* has not yet been divided. **C,** Division of the ansa. A ligature tied to the divided ansa *(arrow)* allows the hypoglossal nerve to be retracted without traumatizing the nerve. **D,** Further access is facilitated by progressively dividing higher external carotid artery branches *(arrow).*

argue that CEA need not be hurried, trainees are supervised in a less stressful environment, and familiarity with shunt insertion means that it is generally easier to operate around the shunt (Figure 36-8B), especially during high exploration. Selective users argue that shunts are only necessary in 10% to 15% of patients, they can cause intimal damage and secondary thromboembolism, and that they get in the way.

It is important to remember that having a shunt in place does not mean it is working. About 3% of shunts malfunction, usually due to impaction on distal ICA coils or kinks.[44] Unless some form of monitoring is available, this is missed. In addition, advocates of selective shunting must accept that awake testing under LRA is the only infallible method for determining who needs a shunt. No other monitoring technique can (or will) provide this information so reliably. Selective shunters must also accept that hemodynamic failure accounts for only 20% of intraoperative strokes.[45] The remainder (due to thromboembolism) still occur unless some other form of monitoring is employed.

The most commonly used shunts are the Javid and the Pruitt-Inahara. The Javid is tapered and held in place with proximal and distal retaining clamps. It has higher flow rates than the Pruitt-Inahara. Its main limitation is the need for more distal dissection to position the retaining clamp. The Pruitt-Inahara has balloons that hold the shunt in position (Figure 36-8B) and facilitate access to the distal ICA. The Pruitt-Inahara does have lower flow rates. However, 90% of patients have flows within 10% of their preclamp value,[46] and no systematic evidence shows that shunt type alters outcome.

Traditional or Eversion Endarterectomy

In a traditional endarterectomy, a Watson-Cheyne dissector is insinuated between the plaque and the media (Figure 36-11A). The plaque is divided proximally, and the dissection plane is continued caudally up the ICA until it either feathers or is transected (Figure 36-11B). The ECA plaque is everted. No evidence shows that tacking sutures alter outcome. In NASCET, tacking sutures were associated with an increased operative risk; however, this could simply mean that a smooth intimal step was more difficult to achieve because of technical problems (high disease, posterior tongue of plaque, excessively thinned wall). Following plaque removal, loose intimal flaps are removed from the endarterectomy zone in a radial direction (Figure 36-12). The arteriotomy is then closed primarily or with a patch (Figure 36-13).

Eversion CEA involves transection of the ICA at its origin (Figure 36-14). The ICA is then everted and the tube of atheroma is expelled. Once the distal limit is exposed, the lesion is excised. The ICA is then shortened, as appropriate, and reanastomosed to the bifurcation after endarterectomy of the distal CCA. Advantages of eversion CEA include no lengthening or kinking of the ICA, and no patching. Clamp time is

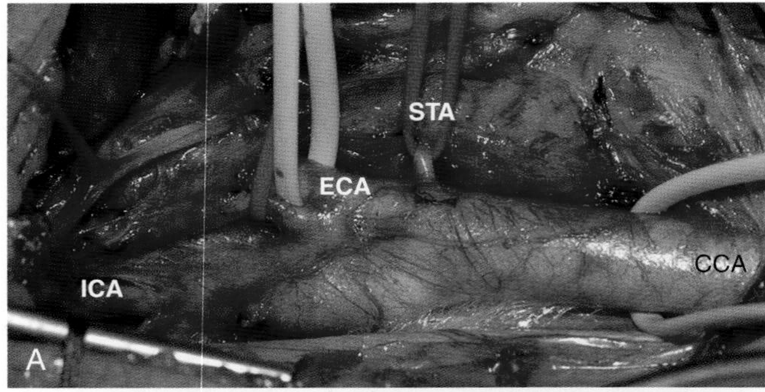

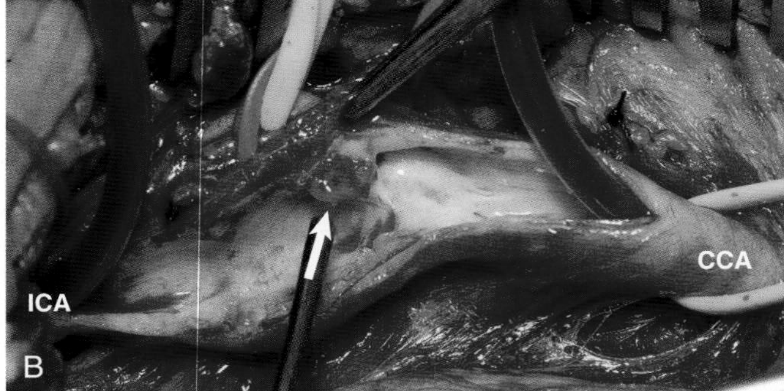

Figure 36-8. **A,** The common carotid artery (CCA), internal carotid artery, external carotid artery, and superior thyroid artery are mobilized but not skeletonized. The aim is to ensure that access is provided above and below the stenosis so that it is possible to insert a shunt easily and atraumatically. **B,** The arteriotomy has been made across the bifurcation, and a Pruitt-Inahara shunt has been inserted. Note the fresh thrombus overlying the stenosis *(white arrow)*. The sling around the CCA is secured around the hub of a West retractor to prevent accidental dislodgment of the proximal balloon of the Pruitt-Inahara shunt. Note that the shunt does not interfere with access to the diseased segment of artery.

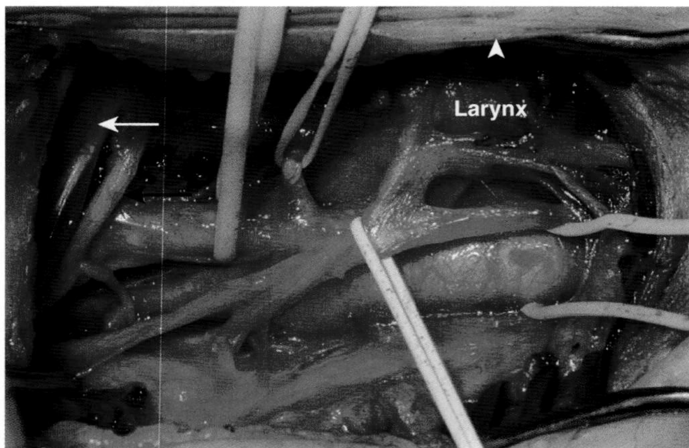

Figure 36-9. Aberrant cranial nerve anatomy. The hypoglossal nerve *(black arrow)* is immediately inferior to digastric *(white arrow)*. The white sling encircles a complex series of aberrant neural structures traversing the bifurcation. These should not be divided.

generally shorter. However, it is not usually possible to insert a shunt until after the endarterectomy has been completed, and the worry is always that a distal intimal flap may go unnoticed. A systematic review[47] has shown no evidence that eversion endarterectomy is preferable to conventional endarterectomy if the arteriotomy is patched.

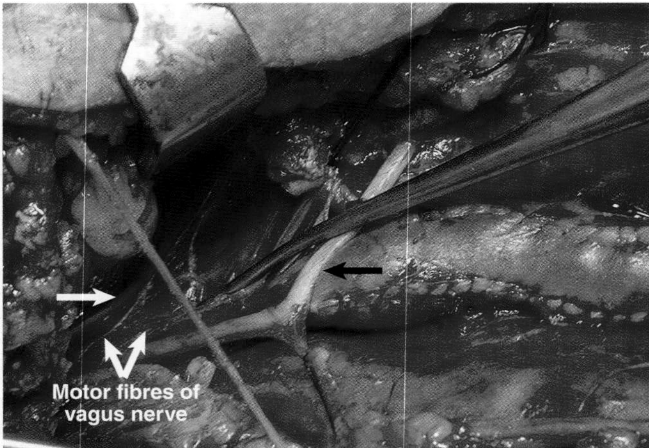

Figure 36-10. Operative view during a high carotid dissection. Between the hypoglossal nerve *(black arrow)* and the glossopharyngeal nerve *(white arrow)* is a thin membrane containing small motor fibers from the vagus nerve. These should be preserved wherever possible. Division of these fibers is one of the commonest reasons for postoperative swallowing problems.

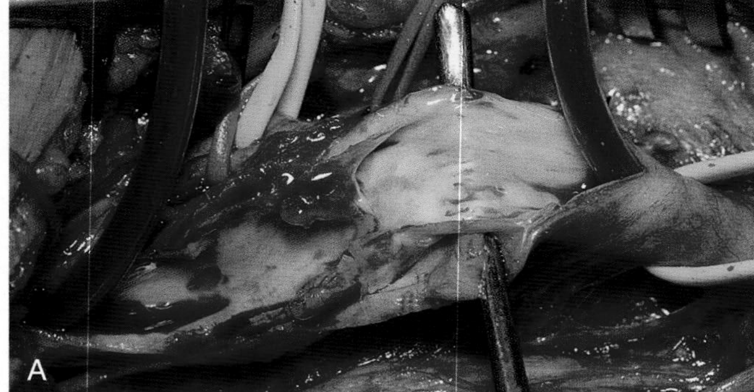

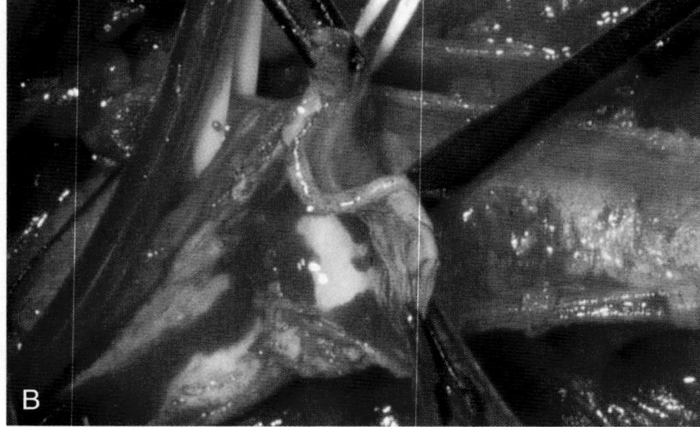

Figure 36-11. **A,** Traditional endarterectomy starts with a Watson-Cheyne dissector insinuated between the plaque and the media in the distal common carotid artery. The plaque is divided over the Watson-Cheyne using a scalpel. **B,** The plaque is then removed by cephalad endarterectomy.

Whether to Patch

The 2004 metaanalysis of randomized trials showed that a policy of routine carotid patching was preferable to routine primary closure (Figure 36-15) and conferred significant

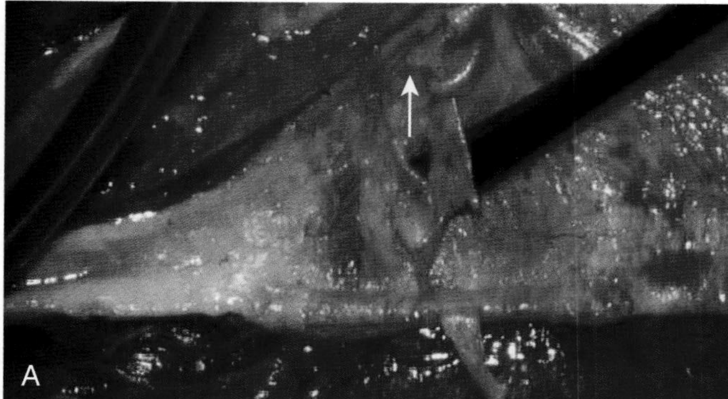

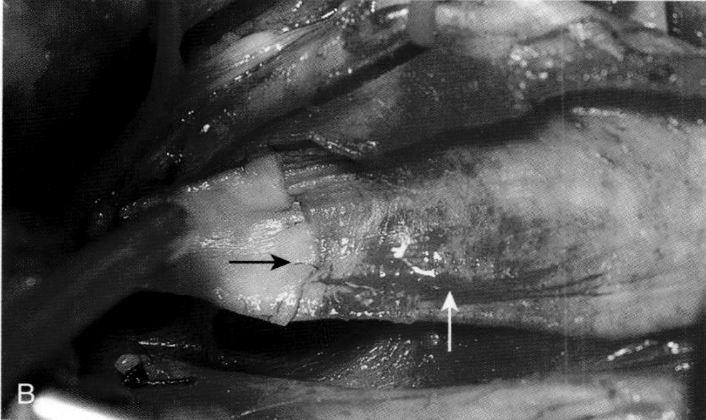

Figure 36-12. The distal intimal step is defined. **A,** Any residual intimal flaps are removed in a radial direction *(arrow)*. Axial (longitudinal) removal of intimal flaps causes a deepening of the endarterectomy plane and may damage the integrity of the arterial wall. **B,** In this case, the distal intimal step has been tacked down *(black arrow)*. Note the bleeding onto the surface of the endarterectomized artery *(white arrow)*. This is derived from "sheared" vasa vasorum, and the ensuing thrombus (unless removed) is an important source of thromboembolism following restoration of flow (see also Figure 36-16).

reductions in early perioperative risks and thrombosis, and a highly significant reduction in late restenosis.[48] No randomized trials have compared routine with selective patching. For those surgeons who prefer a policy of selective patching, criteria usually include female patients, an ICA diameter of less than 5 mm, and an ICA arteriotomy of more than 2 cm. No evidence shows that patch type (prosthetic or vein) affects outcome.[48] Vein patches are susceptible to central rupture

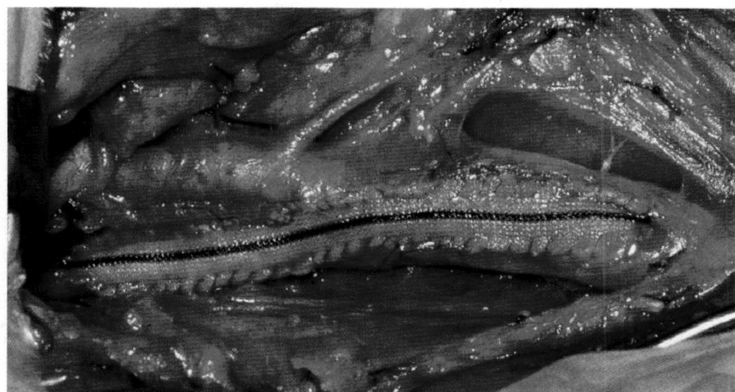

Figure 36-13. Completed endarterectomy with the arteriotomy closed with a thin-walled collagen impregnated polyester patch.

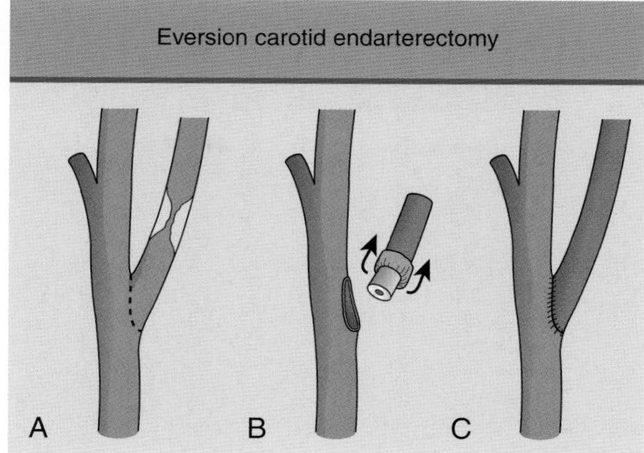

Figure 36-14. Eversion endarterectomy. **A,** The internal carotid artery (ICA) is detached from the bifurcation along the dotted line. **B,** The adventitia/residual media is everted and the core of atheroma expelled. **C,** The ICA can be shortened as appropriate and reanastomosed to the bifurcation after distal common carotid artery (CCA) endarterectomy.

(overall incidence 1%). The risk is increased in women with hypertension but most particularly in those in whom the vein is harvested from the ankle. Prosthetic patches are vulnerable to a 1% incidence of infection (described later).

Monitoring and Quality Control Assessment

Despite awareness that most strokes after CEA follow inadvertent technical error,[49] few surgeons employ any type of completion assessment and no consensus exists about the role of monitoring during carotid surgery. Reasons include the absence of any randomized trials; the lack of accurate audits of the actual causes of perioperative stroke; a tendency to overinterpret single issues, such as the role of the shunt or patch; logistical issues relating to access to equipment and personnel; the mistaken view that one monitoring method is infallible; and most importantly, a failure to ask the right questions.[50]

Each unit has a responsibility to audit its own practice. If it is perceived that there might be a problem, the first question to ask is whether most strokes are intraoperative (i.e., apparent upon recovery from anesthesia) and therefore attributable to an adverse event during the operation. Postoperative strokes occur after normal recovery from anesthesia. Intraoperative strokes (historically the commonest) are predominantly thromboembolic in etiology or hemodynamic (about 20%). Thus, when trying to develop a monitoring protocol, methods must be used that answer the question posed. Table 36-6 presents the chronological sequence from embolus through hemodynamic failure to the onset of a neurological deficit and indicates which monitoring technique detects the underlying problem. For example, performing CEA under LRA is an infallible way of detecting hemodynamic failure during clamping, but it cannot be blamed for failing to warn a surgeon that embolization is occurring. Only transcranial Doppler (TCD) can warn the surgeon of an unstable plaque during dissection or of embolization preceding on-table thrombosis.[51]

A similar approach should apply when evaluating methods for assessing the technical performance of CEA. Table 36-7

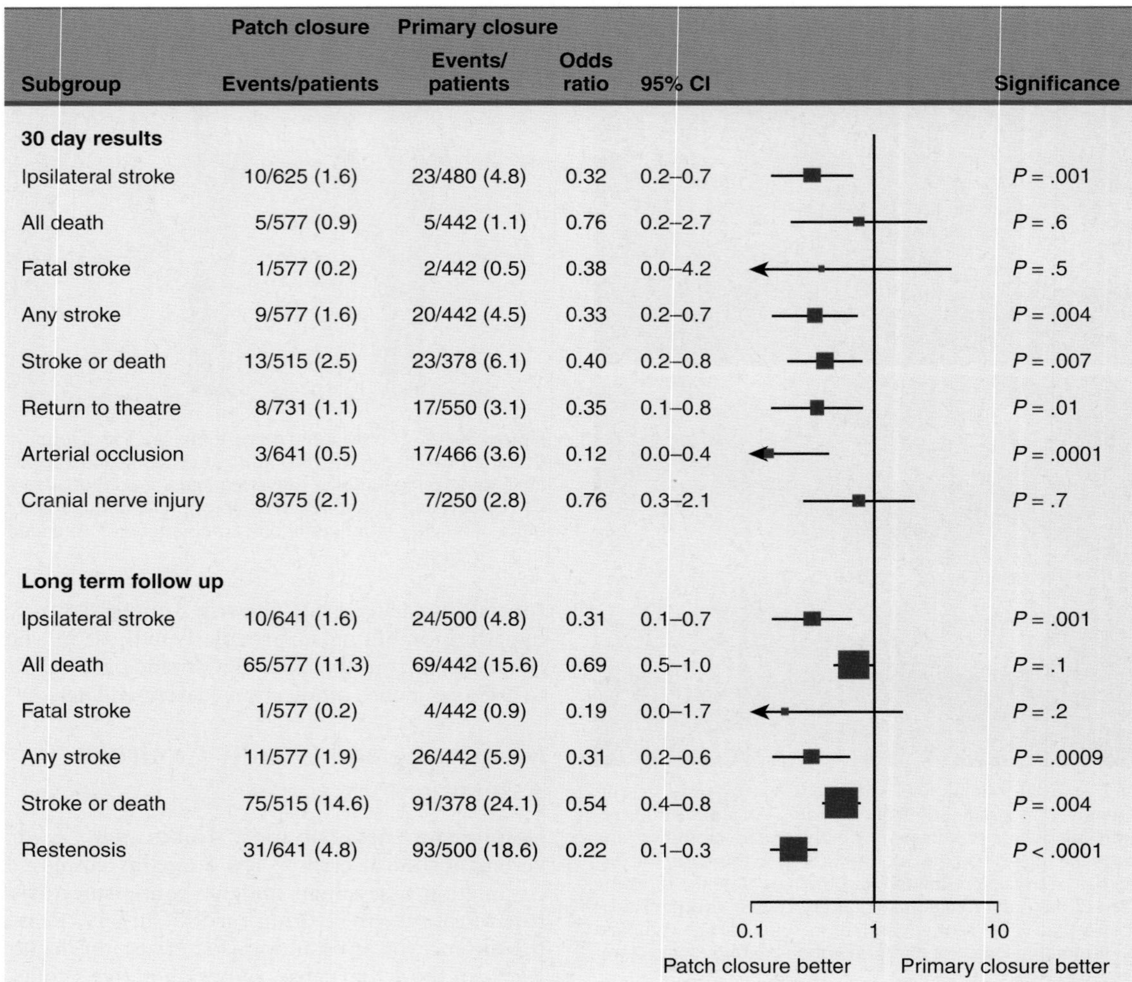

Subgroup	Patch closure Events/patients	Primary closure Events/patients	Odds ratio	95% CI	Significance
30 day results					
Ipsilateral stroke	10/625 (1.6)	23/480 (4.8)	0.32	0.2–0.7	P = .001
All death	5/577 (0.9)	5/442 (1.1)	0.76	0.2–2.7	P = .6
Fatal stroke	1/577 (0.2)	2/442 (0.5)	0.38	0.0–4.2	P = .5
Any stroke	9/577 (1.6)	20/442 (4.5)	0.33	0.2–0.7	P = .004
Stroke or death	13/515 (2.5)	23/378 (6.1)	0.40	0.2–0.8	P = .007
Return to theatre	8/731 (1.1)	17/550 (3.1)	0.35	0.1–0.8	P = .01
Arterial occlusion	3/641 (0.5)	17/466 (3.6)	0.12	0.0–0.4	P = .0001
Cranial nerve injury	8/375 (2.1)	7/250 (2.8)	0.76	0.3–2.1	P = .7
Long term follow up					
Ipsilateral stroke	10/641 (1.6)	24/500 (4.8)	0.31	0.1–0.7	P = .001
All death	65/577 (11.3)	69/442 (15.6)	0.69	0.5–1.0	P = .1
Fatal stroke	1/577 (0.2)	4/442 (0.9)	0.19	0.0–1.7	P = .2
Any stroke	11/577 (1.9)	26/442 (5.9)	0.31	0.2–0.6	P = .0009
Stroke or death	75/515 (14.6)	91/378 (24.1)	0.54	0.4–0.8	P = .004
Restenosis	31/641 (4.8)	93/500 (18.6)	0.22	0.1–0.3	P < .0001

Figure 36-15. Summary estimates of treatment effect from metaanalysis outcomes from seven randomized trials comparing patch angioplasty versus primary closure. The review included 1193 patients (1281 operations). Note that for most outcomes the treatment effect significantly favors routine patch closure rather than routine primary closure. (From Bond R, Rerkasem K, Naylor AR, et al. *J Vasc Surg* 2004;40:1126-1135.)

lists the principal technical errors and those methods best able to identify them. The choice of technique inevitably reflects each center's access to resources and personnel; what is appropriate for one unit may not be effective in another. Surgeons with an operative risk under 3% will feel that change is unnecessary. Others may decide to use one or more monitoring modalities once a review has been made of when most complications occur. It is, however, not acceptable for surgeons with poor outcomes simply to dismiss the concept of monitoring and quality control assessment just because others can achieve complication rates below 2% without them.[51]

Table 36-6
The Role of Monitoring Techniques during Carotid Surgery*

Detection of Embolism	→	Detection of Reduced Perfusion	→	Detection of Loss of Electrical Activity	→	Detection of Neuronal Injury
TCD		Reduced stump pressure Reduced ICA back flow Near-infrared spectroscopy Jugular venous oxygen saturation Xenon-CBF measurement TCD		EEG SSEP		Awake testing

Adapted from Naylor AR, Mackey WC. Editorial comment: is there any evidence that peri-operative monitoring and quality control assessment alter clinical outcome? In: Naylor AR, Mackey WC, eds. *Carotid artery surgery: a problem based approach*. London: WB Saunders; 2000:313-314.
*CBF, cerebral blood flow; EEG, electroencephalography; ICA, internal carotid artery; SSEP, somatosensory evoked potential; TCD, transcranial Doppler.

Table 36-7
The Role of Quality Control Methods during Carotid Surgery*

Embolization	Shunt Malfunction	Luminal Thrombus	Intimal Flap	Distal Stenosis
Immediate: TCD Delayed: EEG SSEP Awake testing	Immediate: TCD Delayed: EEG SSEP Awake testing	Angioscopy Angiography Duplex	Angioscopy Angiography Duplex	Angioscopy Angiography Duplex CW Doppler

Adapted from Naylor AR, Mackey WC. Editorial comment: is there any evidence that peri-operative monitoring and quality control assessment alter clinical outcome? In: Naylor AR, Mackey WC, eds. *Carotid artery surgery: a problem based approach.* London: WB Saunders; 2000:313-314.
*CW Doppler, continuous wave Doppler analysis; EEG, electroencephalography; SSEP, somatosensory evoked potential; TCD, transcranial Doppler.

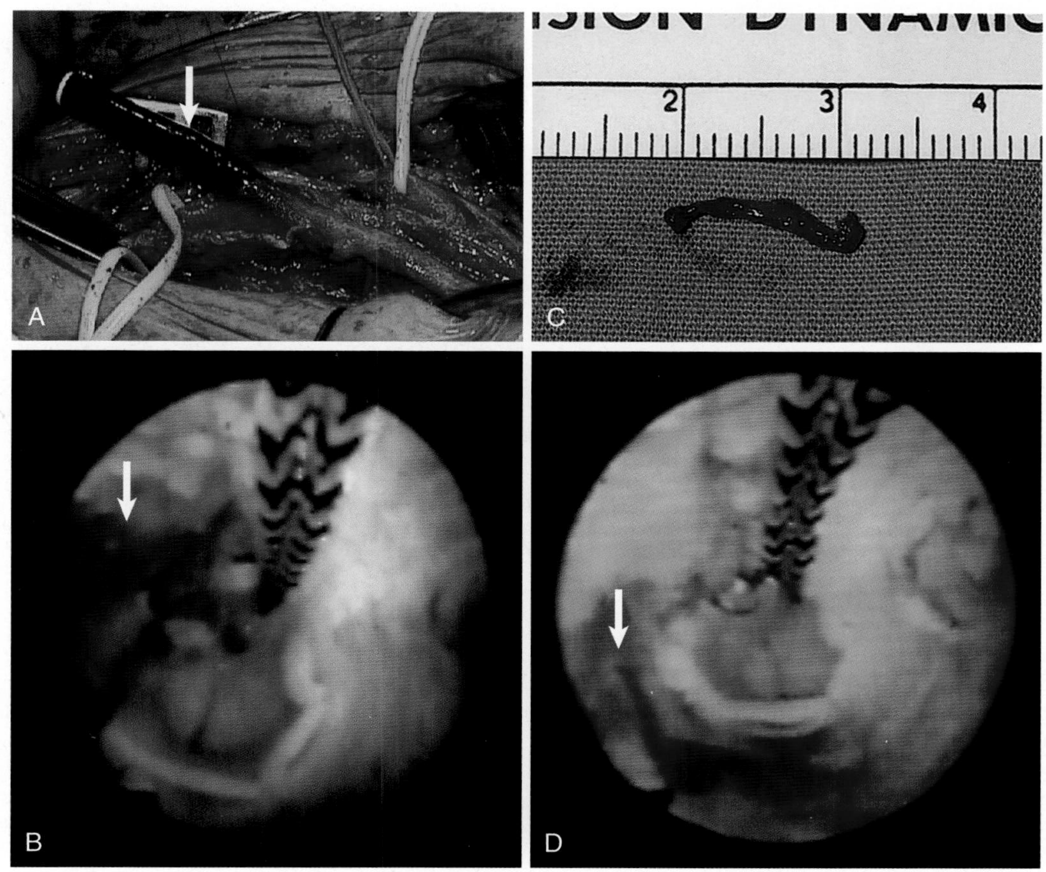

Figure 36-16. Completion angioscopy. **A,** The angioscope (this is actually a hysteroscope) is inserted into the endarterectomy zone before finally completing patch closure *(arrow).* **B,** Thrombus adherent to the proximal common carotid artery *(arrow)* despite prior irrigation with heparinized saline. **C,** Size of thrombus retrieved from panel B. **D,** Bleeding from the vasa vasorum *(arrow)* is the source of these luminal thrombi. (**B** and **C** from Leonard N, Smith JL, Gaunt ME, et al. *Eur J Vasc Endovasc Surg* 1999;17:234-240.)

In Leicester, a combination of monitoring and quality control methods is used (intraoperative TCD, completion angioscopy, and postoperative TCD monitoring). Each has specific questions to answer based on a series of prospective audit studies in 1400 patients.[52] There are only three roles for intraoperative TCD: (1) warning of embolization from unstable plaques during carotid dissection, thus allowing the surgeon to modify the operative technique; (2) providing optimal shunt function by immediately identifying kinking, noting impaction of the distal shunt lumen against a distal ICA coil, and ensuring that the mean middle cerebral artery velocity is more than 15 cm/sec; and (3) rapidly identifying the rare patient who is at risk of developing on-table thrombosis through the detection of increasing rates of embolization while the neck wound is being closed.

Completion angioscopy[53] enables the lumen of the endarterectomy zone to be inspected before flow is restored (Figure 36-16). This is important, as the commonest cause

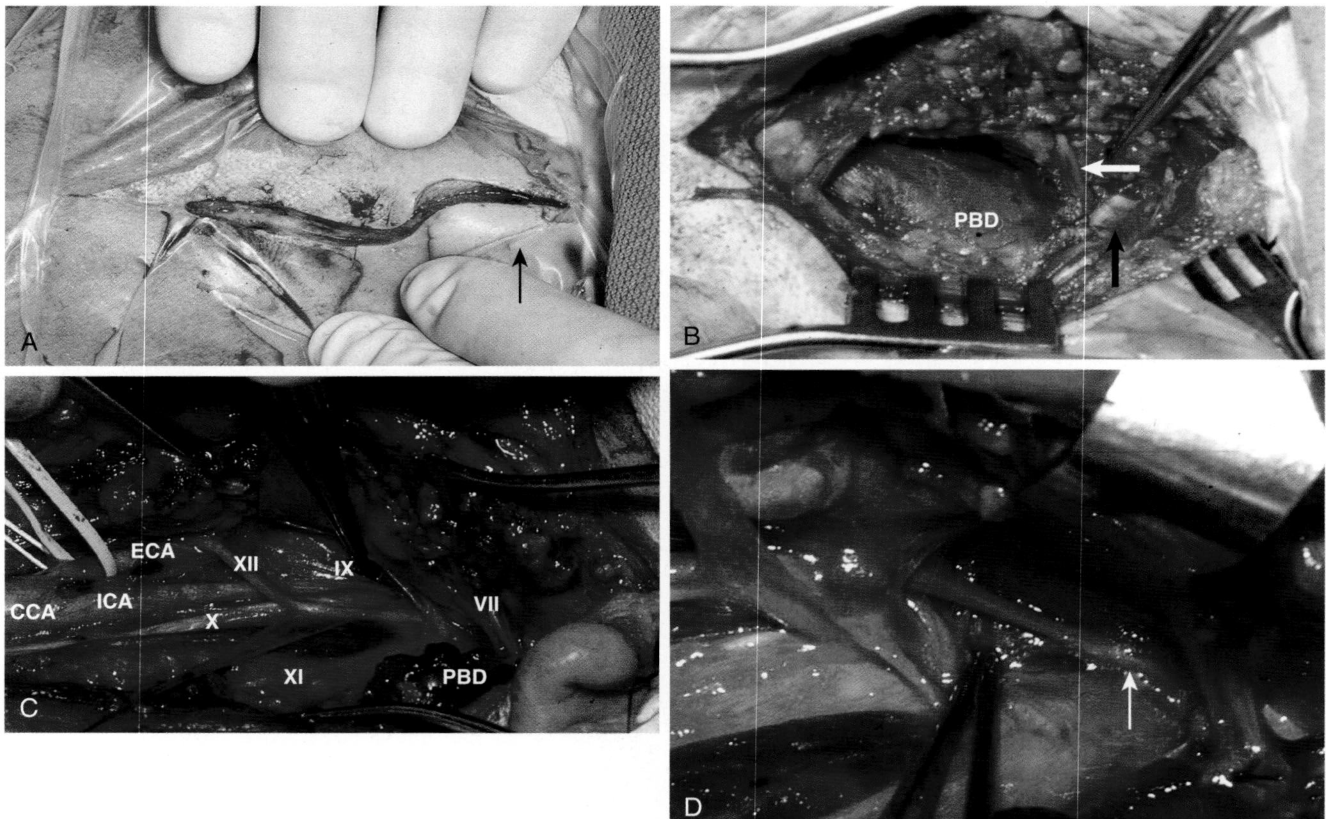

Figure 36-17. An aid to exposing the distal internal carotid artery once the operation is under way (i.e., temporomandibular subluxation is now not possible). In Leicester, this is done as a joint procedure with an ear, nose, and throat specialist. **A,** In this patient who had an infected carotid patch, the incision started above the old wound and then in front of the pinna *(black arrow).* If distal access was necessary during a conventional CEA, the wound is extended similarly. **B,** The parotid gland is mobilized superomedially. Releasing the parotid fascia significantly improves exposure. The tragal pointer is identified *(black arrow),* and dissection continues deeper until the facial nerve is identified *(white arrow)* and then protected. If any difficulty occurs in finding the facial nerve, a further guide is that it is usually just above the superior border of the origin of the posterior belly of digastric (PBD). **C,** Distal dissection and mobilization continues. In this case, the VIIth and IXth through XIIth cranial nerves were exposed. **D,** The styloid apparatus *(white arrow)* was easily exposed without any undue retraction.

of intraoperative stroke seems to be embolization of luminal thrombus following clamp release. This thrombus is derived from bleeding from the sheared vasa vasorum onto the endarterectomized surface (Figures 36-12 and 36-16). Angiography and duplex may also identify luminal irregularities but only after flow has been restored (i.e., it may be too late). Finally, all patients are monitored for 1 hour postoperatively with TCD. This is because early postoperative thrombosis is preceded by increasing rates of embolization, which can then be arrested by incremental infusions of Dextran-40.[52] Since implementing this protocol, the rate of intraoperative stroke has fallen from 4% to 0.3% in the last 1400 patients and no patient has suffered a stroke due to postoperative carotid thrombosis. Previously, this rate was 2.7%. Implementation of this monitoring program has been associated with a 60% reduction in the overall operative risk.[52]

Operative "Challenges"

High Carotid Disease

The surgeon occasionally encounters unexpected high carotid disease, although usually this is anticipated preoperatively. Distal access is facilitated by asking the anesthesiologist to use nasolaryngeal intubation as this opens the angle between mandible and sternomastoid (Figure 36-6B). Remember, it is not possible to undertake temporomandibular subluxation once the operation has started. Further operative measures to gain distal access include division of digastric, mobilization of the hypoglossal nerve, division of the styloid musculature (styloglossus, stylopharyngeus), and finally, styloid process fracture. In my experience, the latter maneuver is not as simple as it sounds.

Exposure (almost to the skull base) can, however, be achieved once the operation is under way (or as a planned strategy from the outset) by working with an otolaryngologist who is familiar with operating at the skull base (Figure 36-17A to D). First, the incision is extended in front of the ear (Figure 36-17A) and the parotid gland is mobilized superomedially. Releasing the parotid fascia considerably improves exposure. The tragal pointer is identified, and dissection continues deeper until the facial nerve is found and then protected. If difficulty occurs in identifying the facial nerve, a further guide is that it is usually situated just above the superior border of the origin of the posterior belly of digastric (Figure 36-17B). Once digastric is divided, exposure continues distally, taking care not to damage the motor fibers leaving the vagus nerve.

With this type of exposure, it is possible to identify several of the more distally placed cranial nerves (Figure 36-17C), as well as the styloid apparatus (Figure 36-17D), without excessive traction. I now use this approach for dealing with high distal disease and large carotid body or glomus tumors.

Hypoplastic ICA

Occasionally, the surgeon encounters a hypoplastic carotid artery. As discussed earlier, this pattern of disease is associated with a very low incidence of late stroke. Accordingly, if this is suspected before opening the vessel, an on-table angiogram should be performed. If a hypoplastic ICA extending to the skull base is confirmed, it is probably best to abandon the procedure and anticoagulate the patient. The rationale is to minimize the risks of thrombus propagation across the circle of Willis in the event of ICA thrombosis. If the artery has been opened, ligation of the hypoplastic ICA and postoperative anticoagulation is appropriate.

Thrombosed ICA

One other rare phenomenon—the thrombosed carotid artery—may confront the surgeon. This manifests itself in two forms. The first is the acutely thrombosed artery, which is avoided if the ICA is rescanned before surgery. If encountered, the artery should be left alone and the procedure abandoned. In practice, the patient must have occluded asymptomatically and attempts to thereafter restore flow could lead to a severe thromboembolic stroke. The second presentation is the partially recanalized ICA. Here, a string of thrombus is adherent to the ICA wall up to the skull base. It is probably unwise to simply pull this thrombus out (unless it is free floating). The two to three times I have encountered this type of problem, the thrombus was quite adherent to the intima throughout its length.

TCD (or awake testing) shows whether middle cerebral artery flow is highly dependent on ipsilateral ICA flow (middle cerebral artery velocity of less than 15 cm/sec during test clamping or new neurological deficit when the carotid is test-clamped under LRA). If this is the case, strenuous attempts should be made to reconstruct the vessel (probably with a vein bypass). If good collateral flow occurs, it is probably safer to ligate the artery and anticoagulate the patient.

Redundant Endarterectomy Zone

Occasionally, the endarterectomy zone may be excessively redundant after CEA and attempts to close the artery predispose the patient to corrugation of the intima or kinking of the bifurcation. Two methods are available for treating this. The first is to resect a segment of redundant intima. Continuity is then restored by a continuous 6:0 Prolene (Ethicon) anastomosis. One of the problems with this strategy is that in a thin-walled endarterectomized vessel (especially in elderly women) sutures can tear out, leaving a bypass as the only remaining option.

The (preferred) alternative is eversion plication. Here, the redundant endarterectomy zone is shortened by everting a segment of the wall outward (Figure 36-18). The first step is to place two stay sutures on either side of the vessel wall, incorporating the redundant segment of artery. The sutures are then tied, which causes the eversion to occur. A continuous 6:0 Prolene suture then completes the anastomosis. The principal advantages are that the distal intimal step can be incorporated into the eversion and the strength and integrity of the arterial wall are not compromised.

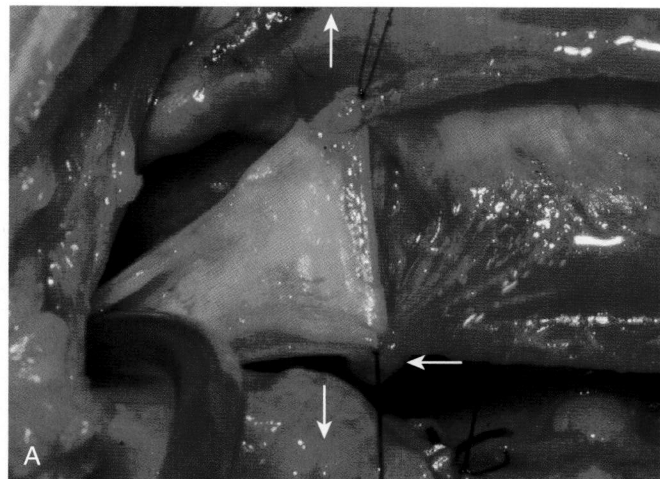

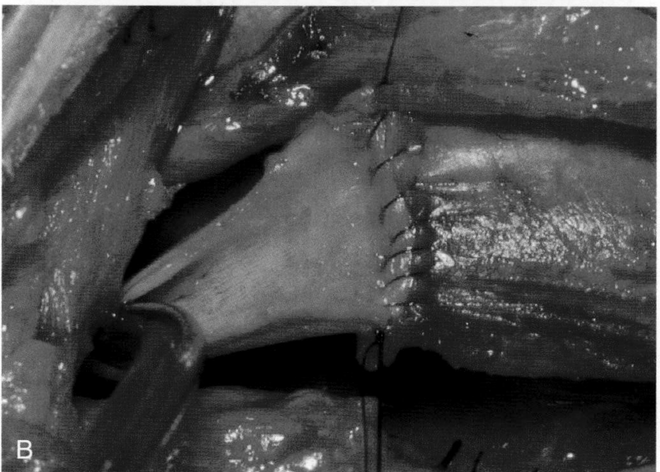

Figure 36-18. Eversion plication of an excessively redundant endarterectomy zone. **A,** Two stay sutures are placed at opposing sides of the wall incorporating the excess redundancy. The sutures are tied and pulled apart *(arrows),* thereby causing eversion of the redundant wall posteriorly *(white arrow).* **B,** The adjacent segments of everted intima and endarterectomized artery are then anastomosed to restore arterial continuity.

Carotid Bypass

Occasionally, it may be necessary to perform a carotid bypass. Both prosthetic material and saphenous vein may be used, and there is no evidence that either is better. My preference is reversed saphenous vein from the groin to avoid the risks of prosthetic infection. If a shunt has been used, this must be removed temporarily. If no shunt has been used, now is the time to prepare one. The flexibility of the Pruitt-Inahara shunt, together with the absence of any need for retaining clamps, makes this an excellent stent for anastomosis and maintenance of distal perfusion. The reversed vein is placed over the distal limb of the shunt, which is reinserted into the distal ICA. The opposed vein and distal ICA are then spatulated and anastomosed (Figure 36-19A). Once completed, it is helpful at this stage to deflate the distal Pruitt-Inahara balloon and carefully retract the shunt to see whether any bleeding points are obvious, especially around the back of the anastomosis. The next step is proximal reconstruction. Options include end-to-end anastomosis with the CCA (this is difficult with a shunt in place), side-to-side anastomosis with the CCA (having oversewn the distal CCA), or reconstruction of the bifurcation. Where possible, the bifurcation should be reconstructed. The first step is to open the back wall of the vein with fine scissors to a point where it is felt that the heel of the anastomosis lies comfortably against the apex of the origin of the ECA (Figure 36-19B). It is then usually straightforward to reconstitute the bifurcation and unnecessary to remove the shunt until the last minute.

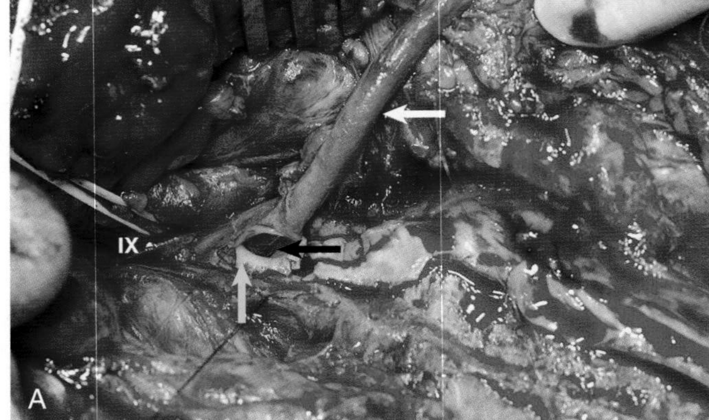

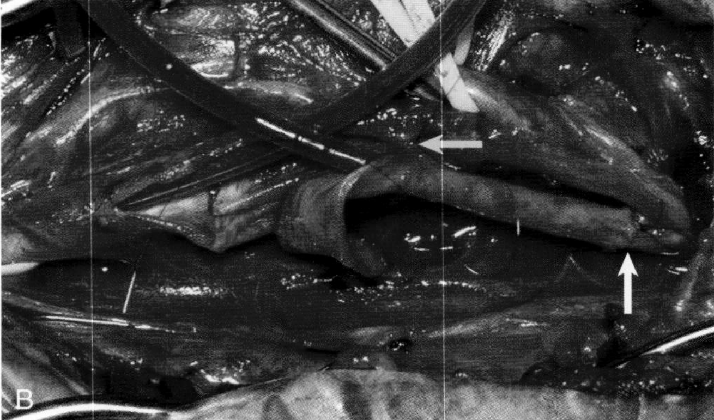

Figure 36-19. Carotid bypass in a patient following excision of an infected carotid patch. **A,** Reversed saphenous vein *(white arrow)* has been placed over the distal limb of a Pruitt-Inahara shunt *(black arrow),* which is then reinserted into the distal internal carotid artery (ICA; *yellow arrow*). The opposed vein and distal ICA are then spatulated and anastomosed just below the glossopharyngeal nerve (IX). The yellow sling is around the ICA above IX. **B,** The proximal component of the vein graft is shortened as necessary and the bifurcation reconstructed with the shunt left in situ. The anastomosis starts with the heel of the opened vein graft being approximated to the external carotid artery origin *(yellow arrow).* The distal anastomosis *(white arrow)* is not from the same patient as in 36-19A.

COMPLICATIONS OF CAROTID SURGERY

Operative Stroke or Death

Tables 36-1 and 36-2 detail the operative risks from the various symptomatic and asymptomatic carotid surgery trials. Surgeons wishing to participate in these trials had to submit their recent track record for scrutiny, and some were excluded from participating. Accordingly, some have criticized ECST and NASCET as not being representative of true clinical practice.

ECST[33] identified three factors on multivariate analysis that were predictive of an increased operative risk: female sex (odds ratio [OR] 2.1), peripheral vascular disease (OR 2.5), and a systolic BP greater than 180 mm Hg (OR 2.2). Similar predictive factors from NASCET[54] included hemispheric as opposed to ocular events (OR 2.3), left versus right CEA (OR 2.3), contralateral occlusion (OR 2.2), ipsilateral infarct on CT or magnetic resonance imaging (OR 1.8), and irregular as opposed to smooth plaque (OR 1.5). In NASCET it was observed that patients taking aspirin at less than 650 mg daily were more likely to suffer an operative stroke.[2] A randomized trial has shown the converse to be true.[35] Randomized evidence suggests that low-dose aspirin (75 to 300 mg) significantly reduces perioperative cardiovascular morbidity or mortality while avoiding the side effects associated with higher-dose therapy.

The combined incidence of intracranial hemorrhage or hyperperfusion stroke is about 1%. Both have similar predisposing factors: severe bilateral extracranial disease, history of hypertension, poor intracranial collateralization, and impaired autoregulation. Current thinking is that the two may be part of a common phenomenon where impaired autoregulation takes some time to reset after CEA, during which time the brain is exposed to increased blood flow. The patient can therefore present with several symptoms, including headache, irritability, drowsiness, seizure, and ultimately stroke, which may be either ischemic or hemorrhagic.

Management of Operation-Related Stroke

Intraoperative Stroke

It is conventional to assume that any patient who recovers from anesthesia with a new neurological deficit may have suffered a stroke due to endarterectomy site thromboembolism. Accordingly, these patients should be reexplored immediately. Delay beyond 1 hour reduces the chances of success.[55] In Leicester, the patient would receive the first of three 8-mg doses of intravenous dexamethasone. Care should be taken to avoid unnecessary neck movement before reexploration, which may precipitate further embolization. If the artery was closed primarily, a patch should now be inserted following thrombectomy. Completion angiography should be performed to exclude persisting technical error and distal mural thrombus. If the thrombus does not clear, extreme care should be employed when passing a number 2/3 Fogarty catheter into the upper reaches of the ICA to minimize the risk of causing a carotid–cavernous sinus fistula. Anecdotal case reports have indicated that there might be a role for catheter-guided thrombolysis in the future.[56]

Postoperative Stroke

Any stroke that occurs in the first 24 hours after surgery should be assumed to be embolic. A CT scan is unlikely to alter decision-making, and this should not delay the patient being returned to operating theater. Any delay beyond 1 hour significantly reduces the chances of a good neurological recovery. Although the stroke may have been due to focal embolism (as opposed to carotid thrombosis), the surgeon has no way of knowing whether an underlying technical error or mural endarterectomy zone thrombus with the potential for further embolization exists.

Any patient who suffers a stroke after 24 hours has elapsed may have suffered an intracranial hemorrhage, hence the need for an emergency CT scan in this situation. Patients with intracranial hemorrhage require careful BP control to avoid the extremes of rising intracranial pressure or hypoperfusion. Patients who report severe headache, seizure, or both in the early postoperative phase require urgent hospitalization. Almost invariably they have grossly elevated BP and are at great danger of intracranial hemorrhage. The mainstay of treatment is rapid control of seizures (titrated intravenous diazepam initially), followed by attempts to reduce the BP (first line is usually titrated intravenous labetolol).

Prevention of Operative Stroke

The introduction of intraoperative monitoring and quality control assessment (described earlier) virtually abolished intraoperative stroke in my institution, but it had no effect on the 2.7% rate of stroke secondary to postoperative carotid thrombosis.[52] Research suggests that patients destined to suffer a stroke due to postoperative carotid thrombosis have increasing rates of embolization before the onset of any neurological deficit.[57,58] This observation has now been corroborated worldwide.[59-62] Increasing embolization can be diagnosed using TCD and arrested by incremental infusion of Dextran-40, which prevents progression to thrombosis.[52] Increasing evidence suggests that postoperative carotid thrombosis may be mediated by factors that enhance platelet function in individual patients, rather than by the actual surgical technique. Evidence supporting this observation includes postoperative embolization being unrelated to patch type[63]; patients undergoing staged bilateral CEAs have similar degrees of embolization after each procedure,[64] and the platelets of patients with higher-rate embolization are significantly more sensitive to adenosine diphosphate.[65] A randomized trial of a single 75-mg dose of clopidogrel administered the night before surgery (in addition to chronic aspirin therapy) conferred a significant reduction in the rate of postoperative embolization.[66] If larger studies corroborate this observation, it may be possible to reduce stroke due to postoperative carotid thrombosis by simply adding one tablet of clopidogrel to the usual preoperative antiplatelet regimen.

Medical Complications

Of NASCET patients, 10% suffered a perioperative medical complication.[67] The commonest were cardiovascular (8%) or respiratory (0.8%). None, however, suffered a pulmonary embolus. Overall, 70% of medical complications were classed as mild, 27% as moderately severe. Only five patients (0.3%) suffered a major medical complication (all myocardial infarction).

Hypertension is a relatively common problem after CEA. Depending on the threshold used, up to 40% of patients may require antihypertensive therapy in the early postoperative period. Some (nonrandomized) evidence indicates that postoperative hypertension is less common if surgery is performed under LRA.[45] Most cases settle within 12 hours.

Cranial Nerve Injury

Cranial nerve injuries were documented in 8.6% of NASCET surgical patients.[54] Almost all were classified as mild, and all recovered within 30 days. None suffered a major cranial nerve injury. The commonest nerves to be injured were the hypoglossal (3.7%), vagus (2.5%), and mandibular branch of the facial nerve (2.2%). No patient in NASCET suffered a glossopharyngeal nerve palsy, presumably reflecting the exclusion of patients with high carotid disease from this study. A recent review by Forsell et al. [68] identified 13 published series (2911 patients) documenting the risk of cranial nerve injury (15% overall) after CEA. The mandibular branch of the facial nerve was injured in about 4%, the glossopharyngeal nerve in 0.5%, the recurrent laryngeal nerve in 5%, and the hypoglossal nerve in 7%.

Surgeons have placed relatively little importance on discussing the potential for cranial nerve injury with patients before carotid surgery. The Forsell series indicates that this stance is no longer acceptable. Most undoubtedly are transient, but the risks and implications of permanent nerve injury must be accepted by patients as they consent to surgery. A severe cranial nerve injury can be just as debilitating as a stroke.

Patch Infection

Prosthetic patch infection complicates 1% of CEA procedures. In a recent review (43 patients), 37% occurred within 2 months of surgery, while 56% occurred after 6 months had elapsed.[69] Early postoperative cases usually present with deep wound infection or false aneurysm formation, and most usually report an earlier wound complication. Published reports of prosthetic patch rupture are extremely rare (four to date) and can occur at any time following operation. Late infections (more than 6 months) tend to present with chronic sinus discharge or false aneurysm formation. Nearly all organisms responsible for prosthetic patch infection (90%) are either staphylococci or streptococci.[69]

Management depends on the mode and urgency of presentation. Preoperative investigation is not usually possible in patients with massive hemorrhage, although it may be useful to have a catheter positioned in the proximal CCA over which an occluding balloon catheter can be positioned. Less urgent cases benefit from duplex or angiographic assessment. Radioisotope-labeled white cell scans are unreliable (a negative scan does not mean no infection has occurred), and no evidence shows that CT results alter outcome. The golden rule is that an abscess overlying a carotid incision must never be incised unless a vascular colleague is present.

Surgical options for treating patch infection include (1) patch removal and autologous venous reconstruction with either patch or bypass; (2) patch removal followed by ligation of the CCA, ICA, and ECA; and (3) debridement and cover with a muscle flap. Ligation should be considered only in patients with a chronically occluded ICA or in the rare patient in whom catastrophic hemorrhage cannot be controlled. Up to 50% of patients who have ligation suffer a stroke. The optimal treatment appears to be patch removal with autologous reconstruction (90% alive, stroke free, and infection free at 2 years). Reconstruction using prosthetic material has a poor outcome and is not to be recommended.[69]

Postoperative Surveillance

With the exception of the management of asymptomatic disease and postoperative surveillance, remarkable similarity is found in transatlantic attitudes regarding the surgical treatment of atherosclerotic carotid artery disease. In the United Kingdom and Scandinavia, few patients undergo serial clinical or ultrasound surveillance. Proponents of surveillance and secondary intervention cite several (highly selective) retrospective studies to support their case. However, this type of data is notoriously unreliable. Nevertheless, quite a few randomized trials undertook planned ultrasound surveillance. A review of these data show no compelling evidence that restenosis correlates with late risk of recurrent ipsilateral stroke. Patients with a restenosis of more than 50% were at no higher risk of suffering a late stroke than those without.[70] In particular, only one ACAS patient (0.12%) underwent reoperation for a symptomatic severe recurrent stenosis, and ACAS found no association between late stroke and recurrent stenosis.[71] Accordingly, it is safe to discharge patients after their routine follow-up at 6 weeks, with instructions to return if any new problems develop. The one possible exception to this practice, however, would be any patient who suffered a neurological deficit (under LRA) or who had middle cerebral artery velocities of less than 15 cm/sec during test clamping. Clearly these patients are at risk of hemodynamic failure should the carotid artery occlude.

NONATHEROMATOUS CAROTID DISEASE

Arteritis

Takayasu's Arteritis

Takayasu's arteritis (TA) is an extremely rare, chronic inflammatory arteritis of unknown etiology. Because of its rarity, few clinicians (especially in the Western world) have acquired substantial experience in its management. TA is predominantly a disease of the aorta and its principal branches (Table 36-8) and comprises varying combinations of occlusion, stenosis, and dilatation. Extracranial carotid involvement can occur on its own (type I) or with multiple disease locations (types IIa, IIb, and V). Accordingly, TA can present with various symptoms and signs (cerebral, coronary, mesenteric, renovascular hypertension, etc.).

The strategy of investigation must, therefore, take account that multiple sites of disease may be present. From the surgical point of view, baseline investigations should include full blood count (looking for anemia, thrombocytosis, and leukocytosis), urea and electrolytes (looking for evidence of end-organ damage to the kidneys), and simple markers of systemic illness (elevated plasma viscosity, erythrocyte sedimentation rate, C reactive protein). If the clinical history or duplex scan (Figure 36-20) suggests a diagnosis of TA, a complete evaluation of the thoracic and abdominal aorta and its principal branches is indicated. Previously this was by contrast angiography, but it has been surpassed by CT angiography.

Table 36-8
Classification of Takayasu's Arteritis

Type 1	Branches of the aortic arch (subclavian, carotid, vertebral)
Type IIa	Ascending aorta Aortic arch + branches
Type IIb	Ascending aorta, aortic arch Aortic arch branches Descending thoracic aorta
Type III	Descending thoracic aorta Abdominal aorta, +/– renal arteries
Type IV	Abdominal aorta +/– renal arteries
Type V	Combination of types IIb and IV

First-line treatment is prednisolone therapy (40 to 60 mg daily). If this fails to control symptoms or the active phase of the disease (which can be monitored using duplex measurement of arterial wall thickness or serial erythrocyte sedimentation rate, C reactive protein, or plasma viscosity), immunosuppression with either methotrexate or cyclophsophamide may be added. In the past, angioplasty was generally avoided in TA because of the long lengths of sclerotic disease involvement. However, anecdotal reports have been made of its application in patients with short-segment disease or carotid involvement, particularly following the introduction of synchronous stenting. Surgical intervention should be reserved, whenever possible, for treating patients who have passed through the active phase of the disease. This is diagnosed by no evidence of worsening constitutional symptoms or end-organ symptoms; reduced erythrocyte sedimentation rate, C reactive protein, or plasma viscosity; and no deterioration in duplex or angiographic occlusions or stenoses. Care should be taken to avoid any anastomosis in arteries involved with TA. Accordingly, carotid bypass should generally derive inflow from the aortic arch rather than the subclavian arteries.

Giant Cell Arteritis

Giant cell arteritis (GCA) is another chronic inflammatory disorder of arteries. Most clinicians are aware of the involvement of branches of the ECA, but GCA can also affect the thoracic and abdominal aorta, carotid and subclavian arteries,

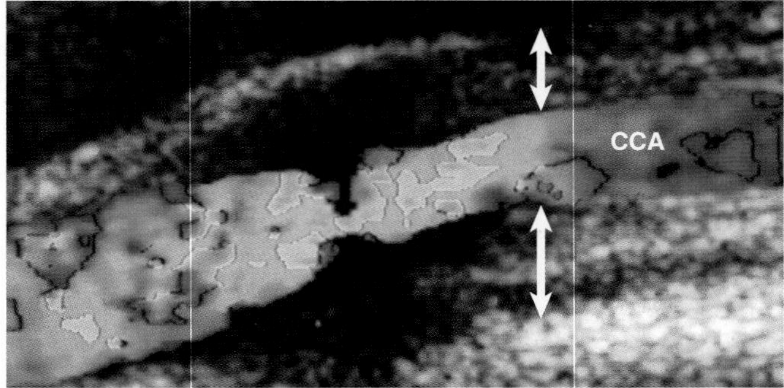

Figure 36-20. Color duplex ultrasound image showing Takayasu's disease in the common carotid artery in a 20-year-old woman who presented with amaurosis fugax and hemispheric transient ischemic attacks. Note the gross thickening of the vessel wall *(arrows)*. This extended down to the aortic arch on magnetic resonance angiography. Severe stenotic or occlusive disease was also present in the contralateral carotid artery, both subclavians, and one vertebral artery.

and femoropopliteal vessels. The symptoms may be similar to those in patients with atherosclerosis (especially as the disease tends to start in patients older than 50 years), but prodromal nonspecific symptoms, jaw claudication, and tenderness over the temporal artery should raise suspicions.

Surgery has little role in the management of cerebral GCA apart from rare occlusive complications presenting with end-organ injury. Stroke or TIA can follow carotid or vertebral artery involvement but is rare. The principal worry is unilateral or even bilateral blindness, which can occur rapidly following occlusion of the posterior ciliary arteries. Any patient in whom there is reasonable suspicion of GCA should have a temporal artery biopsy performed as soon as possible. If any significant delay will occur, oral steroid therapy (20 to 60 mg of prednisolone daily) should be started empirically. Patients with acute blindness should be admitted immediately and receive intravenous corticosteroid therapy. Limited evidence shows that immunosuppression improves the outcome in steroid-resistant patients.

Radiation Arteritis

Exposure to radiation predisposes the patient to an increased risk of carotid stenosis. In the first 3 to 5 years after radiotherapy, the primary injury leads to intimal hyperplasia. These lesions can be quite extensive within segments of the common and internal carotid arteries, but they tend to be smooth. Thereafter, evidence suggests that radiotherapy can predispose a patient toward accelerated atherogenesis.

In clinical practice, the incidence of symptomatic lesions requiring intervention is extremely small. No consensus exists regarding the management of asymptomatic lesions. In the United Kingdom, these patients would probably be treated conservatively unless there was a contralateral occlusion. In North America, surveillance and interventional strategies are less conservative. It would not, however, be appropriate to simply apply the ACAS findings to asymptomatic postradiation stenoses that were nonatherosclerotic.

The risks of surgery are inevitably higher. This is because (1) dissection is made more difficult by the scarring associated with the radiotherapy and any previous radical neck surgery, (2) the normal planes of dissection between intima and media disappear because of radiation-induced fibrosis, (3) the segments of diseased artery can be long and extensive, and (4) the risks of secondary infection (primary arterial, patch) increase because of poor wound healing, especially in the presence of an adjacent tracheostomy.

Surgical options include endarterectomy, patching the stenosis, or formal carotid vein bypass. Surgery has, however, largely been superseded by angioplasty with stenting, which is now probably the first-line treatment.

Carotid Aneurysm

As happens elsewhere in the body, carotid aneurysms (CA) can be true or false. Causes of true CA include atherosclerosis, fibromuscular dysplasia, TA, or GCA. False CA can follow iatrogenic dissection (postangioplasty, post-CEA), spontaneous dissection, or infected prosthetic patch or can be mycotic.

Most CA are treated, primarily because of their potential for embolization or thrombosis in the future. Most are treated surgically, although endovascular intervention may become the treatment of choice, especially for CA located near the skull base.

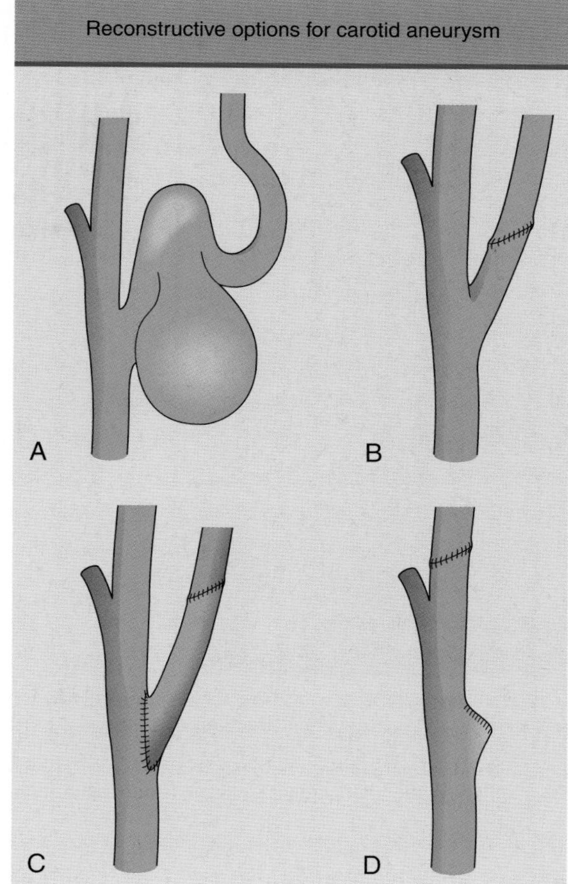

Figure 36-21. Reconstructive options for patients with a true carotid aneurysm include resection **(A)**, end-to-end anastomosis **(B),** interposition vein or prosthetic bypass **(C),** and oversewing the internal carotid artery (ICA) origin with transposition of distal ICA on to external carotid artery **(D).**

The choice of surgical procedure depends on the underlying cause. True atherosclerotic aneurysms tend to be associated with functional elongation of the carotid artery. It may therefore be possible to resect the aneurysm and perform an end-to-end anastomosis (Figure 36-21). If this is not possible or the wall is excessively thinned or infected, a vein bypass can be performed. A final option is to transpose the distal ICA onto the proximal ECA. If no operation is possible and endovascular repair is not considered possible, the only option may have to be carotid ligation. This should be used only as a last resort, as up to 50% of patients suffer a stroke as a consequence.

Carotid Dissection

Carotid artery dissection (CAD) accounts for only about 2% of all strokes. However, one fifth of strokes in young individuals are secondary to CAD, and up to 25% of patients with unexplained stroke following trauma have suffered a dissection. In reality, many cases of CAD are probably misdiagnosed or missed, and the most difficult aspect with regard to planning management is thinking about the diagnosis.

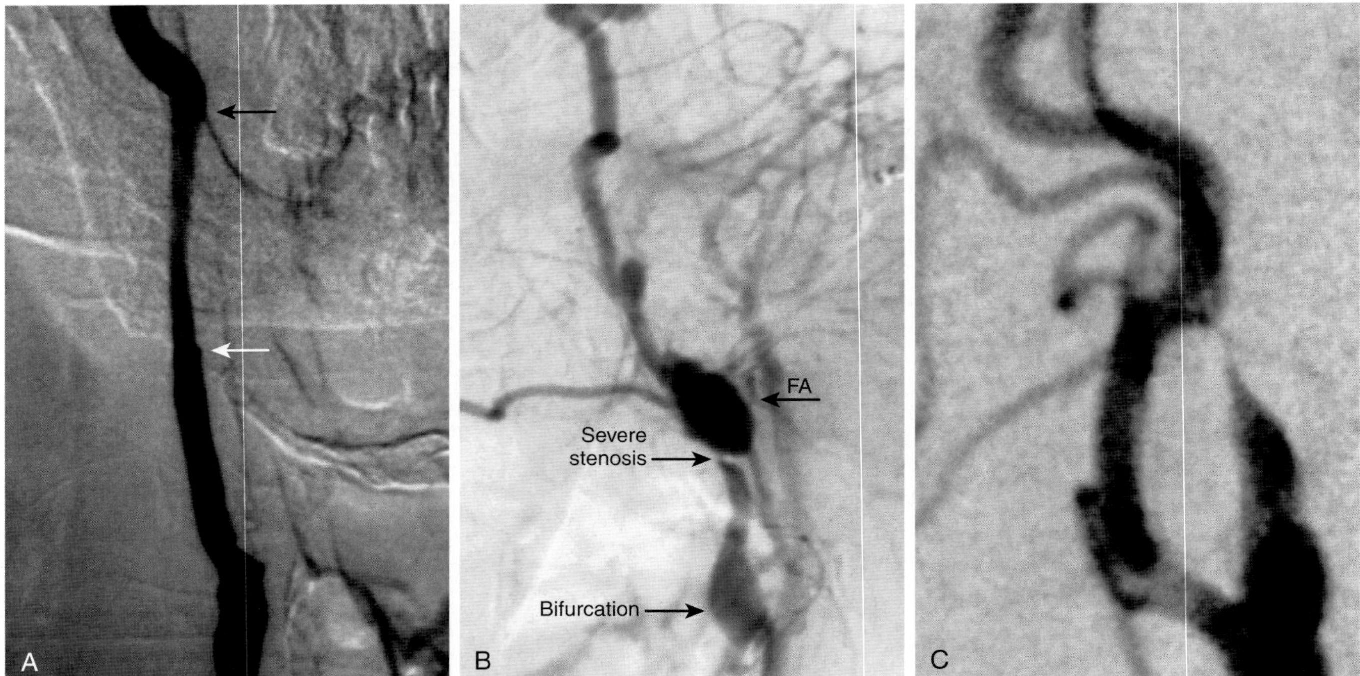

Figure 36-22. Carotid dissection. **A,** Type I: Intimal irregularity with or without stenosis of less than 70% seen in a patient following angioplasty of a recurrent stenosis after carotid endarterectomy. It is presumed that the guide wire caused a dissection entry point *(white arrow)* with reentry higher up *(black arrow)*. **B,** Type II: Stenosis greater than 70% with or without false aneurysm (FA) formation. This 40-year-old male presented with Horner's syndrome and monocular blindness and has both a severe stenosis and a distal FA formation. **C,** Type III: Occlusion, characteristically "flame shaped" and 2 to 3 cm above the bifurcation. Occlusion is due to thrombus in the false channel compressing the true lumen.

CAD can either be asymptomatic or present with one or more of headache, stroke, TIA, painful Horner's syndrome, or cranial nerve paresis (III, IV, or VI). Neurological symptoms follow: (1) ICA occlusion through compression of the true lumen by thrombus in the false lumen, (2) distal embolization from the mural thrombus, and (3) formation of a symptomatic false aneurysm, especially in patients with subadventitial dissection.

Clinical suspicion should guide interpretation of preliminary investigations. Thus, the clinician should be alerted to the possibility of CAD in a young patient with duplex, MRA, or angiography evidence of a carotid occlusion 2 to 3 cm above the bifurcation, or a normal carotid bifurcation but with intimal irregularity or stenosis 2 to 3 cm above it. Angiography is the standard for evaluating suspected CAD, although gadolinium-enhanced MRA may supersede this.

Type I dissection refers to when angiography shows either minor intimal irregularity (Figure 36-22A) or a stenosis less than 70%. Type II dissections show evidence of a severe stenosis greater than 70%, aneurysm formation, or both (Figure 36-22B). Type III dissections classically exhibit a flame-shaped carotid occlusion 2 to 3 cm above the bifurcation (Figure 36-22C). Type I, type III, and most type II dissections should be managed by systemic heparinization followed by warfarinization. The aim is to reduce the risk of secondary dissection, thrombosis, and embolism. Surgery, and possibly endovascular intervention, is reserved for complex cases with recurring symptoms despite best medical therapy and who have amenable lesions. Type II dissections extending to the skull base are particularly difficult to treat if symptoms do not settle with anticoagulation. Options include extracranial–intracranial bypass (but few centers currently offer this service). The optimal management strategy for aneurysm formation after CAD is controversial. In the past, surgery has been recommended, but recent evidence suggests that they may have a more benign prognosis.[72,73] It therefore seems appropriate to recommend conservative management and regular surveillance unless the aneurysm is associated with a severe stenosis, cranial nerve signs, or recurrence of symptoms.

Fibromuscular Dysplasia

Fibromuscular dysplasia predominantly affects the renal arteries of young women. However, about a quarter of all cases involve the carotid or vertebral arteries. Most of those with carotid disease (60%) are bilateral, and typically the middle and upper segments of the ICA are affected. Pathologically, fibromuscular dysplasia can involve any of the three arterial layers. The commonest subtype is medial fibroplasia, which accounts for three quarters of all cases. The arteries of patients with medial fibroplasia typically display a beaded appearance (alternating stenotic webs and dilatations). As seems typical in patients with nonatherosclerotic carotid disease, the presentation of fibromuscular dysplasia is variable, ranging from no symptoms to stroke. Stroke or TIA can be due to thrombosis, embolization, or bleeding because of the association between fibromuscular dysplasia and stenosis formation, false aneurysm formation, distal dissection, and a coassociation with intracranial aneurysms, thereby predisposing patients to subarachnoid hemorrhage.

Newer MRA and CT angiography technology is replacing digital subtraction angiography. Duplex imaging may miss

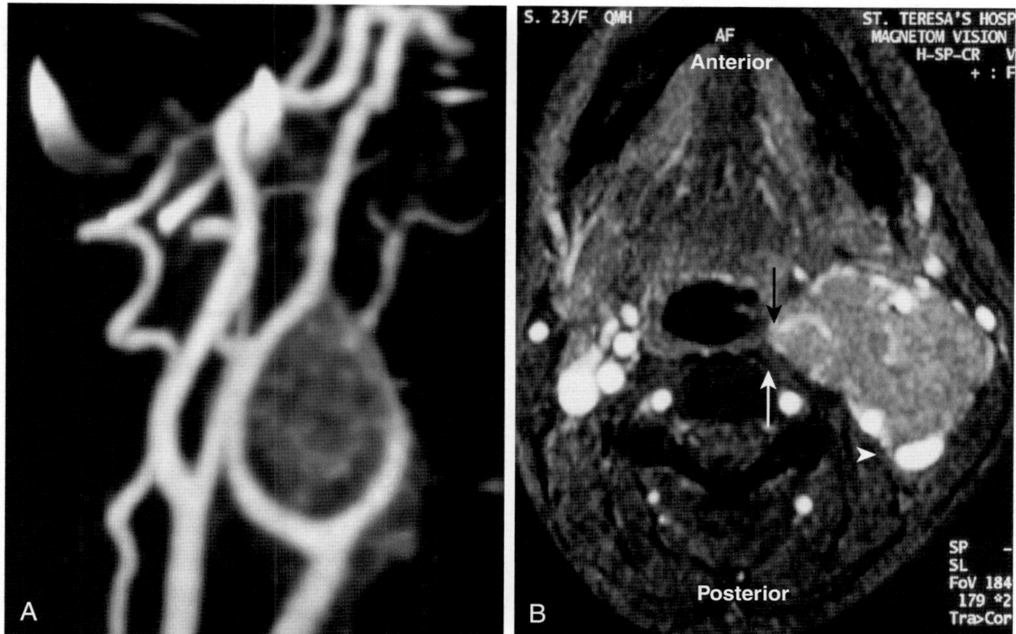

Figure 36-23. Carotid body tumor. **A,** Carotid body tumor causing splaying of the bifurcation on magnetic resonance angiography. **B,** Computed tomography scan showing encroachment of the tumor on the larynx *(black arrow)* and proximity to the pharyngeal mucosa *(white arrow)*. The bulk of the tumor lies anterior to the external carotid artery and internal carotid artery *(arrowhead)*.

high carotid lesions unless the more proximal ICA displays a beaded appearance. Management is usually conservative. No evidence indicates that anticoagulation is preferable to antiplatelet therapy. Patients who become symptomatic should be treated as if they had atherosclerotic disease. Before the advent of endovascular technologies, the standard treatment was either open graduated dilatation or vein bypass. Most, however, are now treated by percutaneous angioplasty, which can be combined with stenting and repeated during the course of follow-up, which should be lifelong.

Carotid Body Tumor

The carotid body is located within the adventitia, posterior to the bifurcation of the carotid artery. Its role is to monitor blood gases and pH. Histologically, it is derived from cells originating from the neural crest ectoderm. A carotid body tumor (CBT) grows within the bifurcation and ultimately causes this to splay (Figure 36-23A). The CBT ultimately presents as a painless swelling or because of pain, compression, or both of adjacent cranial nerves. Stroke or TIA is rare.

Investigation begins with duplex imaging. This usually demonstrates intense vascularity with splaying of the bifurcation. Recognition of the likelihood of CBT warrants either CT or magnetic resonance imaging to exclude bilateral tumors and provide information regarding the overall extent of the lesion. In particular, it is useful to know whether the ICA is encased in tumor (Figure 36-23B).

A case can be made for adopting a conservative approach in elderly patients with relatively small tumors. In the remainder, surgical excision remains the mainstay of management. Some 5% of CBTs are malignant, and 5% are bilateral. CBT surgery should be performed by a surgeon who is experienced at dealing with arteries and bleeding and at performing anastomoses. Surgery is inevitably more difficult the second time, after an inexperienced surgeon has attempted removal. Some surgeons advocate preoperative embolization of the main tumor blood supply so as to minimize operative bleeding. To date, no consensus exists as to whether this alters the outcome. A future option in large tumors may be to place a covered stent within the proximal ECA before surgery. This is because branches of this vessel are the main source of blood to the lesion.

The approach to the bifurcation is just as for CEA. In small tumors, it may be possible to expose each of the important cranial nerves (hypoglossal, vagus) and arteries (CCA, ICA, ECA) without difficulty. The tumor is then gradually removed via dissection that is classically described as being in the subadventitial plane. In reality, the surgeon finds the most superficial plane between artery and tumor and dissection proceeds via a combination of diathermy and a lot of ligatures. The principal blood supply to the tumor is derived from the posterior–inferior aspect of the bifurcation. Occasionally, this vessel can be inadvertently damaged during excision and brisk bleeding ensues. If the injury is small, temporary clamping enables primary closure with interrupted 6:0 Prolene sutures. More extensive injuries may warrant formal arteriotomy, shunt insertion, and even vein bypass. CBT excision can be performed with TCD monitoring. In the event of bleeding, TCD can guide the urgency of shunt deployment. Surgeons should bear in mind that these patients can also have atherosclerotic disease, which can embolize to the brain during injudicious dissection.

Larger CBTs require alternative strategies. First, the patient should be warned of an increased risk of permanent cranial nerve injury. Second, the surgeon should anticipate the need for high dissection. Simple anesthetic and surgical measures were discussed earlier, along with a description of how the upper reaches of the carotid artery can be exposed (Figure 36-17).

Carotid Artery Trauma

Most experience with carotid artery trauma (penetrating or blunt) comes from the major trauma centers in South Africa and North America or during war. Few centers in mainland Europe have significant peacetime exposure to penetrating carotid injuries. Leicester has a large CEA practice, but the vascular unit has only dealt with three penetrating carotid injuries (one iatrogenic) in 15 years.

In the United States, most (80% to 90%) carotid artery injuries are penetrating. In the United Kingdom and Europe, most injuries are blunt. Blunt injuries tend to follow compression or traction to the carotid arteries following rapid deceleration (road traffic accidents). This predisposes the individual to intimal tearing and secondary thrombus formation or distal dissection. The principles of management are similar to those for carotid dissection (described earlier).

Penetrating carotid artery injuries are classified according to their anatomical site. Type I injuries affect the carotid artery between the clavicle and the cricoid cartilage. Type II carotid injuries occur between the cricoid cartilage and the angle of the mandible. Type III injuries affect the carotid artery between the angle of the mandible and the skull base.

The management of carotid artery injuries inevitably depends on the urgency of presentation, the access to imaging and interventional modalities, and the experience of the surgeon. Patients with profuse hemorrhage require immediate exploration, but care must be taken to exclude coexistent trauma such as cervical spine injury. More stable patients warrant imaging wherever possible. Duplex ultrasound has now largely replaced routine angiography as the first-line investigation in patients with a penetrating wound in the type II zone. However, diagnostic angiography is still required in most patients with type I or III injuries because of the reduced accuracy of duplex in these regions. Hospitals with modern imaging facilities will be moving toward CT angiography in this situation, since it is available urgently at all times of the day. Angiography is also often indicated in most type II injuries where duplex suggests an injury that requires surgery. Duplex can, however, be used to survey minor intimal irregularities or small false aneurysms serially, without recourse to angiography.

Individual management decisions inevitably reflect the severity of injury, urgency of presentation, neurological status, and presence of coexisting trauma. As a rule, patients with occluded carotid arteries and either a dense hemiplegia or no neurological symptoms should be treated conservatively. Carotid reconstruction is advocated in patients with less severe neurological deficits, provided they are treated early. The aim is to improve perfusion of a hemodynamically compromised yet viable penumbra around the evolving infarct, without increasing the risk of hemorrhagic transformation.

Various reconstructive options are available, including primary arterial repair, vein patch, transposition of the ICA to the main ECA trunk, and reversed vein bypass. Prosthetic bypass may be necessary in proximal CCA injuries, but the potential for late infection must be remembered. EC-IC bypass might be indicated in patients who would otherwise require carotid ligation. Ligation of the CCA or ICA should only ever be considered in extenuating circumstances. The most likely reason for having to perform ligation is uncontrollable distal hemorrhage in a patient where EC-IC bypass is not possible. Wherever possible, monitoring with TCD may be an invaluable aid in this difficult situation. Newer endovascular techniques now offer the potential for dealing with carotid trauma. Options include insertion of a covered stent (false aneurysms and caroticojugular fistula) or placement of a detachable balloon, which can occlude the cavernous segment of the ICA.

References

1. European Carotid Surgery Trialists Collaborative Group. MRC European Carotid Surgery Trial: interim results for symptomatic patients with severe (70 to 99%) or mild (0 to 29%) carotid stenosis. *Lancet* 1991; 337:1235-1243.
2. North American Symptomatic Carotid Endarterectomy Trial Collaborators. Beneficial effect of carotid endarterectomy in symptomatic patients with high grade stenosis. *N Engl J Med* 1991;325:445-453.
3. Executive Committee for the Asymptomatic Carotid Atherosclerosis Study. Endarterectomy for asymptomatic carotid artery stenosis. *JAMA* 1995;273:1421-1428.
4. Asymptomatic Carotid Surgery Trial Collaborators. The MRC Asymptomatic Carotid Surgery Trial (ACST): Carotid endarterectomy prevents disabling and fatal carotid territory strokes. *Lancet* 2004;363:1491-1502.
5. Barnett HJM, Barnes RW, Clagett GP, et al. Symptomatic carotid artery stenosis: a solvable problem: the NASCET Trial. *Stroke* 1992;23:1050-1053.
6. Wennberg DE, Lucas FL, Birkmeyer JD, et al. Variation in carotid endarterectomy mortality in the Medicare population. *JAMA* 1998;279:1278-1281.
7. Karp HR, Flanders D, Shipp CC, et al. Carotid endarterectomy among Medicare beneficiaries: a statewide evaluation of appropriateness and outcome. *Stroke* 1998;29:46-52.
8. Hsai DC, Krushat WM, Moscoe LM. Epidemiology of carotid endarterectomy among Medicare beneficiaries: 1985-1996 update. *Stroke* 1998;29:346-350.
9. Naylor AR, Rothwell PM, Bell PRF. Overview of the principal results and secondary analyses from the European and the North American randomised trials of carotid endarterectomy. *Eur J Vasc Endovasc Surg* 2003;26:115-129.
10. Donnan GA, Davis SM, Chambers BR, Gates PC. Surgery for prevention of stroke. *Lancet* 1998;351:1372-1373.
11. Walker J, Naylor AR. Ultrasound based diagnosis of "carotid stenosis > 70%": an audit of UK practice. *Eur J Vasc Endovasc Surg* 2006;31:487-490.
12. Rothwell PM, Eliasziw M, Gutnikov SA, et al., for the Carotid Endarterectomy Trialists Collaboration. Analysis of pooled data from the randomised controlled trials of endarterectomy for symptomatic carotid stenosis. *Lancet* 2003;361:107-116.
13. Rothwell PM, Eliasziw M, Gutnikov SA, et al., for the Carotid Endarterectomy Trialists Collaboration. Endarterectomy for symptomatic carotid stenosis in relation to clinical subgroups and timing of surgery. *Lancet* 2004;363:915-924.
14. Rothwell PM, Eliasziw M, Gutnikov SA, et al. Sex difference in the effect of time from symptoms to surgery on benefit from carotid endarterectomy for transient ischaemic attack and minor stroke. *Stroke* 2004;35:2855-2861.
15. Sacco RL, Adams R, Albers G, et al. Guidelines for the prevention of stroke in patients with ischaemic stroke or transient ischaemic attack: a statement for healthcare professionals from the American Heart Association/American Stroke Association Council on Stroke, cosponsored by the Council on Cardiovascular Radiology and Intervention. *Stroke* 2006;37:577-617.
16. Bunch CT, Kresowik TF. Can randomized trial outcomes for carotid endarterectomy be achieved in community wide practice? *Semin Vasc Surg* 2004;17:209-213.
17. EC/IC Bypass Study Group. Failure of extracranial–intracranial arterial bypass to reduce the risk of ischaemic stroke: results of an international randomized trial. *N Engl J Med* 1985;313:1191-1200.
18. Naylor AR, Bell PRF. Stenting for asymptomatic carotid disease: Con. *Semin Vasc Surg* 2008;21:100-107.
19. Young B, Moore WS, Robertson JT, et al. An analysis of peri-operative surgical mortality and morbidity in the Asymptomatic Carotid Atherosclerosis Study. *Stroke* 1996;27:2216-2224.
20. Huber TS, Wheeler KG, Cuddeback JK, et al. Effect of the Asymptomatic Carotid Atherosclerosis Study on carotid endarterectomy in Florida. *Stroke* 1998;29:1099-1105.

21. Alamowitch S, Eliasziw M, Algra A, et al., for the North American Symptomatic Carotid Endarterectomy Trial. Risk, causes and prevention of ischaemic stroke in elderly patients with symptomatic internal carotid artery stenosis. *Lancet* 2001;357:1154-1160.
22. Henderson RD, Eliasziw M, Fox AJ, et al., for the North American Symptomatic Carotid Endarterectomy Trial. Angiographically defined collateral circulation and risk of stroke in patients with severe carotid artery stenosis. *Stroke* 2000;31:128-132.
23. Rothwell PM, Warlow CP. Timing of TIAS preceding stroke: time window for prevention is very short. *Neurology* 2005;64:817-820.
24. Giles MF, Rothwell PM. Risk of stroke after transient ischaemic attack: a systematic review and meta-analysis. *Lancet Neurol* 2007;6:1063-1072.
25. Naylor AR. Time is brain! *Surgeon* 2007;5:23-30.
26. Naylor AR. Delay may increase procedural risk, but at what cost to the patient? *Eur J Vasc Endovasc Surg* 2008;35:383-391.
27. The National Stroke Strategy. Available at. http://www.dh.gov.uk/stroke. Accessed August 13, 2008.
28. Blaisdell WF, Clauss RH, Gailbrath JG, Smith JR. Joint study of extracranial carotid artery occlusion: a review of surgical considerations. *JAMA* 1969;209:1889-1895.
29. Bond R, Rerkasem K, Rothwell PM. Systematic review of the risks of carotid endarterectomy in relation to the clinical indication for and timing of surgery. *Stroke* 2003;34:2290-2303.
30. Naylor AR, Mehta Z, Rothwell PM, Bell PRF. Carotid artery disease and stroke during coronary artery bypass: a critical review of the literature. *Eur J Vasc Endovasc Surg* 2002;23:283-294.
31. Naylor AR, Cuffe R, Rothwell PM, Bell PRF. A systematic review of outcomes following staged and synchronous carotid endarterectomy and coronary artery bypass. *Eur J Vasc Endovasc Surg* 2003;25:380-389.
32. Rodgers A, MacMahon S, Gamble G, et al., for the United Kingdom Transient Ischaemic Attack Collaborative Group. Blood pressure and risk of stroke in patients with cerebrovascular disease. *BMJ* 1996;313:147.
33. Rothwell PM, Warlow CP, for the ECST Collaborative Group. Prediction of benefit from carotid endarterectomy in individual patients: a risk modelling study. *Lancet* 1999;353:2105-2110.
34. Johnson ES, Lanes SF, Wentworth CE, et al. A meta-regression analysis of the dose–response effect of aspirin on stroke. *Arch Intern Med* 1999;159:1248-1253.
35. Taylor DW, Barnett HJM, Haynes RB, et al. Low dose and high dose acetylsalicylic acid for patients undergoing carotid endarterectomy: a randomised trial. *Lancet* 1999;353:2179-2184.
36. CAPRIE Steering Committee. A randomised blinded trial of Clopidogrel versus Aspirin in Patients at Risk of Ischaemic Events (CAPRIE). *Lancet* 1996;348:1329-1339.
37. Payne DA, Hayes PD, Jones CI, et al. Combined effects of aspirin and clopidogrel on platelet function in vivo and in vitro: implications for use in open vascular surgery. *J Vasc Surg* 2002;35:1204-1209.
38. Wilterdink JL, Easton JD. Dipyridamole plus aspirin in cerebrovascular disease. *Arch Neurol* 1999;56:1087-1092.
39. UK Prospective Diabetes Study Group. Effect of intensive blood glucose control with metformin on complications in overweight patients with type II diabetes. *Lancet* 1998;352:854-865.
40. UK Prospective Diabetes Study Group. Tight blood pressure control and risk of macrovascular and microvascular complications in type II diabetics. *BMJ* 1998;317:2035-2038.
41. Heart Protection Study Collaborative Group. MRC/BHF Heart Protection Study of cholesterol lowering with simvastatin in 20536 high-risk individuals: a randomised placebo controlled trial. *Lancet* 2002;360:7-22.
42. Rerkasem R, Bond R, Rothwell PM. Local versus general anaesthesia for carotid endarterectomy. *Cochrane Database Syst Rev* 2004. (2): CD000126.
43. Bond R, Rerkasem K, Counsell C, et al. Routine or selective carotid artery shunting for carotid endarterectomy (and different methods of monitoring in selective shunting). *Cochrane Database Syst Rev* 2002. (2):CD000190.
44. Ghali R, Palazzo EG, Rodriguez DI, et al. Transcranial Doppler intraoperative monitoring during carotid endarterectomy: experience with regional or general anaesthesia, with and without shunting. *Ann Vasc Surg* 1997;11:9-13.
45. Krul JM, van Gijn J, Ackerstaff RG, et al. Site and pathogenesis of infarcts associated with carotid endarterectomy. *Stroke* 1989;20:324-328.
46. Hayes PD, Vainas T, Hartley S, et al. The Pruitt-Inahara shunt maintains mean middle cerebral artery velocities within 10% of pre-operative values during carotid endarterectomy. *J Vasc Surg* 2000;32:299-306.
47. Cao P, De Rango P, Zannetti S. Eversion vs conventional carotid endarterectomy: a systematic review. *Eur J Vasc Endovasc Surg* 2002;23:195-201.
48. Bond R, Rerkasem K, Naylor AR, et al. A systematic review of RCT's of patch angioplasty versus primary closure and different types of patch materials during carotid endarterectomy. *J Vasc Surg* 2004;40:1126-1135.
49. Riles TS, Imparato AM, Jacobowitz GR, et al. The cause of peri-operative stroke after carotid endarterectomy. *J Vasc Surg* 1994;19:206-214.
50. Naylor AR. Prevention of operation related stroke: are we asking the right questions? *Cardiovasc Surg* 1999;7:155-157.
51. Naylor AR, Mackey WC. Editorial comment: is there any evidence that peri-operative monitoring and quality control assessment alter clinical outcome? In: Naylor AR, Mackey WC, eds. *Carotid artery surgery: a problem based approach.* London: WB Saunders; 2000:313-314.
52. Naylor AR, Hayes PD, Allroggen H, et al. Reducing the risk of carotid surgery: a seven year audit of the role of monitoring and quality control assessment. *J Vasc Surg* 2000;32:750-759.
53. Lennard N, Smith JL, Gaunt ME, et al. A policy of quality control assessment reduces the risk of intraoperative stroke during carotid endarterectomy. *Eur J Vasc Endovasc Surg* 1999;17:234-240.
54. Ferguson GG, Eliasziw M, Barr HWK, et al., for the NASCET Trial. The North American Symptomatic Carotid Endarterectomy Trial: surgical results in 1415 patients. *Stroke* 1999;30:1751-1758.
55. Takolander R, Bergentz SE, Bergqvist D. Management of early neurological deficits after carotid thromboendarterectomy. *Eur J Vasc Surg* 1987;1:67-71.
56. Eckstein H-H, Schumacher H, Dorfler A, et al. Carotid endarterectomy and intracranial thrombolysis: simultaneous and staged procedures in ischaemic stroke. *J Vasc Surg* 1999;29:459-471.
57. Gaunt ME, Smith J, Martin PJ, et al. On-table diagnosis of incipient carotid artery thrombosis during carotid endarterectomy using transcranial Doppler sonography. *J Vasc Surg* 1994;20:104-107.
58. Gaunt ME, Smith JL, Martin PJ, et al. A comparison of quality control methods applied to carotid endarterectomy. *Eur J Vasc Endovasc Surg* 1996;11:4-11.
59. Levi CR, O'Malley HM, Fell G, et al. Transcranial Doppler detected cerebral embolism following carotid endarterectomy: high microembolic signal loads predict post-operative cerebral ischaemia. *Brain* 1997;120:621-629.
60. Spencer MP. Transcranial Doppler monitoring and causes of stroke from carotid endarterectomy. *Stroke* 1997;28:685-691.
61. Cantelmo NL, Babikian VL, Samaraweera RN, et al. Cerebral microembolism and ischaemia changes associated with carotid endarterectomy. *J Vasc Surg* 1998;27:1024-1030.
62. Laman DM, Wieneke GH, van Duijn H, van Huffelen AC. High embolic rate after carotid endarterectomy is associated with early cerebrovascular complications, especially in women. *J Vasc Surg* 2002;36:278-284.
63. Hayes PD, Allroggen H, Steel S, et al. A randomised trial of vein versus Dacron patching during carotid endarterectomy: influence of patch type on post-operative embolisation. *J Vasc Surg* 2001;33:994-1000.
64. Hayes PD, Patel F, Bell PRF, Naylor AR. Patients thrombo-embolic potential between bilateral carotid endarterectomies remains stable over time. *Eur J Vasc Endovasc Surg* 2001;22:496-498.
65. Hayes PD, Box H, Tull S, et al. The patients thrombo-embolic response following carotid endarterectomy is related to enhanced platelet sensitivity to ADP. *J Vasc Surg* 2003;38:1226-1231.
66. Payne DA, Jones CI, Hayes PD, et al. Beneficial effects of clopidogrel combined with aspirin in reducing cerebral emboli in patients undergoing carotid endarterectomy. *Circulation* 2004;109:1476-1481.
67. Paciaroni M, Eliasziw M, Kappelle LJ, et al. Medical complications associated with carotid endarterectomy. *Stroke* 1999;30:1759-1763.
68. Forsell C, Bergqvist D, Bergentz SE. Peripheral nerve injuries in carotid artery surgery. In: Greenhalgh RM, Hollier LH, eds. *Surgery for stroke.* London: WB Saunders; 1993:217-234.
69. Naylor AR, Payne D, Thompson MM, et al. Prosthetic patch infection after carotid endarterectomy. *Eur J Vasc Endovasc Surg* 2002;23:11-16.
70. Naylor AR, Chng S, Awad S. Redo carotid intervention: The role of carotid artery stenting. In: Wyatt MG, Watkinson AF, eds. *Endovascular therapies.* Shrewsbury, UK: TFM Publishing; 2006:123-129.
71. Moore WS, Kempczinski RF, Nelson JJ, Toole JF, for the ACAS Investigators. Recurrent carotid stenosis: results of the Asymptomatic Carotid Atherosclerosis Study. *Stroke* 1998;29:2018-2025.
72. Guillon B, Brunereau L, Biousse V, et al. Long-term follow-up of aneurysms developed during extracranial internal carotid artery dissection. *Neurology* 1999;53:117-122.
73. Touze E, Randoux B, Meary E, et al. Aneurysmal forms of cervical artery dissection: associated factors and outcome. *Stroke* 2001;32:418-423.

chapter

37

Endovascular Treatment of Carotid Disease

Jean-Pierre Becquemin, MD, FRCS

Key Points

- The optimal management of carotid stenosis by carotid endarterectomy or carotid artery stenosis (CAS) remains controversial.
- Carotid stenting is technically tricky and requires considerable endovascular expertise; consequently, there is a significant learning curve.
- The safety of CAS can be improved by several means: (1) anatomical assessment of the aortic arch and carotid artery, (2) identification of vulnerable plaque by GSM measurement on Duplex scan of by magnetic resonance imaging, (3) careful selection of patients based on cervical and general risk assessment, (4) proper training and perfect knowledge of the endovascular devices, and (5) advancement of stents and cerebral protection device technology.
- Cerebral protection devices do not prevent all embolic events during CAS.
- Metaanalysis of eight randomized trials demonstrated a trend toward better results with endarterectomy. However, heterogeneity of data, relative small sample of trials, and relative short follow-up leave a room for uncertainty.
- As a result, in symptomatic patients endarterectomy remains the gold standard and in asymptomatic patients further trials are required. For a given patient, indications of CAS must take into account the risk–benefit ratio assessed by a multidisciplinary approach.

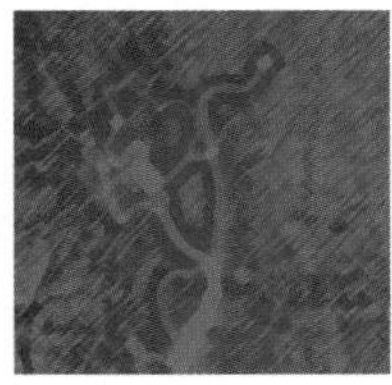

Endovascular treatment of carotid disease is a highly controversial treatment for patients with severe carotid stenosis. Proponents, mostly in the rank of cardiologists, believe that "carotid angioplasty is another nail in the coffin of carotid surgery."[1] Opponents, most of them surgeons, reply by quoting George Bernard Shaw: "When you have a new hammer, everything looks like a nail." The debate will probably continue for some time, since firm evidence is lacking concerning the immediate and long-term benefits of stenting over carotid endarterectomy (CEA). Pooled data from the currently published randomized studies are not in favor of carotid angioplasty stenting (CAS).[2,3] The review of CAS preformed in the United States in 2003 and 2004 is also worrisome, since the in-hospital stroke rate after CAS for asymptomatic patients was twofold higher than after CEA.[4] However, the difference between treatments is slim, and encouraging results from recent clinical series[5-8] indicate that carotid stenting is an alternative for a subset of patients with carotid disease.

The basis of the controversy is no longer the feasibility, which is well demonstrated, but the risk of stroke, which remains the most dramatic complication of all carotid interventions. Most strokes are caused by dislodgment of atherosclerotic debris, which may occur at any time during or even after the procedure.[9] Transcranial Doppler monitoring and brain weight magnetic resonance imaging have shown that carotid stenting produces more microemboli than carotid surgery.[10] The clinical consequences of these observations remain to be assessed since most of these emboli are asymptomatic or produce transient symptoms.

Compared to the first attempts of CAS, substantial technical improvements have been made. Monorail systems with thin catheters, low-profile balloons, stents specifically designed for the carotid territory and cerebral protection devices (CPDs)

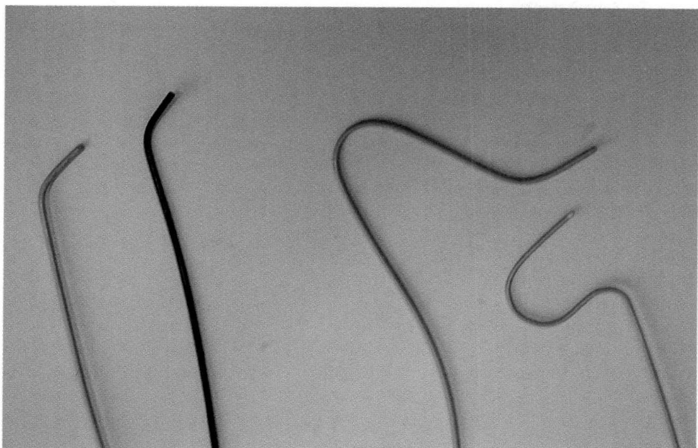

Figure 37-1. Catheters for carotid angioplasty/stenting.

are routinely used. Furthermore, a consensus exists for the adjuvant drug regimens that help avoid acute stent occlusion. Thromboembolic events with the use of urgent rescue techniques also reduce the severity of neurological events. Finally, after the pioneers' learning curve, the technique itself is becoming routine and reproducible.

Carotid angioplasty remains, nevertheless, a relatively sophisticated procedure that needs great care in patient selection, good knowledge of the available devices, good imaging facilities, and excellent skill in endovascular navigation.

MATERIALS, DEVICES, AND TECHNIQUES

This section describes the materials and the techniques that I currently use. Other excellent products are available.

Materials and Devices

Guide Wires

Three types of guide wire are required:

- An angled, 0.035-inch, 2.6-m-long, soft hydrophilic guide wire (Terumo)
- An angled, 0.035-inch, 2.6-m-long, stiff hydrophilic (Terumo) guide wire
- A 0.014-inch soft hydrophilic wire (Spartacor) when using the Spider (EV3) CPD

Catheters

Depending upon the technique used, two types of catheters are required.

Catheter Guide Technique

To gain access to the arterial lumen, a short 5-French (Fr) introducer sheath, 10 cm long, with a valve and a lateral channel is used. Different types of catheters should be available: a vertebral catheter (Terumo) or a JB-2 (Cook) is adequate in 70% of the procedures. For difficult angulated arteries, the left common carotid artery, or both, a glide vertebral catheter, a Simmons or Mani catheter, or both are more appropriate (Figure 37-1). To get the required shape, the Simmons catheter is shaped in the iliac artery opposite from the introducer site; in the renal, superior mesenteric, left subclavian artery; or against the aortic valve. The size of the Simmons or Mani catheter (one of three available sizes) must be chosen to fit the size and shape of the aorta at the level of the arch. Finally, a 7-Fr, 90-cm-long Arrow delivery catheter used to be employed routinely at my institution.

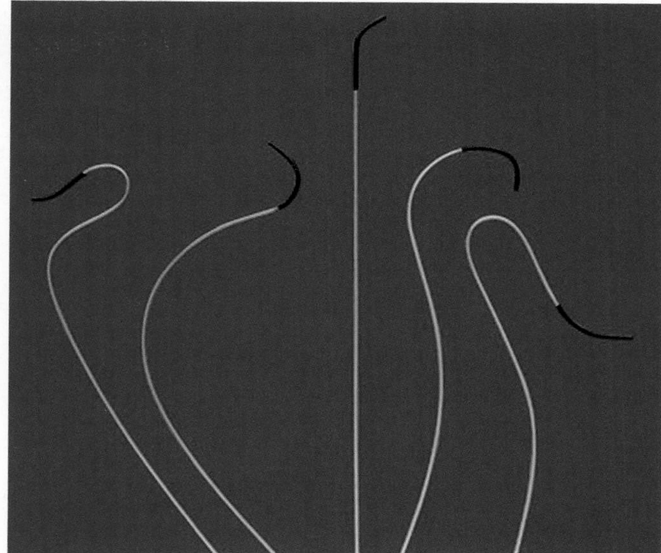

Figure 37-2. Various catheters for the Shuttle introducer sheath.

Long Introducer Sheath Technique

Following wire placement in the femoral artery, a 6-Fr, 80-cm-long Shuttle catheter (Cook) is used. Then, according to the anatomy of the arch and arising vessels, a JB-2 or VTK catheter is used (Figure 37-2).

Balloons

I use monorail balloons (Figure 37-3). For predilatation, a balloon 2 or 3 mm in diameter and 2 to 3 cm in length, such as Crossrail 0.014 (Guidant) or the coronary Speedy or Gazel monorail (Boston Scientific), usually is appropriate. Larger balloons (5 to 6 mm) are also necessary to model the stent after deployment.

Stents

Stainless steel balloon expandable stents such as the Express (Boston Scientific) or Palmaz-blue (Cordis, Johnson and Johnson) are used for lesions located on the proximal carotid artery and or on the innominate trunk. They have two main advantages:

- The stent placement and the crushing of the plaque is a one-shot procedure, which avoids material manipulation.
- The radial force of the stent is among the strongest available.

However, they have several drawbacks:

- The diameter of the balloon with the stent is relatively large, which can be an issue when trying to cross a tight stenosis safely.

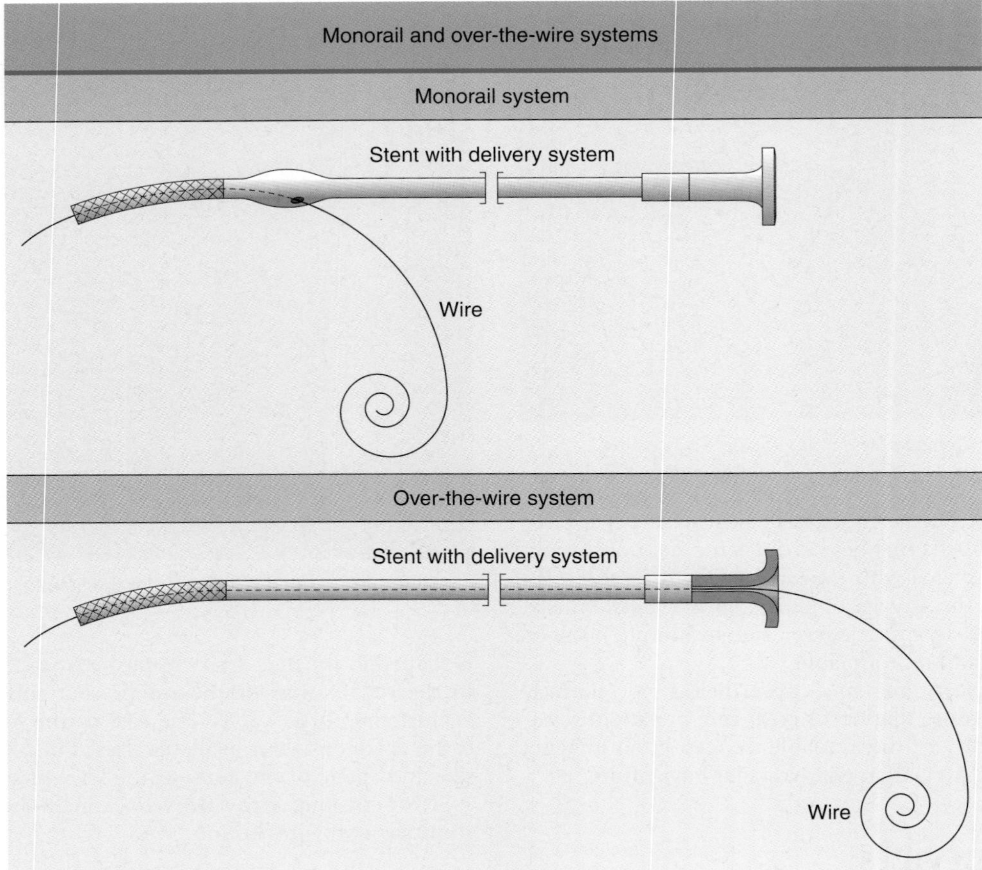

Figure 37-3. Conception of monorail and over-the-wire systems for balloon catheter insertion.

- They are rigid and the stent is not protected by an outer sheath, thereby increasing the risk of plaque dislodgment, stent escape, or blockage.
- Any subsequent external compression may deform the stent.

Self-expanding stents are used routinely for the carotid bifurcation. They are made of stainless steel, such as the carotid Wallstent (Figure 37-4), or of nitinol, such as the Herculink (Guidant), Nextstent (Boston Scientific), AVE (Medtronic), Precise (Cordis; Figure 37-5), Protégé (EV3), or Accunet (Abott).

These stents have good flexibility, are able to cross a tortuous artery, and can match the size discrepancy between the common and the internal carotid arteries. Moreover, the radial forces with these stents are acceptable. Of note is that the carotid Wallstent is more radioopaque than the nitinol stents; this may be of importance when dealing with difficult lesions. Some stents shorten during their release, a phenomenon that

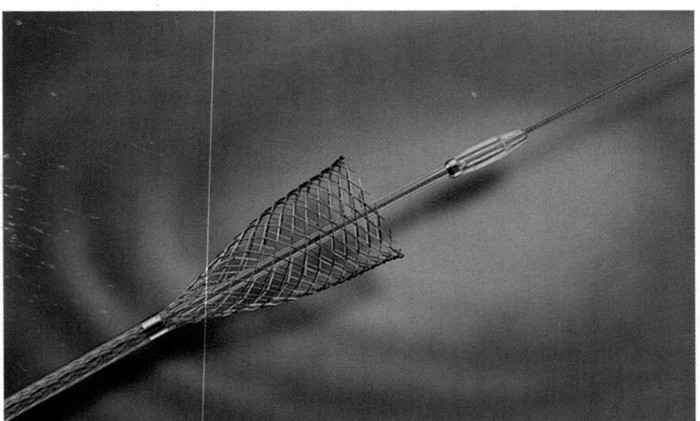

Figure 37-4. Carotid Wallstent from Boston Scientific made of a mesh of stainless steel, producing a closed-cell shape.

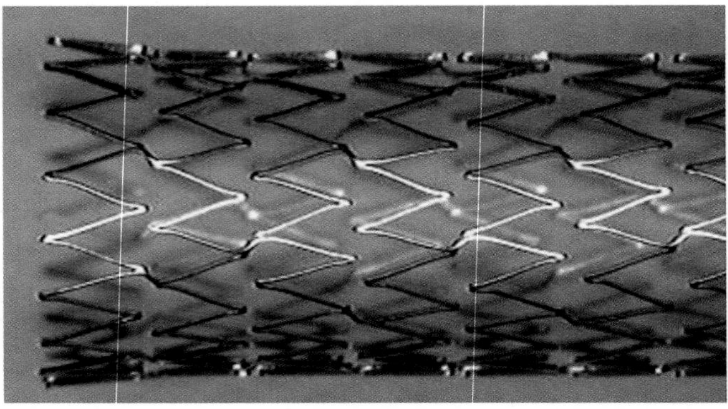

Figure 37-5. Precise nitinol stent from Cordis with an open cells shape.

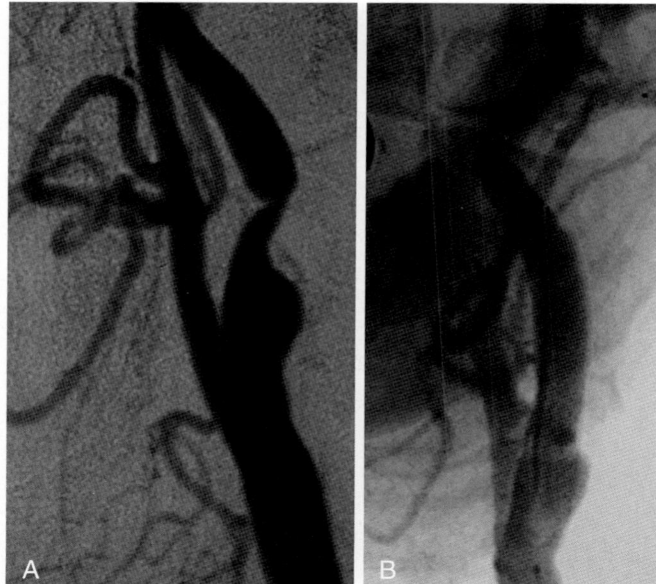

Figure 37-6. Severe carotid stenosis before **(A)** and after **(B)** implantation of a Wallstent.

must be anticipated to allow careful positioning. Each of these stents has pro and cons (Figure 37-6). The carotid Wallstent is more rigid and may not be adequate in tortuous anatomy. On the other hand, the surface free of metal is among the lowest, which has led some investigators to speculate that they may be more efficient in preventing atheromatous debris from being dislodged after stent placement. Nitinol stents have larger surface free of metal, which makes them more flexible and more prone to adapt tortuous anatomy. The downside of this design is the possibility of metal protrusion in the free lumen of the artery with the risk of trapping the wire within the struts. They also may be less efficient in containing the plaque content.[11] So far, however, no randomized data supports this speculation.

Cerebral Protection Devices

There are two types of CPDs. One is based on carotid internal occlusion with a balloon; the other relies on a filter technique.

Percusurge GuardWire System

The Percusurge system (Medtronic) includes a hollow Teflon-coated microcatheter available in 0.014- and 0.018-inch sizes with the balloon close to its distal tip (Figure 37-7). A disposable sealing system enables the balloon to be inflated and deflated. The balloon diameter can be varied from 3.5 to 6 mm. The distal tip of the wire is floppy and radioopaque; radioopaque markers close to the balloon allow its accurate placement above the carotid stenosis. The wire permits exchange of interventional devices, balloons, and stents and placement of an aspiration catheter. Before deflation of the balloon, by decompression with a syringe and slow removal of the aspiration catheter, debris is removed from the carotid artery. The system handles excellently, with good torque and

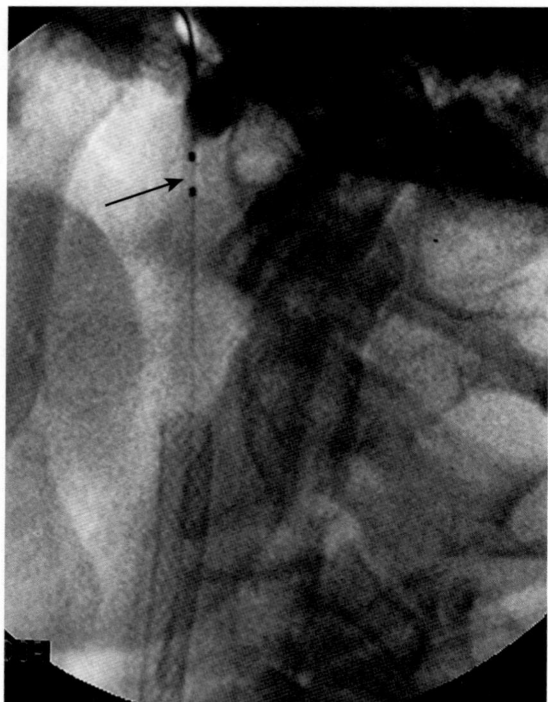

Figure 37-7. Intraoperative view of the Percusurge GuardWire protection device showing the radioopaque markers above the carotid stenosis *(arrow)*.

forward movement. Tight, eccentric, and irregular stenoses can be crossed relatively easily. However, the preparation of the system, notably the sealing system and the aspiration catheter, is relatively sophisticated. Widely used at the beginning of the practice of protected CAS, it has been almost abandoned today.

Parodi Antiemboli System

The Parodi system is based on the principle of reverse flow (Figure 37-8). A guiding catheter with a large balloon is placed in the common carotid artery, proximal to the carotid bifurcation. A lateral channel on the guiding catheter allows, when necessary, a second balloon to be inflated in the external carotid artery. The whole system is linked to a line, which is placed into one of the femoral veins. When the two balloons are inflated, the carotid inflow is stopped and the back flow from the internal carotid is diverted into the venous system. A filter between the arterial and the venous sides traps any debris. Since the flow in the internal carotid is reversed continuously, there is no risk of brain embolization during carotid stenting. However, the system requires a 10-Fr introducer sheath and is relatively cumbersome and complex. In patients with a poor circle of Willis or recent brain ischemic damage, blood flow diversion may not be well tolerated.

MO.MA

Developed in Europe, MO.MA reproduces the principle of the Parodi system.

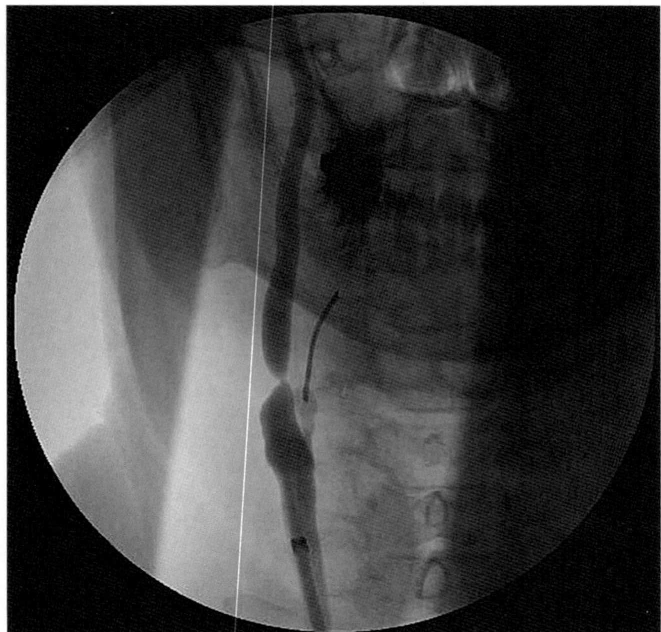

Figure 37-8. The Parodi antiemboli system.

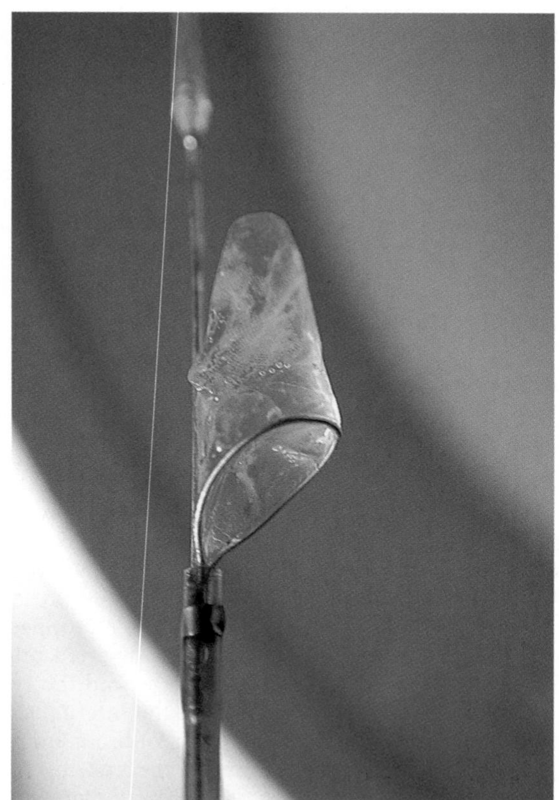

Figure 37-9. EPI filter wire.

EPI Filterwire EZ

Boston Scientific's EPI Filterwire EZ consists of a basket-like, porous membrane at the tip of a 0.014-inch guide wire (Figure 37-9). An outer sheath protects the filter, which is released when the sheath is displaced caudally. The filter has to be deployed about 2 cm above the stenosis in a relatively straight arterial segment. The filter, and particularly its base, should be applied carefully against the arterial wall to offer maximum efficacy. After carotid stent deployment, the filter containing trapped debris is retrieved by pulling it partially within the outer sheath.

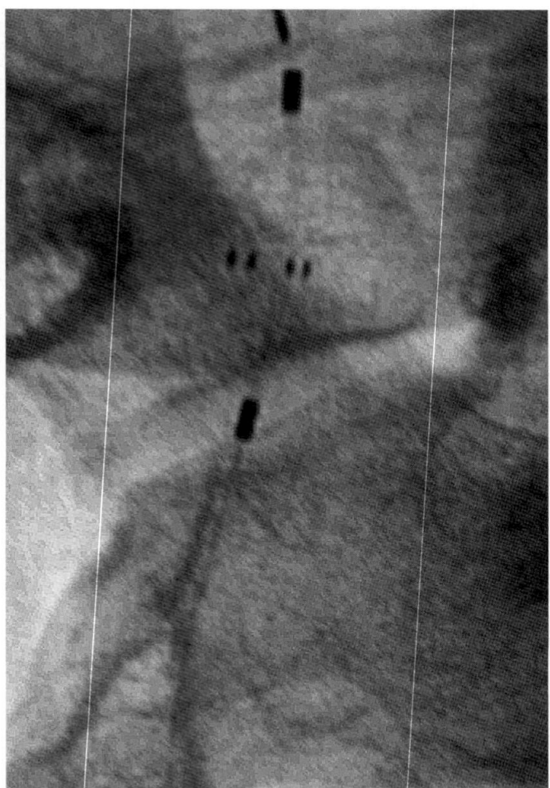

Figure 37-10. Angioguard carotid filter system in position.

Angioguard System

The Angioguard system (Cordis) is also a basket-like filter fixed by longitudinal metallic wires (Figure 37-10). The filter presents micropores, 0.5 mm in diameter. The basket is deployed and captured by pushing or pulling the outer sheath.

Accunet and Neuroshield System

The principles of the Accunet and Neuroshield system (Abbott; Figure 37-11) are similar to the two previously described filters.

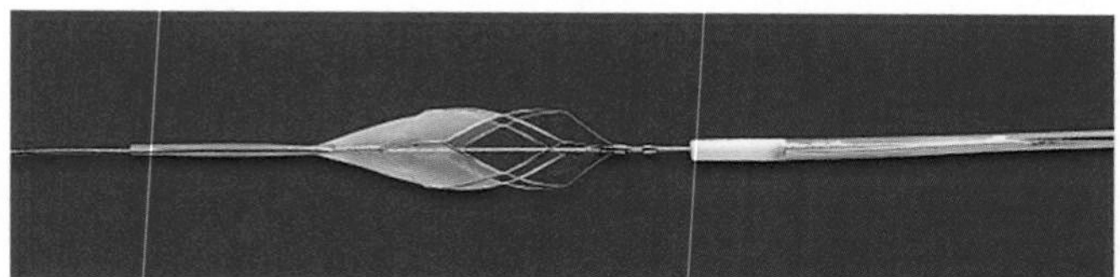

Figure 37-11. The Accunet system.

Spider

The Spider filter (EV3) is made of a small cage of nitinol wires (Figure 37-12). A 0.014-inch guide (I routinely use the Spartacor) is used as a tutor. The 0.018-inch catheter in which the filter is loaded is then pushed over the wire, up to 2 cm above the stenosis. The Spartacor wire is then removed and the filter is pushed in place by the wire attached to the filter. By gently pulling the outer sheath, the filter opens up. The main advantage of the system is the way in which the lesion is crossed—not by the whole system but by an independent and low-profile wire. The catheterism of lesions is easier, and it may be recommended in severely angulated internal carotid arteries and in tight stenosis. The drawback is the need for extra endovascular manipulations.

The main advantage of filters is their relative simplicity. They are indented to keep the carotid blood flow intact during the procedure. However, they have drawbacks:

1. Measurement of flow distal to filter has shown a relative slowdown with certain filters mostly due to the small size of the holes in the filter membrane or free surface of the baskets.
2. They are relatively instable and may move during the maneuvers of carotid stenting.
3. Uncertainty exists about the full apposition of the outer edge of filter on the arterial wall.
4. They may damage the arterial wall.
5. Occasionally, when a large amount of fresh thrombus is trapped in the filter, carotid occlusion may occur. Clots aspiration by an additional catheter is then mandatory to remove the clots and to enable a safe retrieval of the filter.

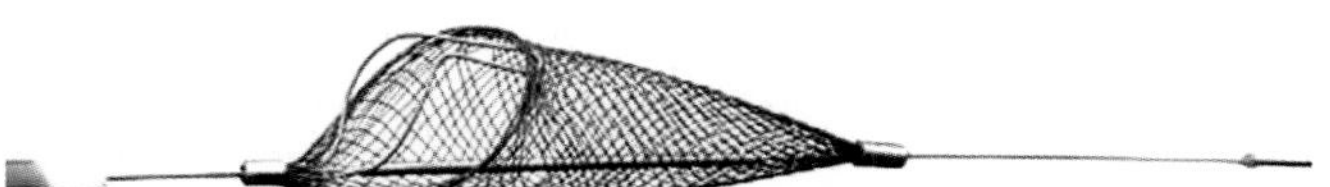

Figure 37-12. The Spider filter.

Techniques of ICA Angioplasty and Stenting

Operating Room Installation

A well-appointed operating room is essential for a successful procedure. The operating table must be radiolucent. Before starting the endovascular maneuver, a clinician must check that no radioopaque bars or wires cross the operating field, including the groin, the whole aorta, the neck, and the skull. Anteroposterior and lateral views must be easily and rapidly obtained, and it must be possible to rotate the C-arm freely around the neck of the patient. The operating team, including the surgeon, the assistant, and the scrub nurse, stand to the right of the patient. A disposable table is placed at the patient's feet (Figure 37-13). This allows positioning of the endovascular devices "in line," limiting the risk of dropping any wires or catheters and septic contamination. The C-arm faces the operating team, with the screen opposite the main operator. The patient is draped in one large sterile sheet with two

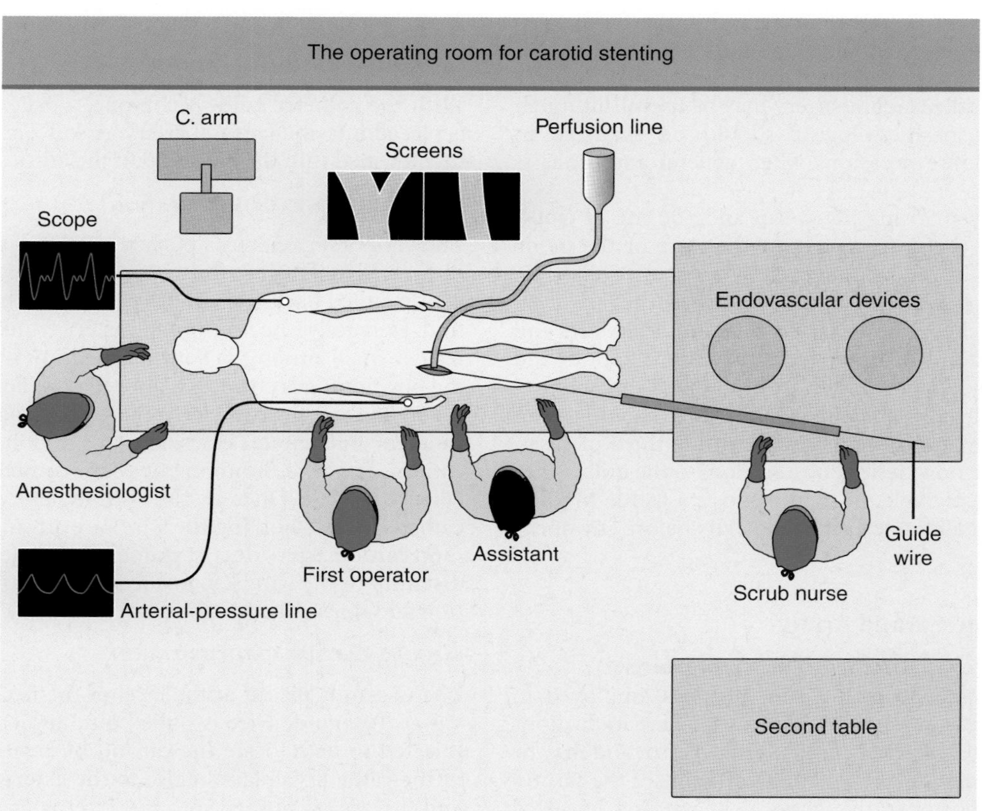

Figure 37-13. Diagram of the operating room for carotid stenting.

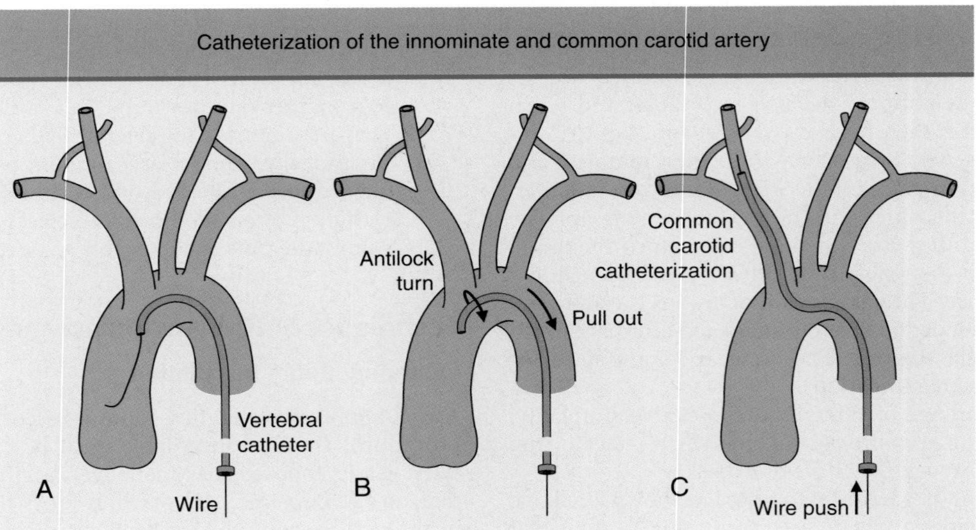

Figure 37-14. Catheterization of the innominate and common carotid artery.

openings in the groin. The groin should have been shaved and washed with antiseptic solution. Various endovascular materials (guide wire, catheters, and stents, all of different sizes and length) should be stored in the vicinity of the operating theater and be easily and rapidly accessible.

Anesthesia, Monitoring, and Medication

Except for combined procedures, patients have carotid procedures under local anesthesia. Since severe bradycardia may occur, continuous cardiac monitoring and intraarterial pressure measurement is essential. Conscious level and motor functions should be surveyed regularly. Transcranial Doppler imaging of the middle cerebral artery may be useful, although not mandatory. Anesthesiologists should be available in the room for the rare occasions when general anesthesia is required urgently.

Patients are given 75 mg of aspirin and 300 mg of clopidogrel on the day before surgery. At the start of the guide wire manipulation, 1 mg/kg of heparin is given intravenously. Heparin is not reversed at the end of the procedure, and low-molecular-weight heparin is started 6 hours afterward and continued for 48 hours. Clopidogrel is given for 1 month and aspirin indefinitely. To prevent severe bradycardia and arterial spasm, 1 mg of atropine may be given before angioplasty or on demand. Bradycardia occurs in about one third of cases, generally with a de novo lesion located close to the bulb. Since this event is unpredictable, in tight stenosis a gentle predilation with a 3-mm balloon tests the reflexivity before any opening of the stent.

Approaches to the Carotid Artery

There are four basic approaches to the carotid artery:

1. Direct percutaneous carotid puncture was employed in the first attempts at carotid angioplasty. Few indications remain, since it is relatively difficult to perform and may be hazardous. Arterial dissection, blind crossing of the carotid stenosis, and postoperative cervical hematoma have led progressively to its abandonment. However, following surgical exposure of the common carotid artery, direct puncture may occasionally be used. The main indication is the presence of tandem lesions, involving the proximal intrathoracic common carotid and the carotid bifurcation.
2. The brachial approach through the humeral artery may be useful when the femoral approach is not adequate, but it has risks of median nerve damage.
3. The radial approach is currently more easily performed due to low-profile material.
4. The femoral approach is routine for my colleagues and I. As mentioned earlier, there are currently two techniques.

Catheter Guide Technique

With the catheter guide technique, a 5-Fr introducer sheath is placed into the femoral artery. A soft Terumo guide wire is then pushed into the aorta, up to the aortic arch.

COMMON CAROTID CATHETERIZATION

The vertebral catheter is pushed up the guide wire. Once the catheter is in the arch, the wire is pulled out and the catheter is gently pulled back while the surgeon exercises clockwise rotation. Generally, the innominate artery trunk is easily catheterized. A small amount of contrast medium is used to check that the positioning is correct (Figure 37-14). For the left common carotid artery, the catheter is pulled back again for a few centimeters. In favorable cases, it jumps into the common carotid ostium. If not, a Simmons or Mani catheter should be used (Figure 37-15). Once in the ostium, the wire and then the catheter (while holding the wire) are advanced into the common carotid artery. It is of prime importance to verify that the distal tip of the wire remains proximal to the carotid bifurcation and does not cross the carotid stenosis blindly.

EXTERNAL CAROTID CATHETERIZATION

The C-arm is placed at the level of the neck to obtain lateral views. The guide wire is pulled out, and contrast medium is injected to help locate the carotid bifurcation. The distal tip of the catheter is placed close to the external carotid ostium, and the wire is pushed into the external carotid artery. Once in place, the vertebral catheter is advanced into the external

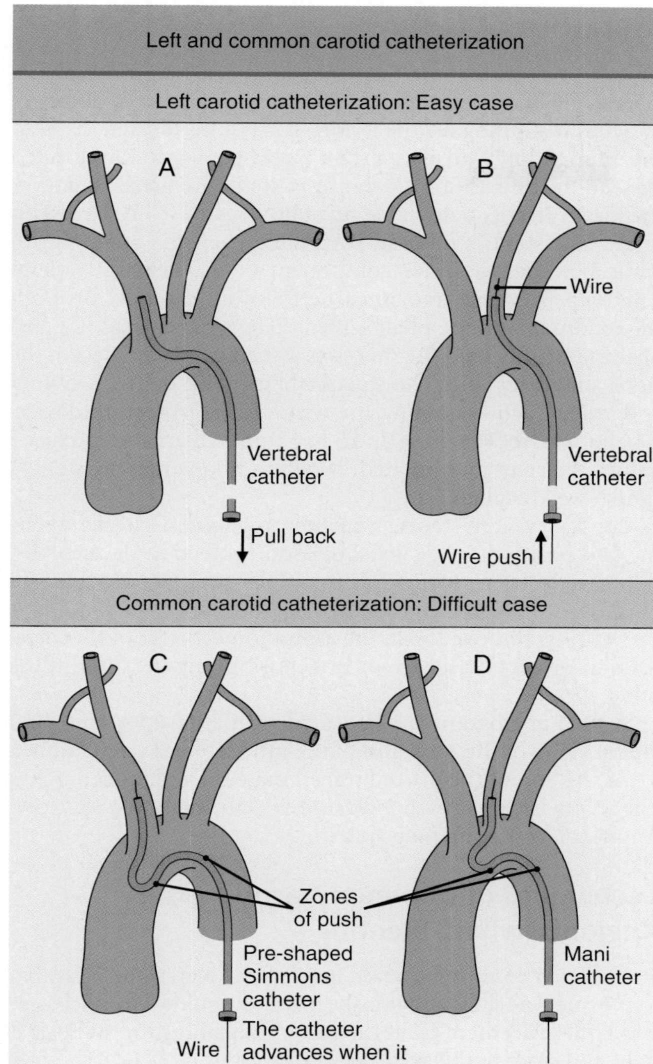

Figure 37-15. Left and common carotid catheterization. **A** and **B,** Catheterization of the left common carotid artery with a vertebral catheter. **C** and **D,** Catheterization of the left common carotid artery with a Simmons and a Mani catheter.

carotid artery. The soft wire is then exchanged for a stiff guide wire, which is blocked into a tributary, the lingual or occipital artery.

DELIVERY CATHETER PLACEMENT

The vertebral catheter is retrieved and replaced by the 7-Fr Arrow catheter. The radioopaque distal tip is placed in the common carotid artery. Then dilatator and wire are pulled out. An angiogram is performed through the Arrow catheter. Images are generally of excellent quality. With the Parodi system, the Arrow catheter is not necessary.

Long Introducer Sheath Technique

With the long introducer sheath technique, a Shuttle catheter is pushed from the femoral artery up to the arch. Then, with an oblique view, an angiogram of the arch is performed by the use of an injector. According to the arch anatomy a VTK or a JB-2 Cook catheter is pushed into the Shuttle (Figure 37-16).

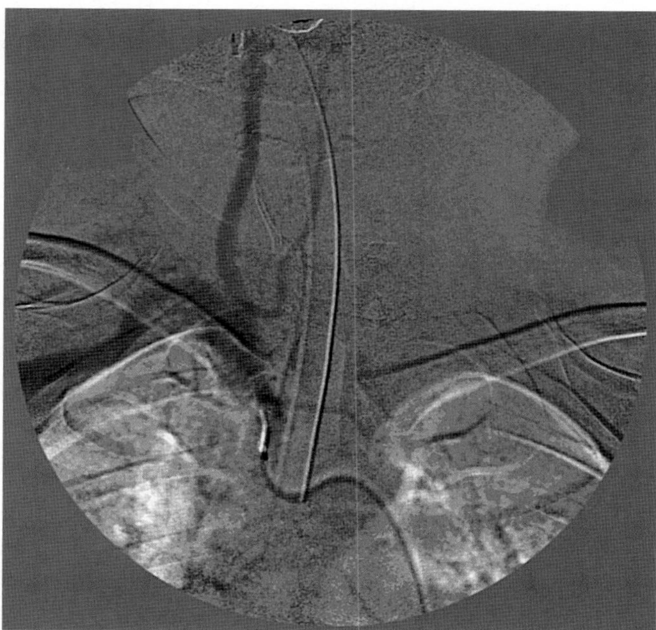

Figure 37-16. Intraoperative view of the Shuttle technique with a VTK catheter.

The distal tips of these catheters are sufficiently rigid to catch the origin of the desired common carotid artery. Then the 0.035-inch soft Terumo wire is pushed upward. Great care must be taken of not inadvertently crossing the lesion. By slightly pushing the VTK catheter and then the Shuttle over it, the surgeon gains access to the middle part of the common carotid artery. In some cases a combination of pushing and pulling the catheters helps the maneuver.

The main advantage of this technique is the limitation of maneuver since external carotid catheterism is unnecessary and no introducer sheath exchanges are used.

CEREBRAL PROTECTION DEVICES PLACEMENT

With the filter devices or the distal protection balloon system, the distal flexible tip of the device is placed proximal to the carotid bifurcation through the introducer sheath (Figure 37-17). Then, using road mapping, the internal carotid artery is catheterized and the stenosis is crossed. This maneuver is generally easy to perform. In the case of an angulated internal carotid artery, the distal tip of the wire must be preshaped. Only a gentle push is employed, to avoid plaque injury. In some cases, the surgeon can facilitate the passage of wire by using an angulated microcatheter. Once the lesion has been crossed, the distal balloon or the filter is deployed about 2 cm above the stenosis.

When a reverse flow system has been chosen, the common carotid and external carotid balloons are inflated and the lesion is crossed with a 0.014-inch standard wire.

PREDILATATION

Predilatation is necessary only for a tight carotid stenosis (more than 95%); this avoids any friction during the crossing by the stent and makes the intrastent balloon angioplasty easier to perform. Without it, it may be impossible to cross the stenosis with the stent or to place the balloon after the release of the stent.

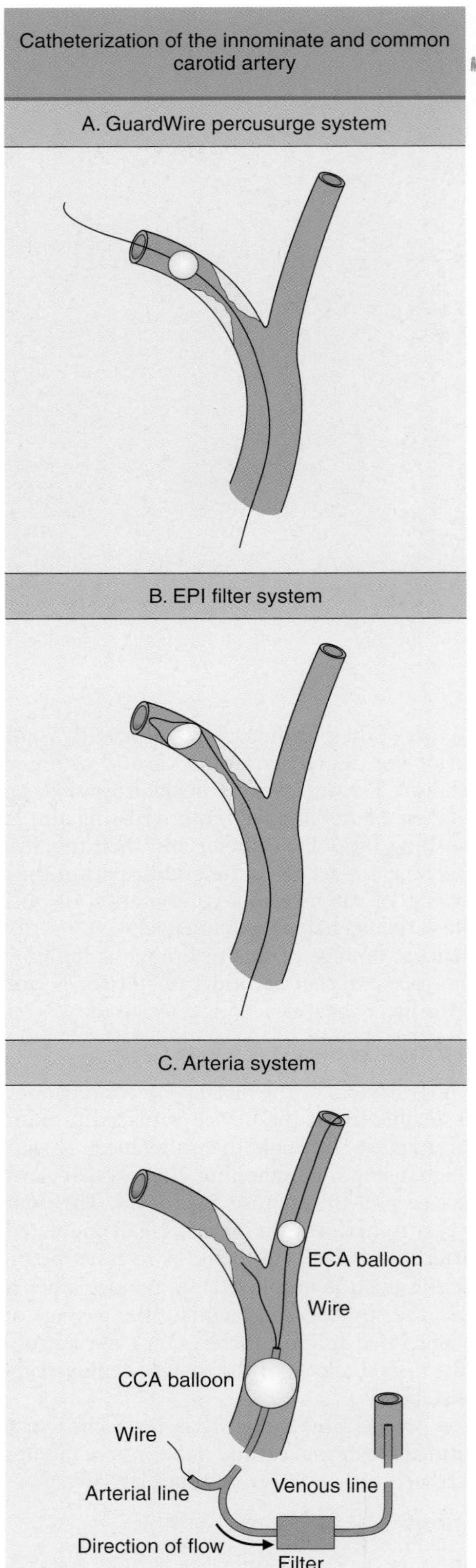

Figure 37-17. Cerebral protection device placement. **A,** Percusurge GuardWire cerebral protection device placement. **B,** Filter placement. **C,** Arteria system placement.

Stenting and Angioplasty

This step is similar to angioplasty and stenting in peripheral arteries (Figure 37-18). I use a relatively long stent (3 or 4 cm), to avoid it slipping off the lesion. For lesions located distal to the bifurcation, 5- to 6-mm stents are used. For lesions located close to the bifurcation, 7- to 8-mm stents are used. Whatever the location, adequate sizing must be assessed from the angiogram. The stent is released by pulling back the outer sheath while holding the inner component of the delivery system. This step is crucial and must be followed carefully on both the roadmap and the plain screens. The smaller field (22 cm) of the C-arm is used for this step. When correctly placed, the stent shows a typical hourglass shape. The delivery system is removed, while holding the wire of the protection device. A balloon, 2 to 3 cm long and 5 to 6 mm in diameter, is placed within the stent and inflated. When radioopaque, the stent is shown well by plain x-ray.

For less visible stents, a further angiogram checks opening and position. With distal balloon protection devices, this step cannot be performed at this time, since the flow is still blocked.

Debris is removed with the aspiration catheter of the distal balloon protection device or by repositioning the filter in the outer sheath.

A final angiogram is performed with anteroposterior and lateral views of the neck and of the intracerebral circulation.

At the end of the procedure, all material is removed. Arterial access is closed with a closure system, such as a Perclose, Angioseal, or Boomerang system.

Techniques of Common Carotid Artery Angioplasty and Stenting

For isolated common carotid lesions, the technique is similar to the one described previously; however, guide wire exchange and CPD placement is all the more difficult as the stenosis is tight and close to the arch (Figure 37-19).

For tandem lesions of the common and internal carotid arteries, the internal carotid is treated in the conventional way; before closing the arteriotomy, the common carotid is punctured with a 5-Fr introducer sheath. Guide wire, balloon, and stent are placed in the proximal common carotid lesion. It is useful to place a pigtail catheter in the aortic arch coming from the groin. It is then easy to survey the correct position of the stent.

Alternatively, the proximal common carotid stenosis can be treated by angioplasty and the internal carotid stenosis by conventional surgical repair. I prefer to start with the conventional repair of the internal carotid and then, before the closure of the artery, puncture the common carotid in a retrograde fashion. Once the endovascular procedure has been completed, debris and clots are flushed through the arteriotomy, which is then repaired by conventional suture.

Case for Routine Stenting

Although the current consensus for carotid angioplasty is to place a stent routinely, the evidence upon which this attitude is based is slim. In the Carotid and Vertebral Artery Transluminal Angioplasty Study (CAVATAS), the percentages of transient ischemic attack or stroke and restenosis

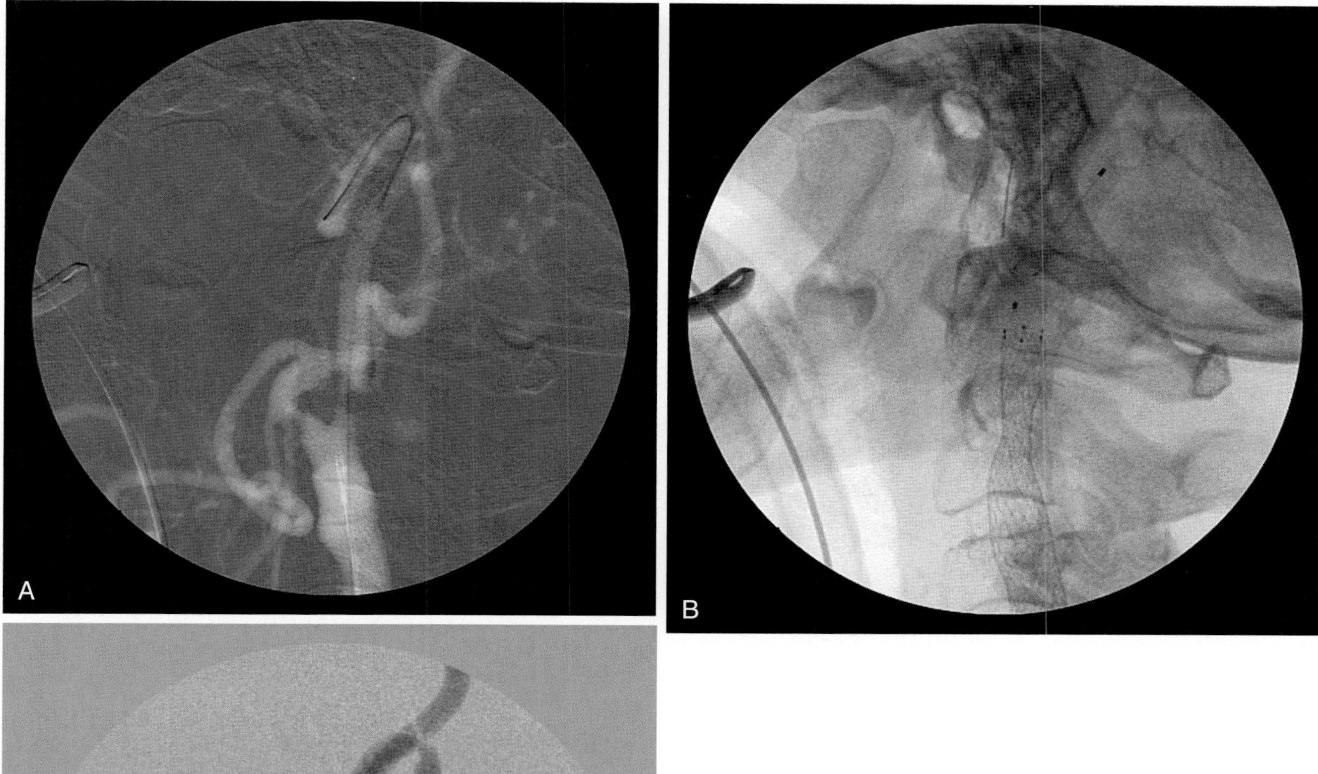

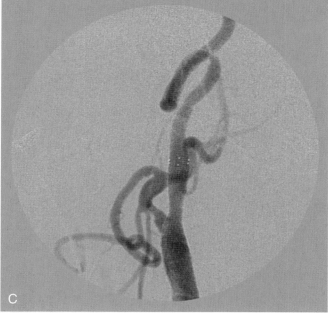

Figure 37-18. Intraoperative views of a difficult case with severe distal tortuosity. **A,** Pretreatment, note the distal tip of the Spartacor catheter in the tortuosity. **B,** Tapered Nitinol stent and Spider filter in place. **C,** Posttreatment.

were similar in the group of patients who had undergone a stent procedure and in the group who had undergone balloon angioplasty alone.[12] With transcranial Doppler assessment, however, Orlandi et al.[13] showed that fewer microemboli were found in the middle cerebral artery in patients in whom a stent was placed compared to those in whom it was not. From a pathological point of view, this finding appears logical. Balloon angioplasty widens the arterial lumen by fracturing the plaque. Thus, atherosclerotic debris and clots contained in the plaque may migrate in the bloodstream. Stents, by permanently crushing the plaque, prevent early recoil. The atherosclerotic material is trapped between the metallic frame and the arterial wall, which may limit migration. The disadvantage of routine stenting is its propensity to develop intimal hyperplasia and excess tissue growth within the struts of the stent, although so far this problem does not seem to be relevant clinically. It may arise from the relatively short length of stent in a relatively high-flow situation.

SELECTION OF ENDOVASCULAR CAROTID TREATMENT

Patient Selection

My current selection criteria are summarized in Table 37-1. However, no evidence, nor consensus, exists on patient selection for carotid angioplasty. Before choosing between carotid

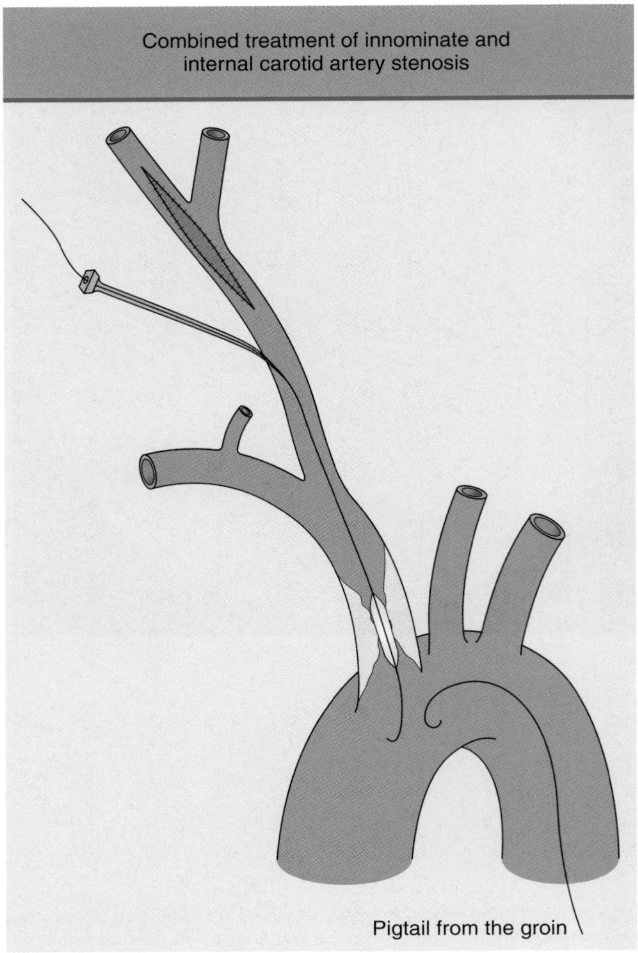

Combined treatment of innominate and internal carotid artery stenosis

Pigtail from the groin

Figure 37-19. Combined treatment of innominate and internal carotid artery stenosis.

Table 37-1
Comparison of Current Selection Criteria for Angioplasty and Stenting or for Surgery for Carotid Stenosis*

	Angioplasty/Stenting	Surgery
Severe coronary disease	+	?
Calcified aortic valve	+/–	+++
Coronary drug-eluted stent	+++	
Renal insufficiency	++	++
Pulmonary disease	+++	+/–
Age >80 years	–	+++
Aortic arch disease	–	+++
Severe angulations	+	+++
Severe tortuosity	+	+++
Aortoiliac disease	+	+++
Hemorrhagic risk	+++	–
Vulnerable plaque	+	+++
Echolucent plaque	–	+++
Circular calcification	–	+++
Floating thrombus	–	+++
Restenosis	+++	+
Postradiation stenosis	+++	+
Inflammatory arteritis	+	++
Atherosclerotic plaque	+++	+++

*–, poor indication; +/++, fair indication; +++, excellent indication.

stenting or surgery, the balance of risks should be examined carefully; this includes general, local, and neurological risk. Also, the risk of technical failure due to anatomical peculiarities must be taken into account.

General Risk

Since surgery is associated with a low mortality (particularly under local anesthetic), it is not easy to predict which patients may benefit from carotid angioplasty rather than surgery.[14] It has been shown that patients with severe coronary, pulmonary, or renal disease have a higher risk of neurological and general complications.[15,16] The Stenting and Angioplasty with Protection in Patients at High Risk for Endarterectomy (SAPPHIRE) Trial has shown that angioplasty and stenting may be less risky in these patients with less myocardial events with CAS than with CEA.[17] On the other hand, in a cardiac patient, angioplasty may be hazardous, since hemodynamic instability is not well tolerated in those with severe coronary disease or with calcified aortic cardiac valve disease. Patients with severe respiratory disorders are probably the least disputable indication, since groin anesthesia is obviously a better option than general or cervical block anesthesia. Patients with renal insufficiency may also benefit from angioplasty, although care should be taken with the risk of contrast nephropathy. In addition, these patients often have unfavorable anatomical lesions.

Local Risk

The risk of cervical nerve injury after surgery is in the range of 7%, although this is usually only temporary.[18,19] This rate is increased to 17% in patients who have had a previous neck operation or neck irradiation.[20] The risk of infection is quite low, except in those patients with a tracheotomy.

Thus, although still challenged by some authors,[21] the consensus is to consider patients with restenosis following a previous CEA, or patients with radiation-induced stenosis (especially those with a tracheostomy), as an accepted indication for carotid stenting (Figure 37-20). Unfortunately, the durability of stenting for this indication is questioned, since severe intrastent restenosis and occlusion has been reported.[22,23]

Neurological Risk

Plaques that are ulcerated, unstable, or full of fresh thrombotic material and floating thrombus are clearly at risk from an endovascular procedure and are probably best treated by open surgery (Figure 37-21). Conversely, fibrotic soft plaque gives rise to less risk. For the usual lesions, (duplex) imaging or magnetic resonance imaging may help detect vulnerable plaques that are at higher risk of procedural events. Computerized calculation of gray-scale median on duplex allows a quantification of the risk.[24]

Contralateral occlusion of the internal carotid artery gives rise to a risk of intolerance to clamping, and a shunt is often required during carotid surgery. These patients may be considered for angioplasty instead.

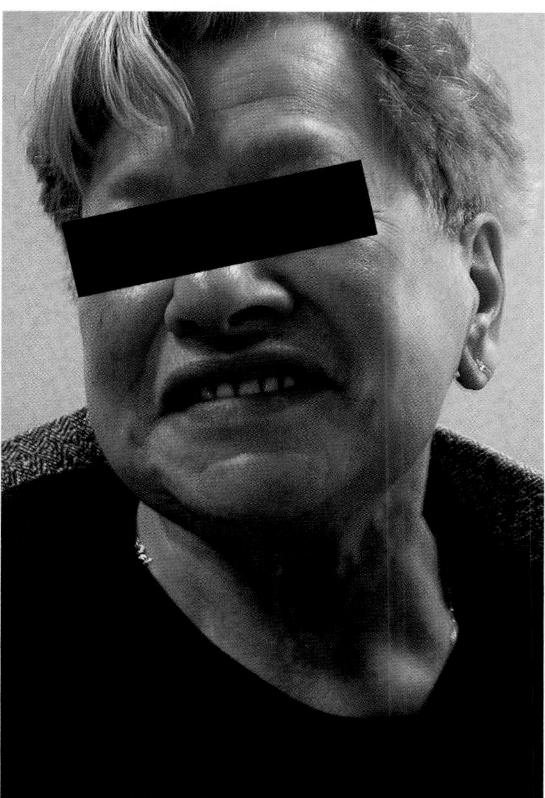

Figure 37-20. A 67-year-old female with a symptomatic left carotid stenosis. She had previously been treated by surgery and radiotherapy for head and neck cancer. This is an accepted indication for carotid stenting.

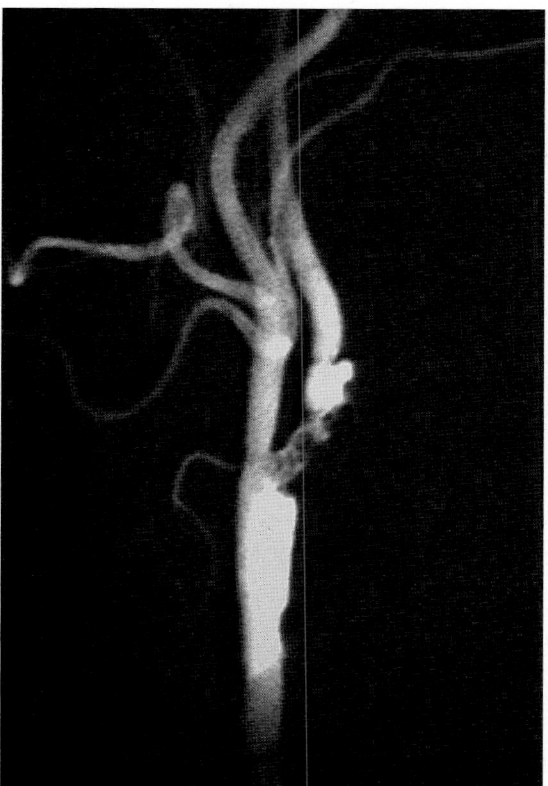

Figure 37-21. Angiography of a carotid bifurcation showing unstable plaque and thrombus. This is a contraindication to carotid stenting.

The status of the aortic arch is an important issue. It has been shown by transesophageal duplex imaging that the aortic arch is often the origin of cerebral emboli (Figure 37-22) and that the frequency of thrombus and significant unstable aortic plaque increase with age.[25-27] In these patients, endovascular treatment, at least from the groin, is not the best option. Cervical approach for CAS may be a useful alternative.[25-28]

Risk of Technical Failure

Angioplasty may fail because of navigation problems or failure of stent deployment. Failure must be anticipated to avoid serious clinical complications.

Iliac stenosis or occlusion is an annoying cause of failure that should be avoidable by preoperative duplex imaging.

Sharp angulations of the aortic arch and common carotid arteries such as seen in type C arch or in bovine arch anatomy also carry risks failure of catheterization (Figure 37-23). The threshold is difficult to define, however, since skilled interventionalists may succeed where the less experienced fail.

Severe common carotid tortuosity may preclude the delivery of the stent.[29] Internal carotid artery tortuosity may also be difficult to deal with, since the positioning of the CPD may be a problem, all the more so because a kink may occur at the distal end of the stent.

Finally, heavy circular calcified plaque or dense fibrotic plaque may be impossible to crush. In this case, if predilatation has not previously been attempted, the stent may remain blocked or partially deployed in the carotid artery.

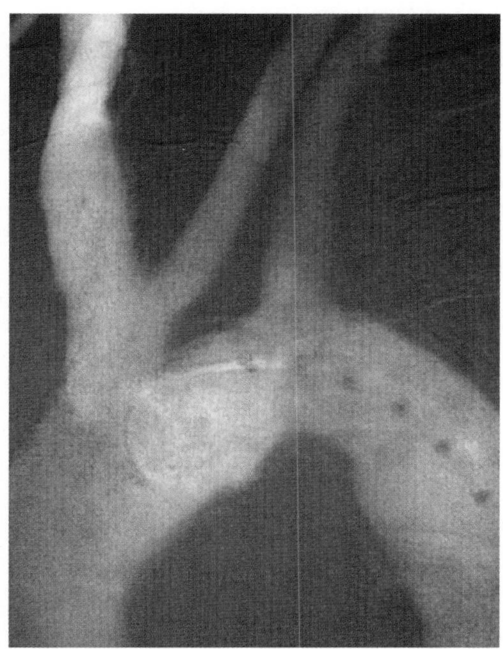

Figure 37-22. Bovine arch that may be difficult for beginners to deal with.

Goals of Therapy

The goal of carotid endovascular therapy is to prevent stroke. Thus, only patients at significant risk of stroke should be treated. Patients with asymptomatic less than 75% stenosis

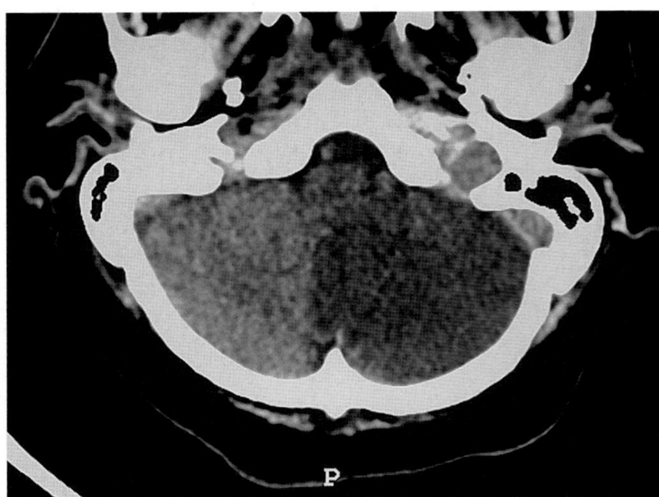

Figure 37-23. Postoperative brain computed tomography scan of a patient successfully treated with a right carotid stent and who developed mild confusion with cerebellum infarct from aortic arch emboli.

Table 37-2
Summary of Evidence Comparing Angioplasty/Stenting and Surgery for Carotid Stenosis*

Author	Patients (*n*)	Grade of Evidence	Clinical Outcome
Naylor[53]	23	Randomized	Surgery > angioplasty
Brooks[54]	104	Randomized	Surgery = angioplasty
CAVATAS[12]	504	Randomized	Surgery = angioplasty
SAPPHIRE[17]	334	Randomized	Surgery < angioplasty
EVA-3S[19]	1200	Randomized	Surgery > angioplasty
SPACE[18]	527	Randomized	Inconclusive
Golledge	33 studies	Systematic review	Surgery > angioplasty
Metaanalysis			Surgery > angioplasty

*CAVATAS, Carotid and Vertebral Artery Transluminal Angioplasty Study; EVA-3S, Endarterectomy versus Angioplasty in Patients with Severe Symptomatic Carotid Stenosis; SAPPHIRE, Stenting and Angioplasty with Protection in Patients at High Risk for Endarterectomy; SPACE, Stent-Supported Percutaneous Angioplasty of the Carotid Artery versus Endarterectomy.

do not require treatment, nor do those with symptomatic less than 60% stenosis, since the natural history of these lesions is benign.

Cost Effectiveness

CEA is a proven procedure with a low mortality–neurological complication rate and durable results. The challenge for carotid angioplasty is at least to equal the results of surgery, even in high-risk patients.

The cost of the materials, including stents, CPDs, and the ancillary materials, is high. In Europe, it can be estimated to be in the range of 2500 Euros. When all costs are taken together (materials, operating theater, physicians' and nurses' time and fees, intensive care unit, and total hospitalization time), the estimated cost in a U.S. institution was $30,140 for angioplasty or stenting and $21,670 for surgery. When complex patients were excluded, the cost was $24,848 for stenting and $19,480 for surgery.[30] However, the calculation of costs may vary from one institution or one country to the other. Brooks et al. showed that, for a community hospital, charges were only slightly higher for stent.[31] Gray et al. found that the costs were higher with surgery ($5409) than with stenting ($3417).[32]

It is expected that the cost of the devices will probably decline if the market increases and if competition occurs among companies selling the devices.

Evidence for Surgery or for Angioplasty/Stenting

Level I evidence comes from randomized studies that tend to favor CEA over CAS, especially in symptomatic patients. However, these figures are challenged by interventionalists and some methodologists, mainly due to the large heterogeneity of patients, devices, and physician expertise in these studies.

To date, six metaanalyses of eight randomized trials are available. Published randomized trials are summarized in Table 37-2.

The following is a summary of the key findings of the larger trials.

Carotid and Vertebral Artery Transluminal Angioplasty Study

The CAVATAS Trial included symptomatic and asymptomatic patients and found no difference in terms of stroke and mortality between CAS and CEA.[12] However, the results of surgery were relatively poor and were not considered to be representative of the surgical standards. On the other hand, CPDs were not used in the angioplasty group, and a stent was placed in only 27% of cases.

Stenting and Angioplasty with Protection in Patients at High Risk for Endarterectomy Trial

The industry-sponsored SAPPHIRE Trial assessed CAS in a group of patients considered high risk for surgery.[17] The authors concluded that CAS was superior to CEA in this subgroup of patients. However, the endpoint of the study combined death, stroke, and myocardial infarction. The higher rate of myocardial infarction in the CEA arm shifted the balance in favor of CAS. The direct relationship between CAS and reduction of myocardial infarction is not clear and may come from multiple factors, of which the use of Clopidogrel only in the CAS arm may have been a significant factor. However, similar reductions in the rate of myocardial infarction have been reported by other investigators.

Endarterectomy versus Angioplasty in Patients with Severe Symptomatic Carotid Stenosis

The Endarterectomy versus Angioplasty in Patients with Severe Symptomatic Carotid Stenosis (EVA-3S) Trial[19] addressed the issue of recently symptomatic patients with a tight carotid stenosis[8] and was funded by a grant from the French Ministry of Health. EVA-3S was stopped prematurely after the inclusion of 527 patients because of safety concerns. The combined death and stroke rate was 9.6% in the CAS group and 3.9% in the CEA group, and the rate of severe stroke and death in the two arms was 3.4% and 1.5%, respectively, with a statistically significant difference.

The main criticism of this study was a relatively low level of expertise in about one third of the interventionalists, which could have contributed to what were considered to be poor results for CAS. However, in the Stent-Supported Percutaneous Angioplasty of the Carotid Artery versus Endarterectomy (SPACE) Trial, in which expertise with CAS may have been higher, the rate of ipsilateral stroke and death after CAS was similar: 4.67%.

SPACE Trial

The SPACE Trial enrolled 1200 symptomatic patients and was terminated prematurely.[18] Although a trend toward better results was found with CEA, no statistical difference was reached after 4 years of recruitment. An updated calculation of sample size showed that at least 2500 patients would be required to achieve an 80% power. This number was inconsistent with the speed of enrolment and the intended end of the study. The authors concluded that the study failed to prove a noninferiority of CAS as compared to CEA.

As far as we are aware, three more randomized trials are ongoing. They may provide further evidence, with more than 8000 patients expected for analysis.

The Asymptomatic Carotid Surgery Trial II is a randomized trial comparing CEA and CAS as treatment for asymptomatic carotid stenosis, where there is substantial uncertainty as to which treatment is more appropriate. The trial is comparing the immediate hazards of the two procedures at 1 month and the stroke rate over the next 5 to 10 years. In all, 5000 patients are planned to be included.

The Carotid Revascularization Endartectomy versus Stenting Trial in the United States is comparing CAS with CEA for the treatment of CAS to prevent recurrent strokes in both symptomatic (who have had a transient ischemic attack or mild stroke within the past 6 months) and asymptomatic patients (who have not had any symptoms in the past 6 months). This trial plans to include 2500 symptomatic and asymptomatic patients. It is scheduled to run until 2011.

The International Carotid Stenting Study (ICSS, CAVATAS 2) is comparing primary stenting with CEA in patients with symptomatic CAS in approximately 1500 patients, using new designs of stents, filters, and CPDs that were not used in the first CAVATAS. This study will include quality-of-life and economic measures as secondary outcomes.

These trials have diminished the enthusiasm for CAS among physicians and led governments on both sides of the Atlantic to limit rather than to expand the indications of CAS. So far, CAS is permitted within trials or in specific indications that we review in the following sections.

High-Risk Patients

Although the definition of high risk for surgery is controversial, CAS is permitted in this setting. The general high-risk definition includes age, severe cardiopathy, pulmonary insufficiency, and renal insufficiency. Cervical high risk includes previous endarterectomy, neck scar or radiation for cancer, tracheotomy, and blocked cervical spine.

Age

Gupta et al.[33] reported excellent results in a group of patients over 65 years of age considered to be inoperable. In contrast, Mathur et al.,[34] Chastain et al.,[26] and Roubin et al.[35] gave strong indications that advanced age (more than 80 years) was an independent predictor of procedural strokes after angioplasty or stenting. The general agreement is to not treat elderly patients with CAS.[36]

Cardiopathy

Waigand et al.[38] and Al-Mubarak et al.[37] reported a series of patients with severe coronary artery disease, mitral incompetence, aortic stenosis, rhythm disorders, or generalized arteriosclerosis treated by carotid stenting. In both series, the mortality rate was zero and the stroke rate minimal. In SAPPHIRE Trial, as well as in cohort studies, including a series from my colleagues and I,[39] there was less elevated Troponin and fewer myocardiac infarctions following CAS. Favorable results with CAS have also been observed in patients who require a combined carotid and cardiac intervention, although pooled data from the literature are less optimistic.[40]

Restenosis

Stenting for restenosis following a previous endarterectomy offers excellent immediate and midterm clinical outcome.[41] New et al.[42] reported a multicenter series of 338 patients (358 arteries). The overall 30-day stroke and death rate was 3.7%. The minor stroke rate was 1.7%, the major nonfatal stroke rate was 0.8%, the fatal stroke rate was 0.3%, and the non-stroke-related death rate was 0.9%. The overall 3-year rate of freedom from all fatal and nonfatal strokes was 96% ± 1% (± standard error).

However, these lesions may be prone to intrastent restenosis. Aburahma et al.[20] reported a comparative series of 83 carotid redo procedures, with 56% restenosis in the stented group versus none in the surgical group ($p < 0.0001$). The rate of restenosis was even higher in the small series from Leger et al.,[22] where 75% of patients developed a severe recurrent stenosis.

Postradiation Angioplasty

Postradiation angioplasty is also an accepted indication for carotid stenting. Unfortunately, only anecdotal cases or short series are available.[43] Although favorable early results are presented, long-term follow-up shows a relatively high percentage of intrastent stenosis.[23]

Apart from the indications of CAS, the ongoing discussion involves the usefulness of CPDs.

No level I evidence is available for the systematic use of cerebral protection during CAS, but level III and IV evidence favors their use.[44]

The risk of emboli during carotid angioplasty has been proved by in vitro testing, intraoperative transcranial Doppler scanning, and debris examination of aspiration and filters. However, clinical consequences are less obvious, and neurological outcome probably depends on particle size. Small particles have no apparent clinical adverse effects, in contrast to medium-sized particles, which may result in transient

Table 37-3
Metaanalysis of Eight Randomized Studies*

Study	CAS *(n/N)*	CEA *(n/N)*	Peto Odds Ratio†	Weight (%)	Peto Odds Ratio†
CAVATAS 2001[12]	25/251	25/253		28.0	1.01 (0.56, 1.81)
Kentucky 2001[54]	0/53	1/51		0.6	0.13 (0.00, 6.56)
Kentucky 2004[55]	0/43	0/42		0.0	Excluded
Leicester 1998[53]	5/11	0/12		2.5	12.88 (1.85, 89.61)
SAPPHIRE 2005[17]	8/167	9/167		10.0	0.88 (0.33, 2.34)
Wallstent 2001	13/107	5/112		10.3	2.76 (1.05, 7.22)
SPACE 2006[18]	46/599	38/584		48.5	1.19 (0.77, 1.86)
EVA-3S[19]	25/263	10/264	0.01 0.1 0.2 0.5 1 2 5 10 100 Favors CAS Favors CEA FavorsCE CEA	29.0	2.5 (1.2, 45.1)
Combined	117/1492	88/1480		100.0	1.8 (0.93, 1.72)

*Metaanalysis of the randomized trials comparing carotid artery stenting (CAS) and carotid endarterectomy (CEA). The endpoint is death or any stroke within 30 days, which was 7.8% overall for CAS and 5.9% for CEA.
†95% confidence intervals are fixed.
***Test for heterogeneity: $chi^2 = 10.46$; $df = 5$; $p < 0.063$.
***Test for overall effect: $z = 1.48$; $p = 0.14$.

Table 37-4
Complications Associated with Carotid Angioplasty and Stenting: The Ways to Prevent and to Manage Them

Complications	Prevention	Treatment
Access		
Iliac blockage	Preoperative duplex	Try contralateral side
Iliac dissection	Gentle manipulation	Try contralateral side
Groin hematoma	Compression, Perclose, Angioseal	Surgery if major bleeding
Difficulty with common carotid catheterization	Patient selection	Appropriate catheter; if still unsuccessful, surgical conversion
Due to angles		
Due to proximal stenosis		
Difficulty crossing internal carotid artery	Patient selection	Try 0.014-inch wire; if still unsuccessful, surgical conversion
Internal Carotid Artery Stenting		
Stent blockage	Choose a stent long enough; use self-expandable stent; drug regimen, avoid fresh hemorrhagic plaque	Surgical conversion
Stent gliding		Put in a second stent
Stent crushing		New dilatation
Stent thrombosis		Thrombolysis or ReoPro
Internal Carotid Artery Angioplasty		
Cardiac arrest	Smooth inflation	Rapid balloon deflation, atropine
Severe bradycardia	Atropine, temporary pacemaker	
Plaque resistance to crushing	Patient selection	Highly resistant balloon
Poststent Complications		
Spasm	Avoid over dilatation	Wait a few minutes, then intravenous atropine
Carotid dissection	Nontraumatic maneuvers	Coronary stenting
Syphon and middle cerebral embolism, thrombosis	Adequate drug regimen	Thrombolysis or ReoPro
Balloon Problems		
Burst	Control pressures	
Blockage at the stent extremities	Use low-profile balloon	Try to modify the position of the wire with a vertebral catheter
Cerebral Protection Problems		
Balloon burst	Choose appropriate size	
Deflation impossible	Check the system before use	Cut the wire
Poor apposition of the filter	Check positioning	Turn the wire
Filter thrombosis	Rapid procedure, adequate drug regimen	Retrieve the filter without closing it
Intolerance to clamping	Use filter	Deflate the balloon, change for filter
Neurological Outcome		
Ischemic events		
Transient ischemic attack	Patient selection	Wait and see
Stroke	Good technique	Urgent treatment according to mechanism
Hemorrhagic events	Blood pressure control	Blood pressure control; stop anticoagulants

ischemic attack or minor stroke. Large particles may provoke a major stroke.[5,6,45-48]

Filters have also shown a good efficacy both in vitro and in clinical series. The Parodi system has also been tested with a good efficacy.

CPDs may fail. With the Percusurge GuardWire device, large particles were associated with a persistent risk of neurological events. Using pre- and postprocedure magnetic resonance angiography, Crawley et al. showed new infarcts in 15% of patients, despite the use of a protection device.[49]

More puzzling is that neurological complication as shown in EVA-3S and in registries may occur before, during, and most surprisingly, within the 48 hours following stent placement.[9,50] Also, emboli may occur in the contralateral hemisphere or in the cerebellum (Figure 37-23). Most of these emboli come from debris in the arch. Since CPDs are effective only once they are in place, the overall benefit may be slim.

In light of these fragmentary, and still controversial, results, should a CPD be used in every case or selectively? Despite the lack of proof, common sense suggests that the best chance for the patient is to avoid any risk of cerebral emboli. Therefore, even if the systems are not ideal, and perhaps not always useful, I prefer to use one routinely.

Which Is the Best Cerebral Protection System?

To date, there is no answer to the question of which cerebral protection system should be used. However, different situations seem to be logical indications for the mechanism of protection. Filters may be the option selected when the patient has poorly developed collateral vessels or previous brain tissue damage. A reversed flow system could be chosen when a severe stenosis or when vulnerable plaques need to be crossed.

COMPLICATIONS

Many complications interfere with the course of carotid angioplasty (Table 37-3). However, most can be prevented by adequate patient selection and technique. Table 37-4 includes possible solutions to difficult situations.

TRAINING

Training is a major issue with CAS. Within the frame of controlled trials such as EVA-3S and Capture trials, where the level of expertise was difficult to prove by statistical assessment, the trend was toward better results in experienced hands. To qualify as experienced, 50 to 75 procedures seem to be considered as a minimum level.[51] This level may be difficult to achieve except in large-volume centers. The development of virtual-reality CAS by computerized means may improve the general expertise with CAS.[52]

SUMMARY

Carotid stenting is a sophisticated procedure whose efficacy is challenged by the excellent results of surgery. Evidence is still lacking concerning the overall benefit in reduction of stroke and death. In recently symptomatic patients with severe stenosis, metaanalysis of randomized trials have shown that surgery is a better choice. In asymptomatic patients, the question remains open and results of ongoing trials are awaited. For the long term, there are clues that, in atherosclerotic lesions at least, stent is as durable as surgery in terms of prevention of stroke and patency. The only obvious and demonstrated advantages are the reduction of cervical nerve injuries and the possibility of treating lesions that are difficult to treat surgically.

Major improvements have recently been made that make carotid stenting safer. The rate of postoperative complications is clearly reduced by technical expertise, better devices, and proper patient selection. It is not known at present whether carotid stenting will become the routine procedure. Further improvements to devices, notably toward simplicity of use, better protection devices, and prevention of intrastent hyperplasia, may increase the number of patients eligible for this technique. Finally, the role of medical treatment and most notably statins may change the practice and current conclusions. In any case, CAS is there to stay, if not as a total replacement of CEA then at least as a complementary tool in the armatarium aimed at preventing strokes.

References

1. White CJ. Another nail in the coffin of carotid endarterectomy. *J Am Coll Cardiol* 2001;38:1596-1597.
2. Ederle J, Featherstone RL, Brown MM. Percutaneous transluminal angioplasty and stenting for carotid artery stenosis. *Cochrane Database Syst Rev* 2007; CD000515.
3. Luebke T, Aleksic M, Brunkwall J. Meta-analysis of randomized trials comparing carotid endarterectomy and endovascular treatment. *Eur J Vasc Endovasc Surg* 2007;34:470-479.
4. McPhee JT, Hill JS, Ciocca RG, et al. Carotid endarterectomy was performed with lower stroke and death rates than carotid artery stenting in the United States in 2003 and 2004. *J Vasc Surg* 2007;46:1112-1118.
5. Hopkins LN, Myla S, Grube E, et al. Carotid artery revascularization in high surgical risk patients with the Nexstent and the Filterwire EX/EZ: 1-year results in the CABERNET Trial. *Catheter Cardiovasc Interv* 2008;71(7):950-960.
6. Iyer SS, White CJ, Hopkins LN, et al. Carotid artery revascularization in high-surgical-risk patients using the carotid Wallstent and Filterwire EX/EZ: 1-year outcomes in the Beach Pivotal Group. *J Am Coll Cardiol* 2008;51:427-434.
7. Gray WA, Yadav JS, Verta P, et al. The Capture Registry: predictors of outcomes in carotid artery stenting with embolic protection for high surgical risk patients in the early post-approval setting. *Catheter Cardiovasc Interv* 2007;70:1025-1033.
8. CaRESS Steering Committee. Carotid revascularization using endarterectomy or stenting systems (CARESS) phase I clinical trial: 1-year results. *J Vasc Surg* 2005;42:213-219.
9. Fairman R, Gray WA, Scicli AP, et al. The Capture Registry: analysis of strokes resulting from carotid artery stenting in the post approval setting: timing, location, severity, and type. *Ann Surg* 2007;246:551-556.
10. Jordan Jr WD, Voellinger DC, Doblar DD, et al. Microemboli detected by transcranial Doppler monitoring in patients during carotid angioplasty versus carotid endarterectomy. *Cardiovasc Surg* 1999;7:33-38.
11. Bosiers M, De DG, Deloose K, et al. Does free cell area influence the outcome in carotid artery stenting? *Eur J Vasc Endovasc Surg* 2007;33: 135-141.
12. Endovascular versus surgical treatment in patients with carotid stenosis in the Carotid and Vertebral Artery Transluminal Angioplasty Study (CAVATAS): a randomised trial. *Lancet* 2001;357:1729-1737.
13. Orlandi G, Fanucchi S, Fioretti C, et al. Characteristics of cerebral microembolism during carotid stenting and angioplasty alone. *Arch Neurol* 2001;58:1410-1413.
14. Yuo TH, Goodney PP, Powell RJ, Cronenwett JL. "Medical high risk" designation is not associated with survival after carotid artery stenting. *J Vasc Surg* 2008;47:356-362.
15. Ouriel K, Hertzer NR, Beven EG, et al. Preprocedural risk stratification: identifying an appropriate population for carotid stenting. *J Vasc Surg* 2001;33:728-732.

16. Jordan Jr WD, Alcocer F, Wirthlin DJ, et al. High-risk carotid endarterectomy: challenges for carotid stent protocols. *J Vasc Surg* 2002;35:16-21.
17. Yadav JS, Wholey MH, Kuntz RE, et al. Protected carotid-artery stenting versus endarterectomy in high-risk patients. *N Engl J Med* 2004;351:1493-1501.
18. Ringleb PA, Allenberg J, Bruckmann H, et al. 30 day results from the space trial of stent-protected angioplasty versus carotid endarterectomy in symptomatic patients: a randomised non-inferiority trial. *Lancet* 2006;368:1239-1247.
19. Mas JL, Chatellier G, Beyssen B, et al. Endarterectomy versus stenting in patients with symptomatic severe carotid stenosis. *N Engl J Med* 2006;355:1660-1671.
20. Aburahma AF, Bates MC, Stone PA, Wulu JT. Comparative study of operative treatment and percutaneous transluminal angioplasty/stenting for recurrent carotid disease. *J Vasc Surg* 2001;34:831-838.
21. Hill BB, Olcott C, Dalman RL, et al. Reoperation for carotid stenosis is as safe as primary carotid endarterectomy. *J Vasc Surg* 1999;30:26-35.
22. Leger AR, Neale M, Harris JP. Poor durability of carotid angioplasty and stenting for treatment of recurrent artery stenosis after carotid endarterectomy: an institutional experience. *J Vasc Surg* 2001;33:1008-1014.
23. Protack CD, Bakken AM, Saad WA, et al. Radiation arteritis: a contraindication to carotid stenting? *J Vasc Surg* 2007;45:110-117.
24. Biasi GM, Froio A, Diethrich EB, et al. Carotid plaque echolucency increases the risk of stroke in carotid stenting: the Imaging in Carotid Angioplasty and Risk of Stroke (ICAROS) study. *Circulation* 2004;110: 756-762.
25. Bazan HA, Pradhan S, Mojibian H, et al. Increased aortic arch calcification in patients older than 75 years: implications for carotid artery stenting in elderly patients. *J Vasc Surg* 2007;46:841-845.
26. Chastain HD, Gomez CR, Iyer S, et al. Influence of age upon complications of carotid artery stenting: UAB Neurovascular Angioplasty Team. *J Endovasc Surg* 1999;6:217-222.
27. Kastrup A, Groschel K, Nagele T, et al. Effects of age and symptom status on silent ischemic lesions after carotid stenting with and without the use of distal filter devices. *AJNR Am J Neuroradiol* 2007.
28. Alvarez B, Ribo M, Maeso J, et al. Transcervical carotid stenting with flow reversal is safe in octogenarians: a preliminary safety study. *J Vasc Surg* 2008;47:96-100.
29. Faggioli G, Ferri M, Gargiulo M, et al. Measurement and impact of proximal and distal tortuosity in carotid stenting procedures. *J Vasc Surg* 2007;46:1119-1124.
30. Jordan Jr WD, Roye GD, Fisher WS III, et al. A cost comparison of balloon angioplasty and stenting versus endarterectomy for the treatment of carotid artery stenosis. *J Vasc Surg* 1998;27:16-22.
31. Brooks WH, McClure RR, Jones MR, et al. Carotid angioplasty and stenting versus carotid endarterectomy: randomized trial in a community hospital. *J Am Coll Cardiol* 2001;38:1589-1595.
32. Gray WA, White Jr HJ, Barrett DM, et al. Carotid stenting and endarterectomy: a clinical and cost comparison of revascularization strategies. *Stroke* 2002;33:1063-1070.
33. Gupta A, Bhatia A, Ahuja A, et al. Carotid stenting in patients older than 65 years with inoperable carotid artery disease: a single-center experience. *Catheter Cardiovasc Interv* 2000;50:1-8.
34. Mathur A, Roubin GS, Iyer SS, et al. Predictors of stroke complicating carotid artery stenting. *Circulation* 1998;97:1239-1245.
35. Roubin GS, New G, Iyer SS, et al. Immediate and late clinical outcomes of carotid artery stenting in patients with symptomatic and asymptomatic carotid artery stenosis: a 5-year prospective analysis. *Circulation* 2001;103:532-537.
36. Baracchini C, Ballotta E. Concerns on carotid stenting in octogenarians. *Eur Heart J* 2007;28:2044-2045.
37. Al-Mubarak N, Roubin GS, Liu MW, et al. Early results of percutaneous intervention for severe coexisting carotid and coronary artery disease. *Am J Cardiol* 1999;84:600-602. A9.
38. Waigand J, Gross CM, Uhlich F, et al. Elective stenting of carotid artery stenosis in patients with severe coronary artery disease. *Eur Heart J* 1998;19:1365-1370.
39. Motamed C, Motamed-Kazerounian G, Merle JC, et al. Cardiac troponin I assessment and late cardiac complications after carotid stenting or endarterectomy. *J Vasc Surg* 2005;41:769-774.
40. Guzman LA, Costa MA, Angiolillo DJ, et al. A systematic review of outcomes in patients with staged carotid artery stenting and coronary artery bypass graft surgery. *Stroke* 2008;39:361-365.
41. Mehta RH, Zahn R, Hochadel M, et al. Comparison of in-hospital outcomes of patients with versus without previous carotid endarterectomy undergoing carotid stenting (from the German ALKK CAS Registry). *Am J Cardiol* 2007;99:1288-1293.
42. New G, Roubin GS, Iyer SS, et al. Safety, efficacy, and durability of carotid artery stenting for restenosis following carotid endarterectomy: a multicenter study. *J Endovasc Ther* 2000;7:345-352.
43. Hernandez-Vila E, Strickman NE, Skolkin M, et al. Carotid stenting for post-endarterectomy restenosis and radiation-induced occlusive disease. *Tex Heart Inst J* 2000;27:159-165.
44. MacDonald S. The evidence for cerebral protection: an analysis and summary of the literature. *Eur J Radiol* 2006;60:20-25.
45. Cheng WY, Stephens M, Lin BP, et al. Particulate debris collected during carotid stenting: are we missing something? *Int J Cardiol* 2007;119: 277-279.
46. Gossetti B, Gattuso R, Irace L, et al. Embolism to the brain during carotid stenting and surgery. *Acta Chir Belg* 2007;107:151-154.
47. Iyer V, De DG, Deloose K, et al. The type of embolic protection does not influence the outcome in carotid artery stenting. *J Vasc Surg* 2007;46: 251-256.
48. Matas M, Alvarez B, Ribo M, et al. Transcervical carotid stenting with flow reversal protection: experience in high-risk patients. *J Vasc Surg* 2007;46:49-54.
49. Crawley F, Stygall J, Lunn S, et al. Comparison of microembolism detected by transcranial doppler and neuropsychological sequelae of carotid surgery and percutaneous transluminal angioplasty. *Stroke* 2000;31: 1329-1334.
50. Mas JL, Chatellier G. Recent carotid stenting trials. *Lancet Neurol* 2007;6:295-296.
51. Verzini F, Cao P, De RP, et al. Appropriateness of learning curve for carotid artery stenting: an analysis of periprocedural complications. *J Vasc Surg* 2006;44:1205-1211.
52. Cates CU. Virtual reality simulation in carotid stenting: a new paradigm for procedural training. *Nat Clin Pract Cardiovasc Med* 2007;4:174-175.
53. Naylor AR, Bolia A, Abbott RJ, et al. Randomized study of carotid angioplasty and stenting versus carotid endarterectomy: a stopped trial. *J Vacs Surg* 1998;28:326-334.
54. Brooks WH, McClure RR, Jones MR, et al. Carotid angioplasty and stenting versus endarterectomy: randomized trial in a community hospital. *J Am Coll Cardiol* 2001;38:1589-1595.
55. Brooks WH, McClure RR, Jones MR, et al. Carotid angioplasty and stenting versus endarterectomy for treatment of asymptomatic carotid stenosis: a randomized trial in a community hospital. *Neurosurgery* 2004;54:318-324.

chapter

38

Surgery for Vertebrobasilar Insufficiency

Edouard Kieffer, MD

Key Points

- Anatomical variations of the vertebral artery (VA) are common, and most of them are clinically relevant.
- Atherosclerotic lesions of the VA are often bilateral and may be associated with lesions of the carotid bifurcations or intrathoracic great vessels that significantly affect the pathophysiology of symptoms and the surgical choices.
- Extrinsic compressions of the VA are anatomically common, although they do not always have a clinical expression.
- Studies using strict criteria for vertebrobasilar transient ischemic attack (TIA) have shown a 5-year stroke rate of 22% to 35%, similar to that of carotid TIA.
- Hemodynamic compromise of the posterior circulation is the primary cause of vertebrobasilar insufficiency (VBI).
- The hindbrain is particularly susceptible to ischemia.
- Reconstruction of the VA may be indicated in three circumstances, of decreasing clinical importance: VBI, concomitant carotid artery disease, and anatomical indications.
- Surgery for thromboembolic VBI should be considered only in patients with TIAs or a small residual deficit.
- The indications for surgery in hemodynamic VBI are quite different: (1) in the presence of significant carotid artery disease, and (2) if medical treatment of incapacitating VBI has been unsuccessful.
- The relationship between clinical symptoms and certain positions of the head and neck should lead to the performance of positional arteriograms.
- Reconstruction of the VA is now possible at the level of any of its four segments.
- The technique of choice for proximal VA reconstruction is transposition of the VA into the common carotid artery.
- Clinical and anatomical results of VA reconstructions have been satisfactory in the most recently reported series.

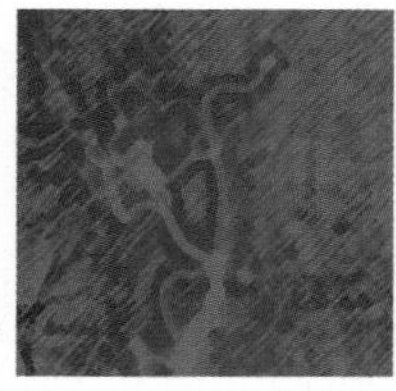

Although more than 40 years have elapsed since the first surgical repairs of proximal vertebral artery (VA) disease,[1,2] VA surgery has not been widely accepted, neither among neurologists nor by many vascular surgeons. However, renewed interest has recently arisen among several groups of workers who have reported series of operated patients with logical indications and good results.[3-23]

Several reasons may explain these difficulties:

- A lot of controversy has surrounded the definition of and criteria for vertebrobasilar insufficiency (VBI), with some neurologists still questioning its individuality as a syndrome.
- Investigators have noticed in some patients an apparent lack of correlation between clinical manifestations and arterial lesions seen at angiography.
- Although occipital, cerebellar, or brainstem infarcts due to vertebral and basilar artery disease have been described precisely for several decades, the prognosis of vertebrobasilar transient ischemic attacks (TIAs) has long been wrongly considered of a benign nature, especially in comparison with those occurring in the carotid territory.

- Angiography of the VA has long suffered a bad reputation due to complications related to the nature of contrast media and direct injections into the VA.
- Besides being limited to the first segment of the artery, VA surgery was deemed difficult and was complicated by a significant number of failures caused by postoperative occlusions.

This chapter attempts to discuss each of the previously mentioned points and present a logical, comprehensive approach to the problems of VA lesions, VBI, and VA reconstruction. It emphasizes the spectrum of anatomical lesions, the pathophysiology of symptoms, and the rationale for surgical indications, as well as the feasibility and safety of VA reconstruction at all levels of the cervical and intracranial courses of the artery.

SURGICAL ANATOMY

The rather complicated anatomical course of the VA may be conveniently divided into four consecutive segments (Figure 38-1).[24,25] The first segment (V1) is in the medial part of the supraclavicular fossa from the subclavian artery to the bony canal of the transverse process of C6. The second segment (V2) runs vertically on the lateral side of the cervical spine, passing through the bony canals from C6 to C2. The third segment (V3) curves laterally and then medially around C1 into the atlantooccipital membrane. The fourth segment (V4) has a short intracranial course toward the opposite VA, forming the basilar artery on the anterior aspect of the brainstem.

Cervical branches of the VA arise exclusively from the V2 and V3 segments. Besides small muscular, osteoarticular, and meningeal branches, radicular arteries follow each of the cervical nerve roots. Some of them—the radiculospinal arteries—may participate in the arterial supply to the spinal cord, together with branches originating from other collaterals of the subclavian artery. Intracranial branches, arising from the V4 segment, include the spinal arteries (anterior and posterior) and the posteroinferior cerebellar artery (PICA), which is the largest collateral branch of the VA.

Anatomical variations of the VA are common, and most of them are clinically relevant. The left VA originates from the aortic arch in 6% to 10% of individuals. In most cases (around 60%), the VAs are not symmetrical (equivalent), with one large (dominant) artery, usually the left, and a small (minor) contralateral artery. While penetration into the bony canal occurs in C6 in 90% of cases, it is either lower (C7) or higher (C5 to C3) in the remaining 10%. The basilar artery may originate only from the dominant VA, while the minor one ends into the ipsilateral PICA. In such cases, the ipsilateral posterior cerebral artery usually originates from the internal carotid artery. Finally, embryological carotid–basilar anastomoses may persist in a small number of individuals.[26] The most common are the trigeminal and hypoglossal arteries. These abnormal anastomoses are usually associated with small VA and hypoplasia or atresia of one or both posterior communicating arteries.

ANATOMICAL LESIONS

Each of the four segments of the VA may be affected by various diseases. Intrinsic, parietal diseases do not differ in nature from those observed in other parts of the body. Extrinsic compressions by bony, muscular, or fibrous elements are more specific of the VA pathology and are therefore studied here in some detail.

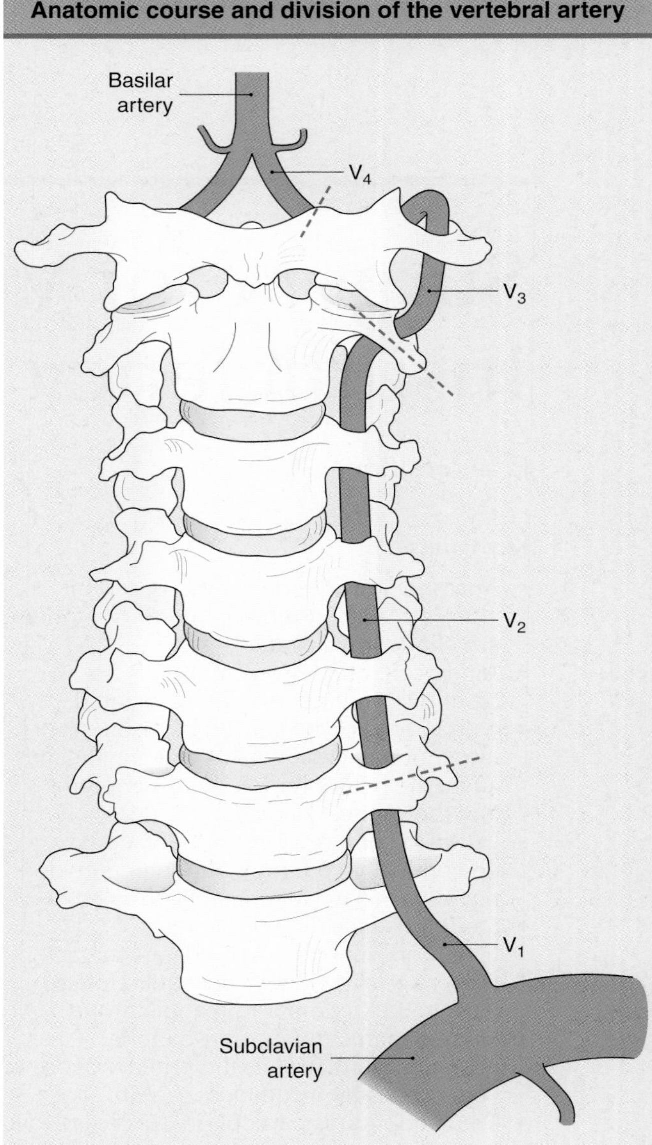

Figure 38-1. Anatomical course and division into four consecutive segments of the vertebral artery running from the subclavian artery to the basilar artery.

Intrinsic Disease

Atherosclerotic Disease

Atherosclerotic lesions are commonly located at the origin of the VA. They are usually in continuity with lesions of the subclavian artery and remain limited to the first centimeter of the artery, except in a few hypertensive, diabetic, or elderly patients. A poststenotic dilatation may be present in cases with tight stenosis. In contradistinction to the usual carotid plaques, intimal ulceration, with or without mural thrombosis, is rarely present. Most plaques of the VA, whether fibrous or calcified, have a smooth surface without intimal damage.[27]

Atherosclerotic disease of the intracranial (V4) segment is second in frequency. It may be associated with lesions of the basilar artery and its branches, emphasizing the need for complete angiographic visualization of both extracranial and intracranial vessels.

The V2 segment is rarely affected by atherosclerotic disease, except in patients with cervical irradiation. It is of utmost surgical importance is that the V3 segment is usually spared from atherosclerosis.[28-30]

Atherosclerotic lesions of the VA are often bilateral and may be associated with lesions of the carotid bifurcations or intrathoracic great vessels, which significantly affect the pathophysiology of symptoms and the surgical choices.

Fibromuscular Disease

Fibromuscular disease is much less common than atherosclerotic disease. It usually affects the V2 segment, V3 segment, or both.[31,32] The most common aspect is that of "strings of beads" with or without an excess in length resulting in buckling or kinking of the artery. Dysplastic aneurysms are rarer. Fibromuscular disease of the VA may be complicated by dissection, arteriovenous (AV) fistula, or thromboembolic manifestations. Associated disease of the internal carotid artery is nearly constant. Intracranial berry aneurysms are found in a small number of patients. Renal and visceral arteries, as visualized by panarteriography, may also be affected.

Arteritis

Takayasu's disease is a nonspecific aortoarteritis that affects mainly the intrathoracic great vessels and subclavian–axillary arteries.[33] Except for its origin from the subclavian artery, the VA is usually spared by arteritis. It may enlarge considerably in cases with bilateral lesions of the carotid arteries and thus become the main arterial supply to the brain. Extensive occlusions of the VA in Takayasu's disease are usually due to secondary thrombosis and not to the disease itself.

Giant cell (temporal) arteritis may affect the VA in a small number of cases.[34]

Trauma

Although routine arteriography for stable patients with penetrating neck trauma may disclose more lesions of the VA than are usually acknowledged, penetrating trauma to the VA remains a rarity.[35-39] Its initial consequences are usually minimal, and patients may remain clinically silent. A self-containing cervical hematoma may compress and occlude the VA or lead to a false aneurysm.[40] AV fistulas are common due to the close relationship between the VA and its surrounding venous plexus.

Blunt trauma to the VA may affect the V2 segment, in conjunction with fractures or dislocations of the spine.[41,42] More often, the V3 segment is the site of traumatic lesions secondary to hyperextension and rotation of the cervical spine resulting from accidental trauma or cervical manipulation with forceful stretching of the VA.[43] Complete or subadventitial rupture occurs rarely. The usual lesion is purely intimal and may lead to thromboembolic complications with or without a traumatic dissection of the VA.

Iatrogenic trauma usually complicates direct puncture following attempts at carotid arteriography or catheterization of the internal jugular vein.[44] An AV fistula is the usual consequence of such trauma. Trauma to the VA has also been reported following surgery of the cervical spine.[45]

Spontaneous Aneurysms, Dissections, and Arteriovenous Fistulas

Spontaneous aneurysms[46-50] and dissections[51-57] are rare lesions that usually affect the V3 segment. Most of them are dysplastic in origin and complicate fibromuscular disease, Ehlers-Danlos syndrome, or neurofibromatosis.

Spontaneous AV fistulas are at least as common as traumatic AV fistulas.[58,59] They are usually located in the V2–V3 segments. Although they may complicate fibromuscular disease, spontaneous AV fistulas, whether single or multiple, are usually congenital in nature. AV malformations are complex lesions that develop in the cervical soft tissues and muscles. In addition to arterial supply from the VA, they are usually fed by other cervical arteries originating from the subclavian and external carotid arteries.

Extrinsic Disease (Compressions)

Close relations of the VA with the cervical spine and fibromuscular elements account for the possibility of extrinsic compressions that are specific of VA disease and may affect any of the segments of the artery.[60-64]

The normal VA is tightly attached to several anatomical elements:

- The VA is connected to the sympathetic chain with the stellate ganglion completely surrounding the proximal VA in the supraclavicular fossa.
- In the V2–V3 segments, the VA is fixed by its adventitia to the periosteum of each transverse foramen and, at the top of the spine, to the upper aspect of the atlas.
- Finally, the VA is tightly fixed to the atlantooccipital membrane as it crosses this structure to enter the dura mater.

The normal VA thus has a certain mobility between these points of fixation:

- In the V1 segment, on each side of the stellate ganglion
- In the V2–V3 segments, between each vertebra

In the V2 segment, the corresponding cervical spine allows only for limited flexion, extension, rotation, and lateral inclination. In sharp contrast, the VA around C1 and C2 is a mobile segment, with an excess in arterial length that has been described as a "safety buckle," allowing for an adaptation of the VA to the considerable amplitude of motion in this area, especially during rotation of the neck.

Extrinsic compressions of the VA are anatomically common, although they do not always have a clinical expression. They may appear late in life due to progressive degenerative disc disease, elevation of the aortic arch, and lengthening of the subclavian artery due to age or hypertension. While some of these compressions may be permanent, most appear or worsen during extreme positions of the neck (rotation, lateral inclination, flexion, and extension).[65,66] The arterial consequences of such compressions vary according to the nature,

Table 38-1
Elements Compressing Vertebral Artery in the Neck

Segment	Elements of Compression	Trigger Position
V1	Stellate ganglion	Ipsilateral rotation and lateral inclination of the neck
	Fibrous band	Same as above and lateral inclination of the neck
	Anterior scalene muscle (with or without thoracic outlet syndrome)	Hyperabduction of the arm
V1–V2 junction	Insertion of longus colli and anterior scalene muscle on C6	Rotation of the neck
	Abnormal entrance into the bony canal:	
	High (C5–C3)	Hyperextension of the neck
	Low (C7)	Same as above and hyperflexion of neck
V2	Cervical spondylosis	Ipsilateral rotation of the neck
	Cervical spine trauma	
	Neural or bony tumor	
V3	Extraosseous course of the vertebral artery	Contralateral rotation of the neck
	Anterior branch of C2 nerve	Same as above
	Hypermotility of C1–C2 joint	Same as above
	Bony canal of the upper aspect of C1	Hyperextension of the neck
V3–V4 junction	Foramen of the atlantooccipital membrane	Hyperextension or hyperflexion of the neck
	Bony abnormalities of the atlantooccipital joint	Same as above

length, and degree of compression. Although the VA may remain normal for years, tight and longstanding compressions may lead to intimal damage with an attending risk of thromboembolic complications.[67-69]

The most significant elements of compression with their topography according to each segment of the VA and their trigger position are indicated in Table 38-1. Although there are many causes of extrinsic compression of the VA,[16,18,60,61,63,67,69-79] two of them deserve special emphasis because of their frequency and clinical importance.

Cervical spondylosis is a classic and common cause of VA compression in the bony canal of the transverse processes.[60,67,69,72,79] Compression is usually limited to one or two of the lower cervical vertebrae (C4 to C6). The two main factors that contribute to disturbances in VA flow are as follows:

- Osteolytic proliferation of the uncinate processes, which pushes the VA toward the back and the outside of its normal pathway
- Shortening of the cervical spine due to degenerative disc disease, which produces an excess in length between each transverse process

The VA compression is progressive and leads to gentle curving of the artery, provided the neck remains in a neutral position. When the neck rotates ipsilaterally, the vertebral interspace tends to become shorter, and tight stenosis or even complete occlusion of the VA may appear (Figure 38-2).

Compression of the VA at the normal V1–V2 junction in C6 has long been described.[74] The VA may be compressed at the cross-insertion of hypertrophic or laterally displaced muscular or tendinous fibers of the longus colli and anterior scalene muscles that insert on the transverse process of the C6 vertebra.[71,73] The compression is usually intermittent and triggered by rotation of the neck. When the V1–V2 junction is at an abnormally located level, extrinsic muscular compressions are more common and may be permanent (Figure 38-3) or intermittent.[63] The usual trigger positions are hyperextension of the neck because of the abnormal arterial pathway, perpendicular or hairpin turn in abnormally low (C7) penetration, and tight and S shaped in abnormally high (C5 to C3) penetration.

PATHOPHYSIOLOGY OF VERTEBROBASILAR INSUFFICIENCY

Postmortem studies and clinical evaluation of patients with VBI have identified two pathological mechanisms: thromboembolism and hemodynamic compromise.[63,80-83] Although these two mechanisms may combine in a few patients, they are usually caused by different anatomical lesions, account for different clinical manifestations, and have different prognostic implications.

Thromboembolic Vertebrobasilar Insufficiency

Although it is the least often involved, thromboembolism may occur in the vertebrobasilar territory much in the same way as it occurs in the carotid territory.[84]

Atherosclerosis does not play a major role in this mechanism because of the usually smooth nature of the atherosclerotic plaques of the VA. Nonatherosclerotic lesions, especially traumatic or spontaneous aneurysms or dissections, are the most common etiologies due to the frequency of intimal disease and the possibility of mural thrombus formation in such lesions.[67,69]

Because of the anatomy of the basilar artery and its branches, most large emboli stop at the top of the basilar artery or in one or both of the posterior cerebral arteries (Figure 38-4). They produce severe and different neurological complications that have been described under the term "top of the basilar syndrome."[82] The smallest emboli may produce TIAs that usually last several hours or reversible ischemic neurological diseases in which neurological symptoms may take several days to a few weeks to disappear.

The distal end of the occlusions may reach different levels depending on anatomical, hemodynamic, and rheological factors. Four types of VA occlusion may be distinguished. Segmental VA occlusions with revascularization at the C1 to C2 level through the "occipital connection"[28,29,63,83] are the most favorable (Figure 38-5). They are usually well compensated by collateral circulation and thus remain accessible to surgical reconstruction by means of a distal bypass. Occlusions may also extend intracranially up to the origin of the PICA, which

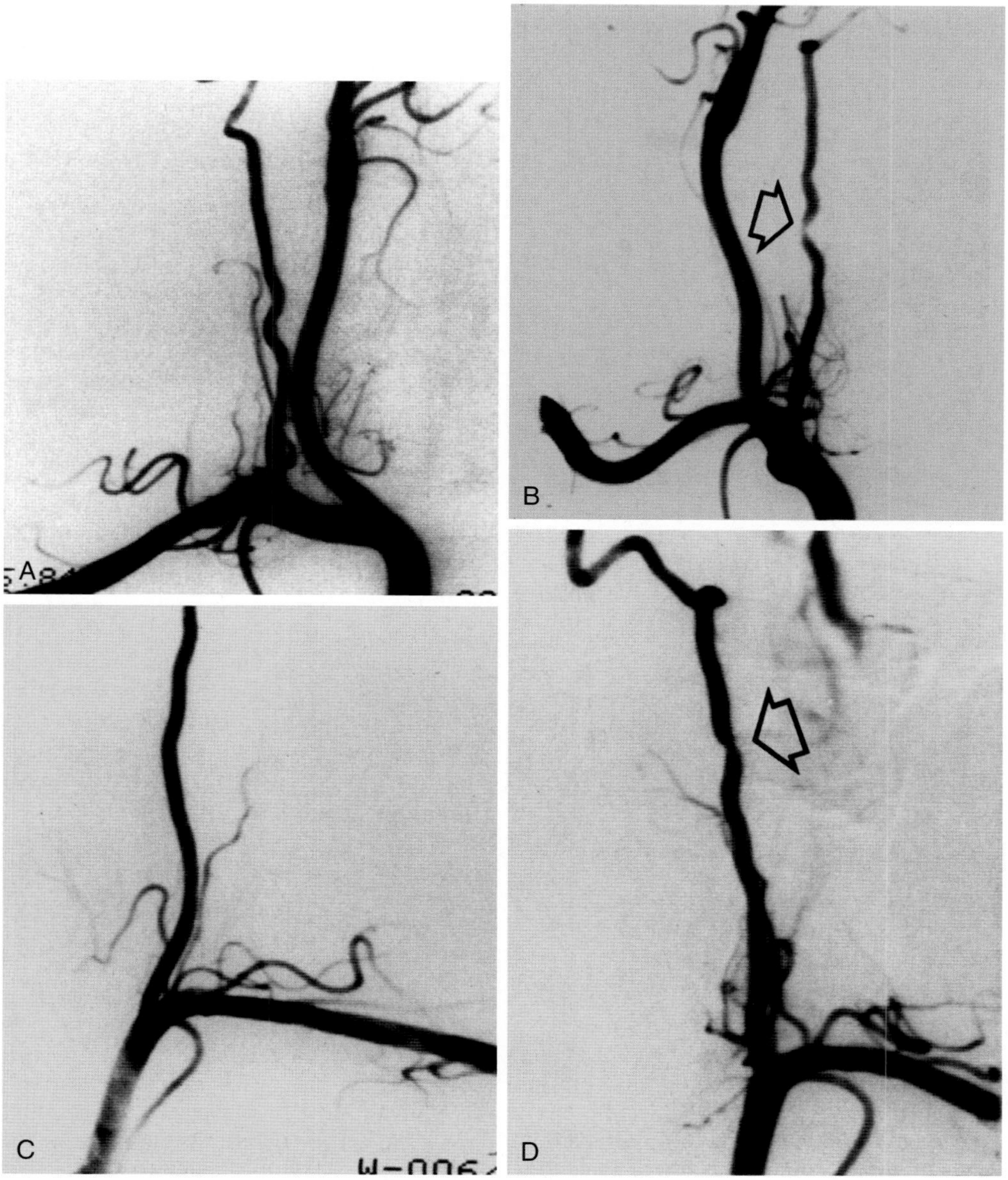

Figure 38-2. Bilateral compression of equivalent vertebral arteries due to spondylosis. While the vertebral arteries are widely patent in neutral positions of the neck **(A, C),** tight stenosis is apparent on both sides *(open arrows)* during ipsilateral rotations of the neck **(B, D).**

remains patent through the opposite VA. Such segmental VA occlusions are compatible with absent or minimal neurological complications.[85,86] In more extensive occlusions that involve the origin of the PICA or the basilar artery itself, neurological complications are usually severe, ranging from limited lateromedullary or cerebellar infarcts to massive infarction of the brainstem. The clinical picture of these vertebrobasilar infarctions has been fully and precisely described for several decades in the classic neurological literature.[87-89]

Although complete or near-complete clinical recovery occurs in about 50% of patients with vertebrobasilar strokes, the early mortality remains as high as 20% to 30%,[90-92] which is significantly more than for carotid strokes. The prognosis for thromboembolic TIA is probably not as good as is usually believed. Studies using strict criteria for vertebrobasilar TIA have shown a 22% to 35% 5-year stroke rate, similar to that of carotid TIA.[93-95]

Hemodynamic Vertebrobasilar Insufficiency

Hemodynamic compromise of the posterior circulation is the primary cause of VBI.[8,63,82-84,96-98] It is usually explained by various factors that may be classified into four main categories (Table 38-2).

Anatomical Factors

The posterior circulation has two anatomical peculiarities that must be considered in the discussion of hemodynamic VBI. First, the basilar artery is normally formed by the union of the two VAs. The direct consequence of this fact is that, provided it is of sufficient diameter, one patent VA is usually enough to ensure satisfactory blood flow to the basilar artery.[3,5,63] The anatomical

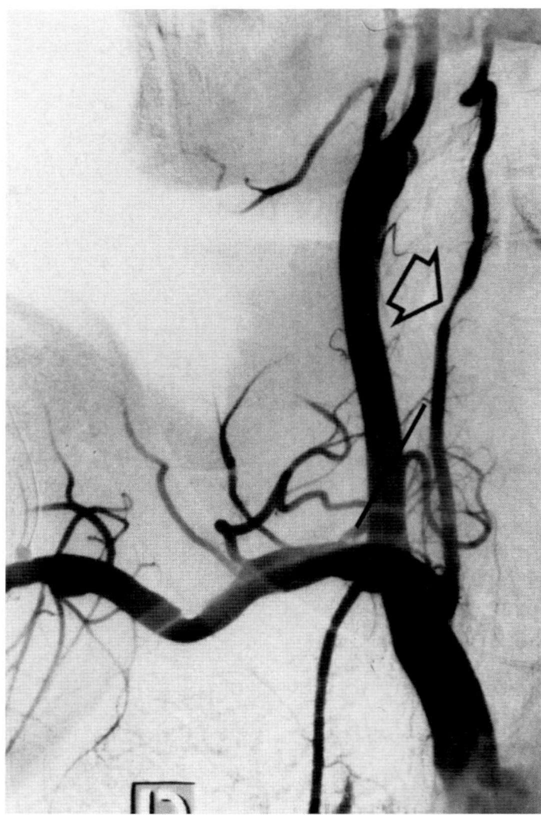

Figure 38-3. Abnormally high penetration of the vertebral artery into the transverse foramen of C4 with tight stenosis due to permanent compression *(open arrow)*.

requisites for hemodynamic VBI are thus bilateral VA disease, unilateral VA disease with contralateral absent or hypoplastic VA, or small contralateral VA ending in the PICA without participating in the formation of the basilar artery (Figure 38-6). These anatomical situations logically constitute the only justified indications for VA reconstruction in hemodynamic VBI.

The second factor to be considered is the continuity of the normal basilar artery with the anterior circulation through the posterior elements of the circle of Willis, namely, both posterior communicating arteries. The two anatomical factors that may therefore increase potential for VBI are as follows:

- Associated carotid artery disease, a finding that is particularly common in atherosclerotic patients
- Congenital absence or hypoplasia of the posterior communicating artery on one or both sides, a finding that is present in approximately 30% of normal individuals (Figure 38-7)

However, these factors are not constantly present in the most severe and indisputable hemodynamic VBI because of the combined influence of other factors that are discussed later. They therefore are not considered indispensable to a justified surgical indication for hemodynamic VBI.

Susceptibility of the Hindbrain to Ischemia

The hindbrain is particularly susceptible to ischemia.[98] There are three main reasons for this. The first is a competition between flow coming from the vertebrobasilar system and that coming from the carotid system through the posterior communicating arteries.[8] This "dead point" is located somewhere in the middle part of the basilar artery varies according to local factors affecting vertebrobasilar flow (such as extrinsic compression), and this may be responsible for rapid variations in brainstem perfusion.[96] This accounts for the apparently paradoxical fact that patency of both posterior communicating arteries is not a protection against VBI. Second, the branches of the basilar artery that perfuse the brainstem are small, terminal arteries, a situation that favors the appearance of watershed ischemia. This also explains why the vestibular nucleus, which is fed by very long, small, and terminal arteries, is one of the most often ischemic structures in patients with hemodynamic VBI. And third, elderly people, especially if hypertensive or diabetic, tend to have poor cerebral autoregulation,[96] which often accounts for the failure of local compensatory mechanisms.

Cardiac and Peripheral Hemodynamic Factors

Cardiac function is an important factor in hemodynamic VBI. Low cardiac output due to cardiac insufficiency, rhythm disturbances, or atrioventricular conduction defects may lower total cerebral blood flow. Similarly, patients with postural (orthostatic) hypotension, either spontaneous or due to medication, also have a tendency to decrease vertebrobasilar blood flow.

Rheological Factors

Anemia, hypoxemia, thrombocytosis, polycythemia, and hyperlipemia are well known contributors to tissue ischemia and may aggravate hemodynamic VBI. Although one of these five factors may largely predominate in an individual patient, they usually combine in different manners to cause hemodynamic VBI.[80] In these cases, symptoms are of short duration and repetitive. They affect mainly the territories that are fed by long terminal arteries. This accounts for the nearly constant vestibular symptoms in hemodynamic VBI because vestibulolabyrinthine arteries are long, terminal branches arising in the midportion of the basilar artery in the vicinity of the hemodynamic dead point. Other symptoms related to brainstem or cerebellar ischemia are due similarly to hypoperfusion in watershed areas of the cerebellum, brainstem nuclei, reticulate substance, long motor or sensory tracts of the brainstem, or upper part of the medulla. Ischemia of the occipital lobe is common when posterior cerebral arteries act as terminal arteries, i.e., in the absence of functioning posterior communicating arteries.

The prognosis of hemodynamic VBI seems to be relatively good. Although the daily repetition of TIAs may become a functional and social handicap, vertebrobasilar strokes are rather rare in this setting. However, the repetition of TIAs and the presence of symptoms related to ischemia of the long tracts of the brainstem should be considered as ominous manifestations and harbingers of vertebrobasilar strokes.

In my opinion, the clinical and prognostic differences between thromboembolic and hemodynamic vertebrobasilar TIAs are of utmost importance and have not been clearly appreciated in the literature.

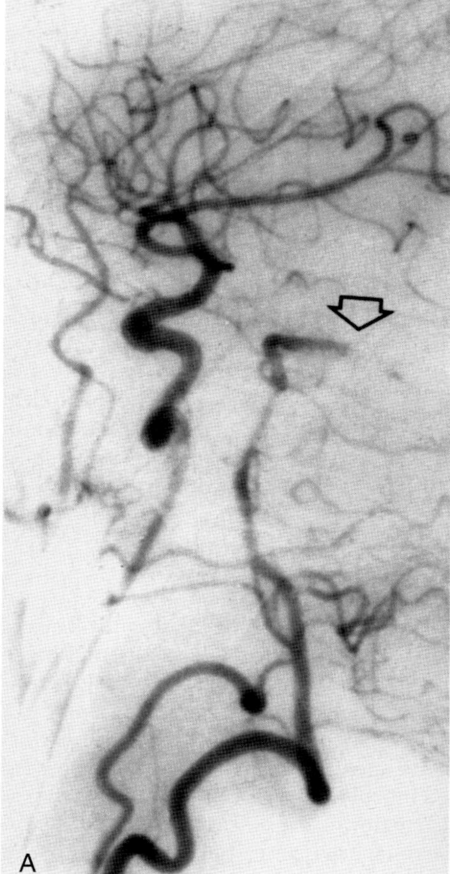

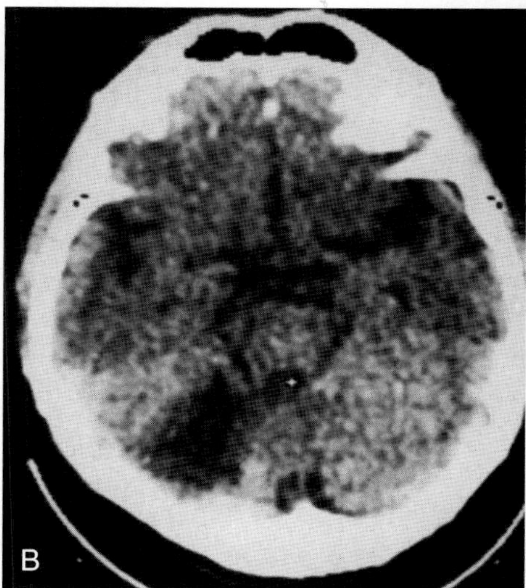

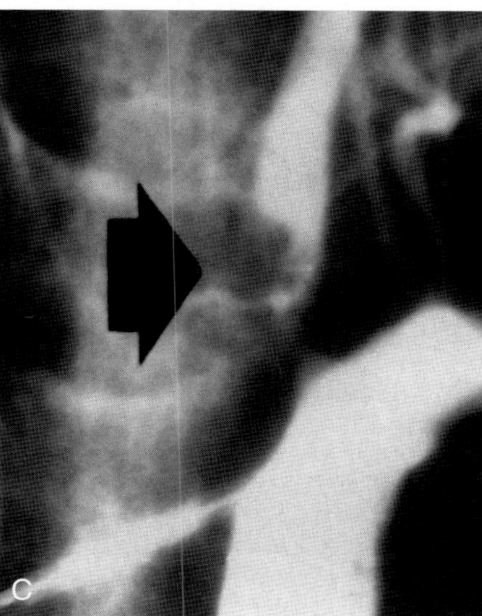

Figure 38-4. Embolic occlusion of the posterior cerebral artery (**A;** *open arrow*) causing large infarction of the occipital lobe **(B)** in a patient with tight stenosis and mural thrombus of the proximal vertebral artery (**C;** *black arrow*).

SURGICAL INDICATIONS

Reconstruction of the VA may be indicated in three circumstances of decreasing clinical importance[62,63,99]:

- VBI
- Concomitant carotid artery disease
- Anatomical indications

Vertebrobasilar Insufficiency

VBI is by far the most common indication for reconstruction of the VA. The rationale for operation is different in thromboembolic as opposed to hemodynamic VBI.

Surgery for thromboembolic VBI should be considered only in patients with TIAs or a small residual deficit. It is aimed at the prevention of further thromboembolic events. Even though the contralateral VA may be widely patent, the presence of an embolic source is a logical indication for surgical treatment using either a direct reconstruction or a distal bypass excluding the lesion.[63] Occlusion of the VA is an indication for surgery only in cases with limited distal extension, leaving the V3 segment accessible for bypass.[28] In patients with more extensive occlusions, surgery may be indicated to reconstruct a large contralateral stenotic VA and therefore to avoid bilateral occlusion with its attending risk of stroke.

The indications for surgery in hemodynamic VBI are quite different (Figure 38-8). My colleagues and I have developed the following practical approach.[63] The patient is fully evaluated for associated medical problems and the presence of significant carotid artery disease. Maximal treatment of medical problems is undertaken and a specific medical treatment of VBI, including antiplatelet and alpha-blocking drugs, is prescribed. Medical management is successful in a good number of patients. Four-vessel arteriography is indicated only in suitable surgical candidates in the following cases:

- In the presence of significant carotid artery disease, with or without symptoms
- If medical treatment of incapacitating VBI has been unsuccessful in a patient without significant carotid artery disease

Four situations may arise according to the degree of VA disease, the association of carotid artery disease, and the possibility for reconstruction of the diseased carotid and vertebral arteries. First, patients with significant, reconstructible carotid artery and VA disease have usually been treated by isolated carotid reconstruction.[100-103] VA reconstruction was performed a few months later if symptoms of VBI persisted. Although many attempts have been made at predicting the clinical results of isolated carotid operations, this usually has not been possible. Failure to cure the symptoms of VBI has

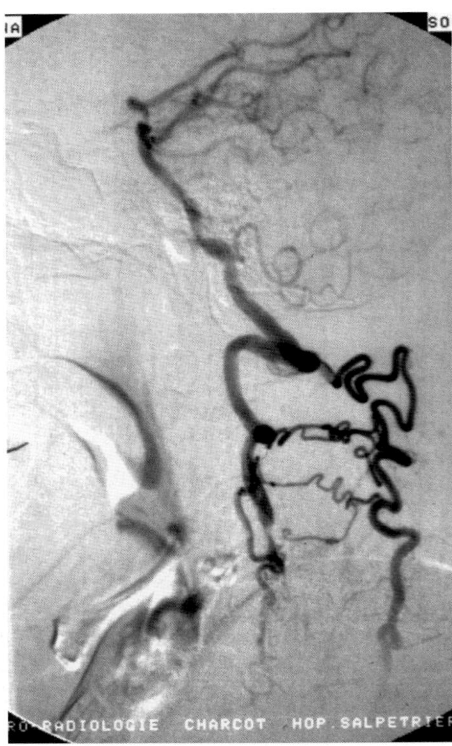

Figure 38-5. Segmental occlusion of the vertebral artery. Patency of the distal cervical vertebral artery is maintained through branches of the ipsilateral subclavian and external carotid arteries.

been noted in 30% to 50% of patients. Associated carotid and vertebral reconstructions in the same operative session solve the problem with a minimal added operative risk and therefore should be performed more widely.[104,105]

Second, patients with VBI and significant carotid artery disease and nonsignificant or nonreconstructible VA disease should have a carotid reconstruction whether or not they have carotid symptoms. This situation may arise in the rare patient with diffuse nonreconstructible VA occlusions or more often in patients with bilateral, small hypoplastic VA, characteristic of hypoplasia of the vertebrobasilar arterial system.

Third, patients with VBI, significant VA lesions, and nonsignificant or nonreconstructible carotid artery lesions should have isolated VA reconstruction (Figures 38-9 and 38-10).

Table 38-2
Factors Compromising Vertebral Artery Flow

	Contributing Factors	Management
Watershed ischemia	Hindbrain	Carotid reconstruction
Autoregulation disturbances	Alpha-blocking medication	Stop drug
Obstruction (permanent or transient)	Vertebral arteries	VA reconstruction
Anemia, hypoxemia, thrombocytosis, polycythemia	Blood	Medical treatment
Orthostatic hypotension	Systemic pressure	Medical treatment
Cardiac failure, rhythm disturbances, arteriovenous conduction defects	Heart	Medical treatment, pacemaker implantation

The presence of nonreconstructible carotid artery disease (such as extensive common and internal carotid artery occlusion or tight stenosis of the carotid siphon) may lead to the use of unusual techniques of reconstruction such as bypass with the proximal anastomosis in the subclavian or external carotid arteries (Figure 38-11).

Finally, in the rare patients with VBI and nonsignificant or nonreconstructible lesions of both the vertebral and carotid arteries, maximal medical management is the only available therapeutic modality.

In each of these cases with hemodynamic VBI, VA reconstruction should be limited to the large "dominant" VA; few patients, if any, need bilateral reconstructions. It should, however, be recognized that one or both of the VA occlusive lesions may not be evident on standard arteriograms because of its positional nature. The relationship between clinical symptoms and certain positions of the head and neck should lead to the performance of positional arteriograms under local anesthesia with the patient in the sitting position.

Carotid Artery Disease without Vertebrobasilar Insufficiency

In the absence of VBI, VA lesions combined with carotid artery disease may become an indication for VA reconstruction in two circumstances. Both of these indications have solely hemodynamic justification and apply only to large, dominant VA.

VA reconstruction may be combined with carotid endarterectomy during the same operation.[4,62] This may be performed with a minimal added morbidity and has the same rationale as simultaneous reconstruction of significant although asymptomatic lesions of the renal or visceral arteries in the course of aortoiliac reconstructions.

More importantly, patients with nonreconstructible carotid artery lesions such as extensive internal carotid artery occlusions without a stenosis of the external carotid artery may be benefitted by the reconstruction of a large diseased VA.[106,107] This may dramatically increase hemispheric cerebral blood flow to a much greater extent than extracranial–intracranial anastomoses do and possibly prevent the appearance or recurrence of hemispheric TIAs or strokes.

Anatomical Indications

VA reconstruction may be indicated in a few asymptomatic patients with isolated VA disease:

- To prevent thromboembolic complications in patients with severe bilateral VA disease
- To treat AV fistulas or malformations—often in conjunction with interventional radiological procedures[59]
- To allow the removal of bony or nervous tumors in proximity to the VA[62,63,108,109]

In most of these patients, a distal bypass to the V3 segment, excluding the proximal part of the VA, allows surgical management or embolization of the proximal lesion.[39]

RECONSTRUCTIVE TECHNIQUES

Reconstruction of the VA is now possible at the level of any of its four segments. The techniques have been described extensively in the literature[18,62,99,110,111] and thus are only briefly discussed here.

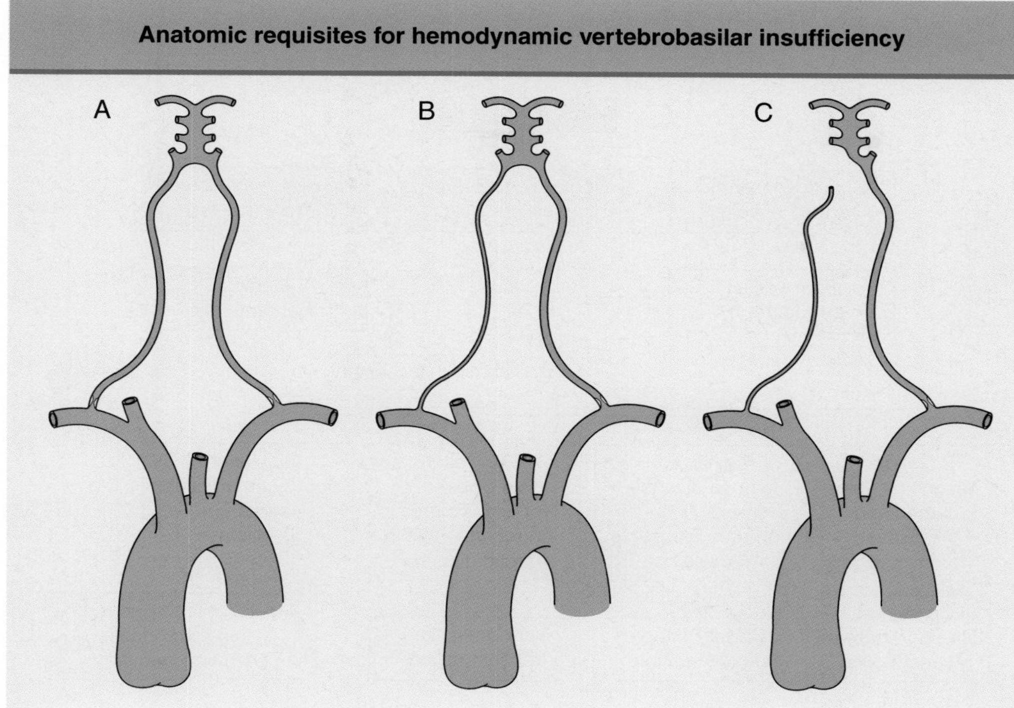

Figure 38-6. Anatomical requisites for hemodynamic vertebrobasilar insufficiency: bilateral vertebral artery disease **(A)**; unilateral vertebral artery disease with a contralateral absent or hypoplastic vertebral artery **(B)**; or a small contralateral vertebral artery ending in the posteroinferior cerebellar artery without participating in the formation of the basilar artery **(C)**.

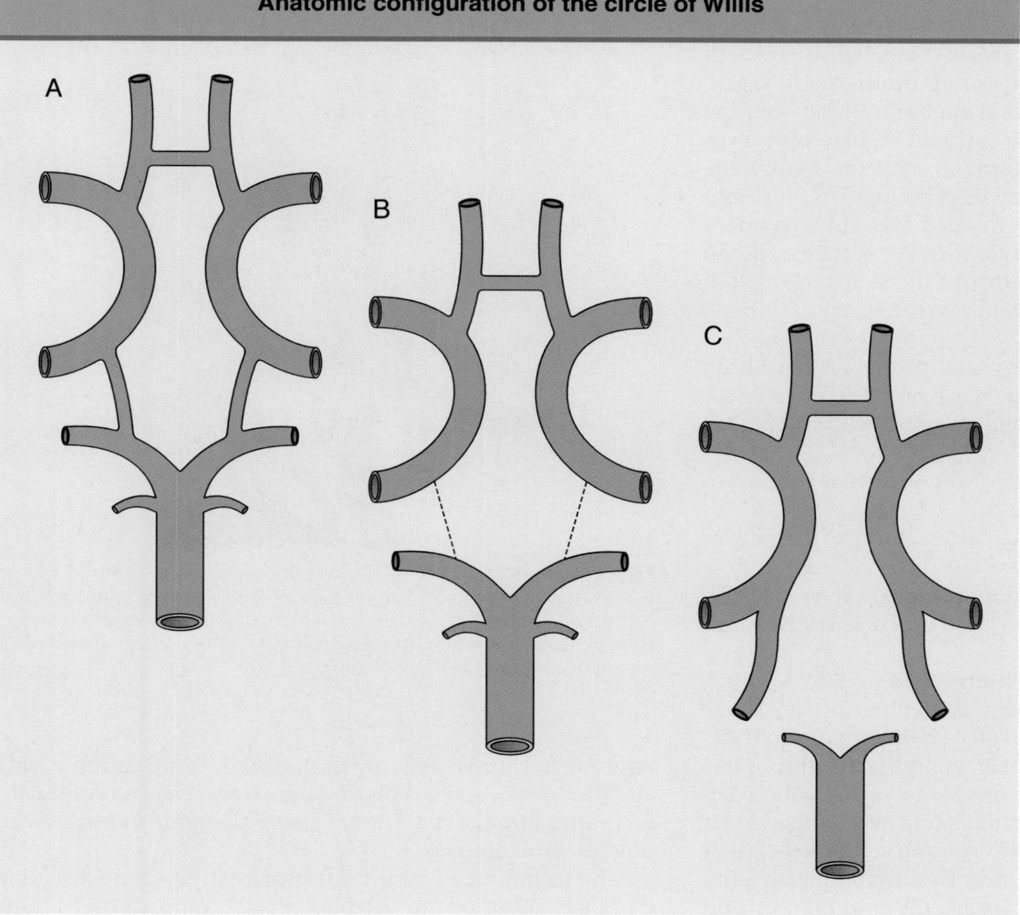

Figure 38-7. Anatomical configuration of the circle of Willis. A normal configuration **(A)** is present in only half of the general population. The most common variations include absence or hypoplasia of one or both of the posterior communicating arteries **(B)** and origin of one or both of the posterior cerebral arteries from the carotid arteries **(C)**.

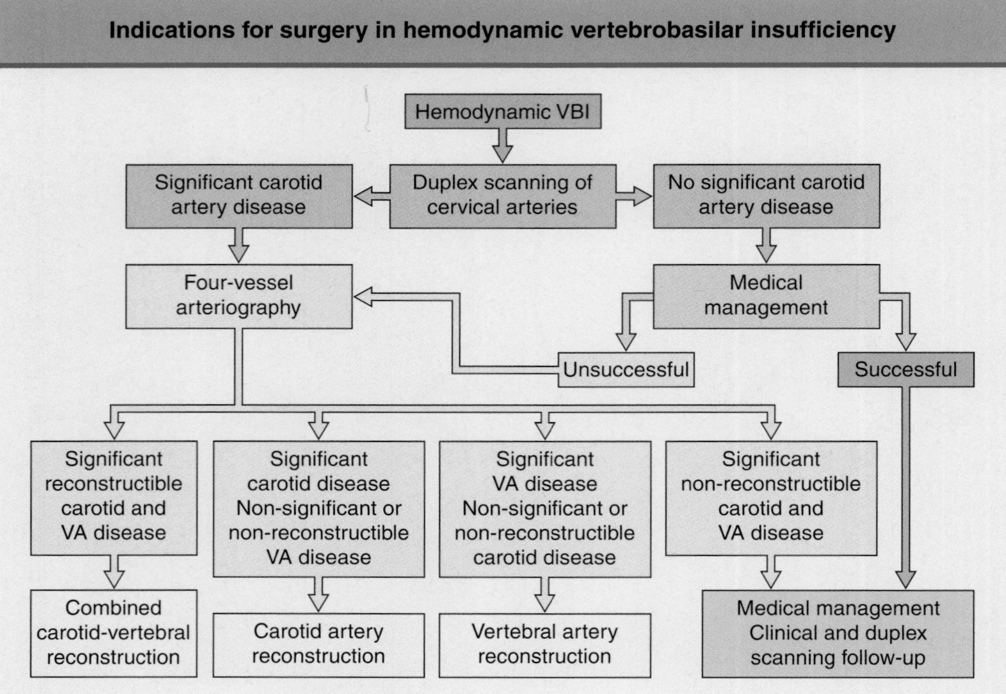

Figure 38-8. Indications for surgery in hemodynamic vertebrobasilar insufficiency (VBI). VA, vertebral artery.

Surgery of the V1 Segment

For the V1 segment, the approach is either through a transverse supraclavicular incision with dissociation of both heads of the sternomastoid muscle or through a low presternomastoid incision. The VA is approached between the common carotid artery and the internal jugular vein, with the vagus nerve being left adjacent to the vein. Lymphatic elements, including the thoracic duct on the left side, and the vertebral vein are carefully divided and cut to avoid a postoperative lymphatic drainage. The VA is then exposed along with the sympathetic chain and the stellate ganglion, which should be preserved to avoid a postoperative Horner's syndrome.

Atherosclerotic lesions at the origin of the VA have been treated using closed (transsubclavian) or open endarterectomy with good results.[22] We seldom use this technique for the following reasons:

- It needs complete exposure of the proximal subclavian and its branches.
- It may lead to an extensive endarterectomy of the subclavian artery, which may necessitate distal tacking sutures.
- It does not take into account the frequent excess in length of the V1 segment, which may lead to postoperative kinking of the VA.
- It entails the risk of a distal intimal flap in the VA, which may be the cause of postoperative stenosis or occlusion.

Similarly, transposition into and venous bypass from the distal subclavian artery[3] are rather complicated procedures since they necessitate complete dissection of the subclavian artery. Moreover, their late results may be compromised by progression of atherosclerotic disease in the subclavian artery itself. In my opinion, these two techniques should be considered only when the ipsilateral common carotid artery is not usable because of occlusion or advanced mural atherosclerosis, severe siphon stenosis, or advanced contralateral carotid occlusive disease, making clamping impossible or potentially dangerous.

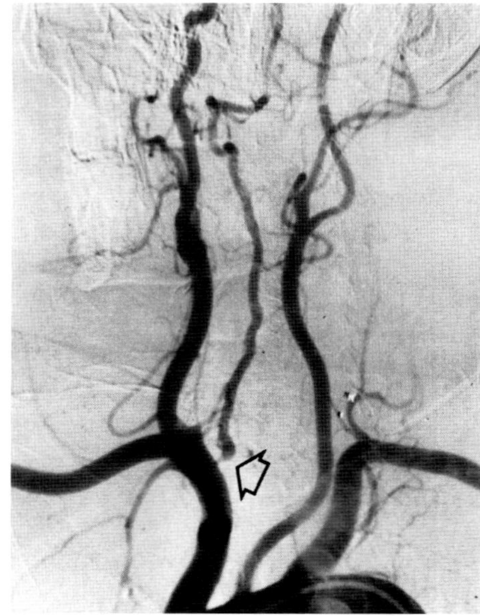

Figure 38-9. Isolated vertebral artery reconstruction. Indication for a vertebral artery reconstruction is logical in this patient with hemodynamic vertebrobasilar insufficiency, absence of the left vertebral artery, tight stenosis of the right proximal vertebral artery *(open arrow),* and nonsignificant carotid artery disease.

The technique of choice for proximal VA reconstruction is transposition of the VA into the common carotid artery

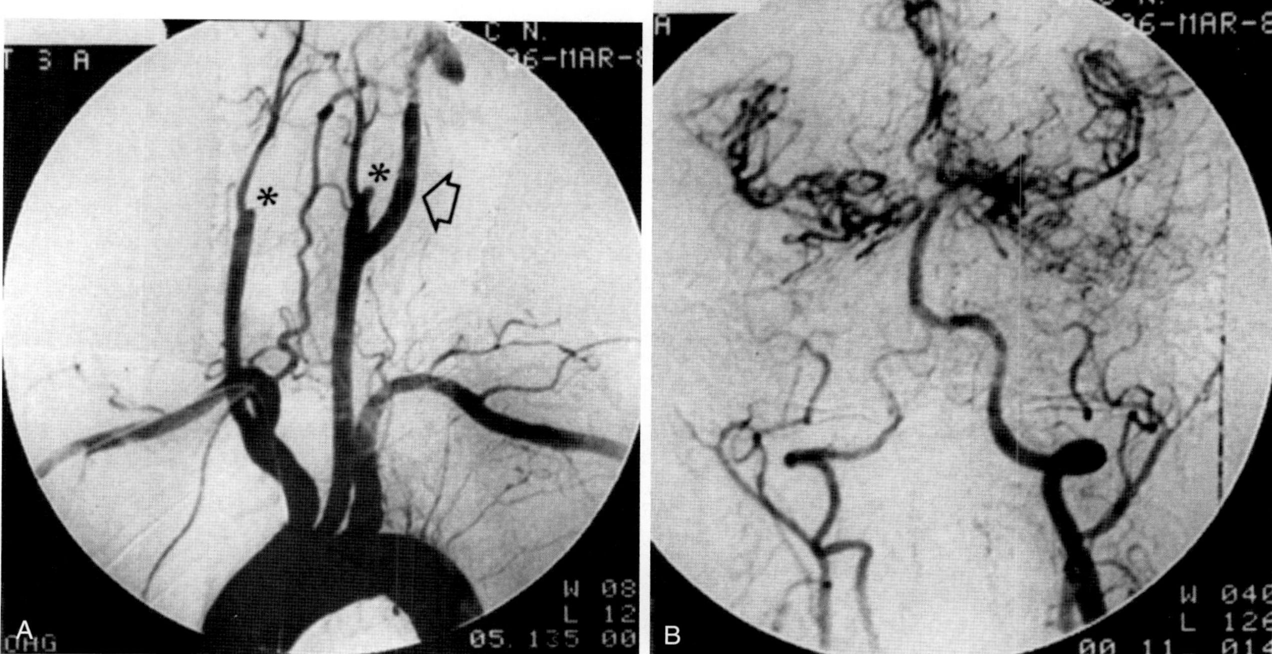

Figure 38-10. Distal vertebral artery reconstruction *(open arrow)* in a patient with bilateral internal carotid occlusion. Both hemispheres are supplied by the vertebral bypass through the basilar artery and both posterior communicating arteries.

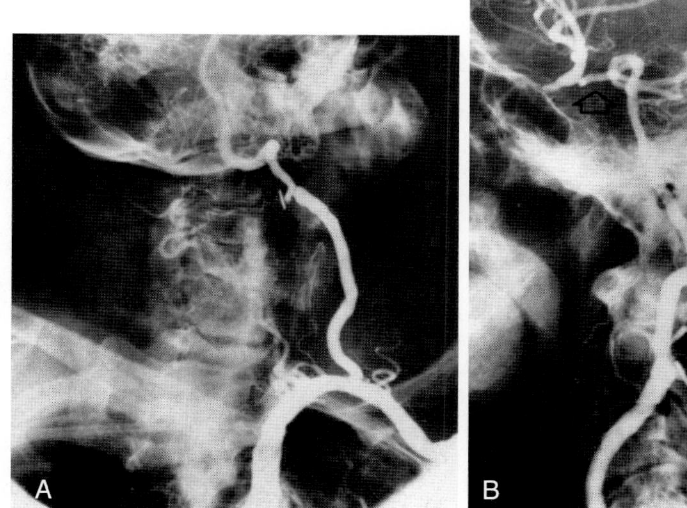

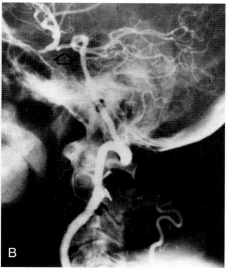

Figure 38-11. Subclavian artery to distal vertebral artery bypass using autogenous saphenous vein graft in a patient with occlusion of the ipsilateral common and internal carotid arteries. The basilar artery supplies the ipsilateral carotid territory through the posterior communicating artery *(open arrow)*.

(Figure 38-12).[9-11,15,62,99,110-112] It is a simple procedure that necessitates only limited exposure of the proximal VA and adjacent common carotid artery. It has the advantage of neglecting the lesions of the subclavian artery. It allows for simultaneous management of excessive length of the VA. Lastly, progression of atherosclerotic disease is seldom encountered in the common carotid artery on late follow-up. Requirements for this technique are a normal common carotid and intracranial internal carotid arteries. Atherosclerotic lesions of the carotid bifurcation should be treated simultaneously using the same presternomastoid incision.[7,104,105,110,111] Clamping of the normal common carotid artery does not entail an added risk of cerebral ischemia because antegrade perfusion of the internal carotid artery is maintained during clamping through the ipsilateral external carotid artery.

Surgery of the V2 Segment

Although tedious and potentially difficult, a direct approach to the VA in the V2 segment is feasible by unroofing the VA in the bony canal of the transverse processes.[113] In this segment,

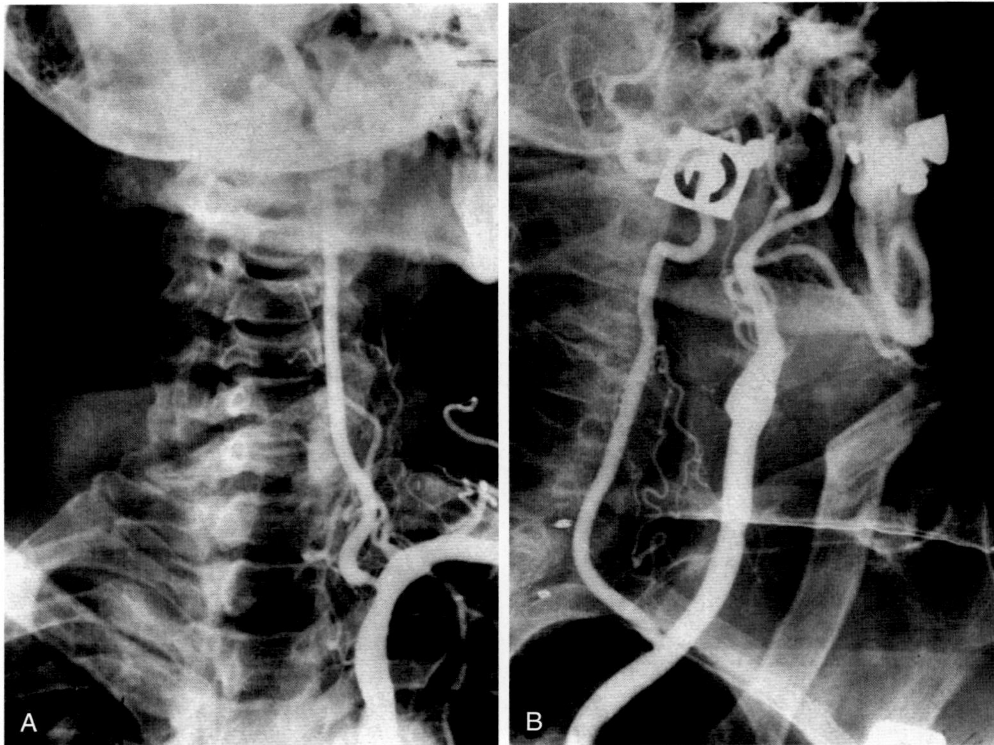

Figure 38-12. Tight stenosis of the proximal vertebral artery **(A)** treated by transposition into the common carotid artery **(B).** While neglecting moderate subclavian artery disease, this procedure is facilitated by an excessive length of the first segment of the vertebral artery.

the VA is surrounded by venous plexus, which has to be coagulated and transsected and may constitute an operative difficulty.

While this approach has been used extensively for direct decompression of the VA in patients with cervical spondylosis, a much simpler distal bypass from the carotid or subclavian to the V3 segment is usually preferred. In our opinion, the only remaining indications for a direct approach of the V2 segment is penetrating trauma to the VA[38] or combined neurological and arterial decompression in patients with cervical spondylosis[72] or tumors.[62,108,109]

Surgery of the V3 Segment

The introduction of a direct approach to the distal cervical VA has been a major advance in the management of VA disease.[6,8,17,28,29,62] The VA is usually approached in the C1 to C2 interspace using a high presternomastoid incision (Figure 38-13). The internal jugular vein is left in the anterior part of the surgical field. The spinal accessory nerve is identified and preserved. The C1 transverse process leads to the underlying C1 to C2 interspace, which is opened by resecting the muscles inserting in the lower aspect of C1. The VA is then dissected from the anterior branch of the C2 nerve and freed from the surrounding venous plexus. Two to three centimeters of healthy VA are available for the distal implantation of a saphenous bypass originating from the common carotid artery (Figure 38-10) or, much less often, from the external carotid, internal carotid, or subclavian artery (Figure 38-11).

Alternative techniques include transposition of the distal VA into the internal carotid artery,[114] transposition of the occipital artery into the VA,[6] or use of an arterial autograft obtained from the proximal V1 segment or from an endarterectomized internal carotid artery.[29] These techniques have the advantage of bypassing all the lesions of the V2 segment, with a distal anastomosis or implantation in a usually healthy portion of the VA.

Rarely, a more distal (above C1) approach to the VA is needed (Figure 38-14).[115] It may be obtained through a posterior extension of the previous incision or through a posterior midline incision with a lateral extension. In both cases, resection of the posterior arch of C1 allows a relatively easy approach to the VA, which can be dissected up to the atlanto-occipital membrane.

Surgery of the V4 Segment

Direct approach to the V4 segment in the posterior fossa is feasible. Successful segmental endarterectomy of the intracranial VA has been reported.[116] However, the usual technique has been extraintracranial revascularization using occipital artery to PICA anastomosis[117] or venous graft from the external carotid artery to the posterior cerebral artery.[118]

CONCLUSION

Although it is not yet widely accepted by the medical community, the concept of hemodynamic VBI appears to be valid. Management of the patients should be performed by a multidisciplinary team including neurologists, neuroradiologists, otolaryngologists, vascular surgeons, neurosurgeons, and other specialists if indicated. Using modern diagnostic tools

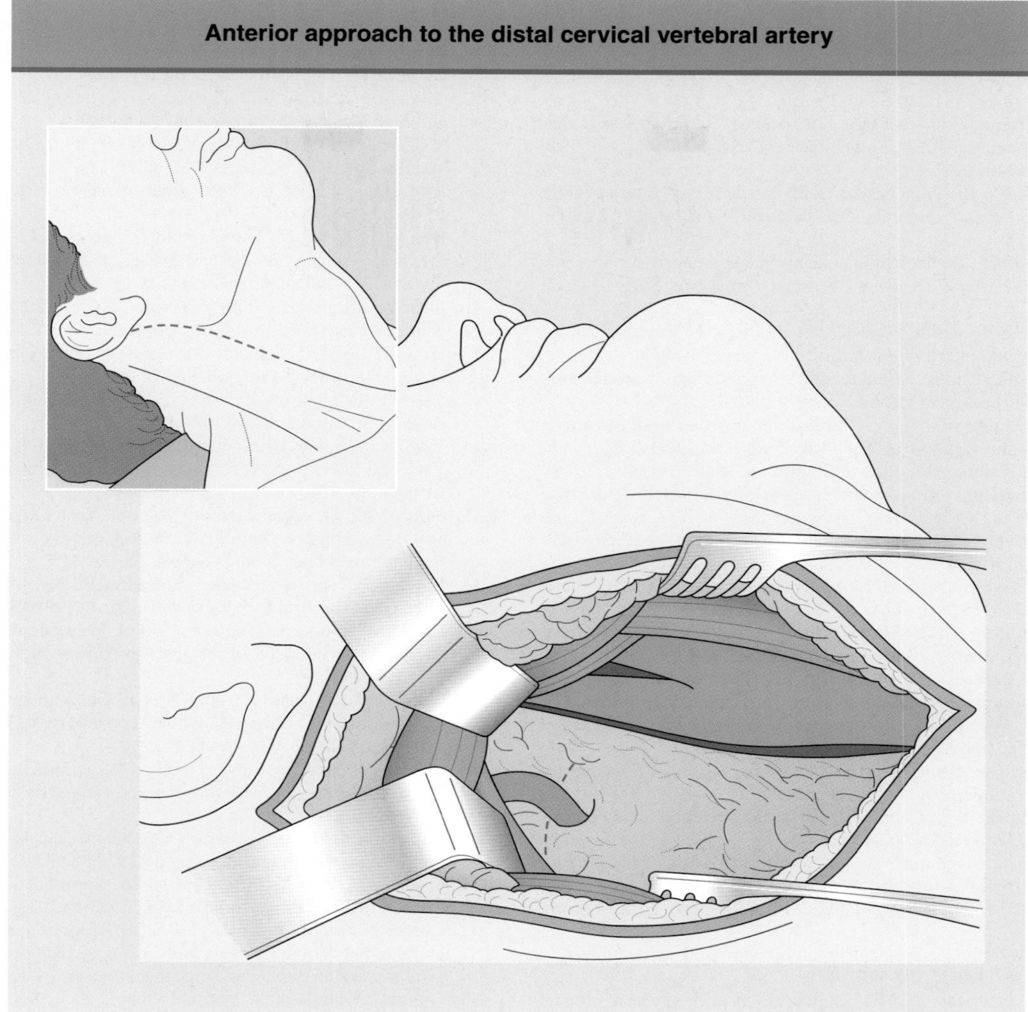

Figure 38-13. Anterior approach to the distal cervical vertebral artery at the level of the C1 to C2 interspace.

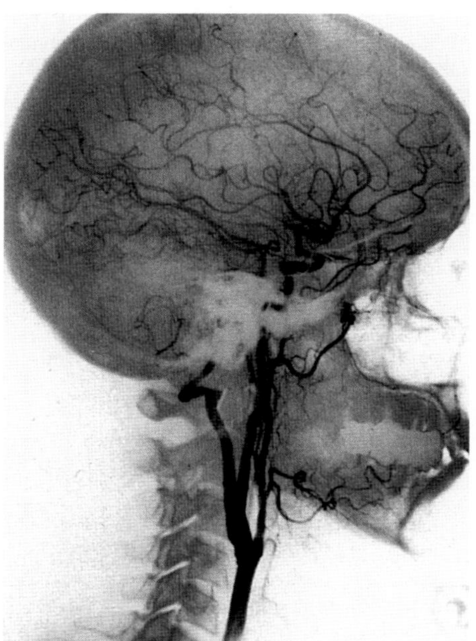

Figure 38-14. Reconstruction of the distal vertebral artery at the C1 level using a saphenous vein graft from the carotid bifurcation.

and logical criteria for diagnosis and indications, as well as precise techniques for surgery, clinical and anatomical results of VA reconstructions have been satisfactory in the most recently reported series.[119] The experience of my colleagues and I now numbers more than 900 VA reconstructions. Mortality for isolated VA procedures has been less than 1%. Early occlusion rate has dropped to less than 4%, with few late occlusions. Cure or maximal improvement of clinical symptoms has been obtained in more than 90% of the patients with hemodynamic VBI.

References

1. Cate WR, Scott Jr HW. Cerebral ischemia of central origin: relief by subclavian–vertebral artery thromboendarterectomy. *Surgery* 1959;45: 19-31.
2. Crawford ES, DeBakey ME, Fields WS. Roentgenographic diagnosis and surgical treatment of basilar artery insufficiency. *JAMA* 1958;168: 509-514.
3. Berguer R, Bauer RB. Vertebral artery reconstruction: a successful technique in selected patients. *Ann Surg* 1981;193:441-447.
4. Berguer R, Feldman AJ. Surgical reconstruction of the vertebral artery. *Surgery* 1983;93:670-675.
5. Berguer R, Flynn LM, Kline RA, Caplan L. Surgical reconstruction of the extracranial vertebral artery: management and outcome. *J Vasc Surg* 2000;31:9-18.

6. Berguer R, Morasch MD, Kline RA. A review of 100 consecutive reconstructions of the distal vertebral artery for embolic and hemodynamic disease. *J Vasc Surg* 1998;27:852-859.
7. Branchereau A, Magnan PE. Results of vertebral artery reconstruction. *J Cardiovasc Surg* 1990;31:320-326.
8. Carney AL. Vertebral artery surgery: historical development, basic concepts of brain hemodynamics, and clinical experience of 102 cases. *Adv Neurol* 1981;30:249-282.
9. Cormier JM, Ricco JB, Francheschi C. 82 cas de réimplantation de la sous-clavière ou de la vertébrale dans la carotide primitive. *Chirurgie* 1979;105:592-596.
10. Deriu GP, Ballotta E, Franceschi L, et al. Surgical management of extracranial vertebral artery occlusive disease. *J Cardiovasc Surg* 1991;32: 413-419.
11. Diaz FG, Ausman JI, de los Reyes RA, et al. Surgical reconstruction of the proximal vertebral artery. *J Neurosurg* 1984;61:874-881.
12. Edwards WH, Mulherin JL. The surgical approach to significant stenosis of vertebral and subclavian arteries. *Surgery* 1980;87:20-28.
13. Edwards WH, Mulherin Jr JL. The surgical reconstruction of the proximal subclavian and vertebral artery. *J Vasc Surg* 1985;2:634-642.
14. Giangola G, Imparato AM, Riles TS, Lamparello PJ. Vertebral artery angioplasty in patients younger than 55 years: long-term follow-up. *Ann Vasc Surg* 1991;5:121-124.
15. Habozit B. Vertebral artery reconstruction: results in 106 patients. *Ann Vasc Surg* 1991;5:61-65.
16. Imparato AM. Vertebral arterial reconstruction: a nineteen-year experience. *J Vasc Surg* 1985;2:626-634.
17. Kieffer E, Praquin B, Chiche L, et al. Distal vertebral artery reconstruction: long-term outcome. *J Vasc Surg* 2002;36:549-554.
18. Pauliukas PA, Barkauskas EM, Shifrin EG, Portnoi IM. Experience with reconstruction of vertebral arteries. In: Caplan LR, Shifrin EG, Nicolaides AN, Moore WS, eds. *Cerebrovascular ischemia: investigation and management.* London: Med-Orion; 1996:577-601.
19. Reul GJ, Cooley DA, Olson SK, et al. Long-term results of direct vertebral artery operations. *Surgery* 1984;96:854-862.
20. Roon AJ, Ehrenfeld WK, Cooke PB, Wylie EJ. Vertebral artery reconstruction. *Am J Surg* 1979;138:29-36.
21. Rosset E, Ayari R, Magnan PE, et al. Long-term results of reconstructions of the vertebral artery. In: Branchereau A, Jacobs M, eds. *Long-term results of arterial interventions.* Armonk, New York: Futura; 1997:67-79.
22. Thevenet A, Ruotolo C. Surgical repair of vertebral artery stenoses. *J Cardiovasc Surg* 1984;25:101-110.
23. Van Schil PE, Ackerstaff RG, Vermeulen FE, et al. Long-term clinical and duplex follow-up after proximal vertebral artery reconstruction. *Angiology* 1992;43:961-968.
24. Argenson C, Francke JP, Sylla S, et al. Les artères vertébrales (segments V1 et V2). *Anat Clin* 1979;2:29-41.
25. Francke JP, Di Marino V, Pannier M, et al. Les artères vertébrales: segments atlanto-axoïdien V3 et intracrânien V4, collatérales. *Anat Clin* 1980;2:229-242.
26. Ouriel K, Green RM, DeWeese JA. Anomalous carotid–basilar anastomoses in cerebrovascular surgery. *J Vasc Surg* 1988;7:774-777.
27. Fisher CM, Gore I, Okabe N, White PD. Atherosclerosis of the carotid and vertebral arteries extracranial and intracranial. *J Neuropathol Exp Neurol* 1965;24:455-476.
28. Berguer R. Distal vertebral artery bypass: technique, the "occipital connection," and potential uses. *J Vasc Surg* 1985;2:621-626.
29. Kieffer E, Rancurel G, Richard T. Reconstruction of the distal cervical vertebral artery. In: Berguer R, Bauer RB, eds. *Vertebrobasilar arterial occlusive disease.* New York: Raven Press; 1984:265-290.
30. Laurian C, Georges B, Houdart R, Cormier JM. Revascularisation de l'artère vertébrale distale (3° segment): indications dans le traitement de l'insuffisance vertébro-basilaire. *Sem Hop Paris* 1984;16:547-552.
31. Chiche L, Bahnini A, Koskas F, Kieffer E. Occlusive fibromuscular disease of arteries supplying the brain: results of surgical treatment. *Ann Vasc Surg* 1997;11:496-504.
32. Stanley JC, Fry WJ, Seeger JF, et al. Extracranial internal carotid and vertebral artery fibrodysplasia. *Arch Surg* 1974;109:215-222.
33. Kieffer E, Natali J. Supraaortic trunk lesions in Takayasu's arteritis. In: Bergan JJ, Yao JST, eds. *Cerebrovascular insufficiency.* New York: Grune & Stratton; 1983:395-415.
34. Thielen KR, Wijdicks EFM, Nichols DA. Giant cell temporal arteritis: involvement of the vertebral and carotid arteries. *Mayo Clinic Proc* 1998;73:444-446.
35. Blickenstaff KL, Weaver FA, Yellin AE, et al. Trends in the management of traumatic vertebral artery injuries. *Am J Surg* 1989;158:101-106.
36. Demetriades D, Theodorou D, Asensio J, et al. Management options in vertebral artery injuries. *Br J Surg* 1996;83:83-86.
37. Golueke P, Sclafani S, Phillips T, et al. Vertebral artery injury: diagnosis and management. *J Trauma* 1987;27:856-865.
38. Meier DE, Brink BE, Fry WJ. Vertebral artery trauma: acute recognition and treatment. *Arch Surg* 1981;116:236-239.
39. Reid JDS, Weigelt JA. Forty-three cases of vertebral artery trauma. *J Trauma* 1988;28:1007-1012.
40. Jean WC, Barrett MD, Rockswold G, Bergman TA. Gunshot wound to the head resulting in a vertebral artery pseudoaneurysm at the base of the skull. *J Trauma* 2001;50:126-128.
41. Biffl WL, Moore EE, Elliott JP, et al. The devastating potential of blunt vertebral arterial injuries. *Ann Surg* 2000;231:672-681.
42. Hayes P, Gerlock AJ, Cobb CA. Cervical spine trauma: a cause of vertebral artery injury. *J Trauma* 1980;20:904-905.
43. Sherman DG, Hart RG, Easton JD. Abrupt change in head position and cerebral infarction. *Stroke* 1981;12:2-6.
44. Van Tets WF, Van Drullemen HM, Tjan GT, Van Berge Henegouwen D. Vertebral arteriovenous fistula caused by puncture of the internal jugular vein. *Eur J Surg* 1992;158:627-628.
45. Smith MD, Emery SE, Dudley A, et al. Vertebral artery injury during anterior decompression of the cervical spine: a retrospective review of ten patients. *J Bone Joint Surg* 1993;75:410-415.
46. Buerger T, Lippert H, Meyer F, Halloul Z. Aneurysm of the vertebral artery near the atlas arch. *J Cardiovasc Surg* 1999;40:387-389.
47. Catala M, Rancurel G, Koskas F, et al. Ischemic stroke due to spontaneous extracranial vertebral giant aneurysm. *Cerebrovasc Dis* 1993;3: 322-326.
48. Hoffman K, Hosten N, Liebig T, et al. Giant aneurysm of the vertebral artery in neurofibromatosis type I: report of a case and review of literature. *Neuroradiology* 1998;40:245-248.
49. Rifkinson-Mann S, Laub J, Haimov M. Atraumatic extracranial vertebral artery aneurysm: case report and review of the literature. *J Vasc Surg* 1986;4:288-293.
50. Thompson JE, Eilber F, Baker JD. Vertebral artery aneurysm: case report and review of the literature. *Surgery* 1979;85:583-585.
51. Caplan LR, Zarins CK, Hemmati M. Spontaneous dissection of the extracranial vertebral arteries. *Stroke* 1985;16:1030-1038.
52. Chiche L, Praquin B, Koskas F, Kieffer E. Spontaneous dissection of the extracranial vertebral artery: indications and long-term outcome of surgical treatment. *Ann Vasc Surg* 2005;19;(1):5-10.
53. Chiras J, Marciano S, Vega Molina J, et al. Spontaneous dissecting aneurysm of the extracranial vertebral artery. *Neuroradiology* 1985;27: 327-333.
54. Mas JL, Bousser MG, Hasboun D, Laplane D. Extracranial vertebral artery dissections: a review of 13 cases. *Stroke* 1987;18:1037-1047.
55. Mokri B, Houser OW, Sandok BA, Piepgras DG. Spontaneous dissections of the vertebral arteries. *Neurology* 1988;38:880-885.
56. Schievink WI. Spontaneous dissection of the carotid and vertebral arteries. *N Engl J Med* 2001;344:898-906.
57. Touzé E, Randoux B, Méary E, et al. Aneurysmal forms of cervical artery dissection: associated factors and outcome. *Stroke* 2001;32:418-423.
58. Cluzel P, Pierot L, Leung A, et al. Vertebral arteriovenous fistulae in neurofibromatosis: report of two cases and review of the literature. *Neuroradiology* 1994;36:321-325.
59. Vinchon M, Laurian C, George B, et al. Vertebral arteriovenous fistulas: a study of 49 cases and review of the literature. *Cardiovasc Surg* 1994;2:359-369.
60. Bauer RB. Mechanical compression of the vertebral arteries. In: Berguer R, Bauer RB, eds. Vertebrobasilar arterial occlusive disease. New York: Raven Press; 1984:45-71.
61. George B, Laurian C. Impairment of vertebral artery flow caused by extrinsic lesions. *Neurosurgery* 1989;24:206-214.
62. George B, Laurian C. *The vertebral artery: pathology and surgery.* Vienna: Springer Verlag; 1987:183-230.
63. Kieffer E, Rancurel G, Branchereau A. Insuffisance vertébrobasilaire par lésion de l'artère vertébrale. *J Mal Vasc* 1985;10(Suppl C):253-313.
64. Toole JF. Positional effects of head and neck on vertebral artery blood flow. In: Berguer R, Caplan LR, eds. *Vertebrobasilar arterial disease.* St. Louis: Quality Medical; 1992:11-14.
65. Hedera P, Bujdakova J, Traubner P. Blood flow velocities in basilar artery during rotation of the head. *Acta Neurol Scand* 1993;88: 229-233.

66. Koskas F, Comizzoli I, Gobin P, et al. Effects of spinal mechanics on the vertebral artery: anatomic basis of positional postural compression of the cervical vertebral artery. In: Berguer R, Caplan LR, eds. *Vertebrobasilar arterial disease.* St. Louis: Quality Medical; 1992:15-28.
67. Alexandrov AV, Norris JW. Recurrent stroke caused by spondylotic compression of the vertebral artery. *Ann Neurol* 1994;35:126-128.
68. Matskevichus ZK, Pauliukas PA. Morphologic changes of the arterial wall at the site of the loops and kinks of the carotid and vertebral arteries. *Arch Pathol* 1990;52:53-58.
69. Sullivan HG, Harbison JW, Vines FS, Becker D. Embolic posterior cerebral artery occlusion secondary to spondylitic vertebral artery compression. *J Neurosurg* 1975;43:618-622.
70. Barton JW, Margolis MT. Rotational obstructions of the vertebral artery at the atlantoaxial joint. *Neuroradiology* 1975;9:117-120.
71. Dadsetan MR, Skerhut HE. Rotational vertebrobasilar insufficiency secondary to vertebral artery occlusion from fibrous band of the longus coli muscle. *Neuroradiology* 1990;32:514-515.
72. Hardin CA. Vertebral artery insufficiency produced by cervical osteoarthritic spurs. *Arch Surg* 1965;90:629-633.
73. Hurvitz SA, Bonecutter GE. Surgical decompression of the first part of vertebral artery for ischemic brainstem dysfunction. *J Cardiovasc Surg* 1999;40:395-400.
74. Husni EA, Bell HS, Storer J. Mechanical occlusion of the vertebral artery: a new clinical concept. *JAMA* 1966;196:474-478.
75. Kojima N, Tamaki N, Fujita K, Matsumoto S. Vertebral artery occlusion at the narrowed "scalenovertebral angle": mechanical vertebral occlusion in the distal first portion. *Neurosurgery* 1985;16:672-674.
76. Lang J, Kessler B. About the suboccipital part of the vertebral artery and the neighboring bone-joint and nerve relationships. *Skull Base Surg* 1991;1:64-72.
77. Mapstone T, Spetzler RF. Vertebrobasilar insufficiency secondary to vertebral artery occlusion from a fibrous band. *J Neurosurg* 1982;56:581-583.
78. Radojevic S, Negovanovic B. La gouttière et les anneaux osseux de l'artère vertébrale de l'atlas (étude anatomique et radiologique). *Acta Anat* 1963;55:186-194.
79. Sheehan S, Bauer RB, Meyer JS. Vertebral artery compression in cervical spondylosis: arteriographic demonstration during life of vertebral artery insufficiency due to rotation and extension of the neck. *Neurology* 1960;10:968-986.
80. Buge A, Rancurel G, Kieffer E, Denvil D. L'insuffisance vertébrobasilaire: revue des critères sémiologiques cérébro-vasculaires et des indications chirurgicales. *Concours Med* 1980;41:102-141.
81. Caplan LR. Vertebrobasilar disease: time for a new strategy. *Stroke* 1981;12:111-114.
82. Caplan LR. Vertebrobasilar occlusive disease. In: Barnett HJM, Stein BM, Mohr JP, Yatsu FM, eds. *Stroke: overview, pathophysiology, diagnosis and management.* Philadelphia: Churchill Livingstone; 1986: 549-619.
83. George B, Laurian C. Vertebro-basilar ischaemia: its relation to stenosis and occlusion of the vertebral artery. *Acta Neurochir Wien* 1982;62:287-295.
84. Caplan LR, Amarenco P, Rosengart A, et al. Embolism from vertebral artery origin occlusive disease. *Neurology* 1992;42:1505-1512.
85. Caplan LR. Occlusion of the vertebral or basilar artery: follow-up analysis of some patients with benign outcome. *Stroke* 1979;10:277-282.
86. Fisher CM. Occlusion of the vertebral arteries causing transient basilar symptoms. *Arch Neurol* 1970;22:13-19.
87. Caplan LR. Patterns of posterior circulation infarctions: correlation with vascular pathology. In: Berguer R, Bauer RB, eds. *Vertebrobasilar arterial occlusive disease.* New York: Raven Press; 1984:15-25.
88. Castaigne P, Lhermitte F, Gautier J, et al. Arterial occlusion in the vertebrobasilar system: a study of 44 patients with post-mortem data. *Brain* 1973;96:133-154.
89. Hauw J-J, Amarenco P, Duyckaerts C, et al. Neuropathologie de l'ischémie vertébro-basilaire. *Sem Hop Paris* 1986;62:2757-2761.
90. Jones Jr HR, Millikan CH, Sandok BA. Temporal profile (clinical course) of acute vertebrobasilar system cerebral infarctions. *Stroke* 1980;11:173-177.
91. McDowell FH, Potes J, Groch S. The natural history of internal carotid and vertebral–basilar artery occlusion. *Neurology* 1961;1:153-157.
92. Patrick BK, Ramirez-Lassepas M, Snyder BD. Temporal profile of vertebrobasilar territory infarction: prognostic implications. *Stroke* 1980;11:643-648.
93. Cartlidge NEF, Whisnant JP, Elveback LR. Carotid and vertebral–basilar transient cerebral ischemic attacks: a community study, Rochester, Minnesota. *Mayo Clin Proc* 1977;52:117-120.
94. Heyman A, Wilkinson WE, Hurwitz BJ, et al. Clinical and epidemiologic aspects of vertebrobasilar and nonfocal cerebral ischemia. In: Berguer R, Bauer RB, eds. *Vertebrobasilar arterial occlusive disease.* New York: Raven Press; 1984:27-36.
95. Whisnant JP, Cartlidge NEF, Elveback LR. Carotid and vertebral–basilar transient ischemic attacks: effects of anticoagulants, hypertension and cardiac disorders on survival and stroke occurrence: a population study. *Ann Neurol* 1978;3:107-115.
96. Naritomi H, Sakai F, Meyer JS. Pathogenesis of transient ischemic attacks within the vertebrobasilar arterial system. *Arch Neurol* 1979;36:121-128.
97. Rosset E, Magnan PE, Branchereau A, et al. Hemodynamic vertebrobasilar insufficiency caused by multiple arterial lesions: results of surgical treatment. *Ann Vasc Surg* 1993;7:243-248.
98. Valerio N, Rosset E, Ede B, et al. Compromised hemodynamics associated with multipedicular lesions of cerebral arteries. *Ann Vasc Surg* 2001;15:219-226.
99. Kieffer E. Chirurgie de l'artère vertébrale. *Encycl Med Chir (Techniques Chirurgicales)* Paris 1984.
100. Branchereau A, Ede B, Magnan PE, et al. Surgery for asymptomatic carotid stenosis: a study of three patient subgroups. *Ann Vasc Surg* 1998;12:572-578.
101. Cardon A, Kerdiles Y, Lucas A, et al. Results of isolated carotid surgery in patients with vertebrobasilar insufficiency. *Ann Vasc Surg* 1998;12:579-582.
102. Humphries AW, Young JR, Beven EG, et al. Relief of vertebrobasilar symptoms by carotid endarterectomy. *Surgery* 1965;57:48-52.
103. Ouriel K, May AG, Ricotta JJ, et al. Carotid endarterectomy for nonhemispheric symptoms: predictors of success. *J Vasc Surg* 1984;1:339-345.
104. Kieffer E, Rancurel G. Surgical management of combined carotid and vertebral disease. In: Berguer R, Bauer RB, eds. *Vertebrobasilar arterial occlusive disease.* New York: Raven Press; 1984:305-311.
105. Malone JM, Moore W, Hamilton R, Smith M. Combined carotid–vertebral vascular disease: a new surgical approach. *Arch Surg* 1980;115: 783-785.
106. Archie JP. Improved carotid hemodynamics with vertebral reconstruction. *Ann Vasc Surg* 1992;6:138-141.
107. Berguer R, McCaffrey JF, Bauer RB. Bilateral internal carotid artery occlusion: its surgical management. *Arch Surg* 1980;115:840-843.
108. Merland JJ, Riche MC, George B, et al. Current trends in the combined radiological and surgical management of vascular malformations, tumors and dysplasia involving the vertebral artery. *J Neuroradiol* 1979;6:269-286.
109. Sen C, Eisenberg M, Casden AM, et al. Management of the vertebral artery in excision of extradural tumors of the cervical spine. *Neurosurgery* 1995;36:106-116.
110. Berguer R, Kieffer E. *Surgery of the arteries to the head.* New York: Springer Verlag; 1992.
111. Edwards WH Sr. Vertebral artery reconstruction: indications and techniques. *Semin Vasc Surg* 1996;9:105-110.
112. Spetzler RF, Hadley MN, Martin NA, et al. Vertebrobasilar insufficiency. I. Microsurgical treatment of extracranial vertebrobasilar disease. *J Neurosurg* 1987;66:648-661.
113. Brink B. Approach to the second segment of the vertebral arteries. In: Berguer R, Bauer RB, eds. *Vertebrobasilar arterial occlusive disease.* New York: Raven Press; 1984:257-264.
114. Koskas F, Kieffer E, Rancurel G, et al. Direct transposition of the distal cervical vertebral artery into the internal carotid artery. *Ann Vasc Surg* 1995;9:515-524.
115. Berguer R. Suboccipital approach to the distal vertebral artery. J Vasc Surg 1999;30:344-349.
116. Allen GS, Cohen RJ, Preziosi TJ. Microsurgical endarterectomy of the intracranial vertebral artery for vertebro-basilar transient ischemic attacks. *Neurosurgery* 1981;8:56-59.
117. Sundt Jr TM, Piedgras DG. Occipital to posterior inferior cerebellar artery bypass surgery. *J Neurosurg* 1978;48:916-928.
118. Sundt Jr TM, Piepgras DG, Houser OW, Campbell JK. Interposition saphenous vein grafts for advanced occlusive disease and large aneurysms in the posterior circulation. *J Neurosurg* 1982;56:205-215.
119. Kline RA, Berguer R. Vertebral artery reconstruction. *Ann Vasc Surg* 1993;7:497-501.

Section IX

Vascular Complications

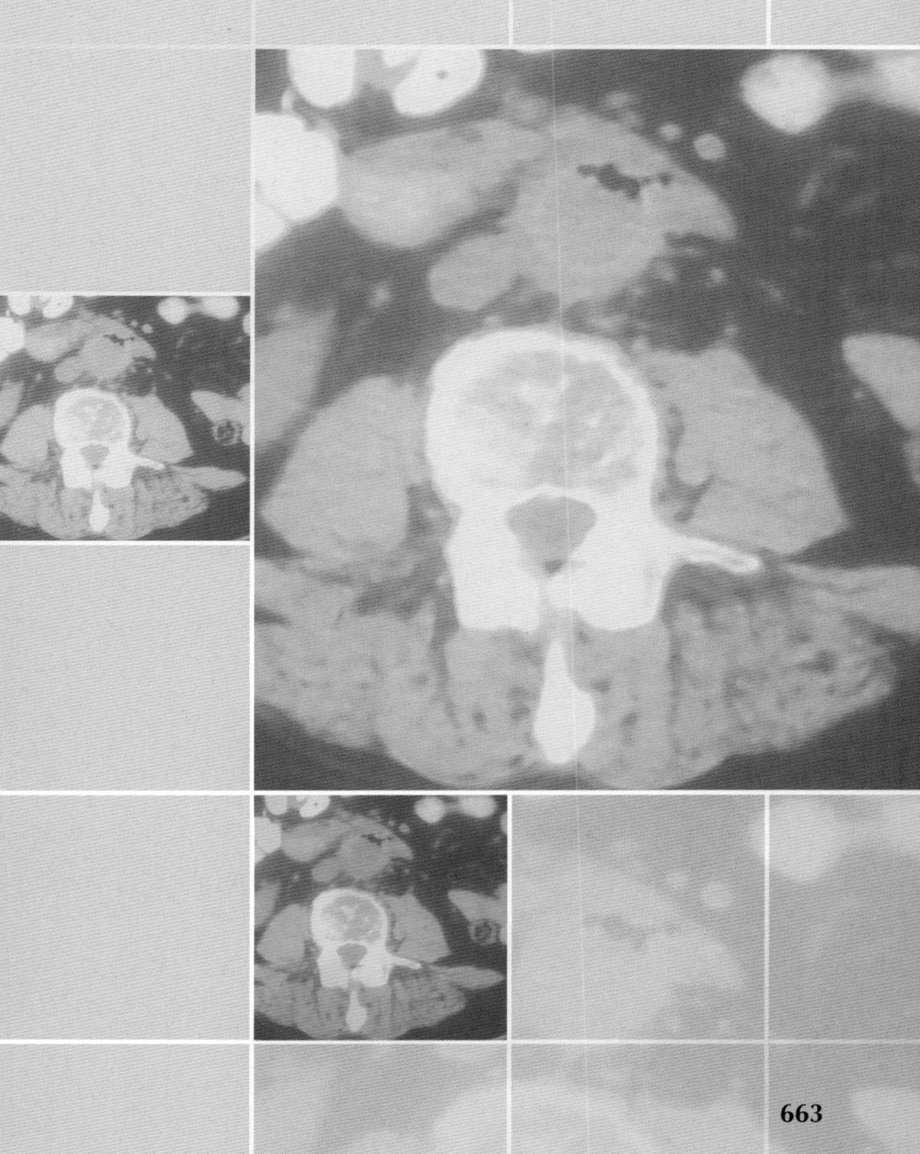

chapter

39

Healing Characteristics and Complications of Prosthetic and Biological Vascular Grafts

Glenn C. Hunter, MD • Kenneth J. Woodside, MD • Joseph J. Naoum, MD

Key Points

- Dacron
- Polytetrafluoroethylene
- Acute complications
- Chronic complications
- Graft dilatation
- Aortic paraanastomotic aneurysms and pseudoaneurysms
- Femoral anastomotic aneurysms and pseudoaneurysms
- Management
- Rupture
- Suture line failure
- Perigraft seroma
- Ureteric obstruction
- Neoplasia
- Reducing graft thrombogenicity
- Modification of anastomotic configuration
- Vein cuffs and patches
- Precuffed (hooded) grafts
- Peripheral endografts
- Venous prosthetic grafts
- Polyurethane
- Human umbilical vein
- Biological grafts
- Bovine xenografts

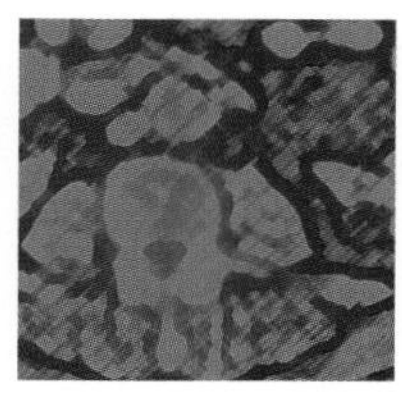

The search for the ideal vascular substitute that mimics a native artery or vein in composition, structure, function, and mechanical properties remains elusive. The saphenous vein, internal thoracic artery, and radial artery are the preferred conduits for bypassing atherosclerotic lesions of the lower extremity and coronary arteries.[1-3] Because of the size disparity and limited availability, no comparable autogenous replacements exist for bypassing occlusive or aneurysmal disease of the aorta, although the femoral vein has been used for aortoiliac or aortofemoral bypass in the setting of prosthetic graft infections. The increasing life span of the population, the persistence of risk factors for atherosclerosis, the increase in complexity of bypass procedures, and the need for revision in approximately one third of patients within 2 years have increased the need for durable prosthetic and biological vascular substitutes that will function satisfactorily throughout the life span of the patient.[4,5]

Among the desirable qualities for prosthetic grafts are that they be impermeable to blood, have long-term mechanical stability, possess nonthrombogenic flow surfaces, and be biocompatible with and incorporated by host tissues. The prosthesis must also be resistant to infection, readily available for elective and emergency use, and easily implantable.[4,6]

Currently, none of the available prostheses manifests all desired characteristics of an ideal arterial or venous replacement. Both polyethylene terephthalate (Dacron) and expanded polytetrafluoroethylene (ePTFE) grafts function well when used to replace large-diameter, high-flow vessels. Cumulative patency rates of bifurcated aortofemoral Dacron grafts range from 85% to 90% at 5 years to 74% and 70% at 10 and 15 years.[7-9] Comparable 5-year patency rates for ePTFE range from 95% to 97%.[10,11] In contrast, the long-term patency rates of small-diameter (6 mm internal diameter) prosthetic grafts

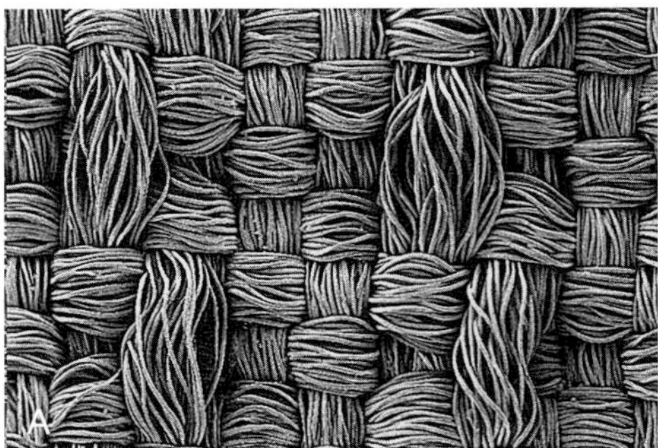

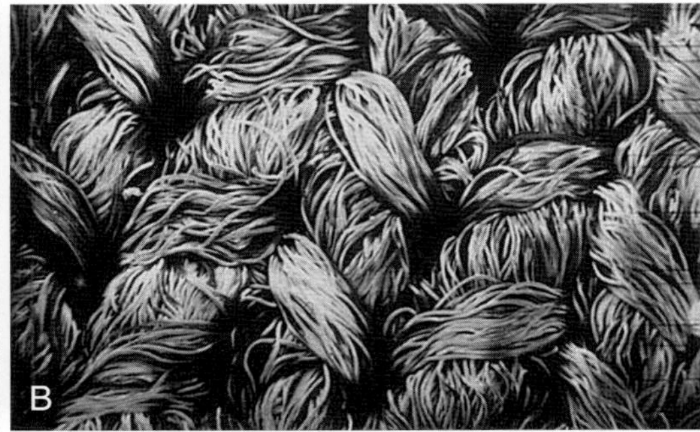

Figure 39-1. Scanning electron photographs demonstrating the surface of a conventional Gelweave woven **(A)** and a Gelseal warp-knitted **(B)** graft.

(SDPG) are lower as a consequence of thrombosis secondary to the thrombogenicity of the graft material, anastomotic neointimal fibrous hyperplasia (NFH), and progression of atherosclerosis. ePTFE, the predominantly used SDPG, and Dacron grafts in the femoropopliteal position have comparable cumulative patency rates at 3 to 5 years, ranging from 37.9% to 71% above knee and 30% to 57% below knee.[12-15]

In this chapter, we provide a brief overview of the fabrication, preparation, healing characteristics, and clinical indications for the use of prosthetic and biological prostheses. The focus of the discussion is on the early and late complications related to grafts fabricated from Dacron, ePTFE, polyurethane, and the commonly used biological grafts: human umbilical vein (HUV) grafts, cryopreserved allografts, and bovine xenografts.

PROSTHETIC GRAFTS

Dacron

Dacron is the most commonly used prosthetic fabric to treat occlusive and aneurysmal disease of the aorta. Dacron grafts are manufactured in either woven or knitted configurations with smooth or veloured surfaces. Following their construction, the tubular fabrics undergo compaction to reduce their initially high porosity, crimping that permanently sets pleats or corrugations in the grafts, and sterilization. Both compaction and crimping require heat and chemical treatments that alter the molecular arrangement, orientation, and crystallinity of the fabric. Prosthetic grafts may be sterilized with dry or moist heat, chemical agents, or irradiation, the preferred method. Each step employed in the fabrication of Dacron grafts affects their durability and healing and contribute to late graft failure.[4]

Woven Grafts

Woven grafts, constructed by interlacing two sets of yarn at right angles to each other, are the strongest prosthetic fabric grafts and account for approximately 45% of large-diameter Dacron grafts implanted annually.[4,6] Nonveloured woven grafts are dimensionally stable, with high tensile strength, and can be fabricated tightly enough that they are impervious to blood. However, early woven grafts were stiff and difficult to handle and suture. The addition of a velour component, incorporating interlaced nontextured yarns perpendicular to the textured ground yarns, reduces the tightness of the weave without altering permeability, resulting in a softer graft that is easier to suture (Figure 39-1A). The tendency of early woven grafts to fray at their cut edges has largely been eliminated by the incorporation of an interlocking stitch in their construction.[16]

Knitted Grafts

Knitted grafts have higher porosity than woven grafts to allow tissue ingrowth and are constructed by one of two processes.[5] Weft-knitted grafts use a single jersey structure that makes them more porous than woven grafts. Warp-knitted grafts are constructed from several sets of yarns interlooped in a zigzag pattern and can be designed to resemble weft-knitted or woven grafts. Because of their interlooped structure, knitted grafts do not run, unravel, or fray at their cut edges like woven grafts (Figure 39-1B). The interlooping yarns used in the construction of knitted grafts permit greater circumferential than longitudinal expansion of the yarn resembling the anisotropic behavior of a normal artery. This property reduces their dimensional stability, predisposing to dilatation when exposed to arterial pressure.[4]

The porosity of knitted grafts (1700 to 3600 ml/min/cm^2) requires that they be made impervious to blood by preclotting[6] or impregnation with collagen,[17,18] gelatin,[17,19-21] or albumin.[21,22] A critical requirement for coated prostheses is that the rate of absorption of the sealant coincides with the precise time frame required for hemostasis. Sealant grafts such as the Hemashield (warp-knitted double velour), Gelseal (knitted), or Gelweave (woven) grafts are particularly advantageous in limiting intraoperative interstitial and anastomotic bleeding in patients undergoing repair of thoracic and abdominal aortic aneurysms. The use of albumin-coated grafts has largely been abandoned because of inconsistencies in their construction and a tendency to embolism.[21]

Polytetrafluoroethylene

ePTFE grafts consist of solid nodes of ePTFE interconnected by longitudinally oriented fibrils that vary in length from 1 to 100 μm depending on the extrusion process. The solid-node fibril structure of ePTFE comprises only 15% to 20% of the volume of the graft material; the remaining void is filled with air (Figure 39-2).[23] Both Gore and Impra ePTFE grafts have an average internodal distance (IND) of about 30 μ in contrast to Atrium grafts that have a dual IND of 60 μ/20 μ. The Gore and Atrium grafts are supported by an external wrap of ePTFE.

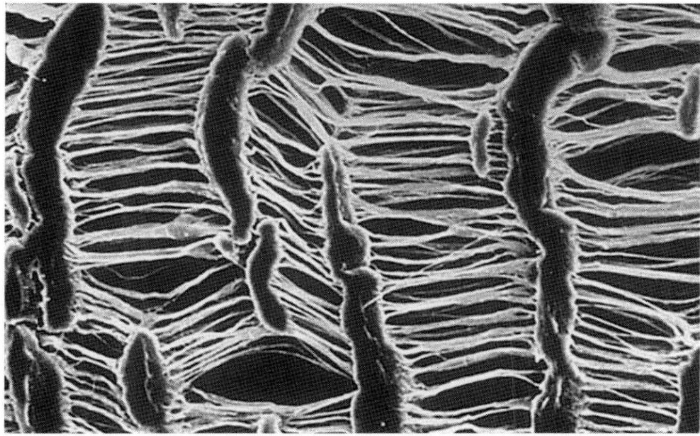

Figure 39-2. Scanning electron photomicrograph demonstrating the node fibril structure of an expanded polytetrafluoroethylene graft.

These grafts, manufactured as either thin-wall (0.4 μm) or standard-wall (0.6 μm) prostheses, are stable, chemical inert, and impervious to blood; hold sutures well; have little propensity to dilate; and are easily thrombectomized.

Healing Characteristics

Prosthetic grafts heal by two distinct cellular processes. The first, anastomotic pannus ingrowth, extends for 1 to 2 cm from the anastomosis and is composed histologically of smooth muscle cells (SMCs) lined by a single layer of endothelial cells (ECs) derived from components of the arterial wall. The second, perigraft fibrous tissue ingrowth, when complete results in encapsulation of the graft. Pannus ingrowth does not provide intrinsic tensile strength; therefore, the anastomosis depends on the suture material for its integrity.[5,24] While some tissue ingrowth is desirable, if excessive it may decrease graft compliance and incorporate adjacent structures such as the ureter into the healing process. The flow surface of a healed Dacron graft is lined by a relatively acellular hypothrombogenic neointima, which uniformly covers the graft except at anastomoses and bifurcations. The thickness of this layer increases progressively if significant outflow obstruction develops, if too large a diameter prosthesis has been used, or if the healing response is excessive. The thickness of the neointima and external fibrous sheath of Dacron grafts is minimal with woven grafts and greatest in veloured grafts. Impaired healing characterized by an incomplete neointimal lining of bifurcated grafts occurs in debilitated patients and in individuals with diabetes.[5]

Anastomotic pannus ingrowth in ePTFE grafts is similar in composition and extent to that seen with Dacron grafts.[25,26] Experimental evidence suggests that some degree of bonding occurs at the anastomoses of ePTFE grafts.[27] The luminal surface of the graft is lined with a thin layer of pseudointima, which becomes transformed into a fibrous sheath. The presence of an external wrap is a physical barrier to tissue ingrowth; therefore, the intervening matrix of the wall of ePTFE grafts becomes filled with relatively acellular proteinaceous material.[28,29] An outer fibrous capsule of varying thickness is present in about 40% of explants by 30 days and, in the absence of infection, progressively increases in thickness with the duration of implantation. Capillary ingrowth extending into the wall of ePTFE grafts has only been observed in human explants with an IND of 60 μ.[30] Endothelialization of prosthetic grafts in humans is limited to anastomotic NFH and has only rarely been described in the body and midportion of prosthetic grafts.[31]

Indications for the Use of Prosthetic Grafts

Aortobifemoral Bypass

Because of differences in their porosity, low-porosity woven grafts (100 to 500 ml/min/cm^2) were the preferred conduit for the elective and emergency repair of thoracic and abdominal aortic aneurysms, whereas knitted grafts were advocated for bypassing aortoiliac and superficial femoral occlusive disease. The versatility in the fabrication of the available coated grafts has made this distinction largely irrelevant.

The indications for ePTFE bifurcated grafts are similar to those for Dacron grafts. The longitudinally extensible configuration (stretch) bifurcated grafts are easier to suture, with less anastomotic suture line bleeding than earlier grafts.[32,33]

Prospective randomized trials have demonstrated equivalent primary (89% versus 91%) and secondary (97% versus 100%) patency rates of bifurcated Dacron and ePTFE grafts but a lower incidence of infection (0% versus 3%) with ePTFE.[10,11,32-34] Prager et al., in a study comparing gelatin (Gel-D)– and collagen (Col-D)–coated Dacron and ePTFE grafts, reported primary patency rates of 77%, 78%, and 79% at 8 years, respectively.[35] Other criteria, such as surgeon preference, propensity to graft dilatation, infectability, suturability, pseudoaneurysm formation, and propensity to anastomotic NFH, are among the factors to be considered when choosing between these two types of prostheses.

Femoropopliteal and Tibial Bypass

Saphenous vein remains the preferred conduit for infrainguinal bypass but is either unavailable because of prior removal or unsuitable due to inadequate diameter, presence of extensive varicosities, or thrombophlebitis in 20% to 30% of patients. Patency rates for femoropopliteal saphenous vein grafts range from 60% to 80% at 5 years.[36-38]

Alternative prostheses available for bypass grafting of infrainguinal atherosclerotic disease in patients who lack a suitable autogenous conduit include ePTFE, Dacron, polyurethane, HUV, and cryopreserved saphenous vein.[12,14,39-41]

ePTFE is the most commonly used alternative prosthetic graft for infrainguinal bypasses in the absence of saphenous vein. Although Dacron is used less often than ePTFE, several studies demonstrate equivalent patency rates for femoropopliteal bypass.[15,42,43] The early patency rates of above-knee prosthetic bypasses are comparable to those of saphenous vein; therefore, some surgeons advocate the use ePTFE or Dacron preferentially and preserve the saphenous vein for later use.[44] However, other authors contend that significant differences in patency are seen between ePTFE and saphenous vein at 5 years (18.4% and 20%) and recommend that saphenous vein be the graft of choice even in the above-knee position.[14,45] The significantly inferior long-term patency rates (12% to 28%)[46,47] for prosthetic crural bypasses without cuffs or arteriovenous fistulas (AVFs), compared to saphenous vein has limited their use to patients who lack suitable saphenous vein or have a life expectancy of less than 2 years.

Dialysis Access

Approximately 330,000 patients undergo chronic hemodialysis in the United States annually. This number is anticipated to increase by 3% per year.[48] The fistula-first initiative has increased the number of Brescia-Cimino and Kaufman AVFs constructed. The goal of the initiative is for 66% of patients to be dialyzed with a fistula by 2010. Arteriovenous grafts (AVGs) constructed between the radial or brachial arteries and the cephalic, basilic, or brachial veins using ePTFE in a straight or looped configuration are the most commonly used prosthetic AVGs for chronic hemodialysis. Primary patency rates range from 56% to 61% and 31% to 36% at 6 and 18 months, respectively, compared to 70% to 74% and 48% to 53% for autogenous vein at the same time points.[49-52]

Axillofemoral and femorofemoral bypass extraanatomical grafts are used to bypass occlusive and aneurysmal lesions of the aorta and iliac arteries in patients who are poor operative candidates because of severe coexisting cardiac or pulmonary disease, hostile abdomens, ostomies, or prosthetic graft infection. Both externally supported ringed Dacron and ePTFE grafts have been used successfully for axillobifemoral or femorofemoral bypass grafting. Primary patency rates of 47% to 71% at 3 to 5 years for axillofemoral grafts have been reported by Johnson et al. and Taylor et al.[53-59] Because of their length, axillofemoral grafts are subject to kinking, resulting in repeated episodes of thrombosis that require multiple thrombectomies to maintain long-term patency. Femorofemoral crossover bypasses are used to treat unilateral iliac occlusive disease and with endovascular aneurysm repair. Primary patency rates of 95% for femorofemoral grafts used with unilimb aortic prostheses and 93%, 83%, and 65% at 2, 5, and 10 years, respectively, for occlusive disease have been reported.[60,61]

Carotid–Subclavian Bypass

Dacron and ePTFE grafts are both used to bypass occlusive or aneurysmal lesions of the innominate, common carotid, subclavian, and axillary arteries and more recently in debranching procedures accompanying endovascular repair of thoracic aortic aneurysms.[62-67] Reported primary patency rates at 1, 5, and 10 years are 100%, 83%, and 47% to 92%, respectively.[68,69] The choice of graft material may affect long-term patency. Saphenous vein, because of its propensity to aneurysmal dilation and tortuousity, has proved inferior to prosthetic grafts in this location.[66] Although ringed ePTFE appears to be superior to Dacron and saphenous vein for carotid subclavian bypass, differences in patency rates of 95%, 84%, and 65% at 5 years were not statistically significant and can likely be attributed to the small sample size.

Cardiac Uses of ePTFE

The current trend in management of infants with congenital heart defects is one-stage corrective repair. However, systemic–pulmonary artery shunts continue to play a vital role in the staged approach or rarely as permanent palliation in the management of infants with a single ventricle and various forms of tetralogy of Fallot with pulmonary atresia.[70] The diameter of the shunt is crucial in regulating pulmonary blood flow and patency. A 1.0-mm deviation from the optimal diameter may result in either too much or too little pulmonary blood flow, which could prove fatal. In a study comparing shunts of different diameters, Opie et al. reported that 61% of 4-mm, 53% of 5-mm, and 100% of 6-mm grafts were functioning.[71]

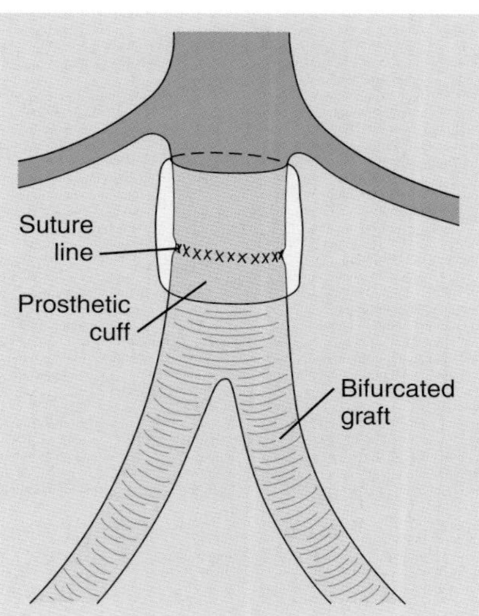

Figure 39-3. Prosthetic cuff technique used to reinforce an aortic anastomosis.

The use of ePTFE for coronary artery bypass grafting has been limited to those patients undergoing second or third coronary artery reoperation, with poor target vessels and no other autogenous alternatives.[72]

Complications of Prosthetic Grafts

The increased use of endovascular procedures to treat aortic aneurysmal and aortoiliac occlusive disease has reduced the number of prosthetic tube and bifurcated grafts surgically implanted. However, because of the large number of grafts implanted over the past 40 to 50 years (predominantly Dacron) and the tendency of complications to increase with time, surgeons need to be aware of the potential complications that may arise and develop effective treatment strategies.

Acute Complications

Perioperative bleeding and graft limb occlusion are the major acute complications of prosthetic grafts. Technical errors, inadequate anticoagulation, inherent graft thrombogenicity, low cardiac output states, and unrecognized thrombophilia are among the factors that contribute to acute graft thrombosis.

BLEEDING

If significant intraoperative bleeding is anticipated, a low-porosity woven or coated fabric graft should be selected. Bleeding from the suture line or rarely through the interstices of the graft are the sources of graft-related blood loss. If anastomotic bleeding persists after placement of additional pledgeted sutures, covering the suture line with a prosthetic cuff or coating the anastomosis with sealant glue may control the bleeding and reinforce the anastomosis (Figure 39-3).[73] In approximately 1 of 200 cases, uncontrollable bleeding occurs through the interstices of the graft, presumably due to an allergic reaction to the graft material. Replacement of the entire prosthesis with one made from different material is usually required to control the blood loss once other sources

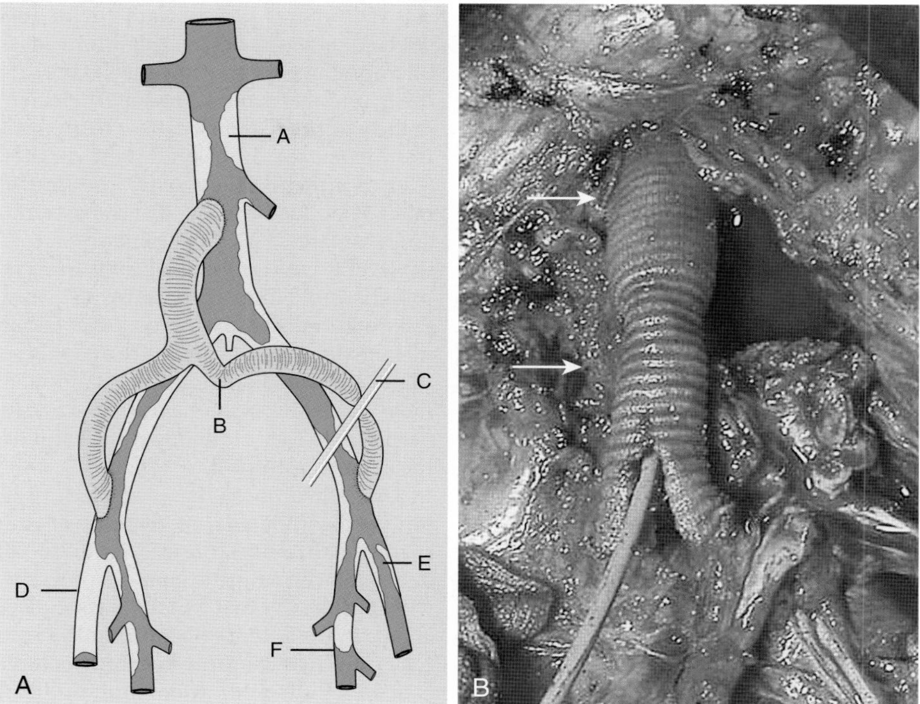

Figure 39-4. A, Potential complications that may involve bifurcated aortic grafts. **B,** Intussusception as a cause of recurrent graft limb occlusion.

of bleeding have been eliminated. In patients requiring combined aortic valve and root replacement, the triplex aortic biological valve conduit, which consists of an inner layer of Dacron and an outer layer PTFE sealed together with an elastomeric membrane, is associated with less needle-hole bleeding and blood loss through the interstices of the conduit.[74]

THROMBOSIS

Graft thrombosis in the early postoperative period occurs in 1.7% to 3.0% of patients undergoing aortic bypass grafting and is almost invariably due to technical imperfections at the distal anastomosis. Other less common causes of graft limb thrombosis are inadequate anticoagulation, heparin-induced platelet aggregation, unrecognized thrombophilia, and low cardiac output.[32,33] All patients should be systemically anticoagulated with heparin (100 U/kg) to achieve and maintain an activated clotting time of more than 250 seconds throughout the duration of the procedure.

The technical defects causing acute occlusion include elevation of a distal intimal flap; narrowing of the anastomotic suture line; thrombus in the graft limb; inadequate runoff through the superficial femoral, profunda femoris, and popliteal arteries; unrecognized inflow disease; kinking or twisting of the graft in the retroperitoneal tunnel; and compression of the graft beneath the inguinal ligament (Figure 39-4). Pallor of the extremity with absence of expected pulses or Doppler signals are the usual clinical findings. The adequacy of pulsatile blood flow through the graft should be assessed in the operating room, and immediate direct evaluation of the involved anastomosis should be undertaken before wound closure if flow is impaired.

Treatment of immediate postreconstruction thrombosis after appropriate anticoagulation consists of thorough inspection of the lumen of the involved anastomosis and runoff vessels. This is best accomplished through an incision in the distal end of the graft or by takedown of the anastomosis and extraction of the thrombus with a balloon thrombectomy catheter. Successful revision may require stabilization of an elevated plaque, extension of a graft limb distally, femorofemoral bypass, or patch angioplasty of the profunda femoris and superficial femoral arteries. A complementary femoropopliteal or infrapopliteal bypass is only required if runoff through the profunda femoris artery is inadequate or there is disease at the trifurcation. Intraoperative balloon angioplasty and stenting of the superficial femoral, popliteal, or tibial arteries is an option in patients with impaired distal runoff and appropriate lesions.

Prevention of early graft limb thrombosis requires an accurate preoperative evaluation of the runoff vessels and precise suturing of the anastomoses. Intraoperatively, the entire length of the graft limb should be assessed to ensure the absence of kinking, twisting, or external compression within the retroperitoneal tunnel. The orifices of the runoff vessels should be inspected and calibrated with dilators, and the distal intima should be secured with tacking sutures to prevent distal dissection. Special attention should be given to the orifice of the profunda femoris artery, which often requires endarterectomy, patch angioplasty, or both or needs extension of the hood of the graft over the profunda orifice as an onlay patch.

Chronic Complications

In a 30-year review of 390 cases of Dacron graft failure, Pourdeyhimi and Wagner[4] reported dilatation in 147 (38%), structural defects in 76 (20%), suture line defects in 56 (14%), and graft infection or bleeding in 30 (8.9%) patients. Ninety percent of chronic graft failures occur within 3 to 5 years of

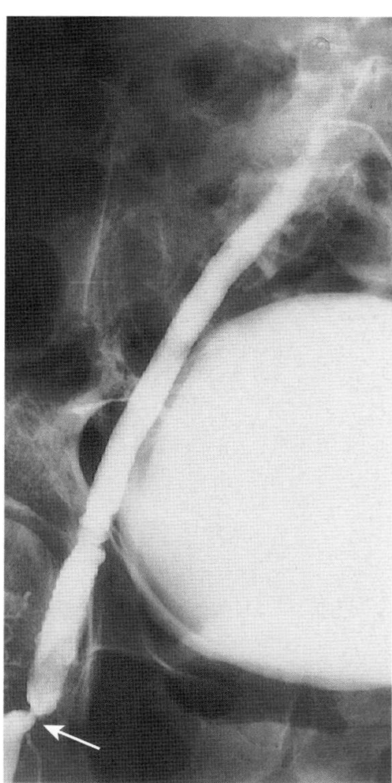

Figure 39-5. Angiogram demonstrating a high-grade stenosis at the distal anastomosis of the right limb of a bifurcated aortic graft.

implantation. Other noninfectious complications associated with late graft failure include anastomotic stenosis, graft dilatation, paraanastomotic aneurysms and anastomotic pseudoaneurysms, suture line failure, perigraft seroma, ureteric obstruction, and neoplasia.

GRAFT LIMB OCCLUSION

Stenosis at either the proximal or the distal anastomosis of prosthetic grafts may contribute to recurrent symptoms and graft occlusion. Residual atherosclerotic plaque, incorrect graft placement, proximal propagation of thrombus, and progression of disease are the usual causes of stenosis above an aortic graft. Progression of atherosclerosis and NFH at the origins of the profunda femoris and superficial femoral arteries are the most common causes of distal anastomotic stenosis (Figure 39-5). Although the symptoms of graft stenosis are usually gradual in onset, occlusion may occur suddenly without antecedent symptoms. The frequency of late limb thrombosis ranges from 5% to 10% after 1 to 5 years and approximates 20% to 30% at 10 years.[7,33,59,75,76] Depending on their level of activity, patients with failing or thrombosed grafts may be asymptomatic or present with recurrent symptoms, a diminution in or loss of previously present pulses, and a concomitant reduction in ankle–brachial indices or the sudden onset of acute ischemia. The severity of ischemia and the health status of the patient dictate the need for and extent of any planned intervention. Computed tomography, magnetic resonance, or digital subtraction angiography can be used to delineate the causative lesion and guide the repair.

The operative management of proximal aortic stenosis may require extension or replacement of the graft after endarterectomy of the severely narrowed aortic segment that was required in 17% of the patients reported by Chiesa.[32] In selected patients, descending thoracic aortofemoral or axillobifemoral bypass grafting may be the safest option. Stenosis of the profunda femoris and superficial femoral arteries, present in 26% of the patients, can be treated with endarterectomy or distal extension of the graft if the runoff through the profunda femoris artery is inadequate.[32] Successful management of stenosis or occlusion at the distal anastomosis can be achieved in approximately 90% of patients.[7,76]

Several endovascular options are available to treat symptomatic graft limb thrombosis as a result of stenosis at the proximal or distal anastomoses of aortic bifurcated grafts. Proximal aortic stenosis can be treated with a balloon-expandable stent or covered stent graft.[77] Balloon angioplasty and placement of kissing stents has been successfully employed to treat occlusive lesions of the superficial and deep femoral arteries at the distal anastomosis.[78]

Once thrombosis has occurred, resolution of the thrombus by thrombolysis, or removal of the clot with surgical or rheolytic thrombectomy is required. Thrombolytic therapy delineates the culprit lesion in approximately 70% of patients with occlusions that last 14 days and is the management of choice in the absence of contraindications to its use.[79,80] Surgical or mechanical thrombectomy is indicated if the extremity is acutely ischemic, when contraindications to thrombolytic therapy exist, or when significant improvement has not occurred after 24 to 48 hours of infusion.

Several therapeutic options are available for managing distal anastomotic stenosis of femoropopliteal grafts. Balloon angioplasty and stenting, atherectomy, cutting balloon angioplasty, and surgical correction are among the available options. The procedure selected must be tailored to the prevailing circumstances in each patient to obtain the optimum result. Surgical options include patch angioplasty, distal extension of the anastomosis, or construction of a new autogenous bypass, which may be the more durable option in younger, good-risk patients. Routine long-term follow-up of these patients is recommended as preemptive surgical or endovascular correction of preocclusive lesions is easier and more likely to be successful than if undertaken once thrombosis has occurred.

GRAFT DILATATION

Graft dilatation, the permanent increase in the diameter of a prosthesis caused by pulsatile stress, occurs with both fabric grafts and arterial homografts. Dilatation of ePTFE grafts is now rarely seen after reinforcement of these grafts by increasing their wall thickness or the application of an external wrap. Significant dilatation of implanted grafts has been documented with all currently available prosthetic materials but occurs most commonly with knitted Dacron grafts.[4,81-87] Dilatation may involve the entire graft or be confined to isolated portions of the prosthesis. The incidence of graft dilatation varies from 0.5% to 3% in reported series and 38% to 42% in case studies. This discrepancy occurs because only symptomatic patients are likely to undergo imaging.[81,88,89]

ETIOLOGY Three etiological factors predispose prosthetic materials to dilatation. Flattening of the crimp when the graft is pressurized, rearrangement of yarns within the textile structure, and yarn fatigue are the important factors implicated in the pathogenesis of graft dilatation (Figure 39-6). Woven grafts, because of their dimensional stability, are more resistant to dilatation than knitted grafts. Dilatation of 10% to 22% can

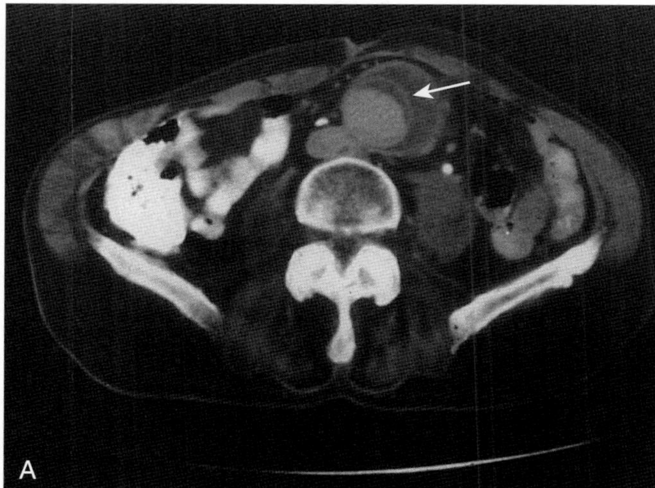

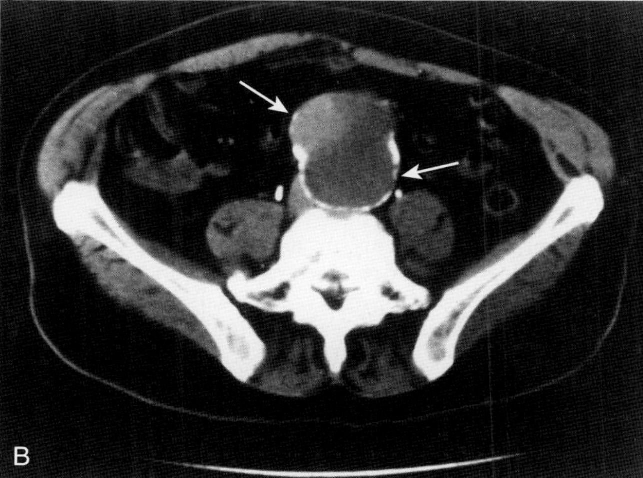

Figure 39-6. Axial abdominal computed tomography scan demonstrating dilatation of an aortic graft *(arrow)* with surrounding thrombus **(A)** and dilation of the aorta at the site of an end–side anastomosis **(B)**.

be expected when knitted grafts are first exposed to arterial pressure.[4] This restores the prosthesis to its preimplantation dimensions reduced by compaction and crimping. The factors contributing to deformation of the fabric structure and yarn fatigue of Dacron grafts are listed in Table 39-1.[82,90]

DIAGNOSIS Dilation of Dacron grafts is a biphasic phenomenon. Early dilatation commences immediately after the graft is exposed to arterial pressure and plateaus within the first year. Late dilatation, caused by yarn slippage or breakage, is usually manifest within 2 to 3 years after implantation. Because of the biphasic nature of graft dilatation, evaluation of patients for abnormal dilatation appears unwarranted within 1 to 5 years after implantation. Late graft dilatation, however, may progress and, once detected, necessitates lifelong monitoring.[81,90]

In most patients, graft dilation is asymptomatic and therefore remains undetected. Graft dilatation should be suspected if widening of the femoral pulse, an anastomotic pseudoaneurysm, or other graft-related complications are detected. B-mode ultrasound, color flow duplex imaging, and computed tomography angiography are the diagnostic imaging studies used to detect graft-related complications such as anastomotic pseudoaneurysm and perigraft collections of fluid or air.[81,91-93]

Table 39-1
Factors Contributing to Fabric Fatigue

Hypertension
Mechanical and chemical degradation
Immune reactions
Manufacturing flaws
Operative trauma

The follow-up of patients with aortic grafts is controversial. Post et al. have recently recommended that aortoiliac grafts be evaluated annually after 10 years in younger patients.[93a] Berman et al. reported a 13.5% incidence of complications in patients followed with computed tomography scans within 43 months of implantation.[81] Because femoral anastomotic complications are more common than those at aortoiliac anastomoses, evaluation of patients with aortoiliac grafts may well be undertaken at less frequent and later intervals. Ideally, color flow duplex imaging of all asymptomatic aortobifemoral grafts seems desirable at 1 and 5 years. If no significant dilatation (more than 20%) of the prosthesis is detected at 5 years, it is unlikely that significant dilatation will occur thereafter, and the frequency of follow-up is reduced or discontinued. However, once dilatation has occurred, continuous surveillance to detect anastomotic pseudoaneurysm and monitor the thickness of the luminal pseudointima is indicated.

COMPLICATIONS The progressive increase in diameter of prosthetic grafts has been implicated in anastomotic aneurysm and pseudoaneurysm formation, graft limb thrombosis, embolization, and rupture of the affected grafts.[82,94,95] Embolization of the pseudointima of a dilated graft is an infrequent potential risk that has not been well documented.

AORTIC PARAANASTOMOTIC ANEURYSMS AND PSEUDOANEURYSMS

Paraanastomotic aneurysms occur at any graft–vessel anastomotic interface.[96-101] The incidence of this complication is underestimated as these lesions are often only detected when they become symptomatic or are discovered incidentally on imaging studies performed for other diagnostic purposes. Paraanastomotic aneurysms occur in 0.5% to 15.0% of patients undergoing aortic reconstruction for aneurysmal or occlusive disease and increase in frequency with time. Paraanastomotic aortic dilatation can result in either true aneurysms or pseudoaneurysms. The incidence of these lesions varies depending on the indication for aortic replacement. Paraanastomotic aneurysms occur most commonly in patients undergoing aortic replacement for aneurysmal disease and result from implantation of the graft into preexisting aortic dilatation, use of too large a diameter prosthesis, endarterectomy of the proximal aorta, placement of the graft below the level of the renal arteries, and ongoing extracellular matrix degradation. The underlying defect in all of these cases is dilatation of the arterial wall and not disruption of the anastomosis. In contrast, anastomotic pseudoaneurysms occur with either end-to-end or end-to-side anastomotic configurations. Endarterectomy of the arterial wall, suture failure, graft type, mismatch in compliance, and infection all contribute to deterioration and disruption of the proximal aortic anastomosis (Figure 39-7).

Most aortic paraanastomotic aneurysms and pseudoaneurysms remain asymptomatic until a herald bleed into a

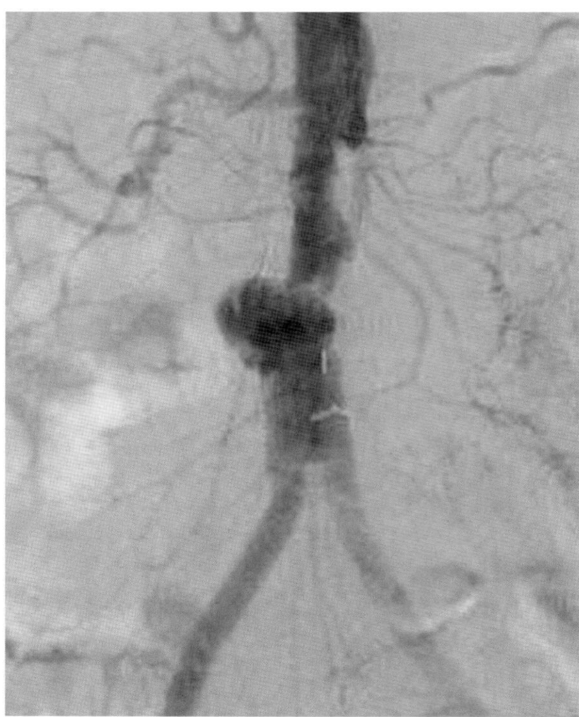

Figure 39-7. Aortogram demonstrating an aortic anastomotic pseudoaneurysm.

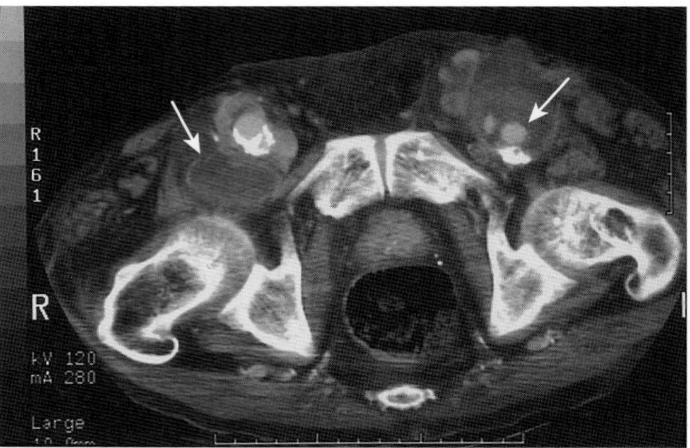

Figure 39-8. Axial computed tomography scan of the pelvis demonstrating bilateral femoral anastomotic pseudoaneurysms. Outline of dilated graft *(right arrow)*; blood in the lumen of the dilated graft *(left arrow)*.

viscus or frank rupture supervenes. The diagnosis is usually confirmed by computed tomography scanning, endoscopy, or both. Careful preoperative evaluation of asymptomatic patients is essential because of the higher morbidity and mortality rates associated with reoperative procedures.[75,76] The size of the aneurysm, the general condition of the patient, and the complexity of the repair are among the factors that need to be considered. Once the aneurysm or pseudoaneurysm has ruptured, resuscitation and emergency intervention are mandatory.

The retroperitoneal approach, if not previously used, provides excellent access for surgical repair of these complex aortic complications. Proximal extension of the graft, with reimplantation of the visceral vessels, is usually required for true aneurysms. When anastomotic aneurysms or pseudoaneurysms are repaired surgically, a specimen of aortic wall should be sent for bacteriological and histological examination. In selected patients, the aortic diameter and proximity to the renal arteries permits endovascular repair.[102] Debranching of the visceral vessels and placement of an aortic endograft form another alternative in appropriate patients. Although endovascular techniques have also been applied to repair of aortic anastomotic pseudoaneurysms, the small but definite risk of an infectious etiology remains a concern. The operative mortality rate for repair of aortic paraanastomotic aneurysms is high, ranging from 20% to 24% for elective procedures and up to 73% once rupture has occurred.[96,100]

Whether aortic paraanastomotic aneurysms and pseudoaneurysms are preventable remains a matter of debate. However, observing the principles of aortic reconstruction may at least reduce the frequency of these complications. The proximal anastomosis should be constructed in healthy aorta and not placed into an obviously aneurysmal segment, and the graft should be placed as close to the renal arteries as possible. If an endarterectomy has been performed, reinforcing the anastomosis with a prosthetic cuff seems prudent.

FEMORAL ANASTOMOTIC ANEURYSMS AND PSEUDOANEURYSMS

Femoral anastomotic aneurysms are uncommon and are usually the result of constructing a graft limb anastomosis to a dilated common femoral artery. Femoral pseudoaneurysms occur with both knitted and woven grafts and account for more than 80% of cases. The reported incidence ranges from 2% to 5% of aortic reconstructive procedures using Dacron[101,103,104] and 1.3% with ePTFE grafts in the absence of infection.[32] Several etiological factors, including weakness of the arterial wall (31%), hypertension (27%), mechanical factors (12%), graft deterioration (12%), impaired wound healing (8%), endarterectomy (7%), and suture failure (3%), have been implicated in the etiology of these lesions[101] (Figure 39-8).

Graft dilatation may also contribute to the development of anastomotic pseudoaneurysms.[82,105,106] The use of a graft of too large a diameter combined with the tendency of knitted grafts to expand when exposed to arterial pressure results in widening of the anastomosis, potentiating anastomotic suture line stress and predisposing the patient to pseudoaneurysm formation.[100] Yarn slippage or breakage at the suture line, more common with older woven grafts, may also be a contributing factor to separation of the graft from the artery.[90] Courbier and Aboukhater[107] have hypothesized that incorporation of the graft by scar tissue beneath the inguinal ligament places undue tension on the anastomosis and predisposes the patient to the development of femoral pseudoaneurysms. They recommend prophylactic partial division of the inguinal ligament.[107] Since most femoral limbs of aortic grafts adhere to the inguinal ligament without pseudoaneurysm formation, routine division of the inguinal ligament does not appear warranted even though the incidence of hernias following this maneuver appears low.

Although femoral pseudoaneurysms are subject to the same complications as true aneurysms, graft limb occlusion due to the accumulation of the pseudointima lining the graft occurs more often than rupture. Graft limb occlusion is usually manifest by the recurrence of ischemic symptoms, a

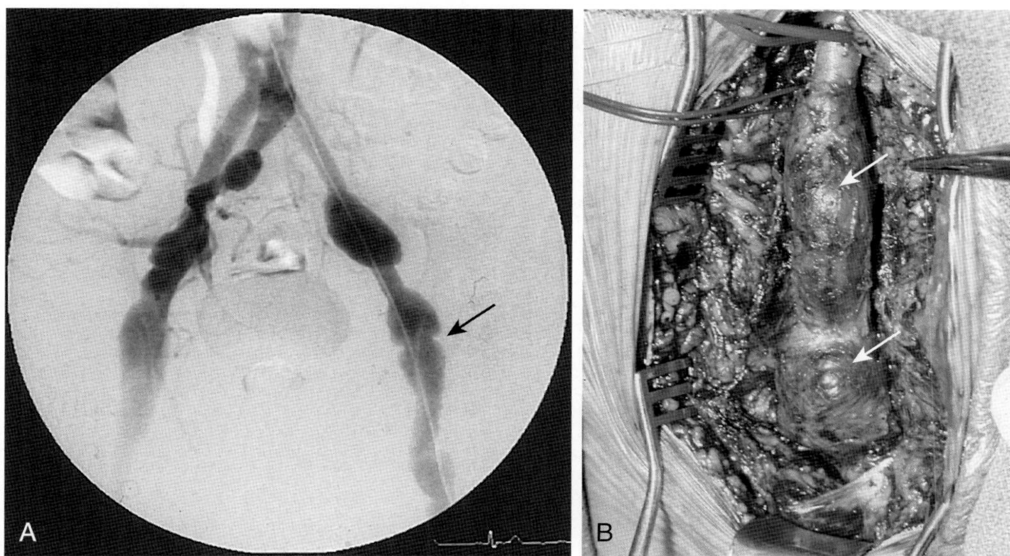

Figure 39-9. A, Angiographic appearance of guideline disruption of the limbs of an end–side aortobifemoral graft. **B,** Guideline disruption.

diminution or absence of peripheral pulses, and a decrease in the ankle–brachial indices. The management of limb occlusion secondary to an anastomotic pseudoaneurysm depends on the size of the pseudoaneurysm and severity of the patient's symptoms. No treatment may be required in asymptomatic patients with small pseudoaneurysms. In patients with limb ischemia, angiography guides treatment planning, the goal of which is to restore flow in the graft limb with thrombolysis or by balloon catheter thrombectomy and replacement of the involved segment of the graft. Resuture of the anastomosis or repair of the pseudoaneurysm with a vein patch is associated with a high recurrence rate and cannot be recommended.[108] The principles of evaluation and management of pseudoaneurysm related to the use of ePTFE grafts are similar to those for anastomotic aneurysms occurring with fabric or biological grafts. Nineteen percent of femoral pseudoaneurysm repairs resulted in recurrent pseudoaneurysms, suggesting degenerative changes in the arterial wall, ongoing impaired healing, and failure of incorporation of the graft.[103,109] Risk factors associated with recurrent femoral anastomotic pseudoaneurysms include local wound complications, female gender, use of woven grafts, and graft dilatation.[103,104,109]

RUPTURE The strength and durability of a textile prosthesis are determined by the properties of the basic polymer, the structure and number of filaments, and the yarn and fabric structure. Grafts manufactured before 1981, made from T-62 yarns with trilobar filaments, were significantly weaker than the current fabric grafts made with nontexturized T-56 yarns with cylindrical filaments.[110] The guideline and remeshing lines are potential sites of weakness in Dacron grafts. The guideline consists of carbon particles, added to the T-56 yarns of both knitted and woven grafts, to allow proper alignment of the graft.[111] The chemical reactions required to insert the guideline weakens the prosthesis, predisposing it to rupture. The remeshing line is formed when two simultaneously knitted bands are joined to form a tubular structure. Both the guideline and the remeshing lines are often the site of rupture. Chakfe et al.[111] found that graft rupture resulting from fractures of the tubular filaments were located in the remeshing line (N = 11), the guideline (N = 6), or both the remeshing and the guideline (N = 3). The contribution of macrophages to disruption of prosthetic grafts is uncertain, but the multinucleate giant cells can be seen engulfing carbon particles and Dacron fibers (Figure 39-9). Ruptures of the prosthesis caused by focal defects within the graft or occasionally disruption of the entire prosthesis are rare but devastating complications. Focal rupture caused by fracture and fragmentation of Dacron fibers or longitudinal tears in grafts manufactured with inadequate tensile strength may result in single or multiple areas of pseudoaneurysm formation (Figures 39-10A and 39-10B). These areas of fabric disruption may result in rupture into a viscus, the retroperitoneum, or the peritoneal cavity and should be repaired when detected.[95,112,113]

Rupture of femoral anastomotic pseudoaneurysms is extremely rare; it is usually noted in patients with very large neglected aneurysms.

MANAGEMENT Patients with significant graft dilatation being considered for surgical or endovascular intervention require careful evaluation because the presence of comorbidities and the complexity of the repair increase operative morbidity and mortality. The treatment of graft dilatation may entail (1) local repair of anastomotic aneurysms or pseudoaneurysms; (2) thrombectomy, profundaplasty, and placement of an interposition graft in patients with graft limb occlusion; (3) femorofemoral crossover graft; or (4) replacement of the entire prosthesis if dilatation is more than 50% of its original diameter or an aortic paraanastomotic aneurysm or pseudoaneurysm is present.

A prosthesis that approximates the diameter of the outflow tract and not the dilated proximal fabric graft should be used to repair anastomotic aneurysms or pseudoaneurysms associated with graft dilatation. ePTFE does not dilate significantly and is the preferred conduit for the repair of noninfected anastomotic femoral pseudoaneurysms.[103] Using a Dacron graft of the same diameter as the dilated primary graft remains a common practice but further aggravates the problem because of its propensity to dilate. When an entire dilated aortic graft is replaced, a segment of the old graft may be left in place

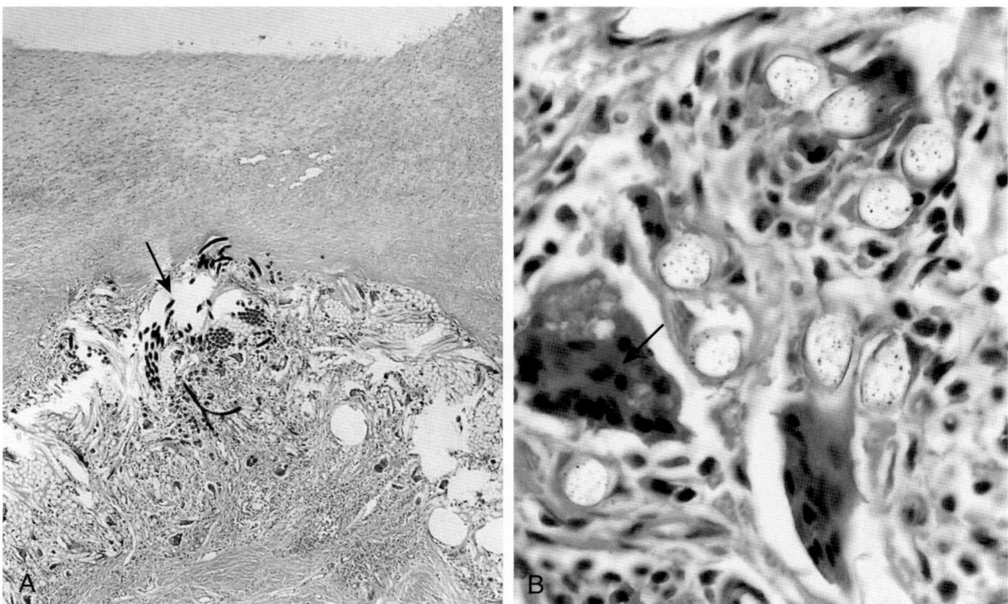

Figure 39-10. Photomicrograph demonstrating macrophages ingesting Dacron fibrils and carbon particles adjacent to the guideline of the limb of a graft (HE 200).

to facilitate replacement of the graft (with limbs tunneled through the dilated graft being replaced) without requiring extensive mobilization of the aorta. Endovascular repair of both aortic and femoral anastomotic aneurysms and pseudoaneurysms should be considered in the absence of infection in patients who have the appropriate anatomy.[39,102]

SUTURE LINE FAILURE

Healing at the graft–anastomotic interface is limited to pannus ingrowth, originating from the arterial wall adjacent to the anastomosis. Although this neointimal tissue extends onto the flow surface of prosthetic grafts, it contributes little tensile strength to the anastomosis. The integrity of a prosthetic graft–artery anastomosis thus depends on the suture material. The desirable qualities of the ideal suture material for vascular anastomoses include long-term durability, high tensile strength, favorable stress–strain relationship, minimal biological reactivity, resistance to infection, low coefficient of friction, and knot security.[114] Braided Dacron, polypropylene, and ePTFE sutures possess many of these characteristics, do not deteriorate over time, are resistant to degradation by hydrolysis or tissue enzymes, and are presently the sutures of choice for constructing vascular anastomoses.[115-121]

Pseudoaneurysms as a result of suture failure with modern sutures are uncommon. However, excessive manipulation of the suture with surgical instruments or inadvertent knotting may mechanically weaken the suture and lead to breakage, anastomotic disruption, and pseudoaneurysm formation.[114] The use of silk, nylon, and polyethylene sutures has been abandoned, but pseudoaneurysms may rarely be encountered in patients who underwent bypass procedures in the early 1960s and 1970s.[118]

Interest has recently been renewed in constructing sutureless anastomoses using rings, clips, adhesives, stents, and laser welding. Each of these devices is associated with technique-related complications. Rigid and noncompliant anastomosis with rings; toxicity, leakage, and aneurysm formation with adhesives; early occlusion with stents; and cost and reduced strength in large-diameter vessels with demand for surgical skills with laser welding are among the disadvantages of these nonsuture techniques. However, the use of vascular clips has improved primary patency rates of both AVFs (67% versus 48%) and AVGs (39% versus 19%) in anastomoses constructed with nonpenetrating clips compared to a running suture techniques at 24 months.[122] Erdmann et al. have demonstrated the feasibility of a side–side arteriovenous anastomosis constructed with magnets in an experimental model.[123] Despite these promising innovations and the apparent early and intermediate advantage of clips in AVF and AVG anastomoses, suturing for the present continues to remain the standard approach.[123]

PERIGRAFT SEROMA

The perigraft reaction is characterized by a painless, fluctuant swelling surrounding a portion of or the entire prosthesis that occurs in 0.2% to 1% of major vascular reconstructions.[124] Extraanatomical grafts seem particularly prone to this complication and account for 60% to 75% of reported cases; grafts in anatomical positions account for the remainder.[124-131] The incidence of perigraft seromas varies from 4.2% in patients with extraanatomical bypasses to 1.2% in those with aortobifemoral bypasses and 0.3% in those with femoropopliteal bypass procedures. Knitted Dacron (54%) and ePTFE (34%) grafts are the prosthetic grafts most often involved.[125] The reported time interval from graft insertion to the presentation of the seroma ranges from 1 to 45 months, (mean of approximately 25 months).[127,131] The etiology of the perigraft fluid accumulation is unknown. The fundamental abnormality is the failure of incorporation of the graft by the host tissues. Fluid transudation through the interstices of the graft, fluid exudation from surrounding tissues, allergic or immune response to the material, mechanical irritation of the host tissue due

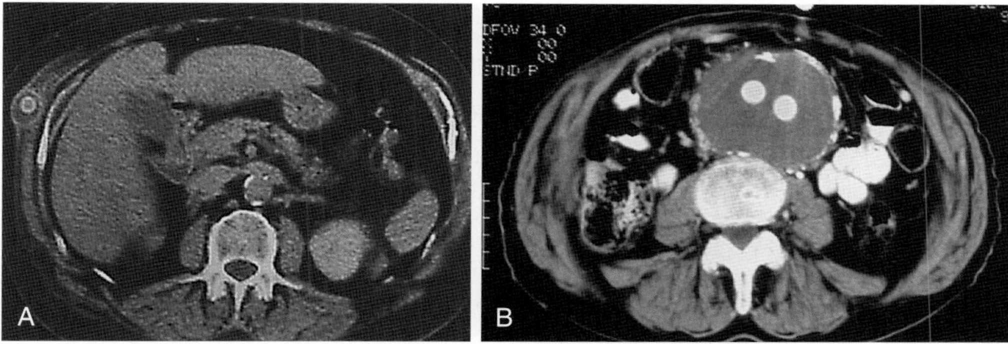

Figure 39-11. Axial abdominal computed tomography scans demonstrating perigraft seromas surrounding a right axillofemoral graft **(A)** and the limbs of an aortic graft **(B).**

to repeated motion of the prosthesis, impaired fibrin formation in the graft interstices due to heparin, and presence of a fibroblast inhibitory factor in the serum are among the proposed etiological factors.[132-134] The serum levels of fibroblast inhibitory factor decline after graft removal or plasmapheresis, implicating the graft material in the pathogenesis of the seroma. Systemic heparinization or flushing ePTFE grafts with heparinized saline, which impairs fibrin formation and sealing of the graft, has been implicated in the development of seromas seen with Blalock-Taussig shunts, but no consistent relationship was found with dialysis access grafts.[135,136] Transudation of fluid through the interstices of aortic endografts has also been implicated in the development of perigraft fluid accumulations and an increase in endotension in these patients. The application of a nonporous external wrap of ePTFE appears to have eliminated this problem (Figure 39-11).

The diagnosis is usually manifest by the presence of fluid accumulation around an extraanatomical or dialysis access graft or by computed tomography scanning of bifurcated grafts. Diagnostic needle aspiration of the fluid for chemical and bacteriological analysis should be performed under sterile conditions. In some patients, the perigraft fluid becomes transformed into a gelatinous material that is difficult to aspirate.

Repeated aspiration is successful in approximately two thirds of patients with perigraft fluid collections and is the treatment of choice in poor-risk patients. However, repeated aspiration predisposes 5% to 12% of patients to infection or thrombosis of the graft.[127] Removal of the graft with its capsule and replacement of it with a prosthesis of different material result in a cure rate of more than 90%. The technique of Lowery et al., in which a communication lined with omentum is fashioned between the graft capsule and the peritoneal cavity, is a reasonable alternative if the fluid is sterile.[137] Whether modulation of fibroblast inhibitory activity by microfibrillar collagen, ginseng, and high-dose vitamin C will prove effective remains to be determined.[132]

URETERIC OBSTRUCTION

Ureteric obstruction is a recognized complication of aortic reconstructive procedures. The etiology of postoperative hydronephrosis includes ureteric ischemia, kinks, scarring from operative dissection, anastomotic aneurysms, graft infection, graft limb thrombosis, and an incidental ureteric tumor. In approximately 1% of patients, dense fibrosis, presumably associated with incorporation of the graft, also encases the ureter as it crosses over the graft and results in hydronephrosis.[138,139] Postoperative hydronephrosis can be categorized as early (within 1 year) or late (after 1 year). Temporary asymptomatic hydronephrosis is present on computed tomography scans in 12% to 30% of patients and mild to moderate permanent ureteral dilation in 2% to 14% of patients following aortic surgery. Ureteral obstruction is more common with anterior placement of the graft limb but can occur with grafts placed posteriorly as well.[140,141]

Hydronephrosis is usually an incidental finding on imaging studies done for other diagnostic purposes but may present with obstructive uropathy or progressive deterioration in renal function. The workup should include biochemical evaluation of renal function and delineation of the site and cause of obstruction by computed tomography.

Encasement of the ureter by perigraft fibrosis can be minimized by precise placement of the limbs of the graft during aortobifemoral bypass grafting. The management of ureteric obstruction depends on the degree of renal impairment, the physical condition of the patient, and the site and severity of the obstruction. In most patients with minor degrees of obstruction, monitoring the patient with ultrasound or computed tomography at 3- to 6-month intervals is all that is required. Severe obstruction with renal impairment is the usual indication for intervention. Therapeutic options include placement of indwelling ureteral stents, excision of the stricture and reimplantation of the ureter, ureterolysis, and rerouting of the graft limb. Graft infection, anastomotic pseudoaneurysms, and graft limb thrombosis remain a concern with both catheter-based interventions and surgical treatment of ureteric obstruction in patients with aortic grafts.[139]

NEOPLASIA

A few case reports note the occurrence of angiosarcoma and malignant fibrous histocytoma in patients with Dacron grafts.[142-147] We are unaware of any reports in the literature of neoplasms associated with the use of ePTFE. The relationship between the presence of Dacron and the development of these sarcomas is not established. Whether these tumors are incidental to the presence of the graft or the prosthetic material is tumorigenic is presently unknown. Although experimental evidence links plastic materials with neoplastic change, the evidence in humans is less convincing. First, the incidence of neoplasms in relation to the number of prosthetic graft implants is extremely low. Second, the time interval from placement of the graft and diagnosis of the angiosarcoma

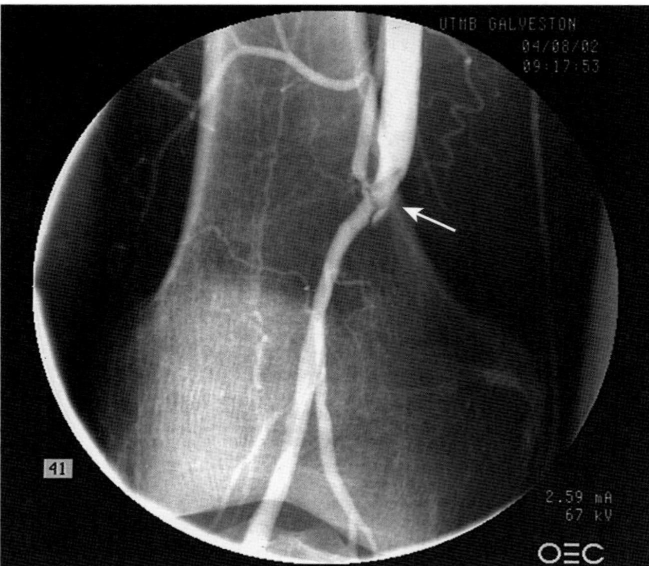

Figure 39-12. Peripheral angiogram demonstrating neointimal hyperplasia at the popliteal anastomosis of an above-knee femoropopliteal graft.

varies considerably. In the case reported by O'Connell et al.,[146] the time interval appears too short to be a causal relationship, suggesting that the tumor was incidental to the presence of the Dacron graft. In contrast, the 12-year interval from placement of the graft to the development of the angiosarcoma in the case reported by Fehrenbacher et al.[145] appears more consistent with a possible cause-and-effect relationship. Nonetheless, even though a direct causal relationship between the use of Dacron grafts and the development of angiosarcomas and histiosarcomas cannot be established with certainty, continued vigilance seems prudent.[148,149]

The diagnosis of aortic sarcomas is seldom made antemortem. Progressively worsening arterial stenosis, vegetative lesions presenting with obstructive or embolic symptoms, aneurysmal dilatation, and anastomotic disruption mimicking a pseudoaneurysm are among the clinical presentations. Computed tomography angiography usually demonstrates an intraluminal filling defect or pseudoaneurysm. Excision or grafting and endarterectomy have been advocated for treatment of these neoplasms. The prognosis of aortic sarcomas remains poor despite the use of adjuvant chemotherapy and radiation, with patient survival usually of only a few months.

Enhancing Small-Diameter Prosthetic Graft Patency

The major causes of failure of SPDG are the inherent thrombogenicity of the graft material and the progression of NFH or atherosclerosis at the distal anastomosis of arterial grafts and the venous anastomosis of AVG (Figure 39-12). The absence of a single unifying etiology for NFH accounts for the multiplicity of suggested approaches described to reduce or eliminate anastomotic NFH and improve the long-term patency of SDPG. Flow surface modification, reconfiguration of the distal anastomosis, and use of antiplatelet agents are among the methods currently used to improve their long-term patency. The use of pharmacological agents to prevent NFH is discussed elsewhere.

Reducing Graft Thrombogenicity

The development of a thrombus-resistant flow surface to improve the patency of SDPGs is a desirable objective. Although several biologically active coatings that inhibit platelet function and other components of the coagulation pathway are under investigation, none of these agents are yet available for clinical use.[150] Whether reducing the thrombogenicity of the graft alone will also reduce or eliminate anastomotic NFH is unknown. Reported methods of modifying the thrombogenicity of the luminal flow surface of prosthetic grafts include carbon coating, heparin bonding, and EC seeding.

Carbon Coating

Carbon impregnation of 25% to 30% of the wall of ePTFE grafts (Carboflow, Impra) reduces surface thrombogenicity and results in statistically significant differences in primary and secondary patency rates of 62.9% and 69.8% for carbon-impregnated grafts compared to 47.4% and 53% for standard ePTFE at 1 year but not at 3 years.[151,152] Although the preceding study and that of Bacourt show some early advantage in primary and secondary patency rates of carbon-coated over standard wall ePTFE, whether these differences will persist over the long-term remains to be determined.[153]

Heparin Bonding

Heparin has been successfully bonded onto the flow surfaces of ePTFE grafts by covalent bonding with glutaraldehyde thermal cross-linking and by a Carmeda BioActive Surface process.[154,155] The objective of attaching heparin to an ePTFE graft is to obtain uniform immobilization and retention of the anticoagulant while maintaining its bioactivity.[154] Thermally bonded heparin grafts are stiff when first implanted but soften as the unbonded gelatin and heparin are released. The Carmeda BioActive Surface process uses a single endpoint covalent bond to immobilize the heparin molecules, allowing the continued binding of heparin on the luminal surface to antithrombin III and retention of its anticoagulant properties. Experimental studies have demonstrated decreased platelet adhesion and reduced thrombogenicity, resulting in improved early and late patency rates of heparin-bonded grafts compared to standard ePTFE prostheses.[156] Heparin bioactivity remains detectable up to 12 weeks after implantation.

In a recent study, Bosiers et al.[157] reported overall primary and secondary patency rates of infrainguinal heparin-bonded ePTFE (Propaten) grafts of 82% and 97% at 1 year, respectively. One-year primary patency rates according to graft location were 84%, 81%, and 74% for above-knee, below-knee, and crural bypasses, respectively. Devine et al.[157a] reported patency rates of heparin-bonded Dacron grafts at 1, 2, and 3 years of 70%, 63%, and 55%, respectively, compared with 56%, 46%, and 42%, respectively, for standard ePTFE.[157] While these initial early and intermediate results using the Propaten and heparin-bonded Dacron grafts for crural bypasses are promising, whether heparin bonding will improve the long-term patency of infrainguinal SDPG remains to be determined. Davidson reported a 20-25% clot free and graft survival advantage over standard wall stretch ePTFE at 3 months.[158]

Endothelial Seeding

Endothelialization of prosthetic grafts in humans, presently limited to the zone of anastomotic pannus ingrowth, is a desirable objective. Potential sources of ECs include anastomotic and transmural ingrowth and fallout endothelialization. Following the initial report by Herring et al.,[159] several investigators have employed autologous EC seeding to improve the patency of SDPG used for dialysis access, coronary artery, and femoropopliteal bypass grafting.[160-170] Endothelialization via transmural ingrowth occurs in experimental canine thoracic grafts but only to a limited extent in humans, with grafts of 60-μ IND.[30] Wu et al.[31] have demonstrated ECs and SMCs remote from the anastomosis in an explant from a patient with a perigraft seroma, confirming that EC fallout from the blood does occur, albeit rarely in humans.

Endothelialization can be enhanced by seeding or sodding (ultraheavy seeding) of prosthetic grafts with ECs harvested from various sources, including HUV and saphenous, jugular, or arm veins. The yield of ECs from these sources is low. Microvascular ECs from breast, omentum, and abdominal wall adipose tissue provide a more substantial source of ECs and, with autologous bone marrow cells, are other sources of ECs. ECs are harvested by either mechanical or chemical digestion or liposuction and from peripheral blood; they are then applied onto the graft surfaces. Cell retention and contamination by myofibroblast-like cells and monocytes remain a problem, especially with microvascular ECs, despite the use of additional purification steps and adhesion-enhancing agents such as fibroblast growth factor and fibronectin.[171,172] ECs and microvascular ECs have been seeded onto ePTFE grafts used for dialysis access and infrainguinal bypass grafting in patients without available autogenous conduits. There appears to be no advantage in patency of seeded or sodded grafts over standard ePTFE in patients undergoing hemodialysis.[160,173] A characteristic finding in sodded dialysis grafts has been the markedly cellular neointima resulting in a significant reduction of luminal diameter of the grafts. In a phase II study, Zilla et al. reported a 72.9% patency rate for 108 EC-seeded femoropopliteal bypass grafts at 3½ years and 66% at 7 years.[164,174] Laube et al. reported a 90.5% patency rate in 21 EC-seeded ePTFE coronary artery bypass grafts followed for a mean of 27.7 months. Postoperative evaluation of the grafts with angiography and angioscopy demonstrated a smooth luminal surface without stenosis or deposition of platelet fibrin thrombi.[175]

While technically feasible, and despite isolated reports of long-term patency, endothelialization of prosthetic grafts has not gained widespread acceptance because of the cumbersome nature of the techniques used and continued proliferation of the neointimal layer, presumably due to contamination by myofibroblasts. Furthermore, variable cellular adhesion and sterility remain concerns with the cell culture-dependent techniques.

Modification of Anastomotic Configuration

Vein Cuffs and Patches

NFH at either the proximal or, more commonly, the distal anastomosis of ePTFE grafts is the major cause of late failure of SDPG. Wall shear plays an important role in the development and biological behavior of anastomotic NFH. Low wall shear stress is associated with prolonged particle residence, predisposing the patient to cellular proliferation, whereas high wall shear stress is accompanied by a significant reduction in SMC proliferation and may actually induce regression of NFH.[176,177] The recognition of the importance of shear stress in the etiology of NFH has resulted in introduction of several technical modifications to alter flow patterns at the distal vessel to PTFE graft anastomosis. The Linton and Taylor patches, vein interposition cuffs such as the Miller and Tyrell cuffs, and precuffed or hooded grafts are all employed to modulate shear stress, reduce NFH, and enhance the patency of crural ePTFE bypasses and dialysis access grafts. Taylor et al. reported patency rates of 74% and 58%, respectively, at 12 and 36 months (Figure 39-13).[178-183] Results of the U.K. prospectively randomized trial comparing infrainguinal ePTFE bypass grafts with and without vein interposition cuffs demonstrated no difference in patency rates for vein cuff versus no vein cuff above-knee bypasses of 80% versus 84%, respectively, at 1 year and 72% versus 70% at 2 years.[180] In contrast, bypasses to the below-knee popliteal artery showed a significant advantage in patency between the cuffed (52%) and noncuffed (29%) grafts at 2 years. These data indicate that vein patches and cuffs may be most beneficial in the below-knee position. Batson et al. showed cumulative patency rates of 74% at 12 months and 65% at 24, 36, and 48 months using the Linton patch.[178] Neville et al., in an evaluation of 80 ePTFE distal bypasses constructed with a vein patch, reported 70% primary patency at 3 years and 62.9% at 4 years.[183] Current data on the value of patches and cuffs in improving ePTFE graft patency are encouraging. Whether the addition of a distal AVF will provide additional improvement in long-term patency awaits further study.

Precuffed (Hooded) Grafts

The results of the hemodynamic studies of Harris and How and the known effect of hemodynamic shear on NFH have led to the introduction of hooded ePTFE grafts.[184] Reporting for the North American Prospective Trial Investigations, Panneton found no significant differences in 30-day and 12-month patency rates between precuffed (Distaflo) and ePTFE grafts with vein modifications.[185] Although the patency rate of precuffed ePTFE was higher than vein cuffed grafts at 24 months (62% versus 44%), these differences did not achieve statistical significance.

Precuffed grafts have also been evaluated as dialysis grafts. In a study of 48 patients, Sorom et al. reported superior graft patency for the cuffed ePTFE compared to the standard wall grafts at 12 months (64% versus 32%) and 24 months (58% versus 21%).[186] The number of interventions was similar between the two prostheses, although the authors reported fewer instances of anastomotic outflow stenosis in the precuffed group.[186] Liu et al. have shown that the average outflow stenosis of AVG was twofold greater with standard wall grafts than in precuffed prostheses.[186,187] These early results with precuffed grafts, although encouraging, await further validation with studies including larger numbers of patients with long-term follow-up. Table 39-2 compares the primary patency rates of modified femoropopliteal grafts.

Anastomotic NFH has not been eliminated despite changes in the geometrical configuration of SPDG with precuffed grafts or vein patches. Energy losses as a result of recirculation in large vortices associated with flow separation that occurs at these sites may contribute to the lack of efficacy from these modifications.[188]

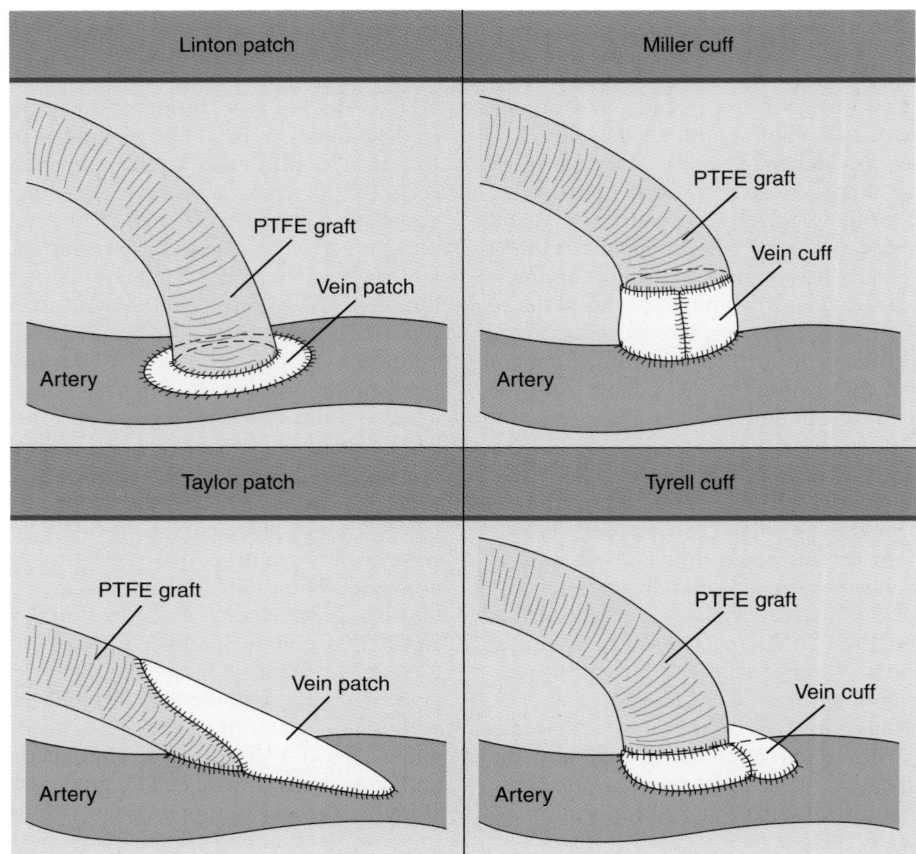

Figure 39-13. Vein patch and graft techniques currently used to improve prosthetic graft anastomotic neointimal fibrous hyperplasia.

Table 39-2
Patency Rates of Modified Femoropopliteal Grafts*

Primary Patency (Years)			
Graft	1	2	3
Heparin-bonded Dacron	70	63	55
ePTFE	56	46	42
Carbon coated	63	43	35
ePTFE	47	36	48
Propaten above knee	90	68	
Propaten below knee	92	81	57
Precuffed	70		54
Vein cuffed	78		

*ePTFE, expanded polytetrafluoroethylene.

Peripheral Endografts

The use of transluminally placed self-expanding stent grafts has recently been extended to treat aortoiliac and femoropopliteal aneurysmal and occlusive disease, as well as AVG complications. The Fluency, Viabahn, and Wallgrafts are the stent grafts currently approved for endovascular use. Both the Fluency and Viabahn stent grafts are made from ultrathin ePTFE reinforced by a self-expanding nitinol skeleton. The nitinol in a Fluency stent graft is encapsulated within the two layers of ePTFE, whereas in Viabahn grafts thin-walled ePTFE is radially reinforced externally with nitinol. The Wallgraft is made from polyester fabric coating a Ni-Co-Ti alloy stent. In a randomized comparison between Viabahn endoprostheses and prosthetic above-knee femoropopliteal bypass grafts, Kedora et al. reported primary patency rates of 84%, 82%, 75.6%, and 73.5% for the stent graft group and 90%, 81.8%, 79.7%, and 74.2% for the surgical group at 3, 6, 9, and 12 months, respectively.[189] Among the factors determining success were graft diameter, absence of calcification, popliteal obstruction or superficial femoral occlusion, use of antiplatelet therapy, and presence of at least one continuous runoff vessel.[190-192] The application of endovascular repair of popliteal aneurysms is becoming more widely accepted. The repair of popliteal aneurysms with Viabahn is associated with primary and secondary patency rates of 77% and 86% and 70% and 76% at 3 and 5 years, respectively.[193] When compared to operative repair, Viabahn has comparable patency rates 100% versus 89% at 1 year and 71.4% versus 88% at 3 years.[194] Thrombosis, stent graft migration, fracture of the struts, and NFH in the stent graft in 26% of limbs were the major complications requiring reintervention. Marin et al.,[195] in a study of the healing characteristics of seven stent grafts retrieved at intervals of up to 6 months from patients with limb-threatening ischemia, observed organizing thrombus on both the luminal and the external surfaces of the implants at 3 weeks. By 6 weeks, the outer surface of the stent graft was firmly adherent to the wall of the native artery, with the neointima lining the lumen of the stent graft extending 2 cm from the graft artery interface. The neointimal layer ranged from 40 to 150 μm in thickness in grafts studied at 3 months. In specimens examined between 3 and 7 months the endograft was well incorporated, with an external capsule. The presence of an external wrap and insertion of the graft into the periadventitial plane elicited a foreign body reaction manifest by multinucleate giant cells. Grafts inserted into the media had less mononuclear and foreign body giant cell reaction than those placed within the periadventitial plane. Atherosclerotic plaque in the iliac or femoral arteries between the stent grafts and the arterial wall were remodeled and histologically consisted entirely of fibrous tissue. In one graft segment, the authors observed extrinsic SMC proliferation of sufficient thickness to indent the stent graft. van Sambeek et al. noted only minimal luminal changes using intravascular ultrasound to interrogate grafts implanted in the superficial femoral arteries of 12 patients.[196] The Gore Viabahn graft has been shown to effective in treating superficial femoral occlusive disease. Whether bonding heparin to the flow surface of these grafts will further reduce their thrombogenicity and improve long-term patency is being evaluated.

Venous Prosthetic Grafts

Vena Caval Obstruction

Both Dacron and ePTFE have been used to treat venous obstruction secondary to trauma, thrombosis or malignancy, and portal venous hypertension.[197] The desirable qualities of graft replacement in the venous system include reduced wall thickness, smooth nonthrombogenic flow surface, and adequate pore size or IND. Kogel et al.[198] reported 43% to 50% 12-month patency rates in polyurethane and modified (60- to 90-μ IND) PTFE canine implants. Endothelialization due to transmural ingrowth was only present in the PTFE grafts. There is not a great deal of information regarding the healing characteristics of prosthetic grafts implanted in the venous system in humans. The patency of unsupported prosthetic grafts to bypass venous occlusive lesions has been limited by low venous distending pressures, slow venous flow, and inherent thrombogenicity of the graft material. The use of externally supported ringed grafts has partially reduced the influence of low distending pressure on graft patency.

Venous bypass should be considered in patients with symptomatic obstruction of the superior vena cava (SVC) or inferior vena cava (IVC) when endovascular interventions are not feasible or have been unsuccessful. Central venous thrombosis, mediastinal fibrosis, and primary or metastatic mediastinal malignancies are the most common causes of SVC obstruction. Occlusion or stenosis of the IVC can result from developmental anomalies, trauma, thrombophilia, iatrogenic injuries associated with liver transplantation, dialysis access, femoral venous catheters, vena caval filters, and invasion by malignancies. Tumors of the liver, kidney, and adrenal gland and retroperitoneal soft tissue sarcomas are particularly prone to invade the IVC. Clinically, SVC and IVC obstruction may be asymptomatic or present with symptoms of venous hypertension manifest as upper or lower extremity edema and chest or abdominal wall venous engorgement.[199,200] Most patients with nonmalignant vena caval obstruction are treated with anticoagulants, thrombolytic therapy, balloon angioplasty, and stenting. Curative resection of invasive tumors may require segmental resection of the IVC or SVC and replacement with ringed 14- to 18-mm ePTFE or Dacron graft. ePTFE grafts used to treat malignancy of the IVC remain patent for periods ranging from 9 to 108 months.[199-201] In a review of SVC reconstruction for nonmalignant disease, Alimi et al.[200] reported 30-day primary and secondary patency rates of 79% and 95%, respectively, for ePTFE used to bypass nonmalignant occlusive disease of the IVC, with secondary patency for the iliocaval or femorocaval grafts of 50% at 2 years. Significant relief of symptoms was obtained in 79% of patients followed long term.[200,202] Anticoagulation with warfarin has not been routinely advocated for patients with venous bypasses for malignant disease. Despite the improved patency of ePTFE used for venous replacement, the assessment of its long-term efficacy is limited by the small number of patients treated.

Portosystemic Shunts

Sarfeh and Rypins popularized the use of partial portosystemic shunts by using 8- and 10-mm ringed, externally supported ePTFE grafts to reduce portal venous pressure while maintaining hepatopetal flow.[203] The introduction of transjugular intraheptic portosystemic shunts has largely eliminated the need for prosthetic portosystemic shunts.

Crossover Grafts

Externally supported ePTFE grafts are also used to bypass symptomatic obstructive lesions of the subclavian and femoral veins. An adjunctive AVF is usually required to maintain flow through the venous bypass. Long-term anticoagulation with warfarin is usually necessary.[202,204,205]

Polyurethane

One of the limitations of both AVF and AVG for hemodialysis is the need for maturation or tissue incorporation before they can be accessed. The time interval from construction to maturation ranges from 6 weeks to 6 months for AVF and 10 to 14 days for AVG. This delay usually necessitates placement of a temporary central venous catheter in patients needing urgent hemodialysis. It is estimated that the average dialysis patient requires approximately 2.3 catheters per patient year, which, in addition to the increased cost, exposes the patient to the risk of complications associated with catheter placement.[206,207]

Polyurethane grafts, such as the Vectra graft, offer the potential for early cannulation and improved hemostasis after cannulation because of their improved sealing capability. The Vectra graft comprises randomly orientated microfibers of varying thickness, ranging from 0.1 to 5.0 μm compared to 0.1 to 1 μm for ePTFE. The favorable characteristics of the Vectra graft are the result of its trilayer design consisting of (1) an inner microporous layer coated with a surface-modifying agent to minimize platelet adhesion; (2) a middle layer of Thoralon to provide strength, flexibility, and sealing properties; and (3) an outer microporous layer to permit tissue ingrowth. The Vectra graft is thinner than reinforced ePTFE (0.46 ± 0.03 μm versus 0.86 ± 0.08 μm) and has somewhat less tensile and bursting strength. Because of their elasticity, polyurethane grafts show more elongation than ePTFE (220% versus 60%) at their breaking point.[208,209]

Polyurethane grafts heal by anastomotic pannus ingrowth and fibrous encapsulation. In a randomized study of 142 patients comparing the Vectra graft with ePTFE, Glickman et al. reported primary patency rates of 55% for Vectra versus 47% for ePTFE at 6 months and 44% versus 36% at 12 months. Secondary patency rates were 87% and 90% for

Vectra and 78% versus 80% for ePTFE at 6 and 12 months, respectively. In addition, 20% to 33% of polyurethane grafts were cannulated within 3 days and 53.9% by 8 days.[210] Glickman et al. reported an 81% cannulation rate at 4 days. No ePTFE grafts were cannulated before 9 days.[206] In a recent comparison between brachiobasilic AVFs and Vectra grafts, Kakkos et al. reported equivalent primary patency rates between the two access modalities but significantly lower primary assisted patency rates for Vectra grafts (70% at 12 months and 58% at 18 months) compared with brachiobasilic AVFs (82% at 12 months and 78% at 18 months).[211] Vectra grafts required a significantly greater number of thrombectomies than autogenous fistulas (45 versus 7). These data suggest that the advantage of early cannulation of Vectra grafts must be balanced against the more frequent need for intervention.

The major advantage of polyurethane vascular grafts used for dialysis is early cannulation. The disadvantages include the need of an outflow vein of more than 3 mm in diameter and a tendency to kinking when routed over curves or areas of muscle bulk. An interposition ePTFE segment may be necessary to negotiate curves or bends. These grafts are technically more difficult to implant with kinking and elongation commonly encountered. To improve the patency of small-diameter polyurethane grafts, Taite et al. have incorporated diazeniumdiolate as a nitric oxide donor into polyurethane and demonstrated a decrease in platelet adhesion and an increase in EC proliferation.[212] In an experimental study evaluating small-caliber polyurethane grafts implanted into rabbits, Ishii et al. found the combination of sirolimus and heparin facilitated endothelial ingrowth without an increase in NFH.[213] In vivo oxidative or hydrolytic degradation of polyurethane graft materials remains a concern.

BIOLOGICAL GRAFTS

Human Umbilical Vein

HUV grafts are prepared from umbilical cords harvested in the delivery room and prepared and cross-linked with glutaraldehyde starch. Soluble proteins and excess Wharton's gel are extracted with ethanol,[214] and a supporting Dacron mesh is applied to the external surface to reduce the risk of aneurysmal dilation. HUV grafts are presently used for femoropopliteal or tibial bypasses and for dialysis access. Reported 5-year primary patency rates for above-knee bypasses are 54%.[14,215] Bypasses to the below-knee popliteal artery and crural vessels have reported secondary patency rates of 71% and 56% (with distal AVFs), respectively.[215-218] Neufang et al. found no differences in patency among above-knee, below-knee, or crural bypasses.[215]

Healing Characteristics

Histologically, the internal elastic membrane of gluteraldehyde-stabilized HUV segments remains intact without an identifiable endothelial lining. After implantation, the internal elastic membrane becomes fragmented. Within a year, the muscle layer, well preserved initially, becomes hyalinized.[216,219] The Dacron mesh becomes incorporated by a fibrous capsule, which increases in thickness with the duration of implantation. HUV explants demonstrate wall thickening with folds and delamination of the lumen, lipid deposition, and thrombus at the anastomosis.[216,219]

Complications

Thrombosis in the early postoperative period occurs in 5% to 16% of popliteal and crural bypasses.[215,218] The principles of treatment of early graft thrombosis are similar to those used to treat acute occlusion of other SDPGs, except that the injudicious application of clamps to the graft should be avoided. Both the proximal and the distal anastomoses should be exposed, the thrombus flushed from the graft with heparinized saline, and the causative lesion corrected.

Anastomotic Stenosis

Late thrombosis of HUV grafts due to NFH or progression of atherosclerosis at the distal anastomosis occurs in 1.8% to 14.7% of patients.[217] Because of the dense fibrotic reaction that often envelops these grafts, the dissection should be limited to the proximal and distal anastomoses. Application of a tourniquet is often invaluable in reoperations on the lower extremity. Thrombus can be removed from HUV grafts by flushing the graft proximally and distally with heparinized saline or by thrombolysis, which delineates the causative lesion and usually limits the dissection to the distal anastomosis. Balloon catheter thrombectomy should be used with caution as it may fracture the luminal surface, predisposing the patient to secondary thrombosis. The treatment of distal anastomotic stenosis may require vein patch angioplasty, extension of the graft to a more distal site, or placement of a new bypass.[217,218] Secondary patency rates of 44% to 56% with flushing and 85% using thrombolysis and limb salvage in 74% of cases can be achieved.[218]

Dilatation

Dilation of HUV grafts is a biphasic phenomenon: early enlargement from a baseline diameter of 4 to 6 mm at implantation to approximately 9 mm is the norm. Uniform diffuse dilation of the graft and mesh has been reported in 21% and focal dilatation or erosion of the graft with rupture of the mesh, resulting in multiple pseudoaneurysms, in 36% to 44% of patients studied with ultrasound beyond 5 years.[217,218,220] Reversal of glutaraldehyde-induced cross-linking and immunological mechanisms have been proposed to explain the progressive increase in diameter resulting in aneurysm formation beyond 5 years.[216] In their most recent series, Dardik et al. report no aneurysms in 283 bypass grafting procedures performed over a 10-year period.[218] The guidelines for excision and grafting of aneurysmal HUV grafts have not been established. It is estimated that graft dilatation of sufficient size to require surgical excision and repair is present in about 6% of grafts implanted beyond 5 years.[216] The studies of Cranely et al.[220] would suggest that resection be considered if the dilated segment exceeds 20 to 30 mm in size. Excision and grafting of segmental aneurysmal change or replacement of the entire graft if diffusely dilated may be necessary.

Anastomotic Aneurysms

Anastomotic aneurysms occur rarely (1.4%) with HUV grafts and appear to develop more often at anastomoses between HUV and Dacron grafts (9%) than between HUV host arteries (0.6%).[216] Serial monitoring with duplex imaging, with examinations increasing in frequency beyond 5 years, is essential if significant dilation is to be detected and treatment instituted before complications occur.

Cryopreserved Allografts

Cryopreserved venous and arterial allografts are currently used for arterial in the absence of autogenous conduits or in the presence of infection. Venous and arterial tissue retrieved from organ donors are sterilized with antibiotics in culture medium and stored in liquid nitrogen and 15% to 20% dimethyl sulfoxide at −120° C to −196° C. Preservation does not alter the structural integrity, the ability to grow in cell culture media, or the ability to produce prostacyclin of cryopreserved vessels. An unresolved question remains concerning the immunogenicity of cryopreserved allografts. Cryopreserved nonvalved allografts induce a strong human leukocyte antigen antibody response in most children. Whether decellularization of these grafts will reduce the levels of class I and class II human leukocyte antigen antibody immune reactions is still unknown.[221]

Dialysis Grafts

Cryopreserved femoral veins are used as dialysis grafts to bypass thrombosed segments of large-diameter veins. Matsuura et al. reported 1-year primary and secondary patency rates of 49% and 75%, respectively, which compared favorably with the 65% primary and 78% secondary patency rates they achieved with brachial artery–to–axillary vein AVG.[222] Although the data are somewhat conflicting, it is recommended that cryopreserved veins be avoided as dialysis grafts in patients awaiting renal transplantation because the significant risk of allosensitization.[223]

Venous Bypass

Anecdotal reports exist of the use of cryopreserved vein to bypass occluded segments of the major veins of the abdomen, thorax, and upper and lower extremities. Cryopreserved venous valves have been evaluated to determine their efficacy in restoring venous competence in patient with chronic venous insufficiency. In a phase I feasibility study in 10 patients, Dalsing et al. reported 6-month valvular patency rates of 67% and 78% and freedom from valvular incompetence at 56% in patients undergoing femoral and popliteal vein valve transplants.[224]

Infrainguinal Bypass

Cryopreserved saphenous veins have been evaluated as an alternative conduit in patients with inadequate or absent autogenous veins for infrainguinal bypass grafting.[40,225,226] Patency rates for femoropopliteal or crural bypass procedures range from 13% to 87% at 1 year and 42% to 78% limb salvage rate at 2 years. The major cause of failure of cryopreserved grafts is thrombosis without demonstrable outflow obstruction. Whether graft thrombosis is the result of the procoagulant effect of shed ECs or ongoing rejection is presently unknown. The use of anticoagulants, immunosuppressive agents, or antiplatelet regimens to prevent graft thrombosis has not proved uniformly successful.[227] Currently, anticoagulation with warfarin sodium and antiplatelet agents is recommended with the addition of prednisone or azothiaprine to suppress the immune response in selected patients.[225] The available data suggest that cryopreserved vein for infrainguinal bypass grafting be reserved for patients with limb salvage or infection with no usable autogenous conduit.

Arterial Allografts

Arterial allografts are used to replace the aortic root, thoracic aorta, or abdominal aorta in patients with bacterial endocarditis, mycotic aneurysms, or infected prosthetic grafts.[228,229] Explanted grafts are acellular with denudation of the endothelial lining a low-grade B-cell lymphocyte infiltrate and fragmentation of the elastic tissue with a collagen layer. In a comparison between prosthetic graft replacement and cryopreserved allografts in patients with aortic infection, Vogt et al. reported lower perioperative (6% versus 18%) mortality and complications rates (24% versus 63%) in patients with allografts compared to those treated with prosthetic grafts.[228] Zhou et al., in a report of 42 patients undergoing treatment for aortic graft infection or mycotic aneurysms, reported a 17% operative mortality rate, a 6% graft occlusion rate, and a 67% 3-year survival in patients treated with cryopreserved aortic allografts.[230] Although few complications of the use of cryopreserved arterial conduits are discussed in the literature, anastomotic disruption due to persistent infection and aneurysmal dilatation (13%) remains an ongoing concern.[229]

Bovine Xenografts

Xenografts prepared from bovine carotid artery, mesenteric vein, or ureter have been used for dialysis access and for femoropopliteal bypass grafting. Poor early patency rates (16% at 1 month and 26% at 14 months), a 6% incidence of aneurysmal dilatation, and a 6% to 7% incidence of infection when used for infrainguinal bypass grafting has limited their use to poor-risk patients with no other alternatives.[41] The primary patency rates for the ProCol (bovine mesenteric vein) graft used for infrainguinal reconstruction was 0% at 3 months in a small series of patients reported by Kovalic et al.[231]

The advantages of using bovine carotid artery grafts for hemodialysis include their availability, ease of implantation, and suitability for immediate access after implantation. Bovine xenografts have patency rates of 76%, 69%, 63%, and 51% at 1 to 4 years.[232-234] In contrast, Mehta et al. reported primary patency of 16% and secondary patency of 39% for bovine carotid artery at 3 years compared with 22% and 54%, for ePTFE grafts.[233,235] Results of the multicenter study comparing bovine mesenteric vein with ePTFE in patients with previously failed prosthetic grafts showed primary patency rates of 35.6% for bovine mesenteric vein versus 28.6% for ePTFE at 1 year.[236] The SynerGraft is a decellularized bovine ureter vascular graft that is not chemically cross linked. During their preparation, cells and cellular debris from tissues are removed without compromising the integrity of the underlying collagen matrix, making them more immunologically compatible. In a study comparing SynerGraft with ePTFE in dialysis patients, Madden et al. found no differences in primary or secondary patency or the number of interventions between the two grafts.[237] Matsuura et al. reported patency rates of 72.6% and 58.6% for SynerGraft compared to 57.4%

for ePTFE at 6 and 12 months, respectively.[238] Explanted SynerGraft demonstrated both acute and chronic inflammation.[239] The late complications of bovine xenografts used for dialysis access include aneurysmal dilation, thrombosis, pseudoaneurysm formation at needle puncture sites, and infection that may result in dissolution of entire segments of the graft.[240] Spark et al. reported aneurysmal dilatation in three of nine and thrombosis in two of the remaining grafts.[239] Thrombosis of bovine heterografts usually requires thrombectomy and revision of the venous anastomosis. Infection in the first month of implantation almost invariably involves both anastomoses, requiring removal of the entire graft. Late infection usually occurs at needle puncture sites and can be treated by replacement of segments of the graft. Dilatation of the entire prosthesis or diffuse pseudoaneurysm formation may require complete removal of the graft. Focal pseudoaneurysms in the absence of infection are managed by local excision of the involved segment and placement of an interposition graft.

Tissue Engineered Grafts

Efforts are ongoing to replicate the functional properties and mechanical strength of blood vessels without relying on permanent synthetic scaffolds. SMCs, ECs, bone marrow mesenchymal cells, and fibroblasts are grown on permanent (Dacron), biodegradable (polyglycolic acid, polylactic acid, or polydioxanone), or nanostructured scaffolds. These tubular structures are either seeded with ECs, embryonic, and adult stem cells or implanted into animals, where they serve as scaffolds for cellular ingrowth.[241-243] Niklason et al. have developed a biodegradable polyglycolic acid mesh scaffold sewn into tubes then seeded with bovine SMCs and ECs under pulsatile conditions. The surface of the polyglycolic acid scaffolds was made more hydrophilic using sodium hydroxide to increase the absorption of proteins and improve SMC attachment. After 8 weeks of culture, ECs could be seeded onto the surface. These engineered vessels display SMC markers and displayed measurable contraction in response to serotonin, endothelin 1 and prostaglandin F2a.[244] Using sheet-based tissue engineering, L'Heureux et al. have assembled blood vessels from fibroblasts cultured under conditions that promote extracellular matrix deposition to produce a cohesive sheet of living cells that can be detached from the culture flask. These sheets can be layered into three-dimensional structures that possess physiological mechanical strength. The vessel consists of a living adventitia, a decellularized internal membrane lined with endothelium. The internal membrane is formed by wrapping the fibroblast sheet around a temporary Teflon-coated stainless steel tube. After maturation, the individual plies are fused to form a cylinder and dehydrated into an acellular substrate for EC seeding. The initial grafts had patency rates of 85% at intervals up to 225 days, when implanted into nude rats, but had a tendency to dilate. In a second study, thicker grafts were implanted with a patency rate of 86%. These grafts were well incorporated, with a smooth lumen, intact anastomosis, and no signs of dilatation.[245]

There remain several limitations to the use of tissue-engineered small-diameter grafts. The cells used have limited proliferative potential and may lose their function during in vitro expansion. Whether the life span of SMCs can be extended by ectopic telomerase reverse transcription subunits remains to be verified.[246] In addition, the vessels do not possess the bursting strength required for arterial grafts without relying on permanent scaffolds. The challenge in vascular engineering is to develop optimal scaffolds and expandable cell sources for the construction of tissue-engineered grafts that are non-thrombogenic, possess sufficient mechanical strength, and confer long-term patency.

References

1. Grondin CM, Campeau L, Lesperance J, et al. Comparison of late changes in internal mammary artery and saphenous vein grafts in two consecutive series of patients 10 years after operation. *Circulation* 1984;70:I208-I212.
2. Motwani JG, Topol EJ. Aortocoronary saphenous vein graft disease: pathogenesis, predisposition, and prevention. *Circulation* 1998;97:916-931.
3. Taylor Jr LM, Edwards JM, Porter JM. Present status of reversed vein bypass grafting: five-year results of a modern series. *J Vasc Surg* 1990;11:193-205. discussion, 206.
4. Pourdeyhimi B, Wagner D. On the correlation between the failure of vascular grafts and their structural and material properties: a critical analysis. *J Biomed Mater Res* 1986;20:375-409.
5. Guidoin R. A biological and structural evaluation of retrieved Dacron arterial prostheses. In: Implant Retrieval: Material and Biological Analysis. Washington, DC: U.S. Department of Commerce/National Bureau of Standards; 1981.
6. Sauvage LR. Biologic behavior of grafts in arterial system. In: Haimovici H, ed. *Vascular surgery*. 3rd ed. East Norwalk, Connecticut: Appleton & Lange; 1989:136-160.
7. Malone JM, Moore WS, Goldstone J. The natural history of bilateral aortofemoral bypass grafts for ischemia of the lower extremities. *Arch Surg* 1975;110:1300-1306.
8. Nevelsteen A, Wouters L, Suy R. Aortofemoral Dacron reconstruction for aorto-iliac occlusive disease: a 25-year survey. *Eur J Vasc Surg* 1991;5:179-186.
9. Szilagyi DE, Elliott Jr JP, Smith RF, et al. A thirty-year survey of the reconstructive surgical treatment of aortoiliac occlusive disease. *J Vasc Surg* 1986;3:421-436.
10. Cintora I, Pearce DE, Cannon JA. A clinical survey of aortobifemoral bypass using two inherently different graft types. *Ann Surg* 1988;208:625-630.
11. Friedman SG, Lazzaro RS, Spier LN, et al. A prospective randomized comparison of Dacron and polytetrafluoroethylene aortic bifurcation grafts. *Surgery* 1995;117:7-10.
12. el-Massry S, Saad E, Sauvage LR, et al. Femoropopliteal bypass with externally supported knitted Dacron grafts: a follow-up of 200 grafts for one to twelve years. *J Vasc Surg* 1994;19:487-494.
13. Green RM, Abbott WM, Matsumoto T, et al. Prosthetic above-knee femoropopliteal bypass grafting: five-year results of a randomized trial. *J Vasc Surg* 2000;31:417-425.
14. Johnson WC, Lee KK. A comparative evaluation of polytetrafluoroethylene, umbilical vein, and saphenous vein bypass grafts for femoral–popliteal above-knee revascularization: a prospective randomized Department of Veterans Affairs cooperative study. *J Vasc Surg* 2000;32:268-277.
15. Abbott WM, Green RM, Matsumoto T, et al. Prosthetic above-knee femoropopliteal bypass grafting: results of a multicenter randomized prospective trial: Above-Knee Femoropopliteal Study Group. *J Vasc Surg* 1997;25:19-28.
16. Quarmby J, Burnand K, Lockhart S, et al. Prospective randomized trial of woven versus collagen-impregnated knitted prosthetic Dacron graft in aortoiliac surgery. *Br J Surg* 1998;85:775-777.
17. Jonas RA, Schoen FJ, Levy RJ, Castaneda AR. Biological sealants and knitted Dacron: porosity and histological comparisons of vascular graft materials with and without collagen and fibrin glue pretreatments. *Ann Thorac Surg* 1986;41:657-663.
18. Quinones-Baldrich WJ, Moore WS, Ziomek S, Chvapil M. Development of a "leak-proof," knitted Dacron vascular prosthesis. *J Vasc Surg* 1986;3:895-903.
19. Adachi H, Mizuhara A, Yamaguchi A, et al. Clinical experience of a new gelatin impregnated woven Dacron graft. *Japan J Artif Organs* 1996;25:214-219.

20. Jonas RA, Ziemer G, Schoen FJ, et al. A new sealant for knitted Dacron prostheses: minimally cross-linked gelatin. *J Vasc Surg* 1988;7:414-419.
21. Kadoba K, Schoen FJ, Jonas RA. Experimental comparison of albumin-sealed and gelatin-sealed knitted Dacron conduits: porosity control, handling, sealant resorption, and healing. *J Thorac Cardiovasc Surg* 1992;103:1059-1067.
22. McGee GS, Shuman TA, Atkinson JB, et al. Experimental evaluation of a new albumin-impregnated knitted Dacron prosthesis. *Am Surg* 1987;53:695-701.
23. Boyce B. Physical characteristics of expanded polytetrafluoroethylene grafts. In: Stanley JC, ed. *Biologic and synthetic vascular prostheses.* New York: Grune & Stratton; 1982:553-561.
24. Wesolowski A. The healing of arterial prostheses: the state of the art. *Thorac Cardiovasc Surg* 1982;30:196-208.
25. Clowes AW, Gown AM, Hanson SR, Reidy MA. Mechanisms of arterial graft failure. 1. Role of cellular proliferation in early healing of PTFE prostheses. *Am J Pathol* 1985;118:43-54.
26. Clowes AW, Kirkman TR, Clowes MM. Mechanisms of arterial graft failure. II. Chronic endothelial and smooth muscle cell proliferation in healing polytetrafluoroethylene prostheses. *J Vasc Surg* 1986;3: 877-884.
27. Quinones-Baldrich WJ, Ziomek S, Henderson T, Moore WS. Primary anastomotic bonding in polytetrafluoroethylene grafts? *J Vasc Surg* 1987;5:311-318.
28. Graham LM, Bergan JJ. Expanded polytetrafluoroethylene vascular grafts: clinical and experimental observation. In: Stanley JC, ed. *Biologic and synthetic vascular prostheses.* New York: Grune & Stratton; 1982: 536-586.
29. Guidoin R, Chakfe N, Maurel S, et al. Expanded polytetrafluoroethylene arterial prostheses in humans: histopathological study of 298 surgically excised grafts. *Biomaterials* 1993;14:678-693.
30. Kohler TR, Stratton JR, Kirkman TR, et al. Conventional versus high-porosity polytetrafluoroethylene grafts: clinical evaluation. *Surgery* 1992;112:901-907.
31. Wu MH, Shi Q, Wechezak AR, et al. Definitive proof of endothelialization of a Dacron arterial prosthesis in a human being. *J Vasc Surg* 1995;21:862-867.
32. Chiesa R, Melissano G, Castellano R, Frigerio S. Extensible expanded polytetrafluoroethylene vascular grafts for aortoiliac and aortofemoral reconstruction. *Cardiovasc Surg* 2000;8:538-544.
33. Prager M, Polterauer P, Bohmig HJ, et al. Collagen versus gelatin-coated Dacron versus stretch polytetrafluoroethylene in abdominal aortic bifurcation graft surgery: results of a seven-year prospective, randomized multicenter trial. *Surgery* 2001;130:408-414.
34. Lord RSA, Nash PA, Raj BT, et al. Prospective randomized trial of polytetrafluoroethylene and Dacron aortic prosthesis. I. Perioperative results. *Ann Vasc Surg* 1988;2:248-254.
35. Prager MR, Hoblaj T, Nanobashvili J, et al. Collagen- versus gelatine-coated Dacron versus stretch PTFE bifurcation grafts for aortoiliac occlusive disease: long-term results of a prospective, randomized multicenter trial. *Surgery* 2003;134:80-85.
36. Allen BT, Reilly JM, Rubin BG, et al. Femoropopliteal bypass for claudication: vein vs. PTFE. *Ann Vasc Surg* 1996;10:178-185.
37. Taylor Jr LM, Porter JM. Clinical and anatomic considerations for surgery in femoropopliteal disease and the results of surgery. *Circulation* 1991;83:I63-I69.
38. Pereira CE, Albers M, Romiti M, et al. Meta-analysis of femoropopliteal bypass grafts for lower extremity arterial insufficiency. *J Vasc Surg* 2006;44:510-517.
39. Dereume JP, van Romphey A, Vincent G, Engelmann E. Femoropopliteal bypass with a compliant, composite polyurethane/Dacron graft: short-term results of a multicentre trial. *Cardiovasc Surg* 1993;1:499-503.
40. Harris RW, Schneider PA, Andros G, et al. Allograft vein bypass: is it an acceptable alternative for infrapopliteal revascularization? *J Vasc Surg* 1993:18:553-560.
41. Rosenberg N. Dialdehyde starch tanned bovine heterografts. In: Sawyer PN, Kaplitt MJ, eds. Vascular grafts. New York: Appleton-Century-Crofts; 1978:261-270.
42. Devine C, Hons B, McCollum C. Heparin-bonded Dacron or polytetrafluoroethylene for femoropopliteal bypass grafting: a multicenter trial. *J Vasc Surg* 2001;33:533-539.
43. Jensen LP, Lepantalo M, Fossdal JE, et al. Dacron or PTFE for above-knee femoropopliteal bypass: a multicenter randomised study. *Eur J Vasc Endovasc Surg* 2007;34:44-49.
44. AbuRahma AF, Robinson PA, Holt SM. Prospective controlled study of polytetrafluoroethylene versus saphenous vein in claudicant patients with bilateral above knee femoropopliteal bypasses. *Surgery* 1999; 126:594-601; discussion, 602.
45. Klinkert P, Schepers A, Burger DH, et al. Vein versus polytetrafluoroethylene in above-knee femoropopliteal bypass grafting: five-year results of a randomized controlled trial. *J Vasc Surg* 2003;37:149-155.
46. Parsons RE, Suggs WD, Veith FJ, et al. Polytetrafluoroethylene bypasses to infrapopliteal arteries without cuffs or patches: a better option than amputation in patients without autologous vein. *J Vasc Surg* 1996;23:347-354; discussion, 355-346.
47. Veith FJ, Gupta SK, Ascer E, et al. Six-year prospective multicenter randomized comparison of autologous saphenous vein and expanded polytetrafluoroethylene grafts in infrainguinal arterial reconstructions. *J Vasc Surg* 1986;3:104-114.
48. National Institute of Diabetes and Digestive Kidney Diseases, ed. USRDS 2001 Annual Data Report. In: U.S. Renal Data System. Bethesda, Maryland: National Institute of Diabetes and Digestive Kidney Diseases, Department of Health and Human Services; 2001.
49. Enzler MA, Rajmon T, Lachat M, Largiader F. Long-term function of vascular access for hemodialysis. *Clin Transplant* 1996;10:511-515.
50. Palder SB, Kirkman RL, Whittemore AD, et al. Vascular access for hemodialysis: patency rates and results of revision. *Ann Surg* 1985;202:235-239.
51. Pherwani AD, Reid JA, Connolly JK. Patency and survival of primary arteriovenous fistulae. In: Henry ML, ed. *Vascular access for hemodialysis-VII.* Chicago: WL Gore & Associates and Precept Press; 2001:47-53.
52. Keuter XH, De Smet AA, Kessels AG, et al. A randomized multicenter study of the outcome of brachial–basilic arteriovenous fistula and prosthetic brachial–antecubital forearm loop as vascular access for hemodialysis. *J Vasc Surg* 2008;47:395-401.
53. el-Massry S, Saad E, Sauvage LR, et al. Axillofemoral bypass with externally supported, knitted Dacron grafts: a follow-up through twelve years. *J Vasc Surg* 1993;17:107-115.
54. Johnson WC, Lee KK. Comparative evaluation of externally supported Dacron and polytetrafluoroethylene prosthetic bypasses for femorofemoral and axillofemoral arterial reconstructions: Veterans Affairs Cooperative Study 141. *J Vasc Surg* 1999;30:1077-1083.
55. Landry GJ, Moneta GL, Taylor Jr LM, Porter JM. Axillobifemoral bypass. *Ann Vasc Surg* 2000;14:296-305.
56. Mii S, Mori A, Sakata H, Kawazoe N. Fifteen-year experience in axillofemoral bypass with externally supported knitted Dacron prosthesis in a Japanese hospital. *J Am Coll Surg* 1998;186:581-588.
57. Rutherford RB, Patt A, Pearce WH. Extra-anatomic bypass: a closer view. *J Vasc Surg* 1987;6:437-446.
58. Taylor Jr LM, Moneta GL, McConnell D, et al. Axillofemoral grafting with externally supported polytetrafluoroethylene. *Arch Surg* 1994;129:588-595.
59. Hertzer NR, Bena JF, Karafa MT. A personal experience with direct reconstruction and extra-anatomic bypass for aortoiliofemoral occlusive disease. *J Vasc Surg* 2007;45:527-535; discussion, 535.
60. Lipsitz EC, Ohki T, Veith FJ, et al. Patency rates of femorofemoral bypasses associated with endovascular aneurysm repair surpass those performed for occlusive disease. *J Endovasc Ther* 2003;10:1061-1065.
61. Mii S, Eguchi D, Takenaka T, et al. Role of femorofemoral crossover bypass grafting for unilateral iliac atherosclerotic disease: a comparative evaluation with anatomic bypass. *Surg Today* 2005;35:453-458.
62. Abou-Zamzam Jr AM, Moneta GL, Edwards JM, et al. Extrathoracic arterial grafts performed for carotid artery occlusive disease not amenable to endarterectomy. *Arch Surg* 1999;134:952-956; discussion, 956-957.
63. Buth J, Penn O, Tielbeek A, Mersman M. Combined approach to stent graft treatment of an aortic arch aneurysm. *J Endovasc Surg* 1998;5: 329-332.
64. Czerny M, Verrel F, Weber H, et al. Collagen patch coated with fibrin glue components. Treatment of suture hole bleedings in vascular reconstruction. *J Cardiovasc Surg (Torino)* 2000;41:553-557.
65. Lauder C, Kelly A, Thompson MM, et al. Early and late outcome after carotid artery bypass grafting with saphenous vein. *J Vasc Surg* 2003;38:1025-1030.
66. Law MM, Colburn MD, Moore WS, et al. Carotid–subclavian bypass for brachiocephalic occlusive disease. Choice of conduit and long-term follow-up. *Stroke* 1995;26:1565-1571.
67. Melissano G, Civilini E, Marrocco-Trischitta MM, Chiesa R. Hybrid endovascular and off-pump open surgical treatment for synchronous aneurysms of the aortic arch, brachiocephalic trunk, and abdominal aorta. *Tex Heart Inst J* 2004;31:283-287.

68. AbuRahma AF, Robinson PA, Jennings TG. Carotid–subclavian bypass grafting with polytetrafluoroethylene grafts for symptomatic subclavian artery stenosis or occlusion: a 20-year experience. *J Vasc Surg* 2000;32:411-418; discussion, 418-419.
69. Cinar B, Enc Y, Kosem M, et al. Carotid–subclavian bypass in occlusive disease of subclavian artery: more important today than before. *Tohoku J Exp Med* 2004;204:53-62.
70. Gold JP, Violaris K, Engle MA, et al. A five-year clinical experience with 112 Blalock-Taussig shunts. *J Cardiovasc Surg* 1993;8:9-17.
71. Opie JC, Traverse L, Hayden RI, et al. Experience with polytetrafluoroethylene grafts in children with cyanotic congenital heart disease. *Ann Thorac Surg* 1986;41:164-168.
72. Weyand M, Kerber S, Schmid C, et al. Coronary artery bypass grafting with an expanded polytetrafluoroethylene graft. *Ann Thorac Surg* 1999;67:1240-1245.
73. Hagberg RC, Safi HJ, Sabik J, et al. Improved intraoperative management of anastomotic bleeding during aortic reconstruction: results of a randomized controlled trial. *Am Surg* 2004;70:307-311.
74. De Paulis R, Scaffa R, Maselli D, et al. A third generation of ascending aorta Dacron graft: preliminary experience. *Ann Thorac Surg* 2008;85:305-309.
75. Goldstone J. Management of late failures of aorto-femoral reconstructions. *Acta Chir Scand Suppl* 1990;555:149-153.
76. Harris PL. Aorto-iliac–femoral re-operative surgery: supplementary surgery at secondary operations. *Acta Chir Scand Suppl* 1987;538:51-55.
77. Ramaiah V, Thompson C, Harvey A, et al. Stenting for proximal para-anastomotic stenosis of an infrarenal aortic bypass graft. *Tex Heart Inst J* 2002;29:45-47.
78. Stricker H, Jacomella V. Stent-assisted angioplasty at the level of the common femoral artery bifurcation: midterm outcomes. *J Endovasc Ther* 2004;11:281-286.
79. Benenati J, Shlansky-Goldberg R, Meglin A, Seidl E. Thrombolytic and antiplatelet therapy in peripheral vascular disease with use of reteplase and/or abciximab: Society for Cardiovascular and Interventional Radiology Consultants' Conference, May 22, 2000, Orlando, FL. *J Vasc Interv Radiol* 2001;12:795-805.
80. Graor RA, Risius B, Denny KM, et al. Local thrombolysis in the treatment of thrombosed arteries, bypass grafts, and arteriovenous fistulas. *J Vasc Surg* 1985;2:406-414.
81. Berman SS, Hunter GC, Smyth SH, et al. Application of computed tomography for surveillance of aortic grafts. *Surgery* 1995;118:8-15.
82. Clagett GP, Salander JM, Eddleman WL, et al. Dilation of knitted Dacron aortic prostheses and anastomotic false aneurysms: etiologic considerations. *Surgery* 1983;93:9-16.
83. Creech OJ, Deterling RA, Edwards S, et al. Vascular prostheses: Report of the Committee for the Study of Vascular Prostheses of the Society for Vascular Surgery. *Surgery* 1957;41:62-80.
84. Hayward RH, White RR. Aneurysm in a woven Teflon graft. *Angiology* 1971;22:90-188.
85. Humphries AW, Hawk WA, DeWolfe VG, Le Fevre FA. Clinicopathologic observations on the fate of arterial freeze-dried homografts. *Surgery* 1959;45:59-71.
86. Knox WG. Peripheral vascular anastomotic aneurysms: a fifteen-year experience. *Ann Surg* 1976;183:120-123.
87. Nunn DB, Freeman MH, Hudgins PC. Postoperative alterations in size of Dacron aortic grafts: an ultrasonic evaluation. *Ann Surg* 1979;189: 741-745.
88. Nunn DB, Carter MM, Donohue MT, Pourdeyhimi B. Dilative characteristics of Microvel and Vasculour-II aortic bifurcation grafts. *J Biomed Mater Res* 1996;30:41-46.
89. Trippestad A. Dilatation and rupture of Dacron arterial grafts. *Acta Chir Scand Suppl* 1985;529:77-79.
90. Berger K, Sauvage LR. Late fiber deterioration in Dacron arterial grafts. *Ann Surg* 1981;193:477-491.
91. Brown OW, Stanson AW, Pairolero PC, Hollier LH. Computerized tomography following abdominal aortic surgery. *Surgery* 1982;91: 716-722.
92. Gooding GA, Effeney DJ, Goldstone J. The aortofemoral graft: detection and identification of healing complications by ultrasonography. *Surgery* 1981;89:94-101.
93. Kalman PG, Rappaport DC, Merchant N, et al. The value of late computed tomographic scanning in identification of vascular abnormalities after abdominal aortic aneurysm repair. *J Vasc Surg* 1999;29:442-450.
93a. Post PN, Kievit J, van Bockel JH. Optimal follow-up strategies after aorto-iliac prosthetic reconstruction: a decision analysis and cost-effectiveness analysis. *Eur J Endovasc Surg* 2004;28:287-295.
94. Lundqvist B, Almgren B, Bowald S, et al. Deterioration and dilatation of Dacron prosthetic grafts. *Acta Chir Scand Suppl* 1985;529:81-85.
95. Rais O, Lundstrom B, Angquist KA, Hallmans G. Bilateral aneurysm of Dacron graft following aorto-femoral graft operation: a case report. *Acta Chir Scand* 1976;142:479-482.
96. Allen RC, Schneider J, Longenecker L, et al. Paraanastomotic aneurysms of the abdominal aorta. *J Vasc Surg* 1993;18:424-432.
97. Curl GR, Faggioli GL, Stella A, et al. Aneurysmal change at or above the proximal anastomosis after infrarenal aortic grafting. *J Vasc Surg* 1992;16:855-860.
98. Edwards JM, Teefey SA, Zierler RE, Kohler TR. Intraabdominal paraanastomotic aneurysms after aortic bypass grafting. *J Vasc Surg* 1992;15:344-353.
99. Locati P, Socrate AM, Costantini E. Paraanastomotic aneurysms of the abdominal aorta: a 15-year experience review. *Cardiovasc Surg* 2000;8:274-279.
100. Mii S, Mori A, Sakata H, Kawazoe N. Para-anastomotic aneurysms: incidence, risk factors, treatment and prognosis. *J Cardiovasc Surg (Torino)* 1998;39:259-266.
101. Szilagyi DE, Smith RF, Elliott JP, et al. Anastomotic aneurysms after vascular reconstruction: problems of incidence, etiology, and treatment. *Surgery* 1975;78:800-816.
102. Zhou W, Bush RL, Bhama JK, et al. Repair of anastomotic abdominal aortic pseudoaneurysm utilizing sequential AneuRx aortic cuffs in an overlapping configuration. *Ann Vasc Surg* 2006;20:17-22.
103. Carson SN, Hunter GC, Palmaz J, Guernsey JM. Recurrence of femoral anastomotic aneurysms. *Am J Surg* 1983;146:774-778.
104. di Marzo L, Strandness EL, Schultz RD, Feldhaus RJ. Reoperation for femoral anastomotic false aneurysm: a 15-year experience. *Ann Surg* 1987;206:168-172.
105. Kim GE, Imparato AM, Nathan I, Riles TS. Dilation of synthetic grafts and junctional aneurysms. *Arch Surg* 1979;114:1296-1303.
106. Kinley CE, Paasche PE, MacDonald AS, Marble AE. Stress at vascular anastomosis in relation to host artery: synthetic graft diameter. *Surgery* 1974;75:28-30.
107. Courbier R, Aboukhater R. Progress in the treatment of anastomotic aneurysms. *World J Surg* 1988;12:742-749.
108. Sharma N, Chin K, Modgill V. Pseudoaneurysms of the femoral artery: recommendation for a method of repair. *JR Coll Surg Edinb* 2001;46:195-197.
109. Ernst CB, Elliott Jr JP, Ryan CJ, et al. Recurrent femoral anastomotic aneurysms: a 30-year experience. *Ann Surg* 1988;208:401-409.
110. Nunn DB. Structural failure of first-generation, polyester, double-velour, knitted prostheses. *J Vasc Surg* 2001;33:1131-1132.
111. Chakfe N, Riepe G, Dieval F, et al. Longitudinal ruptures of polyester knitted vascular prostheses. *J Vasc Surg* 2001;33:1015-1021.
112. Biedermann H, Flora G. Fatigue problems in Dacron vascular grafts. *Int J Artif Organs* 1982;5:205-206.
113. Watanabe T, Kusaba A, Kuma H, et al. Failure of Dacron arterial prostheses caused by structural defects. *J Cardiovasc Surg (Torino)* 1983;24:95-100.
114. Dobrin PB. Surgical manipulation and the tensile strength of polypropylene sutures. *Arch Surg* 1989;124:665-668.
115. Aldrete V. Polypropylene suture fracture. *Ann Thorac Surg* 1984;37:264.
116. Calhoun TR, Kitten CM. Polypropylene suture: is it safe? *J Vasc Surg* 1986;4:98-100.
117. Gayle RG, Wheeler JR, Gregory RT, Snyder Jr SO, Evaluation of the expanded polytetrafluoroethylene (EPTFE) suture in peripheral vascular surgery using EPTFE prosthetic vascular grafts. *J Cardiovasc Surg (Torino)* 1988;29:556-559.
118. Moore WS, Hall AD. Late suture failure in the pathogenesis of anastomotic false aneurysms. *Ann Surg* 1970;172:1064-1068.
119. Myhre OA. Breakage of prolene suture. *Ann Thorac Surg* 1983;36:121.
120. Setzen G, EF Williams III. Tissue response to suture materials implanted subcutaneously in a rabbit model. *Plast Reconstr Surg* 1997;100:1788-1795.
121. Szarnicki RJ. Polypropylene suture fracture. *Ann Thorac Surg* 1983; 35:333.
122. Shenoy S, Miller A, Petersen F, et al. A multicenter study of permanent hemodialysis access patency: beneficial effect of clipped vascular anastomotic technique. *J Vasc Surg* 2003;38:229-235.
123. Erdmann D, Sweis R, Heitmann C, et al. Side-to-side sutureless vascular anastomosis with magnets. *J Vasc Surg* 2004:40.
124. Kaupp HA, Matulewicz TJ, Lattimer GL, et al. Graft infection or graft reaction? *Arch Surg* 1979;114:1419-1422.
125. Ahn SS, Machleder HI, Gupta R, Moore WS. Perigraft seroma: clinical, histologic, and serologic correlates. *Am J Surg* 1987;154:173-178.

126. Bhuta I, Dorrough R. Noninfectious fluid collection around velour Dacron graft: possible allergic reaction. *South Med J* 1981;74:870-872.
127. Blumenberg RM, Gelfand ML, Dale WA. Perigraft seromas complicating arterial grafts. *Surgery* 1985;97:194-204.
128. Bolton W, Cannon JA. Seroma formation associated with PTFE vascular grafts used as arteriovenous fistulae. *Dial Transplant* 1981;10(60):62-63, 66.
129. Buche M, Schoevaerdts JC, Jaumin P, et al. Perigraft seroma following axillofemoral bypass: report of three cases. *Ann Vasc Surg* 1986;1: 374-377.
130. LeBlanc JG, Vince DJ, Taylor GP. Perigraft seroma: long-term complications. *J Thorac Cardiovasc Surg* 1986;92:451-454.
131. Paes E, Vollmar JF, Mohr W, et al. Perigraft reaction: incompatibility of synthetic vascular grafts? New aspects on clinical manifestation, pathogenesis, and therapy. *World J Surg* 1988;12:750-755.
132. Ahn SS, Williams DE, Thye DA, et al. The isolation of a fibroblast growth inhibitor associated with perigraft seroma. *J Vasc Surg* 1994;20:202-208.
133. Schneiderman J, Knoller S, Adar R, Savion N. Biochemical analysis of a human humoral fibroblast inhibitory factor associated with impaired vascular prosthetic graft incorporation. *J Vasc Surg* 1991;14:103-110.
134. Sladen JG, Mandl MA, Grossman L, Denegri JF. Fibroblast inhibition: a new and treatable cause of prosthetic graft failure. *Am J Surg* 1985;149:587-590.
135. Berger RMF, Bol-Raap G, Hop WJ, et al. Heparin as a risk factor for perigraft seroma complicating the modified Blalock-Taussig shunt. *J Thorac Cardiovasc Surg* 1998;116:286-293.
136. Dauria DM, Dyk P, Garvin P. Incidence and management of seroma after arteriovenous graft placement. *J Am Coll Surg* 2006;203:506-511.
137. Lowery Jr RC, Wicker HS, Sanders K, Peniston RL. Management of a recalcitrant periprosthetic fluid collection. *J Vasc Surg* 1987;6:77-80.
138. Johnston KW. Nonvascular complications of vascular surgery. Presented at the 17th Annual Symposium on Current Critical Problems and New Horizons in Vascular Surgery, November 16-18:1990, New York.
139. Wright DJ, Ernst CB, Evans JR, et al. Ureteral complications and aortoiliac reconstruction. *J Vasc Surg* 1990;11:29-37.
140. Frusha JD, Porter JA, Batson RC. Hydronephrosis following aortofemoral bypass grafts. *J Cardiovasc Surg (Torino)* 1982;23:371-377.
141. Thaveau F, Dion YM, Warnier de Wailly G, et al. Early transient hydronephrosis after laparoscopic aortobifemoral bypass grafting. *J Vasc Surg* 2003;38:603-608.
142. Alexander J, Moawad J, Cai D. Primary intimal sarcoma of the aorta associated with a Dacron graft and resulting in arterial rupture. *Vasc Endovasc Surg* 2007;40:509-515.
143. Brand KC. Foreign body tumorigenesis, timing and location of preneoplastic events. *J Natl Cancer Inst* 1971;47:829.
144. Burns WA, Kanhouwa S, Tillman L, et al. Fibrosarcoma occurring at the site of a plastic vascular graft. *Cancer* 1972;29:66-72.
145. Fehrenbacher JW, Bowers W, Strate R, Pittman J. Angiosarcoma of the aorta associated with a Dacron graft. *Ann Thorac Surg* 1981;32:297-301.
146. O'Connell TX, Fee HJ, Golding A. Sarcoma associated with Dacron prosthetic material: case report and review of the literature. *J Thorac Cardiovasc Surg* 1976;72:94-96.
147. Peterson H, Meredith D, Croddock D. Malignant fibrous histiocytoma associated with a Dacron vascular prosthesis. *Ann Thorac Surg* 1989;47:772-774.
148. Goad MEP, Goad DL. Biomedical devices and biomaterials. In: *Handbook of Toxicologic Pathology*, 2nd ed, Vol 1. San Diego: Academic Press Harcourt Science and Technology 2002; 459-477.
149. McGregor D, Baan R, Partensky C, et al. Evaluation of the carcinogenic risks to humans associated with surgical implants and other foreign bodies: a report of an IARC monographic programme meeting. *Eur J Cancer* 2000;36:307-313.
150. Jordan SW, Chaikof EL. Novel thromboresistant materials. *J Vasc Surg* 2007;45(Suppl A):A104-A115.
151. Goegler FM, Kapfer X, Meichelbock W. Crural prosthetic revascularization: randomized, prospective, multicentric comparison of standard and carbon impregnated ePTFE grafts. Presented at the 27th Global Vascular Endovascular Issues Techniques Horizons Symposium, New York 2000, I2.1-I2.3.
152. Kapfer X, Meichelboeck W, Groegler FM. Comparison of carbon-impregnated and standard ePTFE prostheses in extra-anatomical anterior tibial artery bypass: a prospective randomized multicenter study. *Eur J Vasc Endovasc Surg* 2006;32:155-168.
153. Bacourt F. Prospective randomized study of carbon-impregnated polytetrafluoroethylene grafts for below-knee popliteal and distal bypass: results at 2 years—the Association Universitaire de Recherche en Chirurgie. *Ann Vasc Surg* 1997;11:596-603.
154. Iwai Y. Development of a thermal cross-linking heparinization method and its application to small caliber vascular prostheses. *ASAIO J* 1996; 42:M693-M697.
155. Mohamed MS, Mukherjee M, Kakkar VV. Thrombogenicity of heparin and non-heparin bound arterial prostheses: an in vitro evaluation. *JR Coll Surg Edinb* 1998;43:155-157.
156. Lin PH, Chen C, Bush RL, et al. Small-caliber heparin-coated ePTFE grafts reduce platelet deposition and neointimal hyperplasia in a baboon model. *J Vasc Surg* 2004;39:1322-1328.
157. Bosiers M, Deloose K, Verbist J, et al. Heparin-bonded expanded polytetrafluoroethylene vascular graft for femoropopliteal and femorocrural bypass grafting: 1-year results. *J Vasc Surg* 2006;43:313-318; discussion, 318-319.
157a. Devine C, McCollum C. Heparin-bonded Dacron or polytetrafluoroethylene for femoropopliteal bypass: five-year results of a prospective randomized multicenter clinical trial. *J Vasc Surg* 2004;40:924-931.
158. Davidson I. Abstract *Vieth Symposium* November 19, 2008, New York.
159. Herring M, Baughman S, Glover J. Endothelium develops on seeded human arterial prosthesis: a brief clinical note. *J Vasc Surg* 1985;2: 727-730.
160. Swedenborg J, Bengtsson L, Clyne N, et al. In vitro endothelialisation of arteriovenous loop grafts for haemodialysis. *Eur J Vasc Endovasc Surg* 1997;13:272-277.
161. Magometschnigg H, Kadletz M, Vodrazka M, et al. Prospective clinical study with in vitro endothelial cell lining of expanded polytetrafluoroethylene grafts in crural repeat reconstruction. *J Vasc Surg* 1992;15: 527-535.
162. Deutsch M, Meinhart J, Vesely M, et al. In vitro endothelialization of expanded polytetrafluoroethylene grafts: a clinical case report after 41 months of implantation. *J Vasc Surg* 1997;25:757-763.
163. Yu H, Wang Y, Eton D, et al. Dual cell seeding and the use of zymogen tissue plasminogen activator to improve cell retention on polytetrafluoroethylene grafts. *J Vasc Surg* 2001;34:337-343.
164. Zilla P, Deutsch M, Meinhart J, et al. Long-term effects of clinical in vitro endothelialization on grafts. *J Vasc Surg* 1997;25:1110-1112.
165. Sipehia R, Martucci G, Lipscombe J. Transplantation of human endothelial cell monolayer on artificial vascular prosthesis: the effect of growth-support surface chemistry, cell seeding density, ECM protein coating, and growth factors. *Artif Cells Blood Substit Immobil Biotechnol* 1996;24:51-63.
166. Bellón JM, Garcia-Honduvilla N, Escudero C, et al. Mesothelial versus endothelial cell seeding: evaluation of cell adherence to a fibroblastic matrix using 111In oxine. *Eur J Vasc Endovasc Surg* 1997;13:142-148.
167. Shi Q, Wu MH, Hayashida N, et al. Proof of fallout endothelialization of impervious Dacron grafts in the aorta and inferior vena cava of the dog. *J Vasc Surg* 1994;20:546-557.
168. Scott SM, Barth MG, Gaddy LR, Ahl Jr ET, The role of circulating cells in the healing of vascular prostheses. *J Vasc Surg* 1994;19:585-593.
169. Birchall IE, Field PL, Ketharanathan V. Adherence of human saphenous vein endothelial cell monolayers to tissue-engineered biomatrix vascular conduits. *J Biomed Mater Res* 2001;56:437-443.
170. Seifalian AM, Tiwari A, Hamilton G, Salacinski HJ. Improving the clinical patency of prosthetic vascular and coronary bypass grafts: the role of seeding and tissue engineering. *Artif Organs* 2002;26:307-320.
171. Greisler HP, Cziperle DJ, Kim DU, et al. Enhanced endothelialization of expanded polytetrafluoroethylene grafts by fibroblast growth factor type 1 pretreatment. *Surgery* 1992;112:244-254; discussion; 254-255.
172. Zilla P, Bezuidenhout D, Human P. Prosthetic vascular grafts: wrong models, wrong questions and no healing. *Biomaterials* 2007;28:5009-5027.
173. Berman SS, Jarrell BE, Raymond MA, et al. Early experience with ePTFE dialysis grafts sodded with liposuction-derived microvascular endothelial cells. In: Henry ML, Ferguson RM, eds. Vascular access for hemodialysis. Chicago: Precept Press; 1995:292-302.
174. Meinhart J, Deutsch M, Zilla P. Eight years of clinical endothelial cell transplantation: closing the gap between prosthetic grafts and vein grafts. *ASAIO J* 1997;43:M515-M521.
175. Laube HR, Duwe J, Rutsch W, Konertz W. Clinical experience with autologous endothelial cell-seeded polytetrafluoroethylene coronary artery bypass grafts. *J Thorac Cardiovasc Surg* 2000;120:134-141.
176. Kraiss LW, Kirkman TR, Kohler TR, et al. Shear stress regulates smooth muscle proliferation and neointimal thickening in porous polytetrafluoroethylene grafts. *Arterioscler Thromb* 1991(11):1844-1852.
177. Mattsson EJ, Kohler TR, Vergel SM, Clowes AW. Increased blood flow induces regression of intimal hyperplasia. *Arterioscler Thromb Vasc Biol* 1997;17:2245-2249.

178. Batson RC, Sottiurai VS, Craighead CC. Linton patch angioplasty: an adjunct to distal bypass with polytetrafluoroethylene grafts. *Ann Surg* 1984;199:684-693.
179. Taylor RS, Loh A, McFarland RJ, et al. Improved technique for polytetrafluoroethylene bypass grafting: long-term results using anastomotic vein patches. *Br J Surg* 1992;79:348-354.
180. Stonebridge PA, Prescott RJ, Ruckley CV. Randomized trial comparing infrainguinal polytetrafluoroethylene bypass grafting with and without vein interposition cuff at the distal anastomosis: the Joint Vascular Research Group. *J Vasc Surg* 1997;26:543-550.
181. How TV, Rowe CS, Gilling-Smith GL, Harris PL. Interposition vein cuff anastomosis alters wall shear stress distribution in the recipient artery. *J Vasc Surg* 2000;31:1008-1017.
182. Kissin M, Kansal N, Pappas PJ, et al. Vein interposition cuffs decrease the intimal hyperplastic response of polytetrafluoroethylene bypass grafts. *J Vasc Surg* 2000;31:69-83.
183. Neville RF, Tempesta B, Sidway AN. Tibial bypass for limb salvage using polytetrafluoroethylene and a distal vein patch. *J Vasc Surg* 2001;33: 266-272.
184. Harris PL, How TV. Haemodynamics of cuffed arterial anastomoses. *Crit Ischaemia* 1999;9:20-26.
185. Panneton JM. Randomized prospective evaluation of the distally widened (Distaflo™) PTFE graft. Presented at the 27th Global Vascular Endovascular Issues Techniques Horizons Symposium, New York; 2000: IA2.1.
186. Sorom A, Hughes CB, McCarthy JT, et al. Prospective, randomized evaluation of a cuffed expanded polytetrafluoroethylene graft for hemodialysis vascular access. *Surgery* 2002;132:135-140.
187. Liu YH, Hung YN, Hsieh HC, Ko PJ. Impact of cuffed, expanded polytetrafluoroethylene dialysis grafts on graft outlet stenosis. *World J Surg* 2006;30:2290-2294.
188. Heise M, Schmidt S, Kruger U, et al. Flow pattern and shear stress distribution of distal end-to-side anastomoses: a comparison of the instantaneous velocity fields obtained by particle image velocimetry. *J Biomech* 2004;37:1043-1051.
189. Kedora J, Hohmann S, Garrett W, et al. Randomized comparison of percutaneous Viabahn stent grafts versus prosthetic femoral–popliteal bypass in the treatment of superficial femoral arterial occlusive disease. *J Vasc Surg* 2007;45:10-16. discussion, 16.
190. Fischer M, Schwabe C, Schulte KL. Value of the Hemobahn/Viabahn endoprosthesis in the treatment of long chronic lesions of the superficial femoral artery: 6 years of experience. *J Endovasc Ther* 2006:13.
191. Lammer J, Dake MD, Bleyn J, et al. Peripheral arterial obstruction: prospective study of treatment with a transluminally placed self-expanding stent graft—International Trial Study Group. *Radiology* 2000;217: 95-104.
192. Saxon R, Coffman J, Gooding J, Poner D. Long-term patency and clinical outcome of the Viabahn stent graft for femoropopliteal artery obstruction. *J Vasc Interv Radiol* 2007;15:1341-1350.
193. Tielliu I, Verhoeven E, Zeebregts C, et al. Endovascular treatment of popliteal artery aneurysms: is the technique a valid alternative to open surgery? *J Cardiovasc Surg* 2007:48.
194. Antonello M, Frigatti P, Battocchio P, et al. Endovascular treatment of asymptomatic popliteal aneurysm: 8 year concurrent comparison with open repair. *J Cardiovasc Surg* 2007;48:267-274.
195. Marin ML, Veith FJ, Cynamon J, et al. Human transluminally placed endovascular stented grafts: preliminary histopathologic analysis of healing grafts in aortoiliac and femoral artery occlusive disease. *J Vasc Surg* 1995;21:595-604.
196. van Sambeek MR, Hagenaars T, Gussenhoven EJ, et al. Vascular response in the femoropopliteal segment after implantation of an ePTFE balloon-expandable endovascular graft: an intravascular ultrasound study. *J Endovasc Ther* 2000;7:204-212.
197. Soyer T, Lempinen M, Cooper P, et al. A new venous prosthesis. *Surgery* 1972;72:864-872.
198. Kogel H, Vollmar JF, Cyba-Altunbay S, et al. New observations on the healing process in prosthetic substitution of large veins by microporous grafts—animal experiments. *Thorac Cardiovasc Surg* 1989;37: 119-124.
199. Sarkar R, Eilber FR, Gelabert HA, Quinones-Baldrich WJ. Prosthetic replacement of the inferior vena cava for malignancy. *J Vasc Surg* 1998;28:75-83.
200. Alimi YS, Gloviczki P, Vrtiska TJ, et al. Reconstruction of the superior vena cava: benefits of postoperative surveillance and secondary endovascular interventions. *J Vasc Surg* 1998;27:287-301.
201. Illuminati G, Calio FG, D'Urso A, et al. Prosthetic replacement of the infrahepatic inferior vena cava for leiomyosarcoma. *Arch Surg* 2006;141: 919-924; discussion, 924.
202. Jost CJ, Gloviczki P, Cherry Jr KJ, et al. Surgical reconstruction of iliofemoral veins and the inferior vena cava for nonmalignant occlusive disease. *J Vasc Surg* 2001;33:320-327; discussion, 327-328.
203. Sarfeh IJ, Rypins EB. Partial versus total portacaval shunt in alcoholic cirrhosis: results of a prospective, randomized clinical trial. *Ann Surg* 1994;219:353-361.
204. Bergan JJ, Yao JS, Flinn WR, McCarthy WJ. Surgical treatment of venous obstruction and insufficiency. *J Vasc Surg* 1986;3:174-181.
205. Sanders RJ, Rosales C, Pearce WH. Creation and closure of temporary arteriovenous fistulas for venous reconstruction or thrombectomy: description of technique. *J Vasc Surg* 1987;6:504-505.
206. Glickman MH, Stokes GK, Ross JR, et al. Multicenter evaluation of a polytetrafluoroethylene vascular access graft as compared with the expanded polytetrafluoroethylene vascular access graft in hemodialysis applications. *J Vasc Surg* 2001;34:465-473.
207. Rocco MV, Bleyer AJ, Burkart JM. Utilization of inpatient and outpatient resources for the management of hemodialysis access complications. *Am J Kidney Dis* 1996;28:250-256.
208. King MW, Zhang Z, Ukpabi P, et al. Quantitative analysis of the surface morphology and textile structure of the polyurethane Vascugraft arterial prosthesis using image and statistical analyses. *Biomaterials* 1994;15:621-627.
209. Zhang Z, King MW, Guidoin R, et al. Morphological, physical and chemical evaluation of the Vascugraft arterial prosthesis: comparison of a novel polyurethane device with other microporous structures. *Biomaterials* 1994;15:483-501.
210. Jefic D, Reddy PP, Flynn LM, Provenzano R. A single center experience in the use of polyurethane urea arteriovenous grafts. *Nephrol News Issues* 2005;19:44-47.
211. Kakkos S, Andrzejewski T, Haddad JA, et al. Equivalent secondary patency rates of upper extremity Vectra vascular access grafts and transposed brachial–basilic fistulas with aggressive access surveillance and endovascular treatment. *J Vasc Surg* 2008;47:407-414.
212. Taite LJ, Yang P, Jun HW, West JL. Nitric oxide–releasing polyurethane–PEG copolymer containing the YIGSR peptide promotes endothelialization with decreased platelet adhesion. *J Biomed Mater Res B Appl Biomater* 2008;84:108-116.
213. Ishii Y, Sakamoto S, Kronengold RT, et al. A novel bioengineered small-caliber vascular graft incorporating heparin and sirolimus: excellent 6-month patency. *J Thorac Cardiovasc Surg* 2008;135:1237-1245; discussion, 1245-1246.
214. Stanley JC, Lindenauer SM, Graham LM, et al. Biologic and synthetic vascular grafts. In: Moore WS, ed. Vascular surgery: a comprehensive review. Orlando, Florida: WB Saunders; 1990:275-294.
215. Neufang A, Espinola-Klein C, Dorweiler B, et al. Femoropopliteal prosthetic bypass with glutaraldehyde stabilized human umbilical vein (HUV). *J Vasc Surg* 2007;46:280-288.
216. Dardik H, Ibrahim IM, Sussman B, et al. Biodegradation and aneurysm formation in umbilical vein grafts: observations and a realistic strategy. *Ann Surg* 1984;199:61-68.
217. Dardik H, Miller N, Dardik A, et al. A decade of experience with the glutaraldehyde-tanned human umbilical cord vein graft for revascularization of the lower limb. *J Vasc Surg* 1988;7:336-346.
218. Dardik H, Wengerter K, Qin F, et al. Comparative decades of experience with glutaraldehyde-tanned human umbilical cord vein graft for lower limb revascularization: an analysis of 1275 cases. *J Vasc Surg* 2002;35:64-71.
219. Guidoin R, Gagnon Y, Roy PE, et al. Pathologic features of surgically excised human umbilical vein grafts. *J Vasc Surg* 1986;3:146-154.
220. Cranely JJ, Karkow WS, Hafner CD, Flanagan LD. Aneurysmal dilatation in umbilical vein grafts. In: Yao JST, Bergan JJ, eds. Reoperative arterial surgery. New York: Grune & Straton; 1986:343-358.
221. Breinholt JP, Hawkins JA III, Lambert LM, et al. A prospective analysis of the immunogenicity of cryopreserved nonvalved allografts used in pediatric heart surgery. *Circulation* 2000;102:III179-III182.
222. Matsuura JH, Johansen KH, Rosenthal D, et al. Cryopreserved femoral vein grafts for difficult hemodialysis access. *Ann Vasc Surg* 2000;14: 50-55.
223. Benedetto B, Lipkowitz G, Madden R, et al. Use of cryopreserved cadaveric vein allograft for hemodialysis access precludes kidney transplantation because of allosensitization. *J Vasc Surg* 2001;34: 139-142.

224. Dalsing MC, Raju S, Wakefield TW, Taheri S. A multicenter, phase I evaluation of cryopreserved venous valve allografts for the treatment of chronic deep venous insufficiency. *J Vasc Surg* 1999;30:854-864.
225. Buckley CJ, Abernathy S, Lee SD, et al. Suggested treatment protocol for improving patency of femoral–infrapopliteal cryopreserved saphenous vein allografts. *J Vasc Surg* 2000;32:731-738.
226. Harris L, O'Brien-Irr M, Ricotta JJ. Long-term assessment of cryopreserved vein bypass grafting success. *J Vasc Surg* 2001;33:528-532.
227. Farber A, Major K, Wagner WH, et al. Cryopreserved saphenous vein allografts in infrainguinal revascularization: analysis of 240 grafts. *J Vasc Surg* 2003;38:15-21.
228. Vogt PR, Brunner-La Rocca HP, Carrel T, et al. Cryopreserved arterial allografts in the treatment of major vascular infection: a comparison with conventional surgical techniques. *J Thorac Cardiovasc Surg* 1998;116:965-972.
229. Lesèche G, Castier Y, Petit MD, et al. Long-term results of cryopreserved arterial allograft reconstruction in infected prosthetic grafts and mycotic aneurysms of the abdominal aorta. *J Vasc Surg* 2001;34:616-622.
230. Zhou W, Lin PH, Bush RL, et al. In situ reconstruction with cryopreserved arterial allografts for management of mycotic aneurysms or aortic prosthetic graft infections: a multi-institutional experience. *Tex Heart Inst J* 2006;33:14-318.
231. Kovalic AJ, Beattie DK, Davies AH. Outcome of ProCol, a bovine mesenteric vein graft, in infrainguinal reconstruction. *Eur J Vasc Endovasc Surg* 2002;24:533-534.
232. Brems J, Castaneda M, Garvin PJ. A five-year experience with the bovine heterograft for vascular access. *Arch Surg* 1986;121:941-944.
233. Andersen RC, Ney AL, Madden MC, LaCombe MJ. Biologic conduits for vascular access: saphenous veins, umbilical veins, bovine carotid arteries. In: Sommer BG, Henry ML, eds. Vascular access for hemodialysis. Chicago: Pluribus Press; 1989:65-83.
234. Sabanayagam P, Schwartz AB, Soricelli RR, et al. A comparative study of 402 bovine heterografts and 225 reinforced expanded PTFE grafts as AVF in the ESRD patient. *Trans Am Soc Artif Intern Organs* 1980;26:88-92.
235. Mehta S. Statistical summary of clinical results of vascular access procedures for hemodialysis. In: Sommer BG, Henry ML, eds. Vascular Access for Hemodialysis Chicago: W.L. Gore & Associates, Inc. and Precept Press; 1991:145-147.
236. Katzman HE, Glickman MH, Schild AF, et al. Multicenter evaluation of the bovine mesenteric vein bioprostheses for hemodialysis access in patients with an earlier failed prosthetic graft. *J Am Coll Surg* 2005;201:223-230.
237. Madden RL, Lipkowitz GS, Browne BJ, Kurbanov A. A comparison of cryopreserved vein allografts and prosthetic grafts for hemodialysis access. *Ann Vasc Surg* 2005;19:686-691.
238. Matsuura JH, Black KS, Levitt AB, et al. Cellular remodeling of depopulated bovine ureter used as an arteriovenous graft in the canine model. *J Am Coll Surg* 2004;198:778-783.
239. Spark JI, Yeluri S, Derham C, et al. Incomplete cellular depopulation may explain the high failure rate of bovine ureteric grafts. *Br J Surg* 2008;95:582-585.
240. Warakaulle DR, Evans AL, Cornall AJ, et al. Diagnostic imaging of and radiologic intervention for bovine ureter grafts used as a novel conduit for hemodialysis fistulas. *AJR Am J Roentgenol* 2007;188:641-646.
241. Brewster LP, Bufallino D, Ucuzian A, Greisler HP. Growing a living blood vessel: Insights for the second hundred years. *Biomaterials* 2007;28:5028-5032.
242. Hashi CK, Zhu Y, Yang GY, et al. Antithrombogenic property of bone marrow mesenchymal stem cells in nanofibrous vascular grafts. *Proc Natl Acad Sci USA* 2007;104:1920-11915.
243. Wang X, Lin P, Yao Q, Chen C. Development of small-diameter vascular grafts. *World J Surg* 2007;31:682-689.
244. Niklason LE, Gao J, Abbott WM, et al. Functional arteries grown in vitro. *Science* 1999;284:489-493.
245. L'Heureux N, Dusserre N, Konig G, et al. Human tissue–engineered blood vessels for adult arterial revascularization. *Nat Med* 2006;12:361-365.
246. McKee JA, Banik SS, Boyer MJ, et al. Human arteries engineered in vitro. *EMBO Rep* 2003;4:633-638.

chapter

40

Prosthetic Vascular Graft Infection

Linda M. Reilly, MD

Key Points

- Demographics
- Prevention
- Bacteriology
- Pathogenesis
- Presentation
- Extracavitary graft infections
- Intracavitary graft infections
- Diagnosis
- Anatomical imaging modalities
- Computed tomography scanning
- Magnetic resonance imaging
- Sinography
- Endoscopy
- Functional imaging modalities
- Labeled white blood cell scan
- Flourodeoxyglucose–positron emission tomography
- Operative preparation
- Treatment-infected intracavitary (aortic) grafts
- Extraanatomical bypass and infected graft removal
- In situ prosthetic graft replacement
- In situ arterial allograft replacement
- In situ venous autograft replacement
- In situ venous allograft replacement
- Graft preservation
- Outcomes-infected intracavitary (aortic) grafts
- Treatment-infected extracavitary vascular grafts
- Outcomes-infected extracavitary (nonaortic) vascular grafts
- Adjunctive techniques in the management of vascular graft infection
- Muscle flaps
- Negative-pressure wound therapy
- Localized antimicrobial therapy
- Antimicrobial wound irrigation
- Antibiotic-impregnated beads

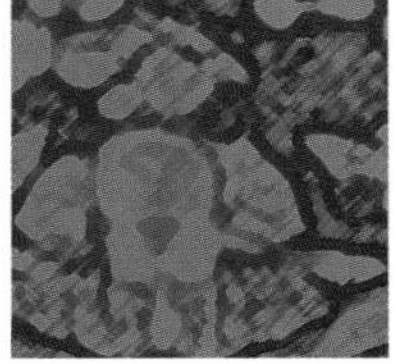

Prosthetic vascular graft infection has always been the diagnosis that no one wants to make. It is a consequence of the treatment of vascular disease with non-tissue conduits. Unlike all other areas of vascular disease, management of prosthetic graft infection has been little altered by the development of and advances in endoluminal technology. Eradication of the infection requires treatment that has significant associated morbidity and mortality, determined predominantly by circumstances that the surgeon has no option to change—the anatomical location of the infected conduit and the clinical status of the patient at the time of presentation. It therefore remains one of the greatest challenges to the skills of the vascular surgeon and poses considerable risk to the health of the patient.

DEMOGRAPHICS

The reported incidence of prosthetic graft infection varies between 0.8% and 6%,[1-5] a frequency that is most influenced by the anatomical location of the involved prosthesis. Prosthetic vascular conduits that have no subcutaneous component have the lowest incidence of infection. Intraabdominal aortoaortic or aortoiliac bypass grafts develop infection in less than 1% of cases.[6,7] Thoracic and thoracoabdominal aortic prosthetic conduits have a reported infection incidence varying between 1% and 2%.[7-11] In contrast, the presence of prosthetic material in the groin increases the rate of infection to 2% to 4%.[7,12] Finally, the longest subcutaneous conduits—those placed in the femoropopliteal, axillofemoral, or axillopopliteal positions—have a reported incidence of infection of 7% to 9%.[13] Although endovascular techniques have not significantly changed the treatment of prosthetic graft infection, accumulated experience to date suggests that endoluminal prosthetic grafts are associated with a lower risk of infection, with reported incidences of less than 1% for aortic prostheses and largely anecdotal reports of infections involving stents and stent grafts in the infrainguinal location.[14-16] All studies acknowledge that reported prosthetic vascular infection rates probably represent a minimal incidence, since complete patient follow-up is necessary to determine the actual rate and such detailed follow-up is rare.

Many factors have been associated with an increased risk of prosthetic vascular graft infection, including patient factors (age, gender, obesity, diabetes, poor glucose control, malnutrition, presence of open skin wounds, immunosuppression, coexistent malignancy), procedural factors (revascularizations that are emergent, reoperative, or lengthy; the presence of a groin incision), and postoperative course factors (sepsis, hypoxemia, hypervolemia, groin wound seroma or hematoma, wound infection, other remote site infections). While several studies have correlated some of these factors with an increased risk of perioperative *wound* infection,[17-19] few studies have actually identified factors that increase the risk of *vascular prosthesis* infection. In a case-controlled study reported by Antonios et al., multivariate analysis identified only groin incision and wound infection as factors increasing the risk of subsequent vascular graft infection. Their study, however, did not include patients undergoing repeat operations, and emergency procedures ($p = 0.09$) and coexistent skin ulcers ($p = 0.07$) showed a near association with increased risk of vascular graft infection.[19] The difficulty in establishing a correlation between any suspected risk factor and subsequent graft infection results from the generally low incidence of graft infection and the necessity for long follow-up to ensure identification of all graft infections.

PREVENTION

Classically, prevention of prosthetic graft infection has focused on the use of antiseptic principles, including meticulous, sterile surgical technique and prophylactic antibiotics. Multiple studies have compared perioperative prophylactic antibiotics with placebo.[20-28] These studies demonstrated a consistent benefit of prophylactic antibiotics in the reduction of wound infection rates.[29] Although no individual study has demonstrated a statistically significant reduction in prosthetic graft infection rates, metaanalysis (fixed-effect model) did show a reduction in early graft infection rates when prophylactic antibiotics were used (relative risk fixed 0.31, 95% confidence interval 0.11 to 0.85, $p = 0.02$).[29] None of these studies provided data about the impact of prophylactic antibiotics on late-appearing graft infections. Other studies have investigated the question of the optimal duration of prophylactic antibiotic administration,[23,30-32] the impact of using broad-spectrum newer-generation antibiotics,[33-36] and the potential benefit of various antibiotic combinations and dosing regimens[22,37-41] on the rate of wound infection and vascular graft infection. The continuation of prophylactic antibiotics beyond 24 hours does not further reduce the rate of either wound infection or graft infection.[29] There is no significant difference in the effect obtained using early- or late-generation antibiotics. None of the tested antibiotic combinations or dosage regimens had any additional impact on the development of wound or prosthetic graft infection.

Preoperative skin antisepsis regimens have also been studied,[42-44] but no additional reduction in wound infection resulted from preoperative bathing with any antiseptic agent when compared to bathing with nonmedicated soap. None of these studies provided data regarding the impact of specific skin preparation techniques on graft infection.

Specific operative protocols for handling of the prosthetic material,[45] as well as postoperative suction groin wound drainage, have also been studied,[46,47] but no reduction in the rate of wound infection was identified and no data regarding subsequent graft infection rates have been provided.

Recently, the use of antimicrobial-bonded (rifampin, silver ion) prosthetic grafts has been investigated. Trials of rifampin bonding have shown no reduction in the rate of either early or late graft infection.[4,48-50] Similarly, silver ion–impregnated prosthetic conduits have not been reported to reduce the incidence of prosthetic graft infection.[7] It is important to bear in mind that the generally low rate of prosthetic graft infection makes it quite difficult to eliminate type 2 error when investigating the impact of any preventive measure on the incidence of graft infection.

BACTERIOLOGY

Gram-positive organisms account for approximately two thirds of all vascular graft infections. In the early era of prosthetic graft implantation, the most common organism recovered from infected grafts was *Staphylococcus aureus.* However, once routine prophylactic antibiotic use was adopted, the spectrum of infecting organisms changed and *Staphylococcus epidermidis* emerged as the most common organism recovered from infected prosthetic grafts.[51] Among gram-negative organisms recovered from infected grafts, the most common are *Escherichia coli, Klebsiella, Proteus, Enterobacter, Pseudomonas, Bacteroides,* and nonhemolytic streptococci. Currently, *S. epidermidis* is recovered from about 45% of graft infections, *S. aureus* from about 40% of infected grafts, and *E. coli* from about 20% of infected prostheses.[52-54] However, when the infected graft is aortic in location, the rate of recovery of coagulase-negative gram-positive organisms declines and that of coagulase-positive gram-positive organisms, as well as the rate of recovery of gram-negative organisms, increases.[55-62] When the aortic graft infection is associated with an aortoenteric fistula, the bacteriology of the infecting organism shifts even more notably to gram-negative organisms.[63]

PATHOGENESIS

The pathways by which prosthetic vascular grafts become infected remain speculative. The two principal mechanisms of graft infection are thought to be bacterial contamination at the time of implantation and hematogenous or lymphogenous transfer of organisms from a remote site.[51,64,65] Hematogenous and lymphogenous seeding may occur early or late after prosthetic graft implantation.

Several potential sources of bacterial contamination are found during implantation of a prosthetic graft. First, the high recovery rate of skin organisms, both *S. epidermidis* and *S. aureus,* from infected vascular conduits supports the theory that direct contamination by contact with skin at the time of graft implantation is a primary mechanism. Second, several studies have documented positive arterial wall cultures in 8% to 45% of specimens tested at the time of clean, elective arterial reconstructive procedures.[66-75] *S. epidermidis* is the organism recovered from these artery cultures in 50% to 70% of cases. While some studies suggested an association between positive arterial wall cultures and subsequent graft infection,[66,70,71] others did not find evidence of such an association.[67,69,72-75] A final potential source of direct prosthesis contamination at the time of graft implantation is the gastrointestinal (GI) tract. Although transudation of intestinal organisms into the peritoneal fluid or the bloodstream, particularly as a result of bowel manipulation during aortic reconstruction procedures, might be expected to yield enteric organisms, *S. epidermidis* is the organism recovered most often.[66,67] However, to date, no study has reported any correlation between this intraoperative finding and subsequent graft infection[66,67,76]

While contamination with a low-virulence organism like *S. epidermidis* at the time of implantation may require a significant interval before the manifestation of clinical symptoms of graft infection, it seems unlikely that all late-appearing graft infections could be traced to contamination at implantation. The possibility of hematogenous or lymphogenous seeding as a mechanism of graft infection may help explain why many graft infections do not appear until years after graft implantation. Laboratory models of prosthetic graft infection have demonstrated that implanted grafts can be seeded with bacterial inocula even many months after implantation. The "infectivity" of the prosthesis by an infection at a remote site is influenced by the interval between implantation and inoculation, as well as the anatomical location of the prosthesis, the graft material, and the organism.[77-81] Many patients undergoing arterial reconstruction have open extremity wounds at the time of implantation of a prosthesis, and it has been hypothesized that this remote site is the source of hematogenous or lymphogenous seeding in the early perioperative period. However, data to support this hypothesis are lacking. In fact, the incidence of open, ischemic, or infected extremity wounds at the time of graft implantation is often in the range of 20% to 50%, which greatly exceeds the rate of graft infection.

The role of hematogenous or lymphogenous seeding in the late postimplantation interval is even more speculative. Since intermittent bacteremia occurs in everyone, this hypothesis fails to differentiate between prostheses that become infected long after implantation and those that do not. The etiology of late graft infection is further confounded by the high incidence of bacterial colonization of clinically uninfected prostheses, explanted at the time of revision for common late complications of vascular reconstructive surgery (thrombosis or false aneurysm formation).[82]

PRESENTATION

The manifestation of a graft infection depends on the interval between graft implantation and infection, the nature of the organism, and the anatomical location of the prosthesis.[52,53,83] Early-appearing graft infections (less than 4 months after implantation) are more likely to involve the graft diffusely and to have systemic manifestations, perhaps because the prosthesis is not yet isolated by the perigraft capsule or because of the nature of the most commonly involved organisms—*S. aureus* and gram-negative organisms. Specific enzymes associated with *S. aureus* infection (catalases, hyaluronidases, coagulases, and proteinases) result in a marked inflammatory reaction, producing suppuration and facilitating local tissue invasion. Gram-negative organisms are somewhat less virulent than *S. aureus* but also cause suppuration and often abscess formation. *Pseudomonas* species, in particular, demonstrate vascular wall invasion, pseudoaneurysm formation, and occasionally arterial wall disruption. In contrast to these organisms, *S. epidermidis,* a common causative organism in late-appearing graft infections, is a low-virulence organism, producing an indolent infection. *S. epidermidis* produces a glycocalyx biofilm ("slime") layer that effectively sequesters the organism, resulting in protection for the organism and a muted host response. These infections tend to manifest years after prosthesis implantation. While the involvement of the graft by these infections may be focal or diffuse, patients are more likely to manifest only focal findings of localized fluid collections (with or without associated cellulitis), recurrent draining wounds, or chronic sinus tracts.

Extracavitary Graft Infections

Extracavitary graft infections (involving femorofemoral, femoropopliteal, or axillofemoral grafts) tend to present early[53] and most commonly demonstrate local signs of infection such as cellulitis, induration, and inflammation. A wound mass or wound drainage is common, as are fever and leukocytosis. A pulsatile wound mass (false aneurysm) occurs less often but is not rare. Few studies delineate the common manifestations of infection involving extracavitary grafts, and unfortunately the available data often include the femoral limb of an aortofemoral bypass graft as an "extracavitary" graft.

Intracavitary Graft Infections

Intracavitary graft infections (involving aortoiliac, aortofemoral, or iliofemoral grafts) tend to present late[53] and have a broader potential spectrum of symptoms (Table 40-1). Infections due to low-virulence organisms most commonly manifest with a focal wound infection, fluid collection, or draining sinus tract. Systemic symptoms are rare. Infections due to high-virulence organisms present with systemic symptoms, but these may vary from quite subtle malaise, discomfort in the region of the prosthesis, and weight loss to obvious fever, leukocytosis, bacteremia, and sepsis. As in the case of extracavitary graft infections, false aneurysms may occur if infection has disrupted an anastomosis (Figure 40-1).

Intracavitary graft infections associated with prosthetic-enteric fistulas or erosions should be considered differently because they more likely represent an initial mechanical problem, followed by contamination, infection, or both of the exposed prosthesis. They present late, not because of a low-virulence causative organism but because the erosion requires time to develop. While at least 65% to 75% of erosions and fistulas have some associated GI blood loss, others are entirely occult and discovered only when treatment of the associated graft infection is undertaken. Prosthetic-enteric fistulas and erosions are most likely to present with fever, leukocytosis, bacteremia, and sepsis, but the overall frequency is still low. The pattern of bleeding results from the type of communication with the GI tract. Erosions tend to present with episodic subacute or chronic low-grade bleeding because the source of bleeding is the eroded edge of the bowel wall. Fistulas

Table 40-1
Spectrum of Clinical Presentation of Intracavitary (Aortic) Graft Infections

		(%)														
Study	*n*	Enteric Fistula or Erosion	Fever	Malaise	Groin Wound Abscess or Infection or Mass	Graft Occlusion	Elevated White Blood Cell Count	Sepsis	Gastrointestinal Bleeding	False Aneurysm	Sinus Tract	Septic Emboli	Other Bleeding	Retroperitoneal Abscess	Abdominal Pain	Acute Ischemia
Armstrong et al.[84]	29	100			4			10	72	4[*]				10	10	
Bandyk et al.[53]	68	37	36		28	2		10	33	28	18	0				
Batt et al.[55]	24	54	38	8	33	4	38	38	25	8[*]					17	4
Becquemin et al.[85]	20	15			80				15	40[†]	10	5	40[‡]			
Daenens et al.[86]	49	No data			20	12		43		22[†]	31	2		4		4
Dorigo et al.[57]	30	100	80				40	27	70	17[*]						
Fiorani et al.[87]	18	50	67		25				39	25[†]	42					
Gabriel et al.[58]	63	0	11		8	17				25	17		6[‡]			
Leseche et al.[60]	23	43	43		61	13	43	43	22	26						13
Menawat et al.[63]	52	100	37	19		17	48		52	6	17	8				33
Seeger et al.[62]	53	19			43	8		23	19	8	2					4
Seeger et al.[88]	36	0			44	11		31		14						11
Young et al.[89]	25	60	24	12	56				40		32					

[*]Proximal.
[†]Femoral.
[‡]Groin bleeding.

involve the artery–prosthesis suture line and tend to present with acute bleeding, including the typical herald bleeding episode, because the source of bleeding is the arterial lumen itself.[90] When the GI tract communication is associated with an anastomotic false aneurysm, infection may be the primary development (causing the false aneurysm), with GI tract erosion secondary to the mass effect of the false aneurysm. Occult graft infection presenting as acute ischemia secondary to graft or graft limb occlusion is rare, as is septic embolization.

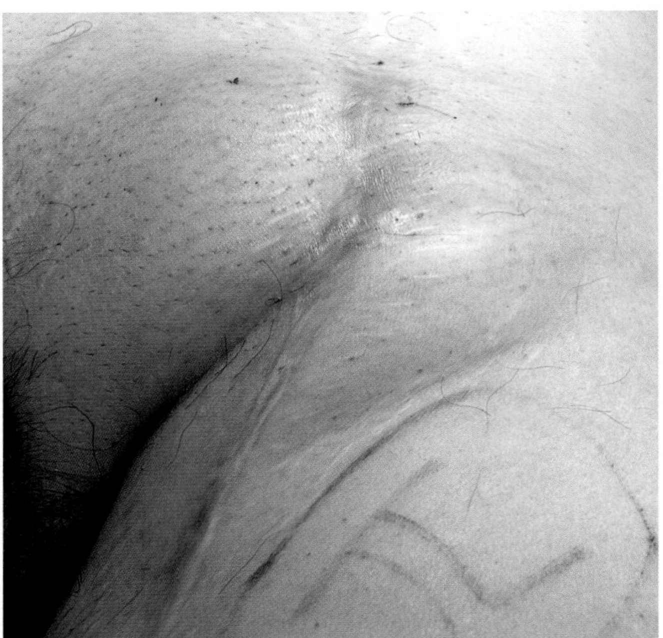

Figure 40-1. Aortobifemoral graft infection manifesting as a left groin mass with overlying erythema.

DIAGNOSIS

The diagnosis of vascular graft infection can be extremely challenging, particularly for intracavitary grafts and for infections caused by low-virulence organisms. Furthermore, optimal treatment requires determination of the extent of involvement of the graft by the infection. Szilagyi et al. established the first descriptive system for graft infection,[91] which has since been modified by Koenig and vonDongen[92] and by Samson et al.[93] (Table 40-2). While these classification systems facilitate comparisons of matched cases of graft infection, they are somewhat confusing. For example, group 1 and 2 "graft infections" in each scheme are not graft infections. Not surprisingly, inclusion of any of these "infections" biases the success of the treatment approach, since there actually was no graft infection.

When the diagnosis of graft infection is clear (exposed prosthesis, purulence surrounding a prosthesis at operative exploration), the goal of further investigation is to establish the extent of graft involvement. When the diagnosis is unclear, then both the presence of infection and the extent of graft involvement are the goals of diagnostic evaluation. All modalities used to evaluate prosthetic graft infection are inferential, since none can actually "see" infection. Rather, each modality looks for changes that are consequences of infection. The ideal diagnostic method would detect a change that is unique to

Table 40-2
Prosthetic Graft Infection Classification Systems

Szilagyi et al.[91]		Koenig and vonDongen[92]		Samson et al.[93]	
Group 1	Infection involves only the dermis	Group 1	Infection extends no deeper than the dermis	Group 1	Infections extend no deeper than the dermis
Group 2	Infection extends into the subcutaneous tissue but does not invade the arterial implant	Group 2	Infection is in the subcutaneous tissue but does not involve the graft	Group 2	Infections involve subcutaneous tissues but do not come into grossly observable direct contact with the graft
Group 3	The arterial implant proper is involved in the infection	Group 3	Infection involves the body of the graft	Group 3	Infections involve the body of the graft but not at an anastomosis
		Stage 1	The body of the graft is infected without the secondary complications of bleeding, thrombosis, and systemic sepsis	Group 4	Infections surround an exposed anastomosis, but bacteremia or anastomotic bleeding has not occurred
		Stage 2	A trickle of bleeding occurs from anastomosis with no thrombosis of graft or systemic sepsis	Group 5	Infections involve a graft-to-artery anastomosis and are associated with septicemia, bleeding, or both at the time of presentation
		Stage 3	Infection is complicated by massive bleeding, systemic sepsis, or bleeding		

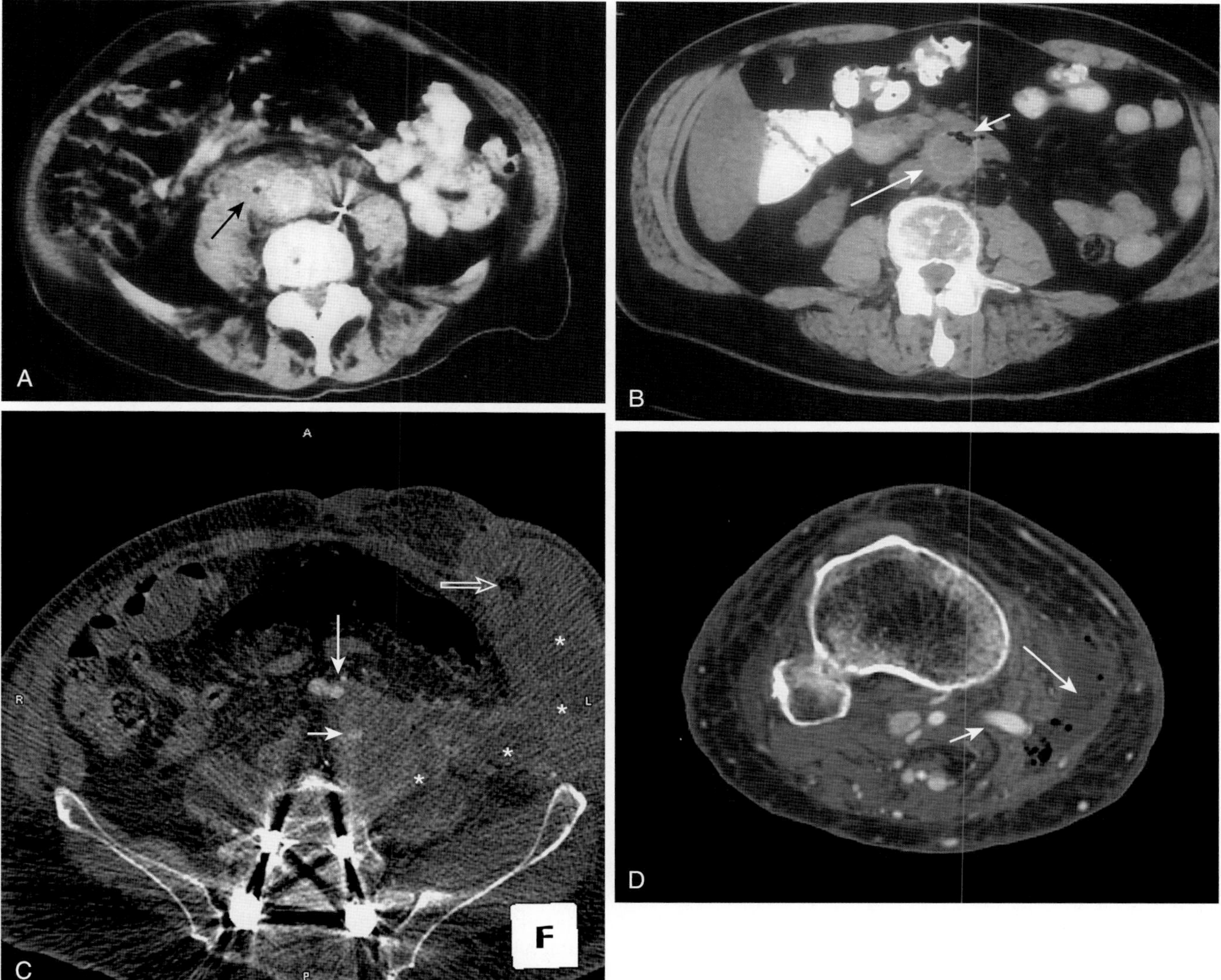

Figure 40-2. Selection of computed tomography (CT) images demonstrating typical findings consistent with vascular graft infection. **A,** CT scan (axial image) showing perigraft fluid with air *(arrow)*. **B,** Computed tomography scan showing thickened perigraft tissue *(large arrow)* and air within the graft and perigraft tissue *(small arrow)*. **C,** CT scan showing left limb of aortobifemoral bypass *(vertical arrow)* surrounded by a large false aneurysm with a small blush of contrast *(small arrow)*. The false aneurysm communicates with a large abscess (*) extending from the retroperitoneum into the left lateral abdominal wall. Note air within the abscess *(large arrow)*. **D,** CT scan of the right leg showing complex abscess containing air at the infrageniculate level *(long arrow)*. Note patent expanded polytetrafluoroethylene bypass graft in continuity with the abscess *(short arrow)*.

the presence of infection. No such diagnostic modality exists; therefore, it is common to use multiple modalities, with the goal of increasing the overall diagnostic accuracy. Diagnostic modalities can be categorized as either anatomical or functional.

Anatomical Imaging Modalities

Computed Tomography Scanning

Computed tomography (CT) scanning is probably the current gold standard among modalities used to diagnose prosthetic graft infection. Findings on CT scan that correlate with graft infection include perigraft fluid, perigraft soft-tissue changes (loss of tissue planes), ectopic gas, presence of a pseudoaneurysm, and focal bowel wall thickening (Figure 40-2). It is evident from this list that many of these findings are not pathognomonic of a graft infection. When CT was first used, reported sensitivity and specificity approached 90% to 100%.[94-96] However, those results were obtained using the criteria listed earlier that probably represent more advanced graft infections. When graft infection is low-grade, CT sensitivity drops to about 50% to 65%.[97,98] The advantages of CT are its ready availability and its ability to assess the remainder of the contents of the anatomical location of the vascular graft. CT also allows the surgeon to define the arterial anatomy (mandatory for planning the reconstruction portion of the procedure) and perform simultaneous interventions (such as needle aspiration). In addition, CT is a study that the vascular surgeon can readily interpret without assistance. The disadvantages of CT scanning include the need for contrast, as well as image artifact induced by metallic implants. Nonetheless, most would

Table 40-3
Accuracy of Imaging Modalities in Vascular Graft Infection*

	(%)			
	Sensitivity	Specificity	Positive Predictive Value	Negative Predictive Value
CT scan[98]	64	86	70	83
MRI[100]	68	97	95	80
Tc-labeled WBC[104]	100	92		
FDG-PET scan[98,111]	91	64	56	93
PET/CT[107]	93	91	88	96
In-labeled WBC[100]	73	87	80	82

*CT, computed tomography; FDG, fluorodeoxyglucose; MRI, magnetic resonance imaging; PET, positron emission tomography; Tc, technetium; WBC, white blood cell.

agree that CT is the initial study of choice to both diagnose and assess the extent of prosthetic vascular graft infection.

Magnetic Resonance Imaging

Magnetic resonance imaging (MRI) has many of the same advantages as CT scanning. It can provide an assessment of the surrounding anatomical area, is readily available, and can define the arterial anatomy. It has the additional advantage that it can differentiate fluid and inflammation from subacute or chronic hematoma, which CT scanning cannot. This probably makes it more useful in assessing the possibility of graft infection in the early postimplantation interval. It does not require contrast administration and has no radiation exposure. Signal voids from metallic clips or calcium may be impossible to differentiate from air. It is more expensive, and unfortunately the recent recognition of nephrogenic systemic fibrosis precludes its use in patients with renal insufficiency, particularly those with diabetes.[99] Reported sensitivity and specificity for MRI are slightly better than those for CT scanning[100] (Table 40-3).

Sinography

Although the presence of a sinus tract is only an occasional finding in a patient with suspected graft infection (Table 40-1), it offers a diagnostic approach that addresses not only the presence of infection but also its extent. Sinography is performed by placing a small catheter in the tract and injecting contrast agent under fluoroscopy. It demonstrates whether or not the tract communicates with the perigraft space and shows how far the contrast agent tracks along the perigraft space, providing definitive evidence of the extent of graft involvement by the infection. Sinography is unique among all diagnostic modalities used to investigate graft infection in that it provides such direct information about the presence and extent of infection.

Endoscopy

Endoscopy is only relevant when evaluating the possibility of infection involving an intracavitary graft and particularly when determining whether or not an associated enteric erosion or fistula occurred. It is most often employed when some evidence exists of GI bleeding, raising suspicion of communication between the graft and the GI tract. Esophagogastroduodenoscopy should be performed with a pediatric colonoscope because the most common site of fistulization or erosion is the third or fourth portion of the duodenum. A standard-length esophagogastroduodenoscopy scope may not be able to examine sufficiently far into the GI tract to reach the area of pathology. Careful examination is required since the spectrum of findings varies from the quite obvious to the subtle (Figure 40-3). Both upper and lower endoscopy should be performed when investigating any aortic graft infection, since involvement of the GI tract can occur at any level (Figure 40-4) and such involvement may be entirely occult. Like sinography, endoscopy can provide direct information about the presence of a graft infection, but it does not provide information about the extent of graft involvement.

Functional Imaging Modalities

Labeled White Blood Cell Scan

The short comings of anatomical studies such as CT and MRI, particularly their inability to differentiate between an abnormality of healing and an abnormality of healing *due to infection* prompted a search for functional tests that could provide this assessment. Nuclear medicine techniques potentially allow infection to be detected on the basis of molecular biology processes. These modalities include labeled white cell scans (using indium or technetium-99m), and fluorodeoxyglucose–positron emission tomography (FDG-PET). Labeled white cell scans were a significant improvement over techniques using gallium as there is little platelet cross labeling, no GI uptake, and therefore a better signal-to-noise ratio.[101-104] However white cells are present in both inflammation and infection, processes that cannot be differentiated using this technique. This is a particular problem in the early postimplantation interval or in the setting of a recent invasive procedure.

Fluorodeoxyglucose–Positron Emission Tomography

A recent addition to the diagnostic armamentarium is FDG-PET.[105-109] In theory, its sensitivity derives from the increased FDG uptake observed in activated inflammatory cells.[110] This, combined with the other advantages of PET (rapid, better spatial resolution), leads to high sensitivity, although this is inevitably associated with a low specificity (high false-positive rate). FDG-PET shares this increased false-positive rate with other nuclear medicine imaging techniques. Studies have suggested the combination of FDG-PET and CT scanning (combining an anatomical modality with a functional one) can overcome this problem, and early results are encouraging[111] (Table 40-3). The Keidar et al. study was also notable for its success in distinguishing adjacent soft-tissue infection from graft involvement.

The diagnosis of vascular graft infection is certainly not easy, particularly for intracavitary grafts. Even the most experienced vascular surgeon using the diagnostic modalities with the highest yield often faces a situation in which the suspicion of graft infection exists but confirmatory data are lacking. As a consequence, in some circumstances operative exploration may be necessary to establish the diagnosis.

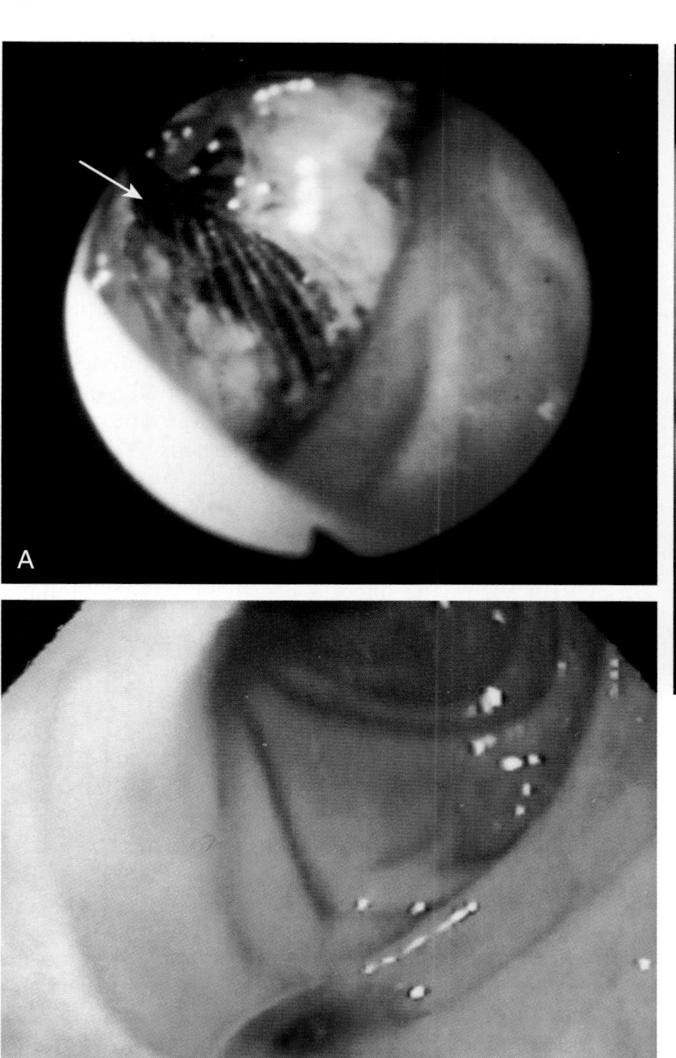

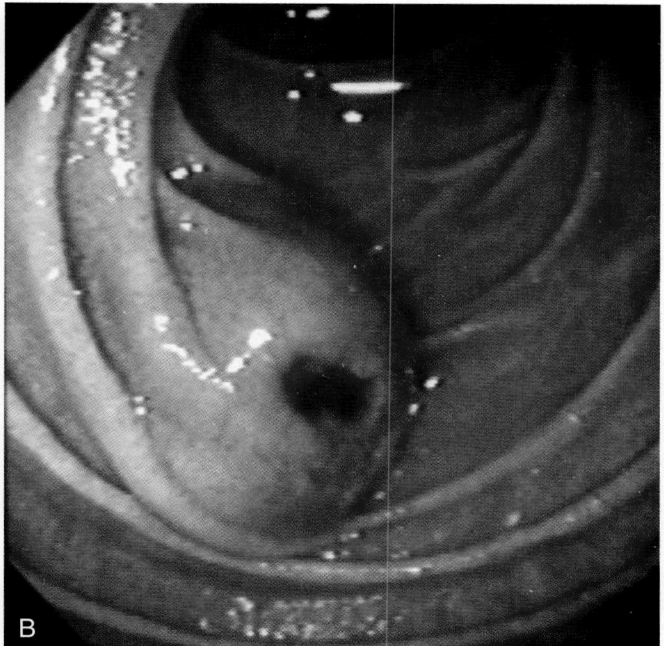

Figure 40-3. Spectrum of esophagogastroduodenoscopy findings in patients with enteric involvement by a prosthetic vascular graft. **A,** Dacron fabric of vascular graft visible in duodenal lumen. **B,** Mass secondary to anastomotic false aneurysm distorting duodenal wall, with associated overlying central mucosal ulceration. **C,** Small ulcer-like duodenal lesion without associated mass or visible graft material.

OPERATIVE PREPARATION

Before treatment, all patients should be placed on appropriately broad antibiotic coverage designed to treat any organisms recovered from wounds, drainage, blood, or tissue, as well as other common infecting organisms. Once intraoperative cultures have delineated the specific organism or organisms responsible for the infection, the antibiotic coverage should be focused accordingly. All patients require delineation of all relevant arterial anatomy to optimally plan the reconstruction. This information may be obtained from the high-quality CT scan obtained during the diagnostic evaluation of the patient. However, if any areas of the arterial anatomy have not been clearly defined, then the patient should undergo catheter angiography as well.

TREATMENT-INFECTED INTRACAVITARY (AORTIC) GRAFTS

Successful treatment of vascular graft infection requires eradication of the infection while maintaining perfusion to the tissue supplied by the infected prosthesis. The traditional treatment approach consisted of removal of the infected prosthesis, with revascularization determined by the adequacy of the remaining perfusion through the native circulation. If the original revascularization was performed for occlusive disease, then native vessel perfusion might be sufficient, but if the original procedure was performed for aneurysmal disease, revascularization after removal of the infected prosthesis would be required. This approach to treatment was associated with mortality rates

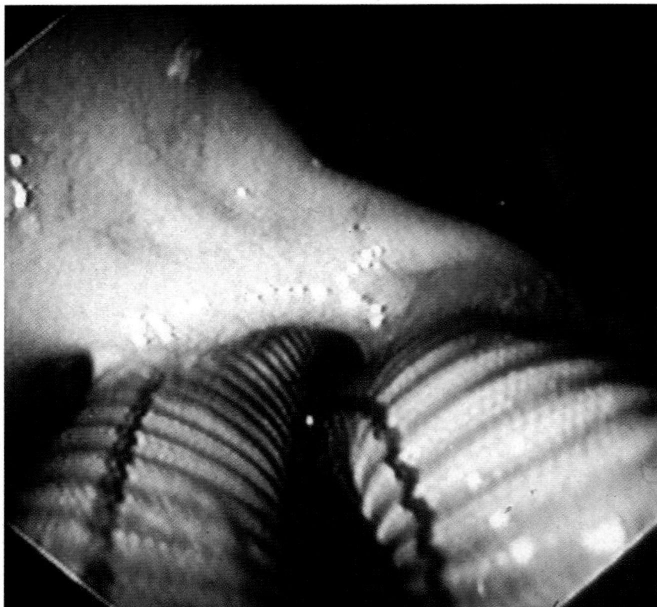

Figure 40-4. Colonoscopic demonstration of both limbs of an aortobifemoral graft within the colon lumen.

of 25% to 50%, as well as major amputation rates of 11% to 30%.[112-114] Such results were not surprising in view of the long periods of extensive ischemia that often resulted and the limited options for revascularization that avoided the infected field. Experience with the technique of extraanatomical bypass was in its infancy, and really only one conduit material was available. The initial improvement in outcomes resulted from advances in conduit materials, the use of tissue conduits, reversal of the sequence of the procedures (performing revascularization before infected graft removal), the staging of lengthy, complex procedures, and finally, improvements in perioperative patient care. Subsequent series of extraanatomical bypass through uninfected fields, infected graft removal, and debridement of the infected tissue reported mortality rates of 7% to 25% and major amputation rates of 5% to 25%.[1,88,115-121] This significant progress still left considerable room for further improvement.

Several other advances soon prompted an almost complete reassessment of the principles long considered basic to successful treatment of infected vascular prostheses. First, the routine use of perioperative antibiotics shifted the most common causative organism in vascular graft infection from the high-virulence *S. aureus* to the low-virulence *S. epidermidis*. Second, reports emerged of the successful treatment of infection involving orthopedic and cardiothoracic implants without complete foreign body removal. Third, the application of tissue-transfer techniques (muscle flaps and myocutaneous flaps) to the management of complex wounds was increasingly successful. Fourth, advances in tissue preservation techniques allowed access to preserved arterial and venous tissue conduits. Finally, prosthetic conduits impregnated with antimicrobial agents became available. As a result of these developments, vascular surgeons began to investigate several alternative approaches to the management of prosthetic graft infection. Currently, the treatment of infected vascular grafts falls into one of five major approaches:

1. Extraanatomical bypass through noninfected tissue fields, followed (either immediately or after an interval of 2 to 5 days) by removal on the infected prosthesis and debridement of the infected tissue beds
2. Removal of the infected prosthetic conduit, followed immediately by in situ reconstruction with another prosthetic graft, with or without antimicrobial impregnation
3. Removal of the infected prosthetic conduit, followed immediately by in situ reconstruction using arterial allograft
4. Removal of the infected prosthetic conduit, followed immediately by in situ reconstruction using venous autograft or allograft
5. Surgical debridement, tissue coverage, and partial or complete preservation of the infected prosthesis

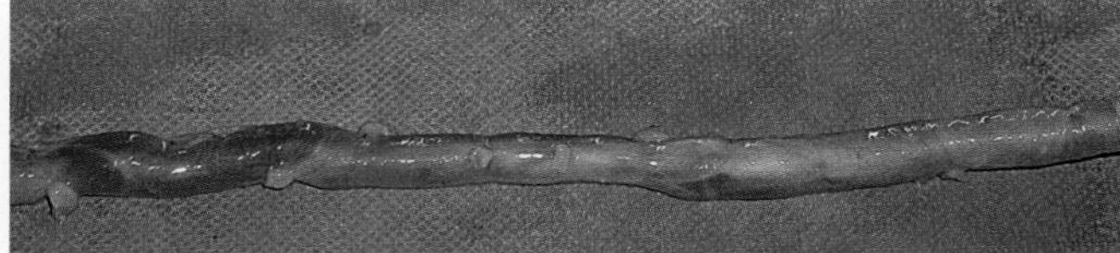

Figure 40-5. Cryopreserved superficial femoral vein conduit.

Extraanatomical Bypass and Infected Graft Removal

The extraanatomical approach is considered the gold standard for the treatment of vascular graft infection, since it completely removes the infected material and the new revascularization is placed through uninfected tissue.[53,57,58,61-63,84,88,115-127] The preferred conduit for the extraanatomical bypass is a prosthetic axillofemoral graft, usually expanded polytetrafluoroethylene, and either a prosthetic or an autogenous cross-femoral conduit, depending on whether infection involves the graft at the femoral level or not. The distal axillofemoral graft anastomosis is performed to the common femoral artery if no groin infection occurs. Otherwise, it is performed to the superficial femoral artery (SFA), if patent, or to the profunda femoral artery if the SFA is occluded. Both the SFA and the profunda femoral artery should be approached lateral to the sartorius muscle to avoid entry into the contaminated femoral triangle. Cross-femoral perfusion is established by direct ilioiliac anastomosis—if the aortic graft is a tube graft and the iliac arteries are not diseased—or by femorofemoral bypass. If direct ilioiliac anastomosis is feasible, it is performed at the time of transabdominal removal of the infected graft, not at the time of extraanatomical revascularization. The femorofemoral conduit is prosthetic in the absence of groin infection. If groin infection is present, then the conduit used is saphenous vein, superficial femoral vein, endarterectomized (previously occluded) SFA, or cryopreserved vein. Currently, our preferred cross-femoral conduit is cryopreserved superficial femoral vein (Figure 40-5), because it is a large conduit, resists infection, and avoids the additional operative time and morbidity involved when an autogenous conduit (vein or artery) is harvested. We always perform the revascularization first, followed by infected graft removal, either under the same anesthetic or after a short interval.

Extraanatomical bypass and infected graft removal is the treatment with the greatest likelihood of complete eradication of the infection. Potential disadvantages include creating long intervals of extensive tissue ischemia if the infected graft is removed first. This can be avoided by creating the new revascularization first.[57,62,63,87,88,122,123] The procedure is complex and lengthy, but this can be mitigated by staging the procedure, performing the new revascularization, and then waiting a few days before removing the infected prosthesis.[57,62,63,87,88,122,124] Additional disadvantages include the creation of an aortic stump with some potential for delayed rupture, the impaired durability of extraanatomical bypasses, and the difficulty of avoiding contamination of the extraanatomical bypass when infection occurs in one or both groins. This latter problem has led some to use bilateral axillounifemoral grafts, or bilateral axillopopliteal bypasses, rather than an construct the axillobifemoral bypass as described earlier.[62,88,123] Unfortunately, those unilateral bypasses demonstrate significantly worse long-term patency rates. To achieve the optimal outcome with this technique, the surgeon should take the following steps:

1. Perform the extraanatomical revascularization first.
2. Use axillobifemoral bypass and avoid unilateral conduits.
3. Preserve as much runoff for the extraanatomical bypass as possible by maintaining flow to the deep femoral artery and to the native iliac arteries. If the infected bypass is an aortofemoral bypass, this requires patching the site of the femoral anastomosis.
4. Use tissue cross-femoral conduits if the infected bypass is aortofemoral in location and infection involves the graft in one or both groins. Options include saphenous vein or superficial femoral vein autografts or allografts, endarterectomized SFA (if chronically occluded), and arterial allografts.
5. Use a staged approach, removing the infected prosthesis after an interval of 2 to 5 days.

In Situ Prosthetic Graft Replacement

Two observations led to the use of in situ prosthetic graft replacement to treat aortic graft infection. The first was that unstable patients bleeding from an aortoenteric fistula, without antecedent or concurrent signs of infection, were occasionally successfully managed with in situ replacement using another prosthetic graft. The second was the emergence of low-virulence pathogens. Since the traditional treatment of infected graft removal and extraanatomical bypass was still associated with significant (although improved) mortality, amputation, extraanatomical bypass infection, and aortic stump disruption rates, the search for a simpler, safer, and more durable approach to aortic graft infection turned to in situ replacement of the infected aortic prosthesis with another prosthesis. It was hoped that this simpler procedure would reduce mortality and that maintaining inline flow would reduce both mortality (avoid aortic stump disruption) and amputation rates. Initially, in situ graft replacement was limited to patients with aortic graft infections secondary to low-virulence pathogens. As experience with the technique accumulated, the indications have expanded to include patients with aortoenteric fistula or erosion. The procedure includes complete infected graft excision, debridement of the surrounding infected and inflamed tissue, intraoperative irrigation with antibiotic or antiseptic, inline replacement with a new prosthetic graft, routing of the graft limbs through new tunnels (when feasible), and 360-degree omental or other tissue coverage of the new prosthesis.[61,63,85,87,89,122,127] Some have recommended placing the new prosthesis through an alternate route that does not bring it into contact with the infected prosthesis, although it seems such an approach would be feasible in only a limited number of cases.[128,129] Some favor use of expanded polytetrafluoroethylene as the conduit material, while others routinely use polyester (Dacron) grafts. Implantation of prostheses impregnated with antimicrobial agents, such as silver ion[55] or antibiotics (rifampin),[53,61,84,89,127,130-135] may result in fewer reinfections, which is the greatest concern about this treatment technique. Intravenous antibiotics are administered for 6 to 8 weeks, and some proponents of this treatment approach also use lifelong suppressive oral antibiotics. If the causative organism is of high virulence or if an associated retroperitoneal abscess is found, this technique is not recommended, as the outcomes are notably worse.[61] The advantages of this technique are that it is a simpler operative procedure, there is no aortic stump, and inline flow is preserved. The potential disadvantages include reinfection of the new prosthesis, anastomotic disruption, the inability to accurately identify the causative organism preoperatively, the need for extended (even lifelong) antibiotic use, and the need for extended monitoring of the new prosthesis.

In Situ Arterial Allograft Replacement

Arterial allografts were actually the first conduits used in vascular reconstruction but were abandoned because of a significant incidence of late degeneration, including dilation, rupture, wall calcification, and thrombosis.[136] The development of prosthetic conduits supplanted arterial allograft conduits in the treatment of vascular disease. Presumably, the experience of cardiac surgeons using aortic homografts in the treatment of infected aortic valves suggested the possibility that arterial allografts could be used to treat infected vascular grafts. However, it is not clear why investigators thought the allograft conduits would have a different clinical course than originally experienced. This approach represented the initial attempt to maintain inline flow after removal of an infected aortic prosthesis, without placing another foreign body in the infected field.[11,56,58,60,126,136-152] In this procedure, the entire infected prosthesis is removed, the perigraft bed is irrigated with antimicrobial agents (antibiotic or povidone-iodine), and the perigraft tissues are debrided. The anastomoses are performed with monofilament sutures, and all aortic allograft branches are repaired with monofilament sutures. The allograft conduit is placed in the field with the lumbar branches on the ventral side to facilitate resuturing if initial suturing is not hemostatic. The allografts are covered with a pedicle omentoplasty in almost all cases. Vogt et al.[151] emphasized several technical points in the handling of arterial allograft conduits:

1. The importance of suturing the side branches, avoiding ties or clips
2. The importance of appropriate conduit length because the tensile strength of these conduits is significantly less than that of prosthetic grafts (although better than fresh arterial allografts)
3. The importance of tension-free anastomoses

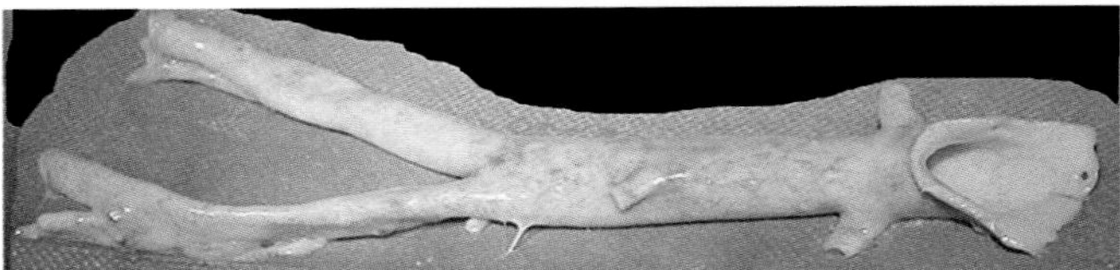

Figure 40-6. Cryopreserved aortoiliac arterial conduit.

4. Liberal reinforcement of the anastomosis with strips of allograft
5. Aggressive and thorough drainage of any adjacent infection

Patients receive a 6- to 8-week course of antibiotics, initially using a parenteral route and then using an oral one. Patients are not placed on immunosuppressive therapy. Initially, freshly harvested arterial allografts were used,[11,138,146] but these conduits again showed a notable tendency to become aneurysmal and to disrupt. Subsequently studies only used cryopreserved arterial allografts as conduits (Figure 40-6). Because of significant issues with availability, use of ABO-matched conduits occurred only in about two thirds of patients. The potential advantages of this technique are that it is a less complex procedure, maintains inline flow, allows complete excision of the infected conduit, and eliminates the use of any prosthetic material in the revascularization and that the arterial conduits demonstrate better resistance to infection than a prosthetic conduit. Potential disadvantages include lack of availability, significant potential for conduit failure (rupture, aneurysmal degeneration, infection, rejection due to immunogenicity), and the need for extended monitoring of the conduit.

In Situ Venous Autograft Replacement

The use of vein conduits has long been a cornerstone of vascular reconstructive surgery. However, the innovation applied to the treatment of aortic graft infection was the use of the superficial femoral vein–popliteal vein complex as a conduit to replace the infected aortic prosthesis, termed the neoaortoiliac system procedure.[2] Prior attempts to use saphenous vein to reconstruct the aortoiliac system generally failed as the saphenous veins were simply not large enough. Failures were both hemodynamic (inadequate caliber to support sufficient flow) and anatomical (kinking, compression, or both along the long course from the infrarenal aortic stump to the femoral artery). The use of the larger superficial femoral–popliteal vein conduits eliminated both of these problems.[2,53,59,84,86,125,153-161] Before the procedure, duplex ultrasonography is used to assess the adequacy of the saphenous vein caliber and the patency of the superficial femoral and popliteal veins. If the saphenous vein caliber is sufficient to warrant use (at least 7 or 8 mm), then vein harvest is planned so that only the saphenous vein or the superficial femoral vein is harvested from a given leg, preserving one of the veins in each leg. Vein harvest is a clean procedure, so any open wounds are excluded from the field during vein conduit harvesting. The saphenous vein is harvested in the standard manner. The superficial femoral vein is harvested through a continuous incision placed along the lateral border of the sartorius muscle. The muscle is reflected medially, and the vein is mobilized. All branches are ligated or suture ligated with monofilament suture on the vein side. The vein is harvested from the level of the profunda femoris vein as far distally into the popliteal vein as needed to obtain adequate length of venous conduit. The profunda vein must be preserved. Also, to prevent thrombus formation in any residual stump of the superficial femoral vein, the superficial femoral vein is transected flush at its junction with the profunda femoris vein and the end is carefully oversewn without impinging on the profunda vein lumen. The harvesting wounds are then closed and sealed. The procedure continues with exposure and mobilization of the infected prosthesis. When the infected prosthesis has been excised and the surrounding infected tissues debrided, the superficial femoral vein is usually placed in a nonreversed orientation to match the largest diameter of the vein with the transected end of the aorta. The vein is usually anastomosed end to end to the aorta. However, if a significant size discrepancy occurs between the superficial femoral vein and the aorta, two segments of superficial femoral vein can be anastomosed to each other and then end to end to the aorta in a pantaloon fashion. Alternatively, the size discrepancy can be managed by oversewing the aorta and anastomosing the vein conduit to the anterior surface of the aorta in the pararenal location. The revascularization can be constructed as an aortobifemoral conduit, an aortounifemoral conduit with a suprapubic femorofemoral limb, or an aortounifemoral conduit with the limb to the contralateral leg originating from the intraabdominal portion of the aortounifemoral graft. The conduits are usually placed in the original tunnels. Some authors use muscle flap coverage of the conduits in the groins, but others do not. The advantages of this approach are maintenance of inline perfusion, complete removal of the infected prosthesis, absence of all prosthetic material, availability of conduit, lack of any conduit immunogenicity issues, and improved resistance of the vein to recurrent infection. The disadvantages are a formidable procedure length, the presence of prior deep venous thrombosis with vein recanalization, the prior harvesting of the saphenous vein, and the consequences of deep vein harvesting—venous hypertension, significant leg edema, venous compartment syndrome, and a need for fasciotomy.

In Situ Venous Allograft Replacement

The technique that my colleagues and I have used to treat most aortic graft infections in the past 5 years is in situ aortic reconstruction using cryopreserved vein allograft conduits. We believe that this technique has the advantages of preserving inline flow, eliminating all prosthetic material and avoiding an aortic stump. It avoids the risk of recurrent infection associated with prosthetic graft reimplantation, the risk of conduit failure and challenge of availability associated with cryopreserved arterial allografts, and the long operative times and venous hypertension morbidity associated with vein autograft harvesting. Although others have reported the use of cryopreserved superficial femoral vein to treat femorofemoral graft infection,[162] and one report details the use of fresh vein allografts to treat intracavitary prosthetic graft infection,[163] no reports exist of the use of cryopreserved vein conduits to treat aortic graft infection. As described earlier, the revascularization can be constructed as an aortobifemoral graft or an aortounifemoral graft with an intraabdominal iliofemoral crossover limb or a suprapubic crossover limb (Figure 40-7). We almost always use sartorius myoplasty to cover the vein grafts in the groin and facilitate groin wound healing (Figure 40-8). To date, we have treated 37 patients with intracavitary aortic graft infections. Forty percent

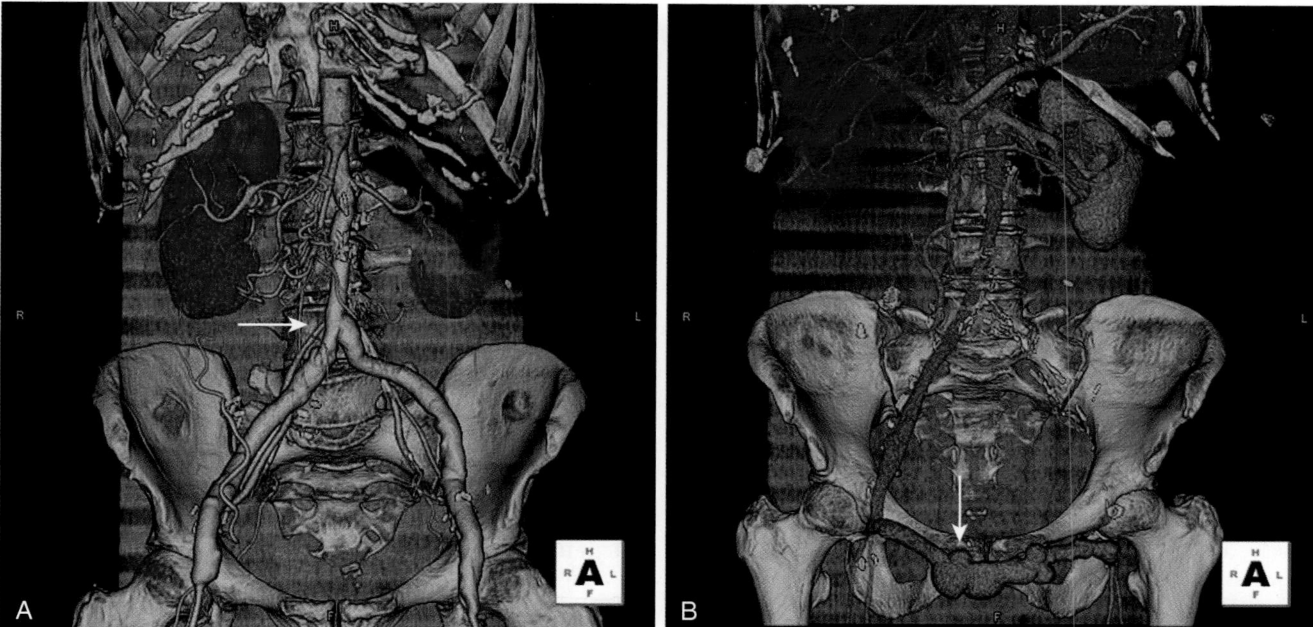

Figure 40-7. Postoperative three-dimensional reconstruction of computed tomography angiograms of inline aortic reconstruction using cryopreserved superficial femoral veins. **A,** Revascularization as an aortobifemoral bypass. Note the more distal location of the intraabdominal anastomosis of the contralateral limb *(arrow)*. **B,** Revascularization as an aortounifemoral bypass with contralateral limb perfusion provided by a femorofemoral conduit. Note the aneurysmal degeneration of the cross-femoral conduit *(arrow),* which was subsequently replaced with a prosthetic graft. Note the lack of aneurysmal degeneration of the retroperitoneal cryovein graft segment.

had an associated enteric erosion or fistula. All infected aortic grafts were completely excised. The perioperative mortality was 16.2% ($n = 6$): 3 from cardiac events, 1 from visceral infarction, 1 from *Candida sepsis*, and 1 probably from a persistent enteric fistula with secondary reinfection of the aortic reconstruction. During mean follow-up of 22 months, no further deaths were related to the graft infection or its treatment, but 7 additional deaths (18.9%) occurred related to underlying comorbidities. Three patients required early reexploration for bleeding from a side branch of the conduit, as we learned the optimal method to secure the side branches. One patient required several graft revisions for recurrent false aneurysm formation at one femoral anastomosis, ultimately successful. Three patients required replacement of the cross-femoral cryovein conduit for aneurysmal degeneration (Figure 40-7B) that developed an average of 34 months postoperatively. In each case, the degenerated conduit was replaced with a prosthetic conduit, as the infection had long been eradicated. We have not seen any aneurysmal degeneration of the retroperitoneal cryovein graft segments, only the subcutaneous and groin segments. No amputations, aortic suture line disruptions, graft stenoses, or graft thromboses occurred during follow-up. We believe that two (5.4%) grafts became infected—the patient who died with a probable persistent enteric fistula and the patient who required several early revisions of a cryovein segment for recurrent false aneurysm formation—although organisms could not be recovered from either conduit.

Graft Preservation

The opposite end of the treatment spectrum for aortic graft infection is complete or partial preservation of the infected prosthesis. This treatment approach requires surgical

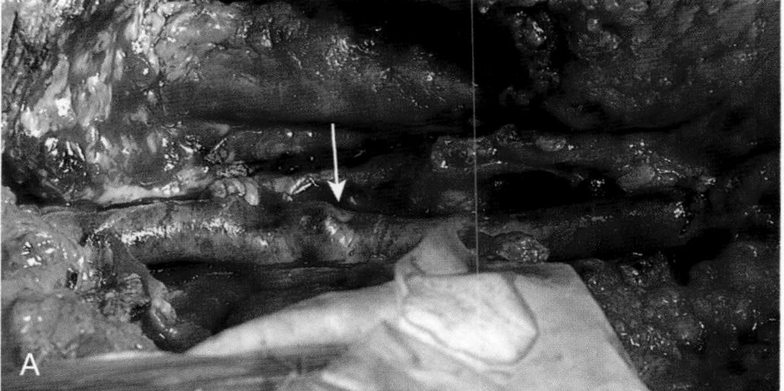

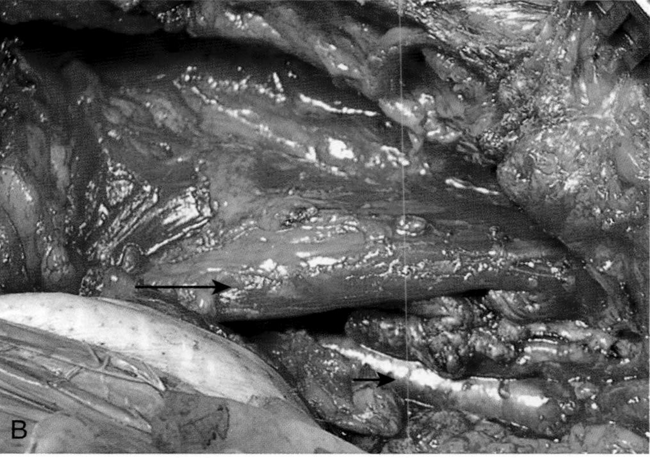

Figure 40-8. A, Intraoperative photograph of the cryovein segment in the groin *(arrow)*. **B,** Intraoperative photograph showing the mobilized sartorius muscle flap *(large arrow)* rotated over the cryovein conduit *(small arrow)*.

exploration and debridement of the infected perigraft tissue, placement of catheters for antibiotic or antiseptic irrigation (usually two to three times per day) and long-term intravenous antibiotics. Patients commonly require an extended stay in the intensive care unit during this treatment, and operative debridement may need to be repeated. Reports of nonresective treatment of vascular graft infection almost always include only extracavitary (nonaortic) infected grafts. When this approach has been applied to aortic grafts, it has almost always been deliberately limited to focal infection involving the femoral region of an aortofemoral bypass graft.[164-170] It is incorrect to consider this equivalent to preserving a pan-infected aortic graft. Akowuah et al. reported eight patients with infection of prosthetic reconstructions of the aortic arch, aortic root, or aortic valve and ascending aorta treated by debridement and irrigation, with a 20% mortality.[171] Calligaro et al. reported nine patients with intraabdominal aortic graft infection who were managed with the nonresective approach described earlier. One patient died perioperatively, and four others ultimately required total or partial graft excision, yielding a treatment success of 44%.[172] All of the patients in Akowuah's series and three of Calligaro's patients developed their graft infection within 30 days of the primary procedure, a feature that increases the likelihood of the success of a nonresective approach.[173] It is important to realize that those factors thought to favor the success of graft preservation—low-virulence infecting organism, absence of perigraft abscess, absence of sepsis, early-appearing infection—are generally not characteristic of intracavitary aortic vascular graft infections.

OUTCOMES-INFECTED INTRACAVITARY (AORTIC) GRAFTS

Several authors have presented literature reviews of the outcomes achieved treating intracavitary vascular graft infection.[2,55,61,83,145,163,174] Table 40-4 summarizes the results of series published within the past 10 years using the therapeutic modalities described earlier to treat infected intracavitary aortic vascular grafts. These data have many shortcomings. First, many published reports include mixed pathologies (patients with primary aortic infection—mycotic aneurysm—as well as patients with infected aortic grafts, and patients with nonaortic graft infections, as well as patients with aortic graft infections), mixed treatment techniques, or both. Yet the outcomes are usually presented in aggregate, not according to the pathology or treatment technique subgroups. As a result, data specific to the management of patients with aortic graft infection and specific to treatment technique are often simply not available.

Second, data reporting is not consistent from study to study. Factors such as the percentage of early- and late-appearing infections, the bacteriology of the infecting organism or organisms, the percentage of culture-negative graft infections, the proportion of grafts with associated enteric erosions or fistulas, the percentage of patients unstable at presentation, the grade of infection, the extent of graft involved by the infection, the sequence of procedures (for patients treated with graft excision and extraanatomical bypass), the anatomy of the revascularization, the amount of graft removed, and the use of adjunctive measures such as muscle flaps are often not reported. Such inconsistencies make it difficult to determine whether the patient group in one study is comparable to that reported in another.

Third, no standardization exists of outcome endpoints. This is most problematic in determining whether persistent infection occurs when in situ reconstruction is the treatment. Patients who die of sepsis may represent failure to eradicate the retroperitoneal infection because of the presence of a conduit in the infected field. Similarly, rupture of the conduit itself (for inline tissue conduits) or rupture of the aortic anastomosis (for inline prosthetic or tissue conduits) may represent persistent infection, but this event is rarely reported as such.

Finally, many recent series report improved outcomes, but almost all of these studies are retrospective, often not consecutive, and lack control groups. In addition, the frequency of vascular graft infection is low enough that the length of time required to accumulate a sufficiently large clinical experience to make any observations ensures that many other changes in patient management span that time interval. This makes it difficult to determine the significance of any apparent improvement in outcomes.

With these limitations in mind, the surgeon can make some observations about the reported outcomes. Extraanatomical bypass and infected graft removal is the treatment with the greatest accumulated experience (n varying between 15 and 50, mean 27). Although outcomes have improved, mortality (11% to 40%) and graft reinfection (3% to 37%) rates remain high. Major amputation (3% to 15%) and aortic stump disruption rates (3% to 24%) have shown significant improvement. This treatment technique is used for patients with the most aggressive and invasive aortic graft infections.

Little experience with in situ prosthetic reconstruction (n varying between 4 and 18, mean 11) has been published, unless an antibiotic-bonded conduit is used (n varying between 8 and 43, mean 17). Both of these in situ reconstruction techniques have lower reported mortality (none to 30%), and very low amputation rates (none to 10%, none in most studies) but a higher rate of conduit reinfection (none to 33%). This treatment is limited to aortic graft infections caused by low-virulence organisms without invasive infection, without abscess, and without enteric fistula or erosion.

The treatment technique most often reported in the last decade is the use of in situ aortic reconstruction with an arterial allograft (n varying between 6 and 179, mean 42). Many of these reports represent interval representation of the expanding work of two or three groups. Mortality rates are not that favorable (9% to 56%), but amputation rates are quite low (none to 8%). However, conduit failure rates, in particular aneurysmal dilation, rupture, and recurrent fistulization, are quite high (Table 40-4). Of note, it is often stated that a benefit of inline reconstruction is the elimination of the risk of aortic stump rupture. Technically, this is true, as there is no aortic stump. However, there is still an aortic anastomotic suture line, at risk for disruption, with bleeding that is every bit as lethal as bleeding from an aortic stump. It is important to note that almost every report of inline arterial allograft reconstruction includes patients whose conduit or anastomosis disrupted with fatal hemorrhage. In Table 40-4, this is represented by a dagger symbol in the aortic stump disruption column.

In situ aortic reconstruction with autogenous superficial femoral–popliteal vein is the last of the major treatment techniques for aortic graft infection and was introduced just a little over a decade ago by Clagett et al.[2] and Nevelsteen et al.[86,159]

Recent published series (n varying from 5 to 49, mean 15) report mortality rates varying between 8% and 33%, with the lowest mortalities attained in the large-volume series (Table 40-4). In general, recurrent infection rates are low. However, reintervention rates for hemodynamically failing conduits are higher than reintervention rates for in situ prosthetic grafts but lower than reintervention rates for aortic allograft failure and for extraanatomical graft failures. Of note, the data regarding venous morbidity are mixed, with some studies reporting a high rate of significant venous morbidity (including the need for fasciotomy and difficult-to-manage venous hypertension), while most studies report only mild to moderate venous morbidity. This procedure has not experienced wider use, most likely because of the length and complexity of the operation, a particular problem in patients who often have significant comorbidities. Finally, the reported results were obtained restricting the use of this technique to aortic graft infection with less virulent organisms, without enteric fistula or erosion and in stable patients.

O'Connor et al.[175] recently published a metaanalysis of reported treatment outcomes using these four most common approaches to the management of aortic graft infection. They demonstrated the highest adverse event rate for extraanatomical bypass and infected graft removal (0.16), followed by in situ autogenous vein (0.10), in situ cryopreserved arterial allografts (0.09), and in situ antibiotic-bonded prosthetic bypass (0.07). Early mortality was highest in the extraanatomical bypass and infected graft removal group and lowest in the in situ antibiotic-bonded prosthetic bypass group. Extraanatomical bypass and infected graft removal and in situ autogenous vein had the highest amputation rates and the highest conduit failure rates, while in situ antibiotic-bonded prosthetic bypass had the lowest amputation and conduit failure rates. In situ arterial allografts and in situ autogenous veins had the lowest rate of reinfection, while in situ antibiotic-bonded prosthetic bypass had the highest reinfection rate. These authors concluded that these results favored the use of any in situ reconstruction approach over extraanatomical bypass and questioned whether it was appropriate for extraanatomical bypass to remain the gold standard for the treatment of infected vascular grafts.

Before accepting these conclusions, consider that the treatment approach with the worst outcomes—extraanatomical bypass and infected graft removal—is generally used to treat the most advanced infections (graft infections with associated enteric fistula or erosions, with perigraft abscess, with anastomotic false aneurysms, and with bleeding), as well as those caused by the most aggressive organisms (*S. aureus, Pseudomonas* species, gram-negative organisms) and most often involves pan-infected aortic prostheses, necessitating complete excision of the infected aortic graft (Table 40-4). In contrast, in situ reconstructions are generally only used and only recommended in the setting of low-virulence organisms, in the absence of any evidence of invasive infection, when no associated enteric fistula or erosion is found, and when only a partial graft excision is needed to manage focal graft infection.

In reality, achieving the optimal outcome for patients with aortic graft infection requires that treatment be individualized for each patient. To do this, the vascular surgeon must be proficient in the use of all potential treatment approaches. Equally importantly, the surgeon must have the judgment to select the modality with the greatest likelihood of success in a given clinical situation. Many factors are important in making this decision. Inline reconstruction is favored in patients with significant infrainguinal occlusive disease and poor runoff. Prosthetic inline reconstruction is only favored in settings with little manifestation of infection and caused by low-virulence organisms. Patients with evidence of invasive arterial infection (false aneurysm or overt bleeding) do better with revascularization from an uninvolved arterial segment and placed in uninvolved tissue. If this is not possible and inline reconstruction must be performed, only tissue conduits should be used. Unstable patients benefit from the most expeditious procedure that controls bleeding, even if this is a temporizing step. Those patients with infections caused by high-virulence organisms should be reconstructed through remote sites, but as in the case of invasive arterial infection, if inline reconstruction is required, only tissue conduits should be used. The failure mode of arterial allografts is degeneration, dilation, and rupture, whereas the failure mode of venous autografts is hemodynamic. In general, the hemodynamic failures are less lethal and easier to treat.

TREATMENT-INFECTED EXTRACAVITARY VASCULAR GRAFTS

Extracavitary vascular reconstruction is performed more often than intracavitary vascular reconstruction—especially in the era of endovascular treatment of aortic aneurysmal and occlusive disease—and the frequency of infection in these predominantly subcutaneous extracavitary conduits is higher than the frequency of infection involving intracavitary (aortic) grafts. Yet only a few published reports focus on the treatment and outcome of treatment of infected extracavitary vascular grafts[12,53,130,164,173,176-181] (Table 40-5). In general, the treatment options described earlier for infected aortic grafts are also the options for treatment of infected nonaortic grafts. However, the limitations imposed by the subcutaneous, extraanatomical location of these grafts often means that infected graft removal and remote bypass through noninfected tissue is not a practical option. The most common treatment approaches are graft excision without revascularization; graft preservation (partial or complete) with wound debridement, with or without muscle flap coverage; and graft excision with in situ revascularization (using either a tissue or prosthetic conduit), also with or without muscle flap coverage.

Graft excision without revascularization may be appropriate if the infected graft is thrombosed or if the indication for the primary revascularization was not critical limb ischemia (rest pain, nonhealing wounds, or gangrene). The technical challenge of excision without revascularization is to maintain flow through the native artery and to prevent the loss of any branches providing critical collateral flow around the occlusion. Maintaining native artery flow means that the arterial defect created by removing the infected graft from each anastomotic site must be patched, preferably with tissue. Some prefer to achieve both of these goals by leaving a short segment of the prosthesis attached at each anastomotic site,[164] often referring to this as partial graft preservation. However, a more common approach is complete excision and closure of the arterial defect at each anastomotic site (after appropriate arterial debridement) with either a tissue patch or a tissue interposition graft. If arterial continuity is not maintained or

Table 40-4
Outcome of Current Treatment of Aortic Graft Infection According to Treatment Modality*

Study	Year	Study Interval	*n*	AEF or AEE (%)	Early (<4 months; %)	CN or S Epi (%)	Unstable (%)	Septic (%)	EAB Anatomy	Sequence or Staging	Mortality (30 day; %)
Extraanatomical Bypass and Infected Graft Removal											
Armstrong et al.[84]	2005	91-04	25	100	0	SGDNR	SGDNR	SGDNR	BiAxUF	Traditional, 7; sequenced, 10; staged, 8	SGDNR
Bandyk et al.[53]	2001	91-00	31	81	SGDNR	SGDNR	SGDNR	SGDNR	SGDNR	Staged, 31	23
Dorigo et al.[57]	2003	90-02	30	100	NR	12	20	NR	AxBiF	Traditional, 14; sequenced, 9; staged, 5	27
Gabriel et al.[58]	2004	97-01	19	0	NR	27	NR	NR	NR	NR	5
Hart et al.[122]	2005	93, 03	15	40	NR	13	NR	40	AxBiF, 10; AxPop, 5	Traditional, 1; staged, 9; unknown, 5	40
Jausseran et al.[123]	1997	80-95	17	76	NR	NR	NR	12	AxBiF	Traditional, 1; sequential, 16	18
Menawat et al.[63]	1997	80-94	40	100	NR	SGDNR	SGDNR	SGDNR	NR	Traditional, 14; sequential, 17; staged, 9	23
Oderich et al.[61]	2006	81-01	43	60	NR	NR	9	NR	AxBiF, 34; BiAxUF, 9	NR	12
Seeger et al.[62]	1999	83-94	40	SGDNR	SGDNR	28	SGDNR	SGDNR	AxUF, 5; AxPop, 11; obturator, 1; BiAxUF, 14; AxBiF, 9	Staged, 23; sequential, 18	27
Seeger et al.[88]	2000	89-99	36	8	NR	NR	NR	31	AxUF, 6; AxUPop, 2; BiAxUPop, 1; BiAxUF, 20; AxUF/AxUPop, 2; AxBiF, 5	Staged, 36	11
Yeager et al.[119]	1999	83-98	50	32	NR	4	NR	NR	SGDNR	Sequential, 50	12
Sicard et al.[125]	1997	90-95	5	NR	NR	0	0	NR	AxBiF, 5	Staged, 5	0
Darling et al.[128]	1997	87-95	12	NR	NR	NR	NR	NR	NR	NR	25
Ten Raa et al.[127]	2002	91-00	18	SGDNR	NR	SGDNR	NR	NR	NR	NR	39
Lavigne et al.[126]	2003	80-94	25	0.32	SGDNR	SGDNR	SGDNR	SGDNR	AxF, 12 AxPop, 4 Obturator, 9	SGDNR	SGDNR

Study	Year	Study Interval	*n*	AEF or AEE (%)	Early (<4 months; %)	CN or S Epi (%)	Unstable (%)	Septic (%)	EAB Anatomy	Sequence or Staging	Mortality (30 day; %)
In Situ Prosthetic											
Bandyk et al.[53]	2001	91-00	9	SGDNR	SGDNR	SGDNR	SGDNR	SGDNR	NA	NA	0
Darling et al.[128]	1997	87-95	16	50	NR	19	0	NR	NA	NA	0
Fiorani et al.[87]	1997	89-95	18	50	NR	NR	0	NR	NA	NA	11
Hart et al.[122]	2005	93-03	8	SGDNR	SGDNR	27	SGDNR	SGDNR	NA	NA	SGDNR
Menawat et al.[63]	1997	80, 94	10	100	NR	NR	NR	NR	NA	NA	30
Oderich et al.[61]	2006	90-01	9	SGDNR	SGDNR	SGDNR	SGDNR	SGDNR	NA	NA	SGDNR
Young et al.[89]	1999	89-98	16	SGDNR	SGDNR	SGDNR	SGDNR	SGDNR	NA	NA	13
Seeger et al.[62]	1999	83-94	4	SGDNR	SGDNR	SGDNR	SGDNR	SGDNR	NA	NA	60

F/U (months)	Partial or Complete Excision	Late Related Mortality (%)	Amputation (%)	Conduit Infection (%)	Conduit Stenosed or Occluded (%)	Conduit Aneurysm or Bleeding (%)	Conduit Revised (%)	Aortic Stump Disruption (%)	Anastomotic Bleeding (%)
51	NR	SGDNR	SGDNR	8	16	SGDNR	SGDNR	4	SGDNR
SGDNR	Complete, 31	SGDNR	10	SGDNR	SGDNR	SGDNR	SGDNR	SGDNR	SGDNR
24	Complete, 30	17	3	7	32	NR	NR	23	NR
NR	Complete, 19	5	5	37	26	NR	NR	5	NR
14	Complete, 15	NR	7	13	NR	NR	NR	7	NR
72	Complete, 17	24	NR	NR	6	NR	12	24	NR
NR	Complete, 40	NR	15	35	18	NR	23	8	
41	Complete, 43	9	9	12	40	NR	NR	9	NR
30	SGDNR	SGDNR	17	10	SGDNR	SGDNR	SGDNR	SGDNR	SGDNR
33	NR	8	11	3	31	NR	NR	3	NR
41	NR	SGDNR	SGDNR	SGDNR	SGNDR	SGDNR	SGDNR	SGDNR	SGDNR
17	NR	0	NR	NR	20	20	20	0	20
51	Complete, 12	NR	8	0	33	NR	NR	NR	NR
SGDNR	Complete, 18	SGDNR	6	6	44	SGDNR	44	0	NR
SGDNR	SGDNR	SGDNR	SGDNR	SGDNR	SGDNR	SGDNR	SGDNR	SGDNR	SGDNR

F/U (months)	Partial or Complete Excision	Late Related Mortality (%)	Amputation (%)	Conduit Infection (%)	Conduit Stenosed or Occluded (%)	Conduit Aneurysm or Bleeding (%)	Conduit Revised (%)	Aortic Stump Disruption (%)	Anastomotic Bleeding (%)
SGDNR	SGDNR	SGDNR	SGDNR	SGDNR	SGDNR	SGDNR	SGDNR	NA	SGDNR
32	NR	13	6	0	25	NR	NR	NA	NR
37	100	0	0	0	11	NR	NR	NA	NR
17	Partial, 8	SGDNR	SGDNR	13	SGDNR	SGDNR	SGDNR	NA	SGDNR
18	Partial, 5; complete, 5	10	10	10	10		10	NA	
SGDNR	SGDNR	SGDNR	SGDNR	33	SGDNR	SGDNR	SGDNR	NA	SGDNR
SGDNR	SGDNR	SGDNR	0	25	SGDNR	SGDNR	SGDNR	NA	SGDNR
SGDNR	SGDNR	SGDNR	0	SGDNR	SGDNR	SGDNR	SGDNR	NA	SGDNR

Continued

Table 40-4
Outcome of Current Treatment of Aortic Graft Infection According to Treatment Modality*—cont'd

Study	Year	Study Interval	*n*	AEF or AEE (%)	Early (<4 months; %)	CN or S Epi (%)	Unstable (%)	Septic (%)	EAB Anatomy	Sequence or Staging	Mortality (30 day; %)
In Situ Antibiotic Bonded Prosthetic											
Armstrong et al.[130]	2007	94-06	13	SGDNR	SGDNR	SGDNR	SGDNR	SGDNR	NA	NA	SGDNR
Bandyk et al.[53]	2001	91-00	16	SGDNR	SGDNR	SGDNR	SGDNR	SGDNR	NA	NA	0
Bandyk et al.[131]	2001	95-99	18	SGDNR	NR	SGDNR	0	0	NA	NA	0
Batt et al.[55]	2003	00-01	24	54	8	33	25	38	NA	NA	17
Hayes et al.[132]	1999	92-97	11	27	18	18	36	9	NA	NA	18
Oderich et al.[61]	2006	90-01	43	SGDNR	SGDNR	SGDNR	SGDNR	SGDNR	NA	NA	SGDNR
Torsello and Sandmann[134]	1997	91-95	12	NR	NR	NR	NR	NR	NA	NA	0
Young et al.[89]	1999	89-98	9	SGDNR	SGDNR	SGDNR	SGDNR	SGDNR	NA	NA	0
Ten Raa et al.[127]	2002	91-00	8	SGDNR	NR	SGDNR	NR	NR	NA	NA	0

Study	Year	Study Interval	*n*	AEF or AEE (%)	Early (<4 months, %)	CN or S Epi (%)	Unstable (%)	Septic (%)	EAB Anatomy	Sequence or Staging	Mortality (30 day; %)
In Situ Arterial Allograft											
Agrifoglio et al.[136]	1997	94-95	24	NR	NR	NR	NR	NR	NA	NA	13
Chiesa et al.[138]	1998	94-96	37	35	NR	NR	NR	SGDNR	NA	NA	14
Chiesa et al.[139]	2002	94-00	68	32	0	NR	NR	NR	NA	NA	16
Desgrange et al.[56]	1998	92-96	15	SGDNR	SGDNR	SGDNR	SGDNR	SGDNR	NA	NA	27
Gabriel et al.[141]	2004	96-00	39	10	NR	SGDNR	SGDNR	SGDNR	NA	NA	15
Gabriel et al.[58]	2004	97-01	44	0	NR	13	NR	NR	NA	NA	9
Kieffer et al.[11]	2001	92-00	11	45	45	18	9	45	NA	NA	18
Kieffer et al.[146]	2004	88-02	179	30	NR	NR	NR	NR	NA	NA	20
Kitamura et al.[142]	2005	98-03	6	SGDNR	NR	SGDNR	SGDNR	SGDNR	NA	NA	50
Lavigne et al.[126]	2003	94-97	18	22	SGDNR	SGDNR	SGDNR	SGDNR	NA	NA	17
Leseche et al.[60]	2001	92-00	23	43	0	NR	NR	NR	NA	NA	17
Locati et al.[143]	1998	94-97	18	17	NR	NR	22	NR	NA	NA	17
Nevelsteen et al.[144]	1998	93-97	25	28	NR	NR	NR	NR	NA	NA	12
Noel et al.[145]	2002	99-01	47	SGDNR	SGDNR	SGDNR	SGDNR	SGDNR	NA	NA	SGDNR
Pirelli et al.[147]	2005	95-04	25	44	NR	NR	NR	NR	NA	NA	56
Ruotolo et al.[148]	1997	88-95	100	27	NR	NR	NR	NR	NA	NA	24
Teebken et al.[149]	2004	00-03	29	21	NR	NR	NR	NR	NA	NA	21
Verhelst et al.[150]	2000	92-98	66	26	17	SGDNR	SGDNR	SGDNR	NA	NA	SGDNR
Vogt et al.[151]	2002	90-99	28	61	NR	SGDNR	SGDNR	SGDNR	NA	NA	SGDNR
Zhou et al.[152]	2006	99-04	36	SGDNR	0	SGDNR	SGDNR	SGDNR	NA	NA	SGDNR

F/U (months)	Partial or Complete Excision	Late Related Mortality (%)	Amputation (%)	Conduit Infection (%)	Conduit Stenosed or Occluded (%)	Conduit Aneurysm or Bleeding (%)	Conduit Revised (%)	Aortic Stump Disruption (%)	Anastomotic Bleeding (%)
SGDNR	SGDNR	SGDNR	SGDNR	SGDNR	SGDNR	SGDNR	SGDNR	NA	SGDNR
SGDNR	SGDNR	SGDNR	SGDNR	SGDNR	SGDNR	SGDNR	SGDNR	NA	SGDNR
SGDNR	Partial, 18	0	0	11	0	NR	11	NA	NR
17	Partial, 6; complete, 18	0	0	4	0	NR	0	NA	0
NR	Complete, 11	18	0	9	0	0	0	NA	9
SGDNR	SGDNR	SGDNR	SGDNR	7	SGDNR	SGDNR	SGDNR	NA	SGDNR
33	Partial, 4; complete, 7	17	0	17	NR	NR	17	NA	NR
SGDNR	SGDNR	SGDNR	0	11	SGDNR	SGDNR	SGDNR	NA	NR
SGDNR	Complete, 8	SGDNR	SGDNR	13	0	NR	NR	NA	NR

F/U (months)	Partial or Complete Excision	Late Related Mortality (%)	Amputation (%)	Conduit Infection (%)	Conduit Stenosed or Occluded (%)	Conduit Aneurysm or Bleeding (%)	Conduit Revised (%)	Aortic Stump Disruption (%)	Anastomotic Bleeding (%)
9	NR	13	4	0	4	8	NR	NA†	NR
15	NR	5	7	NR	18	NR	NR	NA	NR
30	NR	NR	4	NR	16	NR	9	NA	NR
SGDNR	Partial, 5; complete, 10	0	7	NR	7	27	NR	NA†	NR
SGDNR	Complete, 39	3	8	8	26	3	NR	NA†	13
NR	NR	0	7	7	25	NR	14	NA	11
34	NR	9	NR	18	NR	9	9	NA†	NR
46	Complete, 179	2	1	NR	3	8	3	NA†	NR
SGDNR	Partial, 1; complete, 5	0	0	NR	NR	0	0	NA†	33
18	NR	6	0	6	NR	17	6	NA†	17
35	Partial, 10; complete, 13	0	0	0	4	13	17	NA	NR
22	Complete, 18	0	0	0	6	11	17	NA†	0
25	NR	0	SGDNR	SGDNR	SGDNR	24	NR	NA†	NR
SGDNR	SGDNR	SGDNR	SGDNR	SGDNR	SGDNR	SGDNR	SGDNR	NA†	SGDNR
28	NR	NR	8	NR	24	48	NR	NA†	NR
NR	NR	2	3	NR	20	5	15	NA	NR
NR	SGDNR	7	0	NR	3	10	3	NA†	NR
SGDNR	SGDNR	SGDNR	SGDNR	SGDNR	SGDNR	SGDNR	SGDNR	NA†	SGDNR
SGDNR	SGDNR	SGDNR	SGDNR	SGDNR	SGDNR	SGDNR	SGDNR	NA†	SGDNR
SGDNR	SGDNR	SGDNR	SGDNR	SGDNR	SGDNR	SGDNR	SGDNR	NA	SGDNR

Continued

Table 40-4
Outcome of Current Treatment of Aortic Graft Infection According to Treatment Modality*—cont'd

Study	Year	Study Interval	*n*	AEF or AEE (%)	Early (<4 months; %)	CN or S Epi (%)	Unstable (%)	Septic (%)	EAB Anatomy	Sequence or Staging	Mortality (30 day; %)
In Situ Autogenous Vein											
Ali et al.[153]	2008	99-07	26	19	NR	28	NR	NR	NA	NA	15
Bandyk et al.[53]	2001	91-00	10	SGDNR	SGDNR	SGDNR	SGDNR	SGDNR	NA	NA	10
Brown et al.[154]	1999	95-97	5	NR	NR	40	NR	NR	NA	NA	20
Cardozo et al.[155]	2002	95-99	12	NR	NR	42	NR	NR	NA	NA	17
Daenens et al.[86]	2003	90-02	49	0	NR	NR	NR	NR	NA	NA	8
Faulk et al.[156]	2005	99-04	17	NR	NR	NR	NR	NR	NA	NA	12
Franke and Voit[157]	1997	92-95	6	NR	67	17	NR	NR	NA	NA	33
Gibbons et al.[59]	2000	Not stated	4	NR	75	25	NR	NR	NA	NA	25
Gibbons et al.[158]	2003	97-02	9	NR	NR	44	NR	NR	NA	NA	SGDNR
Nevelsteen et al.[159]	1997	90-95	14	21	29	NR	7	NR	NA	NA	14

*AEE, aortoenteric erosion; AEF, aortoenteric fistula; AxBiF, axillobifemoral; AxPop, axillopopliteal; AxUF, axillounifemoral; AxUPop, axillounipopliteal; BiAxUF, bilateral axillounifemoral; CN, culture-negative; DVT, deep vein thrombosis; EAB, extraanatomical bypass; F/U, follow-up; NA, not applicable; NR, not reported; S Epi, staph epidermidis; SGDNR, subgroup data not reported.
†Series includes cases of anastomotic or conduit rupture.

if branches that contribute significantly to collateral perfusion are sacrificed, then even patients whose primary procedure was not performed for critical limb ischemia may develop critical limb ischemia after removal of the infected occluded bypass graft. Because it commonly takes time to assess the degree of limb ischemia in these patients, limb loss often results from this sequence of events.

Graft preservation with wound debridement (often repetitive wound debridement) is often attempted in the setting of infected extracavitary vascular grafts. Quite commonly, rotational muscle flaps are used in this setting to provide well-vascularized tissue to cover the exposed arterial conduit and fill the tissue defect resulting from wound debridement. Adequate debridement of the infected and inflamed tissue is critical to the success of this approach. Some recommend interval (staged) surgical debridement with repetitive wound cultures until wound sterilization has been achieved.[130] Definitive wound closure or coverage is deferred until the wound cultures are negative.

Although graft excision and remote revascularization is usually not an option for infected extracavitary conduits, in situ reconstruction with tissue conduits is a possibility. The major limitation of this technique is tissue conduit availability. The preferred conduit is autogenous vein (greater saphenous vein, if available, or lesser saphenous vein or arm veins). If no autogenous vein conduit is available, an autogenous arterial conduit can be used in certain circumstances. Most often, the only usable arterial conduit is an occluded SFA. This conduit is harvested, endarterectomized, and then used to replace the infected prosthetic conduit. This treatment option is limited by the available length of the SFA, as well as the dissection required to harvest a conduit of adequate length. Cryopreserved vein allograft is a good option when the infected peripheral graft is patent and must be replaced. Although these conduits have limited long-term patency, they achieve the goal of eradication of infection while preserving perfusion. When the conduit fails, the infection is gone and more treatment options are available.

OUTCOMES-INFECTED EXTRACAVITARY (NONAORTIC) VASCULAR GRAFTS

Table 40-5 summarizes the outcomes reported in studies published within the past decade using the preceding techniques to manage extracavitary (nonaortic) vascular graft infection. Excluded from this table are other studies that included 10 or fewer patients with nonaortic infected grafts. In general, infected peripheral vascular grafts pose more threat to limb than to life, which is the opposite of infected aortic grafts. The exception to this is an infected peripheral graft that presents with bleeding[164]; this indicates an invasive arterial infection, a situation that is more likely to have an unfavorable outcome. Amputation rates are usually low, except when most patients in a series are managed with resection without revascularization, which is associated with notably higher limb loss.[177,178,180] Conduit reinfection rates are also quite low, because the most common revascularization technique

F/U (months)	Partial or Complete Excision	Late Related Mortality (%)	Amputation (%)	Conduit Infection (%)	Conduit Stenosed or Occluded (%)	Conduit Aneurysm or Bleeding (%)	Conduit Revised (%)	Aortic Stump Disruption (%)	Anastomotic Bleeding (%)
16	NR	NR	8	12	8	0	0	NA	0
SGDNR	SGDNR	SGDNR	10	SGDNR	SGDNR	SGDNR	SGDNR	NA	SGDNR
16	NR	0	0	0	0	0	0	NA	0
22	Partial, 9; complete, 12	0	25	0	0	0	0	NA[†]	8
41	Complete, 49	0	2	0	4	8	10	NA	0
NR	Complete, 17	NR	0	0	24	6	29	NA[†]	6
23	Complete, 6	0	17	0	17	33	NR	NA[†]	33
NR	Partial, 1; complete, 3	0	0	0	0	0	50	NA	0
22	Partial, 2; complete, 7	SGDNR	0	0	SGDNR	0	SGDNR	NA	0
16	Complete, 14	0	7	0	14	0	14	NA	0

is in situ reconstruction using autologous tissue conduits. In the nonaortic location, the use of in situ prosthetic revascularization is quite rare, contributing to the low reinfection rates.

ADJUNCTIVE TECHNIQUES IN THE MANAGEMENT OF VASCULAR GRAFT INFECTION

Because of the therapeutic challenge posed by vascular graft infection, the use of adjunctive techniques has continued to expand, and in some cases the accumulated experience has led some to consider the adjunctive approach to be definitive. The greatest use of adjunctive therapies has been in the setting of infected extracavitary vascular prostheses or in the setting of infection confined to the femoral portion of an intracavitary graft.

Muscle Flaps

Adequate debridement of the surrounding soft tissue is an essential component of the successful treatment of vascular graft infection, whether the approach is to preserve the involved graft or to excise it and replace it with another tissue or prosthetic conduit. With extracavitary grafts, debridement often leaves a sizeable soft-tissue defect, exposing the graft the surgeon is trying to preserve or necessitating an alternate tissue route for a newly placed conduit. The femoral region is an anatomically constrained space, with limited options for primary closure of a large defect over a "preserved" graft and limited options for an alternate tissue space for a newly placed conduit. Unfortunately, the common consequence of this anatomical limitation has been inadequate debridement, wound closure under tension, and residual dead space, all factors that greatly increase the likelihood of failure. Rotational muscle flaps, developed to reconstruct tissue defects in other settings, provide a solution to this challenge. The muscle is well-vascularized and of adequate bulk to cover the conduit and occupy the dead space created by the combination of infection-induced necrosis and surgical debridement. Although reports exist of muscle flaps used to cover an intracavitary aortic allograft reconstruction[182] and an extraanatomical axillofemoral bypass graft,[183,184] the most common use of muscle flaps has been to treat femoral-level infection involving infrainguinal vascular grafts originating in the groin and suprainguinal vascular grafts terminating in the groin.[130,184-193] Several different muscle flaps have been successfully used to provide tissue coverage in the femoral location, including the sartorius,[130,184,188-193] rectus femoris,[184-186,189,193] rectus abdominis,[184,189] and gracilis[187] muscles. The sartorius flap has been most widely used, even though concern often arises that the adjacent infectious or inflammatory process might involve the sartorius muscle. On the other hand, the concern about using the rectus femoris, and to some extent the gracilis muscle, centers on the almost inevitable presence of atherosclerotic occlusive disease in the femoral arteries, which provide flow to these flaps. Finally, some have reported a significant loss in strength of knee extension after harvesting the gracilis, but this has not been consistently documented.[187] The rectus abdominis muscle is an excellent flap, with significant length and bulk; however, it cannot be used if prior arterial reconstruction procedures have resulted in interruption of the circumflex iliac artery branches. Of note, the contralateral rectus abdominis is always used since this allows rotation on the distally based pedicle, whereas using the ipsilateral muscle would require folding of the pedicle, resulting in greater risk of kinking the vascular pedicle.

Table 40-5
Outcome of Current Treatment of Nonaortic Graft Infection According to Treatment Modality*

Study	n	Infected Graft Location	Excision	Reconstruction	Mortality (%)	Amputation (%)	Conduit Reinfection (%)	Conduit Failure (%)	Conduit Rupture (%)
Armstrong et al.[130]	50	EAB, 19; II, 31	None, 3; partial, 38; complete, 9	In situ autologous, 42; in situ Abx bonded, 3; in situ prosthetic, 2; none, 0; remote, 0			Outcome data not presented by sub-group		
Bandyk et al.[53]	51	EAB, 32; II, 19	None,?; partial,?; complete, 7	In situ autologous, 26; in situ Abx bonded, 6; in situ prosthetic, 9; none, 7; remote, 3	4	4	2	4	NR
Verhelst et al.[150]	26	NR	NR	NR	0	NR	NR	NR	NR
deVirgilio et al.[178]	28	EAB, 28	None, 6; partial, 10; complete, 12	In situ autologous, 8; in situ Abx bonded, 0; in situ prosthetic, 0; none, 12; remote, 8	18	25	11	21	4
Calligaro et al.[164]	106	EAB, 16; II, 90	None, 51; partial, 43; complete, 26	NR	12	13	9	21	5
Calligaro et al.[173]	141	EAB, 17; II, 110	NR	NR	14	13	NR	NR	NR
Castier et al.[176]	15	EAB, 2; II, 13	Complete, 15	In situ allograft, 15	0	0	0	35	12
Chalmers et al.[177]	27	II, 27	None, 7; partial, 0; complete, 20	In situ autologous, 4; none, 23	15	63	NR	NR	NR
Pederson et al.[181]	17	II, 17	None, 11; partial, 0; complete, 6	NR	12	NR	NR	NR	NR
Zetrenne et al.[180]	38	EAB, 14; II, 24	None, 22; partial, 0; complete, 12	In situ (? conduit), 5; none, 27; remote, 6	8	24	NR	NR	NR

*EAB, extraanatomical bypass; II, infrainguinal; Abx, antibiotic; NR, not reported.

Muscle flaps have been used to treat wound healing complications after prosthesis implantation (seroma, lymphocele) by providing coverage of the vascular conduit and elimination of the dead space resulting from wound exploration and debridement. The muscle also provides a route for lymph drainage. Flaps have also been used to cover an infected prosthesis and fill the soft-tissue defect remaining after surgical drainage and debridement of the surrounding wound, when graft preservation is the goal. Finally, muscle flaps have been used to cover new conduits (either prosthetic or tissue) placed in the involved wound after removal of the infected graft. Some authors rotate muscle flaps at the time of the initial debridement, infected graft excision and in situ reconstruction, or both, while others perform serial surgical wound debridement until wound cultures are negative and then perform the rotational myoplasty.[130]

While reported rotational muscle flap mortality rates are quite low, and flap survival rates are quite high, the success of muscle flaps in achieving complete wound healing, graft preservation, limb salvage, and prevention of conduit or anastomotic disruption depends on the clinical presentation, the infecting organism, and the chronicity of the infection[130,184-193] (Table 40-6). Overall, the success of rotational muscle flaps makes it a critical additional tool in the armamentarium of the vascular surgeon who treats infected vascular grafts.

Negative-Pressure Wound Therapy

Negative-pressure wound therapy or vacuum-assisted closure is a newer modality that has been used in the management of open wounds. It was inevitable that it would be applied to the difficult problem of managing complex vascular wounds, particularly after reports that it can control lymph drainage, stimulate granulation tissue growth, and eradicate infection. Kotsis and Lioupis[166] reported its use in eight patients, four of whom had prosthetic vascular graft in the wound. They all achieved successful wound healing, with no bleeding, no need for muscle flaps, and no recurrence of infection at follow-up averaging 17 months. Similarly, Dosluoglu et al.[194] reported successful use in four patients with exposed vascular grafts, with no recurrent infection after 18 months of follow-up. Pinocy et al.[195] initially reported the use of the technique in 24 patients and achieved successful healing in all, with no reappearance of infection an average of 12 months later. Mayer et al.[196] reported successful use of this technique in 29 patients even when the system was applied directly to an exposed artery or vascular graft. In contrast, Svensson et al.[197] reported a mortality of 33%, amputation rate of 25%, and successful wound healing of only 75% in patients who were treated with negative-pressure therapy in the setting of an infected vascular conduit. Six patients developed arterial bleeding or false aneurysms either early ($n = 2$) or late ($n = 4$). They identified

Table 40-6
Muscle Flap Coverage in the Treatment of Infected Vascular Grafts

Study	Year	Patients (*n*)	Grafts (*n*)	Flaps (*n*)	F/U (Months)	Mortality (%)	Graft Salvage (%)	Limb Salvage (%)	Flap Survival (%)
Armstrong et al.[130]	2007	86	86	89	52	2	93	98	98
Akron et al.[185]	2005	33	23	37	No data	6	78	96	100
Schutzer et al.[188]	2005	50	50	50	18	12	98	92	98
Illig et al.[186]	2004	30	30	30	No data	No data	91	80	97
Seify et al.[189]	2005	22	24	26	56	9	33	64	100
Colwell et al.[193]	2004	9	11	9	10	0	82	100	100
Morasch et al.[187]	2004	18	18	20	40	11	89	89	90
Galland et al.[191]	2002	7	11	8	5	0	100	86	100
Graham et al.[184]	2002	21	24	27	36	0	92	71	96
Sladen et al.[190]	1998	25	25	10	26	0	40	100	90
Maser et al.[192]	1997	14	15	15	36	0	100	86	100

the presence of prosthetic graft and gram-negative organisms as prognostic of failure. It seems that this technique is most valuable in aiding wound healing after the local infection has been eradicated by adequate debridement, and graft excision and replacement as needed. It is unlikely to become first-line definitive therapy.

Localized Antimicrobial Therapy

As the treatment of infected vascular grafts began to shift from complete excision and extraanatomical bypass to nonresective graft preservation and in situ revascularization (using either prosthetic or tissue conduits), the critical importance of appropriate and aggressive management of the involved perigraft tissues became evident. Although it is not commonly regarded as an adjunctive technique, surgical wound exploration and debridement is probably the most important step in local control of infection and in preparing the tissue bed for in situ graft replacement. But surgical debridement alone may not achieve wound sterilization. Consequently, two supplemental treatments have been combined with surgical debridement to improve the chance of significantly lowering or even eradicating the bacterial counts in the wounds: antimicrobial wound irrigation and implantation of antibiotic-impregnated beads.

Antimicrobial Wound Irrigation

Wound irrigation with povidone-iodine or wound soaking with mafenide have both been used to sterilize infected or contaminated wounds.[170,179] Unfortunately, the recommended 10% povidone-iodine strength also impairs wound healing and inhibits fibroblasts.[198] This has led to the use of dilute solutions, which are more likely to be ineffective in local bacterial control.[198,199] Some authors recommend combining 10% povidone-iodine with antibiotic irrigation for optimal wound sterilization.[199] Mafenide is at least as effective as undiluted povidone-iodine[200-202] but does not have adverse effects on wound healing and is actually helpful to fibroblast proliferation.[198]

Antibiotic-Impregnated Beads

The difficult problem of osteomyelitis and infection of orthopedic appliances led to the development of antibiotic-impregnated methylmethacrylate bone cement. A derivative of that approach to providing high local concentrations of antimicrobial agents is the use of antibiotic-impregnated beads of methylmethactylate.[203] Recently, some vascular surgeons have begun to use this technique in an attempt to improve the success rates of infected vascular graft preservation.[130] Nielsen et al.[204] reported implanting gentamycin-impregnated beads in 17 patients, with success in 7. One of the patients in whom the treatment failed died of infection (mortality of 6%), and the remaining patients were cured after resection of the infected segment of the prostheses. Stone et al.[168] recently reported the results of their series of 34 patients in whom antibiotic-impregnated beads (predominantly vancomycin) were used as part of a program of wound debridement and pulse-spray antibacterial lavage to sterilize the wound before definitive treatment of the underlying vascular graft infection. Negative wound cultures were achieved in 87% of cases before graft preservation ($n = 16$) or in situ prosthetic replacement ($n = 20$). Mortality was 0% and limb salvage was 100%; however, during follow-up averaging 23 months, 4 “reinfections” (11%) required graft resection. All of these data suggest the potential benefit of this adjunctive technique in optimizing the tissue bed before definitive treatment of the infected graft, but more experience and data are necessary to prove efficacy and define its role.

References

1. Lorentzen JE, Nielsen OM, Arendrup H, et al. Vascular graft infection: an analysis of sixty-two graft infections in 2411 consecutively implanted synthetic grafts. *Surgery* 1985;98:81-86.
2. Clagett GP, Bowers PL, Lopez-Viego MA, et al. Creation of neoaortoiliac system from lower extremity deep and superficial veins. *Ann Surg* 1993;281:19-29.
3. Fletcher JP, Dryden M, Sorrell TC. Infection of vascular prosthesis. *Aust NZ J Surg* 1991;61:432-435.
4. D'Addato M, Curti T, Freyrie A. The rifampin-bonded Gelseal graft. *Eur J Vasc Endovasc Surg* 1997;14(Suppl A):15-17.
5. O'Brien T, Collin J. Prosthetic vascular graft infection. *Br J Surg* 1992;79:1262-1267.
6. Calligaro KD, Veith FJ. Diagnosis and management of infected prosthetic aortic graft. *Surgery* 1991;110:805-813.
7. Ricco J-B. InterGard silver bifurcated graft: features and results of a multicenter clinical study. *J Vasc Surg* 2006;44:339-346.
8. Svensson LG, Crawford ES, Hess KR, et al. Variables predictive of outcome in 832 patients undergoing repairs of the descending thoracic aorta. *Chest* 1993;104:1248-1253.
9. Svensson LG, Crawford ES, Hess KR, et al. Experience with 1509 patients undergoing thoracoabdominal aortic operations. *J Vasc Surg* 1993;17:357-370.

10. Lawrie GM, Earle N, DeBakey ME. Evolution of surgical techniques for aneurysms of the descending thoracic aorta: twenty-nine years experience with 659 patients. *J Cardiovasc Surg* 1994;9:648-661.
11. Kieffer E, Sabatier J, Plissonnier D, Knosalla C. Prosthetic graft infection after descending thoracic–thoracoabdominal aortic aneurysmectomy: management with in situ arterial allografts. *J Vasc Surg* 2001;33: 671-678.
12. Chang JK, Calligaro KD, Ryan S, et al. Risk factors associated with infection of lower extremity revascularization: analysis of 365 procedures performed at a teaching hospital. *Ann Vasc Surg* 2003;17:91-96.
13. Benedetti-Valentini F, Gossetti B, Martinelli O, et al. Extra-anatomic graft infection in the aortofemoral area. *Eur J Vasc Endovasc Surg* 1997;14(Suppl A):71-73.
14. Naylor AR, Hayes PD, Darke S. A prospective audit of complex wound and graft infections in Great Britain and Ireland: the emergence of MRSA. *Eur J Vasc Endovasc Surg* 2001;21:289-294.
15. Ducasse E, Calisti A, Speziale F, et al. Aortoiliac stent graft infection: current problems and management. *Ann Vasc Surg* 2004;18:521-526.
16. Sharif MA, Lee B, Lau LL, et al. Prosthetic stent graft infection after endovascular abdominal aortic aneurysm repair. *J Vasc Surg* 2007;46: 442-448.
17. Lee ES, Santilli SM, Olson MM, et al. Wound infection after infrainguinal bypass operations: multivariate analysis of putative risk factors. *Surg Infect* 2000;1:257-263.
18. Pounds LL, Montes-Walters M, Mayhall CG, et al. A changing pattern of infection after major vascular reconstructions. *Vasc Endovascular Surg* 2005;39:511-517.
19. Antonios VS, Noel AA, Steckelberg JM, et al. Prosthetic vascular graft infection: a risk factor analysis using a case-control study. *J Infect* 2006;53:49-55.
20. Branchereau A, Ondo N'Dong F, La Selve L. Routine antibiotic prophylaxis in reconstructive arterial surgery: a double-blind study. *Presse Medicale* 1987;16:1633-1635.
21. Kaiser AB, Clayson KR, Mulherin Jr JL, et al. Antibiotic prophylaxis in vascular surgery. *Ann Surg* 1978;188:283-289.
22. Walker M, Litherland HK, Murphy J, Smith JA. Comparison of prophylactic antibiotic regimens in patients undergoing vascular surgery. *J Hosp Infect* 1984;5(Suppl A):101-106.
23. Hasselgren PO, Ivarsson L, Risberg B, Seeman T. Effects of prophylactic antibiotics in vascular surgery: a prospective, randomized, double-blind study. *Ann Surg* 1984;200:86-92.
24. Jensen LJ, Aagaard MT, Schifter S. Prophylactic vancomycin versus placebo in arterial prosthetic reconstructions. *Thorac Cardiovasc Surg* 1985;33:300-303.
25. Chester JF, Fergusson CM, Chant AD. The effect of cephradine prophylaxis on wound infection after arterial surgery through a groin incision. *Ann Royal Coll Surg Engl* 1983;65:389-390.
26. Pitt HA, Postier RG, MacGowan AL, et al. Prophylactic antibiotics in vascular surgery: topical, systemic or both? *Ann Surg* 1980;192:356-364.
27. Christenson JT, Eklof B, Hedstrom SA, Kamme C. Prevention of synthetic arterial graft infections by improved hygienic routine and dicloxacillin administration. *Scand J Infect Dis* 1981;13:51-57.
28. Worning AM, Frimodt-Moller N, Ostri P, et al. Antibiotic prophylaxis in vascular reconstructive surgery: a double-blind placebo-controlled study. *J Antimicrob Chemo* 1986;17:105-113.
29. Stewart A, Eyers PS, Earnshaw JJ. Prevention of infection in arterial reconstruction. *Cochrane Database Syst Rev* 2006;3. CD003073.
30. Earnshaw JJ, Slack RC, Hopkinson BR, Makin GS. Risk factors in vascular surgical sepsis. *Ann Royal Coll Surg Engl* 1988;70:139-143.
31. Hall JC, Christiansen KJ, Goodman M, et al. Duration of antimicrobial prophylaxis in vascular surgery. *Am J Surg* 1998;175:87-90.
32. Oostvogel HJ, van Vroonhoven TJ, van der Werken C, Lenderink AW. Single-dose v. short-term antibiotic therapy for prevention of wound infection in general surgery: a prospective, randomized double-blind trial. *Acta Chir Scand* 1987;153:571-575.
33. Edwards Jr WH, Kaiser AB, Tapper S, et al. Cefamandole versus cefazolin in vascular surgical wound infection prophylaxis: cost-effectiveness and risk factors. *J Vasc Surg* 1993;18:470-476.
34. Maki DG, Bohn MJ, Stolz SM, et al. Comparative study of cefazolin, cefamandole and vancomycin for surgical prophylaxis in cardiac and vascular operations: a double-blind randomized trial. *J Thorac Cardiovasc Surg* 1992;104:1423-1434.
35. Edwards Jr WH, Kaiser AB, Kernodle DS, et al. Cefuroxime versus cefazolin as prophylaxis in vascular surgery. *J Vasc Surg* 1992;15:35-41.
36. Marroni M, Cao P, Fiorio M, et al. Prospective, randomized, double-blind trial comparing teicoplanin and cefazolin as antibiotic prophylaxis in prosthetic vascular surgery. *Eur J Clin Microbiol Infect Dis* 1999;18:175-178.
37. Barlow IW, Ausobsky JR, Wilkinson D, Kester RC. Controlled trial of cephradine versus defuroxime in vascular surgery. *Int J Clin Pharma Res* 1989;9:223-227.
38. Risberg B, Drott C, Dalman P, et al. Oral ciprofloxacin versus intravenous cefuroxime as prophylaxis against postoperative infection in vascular surgery: a randomized double-blind, prospective multicentre study. *Eur J Vasc Endovasc Surg* 1995;10:346-351.
39. Kester RC, Antrum R, Thornton CA, Ramsden CH, Harding I. A comparison of teicoplanin versus cephradine plus metronidazole in the prophylaxis of post-operative infection in vascular surgery. *J Hosp Infect* 1999;41:233-243.
40. Dieterich H-J, Groh J, Behringer K, et al. The prophylactic activity of amoxicillin–clavulanate and cefoxitin in vascular surgery: a randomized clinical study. *J Antimicrob Chemo* 1989;24(Suppl B)209-211.
41. Kitzis M, Andreassian B, Branger C. Prophylactic timentin in patients undergoing thoracic or vascular surgery. *J Antimicrob Chemo* 1986;17(Suppl C):183-187.
42. Earnshaw JJ, Berridge DC, Slack RC, et al. Do preoperative chlorhexidine baths reduce the risk of infection after vascular reconstruction? *Eur J Vasc Surg* 1989;3:323-326.
43. Lynch W, Davey PG, Malek M, et al. Cost-effectiveness analysis of the use of chlorhexidine detergent in preoperative whole-body disinfection in wound infection prophylaxis. *J Hosp Infect* 1992;21:179-191.
44. May J, Brooks S, Johnstone D, Macfie J. Does the addition of preoperative skin preparation with povidone-iodine reduce groin sepsis following arterial surgery? *J Hosp Infect* 1993;24:153-156.
45. Zdanowski A, Danielsson G, Jonung T, et al. Intraoperative contamination of synthetic vascular grafts. Effect of glove change before graft implantation: a prospective randomized study. *Eur J Vasc Endovasc Surg* 2000;19:283-287.
46. Dunlop MG, Fox JN, Stonebridge PA, et al. Vacuum drainage of groin wounds after vascular surgery: a controlled trial. *Br J Surg* 1990;77:562-563.
47. Healy DA, Keyser III J, Holcomb III GW, et al. Prophylactic closed suction drainage of femoral wounds in patients undergoing vascular reconstruction. *J Vasc Surg* 1989;10:166-168.
48. Braithwaite BD, Davies B, Heather BP, Earnshaw JJ. Early results of a randomized trial of rifampicin-bonded Dacron grafts for extra-anatomic vascular reconstruction. *Br J Surg* 1998;85:1378-1381.
49. Earnshaw JJ, Whitman B, Heather BP. Two-year results of a randomized controlled trial of rifampicin-bonded extra-anatomic Dacron grafts. *Br J Surg* 2000;87:758-759.
50. D'Addato M, Curti T, Freyrie A. Prophylaxis of graft infection with rifampicin-bonded Gelseal graft: 2-year follow-up of a prospective clinical trial. *Cardiovasc Surg* 1996;4:200-204.
51. Gelabert HA. Primary arterial infections and antibiotic prophylaxis. In: Moore WS, ed. *Vascular surgery: a comprehensive review.* 6th ed. Philadelphia: WB Saunders; 2002:179-199(191).
52. Hicks RCJ, Greenhalgh RM. The pathogenesis of vascular graft infection. *Eur J Vasc Endovasc Surg* 1997;14(Suppl A):5-9.
53. Bandyk DF, Novotney ML, Back MR, et al. Expanded application of in situ replacement for prosthetic graft infection. *J Vasc Surg* 2001;34:411-420.
54. Castelli P, Caronno R, Ferrarese S, et al. New trends in prosthesis infection in cardiovascular surgery. *Surg Infect* 2006;7:S45-S47.
55. Batt M, Magne J-L, Alric P, et al. In situ revascularization with silver-coated polyester grafts to treat aortic infection: early and midterm results. *J Vasc Surg* 2003;38:983-989.
56. Desgrange P, Beaujean F, Brunet S, et al. Cryopreserved arterial allografts used for the treatment of infected vascular grafts. *Ann Vasc Surg* 1998;12:583-588.
57. Dorigo W, Pulli R, Azas L, et al. Early- and long-term results of conventional surgical treatment of secondary aorto-enteric fistula. *Eur J Vasc Endovasc Surg* 2003;26:512-518.
58. Gabriel M, Pukacki F, Checinski P, et al. Current options in prosthetic vascular graft infection: comparative analysis of 63 consecutive cases. *Arch Surg* 2004;389:272-277.
59. Gibbons CP, Ferguson CJ, Edwards K, et al. Use of superficial femoropopliteal vein for suprainguinal arterial reconstruction in the presence of infection. *Br J Surg* 2000;87:771-776.
60. Leseche G, Castier Y, Petit M-D, et al. Long-term results of cryopreserved arterial allograft reconstruction in infected prosthetic grafts and mycotic aneurysms of the abdominal aorta. *J Vasc Surg* 2001;34:616-622.

61. Oderich GS, Bower TC, Cherry Jr KJ, et al. Evolution from axillofemoral to in situ prosthetic reconstruction for the treatment of aortic graft infections at a single center. *J Vasc Surg* 2006;43:1166-1174.
62. Seeger JM, Back MR, Albright JL, et al. Influence of patient characteristics and treatment options on outcome of patients with prosthetic aortic graft infection. *Ann Vasc Surg* 1999;13:413-420.
63. Menawat SS, Gloviczki P, Serry RD, et al. Management of aortic graft-enteric fistulae. *Eur J Vasc Endovasc Surg* 1997;14(Suppl A):74-81.
64. Selan L, Passariello C. Microbiological diagnosis of aortofemoral graft infections. *Eur J Vasc Endovasc Surg* 1997;14(Suppl A):10-12.
65. Angle N, Freischlag JA. Prosthetic graft infections. In: Moore WS, ed. *Vascular surgery: a comprehensive review.* 6th ed. Philadelphia: WB Saunders; 2002:741-750(742).
66. Ernst C, Campbell H, Daugherty M, et al. Incidence and significance of intraoperative bacterial cultures during abdominal aortic aneurysmectomy. *Ann Surg* 1977;185:626-633.
67. Scobie K, McPhail N, Barber G, et al. Bacteriologic monitoring in abdominal aortic surgery. *Can J Surg* 1979;22:368-371.
68. Macbeth G, Rubin J, McIntyre K, et al. The relevance of arterial wall microbiology to the treatment of prosthetic graft infections: graft infection vs arterial infection. *J Vasc Surg* 1984;1:750-756.
69. McAuley C, Steed D, Webster M. Bacterial presence in aortic thrombus at elective aneurysm resection: is it clinically significant? *Am J Surg* 1984;147:322-324.
70. Buckels J, Fielding J, Black J, et al. Significance of positive bacterial cultures from aortic aneurysm contents. *Br J Surg* 1985;72:440-442.
71. Durham J, Malone J, Bernhard V. The impact of multiple operations on the importance of arterial wall cultures. *J Vasc Surg* 1987;5:160-169.
72. Schwartz J, Powell T, Burnham S, et al. Culture of abdominal aortic aneurysm contents: an additional series. *Arch Surg* 1987;122:777-780.
73. Ilgenfritz F, Jordan F. Microbiological monitoring of aortic aneurysm wall and contents during aneurysmectomy. *Arch Surg* 1988;123: 506-508.
74. Brandimarte C, Santini C, Venditti M, et al. Clinical significance of intraoperative cultures of aneurysm walls and contents in elective abdominal aortic aneurysmectomy. *Eur J Epidemiol* 1989;5:521-525.
75. Wakefield T, Pierson C, Schaberg D, et al. Artery, periarterial adipose tissue, and blood microbiology during vascular reconstructive surgery: perioperative and early postoperative observations. *J Vasc Surg* 1990;11:624-628.
76. Russell H, Barnes R, Baker W. Sterility of intestinal transudate during aortic reconstructive procedures. *Arch Surg* 1975;110:402-404.
77. Demirer S, Gecim IE, Aydinuraz K, et al. Affinity of *Staphylococcus epidermidis* to various prosthetic graft materials. *J Surg Res* 2001;99:70-74.
78. Schmitt D, Bandyk D, Pequet A, et al. Bacterial adherence to vascular prostheses. *J Vasc Surg* 1986;3:732-740.
79. Rosenman J, Pearce W, Kempczinski R. Bacterial adherence of vascular prostheses. *J Surg Res* 1985;28:648-655.
80. Moore WS, Malone JM, Keown K. Prosthetic arterial graft material: influence on neointimal healing and bacteremic infectibility. *Arch Surg* 1980;115:1379-1383.
81. LePort C, Goeau-Brissonniere D, LeBrault C, et al. Pseudointimal development and vascular prosthesis susceptibility to bacteremic infection. *Surg Forum* 1974;15:520.
82. Kaebnick H, Bandyk D, Bergamini T, et al. The microbiology of explanted vascular prostheses. *Surgery* 1987;102:756-761.
83. Perera GB, Fujitani RM, Kubaska SM. Aortic graft infection: update on management and treatment options. *Vasc Endovasc Surg* 2006;40:1-10.
84. Armstrong PA, Back MR, Wilson JS, et al. Improved outcomes in the recent management of secondary aortoenteric fistula. *J Vasc Surg* 2005;42:660-666.
85. Becquemin JP, Qvarfordt P, Kron J, et al. Aortic graft infection: is there a place for partial graft removal? *Eur J Vasc Endovasc Surg* 1997;14(Suppl A):53-58.
86. Daenens K, Fournequ I, Nevelsteen A. Ten-year experience in autogenous reconstruction with the femoral vein in the treatment of aortofemoral prosthetic infection. *Eur J Vasc Endovasc Surg* 2003;25:240-245.
87. Fiorani P, Speziale F, Rizzo L, et al. Long-term follow-up after in situ graft replacement in patients with aortofemoral graft infections. *Eur J Vasc Endovasc Surg* 1997;14(Suppl A):111-114.
88. Seeger JM, Pretus HA, Welborn MB, et al. Long-term outcome after treatment of aortic graft infection with staged extra-anatomic bypass grafting and aortic graft removal. *J Vasc Surg* 2000;32:451-461.
89. Young RM, Cherry Jr KJ, Davis PM, et al. The results of in situ prosthetic replacement for infected aortic grafts. *Am J Surg* 1999;178:136-140.
90. Reilly LM, Ehrenfeld WK, Goldstone J, Stoney RJ. Gastrointestinal tract involvement by prosthetic graft infection: the significance of gastrointestinal hemorrhage. *Ann Surg* 1985;202:78-86.
91. Szilagyi DE, Smith RF, Elliott JP, Vrandecic MP. Infection in arterial reconstruction with synthetic grafts. *Ann Surg* 1972;176:321-323.
92. Koenig J, vonDongen RJAM. *Possibilities and results in cardiovascular surgery.* Berlin: Springer; 1980.
93. Samson RH, Veith FJ, Janko GS, et al. A modified classification and approach to the management of infections involving peripheral arterial prosthetic grafts. *J Vasc Surg* 1988;8:147-153.
94. Low RN, Wall SD, Jeffrey RB, et al. Aortoenteric fistula and perigraft infection evaluation with CT. *Radiology* 1990;175:157-162.
95. Mark A, Moss A, Lusby R, Kaiser JA. CT evaluation of complications of abdominal aortic surgery. *Radiology* 1982;145:409-414.
96. Olofsson PA, Aufferman W, Higgins CB, et al. Diagnosis of prosthetic aortic graft infection by magnetic resonance imaging. *J Vasc Surg* 1988;8:99-105.
97. Fiorani R, Speziale F, Rizzo L, et al. Detection of aortic graft infection with leukocyte labeled with technetium 99m-hexametazine. *J Vasc Surg* 1993;17:87-95.
98. Fukuchi K, Ishida Y, Higashi M, et al. Detection of aortic graft infection by fluorodeocyglucose positron emission tomography: comparison with computed tomographic findings. *J Vasc Surg* 2005;42:919-925.
99. Broome DR. Nephrogenic systemic fibrosis associated with gadolinium based contrast agents: a summary of the medical literature reporting. *Eur J Radiol* 2008;66:230-234.
100. Shahidi S, Eskil A, Lundof E, et al. Detection of abdominal aortic graft infection: comparison of magnetic resonance imaging and indium-labeled white blood cell scanning. *Ann Vasc Surg* 2007;21:586-592.
101. Insall RL, Jones NAG, Chamberlain J, et al. A new isotopic technique for detecting prosthetic arterial graft infection: 99mTc-hexametazine-labelled-leukocyte imaging. *Br J Surg* 1990;77:1295-1298.
102. Prats E, Banzo J, Abos ME, et al. Diagnosis of prosthetic vascular graft infection by technetium-99m-HMPAO-labeled leukocytes. *J Nucl Med* 1994;35:1303-1307.
103. Insall RL, Keavey PM, Hawkins T, et al. The specificity of technetium-labelled-leukocyte imaging of aortic grafts in the early postoperative period. *Eur J Vasc Surg* 1991;5:571-576.
104. Liberatore M, Iurilli AP, Ponzo F, et al. Aortofemoral graft infection: the usefulness of 99mTc-HMPAO-labelled leukocyte scan. *Eur J Vasc Endovasc Surg* 1997;14(Suppl A):27-29.
105. Sugawara Y, Braun DK, Kison PV, et al. Rapid detection of human infections with fluorine-18 fluorodeoxyglucose and positron emission tomography: preliminary results. *Eur J Nucl Med* 1998;25:1238-1243.
106. Stumpe KD, Dazzi H, Schaffner A, Von Schulthess GK. Infection imaging using whole-body FDG-PET. *Eur J Nucl Med* 2000;27:822-832.
107. Keidar Z, Engel A, Nitecki S, et al. PET/CT using 2-deoxy-2-[18F]fluoro-D-glucose for the evaluation of suspected infected vascular graft. *Mol Imaging Biol* 2003;5:23-25.
108. Krupnick AS, Lombardi JV, Engels FH, et al. 18-Fluorodeoxyglucose positron emission tomography as a novel imaging tool for the diagnosis of aortoenteric fistula and aortic graft infection: a case report. *Vasc Endovasc Surg* 2003;37:363-366.
109. Stadler P, Bilohlavek O, Spacek M, Michalek P. Diagnosis of vascular prosthesis infection with FDG-PET/CT. *J Vasc Surg* 2004;40:1246-1247.
110. Kaim AH, Weber B, Kurrer MO, et al. Autoradiographic quantification of ^{18}F-FDG uptake in experimental soft-tissue abscesses in rats. *Radiology* 2002;223:446-451.
111. Keidar A, Engel A, Hoffman A, et al. Prosthetic vascular graft infection: the role of 18F-FDG PET/CT. *J Nucl Med* 2007;48:1230-1236.
112. Bunt TJ. Synthetic vascular graft infections. I. Graft infections. *Surgery* 1983;93:733-746.
113. Bunt TJ. Synthetic vascular graft infections. II. Graft-enteric erosions and graft-enteric fistulas. *Surgery* 1983;94:1-9.
114. Liekweg Jr WG, Greenfield LJ. Vascular prosthetic infections: collected experience and results of treatment. *Surgery* 1977;81:225-242.
115. Bacourt F, Koskas F. Axillobifemoral bypass and aortic exclusion for vascular septic lesions: a multicenter retrospective study of 98 cases. *Ann Vasc Surg* 1992;6:119-126.
116. Ricotta JJ, Faggioli GL, Stella A, et al. Total excision and extra-anatomic bypass for aortic graft infection. *Am J Surg* 1991;162:145-149.
117. Reilly LM, Stoney RJ, Goldstone J, Ehrenfeld WK. Improved management of aortic graft infection: the influence of operation sequence and staging. *J Vasc Surg* 1987;5:421-431.

118. O'Hara PJ, Hertzer NR, Beven EG, Krajewski LP. Surgical management of infected abdominal aortic grafts: review of a 25-year experience. *J Vasc Surg* 1986;3:725-731.
119. Yeager RA, Taylor LM, Moneta GL, et al. Improved results with conventional management of infrarenal aortic infection. *J Vasc Surg* 1999;30:76-83.
120. Reilly LM, Altman H, Lusby RJ, et al. Late results following surgical management of vascular graft infection. *J Vasc Surg* 1984;1:36-44.
121. Kuestner LM, Reilly LM, Jicha DL, et al. Secondary aortoenteric fistula: contemporary outcome with use of extra-anatomic bypass and infected graft excision. *J Vasc Surg* 1995;21:184-196.
122. Hart JP, Eginton MT, Brown KR, et al. Operative strategies in aortic graft infections: is complete graft excision always necessary? *Ann Vasc Surg* 2005;19:154-160.
123. Jausseran JM, Stella N, Courbier R, et al. Total prosthetic graft excision and extra-anatomic bypass. *Eur J Vasc Endovasc Surg* 1997;14(Suppl A):59-65.
124. Reid JDS, MacDonald PS. Removing the infected aortofemoral graft using a two-stage procedure with a delay between the stages. *Ann Vasc Surg* 2005;19:862-867.
125. Sicard GA, Reilly JM, Doblas M, et al. Autologous vein reconstruction in prosthetic graft infection. *Eur J Vasc Endovasc Surg* 1997;14(Suppl A):93-98.
126. Lavigne JP, Postal A, Kolh P, Limet R. Prosthetic vascular infection complicated or not by aorto-enteric fistulae: comparison of treatment with and without cryopreserved allograft (homograft). *Eur J Vasc Endovasc Surg* 2003;25:416-423.
127. Ten Raa S, Van Sambeck MR, Hagenaars T, Van Urk H. Management of aortic graft infection. *J Cardiovasc Surg* 2002;43:209-215.
128. Darling III RC, Resnikoff M, Kreienberg PB, et al. Alternative approach for management of infected aortic grafts. *J Vasc Surg* 1997;25:106-112.
129. Matsagas MI, Fatouros M, Mitsis M, et al. Aortobipopliteal bypass grafting for in situ replacement of infected aortobifemoral prosthesis. *Ann Vasc Surg* 2004;18:361-364.
130. Armstrong PA, Back MR, Bandyk DF, et al. Selective application of sartorius muscle flaps and aggressive staged surgical debridement can influence long-term outcomes of complex prosthetic graft infection. *J Vasc Surg* 2007;46:71-78.
131. Bandyk DF, Novotney ML, Johnson BL, et al. Use of Rifampin-soaked gelatin-sealed polyester grafts for in situ treatment of primary aortic and vascular prosthetic infections. *J Surg Res* 2001;95:44-49.
132. Hayes PD, Nasim A, London NJM, et al. In situ replacement of infected aortic grafts with rifampicin-bonded prostheses: the Leicester experience (1992-1998). *J Vasc Surg* 1999;30:92-98.
133. Nasim A, Hayes P, London N, et al. In situ replacement of infected aortic grafts with rifampicin-bonded prostheses. *Br J Surg* 1999;86:695.
134. Torsello G, Sandmann W. Use of antibiotic-bonded grafts in vascular graft infection. *Eur J Vasc Endovasc Surg* 1997;14(Suppl A):84-87.
135. Zegelman M, Gunther G. Infected grafts require excision and extra-anatomic reconstruction. In: Greenhalgh RM, ed. *The evidence for vascular or endovascular reconstruction.* Philadelphia: Saunders; 2002:252-258.
136. Agrifoglio G, Bonalumi F, Scalamogna M, et al. Aortic allograft replacement: north Italy transplant programme (NITp). *Eur J Vasc Endovasc Surg* 1997;14(Suppl A):108-110.
137. Bliziotis IA, Kapaskelis AM, Kasiakou SK, Falagas ME. Limitations in the management of aortic graft infections. *Ann Vasc Surg* 2006;20:669-671.
138. Chiesa R, Astore D, Piccolo G, et al. Homografts in the treatment of prosthetic graft infections: experience of the Italian collaborative vascular homograft group. *Ann Vasc Surg* 1998;12:457-462.
139. Chiesa R, Astore D, Frigerio S, et al. Vascular prosthetic graft infection: epidemiology, bacteriology, pathogenesis and treatment. *Acta Chir Belg* 2002;102:238-247.
140. deGama AD, Rosa A, Soares M, Mouara C. Use of autologous superficial femoral artery in surgery for aortic prosthesis infection. *Ann Vasc Surg* 2004;18:593-596.
141. Gabriel M, Pukacki F, Dzieciuchowicz L, et al. Cryopreserved arterial allografts in the treatment of prosthetic graft infections. *Eur J Vasc Endovasc Surg* 2004;27:590-596.
142. Kitamura T, Morota T, Motomura N, et al. Management of infected grafts and aneurysms of the aorta. *Ann Vasc Surg* 2005;19:335-342.
143. Locati P, Novali C, Socrate AM, et al. The use of arterial allografts in aortic graft infections: a three year experience on eighteen patients. *J Cardiovasc Surg* 1998;39:735-741.
144. Nevelsteen A, Feryn T, Lacroix H, et al. Experience with cryopreserved arterial allografts in the treatment of prosthetic graft infection. *Cardiovasc Surg* 1998;6:378-383.
145. Noel AA, Gloviczki P, Cherry Jr KJ, et al. Abdominal aortic reconstruction in infected fields: early results of the United States cryopreserved aortic allograft registry. *J Vasc Surg* 2002;35:847-852.
146. Kieffer E, Gomes D, Chiche L, et al. Allograft replacement for infrarenal aortic graft infection: early and late results in 179 patients. *J Vasc Surg* 2004;39:1009-1017.
147. Pirelli S, Arici V, Bozzani A, Odero A. Aortic graft infections: treatment with arterial allograft. *Transplant Proc* 2005;37:2694-2696.
148. Ruotolo C, Plissonnier D, Bahnini A, et al. In situ arterial allografts: a new treatment for aortic prosthetic infection. *Eur J Vasc Endovasc Surg* 1997;14(Suppl A):102-107.
149. Teebken OE, Pichlmaier MA, Brand S, Haverich A. Cryopreserved arterial allografts for in situ reconstruction of infected arterial vessels. *Eur J Vasc Endovasc Surg* 2004;27:597-602.
150. Verhelst R, Lacroix V, Vraux H, et al. Use of cryopreserved arterial homografts for management of infected prosthetic grafts: a multicentric study. *Ann Vasc Surg* 2000;14:602-607.
151. Vogt PR, Brunner-LaRocca H-P, Lachat M, et al. Technical details with the use of cryopreserved arterial allografts for aortic infection: influence on early and midterm mortality. *J Vasc Surg* 2002;35:80-86.
152. Zhou W, Lin PH, Bush RL, et al. In situ reconstruction with cryopreserved arterial allografts for management of mycotic aneurysms or aortic prosthetic graft infections: a multi-institutional experience. *Tex Heart Inst J* 2006;33:14-18.
153. Ali AT, Mcleod N, Kalapatapu VR, et al. Staging the neoaortoiliac system: feasibility and short-term outcomes. *J Vasc Surg* 2008;48:1125-1131.
154. Brown Jr PM, Kim VB, Lalikos JF, et al. Autologous superficial femoral vein for aortic reconstruction in infected fields. *Ann Vasc Surg* 1999;13:32-36.
155. Cardozo MA, Frankini AD, Bonamigo TP. Use of the superficial femoral vein in the treatment of infected aortoiliofemoral prosthetic grafts. *Cardiovasc Surg* 2002;10:304-310.
156. Faulk J, Dattilo JB, Guzman RJ, et al. Neoaortic reconstruction for aortic graft infection: need for endovascular adjunctive therapies? *Ann Vasc Surg* 2005;19:774-781.
157. Franke S, Voit R. The superficial femoral vein as arterial substitute in infections of the aortoiliac region. *Ann Vasc Surg* 1997;11:406-412.
158. Gibbons CP, Ferguson CJ, Fligelstone LJ, Edwards K. Experience with femoropopliteal vein as a conduit for vascular reconstruction in infected fields. *Eur J Vasc Endovasc Surg* 2003;25:424-431.
159. Nevelsteen A, Lacroix H, Suy R. Infrarenal aortic graft infection: in situ aortoiliofemoral reconstruction with the lower extremity deep veins. *Eur J Vasc Endovasc Surg* 1997;14(Suppl A):88-92.
160. Tambyraja AL, Wyatt MG, Clarke MJ, Chalmers RTA. Autologous deep vein reconstruction of infected thoracoabdominal aortic patch graft. *J Vasc Surg* 2003;38:852-854.
161. Wojciechowski J, Znaniecki L, Zelechowski P. Superficial femoral vein and superficial femoral artery as replacement for infected axillofemoral graft. *Ann Vasc Surg* 2006;20:544-546.
162. Dosluoglu HH, Kittredge J, Cherr GS. Use of cryopreserved femoral vein for in situ replacement of infected femorofemoral prosthetic artery bypass. *Vasc Endovasc Surg* 2008;42:74-78.
163. Aavik A, Lieberg J, Kals J, et al. Ten years of treating aorto-femoral bypass graft infection with venous allografts. *Eur J Vasc Endovasc Surg* 2008;36:432-437.
164. Calligaro KD, Veith FJ, Schwartz ML, et al. Selective preservation of infected prosthetic arterial grafts: analysis of a 20-year experience with 120 extracavitary-infected grafts. *Ann Surg* 1994;220:461-471.
165. Calligaro KD, Veith FJ. Graft preserving methods for managing aortofemoral prosthetic graft infection. *Eur J Vasc Endovasc Surg* 1997;14(Suppl A):38-42.
166. Kotsis T, Lioupis C. Use of vacuum assisted closure in vascular graft infection confined to the groin. *Acta Chir Belg* 2007;107:37-44.
167. Mirzaie M, Schmitto JD, Tirilomis T, et al. Surgical management of vascular graft infection in severely ill patients by partial resection of the infected prosthesis. *Eur J Vasc Endovasc Surg* 2007;33:610-613.
168. Stone PA, Armstrong PA, Bandyk DF, et al. Use of antibiotic-loaded polymethylmethacrylate beads for the treatment of extracavitary prosthetic vascular graft infections. *J Vasc Surg* 2006;44:757-761.
169. Taylor SM, Weatherford DA, Langan III EM, Lokey JS. Outcomes in the management of vascular prosthetic graft infections confined to the groin: a reappraisal. *Ann Vasc Surg* 1996;10:117-122.
170. Voboril R, Weverova J, Kralove H. Successful treatment of infected vascular prosthetic grafts in the groin using conservative therapy with povidone-iodine solution. *Ann Vasc Surg* 2004;18:372-375.

171. Akowuah E, Narayan P, Angelini G, Bryan AJ. Management of prosthetic graft infection after surgery of the thoracic aorta: removal of the prosthetic graft is not necessary. *J Thorac Cardiovasc Surg* 2007;134:1051-1052.
172. Calligaro KD, Veith FJ, Yuan JG, et al. Intra-abdominal aortic graft infection: complete or partial graft preservation in patients at very high risk. *J Vasc Surg* 2003;38:1199-1205.
173. Calligaro KD, Veith FJ, Schwartz ML, et al. Differences in early versus late extracavitary arterial graft infections. *J Vasc Surg* 1995;22:680-688.
174. Swain TW, Calligaro III KD, Dougherty MD. Management of infected aortic prosthetic grafts. *Vasc Endovasc Surg* 2004;38:75-82.
175. O'Connor S, Andrew P, Batt M, Becquemin JP. A systematic review and meta-analysis of treatments for aortic graft infection. *J Vasc Surg* 2006;44:38-45.
176. Castier Y, Francis F, Cerceau P, et al. Cryopreserved arterial allograft reconstruction for peripheral graft infection. *J Vasc Surg* 2005;41:30-37.
177. Chalmers RTA, Wolfe JHN, Cheshire NJW, et al. Improved management of infrainguinal bypass graft infection with methicillin-resistant *Staphylococcus aureus*. *Br J Surg* 1999;86:1433-1436.
178. deVirgilio C, Cherry Jr KJ, Gloviczki P, et al. Infected lower extremity extra-anatomic bypass grafts: management of a serious complication in high-risk patients. *Ann Vasc Surg* 1995;9:459-466.
179. Zetrenne E, Wirth GA, McIntosh BC, et al. Managing extracavitary prosthetic vascular graft infections. *Ann Plast Surg* 2006;57:677-682.
180. Zetrenne E, McIntosh BC, McRae MH, et al. Prosthetic vascular graft infection: a multi-center review of surgical management. *Yale J Biol Med* 2007;80:113-121.
181. Pederson G, Laxdal E, Hagala M, Aune S. Local infections after above-knee prosthetic femoropopliteal bypass for intermittent claudication. *Surg Infect* 2004;5:174-179.
182. Oelbrandt B, Guelinckx PJ, Nevelsteen A. Use of the superior pedicled rectus abdominis flap to cover infected aortic grafts. *Br J Plast Surg* 2003;56:280-283.
183. Skoll PJ, Kowalczyk J. Superiorly based rectus abdominis wraparound flap for axillofemoral graft sepsis. *Ann Plast Surg* 2001;47:191-193.
184. Graham RG, Omotoso PO, Hudson DA. The effectiveness of muscle flaps for the treatment of prosthetic graft sepsis. *Plast Reconstr Surg* 2002;109:108-113.
185. Akron JD, Smith A, Losee JE, et al. Management of complex groin wounds: preferred use of the rectus femoris muscle flap. *Plast Reconstr Surg* 2005;115:776-783.
186. Illig KA, Alkon JE, Smith A, et al. Rotational muscle flap closure for acute groin wound infections following vascular surgery. *Ann Vasc Surg* 2004;18:661-668.
187. Morasch MD, Sam AD II, Kibbe MR, et al. Early results with use of gracilis muscle flap coverage on infected groin wounds after vascular surgery. *J Vasc Surg* 2004;39:1277-1283.
188. Schutzer R, Hingorani A, Ascher E, et al. Early transposition of the sartorius muscle for exposed patent infrainguinal bypass grafts. *Vasc Endovasc Surg* 2005;39:159-162.
189. Seify H, Moyer HR, Jones GE, et al. The role of muscle flaps in wound salvage after vascular graft infections: the Emory experience. *Plast Reconstr Surg* 2005;117:1325-1333.
190. Sladen JG, Chen JC, Reid JD. An aggressive local approach to vascular graft infection. *Am J Surg* 1998;176:222-225.
191. Galland RB. Sartorius transposition in the management of synthetic graft infection. *Eur J Vasc Endovasc Surg* 2002;23:175-177.
192. Maser B, Vedder N, Rodriguez D, Johansen K. Sartorius myoplasty for infected vascular grafts in the groin: safe, durable and effective. *Arch Surg* 1997;132:525-526.
193. Colwell AS, Donaldson MC, Belkin M, Orgill DP. Management of early groin vascular bypass graft infections with sartorius and rectus femoris flaps. *Ann Plast Surg* 2004;52:49-53.
194. Dosluoglu HH, Schimpf DK, Schultz R, Cherr GS. Preservation of infected and exposed vascular grafts using vacuum assisted closure without muscle flap coverage. *J Vasc Surg* 2005;42:989-992.
195. Pinocy J, Albes JM, Wicke C, et al. Treatment of periprosthetic soft tissue infection of the groin following vascular surgical procedures by means of a polyvinyl alcohol-vacuum sponge system. *Wound Repair Regen* 2003;11:104-109.
196. Mayer DO, Enzler M, Inderbitzi R, et al. Vacuum-assisted closure system with direct contact to native arteries and/or vascular grafts to improve the outcome of perivascular infection (abstract). Available at: http://www.veithsymposium.org/pdf2005/87.pdf. Accessed September 8, 2008.
197. Svensson S, Monsen C, Kolbel T, Acosta S. Predictors for outcome after vacuum assisted closure therapy of peri-vascular surgical site infections in the groin. *Eur J Vasc Endovasc Surg* 2008;36:84-89.
198. Bennett LL, Rosenblum RS, Perlov C, et al. An in vivo comparison of topical agents on wound repair. *Plast Reconstr Surg* 2001;108:675-683.
199. Adams Jr WP, Conner WC, Barton Jr FE, et al. Optimizing breast pocket irrigation: an in vitro study and clinical implications. *Plast Reconstr Surg* 2000;105:334-338.
200. Buehler PK, Reading GP, Jacoby FG, et al. The "Sulfamylon sandwich": a laminated mafenide-saline dressing. *Ann Plast Surg* 1980;5:157-159.
201. Shuck JM, Thorne LW, Cooper CG. Mafenide acetate solution dressings: an adjunct in burn wound care. *J Trauma* 1975;15:595-599.
202. Murphy RC, Kucan JO, Robson MC, et al. The effect of 5% mafenide acetate solution on bacterial control in infected rat burns. *J Trauma* 1983;23:878-881.
203. Henry SL, Galloway KP. Local antibacterial therapy for the management of orthopedic infections: pharmokinetic considerations. *Clin Pharmacokinet* 1995;29:36-45.
204. Nielsen OM, Noer HH, Jergensen LG, Lorentzen JE. Gentamycin beads in the treatment of localized vascular graft infection-long term results in 17 cases. *Eur J Vasc* 1991;5:283-285.

chapter

41

Native Arterial Infections

Luis R. Leon Jr, MD, RVT, FACS • Daniel M. Ihnat, MD, FACS • Joseph L. Mills Sr, MD, FACS

Key Points

- Before the introduction of antibiotics, most infected arterial aneurysms (IAAs) involved the aorta and resulted from endocarditis. Since then, the most common underlying cause has become trauma, the most common bacterium is *Staphylococcus,* and the most common site is the femoral artery.
- IAAs present with various symptoms and may occur in any age group. Nearly all untreated IAAs eventually lead to hemorrhage from rupture.
- A high index of suspicion is warranted in patients with aneurysms associated with a recent prolonged febrile illness, positive blood cultures, loss of calcium in the aneurysm wall, or multilobular morphology or patients who are female.
- When IAA is suspected, blood cultures, a complete blood cell count, and the erythrocyte sedimentation rate should be obtained, followed immediately by institution of antibiotic therapy. Definitive surgical therapy should not be unduly delayed, as the aneurysm could rupture.
- Hemodynamically stable patients with suspected infected aneurysms should undergo radiological evaluation. Contrast-enhanced computed tomography is the initial diagnostic test of choice.
- General management principles for infected aneurysms include control hemorrhage; obtain tissue cultures; widely debride all infected tissues; consider arterial reconstruction with autogenous conduit, preferably through uninfected tissue planes; and continue antibiotic therapy throughout the postoperative period.
- Infected upper extremity aneurysms are rare. Trauma is the most common etiology.

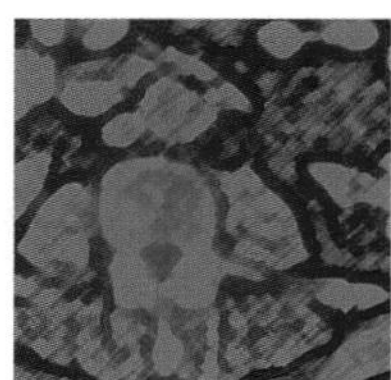

HISTORICAL BACKGROUND

The first account of a nonsyphilitic infected artery was published in 1844 when Rokitansky[1] described arterial wall abscesses in patients with endocarditis. Virkow,[2] Koch,[3] and Tufnell[4] subsequently reported cases of aneurysms felt to be secondary to embolization from endocarditis. The cause of the aneurysm was postulated to be due either to rheumatism[3] or the mechanical forces of the embolus lodged in the artery.[2,4] Goodhart[5] in 1877, was the first to propose that both endocarditis and arterial aneurysms were the result of infection. In 1885, Osler[6] provided the first comprehensive description of infected aneurysms from endocarditis and coined the term mycotic aneurysm. At that time, the term *mycotic* was applied to any infection and did not differentiate bacterial from fungal infections. The use of this term has subsequently created confusion as to whether *mycotic* should be used to describe all infected arterial aneurysms, be limited to infectious processes associated with endocarditis, or be used only for true fungal infections. We prefer the term infected arterial aneurysm (IAA) because of its clarity and simplicity.

In 1887, Eppinger[7] was the first to demonstrate that the bacteria infecting the aortic valve and the concomitant infected aneurysm were identical. He employed the term embolic mycotic aneurysm and believed the infection initially embolized to the adventitia and spread to the media and intima. Subsequently, the concept that the bacteria can infect the artery wall via the vasa vasorum has been generally accepted.

Native arterial infections are a fulminant in nature. Although reports of sterilization of IAAs[8] exist, rapid destruction of the arterial wall often leads to aneurysm rupture before the diagnosis is made. Less commonly, patients develop nonaneurysmal suppurative arteritis, which can also lead to vessel rupture or thrombosis.[9] Before the antibiotic era, IAAs were considered

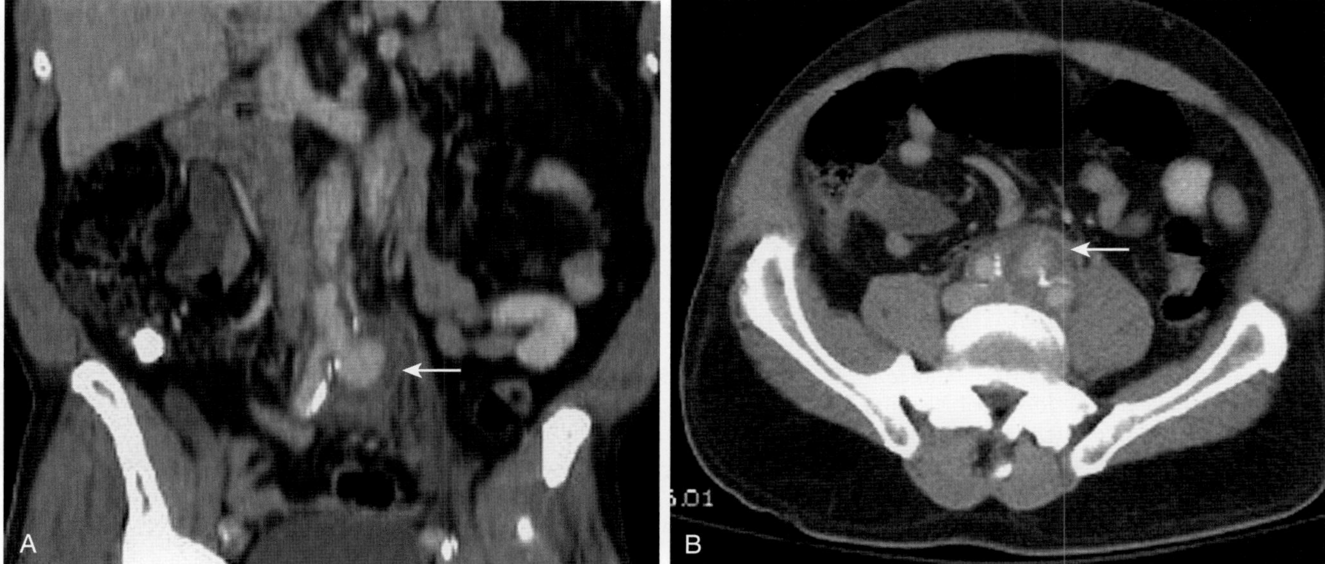

Figure 41-1. Frontal **(A)** and axial **(B)** views from a computed tomography scan demonstrating the contained rupture of an infected left common iliac artery aneurysm *(white arrow)*. The Gram stain of the aneurysm wall revealed three or more white blood cells and three or more Gram-negative rods. The aneurysm wall grew *Klebsiella pneumoniae* and *Enterococci.*

incurable. By 1954, only 10 successfully treated cases of IAAs had been reported.[10] The main determinants of prognosis include the location of the IAA, the presence of rupture, the virulence of the infecting organism, and the patient's immune status.[11-14] IAAs due to Gram-negative organisms are associated with increased mortality and are more likely to present with rupture (Figure 41-1).[11] True fungal infections are rare and typically occur in immunosuppressed patients.[15,16]

BACTERIOLOGY

The pathogenesis of IAAs has significantly changed over the past century. Before the advent of antibiotics, nearly 90% of IAAs were associated with bacterial endocarditis,[17] occurring predominantly in the ascending aorta and arch. The bacteria most commonly grown from the walls of the IAAs were a reflection of those responsible for bacterial endocarditis and included nonhemolytic streptococci, staphylococci, and pneumococci. The introduction and widespread use of antibiotics resulted in a sharp decline in the frequency of endocarditis.[18,19] From approximately 1945 until 1965, the most commonly reported site of IAA was the abdominal aorta and the most frequent organism was *Salmonella.*[20-22] Before 1965, *Salmonella* was responsible for 38% of IAAs and *Staphylococcus aureus* for 19%. Since then, the distribution of responsible organisms has shifted; *Salmonella* decreased in reported frequency to 10%, while *S. aureus* rose to 30%. In parallel with this bacteriological shift, the frequency of endocarditis as the underlying etiology has fallen from 37% to 10% while trauma increased from 10% to 54%, and the femoral artery has become the most commonly involved anatomical site.[23]

The changes in bacterial species and arterial location of IAAs are the result of the increasing incidence of arterial catheterizations, as well as intraarterial injection of street drugs. Intact arterial intima is highly resistant to infection. Therefore, areas of intimal disruption are preferred sites for bacterial seeding, and IAAs are seen in areas of atherosclerotic plaques, bifurcations, trauma, and immediately distal to coarctations.[22,24,25] *Salmonella* species in particular have a strong predilection to infect damaged aortic intima[11-12,21,22,26] and abnormal endocardium.[27] Investigators[28] evaluated patients with positive *Salmonella* blood cultures and found that 25% (10 of 40) of patients older than 50 years of age developed either infected aneurysms or endocarditis. In contrast, none of the 29 patients younger than 50 developed infected aneurysms or endocarditis. This observation provides strong support to the premise that *Salmonella* is prone to infect areas of abnormal arterial intima, especially arteries harboring atherosclerotic plaque.

CLASSIFICATION

Numerous classification systems have been proposed over the past several decades, mostly derived from a combination of historical terminology and etiological factors. Finseth and Abbott[29] proposed the most logical one in 1973:

1. *Primary IAAs* arise from adjacent surrounding areas of infection or trauma, either from direct contact or via lymphatic spread.
2. *Secondary IAAs* arise from septic embolization, either through the vasa vasorum or intraluminally into areas of abnormal intima, such as preexisting aneurysms or atherosclerotic plaques.
3. *Cryptogenic IAAs* arise without a known cause but are believed to occur after an episode of bacteremia.

This classification system is primarily based on etiology and may have some prognostic value. Investigators[13] have suggested that patients with cryptogenic IAAs have a better prognosis compared to those patients with a known source.

CLINICAL PRESENTATION

The clinical presentation may be insidious. Patients often present with fever and vague pain in the anatomical region of the IAA. Once infected, the artery may rapidly become aneurysmal and rupture. Before the antibiotic era, patients with IAAs were typically less than 40 years old. Presently, all age groups are susceptible; however, patients without a recent history of trauma tend to be older and afflicted with peripheral arterial disease. More recent series have reported that the mean age of IAA patients is 55 to 60 years old.[13,20,21] Pain and fever are the most common presenting symptoms, occurring in 75% to 95% of patients; leukocytosis is identified in 65% to 85% of patients[11,13,20-22]; and a palpable aneurysm is detectable in 50% to 65% cases.[11,22] Rupture is also common before diagnosis; 30% to 80% patients with IAAs present with rupture.[13,20-22] Cryptogenic IAAs remain common but are decreasing in incidence. While as many as 50% of patients had cryptogenic IAAs in older reports,[21,22] since 1965, only 22% of reported cases have had no identifiable source.[23] Patients with intraabdominal IAAs often present with vague, nonspecific abdominal or back pain associated with fever and an elevated white blood cell count. A broad differential diagnosis exists for patients presenting with such nonspecific complaints. In contrast, IAAs of the extremities are easier to palpate than intracavitary ones. Often, an extremity IAA can be diagnosed on clinical examination as a tender erythematous peripheral aneurysm, especially if associated with recent arterial trauma.

IAAs may present with various symptoms and may occur in any age group. It is important to remember that nearly all untreated IAAs eventually lead to hemorrhage from rupture. A high index of suspicion is warranted in patients that present with aneurysms associated with a recent prolonged febrile illness, positive blood cultures, loss of calcium in the aneurysm wall, or female gender.[11] If an IAA is suspected, urgent confirmation of the diagnosis and definitive treatment are essential. It is also important to recognize that patients may have multiple IAAs, especially individuals with infective endocarditis.[30]

DIAGNOSIS

Patients with positive blood cultures and an arterial aneurysm should be considered to have an infected aneurysm until proven otherwise. Conversely, negative blood cultures are not sufficient to exclude IAAs. Investigators have noted positive cultures in only 50% to 70% of cases.[11,13,20,22] Furthermore, intraoperative Gram stains of the aneurysm wall are positive in only 20% to 30%.[13,22] An elevated leukocyte count lacks specificity, and the sensitivity may be hindered by concurrent antimicrobial therapy. Erythrocyte sedimentation rates are often elevated but also lack specificity. If the diagnosis is first suspected at operation, Gram stain, cultures, and histological specimens of the aneurysm wall should be obtained. Although not helpful with the intraoperative management, cultures confirm the diagnosis and assist with selection of appropriate antibiotic therapy during the postoperative period. Gram stain is helpful if positive, but a negative result does not exclude IAA. Hemodynamically stable patients with suspected IAA should undergo radiological evaluation. Contrast-enhanced computed tomography (CT) is extremely valuable to detect the presence and morphology of an aneurysm, evidence of arterial inflammation and infection, and the presence of rupture. CT findings indicative of infection include the presence of a saccular aneurysm, irregular lumen, irregular thickened wall, perianeurysmal fluid or gas, hematoma, perianeurysmal enhancement, disruption of intimal calcification, or osteomyelitis in an adjacent vertebral body (Figure 41-2).[31,32]

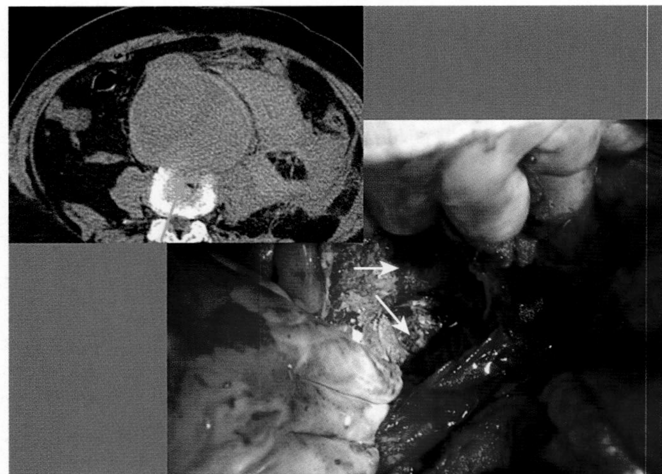

Figure 41-2. Intraoperative photograph of an elderly man who presented with an episode of severe abdominal and back pain associated with syncope. His family reported that he had been complaining of severe low back pain for more than 3 weeks. Computed tomography of the abdomen and pelvis upon arrival showed vertebral body erosion from an 11-cm abdominal aortic aneurysm. Exploratory laparotomy revealed the presence of a large aneurysm (*bottom right;* aneurysm sac shown by horizontal arrow) with a large hole in its posterior wall, *(diagonal arrow)* through which vertebral bodies could be seen. *Staphylococcus aureus* was isolated from cultures of the aneurysm sac and vertebral bodies.

Historically, nonruptured IAAs were definitively diagnosed by angiography. Angiographic findings suggestive of IAAs include a saccular aneurysm in an otherwise-normal-appearing artery or a multilobular aneurysm. Due to increased availability and higher-quality resolution, CT has replaced angiography as the initial diagnostic study of choice. In addition to CT and angiography, nuclear medicine scans have been used to diagnose IAAs.[33] Magnetic resonance angiography has also been used but is more expensive.[34] Ultrasonography is adequate to detect the presence of an aneurysm but lacks a proven ability to detect the presence of infection.

MANAGEMENT

When IAA is suspected, blood cultures, a complete blood cell count, and erythrocyte sedimentation rate should be obtained, followed immediately by institution of antibiotic therapy. Definitive surgical therapy should not be unduly delayed, as the aneurysm could rupture. Management principles unique to specific anatomical locations is discussed in the sections that follow. However, certain general principles apply to all IAAs: (1) control hemorrhage if present; (2) obtain tissue cultures; (3) widely debride all infected tissues; (4) consider arterial reconstruction with autogenous tissue, preferably through uninfected tissue planes; (5) continue antibiotic therapy throughout the postoperative period.

AORTA

IAA of the aorta is uncommon, comprising approximately 3% of abdominal aortic aneurysms[35,36] in autopsy specimens. The incidence is 1% of all aortic and iliac artery aneurysm repairs.[37] Mortality is high; the first survivor[38] was not

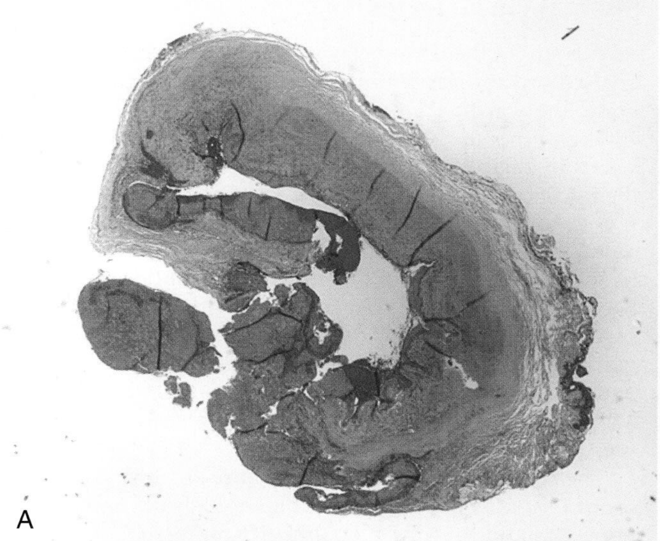

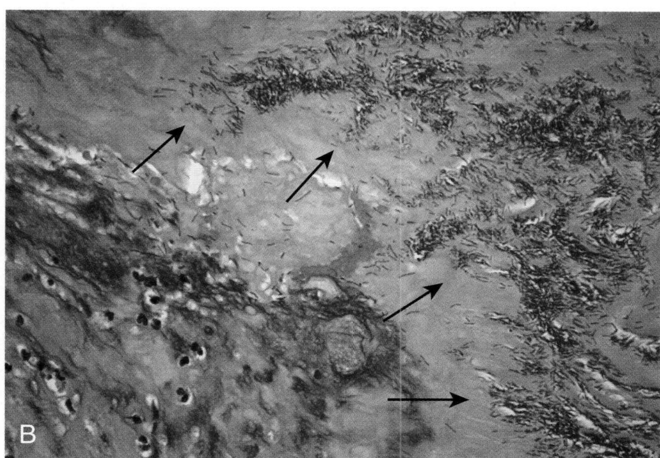

Figure 41-3. Low-power **(A)** and high-power **(B)** microscopic views of an infected brachial artery that ruptured after a repair for thrombosis in a patient with a large open wound from a motor vehicle collision. The Gram stain demonstrated one or more white blood cells and no organisms. The cultures grew *Enterococci.* The microscopic specimen reveals Gram-positive rods *(black arrows)* infiltrating the smooth muscle cells in the right half of the picture **(B).** This is consistent with a clostridial infection.

reported until 1962. Most infected aortic aneurysms are due to *Staphylococcus,* with *Salmonella* being the second most common.[11,13,22,36,39-42] A review of 98 patients in literature[43] revealed that 51% of *Salmonella* infections involved the infrarenal abdominal aorta while only 20% involved the thoracic aorta. As expected, mortality was higher in patients with infected thoracic compared with abdominal aortic aneurysms, 75% versus 47%. In this review, the mean age was 65, and the most common medical comorbidity was diabetes mellitus. Single-center series[13,41] have reported mortality rates of 23% to 31% and noted increased mortality rates for suprarenal compared to infrarenal IAAs and ruptured versus nonruptured IAAs. The traditional treatment for an IAA is to debride all infected tissue, oversew the arterial stump or stumps, and perform revascularization through uninfected tissue planes using autogenous conduit. This is usually not possible for aortic infections, because no suitable autogenous conduits exist that are long enough to tunnel through uninfected tissue planes. The classical method to treat infected aortic aneurysms has been to first perform an axillary–bifemoral bypass[44-46] using an artificial graft, followed by excision of the infected aneurysm. Investigators[41] using this approach have achieved 10% mortality rates, 0% amputation rates, and 0% late aortic or graft infection rates for infected infrarenal aneurysms. Some thoracic aortic segments, such as the arch and ascending aorta, are not amenable to extraanatomical bypass and require in situ replacement with a prosthetic graft. Success with this method has led investigators to attempt in situ replacement of IAAs of the abdominal aorta. Using in situ replacement with Dacron grafts for infected aortic aneurysms in the thoracic, thoracoabdominal, and abdominal aorta, Chan et al.[42] reported a 14% mortality rate and only a 5% reinfection rate. Others[47,48] have used in situ rifampin-bonded gelatin-impregnated Dacron grafts and obtained similar results. In situ replacement with prosthetic graft is reserved primarily for patients with Gram-positive bacterial infections free of frank purulence or in areas not amenable to conventional management. Reports of the use of cryopreserved aortic allografts in infected fields have generally demonstrated inferior results. One multicenter registry[49] noted a 13% mortality rate, 5% amputation rate, and 20% graft complication rate. Another multicenter study[50] demonstrated a high mortality rate (21%), and a high amputation rate (14%) with the use of cryopreserved aortic allografts but fewer graft-related complications. An additional technique that continues to gain popularity is the use of the femoral–popliteal vein as an autogenous in situ conduit. This technique[51] has been reported to have a 10% mortality rate, 5% amputation rate, and 100% primary patency at 5 years. While this conduit is more resistant to recurrent infection than prosthetic and cryografts and has superior patency rates compared to extraanatomical bypass, a small percentage of patients develop significant complications, such as compartment syndrome (12%), deep venous thrombosis (15%), and pulmonary embolus (2.4%).

In addition to open surgical revascularization, some authors have used endoluminal stent grafts to treat infected aortic aneurysms (Figure 41-3). This approach was initially reported[52] using homemade stent grafts in the thoracic aorta of three high-risk patients; no persistent infections were detected, but follow-up was short. While this approach appears to violate traditional surgical tenets by placing an artificial stent graft directly in contact with an infected field, some investigators advocate its use in high-risk patients. Several case reports have been published describing patients with IAAs from *Salmonella, Enterobacter,* methicillin-sensitive *S. aureus,* or *Candida albicans* who were successfully treated with endoluminal stent grafts with follow-up extending to 3 to 4 years.[53-55] One aneurysm treated in this way was noted to have completely resolved after 4 years.[53] Others have reported failure of endoluminal stent graft therapy in the treatment of

IAAs.[56] A recent review[57] of the literature described 48 patients with infected thoracic or abdominal aortic aneurysms treated with endoluminal therapy; 27% were culture negative, 22.9% had persistent infection, 10.4% died within 30 days, and an additional 6.3% died later from residual or recurrent infection. Of these patients, 37% underwent adjunctive procedures such as drainage or debridement of infected periaortic tissue. Patients who presented with rupture, including aortoduodenal fistula and aortobronchial fistula (odds ratio 4.14), or fevers (odds ratio 4.92) were significantly more likely to develop persistent infection.[57] Although these results are clearly inferior to the open surgical options, many of these patients were extremely high risk for open surgery. Until the role for endoluminal therapy is further clarified, its use in treating IAAs should be limited to use as a temporizing procedure until definitive open surgical treatment can be performed or in patients at prohibitive risk for open surgery.

SYPHILIS

Cardiovascular syphilis is now quite rare; however, sporadic cases still occur. Natural history data indicate 75% of untreated patients develop tertiary syphilis after 15 years, with cardiovascular syphilis being the most common manifestation. In fact, 50% of untreated patients have demonstrable cardiovascular involvement after 10 years.[58] The treponema lodges in the vasa vasorum and incites an inflammatory reaction leading to aortitis. Patients subsequently develop aortic insufficiency, coronary ostial stenosis, and less commonly aortic aneurysms. The aortic aneurysms occur most commonly in the ascending and aortic arch and are uncommon below the sixth thoracic vertebral body. Extrathoracic syphilitic aortic aneurysms are extremely rare. Mortality is high in patients with symptomatic syphilitic aneurysms. Antibiotic therapy should be initiated immediately, followed by expeditious definitive surgical therapy.

INFECTED ARTERIAL ANEURYSMS OF MAJOR AORTIC BRANCHES

Innominate Arteries

IAAs affecting the aortic arch branches are uncommon. Lewis and Schrager[59] reported the first case of innominate artery involvement in 1909. Stengel and Wolferth[17] reported only 2 innominate artery cases among a series of 382 IAAs. Kieffer et al.[60] reviewed their single-center 27-year experience. They operated on 27 patients with innominate artery aneurysms, of which the etiology was syphilis in 5 and other infectious agents in 2. Before 1965, innominate aneurysms were most often caused by syphilis, tended to be massive, and were often associated with compression syndromes. The introduction of antibiotics altered this landscape; Takayasu's arteritis and degenerative diseases have supplanted syphilis as common causes of innominate aneurysms. Innominate IAAs can be treated by extraanatomical bypass,[60] especially if the diagnosis is made preoperatively. In situ bypass grafting can also be done in emergent situations by using vein grafts,[61] arterial allografts,[62] or antibiotic-bonded prosthetic grafts.[60] Deep hypothermic circulatory arrest may be required.[60] Currently, branched and fenestrated endovascular grafts for treatment of the suprarenal aorta are still considered experimental.[63]

Subclavian Arteries

Aneurysms of the left subclavian artery are rare, often secondary to thoracic outlet compression from a cervical rib or other bony abnormality.[64] Coselli and Crawford[65] reported only 18 aneurysms of the intrathoracic segment of the subclavian artery in their 17-year review; none were infected. Among their 431 cases of IAAs, Hoover and Lampe[66] only identified 2 cases of infected subclavian arteries. Patra et al.[67] found only 2 cases of infected subclavian–axillary arteries among 58 IAAs (52 patients with IAAs from 19 institutions in France). Baginsky[68] reported a 7-year-old child with three synchronous IAAs in the right subclavian artery, abdominal aorta, and right radial artery. Subclavian IAAs can be caused by syphilis,[69] contiguous invasion by infectious processes such as tuberculosis lymphadenitis,[70] drug injection,[71] or invasive procedures, such as cervical sympathectomy.[72]

The right subclavian artery may have an aberrant origin in about 1% of the population.[73] This anomaly has a well-known association with a diverticulum of Kommerell, an aneurysmal outpouching of the aorta at the origin of the anomalous artery. Infection of such a diverticulum by hemolytic streptococcal endarteritis *(S. pyogenes)* has also been described. Presumably the diverticulum was predisposed to infection due to the turbulent regional blood flow.[74] Subclavian aneurysms are usually asymptomatic; however, they may present with the following: pulsatile mass, distal embolization to the hand or brain, brachial plexopathy, right-sided Horner's syndrome, vocal cord paralysis, hemoptysis, or chest pain.[75,76] Surgical options for subclavian aneurysms include ligation or resection and revascularization with autogenous vein. Endovascular techniques (embolization with metallic coils) have been attempted in situations in which the surgical option is deemed difficult or of prohibitive risk.[77]

Extracranial Cerebral Arteries

Carotid IAAs are caused by contiguous infection from adjacent tissues,[78] arterial trauma as seen in intravenous (IV) drug abusers,[79] and secondarily from septic embolization.[80] They may also rarely be seen after carotid endarterectomy, although this is more likely to follow the use of a prosthetic patch rather than primary or vein patch closure of the arteriotomy.[81] Other less common causes include syphilitic arteritis.[82] Regardless of the cause, the sequelae of carotid IAAs are similar. Platelets and thrombi aggregate inside the dilated lumen and may embolize distally or lead to thrombosis. The aneurysm may exert pressure on neighboring structures, such as cranial nerves; it may also rupture into the oropharynx or through the skin and result in profuse bleeding. Carotid aneurysms can usually be diagnosed clinically; however, carotid tortuosity can be easily confused with aneurysms.

Cerebral angiography remains the gold standard for diagnosis. It also defines associated extra- and intracranial lesions, multiple IAAs, and adequacy of collateral blood supply. Magnetic resonance imaging and CT angiography, however, are increasingly being used for diagnostic confirmation to assess the extent of disease and to plan intervention.

Carotid IAAs are best treated surgically by aneurysm excision and flow restoration. The use of autogenous conduit is preferred. If the artery must be replaced, we prefer autogenous saphenous vein, although Faggioli et al.[83] reported the need to revise two of seven saphenous vein grafts in their small series. Autologous femoral veins have also been successfully used and noted to have an excellent size match for the distal common carotid artery.[84] Femoral vein harvesting is associated with relatively low morbidity.[85] If vascular reconstruction is not possible, ligation and resection can be performed. Ehrenfeld et al.[86] recommended carotid stump pressures as the most reliable predictor of neurological outcomes (using more than 70 and less than 55 mm Hg to reflect adequate and inadequate collateral hemispheric blood flow, respectively). Their conclusions, however, were based on a small number of study subjects. The use of local anesthesia to allow clinical examination during a cross-clamping trial or endovascular carotid balloon occlusion test[87] before surgical exploration have also been described to predict the need for arterial reconstruction (i.e., to determine whether the patient tolerates carotid ligation). Reports also exist of the endovascular treatment of carotid IAAs with covered stents.[88] We prefer to reserve endoluminal treatment of carotid IAAs for patients who are extremely poor surgical risks, since the long-term results of this approach are uncertain and persistent infection requiring removal of carotid stent grafts is likely to prove extremely challenging, often requiring difficult distal exposure to obtain control and vein graft reconstruction.[82]

External carotid IAAs have been seldom reported. A paper from Japan[89] described an infected external carotid artery aneurysm accompanying infectious endocarditis. This lesion was identified in a young male with ocular and neurological symptoms.[89] Similarly, vertebral arterial aneurysms are extremely unusual, accounting for less than 1% of all aneurysms.[90] In one of the largest reported experiences of vertebral artery reconstructions, Berguer et al.[91] performed 100 vertebral procedures in a 14-year period. No case of IAA was found in their series as the indication for the intervention. In one of the few existing reports, vertebral IAA was described as a consequence of a cervicothoracic sympathectomy performed through a supraclavicular approach.[71]

Intracranial Arteries

Intracranial IAAs have also been described. In 1965, Hoover and Lampe published a large review[66] in which the cerebral vessels were affected in 16% of patients. Intracranial infected aneurysms develop more commonly in the anterior than the posterior circulation, commonly affecting the middle cerebral artery.[90] Another report described multiple infected aneurysms in the brain involving both carotid and vertebrobasilar systems in the setting of active infective endocarditis.[92] In Hoover and Lampe's review,[66] only two cases of vertebral artery involvement were noted among their 431 reported cases. When present, they manifest with symptoms of mass effect, neurological symptoms,[71] ischemia, or rupture. The management of these aneurysms is quite difficult, given their deep anatomical location and their intimate relationship with the brain stem and cranial nerves; the associated mortality approaches 70%.[90]

Upper Extremities

Upper extremity involvement by IAAs is rare. Brown et al.[23] reported that about 10% of IAAs affected the upper limbs. They have been associated with trauma (Figure 41-4), endoluminal procedures, or endocarditis. Careful physical examination

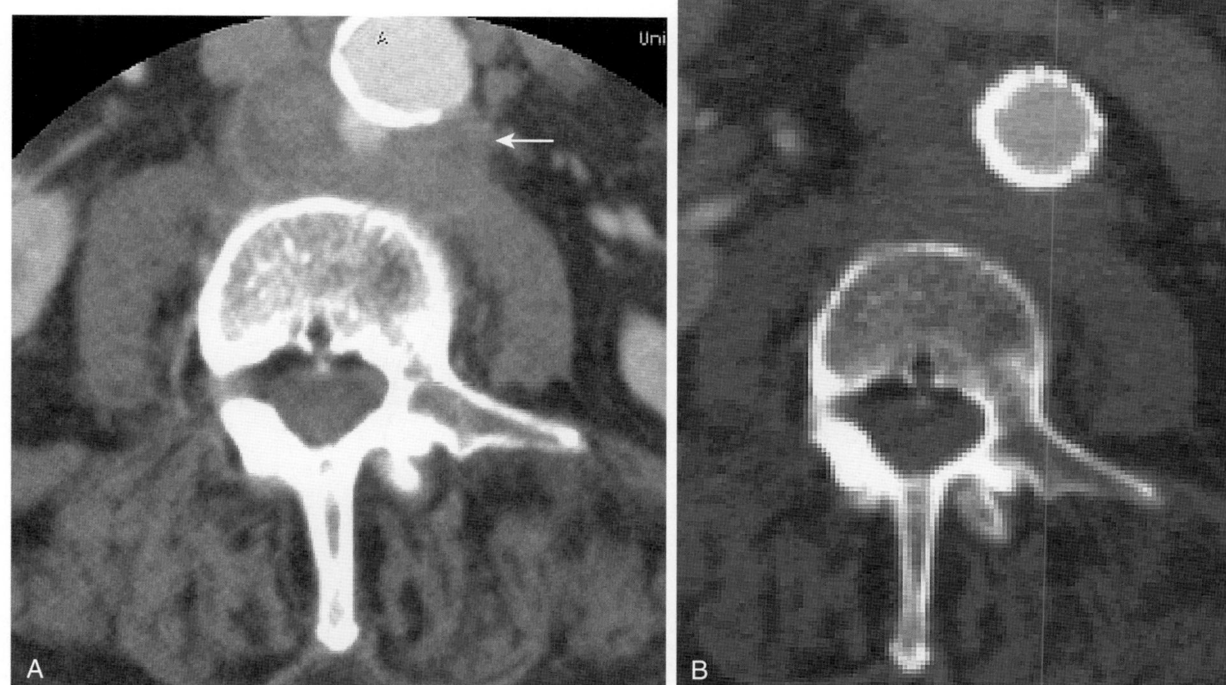

Figure 41-4. A, Computed tomography scan demonstrating an infected aortic aneurysm. A contained rupture with contrast blush is seen posterior to the aorta *(white arrow)*. The patient was treated with an endograft and a prolonged course of antibiotics. **B,** A repeat computed tomography scan 1 month later demonstrates the false aneurysm is sealed.

Table 41-1
Reported Infrapopliteal Infected Arterial Aneurysms*

Study	Year	Age (Years)	Gender	Presentation	History of EC	Etiology	Size	Location	Repair	Follow-up	Outcomes
León et al.[111]	2007	59	Male	Right leg pain and pulsatile mass	Yes	NA	6 cm	Right ATA	RSVG	10 months	Doing well
Kieran et al.[112]	2004	60	Male	Right popliteal fossa pulsatile swelling	Yes	*Staphylococcus aureus*	NA	Right TPT	RSVG	NA	Did well
Larena-Avellaneda et al.[113]	2004	53	Male	Increased limb circumference, sepsis	Yes	*Candida*	Large (size not reported)	Left TPT	Coil embolization	33 months[†]	Doing well
Patra et al.[65]	2001	NA	NA	NA	NA	NA	NA	PTA	NA	NA	NA
Mc Kee and Ballard[114]	1999	15	Male	Pulsatile mass with thrill	Yes	*Brucella canis*	2.6 cm	Right PTA	None (thrombosed)	8 months	Doing well
Mc Kee and Ballard[114]	1999	15	Male	Pulsatile mass with thrill	Yes	*B. canis*	0.8 cm	Right peroneal	None (thrombosed)	8 months	Doing well
Mc Kee and Ballard[114]	1999	15	Male	Pulsatile mass with thrill	Yes	*B. canis*	3.5 cm	Left PTA	RSVG	8 months	ABI = 0.97
Murashia et al[115]	1997	34	Male	Right leg swelling	Yes	*Streptococcus viridans*	4 cm	Right TPT	Both ends closure	18 months	Doing well, no recurrence on ultrasound
Murashia et al[115]	1997	34	Male	Left leg swelling	Yes	*S. viridans*	5.5 cm	Left TPT	Both ends closure	18 months	Doing well, no recurrence on ultrasound
Menanau et al[116]	1995	78	Male	Limb pseudophlebitis	Yes	*Streptococcus bovis*	6 cm	Left PTA	Excision and ligation	3 months	Doing well
Akers et al[117]	1992	49	Male	Leg pain and swelling, pulsatile mass	Yes	*S. viridans*	6 cm	Right TPT	RSVG	9 months	Doing well
Mayall et al[118]	1991	45	Male	NA	Yes	*Streptococcus*	NA	ATA	Excision and ligation	14 years	Doing well
Payne-James[119]	1988	32	Female	Right calf and ankle swelling and pain	Yes	NA	3 cm	ATA	Excision and ligation	2 months[‡]	Doing well
Gedeon[120§]	1973	NA	NA	NA	NA	NA	NA	TPT × 2	NA	NA	NA
Schnider[121]	1954	NA	NA	NA	NA	NA	NA	PT × 5	NA	NA	NA
Tresidder[122]	1953	25	Female	NA	NA	NA	NA	Right PTA	Excision	NA	Satisfactory
Tresidder[122]	1953	25	Female	NA	NA	NA	NA	Left PTA	Excision	NA	Satisfactory
Walker[123¶]	1951	66	Male	NA	NA	NA	NA	Right PTA	Clot evacuation and ligation	3 weeks	Satisfactory result, died from cardiac failure 3 weeks after

Dry[124]	1947	40	Male	Fever, chills, tender and swollen left upper calf	Yes	*Streptococcus*	3.5 × 2.5 cm	Left PTA	None	NA	Died from acute cardiac failure
Herrman[125]	1937	8	Male	Pain in left kneecap, fever, night sweats	Yes	*S. viridans*	NA	Left PTA	None	In house	Leg and brain aneurysm rupture, died
Ossius[126]	1929							PTA			
Stengel and Wolferth[17]	1923	NA	NA	NA	NA	NA	NA	PTA × 8	NA	NA	NA
Richey and Maclachlan[127]	1922	39	Male	Fever, chills, pulsatile mass below knee	Yes	*Streptococcus salivaris*	Small tanger-ine orange	Right PTA × 3	None	2 weeks	Died 2 weeks after PTA aneurysm rupture

*ABI, ankle–brachial index; ATA, anterior tibialis artery; EC, endocarditis; NA, not available; PTA, posterior tibialis artery; RSVG, reversed saphenous vein graft; TPT, tibioperoneal trunk.
†Approximately.
‡At least.
§Gedeon reported four additional cases affecting "arteries of the leg."[121]
¶Cited in Rogers[115] as a personal communication.

is needed to suspect the diagnosis. Splinter hemorrhages and ischemic lesions may be detected as evidence of digital embolization. Recently, to increase awareness of this diagnostic possibility and to characterize its presentation, diagnosis, and therapy, we reviewed the literature concerning upper extremity IAAs.[93] We identified 68 papers reporting 149 cases and analyzed them according to the specific location in the upper limb. The rarity of this condition is evident in that only 12 papers included two cases of upper extremity IAAs, the remainder being single-case reports. The limited number of cases reported in the literature allowed us to draw only a few general conclusions regarding this condition. Endocarditis continues to be the most important overall source of bacteria for these aneurysms, especially in the brachial artery. IV drug abuse was more common in the axillary and brachial artery locations. In the forearm, the high frequency with which intraarterial lines are placed for hemodynamic monitoring has made direct arterial trauma the most important underlying cause. *S. aureus* proved to be the most common bacterial species in all upper extremity locations.

Brachial artery involvement (48%) was reported most often among upper extremity IAAs. A strong male predilection was noted (male-to-female ratio of 8:1), although in many cases the gender was not reported. Patients were also young (mean age at presentation was 41 years). Our review did not identify predominance with respect to side (right to left was 19 to 17). IV drug abusers may deliberately inject into an artery when superficial veins are sclerotic and difficult to access, but more commonly such intraarterial injections occur inadvertently.[94] Forearm IAAs were noted in 37%. The mean age (57 years) at presentation was higher than that of axillary or brachial aneurysms, an expected finding given the difference in the etiologies. Forearm IAAs most often involved the radial artery, an expected finding given the preferential use of this artery for invasive monitoring. An increased risk of infection was associated with radial artery catheterization lasting more than 4 days.[95] When ulnar artery involvement was noted, it was most often in relation to endocarditis.

Treatment of upper limb IAAs showed a generally favorable outcome, with most associated mortality due to the underlying condition (i.e., sepsis or endocarditis) and not to the aneurysm itself. Major adverse outcomes such as permanent neurological deficit or major amputation were rare, likely due to the rich arterial collateralization of this anatomical region and the generally good results of arterial ligation. Behera et al.[96] treated all of their patients with brachial IAAs by excision and ligation; no revascularization was attempted if a Doppler signal was present distally. Using this approach, no upper limb amputations were required. This is particularly true when the infected segment is between the thyrocervical trunk and the subscapular artery or distal to the profunda brachii. When needed, reconstruction should be performed with autogenous vein.[97] Endovascular techniques have also been reported but only anecdotally and in the emergent setting.[98]

We identified eight cases (five males) of IAAs in the hand, with an average age of presentation of 44 years.[93] All IAAs were small and less than 2.5 cm in diameter, not surprising given the anatomical location, which is superficial and visible, limiting the degree of expansion before diagnosis. In these cases, outcomes were favorable with no neurological sequelae or limb loss.

Visceral Arteries

Visceral IAAs are rare and comprise approximately 9% of all IAAs, with the superior mesenteric artery being the most common.[23] Most recent literature consists of individual case reports.[99-102] In 1987, a review[102] of the literature identified only 19 reports of successful treatment of infected superior mesenteric artery aneurysms. Most were treated with simple ligation and excision, several required revascularization, and bowel resection was rarely required. One report[99] described multiple visceral microaneurysms associated with septicemia in an 11-year-old boy. These aneurysms were successfully treated with 6 weeks of antibiotics, without surgical or endoluminal intervention. Others have described the use of gelfoam[100] or metal coils[101] to induce thrombosis of visceral IAAs, followed by a prolonged course of IV antibiotics. Often, patients with visceral IAAs are found to have multiple additional IAAs.[30,99]

Femoropopliteal Arteries

The femoral artery is currently the most common location for IAAs, accounting for 38% in the review of Brown and colleagues.[23] In recent years, an increasing number of IAAs of the femoral artery have been observed following intraarterial drug abuse and trauma.[23,103] It most often presents as an inflamed, tender, pulsatile groin mass but may also present as skin erosion with or without hemorrhage, embolization, compression of adjacent structures, or thrombosis. The ideal method of repair should be selected according to the anatomical location of the aneurysm. When the femoral bifurcation is involved, excision and vascular reconstruction is often needed due to the high rate of amputation (33%) associated with simple excision and ligation.[104,105] In contrast, if the common femoral bifurcation is spared, patients are more likely to tolerate simple ligation (5% limb loss).[106] Treatment must be carefully considered in patients addicted to IV drugs for two reasons: the high rate of graft infection after immediate reconstruction and the common reuse by IV drug abusers of the femoral region for further drug abuse, jeopardizing the vascular reconstruction. An alternative is to ligate the involved arteries and observe the outcome, performing delayed revascularization in those patients who develop ischemia. Anecdotal reports show the use of cryopreserved human allografts and stent grafts in the treatment of infected femoral aneurysms.[107,108] In cases of isolated superficial or deep femoral IAAs, ligation without reconstruction has also been advocated with a low risk of postoperative complications.[109] Others have reported the use of saphenous vein bypasses. Stent graft repair with saphenous vein covered stents has also been used to exclude expanding infected aneurysms in critically ill patients.[110] However, the latter mode of therapy can only be described as anecdotal.

Infrapopliteal Arteries

Infrapopliteal IAAs have only been recognized since 1922. Our review of the literature[111] identified 37 such aneurysms affecting 14 patients with a mean age of 43 years (8 to 78); 86% were adults (Table 41-1).[17,67,111-127] The organisms most often reported are *Streptococcus* species; *Brucella* and *Candida* are also rare causes of IAAs in this location. The reported cases of crural IAAs have been universally associated with bacterial endocarditis, unlike other locations, where trauma is the most common etiology.[23] The crural artery most often affected by aneurysmal disease is the posterior tibial artery, followed by the tibioperoneal trunk. The peroneal artery has reportedly been implicated in only one case. Our group recently reported the third case of anterior tibial artery involvement.[111] Several reports describe a significant delay in diagnosis, probably because these aneurysms must become fairly large before causing symptoms of calf pain, swelling, or a pulsatile mass.

The management of this entity has been almost exclusively surgical by means of ligation of the aneurysm inflow and outflow, with or without aneurysm excision, or vascular reconstruction. The best conduit remains autologous vein. Yao and McCarthy[128] suggested expectant management in aneurysms that are small and asymptomatic. Endovascular techniques have also been described.[113] Major adverse outcomes such as limb loss or exsanguination have not been reported for crural IAAs; however, the follow-up varied widely and was often quite short.

HUMAN IMMUNODEFICIENCY VIRUS–RELATED ANEURYSMS

Patients infected with human immunodeficiency virus (HIV) are now surviving for longer periods due to improvements in their management. The past 25 years has seen an explosive rise in the number of individuals infected with HIV. As the classical causes of morbidity and mortality in this patient population have come under better control, new complications are becoming more prevalent. A growing body of literature focuses on the subject of aneurysmal degeneration of arteries in HIV-infected patients. At least three major mechanisms by which HIV may initiate or predispose to IAAs have been postulated[129]: (1) immunodeficiency allows bacteria that are known to cause IAAs, such as *Salmonella*[130,131] or tuberculosis, to proliferate without immune restraint[132]; (2) one or more of the HIV envelope proteins sufficiently resemble one or more artery-specific antigenic proteins that may trigger an autoimmune response (molecular mimicry); and (3) the HIV virus itself infects arterial cells. Direct infection of aortic fibroblasts by the HIV virus is more likely to be the responsible pathogenetic mechanism than molecular mimicry.

Arterial aneurysms in patients afflicted with HIV have been classified in two groups: IAAs from bacterial or fungal infections and HIV-associated aneurysms as a distinct entity. Marks and Kuskov[133] reported 12 young (12 to 46 years) HIV-positive patients in Zimbabwe without evidence of atherosclerosis, with rapid development of focal necrotizing vasculitis with aneurysm formation and rupture or with slow, progressive development of granulomatous vasculitis. These findings correlate with recent reports in the literature of HIV patients who suffer from vascular lesions such as large artery vasculitis. The sites of vascular involvement included the thoracic, thoracoabdominal, and abdominal aorta and the iliac, femoral, gluteal, popliteal, and subclavian arteries.

Nair et al.[134] analyzed 28 HIV-positive patients (median age 30 years) with 92 arterial aneurysms (range 1 to 10 per patient) treated at a single teaching hospital in a 6-year period. Aneurysms were atypically located and most often involved the carotid (24), superficial femoral (21), and popliteal (9) arteries. These findings correlated with another report from the same investigators; they observed that HIV-related vasculitis affected the small- to medium-sized vessels most often.[135] Histological examination of the aneurysm wall revealed distinctive histological features: the presence of both acute and chronic inflammatory changes, occlusion of the vasa vasorum by inflammatory infiltrate, and prominent vessel wall edema.[135]

Of the 31 symptomatic aneurysms, 25 were treated surgically, including arterial reconstruction in 19 patients and aneurysm resection and ligation in the remainder. Two treatment-related deaths occurred; short-term postoperative outcomes were otherwise favorable.[134] The ideal therapy of these aneurysms should follow the same guidelines as those described for other IAAs. Open,[136,137] endovascular,[136,138] and hybrid approaches[132,138,139] have been described. The most common recommendations for management of HIV-related IAAs include excision of all infected tissue with extraanatomical reconstruction when needed. In situ reconstruction is an acceptable alternative, should the surgeon be unable to create an extraanatomical bypass. To determine the outcome of surgical intervention in patients with HIV-associated vascular disease, Botes and Van Marle[140] identified 109 HIV-positive patients with peripheral vascular disease over a 5-year period. Of these patients, 24 presented with aneurysmal disease and 66 had occlusive disease; the authors analyzed the treatment outcomes based on the mode of presentation. Perioperative mortality was 10.6% for aneurysmal disease compared to 3.6% for occlusive disease. Long-term mortality was also significantly worse for patients with aneurysms. The authors concluded that surgical intervention should be reserved primarily for life-threatening aneurysms due to the higher perioperative and long-term complication rates. Primary amputation may be preferable to bypass surgery in patients with critical limb ischemia.

References

1. Rokitansky CF. Handbuch der pathologischen anatomie. 2nd ed. Austria: 1844:55.
2. Virkow R. Ueber die akute entzuendung der arterian. *Virchows Arch Pathol* 1847;1:272.
3. Koch L. Ueber das Aneurysma der Arteria meseraica. *Inaug. Dissert. Erlangen: JJ Barfus* 1851.
4. Tufnell J. On the influence of vegetation of the valves of the heart in the production of secondary arterial disease. *Dublin QJ Med* 1885;15:371.
5. Goodhart JF. Case of aneurysm from embolism. *Trans Path Soc Lond* 1877;28:106.
6. Osler W. The Gulstonian lectures on malignant endocarditis. *Br Med J* 1885;1:467.
7. Eppinger H. Pathogenesis (Histogenesis und aetiologie) der aneurysmen einschliesslich des aneurysma equi verminosum: pathologisch-anatomische studien. *Arch Klin Chir* 1887;35:1-563.
8. Johansen K, Devin J. Spontaneous healing of mycotic aortic aneurysms. *J Cardiovasc Surg* 1980;21:625-627.
9. Bardin JA, Collins GM, Devin JB, Halasz NA. Nonaneurysmal suppurative aortitis. *Arch Surg* 1981;116:954-956.
10. Barker WF. Mycotic aneurysms. *Ann Surg* 1954;139:84-89.
11. Jarrett F, Darling RC, Mundth ED, Austen WG. The management of infected arterial aneurysms. *J Cardiovasc Surg* 1977;18:361-366.
12. Duncan JM, Cooley DA. Surgical considerations in aortitis. II. Mycotic aneurysms. *Tex Heart Inst J* 1983;10:329-335.
13. Reddy DJ, Shepard AD, Evans JR, et al. Management of infected aortoiliac aneurysms. *Arch Surg* 1991;126:873-878.
14. McCready RA, Bryant MA, Divelbiss JL, et al. Arterial infections in the new millennium: an old problem revisited. *Ann Vasc Surg* 2006;20:590-595.
15. Kyriakides GK, Simmons RL, Najarian JS. Mycotic aneurysms in transplant patients. *Arch Surg* 1976;111:472-476.
16. Wang H, Rammos S, Elwook P. Successful endovascular treatment of a ruptured mycotic intracavernous carotid artery aneurysm in an AIDS patient. *Neurocrit Care* 2007;7:156-159.

17. Stengel A, Wolferth CC. Mycotic bacterial aneurysms of intravascular origin. *Arch Int Med* 1923;31:527-554.
18. Lawrence GH. Surgical management of infected aneurysms. *Am J Surg* 1962;104:355-364.
19. Blum L, Keefer EBC. Clinical entity of cryptogenic mycotic aneurysm. *JAMA* 1964;188:505-508.
20. Bennett DE. Primary mycotic aneurysms of the aorta: report of case and review of the literature. *Arch Surg* 1967;94:758-765.
21. Bennett DE, Cherry JK. Bacterial infection of aortic aneurysms: a clinicopathologic study. *Am J Surg* 1967;113:321-326.
22. Mundth ED, Darling RC, Alvarado RH, et al. Surgical management of mycotic aneurysms and the complications of infection in vascular reconstructive surgery. *Am J Surg* 1968;117:460-468.
23. Brown SL, Busuttil RW, Baker JD, et al. Bacteriologic and surgical determinants of survival in patients with mycotic aneurysms. *J Vasc Surg* 1984;1:541-547.
24. Abbott ME. Statistical study and historical retrospect of 200 recorded cases, with autopsy of stenosis or obliteration of the descending arch. *Am Heart J* 1928;3:574-618.
25. Schneider JA, Rheuban KS, Crosby IK. Rupture of postcoarctation mycotic aneurysms of the aorta. *Ann Thorac Surg* 1979;27:185-190.
26. Zak FG, Strauss L, Saphra I. Rupture of diseased large arteries in the course of enterobacterial *(Salmonella)* infections. *N Engl J Med* 1958;258:824-828.
27. McNally EM, Kennedy RJ, Grace WR. *Salmonella infantis* infection of a pre-existent ventricular aneurysm. *Am Heart J* 1964:541-548.
28. Cohen PS, O'Brien TF, Schoenbaum SC, Medeiros AA. The risk of endothelial infection in adults with *Salmonella* bacteremia. *Ann Intern Med* 1978;89:931-932.
29. Finseth F, Abbott WM. One-stage operative therapy for Salmonella mycotic abdominal aortic aneurysm. *Ann Surg* 1973;179:8-11.
30. Dean RH, Waterhouse G. Mycotic embolism and embolomycotic aneurysms: neglected lessons of the past. *Ann Surg* 1986;204:300-306.
31. Vogelzang RL, Sohaey R. Infected aortic aneurysms: CT appearance. *J Comput Assist Tomogr* 1988;12:109-112.
32. Blair RH, Resnik MD, Polga JP. CT appearance of mycotic abdominal aortic aneurysms. *J Comput Assist Tomogr* 1989;13:101-104.
33. Chen P, Lamki L, Raval B. Indium-111 leukocyte appearance of *Salmonella* mycotic aneurysm. *Clin Nucl Med* 1994;19:646-648.
34. Walsh DW, Ho VB, Haggerty MF. Mycotic aneurysm of the aorta: MRI and MRA features. *J Magn Reson Imaging* 1997;7:312.
35. Parkhurst GF, Decker JP. Bacterial aortitis and mycotic aneurysm of the aorta. *Am J Path* 1955;31:821-835.
36. Somerville RL, Allen EV, Edwards JE. Bland and infected arteriosclerotic abdominal aortic aneurysms: a clinicopathologic study. *Medicine* 1959;207:207-220.
37. Müller BT, Wegener OR, Grabitz K, et al. Mycotic aneurysms of the thoracic and abdominal aorta and iliac arteries: experience with anatomic and extra-anatomic repair in 33 cases. *J Vasc Surg* 2001;33:106-113.
38. Sower ND, Whelan TJ. Suppurative arteritis due to *Salmonella. Surgery* 1962;52:851-858.
39. Ewart JM, Burke ML, Bunt TJ. Spontaneous abdominal aortic infections: essentials of diagnosis and management. *Am Surg* 1983;49:37-50.
40. Katz SG, Andros G, Kohl RD. Salmonella infections of the abdominal aorta. *Surg Gynecol Obstet* 1992;175:102-106.
41. Moneta GL, Taylor LM, Yeager RA, et al. Surgical treatment of infected aortic aneurysm. *Am J Surg* 1998;175:396-399.
42. Chan FY, Crawford ES, Coselli JS, et al. In situ prosthetic graft replacement for mycotic aneurysm of the aorta. *Ann Thorac Surg* 1989;47:193-203.
43. Oskoui R, Davis WA, Gomes MN. *Salmonella aortitis*: a report of a successfully treated case with a comprehensive review of the literature. *Arch Intern Med* 1993;153:517-525.
44. Louw JH. The treatment of combined aortoiliac and femoropopliteal occlusive disease by splenofemoral and axillofemoral bypass grafts. *Surgery* 1964;55:387-395.
45. Cook PA, Ehrenfeld WK. Successful management of mycotic aortic aneurysm: report of a case. *Surgery* 1974;75:132-136.
46. Reilly LM, Stoney RJ, Goldstone J, Ehrenfeld WK. Improved management of aortic graft infection: the influence of operation sequence and staging. *J Vasc Surg* 1987;5:421-431.
47. Gupta AK, Bandyk DF, Johnson BL. In situ repair of mycotic abdominal aortic aneurysms with rifampin-bonded gelatin-impregnated Dacron grafts: a preliminary case report. *J Vasc Surg* 1996;24:472-476.
48. Bandyk DF, Novotney ML, Johnson BL, et al. Use of rifampin-soaked gelatin-sealed polyester grafts for in situ treatment of primary aortic and vascular prosthetic infections. *J Surg Res* 2001;95:44-49.
49. Noel AA, Gloviczki P, Cherry KJ, et al. Abdominal aortic reconstruction in infected fields: early results of the United States cryopreserved aortic allograft registry. *J Vasc Surg* 2002;35:847-852.
50. Zhou W, Lin PH, Bush RL, et al. In situ reconstruction with cryopreserved arterial allografts for management of mycotic aneurysms or aortic prosthetic graft infections. *Tex Heart J* 2006;33:14-18.
51. Clagett GP, Valentine RJ, Hagino RT. Autogenous aortoiliac–femoral reconstruction from superficial femoral–popliteal veins: feasibility and durability. *J Vasc Surg* 1999;25(7):255-270.
52. Semba CP, Sakai T, Slonim SM, et al. Mycotic aneurysms of the thoracic aorta: repair with use of endovascular stent grafts. *J Vasc Interv Radiol* 1998;9:33-40.
53. Berchtold C, Eibl C, Seelig MH, et al. Endovascular treatment and complete regression of an infected abdominal aortic aneurysm. *J Endovasc Ther* 2002;9:543-548.
54. Kpodonu J, Williams JP, Ramaiah VG, Diehrich EB. Endovascular management of a descending thoracic mycotic aneurysm: mid-term follow-up. *Eur J Cardiothoracic Surg* 2007;32:178-179.
55. Ting ACW, Cheng SWK, Ho P, Poon JTC. Endovascular stent graft repair for infected thoracic aortic pseudoaneurysms: a durable option? *J Vasc Surg* 2006;44:701-705.
56. Ishida M, Kato N, Hirano T, et al. Limitations of endovascular treatment with stent grafts for active mycotic thoracic aortic aneurysm. *Cardiovasc Interv Radiol* 2002;25:216-218.
57. Kan CD, Lee HL, Yang YJ. Outcome after endovascular stent graft treatment for mycotic aortic aneurysm: a systemic review. *J Vasc Surg* 2007;46:906-912.
58. Jackman JD. Cardiovascular syphilis. *Am J Med* 1989;87:425-432.
59. Lewis D, Schrager V. Embolomycotic aneurysms. *JAMA* 1909;53:1808.
60. Kieffer E, Chiche L, Koskas F, Bahnini A. Aneurysms of the innominate artery: surgical treatment of 27 patients. *J Vasc Surg* 2001;34:222-228.
61. Hardin CA, Thompson R. Mycotic aneurysm of the innominate artery with supravalvular aortic stenosis. *J Cardiovasc Surg* 1976;17:489-491.
62. Schuch D, Wolff L. Repair of mycotic aneurysm of the innominate artery with homograft tissue. *Ann Thorac Surg* 1991;52:863-864.
63. Chuter TA, Buck DG, Schneider DB, et al. Development of a branched stent-graft for endovascular repair of aortic arch aneurysms. *J Endovasc Ther* 2003;10:940-945.
64. McCollum CH, Da Gama AD, Noon GP, De Bakey ME. Aneurysms of the subclavian artery. *J Cardiovasc Surg* 1979;20:159-164.
65. Coselli JS, Crawford ES. Surgical treatment of aneurysms of the intrathoracic segment of the subclavian artery. *Chest* 1987;91:704-708.
66. Hoover BA II, Lampe WT II. Mycotic aneurysm of the forearm following treated bacterial endocarditis. *Angiology* 1965;16:203-208.
67. Patra P, Ricco JB, Costargent A, et al. for the Association Universitaire de Recherche en Chirurgie, Infected aneurysms of neck and limb arteries: a retrospective multicenter study. *Ann Vasc Surg* 2001;15:197-205.
68. Baginsky A. Septische arteriitis und aneurysma beim kinde. *Berl Klin Wchnschr* 1908;1:144.
69. Khoda J, Sebbag G, Lantsberg L. Syphilitic aneurysm of the subclavian artery: case report. *Vasc Surg* 1993;1:47-51.
70. Hara M, Bransford RM. Aneurysm of the subclavian artery associated with contiguous pulmonary tuberculosis. *Thoracic Cardiovasc Surg* 1963;46:256-264.
71. Miller CM, Sangiuolo P, Schanzer H, et al. Infected false aneurysms of the subclavian artery: a complication in drug addicts. *J Vasc Surg* 1984;1:684-688.
72. Flye MW, Wolkoff JS. Mycotic aneurysm of the left subclavian and vertebral arteries: a complication of cervicothoracic sympathectomy. *Am J Surg* 1971;122:427-429.
73. Goldbloom AA. The anomalous right subclavian artery and its possible clinical significance. *Surg Gynecol Obstet* 1922:378-384.
74. Bisognano JD, Young B, Brown JM, et al. Diverse presentation of aberrant origin of the right subclavian artery: two case reports. *Chest* 1997;112:1693-1697.
75. Olinde AJ. Traumatic subclavian–axillary artery aneurysm. *J Vasc Surg* 1990;11:848-849.
76. Banis JC, Rich N, Whelan TJ. Ischemia of the upper extremity due to noncardiac emboli. *Am J Surg* 1977;134:131-139.
77. Mori K, Saida Y, Kuramoto K, et al. Transcatheter embolization of mycotic aneurysm of the subclavian artery with metallic coils. *J Cardiovasc Surg* 2000;41:463-467.

78. Waggie Z, Hatherill M, Millar A, et al. Retropharyngeal abscess complicated by carotid artery rupture. *Pediatr Crit Care Med* 2002;3:303-304.
79. Ledgerwood AM, Lucas CE. Mycotic aneurysm of the carotid artery. *Arch Surg* 1974;109:496-498.
80. Angle N, Dorafshar AH, Ahn SS. Mycotic aneurysm of the internal carotid artery: a case report. *Vasc Endovascular Surg* 2003;37:213-217.
81. Borazjani BH, Wilson SE, Fujitani RM, et al. Postoperative complications of carotid patching: pseudoaneurysm and infection. *Ann Vasc Surg* 2003;17:156-161.
82. Avellone JC, Ahmad MY. Cervical internal carotid aneurysm from syphilis: an alternative to resection. *JAMA* 1979;241:238-239.
83. Faggioli GL, Freyrie A, Stella A, et al. Extracranial internal carotid artery aneurysms: results of a surgical series with long-term follow-up. *J Vasc Surg* 1996;23:587-594.
84. Modrall JG, Joiner DR, Seidel SA, et al. Superficial femoral–popliteal vein as a conduit for brachiocephalic arterial reconstructions. *Ann Vasc Surg* 2002;16:17-23.
85. Wells JK, Hagino RT, Bargmann KM, et al. Venous morbidity after superficial femoral–popliteal vein harvest. *J Vasc Surg* 1999;29:282-291.
86. Ehrenfeld WK, Stoney RJ, Wylie EJ. Relation of carotid stump pressure to safety of carotid artery ligation. *Surgery* 1983;93:299.
87. Terramani TT, Workman MJ, Loberman Z, et al. Adjunctive endovascular techniques in the management of postoperative carotid artery pseudoaneurysms: useful armamentarium for vascular surgeons—three case reports. *Vasc Endovascular Surg* 2003;37:207-212.
88. Baril DT, Ellozy SH, Carroccio A, et al. Endovascular repair of an infected carotid artery pseudoaneurysm. *J Vasc Surg* 2004;40:1024-1027.
89. Oyanagi M, Sugawara T, Seki H, et al. A case of bacterial aneurysm that occurred in the external carotid artery. *No Shinkei Geka* 2006;34: 175-180.
90. Singh D, Pinjala RK, Purohit AK, et al. Giant mycotic aneurysm of the vertebral artery: a case report. *J Vasc Surg* 2005;42:348-351.
91. Berguer R, Morasch MD, Kline RA. A review of 100 consecutive reconstructions of the distal vertebral artery for embolic and hemodynamic disease. *J Vasc Surg* 1998;27:852-859.
92. Kuki S, Yoshida K, Suzuki K, et al. Successful surgical management for multiple cerebral mycotic aneurysms involving both carotid and vertebrobasilar systems in active infective endocarditis. *Eur J Cardiothorac Surg* 1994;8:508-510.
93. León LR, Psalms SB, Labropoulos N, Mills JL. Infected upper extremity aneurysms: a review. *Eur J Vasc Endovasc Surg* 2008;35:320-331.
94. Yellin AE. Ruptured mycotic aneurysm: a complication of parenteral drug abuse. *Arch Surg* 1977;112:981-986.
95. Swanson E, Freiberg A, Salter DR. Radial artery infections and aneurysms after catheterization. *J Hand Surg* 1990;15:166-171.
96. Behera A, Menakuru SR, Jindal R. Vascular complications of drug abuse: an Indian experience. *Aust NZ J Surg* 2003;73:1004-1007.
97. Benjamin ME, Cohn Jr EJ, Purtill WA, et al. Arterial reconstruction with deep leg veins for the treatment of mycotic aneurysms. *J Vasc Surg* 1999;30:1004-1015.
98. Kurimoto Y, Tsuchida Y, Saito J, et al. Emergency endovascular stent grafting for infected pseudoaneurysm of brachial artery. *Infection* 2003;31:186-188.
99. Kul S, Aydin A, Dinc H, Erduran E. Widespread involvement of hepatic renal and mesenteric arteries with multiple mycotic aneurysms in a child. *Turk J Pediatrics* 2007;39:89-93.
100. Teich S, Tsangaris N, Giordano JH, Druy E. Mycotic aneurysm of the inferior pancreaticoduodenal artery: successful nonoperative management. *South Med J* 1989;82:267-269.
101. Senocac F, Cekirge S, Senocak ME, Karademir S. Hepatic artery aneurysm in a 10-year-old boy as a complication of infective endocarditis. *J Pediatr Surg* 1996;31:1570-1572.
102. Friedman SG, Pogo GJ, Moccio CG. Mycotic aneurysm of the superior mesenteric artery. *J Vasc Surg* 1987;6:87-90.
103. Woodburn KR, Murie JA. Vascular complications of injecting drug misuse. *Br J Surg* 1996;83:1329-1334.
104. Reddy DJ, Smith RF, Elliott Jr JP, et al. Infected femoral artery false aneurysms in drug addicts: evolution of selective vascular reconstruction. *J Vasc Surg* 1986;3:718-724.
105. Johnson JR, Ledgerwood AM, Lucas CE. Mycotic aneurysm: new concepts in therapy. *Arch Surg* 1983;118:577-582.
106. Wright D, Shepard A. Infected femoral artery aneurysms associated with drug abuse. In: Stanley J, Ernst C, eds. *Current therapy in vascular surgery*. Philadelphia: BC Decker; 1990:350-353.
107. Callaert JR, Fourneau I, Daenens K, et al. Endoprosthetic treatment of a mycotic superficial femoral artery aneurysm. *J Endovasc Ther* 2003;10: 843-845.
108. Teebken OE, Pichlmaier MA, Brand S, Haverich A. Cryopreserved arterial allografts for in situ reconstruction of infected arterial vessels. *Eur J Vasc Endovasc Surg* 2004;27:597-602.
109. Manekeller S, Tolba RH, Schroeder S, et al. Analysis of vascular complications in intra-venous drug addicts after puncture of femoral vessels. *Zentralbl Chir* 2004;129:21-28.
110. Papadoulas S, Skroubis G, Marangos MN, et al. Ruptured aneurysms of superficial femoral artery. *Eur J Vasc Endovasc Surg* 2000;19:430-432.
111. León LR, Psalms SB, Stevenson S, Mills JL. Non-traumatic aneurysms affecting crural arteries: case report and review of the literature. *Vascular* 2007;15:102-108.
112. Kieran SM, Cahill RA, Sheehan SJ. Mycotic peripheral aneurysms and intracerebral abscesses secondary to infective endocarditis. *Eur J Vasc Endovasc Surg* 2004;28:565-566.
113. Larena-Avellaneda A, Debus ES, Daum H, et al. Mycotic aneurysms affecting both lower legs of a patient with *Candida endocarditis*—endovascular therapy and open vascular surgery. *Ann Vasc Surg* 2004;18: 130-133.
114. McKee MA, Ballard JL. Mycotic aneurysms of the tibioperoneal arteries. *Ann Vasc Surg* 1999;13:188-190.
115. Murashita T, Yasuda K, Takigami T, et al. Mycotic aneurysm of the bilateral tibioperoneal trunks associated with bacterial endocarditis: a case report. *Int Angiol* 1997;16:176-179.
116. Menanteau B, Gausserand F, Ladam-Marcus V, et al. Mycotic aneurysm of the posterior tibial artery and pseudophlebitis: contribution of color Doppler ultrasonography. *J Radiol* 1995;76:205-208.
117. Akers Jr DL, Fowl RJ, Kempczinski RF. Mycotic aneurysm of the tibioperoneal trunk: case report and review of the literature. *J Vasc Surg* 1992;16:71-74.
118. Mayall JC, Mayall RC, Mayall AC, Mayall LC. Peripheral aneurysms. *Int Angiol* 1991;10:141-145.
119. Payne-James JJ. Infected aneurysm of the anterior tibial artery. *Br J Clin Pract* 1988;42:522-524.
120. Gedeon A. Mycotic aneurysms of the extremities. *J Cardiovasc Surg* 1973;(Spec No):285-287.
121. Tresidder GC, Warren RP. A case of bilateral mycotic aneurysm of the posterior tibial artery treated successfully by excision. *Br J Surg* 1953;41:333-334.
122. Rogers L. Mycotic aneurysms and their treatment. *Ann Royal Coll Surg Engl* 1956;19:257-262.
123. Dry TJ. Mycotic aneurysm of the posterior tibial artery complicating subacute bacterial endocarditis. *Proc Staff Meet Mayo Clin* 1947;22:105.
124. Herrman GV. Bacterial mycotic aneurysm in 8-year-old child. *Am J Dis Child* 1937;53:517.
125. Ossius EA. Subacute bacterial endocarditis. *J Mich State Med Soc* 1929;28:874.
126. Richey WG, Maclachlan WWG. Mycotic embolic aneurysms of peripheral arteries. *Arch Intern Med* 1922;29:131-140.
127. Shnider BI, Cotsona Jr NJ. Embolic mycotic aneurysms, a complication of bacterial endocarditis. *Am J Med* 1954;16:246.
128. Yao JST, McCarthy WJ. Multiple arterial aneurysms: a seven year follow up. *Contemp Surg* 1987;31:73-78.
129. Tilson MD 3rd, Withers L. Arterial aneurysms in HIV patients: molecular mimicry versus direct infection? *Ann NY Acad Sci* 2006;1085: 387-391.
130. Sellami D, Lucidarme O, Lebleu L, Grenier P. Infected aneurysm of abdominal aorta: early CT finding. *J Radiol* 2000;81:899-901.
131. Grotemeyer D, Graupe F, Mackrodt HG, Stock W. *Salmonella enteritidis* infected false aneurysm of the superficial femoral artery in an HIV seropositive patient. *Chirurg* 1998;69:204-206.
132. Bojar RM, Turner MT, Valdez S, et al. Homograft repair of a tuberculous pseudoaneurysm of the ascending aorta. *Chest* 1998;114:1774-1776.
133. Marks C, Kuskov S. Pattern of arterial aneurysms in acquired immunodeficiency disease. *World J Surg* 1995;19:127-132.
134. Nair R, Robbs JV, Naidoo NG, Woolgar J. Clinical profile of HIV-related aneurysms. *Eur J Vasc Endovasc Surg* 2000;20:235-240.
135. Chetty R, Batitang S, Nair R. Large artery vasculopathy in HIV-positive patients: another vasculitic enigma. *Hum Pathol* 2000;31:374-379.
136. Heikkinen MA, Dake MD, Alsac JM, Zarins CK. Multiple HIV-related aneurysms: open and endovascular treatment. *J Endovasc Ther* 2005;12:405-410.

137. Brant-Zawadzki P, Kinikini D, Kraiss LW. Deep leg vein reconstruction for an isolated mycotic common iliac artery aneurysm in an HIV-positive patient. *Vascular* 2007;15:98-101.
138. Patetsios PP, Shutze W, Holden B, et al. Repair of a mycotic aneurysm of the infrarenal aorta in a patient with HIV, using a Palmaz stent and autologous femoral vein graft. *Ann Vasc Surg* 2002;16:521-523.
139. Testi G, Freyrie A, Gargiulo M, et al. Endovascular and hybrid treatment of recurrent thoracoabdominal aneurysms in an HIV-positive patient. *Eur J Vasc Endovasc Surg* 2007;33:78-80.
140. Botes K, Van Marle J. Surgical intervention for HIV related vascular disease. *Eur J Vasc Endovasc Surg* 2007;34:390-396.

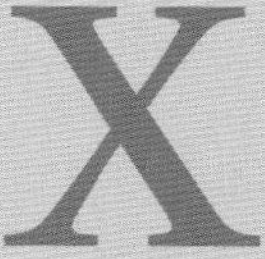

Venous Disease and Lymphedema

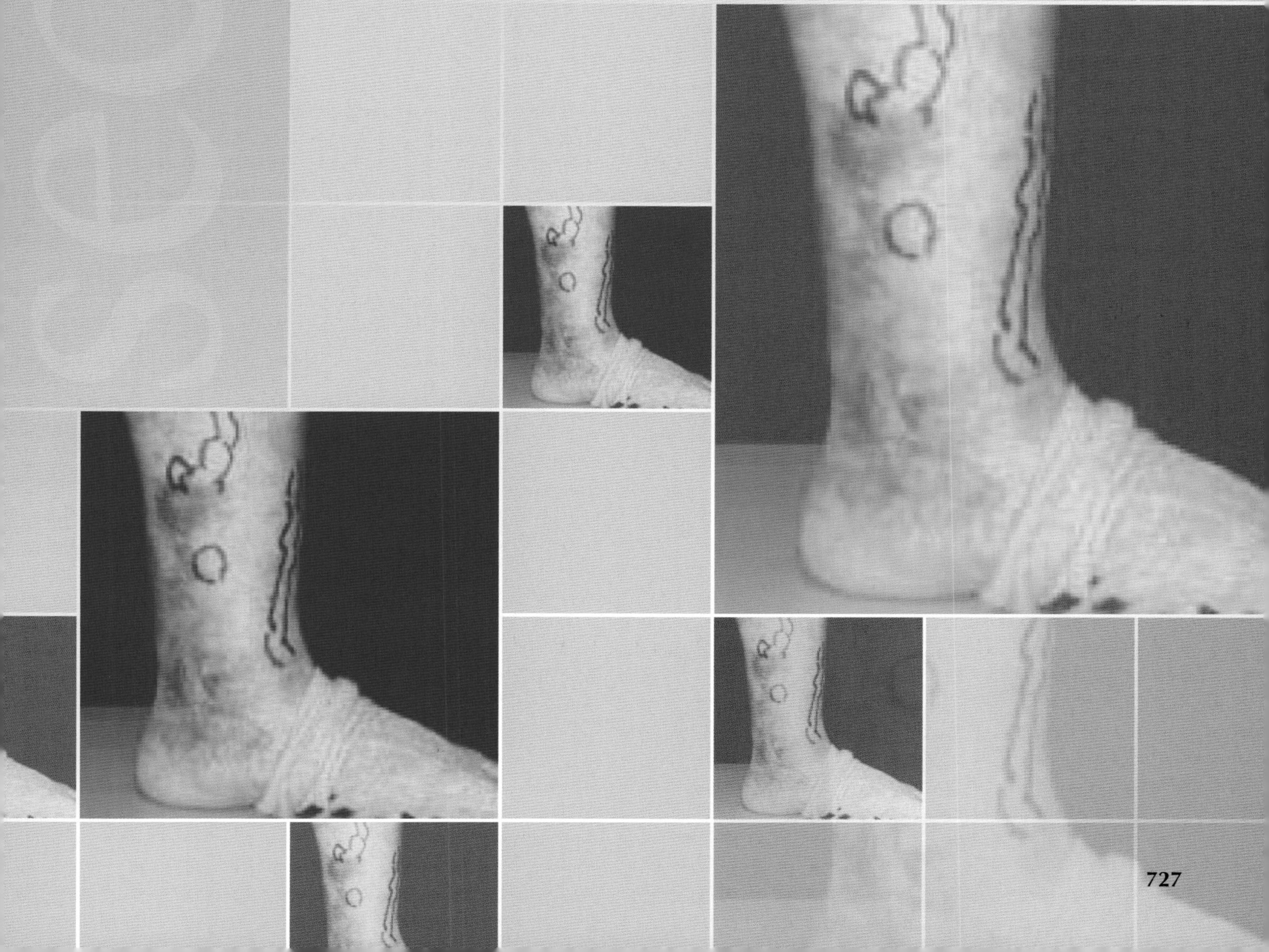

chapter

42

Pathophysiology of Varicose Veins and Chronic Venous Insufficiency

Mark H. Meissner, MD

Key Points

- Chronic venous disorders include a spectrum of clinical manifestations extending from telangiectasias and varicose veins to lipodermatosclerosis and ulceration.
- No single ideal test is available for chronic venous disease, and a combination of physiological and anatomical tests is often required to characterize the extent of disease.
- Varicose veins are present in 25% to 33% and chronic venous insufficiency, with skin changes and ulceration, in 2% to 5% of Western populations.
- Varicose veins have a multifactorial etiology involving the interaction of age, genetic, and environmental factors.
- Varicose veins arise multicentrically, with changes in vein wall architecture preceding the development of valvular incompetence.
- The clinical manifestations of chronic venous insufficiency are due to ambulatory venous hypertension and are mediated by chronic inflammation resulting from altered leukocyte–endothelial interactions.
- Although nonthrombotic iliac obstruction does occur, valvular incompetence, or reflux, is the usual hemodynamic derangement in primary venous disease. Secondary venous disease, usually developing after an episode of acute deep venous thrombosis, may have a combination of reflux and obstruction.
- Reflux in asymptomatic and mildly symptomatic patients is usually isolated and segmental, while that in patients with advanced chronic venous insufficiency is usually multisegmental and often involves the deep, superficial, and perforating veins.

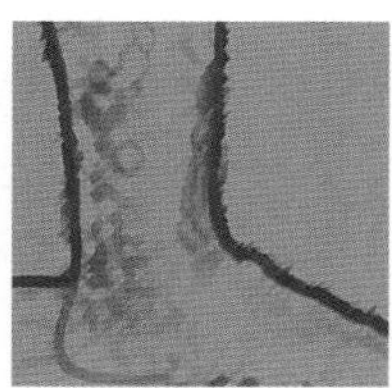

Chronic venous *disorders* include a spectrum of morphological and functional abnormalities of the venous system, ranging from uncomplicated telangiectasias and varicose veins to venous ulceration. The more prevalent disorders, such as telangiectasias, are common in healthy populations and are usually distinguished from chronic venous *diseases,* which are associated with signs and symptoms that are sufficiently severe to require medical attention. Chronic venous insufficiency refers more specifically to those manifestations (edema, skin changes, and ulceration) associated with functional abnormalities of the venous system and sustained venous hypertension.[1] Patients with varicose veins are not classified as having chronic venous insufficiency unless they have associated advanced manifestations of disease.[2] The manifestations of chronic venous disease may result from primary venous insufficiency or be secondary to other disorders, primarily acute deep venous thrombosis (DVT). Regardless of etiology, chronic venous disease has significant socioeconomic consequences and is among the most common problems encountered in surgical practice.

Table 42-1
Clinical Classification of Chronic Venous Disease

Class 0	No visible or palpable signs of venous disease
Class 1	Telangiectasias or reticular veins
Class 2	Varicose veins
Class 3	Edema
Class 4	Skin changes ascribed to venous disease
4a	Pigmentation or eczema
4b	Lipodermatosclerosis or atrophie blanche
Class 5	Skin changes, as defined above, with healed ulceration
Class 6	Skin changes, as defined above, with active ulceration

Adapted from Eklof B, Rutherford RB, Bergan JJ, et al. *J Vasc Surg* 2004;40(6):1248-1252.

It is estimated that chronic venous disease affects up to 1% of the general population[3] and that as many as 164 of every 1000 people seek medical advice for venous problems.[4] In the United States, skin changes and ulceration have been estimated to affect 6 million to 7 million and 400,000 to 500,00 people, respectively.[5]

The social and economic consequences of chronic venous disease are significant. Annual health-care costs for venous ulceration are estimated to be 290 million pounds in the United Kingdom and $1 billion in the United States.[6] Although the costs of wound care alone can exceed $40,000 per patient per year, the time lost from productive activity and the considerable psychological effects of ulceration are as important as the economic costs and are more difficult to measure. Feelings of fear, social isolation, anger, and depression and a negative self-image are more common in patients with venous ulcers than among those undergoing procedures such as cardiac operations.[7]

DIAGNOSTIC CRITERIA

Clinical Manifestations of Chronic Venous Disease

To standardize the reporting and treatment of the diverse manifestations of chronic venous disorders, a comprehensive classification system (CEAP) has been proposed to allow uniform diagnosis and comparison of patient populations. The fundamentals of the CEAP classification include a description of the clinical disease class (C) based on objective signs; the etiology (E); the anatomical (A) distribution of reflux and obstruction in the superficial, deep, and perforating veins; and the underlying pathophysiology (P), whether due to reflux or obstruction.[1,8] Seven clinical disease categories are recognized (Table 42-1): asymptomatic limbs (class 0) and those with telangiectasias (class 1), varicose veins (class 2), edema (class 3), skin changes without ulceration (class 4a and 4b), healed ulcers (class 5), and active ulcers (class 6). The underlying etiology can further be classified as congenital, primary, or secondary. Primary venous disorders are not associated with an identifiable mechanism of venous dysfunction. In contrast, secondary venous disorders result from an anteceded event, usually an episode of acute DVT. When developing after an episode of DVT, manifestations of pain, edema, skin changes, and ulceration are commonly referred to as the postthrombotic syndrome.

Table 42-2
Varicose Veins Diagnostic Criteria

	Telangiectasias	Reticular Veins	Varicose Veins
Size	0.1-1 mm	1-3 mm	>3 mm
Color	Red to purple	Green to blue	None
Palpable	No	No	Yes

Varicose veins are the most common manifestation of primary chronic venous disease. Although various classification systems have been proposed, varicose veins are usually differentiated from reticular veins and telangiectasias[1,9] (Table 42-2). Varicose veins are usually defined as dilated, palpable, tortuous veins greater than 3 mm in diameter that do not discolor the overlying skin. Their saccular, tortuous characteristics distinguish varicose veins from the prominent superficial veins that may be seen in thin, fit individuals. Reticular veins are dilated but nonpalpable, blue, subdermal veins less than 3 mm in diameter and are distinguished from smaller red to purple intradermal telangiectasias. The major saphenous trunks are not usually involved in patients with telangiectasias and reticular veins but often are incompetent with varicose veins. More than 50% of patients have bilateral varicosities, and no particular predilection exists for either leg.[10,11]

The most common reasons for presentation include symptoms attributable to varicose veins (38%), cosmetic considerations (26%), and concern regarding complications.[12] Uncomplicated varicose veins have been associated with symptoms including aching, heaviness, cramps, tingling, and pruritus, the prevalence of which increase with age despite only a limited association with the presence of trunk varicosities.[13-15] No single symptom is pathognomonic for varicose veins, and similar symptoms have been noted in 33% of men and 50% of women without varicose veins.[10] Women are more likely to report venous-associated leg symptoms than men.[16] Symptoms often increase during the course of the day and with prolonged standing. Between 5% and 7% of patients present with complications of their varicose veins, including superficial thrombophlebitis, bleeding, and rarely, skin changes and ulceration.[4,12]

The more severe manifestations of chronic venous disease include edema, skin changes, and ulceration. Early skin changes include hyperpigmentation and corona phlebectatica. Hyperpigmentation results from the accumulation of hemosiderin granules within dermal macrophages after the breakdown of extravasated red blood cells.[17] Corona phlebectatica is recognized as a fan-shaped pattern of intradermal veins over the medial or lateral aspects of the foot and ankle.[1] The subcutaneous tissue later becomes fibrotic and may be associated with cutaneous weeping, scaling, and erythema characteristic of venous eczema. Lipodermatosclerosis refers to the subcutaneous fibrosis and chronic inflammation that result from sustained venous hypertension. Associated physical findings may include a limited range of ankle motion and peripheral neuropathy. Atrophie blanche, characterized by circular, atrophic, white areas of skin, are also considered a manifestation of severe chronic venous disease.

Ulceration is the most advanced stage of chronic venous disease. The differential diagnosis for lower extremity ulcers includes chronic venous disease, arterial disease, collagen vascular diseases, metabolic disorders, and vasculitis. Approximately three quarters of leg ulcers have an underlying venous cause,[18] and among venous ulcers, approximately three quarters involve the medial aspect of the gaiter area. However, venous ulcers may also occur laterally and higher in the calf. More than 95% of medial gaiter ulcers are associated with venous disease, while fewer than 50% of calf ulcers have an underlying venous etiology.[19] Isolated lateral ulcers have been particularly associated with small saphenous incompetence.[20] Although features such as ulcer location and associated lipodermatosclerosis may suggest venous disease, confirmation of a venous etiology requires documentation of venous reflux.

Skin changes and ulceration may be associated with either primary or secondary venous disease, the relative frequency of which depends on the referral population. In some specialty centers, as many as 10% of patients with varicose veins have been reported to have ulcers.[21] Approximately 60% of patients with venous ulceration have no previous history of DVT.[22,23] However, DVT is often occult, and the poor correlation between clinical history and objective evidence of DVT is well recognized.[24] Hanrahan et al.[25] identified a history of DVT or superficial phlebitis in 33% of ulcer patients, with duplex evidence of such an event in 44%. In contrast, Welkie et al.[23] found that duplex imaging of patients with active or healed ulcers increased the number of patients with postthrombotic disease from only 38.3% to 40%.

Venous claudication warrants special consideration. As its manifestations are primarily due to proximal venous obstruction rather than valvular incompetence, it is not ordinarily considered in the spectrum of chronic venous disease. Patients with symptoms of venous claudication complain of lower extremity tightness and bursting pain with vigorous exercise.[26] In contrast to arterial claudication, pain is often less severe and affects the entire limb rather than specific muscle groups. Its onset is more gradual and occurs with a higher intensity of activity. Finally, it may require 15 to 20 minutes of rest, often with leg elevation, for relief. Although muscle blood flow during exercise is reduced in these patients, pain is more likely related to elevated intramuscular pressures than to ischemia.[27] Associated findings may include swelling of the thigh and calf, cyanosis, and prominence of the superficial veins. Patients may have other manifestations of chronic venous disease, including varicose veins and ulceration.[27]

Proposed criteria for the diagnosis of venous claudication include intermittent claudication, iliac vein obstruction, venous hypertension at rest, and increased venous pressure with exercise.[27] Although nonthrombotic iliac lesions are recognized and may be associated with symptoms of pain and edema,[28] venous claudication most often results from persistent iliac vein stenosis or occlusion after an episode of acute DVT. These lesions more commonly occur on the left side[26,27] and are often related to the May-Thurner syndrome or underlying compression of the left iliac vein by the overlying right common iliac artery.[29] Catheter-directed thrombolysis uncovers such lesions in up to one third of limbs with iliofemoral DVT.[30]

Lower Extremity Venous Anatomy

The nomenclature of the lower extremity veins has been recently updated,[31] clarifying many definitions and eliminating most eponyms. The most current nomenclature is used in the following discussion. The venous system of the lower extremities includes the deep veins, which lie beneath the muscular fascia and drain the lower extremity muscles; the superficial veins, which are above the deep fascia and drain the cutaneous microcirculation; and the perforating veins, which penetrate the muscular fascia and connect the superficial and deep veins. Communicating veins connect veins within the same system.[31] The superficial, deep, and most perforating veins contain bicuspid valves consisting of folds of endothelium supported by a thin layer of connective tissue (Figure 42-1).

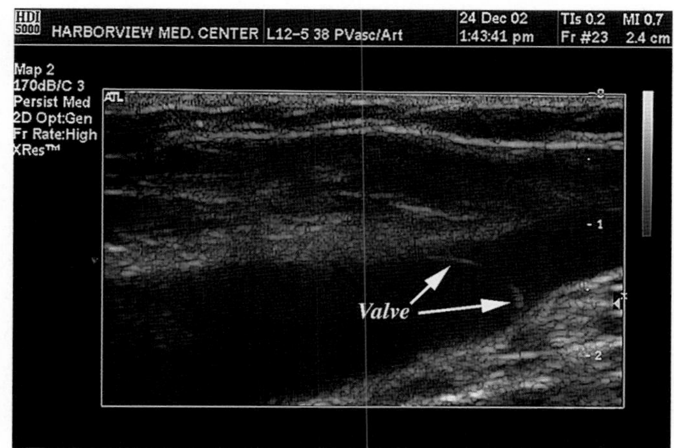

Figure 42-1. B-mode ultrasound of the great saphenous vein showing both cusps of a normal bicuspid valve.

The superficial veins, which include the great and small saphenous veins, drain the skin and subcutaneous tissue (Figure 42-2). The great saphenous vein is duplicated in the thigh in 8% and in the calf in 25% of patients. Usually two main saphenous tributaries appear in the calf, the anterior branch and the posterior arch (Leonardo's) vein, which begins behind the medial malleolus and joins the great saphenous vein just below the knee. A valve is present at the saphenofemoral junction in 94% to 100% of individuals, and 81% have at least one valve in the external iliac–common femoral segment above the junction.[32] The great saphenous vein usually has at least 6 valves, while the small saphenous vein has 7 to 10 closely spaced valves.[33] Varicose great saphenous veins do have slightly fewer valves (mean 6.0 ± 1.7) than normal veins (7.3 ± 2.3),[34] although the relevance of this observation is unclear.

Perforating veins may empty directly into the axial deep veins (direct perforators) or into the venous sinuses of the calf (indirect perforators). Although perforating veins are numerous and variable, four groups are of clinical significance: those of the foot, the medial and lateral calf, and the thigh. The foot perforators are unique in ordinarily directing flow toward the superficial veins.[33,35] The major perforators of the medial calf and thigh have one to three valves that direct flow from the superficial to the deep veins.[33] The medial calf perforators include the paratibial perforators joining the main great saphenous vein or its branches and the posterior tibial perforators that originate in the posterior arch vein. The perforators of the femoral canal connect the great saphenous vein with the distal superficial femoral or proximal popliteal vein. Although several criteria have been used to define an incompetent perforator, the specific diagnostic criteria remain controversial.[36]

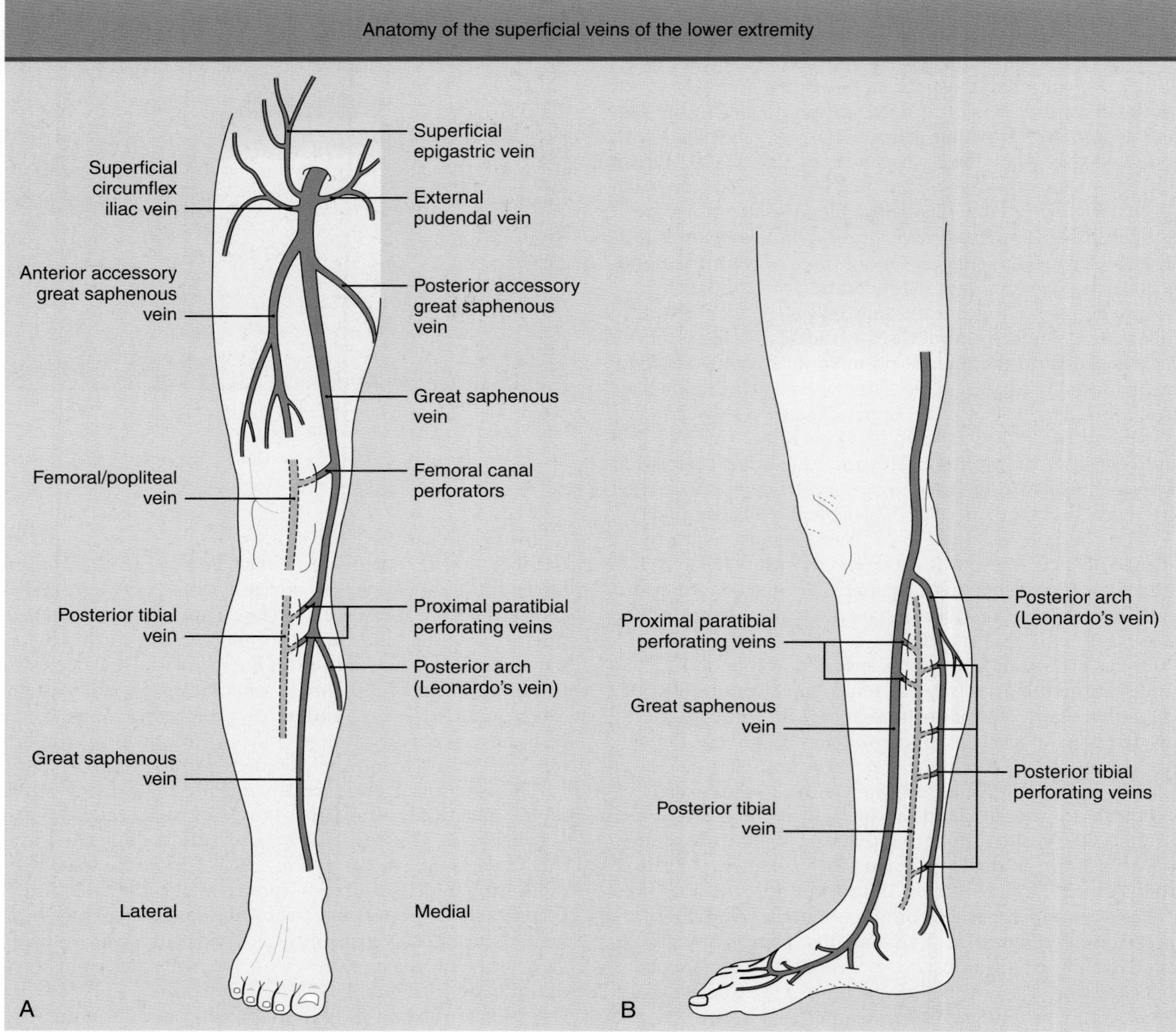

Figure 42-2. Anatomy of the superficial veins of the lower extremity. **A,** Anterior view showing the clinically important femoral canal perforators in the midthigh and paratibial perforators in the calf. **B,** Lateral view showing the posterior tibial and paratibial perforators connecting the posterior arch and greater saphenous veins, respectively, with the posterior tibial vein.

The deep veins of the lower extremity follow the course of the associated arteries, with the number of valves increasing from proximal to distal. The muscular venous sinuses are the principal collecting system of the calf muscle pump. Although also present in the gastrocnemius muscles, the soleal sinuses are of greatest numerical importance. An average of five deep venous valves lie between the inguinal ligament and the popliteal fossa, although the number varies from two to nine.[37] Their arrangement is variable, but generally the inferior vena cava and common iliac veins have no valves; the external iliac and common femoral veins above the saphenofemoral junction have one valve at most; the (superficial) femoral vein above the adductor canal has three or more valves; the distal superficial femoral and popliteal veins have one or two valves; and the tibial–peroneal veins have numerous valves spaced in approximately 2-cm intervals.[33,37] Although the muscle sinusoids are valveless, they often empty into profusely valved, arborizing, draining veins.[37]

Hemodynamics of Chronic Venous Disease

The accumulation of blood in the lower extremity veins while upright is limited by the physical properties of the venous wall, the function of the venous valves, and the action of the calf muscle pump. The valves function to divide the hydrostatic column of blood into segments and to insure antegrade venous flow. Approximately 90% of the venous return in the lower

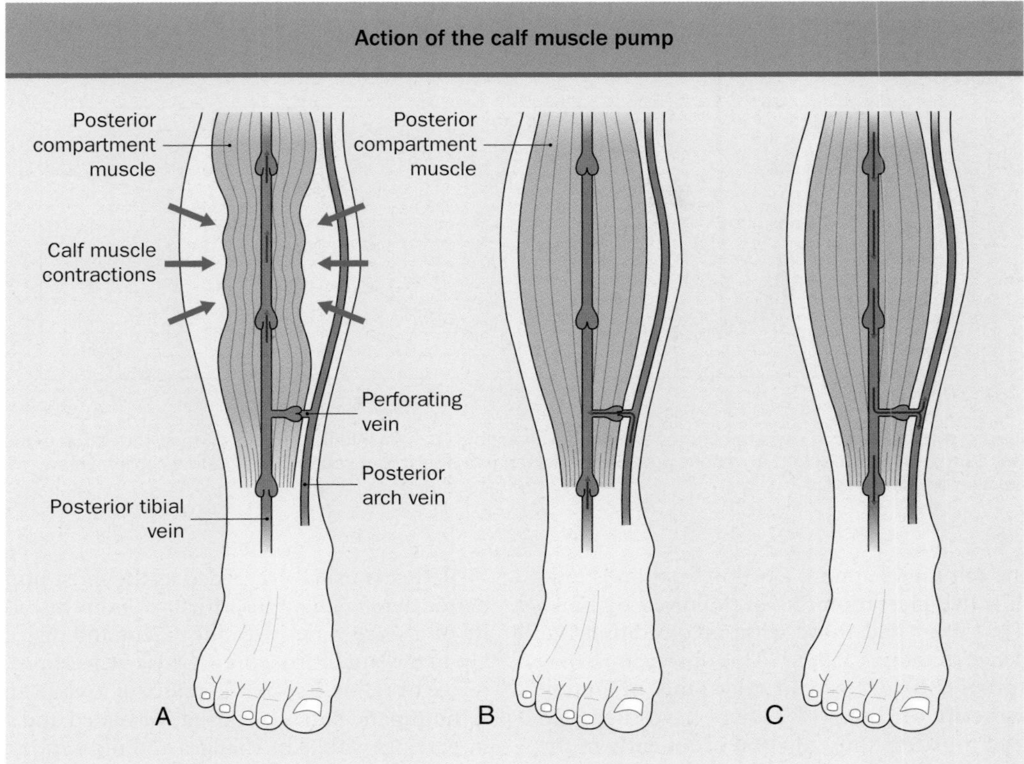

Figure 42-3. Action of the calf muscle pump. **A,** With contraction of the calf muscle (systole), the deep veins are emptied of blood while competent distal and perforating vein valves prevent retrograde flow into the foot and the superficial system. **B,** During the relaxation phase (diastole), competent proximal valves prevent retrograde flow while blood flows from the superficial to the low-pressure deep system through the perforating veins. **C,** In the presence of deep venous reflux, incompetent proximal valves allow rapid venous refilling during the relaxation phase. High deep venous pressures are transmitted from the deep to the superficial system through incompetent perforating veins.

extremities is via the deep veins through the action of the foot, calf, and thigh muscles pumps.[38] The action of these valved pumps critically depends on the deep fascia of the leg, which constrains the muscles during contraction and allows high pressures to be generated within the muscular compartments.

Among the three pumps, the calf pump has the largest capacitance, generates the highest pressures, and is of greatest importance.[35,39] The ejection fraction of the calf muscle pump is approximately 65% in comparison to only 15% for the thigh pump. With contraction of the calf, pressure in the posterior compartment rises to as high as 250 mm Hg,[39] the veins are emptied of blood, and resting venous pressure is lowered as the valves prevent retrograde flow (Figure 42-3A and 42-3B). Pressure in the posterior tibial vein accordingly decreases from 80 to 100 mm Hg to less than 30 mm Hg (Figure 42-4). A reduction in deep venous pressure during the postcontraction relaxation phase favors flow from the superficial to the deep system through the perforating veins. In the presence of competent venous valves, capillary inflow causes a slow rise in deep venous pressure during this phase of activity.

Reflux, or pathological retrograde flow, occurs when the valves are absent or rendered incompetent by either degenerative processes (primary venous disease) or an episode of DVT (secondary venous disease). Under these circumstances, retrograde flow during calf muscle relaxation prevents the usual reduction in pressure and rapid venous refilling occurs from the retrograde flow of blood, as well as slow capillary inflow (Figure 42-3C). High venous pressure may also be transmitted from the deep to the superficial veins through incompetent perforators. The function of the calf muscle pump may also be impaired in patients with chronic venous disease, an observation that is at least partially related to a reduced ankle range of motion.[40]

The clinical manifestations of chronic venous insufficiency are primarily due to ambulatory venous hypertension or failure to adequately lower venous pressure with exercise. Ambulatory venous pressure is determined using a 21-gauge needle to measure the response to 10 tiptoe movements, usually at a rate of 1 per second, in a dorsal foot vein. The ambulatory venous pressure is measured as the lowest pressure achieved at the end of exercise (Figure 42-5). The severity of chronic venous disease is closely related to the magnitude of venous hypertension. Ulceration usually does not occur at ambulatory venous pressures of less than 30 mm Hg, while the incidence is 100% at pressures greater than 90 mm Hg.[41]

The determinants of ambulatory venous pressure are complex and include venous reflux, as well as obstruction and calf muscle pump dysfunction.[42,43] Hemodynamically significant reflux in either the superficial or the deep venous systems is associated with elevated ambulatory venous pressures, as well as short refilling times after exercise ceases. However, for any degree of reflux, the ambulatory venous pressure is worsened by associated venous obstruction. Similarly, abnormal calf muscle pump function is associated with a higher incidence of ulceration and noninvasive indices of venous pressure.[40] Although the relationship with disease severity has not been

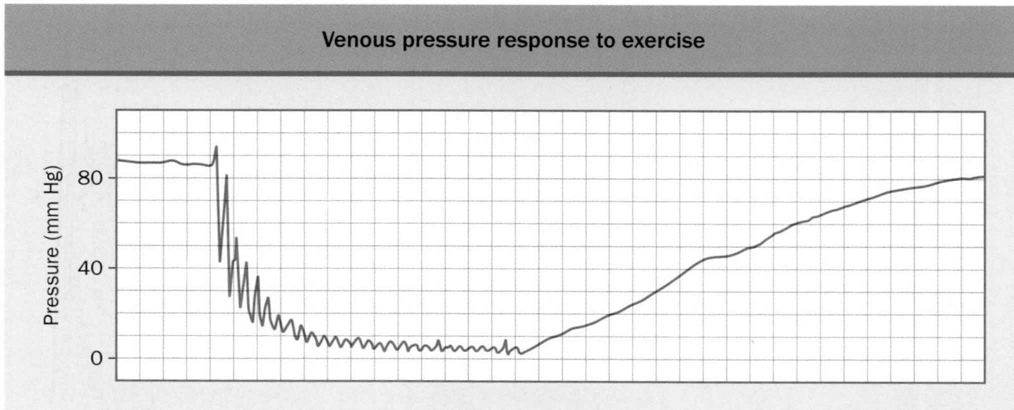

Figure 42-4. Venous pressure response to exercise. During treadmill walking by a patient without venous disease, the action of the calf muscle pump with each step causes a progressive reduction in venous pressure measured in a dorsal foot vein. Arterial inflow causes a slow return to baseline (the venous refilling time) after walking stops.

consistent,[44-46] the calf muscle pump ejection fraction is lowest in limbs with active ulceration (35%), followed by limbs with healed ulcers (49%) and those without ulceration but with duplex evidence of reflux (53%).[47] This observation may be related to the progressive decrease in ankle range of motion with increasing severity of disease.[40] Others have suggested that changes in calf muscle pump function occur early in the development of chronic venous disease and do not worsen with the development of skin changes and ulceration.[23]

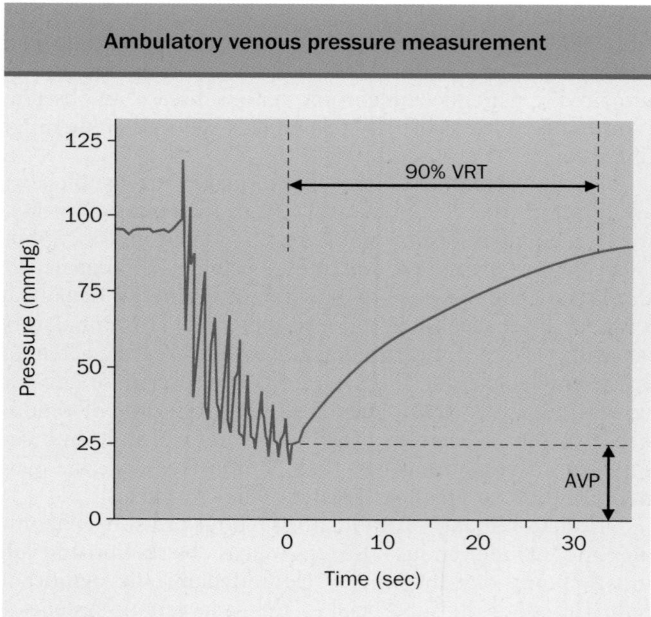

Figure 42-5. Ambulatory venous pressure measurement. In the normal limb, venous pressure as measured in a dorsal foot vein progressively declines with each plantar flexion maneuver. Ambulatory venous pressure represents the pressure at the end of 10 tiptoe maneuvers and is less than 30 mm Hg in normal limbs. The time required for return to baseline is measured as the 90% venous refilling time (VRT). Limbs with hemodynamically significant reflux have an elevated ambulatory venous pressure and rapid 90% VRT.

Reflux is usually regarded as the most important hemodynamic derangement in primary venous disease, and the severity of disease varies with the extent and distribution of reflux. Up to 82% of limbs with varicose veins show noninvasive evidence of reflux.[48,49] While reflux in asymptomatic and mildly symptomatic patients is usually isolated and segmental,[44] that in patients with skin changes and ulceration is usually multisegmental and often involves the deep, superficial, and perforating veins. Approximately two thirds of patients with ulcers have multisystem disease.[25] A combination of superficial and deep venous reflux, with or without documented perforator incompetence, is the most common pattern in these patients (Table 42-3). Reflux in the distal deep venous segments, particularly the popliteal and posterior tibial veins, appears to be important in the pathogenesis of venous ulceration. Although their clinical importance remains controversial and interruption of incompetent perforators does not seem to improve either ulcer healing or recurrence,[36] perforator incompetence does theoretically allow transmission of elevated venous pressure from the deep to the superficial system.

Although venous obstruction is usually not regarded as an important consideration in primary venous disease, primary obstructive lesions of the iliac veins (nonthrombotic iliac vein lesions) do occur and are increasingly recognized. Although historically attributed to the right common iliac artery crossing the left common iliac vein, it is now apparent that such lesions may occur in both the right and the left lower extremities and may involve both the common and the external iliac veins.[28,50] The hemodynamic abnormalities associated with secondary venous disease are more complex, often involving both valvular reflux and venous obstruction. Postthrombotic limbs with edema, hyperpigmentation, or ulceration are more likely to have a combination of reflux and residual obstruction than either abnormality alone[51] (Figure 42-6). Valvular incompetence has usually been presumed to be the more important of these, and postthrombotic symptoms do correlate more closely with a reduction in venous refilling time than with residual abnormalities of venous outflow.[52] However, reports of clinical improvement with correction of iliac vein obstruction,[50] independent of the effects of any residual reflux, raise questions regarding the relative importance of reflux and obstruction and require further investigation.

Table 42-3
Distribution of Reflux in Patients with Venous Ulcers

	Labropoulos et al. ($N = 112$)[22] (%)	Barwell et al. ($N = 593$)[156] (%)	Darke and Penfold ($N = 232$)[24] (%)*	Hanrahan et al. ($N = 95$)[25] (%)
Superficial (S)	23	39		16.8
Perforator (P)	3		4	8.4
Deep (D)	6	8		2.1
S + P	21		39	19.0
S + D	12	43		11.6
P + D	4			4.2
S + P + D	28		35	31.6
No reflux	4	10		6.3
Occlusion or PTS†		2	22	

*Deep venous reflux associated with any other pattern included in S + P + D; superficial incompetence, with or without perforator incompetence, included in S + P.
†PTS, postthrombotic syndrome.

Diagnostic Tests for Chronic Venous Disease

Tests for Venous Reflux

Although most patients with asymptomatic varicose veins require little more than reassurance, the appropriate management of symptomatic chronic venous disease may require both qualitative and quantitative identification and localization of reflux within the lower extremity venous systems. More detailed evaluation of the venous system may be important in establishing an etiology for nonspecific complaints such as pain, swelling, or ulceration; selecting appropriate patients for ablative, extirpative, or reconstructive procedures; assessing hemodynamic improvement after such procedures; and establishing the natural history of chronic venous disease. The evaluation of advanced chronic venous insufficiency is usually more complicated than for simple varicose veins as both reflux and obstruction may involve the deep, superficial, and perforating veins. The ideal diagnostic test for chronic venous disease should be capable of distinguishing primary from postthrombotic disease; identifying both venous obstruction and valvular incompetence; localizing the abnormality to precise segments of the superficial and deep venous systems; and distinguishing among clinical degrees of disease. That is, the test should provide a quantitative measure of reflux that corresponds to the clinical stage of disease.

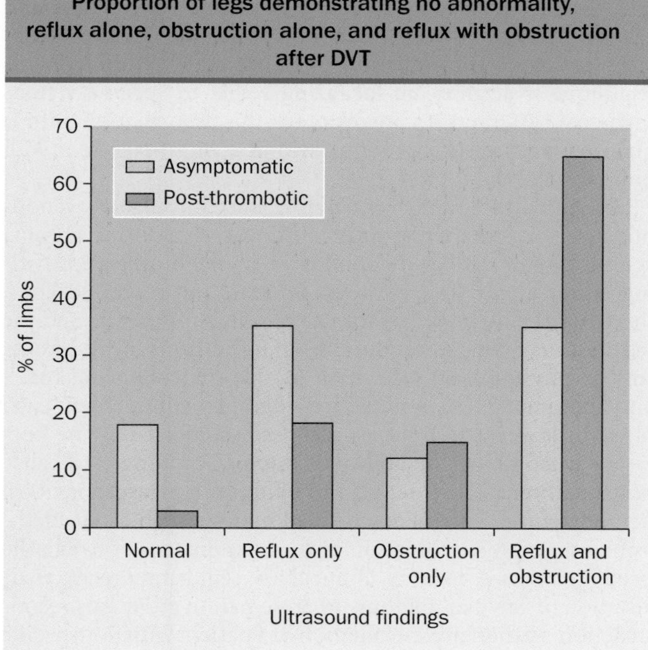

Figure 42-6. Proportion of limbs demonstrating no abnormality (normal), reflux alone, obstruction alone, and reflux with obstruction after deep venous thrombosis. Yellow bars show asymptomatic legs; red bars indicate legs with postthrombotic symptoms. (Adapted from Johnson BF, Manzo RA, Bergelin RO, Strandness DE. *J Vasc Surg* 1995;21:307-313.)

The diagnostic evaluation of the patient with venous disease has evolved from relatively crude noninvasive tests, such as continuous wave Doppler and photoplethysmography, to current standards, including duplex ultrasonography and occasionally air plethysmography. Many of these tests are largely of historical significance and, although useful in understanding the underlying pathophysiology, have little role in the modern management of chronic venous disease.

The Trendelenburg test is perhaps the best-recognized clinical test.[53] The lower extremity veins are drained by elevating the limb to 45 degrees, a tourniquet is applied below the saphenofemoral junction, and the patient is asked to stand. Rapid filling of the distal veins with the tourniquet in place suggests perforator reflux, while rapid filling after the tourniquet is released reflects saphenofemoral incompetence. Although the Trendelenburg test is 91% sensitive for the identification of superficial and perforator reflux, it has a specificity of only 15%.[53] Continuous wave Doppler evaluation of the great and small saphenous veins has historically been used as an adjuvant to the clinical tests. The continuous wave Doppler examination is performed in the standing position, insonating the saphenofemoral and saphenopopliteal junctions as the release of distal calf compression is used to provoke reflux.[54] Reflux that is abolished by compression of the saphenous vein above the knee and is not present in the (superficial) femoral vein is localized to the great saphenous vein. Reflux is similarly localized to the saphenopopliteal junction if it is abolished by distal compression of the small saphenous vein. Although sensitive for the identification of saphenofemoral junction reflux,[53] clinical examination with and without continuous wave Doppler have been noted to lead to selection of inappropriate varicose vein procedures in 20% and 13% of limbs, respectively.[55] Photoplethysmography, based on transmission of infrared light into the skin and measurement of backscattered light by an adjacent photoreceptor, was among the first widely available noninvasive tests for venous disease. The technique generates a recording in which a rapid fall from the baseline occurs with active flexion of the ankle followed by a gradual return with muscular relaxation. The venous refilling time is the time required for return to baseline, and a venous refilling time of 20 seconds has often been considered abnormal. Although simple and inexpensive, photoplethysmography provides little quantitative information. A normal venous refilling time excludes significant valvular incompetence, but the specificity of an abnormal result and the correlation with the quantity of reflux and severity of disease have been limited.

Among the invasive diagnostic tests, descending venography and ambulatory venous pressure have historically been the gold standards for the anatomical localization and hemodynamic quantification of reflux. Although descending phlebography may still have a role in situations such as venous reconstruction, it does have several limitations. It is invasive, the assessment of distal valves may be impossible if proximal valves are competent, and false-positive tests can result from hyperbaric contrast streaming past normal valves. The test also provides limited assessment of the great and small saphenous veins, and the phlebographic grade of reflux correlates only loosely with the severity of disease. In contrast, ambulatory venous pressure measurements are physiological, and to a certain extent, they do correlate with the incidence of ulceration. Unfortunately, this technique also has limitations. Most notably, the test measures only global hemodynamics. It therefore requires reflux at multiple sites, may be insensitive to isolated segmental reflux, and cannot precisely localize reflux to specific venous segments. Ambulatory venous pressure is also influenced by venous obstruction, occasionally making the test difficult to interpret.

Furthermore, since these methods are invasive, they are not easily repeatable and are not appropriate screening tests for many patients with chronic venous disease. This has led to noninvasive alternatives to both anatomical (descending phlebography) and hemodynamic (ambulatory venous pressure) tests. Air plethysmography measures calf volume changes in response to gravity and exercise as a reflection of reflux (Figure 42-7). The calf is placed in a polyvinyl chloride sleeve 35 cm in length, which is then inflated, connected to a pressure transducer, and calibrated with 100 cc of air. After obtaining a baseline recording with the patient supine and leg elevated to 45 degrees, the patient assumes an upright position. The venous volume is recorded as the leg fills. The patient is then instructed to plantar flex on both feet to record the ejected volume followed by 10 tiptoe movements, after which the residual volume is recorded. From this information, it is possible to calculate the venous filling index as the ratio of the 90% filling volume and the 90% venous filling time; the ejection fraction as the ratio of ejected volume to venous volume; and the residual volume fraction as the ratio of residual volume to venous volume. The venous filling index is an index of global venous reflux, while the ejection fraction and the residual volume fraction reflect calf muscle pump function and ambulatory venous pressure, respectively. The incidence of ulceration increases from 0% with a venous filling index of less than 5 ml/sec to 58% for a venous filling index of more than 10 ml/sec.[56] However, as with other global tests of hemodynamics, air plethysmography cannot precisely localize segmental reflux and the residual volume fraction correlates only loosely with the severity of disease.

Venous duplex ultrasonography has become the most widely used test in the diagnosis and management of chronic venous disease. In combining B-mode imaging with the pulsed Doppler, duplex is capable of accurately localizing both venous obstruction and valvular reflux to specific venous segments. Duplex examinations for reflux should always be performed in the standing position. In addition to being physiological, the standing position limits the occurrence of "physiological reflux," in which valves refluxing in the supine position are competent when upright. The duplex criteria for reflux are based on the demonstration of reverse flow in response to a provocative maneuver. Valsalva's maneuver, proximal venous compression, and release of distal compression have been used to elicit reflux. The compression maneuvers may further be performed manually or with standardized pneumatic cuffs. Although acceptable results can be achieved with release of manual distal compression, standardized testing using pneumatic distal cuff deflation is the most accurate and reproducible method of eliciting reflux[57] (Figure 42-8). In evaluating reflux using this technique, the patient stands supported by a frame, with the leg slightly flexed and weight borne by the contralateral extremity. Pneumatic cuffs are inflated distal to the segment of interest, which is then imaged in a longitudinal plane. Doppler signals are recorded as the cuff is inflated and rapidly deflated, simulating muscular contraction and relaxation. Ninety-five percent of normal valves close within 0.5 seconds of cuff deflation[58] (Figure 42-9). Although this technique is accurate in localizing reflux to specific venous segments, attempts to incorporate this information into a quantitative measure of reflux within a limb have met with limited success.

As with descending venography and ambulatory venous pressure measurements, most noninvasive tests for chronic venous disease display the fundamental dichotomy of providing either anatomical or hemodynamic information. Thus, there may be no ideal test for valvular incompetence, and the best test may depend on the clinical indications for the study. Just as physiological tests such as the ankle–brachial index and anatomical tests such as arteriography complement each other in lower extremity arterial assessment, it may be necessary to combine the ability of duplex scanning to localize both anatomical obstruction and reflux with measurements of hemodynamic severity determined by tests such as air plethysmography. A combination of these studies may obviate the need for invasive tests in all but those requiring precise visualization of valvular anatomy in anticipation of venous reconstruction. In the simple evaluation of a patient with nonspecific symptoms, any of the noninvasive tests may be sufficient for the documentation of reflux. However, in some situations, such as planning for an operative procedure, more precise anatomical localization is needed and duplex ultrasonography is the ideal diagnostic test. In contrast, in evaluating the results

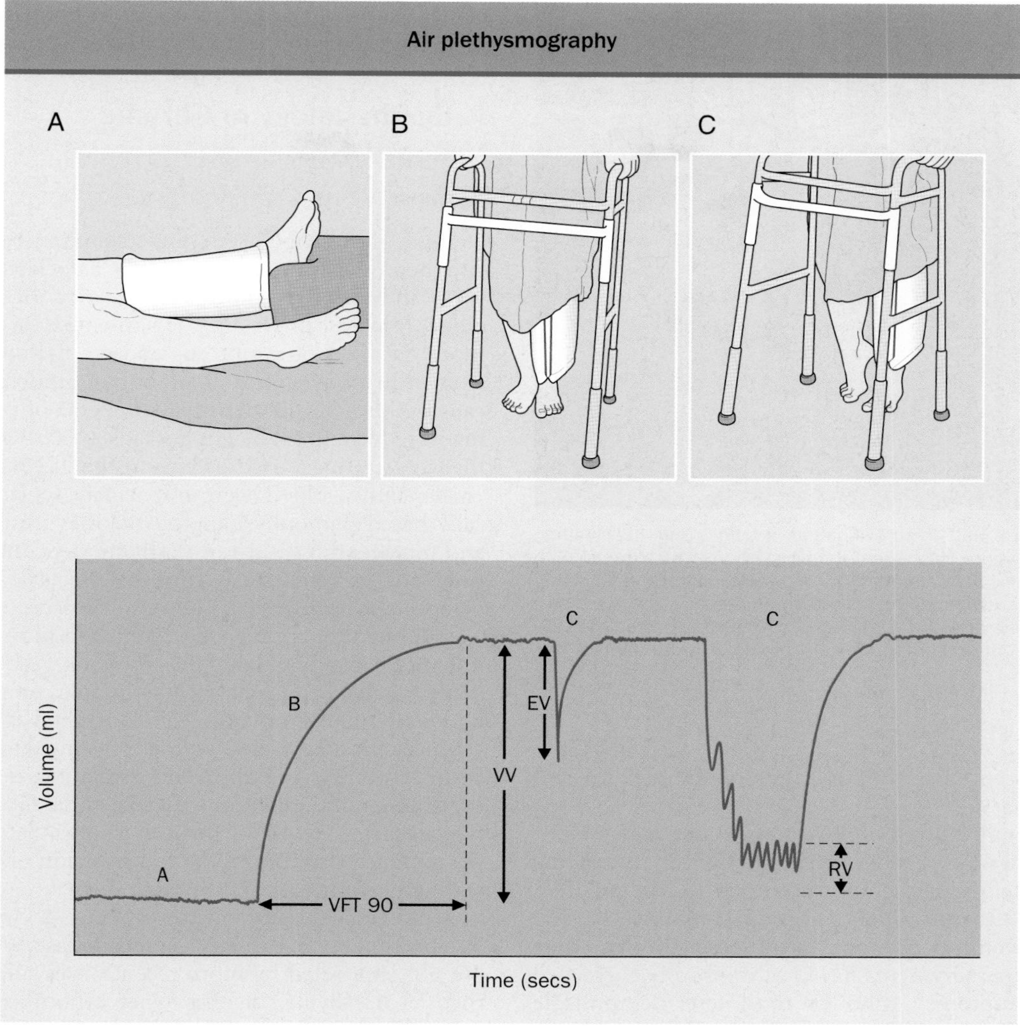

Figure 42-7. Air plethysmography. Patient maneuvers *(top panel)*. Volume tracing *(bottom panel)*. **A,** The calf is placed in a 35-cm polyvinyl chloride sleeve, and after calibration, baseline tracing is recorded in the supine position with the leg elevated. **B,** The patient assumes an upright position, bearing weight on the contralateral limb as the leg fills and the venous volume (VV) is recorded. **C,** The ejected volume (EV) is recorded as the patient plantar flexes on both feet. The residual volume (RV) is recorded after 10 tiptoe maneuvers. See text for details. (Adapted from Christopoulos DG, Nicolaides AN, Szendro G, et al. *J Vasc Surg* 1987;5:148-159.)

of an operative procedure, more quantitative hemodynamic information is necessary, and air plethysmography may be the best test.

Tests for Venous Obstruction

Both duplex ultrasonography and ascending venography have proven accurate in localizing infrainguinal venous obstruction. However, detailed visualization of the iliac segments may be difficult with these techniques. Furthermore, in comparison to intravascular ultrasound, now considered the diagnostic test of choice for iliac venous obstruction, venography has a sensitivity of only 66% for the detection of nonthrombotic iliac vein lesions.[28] Unfortunately, these anatomical studies provide little information regarding the significance of an obstruction in the patient with atypical symptoms or widespread valvular incompetence. Various direct and indirect tests have been proposed to assess the significance of underlying venous obstruction. Most indirect tests rely on plethysmographic techniques (strain gauge, photo-, impedance, and air plethysmography) that, although useful in identifying acute proximal obstruction, may not adequately define the significance of chronic lesions. In comparison to limbs with acute venous obstruction, limbs with chronic obstruction have both a higher outflow and a venous capacity or "dead space."[59]

Direct tests for deep venous obstruction include several pressure measurements. Among these, the resting arm–foot pressure differential and foot pressures after reactive hyperemia (normal is less than 4 mm Hg and is less than 6 mm Hg in fully compensated obstruction) are the most widely used.[60] In combination, the arm–foot and reactive hyperemia tests have been reported to have a sensitivity and a specificity of 91% and 91%, respectively.[61] Measurement of femoral vein pressures may also be useful in defining the importance of an iliac obstruction.[62] Although resting femoral pressures show considerable overlap, the femoral pressure difference (diseased versus healthy limb) after exercise provides reasonable

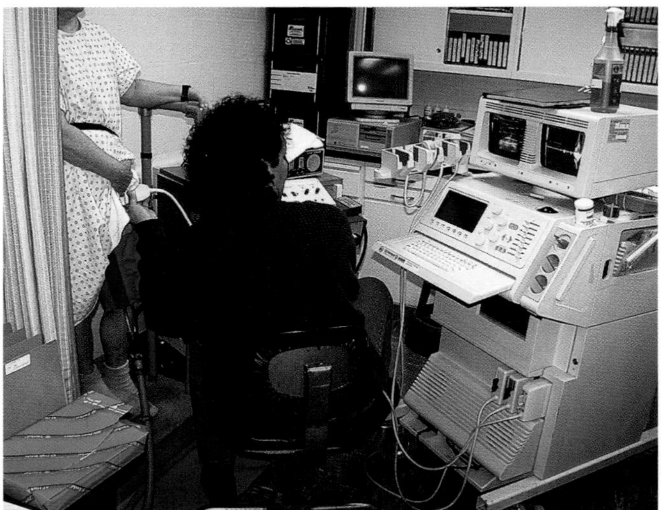

Figure 42-8. Duplex ultrasound evaluation of reflux using the standing cuff deflation technique. The patient stands, supported by a frame, with weight borne on the contralateral limb. Pneumatic cuffs are sequentially applied to the thigh, calf, and foot with inflation pressure varied according to the hydrostatic pressure at that level. Doppler signals in the vein under investigation are recorded at 5 cm proximal to the cuff as it is rapidly deflated.

separation between those with and those without significant iliac obstruction.

Despite the contribution of these tests to our understanding of venous physiology, most have limitations in identifying the patient with clinically significant venous obstruction. Plethysmographic tests are limited by an inconsistent relationship among venous volume, outflow, and disease severity, while direct pressure measurements have not uniformly correlated with clinical symptoms. Although most tests demonstrate adequate specificity, the sensitivity of all tests is limited. None of the current diagnostic tests are able to accurately identify those patients with hemodynamically significant obstruction who will clearly benefit from intervention, and objective clinical improvement often occurs after intervention, despite the lack of improvement in hemodynamic tests.[50]

Pathophysiology of Chronic Venous Disease

Varicose Veins

Despite improvements in understanding the epidemiology and hemodynamic derangements associated with varicose veins and chronic venous insufficiency, the underlying etiology remains uncertain. Treatment is accordingly based more on relief of symptoms and an attempt to correct the altered hemodynamics than on an understanding of the cause. Although the detrimental effects of prolonged standing were recognized by Hippocrates (460 to 377 BC), humoral theories relating varicose veins to the ill effects of "gross" or "melancholy" blood were not widely replaced by scientifically based pathophysiological theories until the eighteenth and nineteenth centuries.[63] Early modern theories presumed that varicose veins arose from the effects of valvular incompetence and venous hypertension. Varicose veins historically were thought to arise in a descending fashion from the saphenofemoral or saphenopopliteal junctions, the saphenofemoral being involved approximately four times more often than the saphenopopliteal junction.[54,64] Congenital absence or incompetence of iliofemoral valves was presumed to cause increased hydrostatic pressure and venous dilation at the level of the saphenofemoral junction with sequential failure of more distal valves.[37] Variants of this theory postulated that varicosities similarly arose from the transmission of venous pressure through incompetent perforating veins.

Unfortunately, little evidence shows a constitutive valvular abnormality in primary venous disease, and these theories are not supported by more recent observations. Descending theories of valvular incompetence cannot explain why truncal varicosities are often found below competent valves, why normal valves are often seen between those exhibiting varices, or why dilation often precedes valvular incompetence.[34,65] Rather than being initiated at the saphenofemoral junction,

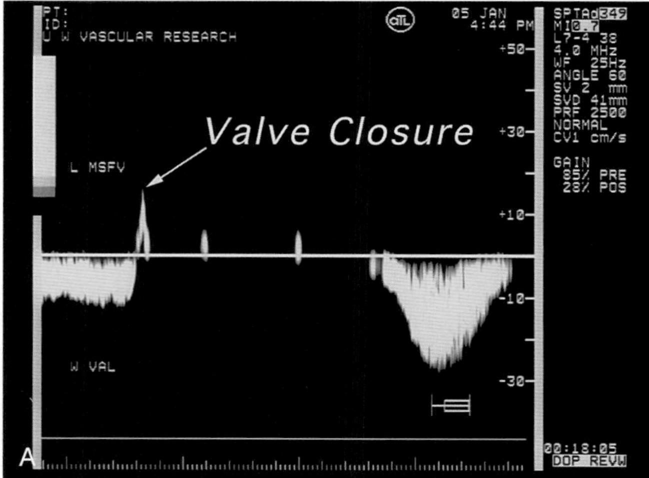

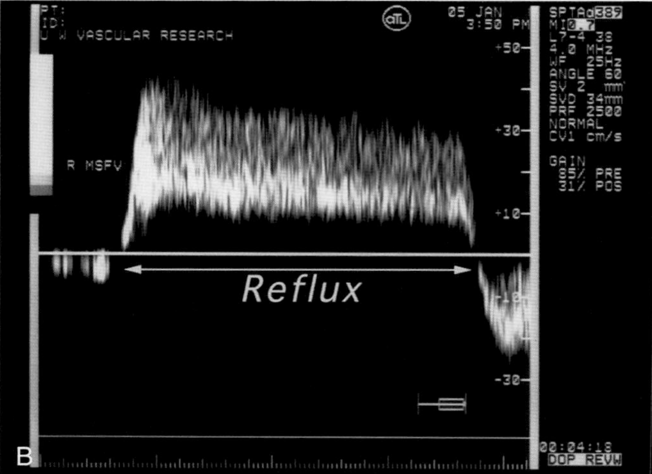

Figure 42-9. Duplex ultrasound detection of reflux in the midsuperficial femoral vein. **A,** No reflux occurs, and valve closure appears as a clearly demarcated period of retrograde flow (above the baseline) of less than 0.5 seconds. **B,** In the presence of valvular incompetence, the duration of reverse flow is greater than 0.5 seconds.

detailed studies of surgical specimens suggest that varices can occur anywhere along the course of the great saphenous vein. Ultrasound-based studies similarly suggest that primary valvular incompetence is a multicentric disease that develops simultaneously in discontinuous venous segments. The below-knee great saphenous segment is most commonly involved (68% of patients), followed by the above-knee segment (55%) and the saphenofemoral junction (32%).[66] It therefore appears that, rather than developing in a descending fashion, primary venous disease can begin as a local, segmental process anywhere in the lower extremity venous system.

It further appears that varicose changes precede the development of overt valvular incompetence[34,67,68] and that valvular dysfunction is a secondary phenomenon. Recent theories have focused on intrinsic structural and biochemical abnormalities of the vein wall. Such "weak wall" theories hypothesize that varicose veins develop because of underlying connective tissue defects and altered venous tone.[32,69-71] While the histological features may be diverse and vary in different regions of the vein, varicose veins demonstrate irregular thickening of the intima, fibrosis between the intima and the adventitia, atrophy and disruption of elastic fibers, thickening of individual collagen fibers, and disorganization of the muscular layers.[38,72-76] These abnormalities are heterogeneously distributed through the great saphenous vein and its tributaries,[73] with some areas appearing hypertrophic while others appear atrophic or normal. Although luminal diameter is increased, overall wall thickness is not changed.[77] That is, although localized areas of thinning may be present, dilation is not associated with generalized atrophy of the venous wall. The saccular dilations constituting the varices are consistently located just to the distal (upstream) side of valve cusps.[34] The configuration of the valve sinus itself is preserved in most varicose segments.

The histological changes suggest that varicose veins have reduced contractility and compliance. Saphenous smooth muscle content, as well as total protein content, is reduced in patients with varicose veins, and effective contraction may be further compromised by fragmentation of the muscle layers.[73,77] The smooth muscle cells are also transformed from a contractile to a secretory phenotype,[78] and corresponding changes occur in the extracellular matrix of both involved and uninvolved venous segments. Varicose saphenous veins show an increased collagen and reduced elastin content with an increased collagen-to-elastin ratio.[67,71] Correspondingly, decreased venous elasticity has been demonstrated both in limbs with overt varices and those without varices but at high risk for their development.[79] Similar connective tissue defects have also been identified in the forearm veins of patients with varicosities.[69] These abnormalities in vein wall architecture likely precede the development of both overt varicosities and valvular incompetence. Reflux is presumed to occur when the weakened vein wall dilates, causing stretching of the commissure between the valve cusps and separation of the valve leaflets.[65] Perhaps not surprisingly, these histological alterations have been correlated with the degree of hemodynamic disturbance present on air plethysmography.[75]

It remains unclear whether the functional, biochemical, and structural changes associated with varicose veins are primary or result from other pathological processes. Several potential mechanisms have been proposed to be responsible for these changes. Some have suggested that hypoxia-induced endothelial activation is responsible for the change in smooth muscle phenotype, leading to an increased synthesis of extracellular matrix.[78] Apoptosis, or programmed cell death, also appears to be downregulated in varicose veins, as evidenced by reduced expression of apoptosis-related proteins.[76] Increased numbers of dysfunctional cells could theoretically account for some observed histological changes. Several changes in enzyme patterns consistent with a decline in energy metabolism and increased lysosomal activity have been reported.[80] Recent theories have focused on systemic alterations in tissue remodeling, including dysregulation of type III collagen production and imbalances in proteolytic enzymes (matrix metalloproteinases, or MMPs) and their inhibitors (tissue inhibitors of metalloproteinases, or TIMPs), leading to weakness and dilation of the venous wall.[71]

Finally, defects in venous tone associated with a loss of vascular reactivity have been postulated to have a primary role in the origin of varicose veins.[73,81] Organ chamber experiments have demonstrated reduced contractility, as well as endothelium-dependent relaxation, in varicose segments. In comparison to control veins, contraction in response to endothelin-1, a potent vasoconstrictor and smooth muscle mitogen, is reduced in both diseased tributaries and grossly uninvolved saphenous veins of patients with varicosities. This decrease in contractility may be due to structural changes, resulting from a loss of contractile proteins, as well as to downregulation of the number of endothelin B receptors.[81] Varicose vein patients also demonstrate imbalances in the humoral mediators of vasoconstriction and venodilation. Plasma levels of endothelin-1 are increased in those with varicose veins and rise disproportionately in response to venous stasis.[82] At least some evidence suggests that such increases are mediated at the transcriptional level within the endothelial cell.[81] Plasma levels of nitric oxide, a potent mediator of vascular relaxation, have variably been found to be either reduced[83] or increased[84] in these patients. Finally, MMP-2 not only may lead to alterations in the extracellular matrix but also may lead to venous relaxation.[71]

Chronic Venous Insufficiency

Although there is little controversy that venous hypertension underlies the manifestations of chronic venous insufficiency, the pathophysiological relationship between venous hypertension and ulceration remains unclear. The histological findings associated with venous hypertension include atrophy and scarring of the dermis with loss of papillary structures at the dermal–epidermal junction.[85] There is associated dilation and convolution of the dermal capillaries, fibrosis of the vein wall and dermis, and a thick amorphous perivascular cuff composed of fibrin, fibronectin, laminin, tenascin, and collagen.[85-89] It was initially presumed that these perivascular cuffs arose from the effects of increased capillary filtration, changes in venous pressure increasing filtration 5 to 10 times more than equivalent changes in arterial pressure.[90] However, more recent data suggest that, although vascular extravasation may be important, the perivascular cuffs are actively assembled by the surrounding connective tissue. These cuffs appear to resolve with compression therapy, and it has been postulated that they represent a protective measure against venous hypertension.[89] These histological changes are associated with a dermal perivascular infiltrate consisting predominantly of lymphocytes, macrophages, and mast cells.[91-93] Scarring of the

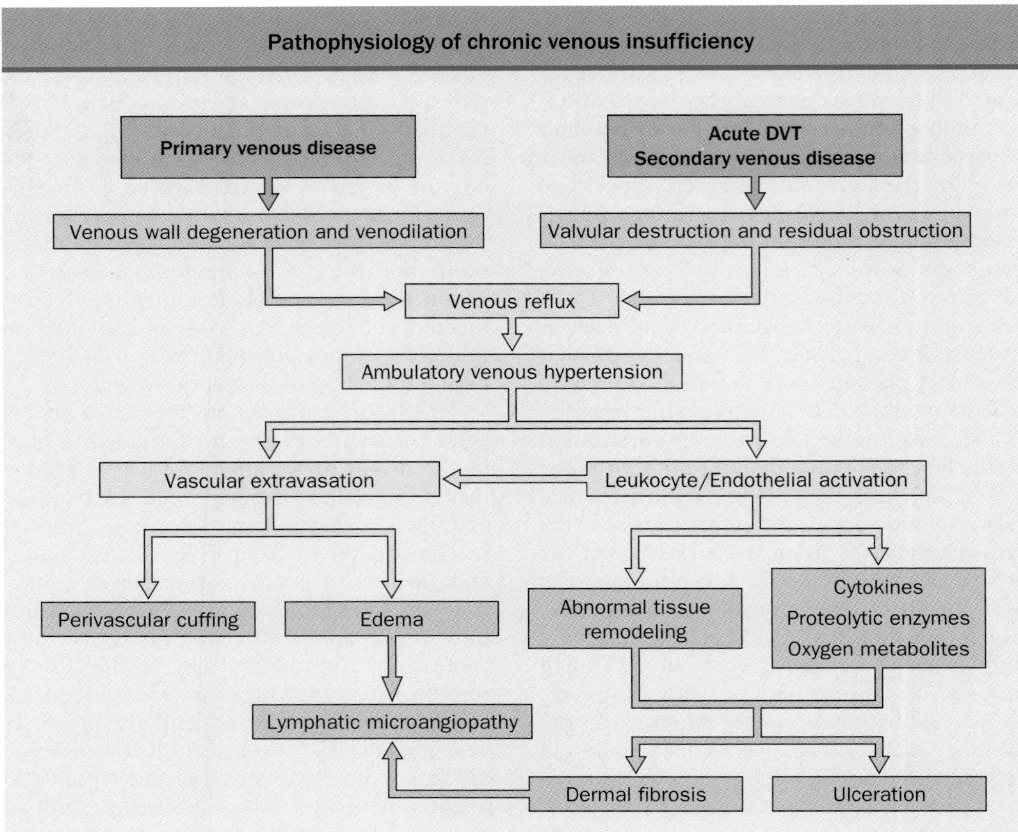

Figure 42-10. Pathophysiology of chronic venous insufficiency. Although both primary and secondary venous disease may lead to advance chronic venous insufficiency, it is now clear that ambulatory venous hypertension leading to a chronic inflammatory state underlies most of the clinical sequelae.

reticular dermis also leads to a lymphatic microangiopathy that likely impairs interstitial fluid exchange.[88]

Unfortunately, investigation of the mechanisms underlying these changes has been limited by the lack of a satisfactory animal model. Early theories suggested venous stasis with slow capillary blood flow and arteriovenous shunting as causes of local cutaneous tissue hypoxia, while later theories focused on the role of venous hypertension in increasing capillary permeability. Although indirect evidence of increased arterial inflow, reduced oxygen extraction, and elevated lower extremity venous oxygen content[79,94] have suggested the existence of arteriovenous fistulae, little evidence supports them as important pathophysiological mechanisms.[35] Browse and Burnand focused on the role of the perivascular cuff and suggested that venous hypertension leads to the transudation of extracellular fluid and the extravasation of macromolecules such as fibrinogen.[90,95] As limbs with lipodermatosclerosis have deficient fibrinolytic activity, any extravascular fibrinogen converted to fibrin is likely to accumulate. The fibrin cuff was postulated to act as a diffusion barrier leading to local tissue hypoxia and impaired cutaneous nutrition. Although extravascular fibrin may be important in the pathophysiology of chronic venous insufficiency, perhaps being chemotactic for fibroblasts and macrophages, downregulating collagen synthesis, or representing a marker for endothelial injury, most data now suggest that it does not act as a diffusion barrier.[96]

Mechanisms concentrating on skin hypoxia alone are too simplistic, and inflammatory processes are emerging as the most important factors in the pathogenesis of chronic venous insufficiency (Figure 42-10). An underlying inflammatory etiology was first suggested by the observation that the ratio of white cells to red cells decreases in the dependent lower extremities, as well as the upper extremities, of patients with chronic venous insufficiency.[87,97,98] This is associated with a dermal leukocyte infiltrate that progressively increases as venous disease becomes more advanced. Leukocytes thus appear to be sequestered in the dependent lower extremities. This phenomenon appears to occur early in the course of chronic venous disease and has been observed both in limbs with varicose veins and with lipodermatosclerosis.[99-101] However, such sequestration resolves promptly on returning to the supine position in limbs with varicose veins but not in those with lipodermatosclerosis.[100]

These observations led to the "white cell trapping" hypothesis of chronic venous insufficiency.[98] Venous hypertension is postulated to reduce flow in the postcapillary venules leading to white blood cell margination and reversible leukocyte adhesion. Trapped leukocytes subsequently become activated, increasing endothelial permeability, migrating extravascularly, and releasing toxic oxygen metabolites, proteolytic enzymes, and cytokines. The number of dermal capillary loops is reduced as they become plugged with white cells,[98] and a perivascular infiltrate of monocytes and macrophages appears in the papillary dermis of lipodermatosclerotic skin.[86,87]

The interaction of leukocytes with the endothelium under conditions of venous hypertension appears to be critical in the pathophysiology of chronic venous disease. Leukocyte adhesion, activation, and migration are mediated by endothelial adhesion receptors, which function as counterligands to those expressed on the leukocytes. It has been speculated that upregulation of endothelial adhesion molecule expression occurs in response to hydrostatic pressure–mediated changes in flow or shear.[91,102] Experimental venous hypertension is associated with endothelial activation and increased circulating levels of adhesion molecules, including endothelial leukocyte adhesion molecule-1, intercellular adhesion molecule-1, and vascular cell adhesion molecule-1.[87,99] Clinically, increased basal levels of adhesion molecules likely reflect chronic endothelial activation.[99] Vascular cell adhesion molecule-1, which mediates the adhesion of monocytes and lymphocytes, shows a greater rise in response to standing among patients with lipodermatosclerosis than in those with varicose veins.[99] Endothelial expression of vascular cell adhesion molecule-1 and intercellular adhesion molecule-1, which mediates leukocyte migration, is also increased in the dermal capillary loops of patients with venous ulcers.[91,103]

Leukocyte activation occurs concurrently with endothelial activation.[99,101,103] Leukocytes normally express adhesion molecules, such as L-selectin, which allow reversible binding to and rolling along the endothelium. Under pathological conditions, L-selectin is shed as a second-stage ligand, CD11b, is expressed, leading to degranulation or extravascular migration. Under conditions of venous hypertension, plasma L-selectin levels increase and circulating CD11b expression decreases as leukocytes are activated and bound to the endothelium.[101] Although primarily a chronic inflammatory process, increases in elastase levels in patients with chronic venous disease also suggest some component of neutrophil activation.[104] Neutrophil adhesion has been demonstrated in saphenous vein segments perfused under hypoxic conditions postulated to resemble those occurring in venous hypertension.[78,105]

The altered connective tissue remodeling observed in chronic venous insufficiency, which includes an imbalance between tissue degradation and repair with increased turnover of the extracellular matrix, may be mediated by chronic inflammation.[85,86] Dermal fibrosis is a fundamental feature of lipodermatosclerosis and is associated with increased content of the cytokine transforming growth factor-β1.[86] This growth factor, likely derived from activated leukocytes, recruits macrophages and fibroblasts into the tissue and leads to the production of extracellular matrix proteins by dermal fibroblasts. transforming growth factor-β1 also regulates the activity of the MMPs,[85,106] a group of proteases that, together with their inhibitors (TIMPs), regulate connective tissue remodeling and degradation of the extracellular matrix. Altered MMP activity, particularly decreased MMP-2 and increased TIMP-1, has been associated with the histological changes observed in varicose veins[107] and has been implicated in the pathogenesis of lipodermatosclerosis and ulceration. Some investigators have identified increased MMP-1, MMP-2, and TIMP-1 messenger RNA and protein expression with corresponding increases in proteolytic activity for type I and type IV collagen in lipodermatosclerotic skin.[85] It has also been postulated that an imbalance between MMP-2 and TIMP-2 may be responsible for fragmentation of dermal elastic fibers and degradation of the epidermal basement membrane and matrix.[85,106]

The precise nature of the injury that initiates chronic inflammation remains unclear. Some have postulated that inflammation derives from the potent chemoattractive properties of extravasated red cells and macromolecules.[108] Others have suggested some role for hypertension induced endothelial injury. Levels of von Willebrand factor, a marker of endothelial injury, are increased in patients with lipodermatosclerosis but not in those with uncomplicated varicose veins.[99]

EPIDEMIOLOGY OF CHRONIC VENOUS DISEASE

Varicose veins are the most common clinical manifestation of chronic venous disease, occurring in one quarter to one third of Western adult populations.[109,110] However, differing terminology, diagnostic criteria, and methodology make it difficult to compare epidemiological data from different studies, and it is generally conceded that the prevalence of varicose veins is underestimated. Up to one third of patients never seek medical attention for their varicose veins or chronic venous insufficiency.[4] Data from interviews and questionnaires may therefore be inaccurate, having a sensitivity of only 47% in men and 67% in women in comparison to physical examination.[11] However, even physical examination has limitations in the absence of clear definitions. Interobserver error in defining the presence of trunk varicosities has been as high as 85% in some studies.[111] Finally, some studies have included only clinically significant varicosities while others have differentiated lesser degrees of disease, such as prominent superficial and reticular veins. Despite these limitations, prevalence figures in Western populations have varied from 10% to 15%, when only pronounced or medically significant varices are considered, to 30% to 50%, when all types of disease are included.[15,111]

Most studies have documented a steep increase in the prevalence of varicose veins with age.[10,11,112] The prevalence increases from 1% and 8% in men and women 20 to 29 years of age to 43% and 72% among those in the seventh decade.[113] Others have estimated similar prevalences of less than 10% among those less than 20 years of age; 25% in men and 40% in women at age 40; and 60% in men and more than 70% in women at age 80.[15] Although few studies have reported incidence estimates, those that have suggest that the incidence of varicose veins may not increase with age. Data from the Framingham study suggest a 2-year incidence of varicose veins averaging 39.4 new cases per 1000 men and 51.9 cases per 1000 women.[114] The increase in prevalence with age may therefore reflect simply an accumulation of cases rather than an increased propensity to develop varicose veins with aging.

Data regarding gender distribution are subject to considerable methodological and age bias. Women are more likely to seek medical attention for varicose veins and are about three times as likely to undergo treatment.[111] Most population-based studies have accordingly reported varicose veins to be two to three times more common in women. Prevalence rates have been reported to be 25% to 46% in women as compared to 7% to 19% among men.[11,112,115] A trend toward a greater prevalence of objectively documented superficial reflux has

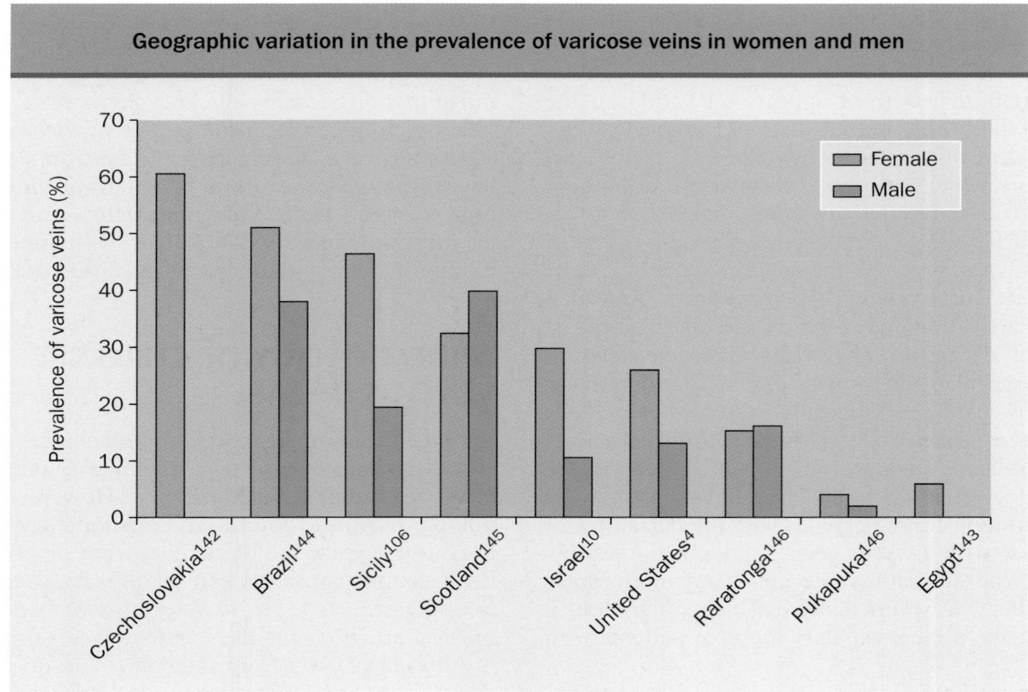

Figure 42-11. Geographical variation in the prevalence of varicose veins in women *(red bars)* and men *(blue bars)*. References are shown in superscript. (Czechoslovakia—Stvrtinova et al.[151]; Egypt—Mekky et al.[152]; Brazil—Maffei et al.[153]; United States—Coon et al.[5]; Israel—Abramson et al.[11]; Sicily—Novo et al.[112]; Scotland—Evans et al.[154]; Rarotonga, Pukapuka—Beaglehole[155].)

been noted in women, although deep venous reflux is more common in men.[116] At least some of these gender differences may arise from a failure to adjust for age.[2,117] Some recent studies have found no gender difference in age-adjusted prevalence. The Edinburgh Vein Study found an overall prevalence of 40% in men and 32% in women.[116] Others have suggested that although reticular veins may be more common in women, the gender distribution of more severe varicose veins is approximately equal.[15]

There do appear to be significant geographical and ethnic differences in both the incidence and the prevalence of varicose veins. Cesarone et al.[4] reported a higher yearly incidence (22 cases per 100 people) in central Italy than observed in the Framingham study in the United States. With respect to prevalence, rates are highest in developed countries and industrial populations,[4,11] while they are generally low in the developing world[118] (Figure 42-11). Even in the same geographical region, prevalence rates are often significantly higher in industrialized areas.[119] Prevalence rates among females have varied from 0.1% in New Guinea to 60.5% in Czechoslovakia.[117,119] Population based studies of Western women have demonstrated more consistent prevalence rates of 25% to 32%.[117] In contrast, rates among women in North and sub-Saharan Africa are one fourth to one fifth of those among European women.[15] However, at least some data suggest that ethnic and regional differences are not preserved among those emigrating at a young age.[15] The etiology of these geographical differences remains unclear. In comparison to Africans, Caucasians do have a relative deficiency of valves. Eighty-one percent of Caucasians have at least one valve in the external iliac–common femoral segment above the saphenofemoral junction in comparison to 100% of Africans.[64] Although an interesting observation, this does not explain the similar prevalence in white and black Americans.[118] It has been suggested that cultural factors, such as diet and exercise, may be more important than genetic or geographical factors.[118]

The epidemiology of the more severe manifestations of venous insufficiency is even less well defined. As many studies rely on self-reporting or are based on patients receiving treatment, incidence and prevalence figures are probably underestimated. In the case of ulceration, it may also be difficult to separate chronic venous ulcers, accounting for approximately 75% of ulcers, from those due to other causes.[117] The best available data suggest that severe chronic venous insufficiency, with skin changes and ulceration, is present in 2% to 5% of Western populations.[15] The prevalence of skin changes has been reported to be 1.2% in Scotland and 3.0% (men) to 3.7% (women) in the United States.[5] The prevalence of active chronic venous ulcers is estimated to be about 0.3% of the adult population in Western countries, corresponding to approximately 500,000 patients in the United States. However, open ulcers constitute only 20% to 25% of the total, and the population prevalence of open and healed ulcers may be closer to 1%.[117,120]

Among patients with advanced chronic venous insufficiency, females generally predominate at all ages, with a female-to-male ratio of 2:1 to 3:1.[3,117,120] Skin changes and ulceration are related to the duration of venous hypertension, and the prevalence of both slowly increases after 30 years of age.[15] The prevalence of skin changes increases from 1.8% in women 30 to 39 years old to 20.7% for women older than 70 years.[5] Initial ulceration occurs after age 50 in 60% of patients.[18] Accordingly, the incidence of venous ulcer is highest in older patients and is estimated to be about 3.5 per 1000 in those over 45 years of age.[121]

RISK FACTORS FOR CHRONIC VENOUS DISEASE

Population-based studies have evaluated the risk factors associated with the development of reflux and varicose veins, often without any clear conclusions[5,11,112,114,115,122] (Table 42-4). The available data suggest that the etiology of varicose veins is multifactorial, involving various initiating, promoting, and contributing factors.[119] Age, genetic factors such as gender and family history, and environmental factors including pregnancy, obesity, and standing occupations have variously been implicated as risk factors for varicose veins. However, the data are often inconsistent and confounded by various selection biases. Age has been among the most consistent and important risk factors in most epidemiological studies.

Nulliparous women appear less likely to develop varicose veins, although no clear relationship exists with the number of pregnancies.[10,11,112] Varicose veins and telangiectasias may occur early in the first trimester of pregnancy, suggesting that hormonal factors rather than simply hydrostatic effects of uterine enlargement may have a role.[113] The effects of estrogen on smooth muscle relaxation and softening of collagen fibers are well recognized, and pregnant patients, as well as those on oral contraceptives, have increased venous distensibility and decreased tone.[123] Estradiol concentrations in postmenopausal women have been related to both increased venous distensibility and presence of truncal varicose veins.[124] However, no studies have yet suggested a relationship between oral contraceptives and varicose veins.

Some have found a higher prevalence of standing vocations among those with telangiectasias or varicose veins.[11,15,113] However, the data are not uniform and it is likely that standing occupations are an aggravating rather than causative factor.[117] Obesity has similarly been a variable risk factor for varicose veins, more often in women than in men.[117,119] In the absence of a consistent relationship with obesity, it has been suggested that there may be a threshold effect above which the risk of varicose veins is increased.[15] A body mass index of greater than 30 kg/m^2 has been associated with a fivefold increased prevalence of varicose veins in postmenopausal women.[123]

Obesity was confirmed to be a risk factor in the Framingham study, although women with varicose veins also had higher systolic blood pressures, were less physically active, and reached menopause at an older age.[114] Men smoked more cigarettes and were less physically active. In addition to previous pregnancy and obesity, the Edinburgh Vein Study found that less oral contraceptive use and mobility at work in women and height and straining at stool in men may be implicated in the development of reflux.[109] Associations with increased intraabdominal pressure have been suggested by others, and varicose veins have inconsistently been associated with constipation, tight undergarments, and inguinal hernias.[11,112] Other population-based studies have found no significant association with social class, smoking, systolic blood pressure, congestive heart failure, diabetes, serum lipids, physical exertion, or hemorrhoids.[11,119]

A hereditary component has also been implicated in the development of varicose veins. As many as 84% of women with telangiectasias or varicose veins have a positive family history.[113] Although varicose veins do appear to be more common among relatives of affected patients, the genetics of this relationship remains unclear.[10] Most data support a polygenic mode of inheritance modified by various external factors.[125,126] Among the putative genes responsible for varicose veins, some data support a role for mutations in the FOXC2 and Notch3 genes.[126,127] Twin studies have demonstrated concordance for varicose veins in 60% to 67% of identical twins in comparison to only 25% to 45% of nonidentical twins.[80,126] The risk of developing varicose veins has been reported to be 90% if both parents suffered from this disease; 25% for males and 62% for females with one afflicted parent; and 20% when neither parent was affected.[128] Risk is further increased if an affected relative is male and if the onset of disease is at an early age.[125] However, others have not found a statistically significant association between family history and development of varicose veins.[114,116,122]

Table 42-4
Risk Factors for Varicose Veins

Consistent Evidence	Inconsistent but Strong Evidence	Weak or Absent Evidence
Age	Female gender	Smoking
Pregnancy	Obesity	Systolic blood pressure
	Family history	Increased intraabdominal pressure
	Industrialized populations	Physical exertion
	Standing vocation	Diabetes
		Serum lipids
		Social class

NATURAL HISTORY OF CHRONIC VENOUS DISEASE

Primary Chronic Venous Disease

Varicose veins and chronic venous insufficiency are slowly progressive, chronic conditions. Although varicose veins without significant valvular incompetence rarely progress to severe chronic venous insufficiency,[4] approximately 10% of varicose veins patients presenting to specialized clinics have ulcers.[21] Unfortunately, as most patients with symptomatic primary disease are treated early after presentation, the rate of progression from uncomplicated varicose veins to skin changes and ulceration remains poorly defined. In one small study of 36 patients in whom varicose vein surgery was deferred for a median of 20 months, no patient developed a new ulcer; new lipodermatosclerosis developed in 1 of 50 limbs at risk; 5 of 16 initially normal contralateral limbs developed new varicosities; and new segmental reflux was seen in 18% of initially effected and 25% of initially normal limbs.[129] However, as the authors noted, this was a select group that was felt likely to remain stable while awaiting operation. Larger studies have suggested skin changes and ulceration may develop in up to 22% and in 4% of patients an average of 4 years after initial presentation.[130]

Few longitudinal studies have evaluated the factors responsible for disease progression. Age is a major determinant of the severity of chronic venous insufficiency, and many factors such as gender and parity lose their significance when adjusted for age. In a case-control study, significant risk factors for venous ulceration, after adjustment for a history of varicose veins and edema, included a history of maternal venous insufficiency, strenuous exercise, and a history of DVT.[131] Other prognostic factors that have been associated with more severe venous insufficiency include obesity, previous lower extremity trauma, exposure to environmental heat, and occupations including being a pensioner or housewife.[132,133] Genetic factors may also play a role in progression to advanced chronic venous disease, and a relationship between the C282Y polymorphism in the hemochromatosis (HFE) gene and the venous ulceration has been described.[126,127]

Despite vagaries in clinical prognostic indicators, the severity of chronic venous disease is clearly related to the magnitude and distribution of reflux, as well as the length of time it has been present. Among those progressing to ulceration, varicose veins have been noted to be present for a mean of 24 years before patients seek treatment.[21] Anatomically, the quantitative extent of reflux determined by duplex better reflects the severity of disease than does standard phlebographic scoring.[134] As discussed earlier, most patients with advanced chronic venous insufficiency have multisystem disease with reflux in the superficial, deep, and perforating veins. From a hemodynamic perspective, the progression of chronic venous disease from mild symptoms to skin changes and ulceration is associated with venous volume expansion, increased reflux, and progressive ambulatory venous hypertension.[23] However, further hemodynamic deterioration was not noted in progression from skin changes to ulceration, perhaps reflecting the importance of microcirculatory changes rather than gross hemodynamic changes in end-stage disease.

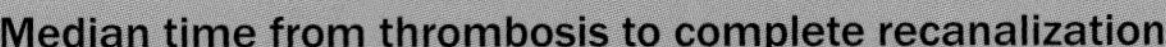

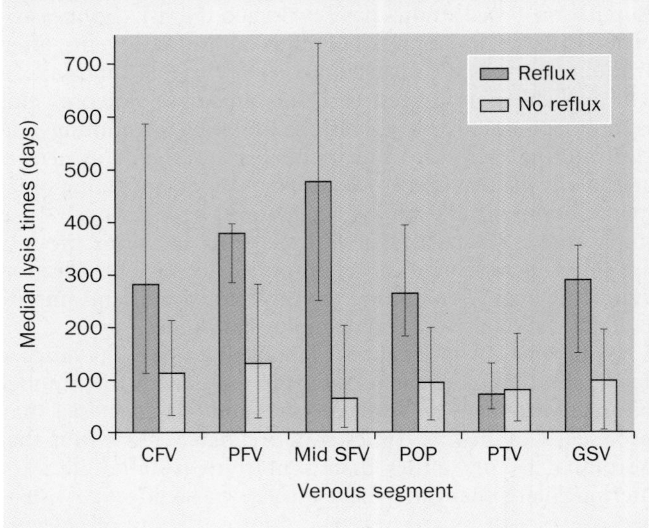

Figure 42-12. Median time (± interquartile range) from thrombosis to complete recanalization, stratified according to ultimate reflux status. Median times are 2.3 to 7.3 times longer among segments developing reflux in all but the posterior tibial veins. Segments: CFV, common femoral vein; GSV, greater saphenous vein; PFV, profunda femoris vein; PPV, popliteal vein; PTV, posterior tibial vein; SFM, midsuperficial femoral vein. (Adapted from Meissner MH, Manzo RA, Bergelin, RO, et al. *J Vasc Surg* 1993;18[4]:596-608.)

Secondary Chronic Venous Disease

The postthrombotic syndrome is a common complication of acute DVT that has often been underemphasized in the medical literature. Among 224 patients followed for 5 years after venographically confirmed DVT, the postthrombotic syndrome developed in 29.6% of those with proximal thrombosis and 30% of those with isolated calf vein thrombosis.[135] Others have reported some postthrombotic symptoms in 29% to 79%, severe manifestations in 7% to 23%, and ulceration in 4% to 6% of patients.[135-139] As acute DVT often has a well-defined, symptomatic starting point, it perhaps affords a better opportunity than primary disease to study the natural history of chronic venous disease. Advances in noninvasive testing have been particularly important in relating changes occurring in the venous system to the development of clinical symptoms.

Rather than remaining static, it is now clear that venous thrombi undergo a dynamic evolution beginning soon after their formation. The processes of thrombus organization and recanalization are beyond the scope of this chapter, but they appear to be largely mediated by inflammatory cells.[140] Approximately 55% of subjects show complete recanalization within 6 to 9 months of thrombosis, with the greatest change in thrombus load over the first 3 to 6 months.[141-143] Reflux results from valvular damage or destruction occurring during the process of recanalization. However, reflux is not a universal consequence of recanalization, and only 33% to 59% of thrombosed venous segments ultimately become incompetent.[144] Factors contributing to the development of valvular incompetence after an episode of acute DVT may include rate of recanalization, degree of recanalization, and recurrent thrombotic events.

Patients with early recanalization have a lower incidence of valvular incompetence. Among 113 patients followed with serial ultrasonography, median times to complete recanalization in segments developing reflux were 2.3 to 7.3 times longer than for corresponding segments not developing reflux[145] (Figure 42-12). Failure of recanalization, or persistent venous obstruction, may also contribute to development of the postthrombotic syndrome. While the detrimental effects of venous obstruction may relate to its direct effect on ambulatory venous pressure, it may also be responsible for the development of reflux in distal segments that were not initially thrombosed. As many as 30% of segments developing reflux after an episode of DVT have not been previously thrombosed, an observation that may be related to the presence of proximal obstruction.[146] Finally, recurrent thrombotic events are highly associated with the development of both reflux and clinical symptoms. Ultrasound documented rethrombosis may occur in up to 31% of limbs,[147] and the incidence of reflux in such segments (36% to 73%) is significantly higher than in those that remain patent (5.7% to 18.2%). Not surprising, the risk of the postthrombotic syndrome is six times greater among patients with recurrent thrombosis.[135] Recurrent thrombotic events have been documented in 45% of patients with postthrombotic symptoms in comparison to only 17% of asymptomatic subjects.[148]

As in the case of primary venous disease, the development of clinical signs and symptoms of the postthrombotic syndrome is related to the global extent of reflux and anatomical distribution of reflux and obstruction.[149] Postthrombotic skin changes are most significantly related to reflux in the popliteal and posterior tibial veins. However, superficial reflux is also commonly associated with the postthrombotic syndrome, being present in 84% to 94% of patients with skin changes and 60% to 100% of patients with ulceration. Although concurrent superficial thrombosis is more common than appreciated, a substantial proportion of superficial reflux is not directly associated with thrombosis, develops at a rate equivalent to that in uninvolved limbs, and likely involves thrombus independent degenerative processes.[150] Finally, unlike most patients with primary venous disease, patients with postthrombotic disease commonly have a component of deep venous obstruction and obstruction of the popliteal vein appears to be clinically most important.[149]

SUMMARY

Chronic venous disease is among the most common disorders encountered by the vascular surgeon. The manifestations of chronic venous disease vary from varicose veins to venous ulceration; may be primary in origin or secondary to other diseases such as DVT; and although primarily due to venous reflux, may have a component of venous obstruction. Among Western populations, varicose veins, skin changes, and ulceration are present in up to 33%, 1% to 3%, and 0.3% of adults, respectively. Although there does appear to be some hereditary predisposition to varicose veins, any inheritance is likely polygenic, with penetrance greatly influenced by environmental factors such as age, place of birth, pregnancy, obesity, and vocation. The factors influencing the progression of chronic venous disease are poorly characterized but clearly include the magnitude, duration, and anatomical distribution of reflux.

Although incompletely understood, it is clear that, rather than developing in a descending fashion, varicose veins are related to intrinsic changes in the venous wall, develop multicentrically, and likely precede the development of reflux as a secondary phenomenon. Despite the variable manifestations, ambulatory venous hypertension underlies all clinical sequelae of chronic venous insufficiency. Furthermore, recent advances in vascular biology have identified the importance of leukocyte–endothelial interactions and chronic inflammation in the etiology of skin changes and ulceration. Although most manifestations of chronic venous disease are due to ambulatory venous hypertension, our ability to correct these hemodynamic derangements remains imperfect. While a surgical approach has proven efficacious in the treatment of varicose veins, modifications of the underlying microcirculatory disturbances and chronic inflammation hold promise as adjuncts in the management of more advanced disease.

References

1. Eklof B, Rutherford RB, Bergan JJ, et al. Revision of the CEAP classification for chronic venous disorders: consensus statement. *J Vasc Surg* 2004;40:1248-1252.
2. Ruckley CV, Evans CJ, Allan PL, et al. Chronic venous insufficiency: clinical and duplex correlations: the Edinburgh Vein Study of venous disorders in the general population. *J Vasc Surg* 2002;36:520-525.
3. Kurz X, Kahn SR, Abenhaim L, et al. Chronic venous disorders of the leg: epidemiology, outcomes, diagnosis and management: summary of an evidence-based report of the VEINES Task Force, Venous Insufficiency Epidemiologic and Economic Studies. *Int Angiol* 1999;18:83-102.
4. Cesarone MR, Belcaro G, Nicolaides AN, et al. "Real" epidemiology of varicose veins and chronic venous diseases: the San Valentino Vascular Screening Project. *Angiology* 2002;53:119-130.
5. Coon WW, Willis PW, Keller JB. Venous thromboembolism and other venous disease in the Tecumseh Community Health Study. *Circulation* 1973;48:839-846.
6. Abenhaim L, Kurz X. The VEINES study (Venous Insufficiency Epidemiologic and Economic Study): an international cohort study on chronic venous disorders of the leg—VEINES Group. *Angiology* 1997;48: 59-66.
7. Phillips T, Stanton B, Provan A, et al. A study of the impact of leg ulcers on quality of life: financial, social, and psychologic implications. *J Am Acad Dermatol* 1994;31:49-53.
8. Porter J, Moneta G. Reporting standards in venous disease: an update. *J Vasc Surg* 1995;21:635-645.
9. Bradbury A, Ruckley CV. Clinical assessment of patients with venous disease. In: Gloviczki P, Yao JST, eds. *Handbook of venous disorders*. 2nd ed. London: Arnold; 2001:71-83.
10. Weddell JM. Varicose veins pilot survey, 1966. *Br J Prev Soc Med* 1969(23):179-186.
11. Abramson JH, Hopp C, Epstein LM. The epidemiology of varicose veins: a survey in western Jerusalem. *J Epidemiol Community Health* 1981;35:213-217.
12. O'Leary DP, Chester JF, Jones SM. Management of varicose veins according to reason for presentation. *Ann R Coll Surg Engl* 1996;78: 214-216.
13. Bradbury A, Evans C, Allan P, et al. What are the symptoms of varicose veins? Edinburgh vein study cross sectional population survey. *BMJ* 1999;318:353-356.
14. Biland L, Widmer LK. Varicose veins (VV) and chronic venous insufficiency (CVI): medical and socioeconomic aspects, Basle study. *Acta Chir Scand Suppl* 1988;544:9-11.
15. Krijnen RMA, de Boer EM, Bruynzeel DP. Epidemiology of venous disorders in the general and occupational populations. *Epidemiol Rev* 1997;19:294-309.
16. Chiesa R, Marone EM, Limoni C, et al. Effect of chronic venous insufficiency on activities of daily living and quality of life: correlation of demographic factors with duplex ultrasonography findings. *Angiology* 2007;58:440-449.
17. Ackerman Z, Seidenbaum M, Loewenthal E, et al. Overload of iron in the skin of patients with varicose ulcers: possible contributing role of iron accumulation in progression of the disease. *Arch Dermatol* 1988;124:1376-1378.
18. Callam MJ, Harper DR, Dale JJ, et al. Chronic ulcer of the leg: clinical history. *Br Med J* 1987;294:1389-1391.
19. Callam MJ, Ruckley CV. Chronic venous insufficiency and leg ulcer. In: Bell PRF, Jamieson CW, Ruckley CV, eds. *Surgical management of vascular disease*. London: WB Saunders; 1992:1267-1303.
20. Bass A, Chayen D, Weinmann EE, et al. Lateral venous ulcer and short saphenous vein insufficiency. *J Vasc Surg* 1997;25:654-657.
21. Hoare MC, Nicolaides AN, Miles CR, et al. The role of primary varicose veins in venous ulceration. *Surgery* 1982;92:450-453.
22. Labropoulos N, Leon M, Geroulakos G, et al. Venous hemodynamic abnormalities in patients with leg ulceration. *Am J Surg* 1995;169: 572-574.
23. Welkie J, Comerota A, Katz M, et al. Hemodynamic deterioration in chronic venous disease. *J Vasc Surg* 1992;16:733-740.
24. Darke SG, Penfold C. Venous ulceration and saphenous ligation. *Eur J Vasc Surg* 1992;6:4-9.
25. Hanrahan LM, Araki CT, Rodriguez AA, et al. Distribution of valvular incompetence in patients with venous stasis ulceration. *J Vasc Surg* 1991;13:805-811.
26. Killewich LA, Martin R, Cramer M, et al. Pathophysiology of venous claudication. *J Vasc Surg* 1984;1:507-511.
27. Qvarfordt P, Eklog B, Plate G, et al. Intramuscular pressure, blood flow, and skeletal muscle metabolism in patients with venous claudication. *Surgery* 1984;95:191-195.
28. Raju S, Neglen P. High prevalence of nonthrombotic iliac vein lesions in chronic venous disease: a permissive role in pathogenicity. *J Vasc Surg* 2006;44:136-143.
29. Hurst DR, Forauer AR, Bloom JR, et al. Diagnosis and endovascular treatment of iliocaval compression syndrome. *J Vasc Surg* 2001;34: 106-113.
30. Mewissen MW, Seabrook GR, Meissner MH, et al. Catheter-directed thrombolysis of lower extremity deep venous thrombosis: report of a national multicenter registry. *Radiology* 1999;211:39-49.
31. Caggiati A, Bergan JJ, Gloviczki P, et al. Nomenclature of the veins of the lower limbs: an international interdisciplinary consensus statement. *J Vasc Surg* 2002;36:416-422.

32. Leu HJ, Vogt M, Pfrunder H. Morphological alterations of non-varicose and varicose veins: a morphological contribution to the discussion on pathogenesis of varicose veins. *Basic Res Cardiol* 1979;74:435-444.
33. Mozes G, Carmichael SW, Gloviczki P. Development and anatomy of the venous system. In: Gloviczki P, Yao JST, eds. *Handbook of venous disorders.* 2nd ed. London: Arnold; 2001:11-24.
34. Cotton LT. Varicose veins: gross anatomy and development. *Br J Surg* 1961;48:589-597.
35. Burnand KG. The physiology and hemodynamics of chronic venous insufficiency of the lower limb. In: Gloviczki P, Yao JST, eds. *Handbook of venous disorders: guidelines of the American Venous Forum.* 2nd ed. London: Arnold; 2001:49-57.
36. O'Donnell TF Jr. The present status of surgery of the superficial venous system in the management of venous ulcer and the evidence for the role of perforator interruption. *J Vasc Surg* 2008;48:1044-1052.
37. Negus D. The surgical anatomy of the veins of the lower limb. In: Dodd H, Cockett FB, eds. *The pathology and surgery of the veins of the lower limb.* 2nd ed. Edinburgh: Churchill Livingstone; 1976:18-49.
38. Goldman MP, Fronek A. Anatomy and pathophysiology of varicose veins. *J Dermatol Surg Oncol* 1989;15:138-145.
39. Ludbrook J. The musculovenous pumps of the human lower limb. *Am Heart J* 1966;71:635-641.
40. Back TL, Padberg FT Jr., Araki CT, et al. Limited range of motion is a significant factor in venous ulceration. *J Vasc Surg* 1995;22:519-523.
41. Nicolaides AN, Hussein MK, Szendro G, et al. The relationship of venous ulceration with ambulatory venous pressure measurements. *J Vasc Surg* 1993;17:414-419.
42. Nicolaides AN. Investigation of chronic venous insufficiency: a consensus statement. *Circulation* 2000;102:E126-E163.
43. Hosoi Y, Zukowski A, Kakkos SK, et al. Ambulatory venous pressure measurements: new parameters derived from a mathematic hemodynamic model. *J Vasc Surg* 2002;36:137-142.
44. Labropoulos N, Giannoukas AD, Nicolaides AN, et al. The role of venous reflux and calf muscle pump function in nonthrombotic chronic venous insufficiency: correlation with severity of signs and symptoms. *Arch Surg* 1996;131:403-406.
45. Cordts PR, Hartono C, LaMorte WW, et al. Physiologic similarities between extremities with varicose veins and with chronic venous insufficiency utilizing air plethysmography. *Am J Surg* 1992;164:260-264.
46. van Bemmelen PS, Mattos MA, Hodgson KJ, et al. Does air plethysmography correlate with duplex scanning in patients with chronic venous insufficiency? *J Vasc Surg* 1993;18:796-807.
47. Araki CT, Back TL, Padberg FT, et al. The significance of calf muscle pump function in venous ulceration. *J Vasc Surg* 1994;20:872-877.
48. Shami SK, Sarin S, Cheatle TR, et al. Venous ulcers and the superficial venous system. *J Vasc Surg* 1993;17:487-490.
49. Sakurai T, Gupta PC, Matsushita M, et al. Correlation of the anatomical distribution of venous reflux with clinical symptoms and venous haemodynamics in primary varicose veins. *Br J Surg* 1998;85:213-216.
50. Neglen P, Hollis KC, Olivier J, et al. Stenting of the venous outflow in chronic venous disease: long-term stent-related outcome, clinical, and hemodynamic result. *J Vasc Surg* 2007;46:979-990.
51. Johnson BF, Manzo RA, Bergelin RO, et al. Relationship between changes in the deep venous system and the development of the postthrombotic syndrome after an acute episode of lower limb deep vein thrombosis: a one- to six-year follow-up. *J Vasc Surg* 1995;21:307-313.
52. Killewich LA, Martin R, Cramer M, et al. An objective assessment of the physiological changes in the postthrombotic syndrome. *Arch Surg* 1985;120:424-426.
53. Kim J, Richards S, Kent PJ. Clinical examination of varicose veins: a validation study. *Ann R Coll Surg Engl* 2000;82:171-175.
54. Hoare MC, Royle JP. Doppler ultrasound detection of saphenofemoral and saphenopopliteal incompetence and operative venography to ensure precise saphenopopliteal ligation. *Aust NZ J Surg* 1984;54:49-52.
55. Singh S, Lees TA, Donlon M, et al. Improving the preoperative assessment of varicose veins. *Br J Surg* 1997;84:801-802.
56. Christopoulos D, Nicolaides AN, Szendro G. Venous reflux: quantification and correlation with the clinical severity of chronic venous disease. *Br J Surg* 1988;75:352-356.
57. van Bemmelen PS, Beach K, Bedford G, et al. The mechanism of venous valve closure. *Arch Surg* 1990;125:617-619.
58. van Bemmelen PS, Bedford G, Beach K, et al. Quantitative segmental evaluation of venous valvular reflux with duplex ultrasound scanning. *J Vasc Surg* 1989;10:425-431.
59. Neglen P, Raju S. Detection of outflow obstruction in chronic venous insufficiency. *J Vasc Surg* 1993;17:583-589.
60. Labropoulos N, Volteas N, Leon M, et al. The role of venous outflow obstruction in patients with chronic venous dysfunction. *Arch Surg* 1997;132:46-51.
61. Raju S, Fredericks R. Venous obstruction: an analysis of one hundred thirty-seven cases with hemodynamic, venographic, and clinical correlations. *J Vasc Surg* 1991;14:305-313.
62. Albrechtsson U, Einarsson E, Eklof B. Femoral vein pressure measurements for evaluation of venous function in patients with postthrombotic iliac veins. *Cardiovasc Intervent Radiol* 1981;4:43-50.
63. Anning ST. The historical aspects. In: Dodd H, Cockett FB, eds. *The pathology and surgery of the veins of the lower limb.* 2nd ed. Edinburgh: Churchill Livingstone; 1976:3-17.
64. Banjo AO. Comparative study of the distribution of venous valves in the lower extremities of black Africans and Caucasians: pathogenetic correlates of prevalence of primary varicose veins in the two races. *Anat Rec* 1987;214:407-412.
65. Alexander CJ. The theoretical basis of varicose vein formation. *Med J Aust* 1972;1:258-261.
66. Labropoulos N, Giannoukas AD, Delis K, et al. Where does venous reflux start? *J Vasc Surg* 1997;26:736-742.
67. Gandhi RH, Irizarry E, Nackman GB, et al. Analysis of the connective tissue matrix and proteolytic activity of primary varicose veins. *J Vasc Surg* 1993;18:814-820.
68. Rose SS, Ahmed A. Some thoughts on the aetiology of varicose veins. *J Cardiovasc Surg* 1986;27:534-543.
69. Vanhoutte PM, Corcaud S, de Montrion C. Venous disease: from pathophysiology to quality of life. *Angiology* 1997;48:559-567.
70. Clarke GH, Vasdekis SN, Hobbs JT, et al. Venous wall function in the pathogenesis of varicose veins. *Surgery* 1992;111:402-408.
71. Raffetto JD, Khalil RA. Mechanisms of varicose vein formation: valve dysfunction and wall dilation. *Phlebology* 2008;23:85-98.
72. Bouissou H, Julian M, Pieraggi MT, et al. Vein morphology. *Phlebology* 1988;3(Suppl 1):1-11.
73. Lowell RC, Gloviczki P, Miller VM. In vitro evaluation of endothelial and smooth muscle function of primary varicose veins. *J Vasc Surg* 1992;16:679-686.
74. Porto LC, Azizi MA, Pelajo-Machado M, et al. Elastic fibers in saphenous varicose veins. *Angiology* 2002;53:131-140.
75. Jones GT, Solomon C, Moaveni A, et al. Venous morphology predicts class of chronic venous insufficiency. *Eur J Vasc Endovasc Surg* 1999;18:349-354.
76. Ascher E, Jacob T, Hingorani A, et al. Expression of molecular mediators of apoptosis and their role in the pathogenesis of lower-extremity varicose veins. *J Vasc Surg* 2001;33:1080-1086.
77. Travers JP, Brookes CE, Evans J, et al. Assessment of wall structure and composition of varicose veins with reference to collagen, elastin and smooth muscle content. *Eur J Vasc Endovasc Surg* 1996;11:230-237.
78. Michiels C, Arnould T, Thibaut-Vercruyssen R, et al. Perfused human saphenous veins for the study of the origin of varicose veins: role of the endothelium and of hypoxia. *Int Angiol* 1997;16:134-141.
79. Clarke GH, Vasdekis SN, Hobbs JT, et al. Venous wall function in the pathogenesis of varicose veins. *Surgery* 1992;111:402-408.
80. Haardt B. A comparison of the histochemical enzyme pattern in normal and varicose veins. *Phlebology* 1987;2:135-158.
81. Barber DA, Wang X, Gloviczki P, et al. Characterization of endothelin receptors in human varicose veins. *J Vasc Surg* 1997;26:61-69.
82. Mangiafico RA, Malatino LS, Santonocito M, et al. Plasma endothelin-1 release in normal and varicose saphenous veins. *Angiology* 1997;48:769-774.
83. Hollingsworth SJ, Tang CB, Dialynas M, et al. Varicose veins: loss of release of vascular endothelial growth factor and reduced plasma nitric oxide. *Eur J Vasc Endovasc Surg* 2001;22:551-556.
84. Schuller-Petrovic S, Siedler S, Kern T, et al. Imbalance between the endothelial cell–derived contracting factors prostacyclin and angiotensin II and nitric oxide–cyclic GMP in human primary varicosis. *Br J Pharmacol* 1997;122:772-778.
85. Herouy Y, May AE, Pornschlegel G, et al. Lipodermatosclerosis is characterized by elevated expression and activation of matrix metalloproteinases: implications for venous ulcer formation. *J Invest Dermatol* 1998;111:822-827.
86. Pappas PJ, You R, Rameshwar P, et al. Dermal tissue fibrosis in patients with chronic venous insufficiency is associated with increased transforming growth factor–β1 gene expression and protein production. *J Vasc Surg* 1999;30:1129-1145.

87. Coleridge Smith PD. Update on chronic venous insufficiency–induced inflammatory processes. *Angiology* 2001;52(Suppl 1):S35-S42.
88. Scelsi R, Scelsi L, Cortinovis R, et al. Morphological changes of dermal blood and lymphatic vessels in chronic venous insufficiency of the leg. *Int Angiol* 1994;13:308-311.
89. Herrick SE, Sloan P, McGurk M, et al. Sequential changes in histologic pattern and extracellular matrix deposition during the healing of chronic venous ulcers. *Am J Pathol* 1992;141:1085-1095.
90. Browse NL, Burnand KG. The cause of venous ulceration. *Lancet* 1982;2:243-245.
91. Hahn J, Junger M, Friedrich B, et al. Cutaneous inflammation limited to the region of the ulcer in chronic venous insufficiency. *Vasa* 1997;26:277-281.
92. Pappas PJ, DeFouw DO, Venezio LM, et al. Morphometric assessment of the dermal microcirculation in patients with chronic venous insufficiency. *J Vasc Surg* 1997;26:784-795.
93. Wilkinson LS, Bunker C, Edwards JC, et al. Leukocytes: their role in the etiopathogenesis of skin damage in venous disease. *J Vasc Surg* 1993;17:669-675.
94. Hopkins NF, Spinks TJ, Rhodes CG, et al. Positron emission tomography in venous ulceration and liposclerosis: study of regional tissue function. *Br Med J (Clin Res Ed)* 1983;286:333-336.
95. Burnand KG, Whimster I, Naidoo A, et al. Pericapillary fibrin in the ulcer-bearing skin of the leg: the cause of lipodermatosclerosis and venous ulceration. *Br Med J (Clin Res Ed)* 1982;285:1071-1072.
96. Van De Scheur M, Falanga V. Pericapillary fibrin cuffs in venous disease. *Dermatol Surg* 1997;23:955-959.
97. Thomas PRS, Nash GB, Dormandy JA. White cell accumulation in dependent legs of patients with venous hypertension: a possible mechanism for trophic changes in the skin. *Br Med J* 1988;296:1693-1695.
98. Coleridge Smith PD, Thomas P, Scurr JH, et al. Causes of venous ulceration: a new hypothesis. *Br Med J (Clin Res Ed)* 1988;296:1726-1727.
99. Saharay M, Shields DA, Georgiannos SN, et al. Endothelial activation in patients with chronic venous disease. *Eur J Vasc Endovasc Surg* 1998;15:342-349.
100. Ciuffetti G, Mannarino E, Paltriccia R, et al. Leucocyte activity in chronic venous insufficiency. *Int Angiol* 1994;13:312-316.
101. Saharay M, Shields DA, Porter JB, et al. Leukocyte activity in the microcirculation of the leg in patients with chronic venous disease. *J Vasc Surg* 1997;26:265-273.
102. Schmid-Schonbein G, Takase S, Bergan JJ. New advances in the understanding of the pathophysiology of chronic venous insufficiency. *Angiology* 2001;52(Suppl 1) S27-S34.
103. Weyl A, Vanscheidt W, Weiss JM, et al. Expression of the adhesion molecules ICAM-1, VCAM-1, and E-selectin and their ligands VLA-4 and LFA-1 in chronic venous leg ulcers. *J Am Acad Dermatol* 1996;34:418-423.
104. Shields DA, Andaz SK, Sarin S, et al. Plasma elastase in venous disease. *Br J Surg* 1994;81:1496-1499.
105. Michiels C, Bouaziz N, Remacle J. Role of the endothelium and blood stasis in the appearance of varicose veins. *Int Angiol* 2002;21:1-8.
106. Saito S, Trovato MJ, You R, et al. Role of matrix metalloproteinases 1, 2, and 9 and tissue inhibitor of matrix metalloproteinase-1 in chronic venous insufficiency. *J Vasc Surg* 2001;34:930-938.
107. Parra JR, Cambria RA, Hower CD, et al. Tissue inhibitor of metalloproteinase-1 is increased in the saphenofemoral junction of patients with varices in the leg. *J Vasc Surg* 1998;28:669-675.
108. Pappas PJ, Duran WN, Hobson RW. Pathology and cellular physiology of chronic venous insufficiency. In: Gloviczki P, Yao JST, eds. *Handbook of venous disorders: guidelines of the American Venous Forum*. 2nd ed. London: Arnold; 2001:58-67.
109. Fowkes FG, Lee AJ, Evans CJ, et al. Lifestyle risk factors for lower limb venous reflux in the general population: Edinburgh Vein Study. *Int J Epidemiol* 2001;30:846-852.
110. Bradbury A, Evans CJ, Allan P, et al. The relationship between lower limb symptoms and superficial and deep venous reflux on duplex ultrasonography: the Edinburgh Vein Study. *J Vasc Surg* 2000;32:921-931.
111. Madar G, Widmer LK, Zemp E, et al. Varicose veins and chronic venous insufficiency disorder or disease? A critical epidemiological review. *Vasa* 1986;15:126-134.
112. Novo S, Avellone G, Pinto A. Prevalence of primitive varicose veins of the lower limb in a randomized population sample of western Sicily. *Int Angiol* 1988;7:176-181.
113. Sadick NS. Predisposing factors of varicose and telangiectatic leg veins. *J Dermatol Surg Oncol* 1992;18:883-886.
114. Brand FN, Dannenberg AL, Abbott RD, et al. The epidemiology of varicose veins: the Framingham Study. *Am J Prev Med* 1988;4:96-101.
115. Sisto T, Reunanen A, Laurikka J, et al. Prevalence and risk factors of varicose veins in lower extremities: mini-Finland health survey. *Eur J Surg* 1995;161:405-414.
116. Evans CJ, Allan PL, Lee AJ, et al. Prevalence of venous reflux in the general population on duplex scanning: the Edinburgh Vein Study. *J Vasc Surg* 1998;28:767-776.
117. Fowkes FG, Evans CJ, Lee AJ. Prevalence and risk factors of chronic venous insufficiency. *Angiology* 2001;52;(Suppl 1):S5-S15.
118. Geelhoed GW, Burkitt DP. Varicose veins: a reappraisal from a global perspective. *South Med J* 1991;84:1131-1134.
119. De Backer G. Epidemiology of chronic venous insufficiency. *Angiology* 1997;48:569-576.
120. Callam MJ, Ruckley CV, Harper DR, et al. Chronic ulceration of the leg: extent of the problem and provision of care. *Br Med J (Clin Res Ed)* 1985;290:1855-1856.
121. Lees TA, Lambert D. Prevalence of lower limb ulceration in an urban health district. *Br J Surg* 1992;79:1032-1034.
122. Franks PJ, Wright DD, Moffatt CJ, et al. Prevalence of venous disease: a community study in west London. *Eur J Surg* 1992;158:143-147.
123. Goodrich SM, Wood JE. Peripheral venous distensibility and velocity of blood flow during pregnancy or during oral contraceptive therapy. *Am J Obstet Gynecol* 1964;90:740-744.
124. Ciardullo AV, Panico S, Bellati C, et al. High endogenous estradiol is associated with increased venous distensibility and clinical evidence of varicose veins in menopausal women. *J Vasc Surg* 2000;32:544-549.
125. Gundersen J, Hauge M. Hereditary factors in venous insufficiency. *Angiology* 1969;20:346-355.
126. Ng MY, Andrew T, Spector TD, et al. Linkage to the FOXC2 region of chromosome 16 for varicose veins in otherwise healthy, unselected sibling pairs. *J Med Genet* 2005;42:235-239.
127. Saiki S, Sakai K, Saiki M, et al. Varicose veins associated with CADASIL result from a novel mutation in the Notch3 gene. *Neurology* 2006;67:337-339.
128. Cornu-Thenard A, Boivin P, Baud JM, et al. Importance of the familial factor in varicose disease: clinical study of 134 families. *J Dermatol Surg Oncol* 1994;20:318-326.
129. Sarin S, Shields DA, Farrah J, et al. Does venous function deteriorate in patients waiting for varicose vein surgery? *J R Soc Med* 1993;86:21-23.
130. Brewster SF, Nicholson S, Farndon JR. The varicose vein waiting list: results of a validation exercise. *Ann R Coll Surg Engl* 1991;73:223-226.
131. Berard A, Abenhaim L, Platt R, et al. Risk factors for the first-time development of venous ulcers of the lower limbs: the influence of heredity and physical activity. *Angiology* 2002;53:647-657.
132. Scott TE, LaMorte WW, Gorin DR, et al. Risk factors for chronic venous insufficiency: a dual case-control study. *J Vasc Surg* 1995;22:622-628.
133. Mota-Capitao L, Menezes JD, Gouveia-Oliveira A. Clinical predictors of the severity of chronic venous insufficiency of the lower limbs: a multivariate analysis. *Phlebology* 1995;10:155-159.
134. Neglen P, Raju S. A comparison between descending phlebography and duplex Doppler investigation in the evaluation of reflux in chronic venous insufficiency: a challenge to phlebography as the "gold standard." *J Vasc Surg* 1992;16:687-693.
135. Prandoni P, Lensing A, Cogo A, et al. The long term clinical course of acute deep venous thrombosis. *Ann Intern Med* 1996;125:1-7.
136. Monreal M, Martorell A, Callejas J, et al. Venographic assessment of deep vein thrombosis and risk of developing post-thrombotic syndrome: a prospective trial. *J Intern Med* 1993;233:233-238.
137. Strandness DE, Langlois Y, Cramer M, et al. Long-term sequelae of acute venous thrombosis. *JAMA* 1983;250:1289-1292.
138. Prandoni P, Villalta S, Polistena P, et al. Symptomatic deep-vein thrombosis and the post-thrombotic syndrome. *Haematologica* 1995;80:42-48.
139. Lindner DJ, Edwards JM, Phinney ES, et al. Long-term hemodynamic and clinical sequelae of lower extremity deep vein thrombosis. *J Vasc Surg* 1986;4:436-442.
140. Meissner MH, Strandness DE. Pathophysiology and natural history of deep venous thrombosis. In: Rutherford RB, ed. *Vascular surgery.* 5th ed. Philadelphia: WB Saunders; 2000:1920-1937.
141. Arcelus JI, Caprini JA, Hoffman KN, et al. Laboratory assays and duplex scanning outcomes after symptomatic deep vein thrombosis: preliminary results. *J Vasc Surg* 1996;23:616-621.
142. Killewich LA, Macko RF, Cox K, et al. Regression of proximal deep venous thrombosis is associated with fibrinolytic enhancement. *J Vasc Surg* 1997;26:861-868.

143. Rosfors S, Eriksson M, Leijd B, et al. A prospective follow-up study of acute deep venous thrombosis using colour duplex ultrasound, phlebography and venous occlusion plethysmography. *Int Angiol* 1997;16:39-44.
144. Markel A, Manzo RA, Bergelin RO, et al. Valvular reflux after deep vein thrombosis: incidence and time of occurrence. *J Vasc Surg* 1992;15:377-384.
145. Meissner MH, Manzo RA, Bergelin RO, et al. Deep venous insufficiency: the relationship between lysis and subsequent reflux. *J Vasc Surg* 1993;18:596-608.
146. Caps MT, Manzo RA, Bergelin RO, et al. Venous valvular reflux in veins not involved at the time of acute deep vein thrombosis. *J Vasc Surg* 1995;22:524-531.
147. Meissner MH, Caps MT, Bergelin RO, et al. Propagation, rethrombosis, and new thrombus formation after acute deep venous thrombosis. *J Vasc Surg* 1995;22:558-567.
148. Beyth RJ, Cohen AM, Landefeld CS. Long-term outcome of deep-vein thrombosis. *Arch Intern Med* 1995;155:1031-1037.
149. Meissner MH, Caps MT, Zierler BK, et al. Determinants of chronic venous disease after acute deep venous thrombosis. *J Vasc Surg* 1998;28:826-833.
150. Meissner MH, Caps MT, Zierler BK, et al. Deep venous thrombosis and superficial venous reflux. *J Vasc Surg* 2000;32:48-56.
151. Stvrtinova V, Kolesar J, Wimmer G. Prevalence of varicose veins of the lower limbs in the women working at a department store. *Int Angiol* 1991;10:2-5.
152. Mekky S, Schilling RS, Walford J. Varicose veins in women cotton workers. An epidemiological study in England and Egypt. *Br Med J* 1969;2:591-595.
153. Maffei FH, Magaldi C, Pinho SZ, et al. Varicose veins and chronic venous insufficiency in Brazil: prevalence among 1755 inhabitants of a country town. *Int J Epidemiol* 1986;15:210-217.
154. Evans CJ, Fowkes FG, Ruckley CV, et al. Prevalence of varicose veins and chronic venous insufficiency in men and women in the general population: Edinburgh Vein Study. *J Epidemiol Community Health* 1999;53:149-153.
155. Beaglehole R. Epidemiology of varicose veins. World J Surg 1986;10:898-902.
156. Barwell JR, Taylor M, Deacon J, et al. Surgical correction of isolated superficial venous reflux reduces long-term recurrence rate in chronic venous leg ulcers. *Eur J Vasc Endovasc Surg* 2000;20:363-368.

chapter 43

Medical Management of Varicose Veins

Manj S. Gohel, MD, MRCS • Amanda Shepherd, MRCS • Maher Hamish, MD, FRCS • Alun H. Davies, MA, DM, FRCS, ILTM

Key Points

- Effective nonsurgical treatments are available for small and large varicose veins.
- Compression therapy can heal venous ulceration, reduce the risk of ulcer recurrence, and prevent progression of chronic venous disease.
- Systemic treatment with flavonoids or oxerutins may reduce the symptoms of venous disease.
- Sclerotherapy is widely considered the optimum treatment for reticular veins and telangectases.
- Foam sclerotherapy is effective in the treatment of residual and recurrent varicosities after surgery.
- The treatment of saphenous reflux with foam sclerotherapy is effective, but multiple treatments may be needed.

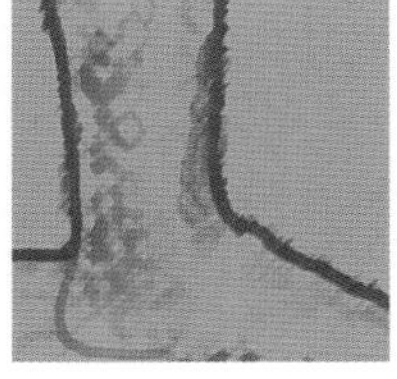

Patients with varicose veins may present with a spectrum of venous disease ranging from minor thread or reticular veins to severe chronic venous hypertension and ulceration. Although surgical options are widely considered the mainstay of therapy for patients with varicose veins, nonsurgical treatment is often beneficial. In many cases, nonsurgical treatment may be adequate to control symptoms, thus avoiding the risks of an operation. In addition, patients may be unwilling to undergo surgery or unsuitable for anesthesia due to concurrent medical illnesses, and in some patients, nonsurgical management may augment operative treatment. The following principal nonsurgical pathways are discussed in this chapter:

- Conservative measures
- Compression
- Medication
- Sclerotherapy

CONSERVATIVE MEASURES

Perhaps the most effective technique for reducing venous hypertension is high elevation as evidenced after even short periods of hospitalization. Patients with chronic venous disease are advised to try and elevate their legs where possible. However, mobilization and regular walking are also essential to encourage calf muscle pump action and prevent the many problems of excessive immobility. The cohort benefits of these measures are unknown as compliance is poor in the elderly and young alike. Assessment of population compliance is difficult to objectively assess. Although the evidence for benefit in venous disease is limited, patient advice should include smoking cessation and nutritional advice in appropriate cases.

COMPRESSION THERAPY

Principles of Compression

The use of compression therapy for patients with venous disease has been described since the time of Hippocrates (460 to 377 BC) and is still a key component of the nonsurgical treatment plan in venous disease.[1] Incompetence of superficial and deep veins of the leg may cause symptoms due to persistent elevation of the venous pressure in the leg, known as venous hypertension.[2] Compression of the limb can help reduce the venous pressure and relieve symptoms. Graduated compression stockings can be effective in symptom control but do not treat the underlying pathology. The effects on the microcirculation include the acceleration of blood flow in the capillaries, improvement of the filtration–absorption ratio in the capillary system, and reduction of tissue edema.

Table 43-1
Compression Classes (European Standard Classification)*

Compression Class	Pressure at Ankle (mm Hg)
A (light)	10-14
I (mild)	15-21
II† (moderate)	22-32
III (strong)	33-46
IV (very strong)	>46

*Compression is based on the pressures exerted at the ankle.
†Class II compression is effective in chronic venous insufficiency. Greater pressures have minimal impact on the reduction of venous volume and may reduce patient compliance.

Venous Ulceration

Wound Dressings

Over the last 25 years, a vast and confusing range of wound dressings have become available. The ideal dressing should provide a moist, clean wound environment; remain nonadherent; absorb exudates and odors; be safe and acceptable to the patient; and be cost effective. Evidence shows that the type of dressing has little influence on healing in venous ulceration, and the dressings used tend to reflect personal preference and familiarity.[3] Simple, nonadhesive gauze used under compression bandaging is thought to be adequate under most circumstances, with adjuvant products only occasionally required for exceptionally wet, painful, or odorous wounds.

Biological Dressings

Over the last decade, numerous skin substitutes have been developed as dressings for chronic wounds. These products are usually cultured from neonatal fibroblasts, with the aim of being the ideal dressing and providing a biological matrix to aid the healing response. Further prospective studies are needed to ascertain whether these products have a role in clinical care.

Topical Growth Factors

Recombinant growth factors including epidermal growth factor and granulocyte macrophage–colony-stimulating factor have been forwarded as beneficial topical agents in chronic wounds. However, clinical studies have been small and demonstrated modest benefits only.[4,5] Some authors have suggested that platelet lysate extracted from autologous blood samples may improve wound healing by providing an abundant local supply of growth factors. However, two randomized studies have failed to demonstrate any benefit for this novel technique.[6,7]

Multilayer Compression

Multilayer bandaging that provides compression graduated from 40 mm Hg at the ankle to 17 mm Hg at the upper calf is widely accepted as the mainstay of treatment for chronic venous ulceration.[8] Continuous-type dressings (such as the classic Unna boot) remain on the patient's leg even during bed rest and are changed once a week (even up to several weeks). More modern compression bandages comprise of nonelastic and elastic components that may vary depending on the size of the leg and the level of compression desired. The graduation in pressure is achieved using a constant stretch on the bandage as the subbandage pressure is inversely proportional to the diameter of the limb. The advantages of these dressings are the high working pressure while walking and the uninterrupted efficacy during the night. The main disadvantages are the problems with personal hygiene and the necessity for trained personnel to change the dressings. Health professionals need to be appropriately trained in the application of bandages to ensure effective and safe treatment.[9,10]

Elastic Compression Stockings

Elastic compression stockings are indicated in maintenance treatment and to reduce the risk of ulcer recurrence in patients with healed ulcers.[11] Elastic stockings should be worn during the day; they may be applied by patients, ideally before getting up in the morning, and are removed just before going to bed at night. Elastic compression stockings are usually available in three lengths—short, normal, and long—and in different compression classes. While custom-made hosiery may provide a better fit for some individuals, for many, readymade stockings are available in different compression classes (Table 43-1). The advantages are the relative ease of application, relatively low cost, and better hygienic conditions. It should be noted that patient compliance with stocking use may be reduced, particularly with elderly patients, although this is difficult to objectively assess.

Pneumatic Compression Therapy

Pneumatic compression systems involve the placement of an inflatable sleeve on the leg that can be inflated in a cyclical pattern. Numerous devices have become commercially available in recent years. Although the use of pneumatic compression has been generally limited to the prevention of deep venous thrombosis, some recent evidence shows that pneumatic compression could be used to augment standard compression therapy in the treatment of patients with venous ulceration.[12]

Efficacy of Compression

Clear evidence indicates that multilayer compression bandaging offers significant clinical benefit for patients with chronic venous ulcers when compared with conservative therapy.[8] Similarly, for patients with healed ulceration, the use of elastic compression stockings can reduce the risk of ulcer recurrence.[11] The level of protection is likely to be greater with higher degrees of compression, although compliance may be lower with tighter stockings.

Fewer studies have evaluated the value of compression therapy in patients with varicose veins without ulceration, and most have assessed the influence of compression therapy, in addition to other treatments. In a randomized, controlled trial to test the efficacy of rutosides, all patients awaiting varicose vein surgery were assigned either placebo alone, rutosides alone, hosiery with placebo, or hosiery with rutosides. Assessment of swelling using a visual analog scale (measured in millimeters) showed that hosiery alone had the greatest effect after 4 weeks of treatment.[13] A randomized, controlled trial by Fraser and colleagues reported a greater reduction in symptoms in patients who used bandages for 6 weeks postsclerotherapy.[14] A 75% reduction in the symptom score was also observed with sclerotherapy and bandages, without any difference among type and duration of bandaging. After sclerotherapy, stockings with ankle pressure of 30 to 40 mm Hg were effective in treating skin changes, and high-pressure stockings were more effective than bandages.[15]

Following varicose vein surgery, a recent randomized trial failed to demonstrate any advantage in wearing stockings for 3 weeks rather than 1 week,[16] although a study by Travers and Makin did demonstrate that the use of stockings for 1 year after surgery dramatically reduced the rate of varicose vein recurrence from 61% to 12%.[17] Although edema is one of the main indications for compression therapy, few studies are available on its efficacy compared with no treatments. Data supporting the use of sequential compression devices in patients with varicose veins are scarce, but a recent controlled study did suggest that there may be an improvement in venous hemodynamic function with sequential leg compression.[18]

Contraindications and Complications of Compression

The main contraindication to the use of compression therapy is arterial insufficiency. The ankle–brachial index should always be assessed to exclude arterial compromise before commencing compression therapy. Compression has been reported to cause phlebitis, blisters, pruritus, and foot swelling when applied too tightly. Compared with stockings, bandages are reported to cause more ankle immobility[19] and a relatively increased risk of thrombosis. Compression of extremities should be performed with caution in patients with severe cardiac failure because of the effect on cardiac preload and output. In pregnancy, compression may influence maternal and fetal heart rate.

MEDICATION FOR VENOUS DISEASE

Types of Venoactive Medication

Systemic drug therapy has been tried for many years in an attempt to reduce symptoms from varicose veins and pharmacologically reduce the chronic skin sequelae of venous hypertension. In Europe, the use of venoactive drugs is generally considered as an adjunct to sclerotherapy or surgery, which are considered more definitive treatments. In general, little level I evidence supports the use of systemic medication for the treatment of varicose veins.

Drugs used for varicose veins may be classified as either venoactive or nonvenoactive. The nonvenoactive drug category has only been used in the management of venous ulcers and includes agents such as stanozalol (lysis of "fibrin-cuff"), pentoxifylline (reduction of white cell activation), ergotamine (vein wall contraction), and aspirin (platelet inhibition). There are two principal categories of venoactive drugs, or phlebotropics: naturally occurring agents and synthetic agents. Their mechanism of action has not been fully elucidated, but they are thought to improve venous tone, assessed by a decrease in venous wall compliance as measured by plethysmography. Increased venous pressure is associated with microcirculatory changes, namely, white cell aggregation and activation, with subsequent release of inflammatory mediators, increased capillary permeability, and microthrombus formation. These agents could also counter these responses by decreasing white cell activation and release of inflammatory mediators, decreasing capillary fragility and permeability, and decreasing blood viscosity.

Results of Clinical Studies

For patients with venous ulcers, several small studies have suggested that pentoxifylline may have a role in accelerating ulcer healing,[20-22] However, a larger randomized study failed to demonstrate a significant effect.[23] Nevertheless, a Cochrane systematic review in 2002 concluded that pentoxifylline may be an effective adjunct to compression for patients with chronic venous ulcers.[24] No randomized studies support the use of stanozolol or ergotamine for the treatment of venous disease.

For patients with varicose veins without ulceration, medications are usually prescribed for symptom relief. The symptoms most often assessed in drug studies are heaviness, fullness, discomfort, cramps, itching, pain, restless legs, sensation of heat, and swelling. Numerous venoactive drugs, including rutin, esculetin, and dihydroergocristine, have been compared to placebo in patients with simple varicose veins, although only limited clinical benefits were observed.[25-27] A placebo-controlled trial of naftazone in primary uncomplicated varicose veins claimed a statistically and clinically significant improvement in disability scores as subjectively assessed on a visual analog scale,[28] and rutosides may be beneficial in relieving the symptoms of varicose veins in pregnancy.[29]

Perhaps the most studied venoactive agent is Daflon (micronized purified flavonoid fraction). A metaanalysis published in 2005 concluded that adjuvant treatment with Daflon conferred an additional 32% chance of healing in patients with chronic venous ulcers.[30] The value of Daflon in relieving other symptoms, including pain, edema, and cramps, has also been reported by a European study of 5000 patients.[31] A recent trial comparing Daflon with oxerutins demonstrated significant clinical and quality-of-life advantages for patients taking oxerutins.[32] These findings are supported by earlier studies that demonstrated hemodynamic benefits in patients treated with oxerutins.[33] Small studies reporting clinical benefits with other venoactive agents, including coumarine rutine, dihydroergocristine, ruscus asculeatus, and calcium dobesilate, have been published.[25,26,34] However, prospective randomized studies and level I evidence are generally lacking, and these agents are not in widespread use. It should also be noted that although pentoxifylline is licensed by the U.S. Food and Drug Administration, most other venoactive medications discussed in this section are not available in the United States.

Risks of Medication

The most commonly reported adverse effects associated with drug therapy are nausea, headache, colicky abdominal pain, and insomnia. Constipation, tiredness, and pruritus are seen in patients taking rutosides.[13,34]

SCLEROTHERAPY

Principles of Sclerotherapy

The basic principle of sclerotherapy is the induction of irritation in the endothelial and subendothelial layers of the wall of the vein, collapsing of the walls so that they lie in apposition

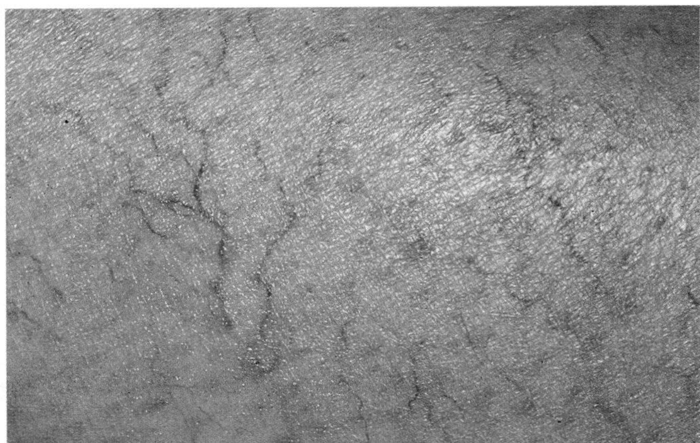

Figure 43-1. Chosen area for treatment.

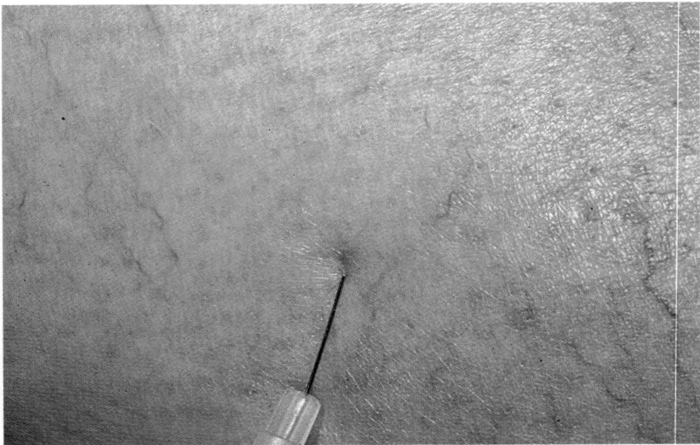

Figure 43-3. Injection of sclerosant.

by compression, and obliteration of the lumen by inflammation and fibrosis. The process of inflammation resolving by fibrosis takes more than 6 months. Sclerosing agents can act either by osmosis, dehydrating and destroying the endothelium (e.g., hypertonic glucose), or by a detergent action on the lipid endothelial cell membrane (e.g., ethanolamine oleate).[35] The second mechanism acts faster than the first. Various techniques have been described, but the development of imaging modalities such as ultrasound and new sclerosing agents have helped in modifying techniques. Sclerotherapy can be used with surgery, either during or after the operation.

Sclerotherapy for Thread or Reticular Veins

Small varicose veins include telangiectasias, reticular veins, and venulectases. Intradermal venulectases (telangiectasias) are intradermal vessels visible to the human eye, measuring 0.1 to 2 mm in diameter. Telangiectasias may be arteriole, venule, or capillary. Reticular varicose veins are dilated subcutaneous veins that do not belong to the main truncal veins or their major tributaries.

The unanimous recommendation of the consensus conference was that sclerotherapy is the preferred treatment option for these types of veins.

Technique

The technique of sclerotherapy for small veins is illustrated in Figures 43-1 to 43-5. The patient is asked to stand or sit for 5 minutes before treatment to encourage venous filling. Alternatively, a blood pressure cuff inflated to 40 mm Hg may be placed above the injection site.

The patient then sits with the leg in a horizontal position on the couch. The skin over the proposed injection site is prepared with an alcohol wipe. Available sclerosing agents include polidocanol (0.2% to 1%), sodium tetradecyl sulfate (1% to 3%), chromated glycerine (25% to 100%), and sodium salicylate (6% to 12%). Small needles with gauges between 25 and 33 are used, and visualization may be enhanced with the use of a magnifying lamp or loupes. A small "test dose" on the first treatment is used to ensure no adverse reactions occur. The needle is advanced into the lumen of the vein, and aspiration of blood back into the syringe is advocated before injection, although this is often not possible when injecting telangiectases. It should be noted that polidocanol is not registered in the United States, but sodium tetradecyl sulfate and ethanolomine oleate are approved by the U.S. Food and Drug Administration.

Some specialists advise using an "air block," in which the vein is injected with air before injection of the sclerosant to empty it of blood.[36] The idea is that less sclerosant is needed,

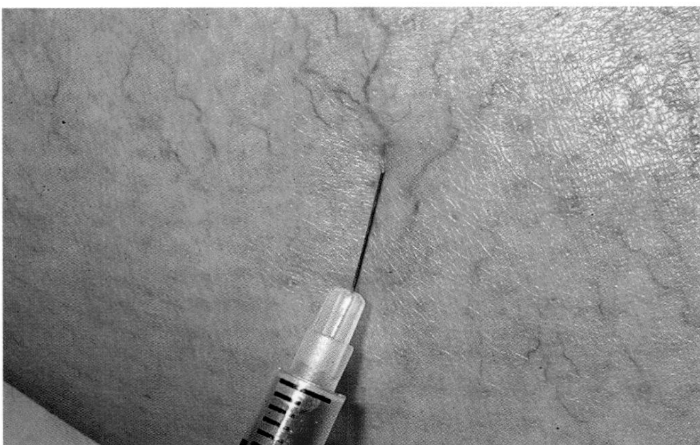

Figure 43-2. Inserting a needle into a vein and obtaining flashback of blood (if possible).

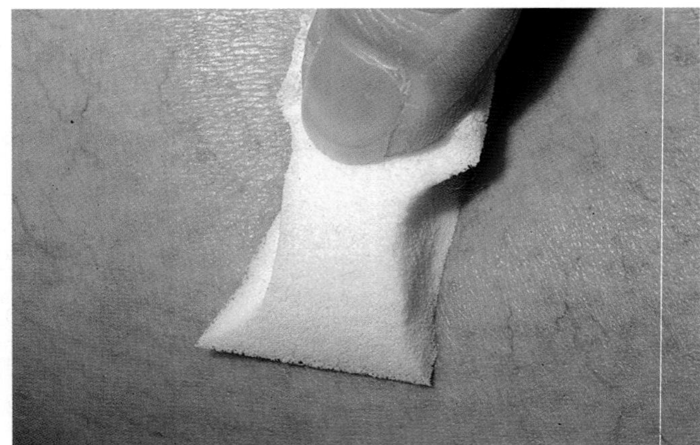

Figure 43-4. Local compression with foam-pad enhancement.

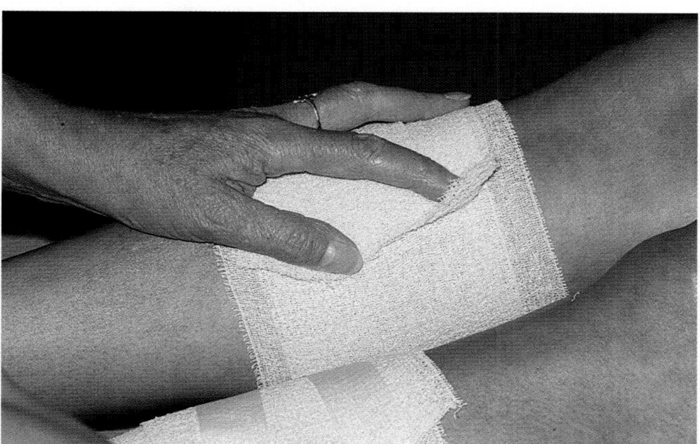

Figure 43-5. Crepe bandage over the sclerotherapy site.

as it is relatively undiluted. Another modification to the technique is the use of a foam sclerosant. A 2-cm^2 area is injected at a time, with a maximum dose of 10 ml of foam used per session. Injection is immediately stopped if any evidence of extravasation appears. Compression can then be applied to the area, although this is not universally practiced. The interval from one session to the next should not be less than 1 week, and the same area should not be revisited within 3 weeks.

Foam Sclerotherapy

The concept of using a foamy sclerosant was first described in 1950, when Orbach first suggested that vigorously shaking the sclerosant 3% sodium tetradecyl sulfate improved the thrombogenic effect.[37] The use of foam has enjoyed a resurgence of interest since the mid-1990s. The conceptual advantage of using foam is the bioavailability. Sclerosant solutions act on venous endothelium that is reached by intravenous injection. Distribution and local concentration depend on the volume and flow rate of blood, which vary with the size of the vein. A progressive dilution in the sclerosant occurs the farther from the point of injection the sclerosant is carried by blood. The concentration also drops off rapidly as the sclerosant fixes to red blood cell membranes, decreasing bioavailability. Microfoam is a drug delivery system that potentially prolongs the time the sclerosant is in contact with the endothelium and achieves a more constant concentration of the sclerosant at the site of action. Foam confers the added advantage of being easily visible on duplex ultrasound. Foam sclerotherapy has been described in the treatment of both small and large varicose veins, including recurrent veins.

Technique

Duplex-guided or echosclerotherapy was first described in 1989 and involves the injection of a vein with sclerosant under ultrasound guidance. The technique has been used in the treatment of greater saphenous, lesser saphenous, and recurrent varicose veins. The main advantages of this technique are ease of treatment and safety. The effect of the sclerosant on the vein wall can be observed immediately as duplex imaging allows estimation of the degree of spasm, length of vein affected, and identification of tributaries, together with control of the deep veins.

Results Following Sclerotherapy

Although sclerotherapy is widely accepted as the optimum treatment for patients with telangiectases, spider veins, and reticular veins, the scientific evidence is limited. A comparison between 1% polidocanol and hypertonic saline demonstrated that both were effective for reticular veins and telangiectases but adverse effects were more common with polidocanol.[38] A study comparing four concentrations of polidocanol in 20 women with telangiectases compared adverse events and improvements based on photographs and suggested that 0.5% polidocanol may be the most effective.[39]

Foam sclerotherapy is an adequate treatment for nonsaphenous varicose veins, local varicose veins, and varicose tributaries of the saphenous trunk without saphenous insufficiency. It is also an ideal choice for treatment of postoperative residual veins and recurrent varicosities. Duplex examination is helpful to exclude primary or recurrent saphenofemoral or saphenopopliteal incompetence in these patients. Several studies have supported the use of compression following sclerotherapy, but scientific evidence suggests that long-term treatment (more than 6 months) is no more effective than shorter treatment. Most scientific evidence for the effect of sclerotherapy on varicose veins is available in the form of studies using it in combination with compression[14,15] and those comparing it with, or using it as an adjunct to, surgery.[40]

A recent randomized trial compared 1% and 3% polidocanol foam for the treatment of greater saphenous vein reflux and concluded that no difference appeared between the groups.[41] The overall 2-year occlusion rate was 68% in this study. A study by Rabe and colleagues demonstrated that 3% foam polidocanol was significantly more effective than 3% liquid polidocanol for greater saphenous vein reflux.[42] Overall, the evidence suggests that early occlusion rates up to 90% are achievable with foam sclerotherapy but multiple treatments may be necessary.[43] Few studies have reported long-term occlusion rates. Better-defined indications like diameter of the saphenous vein, degree of reflux, and selection of patients with short or long saphenous veins might improve the results following sclerotherapy, but presently precise selection criteria remain poorly defined.

Contraindications and Complications of Sclerotherapy

The main contraindication to use of sclerotherapy is known allergy to the agent. The procedure should be performed with caution in the following situations:

- Severe systemic disease
- Recent deep vein thrombosis
- Local or general infection
- Nonambulatory patients
- Severe arterial disorder, especially critical leg ischemia
- Allergic diathesis
- Pregnancy and breast feeding
- Hypercoagulability (protein C and S deficiency and lupus anticoagulant)
- Recurrent deep vein thrombosis

The minor side effects reported after sclerotherapy include pigmentation and local inflammatory reactions. The potential of an adverse cosmetic effect should be explained carefully to every patient before treatment to avoid the distress associated with resulting litigation. Pruritus after injection of polidocanol was reported as often as 35% to 45% in the study by Norris et al.[39] Hyperpigmentation and neovascularization was concentration dependent and seen in 50% to 70% of patients following use of polidocanol. The possible risks of dangerous complications such as thromboembolism, as well as intraarterial injections, may be potentially avoided by careful patient selection and meticulous technique. Other reported complications include thrombosis, superficial phlebitis, night cramps, blisters, and swollen feet. Although deep vein thrombosis, scotoma, and cerebrovascular events have been described following saphenous vein foam sclerotherapy treatment, these are thought to be rare adverse events.

OTHER TREATMENTS

Several other treatment modalities, including physiotherapy, hydrotherapy, and ultrasound therapy, are available, but most of them have not been tested in controlled studies and the available data are not strong enough to draw valid conclusions about their efficacy. Physiotherapy is commonly used. Hydrotherapy provides short-term stimulation, leading to vasoconstriction, diuresis, and vascular–interstitial fluid shift. Ultrasound therapy may be useful as an adjunct in venous ulcer healing.

COSTS OF NONSURGICAL THERAPY FOR VARICOSE VEINS

Venous disorders can be considered an important public health problem. Estimates per country have revealed that the management of venous disorders accounts for 1% to 3% of the total health-care expenditure. The total medical cost for the treatment of venous disorders is thought to exceed 500 million pounds in the United Kingdom. The costs in other European countries such as Germany and France are estimated to be even higher. The true financial burden is likely to be even higher as societal costs and the cost of cosmetic products used by patients are not included in health-care expenditure. Societal costs include loss of productivity due to absence from work, additional costs such as hired help for homemaking activities, and intangible costs.

Studies into the epidemiology, cost effectiveness of different strategies, validity of scoring systems, and diagnostic tests need to be conducted to extend knowledge about venous disorders and improve understanding about the true costs. Randomized clinical trials with long-term follow-up are needed to compare the existing therapies for chronic venous disease and to help define the optimum management strategies.

CONCLUSIONS

Although many would consider surgical intervention as the optimum treatment for patients with venous disease, numerous effective medical options are available. Compression therapy is an essential treatment modality; it can promote healing for patients with chronic venous ulceration and prevent recurrence in patients with healed ulcers. It is also recommended after surgery and sclerotherapy and is effective in preventing skin changes caused by chronic venous hypertension. The use of drug therapy in the management of varicose veins is limited, although some evidence supports the use of flavanoids, oxerutins, and other venoactive medications to reduce symptoms and edema of venous origin. Sclerotherapy is the treatment of choice in telangiectasias, spider veins, and isolated reticular veins. Variations in the availability of venoactive medications and sclerosants in the United States and Europe have limited trial consistency and hindered the development of a consensus in the use of these treatments. Foam sclerotherapy is also an effective and well-tolerated treatment for nonsaphenous varicose veins and recurrent or residual veins after surgery without evidence of venous reflux. Recent evidence has demonstrated that foam sclerotherapy can also be used for the treatment of saphenous vein reflux, although multiple treatments may be necessary to ensure long-term occlusion.

References

1. Anon. De ulceribus and de carnibus. In: Adams EF, ed. *The genuine works of Hippocrates*. London: Sydenham Press; 1949.
2. Nicolaides AN, Hussein MK, Szendro G, et al. The relation of venous ulceration with ambulatory venous pressure measurements. *J Vasc Surg* 1993;17:414-419.
3. Palfreyman SJ, Nelson EA, Lochiel R, Michaels JA. Dressings for healing venous leg ulcers. *Cochrane Database Syst Rev* 2006;3:CD001103.
4. Falanga V, Eaglstein WH, Bucalo B, et al. Topical use of human recombinant epidermal growth factor (h-EGF) in venous ulcers. *J Dermatol Surg Oncol* 1992;18:604-606.
5. Da Costa RM, Ribeiro Jesus FM, Aniceto C, Mendes M. Randomized, double-blind, placebo-controlled, dose-ranging study of granulocyte–macrophage colony stimulating factor in patients with chronic venous leg ulcers. *Wound Repair Regen* 1999;7:17-25.
6. Senet P, Bon FX, Benbunan M, et al. Randomized trial and local biological effect of autologous platelets used as adjuvant therapy for chronic venous leg ulcers. *J Vasc Surg* 2003;38:1342-1348.
7. Stacey MC, Mata SD, Trengove NJ, Mather CA. Randomised double-blind placebo controlled trial of topical autologous platelet lysate in venous ulcer healing. *Eur J Vasc Endovasc Surg* 2000;20:296-301.
8. Cullum N, Nelson EA, Fletcher AW, Sheldon TA. Compression bandages and stockings for venous leg ulcers. *Cochrane Database Syst Rev* 2000;2: CD000265.
9. Callam MJ, Ruckley CV, Dale JJ, Harper DR. Hazards of compression treatment of the leg: an estimate from Scottish surgeons. *Br Med J (Clin Res Ed)* 1987;295:1382.
10. Nelson EA, Ruckley CV, Barbenel JC. Improvements in bandaging technique following training. *J Wound Care* 1995;4:181-184.
11. Nelson EA, Bell-Syer SE, Cullum NA. Compression for preventing recurrence of venous ulcers. *Cochrane Database Syst Rev* 2000;4:CD002303.
12. Kalodiki E, Ellis M, Kakkos SK, et al. Immediate hemodynamic effect of the additional use of the SCD EXPRESS Compression System in patients with venous ulcers treated with the four-layer compression bandaging system. *Eur J Vasc Endovasc Surg* 2007;33:483-487.
13. Anderson JH, Geraghty JG, Wilson YT. Paroven and graduated compression hosiery for superficial venous insufficiency. *Phlebology* 1990;5: 271-276.
14. Fraser IA, Perry EP, Hatton M, Watkin DF. Prolonged bandaging is not required following sclerotherapy of varicose veins. *Br J Surg* 1985;72: 488-490.
15. Scurr JH, Coleridge-Smith P, Cutting P. Varicose veins: optimum compression following sclerotherapy. *Ann R Coll Surg Engl* 1985;67:109-111.
16. Biswas S, Clark A, Shields DA. Randomised clinical trial of the duration of compression therapy after varicose vein surgery. *Eur J Vasc Endovasc Surg* 2007;33:631-637.
17. Travers JP, Makin GS. Reduction of varicose vein recurrence by use of post-operative compression stockings. *Phlebology* 1994;9:104-107.
18. Griffin M, Kakkos SK, Geroulakos G, Nicolaides AN. Comparison of three intermittent pneumatic compression systems in patients with varicose veins: a hemodynamic study. *Int Angiol* 2007;26:158-164.
19. Lentner A, Spath F, Weinert V. Limitation of movement in the ankle and talo-calcaneonavicular joints caused by compression bandages. *Phlebology* 1997;12:25-30.

20. De Sanctis MT, Belcaro G, Cesarone MR, et al. Treatment of venous ulcers with pentoxifylline: a 12-month, double-blind, placebo controlled trial—microcirculation and healing. *Angiology* 2002;53(Suppl 1): S49-S51.
21. Colgan MP, Dormandy JA, Jones PW, et al. Oxpentifylline treatment of venous ulcers of the leg. *BMJ* 1990;300:972-975.
22. Falanga V, Fujitani RM, Diaz C, et al. Systemic treatment of venous leg ulcers with high doses of pentoxifylline: efficacy in a randomized, placebo-controlled trial. *Wound Repair Regen* 1999;7:208-213.
23. Dale JJ, Ruckley CV, Harper DR, et al. Randomised, double blind placebo controlled trial of pentoxifylline in the treatment of venous leg ulcers. *BMJ* 1999;319:875-878.
24. Jull AB, Waters J, Arroll B. Pentoxifylline for treating venous leg ulcers. *Cochrane Database Syst Rev* 2002;1:CD001733.
25. Zuccarelli F. Effacite clinique et tolerance de la coumarine rutine: etude controlee en double aveungle versus placebo. *Gaz Med* 1987;94:1-7.
26. Languillat N, Vecchiali JF, Zuccarelli F, Bouxin A. Essai en double aveungle contre placebo des effets du Vasobral dans les troubels de la permeabilite capillaire lies a l'insuffisance veineuse par le test isotopique de Landis. *Angiologie* 1986;39:1-4.
27. Prerovsky I, Roztocil K, Hlavova A. The effect of hydroxyethylrutosides after acute and chronic oral administration in patients with venous diseases: a double blind study. *Angiologica* 1972;9:408-414.
28. Vayssairat M. Placebo-controlled trial of naftazone in women with primary uncomplicated symptomatic varicose veins. *Phlebology* 1997;12: 17-20.
29. Bamigboye AA, Smyth R. Interventions for varicose veins and leg oedema in pregnancy. *Cochrane Database Syst Rev* 2007;1:CD001066.
30. Smith PC. Daflon 500 mg and venous leg ulcer: new results from a meta-analysis. *Angiology* 2005;56(Suppl 1):S33-S39.
31. Jantet G. Chronic venous insufficiency: worldwide results of the RELIEF study: Reflux Assessment and Quality of Life Improvement with Micronized Flavonoids. *Angiology* 2002;53:245-256.
32. Cesarone MR, Belcaro G, Pellegrini L, et al. Venoruton vs Daflon: evaluation of effects on quality of life in chronic venous insufficiency. *Angiology* 2006;57:131-138.
33. Petruzzellis V, Troccoli T, Candiani C, et al. Oxerutins (Venoruton): efficacy in chronic venous insufficiency—a double-blind, randomized, controlled study. *Angiology* 2002;53:257-263.
34. Widmer L, Biland L, Barras JP. Doxium 500 in chronic venous insufficiency: a double-blind placebo controlled multicentre study. *Int Angiol* 1990;9:105-110.
35. Goldman MP. Sclerotherapy *Treatment of varicose and telangiectatic leg veins*. 2nd ed. St. Louis: Mosby Year Book; 1995.
36. Orbach EJ. Controversies and realities of therapy for varicosis. *Int Surg* 1977;62:149-151.
37. Orbach EJ. The place of injection therapy in the treatment of venous disorders of the lower extremity: with comments on its technique. *Angiology* 1966;17:18-23.
38. McCoy S, Evans A, Spurrier N. Sclerotherapy for leg telangiectasia: a blinded comparative trial of polidocanol and hypertonic saline. *Dermatol Surg* 1999;25:381-385.
39. Norris MJ, Carlin MC, Ratz JL. Treatment of essential telangiectasia: effects of increasing concentrations of polidocanol. *J Am Acad Dermatol* 1989;20:643-649.
40. Neglen P, Einarsson E, Eklof B. The functional long-term value of different types of treatment for saphenous vein incompetence. *J Cardiovasc Surg (Torino)* 1993;34:295-301.
41. Hamel-Desnos C, Ouvry P, Benigni JP, et al. Comparison of 1% and 3% polidocanol foam in ultrasound guided sclerotherapy of the great saphenous vein: a randomised, double-blind trial with 2-year follow-up— "The 3/1 Study." *Eur J Vasc Endovasc Surg* 2007;34:723-729.
42. Rabe E, Otto J, Schliephake D, Pannier F. Efficacy and safety of great saphenous vein sclerotherapy using standardised polidocanol foam (ESAF): a randomised controlled multicentre clinical trial. *Eur J Vasc Endovasc Surg* 2008;35:238-245.
43. Darke SG, Baker SJ. Ultrasound-guided foam sclerotherapy for the treatment of varicose veins. *Br J Surg* 2006;93:969-974.

chapter

44

Surgical Treatment of Varicose Veins

Manju Kalra, MBBS • Peter Gloviczki, MD, FACS

Key Points

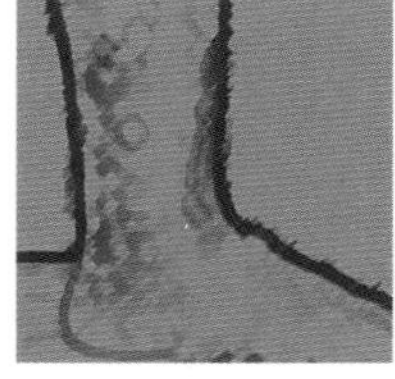

Varicose veins are one of the most prevalent of medical disorders, affecting close to 40 million Americans (10% to 40% of the population), with women affected almost twice as often as men. In some patients, varicosity is a cosmetic problem alone. In most, however, it is a source of discomfort, pain, and swelling, a cause of thrombophlebitis. Varicose veins and associated chronic venous insufficiency may lead to skin changes, ulcers, and disability.[1-3]

TREATMENT OF VARICOSE VEINS

Surgical treatment of varicose veins is aimed at removing unsightly branch veins and treating symptoms of chronic venous disease by reducing ambulatory venous hypertension. It needs to be individualized for each patient based on the results of noninvasive investigation of the venous system. Depending on the underlying pathophysiology in a particular patient, this may be achieved by a combination of the following:

1. Ablation of axial superficial venous reflux
   a. Surgical ablation of saphenous vein reflux
   b. Endovenous ablation of saphenous vein reflux
      i. Thermal ablation (radiofrequency or laser)
      ii. Foam sclerotherapy
2. Removal of varicose veins
   a. Surgical phlebectomy
   b. Sclerotherapy

Ablation of Axial Superficial Reflux

Ablation of gravitational reflux in the great saphenous vein (GSV) or small saphenous vein (SSV) is indicated in patients with varicose veins in whom reflux at the saphenofemoral or saphenopopliteal junction has been identified on duplex ultrasound. Saphenofemoral reflux occurs in 70% of patients with varicose veins. Atypical reflux at other sites or varicosities without gravitational reflux account for the remaining.

For more than a century, ablation of superficial reflux has been performed by high ligation with or without stripping of the GSV or SSV. The treatment of venous disease, especially superficial venous disease, has undergone a radical change over the last 10 years. The superior understanding of venous anatomy and physiology provided by the universal acceptance of duplex ultrasound in the evaluation of venous disease and the introduction of endovenous thermal ablation not only have provided alternatives to traditional saphenous vein stripping but also have challenged the very principles on which this traditional treatment was based. However, the aim of ablating superficial venous reflux, if present, as the first step in the treatment of symptomatic varicose veins remains unchanged. Apart from the attraction of a minimally invasive procedure to ablate superficial venous reflux, with its attendant benefits, advantages of endovenous ablation include a potentially decreased incidence of neovascularization in the groin.

Surgical Ablation of Saphenous Vein Reflux

High ligation of the GSV with stripping has been practiced widely and has been considered the "gold standard" to which other less invasive procedures have been compared. Stripping of the saphenous vein in present-day practice has been limited to the thigh because this eliminates gravitational reflux, which usually extends only to the knee; disconnects thigh perforators; and reduces the incidence of saphenous nerve injury associated with stripping of the below-knee segment. Below-knee calf perforators are not connected directly to the saphenous vein, so no real advantage exists in stripping the vein to the ankle. In occasional cases of gross dilatation of the below-knee segment of the vein with reflux, demonstrated in this situation on duplex ultrasound, stripping may need to be extended to the ankle, usually with the less traumatic inversion technique.

High Ligation and Stripping of the Great Saphenous Vein

High ligation of the GSV is performed through a short (2 to 3 cm), oblique incision in the groin crease situated medial to the femoral pulse. The saphenofemoral junction is identified, as are all tributaries (named and unnamed). The tributaries are dissected out as far as possible and ligated, followed by flush ligation of the saphenous vein, with the surgeon taking care not to impinge upon the underlying femoral vein. A flexible, disposable (Codman) vein stripper is next introduced into the cut end of the vein at the groin and passed to the level of the skin crease at the knee. The saphenous vein is exposed at this level at the medial aspect of the popliteal space, the stripper is pulled through, and the distal end is ligated. Incompetent valves within the GSV allow the stripper to be passed in this manner except occasionally, when it becomes necessary to expose the vein at the knee and pass the stripper antegrade toward the groin. This can be performed through a small incision placed precisely over the vein under ultrasound guidance.

In the event that stripping to the ankle is planned, the GSV is exposed through a small incision anterior to the medial malleolus and carefully dissected away from the saphenous nerve. The vein is ligated around the stripper in the groin with strong, nonabsorbable suture, which is left long, and the stripper is inverted into the saphenous vein (Figure 44-1). The vein is stripped from above downward, and the inverted vein is delivered through the knee incision. Inversion stripping is the preferred method, with decreased resultant trauma to surrounding structures. In the conventional form of stripping, the vein is stripped from the knee to the groin after attaching a head of varying size to the stripper device. Hemorrhage in the tract of the stripped vein is controlled by leg elevation, external pressure, and infiltration of the subcutaneous tissue around the saphenous vein with a tumescent solution of diluted lidocaine and epinephrine before stripping.

In an effort to decrease hemorrhage within the tract, cryostripping has been described. Following high ligation and division of the GSV, a cryoprobe (Erbokryo CA, ERBE, Germany) is inserted into the vein from the groin to the knee, freezing is initiated, and after a few seconds the vein is invaginated with a tug and stripped toward the groin. If indicated, concomitant stab avulsion of varicosities is performed before stripping of the vein so that the leg can be elevated and wrapped in an elastic bandage immediately after stripping. The incisions for the stripping are closed with absorbable sutures and those for stab avulsion with Steri-Strips. The operation is an outpatient procedure, and the patient is permitted to ambulate the same evening.

To avoid stripping and its associated potential complications of nerve injury, pain, and hematoma, high ligation alone was proposed to remove gravitational reflux while preserving the vein. However, reflux has been shown to persist following high ligation alone, and recurrence of varicose veins is more common when compared to high ligation with stripping.[4,5] Persistent patency of the GSV with continued reflux is often associated with recurrent varicose veins.[6,7]

High Ligation and Stripping of the Small Saphenous Vein

Stripping of the SSV is performed in a similar manner, keeping in mind that anatomical variations of the termination of the SSV are common. In 42% of cases, the vein terminates within 5 cm of the knee joint crease, this being the only termination. It may, however, terminate higher in the thigh in the femoropopliteal vein, in the vein of Giacomini (12%), or other unnamed subcutaneous and perforator veins. This anomalous drainage may coexist with a normal saphenopopliteal junction in 50% of cases. Because of this variability in the anatomy of the SSV, it is prudent to mark the saphenopopliteal junction on the skin if the duplex ultrasound is performed immediately before the operation. The procedure is performed through a small transverse incision in the middle of the popliteal fossa with the patient in the prone position. The stripper is inserted in a retrograde fashion, and damage to the sural nerve is avoided by carefully dissecting the distal end of the vein with the stripper within it, separating it from the vein. Reflux in the SSV is commonly segmental, so the distal segment at the ankle can often be spared from stripping.

Endovenous Ablation of Saphenous Vein Reflux

Endovenous Thermal Ablation of the Saphenous Vein

MECHANISM OF ACTION

The mechanism of action of endovenous therapy for GSV ablation involves thermal damage of the vein wall, resulting in destruction of the intima by a process of selective

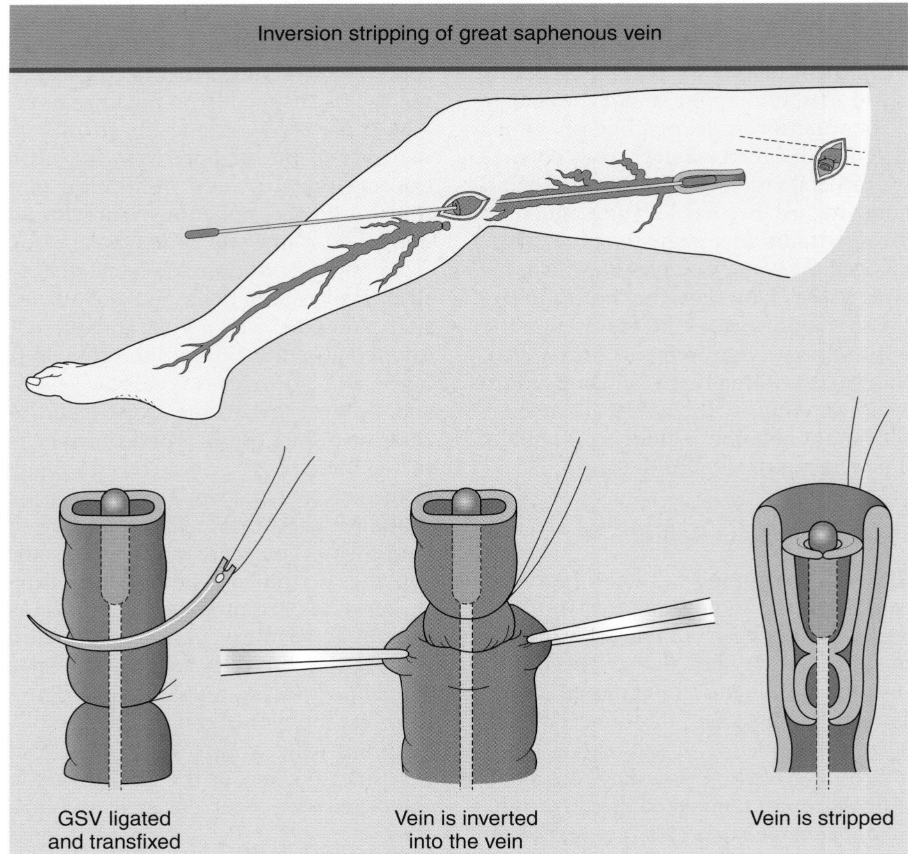

Figure 44-1. Inversion stripping of great saphenous vein (GSV). *Left,* GSV is ligated with a heavy tie, and a transfixing suture is placed around the vein and the stripper. *Middle,* The vein is inverted into the vein by applying tension around the outer wall of the vein. *Right,* The vein is completely inverted and stripped.

photothermolysis and collagen denaturation of the media, with eventual fibrotic occlusion of the vein over time. The two available methods for performing endovenous ablation include radiofrequency ablation (RFA; Closure and Closure-FAST) and endovenous laser treatment (EVLT). The laser system is available in continuous and pulsed modes, as well as in various frequencies, by several manufacturers.

The original RFA catheter uses electromagnetic energy to heat the vein wall by direct contact and therefore requires adjustment of catheter size according to the diameter of the target vein. Radiofrequency-induced resistive heating of the vein wall is controlled by vein wall temperature and impedance feedback. Direct heating of the vein wall occurs to a depth of 1 mm at the site of contact with the catheter, with further heating of the deeper vein wall occurring by conduction. The next-generation ClosureFAST catheter system employs the same basic principle of monitored resistive heating of the vein wall, but the same catheter is suitable for treating veins of all diameters.

The laser probe has a smaller profile, and two mechanisms are postulated for laser-induced thermal damage. The first is indirect heating and damage of the vein wall by intravascular steam-bubble generation by the laser probe, which heats to a temperature of 1000° C, resulting in thrombotic occlusion of the vein. The second involves more direct heating of an empty vein, possibly through a thin film of blood, resulting in direct damage to the vein wall. In the clinical setting, probably a combination of the two mechanisms is responsible for the efficacy of EVLT.

The available lasers include hemoglobin-specific laser wavelengths (810, 940, and 980 nm) and water-specific laser wavelengths (1320 and 1319 nm), with debatable differences in mode of action.[8] Intravascular blood plays a key role in homogeneously distributing the thermal damage throughout the inner vein wall. Proebstle et al. demonstrated the generation of steam bubbles with local and remote injury to the vein wall only in blood filled veins, thermal injury being confined to the site of laser contact in saline-filled veins.[9] The aim of EVLT is to damage the inner vein wall without causing a full thickness burn, which could lead to perforation of the vein with associated bruising or hematoma formation from extravascated blood. In an early animal study comparing endovenous RFA with EVLT, Weiss demonstrated perforation in all laser treated veins on histological examination.[10] Min et al. proposed that vein wall perforation was more likely with the pulsed mode compared to the continuous mode laser.[10a]

PATIENT SELECTION

The indications for endovenous ablation of the saphenous vein are identical to those for surgical high ligation and stripping. The importance of detailed preoperative duplex ultrasound examination cannot be overemphasized. The identification of all refluxing venous segments and their ablation is the key to minimizing recurrence of varicose veins.

Inappropriate vein size (less than 2 mm and more than 15 mm for RFA), a history of superficial thrombophlebitis resulting in a partially obstructed saphenous vein, and the uncommon occurrence of a tortuous GSV on duplex examination should be considered potential contraindications. No absolute contraindications to EVLT exist, including vein diameter although some authors have recently suggested the association of central GSV diameter greater than 15 mm with extension of thrombus into the femoral vein. Other relative contraindications to endovenous saphenous vein ablation include uncorrectable coagulopathy, liver dysfunction limiting local anesthetic use, immobility, pregnancy, and breast feeding.

TECHNIQUE

In comparison to traditional high ligation and stripping of the GSV, the endovenous techniques avoid accessing the groin altogether. The procedure can be performed under local, regional, or general anesthesia, depending on the need for concomitant ancillary procedures. The target vein to be ablated is accessed percutaneously with an 18- to 21-gauge needle under ultrasound guidance at or just below the lowest level of truncal reflux (Figure 44-2A). Placing the patient in reverse Trendelenburg position facilitates this by keeping the vein filled with blood. Guide wire access is obtained through the segment of vein to be treated, followed by insertion of a sheath. The bare laser fiber or RFA probe is introduced through the sheath into the GSV or SSV and advanced centrally to the saphenofemoral or saphenopopliteal junction, respectively. The catheter tip is positioned 1 cm distal to the inferior epigastric vein under ultrasound guidance (Figure 44-2B). When treating the SSV, this position is 10 to 15 mm distal to the saphenopopliteal junction.

The patient is now placed in Trendelenberg position, and the vein is emptied by elevation and compression by instillation of perivenous tumescent anesthesia with dilute anesthetic solution (100 to 300 ml of 0.1% lidocaine with 1 part per 10 million of epinephrine) into the saphenous canal (Figure 44-2C). The importance of adequate tumescent anesthesia has been learned with increasing experience with these techniques. In addition to enhancing contact of the vein wall with the treating catheter for therapeutic effectiveness, it provides analgesia and a heat sink around the treated vein, thereby decreasing heat-related injury to surrounding tissues and reducing the incidence of skin burns and paresthesias. The final position of the catheter is rechecked with duplex ultrasound, and the vein is ablated in a retrograde fashion to just above the puncture site (Figure 44-2D). Subsequently, the catheter is removed and temporary pressure is applied at the entry point. At the end of the procedure, the saphenous vein is reimaged to confirm successful obliteration and absence of thrombus protruding into the saphenofemoral junction (Figure 44-2E). If a patent segment is identified, retreatment is advisable. After GSV treatment, previously marked varicose veins can be treated if indicated, with the preferred method being avulsion or sclerotherapy. The skin incisions are approximated with Steri-Strips, and compression is applied to the extremity from foot to groin with an elastic compression bandage or compression stocking.

Data to support the routine administration of thromboprophylaxis with heparin are not available. Selected patients with a history of thrombophlebitis, deep venous thrombosis, or obesity or subjects older than 50 years of age may benefit from a single dose of low-molecular-weight heparin before the procedure, as these patients are considered to be at an increased risk of proximal extension of thrombus or deep venous thrombosis.[12]

RADIOFREQUENCY ABLATION The original Closure radiofrequency catheter (VNUS Medical Technologies, Sunnyvale, California), the first endovenous thermal ablation technique, was studied first in Europe and approved by the U.S. Food and Drug Administration (FDA) in 1999. The system consists of a bipolar heat generator and collapsible catheter electrodes suitable for use in veins ranging from 2 to 12 mm in diameter. The catheter provides 6- to 8-mm-wide rings of resistive heating of the vein wall and comes in two sizes and designs: 6- and 8-French (Fr), able to treat veins between 2 and 8 mm and 4 to 12 mm in diameter, respectively; it can be advanced over a 0.025-inch guide wire (Figure 44-3A). The 8-Fr catheter consists of two tufts of electrodes with a neutral central element; the 6-Fr catheter a single tuft of collapsible electrodes and a ball-tipped central element. The catheter has a central lumen for heparinized solution infusion (heparin of 5000 IU in 500 ml of normal saline at the rate of 1 drop/sec) to prevent venous thrombosis and accumulation of coagulated blood on the electrodes.

Following percutaneous venous access, positioning of the catheter, and instillation of local tumescent anesthetic, an Esmarch bandage is wrapped around the elevated leg to empty the vein and further enhance contact of the catheter with the vein wall. Additional compression is applied at the saphenofemoral junction to prevent reflux of blood into the vein. The electrodes are unsheathed, and heparinized saline is flushed continuously through the lumen of the catheter. After turning the device on, the vein wall temperature is allowed to equilibrate to the temperature set point (85° C to 90° C) for 15 seconds. Progressive withdrawal of the catheter is performed at a rate of 2.5 to 4 cm/min. The wall temperature is maintained within 3° C of the set temperature, and wattage display below 4 W to ensure the 12- to 16-second exposure needed for the maximal wall contraction. Impedance is kept over 150 ohms for 6-Fr catheters and greater than 100 ohms for 8-Fr catheters. If temperature and impedance exceed the upper or lower set limits, a message is displayed; if the condition persists, the generator shuts itself off. At the end of the procedure, the compression wrap is removed and obliteration of the entire length of the vein is confirmed by ultrasound. Segments not completely occluded are retreated.

This original technique was fairly cumbersome, and the pullback was much slower than the laser ablation method. The catheters were often associated with spasm of the vein and thrombus–coagulum formation despite the continuous heparin infusion, necessitating cessation of treatment, withdrawal, and reintroduction after cleaning.

A new-generation ClosureFAST catheter system was introduced by the same company in 2007 that addressed these problems, and the original system is being phased out. The basic principle of monitored resistive heating of the vein remains the same. The ClosureFAST device consists of a flexible 7-Fr catheter with a distal 7-cm-long heating element covered with a lubricious jacket to prevent sticking (Figure 44-3B). Continuous irrigation is no longer required. It is introduced through a short 8-Fr sheath and is 0.025-inch guide wire compatible.

The contact with the vein wall is achieved by leg elevation, circumferential tumescent anesthetic instillation around the vein, and manual external compression. It is monitored as before by the thermocouple in the catheter and the software in the generator. Following positioning of the catheter 2 cm distal to the saphenofemoral junction, sequential segmental heating of the vein is performed to 120° C in 20-second cycles. On completion of each cycle, the generator automatically shuts off delivery of energy until the catheter is repositioned to treat the next 7-cm segment. Accurate catheter positioning

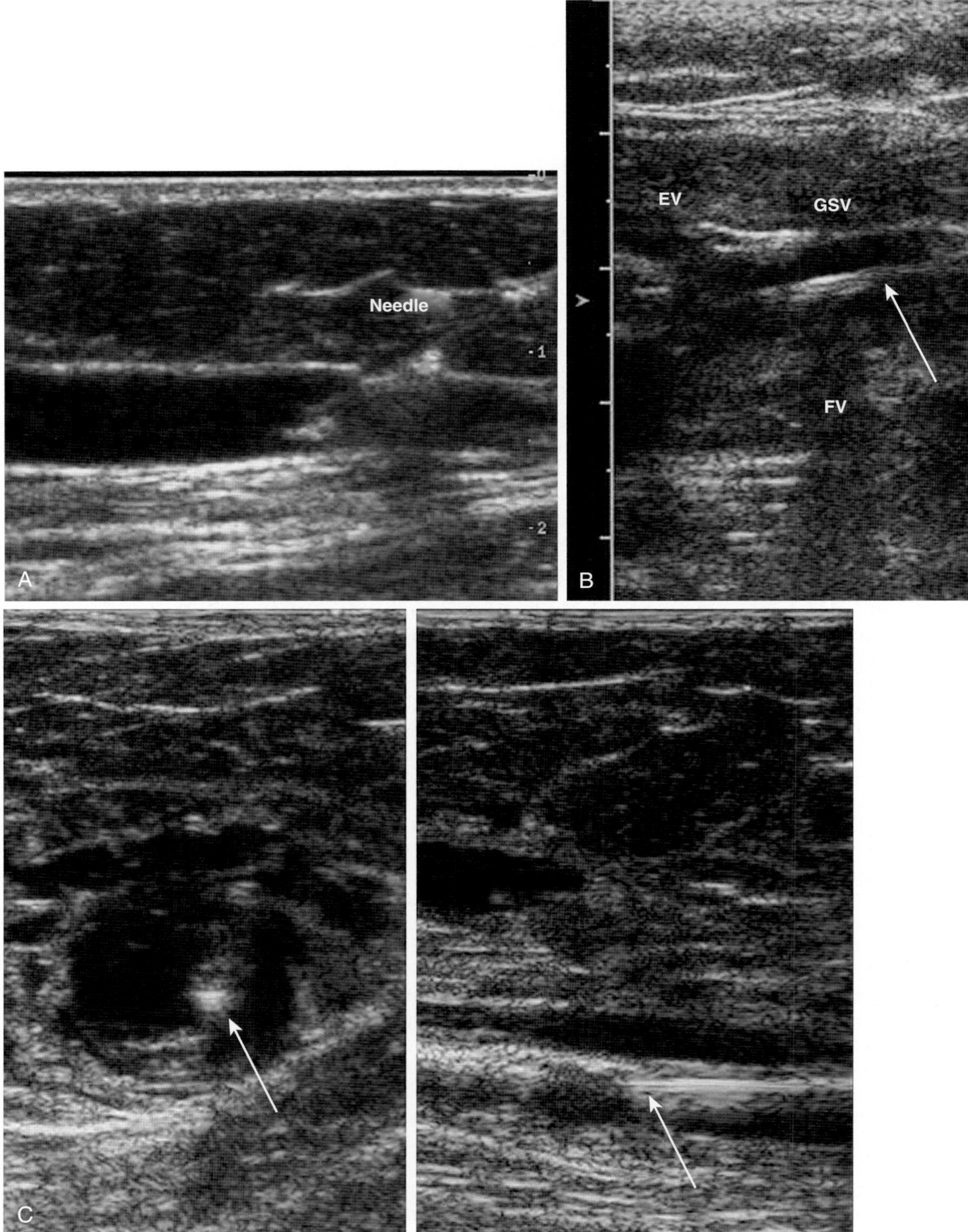

Figure 44-2. A, Longitudinal ultrasound image of percutaneous needle access of great saphenous vein (GSV). **B,** Longitudinal ultrasound image of the saphenofemoral junction demonstrating positioning of the laser fiber *(arrow)* in the GSV distal to the superficial inferior epigastric branch. **C,** Axial and longitudinal ultrasound images of GSV following instillation of tumescent anesthesia into the saphenous canal. Laser fiber with collapsed saphenous vein around it *(arrow)*.

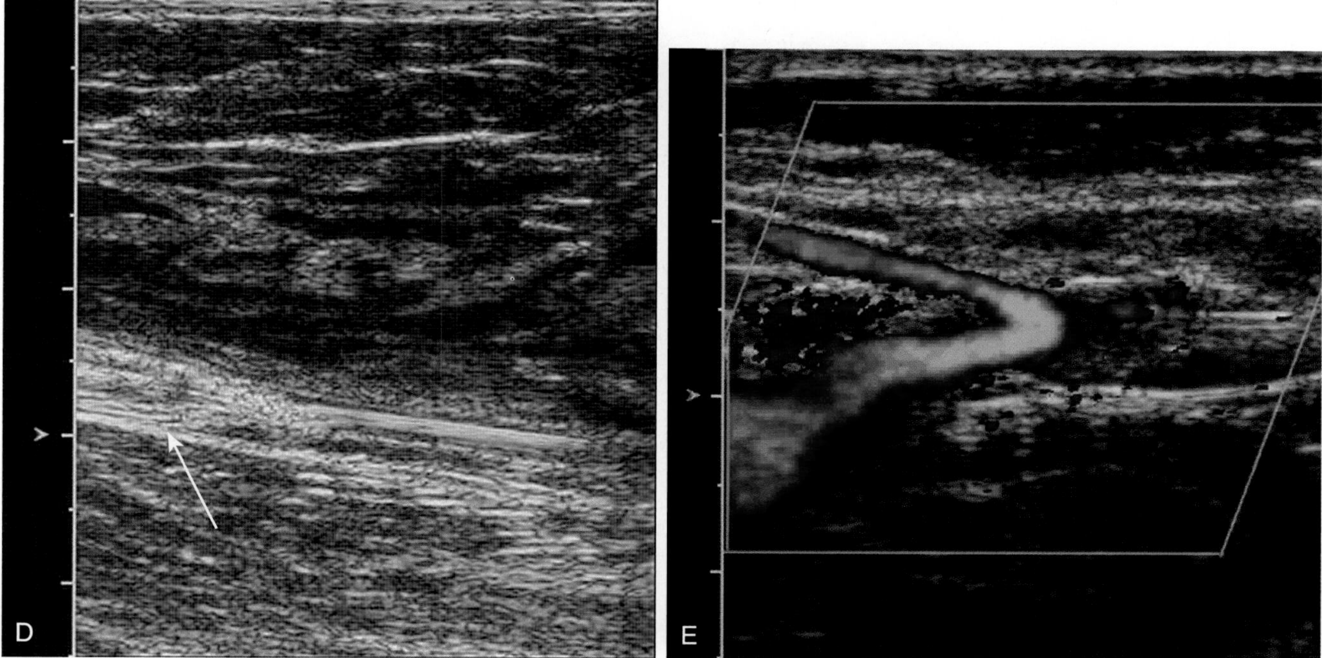

Figure 44-2—cont'd D, Longitudinal ultrasound image of GSV during withdrawal of laser fiber and delivery of laser energy. Intravascular steam bubbles generated by laser thermal energy in a blood-filled environment *(arrow)*. **E,** Longitudinal duplex ultrasound image of the saphenofemoral junction demonstrating normal blood flow in the femoral vein (FV) and inferior epigastric vein (EV), with occlusion of the GSV.

is aided by 6.5-cm increment markings on the shaft to ensure a 0.5-cm overlap of treatment and thus avoid skipping areas of the vein. The first segment is treated twice to ensure closure of the widest segment of vein; veins measuring 2 to 15 mm in diameter are suitable for treatment with this catheter (Figure 44-4). The ClosureFAST system is more user friendly and quicker than the original VNUS device, and the entire length of vein in the thigh can be treated in 3 to 4 minutes.

ENDOVENOUS LASER TREATMENT The first report of endoluminal delivery of laser energy was by Bone.[13] Navarro et al. first reported using endovenous laser to ablate a segment of refluxing GSV.[14] The 810-, 940-, 980-, 1319-, and 1320-nm diode lasers are effective in inducing vessel occlusion.

The tip of a 5-Fr sheath is advanced to the saphenofemoral junction over a 0.035-inch J-tip guide wire. The sheath has markings that facilitate determination of the length of the segment of vein to be treated. A 600-μm-core tip fiber connected to the Diode laser is inserted into the sheath and advanced until the distal marker on the fiber reaches the tip of the introducer sheath (Figure 44-3C). The introducer sheath is then withdrawn 2.5 cm while holding the fiber still until the proximal marker on the fiber reaches the introducer opening, exposing the laser fiber for treatment (Figure 44-5). Laser energy is then delivered (14 W of power in a continuous mode or as per manufacturer instructions). The final position of the laser catheter is rechecked under ultrasound, and the sheath and laser fiber are withdrawn together at a rate of 2 to 3 mm/sec to deliver 50 to 70 Joules/cm of vein. These parameters are for continuous laser treatment with an 810-nm diode laser (Angiodynamics, Queensbury, NY). Manual withdrawal of the laser fiber allows adjustment of the energy delivered to suit the level and size of the venous segment: greater energy for larger, proximal vein and less for distal, superficial vein.

Following completion of laser ablation, patency of the femoral vein and complete occlusion of the GSV are confirmed by ultrasound evaluation. The procedure is faster than the original RFA, and there is no size limitation of the veins that can be treated.

POSTPROCEDURE CARE

A graduated compression stocking (30 to 40 mm Hg) or wrap is applied to the extremity from the base of the toes to the groin and kept on at all times for 2 weeks and when upright or ambulatory thereafter for 6 weeks. Immediate and frequent ambulation is encouraged. Most authors recommend early U.S. evaluation within 72 hours to confirm successful ablation and rule out complications, as well as long-term duplex ultrasound surveillance to assure continued fibrotic occlusion of the vein.

Foam Sclerotherapy of the Great Saphenous Vein

The introduction of duplex ultrasound to the evaluation and treatment of varicose veins in the late 1980s rekindled a waning interest in another endovenous method of treatment, namely, sclerotherapy. Despite improved GSV obliteration rates, ultrasound guidance did not significantly affect the 20% incidence of recanalization.[15] Although the four to five times greater efficacy of "frothed sclerosant with air" was first noted by Orbach[15a] in 1944, it was only in 1997 after Cabrera et al. published results of GSV ablation with the technique in 261 patients that the technique received attention.[16] The increased efficacy of foamed sclerosant is attributed to its ability to displace the blood in the vein, with resultant superior contact of the sclerosant with the vein wall. The air in the foamed mixture prevents the detergent sclerosant from mixing with blood, getting protein bound and inactivated.

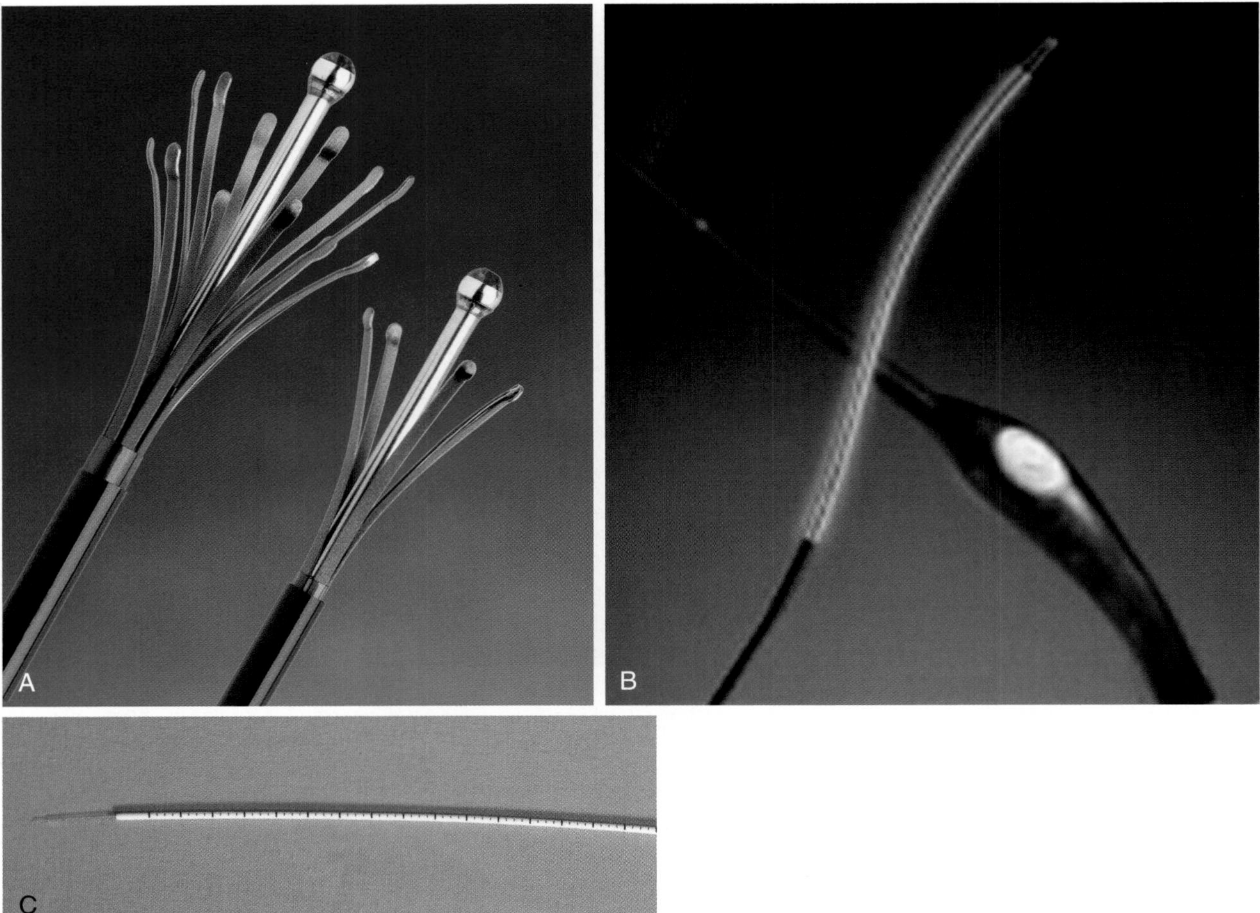

Figure 44-3. **A,** First-generation 8-Fr and 6-Fr Closure catheters with 1-cm-long treatment length. **B,** Next-generation ClosureFAST 7-Fr catheter with 7-cm treatment length. **C,** Endovenous 5-Fr laser probe with heating tip within sheath with external markings.

The technique involves mixing one part of liquid sclerosant (polidocanol or sodium tetradecyl sulfate) with four parts air and injecting it immediately into the incompetent GSV or SSV to be ablated. Tessari described a simple method of creating small-bubble sclerosant foam for immediate use by passing a mixture of air and sclerosant (4:1) between two syringes 20 times with the help of a three-way stopcock.[17] The vein is cannulated distally under ultrasound guidance, and the entire length of vein to be ablated is filled with the foam sclerosant, filling of the proximal vein being aided by elevation of the leg. Kolbel et al. have further refined the technique by injecting the sclerosant foam through a sheath in the GSV introduced percutaneously over a guide wire.[18] The volume of foam to be injected can be calculated from the diameter of the vein as assessed on ultrasound. The communicating branch varicosities should be injected simultaneously to prevent reflux of blood into the treated GSV that might promote subsequent recanalization. Following treatment, a compression bandage or stocking is applied to the leg. Most published results are with the use of operator-made 1% to 3% polidocanol or sodium tetradecyl sulfate foam, the only commercially made product (Varisolve, Provensis, Wrexham, United Kingdom) being studied in the United Kingdom. The only FDA-approved sclerotherapy product in the United States is sodium tetradecyl sulfate in 1% and 3% strengths (Bioniche Life Sciences, Belleville, Ontario, Canada; distributed by Angiodynamics).

Removal of Varicose Veins

In most patients, ablation of the refluxing saphenous vein is not sufficient to eliminate all varicosities. Complete care of the patient with varicose veins requires adjunctive treatment of the varicose tributaries in the form of ambulatory phlebectomy or sclerotherapy.

Stab Avulsion of Varicosities (Ambulatory Phlebectomy)

Stab avulsion of varicosities is performed through 1- to 2-mm incisions overlying the vein clusters marked preoperatively with the patient in the standing position. These incisions are oriented vertically to minimize injury to lymphatic channels, except at the knee or ankle, where they are placed transversely in the skin creases. The incision is deepened through the epidermis and dermis, and the varicose vein is grasped with a crochet or Muller hook. It is delivered through the incision, grasped with a mosquito clamp, extracted gradually, and avulsed (Figure 44-6). As much length of vein as possible is harvested through each incision, and incisions are placed as

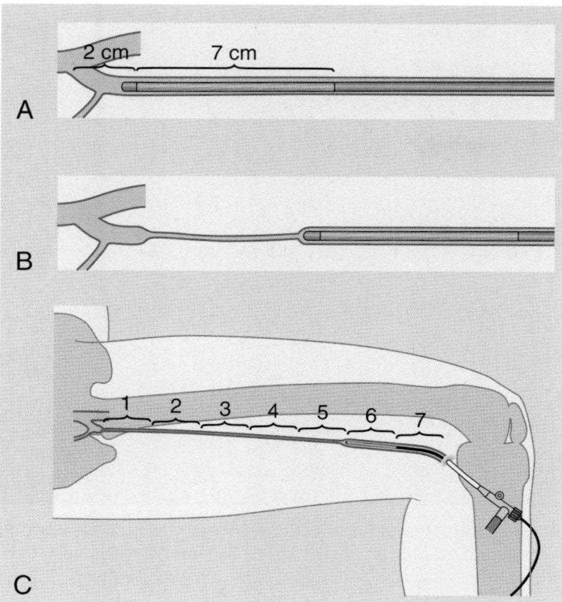

Figure 44-4. Endovenous ablation of the great saphenous vein (GSV) with the ClosureFAST radiofrequency ablation device. **A,** Following percutaneous access of the GSV and placement of the 11-cm-long 7-Fr sheath, the ClosureFAST catheter is introduced and positioned 2 cm distal to the saphenofemoral junction. **B,** The patient is placed in Trendelenburg position, tumescent anesthesia is instilled within the saphenous canal, external compression is applied, and the vein is sequentially heated in 7-cm segments to 120° C in 20-second cycles. The proximal segment of the vein is treated over two consecutive cycles. **C,** The entire length of vein with reflux is ablated, and the catheter and sheath are withdrawn. Hemostasis at the puncture site is achieved with pressure.

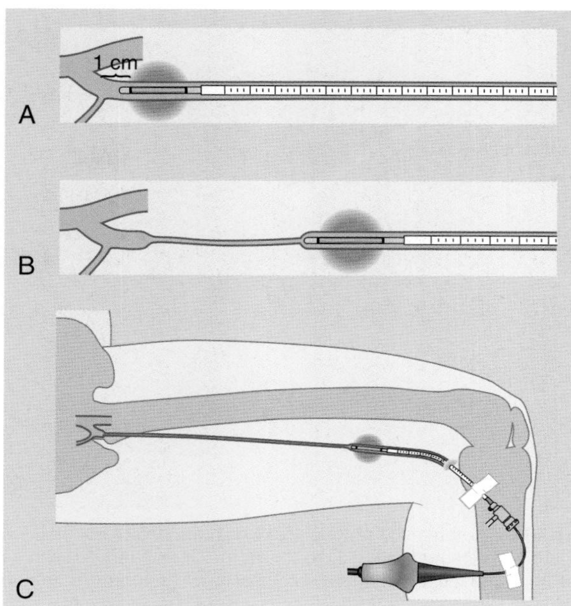

Figure 44-5. Endovenous laser ablation of the great saphenous vein (GSV). **A,** Following percutaneous access of the GSV and placement of the 45-cm-long 5-Fr sheath, the laser fiber is introduced and positioned 1 cm distal to the entry of the inferior epigastric vein. The sheath is withdrawn 2.5 cm to expose the laser fiber. **B,** The patient is placed in Trendelenburg position, tumescent anesthesia is instilled within the saphenous canal, and laser energy is delivered by manual withdrawal of the laser fiber and sheath together at a rate of 2 to 3 mm/sec. **C,** The entire length of vein with reflux is ablated, and the catheter and sheath are withdrawn. Hemostasis at the puncture site is achieved with pressure.

far apart as possible. Small (1 to 2 mm) incisions are closed with Steri-Strips and the larger ones with a single, inverted absorbable suture. A compression bandage is applied at the end of the procedure.

Power suction phlebectomy is a relatively newer, minimally invasive technique of varicosity removal that employs pulverization of the varicose vein clusters with a motorized blade and concomitant suction removal. Tumescent local anesthesia is instilled in the entire area of the varicosities. The TriVex device (Smith and Nephew, Andover, Massachusetts) includes a transillumination probe inserted into a plane deep to the veins to guide accurate maneuvering of the extractor probe. This probe consists of a motorized blade with a lateral cutting edge and a distal blunt tip ensheathed within a tube. Suction draws the vein into the cutting window of the blade and removes the pulverized vein through the inner channel. The control unit allows adjustment of the level of suction and blade movement, as well as simultaneous irrigation with anesthetic solution. It is important to keep the subcutaneous space well instilled with fluid to avoid extravascation of blood with postoperative bruising.

Sclerotherapy of Branch Varicosities

Spider veins and small-branch varicosities, typically less than 4 mm in size, can be treated with sclerotherapy with liquid or foamed sclerosant effectively, in conjunction with or subsequent to ablation of axial superficial venous reflux.

RESULTS OF SUPERFICIAL REFLUX ABLATION

Short-Term Results

Stripping of the GSV to the level of the knee accompanied by high ligation and interruption of all tributaries in the groin is the most accepted surgical method of superficial reflux ablation. Stripping of longer segments increases morbidity, especially the incidence of saphenous neuralgia (7% versus 1.6%), without improving recurrence rates.[19] In addition to the favorable cosmetic result from removal of unsightly varicose veins, the procedure provides relief from the symptoms of venous hypertension. Inversion stripping is less traumatic than conventional stripping and has been shown to be associated with decreased blood loss and lower incidence of saphenous neuralgia, confirmed in a recent randomized, controlled trial.[20] Compared to stripping of the GSV, high ligation alone is associated more commonly with recurrent varicose veins due to the inability of this operation to eradicate axial reflux.[4,21] In most cases, the saphenous vein remains patent in its entirety or segmentally, being fed by connecting thigh perforator veins.

Two recent prospective, randomized trials evaluating cryostripping demonstrated a shorter operative time and less bruising but equivalent postoperative pain, mobility, complications, and improvement in objectively measured quality of life on comparison to conventional stripping.[22,23] With the advent of endovenous ablation techniques, most recent

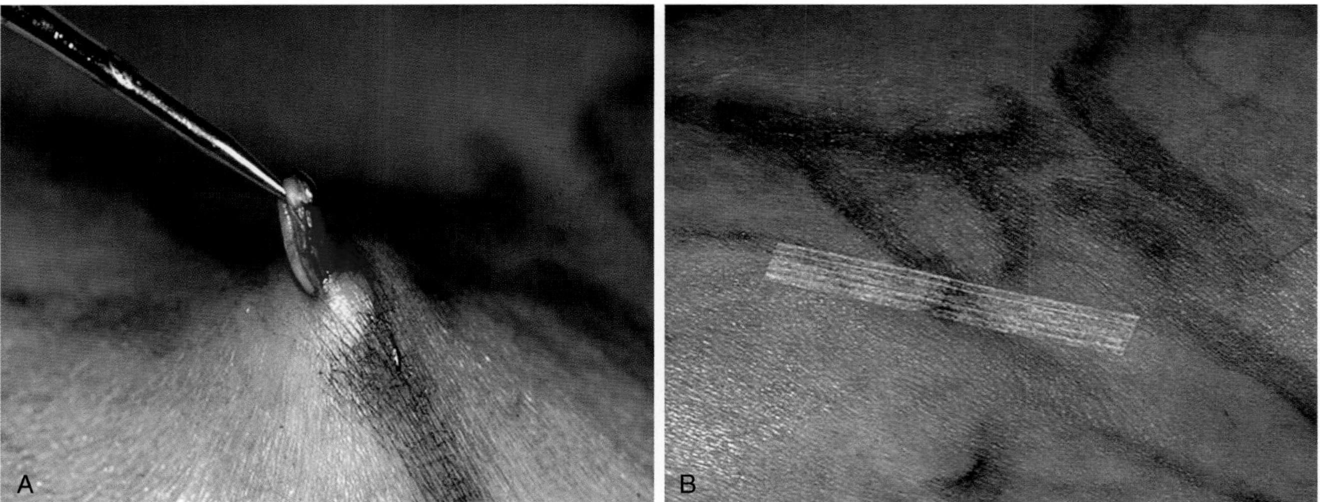

Figure 44-6. Ambulatory phlebectomy of branch varicose veins. **A,** The veins are peroperatively marked on the skin with the patient upright. The veins are hooked up through 1- to 2-mm incisions, grasped with a mosquito clamp, extracted gradually, and avulsed. **B,** Hemostasis is achieved with elevation of the leg and manual compression. The incisions are closed with Steri-Strips.

studies have concentrated on comparing these techniques with the traditional high ligation and stripping. Most practitioners who have used both techniques have observed decreased discomfort and better patient acceptance, with the minimally invasive endovenous procedures.

The original Closure technique of RFA is well tolerated, with minimal short- and long-term morbidity, and results in cessation of duplex-detectable flow in 90% to 96% of limbs (Table 44-1).[12,24-26] Early return to full activity is the norm, and in one study 98% of patients expressed satisfaction with the procedure on a 6-month follow-up survey.[10] Short-term results from the VNUS Closure Registry that enrolled 319 limbs in 286 patients with GSV truncal reflux in veins less than 12 mm diameter from 31 centers in Europe, Australia, and the United States were reported in 2002.[27,28] Partial or complete recanalization in initially successfully treated veins occurred in 12% of limbs by 12 months but without demonstrable reflux on duplex ultrasound.

The clinical benefits of RFA have been demonstrated in four separate randomized clinical studies comparing this technique with conventional stripping.[25,29-31] The EVOLVeS study was a prospective, multicenter, randomized study that included 85 patients randomized to RFA versus high ligation and stripping. Closure resulted in a 91% initial occlusion rate, earlier return to work, less postoperative pain, and better early quality-of-life scores.[25] Complication rates were similar in both groups, but average pain postoperatively was significantly less severe in the endovenous obliteration group. Absence from work was also shorter and physical function was restored faster than in the stripping group, with resultant potential cost saving for society.[29] With increasing experience, the effect of RFA on clinical outcome has been further objectively validated with significant improvement in the venous severity score.[32]

Similarly, early success in terms of ablation of the refluxing vein has been reported as 90% to 98% of patients with EVLT.[10,10a,14] Large, single-center experiences with EVLT have achieved 97% to 98% early occlusion rates and maintained occlusion in 93% of limbs at 3 years.[10a,33,34] Kabnick reported 96% successful occlusion following GSV ablation with the 980-nm laser in an international registry of 5262 patients, and similar efficacy in ablating the GSV has been reported with other wavelengths.[35,36] Some evidence shows that the water-specific laser wavelengths (1320 and 1319 nm) result in less postoperative discomfort; however, no definite evidence supports the use of one laser wavelength over another.[35,37] In addition, a statistically significant improvement in the CEAP classification has been documented following EVLT. In the only prospective, randomized trial comparing EVLT to stripping performed under tumescent anesthesia in 121 patients, Rasmussen et al. reported higher postoperative pain scores in the surgical group but no significant difference in analgesics consumed, time to return to normal activity, or to work. All quality-of-life measure scores appropriately deteriorated early in the postprocedure period but improved significantly by 3 months in both groups.[38]

While RFA and EVLT are similar procedures, employing the principle of endovenous thermal injury to ablate the saphenous vein, some differences exist. In an early report, successful early occlusion of the GSV was similar with the two techniques; 94.4% with EVLT and 90.9% with RFA.[12] The overall local complication rate was significantly higher in the EVLT patients: 20.8% versus 7.6% in the RFA group. Similar observations have been reported by Almeida and Raines, who recently compared experience with RFA and EVLT at a single institution and found a statistically significant difference in occlusion rates in favor of EVLT.[39] On the other hand, Marston et al. reported no significant difference in the frequency of closure of the vein, improvement in venous filling index, CEAP class, and venous clinical severity scores between the two techniques in a study of 80 patients.[40]

Early results of saphenous ablation using the new Closure-FAST system reveal an improvement over the original RFA catheter in terms of ease of use and procedure time, as well as significantly higher short-term occlusion rate. Proebstle et al. reported the first results in 194 patients (252 limbs) with an occlusion rate of the GSV of 99.6% at 6 months on Kaplan-Meier analysis. The average energy delivered to the proximal

Table 44-1
Early Results of Radiofrequency Ablation*

Author	Year	Limbs (*n*)	Occlusion Rate (%)	Skin Burns (%)	Paresthesia (%)	Phlebitis (%)	DVT (%)	PE (%)
Chandler et al.[27]	2000	218	93	2	15	7	2	1
Manfrini et al.[24]	2000	152	91	2	9	10	3	1
Weiss[10]	2002	140	90	0	4	0	0	0
Merchant et al.[28]	2002	318	85	4	15	2	1	1
Rautio et al.[29]	2002	30	83	3	10	6	0	0
Sybrady[83]	2002	26	88	4	19	0	0	0
Lurie et al.[25]	2003	44	90	2	23	4	0	0
Wagner	2004	28	100	0	0	7	4	4
Hingorani et al.[26]	2004	73	96				16	0
ClosureFAST								
Proebstle et al.[41]	2008	252	100	2	3	1	0	0

*DVT, deep vein thrombosis; PE, pulmonary embolism.

7-cm segment of vein was 116 J/cm and to the subsequent 7-cm segments was 68 J/cm, similar to those recommended for successful ablation following EVLT.[41] The venous severity score decreased following treatment from an average of 3.9 ± 2 preoperatively to 1.5 ± 1.8 at 6 months.

Office-based foam sclerosant treatment to ablate axial superficial venous reflux has gained immense popularity over the last few years; however, the need for multiple treatments remains a concern. The earliest series by Cabrera et al.[16] and Frullini[42] reported 80% to 90% occlusion of the GSV. Early occlusion following ultrasound-guided foam sclerotherapy of the GSV has been empirically considered to be superior to treatment with liquid foam for a decade, but the two methods have only recently been directly compared. Hamel-Desnos et al. reported elimination of reflux in the 84% of GSVs treated with foam sclerosant versus 40% of those treated with liquid sclerosant and subsequently equivalent results with 1% and 3% polidocanol foam.[11,43] Other authors similarly found significantly greater incidence of GSV occlusion at 1 year following foam versus liquid sclerotherapy with 3% polidocanol (68% to 69% versus 18% to 27%), as well as sustained hemodynamic benefit and lower incidence of recurrent varicose veins (8% versus 25%).[44,45] Factors unfavorable for a successful outcome include large-diameter veins and use of a low volume of dilute foamed sclerosant.[45,46]

Complications

The most significant complication of saphenous vein stripping is saphenous neuralgia that may occur in 4% to 8% of patients. The incidence can be minimized by limiting the stripping from the groin to the knee. However, van Neer et al. reported persistent reflux in the below-knee GSV in all patients following stripping to the knee alone and residual visible residual varicose veins in 20% of patients.[47] Hematoma, cellulitis, edema, or thrombophlebitis can also occur in the residual thrombosed superficial veins. Deep venous thrombosis or pulmonary embolism is rare.

Minor complications following RFA ablation and EVLT are reported in 3% to 10% of patients and include bruising around the puncture site, bleeding, transient paresthesias, superficial phlebitis, skin burns, or pigmentation (Tables 44-1 and 44-2). Paresthesias have been reported more often following RFA compared to EVLT. In the VNUS Registry, paresthesia was observed in 12.3% of 985 limbs at the initial 1-week follow-up. The incidence decreased to 7.3% by 6 months and was 2.6% at 5 years. Slightly higher paresthesia rates at 6 months have been reported with below-knee GSV treatment (11.6%) and SSV treatment (9.5%).[48] The incidence of skin burns and paresthesias has decreased significantly with increasing experience and routine use of tumescent anesthesia to less than 1%.[49] The risk of thrombophlebitis in branch veins can be avoided by performing concomitant ambulatory phlebectomy. Patients undergoing EVLT often experience a tight, pulling sensation in the medial thigh along the course of the treated GSV secondary to thrombotic occlusion of the vein and thrombophlebitis peaking at 4 to 7 days and lasting 3 to 10 days.[11] This can be significantly minimized by emptying the vein adequately and treating the "empty vein." Although no published reports directly compare postprocedure discomfort following RFA and EVLT, less postoperative bruising and discomfort have been observed with RFA by independent operators. A recently completed prospective trial confirmed this impression in early deliberations.[50] In the first reported series of GSV ablation with the ClosureFAST system, greater than two thirds of patients experienced no pain or tenderness over the treated vein; incidence of ecchymosis was 6% and of paresthesia was 3%, other complications being negligible (Table 44-1).[41]

The more serious complications of deep venous thrombosis and extension of thrombus into the femoral vein have been variously reported in none to 6% of the limbs treated, with one report of 16%.[26] A learning curve shows a decrease in the incidence of all complications with experience (5.5% to 2.3% in our experience).[12,51] The incidence of pulmonary embolism is sufficiently low that the consensus of opinion remains against routine GSV ligation.[52] The reported incidence of deep venous thrombosis is similarly low following SSV ablation, except in one recent report of 5.7% in cohort of 67 patients.[53,54]

Major complications following foam sclerotherapy are rare, are similar to those following conventional liquid sclerotherapy, and are usually short lived. These include urticaria, migraine headaches, scotoma, chest tightness, dry cough, superficial thrombophlebitis, deep venous thrombosis, and skin necrosis.[55] The addition of air to create foam has not been shown to add to the risks of regular sclerotherapy. In fact, foam may decrease some adverse effects because of the increase in effectiveness and thereby the decrease in the volume of sclerosant used.

Table 44-2
Early Results of Endovenous Laser Ablation*

Author	Year	Limbs (n)	Laser Wavelength (nm)	Occlusion Rate (%)	Skin Burns (%)	Paresthesia (%)	Phlebitis (%)	DVT (%)	PE (%)
Navarro et al.[14]	2001	40	810	100.0	0	0	0	0	0
Min[10a]	2003	499	810	98.2	0	5	0	0	0
Proebstle et al.[54]	2003	104	940	90.4	0	10	0	0	0
Perkowski et al.[33]	2004	203	940	97.0	0	0	0	0	0
Puggioni et al.[12]	2005	77	810	94.4	0	5	0	2.30	0
Timperman[36]	2005	100	810	95.0	0	0	0	0	0
Bush et al.[34]	2005	640	940	95.0				0	0
Kabnick[49]	2005	5262	980	96.0				0.27	0.023
Gradman[85]	2005	346	940					0.14	0.013

*DVT, deep vein thrombosis; PE, pulmonary embolism.

Long-Term Results

Traditional surgical treatment of varicose veins with high ligation and stripping is associated with durable relief from symptoms despite the initial morbidity of the procedure. The superior long-term outcome of stripping over high ligation, sclerotherapy, and a combination of the two has been confirmed in prospective, randomized trials.[56,57] At a mean follow-up of 3 to 5 years, 71% to 90% of stripped patients had functional improvement, which was also supported by improved hemodynamic parameters. Significant improvement in quality of life have been demonstrated prospectively by SF-36 as well as venous disease-specific (Aberdeen Varicose Vein Severity Score) questionnaires.[58] A more recent randomized, prospective clinical trial evaluating stripping with or without phlebectomy and conservative treatment in 246 patients with uncomplicated varicose veins found significant improvement in symptoms and quality of life in surgically treated patients to 2 years.[59]

Unlike the guaranteed abolition of the GSV following high ligation and stripping, the fate of the treated vein following endovenous ablation needs to be monitored. Mid- and long-term results following RFA and EVLT have become available in the last few years. At 1 year and beyond, complete disappearance of the GSV or minimal residual fibrous cord with no flow detectable on duplex ultrasound is usual. Nicolini reported 3-year results following RFA in 330 limbs; total occlusion rate was 75%, partial occlusion (less than 5 cm of open segment) 18%, and incomplete occlusion (more than 5 cm of open segment) 7%.[60] Long-term results of the Closure Study Group at 5 years following RFA were published by Merchant and Pichot in 2005 (Table 44-3).[48] The multicenter, prospective registry comprises data from more than 1200 limbs treated. Occlusion rates at 1, 2, and 5 years were 87.1%, 88.2%, and 87.2%, respectively. Duplex ultrasound identified 185 limbs that had one of the following modes of anatomical failure (Figure 44-7):

Type I failure: (nonocclusion) refers to veins that failed to occlude initially and never occluded during the follow-up (12.4%)

Type II failure: (recanalization) refers to veins that were initially occluded but later recanalized, partly or completely (69.7%)

Type III failure: (groin reflux) refers to the situation in which the vein trunk was occluded but reflux was detected at the groin region, often involving an accessory vein (17.8%)

It is important to point out that anatomical failure did not necessarily result in clinical failure. Significant relief from symptoms (pain, fatigue, and edema) was noted in most patients; 70% to 80% of those with anatomical failure remained asymptomatic, compared to 85% to 94% of those with anatomical success. However, when the impact of

Table 44-3
Late Results of Endovenous Ablation of the Great Saphenous Vein*

Author, Year	No. of Limbs	Procedure	Follow-up (Years)	Total Occlusion (%)	Partial Occlusion (%)
Rautio, 2001[86]	33	RFA	1	75	26
Lurie, 2003[25]	44	RFA	2	89	7
Merchant, 2002[28]	319	RFA	2	85	4
Pichot, 2004[74]	65	RFA	2	90	10
Nicolini, 2005[60]	330	RFA	3	75	17
Merchant, 2005[48]	1222	RFA	5	87	8
Min, 2003[10a]	499	EVLT	2	93	
Sadick, 2004[62]	30	EVLT	2	97	
Timperman, 2005[36]	100	EVLT	1	91	4
Proebstle, 2008[41]	252	ClosureFAST	0.5	99	
Ouvry, 2008[78]	47	Polidocanol Foam	3	53	

*EVLT, endovenous laser therapy; RFA, radiofrequency ablation.

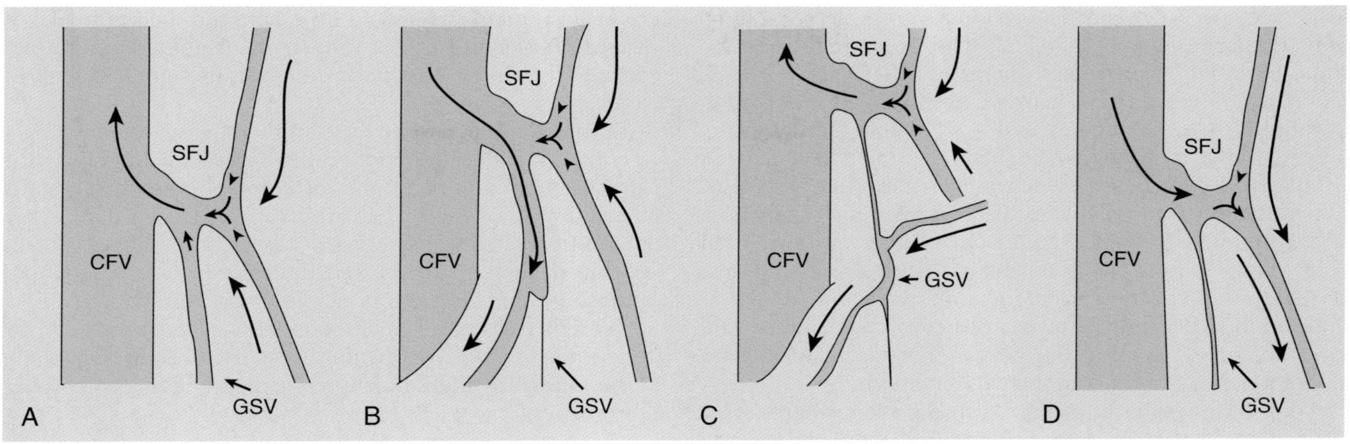

Figure 44-7. Types of anatomical failure following radiofrequency ablation of the great saphenous vein. **A,** Type I failure: (nonocclusion) refers to veins that failed to occlude initially and never occluded during the follow-up. **B,** Type II failure: (recanalization) refers to veins that were initially occluded but later recanalized, partly or completely. **C,** Type III failure: (groin reflux) refers to the situation in which the vein trunk was occluded but reflux was detected at the groin region, often involving an accessory vein. CFV, common femoral vein; GSV, great saphenous vein; SFJ, saphenofemoral junction. (From Merchant RF, Pichot O. *J Vasc Surg* 2005;42[3]:502-509; discussion, 509.)

anatomical failure on varicose vein recurrence was examined, type II and type III failures were found to be risk factors for varicose vein recurrence. In addition, catheter pullback speed and body mass index were the two risk factors associated with RFA anatomical failures. Two-year results of the randomized, controlled trials comparing RFA to high ligation, and stripping reported similar results, with 91.2% versus 91.7% of limbs free of reflux for RFA versus high ligation.[29,61] In the EVOLVeS trial, at 2 years recurrent varicose veins were noted in 14% of the RFA group versus 21% of the surgical group, with a statistically maintained better quality-of-life score in the RFA group.[61]

The excellent early occlusion rates following EVLT have been maintained from 93% to 97% on follow-up to 2 years, with most recurrences occurring by the first 3 months (Table 44-3).[11,62,63] Longer follow-up to 4 years has demonstrated a 95% success rate, with recurrences in reflux occurring secondary to recanalization and not to neovascularization. Sadick and Wasser reported a recurrence rate of 4.3% at 2 years on duplex ultrasound in 94 patients undergoing EVLT and ambulatory phlebectomy.[64] The success of EVLT has been shown to depend on the amount of laser energy delivered with nonocclusion and early reopening of the GSV seen more often with delivery of less than 70 J/cm.[65-67] Most occur early; however, late reopening of the thrombotically occluded veins is known to occur after 2 to 3 years.[63] Overall, long-term occlusion rates have been noticed to be better following EVLT compared to RFA. In a recent retrospective, direct comparative study Almeida and Raines reported primary closure rate by Kaplan-Meier analysis of 85% for RFA (5.5% recanalization) and 92% for EVLT (1.7% recanalization) at 500 days.[39] Early occlusion rates with the new ClosureFAST system are excellent; however, extended results are awaited.

Following treatment of varicose veins, recurrent varicose veins develop in up to 40% of patients on long-term follow-up, the incidence increasing with the length of follow-up. The incidence of recurrence following treatment of secondary varicose veins as high as 65% has been reported.[58,68-70] This seems to be constant regardless of the modality of saphenous vein ablation. Following stripping, a second, previously unrecognized saphenous system or inadequate ligation of the saphenous tributaries accounts for most failures.[58] The significance of removing all tributaries in the groin to primary or even secondary branches was emphasized in 1995 by Ruckley's study of 128 limbs with recurrent varicose veins, which identified a residual inguinal network as an important cause of recurrence.[6] In a contemporary series, even following duplex confirmation of adequate surgical treatment at 3 weeks, recurrent veins occurred in 25% of patients at 5 years, with 13% arising from the saphenofemoral junction, 30% at the saphenopopliteal junction, and 36% associated with both.[68] Hematoma formation within the GSV track has been correlated with subsequent revascularization.[71] Hartmann et al. found junctional recurrences in less than one third of extremities 14 years following high saphenofemoral junction or saphenopopliteal junction ligation and stripping and attributed recurrences to neovascularization and obesity.[69] Neovascularization in the groin has been cited as the predominant cause of recurrent saphenofemoral reflux, is associated with a persistently patent GSV, and occurs more often (52%) following high ligation than high ligation and stripping (23%).[72] However, this entity has been the topic of a longstanding discussion, with recent collective data implicating it as one of the major mechanisms responsible for recurrent saphenofemoral junction reflux. The techniques of RFA and EVLT violate this basic principle of treatment of superficial reflux, namely, high ligation. Proponents of endovenous ablation attribute this neovascularization to postsurgical scarring.

Keeping these concerns in mind, initial GSV ablations with RF were performed in conjunction with high ligation of the GSV. Over the ensuing years, endovenous ablation of the GSV without dissection of the saphenofemoral junction has become the accepted standard of care. Surprisingly, the combined experiences with transcatheter endovenous ablation procedures have shown lower saphenofemoral reflux rates than traditionally reported following surgical ligation and stripping short term and midterm. The theory proposed is that minimizing dissection in the groin and preserving venous drainage in normal, competent tributaries draining the abdominal wall while ablating only the abnormal refluxing segments does not

21. Fligelstone L, Carolan G, Pugh N, et al. An assessment of the long saphenous vein for potential use as a vascular conduit after varicose vein surgery. *J Vasc Surg* 1993;18(5):836-840.
22. Schouten R, Mollen RM, Kuijpers HC. A comparison between cryosurgery and conventional stripping in varicose vein surgery: perioperative features and complications. *Ann Vasc Surg* 2006;20(3):306-311.
23. Menyhei G, Gyevnar Z, Arato E, et al. Conventional stripping versus cryostripping: a prospective randomised trial to compare improvement in quality of life and complications. *Eur J Vasc Endovasc Surg* 2008;35;(2):218-223.
24. Manfrini V, Gasbarro G, Danielsson L, et al. Endovenous Reflux Management Study Group: endovenous management of saphenous vein reflux. *J Vasc Surg* 2000;32:330-342.
25. Lurie F, Creton D, Eklof B, et al. Prospective randomized study of endovenous radiofrequency obliteration (closure procedure) versus ligation and stripping in a selected patient population (EVOLVeS Study). *J Vasc Surg* 2003;38(2):207-214.
26. Hingorani AP, Ascher E, Markevich N, et al. Deep venous thrombosis after radiofrequency ablation of greater saphenous vein: a word of caution. *J Vasc Surg* 2004;40(3):500-504.
27. Chandler J, Pichot O, Sessa C, et al. Treatment of primary venous insufficiency by endovenous saphenous obliteration. *Vasc Surg* 2000;34:201-214.
28. Merchant RF, DePalma RG, Kabnick LS. Endovascular obliteration of saphenous reflux: a multicenter study. *J Vasc Surg* 2002;35(6):1190-1196.
29. Rautio T, Ohinmaa A, Perala J, et al. Endovenous obliteration versus conventional stripping operation in the treatment of primary varicose veins: a randomized controlled trial with comparison of the costs. *J Vasc Surg* 2002;35(5):958-965.
30. Stotter L, Schaaf I, Fendl R, Bockelbrink A. radiowellenobliteraion, invaginierstes stripping oder kryostripping: welches verhfaren belastet den patienten am wenigsten? Eine prospektive, randomisierte vergleichsstudie. *Phlebologie* 2005;34:19-24.
31. Hinchliffe RJ, Ubhi J, Beech A, et al. A prospective randomised controlled trial of VNUS closure versus surgery for the treatment of recurrent long saphenous varicose veins. *Eur J Vasc Endovasc Surg* 2006;31(2):212-218.
32. Vasquez MA, Wang J, Mahathanaruk M, et al. The utility of the Venous Clinical Severity Score in 682 limbs treated by radiofrequency saphenous vein ablation. *J Vasc Surg* 2007;45(5):1008-1014; discussion, 1015.
33. Perkowski P, Ravi R, Gowda RC, et al. Endovenous laser ablation of the saphenous vein for treatment of venous insufficiency and varicose veins: early results from a large single-center experience. *J Endovasc Ther* 2004;11(2):132-138.
44. Yamaki T, Nozaki M, Iwasaka S. Comparative study of duplex-guided foam sclerotherapy and duplex-guided liquid sclerotherapy for the treatment of superficial venous insufficiency. *Dermatol Surg* 2004;30(5):718-722; discussion, 722.
45. Rabe E, Otto J, Schliephake D, Pannier F. Efficacy and safety of great saphenous vein sclerotherapy using standardised polidocanol foam (ESAF): a randomised controlled multicentre clinical trial. *Eur J Vasc Endovasc Surg* 2008;35(2):238-245.
46. Myers KA, Jolley D, Clough A, Kirwan J. Outcome of ultrasound-guided sclerotherapy for varicose veins: medium-term results assessed by ultrasound surveillance. *Eur J Vasc Endovasc Surg* 2007;33(1):116-121.
47. van Neer P, Kessels A, de Haan E, et al. Residual varicose veins below the knee after varicose vein surgery are not related to incompetent perforating veins. *J Vasc Surg* 2006;44(5):1051-1054.
48. Merchant RF, Pichot O. Long-term outcomes of endovenous radiofrequency obliteration of saphenous reflux as a treatment for superficial venous insufficiency. *J Vasc Surg* 2005;42(3):502-509; discussion, 509.
49. Kabnick LS. Endovenous laser system (980 nm) for the treatment of saphenous vein insufficiency: 7611 limbs. ACP 19th Annual Conference, 2005, San Francisco, California.
50. Almeida JI. Current state of endovenous ablation. *Endovasc Today* 2007;6(10):73-76.
51. Mozes G, Kalra M, Carmo M, et al. Extension of saphenous thrombus into the femoral vein: a potential complication of new endovenous ablation techniques. *J Vasc Surg* 2005;41(1):130-135.
52. Gradman WS. Adjunctive proximal vein ligation with endovenous obliteration of great saphenous vein reflux: does it have clinical value? *Ann Vasc Surg* 2007;21(2):155-158.
53. Gibson KD, Ferris BL, Polissar N, et al. Endovenous laser treatment of the small corrected saphenous vein: efficacy and complications. *J Vasc Surg* 2007;45(4):795-801; discussion, 803.
54. Proebstle TM, Gul D, Kargl A, Knop J. Endovenous laser treatment of the lesser saphenous vein with a 940-nm diode laser: early results. *Dermatol Surg* 2003;29(4):357-361.
55. Bergan J, Pascarella L, Mekenas L. Venous disorders: treatment with sclerosant foam. *J Cardiovasc Surg* 2006;47(1):9-18.
56. Rutgers PH, Kitslaar PJ. Randomized trial of stripping versus high ligation combined with sclerotherapy in the treatment of the incompetent greater saphenous vein. *Am J Surg* 1994;168(4):311-315.
57. Neglen P, Einarsson E, Eklof B. The functional long-term value of different types of treatment for saphenous vein incompetence. *J Cardiovasc Surg* 1993;34(4):295-301.

incite neovascularization. The residual saphenofemoral junction tributaries have been reported to be nonrefluxing and clinically insignificant 1 year following EVLT.[73] Pichot et al. reported no incidences of neovascularization 24 months following RFA treatment compared to as high as 60% of groins observed after stripping by Fischer et al.[74,75] A recent study compared the incidence of neovascularization at the saphenofemoral junction following RFA and open high saphenous and stripping of the GSV.[76] In the open surgery group, 6 of 55 (11%) limbs showed clear evidence of tortuous refluxing veins related to the saphenofemoral junction, while none of the 55 limbs in the RFA group showed any neovascularization at the saphenofemoral junction. Further randomized, controlled trials are necessary to confirm these observations.

Long-term results following foam sclerotherapy are scarce, the earliest being those from Cabrera et al.'s original report[16] of more than 80% GSV occlusion to 3 years. Few other authors have reported similar success.[42,77] In a multicenter, randomized, controlled trial comparing foam to liquid sclerotherapy, Ouvry et al. reported only 53% maintained GSV occlusion at 2 years despite early occlusion in 85%.[78] Controversy also exists regarding the ideal concentration of sclerosant foam. Hamel-Desnos et al. reported equivalent results on 2-year follow-up,[43] but other authors noted superior occlusion rates with 3% sclerosant foam (polidocanol or sodium tetradecyl sulfate) at 1 to 3 year follow-up.[79]

Most traditional treatments for symptomatic varicose veins have consisted of ablation of axial reflux in the GSVs, SSVs, or both in conjunction with removal or ablation of branch varicosities. This paradigm has been challenged with the advent of office-based endovenous saphenous vein procedures performed under local anesthesia. Several authors have recommended staged ablation of axial reflux alone followed by intervention on persistent, symptomatic branch veins selectively.[80] Monahan reported spontaneous resolution of 42% of above-knee and 26% of below-knee varicose veins following RFA of the GSV, with most medial varicosities undergoing involution.[81] Almeida and Raines, however, recommended additional need for intervention on branch varicosities for most patients.[39] Simultaneous ablation of large branch varicose veins by stab phlebectomy or sclerotherapy has been felt to improve the GSV occlusion rate following endovenous ablation to 97% at 1 year with complete reflux ablation.[41]

Although ecchymosis, hematomas, paresthesias, and ankle swelling were seen during early experience with power-suction phlebectomy, proponents of the technique report swift and efficacious vein removal with satisfactory results.[82] This technique has not enjoyed widespread acceptance, however, with most operators still employing ambulatory stab phlebectomy or sclerotherapy for the treatment of branch varicose veins.

recanalization of a segment of the vein, and their potential for causing recurrent varicose veins remains unknown. The incidence of groin neovascularization and its significance needs to be determined.

Ultrasound-guided foam sclerotherapy is also emerging as a competitor to other endovenous technique and is particularly useful in superficial and tortuous veins not ideally suited for endovenous thermal ablation, as well as recanalized segments of ablated veins. Surgical treatment remains a valuable option in many patients, and the widespread use of duplex ultrasound, guiding the principle of concomitant treatment of all refluxing segments of the superficial venous system, will undoubtedly improve previously reported results. Only long-term follow-up and uniform reporting standards will provide the answers.

References

1. Stanley JC, Barnes RW, Ernst CB, et al. Vascular surgery in the United States: workforce issues. Report of the Society for Vascular Surgery and the International Society for Cardiovascular Surgery, North American Chapter, Committee on Workforce Issues. *J Vasc Surg* 1996 1/1996;23(1):172-181.
2. Bosanquet N. Costs of venous ulcers: from maintenance therapy to investment programmes. *Phleboblogy Suppl* 1992:44-46.
3. Kalra M, Gloviczki P, Noel AA, et al. Subfascial endoscopic perforator vein surgery in patients with post-thrombotic venous insufficiency: is it justified? *Vasc Endovasc Surg* 2002;36:41-50.
4. McMullin GM, Coleridge Smith PD, Scurr JH. Objective assessment of high ligation without stripping the long saphenous vein. *Br J Surg* 1991;78(9):1139-1142.
5. Munn SR, Morton JB, Macbeth WA, McLeish AR. To strip or not to strip the long saphenous vein? A varicose veins trial. *Br J Surg* 1981;68(6):426-428.
6. Stonebridge PA, Chalmers N, Beggs I, et al. Recurrent varicose veins: a varicographic analysis leading to a new practical classification. *Br J Surg* 1995;82(1):60-62.
7. Darke SG. The morphology of recurrent varicose veins. *Eur J Vasc Surg* 1992;6(5):512-517.
8. Navarro L. Endovenous laser treatment with 810 nm to 980 nm wavelengths: method of action. ACP 19th Annual Conference, 2005, San Francisco, California.
9. Proebstle TM, Lehr HA, Kargl A, et al. Endovenous treatment of the greater saphenous vein with a 940-nm diode laser: thrombotic occlusion after endoluminal thermal damage by laser-generated steam bubbles. *J Vasc Surg* 2002;35(4):729-736.
10. Weiss RA. Comparison of endovenous radiofrequency versus 810 diode laser occlusion of large veins in an animal model. *Dermatol Surg* 2002;28(1):56-61.

10a. Min RJ, Khilnani N, Zimmet SE. Endovenous laser treatment of saphenous vein reflux: long-term results. *J Vasc Interv Radiol* 2003 Aug;14(8):991-996.

11. Hamel-Desnos C, Desnos P, Wollmann JC, et al. Evaluation of the efficacy of polidocanol in the form of foam compared with liquid form in sclerotherapy of the greater saphenous vein: initial results. *Dermatol Surg* 2003;29(12):1170-1175; discussion, 1175.
12. Puggioni A, Kalra M, Carmo M, et al. Endovenous laser therapy and radiofrequency ablation of the great saphenous vein: analysis of early efficacy and complications. *J Vasc Surg* 2005;42(3):488-493.
13. Bone C. Tratamiento endoluminal de las varices con laser de Diodo: estudio preliminary. *Rev Patol Vasc* 1999;5:35-46.

... Min RJ, Bone C. Endovenous laser: a new minimally invasive ... preliminary observations using

...reated by ...548-652.

...avenous air

...nquez MA. ...oduits scle-

64. Sadick NS, Wasser S. Combined endovascular laser plus ambulatory phlebectomy for the treatment of superficial venous incompetence: a 4-year perspective. *J Cosmet Laser Ther* 2007;9;(1):9-13.
65. Proebstle TM, Krummenauer F, Gul D, Knop J. Nonocclusion and early reopening of the great saphenous vein after endovenous laser treatment is fluency dependent. *Dermatol Surg* 2004;30(2 Pt 1):174-178.
66. Timperman PE, Sichlau M, Ryu RK. Greater energy delivery improves treatment success of endovenous laser treatment of incompetent saphenous veins. *J Vasc Interv Radiol* 2004;15(10):1061-1063.
67. Proebstle TM, Moehler T, Herdemann S. Reduced recanalization rates of the great saphenous vein after endovenous laser treatment with increased energy dosing: definition of a threshold for the endovenous fluency equivalent. *J Vasc Surg* 2006;44(4):834-839.
68. Allegra C, Antignani PL, Carlizza A. Recurrent varicose veins following surgical treatment: our experience with five years follow-up. *Eur J Vasc Endovasc Surg* 2007;33(6):751-756.
69. Hartmann K, Klode J, Pfister R, et al. Recurrent varicose veins: sonography-based re-examination of 210 patients 14 years after ligation and saphenous vein stripping. *Vasa* 2006;35(1):21-26.
70. Winterborn RJ, Earnshaw JJ. Crossectomy and great saphenous vein stripping. *J Cardiovasc Surg* 2006;47(1):19-33.
71. Munasinghe A, Smith C, Kianifard B, et al. Strip-track revascularization after stripping of the great saphenous vein. *Br J Surg* 2007;94(7):840-843.
72. Dwerryhouse S, Davies B, Harradine K, Earnshaw JJ. Stripping the long saphenous vein reduces the rate of reoperation for recurrent varicose veins: five-year results of a randomized trial. *J Vasc Surg* 1999;29(4):589-592.
73. Theivacumar NS, Dellagrammaticas D, Beale RJ, et al. Fate and clinical significance of saphenofemoral junction tributaries following endovenous laser ablation of great saphenous vein. *Br J Surg* 2007;94(6):722-725.
74. Pichot O, Kabnick LS, Creton D, et al. Duplex ultrasound scan findings two years after great saphenous vein radiofrequency endovenous obliteration. *J Vasc Surg* 2004;39(1):189-195.
75. Fischer R, Linde N, Duff C, et al. Late recurrent saphenofemoral junction reflux after ligation and stripping of the greater saphenous vein. *J Vasc Surg* 2001;34(2):236-240.
76. Kianifard B, Holdstock JM, Whiteley MS. Radiofrequency ablation (VNUS closure) does not cause neo-vascularisation at the groin at one year: results of a case controlled study. *Surgeon* 2006;4(2):71-74.
77. Coleridge SPW. D. Foam sclerotherapy of saphenous trunk varices. *Phlebology* 2002;17:75.
78. Ouvry P, Allaert FA, Desnos P, Hamel-Desnos C. Efficacy of polidocanol foam versus liquid in sclerotherapy of the great saphenous vein: a multicentre randomised controlled trial with a two-year follow-up. *Eur J Vasc Endovasc Surg* 2008;36:366-370.
79. Ceulen RP, Bullens-Goessens YI, Pi-Van de Venne SJ, et al. Outcomes and side effects of duplex-guided sclerotherapy in the treatment of great saphenous veins with 1% versus 3% polidocanol foam: results of a randomized controlled trial with 1-year follow-up. *Dermatol Surg* 2007;33(3):276-281.
80. Welch HJ. Endovenous ablation of the great saphenous vein may avert phlebectomy for branch varicose veins. *J Vasc Surg* 2006;44(3):601-605.
81. Monahan DL. Can phlebectomy be deferred in the treatment of varicose veins? *J Vasc Surg* 2005;42(6):1145-1149.
82. Cheshire N, Elias SM, Keagy B, et al. Powered phlebectomy (TriVex) in treatment of varicose veins. *Ann Vasc Surg* 2002;16(4):488-494.
83. Sybrandy JE, Wittens CH. Initial experiences in endovenous treatment of saphenous vein reflux. *J Vasc Surg* 2002;36(6):1207-1212.
84. Wagner WH, Levin PM, Cossman DV, et al. Early experience with radiofrequency ablation of the greater saphenous vein. *Ann Vasc Surg* 2004;18(1):42-47.
85. Gradman WS. Proximal great saphenous vein ligation with laser obliteration of saphenous vein reflux: Is there a risk/benefit ratio? *ACP 19th Annual Conference*, 2005; San Francisco, USA; 2005.
86. Rautio TT, Perälä JM, Wiik HT, Juvonen TS, Haukipuro KA. Endovenous obliteration with radiofrequency-resistive heating for greater saphenous vein insufficiency: a feasibility study. *J Vasc Interv Radiol* 2002;13;(6):569-575.

chapter

45

Endovascular Management of Varicose Veins

Cynthia Shortell, MD, FACS • Jovan N. Markovic, MD • Luigi Pascarella, MD

Key Points

- Introduction
- Anatomy of the lower extremity venous system
- Indications for treatment
- Treatment options
- Preoperative evaluation
- Stripping of the great saphenous vein
- Operative technique
- Outcomes and complications
- Radiofrequency ablation
- Description of procedure
- Outcomes and complications
- Endovenous laser ablation
- Description of procedure
- Outcomes and complications
- Sclerotherapy
- Description of procedure
- Conclusion
- Outcomes and complications

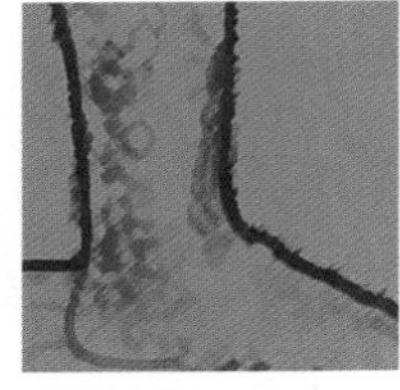

Varicose veins are one of the most common diseases in Western society.[1,2] An estimated 25 million people in the United States have varicose veins; 2 to 6 million have more advanced forms, including swelling and skin changes; and nearly 500,000 have painful venous ulcerations.[3] The term chronic venous insufficiency (CVI) implies a derangement of the lower extremity superficial venous system. Clinical and experimental evidence suggests that valvular incompetence in the superficial venous system is responsible for the onset and progression of venous hypertension and, ultimately, the development of varicose veins and related disorders of the lower extremities.[4,5]

In 1950, Arnoldi defined varicose veins as "any dilated, elongated or tortuous veins, irrespective of size."[6] This simple definition describes the clinical manifestation of telangiectasias, reticular veins, and varicose veins, thus linking them to a common cause. Current experimental investigations have led to the development of a unifying theory regarding the pathophysiology of venous reflux and the manifestations of venous hypertension and CVI.[5] It has been shown that once a condition of venous hypertension has developed, the consequent hemodynamic disruption causes the failure of the venous valves via a blood flow–mediated inflammatory reaction, with activation of leukocytes, diapedesis into the venous parenchyma, release of enzymes, and remodeling of the vascular wall, ending in venous valve destruction and incompetence.[5] This basic pathophysiology has been identified as a common pathway for all manifestations of CVI, including telangiectasias, reticular veins, varicose veins, lipodermatosclerosis, atrophie blanche, and venous ulcers.

Pressure in the veins of the lower extremities is determined by two components. The hydrostatic component represents the weight of the column of the blood, which is transmitted from the right atrium, through valveless vena cava and iliac veins, to the lower extremity veins. The hydrodynamic component represents the pressure produced by skeletal muscle contractions in the lower extremity.[5] It is demonstrated that pressures generated within the muscular compartment approach 100 mm Hg. Competent valves are under the continuous challenge to provide unidirectional blood flow. Consequently, diminished valve competency results in hemodynamic alterations, leading to the CVI and varicosities.[5]

The treatment of venous insufficiency should be always undertaken within the context of a full understanding of the basic molecular and hemodynamic mechanisms underlying this disease. In this instance, the excision or the endovascular

Table 45-1
Summary of Important Changes in Nomenclature of Lower Extremity Veins

Old Terminology	New Terminology
Femoral vein	Common femoral vein
Superficial femoral vein	Femoral vein
Deep vein of the thigh	Profunda femoris vein
Great or long saphenous vein	Great saphenous vein
Smaller or short saphenous vein	Small saphenous vein
Sural veins	Soleal veins
	Gastrocnemius veins
	Medial gastrocnemius vein
	Lateral gastrocnemius vein
	Intergemellar vein
Dodd's perforator	Perforator of the femoral canal
Boyd's perforator	Paratibial perforator (upper third of the leg)
Sherman's perforator (24 cm)	Paratibial perforator (midthird of the leg)
Cockett's perforators	Posterotibial perforators

ablation of an incompetent great saphenous vein (GSV) or other varicose veins, allows the normalization of the hemodynamics of the lower extremity by removing the source of venous hypertension and inflammation.

ANATOMY OF THE LOWER EXTREMITY VENOUS SYSTEM

Proper recognition of anatomical structures and nomenclature of the lower extremity venous system is essential to understanding venous pathophysiology and appropriate treatment.

In 2002, an International Interdisciplinary Consensus on Venous Anatomical Terminology proposed a revision and extension of the *Terminologia Anatomica* of the lower extremity venous system (Table 45-1).[7,8] The new nomenclature should be used in the final mapping of the lower extremity.

For didactic purposes, the venous system of the lower extremity can be divided into deep, superficial, and perforating compartments. The terms *deep*, *superficial*, and *perforating* are used with respect to the anatomical relationship between the venous structures and the deep (muscular) fascia. The deep fascia anatomically divides the lower extremity into two compartments (deep and superficial).[7] The deep compartment lies inferior to the deep fascia. The superficial compartment lies between the skin and the deep fascia. The saphenous compartment is a subdivision of the superficial compartment; it is positioned between deep and superficial (saphenous) fascia (Figure 45-1). The saphenous compartment is an important anatomical subdivision since it is targeted during percutaneous application of tumescent anesthesia.[7]

The superficial veins lie in the superficial compartment without crossing the deep fascia. The deep veins are located in the deep compartment (between the deep fascia and the bones of the lower extremity). Perforating veins connect these two systems by piercing (perforating) the deep fascia. In the past, the term communicating veins was used as a synonym for perforating veins. This terminology has been abandoned, and today this term is reserved for the veins that are connecting veins within the same compartment (without piercing the deep fascia), usually those radiating superficially from the saphenous veins toward the dermis.[8]

The GSV originates from the medial end of the dorsal venous arch of the foot via the medial marginal vein and terminates by joining the common femoral vein proximally to the inguinal ligament, forming saphenofemoral junction (SFJ)

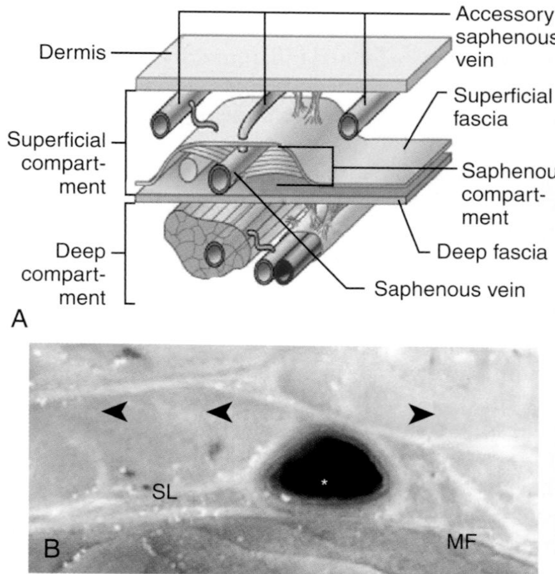

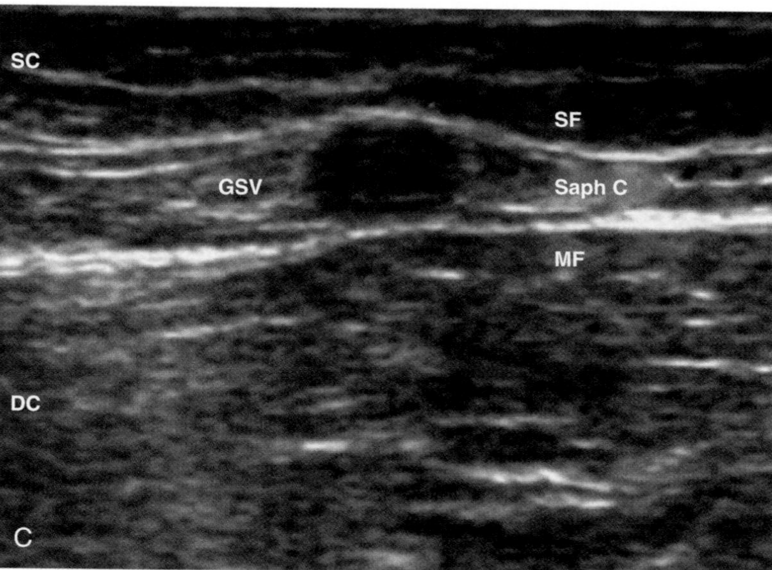

Figure 45-1. A, The saphenous compartment lies between the saphenous fascia and the muscular (deep) fascia. The compartment contains the saphenous vein and the saphenous nerve. **B,** Axial section of cadaveric limb. The saphenous vein and the saphenous compartment are illustrated. MF, muscular fascia; SL, saphenous ligament. **C,** Ultrasound transverse section of the great saphenous vein at midthigh. The saphenous fascia and the muscular fascia appear hyperechoic. The saphenous vein lies within the saphenous compartment. DC, deep compartment; GSV, great saphenous vein; MF, muscular fascia; Saph C, saphenous compartment; SC, superficial compartment; SF, superficial fascia. (**B,** Adapted from Caggiati A, Bergan JJ, Gloviczki P, et al. *J Vasc Surg* 2002;36[2]:416-422. **C,** Adapted from Bergan J. *The vein book.* ch 18. Philadelphia, Elsevier; 2007:175.)

(Figure 45-2). It occupies the anteromedial segment of the leg. Its relative anatomical proximity to the saphenous nerve should be emphasized, since this nerve is a subject to injury during surgical manipulation of the GSV.

INDICATIONS FOR TREATMENT

Indications for surgical treatment are illustrated in Table 45-2. The most common complaint that leads patients to seek medical attention is the appearance of telangiectasias and protuberant varicosities. Typical symptoms include aching, throbbing, leg heaviness, itching, nighttime cramping, and edema and may substantially affect the patient's lifestyle and occupation. Other indications for the treatment include superficial thrombophlebitis of varicose clusters, bleeding from superficial varicose veins, advanced and severe skin changes such as ankle hyperpigmentation, lipodermatosclerosis, atrophie blanche, or onset of a frank ulcer. The treatment of asymptomatic venous insufficiency is somewhat controversial; some experts argue that patients with asymptomatic class 3 and 4 disease should be treated to prevent progression to ulceration and postulate that reflux in normal veins is accelerated when superficial reflux goes untreated.

Table 45-2
Indications for Intervention

- General appearance
- Aching pain
- Leg heaviness
- Easy leg fatigue
- Superficial thrombophlebitis
- External bleeding
- Ankle hyperpigmentation
- Lipodermatosclerosis
- Atrophie blanche
- Venous ulcer

Treatment Options

The ablation of reflux from the deep system to the superficial venous system, including the SFJ, the saphenopopliteal junction, and perforator veins, and the resultant relief of presenting symptoms are the goals of treatment. Several options are available for the treatment of varicose veins:

- GSV stripping or phlebectomies
- Radiofrequency ablation (RFA)
- Endovenous laser ablation (EVLA)
- Sclerotherapy

Regardless of which approach is chosen, the general technical objectives remain the same. The goal of removing the GSV from circulation is to eliminate elevated hydrostatic and hydrodynamic pressures.

Preoperative Evaluation

A meticulous medical history taking and physical examination are important initial steps in the preoperative evaluation. Data concerning family and personal history of venous

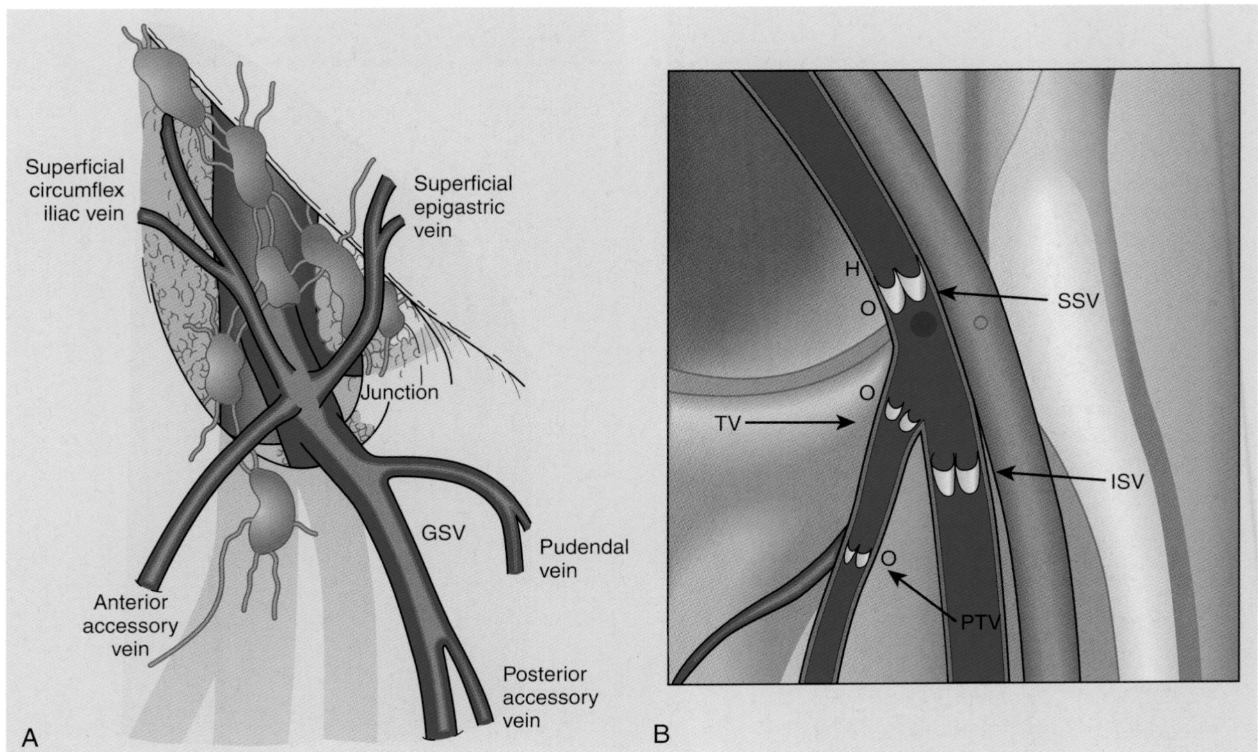

Figure 45-2. A, The saphenofemoral junction (SFJ) includes the great saphenous vein, the superficial iliac circumflex vein, the superficial epigastric vein, and the pudendal veins. **B,** The SFJ with its valves. ISV, infrasaphenic valve; PTV, preterminal valve; SSV, suprasaphenic valve; TV, terminal valve. (**A,** Adapted from Bergan J. *The vein book.* ch 18. Philadelphia, Elsevier; 2007:175. **B,** Modified from the *De venarum ostiolis of Jeronimus Fabricius AB acquapendente,* Venice; 1603. Adapted from Caggiati A, Bergan JJ, Gloviczki P, et al. *J Vasc Surg* 2002;36[2]:416-422.)

Table 45-3
CEAP Classification

Class	Clinical Signs
0	No physical sings of venous disease
1	Telangiectasia
2	Varicosities
3	Edema without skin changes
4	Skin changes (pigmentation, venous eczema, lipodermatosclerosis)
5	Skin changes with healed ulceration
6	Skin changes with active ulceration

disease, length and nature of symptoms, history of deep vein thrombosis, and previous venous treatments should always be carefully obtained. Family history of thrombosis warrants further investigation and possible preoperative anticoagulation therapy. In addition, all existing comorbidities, allergies, and medication history must be documented.

The physical examination should start with height and weight measurement and body mass index calculation. The patient should be examined in an erect position to better identify patterns of telangiectasias, reticular veins, and varicose veins. Cold light transillumination can be particularly useful in identifying reticular veins "feeding" arborization of more superficial telangiectasias. Handheld Doppler's devices can be used to assess reflux in some superficial veins. Observed findings should be classified according to the CEAP classification system (Table 45-3).

Historically, before the advent of vascular ultrasound, clinical tests such as the Trendelenburg test, Schwartz test, and Pethes test were used to diagnose and locate venous reflux disease. In the current clinical practice, their use has been abandoned. Since its inception, duplex ultrasound has provided the physician with practical information to assess venous reflux of the superficial, deep, and perforator systems; thrombotic states; and postthrombotic obstruction. In addition, the use of venous duplex has dramatically improved understanding of the anatomy, physiology, and pathophysiology of the lower extremity venous system.[9] The ultrasound examination is performed with the patient upright. This position maximizes reflux by challenging venous valves and maximally dilates the leg veins. Sensitivity and specificity in detecting reflux are increased by twofold if examination is performed with the patient standing rather than supine.[9] Veins are scanned by moving the probe vertically along their course. Scanning of the entire venous system should be performed in continuity, in the transverse projection, and findings should be recorded on specialized forms (Figure 45-3). During the entire examination, augmentation flow maneuvers, by means of sharp and quick distal manual compression or by use of a pressure cuff, are performed to elicit reflux. The Valsalva maneuver is a reverse flow augmentation stimulus used to assess competence of the SFJ valve.[9]

The presence of reflux through incompetent valves is the most important pathological sonographical sign of CVI. Reflux is measured during the release phase of the augmentation maneuver and during the closed epiglottis (apneic) phase

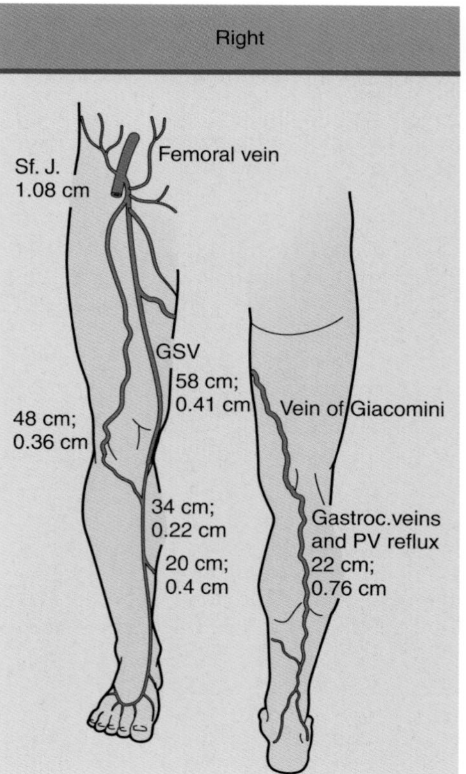

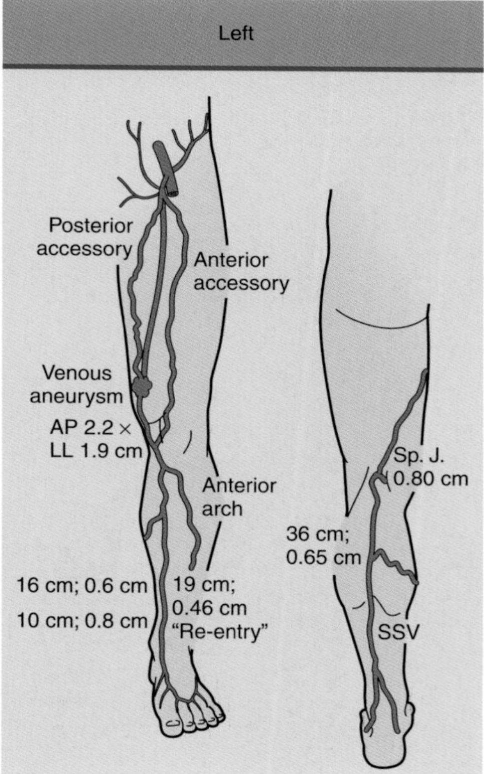

Figure 45-3. This data entry form illustrates the saphenous veins and the most relevant deep veins. Refluxing veins are shown in the heavy black lines. Location of perforating veins can be added, and distance from the floor is measured and indicated. Diameter of perforating veins and venous aneurisms is also noted. (Adapted from Bergan J. *The vein book.* ch 18. Philadelphia, Elsevier; 2007:175.)

of the Valsalva maneuver. It should be noted that retrograde backflow is present in normal veins valves immediately before their closure but a cutoff value of 500 milliseconds (0.5 seconds) defines pathology in the superficial veins, profunda femoris, and deep calf veins.[9] A value of 350 milliseconds is used for perforating veins and 1000 milliseconds for the common femoral, femoral, and popliteal veins.[9] The ultrasound examination should be focused on accurately mapping the entire lower extremity. Duplicated segments, sites of tributary confluence, large perforators, and their confluence with the deep venous system should be noticed and reported.

Stripping of the Great Saphenous Vein

By introducing the first venous stripper in 1904, Charles Mayo opened a new surgical era in the treatment of CVI and varicose veins. The development of this technique can be related to the major understanding that CVI, and its associated symptoms are related to hemodynamic alterations in the lower extremity venous circulation. Stripping of the GSV and excision or avulsion of associated varicose veins became the predominant treatment modality employed to improve hemodynamics of the lower extremity.[10] Several surgical techniques have been proposed and applied. High ligation of the SFJ and the GSV stripping has been demonstrated to be more effective and currently is the most widely accepted surgical option.[10,11]

Operative Technique

Preoperative evaluation, marking the extent of varicose vein clusters (Figure 45-4), and an individual approach to each patient and each limb are of paramount importance to the successful outcome of surgery.

To achieve satisfactory cosmetic results, incisions at the groin and knee level are transverse and should be placed within skin creases. Vertical incisions are reserved for the remainder of the lower extremity, except over the patella, where oblique incisions in skin lines are proven to achieve the best cosmetic results. General or regional anesthesia is required.[10]

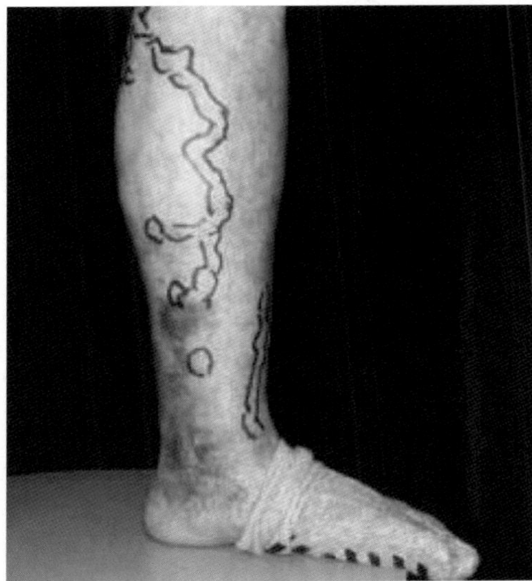

Figure 45-4. Lower extremity preoperative mapping. Truncal varices and associated varicose clusters are noticed. (Adapted from Bergan J, Pascarella L, Mekenas L. *J Cardiovasc Surg [Torino]* 2006;47[1]:9-18.)

Evidence against routine removal of the GSV below the knee resulted in the necessity to individualize the surgical approach for each patient. It was thought that, in the leg, important perforating veins were part of the posterior arch circulation. The introduction of modern imaging modalities (duplex ultrasonography) has discounted this argument. Duplex ultrasonography often demonstrates direct connection between the leg portion of GSV and the perforating veins, justifying the necessity for GSV removal below the knee. Therefore, groin-to-ankle removal of the GSV is a consideration in patients who have infrageniculate pathology. In addition, the close anatomical relation between the saphenous nerve and the GSV below the knee makes this nerve susceptible to injury during the stripping; the saphenous nerve meets the GSV just below the knee, and the two remain inseparable to the level of the medial malleolus. This argument against stripping below the knee has been validated by duplex findings. For this reason, the patient's clinical situation must dictate the level to which the GSV is stripped.[10]

Historically, proper identification and precise division of all tributaries to SFJ within the groin have been important technical issues in the prevention of varicose vein recurrence. Therefore, it was important to draw each of the saphenous tributaries into groin incision and, after placing them on traction, to control primary and even secondary tributaries. The SFJ tributaries were then carefully dissected and ligated. The theory that residual inguinal networks are an important cause of varicose vein recurrence has been questioned by the introduction of ultrasound in the current phlebology practice.[12] This has allowed investigators to detect inguinal networks of new veins that are connected to the junction stump or to the ligated GSV tributaries.[12,13] The neovascularization of previously incised groin, for ligation and stripping of the GSV, has been recognized as major cause for varicose veins recurrence, and it has been identified as the major complication of this technique.[11] Histological findings are suggesting that an inflammatory process, related to the repair of previously dissected tissue, is the underlying etiology for the development of new veins.[11]

The groin incision should be placed either in or 1 cm above the visible skin crease.[10] The dissection of the junction and all GSV tributaries is then performed. After dissection, a disposable plastic stripper is placed into the GSV. A metal stripper can also be used. From cephalad to caudad, the stripper is advanced through incompetent valves to approximately 1 cm medial to the medial border of the tibia and approximately 5 cm distal of the tibial trabeculae. At this level, the stripper can be easily identified via palpation and a small incision is made to dissect the GSV. If a groin-to-ankle procedure is indicated, the stripper is advanced to the level of the medial malleolus. The absence of functioning valves allows, in most cases, the advancement of the stripper to the ankle, where it can be exposed by performing a small skin incision. A transverse phlebotomy allows the delivery of the stripper, whose olive-shaped tip is attached to vein with surgical ties. The stripping is then performed by pulling the stripper gently from above. In nearly all patients, the stripping is supplemented by stab avulsion of clusters of varicose veins that may be connected to the GSV. Since stripping of the GSV induces venous hypertension, it would be technically more challenging to perform stab avulsions once the venous hypertension develops. Therefore, stab avulsion of clusters of varicose veins should be performed

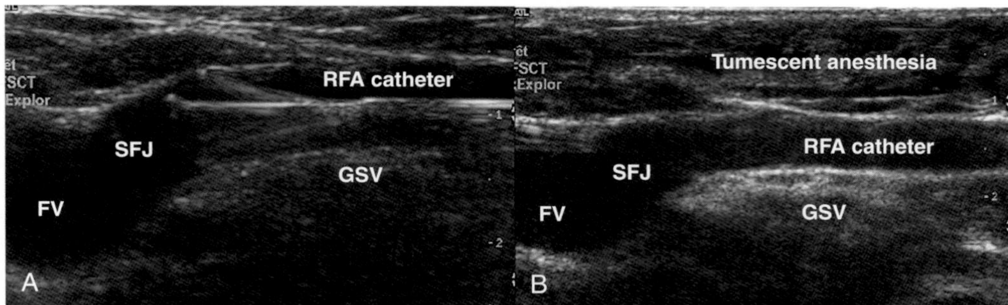

Figure 45-5. A 5-French RFA catheter is shown at the saphenofemoral junction (SFJ) before **(A)** and after **(B)** administration of tumescent anesthesia. FV, femoral vein; GSV, great saphenous vein. Tumescent anesthesia is used for three purposes: to provide analgesia, to prevent skin thermal injuries, and to compress the vein. (Adapted from Pichot O. *Atlas of ultrasound images*. VNUS Medical Technologies; 2002.)

before the actual GSV stripping. Sclerotherapy may also be used as an adjunctive treatment option to remove varicose vein clusters.

Hemostatic tourniquets are applied throughout the entire procedure to reduce bleeding and to decrease the incidence of blood extravasation that is an important cause of skin discoloration and hyperpigmentation.

Outcomes and Complications

Although the surgical approach to varicose veins was the treatment of choice throughout the last century, the high incidence of recurrences and significant morbidity associated with this treatment modality are noteworthy.

Complications of high ligation and stripping of the GSV include pain, hematoma, infection, scarring, and saphenous nerve injury (4% to 7%).[10,11] It should be noted that 4 to 6 weeks of recovery are required before returning to work for individuals who have active jobs (e.g., nurses, hairdressers, or mail carriers). Another disadvantage of the surgical approach to GSV reflux is the high incidence of recurrent varicosities. High ligation and stripping is associated with a 20% rate of recurrent varicosities at 5 years, and up to 24% of patients require additional treatment.[11] Long-term follow-up data on high ligation and stripping are sparse. In 10-year follow-up reviews, the recurrence rate was reported to be between 47% and 60%, with 60% recurrent saphenofemoral incompetence. In about 20% of cases, additional surgery was required.[11]

In a study from Jones et al. in 1996, neovascularization at the SFJ was the most common cause of recurrence 2 years after the stripping.[12] New varicose veins arising from the SFJ were found in 52% of the 113 limbs examined.[12] In a long-term (5 years) follow-up study, neovascularization was present in 68% of the limbs with clinically evident varicose veins.[11]

The effectiveness of high ligation and stripping of the GSV has been also assessed by studying patient satisfaction and quality-of-life improvement. Several methods of measuring quality-of-life improvement have been used. The Aberdeen Varicose Vein Symptom Severity Score (AVVSSS) is a disease-specific questionnaire designed to identify subtle changes in symptom severity. This questionnaire has been used to assess the patient-, technical, and surgeon-related factors that influence the effect of superficial venous surgery on quality of life. About 203 consecutive patients who underwent superficial venous surgery were interviewed and asked to complete the AVVSSS before surgery and at 4 weeks, 6 months, and 2 years following surgery. Multivariate analysis showed that the presence of recurrent or residual varicose veins negatively affected AVVSSS at 6 months, while surgery positively affected AVVSSS at 2 years.[11]

Radiofrequency Ablation and Radiofrequency-Powered Segmental Thermal Ablation

With the U.S. Food and Drug Administration (FDA) approval of RFA (VNUS Closure, VNUS Medical Technologies, San Jose, California) in 1999, a new era of venous therapies began. RFA exposes vascular endothelium to high-frequency alternating current. This exposure is achieved by direct contact of the catheter prongs with the endothelium of the vein. This leads to the loss of vessel wall architecture, disintegration, and carbonization of the vessel. Subsequently, endoluminal obliteration occurs that eliminates hydrostatic and hydrodynamic pressures as the main hemodynamic mechanisms for varicosities.[14]

In addition to the initial preoperative evaluation process performed for surgical therapy, special attention should be paid to the anatomical features of the targeted vein segment, including diameter, tortuous, aneurysmal or sclerotic segments, and anatomical variants. If the preoperative duplex evaluation demonstrates more than a single vein to be incompetent, the most significant vein (with regard to reflux severity and location of pathology) should be treated first, followed by secondary veins. In most cases, this means the GSV treatment first, followed by the SSV; in about 50% of patients, reflux in the SSV resolves following GSV ablation.[15] Treatment of associated accessory varicosities is often delayed, as many accessory veins resolve spontaneously after GSV ablation, SSV ablation, or both.[15] The RFA procedure is performed with the assistance of tumescent anesthesia (a dilute mixture of 1% lidocaine, epinephrine, and sodium bicarbonate) that must be carefully injected into the saphenous sheath under ultrasound guidance.[16] Tumescent anesthesia is used for three purposes: providing analgesia, preventing skin thermal injuries (by physically widening the distance between prongs as the source of heat and skin and acting as a "heat sink") and compressing the vein (to achieve more effective contact between vascular endothelium and catheter prongs; Figure 45-5).[16]

Description of Procedure

Before establishing venous access, the patient is placed in the reverse Trendelenburg position to identify the target vein by ultrasound.[16] The GSV is cannulated via the Seldinger

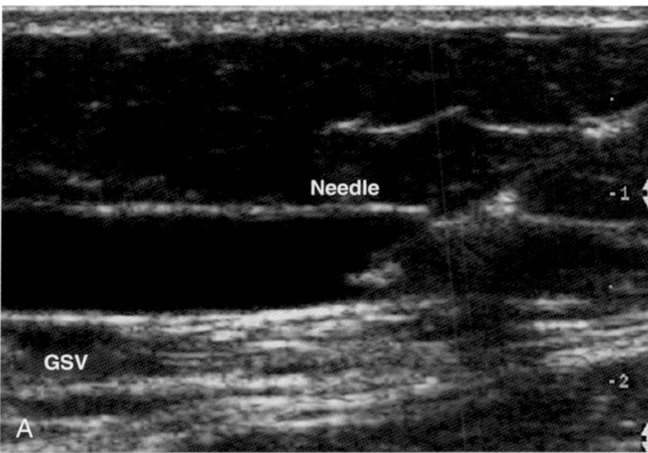

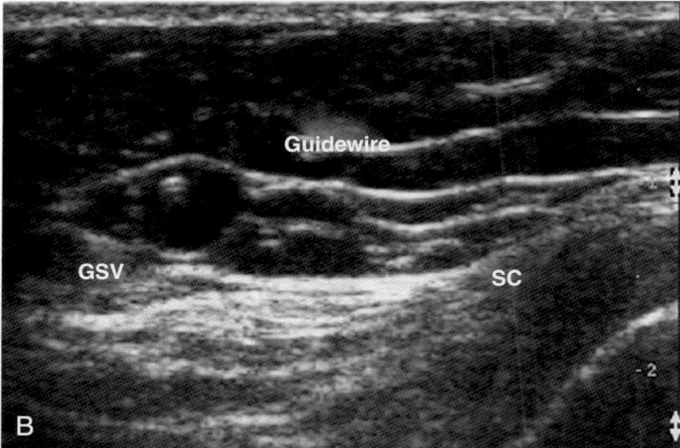

Figure 45-6. A, The great saphenous vein (GSV) is accessed in the distal third via the Seldinger technique. **B,** The RFA catheter is then advanced in the GSV. (Adapted from Pichot O. *Atlas of ultrasound images*. VNUS Medical Technologies; 2002.)

technique around the knee level, as determined by the anatomy of the vein and the location of the varicosities (Figure 45-6A and B). After establishing venous access, the patient is placed in Trendelenburg position and the RFA catheter is inserted into the GSV through a sheath. Under ultrasound

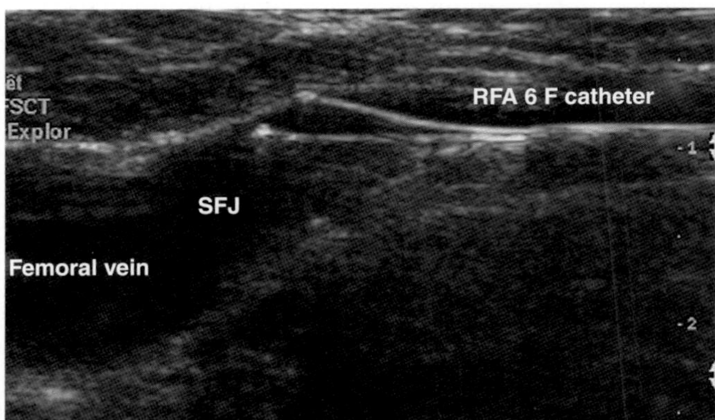

Figure 45-7. The RFA catheter is shown 1 cm distal to the saphenofemoral junction (SFJ) at the level of the superficial epigastric vein. (Adapted from Pichot O. *Atlas of ultrasound images*. VNUS Medical Technologies; 2002).

surveillance, the RFA catheter is then advanced 0.5 to 1 cm distal to the SFJ at the level of the superficial epigastric vein (Figure 45-7).[15] Tumescent anesthesia is percutaneously applied into saphenous sheath along the length of the vein, under ultrasound guidance, achieving depth of greater than 1 cm and adequate "halo" effect.[16] Two types of RFA catheters are available depending on the vessel size. A 6-French (Fr) catheter is used to treat vessels up to 8 mm in diameter, and an 8-Fr catheter is used for vessels 8 mm to 12 mm in diameter. Larger vessels can also be treated with 8-Fr catheters using adjunctive techniques, such as tumescing above the SFJ and externally compressing the vein.[17] The temperature of the probe can be set at 85° C or 90° C. If set at 85° C, the electrode needs to be withdrawn at a rate of 2.5 to 3.0 cm/min. If the temperature is increased to 90° C the speed of electrode withdrawal can be increased to 4.0 cm/min without loss of treatment efficacy.[14]

After the catheter has been withdrawn and the procedure completed, ultrasonography is used to assess the success of venous closure.[16] For this purpose, the patient is returned to a horizontal or reverse Trendelenburg position. If ultrasonography shows the evidence of flow, the procedure can be repeated. Careful evaluation of persistent flow needs to be performed. If the flow is minimal and the vein walls are thickened, a thrombus plug usually forms, resulting in cessation of flow. Under these circumstances, repetition of procedure is unnecessary.[15]

After the RFA procedure, patients are advised to wear compression therapy for 1 week and to ambulate. Patients can resume normal daily activities immediately after the procedure. A follow-up ultrasound is usually done 72 hours after the RFA to confirm procedural success and to exclude the migration, extension, or both of the clot into the common femoral vein.

Outcomes and Complications

A review of 890 patients (1078 limbs) at 1 week, 6 months, and 1, 2, 3, and 4 years showed vein occlusion rates of 97.4%, 91.0%, 88.8%, 86.2%, 84.2%, and 88.8%, respectively.[18] A retrospective review of a single center's experience, where 332 limbs were evaluated 72 hours after RFA treatment, demonstrated complete GSV obliteration in 99% of cases.[15]

In a prospective randomized comparison of RFA versus GSV ligation with stripping (EVOLVeS), immediate success was reported in 95% of patients treated with RFA.[19] Persistent GSV flow had been observed in 16.3% of patients at a 72-hour follow-up scan. Recurrence rates combined at follow-ups performed at 1 and 2 years were 14.3% for the RFA group and 20.9% for the ligation with stripping group.[19,20] In this study, only one case of neovascularization occurred. A technical failure was defined as a cause for GSV to remain patent and incompetent for 2 years.[19,20] At the 2-year follow-up, quality-of-life scores were higher in the RFA group than in the surgical arm.[19,20] The EVOLVeS Trial demonstrated RFA to be at least equivalent to surgery for elimination of GSV reflux and associated varicosities at 2 years.[19,20]

RFA of the GSV is a procedure with low morbidity, low mortality, and virtually no recovery time for the patient. Complications associated with RFA include bruising, focal paresthesia, infection, skin burns, phlebitis, deep vein thrombosis, and pulmonary embolism. Local thrombus at the SFJ and deep vein thrombosis were reported by Merchant et al.

in 0.5% of patients.[18] One of these patients developed pulmonary embolism. Paresthesia rates following RFA, also reported by these authors, were 12.1% at 1 week, 6.7% at 1 month, and 2.0% at 4 years.[18]

Recurrence of varicosities is associated with the persistence of the blood flow in an already-treated vein. Recanalization of the previously formed thrombus and newly formed vessels adjacent to recanalized veins has been identified as the most important cause of recurrence. Varnagy and Labropolous identified "multiple small vessels with arterial signals adjacent to ablated vein segments."[21] It is suspected that these small vessels form multiple small arteriovenous fistulas that ultimately lead to the complete thrombus recanalization.[21]

In the retrospective study from Mayo Clinic, it has been reported that additional RFA treatment was required in 17% of patients at the time of original procedure. This was compared to EVLA, where requirement for an additional treatment was reported to be unnecessary.[22] The same group also reported an immediate complications rate of 7.6% in RFA group, compared to 16.8% in EVLA group. These complications ranged from urinary retention to severe pain.[22]

RFA of the GSV is associated with significantly prolonged procedural time compared to EVLA. In attempt to overcome this disadvantage, a new RFA catheter, using the principle of radiofrequency-powered segmental thermal ablation (RSTA) was developed by VNUS Medical Technologies (Figure 45-8). Initial experience with RSTA documented decreased average procedural time and occlusion rates of 99.6% at 3 days, 3 months, and 6 months after the intervention.[23] These results, when compared with the initial experience with RFA, show significantly shorter procedural time and higher short-term occlusion rates.[23] In addition, the absence of pain was reported in 70.1% of patients at any time after the procedure.[23] This is a potential advantage of RSTA over EVLA, as pain is often reported by the patients treated with EVLA. The most common RSTA side effects reported by the same authors were ecchymosis (6.4%), paresthesia (3.2%), and hyperpigmentation (2%). However, the long-term results for RSTA are unknown, and larger clinical trials are needed before this modification of the RFA can be accurately evaluated in the treatment of varicose veins.

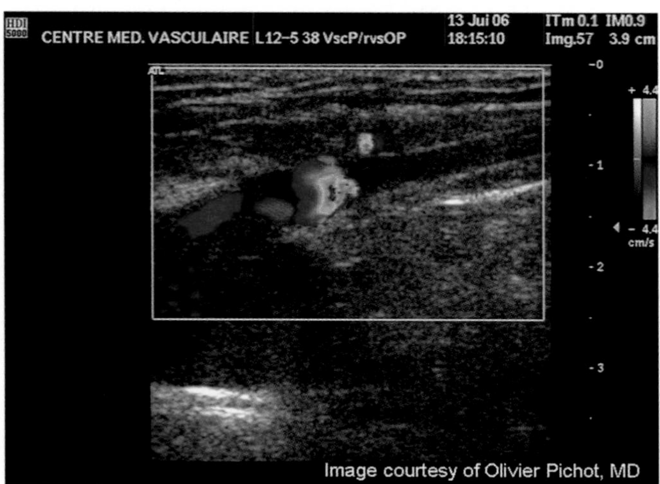

Figure 45-8. Immediate shrinkage of treated vein is seen after RSTA at GSV termination. RSTA, radiofrequency segmental ablation; GSV, great saphenous vein (Courtesy of Oliver Pinchot, MD).

Endovenous Laser Ablation

The technique of using laser energy in the treatment of varicose veins and truncal varicosities was first presented at the International Union of Phlebology in 1999 (Bremen, Germany) by Spanish phlebologist Carlos Bone. However, the first relevant study that brought this technique to the attention of the medical community and patients was published in 2001 by Navarro et al.[24] This was followed by U.S. FDA approval in 2002 of endovenous laser treatment (EVLT). Since EVLT is a registered trademark (Diomed, Andover, Massachusetts), the proper term for this treatment modality is endovenous laser ablation (EVLA).

The mechanism of action by which laser induces vein fibrosis and obliteration is a matter of debate. One theory suggests that laser energy, after being absorbed either by hemoglobin (810, 940, or 980 nm) or water (1320 nm), produces superheated steam blood bubbles within the vein.[25] Generated heat alters the vein architecture from the luminal side, leading to significant shrinkage of the vein wall collagen fibers and consecutive reduction of the vein lumen. In addition, the extensive thermal damage to the endothelium and intima induces thrombotic occlusion of the vein.[25] This occlusion can be visualized on duplex ultrasound as incompressible, hypoechogenic cord within the lumen of the treated vein segment. Although, this theory suggests that boiling bubbles and thrombosis are the part of the mechanism that leads to the vein closure, there appears to be no risk of gas embolism and small risk of deep vein thrombosis associated with EVLA.[25] Another theory suggests that direct heating of the vein wall with the laser beam leads to nonthrombotic vein occlusion.[26] Sufficient heating of the vein is required to induce the wall thickening and subsequent fibrosis and obliteration of the treated vein segment.[26]

Description of Procedure

Patient positioning, preoperative preparation, and perioperative preparation are done as described for RFA. Most commonly, to maintain the minimally invasive characteristics of this technique, the targeted vein is accessed by ultrasound-guided percutaneous needle puncture. Alternatively, the targeted vein could be entered via the stab wound–Mueller hook approach.[24] After cannulation of the targeted vein, a 0.035-inch guide wire is introduced into the vein, and a long sheath (45 or 65 cm, 4- or 5-Fr) is advanced to about 1.5 to 2 cm below the SFJ under ultrasound guidance.[24] The laser fiber is then advanced within the sheath, with only a small segment protruding out of the sheath. The sheath and laser are adjusted so that the laser tip is 1.5 to 2 cm below the SFJ. This differs from RFA, in which the sheath is short and the catheter is advanced "bare."

The success of treatment depends on the amount of energy delivered to the vein wall.[27] Optimal results are achieved with a pullback speed in the range of 0.5 to 3 mm/sec, delivering approximately 80 joules/cm of thermal energy to the vein. Manual compression of the vein can be used to facilitate obliteration of the venous lumen. After the whole length of the vein is treated, ultrasound is used to visualize closure and check for femoral vein clot[26,28] (Figure 45-9). The aftercare and follow-up for EVLA patients are the same as for RFA, including

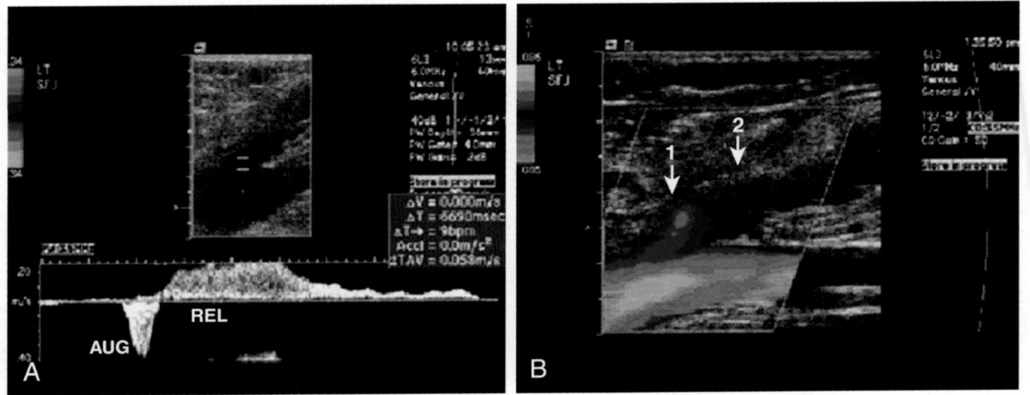

Figure 45-9. Duplex ultrasound examinations of the great saphenous vein (GSV) at the saphenofemoral junction (SFJ) **A,** Pretreatment scan demonstrated an incompetent SFJ after augmentation. **B,** Intraoperative color duplex interrogation showed successful occlusion of the GSV with a patent 3-mm stump *(arrow 1)* and absence of flow within the treated segment *(arrow 2)*. (Adapted from Puggioni, Kalra M, Carmo M, et al. *J Vasc Surg* 2005;42[3]:488-493.)

1 week of compression stocking therapy and follow-up ultrasound at 72 hours.[29]

Outcomes and Complications

The early results of EVLA in the treatment of varicose veins are excellent. A retrospective review of 92 consecutive patients (130 limbs) reported a rate of immediate GSV occlusion of 100%.[21] EVLA has been proven to be safe, with long-term results comparable or superior to traditional stripping. Min et al. published results on 432 patients (499 limbs) that documented GSV occlusion in 98.2% of cases at 1 month and a success rate of 93.4% in 121 of limbs available at 2-year follow-up.[26] Success was defined as the complete disappearance of detectable blood flow in the treated vein segment on duplex ultrasound examination.[26] In a larger clinical trial that included 990 GSVs treated with EVLA, postprocedural duplex ultrasound at 2 weeks revealed recanalization or incomplete occlusion in only 3.3% of cases.[30] A summary of the effectiveness and safety of the EVLA from the period of its introduction until 2004 reported occlusion of the GSV or elimination of reflux in 87% to 100% of cases.[31] In 2007, Sadick and Wasser[32] published their 4-year experience with EVLA combined with ambulatory phlebotomy. Reported recurrence rates were 5.9%, 3.6%, 3.4%, and 0% at 1, 2, 3, and 4 years of follow-up, respectively.[32] In a recent study from France, where 500 patients (511 limbs) were treated with a 980-nm laser, the authors reported occlusion rates of 98.4%, 97.8%, 99.3%, and 97.1% at 1, 2, 3, and 4 years of follow-up, respectively.[33]

Several randomized, controlled trials have been published comparing EVLA and surgical stripping. Darwood et al. compared EVLA with traditional GSV stripping; they showed that both treatment options had the same effectiveness in the elimination of GSV reflux and confirmed that patients treated with EVLA were able to return faster to normal activities and work.[34] The results from the randomized trial recently published by Rasmussen et al.[35] showed similar efficiency and safety of EVLA and stripping, but patients who underwent EVLA had lower rates of postoperative pain and bruising. Another randomized, controlled trial, where 20 patients with bilateral GSV reflux underwent EVLA with high ligation on one extremity and surgical stripping on the other, demonstrated significantly lower rates of bruising and swelling in the EVLA arm of the study.[36] A randomized, controlled trial that included 100 patients reported a significantly smaller hematoma size in patients treated with EVLA (with high ligation) compared to surgical stripping.[37] The same authors reported that short-term quality of life associated with EVLA was at least as good as after stripping.[37]

The sensation of "pulling" along the course of ablated vein is the most commonly described complain following EVLA. The most commonly reported side effects associated with EVLA are pain, ecchymosis, induration, and phlebitis.[31] These side effects are generally self-limited and often resolve without additional therapy.

Major side effects following EVLA are uncommon. However, the extension of the clot into the deep venous system deserves special consideration. A retrospective analysis at the Mayo Clinic reported thrombus protrusion into the femoral vein in 2.3% of cases.[21] Patients were asymptomatic and thrombus extensions were discovered at follow-up ultrasonography. All cases resolved spontaneously with anticoagulation therapy.

Sclerotherapy

Although originally described in 1939, foam sclerotherapy was not initially accepted as a favorable treatment option, leaving the dominant therapeutic role to surgical stripping. The introduction of ultrasound guidance represented a significant advancement that was amplified by Tessari's development of a method for creating microfoam.[38] These advancements contributed to the evolution of ultrasound-guided foam sclerotherapy (UGFS), which has the potential to become a widely applied treatment option among endovascular treatment modalities. The administration of foamed sclerosant was reintroduced in the early 1990s by Cabrera et al.[39] Currently, sclerotherapy is used in the United States and Europe to treat both GSVs and associated varicosities.

Sclerotherapy involves the percutaneous injection of the sclerosing agent into the lumen of an affected vessel. The sclerosing agent causes irreversible chemical injury to the endothelial lining (exposing subendothelial collagen), which initiates platelet aggregation and activation of the intrinsic pathway of the coagulation cascade. Subsequent endofibrosis of the vein leads to endoluminal obliteration, ideally without thrombus formation. Intrinsic (physical) properties of the sclerosants are important factors that affect the efficiency of the treatment.[40] Liquid sclerosants become diluted by intraluminal blood, making it necessary to use higher doses, which in turn increases the possibility of toxicity and side effects. Liquid sclerosants are also less effective in the treatment of large veins. The evolution of foam sclerotherapy offered an advantage in the treatment of varicose veins. Microfoam bubbles displace the intralesional blood (preventing the sclerosant from becoming diluted) and achieve maximal effective exposure between the sclerosing agent and the endothelial lining.[40] These properties make it possible to use smaller doses, decreasing the risk of side effects and toxicity. In addition, the echogenicity of the microfoam bubbles makes them visible on ultrasound surveillance, ensuring that the injection is intraluminal. Today, numerous sclerosing agents are available. Sodium tetradecyl sulfate and polidocanol are the most commonly accepted. Polidocanol has been effectively used in Europe, but the lack of FDA approval limits it usage in the United States.

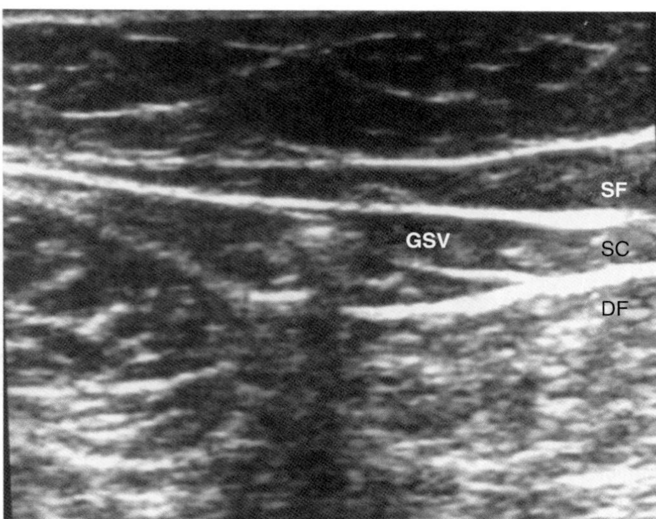

Figure 45-10. Sclerofoam ablation of the great saphenous vein (GSV) can be easily monitored via ultrasound. A solid hyperechogenic core projecting an acoustic shadow on the tissue below is noticed immediately after foam injection. DF, deep fascia; SC, saphenous compartment; SF, superficial fascia. (Adapted from Bergan J. *The vein book*. ch 18. Philadelphia, Elsevier; 2007:175.)

Description of Procedure

There are two methods of foam preparation; Monfreux and Tessari. As mentioned earlier, the Tessari method[38] of mixing is the preferred option for microfoam production. Two syringes, one containing sclerosant and the other filled with atmospheric air (usually in a ratio of 2:1 to 3:1), are attached to a three-way plastic connector. Foam is produced by passing sclerosant between the two syringes. It appears that optimal foam consistency is achieved with 20 passes. The higher the ratio of air-to-liquid sclerosant, the more potent the foam. To improve the safety of the procedure, at the First European Consensus Conference on Foam Sclerotherapy, it was agreed that a maximum volume of 6 to 8 ml of sclerosant per session should be considered safe.[41] Since experience with sclerotherapy showed excellent results and the procedure has been proven to be relatively safe, the maximum recommended volume was increased to 10 ml per session during the Second European Consensus Conference held in 2006.[42]

Local anesthetics can be used to decrease pain and discomfort but are not usually necessary. To empty the superficial venous system and "set" the foam in the leg, the treated extremity should be elevated before sclerosant injection. The SFJ should be externally compressed to prevent advancement of the sclerosant into the deep venous system and to prevent microemboli. When treating the GSV, cannulation is performed under ultrasound guidance as described for EVLA and RFA. When treating varicosities only, either visual or ultrasound guidance may be used. The leg should remain elevated for an additional 10 minutes after injection of the sclerosant to achieve more effective endoluminal obliteration. The whole procedure is performed under ultrasound surveillance (Figure 45-10). The final step is postprocedural placement of compression dressings, left in place by the patient for 1 week. Patients are encouraged to ambulate and return to daily activities immediately after the procedure.

Outcomes and Complications

The first advantage observed with the UGFS was the ability to treat varicose veins regardless of size. As with other endovascular treatment options, UGFS can be performed in an outpatient setting under local anesthesia.

In 2000, Cabrera et al. reported follow-up on 500 limbs treated with polidocanol, with an obliteration rate of 81% after 3 years and disappearance of superficial branches in 96.5%.[39] In 86% of limbs, obliteration was achieved without additional treatments. Two treatments were required in 10.5% and three repetitions in 3.5% of cases. In 2002, Frullini and Cavezzi described 453 patients treated with foam sclerotherapy prepared using the Monfreux and Tessari methods, with immediate success rates of 88.1% and 93.3%, respectively.[40] A multicenter, prospective study conducted in France compared foam with liquid sclerosants in 88 patients.[43] Results demonstrated absence of GSV reflux in 84% after 3 weeks in the group treated with foam sclerotherapy. At 2 months, two recanalizations were reported. At 12 months, no additional recanalizations were observed.[43] A randomized, controlled, multicenter trial that included 106 patients with incompetent GSV demonstrated higher rates of GSV reflux elimination and significantly higher patient satisfaction with the procedure in the group treated with foam sclerotherapy compared to the group in which sclerosant was used in the liquid form.[44] Adverse effects reported from this study were also higher in a group treated with liquid sclerotherapy.[44]

Proper perioperative preparation, care, and technique can significantly reduce the possibility of adverse effects related to UGFS, most importantly with regard to the most debated issue, that of microembolization of foam particles. Complications that occurred on the arterial side of circulation were detected in patients with patent foramen ovale. Specifically, in a series of 869 patients, Bergan reported ocular complications in 4 patients.[45] These complications were not observed after the technique was modified to include elevation of the lower extremity that is being treated. In the study in which 33 consecutive patients with CVI were treated with polidocanol foam sclerotherapy, careful echocardiographical evaluation detected the presence of foam microemboli in the right atrium and ventricle in all 33 cases.[45] In 5 patients, with right to left shunting due the patent foramen ovale, foam microemboli were also detected in the left atrium and ventricle. They were visualized 45 seconds to 15 minutes after the foam was injected, even though procedures were performed with slight leg elevation and external manual compression at the level of the SFJ. However, no neurological defects associated with treatment were reported during the study. An estimated prevalence of patent foramen ovale (which can be the source of paradoxical embolism) in the general population is 26%,[46] but the clinical significance of this with regard to the use of foam sclerotherapy for superficial reflux and varicose veins is unknown.

Other complications associated with foam sclerotherapy are minor and often resolve spontaneously. Extension of the thrombus beyond the SFJ is rare. Perivascular injection of sclerosant may result in local ulceration. The most commonly described side effects associated with sodium tetradecyl sulfate foam sclerotherapy are various allergic reactions and hyperpigmentation. Hyperpigmentation is related to the skin type, and allergic reactions range from urticaria to anaphylaxis. Although allergic reactions related to sodium tetradecyl sulfate are low in incidence, patients susceptible to anaphylactic reactions in general should be treated with special precaution regarding prophylaxis.[47]

Initial experiences with UGFS are encouraging, but further investigation and long-term follow-up studies are needed to accept UGFS as favorable endovascular treatment for varicose veins.

CONCLUSION

Historically, high ligation and GSV stripping has been the mainstay of treatment for varicose veins and CVI associated with superficial reflux disease. Significant morbidity related to bruising and surgical scars and high recurrence rates related to neovascularization have been the major limitations of the surgical approach. In addition, the need for general or regional anesthesia and prolonged recovery time with surgical stripping limited its use. The advent of endovascular techniques has made it possible to treat many more patients with venous disease because of the significant reduction in all these factors and the favorable efficacy profile. Therefore, endovascular procedures are the treatment of choice for most patients with varicose veins associated with superficial reflux. Based on available data, the disadvantages of RFA compared to EVLA include slow pullback time, relatively common need for a second catheter pass, and higher rates of reinterventions. However, the newer iteration of the VNUS catheter (the RSTA) may reduce these distinctions. The advantages of RFA and RSTA include well-tolerated discomfort during and after the procedure by the patient. Randomized, controlled trials comparing EVLA with surgical stripping and RFA with surgical stripping showed that both surgical and endovenous therapies were equally effective but that EVLA and RFA were associated with lower complication rates, reduced postoperative pain, shorter sick leave, faster resumption of normal activities, and higher patient preference. The ability to treat veins regardless of their size, cost effectiveness, and relative procedural simplicity is a significant advantage offered by sclerotherapy, but lack of results regarding safety and durability limits its application in the United States at present.

The decision of which endovascular procedure should be used should be based on the judgment of an experienced practitioner in the context of a discussion of the options with the patient. What is clear today is that all endovascular treatment options represent a significant advancement in the management of varicose veins and superficial reflux, leaving surgical stripping with an important but highly limited role to play. Since the use of endovenous procedures to eliminate venous reflux has been growing exponentially over the last few years, we should expect that advancements in technology will further contribute to the improvement of the endovenous treatments.

References

1. Criqui MH, Denenberg JO, Bergan J, et al. Risk factors for chronic venous disease: the San Diego Population Study. *J Vasc Surg* 2007;46(2):331-337.
2. Beebe-Dimmer JL, Pfeifer JR, Engle JS, Schottenfeld D. The epidemiology of chronic venous insufficiency and varicose veins. *Ann Epidemiol* 2005;15(3):175-184.
3. White JV, Ryjewski C. Chronic venous insufficiency. *Perspect Vasc Surg Endovasc Ther* 2005;17(4):319-327.
4. Pascarella L, Penn A, Schmid-Schonbein GW. Venous hypertension and the inflammatory cascade: major manifestations and trigger mechanisms. *Angiology* 2005;56(Suppl 1):S3-S10.
5. Bergan JJ, Pascarella L, Schmid-Schonbein GW. Pathogenesis of primary chronic venous disease: insights from animal models of venous hypertension. *J Vasc Surg* 2008;47(1):183-192.
6. Arnoldi CC. Treatment of varicose veins of the lower extremities by stripping. *Ugeskr Laeger* 1956;118(35):1015-1017.
7. Caggiati A, Bergan JJ, Gloviczki P, et al. Nomenclature of the veins of the lower limbs: an international interdisciplinary consensus statement. *J Vasc Surg* 2002;36(2):416-422.
8. Caggiati A, Bergan JJ, Gloviczki P, et al. Nomenclature of the veins of the lower limb: extensions, refinements, and clinical application. *J Vasc Surg* 2005;41(4):719-724.
9. Labropoulos N, Tiongson J, Pryor L, et al. Definition of venous reflux in lower-extremity veins. *J Vasc Surg* 2003;38(4):793-798.
10. Bergan JJ. Saphenous vein stripping and quality of outcome. *Br J Surg* 1996;83(8):1027.
11. Winterborn RJ, Earnshaw JJ. Crossectomy and great saphenous vein stripping. *J Cardiovasc Surg (Torino)* 2006;47(1):19-33.
12. Jones L, Braithwaite BD, Selwyn D, et al. Neovascularisation is the principal cause of varicose vein recurrence: results of a randomised trial of stripping the long saphenous vein. *Eur J Vasc Endovasc Surg* 1996;12(4):442-445.
13. Geier B, Olbrich S, Barbera L, et al. Validity of the macroscopic identification of neovascularization at the saphenofemoral junction by the operating surgeon. *J Vasc Surg* 2005;41(1):64-68.
14. Teruya TH, Ballard JL. New approaches for the treatment of varicose veins. *Surg Clin North Am* 2004;84(5):1397-1417, viii-ix.
15. Shortell C, Rhodes JR, Johanssen M, et al. Radiofrequency ablation for superficial venous reflux: improved outcomes in a high volume university setting. Presented at the SVS Annual Meeting, June 12, 2005, Chicago, Illinois.
16. Pichot O, Sessa C, Chandler JG, et al. Role of duplex imaging in endovenous obliteration for primary venous insufficiency. *J Endovasc Ther* 2000;7(6):451-459.
17. Stirling M, Shortell CK. Endovascular treatment of varicose veins. *Semin Vasc Surg* 2006;19(2):109-115.
18. Merchant RF, Pichot O, Myers KA. Four-year follow-up on endovascular radiofrequency obliteration of great saphenous reflux. *Dermatol Surg* 2005;31(2):129-134.
19. Lurie F, Creton D, Eklof B, et al. Prospective randomized study of endovenous radiofrequency obliteration (closure procedure) versus ligation and stripping in a selected patient population (EVOLVeS Study). *J Vasc Surg* 2003;38(2):207-214.
20. Lurie F, Creton D, Eklof B, et al. Prospective randomised study of endovenous radiofrequency obliteration (closure) versus ligation and vein stripping (EVOLVeS): two-year follow-up. *Eur J Vasc Endovasc Surg* 2005;29(1):67-73.
21. Puggioni A, Kalra M, Carmo M, et al. Endovenous laser therapy and radiofrequency ablation of the great saphenous vein: analysis of early efficacy and complications. *J Vasc Surg* 2005;42(3):488-493.
22. Varnagy D, Labropoulos N. The issue of spontaneous arteriovenous fistulae after superficial thrombophlebitis, endovenous ablations, and deep vein thrombosis: an unusual but predictable finding. *Perspect Vasc Surg Endovasc Ther* 2006;18(3):247-250.

23. Proebstle TM, Vago B, Alm J, et al. Treatment of the incompetent great saphenous vein by endovenous radiofrequency powered segmental thermal ablation: first clinical experience. *J Vasc Surg* 2008;47(1):151-156.
24. Navarro L, Min R, Boné C. Endovenous laser: a new minimally invasive method of treatment for varicose veins—preliminary observations using an 810-nm diode laser. *Dermatol Surg* 2001;27:117-122.
25. Proebstle TM, Lehr HA, Kargl A, et al. Endovenous treatment of the greater saphenous vein with a 940-nm diode laser: thrombotic occlusion after endoluminal thermal damage by laser generated steam bubbles. *J Vasc Surg* 2002;35:729-736.
26. Min RJ, Khilnani N, Zimmet SE. Endovenous laser treatment of saphenous vein reflux: long-term results. *J Vasc Interv Radiol* 2003;14(8):991-996.
27. Proebstle TM, Gul D, Kargl A, Knop J. Non-occlusion and early reopening of the great saphenous vein after endovenous laser treatment is fluency dependent. *Dermatolog Surg* 2004;30:174-178.
28. Min RJ, Khilnani NM. Lower-extremity varicosities: endoluminal therapy. *Semin Roentgenol* 2002;37(4):354-360.
29. Min RJ, Khilnani NM. Endovenous laser treatment of saphenous vein reflux. *Tech Vasc Interv Radiol* 2003;6(3):125-131.
30. Ravi R, Rodriguez-Lopez JA, Traylor EA, et al. Endovenous ablation of incompetent saphenous veins: a large single-center experience. *J Endovasc Ther* 2006;13:244-248.
31. Mundy L, Merlin TL, Fitridge RA, Hiller JE. Systematic review of endovenous laser treatment for varicose veins. *Br J Surg* 2005;92:1189-1194.
32. Sadick NS, Wasser S. Combined endovascular laser plus ambulatory phlebectomy for the treatment of superficial venous incompetence: a 4-year perspective. *J Cosmet Laser Ther* 2007;9:9-13.
33. Desmyttère J, Grard C, Wassmer B, Mordon S. Endovenous 980-nm laser treatment of saphenous veins in a series of 500 patients. *J Vasc Surg* 2007;46(6):1242-1247.
34. Darwood RJ, Theivacumar N, Dellagrammaticas D, et al. Randomized clinical trial comparing endovenous laser ablation with surgery for the treatment of primary great saphenous varicose veins. *Br J Surg* 2008;95(3):294-301.
35. Rasmussen LH, Bjoern L, Lawaetz M, et al. Randomized trial comparing endovenous laser ablation of the great saphenous vein with high ligation and stripping in patients with varicose veins: short-term results. *J Vasc Surg* 2007;46(2):308-315.
36. Medeiros CAF, Luccas GC. Comparison of endovenous treatment with an 810 nm laser versus conventional stripping of the great saphenous vein in patients with primary varicose veins. *Dermatol Surg* 2005;31:1685-1694.
37. Kalteis M, Berger I, Messie-Werndl S, et al. High ligation combined with stripping and endovenous laser ablation of the great saphenous vein: early results of a randomized controlled study. *J Vasc Surg* 2008;47(4):822-829.
38. Tessari L, Cavezzi A, Frullini A. Preliminary experience with a new sclerosing foam in the treatment of varicose veins. *Dermatol Surg* 2001;27(1):58-60.
39. Cabrera J, Cabrera J, Garcia-Olmedo MA. Treatment of varicose long saphenous veins with sclerosant in microfoam form: long term outcomes. *Phlebology* 2000;15:19-23.
40. Frullini A, Cavezzi A. Sclerosing foam in the treatment of varicose veins and telangiectases: history and analysis of safety and complications. *Dermatol Surg* 2002;28(1):11-15.
41. Breu FX, Guggenbichler S. European consensus meeting on foam sclerotherapy, April, 4-6, 2003, Tegernsee, Germany. *Dermatol Surg* 2004;30:709-717.
42. Breu FX, Guggenbichler S. Wollmann J-C. 2nd European consensus meeting on foam sclerotherapy, April 28-30, 2006, Tegernsee, Germany. *Vasa* 2008:37.
43. Bergan J, Pascarella L, Mekenas L. Venous disorders: treatment with sclerosant foam. *J Cardiovasc Surg (Torino)* 2006;47(1):9-18.
44. Rabe E, Otto J, Schliephake D, Pannier F. Efficacy and safety of great saphenous vein sclerotherapy using standardised polidocanol foam (ESAF): a randomised controlled multicentre clinical trial. *Eur J Vasc Endovasc Surg* 2008;35(2):238-245.
45. Ceulen RP, Sommer A, Vernooy K. Microembolism during foam sclerotherapy of varicose veins. *N Engl J Med* 2008;358(14):1525-1526.
46. Meier B, Lock JE. Contemporary management of patent foramen ovale. *Circulation* 2003;107(1):5-9.
47. Bergan J, Pascarella L, Mekenas L. Venous disorders: treatment with sclerosant foam. *J Cardiovasc Surg (Torino)* 2006;47(1):9-18.

chapter

46

Surgical Treatment of Chronic Venous Insufficiency

Joseph J. Ricotta II, MD • Peter Gloviczki, MD, FACS

Key Points

- Goals of surgical treatment
- Preoperative evaluation
- Ablation of perforator vein reflux
- Ablation of deep vein reflux
- Valvuloplasty
- Valve transposition or transplantation
- Treatment of deep venous obstruction
- Endovascular treatment
- Surgical treatment

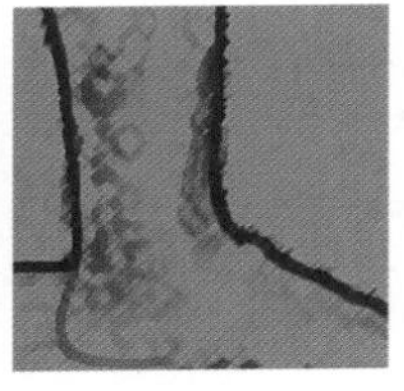

Chronic venous disorders include venous problems ranging from spider veins and simple varicosities to venous ulcers. The term chronic venous insufficiency (CVI) implies a functional abnormality of the venous circulation and is reserved for the advanced forms of chronic venous disease that include venous edema, lipodermatosclerosis, or other skin changes and healed or active venous. In the United States, 10% to 35% of adults have some form of CVI. CVI with advanced skin change and ulcers affects approximately 2% of the population in Western countries, with a prevalence comparable to that of diabetes.[1] Venous ulcers are the most common form of leg ulcers, and their incidence has remained unchanged over the last 25 years. The cost to health-care systems of chronic venous disease is massive: 5% of patients lose their jobs as a result of the disease, and 4.6 million U.S. workdays are lost each year. As a result, the population-based costs to the U.S. government for CVI treatment are estimated to exceed $1 billion per year.[2]

GOALS OF SURGICAL TREATMENT

Surgical treatment of CVI is aimed at removing unsightly varicose veins, preventing recurrence of varicosities, and treating signs and symptoms of chronic venous disease, such as venous claudication, limb swelling, eczema, pain, and ulceration (Figure 46-1).

The main goal of surgical treatment is to correct the underlying abnormal venous physiology. Surgical correction of the abnormal ambulatory venous pressure is mandatory to achieve lasting relief of symptoms. The relationship between venous ulceration and ambulatory venous pressure was described by Beecher et al. as early as 1931.[19] Subsequent studies have confirmed that ambulatory venous pressure has not only diagnostic but also prognostic significance in CVI.[3] Reflux caused by valvular incompetence is predominantly responsible for high ambulatory venous pressure in CVI. The CEAP classification[4,5] listed the three etiologies of CVI: congenital, primary, and secondary (Table 46-1). Primary valvular incompetence (PVI) may involve the superficial, perforator, and deep veins. It is classified as primary in the absence of documented deep venous thrombosis (DVT) by history or evidence of postthrombotic changes in the deep veins on duplex examination or venography. Secondary incompetence is often limited to the deep and perforating veins and usually occurs following one or more episodes of DVT. Deep venous obstruction secondary to DVT is a less common cause of advanced CVI (less than 10%), resulting more often in leg swelling and venous claudication.[6] The rare combination of iliac vein obstruction with reflux below the common femoral vein in a postthrombotic leg results in a complex lesion with severe consequences.

PVI accounts for approximately 70% of advanced CVI (class 4 to 6), with the remainder occurring in legs following DVT.[7,8] Severe isolated incompetence of the superficial system may also lead to high ambulatory pressures and the development of ulcers, but most patients with a venous ulcer have multisystem (superficial, deep, perforator) incompetence, involving at least two of the three venous systems.[9,10] A duplex ultrasound study in 91 legs with venous ulcerations from Boston University revealed isolated superficial vein incompetence in only 17%.[11] Incompetent calf perforators in conjunction

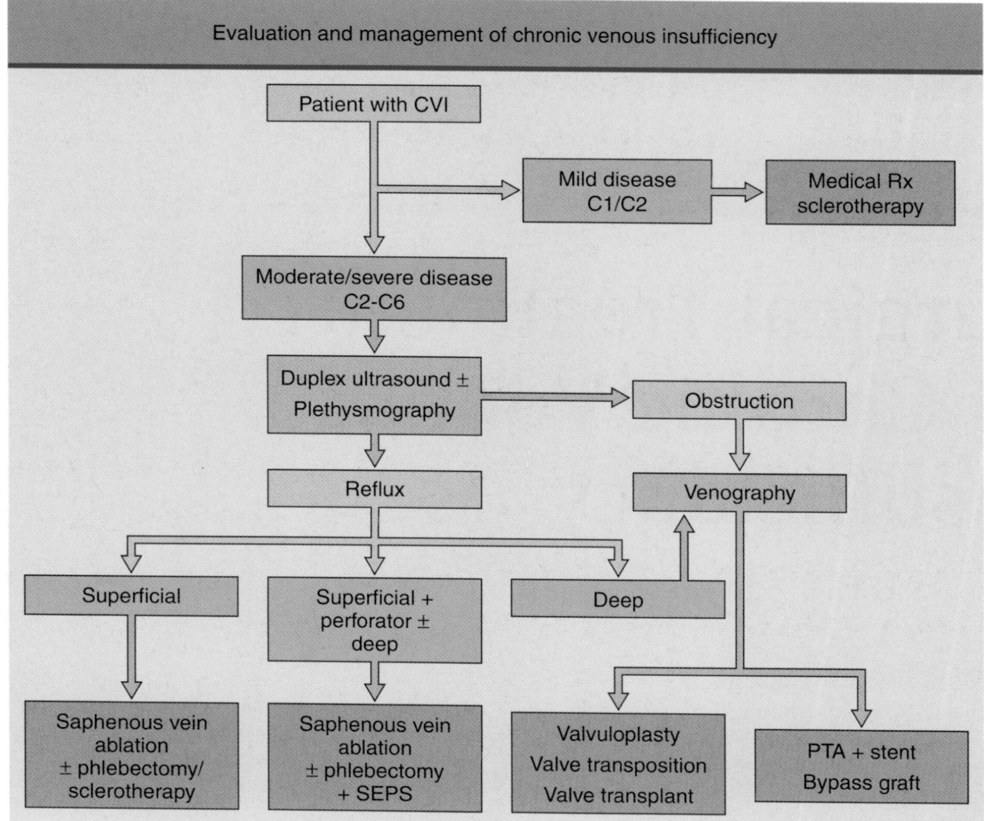

Figure 46-1. Evaluation and management of chronic venous insufficiency.

with superficial or deep reflux have been reported in 66% of legs with venous ulceration, and they occur more often in advanced disease with skin change.[12] Deep venous incompetence can occur in as many as 80% of patients with a venous ulcer (Table 46-2).[9,12]

PREOPERATIVE EVALUATION

The initial evaluation of a patient with CVI is a clinical examination supplemented by a handheld continuous-wave Doppler exam. The extent of further investigation and treatment planning is dictated by the severity of the clinical stage of chronic venous disease as assessed by the CEAP classification and the degree to which the patient is willing to accept a change in lifestyle. In the event of spider veins or telangiectasias (class 1) causing only cosmetic concerns, and no reflux on clinical or continuous-wave Doppler examination, no further investigation is necessary. If reflux is suspected clinically, a duplex ultrasound is warranted. Patients with varicose veins alone (class 2) and those with moderate or advanced CVI (class 3 to 6) who are potential surgical candidates require a complete workup in the vascular laboratory. Patients who are not surgical candidates because of advanced age or multiple comorbidities and are only offered conservative treatment do not merit a detailed workup. Noninvasive workup begins with duplex examination, which is all that is required in patients with varicose veins with no edema or skin changes (class 2).[13] Plethysmography is indicated to evaluate the impact of the anatomical abnormalities found on duplex on the pathophysiology of the venous system. At this stage, it is possible to complete the remaining elements of the CEAP classification and provide a comprehensive description of the patient's venous problem, (clinical, etiological, anatomical, and pathophysiological). The CEAP classification provides description of venous disease in a uniform, reproducible language; allows an objective evaluation of the effect of treatment; and facilitates comparison of treatment modalities across centers. It is imperative that every patient undergoing surgical treatment for CVI today have a venous disease studied adequately and defined according to these criteria. With the level of sophistication of present-day duplex scans, contrast venography is rarely indicated. We recommend performing contrast venography in patients with suspected significant deep venous obstruction and in those who may undergo treatment for deep vein valvular incompetence.

Duplex Scan

The duplex scan that combines B-mode imaging, color flow, and pulsed Doppler is the most valuable test in the evaluation of venous disease today. Direct visualization provides information on the patency and wall characteristics of each venous segment and the morphology of the valves. Systematic interrogation of the superficial, deep, and perforator systems provides an anatomical map of the veins of the lower limb. It helps determine whether obstruction, reflux, or a combination

Table 46-1
CEAP Classification of Lower Extremity Chronic Venous Disease

C = Clinical Signs (Class 0-6)
C0: No visible or palpable sign of venous disease
C1: Telangiectases, reticular veins, and malleolar flare
C2: Varicose veins
C3: Edema without skin changes
C4: Skin changes attributed to venous disease (e.g., pigmentation, venous eczema, lipodermatosclerosis)
C5: Healed venous ulcer
C6: Active venous ulcer

E = Etiological Classification
Congenital (E_C): Cause of venous disease present since birth
Primary (E_P): Chronic venous disease of undetermined cause
Secondary (E_S): Chronic venous disease with known cause (postthombotic, posttraumatic, other)

A = Anatomic Distribution
A_{S1-5}: Superficial veins
A_{D6-16}: Deep veins
A_{P17-18}: Perforating veins

P = Pathophysiology Dysfunction
P_R: Reflux
P_O: Obstruction
$P_{R,O}$: Reflux and obstruction

of the two is responsible for causing the symptoms and signs of CVI. In most cases, it is possible to differentiate PVI from postthrombotic syndrome on duplex scanning. The presence and site of valvular incompetence is identified by documenting retrograde flow on the Valsalva maneuver or release of a distal tourniquet with the patient standing. Retrograde flow that lasts longer than 0.5 seconds or the duration of antegrade flow signifies valvular incompetence.[17] Perforator veins are identified visually and incompetence confirmed by bidirectional flow on manual calf compression. Candidates for subfascial endoscopic perforator vein surgery (SEPS) should have the sites of incompetent perforators marked on the skin the day before surgery. Duplex examination can provide qualitative information about the anatomical presence of obstruction or reflux; however, it cannot quantitate it or assess its hemodynamic significance.

Plethysmography

Duplex scanning identifies the presence and location of reflux or obstruction in the venous system, but plethysmography is required to quantitate the pathophysiological abnormality identified. Various plethysmographic techniques (air, strain gauge, impedance) quantitate the degree of reflux, obstruction, or calf muscle dysfunction by measuring a change in calf volume on various maneuvers. Venous outflow obstruction is assessed by determining the outflow fraction, which is the venous outflow volume in 1 second divided by the total calf volume. Valvular reflux is measured by estimating the venous filling index, the rate of filling through 90% of venous volume. Calf muscle pump function is assessed by measuring the ejection fraction and the residual volume fraction of calf venous volume following calf muscle contraction. However, these techniques provide information about the hemodynamics of the entire limb without the ability to localize the abnormality. It is especially useful in patients in whom both reflux and partial obstruction are elicited on duplex scanning, where it helps identify the dominant pathology. Repeated plethysmographic examination, because of its quantitative nature, can be used to monitor the progression of venous disease, as well as the response to surgical treatment.

Venography

Ascending venography is performed in the semierect, non-weight-bearing position by injecting intravenous contrast into a dorsal foot vein after placing a tourniquet at the ankle to

Table 46-2
Distribution of Valvular Incompetence in Patients with Advanced Chronic Venous Disease*

Author	Year	Limbs *(n)*	Sup *n* (%)	Perf *n* (%)	Deep *n* (%)	Sup + Perf *n* (%)	Sup + Perf + Deep *n* (%)
Schanzer and Peirce[14]	1982	52	3 (6)	20 (38)	4 (8)	11 (21)	14 (27)
Negus and Friedgood[15]	1983	77	0 (0)	0 (0)	0 (0)	35 (46)	42 (54)
Sethia[95]	1984	60	0 (0)	5 (8)	20 (33)	17 (28)	18 (30)
van Bemmelen[96]	1991	25	0 (0)	0 (0)	2 (8)	3 (12)	20 (80)
Hanrahan et al.[11]	1991	91	16 (17)	8 (8)	2 (2)	18 (19)	47 (49)
Darke[16]	1992	213	0 (0)	8 (4)	47 (22)	83 (39)	75 (35)
Lees[97]	1993	25	3 (12)	0 (0)	3 (12)	10 (40)	9 (36)
Shami[98]	1993	59	0 (0)	0 (0)	19 (32)	31 (53)	9 (15)
van Rij et al.[9]	1994	120	48 (40)	6 (5)	10 (8)	31 (26)	25 (21)
Myers et al.[12]	1995	96	15 (16)	2 (2)	7 (8)	25 (26)	47 (49)
Labropoulos et al.[10]	1996	120	26 (22)	1 (1)	5 (4)	23 (19)	65 (54)
Gloviczki et al.[7]	1999	146	0 (0)	7 (5)	0 (0)	66 (45)	73 (50)
Total Limbs *n* (%)		1084	111 (10)	57 (5)	119 (11)	353 (32)	444 (41)

*Deep, deep vein incompetence; Perf, perforator incompetence; Sup, superficial incompetence.

prevent filling of the superficial veins. Thenatomy of calf and thigh veins is accurately demonstrated, obstructed segments and collaterals are readily visualized, and the presence and site of incompetent perforators can be identified. It is the best available test to differentiate between PVI and postthrombotic syndrome and remains fundamental to planning deep venous reconstruction.

Descending venography is necessary to identify the location of venous valves and evaluate their degree of incompetence before venous valve reconstruction. Contrast is injected into the external iliac vein via a catheter inserted through the contralateral groin, and images are recorded on videotape with and without Valsalva maneuver. Severity of venous reflux can be classified according to Kistner's grades 0 to 4 (0: no incompetence; 1: reflux into the proximal superficial femoral vein, or SFV; 2: reflux limited to the thigh; 3: reflux into the popliteal vein and proximal calf; 4: reflux to the distal calf or ankle).[17] Patients with reflux extending below the knee are suitable candidates for venous valve reconstruction or transplantation. Descending venography alone may fail to demonstrate significant superficial femoral or popliteal reflux in the presence of a competent common femoral vein valve.

Ambulatory Venous Pressure Measurement

Rarely performed these days in its original form, the ambulatory venous pressure measurement provides an objective assessment of venous hemodynamics and the degree of CVI. A dorsal foot vein is cannulated, and the pressure is measured in the standing position before, during, and after 10 tiptoe exercises. Normal ambulatory venous pressure ranges from 20 to 30 mm Hg, or a greater than 50% decrease from the resting state, which is usually 80 to 90 mm Hg. A refill time of greater than 20 seconds is considered normal. With the availability of noninvasive venous testing such as duplex imaging and plethysmography, the clinical application of ambulatory venous pressure measurement has diminished.

Direct cannulation of the femoral vein to measure the pressure gradient across an iliac lesion is used to assess the hemodynamic significance of a proximal venous occlusion. A pressure gradient of 5 mm Hg, or a twofold increase in venous pressure, following foot exercise suggests hemodynamically significant venous obstruction.

SURGICAL TREATMENT

Surgical treatment aims to alleviate symptoms of CVI and promote ulcer healing by reducing ambulatory venous hypertension. It needs to be individualized for each patient based on the results of both noninvasive and invasive investigation of the venous system as described earlier. Depending on the underlying pathophysiology in a particular patient, this may be achieved by the following:

1. Ablation of superficial reflux
   a. Ablation of saphenous vein reflux
   b. Removal of varicose veins (phlebectomy)
2. Ablation of perforator vein reflux
3. Ablation of deep venous reflux
4. Treatment of deep venous obstruction

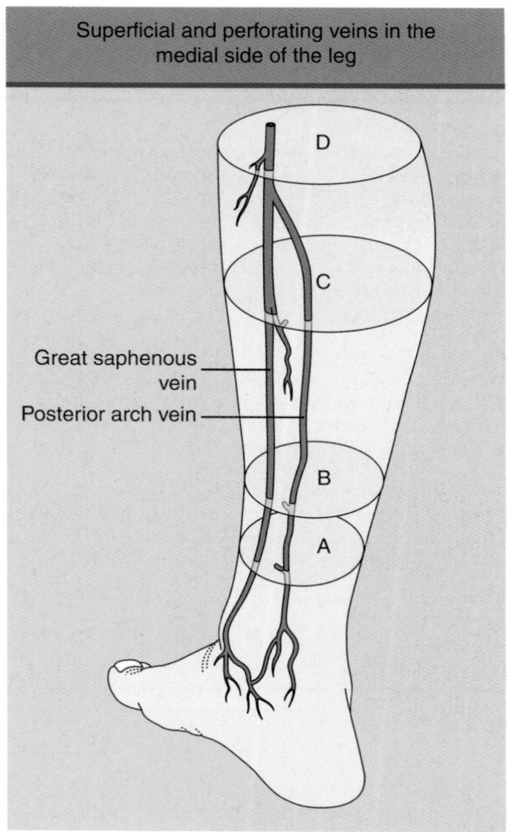

Figure 46-2. Superficial and perforating veins in the medial side of the leg. (From Mozes G, Gloviczki P, Menawat SS, et al. *J Vasc Surg* 1996;24:800-808.)

Ablation of Superficial Reflux

Ablation of saphenous vein reflux and removal of varicose veins is comprehensively addressed in Chapter 44.

Perforator Vein Interruption

Anatomy of Perforating Veins

Perforating veins connect the superficial to the deep venous system, either directly to the main axial veins (direct perforators) or indirectly to muscular tributaries or soleal venous sinuses (indirect perforators). In most calf and thigh perforators, venous valves assure unidirectional flow, from superficial to deep veins. Perforating veins of the foot, on the other hand, are valveless, and flow occurs paradoxically from the deep to the superficial venous system.[18,19]

The most significant medial calf perforators, termed the posterior tibial or Cockett's perforators, do not originate from the great saphenous vein (GSV) but connect the posterior arch vein (Leonardo's vein) to the paired posterior tibial veins (Figure 46-2). This observation is extremely important as, although the posterior arch vein does connect to the GSV just below the knee, stripping it does not affect flow through these perforators. Three groups of perforators have been identified: the upper, middle and lower posterior tibial perforators, or Cockett I, II, and III. The Cockett I perforator is located posterior to the medial malleolus and may be difficult to reach endoscopically. The Cockett II and III perforators are located

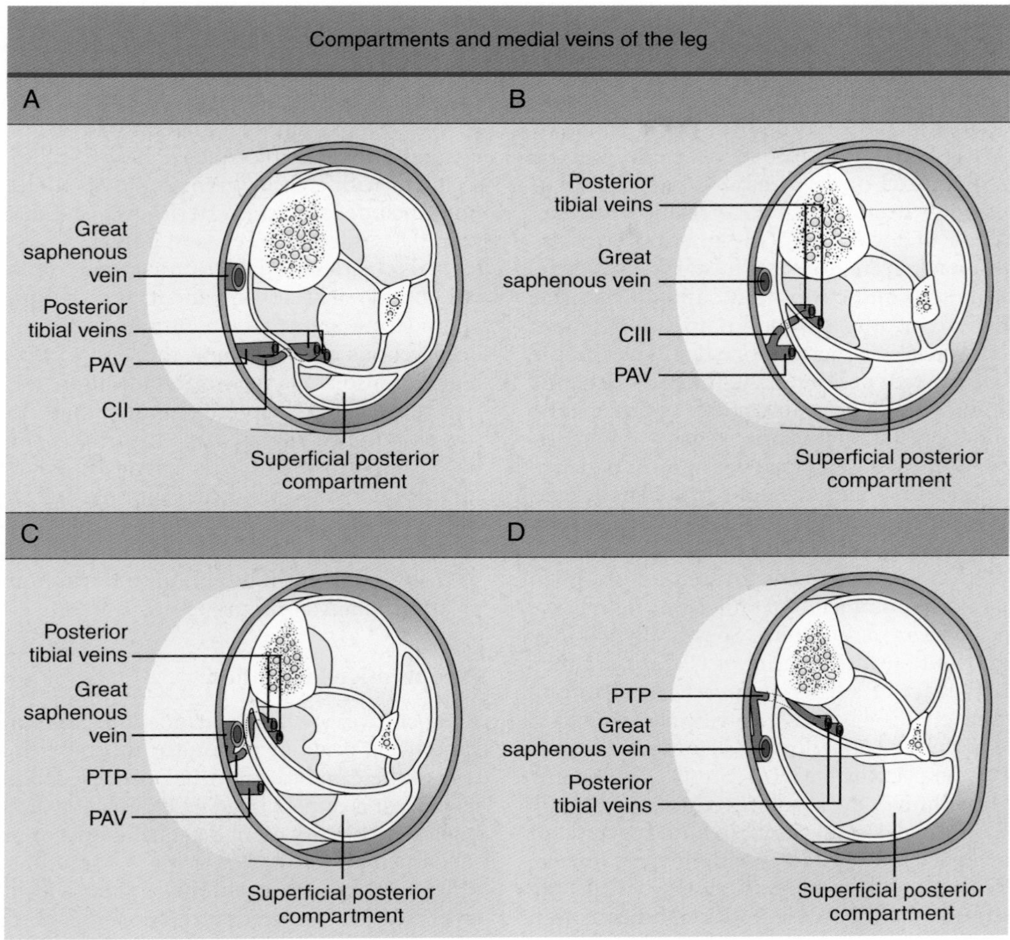

Figure 46-3. Compartments and medial veins of the leg. Cross sections are at the levels of Cockett II (CII; **A**), Cockett III (CIII; **B**), 24 cm **(C)**, and proximal paratibial perforating veins **(D)**. GSV, great saphenous vein; PAV, posterior arch vein; PTP, paratibial perforator; PTVs, posterior tibial veins; SPC, superficial posterior compartment. (From Mozes G, Gloviczki P, Menawat SS, et al. *J Vasc Surg* 1996;24:800-808.)

7 to 9 cm and 10 to 12 cm, respectively, proximal to the lower border of the medial malleolus (Figure 46-3).[20] All are found in "Linton's line," 2 to 4 cm behind the medial edge of the tibia. [18] The paratibial perforators connect the GSV and its tributaries to the posterior tibial and popliteal veins. They are found in three groups, all located 1 to 2 cm posterior to the medial tibial border, 18 to 22 cm, 23 to 27 cm, and 28 to 32 cm from the inferior border of the medial malleolus. Three additional direct perforating veins connect the GSV to the popliteal vein and SFV: Boyd's perforator, just distal to the knee, and Dodd's and Hunterian perforators in the thigh. Boyd's perforator may be reached endoscopically, while stripping of the GSV interrupts the drainage of Dodd's and Hunterian perforators, except in 8% of individuals who have a duplicated saphenous system. In cadaver dissections, Mozes et al. noted that only 63% of all medial perforators were directly accessible from the superficial posterior compartment.[18] These comprise 32% of the midposterior tibial (Cockett II), 84% of the upper posterior tibial (Cockett III), and 43% of lower paratibial perforating veins; the remaining perforators traverse the intermuscular septum dividing the deep and superficial compartments or reside solely within the posterior deep compartment.[18] To interrupt all incompetent perforating veins, two additional areas require exploration: the deep posterior compartment and the intermuscular septum in Linton's line. In the calf, anterior and lateral perforators are also found that may gain clinical significance in patients with lateral ulceration. The anterior perforators connect tributaries of the great and small saphenous veins directly to the anterior tibial veins. The lateral perforating veins connect the small saphenous vein to the peroneal veins (Bassi's perforator).

Significance of Perforating Veins

The consensus of opinion is that venous hypertension in an erect subject and during ambulation is the most important factor responsible for the development of skin change and venous ulceration in CVI. The relationship between venous ulceration and ambulatory venous pressure was first described by Beecher et al. in 1931.[19] Subsequent studies have confirmed that ambulatory venous pressure not only has diagnostic but also has prognostic significance in CVI. Negus and Friedgood described pressures in the supramalleolar network well above 100 mm Hg during calf muscle contraction.[15] The importance of incompetent perforators is also supported by the observation that skin change and venous ulcers almost always develop in the gaiter area of the leg (the area between the distal edge of the soleus muscle and the ankle), where large incompetent medial perforating veins are located.

Most patients with a venous ulcer have multisystem (superficial, deep, perforator) incompetence, involving at least two of the three venous systems. Incompetent calf perforators in conjunction with superficial or deep reflux occur in 56% to 73% of legs with venous ulceration.[7,21] A correlation between the number and size of incompetent perforating veins, as detected by duplex imaging, and the severity of CVI was demonstrated by Labropoulos and coworkers.[10] In patients with advanced disease, more incompetent perforators were found, and their diameters were also larger. Despite this evidence, the contribution of incompetent perforators to the hemodynamic derangement in limbs with CVI remains a topic of debate. The problem is that functional studies cannot reliably differentiate perforator from deep vein incompetence in most patients, so the task of documenting hemodynamic problems related directly to perforator incompetence, even if confirmed with duplex imaging, remains difficult.

The crucial question that remains is focused not so much on the hemodynamic significance but rather on the relative clinical significance of perforating veins. Specifically, do they independently contribute to the severity of CVI, or are they merely a secondary effect of advanced superficial incompetence, deep incompetence, or both? A statistically significant decrease occurred in the rate of perforator incompetence over 12 months in 261 patients in the ESCHAR Study after superficial venous surgery, although the absolute reduction was only from 51% to 42%.[21] Mendes et al. similarly found reversal of perforator incompetence in 71% of legs with no deep incompetence treated with superficial surgery alone,[22] while the Edinburgh group found that 72% of legs with significant deep venous involvement still had persistent perforator incompetence after isolated superficial venous surgery.[23]

Indications for Perforator Interruption

The contribution of incompetent perforating veins to the hemodynamic abnormality in legs with CVI remains a topic of debate. Venous ulcers almost always develop in the gaiter area of the leg where large incompetent medial perforating veins are located. Direct estimation of their hemodynamic significance is difficult, since isolated perforator vein incompetence in CVI is rare[10] and incompetent perforators have been observed in as many as 21% of normal legs. Several authors have demonstrated a correlation between the number and size of incompetent perforating veins detected by duplex ultrasonography and the severity of CVI.[24] Delis et al. quantified perforator incompetence based on diameter, flow velocities, and volume flow and stressed that incompetent perforators sustain further hemodynamic impairment in the presence of deep reflux.[25]

The presence of incompetent perforators in a patient with advanced CVI (clinical classes 4 to 6, i.e., lipodermatosclerosis, healed ulceration, or active ulceration) and low operative risk constitutes a potential indication for perforator ligation. This includes patients with isolated perforator incompetence, as well as those with combined superficial, deep, and perforator incompetence. In the latter group, combined superficial and perforator reflux ablation is a reasonable approach to provide maximum benefit; however, the procedures may be staged in selected patients, reserving perforator interruption for persistent ulceration. Patients with varicose veins (C2 to C3) should be considered for perforator ligation only if varices recur following treatment of superficial incompetence.

While most authors prefer to perform open perforator ligation only after ulcers have healed, SEPS may be done in a patient with a clean, granulating open ulcer. Contraindications include associated arterial occlusive disease (ABPI of less than 0.8), infected ulcer, and a nonambulatory or medically high-risk patient. Diabetes, renal failure, liver failure, morbid obesity, or ulcers in patients with rheumatoid arthritis or scleroderma are relative contraindications. The presence of deep venous obstruction at the level of the popliteal vein or higher is also a relative contraindication. Patients with extensive skin changes, large circumferential ulcers, recent DVT, severe lymphedema, or large legs may not be suitable. SEPS has been performed for recurrent disease after previous perforator interruption; however, it is technically more demanding in this situation. Due to the limited space in the lateral subfascial compartment, legs with lateral ulceration should be managed by open perforator interruption or percutaneous ablation, where appropriate.

Preoperative Evaluation

Preoperative evaluation includes imaging studies to document superficial, deep, or perforator incompetence or a combination of these and to guide the operative intervention. The preferred test is duplex imaging that has 100% specificity and the highest sensitivity of all diagnostic tests to predict the sites of incompetent perforating veins.[26] Ascending and descending phlebography is reserved for patients with underlying occlusive disease or recurrent ulceration after perforator division in whom deep venous reconstruction is being considered. Preoperative duplex mapping assists the surgeon in identifying all incompetent perforators at the time of operation. Duplex imaging is performed with the patient on a tilted examining table and the affected leg in a near-upright, non-weight-bearing position. Perforator incompetence is defined by retrograde (outward) flow lasting greater than 0.3 seconds or longer than antegrade flow during the relaxation phase after release of manual compression. Identified perforators are marked on the skin with a nonerasable pen.

In addition, a functional study such as strain-gauge or air plethysmography is performed before and after surgery to quantitate the degree of incompetence, identify abnormalities in calf muscle pump function, aid in the exclusion of outflow obstruction, and assess hemodynamic results of surgical intervention.

Surgical Technique

Open Technique of Perforator Interruption

Linton's original radical operation of subfascial ligation[27] that included long medial, anterolateral, and posterolateral calf incisions was abandoned because of a high rate of wound complications. In a subsequent report published in 1953, Linton advocated only a long medial incision from the ankle to the knee to interrupt all medial and posterior perforating veins.[30,30a] Several authors proposed modifications to Linton's open procedure to limit wound complications. Cockett advocated ligation of the perforating veins above the deep fascia.[28]

The importance of ligating the perforating veins subfascially was emphasized by Sherman, as they branch extensively once they penetrate the deep fascia.[18] Further modifications included the use of shorter medial incisions or a more posteriorly placed stocking seam–type incision.[29] DePalma observed good results and limited wound complications using multiple, parallel bipedicled flaps placed along skin lines to access and ligate the perforating veins above or below the fascia.[30]

Linton[27] and Cockett[28] both reported benefit from open perforator ligation, and this was supported later by data from several other investigators. In larger series, however, ulcer recurrence rates averaged 24%. Burnand et al. reported a 55% ulcer recurrence rate in their patients, with 100% recurrence in a subset of 23 patients with postthrombotic syndrome.[31] Although these data provided compelling evidence against perforating vein ablation, ulcer recurrence in the other patients in the same study, without damage to the deep veins, was only 6%.

The concept of ablating incompetent perforating veins from a site remote from diseased skin was first introduced by Edwards in 1976.[32] He designed a device called the phlebotome, which was inserted through a medial incision just distal to the knee, pushed deep to the fascia, and advanced to the level of the medial malleolus. Resistance was felt as perforators were engaged and subsequently disrupted with the leading edge. Other authors have subsequently reported successful application of this device, passed in either the subfascial or the extrafascial plane.

Interruption of perforators through stab wounds and hook avulsion is another possibility; accuracy of this blind technique is improved if duplex imaging is used. Suture ligation of perforators without making skin incisions is another reported technique. With the widespread use of ultrasound guided techniques, it is possible to localize perforators and do a small, direct cutdown, thus minimizing the extent of the operation. Sclerotherapy of perforating veins is an emerging technique that avoids some of the hazards of surgery.

Techniques of Subfascial Endoscopic Perforator Vein Surgery

First introduced by Hauer in 1985, interruption of incompetent perforators using endoscopic instruments may now be performed through small ports placed remotely from the active ulcer.[33-35] Since its introduction, two main techniques have been developed. The first, practiced mostly in Europe, is a refinement of the original work of Hauer[33] with further development by Bergan[34] and by Pierik et al.[26] This single port technique started using available light sources such as mediastinoscopes and bronchoscopes. With time, a specially designed instrument was devised that uses a single telescope with channels for the camera and working instruments; this can make visualization and dissection in the same plane difficult. Recent developments include the use of carbon dioxide insufflation into the subfascial plane.

The second technique, using instrumentation from laparoscopic surgery, was introduced in the United States by O'Donnell,[36] and developed simultaneously at the Mayo Clinic[37] and by Conrad in Australia.[38] This two-port technique employs one port for the camera and a separate port for instrumentation, thereby making it easier to work in the limited subfascial space. To provide a bloodless field, the limb is first exsanguinated with an Esmarque bandage and a thigh tourniquet is inflated to 300 mm Hg (Figure 46-4A). A 10-mm endoscopic port is next placed in the medial aspect of the calf 10 cm distal to the tibial tuberosity and proximal to the diseased skin. Balloon dissection is used to widen the subfascial space and facilitate access after port placement (Figure 46-4B). The distal 5-mm port is then placed halfway between the first port and the ankle (about 10 to 12 cm apart) under direct vision with the camera (Figure 46-4C). The 10-mm camera withstands the torque better than a 5-mm device and reaches all the way to the medial malleolus. Carbon dioxide is insufflated into the subfascial space, and pressure is maintained around 30 mm Hg to improve visualization and access to the perforators. Using laparoscopic scissors inserted through the second port, the remaining loose connective tissue between the calf muscles and the superficial fascia is divided.

The subfascial space is widely explored from the medial border of the tibia to the posterior midline and down to the level of the ankle. All perforators encountered are divided with the harmonic scalpel, electrocautery, or sharply between clips (Figure 46-4D). A paratibial fasciotomy is next made by incising the fascia of the posterior deep compartment close to the tibia to avoid any injury to the posterior tibial vessels and the tibial nerve. The Cockett II and Cockett III perforators are often located within an intermuscular septum, and this has to be incised before identification and division of the perforators can be accomplished. The medial insertion of the soleus muscle on the tibia may also have to be exposed to visualize proximal paratibial perforators. By rotating the ports cephalad and continuing the dissection up to the level of the knee, the more proximal perforators can also be divided. While paratibial fasciotomy can aid in distal exposure, reaching the retromalleolar Cockett I perforator endoscopically is not usually possible, and if incompetent, a separate small incision is needed over it to gain direct exposure.

After completion of the endoscopic portion of the procedure, the instruments and ports are removed, the carbon dioxide is manually expressed from the limb, and the tourniquet is deflated. Next, 20 ml of 0.5% bupivacaine solution is instilled into the subfascial space for postoperative pain control. Stab avulsion of varicosities, in addition to high ligation and stripping of the GSV, small saphenous vein, or both, if incompetent, is performed. The wounds are closed, and the limb is elevated and wrapped with an elastic bandage. Elevation is maintained at 30 degrees postoperatively for 3 hours, after which ambulation is permitted.

Unlike the in-hospital stay after an open Linton procedure, this is an outpatient procedure and patients are discharged the same day or next morning following overnight observation. Restrictions are the same as with GSV stripping. Patients are allowed to return to work in 10 days to 2 weeks. Proebstle et al. has reported performing SEPS successfully under tumescent local anesthesia alone in 78% of patients.[39]

Ultrasound-Guided Ablation of Incompetent Perforator Veins

Ultrasound-guided ablation of the saphenous vein is discussed in Chapter 44. Using similar techniques, these office-based therapies of radiofrequency ablation, endovenous laser ablation, and ultrasound-guided foam sclerotherapy have likewise been applied to the treatment of perforator veins in the setting of CVI. Radiofrequency and laser ablation can be more demanding technically than saphenous vein ablation due to the short and often tortuous nature of these perforators[40,41] (Figure 46-5). Whiteley et al. treated 545 perforators with radiofrequency ablation and observed a 93% occlusion rate in 82 cases followed up to 1 year.[42]

Proebstle and colleagues[41] treated 67 perforating veins using 940-nm diode laser and a Nd:YAG laser with 1320 nm and laser fibers of 600-microm diameter. Perforators were accessed through ultrasound-guided puncture using 1560- and 18-gauge cannulas, respectively. Laser energy was delivered in a pulsed fashion using 5- and 30-W laser powers. By day 1, 66 of 67 veins occluded; side effects were moderate. Recurrence after laser treatment of perforating veins is not known.

Although SEPS is the most common way to treat incompetent perforating veins, ultrasound-guided ablation and sclerotherapy have several potential advantages. They are truly minimally invasive procedures that can be performed in an office setting. Unlike SEPS, the approach is not limited by perforating vein location, and the perforators can be accessed at various positions that are not accessible with SEPS, including the more proximal Boyd's, Dodd's, midthigh Hunterian, and lateral perforators. In addition, these procedures allow the flexibility of repeat treatment for persistent or newly developed incompetent perforators, which can be quite difficult with SEPS because of disturbed tissue planes.

Results of Perforator Ablation

Clinical Results

In their seminal papers, Linton and Cockett reported the initial clinical benefits of open perforator ligation.[27,28] Table 46-3 summarizes the results from 10 reports of open perforator ablation in nearly 600 legs performed since the 1970s. The ulcer healing rate was excellent at 89%. Ulcer recurrence was 23% over 2 to 5 years, but most of these reports originated before present-day reporting standards and the patient populations are likely heterogeneous. Burnand et al. questioned the value of open perforator ablation into question with their report of a 55% ulcer recurrence rate.[31] The long recovery combined with a significant wound complication rate of 25% led to abandonment of open perforator ligation. The debate was concluded by Pierik et al. after their randomized trial comparing open and endoscopic perforator ablation. The study was terminated early due to the high (53%) wound

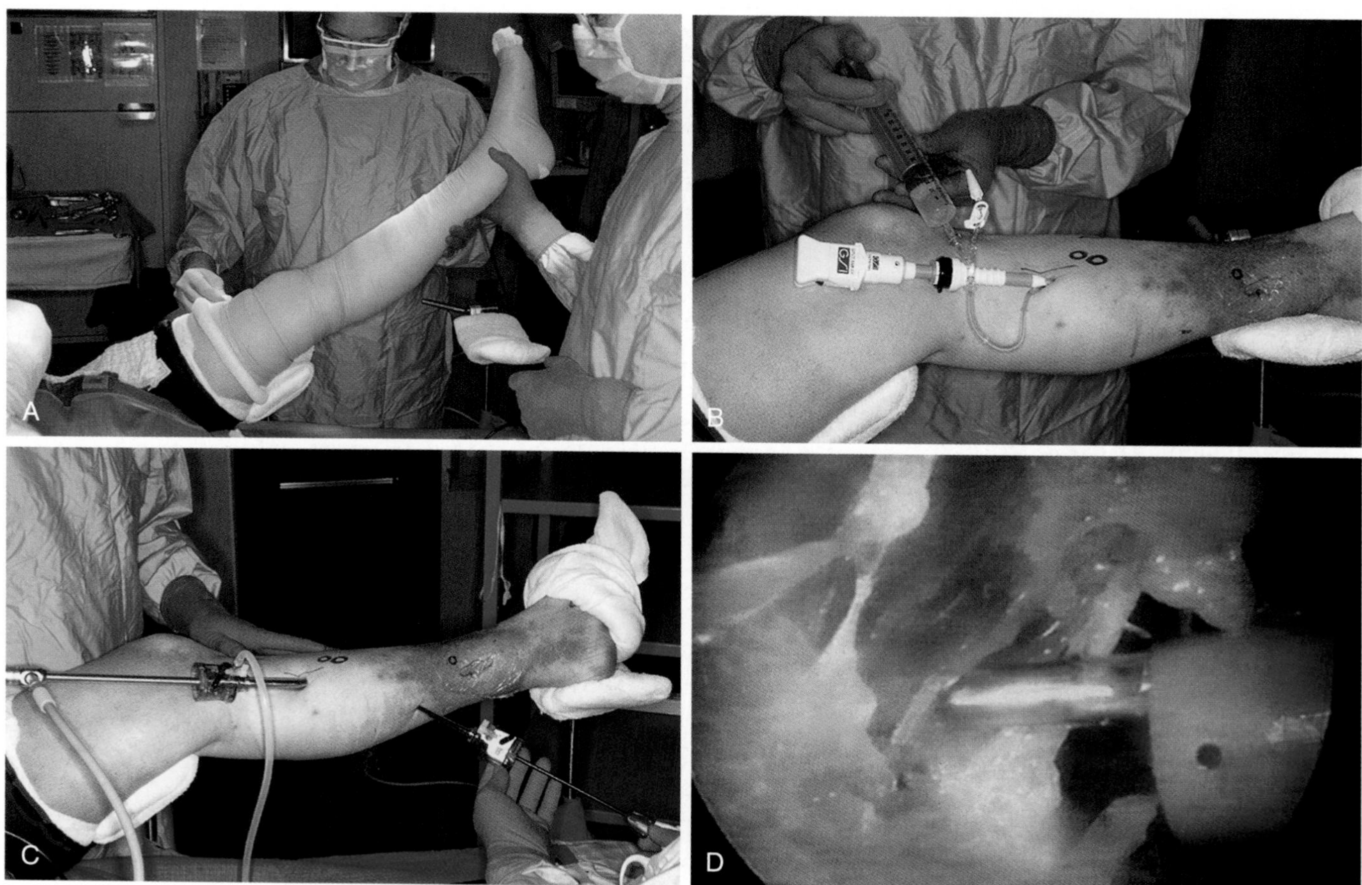

Figure 46-4. Two-port technique of subfascial endoscopic perforator vein surgery (SEPS). **A,** A thigh tourniquet inflated to 300 mm Hg is used to create a bloodless field. **B,** Balloon dissection is used to widen the subfascial space. **C,** SEPS is performed using two ports: a 10-mm camera port and a 5- or 10-mm distal port inserted under video control. Carbon dioxide is insufflated through the camera port into the subfascial space to a pressure of 30 mm Hg to improve visualization and access to perforators. **D,** The subfascial space is widely explored from the medial border of the tibia to the posterior midline and down to the level of the ankle, and all perforators are interrupted using clips or harmonic scalpel. (From Gloviczki P, Canton LG, Cambria RA, Rhee RY. Subfascial endoscopic perforator vein surgery with gas insufflation. In: Gloviczki P, Bergan JJ, eds. *Atlas of endoscopic perforator vein surgery*. London: Springer-Verlag, 1998:125-138.)

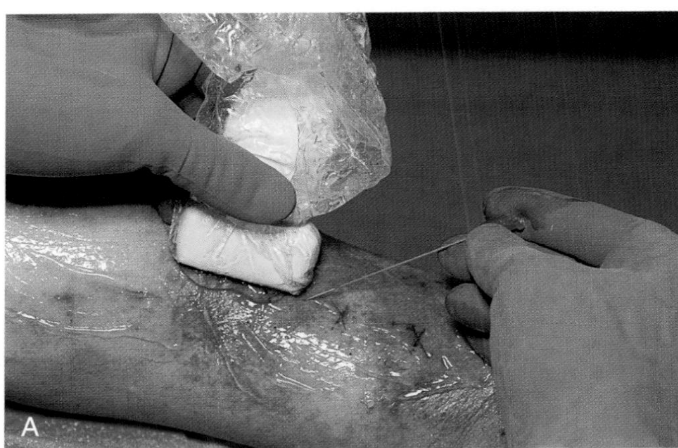

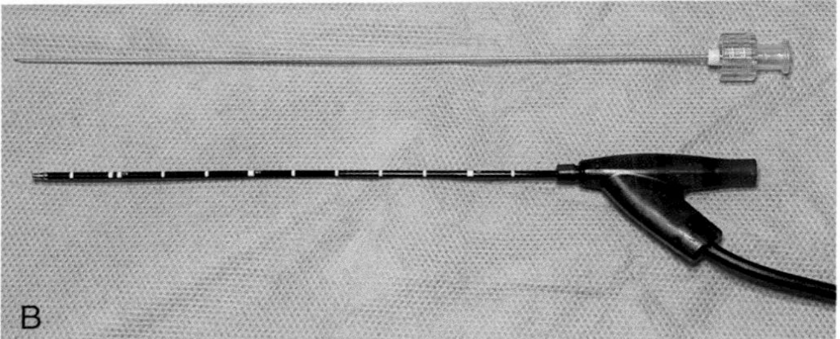

Figure 46-5. Radiofrequency ablation of an incompetent perforator vein.

complication rate in the open group compared to none in the SEPS group; no ulcers recurred in either group over a mean follow-up of 21 months.[26]

With the advent of SEPS, the wound complication rates and prolonged recovery were no longer major concerns as documented by multiple reports from centers in both Europe and North America.[12,34,42-44] These series also documented the safety and efficacy of SEPS, with rapid ulcer healing and low early recurrence rates. With extended follow-up, however, ulcer recurrence rates after SEPS are comparable to those seen historically with open perforator ablation. In reporting late results of their prospective randomized study comparing SEPS to open perforator ligation, Pierik et al. noted no significant difference in ulcer recurrence: 22% versus 12% respectively.[26] The midterm (24 months) results of the North American (NASEPS) registry, reporting on SEPS performed in 17 U.S. centers, demonstrated an 88% cumulative ulcer healing rate at 1 year.[7] The median time to ulcer healing was 54 days. The cumulative rate of ulcer recurrence was 16% at 1 year and 28% at 2 years. In the largest series from a single institution, Nelzen et al reported on prospectively collected data from 149 SEPS procedures in 138 patients.[46] During a median follow-up of 32 months, 32 of 36 ulcers healed, more than half (19 of 36) within 1 month. Three ulcers recurred, one of which subsequently healed during follow-up. Table 46-4 summarizes data from 13 separate reports in more than 800 legs. The ulcer healing rate of 90% is indistinguishable from that seen after open perforator ablation. The crude ulcer recurrence rate was also comparable at 11%, although the follow-up was slightly less in the SEPS series ranging from just under 1 year to almost 4 years.

TenBrook and colleagues undertook a systematic review and a combined statistical analysis of the reported series on SEPS that included a total of 1140 legs.[47] They found similar results to those listed in Table 46-4 but identified that the presence of a large ulcer (more than 2 cm), secondary etiology of the venous disease, and presence of persistent incompetent perforating veins postoperatively were all risk factors for nonhealing of the ulcers. Interestingly, the presence of deep venous incompetence was not a risk factor for nonhealing of the ulcers or recurrence. Kalra et al. for the Mayo Clinic specifically examined the results in these postthrombotic legs.[8] Although the 5-year ulcer recurrence was significantly higher in this subgroup (primary 15% versus secondary 56%), the patients still gained clinical benefit as measured by improved Venous Clinical Severity Scores, as well as an apparent ease in treating the smaller, superficial ulcers compared to their preoperative state.

The Dutch SEPS Trial was a randomized multicenter trial prospectively comparing surgical treatment (SEPS with or without superficial reflux ablation) to medical treatment (ambulatory venous compression) in patients with a venous ulcer.[47] The study included 200 patients. The ulcer healing rate of 83% and the recurrence rate after surgery of 22% at

Table 46-3
Clinical Results of Open Perforator Interruption for the Treatment of Advanced Chronic Venous Disease

Author	Year	Limbs Treated *(n)*	Limbs with Ulcer *(n)*	Wound Complications *n* (%)	Ulcer Healing *n* (%)	Ulcer Recurrence *n* (%)†	Mean Follow-Up (Years)
Silver[99]	1971	31	19	4 (14)	—	— (10)	1-15
Thurston[100]	1973	102	0	12 (12)	*	11 (13)	3.3
Bowen	1975	71	8	31 (44)	—	24 (34)	4.5
Burnand et al.[31]	1976	41	0	—	*	24 (55)	—
Negus and Friedgood[15]	1983	108	108	24 (22)	91 (84)	16 (15)	3.7
Wilkinson[101]	1986	108	0	26 (24)	*	3 (7)	6
Cikrit[102]	1988	32	30	6 (19)	30 (100)	5 (19)	4
Bradbury[103]	1993	53	0	—	*	14 (26)	5
Pierik et al.[26]	1997	19	19	10 (53)	17 (90)	0 (0)	1.8
Sato et al.[43]	1999	29	19	13 (45)	19 (100)	13 (68)	2.9
Total		594 (100)	203 (34)	126/497 (25)	157/176 (89)	110/471 (23)	—

*Only class 5 (healed ulcer) patients were admitted in the study.
†Recurrence was calculated where data were available, and the percentage accounts for the patients lost to follow-up.

Table 46-4
Clinical Results of Subfascial Endoscopic Perforator Vein Surgery for the Treatment of Advanced Chronic Venous Disease

Author	Year	Limbs Treated (*n*)	Limbs with Ulcer (*n*)*	Concomitant Saphenous Ablation *n* (%)	Wound Complications *n* (%)	Ulcer Healing *n* (%)	Ulcer Recurrence *n* (%)‡	Mean Follow-Up (Months)
Jugenheimer[104]	1992	103	17	97 (94)	3 (3)	16 (94)	0 (0)	27
Pierik[105]	1995	40	16	4 (10)	3 (8)	16 (100)	1 (2.5)	46
Bergan et al.[34]	1996	31	15	31 (100)	3 (10)	15 (100)	(0)	—
Wolters[106]	1996	27	27	0 (0)	2 (7)	26 (96)	2 (8)	12-24
Padberg et al.[45]	1996	11	0	11 (100)	—	†	0 (0)	16
Pierik et al.[26]	1997	20	20	14 (70)	0 (0)	17 (85)	0 (0)	21
Gloviczki et al.[7]	1999	146	101	86 (59)	9 (6)	85 (84)	26 (21)	24
Illig[107]	1999	30	19	—	—	17 (89)	4 (15)	9
Sato et al.[43]	1999	27	20	17 (63)	2 (7)	18 (90)	5 (28)	8
Nelzen[108]	2001	149	36	132 (89)	11 (7)	32 (89)	3 (5)	32
Kalra et al.[8]	2002	103	42	74 (72)	7 (6)	38 (90)	15 (21)	40
Iafrati[109]	2002	51	29	33 (65)	3 (6)	22 (76)	6 (13)	38
Baron[110]	2004	98	53	36 (42)	—	53 (100)	0 (0)	—
Total Limbs *n* (%)		836 (100)	395 (47)	535/789 (68)	50/680 (7)	355/395 (90)	62/580 (11)	—

*Only class 6 (active ulcer) patients are included.
†only class 5 (healed ulcer) patients were admitted in this study.
‡Recurrence was calculated for class 5 and 6 limbs only, where data were available, and the percentage accounts for the patients lost to follow-up.

29 months in this trial were comparable to previous results. In the conservative group, ulcers healed in 73% and recurred in 23% of legs. Ulcer size and duration were independent factors adversely affecting both healing and recurrence rates. On extended follow-up, the authors reported that ulcer-free rate was significantly greater in the surgical group (72% versus 53%), as was the ulcer-free period.[48]

It must be emphasized that two thirds of patients reported in the preceding studies also underwent saphenous vein stripping and branch varicosity avulsion, making it difficult to ascertain how much clinical improvement can be attributed to SEPS alone. Patients undergoing SEPS and accessory vein avulsion without saphenous stripping have been shown to have significant clinical improvement, as measured by Venous Clinical Severity Scores. The NASEPS registry demonstrated improved ulcer healing in legs that underwent SEPS with saphenous vein stripping, compared to legs that underwent SEPS alone: 3- and 12-month cumulative ulcer healing rates of 76% and 100% versus 45% and 83%, respectively.[7] Ulcer recurrence at 3 years was not significantly different between the two groups. Although this is indirect evidence, it does support the clinical benefit of treating perforator incompetence. In an analysis of 103 legs in patients at the Mayo Clinic,[8] ulcer healing was significantly delayed in legs that had SEPS alone, compared to legs that had SEPS with superficial reflux ablation: 90-day cumulative ulcer healing rates were 49% versus 90%, respectively. Cumulative ulcer recurrence at 5 years was also higher after SEPS alone (53%), compared to SEPS with additional superficial reflux ablation (19%). However, all limbs in the SEPS alone group had recurrent or persistent ulcers after previous saphenous stripping, and more patients had secondary postthrombotic change in this group.

In addition, ongoing controversy surrounds the hemodynamic improvement that can be attributed to perforator interruption. Because perforator incompetence is often treated with ablation of superficial reflux, postoperative hemodynamic measurements reflect the results of a combined operation. Akesson et al. demonstrated a significant reduction in ambulatory venous pressure after saphenous stripping in patients with recurrent venous ulcers, but the improvement in mean ambulatory venous pressure did not reach significance after further perforator interruption.[50] In a classical study, however, using ambulatory venous pressure measurements, Schanzer and Pierce documented significant hemodynamic improvements after isolated perforator interruption in 22 patients.[14] These results were confirmed in a study by Padberg and colleagues,[45] using foot volumetry and duplex imaging. At a median follow-up of 66 months, in patients with no ulcer recurrence, both expulsion fraction and half-refilling times had improved significantly. When strain-gauge plethysmography was used to quantitate calf muscle pump function and venous incompetence before and 6 months after SEPS[45], a significant improvement occurred in both modalities in 31 legs. Of the 31 legs, 24 underwent saphenous stripping in addition to SEPS. Although the 7 legs treated by SEPS alone had significant clinical benefits, the hemodynamic improvements did not reach statistical significance.

Further research is needed to determine the best preoperative test with which to predict the hemodynamic effects of treating incompetent perforators, which would help select patients for SEPS. The evolution of less-invasive techniques, often performed in the office setting under local anesthetic, have started the concept of treating venous incompetence in the leg in a stepwise fashion. Proebstle et al. have reported a 98.5% technical success rate of perforator vein ablation using endovenous laser therapy with perforator vein occlusion in 66 or 67 patients within 24 hours of the procedure and no significant associated complications or side effects.[41]

Masuda et al. reported their results with ultrasound-guided sclerotherapy with sodium morrhuate in 80 legs with predominantly perforator incompetence alone.[44] After treatment, there was a significant improvement in Venous Clinical Severity Scores and an 86.5% ulcer healing rate, with a mean time to healing of 36 days. The ulcer recurrence rate was 32% after a mean of 20 months, despite only a 15% compliance with compression hose. These results are similar to those seen in the NASEPS registry. Based on available data, it seems likely that the clinical outcome and hemodynamic benefit of perforator vein ligation is likely to be similar regardless of the method of ablation: open, endoscopic, or endovenous.

Correction of Deep Venous Reflux

Indications

Since the first direct venous valve reconstruction by Kistner in 1968, several techniques have been developed to repair incompetent venous valves.[52] Today, several procedures exist to treat patients with advanced CVI and deep vein valve incompetence, but only a relatively small number of venous surgeons perform them. If deep venous reflux is confirmed on noninvasive evaluation and the patient is a surgical candidate, venography is undertaken to assist in planning the operative procedure. Ascending venography is performed first to exclude the presence of significant outflow obstruction. Next, descending venography is done to confirm the presence, location, and magnitude of valvular reflux in the entire extremity. Descending venography also differentiates the floppy, elongated valves and dilatation of the vein seen in PVI from the thickened, shortened valves with luminal narrowing characteristic of postthrombotic syndrome. Patients with reflux down through popliteal veins into the tibial veins (Kistner grade 3 or 4), in association with symptoms and signs of advanced CVI, are candidates for correction of deep venous reflux.

Patients with PVI could have either internal or external valvuloplasty. Vein valves are often destroyed in postthrombotic legs, and direct valve repair is usually not feasible. Options available include valve transposition or transplantation and attempts at de novo valve reconstruction.

Despite demonstrable reflux in multiple valves in the deep system, only one valve is usually repaired, typically the first valve of the SFV. If the profunda femoris vein valve is also incompetent, it too should be repaired. Alternatively, repair of an incompetent valve at the popliteal vein level can prevent reflux into the popliteal and tibial veins.

Valvuloplasty

Internal valvuloplasty is usually done for surgical ablation of deep venous reflux secondary to PVI. First described by Kistner, modifications to the technique have been reported by Raju and Sottiurai.[52-54] The procedure is performed through a standard groin incision with dissection of the femoral and saphenous veins. The valve attachment lines should be identified clearly on the vein wall before a venotomy is performed. In patients with a thickened, fibrotic femoral vein, this may require adventitial dissection to expose the position of the valve leaflets. Once the position of the valve is determined and it is confirmed to be incompetent on the strip test, proximal and distal control of the vein segment is obtained. Following systemic heparinization, internal valvuloplasty involves plication of the valve cusps under direct vision with interrupted 7-0 prolene sutures. Raju and Fredericks estimated that decreasing the length of the valve leaflets by approximately 20% is sufficient to restore competence.[53] The original method described by Kistner involves direct transcommisural exposure of the valve cusps via a longitudinal venotomy (Figure 46-6A). A transverse venotomy situated just above the valve is recommended by Raju to avoid possible narrowing of a longitudinal suture line across the valve (Figure 46-6B). However, accurate positioning of the transverse venotomy is essential to obtain an adequate view of the valve leaflets. Sottiurai proposed a T-shaped venotomy with addition of a longitudinal limb extending down to the level of, but not across, the valve annulus (Figure 46-6C).[54] Competence of the repaired valve is confirmed by the strip test or duplex imaging. Anticoagulation and intermittent pneumatic compression is employed perioperatively to reduce the incidence of DVT.

External valvuloplasty, originally suggested by Kistner, is a simpler technique that avoids a venotomy. Partial thickness transmural plicating sutures are placed from the outside to narrow the widened commisural angles (Figure 46-7). Although a venotomy and full heparinization are avoided, lack of direct visualization makes this repair anatomically less precise.

Angioscope-assisted valvuloplasty was reported by Gloviczki et al. in 1991, whereby through and through-transluminal sutures are inserted from the outside to narrow the commisures, while viewing the valve leaflets with an angioscope positioned above the valve via a tributary of the saphenous vein (Figures 46-8 and 46-9).[55] Heparinization and control of the vein are required, as for internal valvuloplasty. Blood is flushed out of the isolated segment and heparinized saline instilled to facilitate visualization. Competence is checked progressively during the repair by rapid flooding of the valve leaflets with heparinized saline from above. Raju and Hardy prefer to insert the angioscope through a venotomy close to the valve station and use it to visualize the valve leaflets before and after placement of full-thickness plicating sutures from the outside. The angioscope cannot be used during placement of the sutures,[56] but dissection can be limited and operative time shortened with this method.

Venoplastic procedures have been employed in circumstances where extreme widening of the commisural angle raises concerns that invagination of too much tissue to gain valve competence during a standard internal or external valuloplasty can narrow the femoral vein. A longitudinal-transverse or inverted "Y-V" venoplasty is performed above the valve commisure after heparinization and vascular control. This results in narrowing of the commisure by pulling up and tightening the valve cusps without direct placement of sutures in them. This maneuver also widens and deepens the valve sinuses somewhat, contributing to valve competence. The procedure is recommended by Raju and Hardy for small veins, as well as in obese patients who may have compromised exposure of the valve for standard intraluminal valvuloplasty.[56]

De novo valve reconstruction was first described by Durango in 1993, whereby new valve cusps were created from excised saphenous vein and sutured into an appropriate host vein.[57] The adventitia and part of the media are removed from the harvested vein segment to provide thin and supple tissue. U-shaped cusps are created from this and the corners oriented and anchored with mattress sutures tied externally to create a bicuspid valve. The rest of the edge of the leaflet is sutured in a continuous manner with 7-0 prolene. Raju and Hardy modified the technique to orient the valves with the intimal surface outward in an effort to reduce the incidence of thrombosis in the sinus where blood flow is relatively sluggish.[56] They also

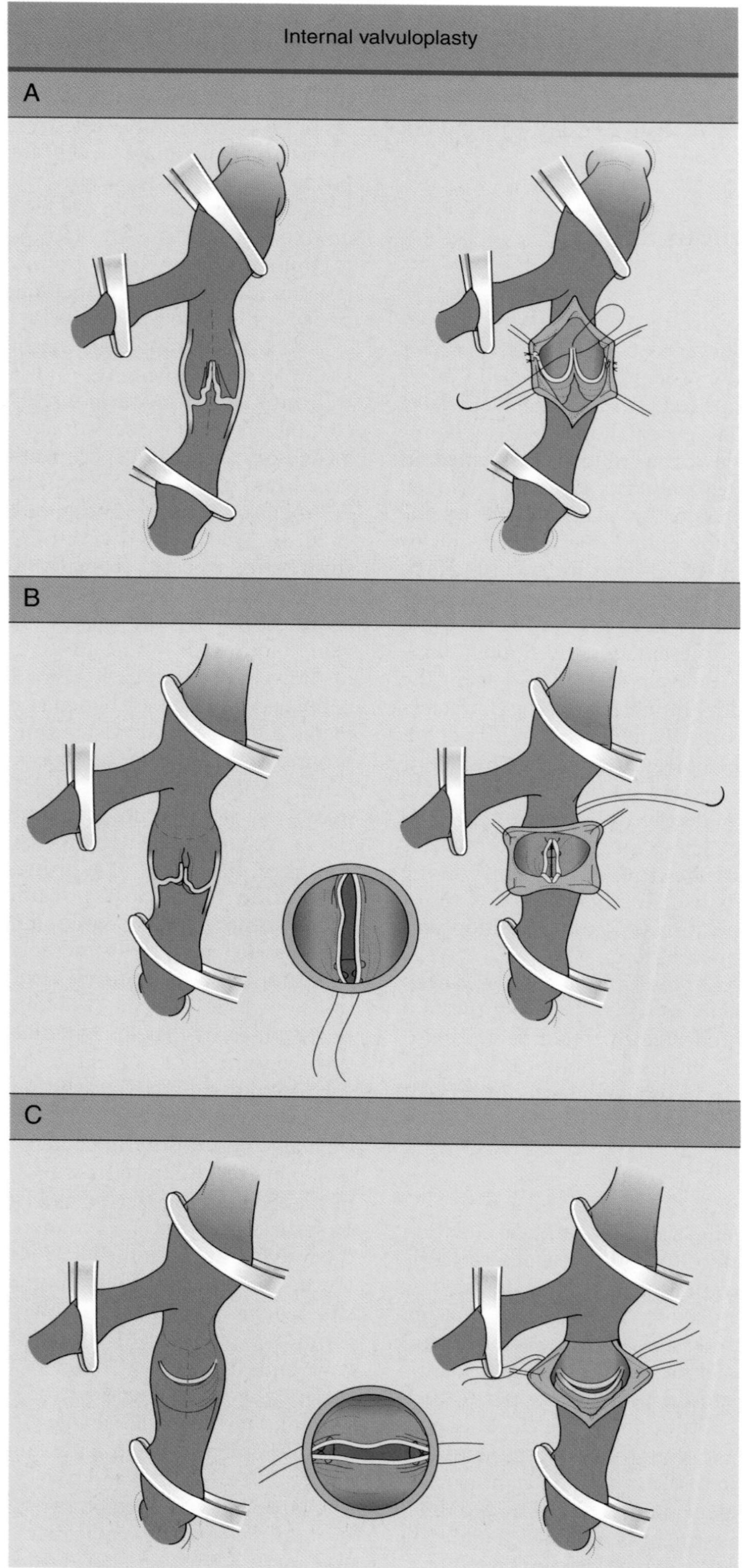

Figure 46-6. Internal valvuloplasty. **A,** The Kistner transcommissural approach allows for visualization of the venous valves. Care must be taken to prevent damage to the valve cusps during the longitudinal venotomy. The transcommissural incision and the valve undergoing repair are pictured. **B,** The Raju supracommissural approach minimizes the potential of valve cusp damage but sacrifices some excellent exposure afforded by the transcommissural approach. Illustrated is the valve structure during incision and valvuloplasty. **C,** The Sottiurai supra-T commissural approach improves the visualization of the valve mechanism by extending the supracommissural incision parallel to the vein in a T shape. (From Nachreiner RD, Bhuller AS, Dalsing MC. Surgical repair of incompetent venous valves. In: *Handbook of venous disorders*. 2nd ed. London: Arnold Publishing; 2000.)

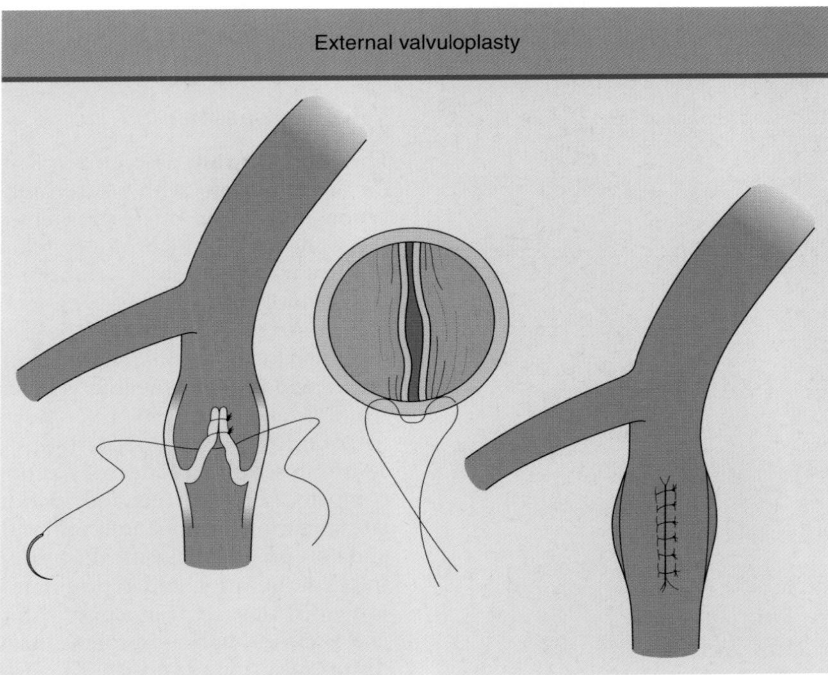

Figure 46-7. External valvuloplasty eliminates the need for venotomy. External suture placement is aimed at tightening the commissural angle. (From Nachreiner RD, Bhuller AS, Dalsing MC. Surgical repair of incompetent venous valves. In: *Handbook of venous disorders.* 2nd ed. London: Arnold Publishing; 2000.)

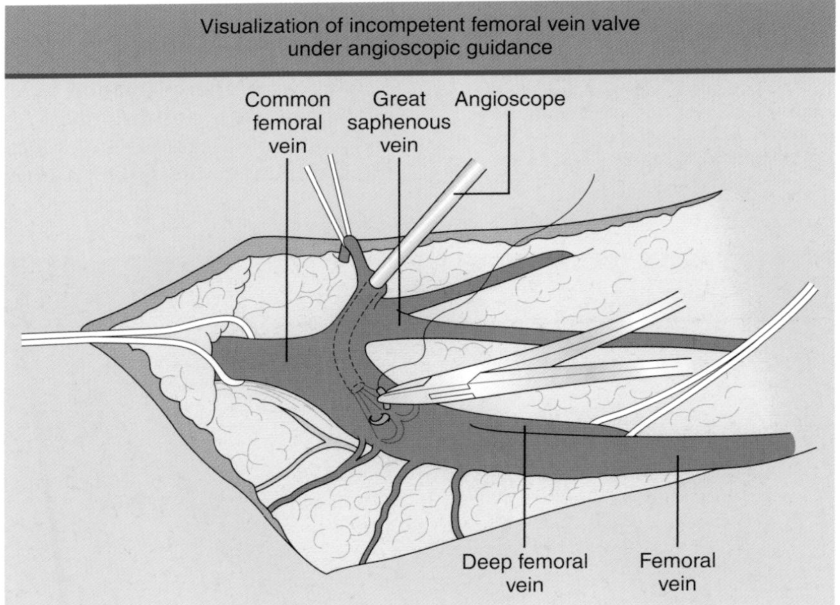

Figure 46-8. Visualization of incompetent femoral vein valve under angioscopic guidance. (From Gloviczki P, Merrell SW, Bower TC. *J Vasc Surg* 1991;14:645-648.)

recommend using the axillary or other deep vein or a tributary as the donor to create thinner leaflets compared to the saphenous vein. The technique has not been used widely so far. The complexity of the repair precludes its use except in circumstances where valvuloplasty is not feasible and no competent valve is available for transfer.

External banding with a prosthetic sleeve is an option in a few valves with early reflux. It is suitable for valves with reflux secondary to vein dilatation that become competent intraoperatively on the strip test when the vein constricts in response to dissection. A 2- to 3-cm fascial, Dacron, silastic, or polytetrafluoroethylene (PTFE) strip is wrapped around the vein segment containing the valve to narrow the annulus. It is tightened around the vein, sutured shut longitudinally, and then anchored to the adventitia to prevent displacement. External banding has been used to complement internal or

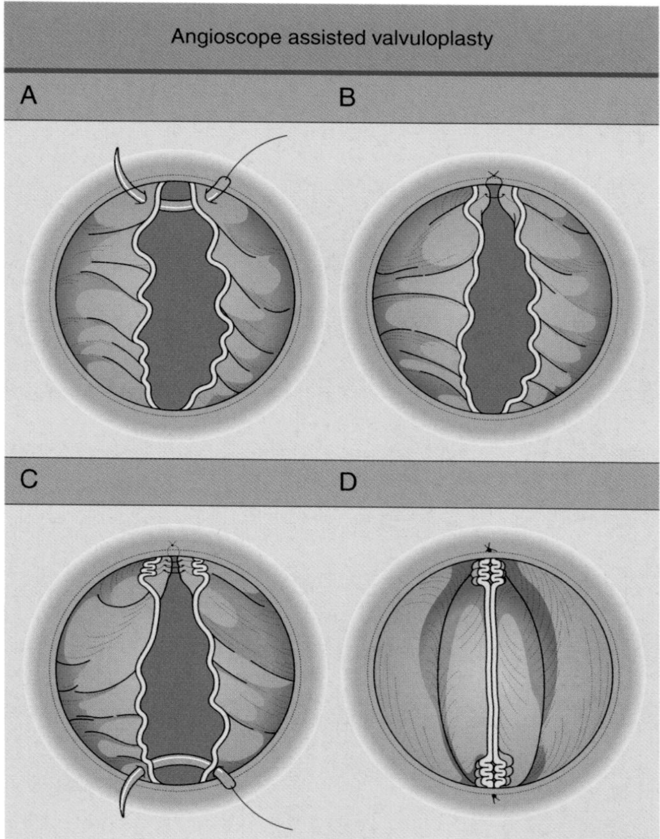

Figure 46-9. **A,** Angioscopic view of needle passage thorough the incompetent valve leaflets. **B,** Assessment of valve redundancy after each suture placement. **C,** Suture placement on both commissures to achieve complete valvular competence. **D,** Angioscopic view of competent valve. (From Gloviczki P, Merrell SW, Bower TC. *J Vasc Surg* 1991;14:645-648.)

external valvuloplasty where dilatation of the vein is suspected to contribute to incompetence.

Valve Transposition

This procedure was described by Kistner and Sparkuhl in 1979 for use in patients with postthrombotic syndrome with deep venous reflux and one competent valve at the groin: either the saphenous or the profunda femoris valve.[58] The principle of valve transposition or venous segment transfer is to interpose a competent valve-bearing venous segment into the deep venous system at the level of the groin. The simplest option is diconnection of the SFV and anastomosis of the distal segment end to end to the saphenous vein with a competent saphenofemoral valve (Figure 46-10). Often, the GSV is either incompetent or has been stripped. In this situation, the SFV may be anastomosed end to side to the profunda femoris vein below a competent PFV. Kistner and Sparkuhl subsequently reported late fatigue of the saphenous vein with recurrence of symptoms and now preferentially use the profunda femoris vein.[58] Under full heparinization and appropriate vascular control, the SFV is divided close to its junction with the PFV and the proximal end is closed with 5-0 prolene, taking care not to narrow or distort the profunda orifice. The distal end is anastomosed end to side to the profunda femoris or end to end to its first branch using interrupted sutures of 7-0 prolene or the triangulation technique of Carrel. Competence of the transposed segment is confirmed by the strip test, duplex ultrasound, or both.

Valve Transplantation

Venous valve transplantation is the next available option in patients with postthrombotic syndrome whose pattern and extent of disease precludes local valve reconstruction or transposition in the groin. Autogenous transplantation of

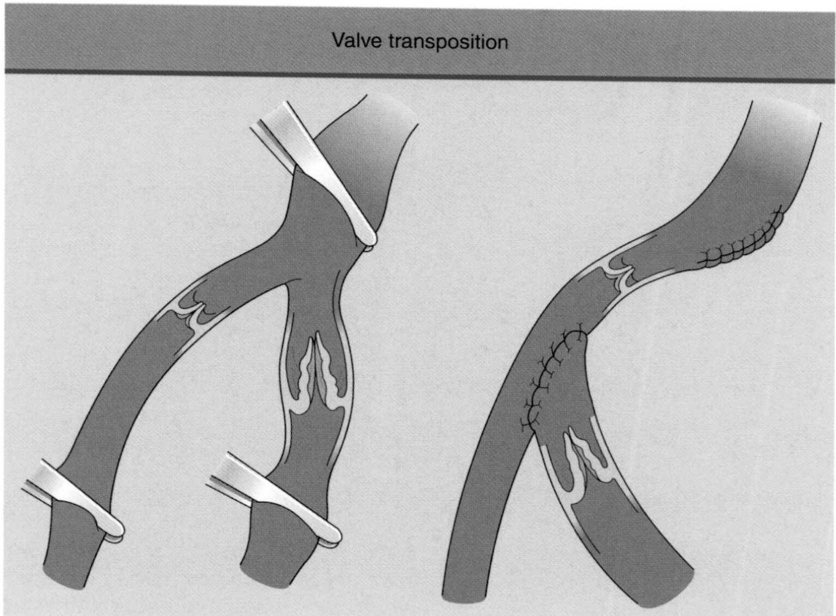

Figure 46-10. Transposition of the superficial femoral vein (SFV) after ligation distal to its junction with the common femoral vein (CFV) involves implantation of the translocated SFV distal to a competent valve lying within the profunda femoral vein (PFV). (From Dalsing MC, Nachreiner RD, Bhuller A. *Role of venous valvular surgery in chronic venous insufficiency in vascular surgery: year 2000*. New York: McGraw-Hill; 2000.)

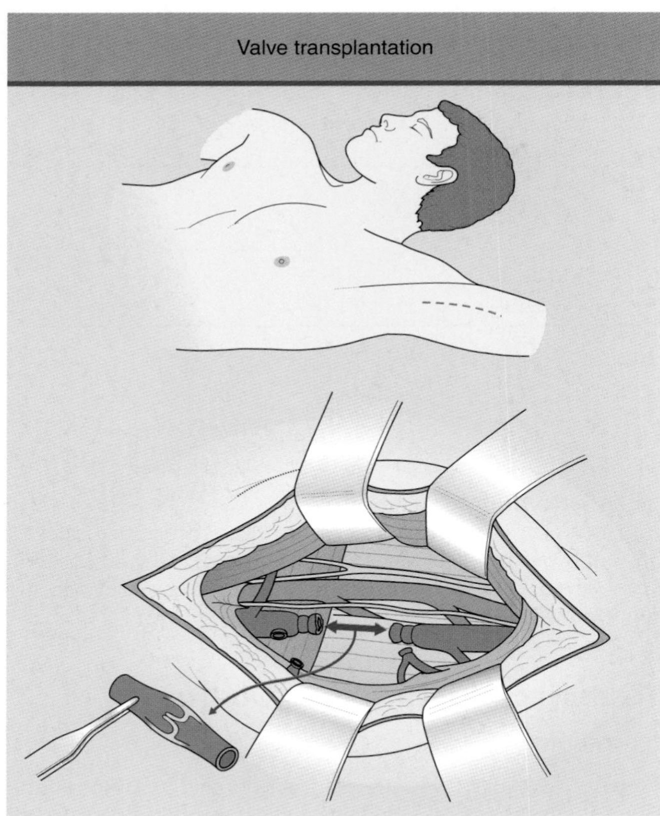

Figure 46-11. Transplantation can be performed by harvesting an axillary venous segment containing a competent valve or a valve that has been made competent by valvuloplasty. (From Dalsing MC. Chronic venous disease. In: Greenfield L, Lilemoe K, Mulholland M, et al, eds. *Surgery: scientific principle and practice.* 3rd ed. Philadelphia: Lippincott Williams & Wilkins; 2001:23.)

a competent valve from the arm to the leg was introduced by Taheri et al. in 1982 (Figure 46-11).[59] The original procedure involved transplant of a brachial vein segment containing a competent valve to replace a short segment of SFV. A 4- to 8-cm segment of brachial vein is harvested through a longitudinal incision in the arm after confirming the presence of a competent valve within it by preoperative duplex imaging. The SFV vein is prepared as before over a length of 10 to 12 cm. A 2- to 3-cm segment of the SFV 4 to 5 cm distal to the profunda femoris junction is excised; approximately half the length of vein segment to be implanted. The brachial vein segment is anastomosed as an interposition graft into the SFV. The anastomoses are performed in a triangulated manner or with interrupted 7-0 prolene sutures, the distal followed by the proximal. Raju and Hardy adopted the technique but preferred to use the axillary vein as the donor vein segment, citing better size match with the SFV.[56] Despite this, some dilatation of the transplanted vein segment still occurred, just as Taheri et al noted in the brachial vein.[59] To circumvent this problem, they suggested an external Dacron wrap around the transplanted segment to prevent late recurrence of reflux. They also reported incompetence in situ in 44% of axillary vein valves explored for harvesting; 14% of explored patients had bilateral axillary vein valvular incompetence. In this situation, they proceeded to perform bench repair of the axillary vein valve by external valvuloplasty before transplantation, but disappointing early results prompted them to change to transcommisural repair in recent years. O'Donnell et al. further adapted the technique to transplant an axillary vein segment into the popliteal vein in an effort to provide a better size match and prevent delayed dilatation of the transplanted vein segment.[60] They also proposed that correcting reflux at the popliteal level was more critical based on its relation to the calf muscle pump.

Results of Deep Vein Valve Reconstruction

Operative mortality after deep venous repair is negligible, with most series having no deaths. The considerable concern regarding the risk of DVT and pulmonary embolism following direct surgical intervention on the deep venous system has not materialized. The incidence of DVT has been reported as 0% to 11% in series with long-term follow-up.[53,61] Not unexpectedly, the rate is higher following repairs in postthrombotic legs compared to legs with primary valvular insufficiency.[62] The incidence of wound hematoma is directly related to the use of heparin and occurs in 2% to 16% of cases with half requiring operative evacuation.[61,63,64] Early intervention is extremely important to prevent the hematoma from compressing the repair and causing secondary thrombosis. Wound seromas, infection, and lymphatic leak each occur in 2% to 4% of patients.

Several authors have reported clinical success in 70% to 90% of patients on midterm follow-up (2 to 4 years) following valve repair for primary venous insufficiency (Table 46-5).[56,68-70]

Table 46-5
Results of Valvuloplasty*

Author	Year	Limbs *(n)*	Limbs with Ulcer *(n)*	Clinical Success *n* (%)	Valve Competency Rate *n* (%)	Ulcer Recurrence *n* (%)	Mean Follow-Up (Months)
Eriksson[111]	1990	27	NA	19 (70)	19 (70)	NA	6-108
Masuda and Kistner[61]	1994	32	0†	23 (73)	25 (77)	NA	126
Raju et al.[65]	1996	258	137	NA‡	(62)§	36 (26)	12-144
Sottiurai[66]	1997	143	NA	NA	107 (75)	NA	9-168
Perrin[67]	2000	85	35	65 (80)	67 (79)	8 (23)	12-168

*NA, not available.
†Only class 3 (96%) and class 2 (4%) limbs were included in the study.
‡Clinical improvement was found in 55% of patients with no ulcer (class 4).
§Includes overall competency rate following all valve repairs.

Table 46-6
Results of Valve Transplantation*

Author	Year	Limbs (n)	Limbs with Ulcer (n)	Clinical Success n (%)	Valve Competency Rate n (%)	Ulcer Recurrence n (%)	Mean Follow-Up (Months)
Eriksson[69]	1990	35	NA	32 (90)	NA	(18)	60
Raju et al.[65]	1996	44	44	16 (36)	16 (33)	(54)	24
Iafrati[112]	1997	15	NA	14 (92)	NA	(21)	64
Taheri[113]	1997	102	NA	46 (45)	NA	NA	60
Sottiurai[66]	1997	33	31	13 (39)	13 (39)	17 (55)‡	74
Perrin[67]	2000	32	23	20 (62)	9 (39)†	9 (39)	12-124

*NA, not available.
†Postoperative thrombosis occurred in 12 valves and reflux in 6.
‡Ulcers recurred in 14 limbs and failed to heal in two limbs.

Of these, 70% of patients with a good outcome, about half were asymptomatic without elastic support, and the other half continued to require compression to remain symptom free. Masuda and Kistner recently reported persistence of these findings on longer follow-up (up to 21 years), with stabilization of the results in all groups of patients by 6 years.[61] The study included 51 patients undergoing various deep venous reconstructive procedures: 43% with PVI, 31% with PTS, and 26% with combined disease. Cumulative clinical success was significantly better in patients with PVI who underwent valve repair (73%) compared to patients with PTS who underwent valve transposition or transplant (43%). Patients with a mixed pattern of disease, with proximal PVI and distal PTS, fared somewhere between. At 10 years, the cumulative clinical success rate in the entire group was 60%. However, ulcers recurred in 15 of 29 patients with class 5 and 6 disease; 5 patients had multiple ulcer recurrences. In most of these, ulcers were related to neglect or trauma, were smaller, and healed again easily.

Clinical outcome in all series has correlated closely with the eventual state of valve competence; patients with sustained competence demonstrated on duplex remained asymptomatic, and patients with recurrence of symptoms invariably had failure of the reconstruction.[56,61] Modest improvement in hemodynamic parameters following valve repair has been reported by several authors.[56,61-63] In all series, hemodynamic improvement failed to reach the same levels as clinical improvement. Masuda et al reported improvement in ambulatory venous pressures in legs classified as class 0 or 1 but still not a return to normal.[44] This is not surprising as valve repair only corrects the abnormality at one level in legs that often have global abnormalities. The pathophysiological improvement may be sufficient to relieve symptoms but not enough to affect plethysmographic and venous pressure measurements.

Chances of success decrease with increasing complexity of the deep venous reconstruction. Available series in the literature report a crude ulcer healing rate of 79% following valve transfer in 157 patients (Table 46-6).[67,71,72] Cumulative ulcer-free interval at 6 years ranged from 50% to 65%. The overall mean occlusion rate of valve transplants in 250 legs studied with ascending venography was 5.6%, but was as high as 38% in 32 procedures in the series of Perrin et al.[67] Improvement in venous pressure measurement and air plethysmography has been equivocal. Raju et al. reported a decrease in the venous filling index from 6 ml/sec to 4 ml/sec.[61,67] Results of valve transposition are comparable, with ulcer recurrence rates of 35% and occlusion of the reconstruction in 10% of legs.[61,67] Only seven patients with de novo valve reconstruction are reported with acceptable clinical results.[56]

Treatment of Deep Venous Obstruction

Indications

Patients with deep venous obstruction and symptoms and signs of advanced CVI who have failed conservative treatment and all other simpler surgical procedures may be considered for intervention on the deep venous system. Deep venous obstruction is a rare cause of CVI, occurring in fewer than 10% of patients.[1] Standard hemodynamic tests are unreliable in diagnosing deep venous outflow obstruction, having a high positive but low negative predictive value. Raju et al have suggested that deep venous obstruction accounts for a larger percentage of patients with CVI than previously believed, up to 40% of patients in their practice.[65] Careful attention to the patient's symptoms and a high degree of suspicion are essential to avoid missing the diagnosis. The presence of skin changes and venous ulcers make the diagnosis easy; however, most patients present with leg swelling and disabling venous claudication.

DVT is the most common cause of venous obstruction. In symptomatic patients, recanalization of the thrombosed veins is incomplete and collateralization inadequate. May and Thurner[114] observed secondary changes, such as an intraluminal web or "spur" in the proximal left common iliac vein in 20% of the patients during 430 autopsies, recognized now as a predisposing factor for left iliofemoral vein thrombosis. Other causes include iatrogenic trauma, retroperitoneal fibrosis, radiation injury, cysts, and rarely aneurysms. In addition to duplex imaging, ascending venography may be needed to visualize the deep veins system of the affected leg, as well as the iliac veins and inferior vena cava in every patient. Descending venography is performed to identify the presence of concomitant reflux often seen in PTS. Venous pressures are measured to assess the severity of the occlusion; a pressure difference of 5 mm Hg between the two femoral veins in unilateral iliac disease or between the femoral and the central veins or a 5 mm Hg increase in femoral vein pressure after exercise indicates a hemodynamically significant lesion.

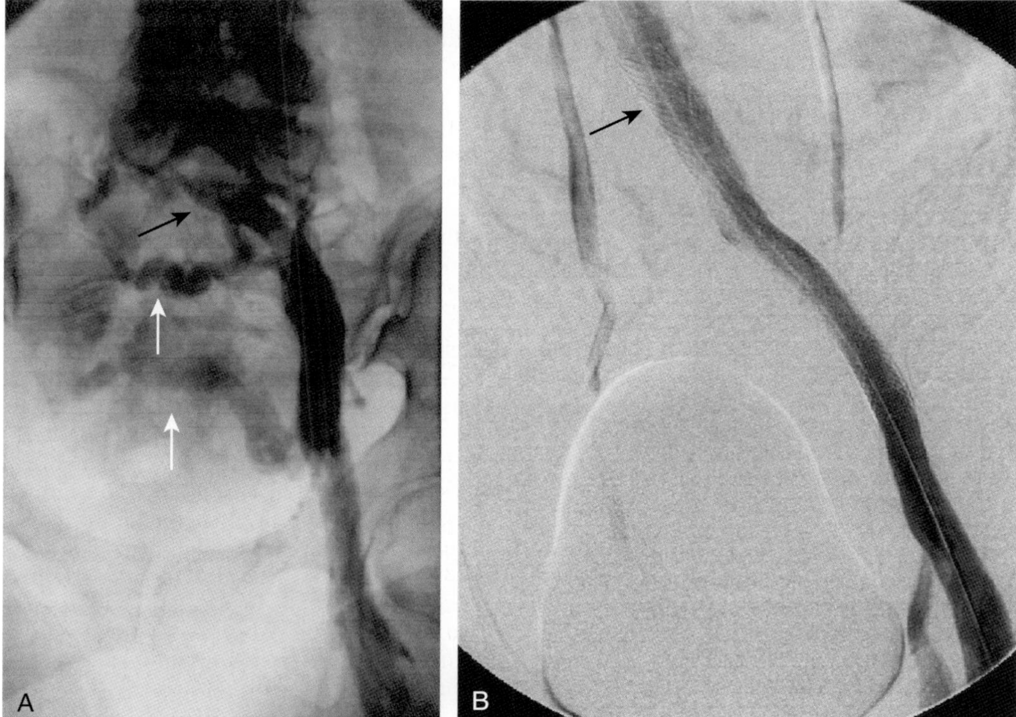

Figure 46-12. Iliac vein stenting. **A,** Ascending venogram of left lower extremity of a 33-year-old woman with May-Thurner syndrome showing occlusion of the common femoral vein *(dark arrow)* with transpelvic collaterals *(white arrows)* and postthrombotic changes in the common femoral and external iliac veins. **B,** Ascending venogram following insertion of two Wallstents (14 × 40 mm and 14 × 60 mm) across the common iliac vein extending into the inferior vena cava *(arrow)*.

Endovascular Treatment

Endovascular treatment of iliac vein occlusion over the last decade has significantly decreased the number of patients subjected to operative procedures. Initial experience was with balloon dilatation of residual stenoses following thrombolytic therapy for acute iliofemoral DVT. In recent years, the same principles have been applied to the management of chronic iliac vein stenoses and even occlusion.

Procedure

Baseline diagnostic ascending venography is performed through a transfemoral route; however, the importance of visualizing the distal femoropopliteal and tibial segments has been emphasized. Tandem distal thromboses with compromised inflow are factors associated with early failure of iliac vein stenting. Several authors have stressed the importance of improving inflow by additional thrombolysis of the distal venous tree.[73,74] For the therapeutic procedure to disobliterate the iliac vein, the patient is positioned supine with an indwelling bladder catheter. Access is usually gained through the popliteal vein or a tributary under ultrasound guidance or through injection of contrast through a foot vein. This significantly decreases the risk of puncture site hematoma. A sheath is inserted into the vein, and the lesion is traversed with a guide wire, if possible. Some authors have described using local thrombolysis for 24 to 48 hours to soften the chronic thrombus and facilitate passage of guide wires and catheters. Others have recanalized short, subtotal occlusions without employing lytic therapy. Raju et al[72] have performed iliac vein stenting in 400 patients without any pretreatment thrombolysis or posttreatment anticoagulation.[73-75] Once the target lesion is crossed, a stiffer exchange wire is passed, after which sequential dilation of the iliac vein and vena cava is performed with 8- to 14-mm balloons (Figure 46-12). The low pressure venous system is amenable to balloon dilatation, and a previously occluded vein can be dilated to 14 to 16 mm (with careful attention to wall resistance). No venous ruptures have been reported. Immediate recoil is the rule in most cases, and routine stenting is recommended. The flexibility of self-expanding Wallstents makes them particularly suitable for venous stenting; however, several other stents have been employed.[73] The entire length of the lesion is stented; concomitant stenting of the femoral vein has been recommended to improve inflow in this situation. Intravascular ultrasound can improve the accuracy of stent placement. Anticoagulation is continued for 6 months in most and indefinitely in selected patients.

Results

The most common complication of venous stenting is puncture site hematoma. The rate can be reduced with ultrasound-guided access. Major bleeding requiring transfusion is reported in up to 25% of patients. Early rethrombosis occurs in 10% and pulmonary embolism in less than 1% of patients. Death due to pulmonary embolism, intracranial and retroperitoneal hemorrhage, myocardial infarction, and sepis are all rare but reported complications in less than 1% of patients. Most patients in most reported series have had an acute DVT; not unexpectedly, they fare better than patients with chronic venous occlusion. The best results are in patients with short, focal lesions similar to the results of stenting in the arterial system. Patients with May-Thurner syndrome and no evidence of previous DVT get a better result than those complicated by thrombosis. Initial technical success in series reporting treatment of acute and chronic lesions is more than 90%; patency at 1 year ranges from 79% to 94%.[65,76,77] Nazarian et al. reported 1 year primary and secondary patency rates of 50% and 81% in a varied group of patients, with mostly chronic occlusion.[78] The only series reporting exclusively on chronic venous occlusions is from Raju et al., with 304 limbs (142 nonthrombotic and 162 postthrombotic) undergoing stenting without thrombolysis.[79] Primary and secondary patency rates at 2 years were 71% and 97%; patency in legs with nonthrombotic disease was 90% versus 70% in postthrombotic legs. In most instances, resolution of symptoms parallels patency of the stented vein. However, reported cumulative ulcer healing rates are 68% and 2-year ulcer-free survival is 62%.[79]

Neglén and colleagues[80] presented the largest series so far of 982 chronic nonmalignant lesions of the femoroiliocaval vein that were treated with angioplasty and stenting under intravascular ultrasound guidance. Stenting was performed with no mortality and low morbidity. Early thrombotic events were rare (1.5%). At 72 months, primary, assisted primary, and secondary cumulative patency rates were 79%, 100%, and 100% in nonthrombotic disease and 57%, 80%, and 86% in thrombotic disease, respectively. Severe in-stent restenosis (more than 50%) occurred only in 5% of the limbs at 5 years. Clinical improvement was excellent; stenting decreased both leg pain and swelling and improved quality-of-life scores.

Initial success, intermediate results, and in the experience of Neglén et al.,[80] long-term results of venous stenting are encouraging. The obvious advantage of minimal invasiveness and low complication rate make iliac vein stenting an obvious first choice in most patients. Unsuccessful or failed stenting does not preclude the subsequent performance of an open surgical procedure.

Surgical Treatment

Surgical treatment is indicated for patients with disabling symptoms who are refractory to all other forms of treatment. In the infrainguinal location, autologous grafts have the best chance of long-term success. If available, the ipsilateral or contralateral GSV is the conduit of choice, followed by arm vein. Harvesting the contralateral SFV in the postthrombotic leg is best avoided unless necessary because of potential morbidity. Externally supported extended PTFE is currently the best choice for prosthetic replacement of large veins where autologous vein is not available.

Factors responsible for poor patency in venous grafts include low flow and pressure, external compression, and hypercoagulability. Some surgeons consider thrombophilia a contraindication to venous bypass surgery. All procedures are performed under the cover of intra- and postoperative anticoagulation and intermittent pneumatic compression. Many authors have confirmed that a distal arteriovenous fistula, first suggested by Kunlin[80a] in 1953, improves the patency of grafts placed in the venous system. However, elevated cardiac output secondary to a large fistula may potentially accentuate the venous outflow obstruction and cause worsening of symptoms until the fistula is taken down. A femoral arteriovenous fistula is recommended for prosthetic grafts anastomosed to the femoral vein and iliocaval grafts longer than 10 cm. The fistula is closed surgically or by endovascular embolisation 3 to 6 months after the operation, although fistulas that cause no symptoms can be left indefinitely. A small silastic sheet wrapped around the fistula facilitates its localization at time of surgical closure. Palma procedures can be done without a fistula in patients with a high pressure gradient (10 to 20 mm Hg), but those with a lower pressure gradient and those with low initial flow (less than 100 ml/min) benefit from temporary fistula formation.

Saphenopopliteal Bypass

First advocated by Warren and Thayer[80b] in 1954 and reintroduced by Husni[81] and May,[82] saphenopopliteal bypass (May-Husni operation) is indicated for patients with occlusion of the superficial femoral or proximal popliteal veins.

In the original operation, the ipsilateral saphenous vein was used for conduit. A single distal anastomosis is performed, usually end to side, between the mobilized and divided saphenous vein and the distal popliteal vein, using running 6-0 or 7-0 prolene sutures. An end-to-side arteriovenous fistula can be constructed at the ankle between the posterior tibial artery and one of the paired posterior tibial veins or the saphenous vein. Alternatively, a bypass graft may be performed with free contralateral saphenous or arm vein.

Cross-Pelvic Venous Bypass (Palma-Dale Procedure)

Initially described by Palma in Uruguay and popularized by Dale in the United States the Palma-Dale procedure has remained a useful technique for venous reconstruction in patients with chronic unilateral iliac vein obstruction of any etiology.[83,84] A prerequisite for the procedure is a normal contralateral iliofemoral venous system to assure venous drainage. Absence of distal deep venous obstruction or reflux is associated with superior results.

Patients with unilateral iliac vein obstruction and minimal if any infrainguinal disease are the best candidates for saphenous vein transposition (Palma procedure; Figure 46-13). Unfortunately, many patients with postthrombotic syndrome have extensive femoral venous obstruction, and patients with poor inflow to the groin have less chance of a durable result. The contralateral saphenous vein is mapped with duplex ultrasound and marked on the skin preoperatively for bypass. The vein should be 5 to 6 mm for a good conduit. The common femoral vein on the affected side is exposed first through a 5- to 7-cm-long longitudinal groin incision. The collateral veins are preserved if possible. If an arteriovenous fistula is planned, the proximal superficial femoral artery is also dissected. The GSV of the contralateral leg is dissected through a 3- to 4-cm-long longitudinal or oblique incision in the groin crease, starting just medial to the femoral artery pulse. Tributaries of the saphenous vein are ligated and divided, and adequate saphenous vein is mobilized. A short, second upper-thigh incision is made to dissect a total of 20 to 25 cm of GSV. After heparinization, the saphenous vein is ligated, divided distally, and pulled up to the groin incision. Alternatively, the GSV can be harvested endoscopically. The saphenofemoral junction is dissected, but the vein is not divided proximally. Before tunneling, a small side-biting vascular clamp is placed on the common femoral vein and the saphenous vein is distended with heparinized papaverine solution

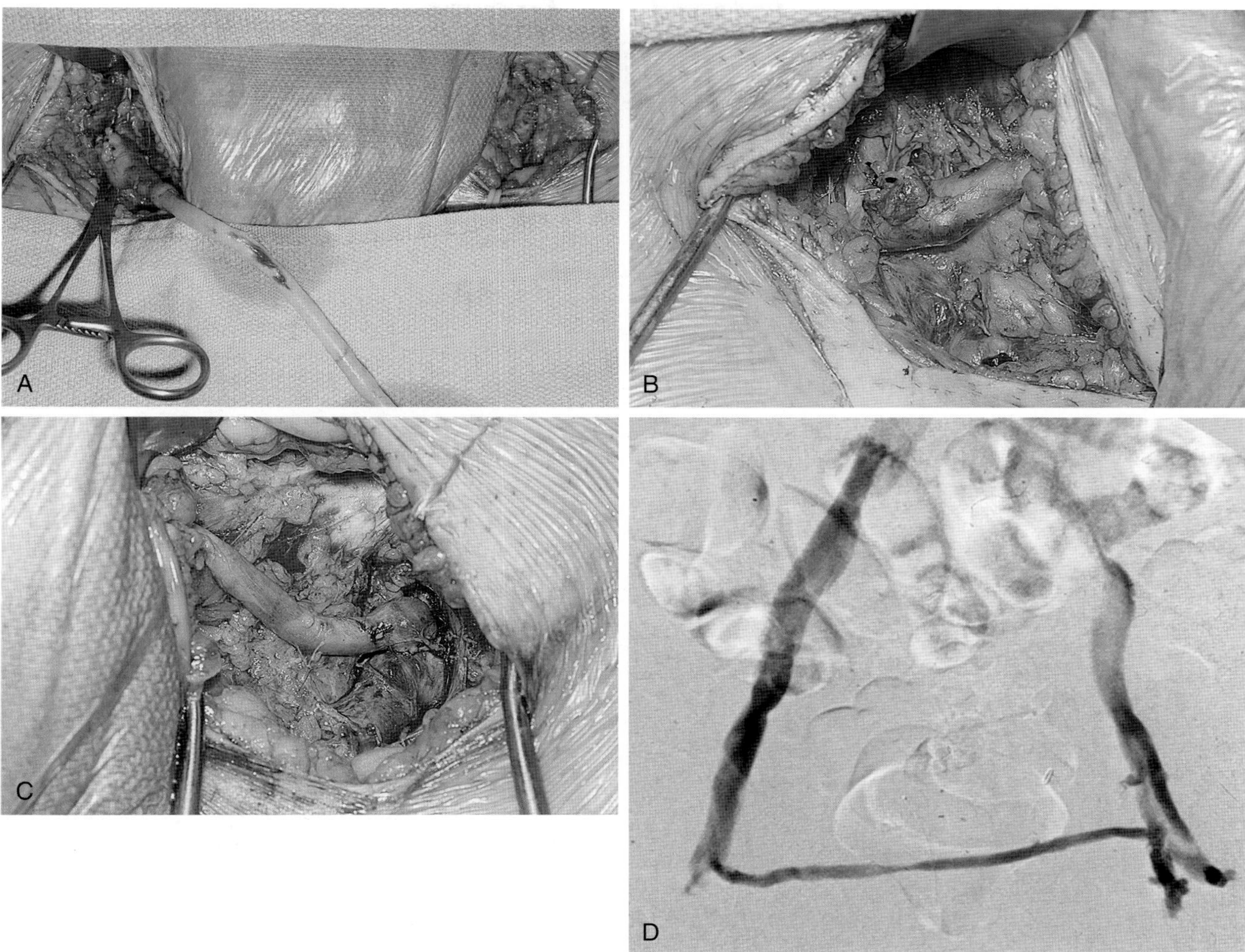

Figure 46-13. **A,** Preparation of the right great saphenous vein before a suprapubic saphenous vein transposition (Palma procedure). Bilateral groin incisions were performed to expose the left common femoral vein and the right saphenofemoral junction. The right saphenous vein was harvested through short incisions in the thigh, and a clamp is placed to occlude the saphenous vein and partially the common femoral vein. The vein is distended with heparinized papaverine solution before tunneled to the left side for anastomosis with the femoral vein. **B,** The right saphenofemoral junction after tunneling the vein to the left side in the suprapubic space. Note excellent inflow without kink in the saphenous vein. **C,** Anastomosis of the saphenous vein with the left common femoral vein. **D,** Postoperative veography confirms patent saphenous vein graft.

(Figure 46-13A). This is an important part of the procedure since the saphenous vein is usually in spasm and distention increases the size of the conduit. The suprapubic tunnel has to be wide to avoid external constriction of the vein graft and is made proximal to the external opening of the inguinal canal to avoid any injury to the spermatic cord structures in men. If a kink occurs in the vein at the saphenofemoral junction after tunneling, sometimes it is necessary to disconnect the GSV with a 2-mm cuff from the common femoral vein and reanastomose it with a running 6/0 polypropylene suture, after turning it upward through 180 degrees. The common femoral vein of the affected limb is then cross-clamped with soft vascular clamps and opened longitudinally over about 2 cm. The anastomosis between the GSV and the femoral vein is performed with running 6/0 or 7/0 polypropylene sutures. If the vein is small, interrupted sutures can be employed. If the vein is less than 5 mm in diameter, or the pressure difference between the two femoral veins is less than 3 mm Hg, femoral arteriovenous fistula is indicated. This is performed between the SFV and the hood of the saphenous vein using a separate reversed segment of the right GSV. An alternative is to use a segment of 4×7 mm PTFE graft to create a 4- or 5-mm-diameter fistula.

Although few large series have been reported, overall patency of Palma grafts in nine series including 412 operations ranged between 70% and 83% at 3 to 5 years.[84-87] Results were better in patients who had no or minimal infrainguinal venous disease and in those with May-Thurner syndrome without previous deep vein thrombosis.

Femorofemoral Prosthetic Bypass

When the saphenous vein is small or not available, crossover femoral venous prosthetic bypass with an 8- or 10-mm externally supported extended PTFE is a good alternative (Figure 46-14). The femoral veins are exposed bilaterally, the extended PTFE graft is positioned in the subcutaneous suprapubic tunnel, and an end-to-side anastomosis is performed

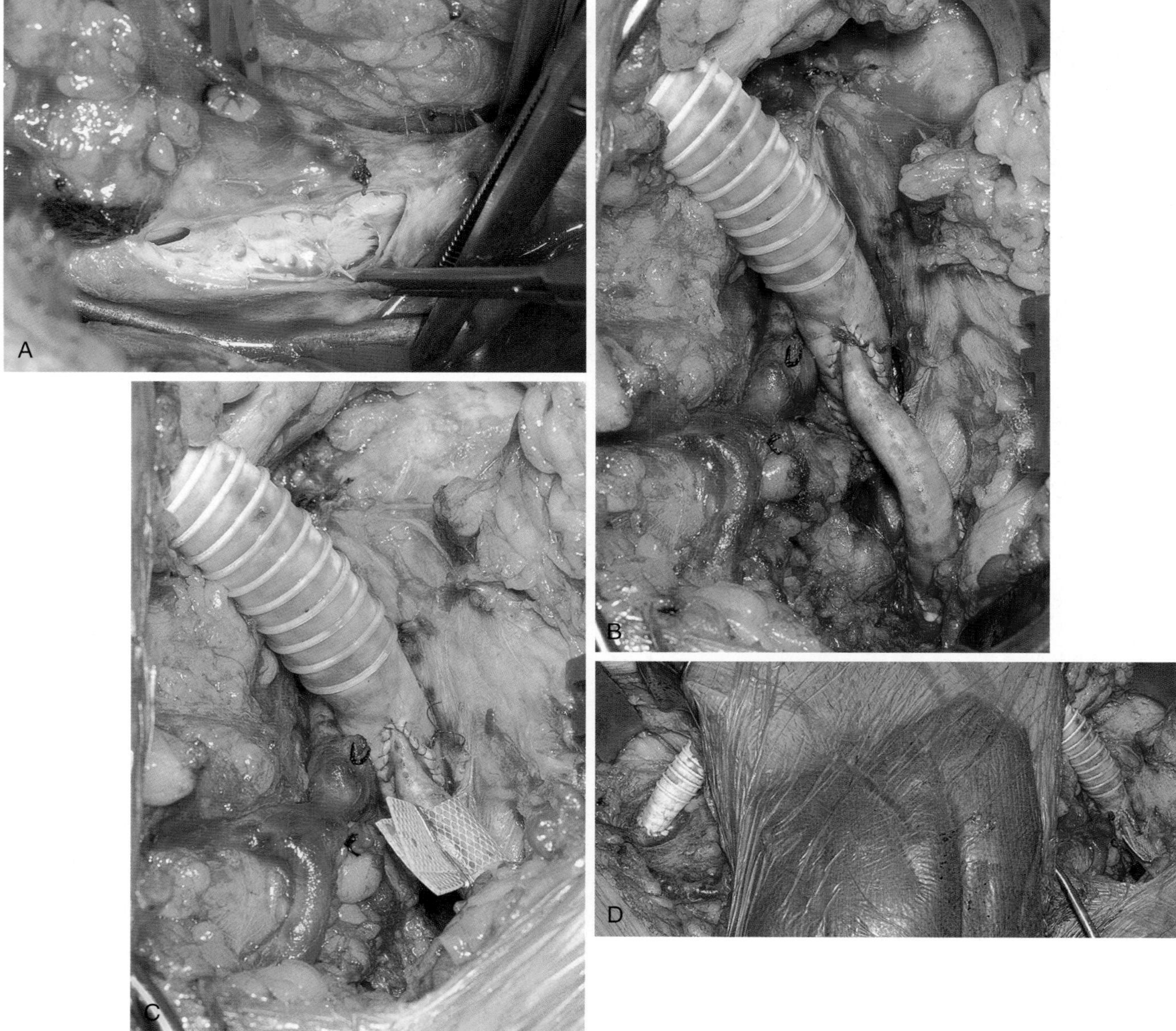

Figure 46-14. A, Partially recanalized femoral vein found after venotomy. Endophlebectomy was performed to remove the organized thrombus and improve inflow into a femorofemoral crossover venous polytetrafluoroethylene (PTFE) bypass. **B,** A PTFE arteriovenous fistula was performed between the superficial femoral artery and the hood of the cross-femoral PTFE graft. **C,** A small silastic sheath is placed around the fistula and marked with metal clips for easy identification at reoperation when the fistula is closed. **D,** Completed left-to-right femoral crossover PTFE graft with an arteriovenous fistula.

to the common femoral veins on each side. It is not unusual to need endophlebectomy of the partially recanalized femoral vein to optimize inflow into the graft (Figure 46-14A). A distal arteriovenous fistula on the affected side is routinely added to the procedure using a 4- to 5-mm PTFE graft between the PTFE graft and the superficial femoral artery (Figure 46-14B). Sotturai recommends cutting out a small window rather the just making a longitudinal cut in the cross-femoral graft at the hood of the femoral anastomosis to optimize inflow and decrease intimal hyperplasia.[66] A small silastic sheath is placed around the fistula and marked with metal clips, and a large prolene stitch is positioned under the skin (Figure 46-14C). When surgery is undertaken to close the fistula after 3 to 9 months, it is easy to find by following the thread; the silastic sheath that prevents any ingrowth into the PTFE graft.

The patency rates of extended PTFE grafts in this location are extremely variable, ranging between 0% and 100%.[66] At the Mayo Clinic, long-term patency is about 50%, and preference is given to saphenous crossover grafts, where possible.[66,87-89]

Femoroiliocaval Reconstructions

Anatomical inline iliac or iliocaval reconstruction is indicated for unilateral disease, when autologous vein is not available, or for bilateral iliac, iliocaval, or inferior vena cava occlusion.

The femoral vessels (for the arteriovenous fistula or for the site of the distal anastomosis) are exposed at the groin through

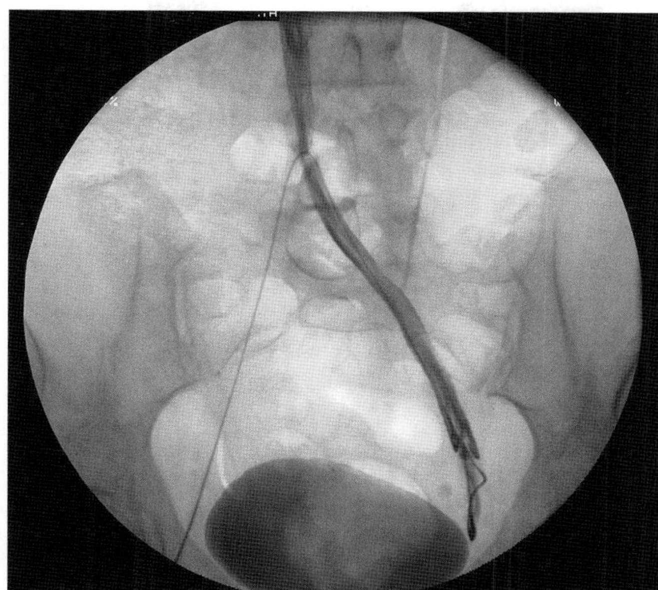

Figure 46-15. Patent left femorocaval extended PTFE bypass graft in a 54-year-old woman 11.7 years after graft placement. (From Jost CJ, Gloviczki P, Cherry KJJ, et al. *J Vasc Surg* 2001;33(2):320-327.)

a vertical incision. The iliac vein or the distal segment of the inferior vena cava is exposed through a right oblique flank incision using the retroperitoneal approach. The iliocaval segment is usually reconstructed with a 14-mm and the femorocaval segment with a 10- or 12-mm extended PTFE graft (Figure 46-15). The arteriovenous fistula is constructed first in patients who undergo a long iliocaval bypass using a tributary of the GSV. During femorocaval bypass, the proximal and distal anastomoses are performed before the fistula is created and then the circulation is opened through the graft. A small polyethylene catheter is placed at the level of the distal anastomosis for infusion of low-dose heparin (500 U/hour).

Results of Deep Venous Bypass

Although the first successful venous reconstruction was reported more than 40 years ago by Warren and Thayer,[80b] results of surgical treatment for venous obstruction have been less than satisfactory for many years. Some improvement has been made in diagnosis, patient selection, and surgical technique over the last two decades. The original May-Husni transposition is rarely performed, and popliteofemoral bypasses are infrequent. In nine series that included 218 operations, functional improvement was reported in 77%.[84,85,90] In an earlier review of 59 operations, Smith and Trimble[91] reported clinical success in 76% of the patients. Crude patency rates at variable follow-up ranged from 5% to 100%, but only four of nine studies reported on late imaging of the grafts to ascertain patency.[85,86,90,91]

Patency rates of 412 Palma operations, published in nine series, were somewhat better, with clinical improvement in 63% to 89% and patency rates between 70% and 85% (Table 46-7). However, follow-up was variable, and objective graft assessment with imaging was rarely employed. Husni reported patency of 47 of 67 grafts, followed from 6 months to 15 years.[81] Four-year patency of the 18 Palma grafts performed at the Mayo Clinic was 83%.[66] Extended PTFE grafts in this location are not so good, with early occlusion of all three grafts implanted at the Mayo Clinic and five of six grafts performed by Eklof et al.[92] However, Comerota et al.[93] reported patency in two of three grafts at 40 and 63 months. Gruss et al. have the largest experience with extended PTFE graft in this position. These authors reported an 85% (27 of 32) patency rate in a long-term follow-up study.[84,85] Based on his results and those of others, Gruss now recommends using externally supported extended PTFE grafts with arteriovenous fistula for all cross-pubic venous bypasses.

An alternative is inline femorocaval bypass for patients without suitable saphenous vein for a Palma procedure. Secondary patency of 13 iliocaval or femorocaval extended PTFE bypasses was, however, only 54% (Table 46-8). Sottiurai et al. reported patency in 9 of 13 femorocaval extended PTFE bypass grafts at 1 year.[94] Overall open venous reconstruction for iliofemoral or inferior vena caval obstruction offers 3-year patency rates of 62%.

CONCLUSION

Optimal treatment of patients with CVI and venous ulcers is not yet established. Surgical treatment focuses on removing varicose veins in milder cases and restoring venous function to reduce ambulatory venous hypertension in patients with more advanced chronic venous disease.

Treatment of perforating vein incompetence in patients with advanced chronic venous disease remains controversial. The debate has continued due to the lack of studies that address isolated treatment of perforator incompetence. Use of more radical open perforator ablative techniques is now of historical interest only. Treatment of superficial axial reflux is clearly beneficial in patients with advanced CVI. The addition of perforator ablation by SEPS appears to add to the overall hemodynamic and clinical benefit, although the exact degree of advantage remains undetermined. Based on available data, patients who benefit most from SEPS are those with ulcers due to PVI of the superficial, perforating, and deep veins. These patients have accelerated ulcer healing and an estimated 80% to 90% chance of freedom from ulcer recurrence in the long-term. SEPS is also controversial in patients with postthrombotic syndrome, as only 50% are free from ulcer recurrence in the long term. Despite the increasing popularity of office-based endovenous techniques for perforator ablation, they are still in their infancy and clinical efficacy needs to be proven before they can be endorsed as alternatives to SEPS.

Deep vein valve reconstructions continue to be challenging and rarely performed. Still, good clinical outcome has been reported in up to 80% of patients undergoing direct valve reconstructions. Results of vein transplantations and transpositions are less good, although benefit has been reported in 50% of patients.

Endovascular stenting is used increasingly for iliac vein obstruction, and it is the first option for treatment of symptomatic patients. For patients with unilateral iliac vein obstruction who are not suitable for or who fail endovascular treatment, the Palma procedure remains the best open surgical technique for autologous reconstruction. Patients with recurrent or persistent symptoms and significant disability should be considered for femoroiliac or femorocaval bypass grafts. Expanded PTFE is currently the best prosthetic material

Table 46-7
Results of Femorofemoral Crossover Bypass*

Author	Year	Limbs (*n*)	Follow-Up (Years)	Postoperative Imaging (%)	Patency Rate (%)	Clinical Improvement (%)	Graft Material
Palma and Esperon[83]	1960	8	Up to 3	13	NA	88	Vein
May[82]	1981	66	NA	NA	73	NA	Vein
Dale[115]	1979	56	NA	NA	NA	80	Vein
Husni[81]	1983	85	0.5 to –15	NA	70	74	Vein (n = 83) PTFE (n = 2)
Halliday[116]	1985	47	Up to 18	72	75 cumulative)	89	Vein
Danza et al.[86]	1991	27	NA	NA	NA	81	Vein
AbuRahma et al.[85]	1991	24	5.5	100	75	63	Vein
Gruss[84]	1997	19	NA	NA	71	82 overall	Vein
		32	NA	NA	85		PTFE
Jost et al.[87]	2001	21	3.5	100	75	67 overall†	18 vein, 3 extended PTFE

*NA, not available; PTFE, polytetrafluoroethylene.
†Includes outcome for all deep venous bypasses.

Table 46-8
Results of Femorocaval or Iliocaval Bypass*

Author	Year	Limbs (*n*)	Follow-Up (Months)	Imaging (%)	Patency Rate (%)	Clinical Improvement (%)	Graft Material
Husfeldt[117]	1979	4	4 to 30	100	100	100	ePTFE
Dale[118]	1984	3	1 to 30	100	100	100	ePTFE
Alimi[119]	1997	8	Mean 19.5	100	88	88	ePTFE
Sottiurai[70]	1997	45	11 to 139	100‡	93†	89§	ePTFE
Jost et al.[87]	2001	18	42	100	56	67	13 ePTFE, 5 spiral vein

*ePTFE, extended polytetrafluoroethylene.
†Includes 6 femoroiliac, 26 femorofemoral, 8 femorocaval, and 5 femorofemoralcaval grafts.
‡Postoperative duplex scan, followed by annual air plethysmography and selective venography.
§An additional 8 patients (18%) developed recurrent ulcers during follow-up.

for reconstruction of the vena cava and short, large-diameter grafts have the best long-term patency. However, patients with significant infrainguinal venous disease have a lower chance of long-term success. While endovascular techniques may limit the need for surgical treatment in the future, carefully selected patients with symptomatic large vein obstruction will continue to enjoy durable benefit from open surgical venous reconstruction.

References

1. Stanley JC, Barnes RW, Ernst CB, et al. Vascular surgery in the United States: workforce issues—Report of the Society for Vascular Surgery and the International Society for Cardiovascular Surgery, North American Chapter, Committee on Workforce Issues. *J Vasc Surg* 1996;23:172-181.
2. Bosanquet N. Costs of venous ulcers: from maintenance therapy to investment programmes. *Phleboblogy* 1992;1(Suppl):44-46.
3. Nicolaides AN, Hussein MK, Szendro G, et al. The relation of venous ulceration with ambulatory venous pressure measurements. *J Vasc Surg* 1993;17:414-419.
4. Nicolaides AN, Bergan JJ, Eklof B, et al., and the American Venous Forum Consensus Committee. Classification and grading of chronic venous disease in the lower limbs: a consensus statement. In: *Handbook of venous disorders*. London: Chapman and Hall; 1996:652-660.
5. Porter JM, Moneta GL. Reporting standards in venous disease: an update—International Consensus Committee on Chronic Venous Disease. [Comments.] *J Vasc Surg* 1995;21:635-645.
6. Raju S. Venous insufficiency of the lower limb and stasis ulceration: changing concepts and management. *Ann Surg* 1983;197:688-697.
7. Gloviczki P, Bergan JJ, Rhodes JM, et al. Mid-term results of endoscopic perforator vein interruption for chronic venous insufficiency: lessons learned from the North American subfascial endoscopic perforator surgery registry—The North American Study Group. *J Vasc Surg* 1999;29:489-502.
8. Kalra M, Gloviczki P, Noel AA, et al. Subfascial endoscopic perforator vein surgery in patients with post-thrombotic venous insufficiency: is it justified? *Vasc Endovasc Surg* 2002;36:41-50.
9. van Rij AM, Solomon C, Christie R. Anatomic and physiologic characteristics of venous ulceration. *J Vasc Surg* 1994;20:759-764.
10. Labropoulos N, Delis K, Nicolaides AN, et al. The role of the distribution and anatomic extent of reflux in the development of signs and symptoms in chronic venous insufficiency. *J Vasc Surg* 1996;23:504-510.
11. Hanrahan LM, Araki CT, Rodriguez AA, et al. Distribution of valvular incompetence in patients with venous stasis ulceration. *J Vasc Surg* 1991;13:805-812.
12. Myers KA, Ziegenbein RW, Zeng GH, Matthews PG. Duplex ultrasonography scanning for chronic venous disease: patterns of venous reflux. *J Vasc Surg* 1995;21:605-612.
13. van Bemmelen PS, Bedford G, Beach K, Strandness DE. Quantitative segmental evaluation of venous valvular reflux with duplex ultrasound scanning. *J Vasc Surg* 1989;10:425-431.
14. Schanzer H, Peirce EC. A rational approach to surgery of the chronic venous statis syndrome. *Ann Surg* 1982;195:25-29.
15. Negus D, Friedgood A. The effective management of venous ulceration. *Brit J Surg* 1983 10/1983;70(10):623-627.
16. Darke SG. The morphology of recurrent varicose veins. [Comments.] *Eur J Vasc Surg* 1992;6:512-517.
17. Kistner RL, Ferris EB, Randhawa G, Kamida C. A method of performing descending venography. *J Vasc Surg* 1986;4:464-468.

18. Sherman RS. Varicose veins: further findings based on anatomic and surgical dissections. *Ann Surg* 1949;130:218-232.
19. Beecher HK, Field ME, Krogh A. The effect of walking on the venous pressure at the ankle. *Skand Arch F Physiol* 1936;73:133-140.
20. Mozes G, Gloviczki P, Menawat SS, et al. Surgical anatomy for endoscopic subfascial division of perforating veins. *J Vasc Surg* 1996;24:800-808.
21. Barwell JR, Davies CE, Deacon J, et al. Comparison of surgery and compression with compression alone in chronic venous ulceration (ESCHAR study): randomised control trial. *Lancet* 2004;363:1854-1859.
22. Mendes RR, Marston WA, Farber MA, et al. Treatment of superficial and perforator vein incompetence without deep venous insufficiency: is routine perforator ligation necessary? *J Vasc Surg*. 2003;38:891-895.
23. Stuart WP, Adam DJ, Allan PL, et al. Saphenous surgery does not correct perforator incompetence in the presence of deep venous reflux. *J Vasc Surg* 1998 11/1998;28(5):834-838.
24. Stuart WP, Adam DJ, Allan PL, et al. The relationship between the number, competence, and diameter of medial calf perforating veins and the clinical status in healthy subjects and patients with lower-limb venous disease. *J Vasc Surg* 2000;32:138-143.
25. Delis KT, Husmann M, Kalodiki E, et al. In situ hemodynamics of perforating veins in chronic venous insufficiency. *J Vasc Surg* 2001;33: 773-782.
26. Pierik EG, van Urk H, Hop WC, Wittens CH. Endoscopic versus open subfascial division of incompetent perforating veins in the treatment of venous leg ulceration: a randomized trial. *J Vasc Surg* 1997;26:1049-1054.
27. Linton RR. The operative treatment of varicose veins and ulcers, based upon a classification of these lesions. *Ann Surg* 1938;107:582-593.
28. Cockett FB, Jones BD. The ankle blow–out syndrome: a new approach to the varicose ulcer problem. *Lancet* 1953;i:17-23.
29. Lim RCJ, Blaisdell FW, Zubrin J, et al. Subfascial ligation of perforating veins in recurrent stasis ulceration. *Am J Surg* 1970;119:246-249.
30. DePalma RG. Surgical therapy for venous stasis: results of a modified Linton operation. *Am J Surg* 1979;137:810-813.
30a. Howard PM, Harris AE, Price RR. Venous and lymphatic stasis of the lower extremity—treatment of chronic changes by a modified Linton procedure. *Rocky Mt Med J* 1967;64(1):47-49.
31. Burnand K, Thomas ML, O'Donnell T, Browse NL. Relation between postphlebitic changes in the deep veins and results of surgical treatment of venous ulcers. *Lancet* 1976;1:936-938.
32. Edwards JM. Shearing operation for incompetent perforating veins. *Br J Surg* 1976;63:885-886.
33. Hauer G. Endoscopic subfascial discussion of perforating veins—preliminary report. [German.] *Vasa* 1985;14:59-61.
34. Bergan JJ, Murray J, Greason K. Subfascial endoscopic perforator vein surgery: a preliminary report. *Ann Vasc Surg* 1996;10:211-219.
35. Gloviczki P, Bergan JJ, Menawat SS, et al. Safety, feasibility, and early efficacy of subfascial endoscopic perforator surgery: a preliminary report from the North American registry. *J Vasc Surg* 1997;25:94-105.
36. O'Donnell TF. Surgical treatment of incompetent communicating veins. In: *Atlas of venous surgery*. Philadelphia: WB Saunders; 2000:111-124.
37. Gloviczki P, Cambria RA, Rhee RY, et al. Surgical technique and preliminary results of endoscopic subfascial division of perforating veins. *J Vasc Surg* 1996;23:517-523.
38. Conrad P. Endoscopic exploration of the subfascial space of the lower leg with perforator interruption using laparoscopic equipment: a preliminary report. *Phlebology* 1994;9:154-157.
39. Proebstle TM, Weisel G, Paepcke U, et al. Light reflection rheography and clinical course of patients with advanced venous disease before and after endoscopic subfascial division of perforating veins. *Dermatol Surg* 1998;24:771-776.
40. Peden E, Lumsden A. Radiofrequency ablation of incompetent perforator veins. *Perspect Vasc Surg Endovasc Ther* 2007;1:73-77.
41. Proebstle TM, Herdemann S. Early results and feasibility of incompetent perforator vein ablation by endovenous laser treatment. *Dermatol Surg* 2007;33(2):162-168.
42. Whiteley MS, Holstock JM, Price BA, et al. Radiofrequency ablation of refluxing great saphenous systems, Giacomini veins and incompetent perforating veins using VNUS closure and TRLOP technique. *Phlebology* 2003;18:52.
43. Sato DT, Goff CD, Gregory RT, et al. Subfascial perforator vein ablation: comparison of open versus endoscopic techniques. *J Endovasc Surg* 1999;6:147-154.
44. Masuda EM, Kessler DM, Lurie F, et al. The effect of ultrasound-guided sclerotherapy of incompetent perforator veins on venous clinical severity and disablility scores. *J Vasc Surg* 2006;43:551-557.
45. Padberg FTJ, Pappas PJ, Araki CT, et al. Hemodynamic and clinical improvement after superficial vein ablation in primary combined venous insufficiency with ulceration. [Comments.] *J Vasc Surg* 1996;24:711-718.
46. Nelzen O. Prospective study of safety, patient satisfaction and leg ulcer healing following saphenous and subfascial endoscopic perforator surgery. [comments.] *Br J Surg* 2000;87:86-91.
47. TenBrook JA, Iafrati MD, O'Donnell TF, et al. Systematic review of outcomes after surgical management of venous disease incorporating subfascial endoscopic perforator surgery. *J Vasc Surg* 2004;39(3)583-589.
48. van Gent WB, Hop WC, van Praag MC, et al. Conservative versus surgical treatment of venous leg ulcers: A prospective, randomized, multicenter trial. *J Vasc Surg* 2006;44(3):563-571.
49. van Gent Wb HW, Van Praag MC, Mackaay AJ, et al. Conservative versus surgical treatment of venous leg ulcers: a prospective, randomized, multicenter trial. *Perspect Vasc Surg Endovasc Ther* 2006;18(4):347-349.
50. Akesson H, Brudin L, Cwikiel W, et al. Does the correction of insufficient superficial and perforating veins improve venous function in patients with deep venous insufficiency? *Phlebology* 1990;5:113-123.
51. Rhodes JM, Gloviczki P, Canton LG, et al. Endoscopic perforator vein division with ablation of superficial reflux improves venous hemodynamics. *J Vasc Surg* 1998;28:839-847.
52. Kistner RL. Surgical repair of the incompetent femoral vein valve. *Arch Surg* 1975;110:1336-1342.
53. Raju S, Fredericks R. Valve reconstruction procedures for nonobstructive venous insufficiency: rationale, techniques, and results in 107 procedures with two- to eight-year follow-up. *J Vasc Surg* 1988;7:301-310.
54. Sottiurai VS. Technique in direct venous valvuloplasty. *J Vasc Surg* 1988;8:646-648.
55. Gloviczki P, Merrell SW, Bower TC. Femoral vein valve repair under direct vision without venotomy: a modified technique with use of angioscopy. *J Vasc Surg* 1991;14:645-648.
56. Raju S, Hardy JD. Technical options in venous valve reconstruction. *Am J Surg* 1997;173:301-307.
57. Durango E. Creation of new venous valves. Second Meeting of Cardiovascualr Surgeons and First Ecuadorian Course on Angiology and Vascular Surgery, 1993, Quito, Ecuador.
58. Kistner RL, Sparkuhl MD. Surgery in acute and chronic venous disease. *Surgery* 1979;85:31-43.
59. Taheri SA, Lazar L, Elias S. Status of vein valve transplant after 12 months. *Arch Surg* 1982;117:1313-1317.
60. O'Donnell TFJ, Mackey WC, Shepard AD, Callow AD. Clinical, hemodynamic, and anatomic follow-up of direct venous reconstruction. *Arch Surg* 1987;122:474-482.
61. Masuda EM, Kistner RL. Long-term results of venous valve reconstruction: a four- to twenty-one-year follow-up. *J Vasc Surg* 1994;19:391-403.
62. Cheatle TR, Perrin M. Venous valve repair: early results in fifty-two cases. *J Vasc Surg* 1994;19:404-413.
63. Welch HJ, McLaughlin RL, O'Donnell TF Jr. Femoral vein valvuloplasty: intraoperative angioscopic evaluation and hemodynamic improvement. *J Vasc Surg* 1992;16:694-700.
64. Jamieson WG, Chinnick B. Clinical results of deep venous valvular repair for chronic venous insufficiency. *Canad J Surg* 1997;40:294-299.
65. Raju S, Fredericks RK, Neglén PN, Bass JD. Durability of venous valve reconstruction techniques for "primary" and postthrombotic reflux. *J Vasc Surg* 1996;23:357-366.
66. Sottiurai VS. Venous bypass and valve reconstruction: indication, technique and results. *Phlebology* 1997;25:183-188.
67. Perrin M. Reconstructive surgery for deep venous reflux: a report on 144 cases. *Cardiovasc Surg* 2000;8:246-255.
68. Perrin M. Introduction: surgery of the venous valve. [French.] *Journal des Maladies Vasculaires* 1997;22:96.
69. Eriksson I, Almgren B. Surgical reconstruction of incompetent deep vein valves. *Upsala J Med Sci* 1988;93:139-143.
70. Sottiurai VS. Results of deep vein reconstruction. *Vasc Surg* 1997;31: 276-278.
71. Bry JD, Muto PA, O'Donnell TF, Isaacson LA. The clinical and hemodynamic results after axillary-to-popliteal vein valve transplantation. *J Vasc Surg* 1995;21:110-119.

72. Raju S, Neglén P, Doolittle J, Meydrech EF. Axillary vein transfer in trabeculated postthrombotic veins. *J Vasc Surg* 1999;29:1050-1062.
73. Thorpe PE. Endovascular therapy for chronic venous occlusion. *J Endovasc Surg* 1999;6:118-119.
74. Bjarnason H, Kruse JR, Asinger DA, et al. Iliofemoral deep venous thrombosis: safety and efficacy outcome during 5 years of catheter-directed thrombolytic therapy. *J Vasc Intervent Radiol* 1997;8:405-418.
75. Neglén P, Raju S. Balloon dilation and stenting of chronic iliac vein obstruction: technical aspects and early clinical outcome. [Comments.] *J Endovasc Ther* 2000;7:79-91.
76. O'Sullivan GJ, Semba CP, Bittner CA, et al. Endovascular management of iliac vein compression (May-Thurner) syndrome. *J Vasc Intervent Radiol* 2000;11:823-836.
77. Hurst DR, Forauer AR, Bloom JR, et al. Diagnosis and endovascular treatment of iliocaval compression syndrome. *J Vasc Surg* 2001;34: 106-113.
78. Nazarian GK, Austin WR, Wegryn SA, et al. Venous recanalization by metallic stents after failure of balloon angioplasty or surgery: four-year experience. *Cardiovasc Intervent Radiol* 1996;19:227-233.
79. Raju S, Owen SJ, Neglén P. The clinical impact of iliac venous stents in the management of chronic venous insufficiency. *J Vasc Surg* 2002;35: 8-15.
80. Neglén P, Hollis KC, Olivier J, Raju S. Stenting of the venous outflow in chronic venous disease: long-term stent-related outcome, clinical, and hemodynamic result. *J Vasc Surg* 2007;46:979-990.
80a. Kunlin J. The reestablishment of venous circulation by graft in the case of traumatic obliteration or thrombophlebitis; 18 cm graft between the internal saphenus and external iliac veins; thrombosis after three weeks of successful blood passage. *Mem Acad Chir* (Paris) 1953;79(4-5):109-111.
80b. Warren R, Thayer TR. Transplantation of the saphenous vein for post-phlebitic stasis. *Surgery* 1954;35(6):867-878.
81. Husni EA. Reconstruction of veins: the need for objectivity. *J Cardiovasc Surg* 1983;24:525-528.
82. May R. The Palma operation with Gottlob's endothelium perserving suture. In: May R, Weber J, editors. *Pelvic and abdominal veins: progress in diagnosis and therapy*. Amsterdam: Excerpta Medica; 1981:192-197.
83. Dale WA. Crossover vein grafts for relief of iliofemoral venous block. *Surgery* 1965;57:608-612.
84. Gruss JD, Hiemer W. Bypass procedures for venous obstruction: Palma and May-Husni bypasses, Raju perforator bypass, prosthetic bypasses, and primary and adjunctive arteriovenous fistulae. In: Raju S, Villavicencio JL, eds. *Surgical management of venous disease*. Baltimore: Williams & Wilkins; 1997:289-305.
85. AbuRahma AF, Robinson PA, Boland JP. Clinical, hemodynamic, and anatomic predictors of long-term outcome of lower extremity venovenous bypasses. [Comments.] *J Vasc Surg* 1991;14:635-644.
86. Danza R, Navarro T, Baldizan J. Reconstructive surgery in chronic venous obstruction of the lower limbs. *J Cardiovasc Surg* 1991;32:98-103.
87. Jost CJ, Gloviczki P, Cherry KJJ, et al. Surgical reconstruction of iliofemoral veins and the inferior vena cava for nonmalignant occlusive disease. *J Vasc Surg* 2001;33:320–327.
88. Gloviczki P, Cho JS. Surgical treatment of chronic occlusions of the iliocaval veins. In: Rutherford RB, ed. *Rutherford's vascular surgery*. 6th ed. Philadelphia: Elsevier; 2005:2303-2320.
89. Bower TC, Nagorney DM, Cherry Jr KJ, et al. Replacement of the inferior vena cava for malignancy: an update. *J Vasc Surg* 2000;31:270-281.
90. Lalka SG, Lash JM, Unthank JL, et al. Inadequacy of saphenous vein grafts for cross-femoral venous bypass. *J Vasc Surg* 1991;13:622-630.
91. Smith DE, Trimble C. Surgical management of Obstructive venous disease of the lower extremity. In Rutherford RB, ed. *Vascular surgery*. Philadelphia: WB Saunders; 1977:1247-1268.
92. Eklof BG, Kistner RL, Masuda EM. Venous bypass and valve reconstruction: long-term efficacy. [Review] [43 refs]. *Vasc Med* 1998;3:157-164.
93. Comerota AJ, Aldridge SC, Cohen G, et al. A strategy of aggressive regional therapy for acute iliofemoral venous thrombosis with contemporary venous thrombectomy or catheter-directed thrombolysis. [Comments.] *J Vasc Surg* 1994;20:244-254.
94. Sottiurai VS, Gonzales J, Cooper M, et al. A new concept of arteriovenous fistula in venous bypass requiring no fistula interruption: surgical technique and long-term results. J Cardiovasc Surg 2002.
95. Sethia KK, Darke SG. Long saphenous incompetence as a cause of venous ulceration. *Br J Surg* 1984;71:754-755.
96. van Bemmelen PS, Bedford G, Beach K, Strandness Jr DE. Status of the valves in the superficial and deep venous system in chronic venous disease. *Surgery* 1991;109:730-734.
97. Lees TA, Lambert D. Patterns of venous reflux in limbs with skin changes associated with chronic venous insufficiency. *Br J Surg* 1993;80:725-728.
98. Shami SK, Sarin S, Cheatle TR, et al. Venous ulcers and the superficial venous system. *J Vasc Surg* 1993;17:487-490.
99. Silver D, Gleysteen JJ, Rhodes GR, et al. Surgical treatment of the refractory postphlebitic ulcer. *Arch Surg* 1971;103:554-560.
100. Thurston OG, Williams HT. Chronic venous insufficiency of the lower extremity. Pathogenesis and surgical treatment. *Arch Surg* 1973;106:537-539.
101. Wilkinson Jr GE, Maclaren IF. Long term review of procedures for venous perforator insufficiency. *Surg Gynecol Obstet* 1986;163:117-120.
102. Cikrit DF, Nichols WK, Silver D. Surgical management of refractory venous stasis ulceration. *J Vasc Surg* 1988;7:473-478.
103. Bradbury AW, Stonebridge PA, Callam MJ, et al. Foot volumetry and duplex ultrasonography after saphenous and subfascial perforating vein ligation for recurrent venous ulceration. *Br J Surg* 1993;80:845-848.
104. Jugenheimer M, Junginger T. Endoscopic subfascial sectioning of incompetent perforating veins in treatment of primary varicosis. *World J Surg* 1992;16:971-975.
105. Pierik EGJM, Wittens CHA, van Urk H. Subfascial endoscopic ligation in the treatment of incompetent perforator veins. *Eur J Vasc Endovasc Surg* 1995;5:38-41.
106. Wolters U, Schmit-Rixen T, Erasmi H, et al. Endoscopic dissection of incompetent perforating veins in the treatment of chronic venous leg ulcers. *Vasc Surg* 1996;30:481-487.
107. Pierik EG, van Urk H, Wittens CH. Efficacy of subfascial endoscopy in eradicating perforating veins of the lower leg and its relation with venous ulcer healing. *J Vasc Surg* 1997;26:255-259.
108. Nelzen O. Prospective study of safety, patient satisfaction and leg ulcer healing following saphenous and subfascial endoscopic perforator surgery. *Br J Surg* 2000;87:86-91.
109. Iafrati MDPG, O"Donnell TF, Estes J. Is the nihilistic approach to surgical reduction of superficial and perforator vein incompetence for venous ulcer justified? *J Vasc Surg* 2002;36:1167-1174.
110. Baron HC, Wayne MG, Santiago CA, Grossi R. Endoscopic perforator vein surgery for patients with severe chronic venous insufficiency. *Vasc Endovasc Surg* 2004;38:439-442.
111. Eriksson I, Almgren B. Surgical reconstruction of incompetent deep vein valves. *Ups J Med Sci* 1988;93(2):139-143.
112. Iafrati M, O'Donnell TF. Surgical reconstruction for deep venous insufficiency. *J Mal Vasc* 1997;22(3):193-197.
113. Taheri SA. Vein valve transplantation. *Vasc Surg* 1997;31:278-281.
114. May R, Thurner JZ. A vascular spur in the vena iliaca communis sinistra as a cause of predominantly left-sided thrombosis of the pelvic veins. *Kreislaufforsch* 1956;45:912-922.
115. Dale WA. Reconstructive venous surgery. *Arch Surg* 1979;114(11):1312-1318.
116. Halliday AW, Mansfield AO. Congenital arteriovenous malformations. *Br J Surg* 1993;80(1):2-3.
117. Husfeldt KJ, Gall FP, Schulz HP, et al. Vein substitution using PTFE prosthesis–results of animal experiments and initial clinical experiences. German. *Chir Forum Exp Klin Forsch* 1979:11-15.
118. Dale WA, Harris J, Terry RB. Polytetrafluoroethylene reconstruction of the inferior vena cava. *Surgery* 1984;95:625-630.
119. Alimi YS, DiMauro P, Fabre D, et al. Iliac vein reconstructions to treat acute and chronic venous occlusive disease. *J Vasc Surg* 1997;25: 673-681.

chapter 47

Venous Thrombosis and Pulmonary Thromboembolic Disease

Brad H. Thompson, MD • Kong Teng Tan, MD • Edwin J.R. van Beek, MD, PhD

Key Points

- Deep venous thrombosis (DVT) and pulmonary embolism (PE) are a single clinicopathological entity (venous thromboembolic disease, or VTE).
- The incidence is 1 case of DVT and 0.5 case of PE per 1000 population per year in the Western world.
- In a hospital setting, 15% of medical and 30% to 50% of surgical patients develop VTE if no thromboprophylaxis is initiated.
- Clinical features are nonspecific and inaccurate, resulting in misdiagnosis of VTE in many patients.
- Serious immediate and long-term complications occur; untreated PE has 30% to 40% mortality, and up to 50% of patients with DVT develop postthrombotic syndrome.
- Several diagnostic algorithms can prove or rule out the diagnosis of VTE safely. Of these, computed tomography pulmonary angiography is now most commonly employed with clinical risk assessment and plasma D-dimer testing.
- Anticoagulation is the cornerstone of treatment, but thrombolysis is an option for life-threatening VTE.
- Of patients with suspected VTE, 70% do not have this condition and treatment should be withheld.

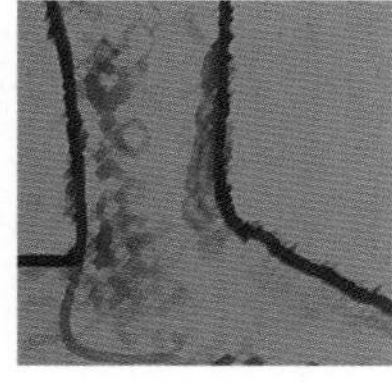

Approximately 3 in 1000 people suffer from symptoms suggesting acute pulmonary embolism (PE) every year, and the prevalence of deep venous thrombosis (DVT) in the United States is estimated at 2 million cases per year.[1] About 30% to 50% of these patients have concurrent PE, and 10% of these die within the first hour of presentation.[2] If untreated, the mortality rate may be as high as 26%. In the United States, PE is reported to have caused more deaths than motor vehicle accidents, which accounted for 43,536 fatalities in 1993.

DVT and PE were considered separate clinicopathological entities until relatively recently. However, numerous autopsy studies have demonstrated a strong association between PE and concurrent DVT.[3] Of patients with proven PE, 70% also have lower extremity DVT, while 50% of patients with documented DVT have PE.[4] In addition, clinical outcomes are similar in patients with DVT with or without PE. Ample evidence suggests that both DVT and PE should be considered as a single medical condition often requiring similar therapeutic interventions.

PE commonly develops as a complication during hospitalization in nonambulatory, severely ill patients. The clinical presentation of PE is often nonspecific, with symptoms that suggest alternative diagnoses. In other patients, the event may be clinically silent or unsuspected, being masked by other comorbid conditions. Autopsy studies have shown repeatedly that PE is regularly missed, especially in the elderly and those with concurrent cardiorespiratory diseases. A timely diagnosis, however, is paramount, as the likelihood of recurrent, potentially fatal pulmonary thromboembolic disease is 30%.

Thromboprophylactic measures introduced over the last few decades have positively affected the incidence of venous thromboembolic disease (VTE). A necropsy series, covering the period 1965 to 1990, from a London teaching hospital showed that the percentage of fatal PE fell progressively from 6.1% to 2.1%.[5] However, the incidence of DVT in nonsurgical patients remains unchanged.[6] To date, there is ongoing discussion and controversy relating to the diagnosis, prophylaxis, and treatment of VTE.[7,8]

EPIDEMIOLOGY

The true prevalence of VTE is difficult to determine, since acute VTE and PE represent entities that are often occult, not suspected, or overlooked. In others, the symptoms of PE are attributed to other cardiopulmonary disorders such as angina or pneumonia. A retrospective population-based survey found an average annual incidence of 48 primary and 36 recurrent cases of DVT, plus 23 cases of pulmonary emboli per 100,000 residents.[9] Figures from Vital Statistics and from the National Hospital Discharge Survey in the United States from 1970 to 1985 showed an age-adjusted rate for PE in 51 per 100,000 and venous thrombosis in 79 per 100,000 inhabitants.[10] A 25-year population-based study of 2218 patients in Olmsted County, Minnesota, from 1966 to 1990 showed an annual incidence of VTE of 117 per 100,000 (DVT, 48 per 100,000; PE, 69 per 100,000).[6] Furthermore, the incidence of VTE was higher in men than in women (ratio 1.2:1). Reviewing the epidemiological studies, a fair estimate of the annual incidence of DVT and PE in the Western world is about 1 and 0.5 cases per 1000 population, respectively.

A more recent study showed that the incidence of VTE demonstrated by venography or duplex ultrasonography in hospitalized, acutely ill medical patients who did not receive any anticoagulation was 14.9%.[11] In another study of postoperative neurosurgical patients who received compression stockings as the only measure of thromboprophylaxis, an incidence of 43 of 129 patients (33%) was demonstrated.[12]

Autopsy studies, as expected, showed higher incidences of PE (50% to 60%), especially when the lung specimens were examined in detail. However, it should be remembered that, in most cases, the emboli were small and unlikely to be the main cause of death, although they may have contributed indirectly.[13] The true incidence of PE as a cause of death is not known. Studies in the 1970s suggested that 7% of deaths in hospital were secondary to PE. This result was probably inaccurate, as subsequent investigations refuted this finding. Most recent autopsy series quote a more conservative estimate of 1% to 3%.[14]

In conclusion, although the exact incidence of VTE is obscure, it is estimated to affect 1.5 million patients per year in the Western world and, without doubt, is a major cause of morbidity and mortality.

PATHOPHYSIOLOGY

The pathophysiology of VTE includes the causes of thrombogenesis and the pathophysiological sequela of DVT and PE.

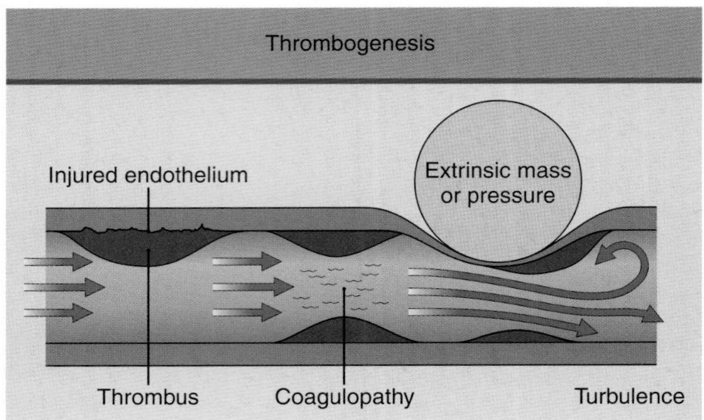

Figure 47-1. Thrombogenesis. Virchow's triad: (1) endothelial abnormalities, (2) coagulopathy, and (3) stasis of blood flow.

Thrombogenesis

The triad of German pathologist Rudolf Virchow (1821 to 1902) provides a compartmentalized approach for causative factors required for intravascular thrombosis (DVT). The three components of Virchow's triad (Figure 47-1) are as follows:

- Endothelial abnormality
- Stasis of blood flow
- Hypercoagulability of blood

Although a single component of the triad may be sufficient to instigate intravascular thrombosis, most cases involve defects of multiple components of Virchow's triad.

The most common site of venous thrombosis occurs in the deep veins of the leg. Additional sites include veins of the pelvis and the inferior vena cava (IVC). Thrombosis within the superior vena cava and upper extremity DVT are increasing in prevalence due to increased use of indwelling central venous catheters and lines.[15] The likelihood of occurrence of embolic disease to the lungs is highest from centrally located DVT (cava) and right heart, with a slightly lower incidence for PE from clot originating from more peripheral veins.[16] Thrombosis of the iliofemoral veins is estimated to result in PE in 30% to 50% of cases and, when combined with popliteal vein thrombosis, to account for more than 90% of all cases of PE.[2]

Endothelial Abnormalities

The endothelial lining of blood vessels provides a smooth nonthrombotic surface for normal laminar blood flow. Of the three components of Virchow's triad, endothelial injury appears to be the least important factor for the development of venous thrombosis.[17] Endothelial injury most often occurs with direct vascular trauma, occurring from blunt force, vessel manipulation (hip replacement), or venous catherization.[18] Endothelial injury can also occur from localized cytotoxic effects from intravascularly administered drugs like chemotherapeutic agents and iodinated contrast material. The reported incidence of DVT following venography using ionic contrast media ranges from 9% to 30%[19] and this can be reduced to 3% using newer nonionic contrast agents.[20] Systemic illness such as autoimmune diseases or septicemia can also damage the endothelium by immune

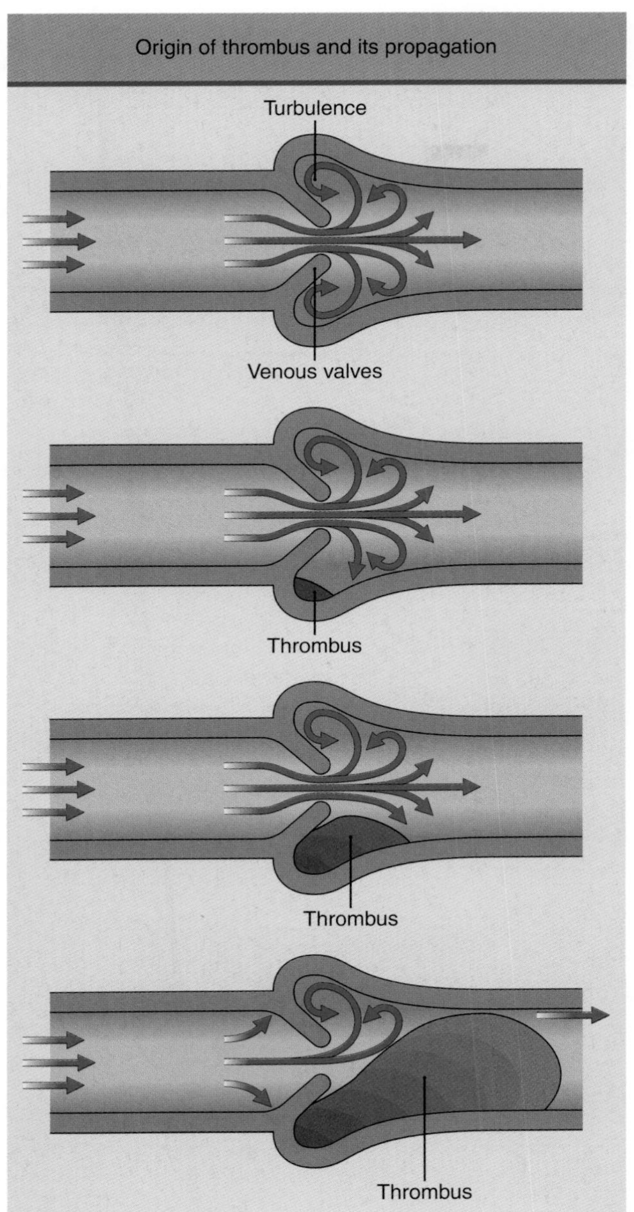

Figure 47-2. Origin of thrombus and its propagation. Thrombus forms in the valve pockets secondary to venous stasis. Subsequent deposition of fibrin-platelet layers leads to propagation of the thrombus.

complex deposition (type III reaction), resulting in vasculitis and subsequent venous thrombosis.[17] Regardless of the cause, endothelial injury promotes localized platelet adhesion to the endothelial surface, along with activation of the clotting cascade.

Blood Flow (Stasis)

Venous stasis is the predominant causative factor for the development of thrombosis. Normal blood flow in the venous system depends on factors such as adequate cardiac output, low venous resistance, and augmentation of venous blood flow from muscular contractions. Cardiac failure, intraabdominal masses (pregnancy or tumor), immobilization, or external compression such as casting material or bandages are often initiators for venous thrombosis. Intravascular devices such as venous catheters, pacing wires, and caval filters can also disrupt normal blood flow and promote thrombus formation.[15] Once thrombosis develops, the initiation point is commonly around the site of valves, where eddy currents produce localized pools of relatively stagnant flow (Figure 47-2).

Table 47-1
Causes of Hypercoagulability

Inherited
Common
Factor V Leiden
Prothrombin gene mutation (G20110A)
Homozygous C677T mutation in methylene
Tetrahydrofolate reductase gene
Rare
Antithrombin deficiency
Protein S deficiency
Protein C deficiency
Dysfibrinogenemia
Homozygous homocystinuria
Acquired
Age
Surgery and trauma
Immobilization
Malignant disease
Previous venous thromboembolism
Pregnancy and puerperium
Oral contraceptive and hormone replacement therapy
Antiphospholipid antibodies
Unknown (Probably Multifactorial)
Elevated levels of factor VIII, IX, and XI and fibrinogen

Blood Hypercoagulability

In a normal person, plasma coagulation factors exist in a nonactivated state. Upon activation, the intrinsic regulating system prevents excessive activation that could lead to a hypercoagulable state like disseminated intravascular coagulopathy. Many etiologies are responsible for hypercoagulable conditions that can be inherited or acquired (Table 47-1).

Pathophysiological Consequences of Deep Venous Thrombosis

As part of the normal coagulation process, local vasoconstriction along with thrombus development results in narrowing of the vascular lumen (Figure 47-3). This increases the resistance to blood flow, resulting in the recruitment of collateral vessels that are commonly demonstrated by angiograms, venography, and computed tomography (CT). Once hemostastasis has been achieved, the thrombus undergoes degradation by lysis, fragmentation, embolization, organization, or a combination of these. Thrombus that is not dissolved by the fibrinolytic process or has not embolized slowly contracts and becomes adherent to the endothelium. This process, which is referred to as organization, instigates a local inflammatory response in the vessel wall, promoting proliferation of granulation tissue and converting the clot into localized scar tissue. Fibrinolysis eventually restores lumen caliber and patency.

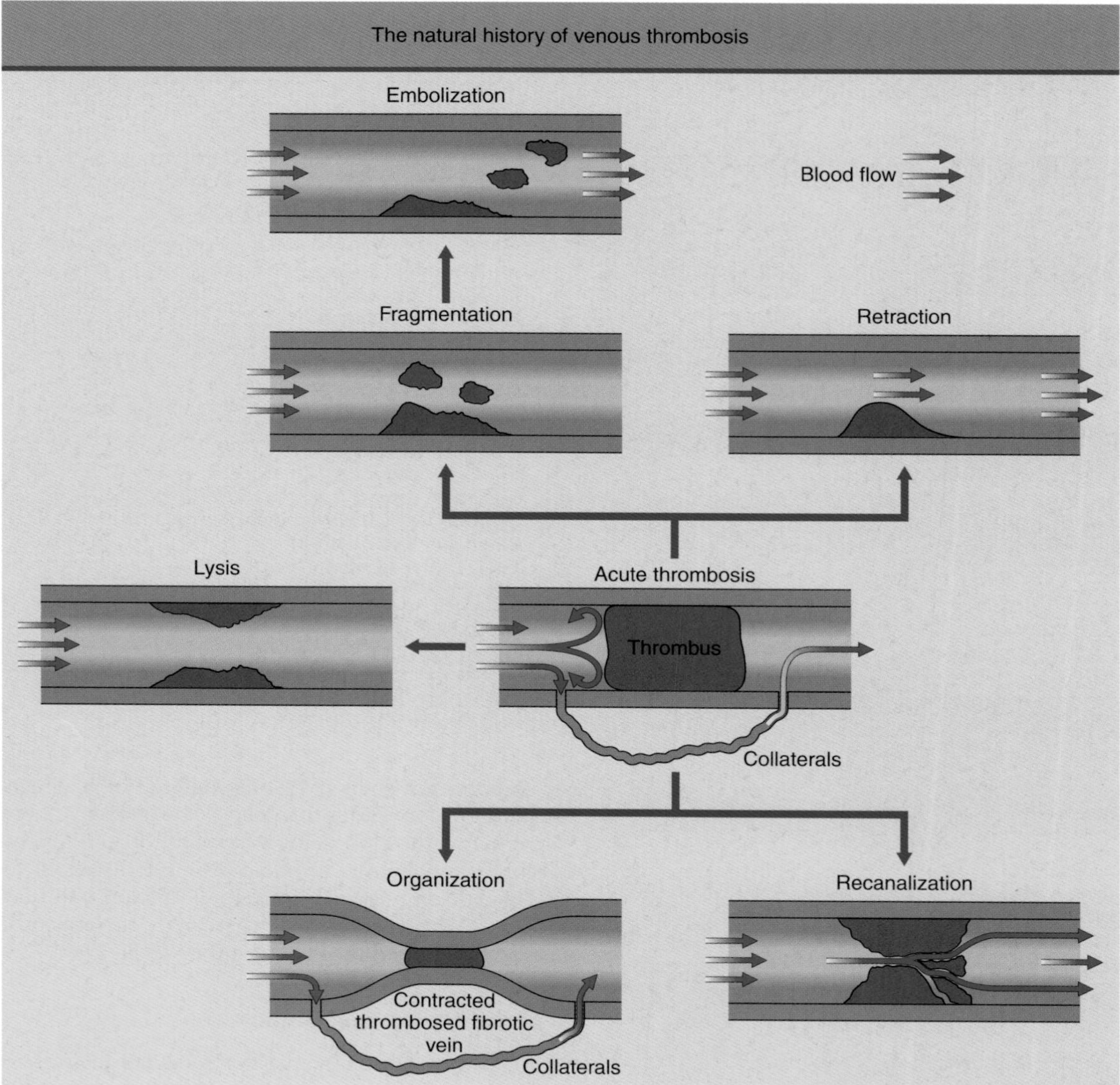

Figure 47-3. Natural history of venous thrombosis. The vein may remain occluded, with venous return restored through collateral veins. If the vein recanalizes, the valves are often destroyed, leaving venous incompetence.

Lysis failure can result in a permanently occluded venous segment. In addition, any thrombosis occurring adjacent to venous valves may elicit a localized inflammatory reaction, resulting in a postthrombotic syndrome that in turn results in venous obstruction, reflux, and stasis. This syndrome occurs in half to two thirds of patients with DVT.[21]

Pathophysiological Consequences of Pulmonary Embolism

The immediate effects due to clot embolization to the pulmonary arterial system are twofold:

- Obstruction of blood flow distal to the clot
- Rapid increase in pulmonary arterial and right heart pressures

The hemodynamic effects of PE depend on the size and number of emboli (thrombotic burden) and the cardiopulmonary reserve of the patient.

Pulmonary Consequences of Pulmonary Embolism

In most cases of acute PE, the blood supply to lung tissue distal to the clot is maintained through collateral flow from bronchial arteries. PE of sufficient size to completely occlude pulmonary blood flow can result in infarction of the pulmonary parenchyma, but this phenomenon is encountered in only 10% to 15% of cases.[2] Infarction is common when emboli occlude smaller peripheral branch vessels and in patients with coexisting malignancy or cardiopulmonary disease.[22]

Acute PE can also produce transient local bronchoconstriction, which can last 4 to 6 hours. Although this is rarely suspected clinically, it is commonly identified by physiological testing in most patients.[23] Serotonin and histamine release by platelets incorporated into the embolus are thought to be the chemical mediators responsible for this phenomenon.

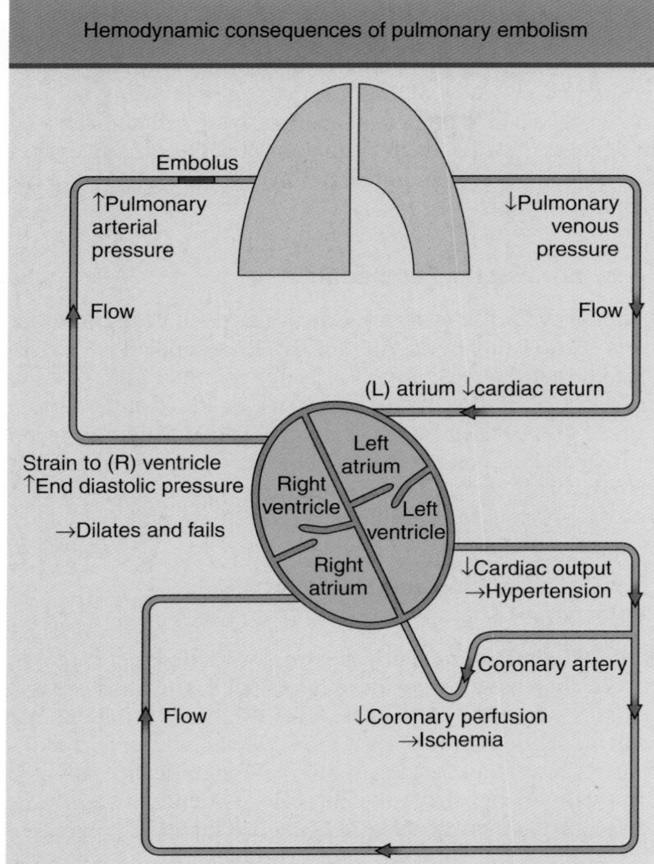

Figure 47-4. Hemodynamic consequences of pulmonary embolism. A large embolus increases pulmonary arterial pressure and therefore increases the work of the right (R) ventricle. However, the cardiac return to the left (L) atrium decreases, leading to poor cardiac output and decreased systemic and coronary perfusion, which in turn may lead to cardiac ischemia.

Atelectasis is also a common radiographic observation in regions of ischemic lung and likely secondary to a combination of decreased surfactant production and regional bronchoconstriction.[24,25] In patients with acute massive PE who also develop right heart failure and systemic hypotension, impaired gas exchange in the ischemic areas of lung can lead to hypercarbia. In such cases, compensatory hyperventilation in areas of normally perfused lung can paradoxically produce hypocapnia.[26]

Hemodynamic Consequences of Pulmonary Embolism

Several factors influence the hemodynamic consequences of acute PE (Figure 47-4). First, hemodynamic effects are related to the number and size of emboli. Second, the cardiopulmonary reserve of the patient has important implications on the consequences and clinical outcome of acute PE. Smaller emboli, which often do not produce any cardiovascular perturbations, may do so if the patient has comorbid conditions, such as pneumonia, structural lung disease, or impaired cardiac function. Larger emboli often cause cardiopulmonary effects (hypotension, tachycardia, and pulmonary hypertension) that are more often fatal. It has been estimated that a 50% occlusion of the pulmonary vascular bed would be required before pulmonary arterial pressure would increase in a healthy individual.[27] For example, cross-clamping of a main pulmonary artery is usually well tolerated, resulting in only a minimal increase in pulmonary arterial pressure. In contrast, a large PE obstructing a main pulmonary artery often has major hemodynamic consequences due to release of vasoactive substances from endothelium and platelets, such as serotonin, endothelin-1, and thromboxane A2. These mediators are thought to be responsible for the local vasoconstrictive effects of thromboemboli.

Vascular occlusion and vasoconstriction increases pulmonary wedge pressures with a concomitant increase in end-diastolic pressure in the right ventricle. With acute PE, ventricular afterload or impedance of the right ventricle increases along with pulmonary arterial pressure, thereby placing additional stress on the heart. According to the Frank-Starling law, the stroke volume or ventricular performance should increase normally as preload increases. This mechanism works by increasing the heart rate and myocardial contractility, primarily through sympathetic stimulation. Right ventricular myocardial mass is relatively small and responds poorly to a sudden obstruction to flow. If right ventricular contractility cannot increase, the end diastolic right ventricular pressure rises and the ventricle dilates. A corresponding fall in cardiac output can lead to hypotension, risking impaired cerebral and coronary perfusion. In patients with large clot burdens and underlying cardiac insufficiency, this phenomenon can be accelerated leading to cardiac ischemia and death.[28] In patients with chronic thromboembolic disease, pulmonary arterial pressures can become substantially increased, resulting eventually in pulmonary hypertension with right ventricular hypertrophy.

Risk Factors for Venous Thromboembolic Disease

Old Age

Age is a major risk factor of VTE. The prevalence of VTE increases steadily with age, after adjusting for other risk factors.[6,9] Furthermore, the case-fatality index of PE is far higher in the elderly. In addition, a strong association occurs between likelihood of postoperative DVT and advancing patient age.

Prior Venous Thromboembolism

Although a previous history of VTE is an independent risk factor in the development of future VTE, most patients who have recurrent DVT or PE have other identifiable risk factors, such as thrombophilia or carcinoma. A previous thromboembolic episode also places patients at a particularly high risk for recurrence should they undergo surgery or become pregnant or immobilized.[29] Therefore, it is crucial that this group of patients have appropriate thromboprophylaxis to minimize the risk of recurrence.

Immobilization

Immobilization is significant risk factor for the development of DVT and subsequent PE. Warlow et al., using radiolabeled fibrinogen, demonstrated this in a study group of patients with unilateral lower extremity paralysis.[30] They found that DVT

Table 47-2
Incidence of Venous Thromboembolism in Patients Following Surgery or Trauma*

	Calf DVT	Proximal DVT	Fatal PE
High risk	40-80%	10-30%	>1%
• Surgical patients with history of venous thromboembolism			
• Major pelvic or abdominal surgery for malignancy			
• Major trauma			
• Major lower limb orthopedic surgery			
Moderate risk	10-40%	1-10%	0.1-1%
• General surgery in patients >40 years			
• Patients on oral contraception			
• Neurosurgical patients			
Low risk	<10%	<1%	<0.1%
• Uncomplicated surgery in patients <40 years without any other risk factors			
• Minor surgery in patients >40 years without any other risk factors			

*DVT, deep vein thrombosis; PE, pulmonary embolism.

developed in 60% of the paralyzed limb compared with only 7% of the contralateral normal leg, which was used as a control. Prolonged immobilization during air travel has also been established as risk factor for DVT. Scurr et al. demonstrated a strong relationship between DVT and prolonged air travel in a randomized controlled trial.[31] None of the study participants who wore below-knee elastic compression stockings developed DVT, compared to the 10% (12 of 116) of those who flew without. In the LONFLIT3 (venous thromboembolism in air travel) study, DVT was identified in 4.8% of the control group, 3.6% of subjects taking aspirin, and no members of the group who received one dose of enoxaparin.[32]

Hospitalization and Surgery

Patients hospitalized with severe trauma or major surgery are at higher risk for VTE.[33-35] The incidence of VTE (Table 47-2) depends on numerous factors, including age, prior VTE, obesity, malignancy, and type of surgery. Without thromboprophylaxis, major orthopedic and abdominal or pelvic surgery is associated with a 40% to 80% risk of calf DVT, with most DVT in the first 5 days following surgery. Following major trauma, more than 50% of patients develop DVT, with 20% localized to the iliofemoral venous system.[35] In this patient population, The incidence of fatal PE is 1%.[33,34] The published incidence of VTE in hospitalized nonsurgical patients without thromboembolic prophylaxis ranges from 9% to 30%.[36] Patients with cardiac failure, myocardial infarction, and neurological diseases are at highest risk of developing VTE, with reported incidences of up to 70%, 30%, and 50%, respectively.[37] Hence, if no contraindication is found, it is essential for these patients to receive thromboprophylaxis on admission.

Malignancy

Malignancies are a known risk factor for the development of VTE, probably resulting from activation of the coagulation cascade producing a procoagulant state.[38] Furthermore, the risk in these patients increases twofold if they have coexisting risk factors such as recent surgery, immobilization, or cytotoxic chemotherapy.[39] Patients presenting with idiopathic spontaneous DVT or venous thromboembolic events, with no known risk factors, often have an underlying and undiagnosed malignancy.[40] A thorough evaluation of common cancer sites (breast, colon, lung, and prostate) may successfully reveal the primary tumor.

Pregnancy and the Puerperium

Although VTE is a leading cause of maternal death, it is still rare.[41] Two studies, in the United Kingdom and Sweden, showed that the risk for VTE remains minimal until close to delivery.[42,43] The relative risk of DVT or PE (compared to a control group) then increases dramatically during near term, with a fiftyfold greater risk at delivery. The most important maternal risk factors include multiparity, coexisting cardiac disease, previous VTE, and inherited thrombophilia.

Oral Contraception and Hormone Replacement Therapy

Although oral contraceptives are associated with a three- to sixfold increased risk of developing VTE, the absolute risk remains minimal.[44] Aggregate risk is highest during the first year of administration but ceases when therapy is discontinued. Lower-dose estrogen pills have significantly affected further lowering of the overall VTE. Patients on hormone replacement therapy have a two- to threefold increased risk of VTE, but like oral contraceptives, the absolute risk remains minimal and is confined to the first year of treatment.[45] When considering hormone replacement therapy, it is important to elicit a history of prior VTE, as the risk increases tenfold for recurrent disease once therapy is initiated.[46]

Superficial Thrombophlebitis

Superficial thrombophlebitis is an independent risk factor for the development of DVT. Approximately 1 in 20 patients with untreated thrombophlebitis develop DVT.[47]

Antiphospholipid Antibody Syndrome

Antiphospholipid antibodies such as anticardiolipin and lupus anticoagulant antibodies are a heterogeneous group of immunoglobulins directed against negatively charged phospholipids, protein–phospholipid complexes, and plasma proteins. Although these antibodies can be present in patients with systemic lupus erythematosus, they are also often found in other autoimmune disorders and in healthy people without any underlying disease.[48] The antiphospholipid antibody syndrome is an autoimmune disorder consisting of antiphospholipid antibodies and frequent venous and arterial clotting, along with miscarriages and thrombocytopenia.[49] Antiphospholipid antibody syndrome accounts for 15% to 20% of DVT in patients under 50 and is more common in women. Lower extremity DVT is the most common presentation of antiphospholipid antibody syndrome, although thrombosis of unusual venous sites such as the dural sinuses may also occur.[50]

Antiphospholipid antibodies occur in approximately 2% of the population and in 30% to 50% of patients with systemic lupus erythematosus.[51-53] The frequency of VTE in patients with systemic lupus erythematosus and positive antiphospholipid antibodies is about 50%, with half of those patients also having PE.[53] In patients without systemic lupus erythematosus, the relationship between these antibodies and venous thrombosis is complex. A strong association occurs between lupus anticoagulant antibody and venous thrombosis, but in contrast, the association of anticardiolipin antibody and thrombosis is less certain.

The risk of recurrent DVT in patients with positive antiphospholipid antibodies following discontinuation of anticoagulation therapy is three times higher than normal. Furthermore, patients with antiphospholipid antibody syndrome may have resistance to standard anticoagulant therapy, which requires higher doses to achieve adequate prophylaxis against DVT.[54]

Inherited Thrombophilia

The thrombophilic syndromes include antithrombin deficiency, protein C deficiency, protein S deficiency, and resistance to activated protein C. The true prevalence of inherited thrombophilia is currently unknown. Inherited thrombophilia should be suspected in any patient with recurrent VTE, a positive family history of venous thrombotic disease, a first event when under 45 years of age, or no obvious risk factors. The most common inherited thrombophilia is due to substitution of adenine for guanine at nucleotide 1691 of factor V gene, resulting in resistance to activated protein C. The resulting protein is known as factor V Leiden.[55] Mutation of prothrombin gene (G20210A) was recently discovered to be a common form of inherited thrombophilia and is due to a substitution of adenine for guanine at nucleotide 20210, leading to an elevated prothrombin time.[56] Hyperhomocysteinemia causes a unique form of thrombophilia that predisposes to both arterial and venous thrombosis.[57] The C677T mutation in the methylene tetrahydrofolate reductase gene, leading to hyperhomocysteinemia, is relatively common, but its role in venous thrombosis is uncertain.[58] Homozygous homocystinuria is a rare form of hyperhomocysteinemia, with clinical features of severe arterial and venous thrombosis presenting at a young age.

High levels of factor VIII, IX, and XI and fibrinogen are also associated with an increased risk of venous thrombosis, but the exact basis for the elevated levels is still unknown and is likely to be caused by a combination of both genetic and acquired disorders.

Epidemiology and Clinical Features of Inherited Thrombophilia

Factor V Leiden and G20210A mutation of prothrombin genes are common in Caucasians, with a prevalence of 5% and 3%, respectively. They are rare in the Asian and African populations.[59] Protein C, protein S, and antithrombin deficiency are relatively rare autosomal dominant transmitted disorders. The diagnosis of inherited thrombophilia should be considered in any patient with VTE, especially since the incidence for thrombophilia is higher than in the normal population (Table 47-3). Of patients with VTE, 20% have factor V Leiden and 7% have the G20210A prothrombin mutation.[60] In most patients, the thromboembolic event is precipitated by surgery or immobilization or occurs during pregnancy.

Table 47-3
Incidence of Inherited Thrombophilia in Normal Subjects and Patients Who Have Venous Thromboembolic Disease (VTE)

Thrombophilia	General Population (%)	Patients with VTE (%)
Factor V Leiden	5	20
Prothrombin G20210A	3	7
Elevated factor VIII*	6-8	10-15
Protein C deficiency	0.2-0.5	3
Protein S deficiency	0.2-0.5	3
Antithrombin deficiency	0.02	1
Hyperhomocysteinemia*	5	10

*Likely to be multifactorial.

Patients with protein C, protein S, or antithrombin deficiencies have a greater than 50% risk for developing VTE in their lifetime. Although these disorders are generally inherited, they have also been observed in patients with liver disease, disseminated intravascular coagulopathy, or sepsis and those on coumadin therapy.

Patients who are homozygous for any inherited form of thrombophilia, or who have more than one type of inherited thrombophilia, are at far higher risk of developing VTE. In addition, the age of presentation is earlier and they have a higher recurrence rate for VTE, even despite adequate anticoagulant therapy.

Women with inherited thrombophilia are at high risk of developing VTE during pregnancy or the puerperium. Up to 60% of women with antithrombin deficiency and up to 20% with either protein C or protein S deficiency develop VTE during their pregnancy or in the postpartum period.[61]

The administration of oral contraception to women with inherited thrombophilia increases the risk of venous thrombosis by as much as tenfold.[62] Screening for inherited thrombophilia before initiating oral contraception, however, should be done in women with a history of VTE, remembering that 10% of white women carry the defective gene.[60] Screening should be limited to women with a personal or family history of VTE.

Mechanisms of Thrombosis in Inherited Thrombophilia

Regulation of thrombin activation and neutralization plays a central role in most inherited coagulopathies. In the normal coagulation cascade, prothrombin is converted to thrombin by factors Xa and Va. Thrombin hydrolyses the peptide bonds of fibrinogen, releasing fibrinopeptides A and B, which allow polymerization of fibrinogen molecules to form fibrin. The inhibitory mechanisms of coagulation are complex (Figure 47-5). Antithrombin is the most potent inhibitor of coagulation. It inactivates serine proteases (thrombin, factor XIa, factor IXa, and factor Xa) by forming a stable complex with them, which is greatly potentiated by heparin. Activated protein C is generated from its vitamin K–dependent precursor by the action of thrombin. Thrombin binds to thrombomodulin, which is an endothelium receptor, and

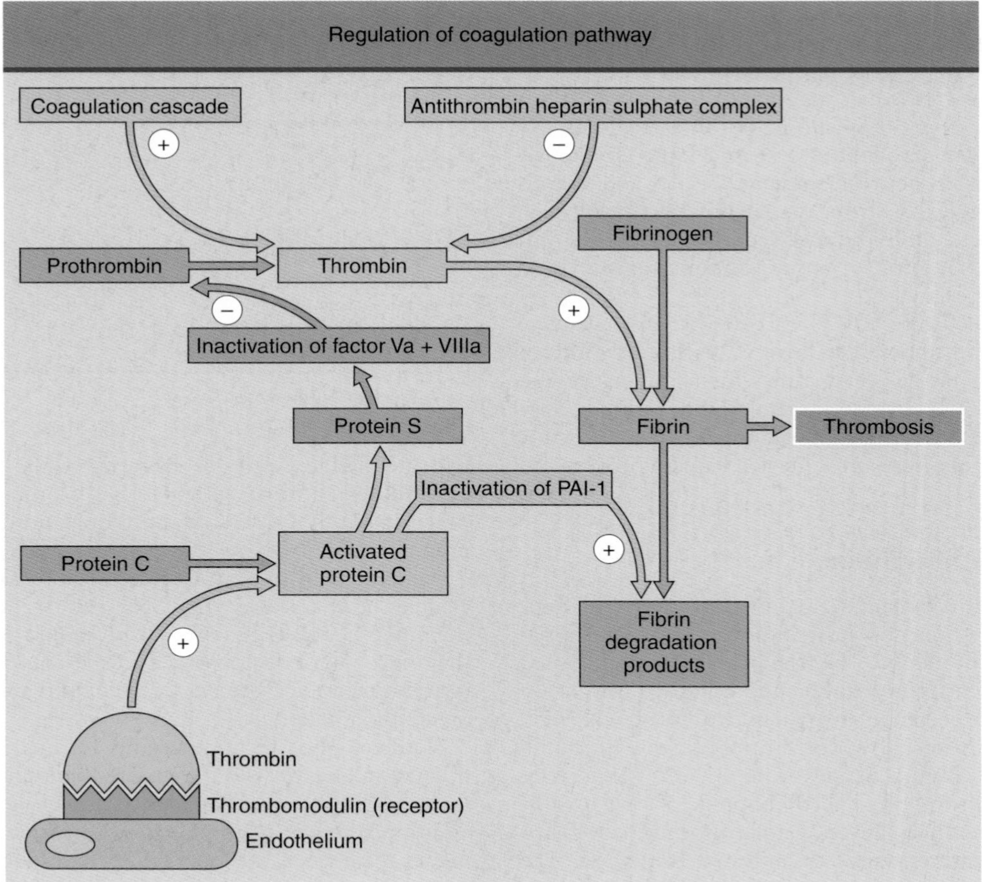

Figure 47-5. Regulation of coagulation pathway. PAI-1, plasminogen activator inhibitor-1.

activates protein C. Activated protein C inhibits factors Va and VIIIa in the presence of free protein S, thereby preventing the formation of thrombin. Protein C also causes inactivation of plasminogen activator inhibitor-1 (which inactivates tissue plasminogen activator), thereby promoting fibrinolysis. Furthermore, free protein S itself has an anticoagulant property. Any reduction in the activity of antithrombin, protein C, or protein S therefore increases the risk of VTE (Figure 47-6).

Resistance to activated protein C, caused by mutation of factor V, is the most common inherited thrombophilia. Factor Va converts prothrombin to thrombin. The mutant factor Va is resistant to the proteolytic activity of activated protein C, thus leading to uninhibited production of thrombin from prothrombin.

Investigation for Suspected Inherited Thrombophilia

Inherited thrombophilia should be suspected in patients with spontaneous venous or arterial thrombosis or those who have met one of the following criteria:

- Age less than 45 years
- Recurrent episodes of VTE
- Family history of VTE
- Thrombosis at unusual venous sites such as dural sinuses
- Recurrent miscarriages[60]

Any individual meeting these criteria should be tested for the common inherited thrombophilias, namely, G20210A prothrombin gene mutation, factor V Leiden, homocysteinemia, elevated factor VIII, and antiphospholipid antibody syndrome. Additional testing may be required to identify the less common protein C, protein S, and antithrombin deficiencies.

Clinical Features of Venous Thromboembolic Disease

Lower Extremity Deep Venous Thrombosis

Depending on location, the clinical manifestations of DVT can be local, distant, or systemic. The local symptoms of DVT are as follows:

- Swelling
- Pain, especially with Homan's maneuver
- Red–blue skin discoloration
- Localized erythema

The magnitude of these clinical features obviously depends on clot size and location. Leg pain experienced during dorsiflexion of the foot (Homan's sign) suggests the diagnosis of DVT in or below the popliteal vein. Unexplained pyrexia, especially in immobile or postoperative patients, is commonly present in cases of acute DVT. Unfortunately, clinical signs and symptoms alone are not reliable markers for DVT. Confirmatory testing is generally required to confirm clot

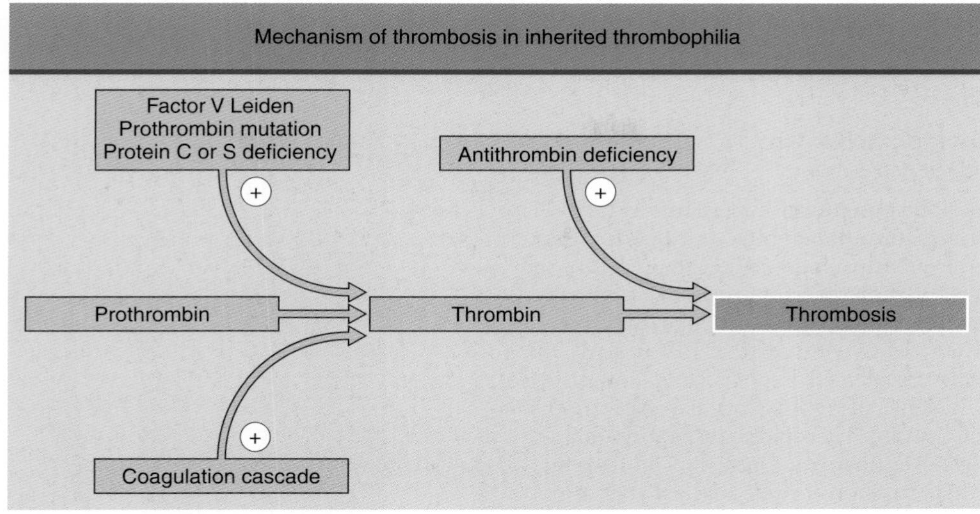

Figure 47-6. Mechanism of thrombosis in inherited thrombophilia. (From Seligsohn U, Lubetsky A. *N Engl J Med* 2001;344:1222-1231.)

in any patient presenting with clinical findings that suggest acute DVT.

Upper Extremity Deep Venous Thrombosis

Upper extremity DVT is less common that lower extremity DVT, occurring in 2% to 5% of the population. Arm DVT is most commonly encountered in association with indwelling mechanical devices such as pacer leads or central venous catheters (30% to 40% of cases). Venous thrombosis may also occur in conditions of venous compression or obstruction due to lymphadenopathy or tumors of the arm or lung (Pancoast).[15] Upper extremity DVT is also associated with repetitive arm movement or prolonged abduction (Paget-Schroetter syndrome, or effort syndrome). Inherited thrombophilia or malignancy should also be considered in any patient with arm thrombosis yet without other identifiable risk factors.[63] Recent studies have shown that acute upper extremity DVT is associated with a 10% to 30% risk for PE (similar to leg DVT), and a 10% to 15% recurrence once anticoagulation therapy is terminated.[64] Up to 50% of patients continue to have symptoms due to venous obstruction.[63-65]

Table 47-4
Classification of Pulmonary Embolism*

Pulmonary Embolism	History	Pathophysiology	Therapy
Acute massive	Acute	Circulatory collapse	Thrombolysis, thrombectomy
Acute submassive	Acute	Stable, echocardiographic signs of RV overload	Thrombolysis?, heparin
Acute nonmassive	Acute	Stable	Heparin
CTEPH	Chronic	RV overload	Medical or elective thromboendarterectomy

*CTEPH, chronic thromboembolic pulmonary hypertension; RV, right ventricle.

Pulmonary Embolization

A qualitative classification scheme for PE can be created based on the quantity of embolized clot and its incipient hemodynamic effects. (Table 47-4).

Acute Massive Pulmonary Embolism

Extensive pulmonary embolic disease resulting in 50% or more occlusion of the pulmonary arterial circulation often has severe cardiopulmonary and hemodynamic effects. In patients with large embolic clot burdens, severe acute dyspnea (70%), syncope, and cardiopulmonary collapse are common presenting symptoms. Patients may present with angina, reflecting a sudden drop in myocardial perfusion that results from acute cardiac dysfunction (see the Pathophysiology section).[27,28] Sudden death occurs in 10% of patients with massive PE, often within the first hour. Patients who survive may require rapid intervention with thrombectomy or thrombolysis.

Acute Submassive Pulmonary Embolism

Patients with submassive PE have stable hemodynamic parameters but show evidence of right ventricular strain relating to rapid increases in pulmonary arterial pressures. Echocardiography is preferred modality to detect right ventricular strain,[67,68] although right ventricular dilatation with bowing of the interventricular septum toward the left ventricle also suggests this diagnosis on CT. Treatment for PE with right ventricular strain requires anticoagulation, along with possible thrombolytic therapy depending on the hemodynamic indices.

Acute Nonmassive Pulmonary Embolism

Some patients with PE that obstructs less than 50% of the pulmonary circulation may be asymptomatic; others present with symptoms of tachypnea, hypocapnia, dyspnea, acute pleuritic chest pain, or a combination of these.[69] Hemoptysis may signal areas of lung ischemia, infarction, or both. Clinical examination is often unremarkable, but pleural rubs, pleural effusions, and atelectasis or consolidation suggest the diagnosis of acute PE, especially in the right clinical setting. Pyrexia is a common clinical observation that can occasionally lead to an erroneous diagnosis of pneumonia.

Chronic Thromboembolic Disease with Pulmonary Hypertension

Chronic thromboembolic pulmonary hypertension (CTEPH) is caused by either large thromboembolic burdens or recurrent PE. With long-term occlusion of greater than 50% of the pulmonary arterial circulation, pulmonary vascular pressures increase, leading eventually to right ventricular dysfunction or strain. Clinically, patients with chronic PE present with progressive dyspnea, unexplained hypoxia, and diminished exercise tolerance. Evidence of right ventricular hypertrophy, such as a parasternal heave or tricuspid regurgitation, may be identified on physical examination. Chest film findings suggesting pulmonary hypertension include marked central pulmonary arterial enlargement with vascular pruning. However, these radiographic findings are neither sensitive nor specific for chronic PE. Right ventricular hypertrophy and strain are best detected with electrocardiography or CT.

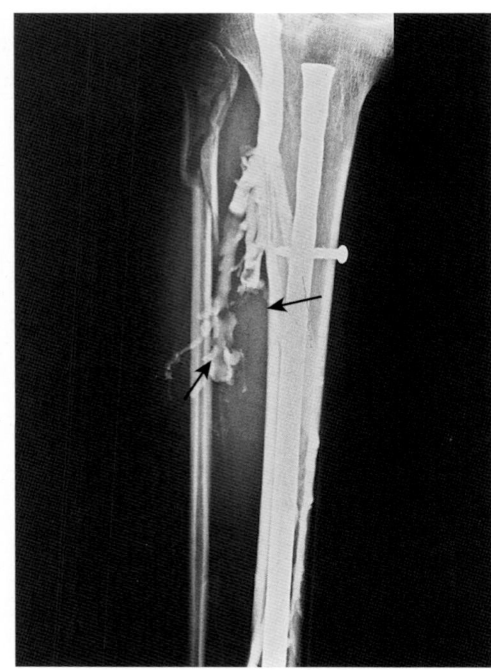

Figure 47-7. Venogram of a patient with intramedullary nail for fractured tibia, showing multiple filling defects in the calf veins consistent with deep venous thrombosis.

INVESTIGATIONS OF DEEP VENOUS THROMBOSIS

Many diagnostic tests have been used for the diagnosis of DVT, but only a few are currently in widespread use. Many of these modalities, namely, venography, ultrasound, CT, and magnetic resonance imaging (MRI) are all capable of demonstrating the thrombus. Plethysmography and Doppler ultrasonography can demonstrate venous flow obstruction resulting from DVT. Radiolabeled fibrinogen as a biomarker for thrombus has been investigated and used as a tool for identifying DVT but is no longer offered due to its poorer sensitivity and cost relative to Doppler ultrasound. D-dimer testing is a widely used assay that can be useful as a screening test in patients with suspected DVT, but it has low specificity for DVT because many other medical conditions may also produce elevated blood D-dimer levels.

D-Dimer Assay

D-dimer is a degradation product resulting from proteolysis by plasmin of cross-linked fibrin. Several commercial assays can be used to either qualitatively or quantitatively measure D-dimer levels in blood. Traditional enzyme-linked immunosorbent assay (ELISA) is time consuming to perform and as such not very useful from a point-of-care perspective. Whole-blood agglutination testing (SimpliRED) is quick and similar to automated systems using enzyme-linked fluorescent assays and latex-enhanced light scattering immunoassays, with testing completed within 15 to 30 minutes.[70,71] The ELISA assay is more accurate than latex agglutination, with a sensitivity of 98% (more than 500 μg/L).[71,72] A new rapid ELISA test, with similar accuracy to the classical ELISA test, has been developed.[73] While the latex agglutination test is quicker to perform, this test is not favored over ELISA due to lower accuracy.[72,74] One significant limitation of all available D-dimer tests is a lack of result normalization, along with varying specificities and sensitivities for both VTE and PE. In general, the sensitivities range from 44% to 72% for DVT and 44% to 70% for PE. While a negative D-dimer test has an excellent negative predictive value, a positive test is neither specific nor necessarily diagnostic for DVT, as numerous other medical conditions may also elevate D-dimer levels. Elevated levels of D-dimer are especially common in patients with myocardial ischemia, sepsis, and postoperative states without DVT. Accordingly, specificity decreases in older patients, those with known malignancies, and patients in the immediate peripartum period. Despite these limitations, D-dimer assays are routinely used as a first test on patients with suspected DVT. Negative D-dimer testing in patients with low or immediate probability for DVT generally obviates the need for additional testing.[75]

Venography

Venography involves opacification of the venous system of an affected limb by injecting iodinated contrast material, usually through a peripheral foot or hand vein. Clot is depicted as an intraluminal filling defect or defects (Figure 47-7). Additional venographic findings that may be observed include nonopacification of the deep veins and demonstration of abnormal venous collaterals. In experienced hands, the accuracy of venography is more than 90%.[76]

With a failure rate as high as 20%, disadvantages of venography include lack of suitable venous access for injection. The use of iodinated contrast is also not advised in patients with history of contrast allergy or in patients with impaired renal function. Venography is fraught with technical limitations, primarily due to suboptimal enhancement of the pelvic veins and deep venous system of the leg. Generally, progressive dilution of contrast material as it proceeds superiorly from point of injection often renders evaluation of the venous system of

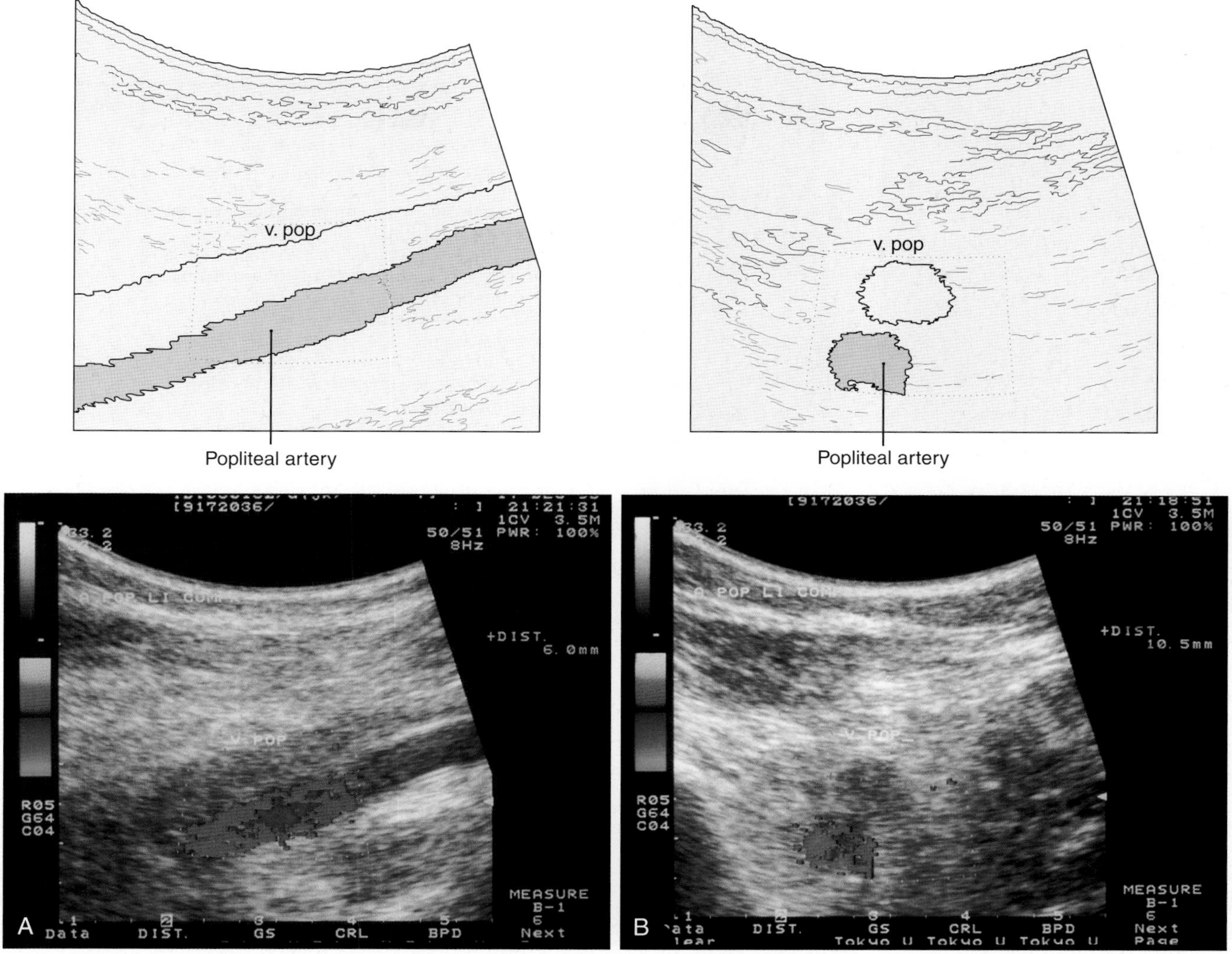

Figure 47-8. Venous thrombosis. **A,** Duplex examination of the popliteal fossa in longitudinal section, showing an echogenic popliteal vein with no demonstrable flow consistent with thrombosis. **B,** Transverse section of the popliteal fossa with compression, showing incompressible popliteal vein.

the upper leg and pelvis indeterminate. While venography may still be considered the gold standard for the diagnosis of DVT, it has largely fallen out of use, primarily in favor of the noninvasive Doppler ultrasound examination.

Ultrasonography

Sonography is now the primary modality for the evaluation of DVT, mainly due to its accuracy, portability, and lack of ionizing radiation.[77] Ultrasound permits direct visualization of the thrombus, as well as documentation of altered vascular hemodymamics by Doppler (Figure 47-8). Absence of blood flow, lack of venous phasic flow, and diminished response to Valsalva maneuvering or augmentation by calf compression are all associated Doppler findings characteristic of DVT. The accuracy of ultrasound exceeds 95% in many studies.[78,79]

Disadvantages of ultrasound include scan variability and quality depending on operator skill. Evaluation of larger patients may also impair image quality and sensitivity. Furthermore, the accuracy of detecting DVT in calf or pelvic veins is often quite limited with ultrasound; documentation of the superior extent of clot in the femoral or saphenous systems may be difficult with ultrasound due to limited acoustic windows in the deep pelvis.

Magnetic Resonance Imaging Venography

Direct visualization of thrombus with MRI venography provides another diagnostic option in patients with suspected DVT. Unlike traditional venography, MRI can rapidly produce multiplanar images and three-dimensional reconstructions of the entire venous system (Figure 47-9), and it can do so without ionizing radiation or contrast. Published studies have shown MRI to be reliable and accurate in the diagnosis of venous thrombosis, with sensitivities and specificities exceeding 90%.[80-82] In addition, MRI may be better suited than either ultrasound or conventional venography in demonstrating DVT in pelvic veins. Despite these advantages, MRI is not in wide use as a first-line imaging tool for DVT because of the ease, convenience, and lower cost of ultrasound. A relatively recent technique is capable of detection venous thrombosis

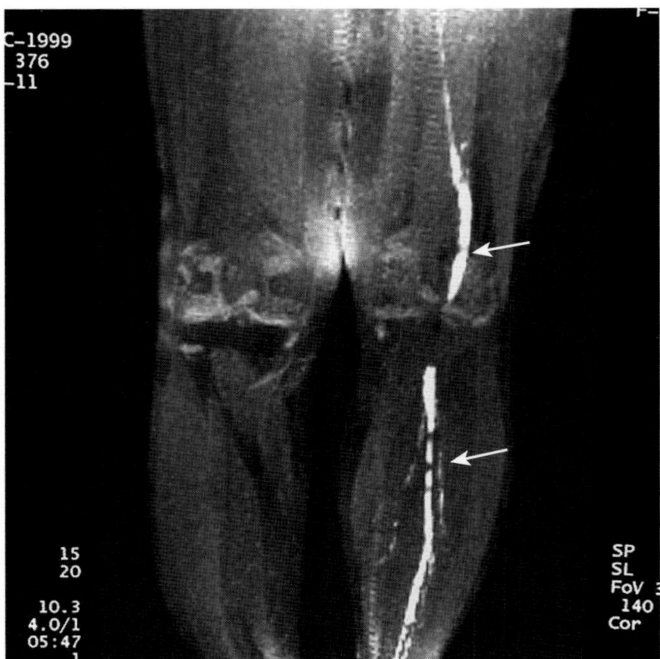

Figure 47-9. Magnetic resonance image of deep vein thrombosis.

Table 47-5
Modified Wells Criteria for Deep Vein Thrombosis (DVT)

Criteria	Score
Active cancer (receiving treatment within previous 6 months or receiving palliative treatment)	1
Paralysis, paresis, or recent immobilization of lower extremities	1
Recently bedridden for ≥3 days, or major surgery within 12 weeks requiring any type anesthesia	1
Localized tenderness along distribution of deep venous system	1
Entire leg swollen	1
Calf swelling ≥3 cm increased compared to asymptomatic leg (measured 10 cm below tibial tuberosity)	1
Pitting edema confined to symptomatic leg	1
Collateral superficial veins (nonvaricose)	1
Previously documented DVT	1
Alternative diagnosis at least as likely as DVT	−2
Intermediate risk	1-2
Low risk	≤0
Likely	≥2
Unlikely	<2

From Wells PH, Anderson DR, Rodger M. *N Engl J Med* 2003;349:1227-1235.

without the need for contrast injection, and this technology is likely to find its way into clinical practice due to its relative simplicity.[83]

Helical or Spiral Computed Tomography

Multidetector CT venography has been investigated as an alternative means of directly visualizing clot in the venous system of the leg, thigh, and pelvis. Using foot venapuncture and contrast injection to opacify the leg veins in a manner similar to conventional leg venography, helical CT can provide diagnostic images of the venous system.[84]

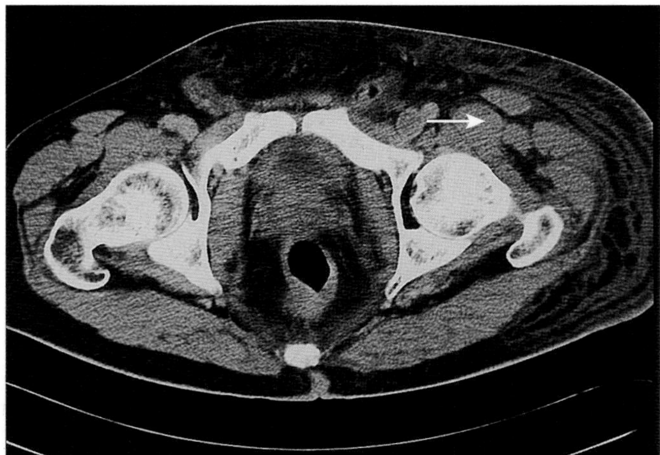

Figure 47-10. Computed tomography of a patient with deep vein thrombosis of the left femoral vein *(arrow)*. The vein is not opacified or distended in comparison to the right femoral vein. Extensive subcutaneous edema appears on the left.

Lower limb CT venography (Figure 47-10) has also been performed following CT pulmonary angiography in patients suspected of having VTE.[85] Disadvantages of CT are similar to those of venography, namely, radiation, cost, and risk of nondiagnostic examination, which is usually due to suboptimal contrast enhancement of the deep leg and pelvic veins. This shortcoming is most often encountered with upper extremity contrast injections when the examination is coupled with a CT pulmonary angiogram evaluation for PE.

Other Methods

Impedance plethysmography can indirectly identify DVT by documenting reduced venous blood. This modality has 90% accuracy in detecting proximal DVT, but the sensitivity rate drops to less than 60% for calf vein thrombosis. Although useful, this test has been largely replaced with Doppler ultrasonography, which is considered more accurate.[78] Other methods that have been used in the past, such as radioisotope-labeled fibrinogen, thermography, and light reflection rheography, are diagnostic tests no longer used in the workup of suspected DVT.

DIAGNOSTIC STRATEGIES FOR DEEP VENOUS THROMBOSIS

Clinically Suspected First Episode of Deep Vein Thrombosis

From a point-of-care perspective, the initial investigation into suspected DVT should depend on assessment of risk or likelihood of venous thrombosis using the (revised) Wells criteria (Table 47-5).[86-87] The negative predictive value of a low Wells score is 96%, and the negative likelihood ratio is 0.25.[88] Individual calculation of risk and likelihood can be accomplished using the Wells score plus D-dimer assay. A Wells score of less than 2 and a negative D-dimer effectively excludes DVT (recurrence rate 0.7%, confidence interval 0.3% to 1.3%).[89-90] With a Wells score more than 2, or if the D-dimer is elevated, additional testing is required. For most cases, this entails ultrasound, which has a sensitivity of 95% and a specificity of 96% for DVT.[91] Even in the presence of an abnormal D-dimer assay, the probability of DVT is less than 1% with a normal ultrasound examination. Repeat ultrasound is advised in cases when initial sonograms are negative despite a strong clinical suspicion for DVT or when the Wells score is more than 3.[92]

Diagnosis of Recurrent Deep Vein Thrombosis

After a documented DVT, the 5-year incidence of recurrent venous thromboembolic events is 25% and is 36% after a second DVT. The 5-year cumulative incidence of fatal PE is 2.6% after a first DVT.[93] Unfortunately, the diagnosis of recurrent DVT, especially in leg veins, is problematic primarily due to residual venous abnormalities that persist following the initial event. In 50% of patients, compression ultrasound remains abnormal 1 year after the first DVT.[94,95] Extension of thrombosis and an increase in the diameter of an incompressible segment of vein by more than 4 mm have been suggested as features of recurrent thrombosis. Hence, during serial ultrasound examinations, it is important that exact anatomical correlation is achieved in affected segments and that clot extent is carefully documented.[96]

TREATMENT OF DEEP VENOUS THROMBOSIS

Three main objectives are involved in the treatment of DVT, and the type of intervention depends on the clinical setting. The first goal is to prevent propagation or embolization of thrombus. In most patients, this can be accomplished with proper anticoagulative drug therapy. The primary action of anticoagulants, heparins, and oral vitamin K antagonists is to prevent the formation of new thrombus while the host fibrinolytic system eliminates the clot. The second goal is to reduce the risk of postthrombotic sequelae. Coumadin reduces the risk of recurrent thrombotic events while clot lysis and organization occurs. Finally, in patients who have DVT and PE, options such as caval filter placement, venous interruption, thrombectomy, and long-term anticoagulant therapy should be considered.

Valve damage within thrombosed venous segments commonly occurs following clot lysis and recanalization. The incidence of postthrombotic syndrome can be reduced with a more aggressive approach in the management of acute DVT by either thrombolysis or thrombectomy.

Thrombolysis

In acute DVT, considerable debate occurs about the indication for thrombolysis. Current research suggests that thrombolysis may benefit two groups of patients: those with venous gangrene at risk for limb loss and those with extensive iliofemoral clot who are at higher risk for postthrombotic syndrome.[97] Fibrinolytic therapy is effective primarily on thrombi less than 7 days old. Thrombolytics work less effectively as clots mature and undergo organization.[98] Thrombolysis of simple calf vein thrombosis generally is not indicated since this condition rarely results in postthrombotic syndrome.

Contraindications to Thrombolysis

Since the principal complication of thrombolysis is spontaneous hemorrhage, contraindications to its use include the following[99]:

- Recent surgery (a minimum of 7 days after surgery is recommended before initiation of thrombolysis)
- Bleeding diatheses
- Patients on coumadin (Patients may require vitamin K before thrombolysis)
- History of previous gastrointestinal bleeding, unless the cause of the bleeding has been treated
- Stroke within 2 months
- Pregnancy
- Severe hypertension

Intravenous Thrombolytic Regimens

The drug streptokinase acts by stimulating the conversion of plasminogen to plasmin. This agent, which is derived from β-hemolytic streptococci, is antigenic. Following administration, host antibodies may eventually neutralize its therapeutic action rendering especially to repeated administration. Streptokinase is given intravenously, starting with a loading dose of 250,000 units over 30 to 60 minutes to neutralize in situ antibodies.[100] This is followed by a maintenance dose of 100,000 units per hour for 24 to 48 hours, or longer depending on clinical findings and extent of disease.

Recombinant tissue plasminogen activator is produced by cultured eukaryotic cells and has structural and biochemical properties identical to those of native tissue plasminogen activator. Original protocols in use for acute myocardial infarction have proven as effective in the lysis of acute DVT. A 100-mg dose of recombinant tissue plasminogen activator given intravenously over 3 hours can be sufficient to provide rapid thrombolysis. Lower-dose infusion rates of between 1 and 5 mg/hour can be given intravenously for 24 to 48 hours. Thrombolytic agents provide superior clot lysis compared to conventional IV heparin therapy, with best responses occurring when the clot is nonocclusive.[101] A recent study showed that a higher dosage of thrombolytic agent could achieve better short- and long-term vein patency but at the cost of higher complication rates.[102]

Complications of Intravenous Thrombolysis

Before initiation of any thrombolytic therapy, a clotting profile should be ordered to identify any potential coagulopathies or bleeding diathesis. Despite such precautions, hemorrhagic complications from lytic therapy occur in up to 60% of patients, with serious hemorrhage occurring in approximately 10%. Intracranial hemorrhage is the most feared complication and occurs in up to 2% of patients.[103]

The major risk factors for intracranial hemorrhage from thrombolytic therapy are age, hypertension, and previous cerebrovascular disease.[104] The management of any major hemorrhagic events consists of discontinuing lytic therapy, rapid transfusion, replacement of coagulation factors (especially fibrinogen), and administration of antifibrinolytic agents such as tranexamic acid. An increased risk for PE has also been identified from thrombolytic treatment, likely related to clot fragmentation.[102]

Due to the disappointing benefit–risk ratio of thrombolytic therapy for isolated deep vein thrombosis, this therapy has been largely abandoned and replaced by catheter-directed methods to allow for direct clot infusion and clot lysis.

Catheter-Directed Thrombolysis

By directly catheterizing the affected vessel or vessels and infusing the thrombolytic drug directly into the clot, catheter-directed thrombolysis can be a more effective method to achieve thrombolysis.[105] Low-dose, large-volume thrombolytic agent is administered by continuous infusion or by the pulse-spray technique (0.5 to 1 mg of tissue plasminogen activator in 100 ml of 0.9% NaCl per hour). Periodic venography is performed every 12 hours to assess the progress of lysis. Once lysis is complete, this method also provides access when additional interventional therapy is warranted to treat the precipitating cause for DVT, such as vascular stenosis. Catheter-directed thrombolysis has a reported 1-year patency rate of 80% for iliac vein thrombosis and 50% for femoral vein thrombosis and is associated with a lower complication rate than that reported with systemically administered drug therapy.[106]

Although thrombolysis may result in higher radiologically proven vein patency rates in comparison to anticoagulation, the long-term result is uncertain. Given the inherent risk for serious complications associated with systemic thrombolysis, catheter-directed thrombolysis represents an attractive albeit more invasive alternative therapy.

Thrombectomy

Percutaneous Mechanical Thrombectomy

The indications for mechanical thrombectomy are identical to those for thrombolytic therapy.[107] Several percutaneous thrombectomy devices are available for clinical use. The principle mechanism of these devices is to macerate the clots by mechanical means. For example, high-frequency rotating wires or cages are used in the Arrow-Trerotola device (Arrow International), while Angiojet (Possis Medical) uses high-pressure water jets to disrupt the thrombus. Although these devices allow more rapid removal of clots and restoration of blood flow, catheter-directed thrombolysis is still often required to remove the thrombus, albeit for a shorter treatment duration. Clinical scenarios in which mechanical thrombectomy devices are most beneficial are in patients who developed iliofemoral DVT in the early postoperative period, where thrombolysis is contraindicated, and in patients with venous gangrene or superior vena cava syndrome, where rapid blood flow restoration is crucial. However, these devices are costly, can be difficult to use, and are not widely available except in large institutions.

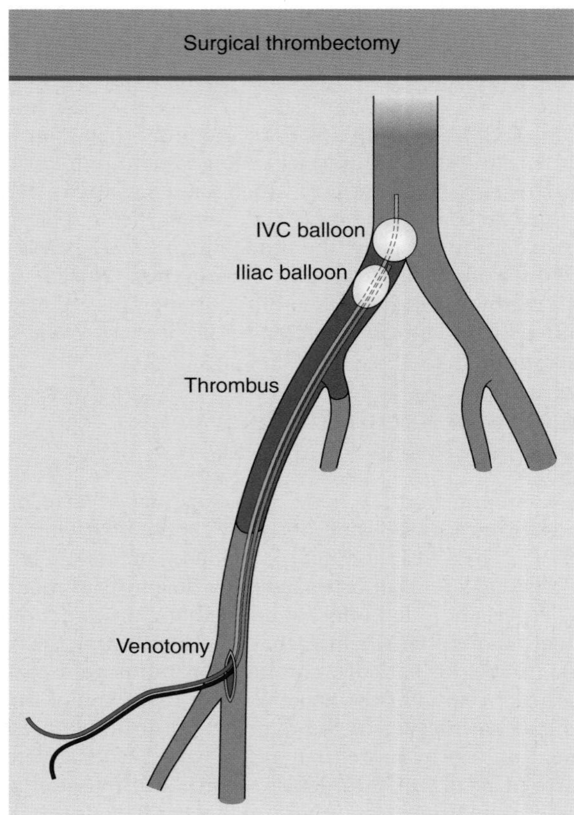

Figure 47-11. Surgical thrombectomy.

Surgical Thrombectomy

Although the surgical thrombectomy method remains a true surgical procedure, the appeal of this particular technique has increased with the introduction of catheter designs that have made thrombectomy easier and less invasive to perform. While both lytic therapy and thrombectomy offer superior results compared to traditional systemic anticoagulation, thrombolysis is generally preferred to the more invasive thrombectomy.[108,109] However, percutaneous thrombectomy may offer a distinct critical time advantage for limb salvage compared to lysis, especially when additional interventions such as angioplasty or stent placement are anticipated.

Technique of Surgical Thrombectomy–Iliac Vein

The surgical thrombectomy procedure, which is performed under general anesthesia, is divided into three components (Figure 47-11).[97]

EXPOSURE AND PREVENTION OF CLOT EMBOLIZATION

After a longitudinal incision is made from the inguinal ligament, the common femoral vein and its tributaries are dissected and exposed, with the surgeon being careful not to embolize thrombus proximally. A longitudinal incision is then made in the common femoral vein distal to the clot, with evacuation of any identifiable clot. Once the regional thrombus has been removed, a balloon catheter large enough to occlude the IVC is passed up into the IVC. With the balloon inflated, the catheter is pulled slowly downward until it lodges against the proximal end of the common iliac vein. This prevents clot embolization while trying to clear the iliac vein thrombus.

EVACUATION OF ILIAC VEIN THROMBUS

A second inflated balloon catheter that has been positioned next to the first balloon is pulled back to the venotomy site. This is repeated as necessary to evacuate all thrombus from the vessel. Intraoperative venography is then performed to evaluate for any residual clot. This procedure is needed to remove any residual thrombus.

CLEARANCE OF THROMBUS BELOW THE VENOTOMY SITE

Thrombus in the vein distal to the venotomy can be removed by applying compression along the leg from ankle, working along the vein in a cephalad direction and extruding any existing clot. A separate venotomy incision can be made in the popliteal vein, permitting evacuation of clot and again using the balloon catheter technique.

Anticoagulant Regimen for Acute Deep Vein Thrombosis

Anticoagulants can be divided into two types, depending on the method of administration: parenteral anticoagulants (heparin based) and oral anticoagulants. Acutely, the standard treatment for uncomplicated acute DVT is administration of IV heparin, thereby achieving immediate anticoagulation followed by maintenance oral anticoagulation with coumadin. Heparin therapy can then be discontinued once therapeutic levels of anticoagulation have been achieved, usually in 3 to 5 days.

Unfractionated Heparin

Heparin is produced endogenously, primarily by mast cells. Its main function is to inhibit the activity of thrombin. Unfractionated heparin (UFH) can be given either intravenously (bolus or continuous infusion) or subcutaneously. Continuous IV administration has a better pharmacokinetic profile than does the bolus technique because of a very short half-life (approximately 1 hour). Several studies have shown that continuous administration results in fewer complications relating to spontaneous bleeding.[110]

Dose

Effective dosing of heparin can be determined by serial measurements of the accelerated partial thromboplastin time (APTT). Therapeutic doses should elevate the APTT to twice the normal value. To best accomplish this goal, a loading dose of 5000 IU is given intravenously, followed by 20,000 to 40,000 IU every 24 hours. The APTT should be monitored twice daily during the initial days of therapy and once a day after an acceptable APTT has been achieved. A "weight-based" nomogram can be used to calculate the dose required to achieve satisfactory anticoagulation.[111]

Complications

BLEEDING

Bleeding is the most serious complication of heparin therapy and occurs in approximately 3% to 4% of treated patients.[112] The risk for bleeding is dose related, with greatest risk in elderly patients. Spontaneous bleeding requires immediate cessation of heparin, and if needed the effects can be quickly reversed with administration of protamine sulfate.

HEPARIN-INDUCED THROMBOCYTOPENIA

Heparin-induced thrombocytopenia (HIT) occurs in 2% of patients on UFH and is due to the production of antiplatelet antibodies to heparin.[113] HIT manifests after 3 to 5 days of treatment or earlier if patients have previous exposure to heparin. HIT usually causes serious bleeding but paradoxically may result in thromboembolic complications as a result of platelet aggregation. It is a serious condition, with a mortality rate of 10% to 30%. Patients on UFH for more than 3 days should have their platelet counts monitored daily, together with serial APTT testing. Increasing requirements for heparin (decreasing APTT) and a falling platelet level suggest HIT. If HIT occurs, heparin should be discontinued and replaced with another anticoagulant.[114] Low-molecular-weight heparins (LMWHs) should not be given to patients with known HIT, because they have a higher degree of in vitro cross-reactivity with the antibody. Treatment with Danaparoid sodium, which cross-reacts minimally with heparin antibodies in vitro, has been used successfully in this setting. Alternatively, direct thrombin inhibitors such as hirudin, bivalirudin, or argatroban can be used.[115] The use of heparin in patients with a history of HIT should be restricted to those with a compelling indication, such as cardiac or vascular surgery; it should be considered only if heparin-dependent antibodies cannot be detected by a sensitive assay.

OSTEOPOROSIS

Osteoporosis can occur in patients who have maintenance heparin treatment for 6 months or longer. The effect is dose related and rarely occurs when doses below 10,000 IU per day are used.

Low-Molecular-Weight Heparin

LMWHs are fragments of UFH produced by controlled enzymatic or chemical depolymerization composed of chains, with a mean molecular weight of about 5000 IU. Both UFH and LMWHs exert their anticoagulant activity by activating antithrombin. LMWHs have several pharmacological advantages over UFH, including increased bioavailability, substantially reduced protein binding, and a prolonged half-life, allowing for once-daily dosing.[116] These agents also have decreased interactions with platelets, which may reduce the risk of bleeding and HIT. Furthermore, outpatient treatment is safer and monitoring is generally not required. These agents are now the treatment of choice in many medical centers and are a cornerstone of ambulant management regimens for DVT.

Dose

LMWHs can be given by either subcutaneous or IV injections. Subcutaneous injection is more widely accepted because it has a better pharmacokinetic profile. The half-life of LMWHs is two to four times longer than that of UFH, ranging from 2 to 4 hours following IV injection and from 3 to 6 hours after subcutaneous injection. The dose depends on the type of LMWH used, the weight of the patient, and the indication for treatment. The dose of LMWH used for treating VTE is double

Table 47-6
Dose of Low-Molecular-Weight Heparins (LMWHs) for Venous Thromboembolism

LMWH	Prophylaxis	Treatment
Certoparin	3000 units daily	Unlicensed
Dalteparin	2500-5000 units daily	46-56 kg, 10,000 units daily 57-68 kg, 12,500 units daily 69-82 kg, 15,000 units daily >82 kg, 18,000 units daily
Enoxaparin	2000-4000 units daily	1.5 mg/kg once daily
Reviparin	1432 units daily	Unlicensed
Tinzaparin	3500-4500 units daily	175 units/kg daily

that used for DVT prophylaxis (Table 47-6). As with UFH, treatment is continued until adequate oral anticoagulation is achieved.

Complications

LMWHs have been shown in several trials to be at least as safe as UFH for the prevention and treatment of VTE. The incidences of thrombocytopenia and osteoporosis are significantly lower with LMWHs.[117,118] When need arises, it should be remembered that protamine sulfate only partially reverses the anticoagulant effects of LMWHs; if serious bleeding complications occur, treatment with fresh frozen plasma may be required.

Clinical Effectiveness

Several studies have suggested that LMWHs are more effective than IV UFH in preventing progression of VTE in patients with acute PE or DVT and do so with fewer complications. In addition, published data recently have shown that LMWHs are more effective in reducing thrombus size in comparison to UFH.[119] Cost-benefit analysis also favors LMWHs, with a potential 60% reduction in cost that can be realized through outpatient-based therapy.[120]

Oral Anticoagulants

The two types of oral anticoagulants are the coumarins (warfarin, dicoumarol, and nicoumalone) and the indanediones. The latter are rarely used due to their frequent side effects. These agents are well absorbed in the gastrointestinal tract and highly bound to plasma albumin. These drugs are metabolized by the liver and excreted in hydroxylated form by the kidney. The half-life of warfarin is as long as 42 hours, thus leading to a more stable anticoagulant effect. These drugs inhibit the actions of vitamin K in the synthesis of procoagulant factors (factors II, VII, IX, and X) and anticoagulant factors (proteins C and S). Prothrombin time effectively measures the efficacy of treatment and is expressed as the international normalized ratio (INR; ratio of the patient's prothrombin time to the laboratory control).

Dose

Once initial anticoagulation has been established with IV heparin, the standard protocol for oral anticoagulation is a loading dose, followed by a maintenance doses, titrated in concert with the INR. The INR should be measured twice a day, with doses adjusted accordingly to achieve a therapeutic level (INR between two and three times normal). Once a therapeutic INR value is achieved, usually after 4 to 5 days of treatment, parenteral doses of IV anticoagulation are used. INR monitoring should be performed two to three times weekly for the first 2 weeks and once weekly thereafter. For those on long-term treatment, once or twice monthly testing is adequate, depending on the stability of the patient's INR.

Complications

HEMORRHAGE

Hemorrhage is the primary complication of all oral anticoagulant therapy, with a mortality rate of approximately 1 per 100 treatment-years. Nonfatal bleeding occurs in 4 to 16 per 100 treatment-years.[121,122] Major risk factors for bleeding include age, especially in patients older than 80, and when the INR exceeds 2. Most cases of bleeding occurs in the first 3 months of therapy.[123,124] Treatment for bleeding includes cessation of drug therapy, volume replacement, and administration of vitamin K, which usually returns the prothrombin time to normal in 4 to 6 hours. In cases of severe bleeding, fresh frozen plasma replacement may be necessary.

DRUG INTERACTION

Oral anticoagulants interact with a range of drugs, affecting drug absorption rates, metabolism, and binding to albumin. These interactions may result in an increase or a decrease in the anticoagulant effect of oral therapies. The most common drug interactions are encountered in patients receiving antibiotics, steroids, and aspirin.

SKIN NECROSIS

Skin necrosis is a rare complication of coumadin therapy, with an incidence of 0.01% to 0.1%. This phenomenon is more common in women and those with inherited thrombophilias. It is important not to confuse this condition with venous gangrene, which can have a similar clinical presentation.[125]

Thrombin Inhibitors

Various direct thrombin inhibitors have been introduced over the last few years. Desirudin and lepirudin are recombinant derivatives of the leech enzyme hirudin, which is one of the most potent antithrombotic agents developed. These drugs are more effective than heparin in the management of acute coronary syndromes, but their role in the treatment of VTE is still unknown.[126] Fondaparinux and ximelagatran are as effective and safe as LMWHs in preventing venous thromboembolic events in surgical patients.[127,128] Furthermore, these agents can be useful in the management of patients with HIT.[115]

Duration of Oral Anticoagulation Therapy

The optimal duration of oral anticoagulation depends on the balance between the risk of recurrent thrombosis if anticoagulants are stopped and the risk of bleeding on treatment (Table 47-7). Trials comparing short- and long-term anticoagulant treatment have suggested that long-term anticoagulation significantly reduces the incidence of recurrence of

Table 47-7
Frequency of Signs on Chest Radiography in Patients with Pulmonary Embolism

Signs	Frequency (%)
Atelectasis or consolidation	70
Pleural effusion	50
Elevation of hemidiaphragm	20
Decreased pulmonary vasculature	20
Distension of proximal vessels	15

thromboembolic disease but at the cost of higher complication rates.[129,130] The risk of recurrence is lower if DVT was precipitated by a major reversible risk factor such as surgery. Patients with idiopathic DVT (no apparent risk factor) and those with persistent risk factors (i.e., malignancy or inherited thrombophilia) have a higher risk of recurrence. When the risk of recurrence risk is low, 3 months of anticoagulation is recommended. Longer periods of treatment are required (6 months or longer) when the risk is high, always balancing the risk of recurrence with the risk of hemorrhage individually for each patient.[131,132]

LMWH preparations, at doses intermediate to those used for the acute treatment of VTE, are an alternative to oral anticoagulation during the maintenance phase of treatment. Studies have shown that they are as effective as warfarin, with similar or fewer hemorrhagic complications.[133,134] UFH given subcutaneously at a dose of 5000 IU twice a day does not appear useful in preventing recurrent disease,[135] but is effective if given in adjusted doses (APTT twice normal).[136]

Finally, routine wearing of a below-knee graduated compression stocking for 2 years after an acute DVT has been shown to decrease the risk of postthrombotic syndrome by 50%, although it does not influence the rate of recurrent DVT.[137,138]

INVESTIGATION OF SUSPECTED PULMONARY EMBOLUS

While a diagnosis of PE is commonly considered in patients presenting with chest pain and shortness of breath, only 15% to 30% of suspected cases are proven to have the disease.[139] The primary clinical dilemma stems from myriad disorders with presentations that mimic the presentation of acute PE. The risks associated with anticoagulative therapy make it imperative that the diagnosis be accurately confirmed or excluded. Requiring a thorough and complete investigation, the workup of suspected PE should be logical and deliberate and should use a strategy that is both accurate and cost effective.[91,140] The primary goal rests with establishing with definitive proof that the disease is either present or finding an alternative disease that is responsible for the patient's symptomatology. Considering the inherent risks of anticoagulation, an erroneous diagnosis could be catastrophic. In the end, the diagnosis (or exclusion) of PE is only achieved successfully and efficiently using a strategy that requires a judicious use of both laboratory and diagnostic imaging, with choices largely predicated on the level of suspicion based on physical examination and clinical findings.

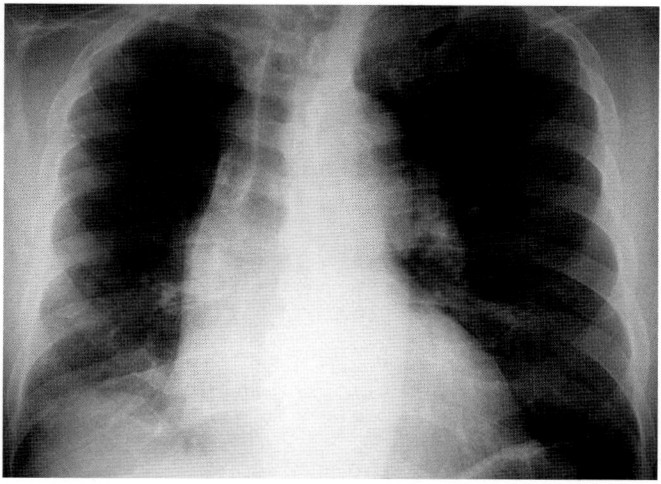

Figure 47-12. Chest x-ray: Westermark's sign. Distension of the pulmonary artery, decreased pulmonary vascularity.

Modalities Useful in the Diagnosis of Acute Pulmonary Embolism

Chest Radiography

While most patients with proven PE have abnormal chest radiographs, these abnormalities are not specific for the disease (Table 47-7). Furthermore, a normal chest film does not exclude the diagnosis, even in cases of massive PE. Specific radiographic evidence that suggests the diagnosis of PE includes diminished pulmonary vascularity (i.e., oligemia or Westermark's sign; Figure 47-12) or pulmonary infarction (Hampton's hump). Unfortunately, while these findings are valuable, they are rarely encountered.[141,142] In the clinical setting of possible acute PE, the primary value of chest radiography is to exclude cardiopulmonary conditions that may explain clinical finding, and it is warranted in every patient presenting with sudden dyspnea, chest pain, or both.

Electrocardiography

Generally, the electrocardiogram (EKG) is normal in acute PE (approximately 70%), and as with radiographs, a normal result cannot be used to exclude PE.[142] Sinus tachycardia is the most common EKG abnormality in acute PE; other tachyarrhythmias are less common. In massive PE, the EKG is often abnormal, with nonspecific ST wave changes. The classical EKG findings of $S_1Q_3T_3$ (Figure 47-13) and T wave inversion in the right ventricular leads, with right axis deviation, are occasionally seen in PE. In chronic thromboembolic disease, changes compatible with right ventricular hypertrophy may be evident. The main role of the EKG is to exclude other conditions associated with acute chest pain, such as myocardial infarction and pericarditis.

Blood Gas Analysis

While PE may be associated with hypoxemia, 25% of patients with proven PE have normal arterial oxygen saturation. Measuring the alveolar–arterial oxygen gradient may be more accurate than measuring the arterial oxygen pressure in the diagnosis of PE, but the results from clinical trials are disappointing.[143]

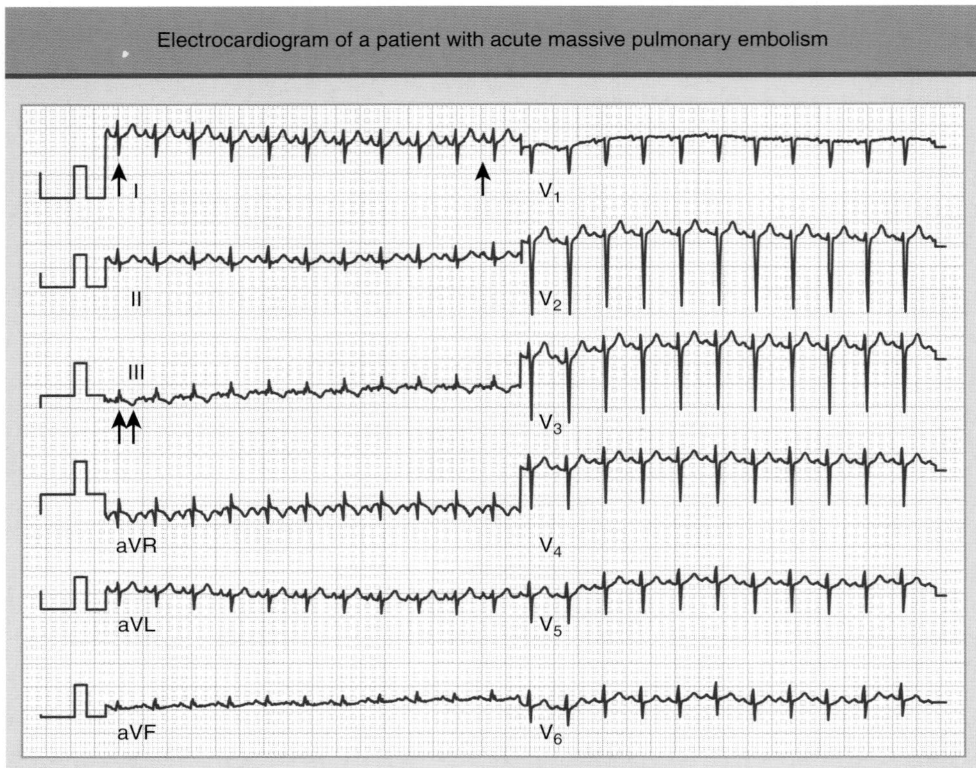

Figure 47-13. Electrocardiogram of a patient with acute massive pulmonary embolism showing the classical but rare $S_1Q_3T_3$ changes *(arrows)*.

D-Dimer

The clinical value of D-dimer assays in PE is similar to that of DVT. Lack of specificity and variation in standardization make positive assay results difficult to interpret. Furthermore, while the negative predictive value is valuable, a normal assay does not exclude subsegmental embolism.[144] Regardless, a negative D-dimer may appear to provide sufficient evidence to effectively exclude PE, thus obviating additional testing and anticoagulation therapy.[145-147]

Echocardiography

Echocardiography has utility in the assessment of patients with acute symptoms of unexplained chest pain and dyspnea. Echocardiography can provide a simultaneous assessment of the heart, pericardium, and proximal great vessels. Since the examination can be performed portably, echocardiograms are a valuable tool in the initial assessment of patients with sudden cardiovascular collapse, documenting disorders such as pericarditis, aortic dissection, and PE in the proximal pulmonary arterial circulation. In addition, echocardiography can provide information about cardiac function and morphology, which is difficult by traditional CT. With massive PE, echocardiography can provide better insight into right ventricular dynamics and pulmonary blood flow. Features on echocardiography characteristic of massive PE include right ventricular dilatation and dysfunction (Figure 47-14), pulmonary artery dilatation, tricuspid regurgitation, and blood flow perturbation in the right ventricle.[66]

Lung Scintigraphy (Ventilation and Perfusion Scan)

Consisting of two separate examinations, namely, perfusion and ventilation imaging, V/Q scans have been validated as a useful tool to confirm or exclude PE. Perfusion imaging is performed following IV injection of technetium-labeled macroaggregated albumin (Figure 47-15). Perfusion defects relating to occlusion of the pulmonary arteries by clot appear as photopenic regions. Ventilation imaging performed by inhalation of radiolabeled xenon gas evaluates for regional defects in lung aeration. A diagnosis of PE is suggested when areas of ventilation–perfusion mismatch are demonstrated (Figure 47-16). A final diagnosis of PE requires satisfaction of criteria set forth by the Prospective Investigation of Pulmonary Embolism Diagnosis study, using a classification scheme of normal, high probability, or nondiagnostic examinations.[148-150]

Lung scintigraphy can refute or confirm the diagnosis of PE with greater than 85% certainty in the high probability (25% of all cases) or low probability or normal groups (25% of all cases). The remaining 50% of patients who have inconclusive scintigraphic require further evaluation. Indeterminate examinations are unfortunately common, especially in patients with coexisting cardiopulmonary disease such as pneumonia or large pleural effusions. In this group, which historically encompasses 50% of all V/Q scans, additional testing is required to establish to confirm or exclude the diagnosis.

The advantages and disadvantages of lung scintigraphy are as follows:

Advantages

- Safe
- Noninvasive
- Commonly available examination in most hospitals

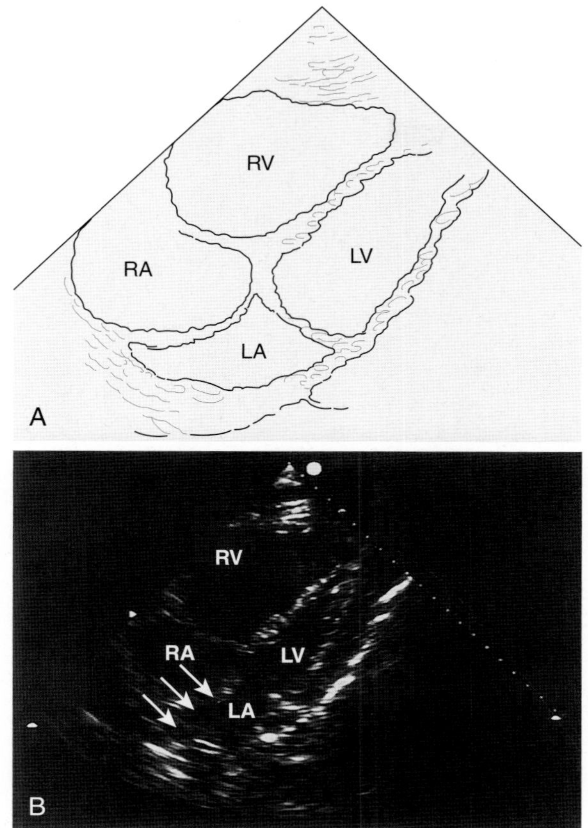

Figure 47-14. Four-chamber echocardiogram of a patient with acute massive pulmonary embolism. The interatrial septum bulges to the left *(arrows),* and the right ventricle is dilated in keeping with significant pulmonary outflow obstruction.

Disadvantages

- Complex diagnostic criteria and classification[148]
- High number of nondiagnostic results, especially in patients with preexisting respiratory disease (up to 50% of cases)
- 30% false-negative and 10% false-positive rate in low probability and high probability scans, respectively
- Image interpretation difficult due to poor image resolution
- Inferred diagnosis of PE; thrombus is not directly visualized as it is with CT or angiography
- Questionable utility in patients with significant coexisting pulmonary or pleural abnormalities on chest radiographs

A recent metaanalysis evaluated the diagnostic accuracy of lung scintigraphy.[151] The negative predictive value of V/Q scans is nearly 100%. Specifically, a normal perfusion study excludes the diagnosis of PE in nearly 100%. Conversely, a high-probability lung scan has sufficient specificity to warrant appropriate anticoagulation therapy. Definitive tests such as CT or angiography may be required in select cases where inherent bleeding risks from anticoagulation therapy exist, i.e., intracranial aneurysm or when anticoagulation therapy is deemed risky (gastrointestinal bleed).

Pulmonary Angiography

Through its ability to directly demonstrate arterial thrombus, pulmonary angiography has been traditionally considered the gold standard for PE. In practice, the invasiveness and radiation of angiography usually relegated this examination

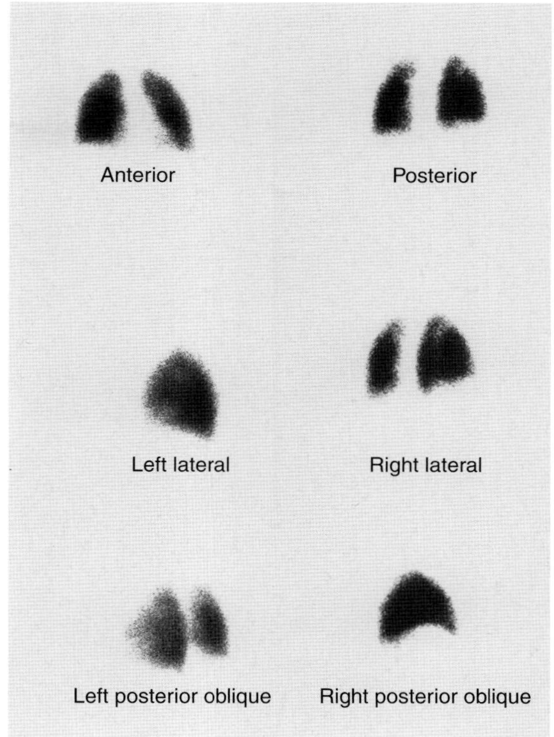

Figure 47-15. Normal-perfusion lung scintigraphy.

to patients with equivocal or indeterminate V/Q scans. The sensitivity of conventional pulmonary angiography remains highly dependent on the skill of the angiographer and diligence to completely interrogate the entire pulmonary vascular system.[152] To do so, pulmonary angiography requires multiple contrast injections in several projections, looking for the characteristic intraluminal filling defect (Figure 47-17). The disadvantages of pulmonary angiography relate to its invasive complexity, expense, and operator expertise. Furthermore, right heart catheterization may cause cardiac arrhythmias. With current estimates of mortality and morbidity at 0.03% and 0.47%, respectively, this examination has largely been usurped with helical CT, but it maintains some utility when arterial access is needed for therapeutic interventions such as embolectomy, thrombolysis, or vena cava filter placement.

Helical Computed Tomography

With the technological advantages afforded by helical CT, the popularity of pulmonary angiography has declined and is primarily reserved in cases with a high suspicion of PE despite a negative or inconclusive CT or in patients with a bona fide contraindication for long-term anticoagulation. Helical or multidetector CT has also replaced lung scintigraphy as an initial test for PE at most medical centers. Advances and refinement of scanner technology now provide accurate documentation of thrombus to the subsegmental arterial level (Figure 47-18). Helical CT not only is capable of visualizing the clot directly (Figure 47-18) but also can provide alternative diagnoses that may explain the patient's clinical presentation.

The imaging protocol varies according to the CT system used. A 130- to 150-ml contrast bolus is infused, with scanning beginning during peak pulmonary arterial enhancement.

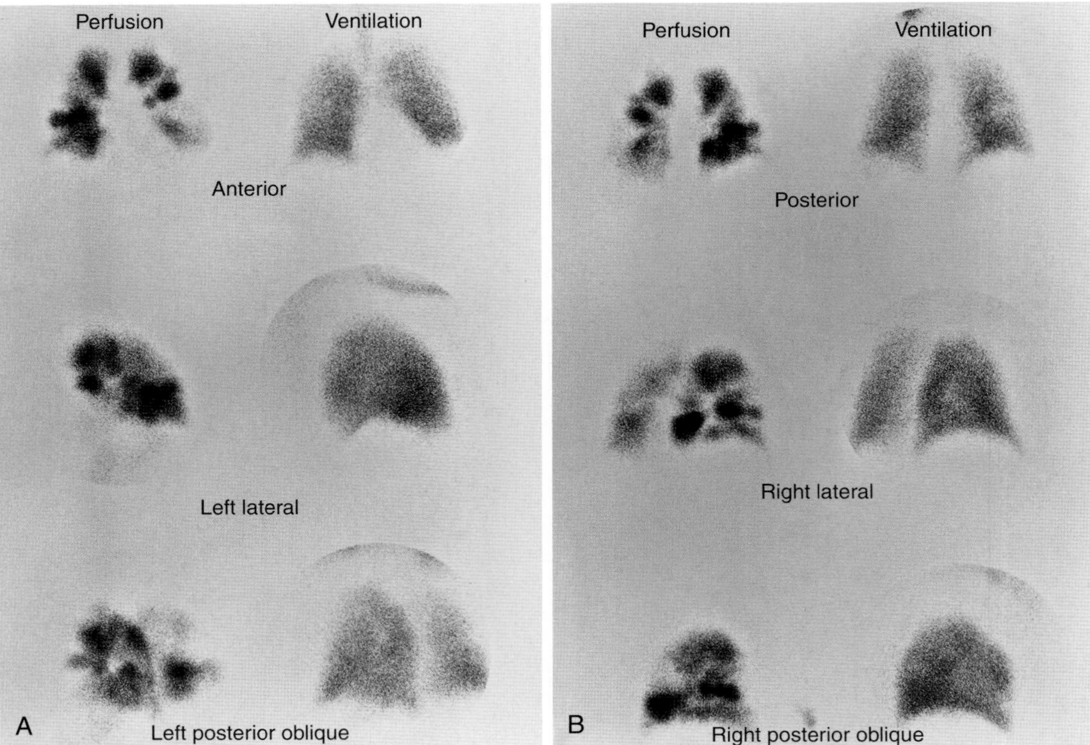

Figure 47-16. Ventilation perfusion scintigraphy showing multiple large, unmatched defects between ventilation and perfusion secondary to multiple pulmonary embolism.

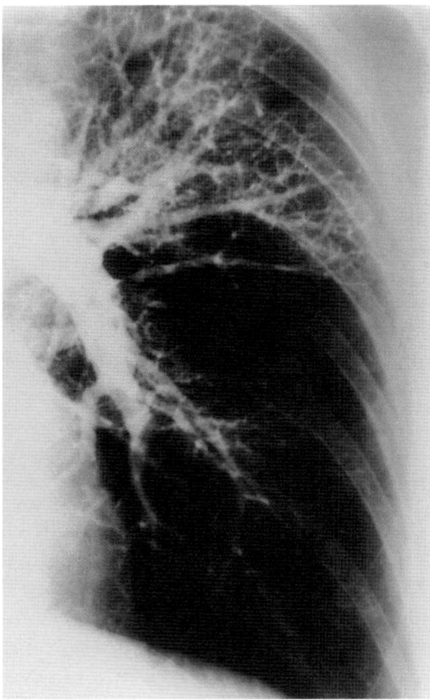

Figure 47-17. Selective left pulmonary angiogram showing marked hypoperfusion of the lower lobe secondary to multiple embolism.

Peak arterial enhancement and initiation of scanning is accomplished using bolus tracking software, which triggers imaging at a predetermined Hounsfield measurement. Using slice thicknesses of 1.5 to 2 mm, the entire chest from thoracic inlet to upper abdomen can be accomplished during one breath-hold. Newer 64-plus slice scanners can provide isotropic resolutions of 0.5 mm^3. Given the attributes of scan reproducibility, relative ease, and speed of acquisition, helical CT is the examination of choice for the investigation of PE, with reported sensitivity and specificity greater than 90%.[146,149,151,153]

Magnetic Resonance Imaging

MRI (Figure 47-19) has great potential for noninvasive imaging for PE. It is sensitive in demonstrating pulmonary arterial thrombi down to the segmental arterial level.[154,155] The largest study to date evaluated 141 patients with abnormal perfusion lung scans and reported that magnetic resonance angiography had similar accuracies to single-slice helical CT.[155] The role of MRI is still limited to trial patients, but rapid advancements in technology (shorter acquisition time and better image quality) may augment its utility. An example is the development of techniques for assessment of pulmonary vasculature, including magnetic resonance perfusion imaging, which has potential for more detailed evaluation of clot obstruction and the clinical implications this may have on physiological parameters.[156]

DIAGNOSTIC STRATEGIES FOR PULMONARY EMBOLISM

The clinical signs and symptoms of pulmonary embolus are generally too nonspecific to be relied on solely to render a diagnosis. Symptoms of chest pain, cough, and hemoptysis are often encountered in conditions such as pneumonia,

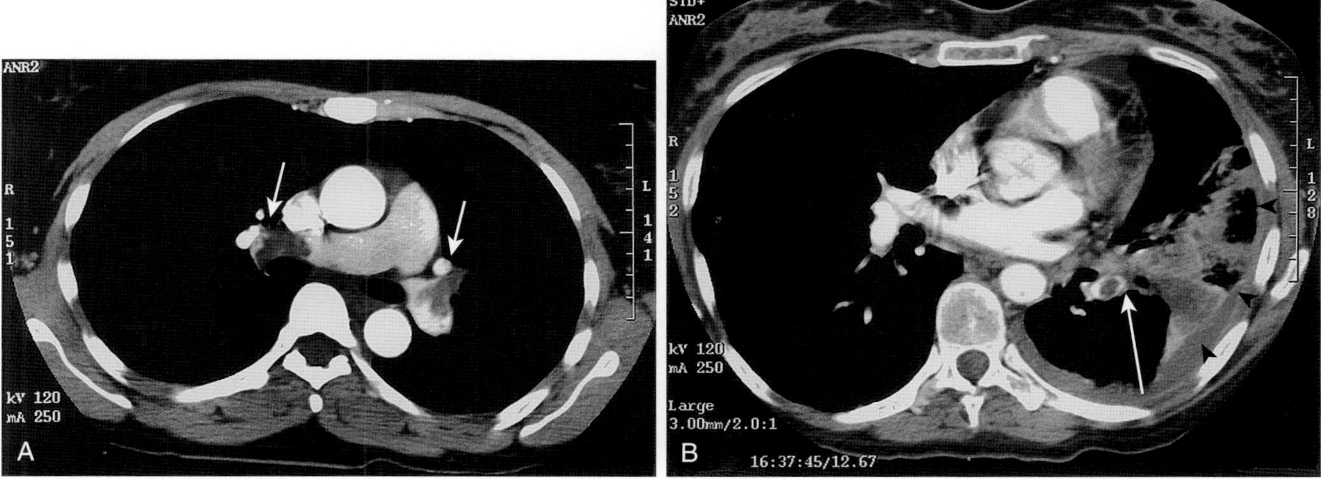

Figure 47-18. Computed tomography. **A,** Large central pulmonary emboli *(arrows)*. **B,** Peripheral embolism *(arrow)* with secondary consolidation or infarction of the lung *(arrow head)*.

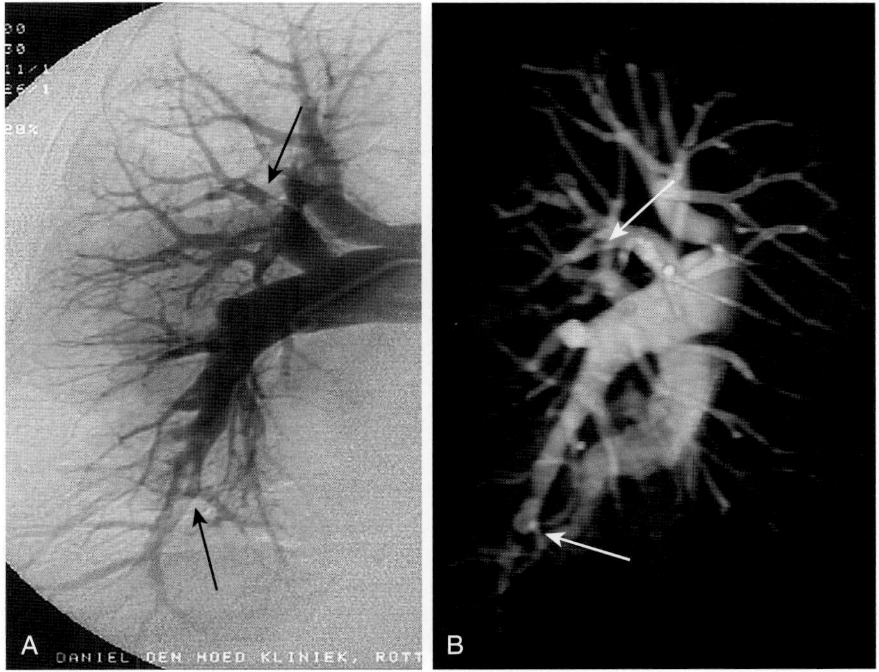

Figure 47-19. Magnetic resonance imaging of pulmonary embolism. **A,** Pulmonary angiogram. **B,** Magnetic resonance pulmonary angiogram in same patient.

cancer, and congestive heart failure. After initial plain films are used to exclude obvious cardiopulmonary disorders, use of either the simplified Wells criteria[157,158] or the revised Geneva score[159,160] (Table 47-8) to establish relative likelihood of PE should be initiated in all cases of suspected PE, thereby assisting with stratification of patients into low-, intermediate-, and high-risk categories. Using the Wells criteria, the negative predictive value of a low probability score is 97%.[161] Although scores of more than 2 have insufficient specificity to be solely relied on for a definitive diagnosis, the criteria's primary value is to identify cases for which additional testing is required, namely, D-dimer assay, measurement of arterial oxygen saturation, EKG, and with sufficient suspicion, confirmatory imaging.

Once a likelihood assessment for PE has been established, subsequent D-dimer assay is a logical next test for those at intermediate or high risk (Figure 47-20). From a point-of-care perspective, as an initial test, D-dimer excludes the diagnosis of PE in approximately 30% to 40% of patients (D-dimer of less than 500 mg/L) and is useful in the outpatient setting. In the hospital setting, however, underlying medical conditions that often result in elevated D-dimer assays may render this test difficult to interpret (Figure 47-21). D-dimer levels greater than 500 mg/L mandate further evaluation with either

Table 47-8
Main Clinical Scores for Classification of Likelihood of Pulmonary Embolism*

Original		Simplified	
Wells Scores			
Previous DVT or PE	1.5		1
Heart rate >100 beats per minute	1.5		1
Recent surgery or immobilization	1.5		1
Clinical signs of DVT	3		1
Alternative diagnosis less likely than PE	3		1
Hemoptysis	1		1
Cancer	1		1
Low probability	0-1	Unlikely	≤1
Intermediate probability	2-6	Likely	>1
High probability	≥7		
Original		**Revised**	
Geneva Scores			
Previous DVT or PE	2		3
Heart rate >100 beats per minute	1	Age >65 years	1
Recent surgery	3	Surgery (general anesthesia) or lower limb fracture within 1 month	2
Age (years):		Active malignant condition (solid or hematological malignant condition, currently active or considered cured <1 year)	2
60-79	1		
≥80	2		
Partial CO_2:			
<6.5 kPa	2		
4.8-5.9 kPa	1		
Partial O_2:			
<6.5 kPa	4	Unilateral lower limb pain	3
6.5-7.99 kPa	3	Hemoptysis	2
		Heart rate (beats per minute):	
8-9.49 kPa	2	75-94	3
9.5-10.99 kPa	1	≥95	5
Atelectasis	1	Pain on lower-limb deep venous palpation and unilateral edema	4
Elevated hemidiaphragm	1		
Low probability	0-4		0-3
Intermediate probability	5-8		4-10
High probability	≥9		≥11

*CO_2, carbon dioxide; DVT, deep vein thrombosis; kPa, kilopascal; PE, pulmonary embolism.

helical CT or lung scintigraphy. Alternatively, ultrasound examination may be considered as an initial investigation for bed-ridden or nonambulatory inpatients, since approximately 90% of PE originates from the venous system of the lower extremity. However, a normal leg sonogram does not exclude PE, since approximately 50% of patients with proven PE have normal duplex scans.[162] In such cases, pelvic or calf veins are likely sources of emboli but are notoriously difficult to evaluate satisfactorily by ultrasound. Despite the obvious advantages of helical CT pulmonary angiography, V/Q scans remain a viable option, especially in patients with contrast allergies or renal insufficiency. Transthoracic echocardiography should be considered when symptoms, laboratory, and EKG results suggest alternative diagnoses such as heart failure, pericarditis, or aortic dissection. Identification of right heart dysfunction by echo may suggest a diagnosis of acute massive PE, necessitating confirmation with helical CT.

Documentation of Recurrent Pulmonary Embolism

The incidence of recurrent PE ranges from 2.5% to 8%.[163,164] Provide that a baseline examination exists, repeat CT or V/Q scans can be used to document new thromboembolic disease or new perfusion abnormalities indicative of recurrent disease. Helical CT also has utility in providing additional morphological information about response to therapy, especially relating to clot lysis and arterial recannulation. CT is also instrumental in identifying laminated or calcified pulmonary arterial thrombi characteristic of chronic PE.

TREATMENT OF PULMONARY EMBOLISM

Treatment of PE can be predicated on the extent and burden of clot within the pulmonary arterial system, with treatment options based on the following disease categories (previously described under the Pulmonary Embolization section):

- Acute massive PE
- Acute submassive PE
- Acute nonmassive PE
- Chronic thromboembolic disease with pulmonary hypertension

Acute Massive Pulmonary Embolism

The symptoms of massive PE can be variable, ranging from moderate systemic hypotension to full cardiac arrest. The immediate goals of treatment are to maintain blood pressure cardiac output and oxygen saturation. Oxygen saturation can be improved by oxygen delivery via mask or nasal prongs. Mechanical ventilation may be necessary to improve oxygenation, with ventilation pressures set as low as possible to prevent further impairment of right heart venous return that is common with massive PE.[26,27,165] Rapid frequency ventilation with a low tidal volume may assist in maintaining cardiac output.

Fluid resuscitation in patients with massive PE remains controversial. Experimental studies using animals with massive PE and hypotension showed a negative response to fluid resuscitation. Massive PE is commonly associated with right heart strain, and fluid replacement risks further deterioration of right heart function. However, a few small clinical studies have shown that the cardiac index in some patients improves some small boluses of IV fluid (500 cc).[166,167]

A small study showed a beneficial effect of using β-adrenergic agonists like IV dobutamine and dopamine. These drugs, which improve cardiac index, systemic blood pressure, and mean pulmonary arterial pressure, can be useful in patients with massive PE.[168] The role of epinephrine and norepinephrine in

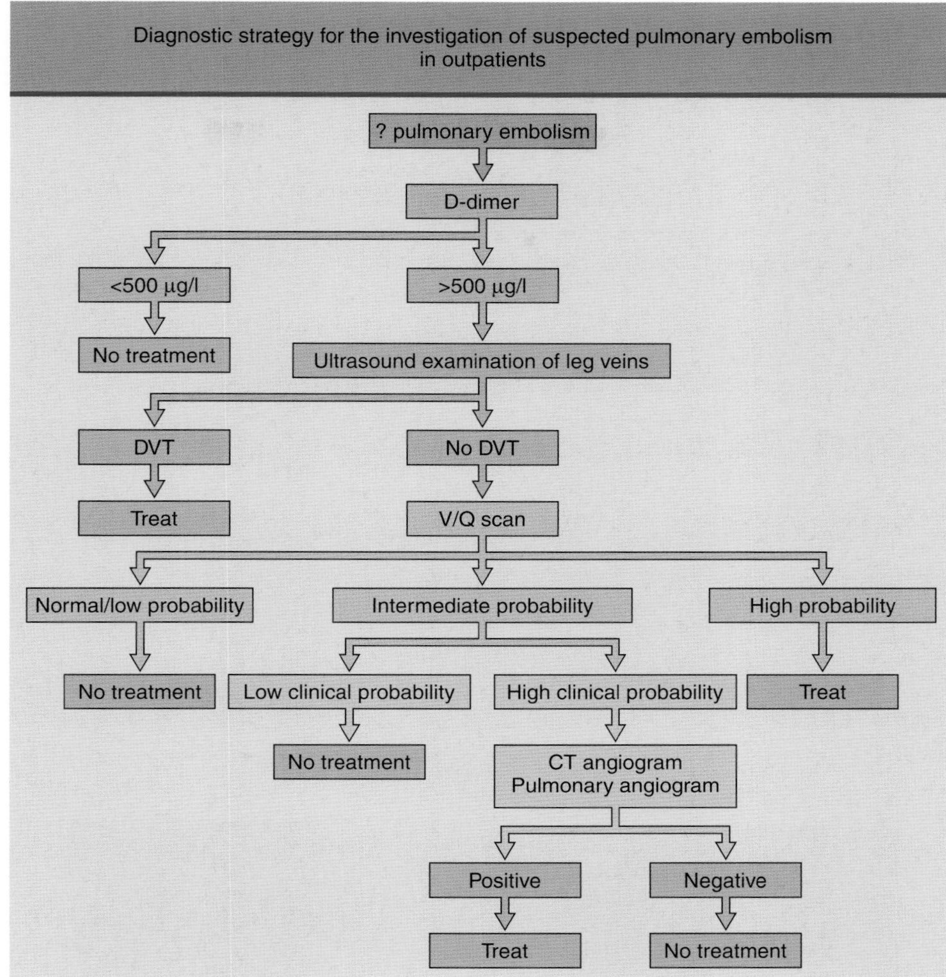

Figure 47-20. Diagnostic strategy for the investigation of suspected pulmonary embolism in outpatients. (Modified from Perrier A. *Lancet* 1999;353: 190-195.)

massive PE is unclear, and the use of these agents should probably be limited to patients with profound hypotension that is refractory to initial therapy.[169]

Massive PE may elicit a rapid release of potent vasoconstrictive substances such as thromboxane A2 and endothelin-1.[170] Antagonizing the effects of these mediators has been shown to dramatically improve hemodynamic parameters in experimental PE in animals.[171] Inhalation of nitric oxide, which is a selective pulmonary vasodilator, lowers pulmonary arterial resistance, thereby improving cardiac output and oxygenation in patients with massive PE.[172]

Thrombolytic treatment is reserved for patients with severe cardiopulmonary collapse, hypotension (systolic pressure of less than 90 mm Hg), oliguria, or hypoxia. The goal of IV thrombolytic treatment is to quickly decrease clot burden (Figure 47-22), thereby decreasing pulmonary arterial resistance. In addition, lysis therapy may provide an additional benefit by eliminating the primary source of thrombus, preventing recurrent embolic disease. Administration of systemic thrombolytic agents is generally more practical compared to catheter-directed thrombolysis, which is best reserved for cases in which pulmonary angiography is deemed necessary.[173] Compared to heparin therapy, thrombolysis improves cardiac index and reduces the pulmonary arterial pressure more rapidly but with an increased risk of hemorrhagic complications (22% versus 8%).[174,175] Finally, thrombolytic treatment are not generally indicated in patients with nonmassive PE, and its use in patients with submassive PE is unclear.

The indication for embolectomy for massive PE is primarily reserved for patients with contraindications to thrombolytic therapy or those who respond poorly to thrombolysis. Embolectomy can be performed either surgically or percutaneously using recently developed embolectomy devices. This procedure, which is not in common use, is generally performed on only a few patients per year. While effective, surgical thrombectomy is associated with high perioperative morbidity and mortality rates (30% to 50%). However, the long-term outlook for survivors is good, with 70% of patients alive after 8 years. Furthermore, recent refinements in anesthesia and circulatory bypass techniques may allow excellent long-term outcome in patients who develop thromboembolic pulmonary hypertension necessitating thromboendarterectomy.[176]

As an alternative to surgical embolectomy, percutaneous catheter-directed embolectomy is generally easier and quicker to perform. Several devices are available, all capable of quickly

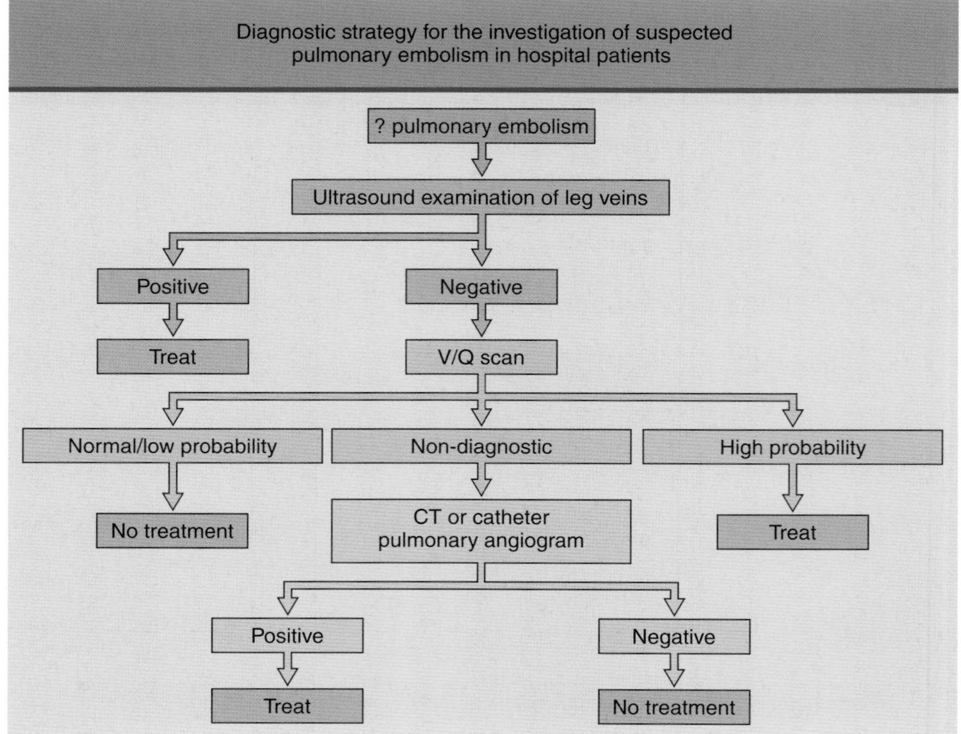

Figure 47-21. Diagnostic strategy for the investigation of suspected pulmonary embolism in hospital patients.

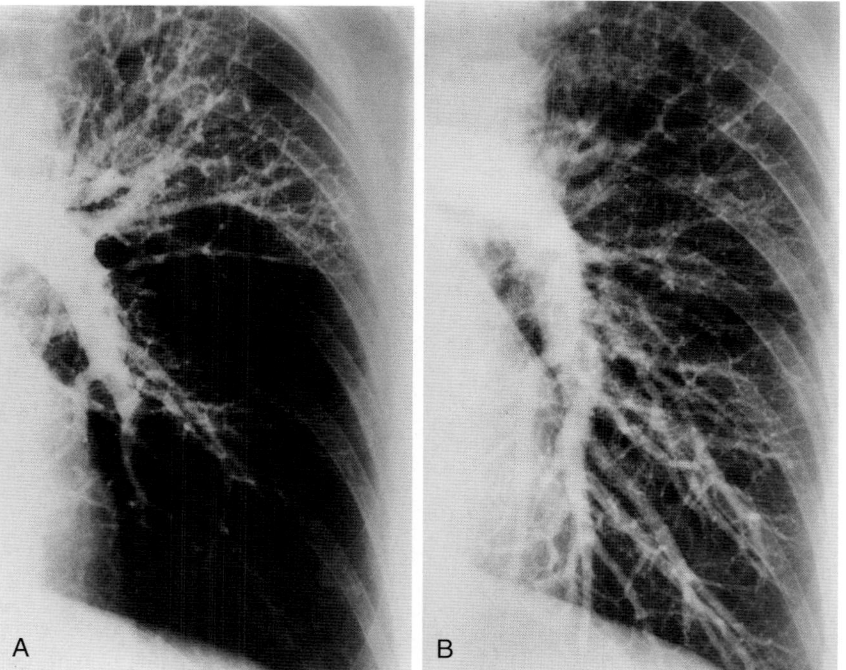

Figure 47-22. Thrombolytic treatment for pulmonary embolism. **A,** Initial angiogram shows hypoperfusion of the left lower lobe. **B,** Following systemic administration of streptokinase, the pulmonary circulation is restored to normal.

restoring pulmonary circulation (Figure 47-23). The efficacy of percutaneous thrombectomy can be augmented with administration of thrombolytics, which speeds up clot fragmentation. A recent review has described the various devices available.[177]

Once a diagnosis of massive PE has been established and effectively treated, anticoagulation therapy should be maintained to decrease the risk of recurrent PE. The precise duration is always a balance between the risk of recurrent embolism and the incipient complications of anticoagulation (Table 47-9).

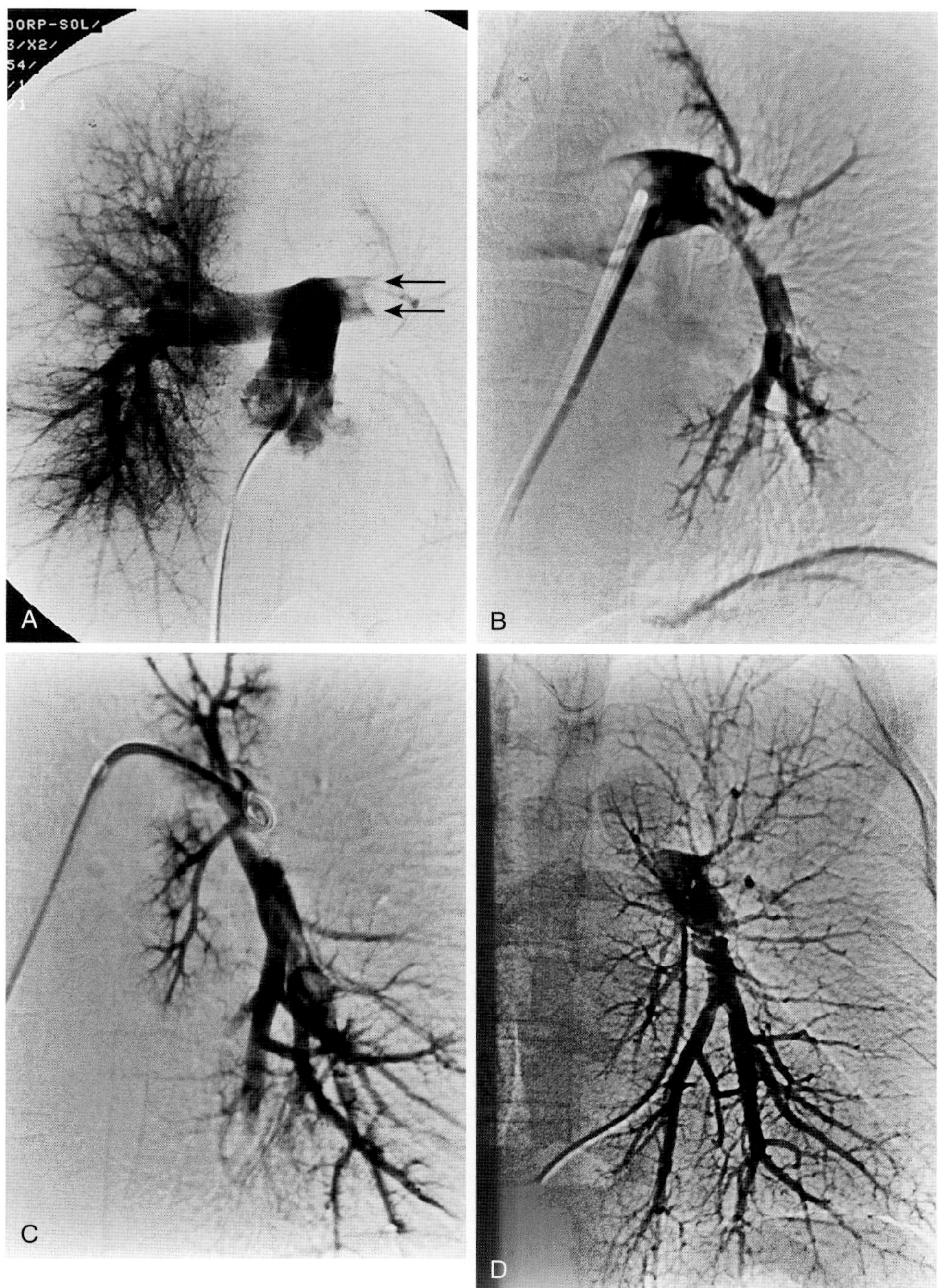

Figure 47-23. Massive pulmonary embolism treated initially by mechanical thrombectomy (Hydrolyser catheter) and followed by thrombolysis. **A,** Catheter pulmonary angiogram showing a large left pulmonary embolus *(arrows)*. **B,** Partial fragmentation of the embolus by mechanical thrombectomy (Hydrolyser). **C,** Lysis of embolus by streptokinase administered via the pigtail catheter in the left main pulmonary artery. **D,** Pulmonary angiogram at 2 weeks following mechanical thrombectomy and thrombolysis, with almost complete disappearance of the thrombus.

Acute Submassive Pulmonary Embolism

Debate relates to the most effective therapy in patients with submassive PE. While these patients are usually hemodynamically stable, many exhibit right ventricular dysfunction (strain). Right ventricular strain is associated with an unfavorable prognosis and has spurred discussion about whether more aggressive treatments should be initiated in these patients.[67,178] Generally, most patients with submassive PE are treated conservatively with IV anticoagulation.

Acute Nonmassive Pulmonary Embolism

As soon as the diagnosis of PE is clinically suspected, heparin therapy should be started pending results of confirmatory diagnostic tests. If UFH is used, the protocol is identical as

Table 47-9
Duration of Anticoagulation for Venous Thromboembolic Disease*

Risk of Recurrent DVT	Duration
Low	3 months
• Provoked DVT or PE (e.g., surgery or trauma)	
• Heterozygous for factor V Leiden	
• Heterozygous or homozygous for prothrombin G10120A mutation	
Intermediate	>6 months
• Unprovoked or idiopathic DVT or PE	
• First episode of recurrence (DVT or PE)	
• Persistent risk factor (malignancy, oral contraceptives, immobilization)	
• Protein C or S deficiency	
High	Indefinite
• Inherited thrombophilia	
• Homozygous for factor V Leiden	
• More than one thrombophilia	
• Antithrombin deficiency	
• Antiphospholipid antibodies	
• Recurrent DVT or PE ≥ 2	

*DVT, deep vein thrombosis; PE, pulmonary embolism.

for treatment of DVT (see the Treatment of Deep Venous Thrombosis section). LMWHs are now considered safe and are widely used in place of UFH at most medical centers.[179,180] Long-term oral anticoagulation is mandatory in the management of PE, and with effective therapy, mortality rates have dropped from 25% to less than 5%.[181] Oral anticoagulation should be begun immediately following confirmation of PE, and once therapeutic levels of anticoagulation are achieved (INR is two to three times normal), heparin can then be discontinued. The duration of coumadin treatment depends on the etiology of the PE (Table 47-9).

Placement of a vena cava filter is advised in patients who have recurrent PE despite adequate anticoagulation or in those individuals who cannot receive long-term anticoagulation. Currently, the use of cava filters is gaining popularity, with approximately 40,000 devices placed annually. While a host of filter configurations are available, all of these devices block passage of emboli to the lungs while allowing blood flow (Figure 47-24). In addition, temporary filters can be deployed in patients who have a short-term high risk for PE, with eventual removal once the risk is over.[182]

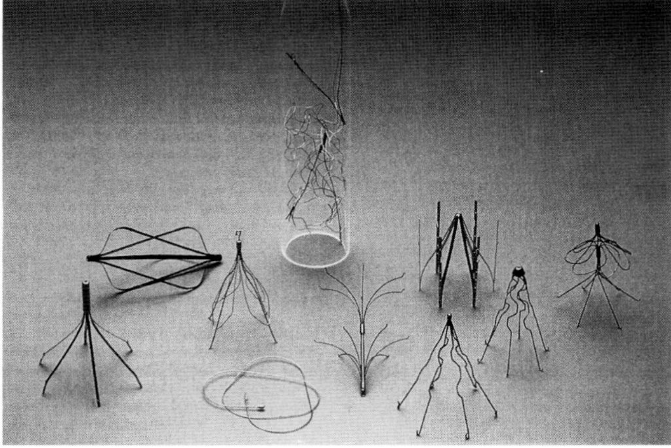

Figure 47-24. Types of vena cava filters. *Back row, left to right:* Antheor, Gunther tulip, Bird's nest, Vena Tech LGM, and Simon Nitonol. *Front row, left to right:* Keeper, Dil, FCP, Greenfield titanium, and Greenfield steel. (From Oudkerk, Van Beek EJR, Ten Cate JW, et al. *Pulmonary embolism.* Berlin: Blackwell Wissenschafts-Verlag; 1999.)

The placement of an IVC filter generally requires access to the IVC via a right common femoral vein or right internal jugular vein approach. Before placement of any filter, an inferior vena cavagram (Figure 47-25) should be performed not only to demonstrate caval anatomy, and the diameter of the IVC, but also to exclude coexisting thrombus. One anatomical abnormality that must be excluded in a patient with recurrent DVT is a duplicated IVC (Figure 47-26), which requires placement of a second filter to achieve adequate protection from VTE.

To prevent renal vein thrombosis, IVC filter placement should be located inferior to the renal veins (Figure 47-27). A suprarenal location may be necessary when there is a thrombus in the renal veins or more proximal IVC. A suprarenal placement may also be required in pregnant females who have caval compression from gravid uterus. Deployment of shorter filter configurations such as the Greenfield, Guenther tulip, or Vena Tech LGM designs within the superior vena cava may provide necessary protection in patients with VTE originating from an upper extremity.[183,184]

With correct filter placement, the incidence of PE is reduced to about 2% to 3%. The prevention of PE with a filter, coupled with anticoagulation, appears greatest during the first several weeks when compared to anticoagulant therapy alone (incidence of PE 1.1% versus 4.8%). At 2 years however, the efficacy of both regimens were equal in preventing PE.[185] These results suggest that removable filters may be a reasonable alternative to treat VTE without the inherent complications associated with permanent indwelling filters. Care must be taken when removing such a filter, as emboli may be present within the filter (Figure 47-28).

The incidence of complications from vena cava filters is 5% to 10%, and deaths directly related to a caval filter are rare.[186,187] Reported complications from IVC filters include the following:

- Insertion site thrombosis (10%)—Femoral vein thrombosis occurs in 30% of patients, but this risk has diminished with smaller-catheter delivery designs.[188]
- Filter migration—Rarely, a filter may dislodge and migrate proximally, occasionally lodging in the heart or pulmonary arteries. In such cases, snaring and retrieval of the filter usually is indicated.
- IVC thrombosis—The reported incidence for caval thrombosis due to a filter is about 10%. Most patients who experience caval thrombosis remain asymptomatic due to development of venous collateralization. Confirmation of this diagnosis usually requires sonography or venography, and this complication may lead to the post-thrombotic syndrome in some patients.
- Caval penetration—Perforation of the cava occurs in 20% of patients either during or after filter placement. This phenomenon, which is due to perforation of the caval wall by anchoring filter struts, rarely leads to clinical symptoms.

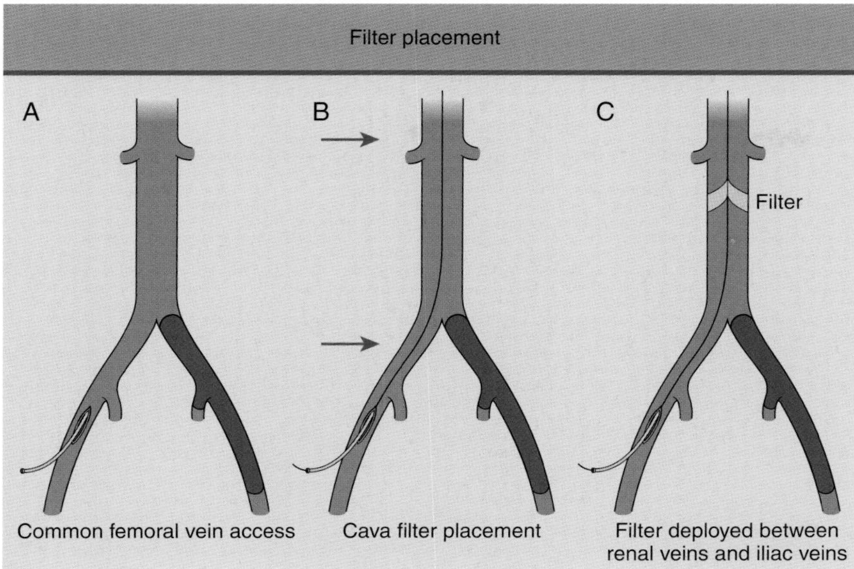

Figure 47-25. Filter placement. **A,** Common femoral vein access. A sheath is inserted, and a cavagram is performed. **B,** Cava filter placement. The position of the renal veins and the bifurcation of the inferior vena cava are marked by metal clips on the surface of the skin. A guide wire is placed above the renal veins. **C,** The filter is deployed between the renal veins and the iliac veins.

PHLEGMASIA CERULEA DOLENS AND VENOUS GANGRENE

Complications of DVT include phlegmasia cerulea dolens (PCD) and venous gangrene. PCD is a rare condition that occurs in less than 1% of patients with DVT. In 50% of patients, PCD progresses to venous gangrene.[189] Both are serious medical conditions; they may require eventual amputation in 30% to 50% of patients, and they have overall high mortality rates of 20% to 40%.[189,190]

Pathophysiology

The pathophysiology of both PCD and venous gangrene relates to complete occlusion of the venous drainage, leading to dramatic increases in capillary hydrostatic pressure with subsequent exudation of large amounts of fluid out into the interstitial space.[191] Up to 90% of patients who develop PCD have an underlying malignancy.[192] In half of these, the malignancy is occult, resulting in a hypercoagulable state that is responsible for the development of DVT. Other risk factors

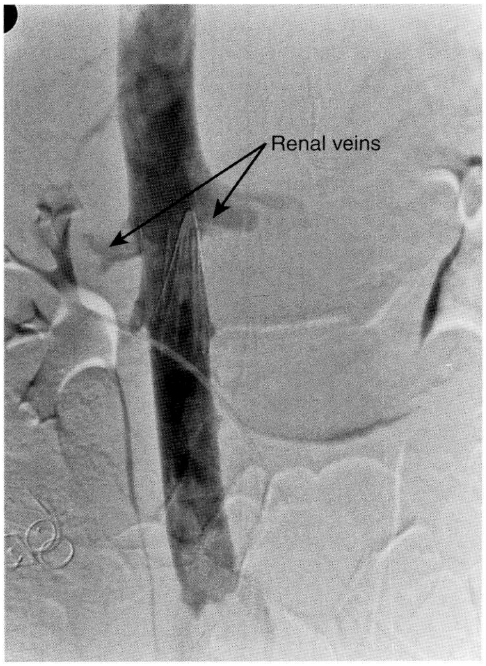

Figure 47-26. Coronal reformat of computed tomography scan showing bilateral inferior vena cava *(arrows).*

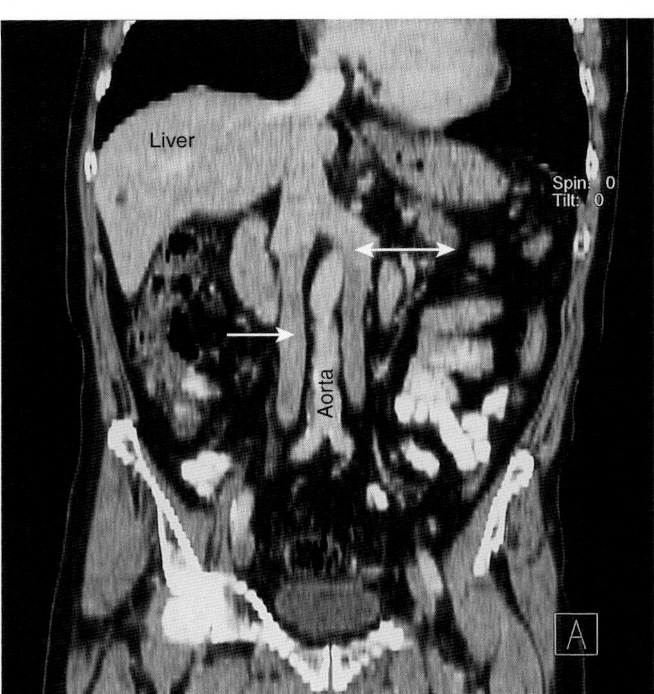

Figure 47-27. Position of a caval filter (LCM, Vena Tech). The filter should be positioned in the infrarenal section of the inferior vena cava (arrows mark the position of renal veins).

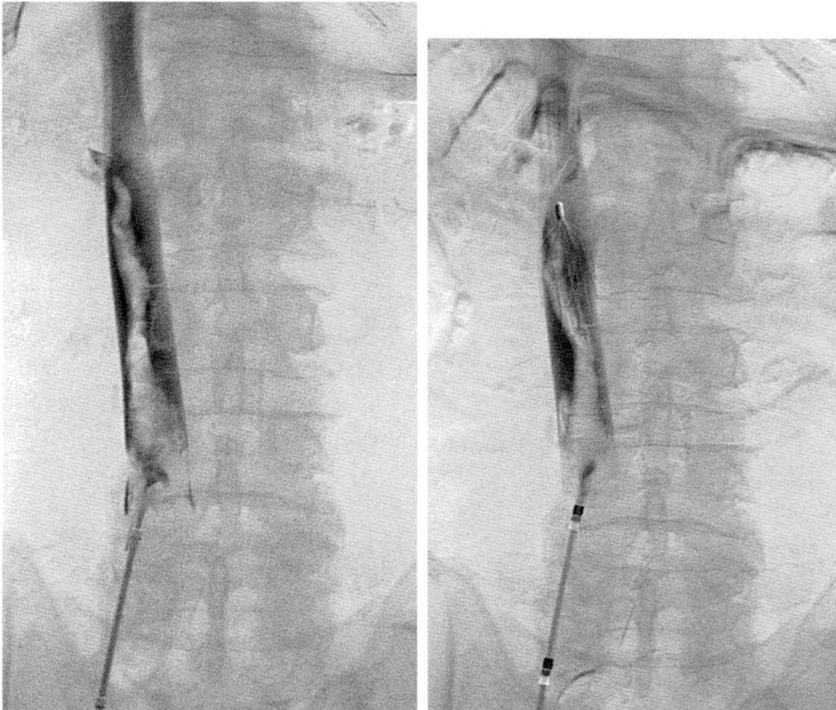

Figure 47-28. Removal of retrievable filter containing significant embolic material.

for PCD include immobilization from surgery, trauma, and inherited thrombophilia.

The requisite development of severe soft-tissue edema in PCD results in a corresponding increase in the interstitial pressure to 25 to 45 mm Hg (normal pressure is 0 to 10 mm Hg), eventually leading to decreased tissue perfusion and to ischemia from compression of small arteries.[193] The characteristic clinical features of PCD include soft-tissue edema, pain, and cyanosis of the affected extremity (Figure 47-29).[194] Once severe soft-tissue edema develops, eventual skin blistering and cyanosis follows, usually progressing up the extremity and occasionally involving the trunk. The diagnosis of PCD is typically based on the clinical signs and symptoms. In these cases, Doppler ultrasound examination provides a rapid and accurate means to confirm the diagnosis and to localize the thrombosis within the affected extremity. Contrast-enhanced CT may be necessary to assist in the identification of centrally located venous clot within pelvic veins or cava (Figure 47-30). The rapidity of onset and the progression of the disease are variable. Some cases of PCD are fulminate with rapid development of gangrene in 1 to 2 days, while others may present initially with a simple DVT that slowly progresses to venous gangrene. Venous gangrene occurs mostly in the elderly but is reported across all age groups.[193] Hypotension and shock due to massive extravasation of intravascular fluid have also been reported with PCD.

Treatment

The mainstay of treatment of PCD is the prevention of clot propagation, maintenance of vascular perfusion, preservation of tissue viability, and prevention of postthrombotic syndrome.[195] Initial treatment should consist of fluid resuscitation, heparin, and elevation of the affected extremity. These treatments may be adequate in most patients who have not yet developed gangrene.[195] Unresponsive cases may require more aggressive interventions such as catheter-directed thrombolysis. Continuous infusion of thrombolytics directly into the clot has become a preferred treatment for severe cases of PCD. Simultaneous arterial infusion of thrombolytic agents has also been used in severe cases.[196] Neither systemic IV thrombolytic therapy nor surgical thrombectomy appears to be a viable treatment for PCD, due to overall poorer results.

VENOUS THROMBOEMBOLISM IN PREGNANCY

Venous thromboembolism, although uncommon, is a major cause of maternal mortality.[41] The incidence of VTE is estimated to be approximately 0.1% of all pregnancies.[197] The greatest risk for PE occurs late in pregnancy and during the immediate postpartum period, with a slightly higher risk for PE in females who deliver by cesarean section.[42,43]

Diagnosis

Although inherent risks exist for fetal exposure to ionizing radiation during CT angiography, with appropriate shielding of the abdomen and pelvis, the exposure risk is minimal (5 mGy).[198] Sonography of lower extremities in patients with suspected DVT or V/Q imaging is a viable alternative in making the diagnosis of VTE, although CT is now preferred over scintigraphy at most institutions.

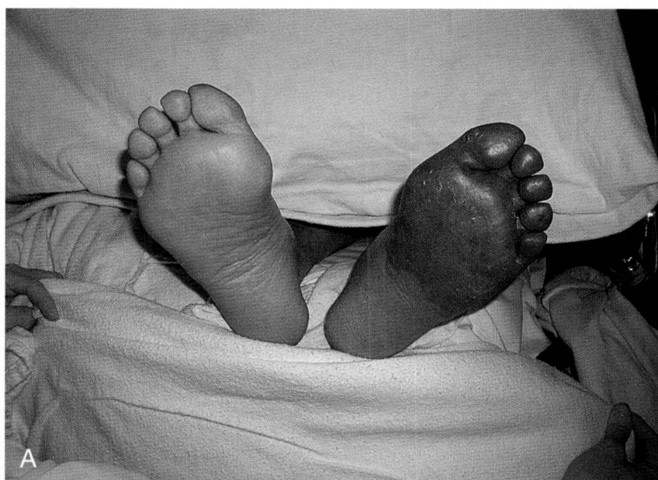

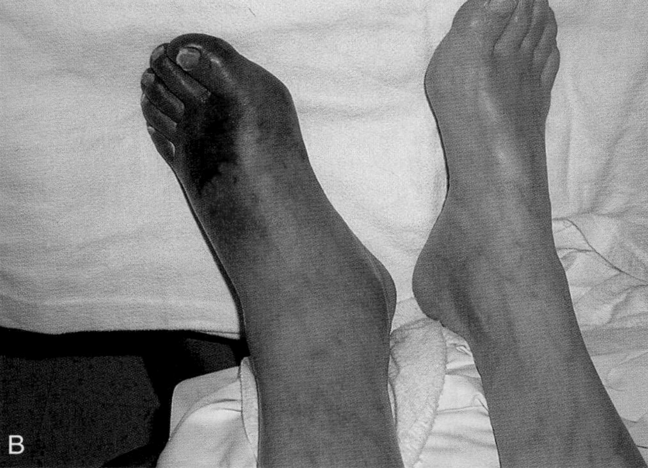

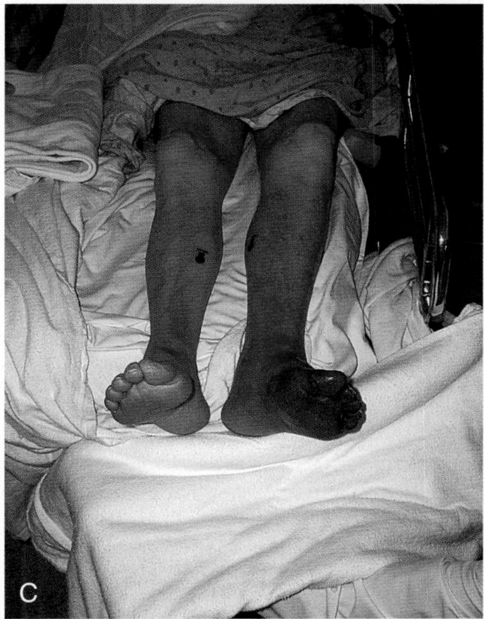

Figure 47-29. This patient had advanced metastatic lung cancer and hypercoagulability, with phlegmasia cerulea dolens and early venous gangrene. Ultrasound showed extensive obstructive, acute femoral, and popliteal vein thrombosis.

Treatment

Coumadin should not be used in pregnancy because of potential teratogenic effect on the fetus.[199] UFH and LMWHs are both effective drugs, but because LMWH does not cross the placenta, it has the advantage of fewer complications.[199,200] Placement of vena cava filters has been used with good results and provides a reasonable alternative to drug therapy.[201]

Anticoagulation protocols for pregnancy both before and after delivery are identical to those used for PE and DVT. Warfarin is not excreted in any significant amount in breast milk and can be considered safe during lactation.

PREVENTION OF VENOUS THROMBOEMBOLISM

Prevention against the development of DVT must always be considered in hospitalized patients and those individuals with a history of prior VTE. Although a range of methods have been shown to be effective in preventing VTE, thromboprophylaxis is not commonly in use at many hospitals. The practice of routine thromboprophylaxis varies widely across hospitals, ranging from 28% to 100% of respondents.[202] A Scottish study revealed that 56% of patients who died of PE did not receive prophylaxis, despite having significant risk factors and no contraindication to anticoagulation prophylaxis.[203]

Methods of Prophylaxis for Venous Thromboembolic Disease

While rapid mobilization of hospitalized patient is an effective and easy means to diminish the risk of VTE, many conditions make this option impractical. In most hospital situations, other forms of prophylaxis must be initiated, usually employing both mechanical and pharmacological methods to achieve optimal protection against VTE.

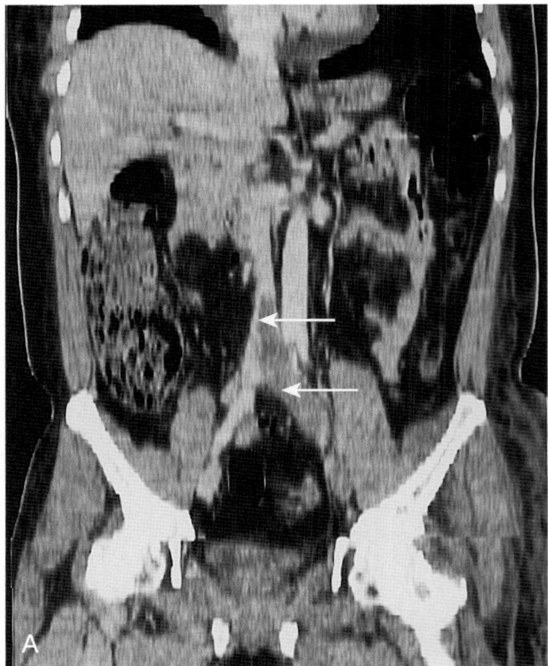

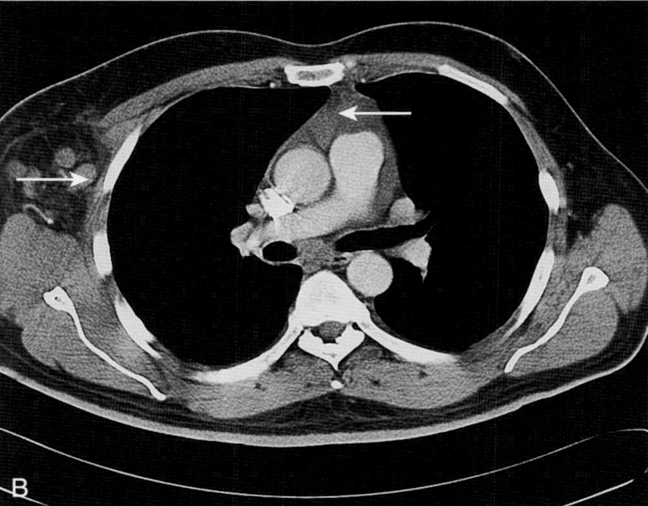

Figure 47-30. Computed tomography (CT) examination of a patient who presented with left leg venous gangrene and was subsequently found to have lymphoma. **A,** Coronal reformat demonstrating extensive thrombosis of the inferior vena cava and left iliac vein *(arrows)*. **B,** CT of the thorax of the same patient showing lymphadenopathy in the right axilla and anterior mediastinum *(arrows)*.

Mechanical Protection against Venous Thromboembolic Disease

Both graduated compression stockings and intermittent lower extremity compression pneumatic devices have been shown to be effective in preventing VTE without the risks associated with anticoagulation.[138,204] These techniques are particularly useful in cases for which anticoagulants are contraindicated.

Pharmacological Methods

Three main types of pharmacological therapies are available:

- Oral anticoagulant (vitamin K antagonists)
- Heparin (UFH or LMWHs)
- Aspirin

Vitamin K Antagonists

While Vitamin K agents are effective in preventing DVT, they have a delayed onset of action, have a long half-life, and require regular monitoring of coagulation profiles.[205] This therapy should be considered for VTE prophylaxis in patients with a higher risk of DVT due to immobilization.

Heparin

The incidence of VTE is inversely related to the dose and frequency of administration of anticoagulation.[206] Subcutaneous heparin (5000 IU) given two or three times daily during hospitalization reduces the incidence of VTE by a factor of three. LMWHs are as effective as heparin and have an added benefit of once-daily administration.

Aspirin

Although thromboprophylaxis with aspirin is useful,[207] it is not as effective as heparin or warfarin.[208] Therefore, aspirin therapy alone is deemed insufficient for most hospitalized patients but can be used as a supplement with other treatments, especially in patients at high risk of VTE. Advantages of aspirin relate to its low cost and ease of administration.

Recommendations for Prophylaxis

Rather than using a standardized thromboprophylaxis regimen for all patients, therapy should be tailored individually, depending on the relative risk for VTE (Tables 47-2 and 47-9). The risk can be divided into three categories (Table 47-2). Patients at low risk do not require prophylaxis, but early mobilization is encouraged. For the moderate risk group, either heparin (UFH or LMWH) or a lower extremity pneumatic compression or compression stocking is usually sufficient. Patients in the high-risk category need both mechanical and pharmacological prophylaxis.

SUMMARY

VTE is a common disease with potentially fatal results. As a common complication in critically ill, hospitalized, or immobile patients, effective precaution against DVT is of paramount importance. Furthermore, close clinical surveillance of incipient complications associated with DVT, such as PE, make it imperative that a thorough risk assessment for VTE be performed in any at-risk patient presenting with any unexplained cardiopulmonary symptomatology that suggests the diagnosis.

References

1. Hirsh J, Hoak J. Management of deep vein thrombosis and pulmonary embolism: a statement for health professionals. Council on Thrombosis (in consultation with the Council on Cardiovascular Radiology), American Heart Association. *Circulation* 1996;93:2212-2245.
2. Moser KM. Venous thromboembolism. *Am Rev Respir Dis* 1990;141:235-249.
3. Salzman EW, Hirsh J. The epidemiology, pathogenesis and natural history of venous thrombosis. In: Colman RW, Hirsh J, Marder V, eds. *Thrombosis and haemostasis: basic principles and clinical practice*. Philadelphia: JB Lippincott; 1993:1275-1296.
4. Huisman MV, Büller HR, ten Cate JW, et al. Unexpected high prevalence of silent pulmonary embolism in patients with deep venous thrombosis. *Chest* 1989;95:498-502.
5. Cohen AT, Edmondson RA, Phillips MJ, et al. The changing pattern of venous thromboembolic disease. *Haemostasis* 1996;26:65-71.
6. Silverstein MD, Heit JA, Mohr DN, et al. Trends in the incidence of deep vein thrombosis and pulmonary embolism: a 25-year population-based study. *Arch Intern Med* 1998;158:585-593.
7. Turton EP, Coughlin PA, Berridge DC, Mercer KG. A survey of deep venous thrombosis management by consultant vascular surgeons in the United Kingdom and Ireland. *Eur J Vasc Endovasc Surg* 2001;21:558-563.
8. van Erkel AR, van den Hout WB, Pattynama PM. International differences in health care costs in Europe and the United States: do these affect the cost-effectiveness of diagnostic strategies for pulmonary embolism? *Eur Radiol* 1999;9:1926-1931.
9. Anderson FA, Wheeler HB, Goldberg RJ, et al. A population-based perspective of hospital incidence and case-fatality rates of deep venous thrombosis and pulmonary embolism: the Worcester DVT study. *Arch Intern Med* 1991;151:933-938.
10. Gillum RF. Pulmonary embolism and thrombophlebitis in the United States, 1970-1985. *Am Heart J* 1987;114:1262-1264.
11. Samama MM, Cohen AT, Darmon JY, et al. A comparison of enoxaparin with placebo for the prevention of venous thromboembolism in acutely ill medical patients: prophylaxis in Medical Patients with Enoxaparin Study Group. *N Engl J Med* 1999;341:793-800.
12. Agnelli G, Piovella F, Buoncristiani P, et al. Enoxaparin plus compression stockings compared with compression stockings alone in the prevention of venous thromboembolism after elective neurosurgery. *N Engl J Med* 1998;339:80-85.
13. Morrell MT, Dunnill MS. The post-mortem incidence of pulmonary embolism in a hospital population. *Br J Surg* 1968;55:347-352.
14. Karwinski B, Svendsen E. Comparison of clinical and post-mortem diagnosis of pulmonary embolism. *J Clin Pathol* 1989;42:135-139.
15. Horattas MC, Wright DJ, Fenton AH, et al. Changing concepts of deep venous thrombosis of the upper extremity: report of a series and review of the literature. *Surgery* 1988;104:561-567.
16. Lohr JM, James KV, Deshmukh RM, Hasselfeld KA. Calf vein thrombi are not a benign finding. *Am J Surg* 1995;170:86-90.
17. Thomas DP. Venous thrombogenesis. *Ann Rev Med* 1985;36:39-50.
18. Stamatakis D, Kakkar VV, Sagar S, et al. Femoral vein thrombosis and total hip replacement. *BMJ* 1977;2:223-225.
19. Hull R, Hirsh J, Sackett DL, et al. Cost effectiveness of clinical diagnosis, venography and non-invasive testing in patients with symptomatic deep vein thrombosis. *N Engl J Med* 1981;304:1561-1567.
20. AbuRahma AF, Powell M, Robinson PA. Prospective study of safety of lower extremity phlebography with nonionic contrast medium. *Am J Surg* 1996;171:255-260.
21. Stain M, Schonauer V, Minar E, et al. The post-thrombotic syndrome: risk factors and impact on course of thrombotic disease. *J Thromb Heaemost* 2005;3:2671-2676.
22. Schraufnagel DE, Tsao M, Yao YT, et al. Factors associated with pulmonary infarction: a discriminant analysis study. *Am J Clin Pathol* 1985;84:15-18.
23. Sasahara AA, Cannilla JE, Morse RL, et al. Clinical and physiologic studies in pulmonary thromboembolism. *Am J Cardiol* 1967;20:10-20.
24. Nakos G, Kitsiouli EI, Lekka ME. Bronchoalveolar lavage alterations in pulmonary embolism. *Am J Respir Crit Care Med* 1998;158:1504-1510.
25. Gorham LW. A study of pulmonary embolism. II. The mechanism of death; based on a clinicopathological investigations of 100 cases of massive and 285 cases of minor embolism of the pulmonary artery. *Arch Intern Med* 1961;108:189-207.
26. Soloff LA, Rodman T. Acute pulmonary embolism: review. *Am Heart J* 1967;74:710-724.
27. McIntyre KM, Sasahara AA. The ratio of pulmonary arterial pressure to pulmonary vascular obstruction: index of pre-embolic cardiopulmonary status. *Chest* 1977;71:692-697.
28. Ramirez-Rivera A, Gutierrez-Fajardo P, Jerjes-Sanchez C, et al. Acute right myocardial infarction without significant obstructive coronary lesions secondary to massive pulmonary embolism. *Chest* 1993;104:80S.
29. Flordal PA, Bergqvist D, Burmark US, et al. Risk factors for major thromboembolism and bleeding tendency after elective general surgical operations. *Eur J Surg* 1996;162:783-789.
30. Warlow C, Ogston D, Douglas AS. Venous thrombosis following strokes. *Lancet* 1972;1:1305-1306.
31. Scurr JH, Machin SJ, Bailey-King S, et al. Frequency and prevention of symptomless deep-vein thrombosis in long-haul flights: a randomised trial. *Lancet* 2001;357:1485-1489.
32. Cesarone MR, Belcaro G, Nicolaides AN, et al. Venous thrombosis from air travel: the LONFLIT3 study: prevention with aspirin vs low molecular weight heparin (LMWH) in high-risk subjects—a randomized trial. *Angiology* 2002;53:1-6.
33. Turpie AGG, Levine MN, Hirsh J, et al. A randomized controlled trial of a low molecular weight heparin (enoxaparin) to prevent deep vein thrombosis in patients undergoing elective hip surgery. *N Engl J Med* 1986;315:925-929.
34. Clagett GP, Anderson FA, Heit J, et al. Prevention of venous thromboembolism. *Chest* 1995;108:312-334.
35. Geerts W, Code KL, Jay RM, et al. A prospective study of venous thromboembolism after major trauma. *N Engl J Med* 1994;331:1601-1606.
36. Thromboembolic Risk Factors Consensus Group. Risk of and prophylaxis for venous thromboembolism in hospital patients. *Br Med J* 1992;79:1-17.
37. Mismetti P, Juillard-Delsart D, Tardy B, et al. Evaluation of the risk of venous thromboembolism in the medical patients. *Therapie* 1998;53:565-570.
38. Luzzatto G, Schafer AL. The prethrombotic state in cancer. *Semin Oncol* 1990;17:147-159.
39. Sue-Ling HM, Johnston D, McMahon MU, et al. Preoperative identification of patients at high risk of deep venous thrombosis after elective major abdominal surgery. *Lancet* 1986;1:1173-1176.
40. Baron JA, Gridley G, Weiderpass E, et al. Venous thromboembolism and cancer. *Lancet* 1998;351:1077-1080.
41. Rochat RW, Koorin LM, Atrash HK, et al. Maternal mortality in the United States: report from the Maternal Mortality Collaborative. *Obstet Gynecol* 1988;72:91-97.
42. Simpson EL, Lawrenson RA, Nightingale AL, et al. Venous thromboembolism in pregnancy and the puerperium: incidence and additional risk factors from a London perinatal database. *BJOG* 2001;108:56-60.
43. Salonen Ros H, Lichtenstein P, Bellocco R, et al. Increased risks of circulatory diseases in late pregnancy and puerperium. *Epidemiology* 2001;12:456-460.
44. Vandenbroucke JP, Rosing J, Bloemenkamp KWM, et al. Oral contraceptives and the risk of venous thrombosis. *N Engl J Med* 2001;344:1527-1535.
45. Hoibraaten E, Abdelnoor M, Sandset PM. Hormone replacement therapy with estradiol and risk of venous thromboembolism: a population based case control study. *Thromb Haemost* 1999;82:1218-1221.
46. Lowe G, Woodward M, Vessey M, et al. Thrombotic variables and risk of idiopathic venous thromboembolism in women aged 45-64 years: relationships to hormone replacement therapy. *Thromb Haemost* 2000;83:530-535.
47. van Weert H, Dolan F, de Vries C, ter Riet G, Büller H. Spontaneous superficial thrombophlebitis: does it increase risk for thromboembolism? *J Fam Pract* 2006;55:52-57.
48. Finazzi G, Brancaccio V, Moia M, et al. Natural history and risk factors for thrombosis in 360 patients with antiphospholipid antibodies: a four year prospective study from the Italian registry. *Am J Med* 1996;100:530-536.
49. Ondi-Ros J, Perez-Pemaa P, Monasterio J. Clinical and therapeutic aspects associated to phospholipid binding antibodies (lupus anticoagulant and anticardiolipin antibodies). *Haemostasis* 1994;24:165-174.
50. Provenzale JM, Ortel TL. Anatomic distribution of venous thrombosis in patients with antiphospholipid antibody: imaging findings. *AJR Am J Roentgenol* 1995;165:365-368.

51. Love PE, Santoro SA. Antiphospholipid antibodies, anticardiolipin and the lupus anticoagulant in systemic lupus erythematosus (SLE) and in non-SLE disorders. *Ann Intern Med* 1990;112:682-698.
52. Simioni P, Prandoni P, Zanon E, et al. Deep venous thrombosis and lupus anticoagulant: a case control study. *Thromb Haemost* 1996;76:187-189.
53. Hanly JG. Antiphospholipid syndrome: an overview. *CMAJ* 2003;169:1675-1682.
54. Prandoni P, Simioni P, Girolami A. Antiphospholipid antibodies, recurrent thromboembolism, and intensity of warfarin anticoagulation. *Thromb Haemost* 1996;75:859.
55. Bertina RM, Koeleman BP, Koster T, et al. Mutation in blood coagulation factor V associated with resistance to activated protein C. *Nature* 1994;369:64-67.
56. Poort SR, Rosendaal FR, Reitsma PH, Bertina RM. A common genetic variation in the 3¢-untranslated region of the prothrombin gene is associated with elevated plasma prothrombin levels and an increase in venous thrombosis. *Blood* 1996;88:3698-3703.
57. Mudd SH, Skovby F, Levy HL, et al. The natural history of homocystinuria due to cystathionine β-synthase deficiency. *Am J Hum Genet* 1985;37:1-31.
58. Alhenc-Gelas M, Arnoud E, Nicaud V, et al. Venous thromboembolic disease and the prothrombin, methylene tetrahydrofolate reductase and factor V genes. *Thromb Haemost* 1999;81:506-510.
59. Klatsky AL, Armstrong MA, Poggi J. Risk of pulmonary embolism and/or deep venous thrombosis in Asian-Americans. *Am J Cardiol* 2000;85:1334-1337.
60. Seligsohn U, Lubetsky A. Medical progress: genetic susceptibility to venous thrombosis. *N Engl J Med* 2001;344:1222-1231.
61. Girling J, de Swiet M. Inherited thrombophilia and pregnancy. *Curr Opin Obstet Gynaecol* 1998;10:135-144.
62. Vandenbroucke JP, Koster T, Briët E, et al. Increased risk of venous thrombosis in oral contraceptive users who are carriers of factor V Leiden mutation. *Lancet* 1994;344:1453-1457.
63. Baarslag HJ, Koopman MMW, Hutten B, et al. Long-term follow-up of patients with deep vein thrombosis of the upper extremity: survival, risk factors and post-thrombotic syndrome. *Eur J Intern Med* 2004;15:503-507.
64. Prandoni P, Polistena P, Bernardi E, et al. Upper extremity deep vein thrombosis: risk factors, diagnosis and complications. *Arch Intern Med* 1997;157:57-62.
65. Monreal M, Raventos A, Lerma R, et al. Pulmonary embolism in patients with upper extremity DVT associated to venous central lines: a prospective study. *Thromb Haemost* 1994;72:548-550.
66. ESC Task Force on Pulmonary Embolism. Guidelines on management of acute pulmonary embolism. *Eur Heart J* 2000;21:1301-1336.
67. Ribeiro A, Lindmarker P, Juhlin-Dannfelt A, et al. Echocardiography Doppler in pulmonary embolism: right ventricular dysfunction as a predictor of mortality rate. *Am Heart J* 1997;134:479-487.
68. Ribeiro A, Lindmarker P, Johnsson H, et al. Pulmonary embolism: one-year follow-up with echocardiography Doppler and five-year survival analysis. *Circulation* 1999;99:1325-1330.
69. Stein PD, Goldhaber SZ, Henry JW, Miller AC. Arterial blood gas analysis in the assessment of suspected acute pulmonary embolism. *Chest* 1996;109:78-81.
70. Haas FJL, Kamphuisen PW. The role of D-dimer in the diagnosis of deep venous thrombosis and pulmonary embolism. *Imaging Decisions* 2007;11(3):23-28.
71. Bounameaux H, de Moerloose P, Perrier A, Reber G. Plasma measurement of D-dimer as diagnostic aid in suspected venous thromboembolism: an overview. *Thromb Haemost* 1994;71:1-6.
72. van Beek EJR, van den Ende A, Berckmans RJ, et al. A comparative analysis of D-dimer assays in patients with suspected pulmonary embolism. *Thromb Haemost* 1993;70:408-413.
73. De Moerloose P, Desmarais S, Bounameaux H, et al. Contribution of a new, rapid, individual and quantitative automated D-dimer ELISA to exclude pulmonary embolism. *Thromb Haemost* 1996;75:11-13.
74. Goldhaber SZ, Simons GR, Elliot CG, et al. Quantitative plasma D-dimer levels among patients undergoing pulmonary angiography for suspected pulmonary embolism. *JAMA* 1993;270:2819-2822.
75. Michiels JJ, Freyburger G, van der Graaf F, et al. Strategies for the safe and effective exclusion and diagnosis of deep vein thrombosis by the sequential use of clinical score, D-dimer testing, and compression ultrasonography. *Semin Thromb Hemost* 2000;26:657-667.
76. Hull R, Hirsch J, Sackett DL. Clinical validity of a negative venogram in patients with clinically suspected venous thrombosis. *Circulation* 1981;64:622-625.
77. Lensing AW, Prandoni P, Brandjes D, et al. Detection of DVT by real-time B-mode ultrasonography. *N Engl J Med* 1989;320:342-345.
78. Heijboer H, Büller HR, Lensing AW, et al. A comparison of real-time compression ultrasonography with impedance plethysmography for the diagnosis of DVT in symptomatic outpatients. *N Engl J Med* 1993;329:1365-1369.
79. Lensing AWA, Kraaijenhagen R, van Beek EJR, Büller HR. Diagnosis of venous thrombosis. In: Oudkerk M, van Beek EJR, ten Cate JW. *Pulmonary embolism*. Berlin: Blackwell Science; 1999:47-55.
80. Montgomery KD, Potter HG, Helfet DL. Magnetic resonance venography to evaluate the deep venous system of the pelvis in patients who have an acetabular fracture. *J Bone Joint Surg Am* 1995;77:1639-1649.
81. Evans AJ, Sostman HD, Witty LA, et al. Detection of deep venous thrombosis: prospective comparison of MR imaging and sonography. *J Magn Reson Imaging* 1996;6:44-45.
82. Sampson FC, Goodacre SW, Thomas SM, van Beek EJR. The accuracy of MRI in diagnosis of suspected deep vein thrombosis: systematic review and meta-analysis. *Eur Radiol* 2007;17:175-181.
83. Fraser DG, Moody AR, Morgan PS, et al. Diagnosis of lower-limb deep venous thrombosis: a prospective blinded study of magnetic resonance direct thrombus imaging. *Ann Intern Med* 2002;136:89-98.
84. Thomas SM, Goodacre SW, Sampson FC, Van Beek EJR. Diagnostic value of computed tomography (CT) for deep vein thrombosis: results of a systematic review and meta-analysis. *Clin Radiol* 2008;63:299-304.
85. Loud PA, Katz DS, Bruce DA, et al. Deep venous thrombosis with suspected pulmonary embolism: detection with combined CT venography and pulmonary angiography. *Radiology* 2001;219:498-502.
86. Wells PS, Anderson DR, Bormanis J, et al. Value of assessment of pretest probability of deep-vein thrombosis in clinical management. *Lancet* 1997;350:1795-1798.
87. Wells PH, Anderson DR, Rodger M. Evaluation of D-dimer in the diagnosis of suspected deep venous thrombosis. *N Engl J Med* 2003;349:1227-1235.
88. Goodacre S, Sutton AJ, Sampson FC. Meta-analysis: the value of clinical assessment in the diagnosis of deep venous thrombosis. *Ann Intern Med* 2005;143:129-139.
89. ten Cate-Hoek AJ, Prins MH. Management studies using a combination of D-dimer test result and clinical probability to rule out venous thromboembolism: a systematic review. *J Thromb Haemost* 2005;3:2465-2470.
90. Fancher TL, White RK, Kravitz RL. Combined rapid D-dimer testing and estimation of clinical probability of deep vein thrombosis: systematic review. *BMJ* 2004;329:821.
91. Kamphuisen PW, Oudkerk M. Diagnosis of deep-vein thrombosis and pulmonary embolism: new guideline of the Dutch Institute for Health Care Improvement. *Imaging Decisions* 2007;11(3):3-7.
92. Cogo A, Lensing AW, Koopman MM, et al. Compression ultrasonography with clinically suspected deep vein thrombosis: prospective cohort study. *BMJ* 1998;316:17-20.
93. Hansson PO, Sorbo J, Eriksson H. Recurrent venous thromboembolism after deep vein thrombosis: incidence and risk factors. *Arch Intern Med* 2000;160:769-774.
94. Murphy TP, Cronan JJ. Evolution of deep venous thrombosis: a prospective evaluation with US. *Radiology* 1990;177:543-548.
95. Heijboer H, Jongbloets LM, Büller HR, et al. The clinical utility of real-time compression ultrasound in the diagnostic management of patients with recurrent venous thrombosis. *Acta Radiol* 1992;33:297-300.
96. Huisman MV. Recurrent venous thromboembolism: diagnosis and management. *Curr Opin Pulm Med* 2000;6:330-334.
97. Browse NL, Burnand KG, Irvine AT, Wilson NM. *Diseases of the veins*. London: Arnold; 1999; 319-358.
98. Chavatzas D, Martin P. A study of streptokinase in deep vein thrombosis of the lower extremities. *Vasa* 1975;4:68-72.
99. British National Formulary March 2002; No. 43: section 2.10.2.
100. Schulman S, Lockner D, Granqvist S, et al. A comparative randomized trial of low dose versus high dose streptokinase in deep vein thrombosis of the thigh. *Thromb Haemost* 1984;51:261-265.
101. Thery C, Bauchartt JJ, Lesenne M, et al. Predictive factors of effectiveness of streptokinase in deep venous thrombosis. *Am J Cardiol* 1992;69:117-122.
102. Schweizer J, Kirch W, Koch R, et al. Short and long-term results after thrombolytic treatment of deep venous thrombosis. *J Am Coll Cardiol* 2000;36:1336-1343.

103. Kanter DS, Mikkola KM, Patel SR, et al. Thrombolytic therapy for pulmonary embolism: frequency of intracranial haemorrhage and associated risk factors. *Chest* 1997;111:1241-1245.
104. Mikkola KM, Patel SR, Parker JA, et al. Increasing age is a major risk factor for haemorrhagic complications following pulmonary embolism thrombolysis. *Am Heart J* 1997;134:69-72.
105. Comerota AJ, Throm RE, Mathias SD, et al. Catheter-directed thrombolysis for iliofemoral deep vein thrombosis improves quality of life. *J Vasc Surg* 2000;32:130-137.
106. Bjarnason H, Kruse JR, Asinger DA, et al. Iliofemoral deep venous thrombosis: safety and efficacy outcome during 5 years of catheter-directed thrombolytic therapy. *J Vasc Interv Radiol* 1997;8:405-418.
107. Delomez M, Beregi JP, Willoteaux S, et al. Mechanical thrombectomy in patients with deep venous thrombosis. *Cardiovasc Intervent Radiol* 2001;24:42-48.
108. Ganger KH, Nachbur BH, Ris HB, et al. Surgical thrombectomy versus conservative treatment for deep venous thrombosis; functional comparison of long-term results. *Eur J Vasc Surg* 1989;3:529-538.
109. Hold M, Bull PG, Raynoschek H, Denck H. Deep venous thrombosis: results of thrombectomy versus medical therapy. *Vasa* 1992;21:181-187.
110. Glazier RL, Crowell EB. Randomized prospective trial of continuous or intermittent heparin therapy. *JAMA* 1976;236:1365-1367.
111. Raschke RA, Reilly BM, Guidry JR, et al. The weight-based heparin dosing nomogram compared with a "standard care" nomogram: a randomized controlled trial. *Ann Intern Med* 1993;119:874-881.
112. Zidane M, Schram MT, Planken EW, et al. Frequency of major hemorrhage in patients treated with unfractionated intravenous heparin for deep vein thrombosis or pulmonary embolism: a study in routine clinical practice. *Arch Intern Med* 2000;160:2369-2373.
113. Warkentin TE, Levine MN, Hirsh J, et al. Heparin-induced thrombocytopenia in patients treated with low-molecular-weight heparin or unfractionated heparin. *N Engl J Med* 1995;332:1330-1335.
114. Walenga JM, Bick RL. Heparin-induced thrombocytopenia, paradoxical thromboembolism, and other side effects of heparin therapy. *Med Clin North Am* 1998;82:635-658.
115. Lewis BE, Wallis DE, Berkowitz SD, et al. Argatroban anticoagulant therapy in patients with heparin-induced thrombocytopenia. *Circulation* 2001;103:1838-1843.
116. Weitz JI. Low-molecular-weight heparins. *N Engl J Med* 1997;337:688-698.
117. Warkentin TE, Levine MN, Hirsh J, et al. Heparin-induced thrombocytopenia in patients treated with low-molecular-weight heparin or unfractionated heparin. *N Engl J Med* 1995;332:1330-1335.
118. Monreal M, Lafoz E, Olive A, et al. Comparison of subcutaneous unfractionated heparin with a low molecular weight heparin (Fragmin) in patients with venous thromboembolism and contraindications to coumarin. *Thromb Haemost* 1994;71:7-11.
119. Breddin HK, Hach-Wunderle V, Nakov R, et al. Effects of a low molecular weight heparin on thrombus regression and recurrent thromboembolism in patients with deep vein thrombosis. *N Engl J Med* 2001;344:626-631.
120. Bossuyt PM, Prins MH. Does low-molecular-weight heparin reduce the costs of venous thromboembolism treatment? *Haemostasis* 2000;30:136-140.
121. van der Meer FJM, Rosendaal FR, Vandenbroucke JP, Briët E. Bleeding complications in oral anticoagulant therapy: an analysis of risk factors. *Arch Intern Med* 1993;153:1557-1562.
122. Levine MN, Raskob G, Landefeld S, Hirsh J. Hemorrhagic complications of anticoagulant treatment. *Chest* 1995;108(Suppl 4): 276S-290S.
123. Fihn SD, McDonell M, Martin D, et al. Risk factors for complications of chronic anticoagulation: a multicenter study. Warfarin Optimized Outpatient Follow-up Study Group. *Ann Intern Med* 1993;118:511-520.
124. Fihn SD, Callahan CM, Martin DC, et al. The risk for and severity of bleeding complications in elderly patients treated with warfarin: the National Consortium of Anticoagulation Clinics. *Ann Intern Med* 1996;124:970-979.
125. Chan YC, Valenti D, Mansfield AO, Stansby G. Warfarin induced skin necrosis. *Br J Surg* 2000;87:266-272.
126. Direct Thrombin Inhibitor Trialists' Collaborative Group. Direct thrombin inhibitors in acute coronary syndromes: principal results of a meta-analysis based on individual patients' data. *Lancet* 2002;359:294-302.
127. Heit JA, Colwell CW, Francis CW, et al. Comparison of the oral direct thrombin inhibitor ximelagatran with enoxaparin as prophylaxis against venous thromboembolism after total knee replacement. *Arch Intern Med* 2001;161:2215-2221.
128. Bauer KA, Eriksson BI, Lassen MR, Turpie AG. Fondaparinux compared with enoxaparin for the prevention of venous thromboembolism after elective major knee surgery. *N Engl J Med* 2001;345:1305-1310.
129. Schulman S, Rhedin AS, Lindmarker P, et al. A comparison of six weeks with six months of oral anticoagulant therapy after a first episode of venous thrombosis: duration of Anticoagulation Trial Study Group. *N Engl J Med* 1995;332:1661-1665.
130. Kearon C, Gent M, Hirsh J, et al. A comparison of three months of anticoagulation with extended anticoagulation for a first episode of idiopathic venous thromboembolism. *N Engl J Med* 1999;340:901-907.
131. Couturaud F, Kearon C. Long-term treatment for venous thromboembolism. *Curr Opin Hematol* 2000;7:302-308.
132. Schulman S, Granqvist S, Holmström M, et al. The duration of oral anticoagulant therapy after a second episode of venous thromboembolism. *N Engl J Med* 1997;336:393-398.
133. Lopaciuk S, Bielska-Falda H, Noszczyk W, et al. Low molecular weight heparin versus acenocoumarol in the secondary prophylaxis of deep vein thrombosis. *Thromb Haemost* 1999;81:26-31.
134. Pini M, Aiello S, Manotti C, et al. Low molecular weight heparin versus warfarin in the prevention of recurrences after deep vein thrombosis. *Thromb Haemost* 1994;72:191-197.
135. Hull R, Delmore T, Genton E, et al. Warfarin sodium versus low-dose heparin in the long-term treatment of venous thrombosis. *N Engl J Med* 1979;301:855-858.
136. Hull R, Delmore T, Carter C, et al. Adjusted subcutaneous heparin versus warfarin sodium in the long-term treatment of venous thrombosis. *N Engl J Med* 1982;306:189-194.
137. Brandjes DP, Büller HR, Heijboer H, et al. Randomised trial of effect of compression stockings in patients with symptomatic proximal vein thrombosis. *Lancet* 1997;349:759-762.
138. Wells PS, Lensing AWA, Hirsch J. Graduated compression stockings in the prevention of postoperative VTE: a meta-analysis. *Arch Intern Med* 1994;154:67-72.
139. Perrier A, Desmarais S, Miron MJ, et al. Noninvasive diagnosis of venous thromboembolism. *Lancet* 1999;353:190-195.
140. Oudkerk M, van Beek EJ, van Putten WL, Büller HR. Cost-effectiveness analysis of various strategies in the diagnostic management of pulmonary embolism. *Arch Intern Med* 1993;153:947-954.
141. Miniati M, Prediletto R, Formichi B, et al. Accuracy of clinical assessment in the diagnosis of pulmonary embolism. *Am J Respir Crit Care Med* 1999;159:864-871.
142. Stein PD, Henry JW. Clinical characteristics of patients with acute pulmonary embolism stratified according to their presenting syndromes. *Chest* 1997;112:974-979.
143. Stein PD, Goldhaber SZ, Henry JW. Alveolar–arterial oxygen gradient in the assessment of acute pulmonary embolism. *Chest* 1995;107:139-143.
144. Sijens PE, van Ingen HE, van Beek EJ, et al. Rapid ELISA assay for plasma D-dimer in the diagnosis of segmental and subsegmental pulmonary embolism: a comparison with pulmonary angiography. *Thromb Haemost* 2000;84:156-159.
145. Wells PS, Anderson DR, Rodger M, et al. Excluding pulmonary embolism at the bedside without diagnostic imaging: management of patients with suspected pulmonary embolism presenting to the emergency department by using a simple clinical model and D-dimer. *Ann Intern Med* 2001;135:98-107.
146. Perrier A, Roy PM, Sanchez O, et al. Multidetector row computed tomography in suspected pulmonary embolism. *N Engl J Med* 2005;352:1760-1768.
147. Wells PS, Anderson DR, Rodger M, et al. Excluding pulmonary embolism at the bedside without diagnostic imaging: management of patients with suspected pulmonary embolism presenting to the emergency department by using a simple clinical model and D-dimer. *Ann Intern Med* 2001;135:98-107.
148. Gottschalk A, Sostman HD, Coleman RE, et al. Ventilation–perfusion scintigraphy in the PIOPED study. Part II. Evaluation of the scintigraphic criteria and interpretations. *J Nucl Med* 1993;34:1119-1126.
149. Stein PD, Fowler SE, Goodman LR, et al. Multidetector computer tomography for acute pulmonary embolism. *N Engl J Med* 2006;354:2317-2327.
150. Hull RD, Raskob GE. Low-probability lung scan findings: a need for change. *Ann Intern Med* 1991;114:142-143.

151. van Beek EJR, Brouwers EMJ, Bongaerts AH, Oudkerk M. Lung scintigraphy and helical computed tomography in the diagnosis of pulmonary embolism: a meta-analysis. *Clin Appl Thromb Hemost* 2001;7:87-92.
152. van Beek EJR, Brouwers E, Song B, et al. Clinical validity of a normal pulmonary angiogram in patients with suspected pulmonary embolism: a critical review. *Clin Radiol* 2001;56:838-842.
153. Rathbun SW, Raskob GE, Whitsett TL. Sensitivity and specificity of helical computed tomography in the diagnosis of pulmonary embolism: a systematic review. *Ann Intern Med* 2000;132:227-232.
154. Gupta A, Frazer CK, Ferguson JM, et al. Acute pulmonary embolism: diagnosis with MR angiography. *Radiology* 1999;210:353-359.
155. Oudkerk M, van Beek EJR, Wielopolski P, et al. Comparison of contrast-enhanced MRA and DSA for the diagnosis of pulmonary embolism: results of a prospective study in 141 consecutive patients with an abnormal perfusion lung scan. *Lancet* 2002;11(359):1643-1647.
156. Pedersen MR, Fisher MT, van Beek EJR. MR imaging of the pulmonary vasculature: an update. *Eur Radiol* 2006;16:1374-1386.
157. Wells PS, Anderson DR, Rodger M, et al. Derivation of a simple clinical model to categorize patients probability of pulmonary embolism: increasing the model's utility with the SimpliRED D-dimer. *Thromb Haemost* 2000;83:416-420.
158. Gibson NS, Sohne M, Kruip MJH, et al. Further validation and simplification of the Wells clinical decision rule in pulmonary embolism. *J Thomb Haemost* 2007;5(Suppl 2). P-M-535 [abstract].
159. Wicki J, Perneger TV, Junod AF, et al. Assessing clinical probability of pulmonary embolism in the emergency ward: a simple score. *Arch Intern Med* 2001;161:92-97.
160. Le Gal G, Righini M, Roy PM, et al. Prediction of pulmonary embolism in the emergency department: the revised Geneva score. *Ann Intern Med* 2006;144:165-171.
161. Tamariz LJ, Eng J, Segal JB. Usefulness of clinical prediction rules for the diagnosis of venous thromboembolism: a systematic review. *Am J Med* 2004;117:676-684.
162. Turkstra F, Kuijer PMM, van Beek EJR, et al. Value of compression ultrasonography for the detection of deep venous thrombosis in patients suspected of having pulmonary embolism. *Ann Intern Med* 1997;126:775-781.
163. Prandoni P, Noventa F, Ghirarduzzi A, et al. The risk of recurrent venous thromboembolism after discontinuing anticoagulation in patients with acute proximal deep vein thrombosis or pulmonary embolism: a prospective cohort study in 1626 patients. *Haematologica* 2007;92:199-205.
164. Douketis JD, Gu CS, Schulman S, et al. The risk for fatal pulmonary embolism after discontinuing anticoagulant therapy for venous thromboembolism. *Ann Intern Med* 2007;147:766-774.
165. Jardin F, Gurdjian F, Desfonds P, et al. Hemodynamic factors influencing arterial hypoxemia in massive pulmonary embolism with circulatory failure. *Circulation* 1979;59:909-912.
166. Ozier Y, Dubourg O, Farcot JC, et al. Circulatory failure in acute pulmonary embolism. *Intens Care Med* 1984;10:91-97.
167. Mercat A, Diehl JL, Meyer G, et al. Hemodynamic effects of fluid loading in acute massive pulmonary embolism. *Crit Care Med* 1999;27:540-544.
168. Jardin F, Genevray B, Brun-Ney D, Margairaz A. Dobutamine: a hemodynamic evaluation in pulmonary embolism shock. *Crit Care Med* 1985;13:1009-1012.
169. Layish DT, Tapson VF. Pharmacologic hemodynamic support in massive pulmonary embolism. *Chest* 1997;111:218-224.
170. Smulders YM. Pathophysiology and treatment of haemodynamic instability in acute pulmonary embolism: the pivotal role of pulmonary vasoconstriction. *Cardiovasc Res* 2000;48:23-33.
171. Weimann J, Zink W, Gebhard MM, et al. Effects of oxygen and nitric oxide inhalation in a porcine model of recurrent microembolism. *Acta Anaesthesiol Scand* 2000;44:1109-1115.
172. Capellier G, Jacques T, Balvay P, et al. Inhaled nitric oxide in patients with pulmonary embolism. *Intens Care Med* 1997;23:1089-1092.
173. Verstraete M, Miller GAH, Bounameaux H, et al. Intravenous and intrapulmonary recombinant tissue–type plasminogen activator in the treatment of acute massive pulmonary embolism. *Circulation* 1988;77:353-360.
174. Goldhaber SZ, Haire WD, Feldstein ML, et al. Alteplase versus heparin in acute pulmonary embolism: randomised trial assessing right-ventricular function and pulmonary perfusion. *Lancet* 1993;341:507-511.
175. Jerjes-Sanchez C, Ramirez-Rivera A, De Lourdes Garcia M, et al. Streptokinase and heparin versus heparin alone in massive pulmonary embolism: a randomized controlled trial. *J Thromb Thrombolys* 1995;2:227-229.
176. Thistlethwaite PA, Kemp A, Du L, et al. Outcomes of pulmonary endarterectomy for treatment of extreme thromboembolic pulmonary hypertension. *J Thorac Cardiovasc Surg* 2006;131:307-313.
177. Uflacker R. Interventional therapy for pulmonary embolism. *J Vasc Interv Radiol* 2001;12:147-164.
178. Goldhaber SZ, Haire WD, Feldstein ML, et al. Alteplase versus heparin in acute pulmonary embolism: a randomized trial assessing right-ventricular function and pulmonary perfusion. *Lancet* 1993;341: 507-511.
179. Investigators Columbus. Low molecular weight heparin in the treatment of patients with venous thromboembolism. *N Engl J Med* 1997;337:657-662.
180. Simonneau G, Sors H, Charbonnier B, et al. A comparison of low molecular weight heparin with unfractionated heparin for acute pulmonary embolism. *N Engl J Med* 1997;337:663-669.
181. Barritt DW, Jordan SC. Clinical features of pulmonary embolism. *Lancet* 1961;1:729-732.
182. Bovyn G, Gory P, Reynaud P, et al. The tempofilter: a multicenter study of a new temporary caval filter implantable for up to six weeks. *Ann Vasc Surg* 1997;11:520-528.
183. Spence LD, Gironta MG, Malde HM, et al. Acute upper extremity deep venous thrombosis: safety and effectiveness of superior vena caval filters. *Radiology* 1999;210:53-58.
184. Ascher E, Hingorani A, Tsemekhin B, et al. Lessons learned from a 6 year clinical experience with superior vena cava Greenfield filters. *J Vasc Surg* 2000;32:881-887.
185. Decousus H, Leizorovicz A, Parent F, et al. A clinical trial of vena cava filters with prevention of pulmonary embolism in patients with proximal deep vein thrombosis. *N Engl J Med* 1998;338:409-415.
186. Ballew KA, Philbrick JT, Becker DM. Vena cava filter devices. *Clin Chest Med* 1995;16:295-305.
187. Athanasoulis CA, Kaufman JA, Halpern EF, et al. Inferior vena caval filters: review of a 26 year single center clinical experience. *Radiology* 2000;216:54-66.
188. Greenfield LJ, Delucia A III. Endovascular therapy of venous thromboembolic disease. *Surg Clin North Am* 1992;72:969-989.
189. Stallworth JM, Bradham GB, Kletke RR, Price RG Jr. Phlegmasia cerulea dolens; a 10 year review. *Ann Surg* 1965;161:802-811.
190. Brockman SK, Vasko JS. Phlegmasia cerulea dolens. *Surg Gynecol Obstet* 1965;121:1347-1356.
191. Brockman SK, Vasko JS. The pathological physiology of phlegmasia cerulea dolens. *Surgery* 1966;59:997-1007.
192. Anderson LA. Ischemic venous thrombosis: its hidden agenda. *J Vasc Nurs* 1999;17:1-5.
193. Hirschmann JV. Ischaemic forms of acute venous thrombosis. *Arch Dermatol* 1987;123:933-936.
194. Perkins JMT, Magee TR, Galland RB. Phlegmasia caerulea dolens and venous gangrene. *Br J Surg* 1996;83:19-23.
195. Hood DB, Weaver FA, Modrall JG, Yellin AE. Advances in the treatment of phlegmasia cerulea dolens. *Am J Surg* 1993;166:206-210.
196. Wlodarczyk ZK, Gibson M, Dick R, Hamilton G. Low dose intra-arterial thrombolytic therapy in the treatment of phlegmasia caerulea dolens. *Br J Surg* 1994;81:370-372.
197. Danilenko-Dixon DR, Heit JA, Silverstein MD, et al. Risk factors for deep vein thrombosis and pulmonary embolism during pregnancy or post partum: a population-based, case-control study. *Am J Obstet Gynecol* 2001;184:104-110.
198. Ginsberg JS, Hirsh J, Rainbow AJ, et al. Risks to fetus of radiological procedures used in the diagnosis of maternal venous thromboembolic disease. *Thromb Haemost* 1989;61:189-196.
199. Burns MM. Emerging concepts in the diagnosis and management of venous thromboembolism during pregnancy. *J Thromb Thrombolys* 2000;10:59-68.
200. Lepercq J, Conard J, Borel-Derlon A, et al. Venous thromboembolism during pregnancy: a retrospective study of enoxaparin safety in 624 pregnancies. *BJOG* 2001;108:1134-1140.
201. AbuRahma AF, Boland JP. Management of deep vein thrombosis of the lower extremity in pregnancy: a challenging dilemma. *Am Surg* 1999;65:164-167.
202. Geerts WH, Heit JA, Clagett GP, et al. Prevention of venous thromboembolism. *Chest* 2001;119(Suppl):132S-175S.
203. Gillies TE, Ruckley CV, Nixon SJ. Still missing the boat with fatal pulmonary embolism. *Br J Surg* 1996;83:1394-1395.
204. Butson ARC. Intermittent pneumatic calf compression for prevention of deep venous thrombosis in general abdominal surgery. *Am J Surg* 1981;142:525-527.

205. Taberner DA, Poller L, Burslem RW, et al. Oral anticoagulants controlled by the British comparative thromboplastin versus low-dose heparin in prophylaxis of deep venous thrombosis. *BMJ* 1978;1:272-274.
206. Koch A, Bouges S, Ziegler S, et al. Low molecular weight heparin and unfractionated heparin in thrombosis prophylaxis after major surgical intervention: update of previous meta-analyses. *Br J Surg* 1997;84:750-759.
207. Anonymous. Prevention of pulmonary embolism and deep vein thrombosis with low dose aspirin: Pulmonary Embolism Prevention (PEP) trial. *Lancet* 2000;355:1295-1302.
208. Westrich GH, Haas SB, Mosca P, Peterson M. Meta-analysis of thromboembolic prophylaxis after total knee arthroplasty. *J Bone Joint Surg Br* 2000;82:795-800.

chapter 48

Soft-Tissue Vascular Malformations

Gilles Soulez, MD, MSc • Josée Dubois, MD • Vincent L. Oliva, MD

Key Points

- Classification of vascular malformation
- Histology and genetics
- Investigation of vascular malformation
- Clinical examination
- Imaging studies
- Radiography
- Doppler ultrasound
- Magnetic resonance imaging
- Computed tomography scan
- Angiography and phlebography
- Low-flow vascular malformations
- Venous malformations
- Clinical presentation
- Coagulopathy
- Pathology
- Imaging
- Plain films
- Doppler ultrasound
- Computed tomography scan
- Magnetic resonance imaging
- Direct percutaneous phlebography
- Peripheral phlebography
- Arteriography
- Treatment
- Medical treatment
- Sclerotherapy
- Surgical resection
- Laser therapy
- Capillary malformations
- Lymphatic malformations
- High-flow malformations
- Arteriovenous malformations
- Associated syndromes
- Syndromes associated with vascular stains and low-flow vascular malformation
- Syndromes associated with vascular stains and high-flow malformation
- Syndromes without vascular stain associated with venous, lymphatic, or mixed malformations
- Conclusion

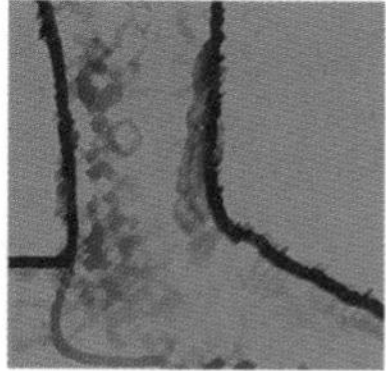

Vascular malformations comprise a spectrum of lesions involving all parts of the body. In the past, diagnosis and treatment of vascular abnormalities were hampered by considerable confusion due to the use of complex hybrid terminology. A biological classification has helped resolve the confusion regarding terminology in the field of vascular anomalies. On the basis of cellular kinetics and clinical behavior, Mulliken and Glowacki proposed in 1982 the most helpful classification for vascular abnormalities.[1,2] They classified vascular anomalies in two major categories: vascular tumors (lesions that arises by endothelial hyperplasia) and vascular malformations (lesions that arise by dysmorphogenesis and exhibit normal endothelial turnover).

Hemangioma is the most common vascular tumor, occurring in the skin of 4% to 10% of infants.[2] Infants have early rapid growth during the first year of life and stabilize at 2 years, followed by slow regression from 2 to 7 years of age. The term hemangioma must be applied only to this pediatric entity.

Vascular malformations are localized or diffuse errors of embryonic developments at some stage of either vasculogenesis or angiogenesis. They presumably are present at birth, although they may not become evident until adolescence or adulthood, and they persist throughout life. They are the most often encountered vascular anomalies in adult patients.[2] Malformations, unlike hemangiomas, do not regress spontaneously and can result in venous stasis, ischemia, localized consumptive coagulopathy, and skeletal anomalies. Boys and girls are equally affected.

We review in this chapter the clinical and imaging features of vascular malformations and discuss the available therapeutic options and their relative indications.

Table 48-1
Vascular Anomalies*

Vascular Tumors	Vascular Malformations	
Hemangioma	Simple	Combined
Proliferative phase	Capillary malformation	AVF, AVM, CVM, CLVM
Involutive phase	Lymphatic malformation (macro, micro, mixed)	LVM, CAVM, CLAVM
Others	Venous malformation	

*AVF, arteriovenous fistula; AVM, arteriovenous malformation; CAVM, capillary–arteriovenous malformation (Parkes Weber syndrome); CLAVM, capillary–lymphatic–arteriovenous malformation; CLVM, capillary–lymphatic–venous malformation (Klippel-Trénaunay syndrome); CVM, capillary–venous malformation; LVM, lymphatic–venous malformation.

CLASSIFICATION OF VASCULAR MALFORMATION

Vascular malformation classification based on the histological appearance of the abnormal channel, flow characteristics, and clinical behavior was updated during the 1992 meeting of the International Society for the Study of Vascular Anomalies (Table 48-1).[3]

Vascular malformations are classified as low-flow malformations, including capillary malformations, venous malformations, lymphatic malformations, capillary–venous malformations (CVM), and capillary–lymphatic–venous malformations (CLVM), and as high-flow malformations, including arteriovenous fistula (AVF) and arteriovenous malformations (AVM).

HISTOLOGY AND GENETICS

Vascular malformations result from morphological errors in vascular development. On histological examination, vascular malformation cells are stable, with a slow (normal) turnover and a flat endothelium with a normal thin basal membrane. They have mixtures of dilated sinusoidal lymphatic, venous, and arterial vessels. In addition, vascular malformations are thin walled, having a large lumen lined with a thin layer of pericytes and smooth muscle.[4]

Most vascular malformations are sporadic, but some exhibit Mendelian autosomal dominant inheritance. Molecular studies suggest that vascular malformation are caused by dysfunction of the signaling process that regulate proliferation, differentiation, maturation, and apoptosis of vascular cells.[5] A locus for autosomal dominant multiple cutaneous and mucosal venous malformations, VMCM1, was identified on chromosome 9p21.[6] This mutation causes ligand-independent activation of an endothelial cell–specific receptor tyrosine kinase TIE2.[7] This mutation is likely to occur in vascular malformations. Familial forms of venous malformations with glomus cells (glomangiomas) have also been linked to loss-of-function mutations in glomulin on chromosome 1p21-p22.[8]

On histology, capillary malformations or "port-wine stains" are characterized by dilated, increased number, or both of capillary-like vessels. Autosomal dominant inheritance of capillary malformations allowed mapping of CMC1 locus on 5q13-22.[9] Discovery of the causative gene revealed an unrecognized clinical entity, named capillary malformation–AVM.[10] Families not linked to CMC1 suggest locus heterogeneity.[9] Mutations in RASA1 were identified in six families with inherited atypical cutaneous capillary malformations.[10] Some individuals with this mutation had an additional high-flow lesion, AVM, or Parkes Weber syndrome.[9]

Theories surrounding the genesis of lymphatic malformations include abnormal sequestration of lymphatic sacs, failure of communication of the lymphatic tissues with peripheral draining channels, and abnormal budding of lymphatics in embryogenesis.[4] Lymphatic malformations are usually congenital and often enlarge when infected. No evidence for inheritance exists, suggesting that the possible genetic causes are compatible with life only as somatic mutations in a restricted area of the lymphatic network. They can be associated with Turner syndrome.[11,12] Several candidate genes may be responsible for lymphatic malformations. Vascular endothelial growth factor receptor-3 (VEGFR-3) and its ligands VEGF-C and VEGF-D are clearly involved in lymphangiogenesis.[13] Genetic studies of families with autosomal dominantly inherited congenital lymphedema (Milroy's disease) have proven a nonconservative mutation in the gene expressing VEGFR-3 on chromosome 5q.[14]

Hereditary hemorrhagic telangiectasia, also named Rendu-Osler-Weber disease, is an autosomal dominant disease linked to two causative genes. The mutated gene for hereditary hemorrhagic telangiectasia type 1 has been identified as endoglin, which encodes an endothelial membrane glycoprotein binding the transforming growth factor-β on chromosome 9q33-34.[9] Another locus for hereditary hemorrhagic telangiectasia type 2 maps for chromosome 12q11-14, the site of the activin receptor–like kinase 1 gene of endothelium.[9]

INVESTIGATION OF VASCULAR MALFORMATION

Clinical Examination

Vascular malformations usually present during childhood. Since they are often stimulated by hormonal influences, such as puberty or pregnancy, patients are often seen for the first time in their late teen years or later. Depending on the type of malformation, patients can present with numerous symptoms, including apparition or worsening of a soft-tissue mass, pain, heaviness, pulsation, hemorrhage, distal ischemia, skin discoloration, skin atrophy, and congestive heart failure.[15] On physical examination, the clinician should assess the coloration of the skin, the softness of the mass, the presence of a thrill and of dilated veins and the variation of the mass with the Valsalva maneuver. Scars of previous surgeries should be noted. Examination should include inspection of the whole skin and of the mucous membrane for the presence of telangiectasia or dysplastic veins. Limb-length discrepancy and presence of lymphedema should be noted.

Imaging Studies

Radiography

Radiography can demonstrate the presence of phleboliths, which are typical of venous malformation (Figure 48-1). In a complex syndrome, they can show evidence of hemihypertrophy. Lytic or permeative changes in bone can be

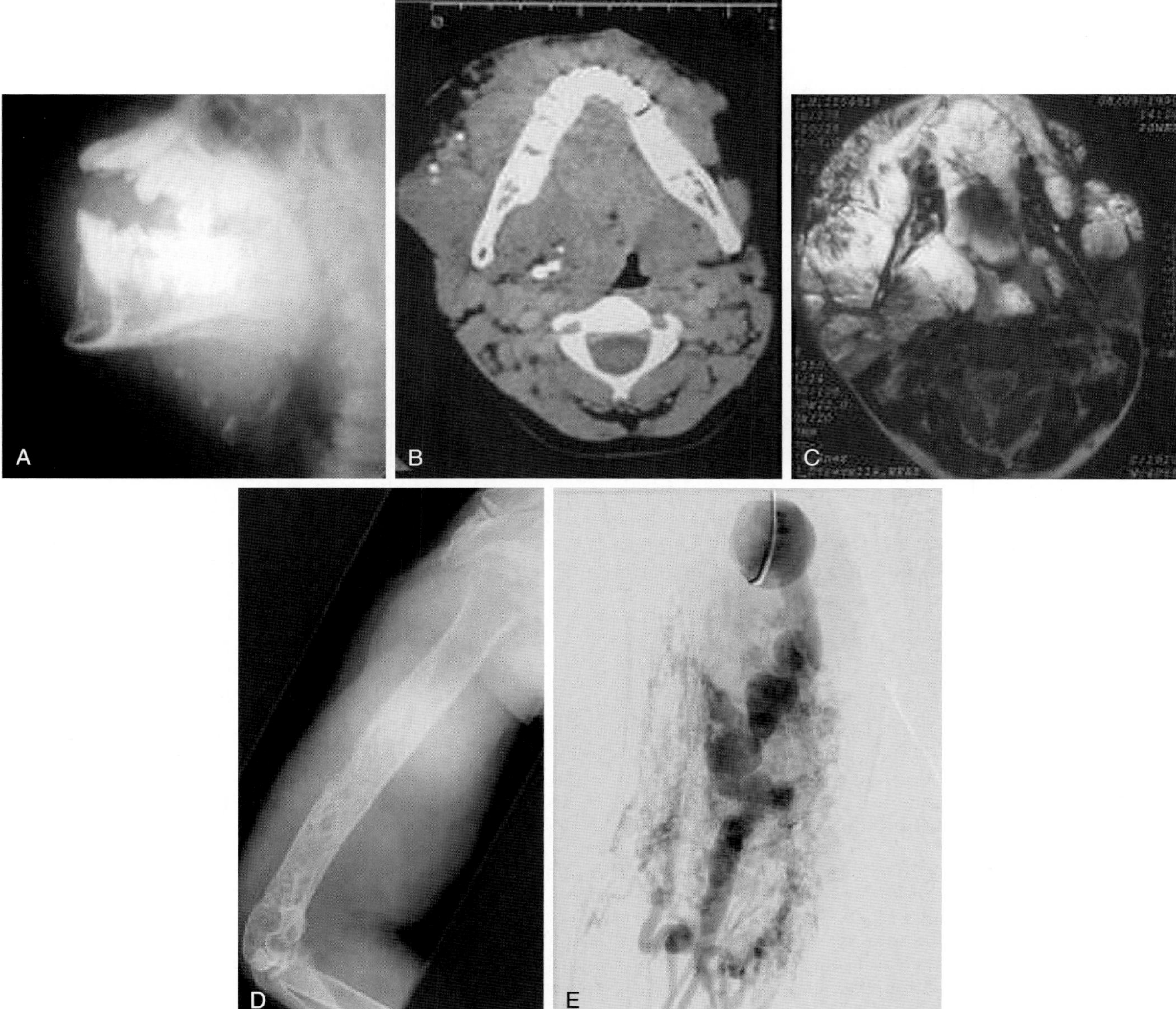

Figure 48-1. **A,** Lateral x-ray of the neck. A large soft-tissue mass around the mandible is seen. The presence of phleboliths is characteristic of a venous malformation. **B,** Computed tomography scan of the face in the same patient. A large soft-tissue mass involving the cheek, the lower lip, the tongue, and the parapharyngeal space is seen. Multiple phleboliths are seen. **C,** T_2-weighted axial magnetic resonance sequence in the same patient, showing a large mass with a strong hypersignal infiltrating the right hemiface, the maxillary and parapharyngeal space, the lower lip, and the tongue and extending into the left portion of the maxillary space, suggesting an extensive venous malformation. **D,** Conventional x-ray of the left arm in another patient, showing multiple serpiginous bone erosions surrounded by sclerotic borders within the humeral bone and a soft-tissue mass suggestive of a vascular anomaly. **E,** Selective catheter angiography of the left axillary artery in the same patient, confirming a high-flow arteriovenous malformation of the arm.

seen in arteriovenous, lymphatic, or venous malformations (Figure 48-1).[15]

Doppler Ultrasound

Doppler ultrasound is the first examination to perform when a vascular malformation is suspected. This inexpensive and noninvasive examination allows differentiation of low-flow and high-flow lesions. Ultrasound also shows whether the lesions are easily accessible for direct puncture to perform sclerotherapy or direct embolization.

Magnetic Resonance Imaging

Magnetic resonance imaging (MRI) is the best method to evaluate the extension of the malformation and its relationship to adjacent structures.[16] It provides an excellent contrast resolution to delineate venous and lymphatic malformations. The presence of flow void on T_1- and T_2-weighted sequence is typically seen in AVMs.[17] The examination should include spin echo T_1- and T_2-weighted sequence with fat suppression. Gradient echo sequence allows differentiation of low-flow from high-flow lesions.[18] In peripheral malformation, fat suppression with short T_1 (inversion-time) inversion recovery

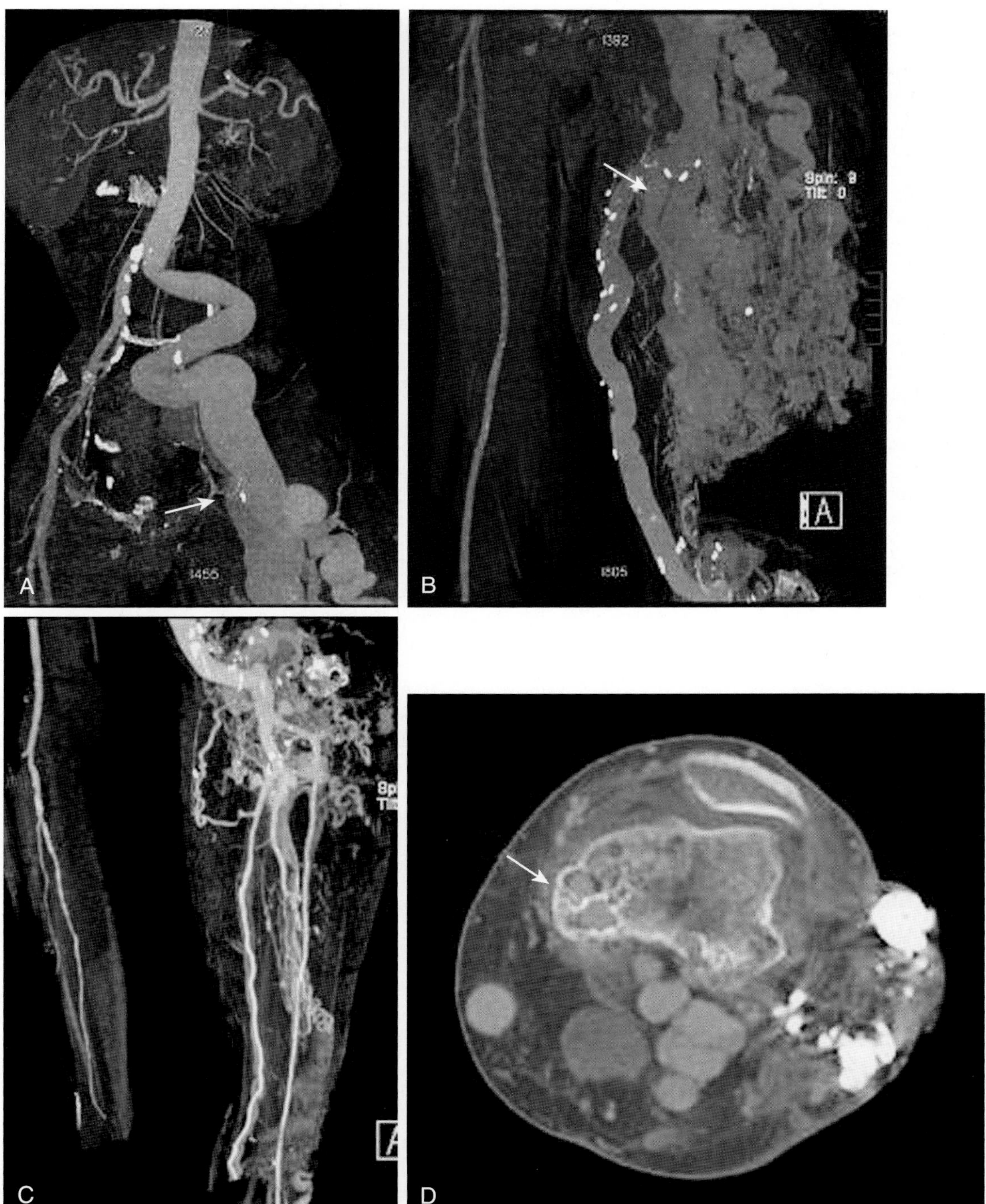

Figure 48-2. Patient with an arteriovenous malformation of the left knee who underwent (in another institution) a ligation of the superficial femoral artery and a femoropopliteal bypass. Clinical deterioration with apparition of an edema of the leg and bleeding episodes from the lateral portion of the knee. **A,** Maximum intensity projection (MIP) of a computed tomography angiography (CTA) examination on the pelvis showing an aneurysmal dilatation of the left external iliac and femoral arteries inducing a compression on the left common femoral vein *(arrow)*. **B,** MIP of a CTA examination on the femoropopliteal station showing the enlarged femoropopliteal bypass and an extensive recruitment of the arteriovenous malformation through the branches of the femoral profundi artery and the distal superficial femoral artery distally to the ligation site *(arrow)*. **C,** MIP of a CTA examination on the infrapopliteal station showing a recruitment of the genicular and tibial recurrent arteries. **D,** Axial image of a CTA examination of the same patient on the distal portion of the femoral bone, showing bone erosion and infiltration by the arteriovenous malformation *(arrow)*.

(STIR) T_2-weighted sequences are very sensitive to demonstrate the extension of venous and lymphatic malformations (LVMs; Figure 48-2). A T_1 sequence with fat suppression after gadolinium enhancement is helpful to evaluate the circulating portion of the malformation. Finally, a three-dimensional gadolinium-enhanced sequence with angiographic reconstruction is helpful to evaluate the vascularization of the malformation.[19] More recently, time-resolved magnetic resonance angiography sequences have been used to appreciate the dynamic circulation of AVM.[20,21]

Computed Tomography Scan

Computed tomography (CT) plays a limited role for the evaluation of vascular anomalies given the inherent lack of soft-tissue detail with CT, and it results in significant exposure to unnecessary ionizing radiation.[16,22] Although last generation, multidetector CT can be valuable to obtain a tridimensional reformation and assess aneurismal dilatation, bone erosion in AVMs, and phleboliths in venous malformations (Figures 48-1 and 48-2).

Angiography and Phlebography

Angiography is indicated in cases of high-flow malformation to demonstrate the degree of arteriovenous shunting, the presence of macrofistulas or microfistulas, and the lesion's nidus. It can also determine whether embolization is feasible and safe.[16,22] Selective and hyperselective angiography is mandatory before initiating any endovascular or surgical treatment of AVMs. Angiography is also useful in complex malformation to demonstrate presence of AVF or capillary staining.

Phlebography by direct puncture of the malformation is useful before sclerotherapy of venous malformation to evaluate the extent of the malformation and its venous drainage (Figure 48-3).[16,22] Lymphography and lymphoscintigraphy, although useful for the assessment of lymphedema, are rarely used in the evaluation and treatment of lymphatic malformations.[4]

LOW-FLOW VASCULAR MALFORMATIONS

Low-flow vascular malformations include primarily venous, capillary, lymphatic, and various combined malformations.

Venous Malformations

A venous malformation is classified as a simple malformation with slow flow and an abnormal venous network. The old denomination "cavernous hemangioma" is no longer appropriate and must be abandoned. Venous malformations are the most prevalent vascular malformation and have a propensity for the head and neck region, but they can be found anywhere in the body.[2,22,23]

Clinical Presentation

Venous malformations are characterized by a soft, compressible, nonpulsatile tissue mass. The overlying skin usually has a bluish tint, but occasionally it may appear normal (Figure 48-3). The main locations are the head and neck (40%), trunk (20%), and extremities (40%). Characteristically, venous malformations expand after Valsalva maneuver or if they are in a dependent position and may be flattened by pressure. Over time, they tend to grow proportionally with the growth of patients. They often enlarge during puberty and pregnancy (hormonal influence) and do not regress. Symptoms are related to size and location. Although most venous malformations are in the skin and subcutaneous tissues, they also often involve underlying muscle, bone, and abdominal viscera. Most venous malformations are solitary, but multiple cutaneous or visceral lesions can occur.

Deep cutaneous or intramuscular lesions usually cause discomfort, often at the end of the day or with exertion. Intraoral venous malformations can bleed, distort dentition, cause speech problems, or obstruct the upper airway and pharynx.[2] Swelling and pain are common in venous malformations. Phlebothrombosis is also a common and painful occurrence for the patient.[24]

Familial multiple glomangiomas present as multiple, often tender, blue nodular dermal lesions in the skin located on the extremities.[25] They involve skin, subcutis, and rarely mucosa. They are commonly multifocal, often hyperkeratotic, and painful on palpation. They cannot be completely emptied by compression.[26]

Only symptomatic venous malformations or lesions causing important aesthetic prejudice should be treated.

Coagulopathy

A coagulation profile should be performed for any patient with an extensive venous malformation, especially one with a history of easy bruising or bleeding. Stagnation within a venous malformation can cause localized intravascular coagulopathy (LIC).[3,27] Local activation of the coagulation is caused by altered endothelium within the vascular malformation or secondary to venous stasis and acidosis. In a series of 24 patients with diffused limb venous malformations, Mazoyer et al. have found evidence of LIC characterized by a decrease in fibrinogen (0.5 to 1 g/L), an increase in D-dimers (2 to 64 μg/ml), and the presence of a soluble complex of fibrin.[27] Platelet counts were normal or slightly decreased.[27] A correlation occurred between the size of the venous malformation and the severity of LIC. Conversion of LIC to disseminated intravascular coagulation, with bleeding related to factor consumption and multiorgan failure related to disseminated microvascular thrombosis, can be observed after sclerotherapy, surgery, bone fracture, prolonged immobilization, and pregnancy or even be triggered by menstruation. Worsening of LIC can translate in pain exacerbation, thrombosis, and bleeding at wound sites or during surgery.[27] Consumptive coagulopathy must be detected before any treatment and can be treated with low-molecular-weight heparin and an elastic stocking to limit venous stasis.[3,27]

Pathology

Histopathological examination of venous malformations shows thin-walled, dilated, spongelike channels varying in size from capillary to cavernous dimensions, with sparse smooth muscle cells, adventitial fibrosis, thrombosis, and phleboliths.[3] Smooth-muscle actin staining reveals muscle in clumps instead of the normal smooth muscular architecture. The mural muscular abnormality is probably responsible for the gradual expansion.[3] Histologically, glomangioma is characterized by abnormally differentiated venous smooth muscle cells called glomus cells in the walls of distended venous channels.[9]

Imaging

Plain Films

Plain films usually show a soft-tissue mass with occasional phleboliths and sometimes adjacent skeletal anomalies (Figure 48-1).

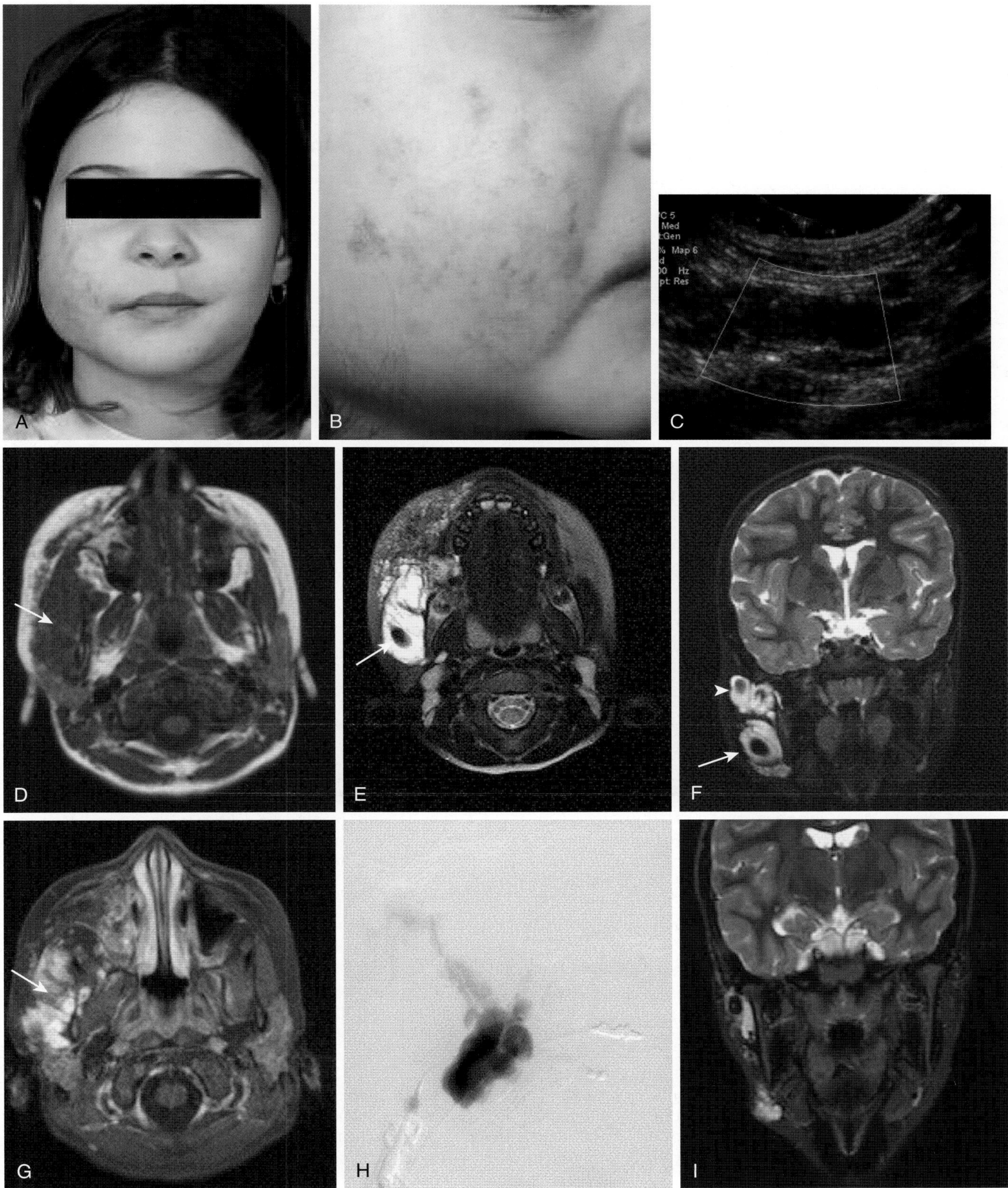

Figure 48-3. Venous malformation of the face. **A,** A soft-tissue lump is observed on the right cheek. **B,** The bluish discoloration of the overlying skin is suggestive of a venous malformation. **C,** Color Doppler ultrasound examination of the right cheek showing an infiltration of soft tissue by a hypoechoic mass with slow flow. **D,** Axial T_1-weighted spin echo magnetic resonance sequence of the maxillary area showing an infiltration of the masseter muscle and subcutaneous fat of the cheek by a soft-tissue mass with a isointense signal *(arrows)*. **E** and **F,** Axial and coronal T_2-weighted magnetic resonance acquisitions showing the malformation with a hyperintense signal. Several areas of hyposignal corresponding to phlebolitis can be seen within the malformation *(arrows)*. **G,** T_1-weighted axial acquisition after contrast injection showing a partial filling of the malformation *(arrow)*. **H,** Percutaneous phlebography performed during a sclerotherapy session showing a cavitary venous malformation. No drainage in central veins is observed. **I,** Coronal T_2-weighted acquisition performed after completion of several sclerotherapy sessions showing an important size reduction of the malformation.

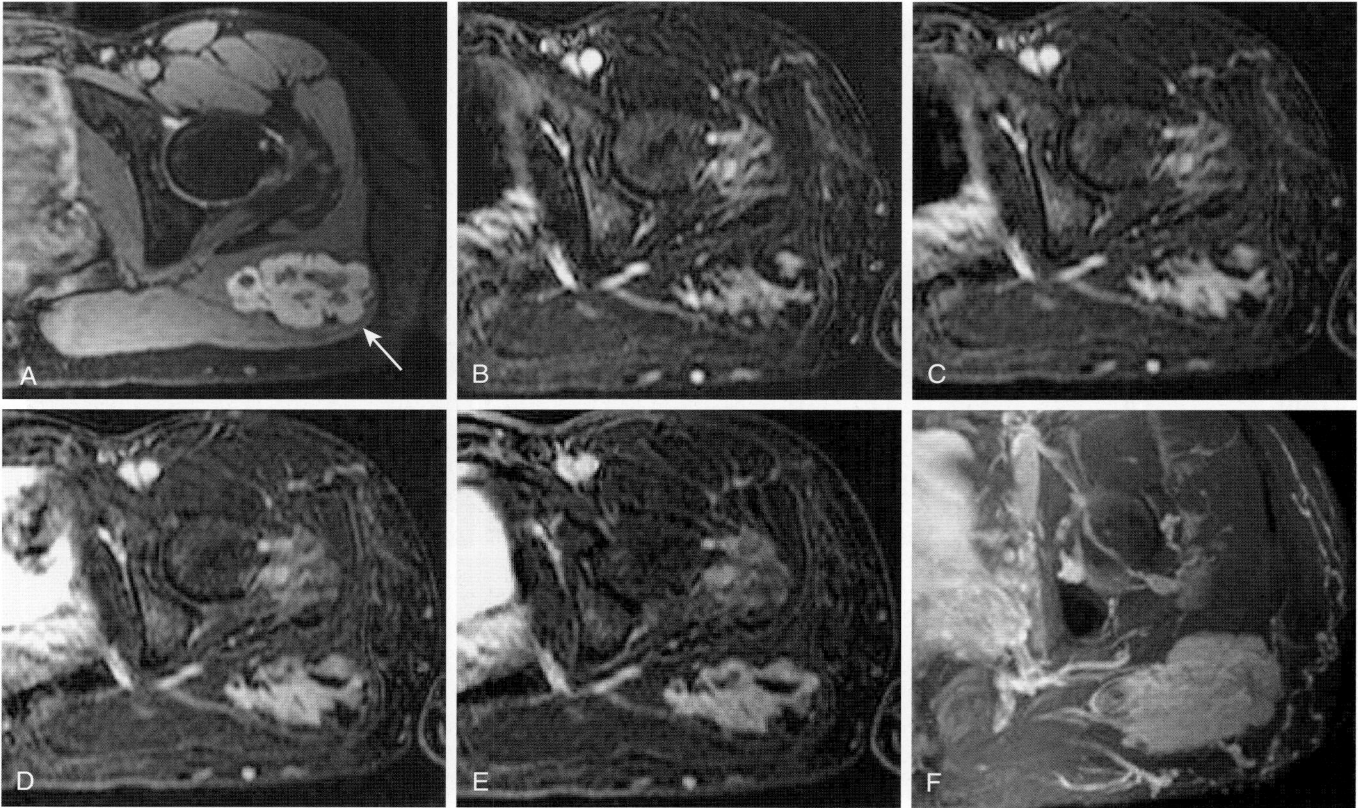

Figure 48-4. Patient presenting a venous malformation of the left buttock. **A,** Axial T_2-weighted magnetic resonance acquisition (multiple-echo data image combination sequence) showing a hyperintense soft-tissue mass in the left gluteal muscle with several phleboliths *(arrow)*. Dynamic volumetric interpolated breath-hold examination acquisition performed after contrast injection at 1 **(B),** 2 **(C),** 5 **(D),** and 10 **(E)** minutes showing a progressive filling of the malformation by gadolinium. **F,** Maximum intensity projection reformation showing the connection of the venous malformation with superficial draining veins.

Doppler Ultrasound

Doppler ultrasound is essential to differentiate venous malformations from other vascular abnormalities. Ultrasonic examination should be performed with a high-frequency linear array transducer (5 to 10 MHz). Exploration begins with a gray-scale examination to delineate the margins of the malformation. Usually, venous malformations appear as compressible hypoechoic or heterogeneous lesions in 80% of the patients (Figure 48-3).[23,28] Anechoic channels can be demonstrated in less than 50% of the cases. Sometimes, isoechoic thickening of the subcutaneous tissues without a solid mass or discernible channels is the only feature. Hyperechoic foci with posterior acoustic shadowing related to phleboliths can be shown in less than 20% of the cases.[23]

In most cases, Doppler ultrasound shows a monophasic low-velocity flow. In 20% of the lesions, no flow can be demonstrated. Flow can be demonstrated by using dynamic maneuvers like Valsalva or manual compression. The absence of flow may reflect thrombosis or be caused by equipment limitation.[23]

Computed Tomography Scan

CT examination usually demonstrates the extension of the lesion, but the contrast resolution is less than with MRI. Venous malformations are hypodense, isodense, or heterogeneous lesions enhancing peripherally and slowly after bolus injection. Phleboliths are more clearly depicted on CT scan images. Fatty components can sometimes be demonstrated on CT scan. If both imaging modalities (CT scan and MRI) are available, MRI is more accurate in assessing the extension of venous malformations.

Magnetic Resonance Imaging

MRI is an excellent modality to define the extension of the lesions and their relationship to adjacent structures. The examination protocol should begin with a spin echo or fast spin echo T_1-weighted sequence for basic anatomical evaluation. The extension of the malformation should be assessed with a T_2-weighted sequence with fat suppression. Fat suppression with a short inversion-time inversion recovery T_2-weighted sequence with a 512 matrix is well suited for this purpose. T_2-weighted gradient echo sequences can also be used to demonstrate calcification or hemosiderin. On gradient echo sequence, the absence of signal in the blood vessel in the vicinity of the malformation suggest a low-flow malformation.[18]

A fast spin echo T_1-weighted sequence with fat suppression should be performed after gadolinium injection to evaluate the perfusion of the malformation. In our institution, we perform a dynamic perfusion study at 1, 2, 5, and 10 minutes after contrast infusion using a volumetric interpolated breath-hold examination sequence (Figure 48-4). These contrast-enhanced three-dimensional acquisitions are also useful to appreciate the drainage of the malformation in the venous system.[29]

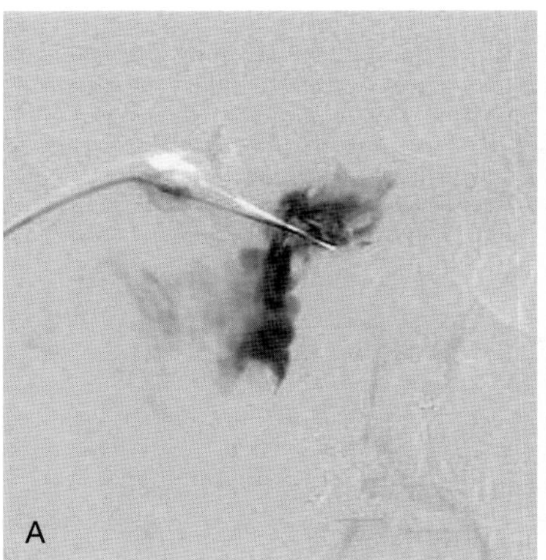

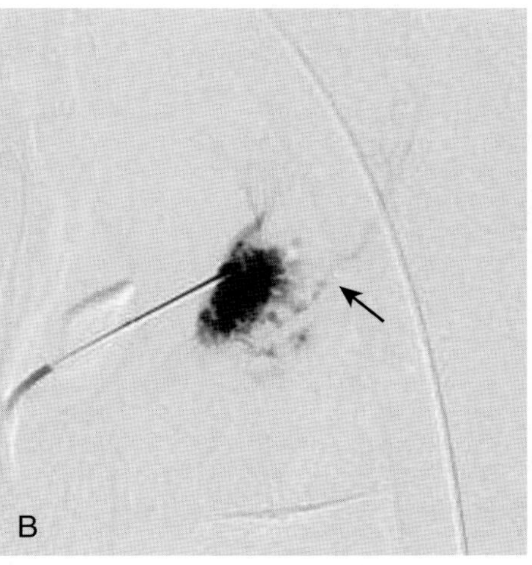

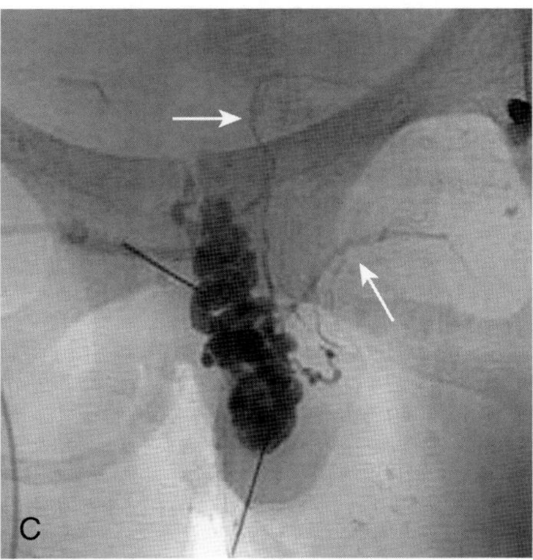

Figure 48-5. Illustration of the common features observed on percutaneous phlebography of venous malformation. **A,** Venous malformation of the right hemiface. Percutaneous phlebography of the infraorbital portion showing a cavitary pattern. **B,** Venous malformation of the left mandibule and lower lip. Percutaneous phlebography of the manibular portion in the same patient showing a honeycomb pattern with a late venous drainage *(arrow)*. **C,** Venous malformation of the left major labia (different patient). Percutaneous phlebography showing an opacification of dysplastic veins draining into normal veins *(arrows)*.

Usually, venous malformations are hypointense or isointense on T_1-weighted sequences. In cases of hemorrhage or thrombosis, a heterogeneous signal can be observed on T_1 sequences. Abnormal veins can be observed in the area of the malformation. On T_2-weighted sequences, venous malformations display a bright signal. Areas of hyposignal can be observed related to thrombosis, septation inside the malformation, or phleboliths. On T_2-weighted sequences, the extension of the malformation into adjacent structures is usually clearly delineated (Figures 48-3 and 48-4).

After sclerotherapy, venous malformations present a heterogeneous signal on either T_1- or T_2-weighted sequences. A delay of up to several months is necessary to evaluate the therapeutic response after sclerotherapy, allowing time for the transient inflammatory reaction to resolve. In most cases, progressive shrinkage of the malformation is observed. Postgadolinium sequences are useful to demonstrate residual perfusion of the malformation and to direct additional treatment.

MRI is sensitive for identifying and assessing the extension of venous malformations, but it is not very specific. Findings must be correlated to the clinical examination and Doppler findings to secure the diagnosis. In cases of atypical clinical or imaging findings, percutaneous phlebography must be performed to confirm the diagnosis. If phlebography is not conclusive, then percutaneous or surgical biopsies must be performed to rule out malignant disease.[15]

Direct Percutaneous Phlebography

Direct percutaneous phlebography can be performed as a diagnostic procedure in cases of atypical venous malformations. It is often performed as the initial step during a sclerotherapy session. Direct puncture of the malformation is performed with a 20- or 21-gauge needle. Ultrasound can be useful for guiding the puncture, especially if the malformation is located deeply in the soft tissues. The needle is connected to a syringe through extension tubing and is progressively withdrawn while applying slight suction. Once blood return is observed, a small amount of low-osmolarity iodinated contrast is injected to obtain a phlebogram.

Three phlebographic patterns can be observed with venous malformation opacification (Figure 48-5)[16,30]:

- The most common appearance is a cavitary pattern with late filling of venous drainage without evidence of abnormal veins.
- The second pattern is a spongy appearance with small honeycomb cavities and late venous drainage.
- The third form is rapid opacification of dysmorphic veins.

Another four-stage classification reported by Puig et al. distinguish type I lesions, representing isolated malformations without discernible venous drainage; type II lesions draining into normal veins; type III lesions draining into dysplastic veins; and type IV lesions consisting primarily or solely of venous ectasia.[31,32]

Peripheral Phlebography

In most cases, peripheral limb phlebography is not helpful for the diagnosis of upper or lower limb venous malformations because most of them are not opacified by peripheral phlebography. In cases with venous malformations composed of dysmorphic veins, it is helpful to demonstrate the venous drainage of the malformation.

Arteriography

Arteriography is usually not required for the diagnosis of venous malformations. It can be normal or can demonstrate dysmorphic veins on the late venous opacification phase. It can be useful in cases of complex malformations such as CVMs or to demonstrate microfistulas. The physiopathology and clinical significance of these microfistulas are unclear. They are probably related to an inflammation secondary to vein thrombosis inducing a local hypervascularization (Figure 48-6).

Treatment

Medical Treatment

Asymptomatic venous malformation should be treated conservatively. The patient must be aware of a potential worsening of the malformation during puberty or pregnancy. Trauma must be avoided on the malformation. Extensive

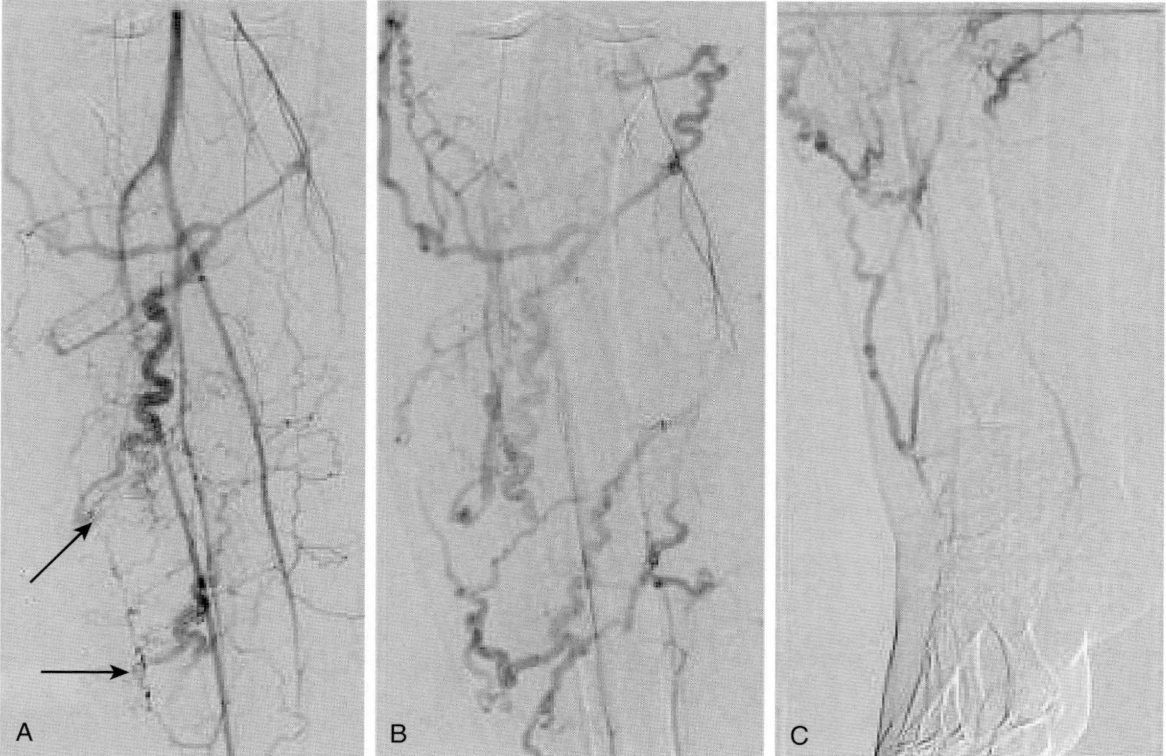

Figure 48-6. Patient presenting with Klippel-Trénaunay syndrome. Since a high-flow Doppler signal was detected in several superficial veins of the calf, an angiography was performed. Multiple microfistulas *(arrows)* arise from the anterior, posterior tibial, and peroneal arteries draining into superficial veins. These microfistulas are probably related to an inflammation secondary to recurrent venous thrombophlebitis. The patient was treated conservatively (nonsteroidal anti-inflammatory drug and elastic stocking).

lower or upper extremity venous malformations should first be treated with elastic stockings. Low-dose aspirin seems to minimize phlebothromboses. Preoperative control of intravascular coagulopathy with low-molecular-weight heparin should be considered before the resection of large venous malformations.[27]

Sclerotherapy

Treatment of venous malformations is indicated when they cause aesthetic problems, pain, or functional problems. Absolute ethanol and sodium tetradecyl sulfate are the most commonly used agents in the United States.[33] Absolute ethanol (dehydrated alcohol, injection USP, 100% v/v; Sandoz Canada, Boucherville, Quebec) is the most destructive sclerosant; it is assumed that it has the lowest recurrence rate. Injection of ethanol produces marked tissue swelling because of intralesional thrombosis and edema.[33] It is painful and necessitates general anesthesia in most cases. Absolute ethanol can be opacified with metrizamide powder; however, this powder can induce permanent skin staining. Intravascular ethanol administration can cause precapillary pulmonary arterial vasospasm, leading to sustained pulmonary hypertension in nearly a third of patients and then to cardiopulmonary collapse and death.[34] Bronchospasm, pulmonary embolus, hyperthermia, death, and intoxication have also been reported.[34] As a guideline, ethanol administration should not exceed 1 ml/kg at any one visit.[35] A less-diffusible alcohol gel solution was developed and gave interesting preliminary results, although no large series reports long-term efficacy.[36]

A detergent sclerosing agent such as sodium tetradecyl sulfate (Thromboject 1% and 3%, Omega, Montreal, Quebec), 1% polidocanol (Aethoxysclerol, Kreussler, Wiesbaden, Germany), or ethanolamine oleate (Ethamolin 5%; Questcor Pharmaceuticals, Union City, California) causes injury by altering the surface tension surrounding endothelial cells. Sodium tetradecyl sulfate is likely less toxic than ethanol because of lower reported rates of skin necrosis, nerve impairment, and systemic complications.[34] Polidocanol has some anesthetic properties and is well tolerated during injection; however, its sclerosing efficacy could be less than sodium tetradecyl sulfate and alcohol.[37] Ethanolamine oleate is a salt of unsaturated fatty acid originally used in gastroesophageal varices as a result of its ability to induce thrombosis by damage to the vascular wall. Compared with ethanol, ethanolamine oleate has less effect on deeper layers of the vascular wall, has no penetrative effect, and is safer to use in situations where vascular structures are close to nerves.[38] This material can cause renal insufficiency, intravascular hemolysis, and hepatotoxicity.

More recently, the technique of foam sclerotherapy using a mix of one of these three last agents (sotradecyl sulfate, ethanolamine oleate, or polidocanol) with lipiodol and room air has been gaining popularity.[39-42] In a recent randomized trial comparing foam versus liquid sclerotherapy, better efficacy using foam sclerotherapy with a lower sclerosing agent dose was reported.[43]

Ethibloc (Ethicon, Norderstedt, Germany), a mixture of zein (a corn protein), alcohol, and contrast medium, is commonly used in Europe and good results have been reported.[30,44]

Since this solution is viscous, it remains static within the lesion and could have less risk of migration in central veins.[30] The main drawback of this agent is its propensity to induce cutaneous fistulization with extrusion of the agent.[30]

Sclerotherapy should be performed by a skilled interventional radiologist under fluoroscopic control. The amount of sclerosing agent required is evaluated by a preliminary phlebography. It is important to avoid filling of drainage veins with the sclerosing agent. When using foam, sclerotherapy injection can be performed using roadmap fluoroscopy to get a substracted fluoroscopy and improve the visualization of sclerosing agent diffusion. A tourniquet or manual compression can be useful in minimizing the passage of the sclerosing agent into the systemic circulation. After alcohol injection, this compression must be released progressively to avoid rapid release of alcohol in the pulmonary circulation.

The feasibility of performing sclerotherapy under magnetic resonance guidance was reported.[45] This approach could be interesting in lesions deeply located and poorly seen under ultrasound, such as intramuscular lesions. C-arm–CT acquisition could be useful adjunct in the angiographic suite to guide needle puncture and assess diffusion of the sclerosing agent within the malformation (Figure 48-7).[46] The main complications of sclerotherapy are cutaneous necrosis and neural toxicity, especially with alcohol.[47] Cutaneous necrosis or blistering is more common when the malformation is blue, indicating extension in the superficial dermis.[33] Systemic complications are rare, are related to the systemic passage of alcohol, and include hemolysis with potential renal toxicity and cardiac arrest.[48] It is recommended to perform sclerotherapy with alcohol with careful monitoring in the presence of an anesthesiologist. Anaphylactic reaction to sodium tetradecyl sulfate injection and cardiac arrest after polidocanol injection have also been reported.[49,50]

Sclerotherapy induces an inflammatory reaction that worsens the symptoms during the week following the intervention. Analgesic and anti-inflammatory (nonsteroidal anti-inflammatory drugs or corticoids) medication must be given to minimize the symptoms. A delay of 1 to 3 months should be observed between each sclerotherapy session.

Venous anomalies have a propensity for recanalization and recurrence. We have observed better results of sclerotherapy with cavitary lesions and dysmorphic vein patterns; furthermore, dysmorphic vein patterns are more prone to recurrence. Spongy patterns, especially when intramuscular, are more difficult to treat.[16] Success rates varying between 30% and 95% have been reported.[34] The variation in sclerotherapy technique also criteria used to define success can explain this variability.

Surgical Resection

Surgery is generally contemplated after sclerotherapy when treatment is incomplete or when an aesthetic prejudice requires correction.[51] Since sclerotherapy may be less effective and compression garments may increase discomfort, the treatment of choice for glomuvenous malformations is surgical resection, which sometimes can be associated with sclerotherapy.[13]

Laser Therapy

Laser therapy can be useful in superficial forms of venous malformations and in oromucosal lesions. Intense, pulsed dye laser is effective for small superficial cutaneous lesions.[52-54] Satisfactory results with minimal scarring, especially to treat skin discoloration, have been reported, but recurrences and repeated treatments are common.[52] When used as a pretreatment, the nd-YAG laser, which has a deeper penetration, can induce shrinkage of the tissue and dermal fibrosis that facilitates the surgical handling of the skin and reduces the risk of skin loss in surgery and sclerotherapy. For deeper lesions, laser probes can be inserted subcutaneously.

Capillary Malformations

Capillary malformations are intradermal vascular anomalies.[55] They were previously named port-wine stains, but this denomination should be abandoned. Capillary malformation should not be confused with macular stain (nevus flammus neonatorium).[56] These pale pink macular stains are composed of ectatic dermal capillaries. They occur in 35% to 50% of newborns and usually regress.[56] Capillary malformations are pink and flat at birth and become more purple, with a tendency to darken, thicken, and become more nodular with age.[57,58] Capillary malformations have irregular borders; they usually involve the face but can occur anywhere on the body. It is important to eliminate complex anomalies that can be associated with capillary malformations such as Sturge-Weber, Klippel-Trénaunay, Parkes Weber, Cobb, and Proteus syndromes. Cutaneous capillary malformations are often associated with hypertrophy of soft tissue and underlying skeleton and glaucoma.[2,58,59] Less common anomalies associated with capillary malformations include underlying spinal dysraphism, which may occur not only in the classic lumbar location but also in the cervical area, when the stain is associated with an underlying mass or pit.[60,61]

Since capillary malformations are superficial, imaging studies are not helpful in making the diagnosis. The role of imaging studies is to eliminate an associated arteriovenous or venous malformation hidden underneath the capillary malformation. In this setting, an ultrasound examination is often recommended.

Capillary malformations causing little esthetic prejudice can be treated conservatively. If the indication is to treat, pulsed dye laser is the treatment of choice.[62] Significant improvement is observed in 70% of patients, and results are better in facial lesions.[2] A recent report promoted the use of intense pulsed light for the treatment of capillary malformations, especially those resistant to prior management with pulsed dye laser therapy.[63] Soft-tissue lesions and skeletal hypertrophy can require surgical correction.

Lymphatic Malformations

We do not discuss lymphedema in this chapter and instead focus on localized congenital lymphatic malformations. These lymphatic malformations are often referred to as lymphangiomas. Lymphatic malformations are usually present at birth (65% to 75%), but sometimes they become evident during childhood or adolescence.[13] There is two clinical types of lymphatic malformation: the macrocystic type (cyst size of more than 2 cm^3; Figure 48-8), misnamed cystic hygroma, and the microcystic type (cyst size less than 2 cm^3; Figure 48-9), which is more infiltrative with clear or hemorrhagic vesicles on top.[3,64] These two types can be combined. Histologically, lymphatic malformations consist of chyle-filled cysts lined with endothelium.[65] Combined LVMs are common.

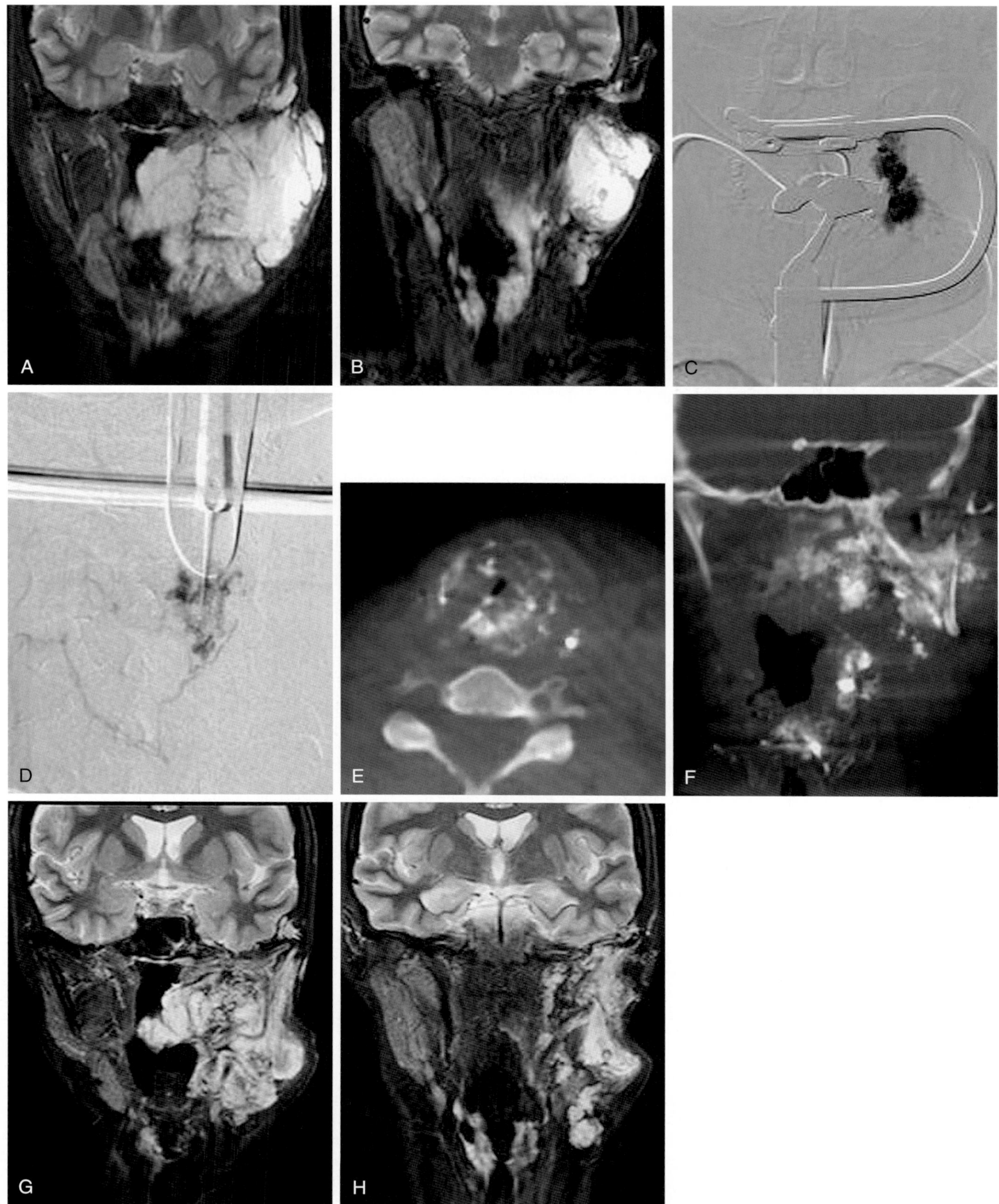

Figure 48-7. Patient presenting a voluminous venous malformation of the left hemiface with symptoms of dysphagia and dyspnea in supine position. **A** and **B,** Magnetic resonance imaging examination showing the extension of the malformation in the nasopharynx, oropharynx, and vocal cords. **C** and **D,** A tracheostomy was performed, and a first sclerotherapy session was directed at the oropharynx, larynx, and vocal cords regions. **E** and **F,** Coronal and axial reformations of C-arm–computed tomography acquisitions showing the diffusion of the sclerosant foam within the malformation. **G** and **H,** Control magnetic resonance imaging examination after three sclerotherapy sessions showing a significant reduction of the venous malformation in the nasopharynx, oropharynx, and larynx compared to the preoperative examination. The patient had an excellent clinical evolution with significant improvement of the lesion in the larynx and vocal cords documented on endoscopy.

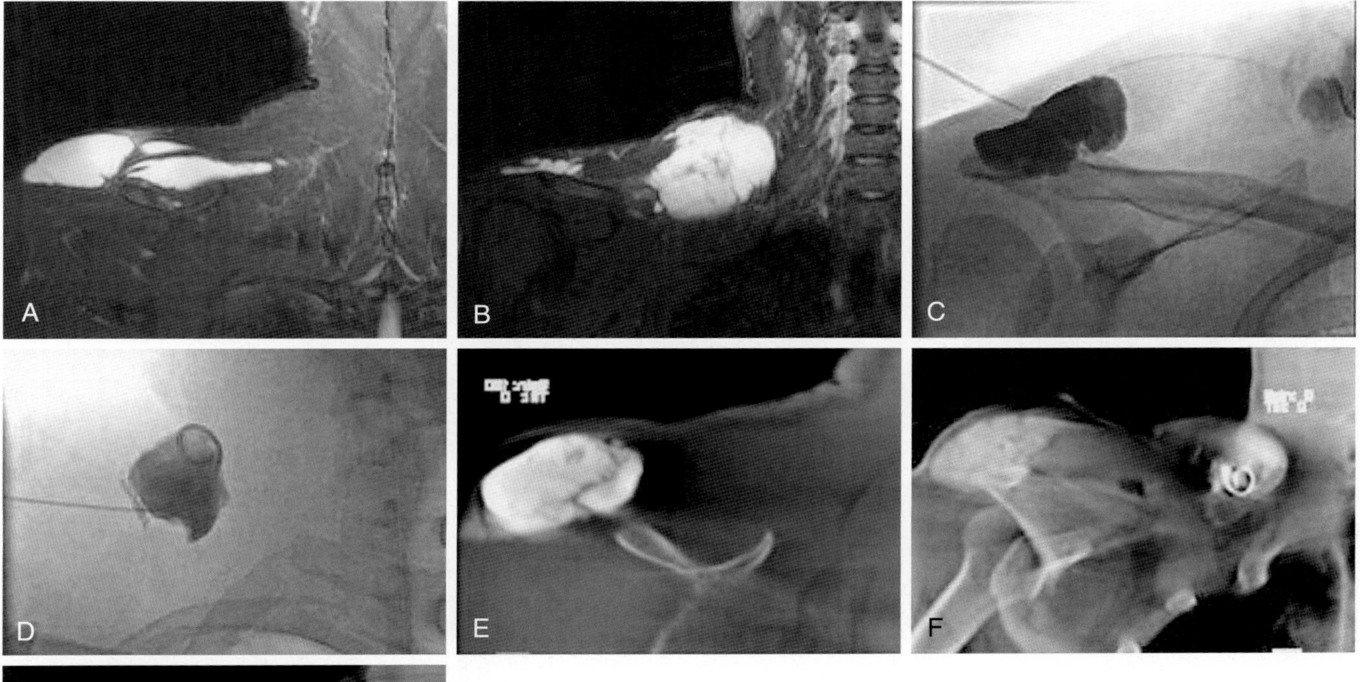

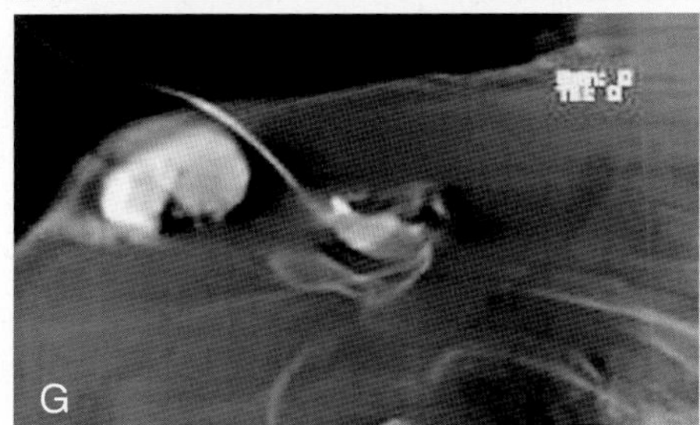

Figure 48-8. Patient presenting a macrocystic lymphangioma of the right cervicothoracic region. **A** and **B,** Coronal short inversion-time inversion recovery magnetic resonance imaging (MRI) acquisitions showing three main cystic components. **C** and **D,** Under ultrasound and fluoroscopic guidance, only two cystic components were drained and injected with Ethibloc mixed with absolute ethanol. **E** and **F,** C-arm–computed tomography acquisition showing that the middle cystic component seen on MRI was not injected. **G,** After careful ultrasound examination, the middle cystic component was located into the supraspinatus muscle and injected successfully.

The most common locations for lymphatic malformations are the cervicofacial region and the axilla and upper chest area. Less common locations include intrathoracic, retroperitoneum, or intraabdominal viscera; buttock; and anogenital areas.[66-69]

These lesions are located beneath a normal or bluish skin. Spontaneous shrinkage can occur, but sudden enlargement can happen secondary to infection or bleeding.[70] Cervicofacial lymphatic malformations can be associated with overgrowth of the mandibular body.[71] Diffuse thoracic lymphatic malformations can manifest as recurrent pleural or pericardial chylous effusion. Chronic protein-losing enteropathy with hypoalbuminemia can be observed in cases of involvement of the gastrointestinal tract. Involvement of an extremity can cause swelling and skeletal overgrowth.[2]

On plain film radiography, a soft-tissue mass can be noted. Distorsion or hypertophy of bone is occasionally noted.[70] Rarely, in diffuse soft-tissue and skeletal lymphatic malformations, progressive osteolysis, especially on the clavicular bone, has been reported. This is called Gorham-Stout syndrome.[72]

On ultrasound, macrocystic lesions appear as a multiloculated cystic mass with no flow except in the septa, where high-resistive-index vessels can be depicted[28] (Figure 48-10). Microcystic lymphangiomas are hyperechoic without flow.[70]

On MRI, the characteristic finding is the presence of a heterogeneous fluid-filled mass with an iso or hyposignal on T_1-weighted sequence and hypersignal on T_2-weighted sequence. Sometimes a high signal on T_1 sequence or a fluid level can be observed in cases of cyst with a high protein or a hemorrhagic content.[18] Pure lymphatic malformations present no or minimal enhancement of septation, whereas combined LVMs show enhancement of the lymphatic space.[18]

Macrocystic lymphangiomas can be treated by either surgery or sclerotherapy. Usually, macrocystic lymphatic malformations present a good response after sclerotherapy. Different sclerosing agent have been used: In North America, ethanol, sodium tedradecyl sulfate, and doxycycline; in Europe and Canada, alcoholic solution of zein (Ethibloc)[73,74]; and in Japan, OKT3 (picibanil, a killed strain of group A Streptococcus pyogenes) have been used.[75] It is hypothesized that OKT3 works by inducing apoptosis of lymphatic endothelium or stimulating the production of soluble cytokines, which in turn induce a local cellular inflammatory reaction.[76] More recently, bleomycin has been used in macrocystic and mixed malformations with a success rate varying between 70% and 95%.[77-82] Since it is administrated locally, bleomycin is absorbed systemically at very low levels.[34] Although systemic bleomycin administration may be suspected in the development of fatal pulmonary fibrosis even in low doses, no definitive cases of this complication have been identified during local administration for lymphatic malformations.[34]

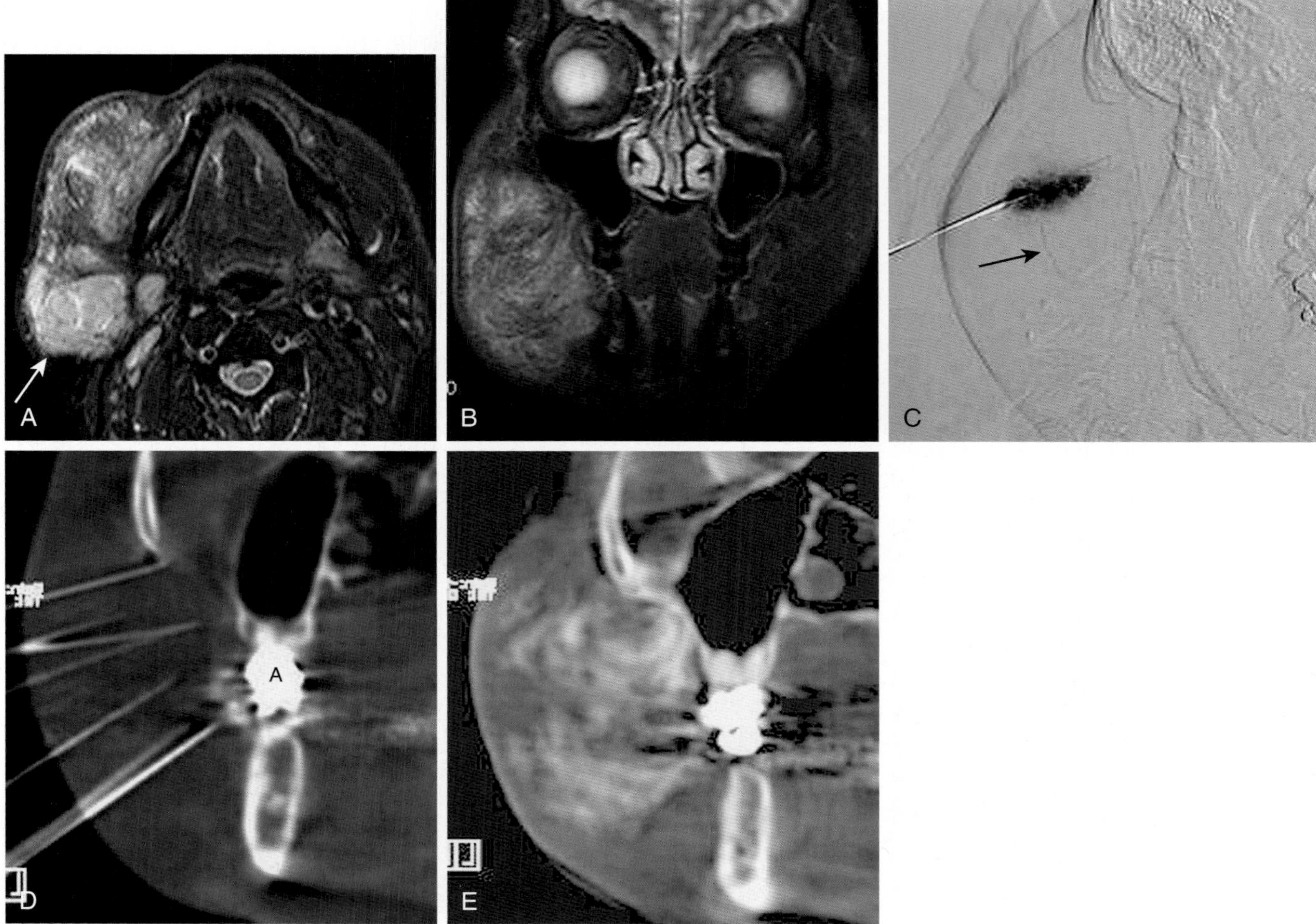

Figure 48-9. Patient presenting a microcystic lymphangioma and venous malformation involving the right hemiface. **A** and **B,** Coronal and axial short inversion-time inversion recovery acquisition showing an extensive infiltrative microcystic lymphangioma. On the axial image, we can delineate the posterior aspect of the lesion corresponding to the venous malformation component *(arrow)*. **C,** After direct puncture guided by ultrasound, small contrast infusion demonstrates tiny cysts with small venous drainage *(arrow)*. **D,** C-arm–computed tomography acquisition performed after needle placement showing adequate coverage of the lesion. **E,** C-arm–computed tomography acquisition after bleomycin infusion showing adequate filling of the lesion.

Microcystic lymphangiomas do not respond well to sclerosant therapy although, good response using bleomycin and OKT3 has been reported by several authors.[76,80] Microcystic lymphangiomas should be managed conservatively; however, if a treatment is required, a surgical approach is preferred. A recurrence rate of 40% after incomplete excision and 17% after macroscopically complete excision has been reported.[69] The role of bleomycin sclerotherapy combined with surgery remains to be defined.

HIGH-FLOW MALFORMATIONS

Arteriovenous Malformations

AVMs represent a direct connection between the arterial and the venous systems.[1,35] AVMs are usually present at birth but may not be clinically evident. They become evident in childhood and are often exacerbated during puberty or pregnancy.[83,84] A purple or red coloration of the skin can be seen that can be confused with a cutaneous port-wine stain. Closer examination reveals increased temperature, dilated veins, and a thrill that is usually noted at palpation.[85] These lesions can be dangerous when they are in evolution. Cutaneous ischemia with ulceration or infection and hemorrhage are the most common local complications. If the malformation is extensive, high-output cardiac failure can be seen.[3] Schobinger reported a clinical staging system to grade the evolution of AVMs[2,84]:

Stage I (quiescence)—pink-bluish stain, warmth, and arteriovascular shunting on Doppler ultrasound examination

Stage II (expansion)—same as stage I plus enlargement, pulsations, thrill and bruit, and tortuous or tense veins

Stage III (destruction)—same as stage II plus dystrophic skin changes, ulceration, bleeding, persistent pain, or tissues necrosis

Stage IV (decompensation)—same as stage III plus cardiac failure

Doppler ultrasound is the best examination to diagnose AVMs. The lesion is made of multiple feeding arteries with increased diastolic flow and an increase venous return with a systolodiastolic flow (Figure 48-11). Power or color

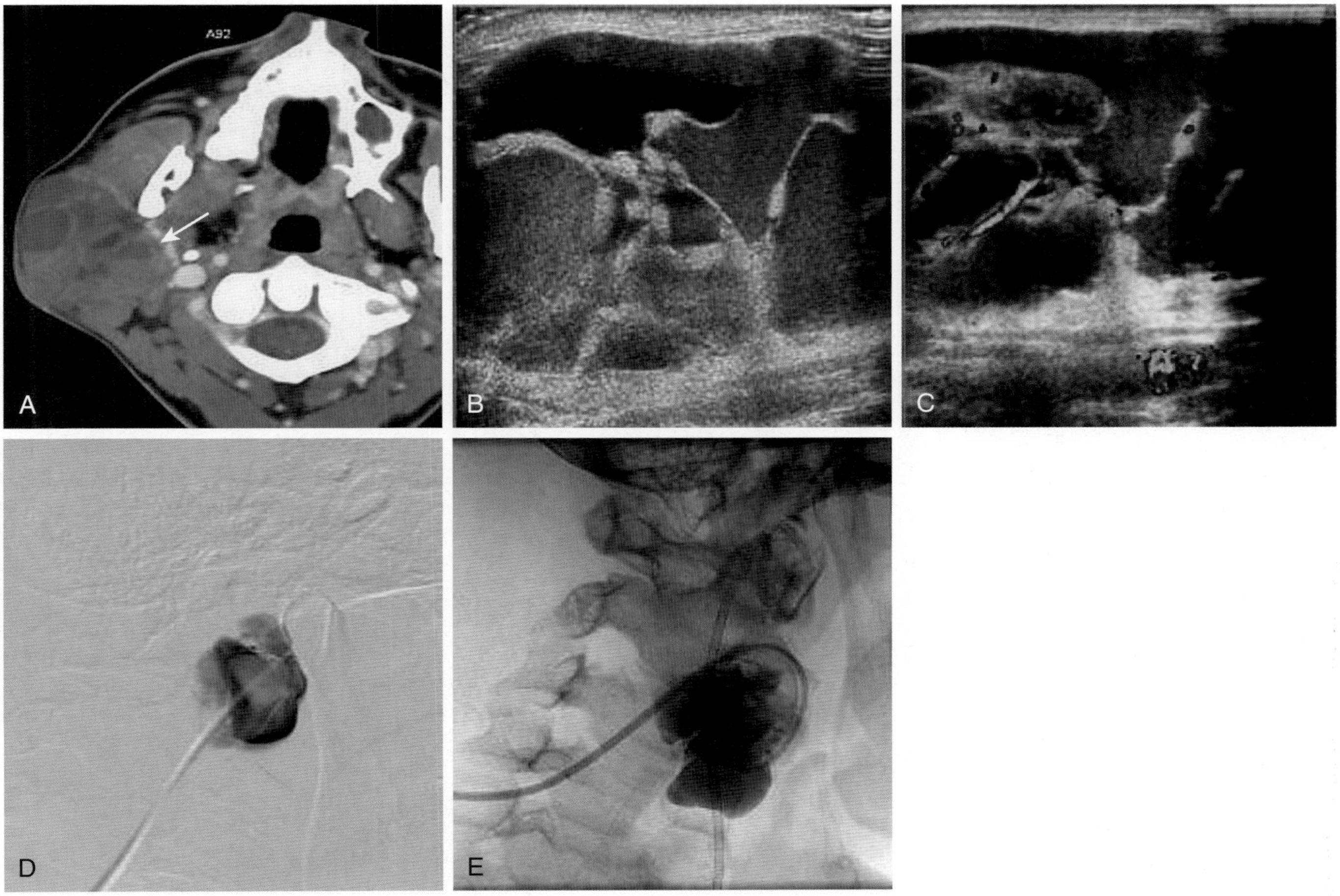

Figure 48-10. Patient presenting with a mass of the right parotid region with sudden pain and enlargement. **A,** Computed tomography scan of the mandibular area showing a large mass in the right parotid region with presence of several fluid level *(arrow),* suggesting a hemorrhagic component. **B,** Gray-scale ultrasound examination confirming a complex cystic mass with hyperechoic content located in a dependent position, also suggesting presence of blood. **C,** Doppler ultrasound examination showing high-resistance arterial flow within the septa. **D** and **E,** The cyst was successfully aspirated by positioning two drains and was sclerosed with absolute ethanol.

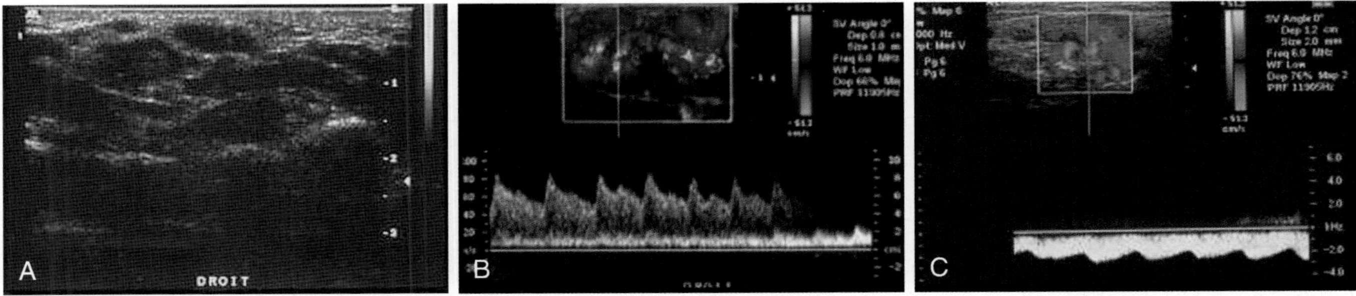

Figure 48-11. Arteriovenous malformation of the hand. **A,** Gray-scale ultrasound of the hand. Multiple dilated hypoechoic channels are seen. **B,** Color Doppler ultrasound. A high-flow malformation is present. A diastolic flow is observed after duplex insonation of an arterial feeder, indicating the presence of arteriovenous fistula. **C,** Diagnosis of an arteriovenous malformation is confirmed by the presence of a systolodiastolic flow within a draining vein.

Doppler examination is helpful to delineate the network of the malformation.

MRI is the best examination to evaluate the extension of the malformation in adjacent structures, especially for bone involvement. MRI findings include dilated feeding and draining vessels with little tissue matrix and no venous lakes.[17] Signal voids are typically observed in these vessels on both T_1- and T_2-weighted spin echo sequence (Figure 48-12), whereas a hypersignal is observed on gradient echo and angiographic sequence, indicating a high-flow lesion.[18] Gadolinium-enhanced magnetic resonance angiography is helpful to evaluate feeding arteries and draining veins (Figure 48-12). The presence of an early venous filling is typically seen in AVMs; using time-resolved magnetic resonance angiography sequences, it now possible to evaluate the dynamic opacification of AVM.[21,86-89] Since these sequences have a high temporal

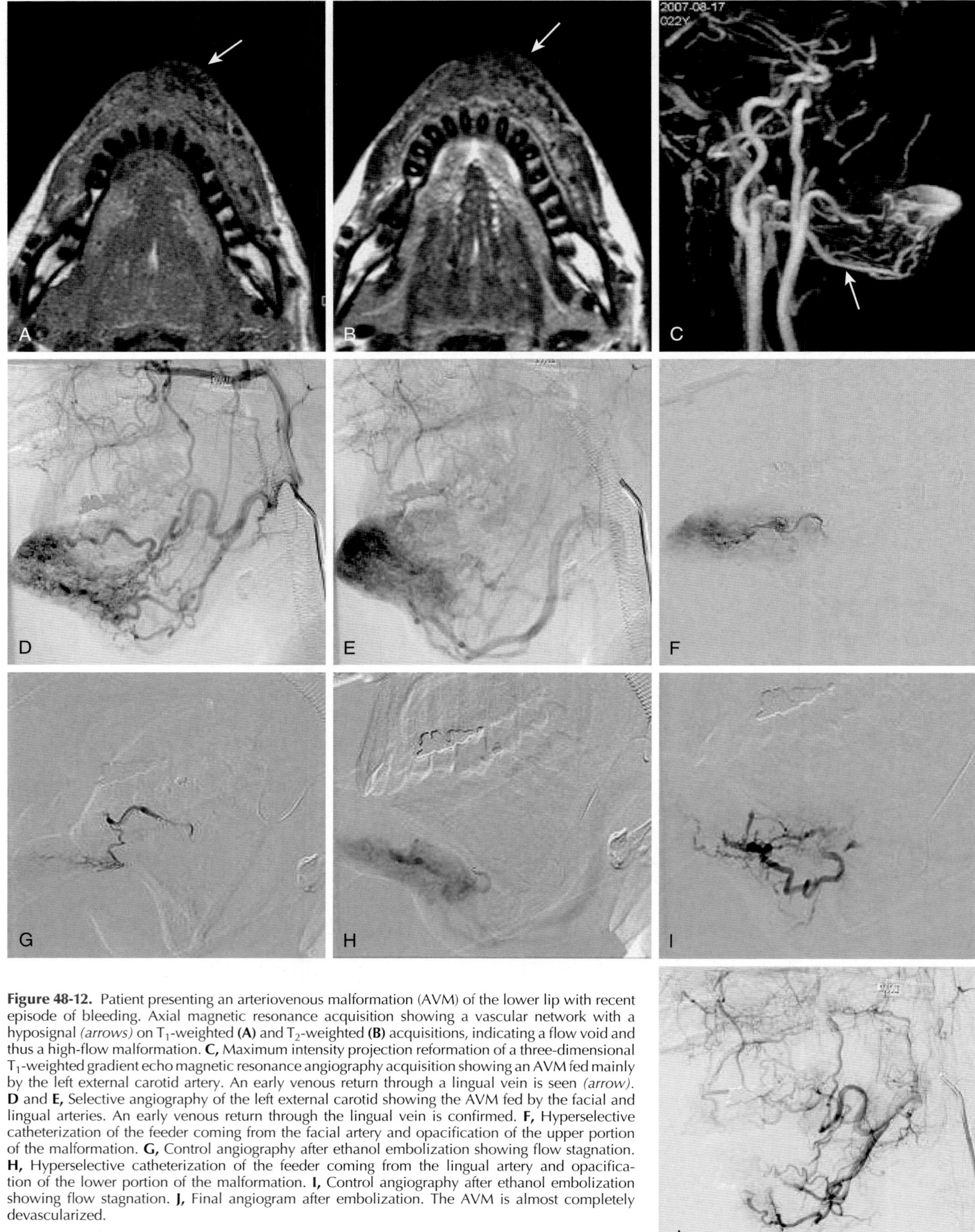

Figure 48-12. Patient presenting an arteriovenous malformation (AVM) of the lower lip with recent episode of bleeding. Axial magnetic resonance acquisition showing a vascular network with a hyposignal *(arrows)* on T_1-weighted **(A)** and T_2-weighted **(B)** acquisitions, indicating a flow void and thus a high-flow malformation. **C,** Maximum intensity projection reformation of a three-dimensional T_1-weighted gradient echo magnetic resonance angiography acquisition showing an AVM fed mainly by the left external carotid artery. An early venous return through a lingual vein is seen *(arrow)*. **D** and **E,** Selective angiography of the left external carotid showing the AVM fed by the facial and lingual arteries. An early venous return through the lingual vein is confirmed. **F,** Hyperselective catheterization of the feeder coming from the facial artery and opacification of the upper portion of the malformation. **G,** Control angiography after ethanol embolization showing flow stagnation. **H,** Hyperselective catheterization of the feeder coming from the lingual artery and opacification of the lower portion of the malformation. **I,** Control angiography after ethanol embolization showing flow stagnation. **J,** Final angiogram after embolization. The AVM is almost completely devascularized.

resolution, a compromise is made on spatial resolution, which is lower than conventional three-dimensional magnetic resonance angiography, using parallel imaging techniques.

Catheter angiography is mandatory before any therapeutic interventions. It allows precise evaluation of the feeding arteries and draining veins of the malformation and determination of the feasibility of embolization. The angiographic characteristics of AVMs are dilatation and lengthening of afferent arteries, with early opacification of enlarged veins[83] (Figure 48-12). Selective and superselective catheterizations are necessary to demonstrate the full extent of these high-flow malformations and to allow precise mapping of feeding and draining vessels.

Treatment of AVMs is complex and should be reserved for symptomatic cases. It is rarely indicated during infancy or childhood. Sometimes, stage I and II malformations can be treated if they are well localized. Stage III and IV lesions should be treated because of the risk of progression and serious hemorrhage.[2,84] Extensive stage I lesions should be managed conservatively with compressive garments because extensive resection and complex reconstruction of the lesion can be worse than the lesion itself and recurrence is likely.[84,90]

The ideal treatment is selective embolization followed by complete resection, if possible. The preferred agents for embolization are absolute alcohol and N-butyl cyanoacrylate because these liquid agents can be injected within the nidus of the malformation. Glue can migrate through the AVF into the pulmonary circulation and has a propensity to recanalize.[34] Alcohol is the most definitive sclerosant agent and gives the best clinical results, although it may induce nerve injury and skin necrosis in 15% of the cases.[91] It can be injected after hyperselective catheterization of the feeding arteries or by direct puncture of the nidus of the AVM. Direct puncture is preferred if arterial access is complicated or if selective arterial embolization carries a risk of distal embolization in normal vessels.[92,93] A vascular channel within the nidus of the lesion is punctured under fluoroscopic, ultrasound, or both types of guidance.[35] Flow reduction techniques increase concentration and dwell time and allow greater control of distribution of sclerosant within the nidus. In this regard, a balloon catheter can be positioned at the arterial inflow or outflow. Similarly, tourniquets or pneumatic cuffs can be inflated upstream or downstream of the extremity AVMs.[34] Permanent occlusion can be performed using coils or cyanoacrylate adhesives to collateral arterial pathways in an effort to reduce arterial inflow and the amount of sclerosant necessary.[91]

Large coils also can be placed within the collateral or main venous drainage to assist flow reduction.[91] Thereafter, multisession direct sclerotherapies are performed with ethanol to treat the nidus of the AVM. A small volume of alcohol should be injected at once (1 to 3 ml); the volume and rate of injection should be based on flow evaluation following a digital subtraction angiography acquisition using same catheter position and adjunct flow control maneuver. After each alcohol injection, the operator should wait 5 minutes, allowing time for endothelial damage to become evident, and should repeat angiography before undergoing another bolus ethanol administration.[91] The procedure is repeated until significant slowing of the flow can be seen on digital subtraction angiography acquisition (Figure 48-12). It is important to stop alcohol injection when normal arterial branches become visible. Pulmonary arterial pressure is monitored during ethanol administration, and vasodilator therapy is administered if pulmonary arterial pressures increase to greater than 25 mm Hg compared to baseline values.[34]

Complications are skin necrosis, nerve injury, distal emboli, pulmonary emboli of coils, or glue. As for venous malformations, fatal cardiac arrest has been reported with alcohol sclerotherapy. The success of combined embolization and surgical resection is better for stage I or II well-localized AVMs.[84,90] In extensive AVMs, palliative embolization has shown to be helpful in controlling symptoms, but surgical resection cannot be considered in most cases.[91] With alcohol embolization alone, Do et al. have reported a 68% success rate (cure and improvement).[91]

ASSOCIATED SYNDROMES

Some combined or complex malformations are associated with various syndromes.

Syndromes Associated with Vascular Stains and Low-Flow Vascular Malformation

Sturge-Weber syndrome is a nonheritable cutaneous disorder consisting of an unilateral facial port-wine stain in the trigeminal area, an ipsilateral leptomeningeal malformation, and a malformation of the choroid of the eye; atrophy and calcifications in the subjacent cerebral cortex; seizures; hemiparesis and visual field defects controlateral to the brain lesion; mental retardation of variable degree; and sometimes buphthalmos or glaucoma.[94]

Klippel-Trénaunay syndrome is a CLVM associated with soft-tissue and skeletal hypertrophy of one or more limbs.[95,96] The presence of two of the three cardinal features is sufficient to make a Klippel-Trénaunay syndrome diagnosis.[95] The lower limb is more often involved, with possible extension of the malformation into the perineum or sometime in the abdomen. The upper limb, the trunk, or the neck is rarely involved.[97] The cutaneous vascular malformation is always present at birth and is a capillary malformation most often of the port-wine type. The varicosities occur ipsilateral to the port-wine stain and become apparent during childhood. These anomalous veins have deformed, insufficient, or absent valves and are commonly associated with fibromuscular dysplasia.[98] The pathognomonic marginal vein of Servelle is often identified in the subcutaneous fat of the lateral calf and thigh, and it can communicate with the deep venous system at various levels (Figure 48-13). Contrast venography is useful in selected patients to depict the route of drainage and the feasibility of resecting or sclerosing varicosities.[2] The etiology of limb bone overgrowth is unclear. Beside bone overgrowth, limb hypertrophy is predominantly made of fat. Family studies have suggested multifactorial inheritance.[99] Lymphedema can be associated, resulting from malformations and hypoplasias of the lymphatic vessels.[100]

Syndromes Associated with Vascular Stains and High-Flow Malformation

The CAVMs correspond to the Parkes Weber syndrome, which combines AVFs, congenital varicose veins, and a cutaneous capillary malformation associated with a limb hypertrophy.[3]

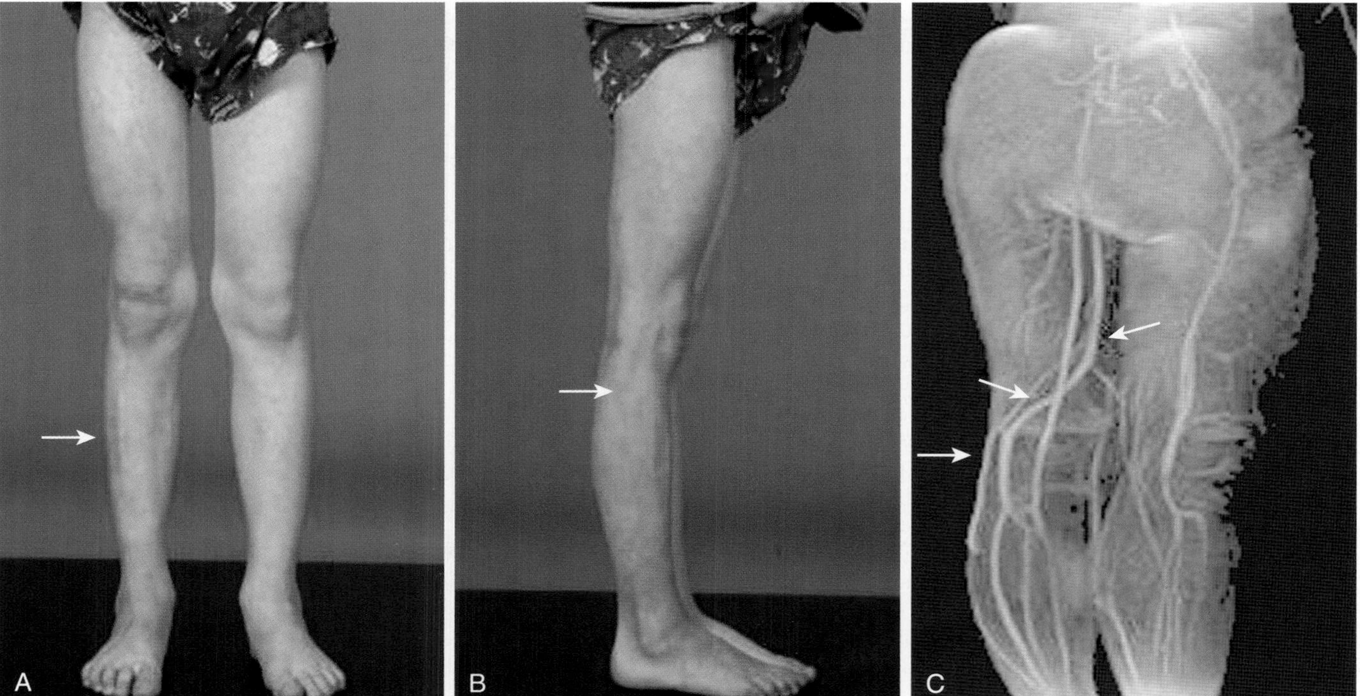

Figure 48-13. Patient with Klippel-Trénaunay syndrome. **A** and **B,** Presence of the marginal vein of Servelle in the lateral portion of the calf *(arrow)*. **C,** On magnetic resonance phlebography, an atrophy of the deep venous system is seen at the infrapopliteal level. The marginal vein of Servelle is draining into the internal saphenous vein *(arrows)*.

Unlike CLVM, the soft-tissue overgrowth in the limb in CAVM is shown by MRI to be both muscular and bony. The enlarged limb muscles and bones exhibit an abnormal signal and enhancement. Magnetic resonance angiography and magnetic resonance venography show generalized arterial and venous dilation. The AVFs are multiple, small, and confined to the affected limb. The lower limb is more often affected than upper limb.[2]

AVMs can be associated with Rendu-Osler-Weber syndrome, which consists of diffuse mucosal telangiectasia involving the nasopharynx, the gastrointestinal tract, and sometimes urinary and genital mucosa; AVFs; and arterial aneurysms involving the pulmonary, hepatic, and digestive arteries.[101]

Capillary malformation–AVM syndrome is a recently described hereditary disorder that is characterized by cutaneous capillary malformation occurring in association with high-flow vascular lesions (AVMs or AVFs). This condition is caused by mutations in the RASA1 gene. Some of these patients have the clinical features of Parkes Weber syndrome. The capillary malformations are often small pink–red macules that may be widely distributed over the skin surface. Larger solitary capillary malformations are also reported in this condition.[102]

Cobb syndrome is a rare nonhereditary disorder that involves the association of spinal "angiomas" or AVMs with congenital, cutaneous vascular lesions. It is not a true capillary malformation (port-wine stain) but a quiescent Schobinger stage I AVM in the same dermatome. The cutaneous vascular lesions are associated with a spinal cord angioma or AVM that may result in variable neurological complications.[102,103]

Syndromes without Vascular Stain Associated with Venous, Lymphatic, or Mixed Malformations

Blue rubber bleb nevus syndrome[104,105] is a rare disorder that associates multiple dome-shaped cutaneous venous malformations of the skin with multiple gastrointestinal venous malformations that can present with bleeding and anemia. It is a sporadic disease, but familial cases have been reported. Histopathology reveals large blood-filled spaces or sinuses lined by single or multiple layers of endothelial cells. Multiple cutaneous lesions on the trunk, palms, and soles of the feet may be markers for blue rubber bleb nevus syndrome.[2,104] The gastrointestinal lesions can result in hemorrhage, intussusception, and volvulus.[4]

Maffucci syndrome is a nonheritable syndrome considered as a mesodermal dysplasia that consists of diffuse asymmetrical enchondromatosis involving preferentially metacarpal and phalanges of the hand and metatarsal bones of the feet associated with multiple venous or lymphatic malformations or LVMs.[58]

Proteus syndrome associates multiple subcutaneous hamartomatous tumors, verrucous pigmented nevi with a hemihypertrophy, a partial gigantism involving the extremities (foot, hand), an intraabdominal lipomatosis, a pachydermia involving the palmar and plantar aspects of the hand and foot, a hypertrophy of vertebral bodies, and a macrocrania with LVMs. Its inheritance is unclear.[106-109]

Bannayan-Riley-Ruvalcaba syndrome is an autosomal dominant condition with a variable clinical phenotype.

The predominant clinical features are macrocephaly, developmental delay, pseudopapilledema, pigmented macules on the glans penis, and hamartomatous growths, including subcutaneous and visceral lipomas, gastrointestinal polyposis, and capillary and combined malformations.[102]

CONCLUSION

Good knowledge of the classification and clinical characteristics of the vascular malformation is necessary to take charge of patients. Doppler ultrasound and MRI are the two main imaging modalities allowing classification of the malformation. Before making a diagnosis, good knowledge of clinical history is crucial when reading these imaging studies. A multidisciplinary team composed of a plastic surgeon, an interventional radiologist, and a dermatologist is necessary to be able to offer to the patient the best treatment or treatment sequence. It is important to focus on the patient's symptoms, treat the patient only when indicated, and try to avoid unnecessary intervention that can worsen the patient's condition, especially in cases of AVMs. With current trends, percutaneous management of vascular malformations has become the mainstay of therapy. Better knowledge of the genetic and molecular biology related to these diseases will probably offer new therapeutic opportunities.

References

1. Mulliken JB, Glowacki J. Classification of pediatric vascular lesions. *Plast Reconstr Surg* 1982;70:120-121.
2. Mulliken JB, Fishman SJ, Burrows PE. Vascular anomalies. *Curr Probl Surg* 2000;37:517-584.
3. Enjolras O. Classification and management of the various superficial vascular anomalies: hemangiomas and vascular malformations. *J Dermatol* 1997;24:701-710.
4. Arneja JS, Gosain AK. Vascular malformations. *Plast Reconstr Surg* 2008;121:195e-206e.
5. Vikkula M, Boon LM, Mulliken JB, Olsen BR. Molecular basis of vascular anomalies. *Trends Cardiovasc Med* 1998;8:281-292.
6. Boon LM, Mulliken JB, Vikkula M, et al. Assignment of a locus for dominantly inherited venous malformations to chromosome 9p. *Hum Mol Genet* 1994;3:1583-1587.
7. Vikkula M, Boon LM, Carraway KL III, et al. Vascular dysmorphogenesis caused by an activating mutation in the receptor tyrosine kinase TIE2. *Cell* 1996;87:1181-1190.
8. Boon LM, Brouillard P, Irrthum A, et al. A gene for inherited cutaneous venous anomalies ("glomangiomas") localizes to chromosome 1p21-22. *Am J Hum Genet* 1999;65:125-133.
9. Brouillard P, Vikkula M. Genetic causes of vascular malformations. *Hum Mol Genet* 2007;16(Spec No. 2):R140-R149.
10. Eerola I, Boon LM, Mulliken JB, et al. Capillary malformation–arteriovenous malformation, a new clinical and genetic disorder caused by RASA1 mutations. *Am J Hum Genet* 2003;73:1240-1249.
11. Chervenak FA, Isaacson G, Blakemore KJ, et al. Fetal cystic hygroma: cause and natural history. *N Engl J Med* 1983;309:822-825.
12. Langer JC, Fitzgerald PG, Desa D, et al. Cervical cystic hygroma in the fetus: clinical spectrum and outcome. *J Pediatr Surg* 1990;25:58-61; discussion, 61-52.
13. Garzon MC, Huang JT, Enjolras O, Frieden IJ. Vascular malformations: part I. *J Am Acad Dermatol* 2007;56:353-370. quiz, 371-354.
14. Ferrell RE. Research perspectives in inherited lymphatic disease. *Ann NY Acad Sci* 2002;979:39-51. discussion, 76-39.
15. Simons ME. Peripheral vascular malformations: diagnosis and percutaneous management. *Can Assoc Radiol J* 2001;52:242-251.
16. Dubois J, Soulez G, Oliva VL, et al. Soft-tissue venous malformations in adult patients: imaging and therapeutic issues. *Radiographics* 2001;21:1519-1531.
17. Hovius SE, Borg DH, Paans PR, Pieterman H. The diagnostic value of magnetic resonance imaging in combination with angiography in patients with vascular malformations: a prospective study. *Ann Plast Surg* 1996;37:278-285.
18. Siegel MJ. Magnetic resonance imaging of musculoskeletal soft tissue masses. *Radiol Clin North Am* 2001;39:701-720.
19. Dobson MJ, Hartley RW, Ashleigh R, et al. MR angiography and MR imaging of symptomatic vascular malformations. *Clin Radiol* 1997;52:595-602.
20. Ohgiya Y, Hashimoto T, Gokan T, et al. Dynamic MRI for distinguishing high-flow from low-flow peripheral vascular malformations. *AJR Am J Roentgenol* 2005;185:1131-1137.
21. Taschner CA, Gieseke J, Le Thuc V, et al. Intracranial arteriovenous malformation: time-resolved contrast-enhanced MR angiography with combination of parallel imaging, keyhole acquisition, and k-space sampling techniques at 1.5 T. *Radiology* 2008;246:871-879.
22. Abernethy LJ. Classification and imaging of vascular malformations in children. *Eur Radiol* 2003;13:2483-2497.
23. Trop I, Dubois J, Guibaud L, et al. Soft-tissue venous malformations in pediatric and young adult patients: diagnosis with Doppler US. *Radiology* 1999;212:841-845.
24. Wirth GA, Sundine MJ. Slow-flow vascular malformations. *Clin Pediatr (Phila)* 2007;46:109-120.
25. Rudolph R. Familial multiple glomangiomas. *Ann Plast Surg* 1993;30:183-185.
26. Boon LM, Mulliken JB, Enjolras O, Vikkula M. Glomuvenous malformation (glomangioma) and venous malformation: distinct clinicopathologic and genetic entities. *Arch Dermatol* 2004;140:971-976.
27. Mazoyer E, Enjolras O, Laurian C, et al. Coagulation abnormalities associated with extensive venous malformations of the limbs: differentiation from Kasabach-Merritt syndrome. *Clin Lab Haematol* 2002;24:243-251.
28. Paltiel HJ, Burrows PE, Kozakewich HP, et al. Soft-tissue vascular anomalies: utility of US for diagnosis. *Radiology* 2000;214:747-754.
29. Li W, David V, Kaplan R, Edelman RR. Three-dimensional low dose gadolinium-enhanced peripheral MR venography. *J Magn Reson Imaging* 1998;8:630-633.
30. Dubois JM, Sebag GH, De Prost Y, et al. Soft-tissue venous malformations in children: percutaneous sclerotherapy with Ethibloc. *Radiology* 1991;180:195-198.
31. Puig S, Aref H, Chigot V, et al. Classification of venous malformations in children and implications for sclerotherapy. *Pediatr Radiol* 2003;33:99-103.
32. Puig S, Casati B, Staudenherz A, Paya K. Vascular low-flow malformations in children: current concepts for classification, diagnosis and therapy. *Eur J Radiol* 2005;53:35-45.
33. Berenguer B, Burrows PE, Zurakowski D, Mulliken JB. Sclerotherapy of craniofacial venous malformations: complications and results. *Plast Reconstr Surg* 1999;104:1-11; discussion, 12-15.
34. Legiehn GM, Heran MK. Classification, diagnosis, and interventional radiologic management of vascular malformations. *Orthop Clin North Am* 2006;37:435-474, vii-viii.
35. Yakes WF, Rossi P, Odink H. How I do it: arteriovenous malformation management. *Cardiovasc Intervent Radiol* 1996;19:65-71.
36. Dompmartin A, Labbe D, Theron J, et al. The use of an alcohol gel of ethyl cellulose in the treatment of venous malformations. *Rev Stomatol Chir Maxillofac* 2000;101:30-32.
37. Suzuki N, Nakao A, Nonami T, Takagi H. Experimental study on the effects of sclerosants for esophageal varices on blood coagulation, fibrinolysis and systemic hemodynamics. *Gastroenterol Jpn* 1992;27:309-316.
38. Mitsuzaki K, Yamashita Y, Utsunomiya D, et al. Balloon-occluded retrograde transvenous embolization of a pelvic arteriovenous malformation. *Cardiovasc Intervent Radiol* 1999;22:518-520.
39. Rao J, Goldman MP. Stability of foam in sclerotherapy: differences between sodium tetradecyl sulfate and polidocanol and the type of connector used in the double-syringe system technique. *Dermatol Surg* 2005;31:19-22.
40. Siniluoto TM, Svendsen PA, Wikholm GM, et al. Percutaneous sclerotherapy of venous malformations of the head and neck using sodium tetradecyl sulphate (sotradecol). *Scand J Plast Reconstr Surg Hand Surg* 1997;31:145-150.
41. Yamaki T, Nozaki M, Fujiwara O, Yoshida E. Duplex-guided foam sclerotherapy for the treatment of the symptomatic venous malformations of the face. *Dermatol Surg* 2002;28:619-622.
42. Choi YH, Han MH, O-Ki K, et al. Craniofacial cavernous venous malformations: percutaneous sclerotherapy with use of ethanolamine oleate. *J Vasc Interv Radiol* 2002;13:475-482.
43. Yamaki T, Nozaki M, Sakurai H, et al. Prospective randomized efficacy of ultrasound-guided foam sclerotherapy compared with ultrasound-guided liquid sclerotherapy in the treatment of symptomatic venous malformations. *J Vasc Surg* 2008;47:578-584.

44. Gelbert F, Enjolras O, Deffrenne D, et al. Percutaneous sclerotherapy for venous malformation of the lips: a retrospective study of 23 patients. *Neuroradiology* 2000;42:692-696.
45. Hayashi N, Masumoto T, Okubo T, et al. Hemangiomas in the face and extremities: MR-guided sclerotherapy—optimization with monitoring of signal intensity changes in vivo. *Radiology* 2003;226:567-572.
46. Wallace M, Kuo M, Glaiberman C, et al. Three-dimensional C-arm cone beam computed tomography imaging: applications in the interventional suite. *J Vasc Interv Radiol* 2008;19(6):799-813.
47. Lee BB, Do YS, Byun HS, et al. Advanced management of venous malformation with ethanol sclerotherapy: mid-term results. *J Vasc Surg* 2003;37:533-538.
48. Lee BB, Bergan JJ. Advanced management of congenital vascular malformations: a multidisciplinary approach. *Cardiovasc Surg* 2002;10:523-533.
49. de Lorimier AA. Sclerotherapy for venous malformations. *J Pediatr Surg* 1995;30:188-193; discussion, 194.
50. Marrocco-Trischitta MM, Guerrini P, Abeni D, Stillo F. Reversible cardiac arrest after polidocanol sclerotherapy of peripheral venous malformation. *Dermatol Surg* 2002;28:153-155.
51. Loose DA. Surgical management of venous malformations. *Phlebology* 2007;22:276-282.
52. Derby LD, Low DW. Laser treatment of facial venous vascular malformations. *Ann Plast Surg* 1997;38:371-378.
53. Raulin C, Werner S. Treatment of venous malformations with an intense pulsed light source (IPLS) technology: a retrospective study. *Lasers Surg Med* 1999;25:170-177.
54. Sarig O, Kimel S, Orenstein A. Laser treatment of venous malformations. *Ann Plast Surg* 2006;57:20-24.
55. Spring MA, Bentz ML. Cutaneous vascular lesions. *Clin Plast Surg* 2005;32:171-186.
56. Tan KL. Nevus flammeus of the nape, glabella and eyelids: a clinical study of frequency, racial distribution, and association with congenital anomalies. *Clin Pediatr (Phila)* 1972;11:112-118.
57. Kauvar AN, Wang RS. Laser treatment of cutaneous vascular anomalies. *Lymphat Res Biol* 2004;2:38-50.
58. Esterly NB. Cutaneous hemangiomas, vascular stains and malformations, and associated syndromes. *Curr Probl Pediatr* 1996;26:3-39.
59. Marler JJ, Mulliken JB. Current management of hemangiomas and vascular malformations. *Clin Plast Surg* 2005;32:99-116, ix.
60. Davis DA, Cohen PR, George RE. Cutaneous stigmata of occult spinal dysraphism. *J Am Acad Dermatol* 1994;31:892-896.
61. Enjolras O, Boukobza M, Jdid R. Cervical occult spinal dysraphism: MRI findings and the value of a vascular birthmark. *Pediatr Dermatol* 1995;12:256-259.
62. Tan OT, Sherwood K, Gilchrest BA. Treatment of children with port-wine stains using the flashlamp-pulsed tunable dye laser. *N Engl J Med* 1989;320:416-421.
63. Bjerring P, Christiansen K, Troilius A. Intense pulsed light source for the treatment of dye laser resistant port-wine stains. *J Cosmet Laser Ther* 2003;5:7-13.
64. Brock ME, Smith RJ, Parey SE, Mobley DL. Lymphangioma: an otolaryngologic perspective. *Int J Pediatr Otorhinolaryngol* 1987;14:133-140.
65. Koeller KK, Alamo L, Adair CF, Smirniotopoulos JG. Congenital cystic masses of the neck: radiologic–pathologic correlation. *Radiographics* 1999;19:121-146. quiz, 152-123.
66. Fordham LA, Chung CJ, Donnelly LF. Imaging of congenital vascular and lymphatic anomalies of the head and neck. *Neuroimaging Clin North Am* 2000;10:117-136, viii.
67. Brown RL, Azizkhan RG. Pediatric head and neck lesions. *Pediatr Clin North Am* 1998;45:889-905.
68. Godin DA, Guarisco JL. Cystic hygromas of the head and neck. *J La State Med Soc* 1997;149:224-228.
69. Alqahtani A, Nguyen LT, Flageole H, Shaw K, Laberge JM. 25 years' experience with lymphangiomas in children. *J Pediatr Surg* 1999;34:1164-1168.
70. Dubois J, Garel L, Grignon A, et al. Imaging of hemangiomas and vascular malformations in children. *Acad Radiol* 1998;5:390-400.
71. Padwa BL, Hayward PG, Ferraro NF, Mulliken JB. Cervicofacial lymphatic malformation: clinical course, surgical intervention, and pathogenesis of skeletal hypertrophy. *Plast Reconstr Surg* 1995;95:951-960.
72. Gorham LW, Stout AP. Massive osteolysis (acute spontaneous absorption of bone, phantom bone, disappearing bone): its relation to hemangiomatosis. *J Bone Joint Surg Am* 1955;37-A:985-1004.
73. Dubois J, Garel L, Abela A, et al. Lymphangiomas in children: percutaneous sclerotherapy with an alcoholic solution of zein. *Radiology* 1997;204:651-654.
74. Molitch HI, Unger EC, Witte CL, vanSonnenberg E. Percutaneous sclerotherapy of lymphangiomas. *Radiology* 1995;194:343-347.
75. Ogita S, Tsuto T, Nakamura K, et al. OK-432 therapy in 64 patients with lymphangioma. *J Pediatr Surg* 1994;29:784-785.
76. Sung MW, Lee DW, Kim DY, et al. Sclerotherapy with picibanil (OK-432) for congenital lymphatic malformation in the head and neck. *Laryngoscope* 2001;111:1430-1433.
77. Baskin D, Tander B, Bankaoglu M. Local bleomycin injection in the treatment of lymphangioma. *Eur J Pediatr Surg* 2005;15:383-386.
78. Muir T, Kirsten M, Fourie P, et al. Intralesional bleomycin injection (IBI) treatment for haemangiomas and congenital vascular malformations. *Pediatr Surg Int* 2004;19:766-773.
79. Orford J, Barker A, Thonell S, et al. Bleomycin therapy for cystic hygroma. *J Pediatr Surg* 1995;30:1282-1287.
80. Zhong PQ, Zhi FX, Li R, et al. Long-term results of intratumorous bleomycin-A5 injection for head and neck lymphangioma. *Oral Surg Oral Med Oral Pathol Oral Radiol Endod* 1998;86:139-144.
81. Zulfiqar MA, Zaleha AM, Zakaria Z, Amin T. The treatment of neck lymphangioma with intralesional injection of bleomycin. *Med J Malaysia* 1999;54:478-481.
82. Sanlialp I, Karnak I, Tanyel FC, et al. Sclerotherapy for lymphangioma in children. *Int J Pediatr Otorhinolaryngol* 2003;67:795-800.
83. Burrows PE, Laor T, Paltiel H, Robertson RL. Diagnostic imaging in the evaluation of vascular birthmarks. *Dermatol Clin* 1998;16:455-488.
84. Kohout MP, Hansen M, Pribaz JJ, Mulliken JB. Arteriovenous malformations of the head and neck: natural history and management. *Plast Reconstr Surg* 1998;102:643-654.
85. Vander Kam V, Achauer BM. Arteriovenous malformations: a team approach to management. *Plast Surg Nurs* 1995;15:53-57.
86. Reinacher PC, Stracke P, Reinges MH, et al. Contrast-enhanced time-resolved 3-D MRA: applications in neurosurgery and interventional neuroradiology. *Neuroradiology* 2007;49(Suppl 1):S3-S13.
87. Saleh RS, Lohan DG, Villablanca JP, et al. Assessment of craniospinal arteriovenous malformations at 3T with highly temporally and highly spatially resolved contrast-enhanced MR angiography. *AJNR Am J Neuroradiol* 2008.
88. Wu Y, Kim N, Korosec FR, et al. 3D time-resolved contrast-enhanced cerebrovascular MR angiography with subsecond frame update times using radial k-space trajectories and highly constrained projection reconstruction. *AJNR Am J Neuroradiol* 2007;28:2001-2004.
89. Ziyeh S, Strecker R, Berlis A, et al. Dynamic 3D MR angiography of intra- and extracranial vascular malformations at 3T: a technical note. *AJNR Am J Neuroradiol* 2005;26:630-634.
90. Upton J, Coombs CJ, Mulliken JB, et al. Vascular malformations of the upper limb: a review of 270 patients. *J Hand Surg [Am]* 1999;24:1019-1035.
91. Do YS, Yakes WF, Shin SW, et al. Ethanol embolization of arteriovenous malformations: interim results. *Radiology* 2005;235:674-682.
92. Han MH, Seong SO, Kim HD, et al. Craniofacial arteriovenous malformation: preoperative embolization with direct puncture and injection of n-butyl cyanoacrylate. *Radiology* 1999;211:661-666.
93. Lee CH, Chen SG. Direct percutaneous ethanol instillation for treatment of venous malformation in the face and neck. *Br J Plast Surg* 2005;58:1073-1078.
94. Enjolras O, Riche MC, Merland JJ. Facial port-wine stains and Sturge-Weber syndrome. *Pediatrics* 1985;76:48-51.
95. Jacob AG, Driscoll DJ, Shaughnessy WJ, et al. Klippel-Trénaunay syndrome: spectrum and management. *Mayo Clin Proc* 1998;73:28-36.
96. Gloviczki P, Driscoll DJ. Klippel-Trénaunay syndrome: current management. *Phlebology* 2007;22:291-298.
97. Cohen MM Jr.. Klippel-Trénaunay syndrome. *Am J Med Genet* 2000;93:171-175.
98. Lie JT. Pathology of angiodysplasia in Klippel-Trénaunay syndrome. *Pathol Res Pract* 1988;183:747-755.
99. Aelvoet GE, Jorens PG, Roelen LM. Genetic aspects of the Klippel-Trénaunay syndrome. *Br J Dermatol* 1992;126:603-607.
100. Baskerville PA, Ackroyd JS, Lea Thomas M, Browse NL. The Klippel-Trénaunay syndrome: clinical, radiological and haemodynamic features and management. *Br J Surg* 1985;72:232-236.
101. Guttmacher AE, Marchuk DA, White Jr RI. Hereditary hemorrhagic telangiectasia. *N Engl J Med* 1995;333:918-924.
102. Garzon MC, Huang JT, Enjolras O, Frieden IJ. Vascular malformations. II. Associated syndromes. *J Am Acad Dermatol* 2007;56:541-564.
103. Jessen RT, Thompson S, Smith EB. Cobb syndrome. *Arch Dermatol* 1977;113:1587-1590.

104. Moodley M, Ramdial P. Blue rubber bleb nevus syndrome: case report and review of the literature. *Pediatrics* 1993;92:160-162.
105. Fretzin DF, Potter B. Blue rubber bleb nevus. *Arch Intern Med* 1965;116:924-929.
106. Wiedemann HR, Burgio GR. Encephalocraniocutaneous lipomatosis and Proteus syndrome. *Am J Med Genet* 1986;25:403-404.
107. Clark RD, Donnai D, Rogers J, et al. Proteus syndrome: an expanded phenotype. *Am J Med Genet* 1987;27:99-117.
108. Samlaska CP, Levin SW, James WD, et al. Proteus syndrome. *Arch Dermatol* 1989;125:1109-1114.
109. Darmstadt GL, Lane AT. Proteus syndrome. *Pediatr Dermatol* 1994;11:222-226.

chapter

49

Lymphedema

Catharine L. McGuinness, MS, FRCS • Kevin G. Burnand, MBBS, MS, FRCS

Key Points

- Lymphedema is swelling that occurs as a result of impaired clearance of tissue fluid by lymphatic vessels.
- Lymphedema usually affects the legs, but swelling of the arms, genitals, and face also occurs.
- Lymphedema can be primary, when it appears to be caused by genetic abnormalities, or secondary, when the lymphatic vessels have been damaged by a separate pathology.
- Primary lymphedema is associated with other congenital syndromes and abnormalities.
- The clinical onset of primary lymphedema is variable, but in most cases it causes mild leg swelling.
- Mild lymphedema should be treated by compression and avoidance of skin and subcutaneous infections.
- Severe lymphedema can be treated by surgical bypass or reduction surgery.
- The rare conditions associated with megalymphatics can be treated by detailed investigation and tailored surgical operations.
- Drug treatments are not of major clinical value.
- Lymphangiosarcoma and other malignancies are rare but important sequelae of chronic lymphedema.

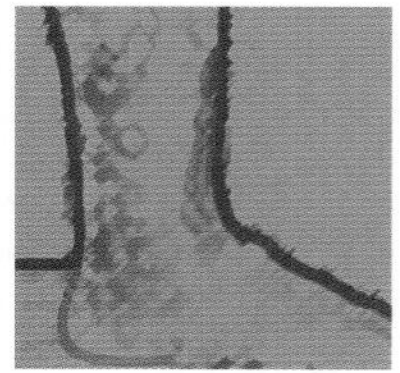

Lymphedema is the term given to excessive accumulation of interstitial fluid as a consequence of defective lymphatic drainage. This results in a "brawny" or firm edema, which most commonly affects the legs, perhaps influenced by the increased hydrostatic pressure from gravity. Most individuals affected by lymphatic edema have a recognized cause, and the lymphedema is therefore called secondary.

Recent developments in genetic techniques, together with mapping of the human genome, have led to a major advance in the understanding of the factors responsible for lymphatic development and, as a consequence, the mechanisms responsible for some subtypes of primary lymphedema.

ETIOLOGY

Although, by definition, the cause of primary lymphedema is not known, genetic predisposition clearly influences its development. A few babies have lymphedematous limbs at birth, and these infants have abnormal lymphatics and a dominant mode of inheritance (Milroy's disease).

Milroy originally described a large North American family who had a dominantly inherited pattern of congenital lymphedema and suggested that a genetic cause existed for this condition.[1] Linkage studies carried out in families with Milroy's phenotypes in North America and the United Kingdom identified that the condition was mapped to the telomeric part of chromosome 5q, in the region 5q34-q35. This region contains the gene for vascular endothelial growth factor receptor-3 (VEGFR-3), which encodes a receptor, tyrosine kinase, specific for lymphatic vessels. Defective VEGFR-3 signaling seems to be the cause of congenital hereditary lymphedema linked to 5q34-q35.[1a,2-5]

VEGF is a key regulator of blood vessel development in embryos and angiogenesis in adult tissues. Unlike VEGF-A, the related VEGF-C stimulates the growth of lymphatic vessels through its specific lymphatic endothelial receptor VEGFR-3. It has been shown that targeted inactivation of the gene encoding VEGFR-3 causes defective blood vessel development in early mouse embryos, leading to embryonic death.[6] Abnormalities in the VEGFR-3 gene are responsible for Milroy's disease.

Because the signaling pathway between VEGF-C and VEGF-D and their receptor, VEGFR-3, has been shown to be essential for lymphangiogenesis, it has been suggested that gene therapy may be used to stimulate lymphatic growth and function and to treat tissue edema.[7,8] VEGF-C gene transfer to the skin of mice with lymphedema induced a regeneration of the cutaneous lymphatic vessel network.[7]

In the more common Meig's disease, where mild lymphedema develops around the teenage years, numerous studies have indicated about a one in three risk of inheriting the condition; three times more women are affected than men. The genetic abnormality responsible for the condition has not yet been elucidated.

Hereditary "lymphedema–distichiasis" is a rare autosomal dominant disorder that presents as primary lymphedema of the limbs, with a variable age of onset, and distichiasis (extraaberrant growth of eyelashes from the meibomian gland often abutting the conjunctiva and cornea). Photophobia, exotropia, ptosis, congenital ectropion, and congenital cataracts are additional eye findings. Fourteen families in the United Kingdom, attending Moorfield's, St Thomas', and St George's hospitals, with this syndrome provided another important clue into the genetic origin of primary lymphedema. Confirmation of the phenotype by isotope lymphography and blood taken from affected individuals showed that the condition was mapped to the q24 position on chromosome 16. The FOXC2 gene is present in this region. Truncating mutations in this forkhead transcription factor gene have been shown to be responsible for these developmental abnormalities. Numerous other clinical associations have been reported, including congenital heart disease, varicose veins, cleft palate, and spinal extradural cysts. Lymphatic imaging has confirmed the earlier suggestion that lymphedema–distichiasis is associated with a normal or increased number of lymphatic vessels rather than the hypoplasia or aplasia seen in other forms of primary lymphedema.[9-12] Patients with this condition have been shown to have defective valves in their deep and superficial veins, as well as their lymphatics.[13]

Lymphedema is also associated with other syndromes known to be a consequence of chromosomal abnormalities, for example, Pierre Robin syndrome (micrognathia and skeletal anomalies), Noonan's syndrome, yellow nail syndrome (characterized by primary lymphedema, recurrent pleural effusion, and yellow discoloration of the nails), Aagenaes syndrome (cholestasis and lymphedema), and autosomal dominant microcephaly–lymphedema–chorioretinal dysplasia syndrome.[14-17] A lymphedema critical region in the X chromosome has now been identified in Turner syndrome.[18]

Another gene of interest is the homeobox gene, Prox1, which is expressed in a subpopulation of endothelial cells that give rise to the lymphatic system by budding and sprouting. The anterior cardinal veins of embryos are the initial site where the first lymphatic sacs bud off. Lymphatic development is absent in Prox1 nullizygous embryos, where budding and sprouting are arrested, although vasculogenesis and angiogenesis of the vascular system are unaffected. These findings suggest that Prox1 is a specific and crucial regulator of the development of the lymphatic system and that the vascular and lymphatic systems develop independently.[19,20]

It is still not known how and why the lymphatic system is damaged or malformed in some patients. Some degree of inheritance can be demonstrated in about one third of all patients with primary lymphedema. Congenital abnormality or absence of the lymphatics does not explain why lymphedema develops relatively late in most patients, the most common age of onset being between 10 and 25 years.

Possibly, the constituents of the lymph draining through the lymphatics may damage the lymphangioles or lymph nodes. Lymph may contain large amounts of fibrinogen under certain circumstances, and this may coagulate and block the lymphatics; abnormal lymph may also cause nodal fibrosis, which may lead to "die back" or disappearance of the lymphangioles. The primary disease may therefore be in the node, and this may cause the lymphatic hypoplasia. Anticoagulant therapy has been reported to produce improvement in patients with lymphedema, lending some support to the concept that hypercoagulability of lymph may be harmful. The benzopyrone drugs, which have been reported to reduce lymphedema clinically, increase proteolysis by macrophages and the number of macrophages.[21] Molecules as yet unrecognized within lymph may also be harmful to nodes and lymphatic vessels. None of these explanations account for the development of hyperplastic or dilated lymphatics.

It is now apparent that several genes are responsible for the development of primary lymphedema, as they appear to control the lymphangiogenesis that occurs in the embryo and, perhaps, throughout other stages of life. A full knowledge and understanding of these genes may lead to better genetic counseling, improved diagnosis, and possibly, genetic manipulation to improve lymphatic growth.

ANATOMY AND PHYSIOLOGY

In embryonic life, four cystic spaces appear, one on each side of the neck and one in each groin. Lymphatic vessels (lymphangioles) connect these spaces and carry lymph from the legs and abdomen to the cisterna chyli. On the left side, the thoracic duct transports lymph to the left internal jugular vein. On the right, another lymphatic trunk drains lymph from the right arm and right side of the head and neck to the right internal jugular vein. Lymph nodes develop along the course of these lymphatic pathways.

Developmental abnormalities include lymphatic aplasia, megalymphatics, cystic hygromata, lymphatic and nodal hypoplasia and hyperplasia, and lymphangiomas.

PATHOPHYSIOLOGY

In addition to the excessive accumulation of interstitial fluid as a result of impaired drainage, lymphedema involves reduced transport of autologous and foreign proteins. The parenchymal and immune cells secrete cytokines, which may be responsible for the proliferation of fibroblasts and epithelial cells that cause the sclerotic changes in the skin and subcutaneous tissues.

The lymphatic system has two main functions. First, it returns any large molecules and interstitial fluid that escapes from the circulation to the intravascular compartment. Albumin, globulins, fibrinogen, coagulation factors, and fibrinolytic activators all pass through the lymphatics. The second major function is to return lymphocytes from the lymph back in to the bloodstream. Most exogenous antigens are presented to the central lymphoid system for the first time via the lymphatics. Recognition of antigens, with subsequent proliferation of specific clones of lymphocytes, takes place in the lymph nodes. Activated lymphocytes then pass into the circulation and thus to the other lymphatic tissues throughout the body.

The interstitial space has a negative pressure, and this, in combination with the hydrostatic pressure of the capillaries, encourages fluid to escape from the vascular compartment, overcoming the oncotic pressure of the intravascular plasma

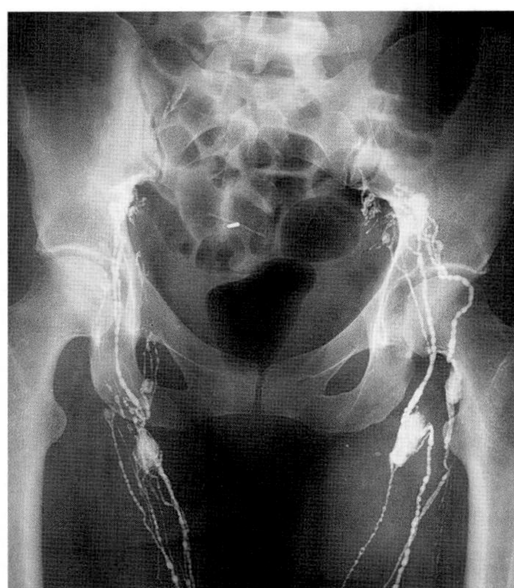

Figure 49-1. A plain x-ray after bipedal lymphangiography, demonstrating a paucity of lymphatics draining the iliac nodes in a patient with primary lower limb lymphedema.

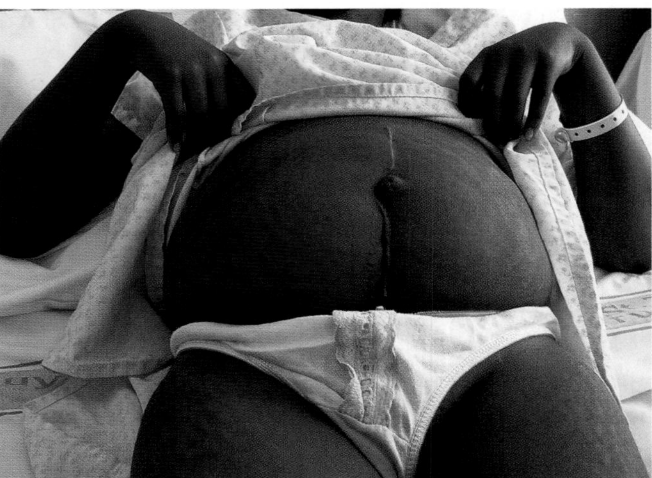

Figure 49-2. Chylous ascites in a young girl with widespread bowel lymphangiectasia, which was treated by small bowel resection of the most severe bowel segment and insertion of a Denver shunt.

proteins. The intraluminal pressure of the lymph system is similar to that of the interstitial fluid; therefore, lymph capillaries must actively absorb proteins through their pores. The mechanism by which this is achieved is not known.

The lymphatic capillaries have large pores that allow large molecules to enter the lumen and many valves that prevent the reflux of lymph. Lymphatics have some circular smooth muscle in their wall and are capable of contraction. The combination of inherent contractility and valves ensures that lymph is propelled along the lymphatics and into the veins. Other factors that may influence lymphatic drainage include compression from surrounding arteries and the negative pressure in the thoracic cavity, encouraging lymph flow upward into the thorax from the abdomen.

CLASSIFICATION AND SUBDIVISIONS

Lymphedema is subdivided into primary and secondary lymphedema, the latter being the most common. Secondary lymphedema is the result of some recognized pathological process disrupting the lymphatic drainage. Primary or idiopathic lymphedema is by comparison much rarer, although its precise prevalence or incidence is not known. Many mildly affected subjects may never attend physicians, and at present, good population-based studies with objective confirmatory tests are lacking. It is possible that people with mild lymphedema may develop ankle swelling after prolonged standing or sitting, which does not lead them to seek medical advice.

Primary Lymphedema

Subdivisions of primary lymphedema have been made on the basis of the anatomical lymphatic abnormalities. The lymphatic channels may be absent or severely hypoplastic, being few in number and disappearing more proximally (Figure 49-1). They may also be excessive in number although defective in function: such lymphatic hyperplasia is usually associated with excessive numbers of lymph nodes. The lymphatics may be dilated and ectatic (megalymphatics), and this abnormality is often associated with chylous ascites (Figure 49-2), chylothorax, and lymphatic reflux. Finally, the lymphatics may be obstructed; in primary lymphedema, this is often associated with fibrosis within the lymph nodes.

Primary lymphedema is associated with many other congenital abnormalities including vascular deformities, gonadal dysgenesis, congenital heart disease, hypogammaglobulinemia, autoimmune hypothyroidism, nephropathy, glaucoma, xanthomatosis, esotropia, nail dystrophy, and cleft palate.[22-28]

Secondary Lymphedema

All patients presenting with lymphedema must have a possible cause excluded by careful examination and special tests, where necessary.

Filariasis

This helminthic infection known as filariasis is the most important cause of lymphedema worldwide. Three filarial worms cause lymphatic filariasis: *Wuchereria bancrofti, Brugia malayi,* and least often, *Brugia timori.* Infection results from a bite from an infected arthropod. The larvae mature into adult worms within the human host, and the female produces microfilariae that are then transmitted to other biting insects, thus completing the life cycle. Approximately 80 million people in 76 countries are infected with filarial parasites. *W. bancrofti* accounts for about 90% of infections and *B. malayi* for most of the remaining cases. About two thirds of infected people live in China, India, or Indonesia.

Worms enter the lymphatics and lodge in the lymph nodes; these become fibrotic, causing obstruction to the lymphatic pathways, which are often grossly dilated. This results in severe swelling of the limbs (usually the legs), called elephantiasis.

A strongly positive complement fixation test suggests active or past filariasis. The diagnosis is confirmed by finding microfilariae, which enter the blood in large numbers at night.

Treatment with diethylcarbamazine destroys the filariae but cannot reverse established lymphedema, although progression

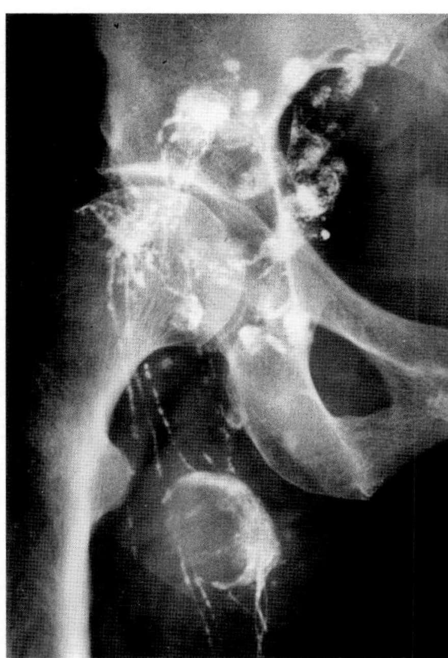

Figure 49-3. A lymphangiogram performed to investigate lymphedema of the right leg, which demonstrates malignancy in the right groin nodes. In this case, malignant melanoma deposits in the proximal nodes were the cause of secondary lymphedema.

of the disease may be slowed or prevented. Established lymphedema is treated by the same methods as those used to treat primary lymphedema.[29-31]

Nonfilarial Elephantiasis

Podoconiosis is a form of endemic nonfilarial elephantiasis that has been reported in certain parts of East Africa and Ethiopia where filariasis does not exist. It is thought that the condition is the result of an obstructive lymphopathy caused by aluminosilicate and silica absorbed from soil through the soles of the feet. The silica causes a dense fibrotic reaction in the inguinal nodes of barefoot tribesmen.

Malignancy

Any malignant process that spreads to the lymph nodes can cause secondary lymphedema, but it is more common after surgical resection or radiotherapy directed at nodal deposits of tumor. Hodgkin's disease and the non-Hodgkin's lymphomas occasionally present with lymphedema, which may also complicate malignant melanomas and testicular seminomas (Figure 49-3). The mass effect of large tumors can also obstruct lymph flow.[32]

Surgical Block Dissection

The block dissection operation is usually carried out to treat malignancies affecting lymph nodes, although in many cases it forms part of a staging or prophylactic procedure. The carcinomas commonly treated by block dissections are those of the breast and uterus.[33] Malignant melanoma and testicular tumors are also often treated by block dissection or irradiation.

Radiotherapy

Radiotherapy was a common cause of secondary lymphedema of the arm in patients with breast carcinoma in the 1970s and 1980s, especially when given after an axillary clearance. The combination of radiotherapy and surgery carries a higher risk of lymphedema than either treatment in isolation. Radiotherapy results in nodal fibrosis, which causes obstruction of the lymphatic vessels. Recurrent tumor in an irradiated field may also be responsible for lymphedema that develops some years after treatment of the primary disease.

Trauma

Severe trauma occasionally causes tissue loss that includes lymph nodes or lymphatic channels. This is particularly common after severe degloving injuries.

Chronic Infection

Although tuberculosis has often been cited as a cause of lymphedema, it is uncommon today.[34]

Chronic Inflammation

Severe rheumatoid disease, psoriatic arthritis, and severe chronic eczema are recognized causes of lymphedema. Chronic stimulation of the lymph nodes in these patients results in fibrosis and mild obstruction to the lymphatic drainage.[35-38]

Acute Infection

Severe cellulitis can occasionally damage the local subcutaneous lymphatics and cause mild lymphedema. Patients with subclinical primary lymphedema may also develop a secondary cellulitis: the two presentations can be difficult to distinguish.

Self-Induced

Self-induced lymphedema is a quite common form of Munchausen's syndrome, produced by repeated tight application of a tourniquet (Figure 49-4). Total disuse of a limb can also cause swelling: this form of self-induced lymphedema should be suspected if passive movement of the limb is not possible (Figure 49-5). Lymphograms are usually normal or only mildly abnormal. The cause should be suspected if a sharp cutoff to the lymphedema is demarcated by a rut from application of the tourniquet. Patients should be informed of the doctor's suspicions and referred for psychiatric advice.

CLINICAL FEATURES

Primary lymphedema is more common in the legs than in the arms. Although this is partly explained by the influence of gravity, anatomical abnormalities are rarely present in the lymphatics of the arm.

The swelling may affect one or both legs, the lower abdomen, the genital region, one or both arms, and rarely, the face or chest. In the legs, swelling usually develops around the ankle and on the dorsum of the foot, and it spreads proximally. In most patients, the edema does not spread above the knee. Severe edema of the whole leg, including the buttock, suggests

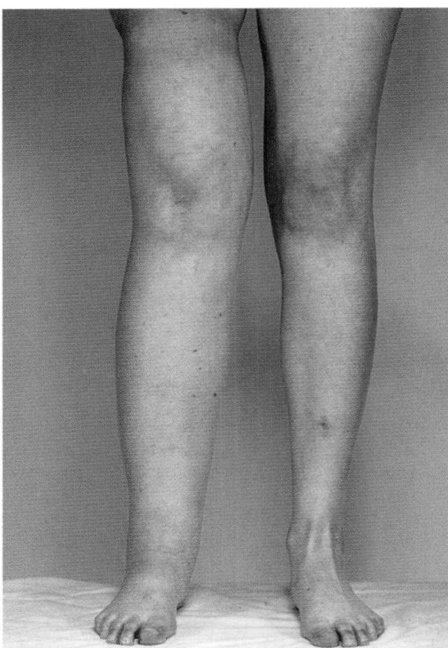

Figure 49-4. Self-induced right leg lymphedema. The indentation from the tourniquet used by the patient to effect the swelling can be seen in the upper thigh.

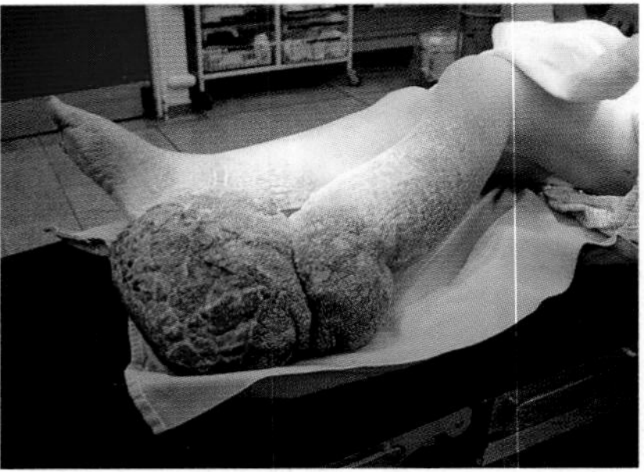

Figure 49-5. Self-induced left foot lymphedema. In this case, the swelling was produced by a combination of compression of the medial thigh by the contralateral knee, total disuse, and dependency. The patient had a through-knee amputation.

a proximal nodal lymphatic occlusion. There are exceptions to this rule, however, and patients with proximal lymphatic occlusions may have no edema of the ankle or foot.

Because lymphatic edema is chronic and has often been present for many years, it stimulates a fibrotic reaction in the subcutaneous tissues, making them more resistant to deformation than does "acute edema" associated with cardiac failure or hypoproteinemia. Prolonged digital pressure, however, always produces a "pit." The diagnosis of lymphedema must be questioned, and another cause for the swelling should be sought if pitting cannot be demonstrated.

The onset of the swelling is usually insidious, and the amount of swelling may fluctuate initially. Even when lymphedema becomes fixed, most patients report that the swelling decreases during sleep and is maximal at the end of the day. The onset can occasionally be sudden and progression rapid. This is often associated with cellulitis, which can be both a cause and a result of the lymphedema. Patients with sudden severe swelling usually have a proximal lymphatic occlusion and may have an underlying cause for the condition. Patients with malignant obstruction of both the veins and the lymphatics often develop a severe brawny edema of rapid onset; this can cause intractable pain, which may be difficult to alleviate. Some patients develop marked cutaneous thickening, which can progress to lymphatic warts (condylomata) and multiple coarse papillae. Other patients are troubled by repeated attacks of cellulitis. The infecting agent may enter through the hyperkeratotic skin or through cracks in the interdigital clefts that occur in athlete's foot.

Occasionally, patients develop numerous vesicles in the skin that may leak clear lymph or chyle. These vesicles usually indicate that megalymphatics and lymphatic reflux are present. Vesicles typically arise over the upper thighs or on the external genitalia (Figure 49-6), and they may also act as a portal of entry for bacteria. Occasionally, the lymph leakage from these vesicles is severe enough to be a major source of embarrassment and irritation.

Severe edema of the male genitalia is both embarrassing and uncomfortable, interfering with work and sexual relationships. When the penis is almost hidden inside a grossly swollen scrotum, penetration may be impossible and urination may be difficult. Leaking vesicles and recurrent attacks of cellulitis often complicate the condition. Women with genital edema usually have fewer problems, but massive labial swelling can occur.

Lymph can leak into both the abdominal and the pleural cavities, causing chylous ascites and pleural effusions. Patients present with abdominal distension, dyspnea, or both. These problems are usually the result of leakage from refluxing megalymphatics. Chyluria and chylous leakage from the vagina (chylometrorrhea) are rare complications. Protein-losing enteropathy can cause severe weight loss, and chylous leakage from the serosal surface of the bowel may increase the ascites.

Lymphedema may occasionally affect the arm, including the fingers, and unilateral pectoral swelling can also occur.

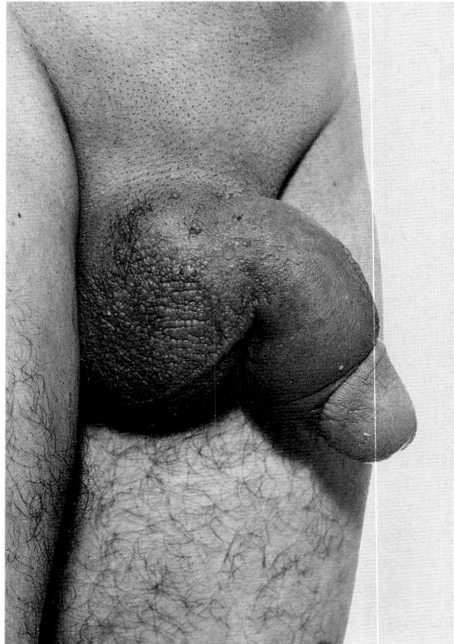

Figure 49-6. Skin vesicles seen around a lymphedematous penis.

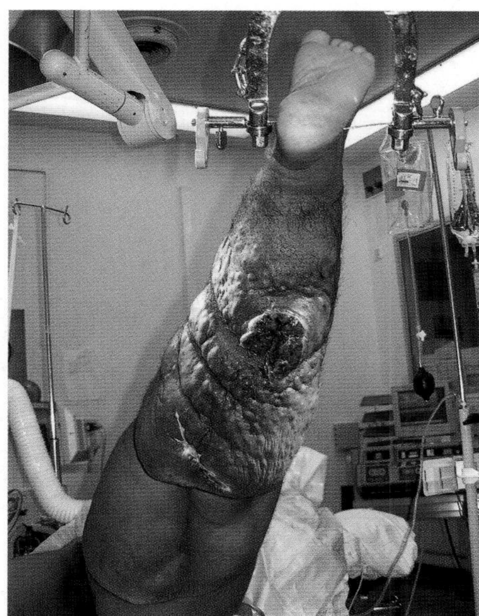

Figure 49-7. Lymphangiosarcoma in a young female with longstanding severe primary lymphedema. The area of ulceration had been present for a few months. Biopsy confirmed sarcoma, and the patient underwent amputation (a disarticulation of the hip).

Edema of the face usually presents as swelling of the eyelids, which are the most lax tissues in this region.

Patients with lymphedema usually seek advice because they want to know the reason for the swelling, which can cause major cosmetic embarrassment, even though it is often only of nuisance value. Severe swelling may make it impossible to put on normal shoes, and if the leg continues to swell, its weight interferes with normal walking. Recurrent attacks of cellulitis may also be a major problem, causing the patient to lose time off school or work. Severe attacks may require admission to hospital for intravenous antibiotics and may even be life threatening.

Several tumors are associated with lymphedema. Lymphangiosarcoma (Stewart-Treves syndrome) rarely develops in legs following longstanding lymphedema (Figure 49-7); it is more common in patients with secondary lymphedema.[39,40] Squamous cell carcinoma, cutaneous plasmacytoma, angiosarcoma, and Kaposi's sarcoma have all been reported in lymphedematous limbs.[41-46]

A detailed medical and family history should exclude secondary causes of lymphedema and may suggest a genetic cause of the primary condition.

Physical examination confirms the presence of "pitting," excludes other causes of limb swelling, and reveals any associated abnormalities. Examination of the feet may confirm the presence of "square toes," which result from footwear preventing toe expansion. An inability to pinch the skin together over the dorsum of the second toe (Stemmer's sign) supports a diagnosis of lymphedema. It is important to inspect the web spaces between the toes for fungal infection, which is especially common in lymphedematous legs and is an important portal of entry for bacteria that cause recurrent cellulitis.

The skin should be carefully examined for papillae and vesicles, and the circumference of the limbs should be measured at several levels, above and below fixed bony points. This allows comparison over time and the results of therapy to be evaluated. The length of the limbs should also be recorded and the presence of any abnormal veins noted. The abdomen and chest should be carefully examined for ascites or effusions. The groins, axillae, and neck should be palpated for pathologically enlarged lymph nodes. Rectal and vaginal examinations are indicated if a pelvic malignancy is suspected.

The history and physical examination should indicate whether the patient has primary or secondary lymphedema, but unequivocal confirmation of the diagnosis is desirable. Other investigations are necessary if the swelling is not considered to be the result of lymphedema.

DIFFERENTIAL DIAGNOSIS

Venous edema can sometimes be difficult to differentiate from lymphedema, especially if it is caused by the iliac vein compression syndrome, when there is often little in the way of superficial venous engorgement. The presence of dilated collateral veins, varicose veins, and lipodermatosclerosis of the calf skin suggest the likelihood of venous edema, as does a past history of deep vein thrombosis. Other causes of bilateral limb edema include cardiac disease, nephrotic syndrome, hypoproteinemia, fluid overload during intravenous therapy, and chronic liver disease. These disorders can be excluded by a careful physical examination and appropriate blood tests. Klippel-Trénaunay and Parkes Weber syndromes also cause limb enlargement. The former is associated with bony and soft tissue overgrowth, superficial varicosities in an unusual distribution, and a large capillary nevus. Some patients with Klippel-Trénaunay have a lymphatic element to the vascular malformation, although this is usually mild.

Patients with Parkes Weber syndrome (multiple congenital arteriovenous malformations throughout a limb) often have an oversized limb with evidence of venous hypertension (varicosities, nevi, and lipodermatosclerosis). Multiple machinery murmurs can be heard at many sites, and it should be possible to elicit the Branham-Nicoladoni sign (occlusion of the arterial inflow to the fistula by a tourniquet causes a slowing of the pulse rate).

True gigantism (Robertson's giant limb) is a rare disorder in which all tissues (muscles and bones) are hypertrophied.

A common misdiagnosis is that of lipoidosis or "lipodystrophy," a genetic condition that results in abnormal fat deposition, usually in proximal limbs. It can be excluded because the fat does not pit and the dorsum of the foot is unaffected and therefore not swollen (Figure 49-8).

Premenstrual edema is mild and has an obvious cyclical history, and rapidly growing soft tissue tumors rarely cause diagnostic problems.

Before making a diagnosis of one of these rare conditions, for which venography, computed tomography, magnetic resonance imaging, and arteriography may be required, it is often simpler to exclude a diagnosis of lymphedema by isotope lymphography.[47]

DIAGNOSTIC TECHNIQUES

Investigations

A full blood count, erythrocyte sedimentation rate, and chest radiographs are usually requested, and measurement of serum protein, blood urea, creatinine, electrolytes, and liver function tests should be obtained in all patients with bilateral edema. An electrocardiogram and echocardiogram may be helpful if cardiac edema is suspected.

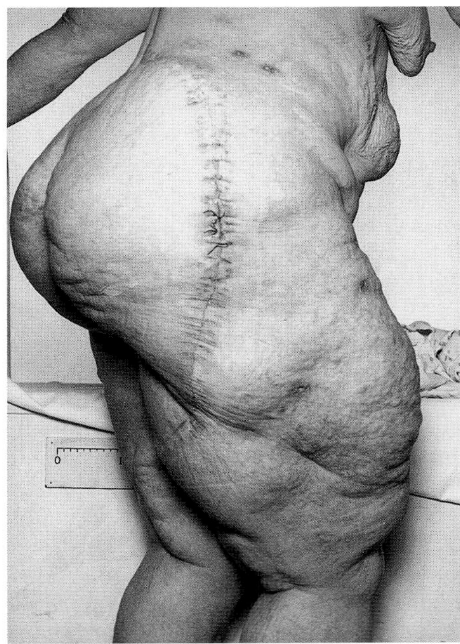

Figure 49-8. Lipodystrophy characterized by an abnormal propensity for the deposition of fat around the thighs and buttocks.

Isotope Lymphography

Isotope lymphography has replaced contrast lymphangiography as the primary diagnostic technique. Rhenium sulfur colloid is specifically taken up by lymphatics and allows the presence of lymphedema to be confirmed by a simple outpatient investigation with a reasonable degree of accuracy. Normally, 0.3% of the injected dose arrives in the groin within 30 minutes, and more than 0.6% arrives within 1 hour. An excessive uptake occurs in patients with venous edema, often above 3% at 30 minutes, and this test can therefore distinguish between venous and lymphatic edema, although a "grey area" of overlap exists. γ-Camera pictures provide information that the isotope is reaching the lymph nodes of the groin, and delayed images may show a failure of progression, indicating proximal obstruction. This should be confirmed by contrast lymphography, as should any equivocal findings. Isotope lymphography is a moderately sensitive test for lymphedema but may mistakenly classify some normal legs as lymphedematous. It often correctly identifies patients who are suitable for lymphatic bypass surgery.[48]

Contrast Lymphangiography

Contrast lymphangiography is sometimes indicated to confirm the diagnosis when the isotope test is equivocal and to determine whether the lymphatic obstruction is suitable for bypass. It is also indicated in patients with chylous ascites or megalymphatics with dermal leakage to show the extent of the lymphatic abnormality and indicate where leakage is occurring. Contrast is infused directly into the peripheral lymphatics of the arm or leg, which are visualized through an operative microscope after subcutaneous injection of dye into the web spaces (Figure 49-9). Patients are admitted to hospital for contrast lymphography, and general anesthesia is usually necessary as few patients can keep sufficiently still for the time required to obtain the radiographs. Before the test, patients often require bed rest and leg elevation in hospital for a few days to reduce foot edema and make lymphatic cannulation easier. Lymphangiography does, however, provide precise information on the presence of lymphatic hypoplasia, the extent of the megalymphatics, and the site of the lymphatic obstruction.

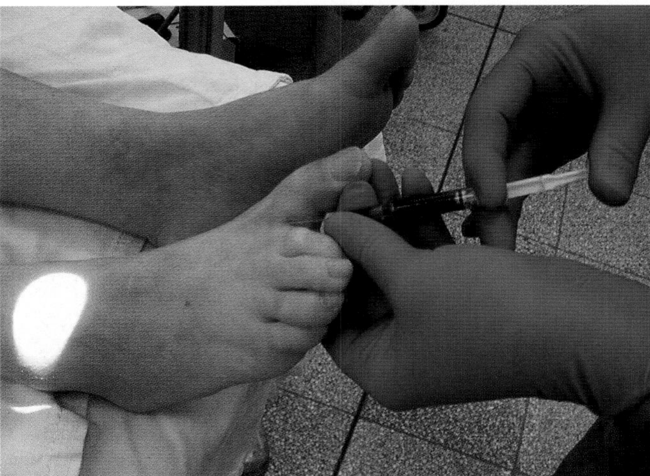

Figure 49-9. Contrast lymphangiography. Patent blue–green dye is injected into the web spaces before lymphangiography.

Contrast lymphangiography remains the investigation against which other techniques are judged. It is still essential before lymphatic bypass is considered and is of some value in assessing prognosis.

Magnetic resonance imaging of a limb can show dilated subcutaneous lymphatics but cannot define the site of lymphatic obstruction. Magnetic resonance imaging alone, or in combination with superparamagnetic contrast agents (lymphangiomagnetograms) or fat subtraction (suppression), has the potential to yield further information. Ultrasound imaging, computed tomography, and magnetic resonance imaging can all demonstrate enlarged lymph nodes, and guided biopsies of lymph nodes can be taken if malignancy is suspected. Needle or Tru-Cut biopsies are probably safer as a preliminary procedure, since removal of large solitary fibrotic nodes may worsen existing lymphedema. A calcium chloride test may be helpful when protein-losing enteropathy is suspected.

Fluorescent microangiolymphography and an injection of intradermal brominated fluorocarbon can be used to identify lymph nodes. These noninvasive imaging techniques can be used to monitor and document the efficacy of treatments designed to remedy defective lymph transport in chylous reflux syndrome. They can also be used to delineate incompetent lymphangiectatic or lymphangiomatous truncal elements so that they can be sclerosed successfully using percutaneous computer-guided catheters.[49]

MANAGEMENT

Distal Hypoplasia: Meig's Disease

Young women with mild lymphedema of gradual onset usually have distal lymphatic hypoplasia: the time taken for the isotope to reach the groin nodes is prolonged, but onward passage is normal. This type of lymphedema is often inherited

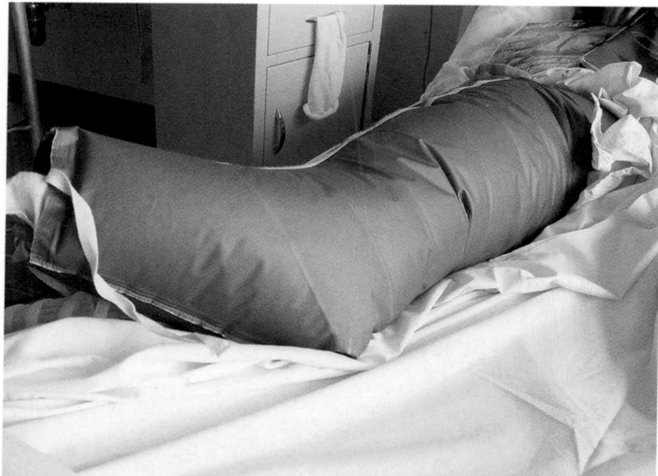

Figure 49-10. A pneumatic massaging device.

(in around a third of patients) and rarely becomes severe or extends above the knee. It is often bilateral, but one leg may be affected several years before the other. Rarely, the arms are also involved.[50]

Physical Methods

Patients with distal lymphatic hypoplasia rarely require surgery. They should be given advice on leg elevation, especially in the evenings and at night. Some patients obtain benefit from regular massage or mechanical compression, combined with wearing graduated elastic compression stockings during waking hours. Pneumatic massaging devices are available, and sequential segmental machines such as the Lymphopress are probably more effective than single-chamber boots (Figure 49-10). These may be worn in the evenings or in bed at night, although they may interfere with sleep.[51]

Correctly fitted graduated compression stockings (30 to 50 mm Hg at the ankle, decreasing up the leg) only need to be prescribed to knee level if the lymphedema is distal in distribution. Elastic compression stockings do not cure lymphedema, but they reduce fluid accumulation during the day and often produce considerable symptomatic relief. They are poorly tolerated in warm climates, and young men and women tend to be conscious of their appearance. Many patients with mild lymphedema require little in the way of active treatment apart from reassurance and a prescription for elastic stockings. Weight reduction and physical exercise are often beneficial and never harmful. Concentrated compression therapy and massage that reduces the size of lymphedematous legs can be maintained if the patient obsessively wears good elastic stockings or repeatedly applies tight bandages.[52]

Drug Therapy

Diuretics are of little value in lymphedema as they do not selectively remove fluid from the lymphedematous tissues and may cause side effects when used for prolonged intervals. Paroven (hydroxyrutosides) and the benzopyrones may reduce swelling, but both of these compounds only have a small clinical effect.[53-55]

Autologous lymphocyte infusion, which was reported to relieve swelling, has not proved to be of any long-term benefit. It was thought that cytokines produced by lymphocytes would mediate proteolysis by macrophage proteinases in the lymphedematous leg. This would remove the excess protein and relieve edema.[56,57]

Antibiotics (flucloxacillin, amoxicillin, or one of the cephalosporins) should be prescribed for cellulitis. Low-dose prophylactic antibiotics should be used if patients are troubled by repeated attacks, as prevention of cellulitis may reduce progression of the swelling.[58]

Athlete's foot must be treated by appropriate antifungal medication with Lamasil. Careful podiatry prevents infection and avoids an important portal of entry for virulent bacteria.

Patients with Severe Whole Limb Lymphedema

Surgery may be considered for patients with severe lymphedema (often associated with proximal obstruction) where the whole limb is swollen and interferes with mobility or is tremendously unsightly. Most patients have a poor result from prolonged conservative treatment, as described earlier.

Surgery

In a small proportion of patients, preoperative contrast lymphangiography discloses a proximal lymphatic obstruction in the ilioinguinal region, with normal distal leg lymphatics. These patients (1% to 3% of all those seen) can expect to benefit from some form of lymphatic bypass operation. Many patients have been selected for investigation because the foot is "spared" from edema and the isotope suggests that the contrast reaches the groin but fails to pass to the iliac nodes.

Lymphatic Bypass

Several methods have been used to join obstructed lymphatics to the venous system. Many of these techniques are of historical interest only, such as the omental pedicle and the skin bridge devised by Gillies, which was sutured to the obstructed lymph nodes in the groin.[58a] Direct anastomosis of lymph nodes to veins was originally performed by Niebulowitz, but fibrosis and low flow resulted in a high failure rate.[58b] Degni used a special needle to insert lymphatics into the lumen of the vein, but the imprecise nature of this procedure has prevented its widespread acceptance.[58c] The advent of the operating microscope made it possible to divide obstructed lymphatics and anastomose them directly to veins. The results, however, have generally been disappointing. At least three or four lymphatics should be attached to the femoral vein in the groin in the hope that one or two anastomoses will remain patent. Although centers throughout the world advocate microvascular techniques for the treatment of lymphedema, lack of evidence of long-term efficacy has resulted in little interest in the United Kingdom.[59-65]

Kinmonth and associates developed the mesenteric bridge procedure as an alternative to direct lymphovenous anastomosis.[65a] This operation uses the copious submucosal lymphatic plexus and the mesenteric lymphatics to drain lymph from obstructed nodes in the ilioinguinal region. About 5 cm of the terminal ileum is resected on its mesenteric pedicle, as for an ileal conduit, taking great care to maintain the mesenteric lymphatic drainage. The small bowel is reanastomosed behind the pedicle. The isolated segment is then opened along its antimesenteric border, and the mucosa is stripped off the submucosa by a combination of sharp and blunt dissection after a submucosal injection of a solution of adrenaline in saline (1:400,000). The isolated pedicle is then brought down to the first normal group of lymph nodes below the level of the obstruction, and sutured over them after they have been bivalved. Connections develop between the divided nodes and the submucosal plexus so that lymph from the legs drains up the pedicle into the mesenteric lymph nodes and eventually into the thoracic duct.

This operation has been performed on more than 40 patients at St Thomas' Hospital, London, and has produced good results in approximately half of them. Unfortunately, no means exists of predicting which patients will benefit from the procedure. Young patients appear to fare better, and the distal leg lymphatics must still be functioning if a successful result is to be achieved. Resolution is poor if legs are too swollen, but the swelling must be severe enough to justify major abdominal surgery. Perhaps for this reason, lymphatic bypass surgery is appropriate for few patients.

Reduction Operations

Absence of any functioning lymphatics in the leg precludes bypass surgery, and limb "reduction" is the only other surgical option.

Four types of excisional operation have been described to reduce the size of lymphedematous legs. The Sistrunk operation consists of the excision of a large wedge or ellipse of skin and subcutaneous tissue, which is then closed by skin sutures. In Homan's reduction, skin flaps are elevated from the subcutaneous fat, excising the underlying subcutaneous tissue and redundant skin. The skin flaps are then sutured back in place (Figure 49-11).

Thompson modified Homan's operation by suturing one of the skin flaps to the deep fascia. Denudation of the superficial layers of the flap stops hair growth and prevents pilonidal sinus formation. The second flap is then sutured over the top of the denuded skin. This operation has now largely been abandoned: because it leaves unsightly scars, it is often complicated by pilonidal sinus formation, and the results appear to be no better than those of the simpler Homan's procedure. The theoretical benefit that cutaneous lymphatics could connect to the deep lymphatics through the buried flap has not been realized in practice.

Both Homan's and Thompson's operations can be complicated by skin flap necrosis and poor healing, particularly at the corners of the flaps. Great care needs to be taken to maintain the blood supply of the flaps, which must not be cut too thin. Flap reduction of the calf and foot is normally combined with a Sistrunk operation on the thigh if the whole leg is to be reduced in size.

Charles invented an operation to remove the severely thickened skin in patients with filariasis in India. He excised all the diseased skin and the waterlogged subcutaneous tissue down to, and often including, the deep fascia, from just above the ankle to just below the knee. The periosteum over the tibia was left intact, and split skin grafts were then taken from normal donor skin (the opposite normal leg or the abdomen, back, and buttocks) and used to cover the deep fascia or muscle.

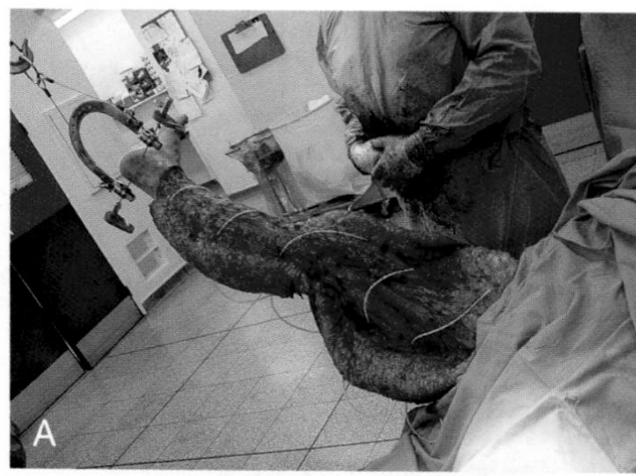

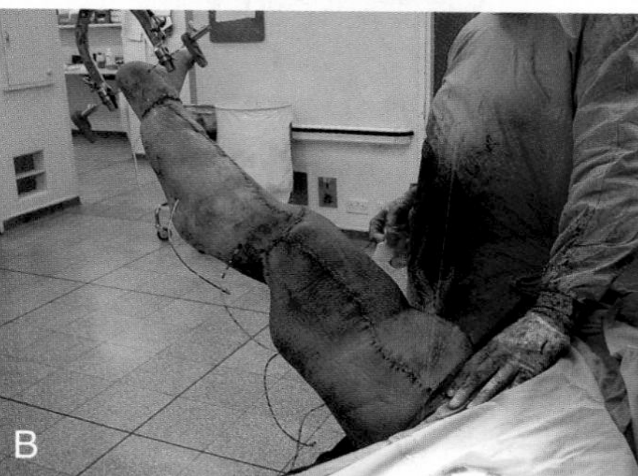

Figure 49-11. Homan's reduction. **A,** Intraoperative Homan's procedure, showing the extent of dissection used to elevate the skin and subcutaneous flaps. **B,** The same patient at the end of the procedure.

This operation produces the best reduction in leg size but often does so at the expense of cosmesis (Figure 49-12). The ankle and knee area have to be tailored carefully to avoid a pantaloon effect, and thigh reduction is also often necessary. Some patients have a poor acceptance of split skin grafts and require multiple operations to achieve complete healing. Other patients develop severe hyperkeratotic scars with warty excrescences, which produce deformity in the operated leg. These can be treated by shaving off the warty nodules and thickened scars with a scalpel or skin graft knife; additional skin grafts are then occasionally needed to cover denuded areas. Final results are often satisfactory, especially in a grossly enlarged leg with abnormal calf skin (Figures 49-13 and 49-14).

Liposuction

It should be possible to remove large quantities of edematous fat from the subcutaneous tissue by a liposuction technique, but it has proved disappointing in patients with severely swollen legs from primary lymphedema. Brorson has reported excellent long-term results in patients with secondary edema of the arm after mastectomy.[66] These results must be confirmed by others.

LYMPHEDEMA OF OTHER SITES

Genital Lymphedema

Minor scrotal and penile lymphedema can be tolerated without specific treatment, although support garments may be helpful. Severe scrotal edema is best treated by excisional reduction surgery in which a large central segment is excised from the scrotum, preserving the spermatic cords and testicles. The flaps are then primarily sutured using an absorbable material

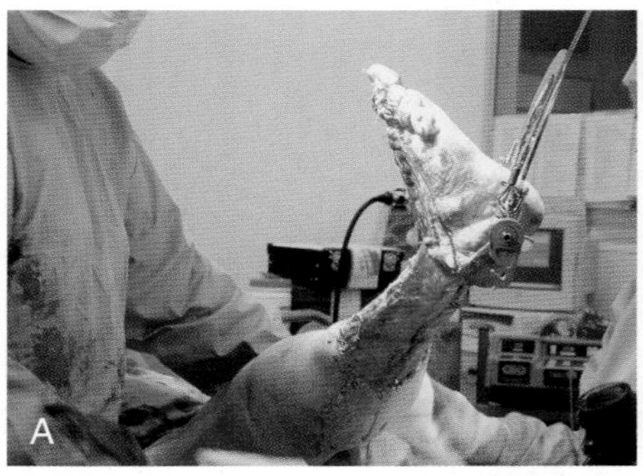
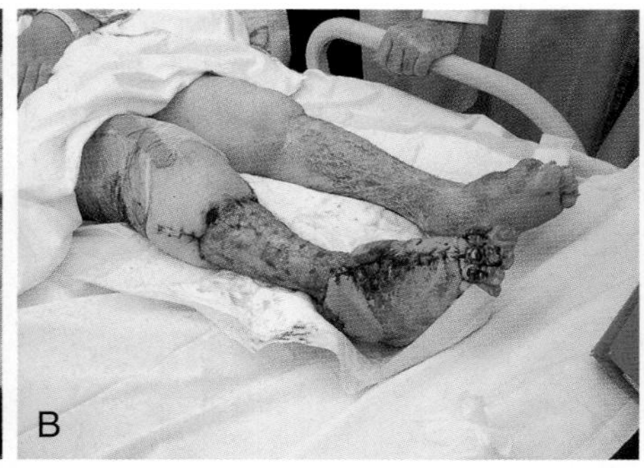
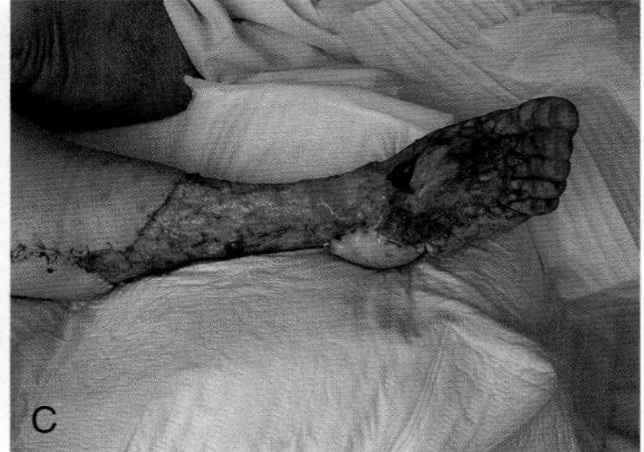

Figure 49-12. Charles' reduction. **A,** At the end of Charles' reduction. Skin grafts have been taken from the ipsilateral thigh, and the foot has been reduced by a Homan's-type procedure. **B,** The appearance of a Charles procedure on the fifth postoperative day, when the dressings are removed. The patient previously had her left leg reduced by a Charles operation. **C,** This patient has had a Charles operation and skin grafting to the dorsum of the foot.

and the scrotum is drained. Mobilization of the testes with gentle abrasion of their surfaces may encourage adhesions to form, allowing lymph to drain via the testicular lymphatics and aiding the scrotal reduction (Figure 49-15).

The penis may be reduced by simple excisional procedures, combined with circumcision if necessary. Alternatively, surgical excision of the affected tissue and split-skin grafting (Charles' reduction) is effective for severe lymphedema of the scrotum and penis. Both scrotal and penile reduction operations produce gratifying results for the patient.[67-69]

Massive labial swelling can also be treated by simple excision.

Eyelids and Upper Limb

Eyelid swelling can be treated by lid reduction,[70,71] but management of lymphedema of the head and neck is usually by manual lymphatic drainage.[72]

Arm swelling can be treated by liposuction or a Homan's type of limb reduction. This can be performed on both the inner and the outer sides of the arm. Patients with postmastectomy edema must be assessed carefully to ensure that the venous drainage is satisfactory and to be certain that no evidence exists of recurrent axillary nodal disease. Both venous obstruction and recurrent malignancy are contraindications to arm reduction. Postoperatively, an elasticated sleeve should be worn to try to prevent recurrent swelling.

Chylous Reflux

Some patients have dilated valveless megalymphatics that allow the reflux of lymph (often chyle) against the expected direction of flow. These dilated lymphatics often end in cutaneous vesicles, which are visible in the skin or may rupture into body cavities such as the pleura, peritoneum, kidney, bladder, uterus, or vagina. Rupture results in the accumulation

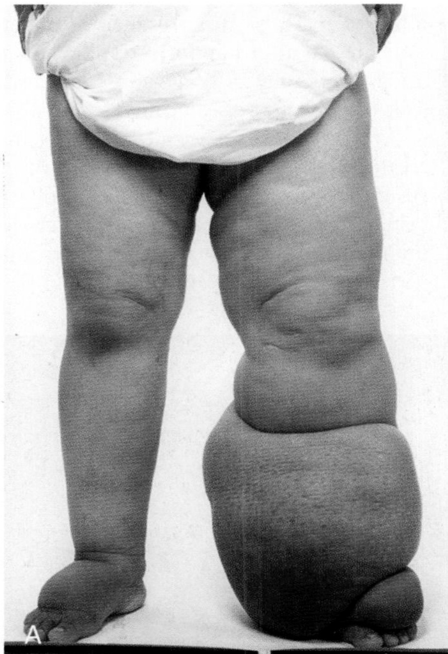
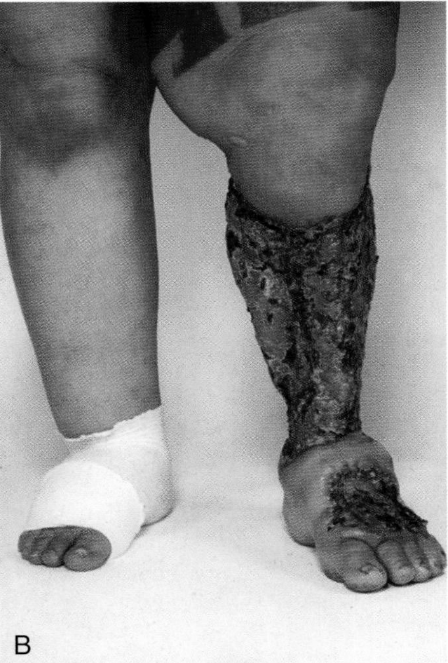

Figure 49-13. Before and 2 weeks after Charles' reduction of the lower leg and foot.

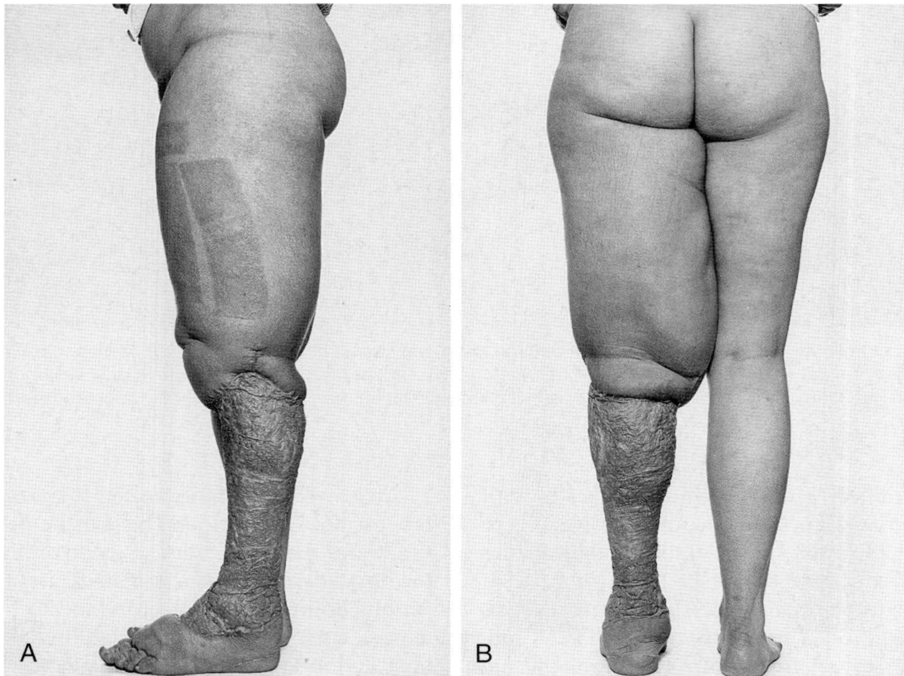

Figure 49-14. Results of Charles' reduction at 6 months.

of lymph or chyle in the relevant cavity (chylothorax, hydrothorax, chylous ascites, chyluria), and chylous discharge onto the skin surface or mucosa is common. Accumulation of chyle in the pleural and peritoneal cavities produces severe symptoms, and patients often become dyspneic and distended. Some patients have a more generalized lymphatic abnormality associated with lymphedema of the limbs. Patients with megalymphatics often also have leakage of lymph from the mucosal or serosal surfaces of the bowel, leading to hypoproteinemia or ascites, respectively. Primary intestinal lymphangiectasia is characterized by widespread dilation of the small bowel lymphatics and a protein-losing enteropathy (with loss of lymph into the bowel lumen), which can cause weight loss and hypoproteinemia that further exacerbates accumulation of fluid in the body cavities and tissues.[73]

The diagnosis of chylous ascites or a chylothorax must first be confirmed by aspiration of the fluid, which is then tested for chylomicrons, although the milky appearance is usually obvious. The condition may be suspected if lymphedema of the extremities pre-exists, and it is especially likely if vesicles with lymphatic leakage are present. In quite a few patients, the condition develops de novo. Chylothorax and chylous ascites must be distinguished from malignant ascites or a malignant effusion: cytological examination of the aspirate may help exclude or confirm the presence of malignant cells. Computed tomography and ultrasound can demonstrate or rule out enlargement of the abdominal or mediastinal lymph nodes. Enlarged nodes suggest the possibility of a lymphoma or secondary malignant spread. Guided biopsy, laparoscopy, or laparotomy may be necessary to confirm these diagnoses. Contrast lymphography demonstrates lymphadenopathy, filling defects, or the presence of megalymphatics. It is only indicated if the diagnosis remains in doubt. Contrast lymphography may also demonstrate and localize a lymphatic leak, which can be sealed surgically.[74,75]

Lymphedema associated with megalymphatics rarely requires reduction surgery, but the complications of lymphatic vesicles, recurrent infections, lymphatic discharge onto the skin, chylous ascites, chyluria, and chylothorax often demand intervention. Leakage of chyle or lymph may be prevented by

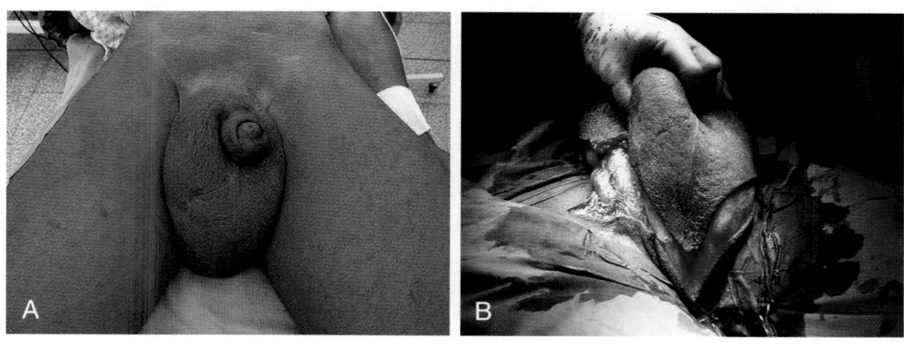

Figure 49-15. A, Genital lymphedema. **B,** Scrotal reduction.

ligating or underrunning the dilated lymphatic channels, but this carries the risk of causing lymphatic obstruction, which worsens the leg swelling. Despite this, many patients benefit from ligation of dilated lymphatics and sealing off of any obvious site of fistulation.

Chromium chloride studies and a small bowel enema may provide useful information before a laparotomy is performed, if a patient with chylous ascites or chylothorax has no obvious leak on the lymphangiogram. At laparotomy, the posterior abdominal wall over the main lymphatic pathways must be inspected carefully for the presence of leakage, and the whole of the intestine should be examined. If the surface of the small bowel is grossly abnormal and leaking lymph, the involved or most abnormal segment should be resected. The ascites can be returned back into the venous system using a Denver shunt if this fails. Although these shunts work well in patients with other types of ascites, chyle often blocks the tubing or the valve and produces an early occlusion of the shunt. Many patients improve with simple avoidance of fat and prescription of medium-chain triglycerides combined with diuretics.

Chylothorax may respond to aspiration but often recurs and is best prevented by pleurodesis by surgical removal of the pleura. A small mortality is associated with this procedure, and some patients die from fluid- or lymph-overloaded lungs as the lymphatics draining the lung become obstructed when they are no longer able to empty into the pleural cavity.

The prognosis of many patients with severe problems from their megalymphatics can be helped by some of the procedures outlined earlier. Cutaneous vesicles may simply be excised or touched with diathermy or cautery, but they tend to recur. Recurrent infections should be treated by a prolonged course of broad-spectrum antibiotics.

Lymphangioma Circumscriptum

These cutaneous vesicles and associated subcutaneous swellings are considered to be hamartomas or localized abnormalities of the cutaneous lymphatic drainage. They present as several clear or slightly hemorrhagic cutaneous vesicles, often associated with subcutaneous thickening in the underlying fat. Whimster thought that lymphangioma circumscriptum was the result of defective lymphatic drainage from the subcutaneous tissue, where several cisterns "pump" lymph back into the overlying skin. These areas should be excised if they are unsightly or painful.[75a] They often occur on the trunk, and it is important to excise a generous amount of subcutaneous tissue well beyond the ellipse of skin bearing the vesicles to remove the subcutaneous bladders described by Whimster. It is often quite difficult to excise all skin lesions, and they have a propensity to recur: excisional surgery is only required if they are symptomatic.[76]

Cystic Hygroma

Cystic hygroma is a developmental abnormality of the lymphatic system in which lymphatic fluid collects in a cystic space that is often multilocular and situated at the base of the neck, often extending into the axilla. It commonly appears in childhood and presents as a soft, brilliantly translucent swelling in the base of the neck. Aspiration and injection of sclerosant may be attempted, but the multiloculated swellings often recur and may require surgical excision. Cystic hygromas must be dissected with great care as several important structures lie adjacent to them.

Mesenteric Cysts

Localized lymphatic cysts within the mesentery appear as well-circumscribed mobile lumps within the abdomen. The diagnosis can be confirmed by ultrasound or computed tomography. They are treated by resection, often in association with the overlying area of small bowel. Although harmless, they may reach a considerable size if left untreated.

SUMMARY

Most patients with lymphatic disorders can be managed conservatively. Few patients are suitable for bypass surgery: when surgery is indicated, an enteromesenteric bridge is probably the best form of bypass, having an excellent result in about half of the patients. Bypass surgery should be reserved for patients with severe leg swelling that interferes with limb function. Patients with gross leg swelling and severe skin changes are best treated by Charles' reduction, combined with a local excision of thigh tissue. Homan's operation should be reserved for those with a moderate to severe degree of swelling interfering with limb function after a prolonged course of conservative treatment. Patients with secondary lymphedema caused by malignancy often have associated venous edema. The results of reduction surgery under these circumstances are extremely poor.

References

1. Milroy WR. An undescribed variety of hereditary oedema. *NY Med J* 1892;56:505-508.

1a. Karkkainen MJ, Ferrell RE, Lawrence EC, et al. Missense mutations interfere with VEGFR-3 signalling in primary lymphoedema. *Nat Genet* 2000;25:153-159.

2. Karkkainen MJ, Saaristo A, Jussila L, et al. A model for gene therapy of human hereditary lymphedema. *Proc Natl Acad Sci USA* 2001;98: 12677-12682.
3. Irrthum A, Karkkainen MJ, Devriendt K, et al. Congenital hereditary lymphedema caused by a mutation that inactivates VEGFR3 tyrosine kinase. *Am J Hum Genet* 2000;67:295-301.
4. Holberg CJ, Erickson RP, Bernas MJ, et al. Segregation analyses and a genome-wide linkage search confirm genetic heterogeneity and suggest oligogenic inheritance in some Milroy congenital primary lymphedema families. *Am J Med Genet* 2001;98:303-312.
5. Evans AL, Brice G, Sotirova V, et al. Mapping of primary congenital lymphedema to the 5q35.3 region. *Am J Hum Genet* 1999;64:547-555.
6. Dumont DJ, Jussila L, Taipale J, et al. Cardiovascular failure in mouse embryos deficient in VEGF receptor-3. *Science* 1998;282:946-949.
7. Saaristo A, Veikkola T, Tammela T, et al. Lymphangiogenic gene therapy with minimal blood vascular side effects. *J Exp Med* 2002;196: 719-730.
8. Karkkainen MJ, Jussila L, Ferrell RE, et al. Molecular regulation of lymphangiogenesis and targets for tissue oedema. *Trends Mol Med* 2001;7: 18-22.
9. Brice G, Mansour S, Bell R, et al. Analysis of the phenotypic abnormalities in lymphoedema–distichiasis syndrome in 74 patients with FOXC2 mutations or linkage to 16q24. *J Med Genet* 2002;39:478-483.
10. Erickson RP, Dagenais SL, Caulder MS, et al. Clinical heterogeneity in lymphoedema–distichiasis with FOXC2 truncating mutations. *J Med Genet* 2001;38:761-766.
11. Bell R, Brice G, Child AH, et al. Analysis of lymphoedema–distichiasis families for FOXC2 mutations reveals small insertions and deletions throughout the gene. *Hum Genet* 2001;108:546-551.
12. Rosbotham JL, Brice GW, Child AH, et al. Distichiasis–lymphoedema: clinical features, venous function and lymphoscintigraphy. *Br J Dermatol* 2000;142:148-152.

13. Mellor RH, Brice G, Stanton AWB, et al. Mutations in FOXC2 are strongly associated with primary valve failure in veins of the lower limb. *Circulation* 2007;115:1912-1920.
14. Casteels I, Devriendt K, Van Cleynenbreugel H, et al. Autosomal dominant microcephaly–lymphoedema–chorioretinal dysplasia syndrome. *Br J Ophthalmol* 2001;85:499-500.
15. D'Alessandro A, Muzi G, Monaco A, et al. Yellow nail syndrome: does protein leakage play a role? *Eur Respir J* 2001;17:149-152.
16. Hashem FK, Ahmed S. Idiopathic scrotal lymphedema in Down's syndrome. *Aust NZ J Surg* 1999;69:75-77.
17. Aagenaes O. Hereditary cholestasis with lymphedema: new cases and follow-up from infancy to adult age. *Scand J Gastroenterol* 1998;33:335-345.
18. Boucher CA, Sargent CA, Ogata T, Affara NA. Breakpoint analysis of Turner patients with partial Xp deletions: implications for the lymphoedema gene location. *J Med Genet* 2001;38:591-598.
19. Wigle JT, Oliver G. Prox1 function is required for the development of the murine lymphatic system. *Cell* 1999;98:769-778.
20. Wigle JT, Harvey N, Detmar M, et al. An essential role for Prox1 in the induction of the lymphatic endothelial cell phenotype. *EMBO J* 2002;21:1505-1513.
21. Casley-Smith JR, Casley-Smith JR. The effects of O-(β-hydroxy-ethyl)-rutosides (HR) on acute lymphoedema in rats' thighs, with and without macrophages. *Microcirc Endothelium Lymphatics* 1990;6:457-463.
22. Jones AL, Webb DJ. Selective IgA deficiency, hypothyroidism and congenital lymphoedema. *Scott Med J* 1996;41:22-23.
23. Usta M, Dilek K, Ersoy A, et al. A family with IgA nephropathy and hereditary lymphedema praecox. *J Intern Med* 2002;251:447-451.
24. Karg E, Bereczki C, Kovacs J, et al. Primary lymphoedema associated with xanthomatosis, vaginal lymphorrhoea and intestinal lymphangiectasia. *Br J Dermatol* 2002;146:134-137.
25. Fatinni Y, Asindi A, Al Falki Y, et al. Possible new autosomal recessive syndrome of congenital lymphoedema, nail dystrophy and esotropia in a Saudi family. *Acta Paediatr* 2001;90:151-153.
26. Benson PF, Taylor AI, Gough MH. Chromosome anomalies in primary lymphoedema. *Lancet* 1967;1:461-462.
27. Haugen OH, Krohn J. Bilateral congenital glaucoma in a child with hydrops fetalis, congenital pulmonary lymphangiectasia, and lymphoedema. *J Pediatr Ophthalmol Strabismus* 2000;37:44-46.
28. Tatnall FM, Sarkany I. Primary facial lymphoedema with xanthomas. *J R Soc Med* 1988;81:113-114.
29. Bockarie MJ, Tavul L, Kastens W, et al. Impact of untreated bednets on prevalence of *Wuchereria bancrofti* transmitted by *Anopheles farauti* in Papua New Guinea. *Med Vet Entomol* 2002;16:116-119.
30. Ngwira BM, Jabu CH, Kanyongoloka H, et al. Lymphatic filariasis in the Karonga district of northern Malawi: a prevalence survey. *Ann Trop Med Parasitol* 2002;96:137-144.
31. Molyneux DH, Taylor MJ. Current status and future prospects of the Global Lymphatic Filariasis Programme. *Curr Opin Infect Dis* 2001;14:155-159.
32. Mogulkoc N, Onal B, Okyay N, et al. Chylothorax, chylopericardium and lymphoedema: the presenting features of signet-ring cell carcinoma. *Eur Respir J* 1999;13:1489-1491.
33. Sparaco A, Fentiman IS. Arm lymphoedema following breast cancer treatment. *Int J Clin Pract* 2002;56:107-110.
34. Ramesh V, Ramesh V. Lymphedema of the genitalia secondary to skin tuberculosis: report of three cases. *Genitourin Med* 1997;73:226-227.
35. Schmit P, Prieur AM, Brunelle F. Juvenile rheumatoid arthritis and lymphedema: lymphangiographic aspects. *Pediatr Radiol* 1999;29:364-366.
36. Bohm M, Riemann B, Luger TA, Bonsmann G. Bilateral upper limb lymphoedema associated with psoriatic arthritis: a case report and review of the literature. *Br J Dermatol* 2000;143:1297-1301.
37. Gach JE, King CM. Constitutional pompholyx eczema complicated by secondary lymphoedema. *Acta Derm Venereol* 2001;81:437-438.
38. Fitzgerald DA, English JS. Lymphoedema of the hands as a complication of chronic allergic contact dermatitis. *Contact Dermatitis* 1994;30:310.
39. Stewart FW, Treves N. Lymphangiosarcoma in post mastectomy lymphedema: a report of six cases in elephantiasis chirurgica. *Cancer* 1948;1:64-81.
40. Aygit AC, Yildirim AM, Dervisoglu S. Lymphangiosarcoma in chronic lymphoedema: Stewart-Treves syndrome. *J Hand Surg [Br]* 1999;24:135-137.
41. Lister RK, Black MM, Calonje E, Burnand KG. Squamous cell carcinoma arising in chronic lymphoedema. *Br J Dermatol* 1997;136:384-387.
42. Echenique-Elizondo M, Elorza J. Squamous-cell carcinoma on long-lasting lymphoedema. *Lancet Oncol* 2002;3:319.
43. Corazza M, Lombardi A, Strumia R, et al. Primary cutaneous plasmacytoma on chronic lymphedema. *Eur J Dermatol* 2002;12:191-193.
44. Atillasoy ES, Santoro A, Weinberg JM. Lymphedema associated with Kaposi's sarcoma. *J Eur Acad Dermatol Venereol* 2001;15:364-365.
45. Schwartz RA, Cohen JB, Watson RA, et al. Penile Kaposi's sarcoma preceded by chronic penile lymphoedema. *Br J Dermatol* 2000;142:153-156.
46. Azurdia RM, Guerin DM, Verbov JL. Chronic lymphedema and angiosarcoma. *Clin Exp Dermatol* 1999;24:270-272.
47. Parkes Weber F. Angioma formation in connection with hypertrophy of limbs and hemihypertrophy. *Br J Dermatol* 1907;19:231.
48. Burnand KG, McGuinness CL, Lagattolla NR, et al. Value of isotope lymphography in the diagnosis of lymphoedema of the leg. *Br J Surg* 2002;89:74-78.
49. Witte CL, Witte MH. Diagnostic and interventional imaging of lymphatic disorders. *Int Angiol* 1999;18:25-30.
50. Mortimer PS. Managing lymphedema. *Clin Exp Dermatol* 1995;20:98-106.
51. Chen AH, Frangos SG, Kilaru S, Sumpio BE. Intermittent pneumatic compression devices; physiological mechanisms of action. *Eur J Vasc Endovasc Surg* 2001;21:383-392.
52. Mason M. Bandaging and subsequent elastic hosiery is more effective than elastic hosiery alone in reducing lymphedema. *Aust J Physiother* 2001;47:153.
53. Casley-Smith JR. Changes in the microcirculation at the superficial and deeper levels in lymphoedema: the effects and results of massage, compression, exercise and benzopyrones on these levels during treatment. *Clin Hemorheol Microcirc* 2000;23:335-343.
54. Casley-Smith JR. Benzo-pyrones in the treatment of lymphoedema. *Int Angiol* 1999;18:31-41.
55. Piller NB, Morgan RG, Casley-Smith JR. A double-blind, cross-over trial of O-(β-hydroxyethyl)-rutosides (benzo-pyrones) in the treatment of lymphoedema of the arms and legs. *Br J Plast Surg* 1988;41:20-27.
56. Nagata Y, Murata R, Mitsumori M, et al. Intraarterial infusion of autologous lymphocytes for the treatment of refractory lymphedema: preliminary report. *Eur J Surg* 1994;160:105-109.
57. Knight KR, Ritz M, Lepore DA, Booth R, Octigan K, O'Brien BM. Autologous lymphocyte therapy for experimental canine lymphedema: a pilot study. *Aust NZ J Surg* 1994;64:332-337.
58. Woo PC, Lum PN, Wong SS, Cheng VC, Yuen KY. Cellulitis complicating lymphedema. *Eur J Clin Microbiol Infect Dis* 2000;19:294-297.

58a. Gilles HD, Fraser FR. The treatment of lymphoedema by plastic operations. *Br Med J* 1935;1:96-98.

58b. Niebulowitz J, Olszewski W. Surgical lymphatico-venous shunts in patients with secondary lymphoedema. *Brit J Surg* 1968;55:440-443.

58c. Degni M. New technique of lymphatic-venous anastomosis (buried type) for the treatment of lymphedema. *Vasa* 1974;3(4):479-483.

59. Campisi C, Boccardo F. Role of microsurgery in the management of lymphedema. *Int Angiol* 1999;18:47-51.
60. Campisi C, Boccardo F. Frontiers in lymphatic microsurgery. *Microsurgery* 1998;18:462-471.
61. Binoy C, Rao YG, Ananthakrishnan N, et al. Omentoplasty in the management of filarial lymphedema. *Trans R Soc Trop Med Hyg* 1998;92:317-319.
62. Chen HC, O'Brien BM, Rogers IW, et al. Lymph node transfer for the treatment of obstructive lymphoedema in the canine model. *Br J Plast Surg* 1990;43:578-586.
63. Ipsen T, Pless J, Frederiksen PB. Experience with microlymphaticovenous anastomoses for congenital and acquired lymphedema. *Scand J Plast Reconstr Surg Hand Surg* 1988;22:233-236.
64. Dimakakos PB, Arkadopoulos N. E Kondoleon: the man behind the procedure. *Int Angiol* 2000;19:84-88.
65. Rao YG, Ananthakrishnan N, Pani SP, et al. Factors influencing response to lymphonodovenous shunt in filarial lymphedema. *Natl Med J India* 1999;12:55-58.

65a. Kinmonth JB, Hurst PA, Edwards JM, Rutt DL. A gut and mesentery pedicle for bridging lymphatic obstruction. *Brit J Surg* 1978;65:829-833.

66. Brorson H. Liposuction gives complete reduction of chronic large arm lymphoedema after breast cancer. *Acta Oncol* 2000;39:407-420.
67. Bolt RJ, Peelen W, Nikkels PG, de Jong TP. Congenital lymphoedema of the genitalia. *Eur J Pediatr* 1998;157:943-946.
68. Ollapallil JJ, Watters DA. Surgical management of elephantiasis of male genitalia. *Br J Urol* 1995;76:213-215.
69. Hegemann B, Helmbold P, Marsch WC. Genital inflammatory lymphoedema: peculiar microvascular long-distance metastasis of gastric carcinoma. *Br J Dermatol* 2001;144:419-420.

70. Kabir SM, Raurell A, Ramakrishnan V. Lymphoedema of the eyelids. *Br J Plast Surg* 2002;55:153-154.
71. Austin MW, Patterson A, Bates RA. Conjunctival lymphoedema in Turner's syndrome. *Eye* 1992;6(Pt 3):335-336.
72. Withey S, Pracy P, Wood S, Rhys-Evans P. The use of a lymphatic bridge in the management of head and neck lymphoedema. *Br J Plast Surg* 2001;54:716-719.
73. Ballinger AB, Farthing MJ. Octreotide in the treatment of intestinal lymphangiectasia. *Eur J Gastroenterol Hepatol* 1998;10:699-702.
74. Browse NL, Wilson NM, Russo F, et al. Aetiology and treatment of chylous ascites. *Br J Surg* 1992;79:1145-1150.
75. O'Driscoll JB, Chalmers RJ, Warnes TW. Chylous reflux into abdominal skin simulating lymphangioma circumscriptum in a patient with primary intestinal lymphangiectasia. *Clin Exp Dermatol* 1991;16:124-126.
75a. Whimster IW. The pathology of lymphangioma circumscriptum. *Br J Dermatol* 1976;94(5):473-486.
76. Konen O, Rathaus V, Dlugy E, et al. Childhood abdominal cystic lymphangioma. *Pediatr Radiol* 2002;32:88-94.

Index

A

Page numbers followed by f indicate figures; t, tables; b, boxes. Special indicators are not listed when content is on multiple inclusive pages. Special indicators are listed separately from page content as appropriate.

B

C

D

E

J

K

L

M

N

O

P

Q

R

S

T

U

V

W

X

Y

Z